PRONUNCIATION

You can use this dictionary to learn how to pronounce medical terms. The pronunciation appears in parentheses between the term and the beginning of its definition. The pronunciation of terms defined in this dictionary is indicated with letters of the English alphabet rather than with phonetic symbols. The following key shows the sounds represented by these letters.

VOWELS

ā	day, care, trait, gauge	ĕ	erythrocyte, genesis, system, lower	ū	prune, fruit, genu, food
a	mat, damage, far	ī	isle, lie, pyre, bacilli	yū	cube, urine, beauty, value
ă	about, hepatitis, data, tartar	i	igloo, hip, irritate	u	put, wool
ah	father, what	ĭ	pencil, circus	ŭ	upset, putt, murmur, tough
aw	raw, fall, cause	ō	oval, form, go		
ē	ego, here, bead, beet, artery	o	got, bought		
e	bed, head, therapy, teratoma	ŏ	oven, bottom, motor		
		ow	cow, hour		
		oy	boy, oil		

CONSONANTS

b	bad, tab		wherein the ending of that word is pronounced as if swallowed.	r	rot, atropy, tar
ch	child, itch			s	so, distill, mess (cf z); center, council (cf k)
d	dog, bad	j	jade; gender, rigid, edge (cf g)	sh	show, wish; social
dh	this, smooth (cf. th)	k	cut, tic; tachycardia (cf. ch)	t	ten, batter, put
f	fit, defect; phase, hyphen; tough	ks	extra, tax	th	thin, with (cf dh)
g	got, bag	kw	quick, aqua	v	vote, oven, nerve
h	hit, behold	l	law, kill	w	we, awake, tow
[h]	Denotes an approximation of a tone used in French words whereby the sound is pulled to the back of the tongue. The closest equivalent in English is found in the word "zone"	m	me, timid, bum	y	yes, payload
		n	no, tender, run	z	zero; disease, faces (cf s); xiphoid (cf ks)
		ng	ring	zh	azure, vision, measure
		p	pan, upset, top		

BUILDING BLOCKS OF MEDICAL LANGUAGE

Prefixes, suffixes, and combining forms make up 90 to 95 percent of medical vocabulary. Throughout the A–Z section these terms are marked with the ♻ symbol.

- ♻ **ab-** from, away from, off
- ♻ **abs-** from, away from, off
- ♻ **alge-** pain
- ♻ **cardi-** 1 heart; 2 esophageal opening of stomach
- ♻ **cardio-** 1 heart; 2 esophageal opening of stomach
- ♻ **cata-** down
- ♻ **cephal-** the head
- ♻ **chem-** 1 chemistry, 2 drug
- ♻ **chemo-** 1 chemistry, 2 drug
- ♻ **cyst-** 1 bladder; 2 cyst; 3 cystic duct
- ♻ **cysti-** 1 bladder; 2 cyst; 3 cystic duct
- ♻ **cysto-** 1 bladder; 2 cyst; 3 cystic duct
- ♻ **cyt-** cell
- ♻ **-cyte** cell
- ♻ **cyto-** cell
- ♻ **dactyl-** finger, toe

STEDMAN'S
Pocket Medical Dictionary

FIRST EDITION

⊞ Wolters Kluwer | Lippincott Williams & Wilkins
Health

Philadelphia · Baltimore · New York · London
Buenos Aires · Hong Kong · Sydney · Tokyo

Publisher: Julie K. Stegman
Product Director: Eric Branger
Product Manager: Tiffany Piper
Chief Copyeditor: Raymond Lukens
Copyeditor & Pronunciations: Kristi Lukens
Typographic Design: Parkton Art Studio, Inc.
Compositor: Absolute Service, Inc.
Manufacturing Coordinator: Margie Orzech

DISCLAIMER
Care has been taken to confirm the accuracy of the information present and to describe generally accepted practices. However, the authors, editors, and publisher are not responsible for errors or omissions or for any consequences from application of the information in this book and make no warranty, expressed or implied, with respect to the currency, completeness, or accuracy of the contents of the publication. Application of this information in a particular situation remains the professional responsibility of the practitioner; the clinical treatments described and recommended may not be considered absolute and universal recommendations.

The authors, editors, and publishers have exerted every effort to ensure that drug selection and dosage set forth in this text are in accordance with current recommendations and practice at the time of publication. However, in view of ongoing research, changes in government regulations, and the constant flow of information relating to drug therapy and drug reactions, the reader is urged to check the package insert for each drug for any change in indications and dosage and for added warnings and precautions. This is particularly important when the recommended agent is a new or infrequently employed drug.

Some drugs and medical devices presented in this publication have Food and Drug Administration (FDA) clearance for limited use in restricted research settings. It is the responsibility of the health care provider to ascertain the FDA status of each drug or device planned for use in their clinical practice.

Library of Congress Cataloging-in-Publication Data
Stedman, Thomas Lathrop, 1853-1938.
    Stedman's pocket medical dictionary. — 1st ed.
        p. ; cm.
    Terms from: Stedman's medical dictionary for the health professions and nursing, 6th ed., 2008 and Stedman's medical dictionary, 28th ed., 2006.
    Includes bibliographical references and index.
    ISBN 978-0-7817-7950-0 (alk. paper)
    1. Medicine—Dictionaries. I. Stedman, Thomas Lathrop, 1853-1938. Stedman's medical dictionary for the health professions and nursing. II. Stedman, Thomas Lathrop, 1853-1938. Stedman's medical dictionary. III. Title IV. Title: Pocket medical dictionary.
    [DNLM: 1. Medicine—Dictionary—English. W 13 S812sp 2009]
    R121.S822 1987
    610.3—dc22
                                                    2009005282

Contents

A Message from the Publisher

Stedman's, first produced as Dunglison's *New Dictionary of Medical Science and Literature* in 1833, has a long standing tradition of excellence. With this edition of *Stedman's Pocket Medical Dictionary,* we strove to continue this reputation of excellence, providing our readers with a complete and comprehensive reference in a portable, pocket size.

Stedman's Pocket Medical Dictionary provides students, educators, and practitioners access to the core language of medicine, health professions, and nursing. This edition features more than 38,000 terms drawn from *Stedman's Medical Dictionary for the Health Professions and Nursing, 6th Edition* and *Stedman's Medical Dictionary, 28th Edition.*

Exciting Electronic Additions

Stedman's Pocket Medical Dictionary also includes a free download featuring the entire content of the dictionary in an easy-to-use, searchable interface. To enhance this content, we have included over 650 images with the ability to copy and paste the images to the reader's computer and to reuse them in presentations and documentation. We have also included audio pronunciations for over 34,000 terms, enabling readers to not only read the written pronunciation but hear how the term is pronounced. In addition, we have included appendices and videos for key terms to aid in comprehension. These videos come from *Acland's DVD Atlas of Human Anatomy,* and we are proud to have them as a featured component of our electronic dictionary.

This download is available on our thePoint site, thePoint.lww.com/ StedPocket1e. There readers will also find appendices available as PDFs and an additional 300 LifeART™ images.

Acknowledgments

As always, we at Lippincott Williams & Wilkins are grateful to all of our consultants from the medical, nursing, and health professions disciplines for their help in reviewing, writing, and revising the thousands of entries in this dictionary. Without them, none of the terminology presented here would be relevant or useful.

The development of *Stedman's Pocket Medical Dictionary* has greatly benefited from the experience and expertise of Raymond Lukens, Chief Copyeditor, whose patience, dedication, and hard work have given this edition an unparallel level of quality. A key ingredient to making sure we are successful is making sure we listen to our customers. We are indebted to our colleagues at Lippincott Williams & Wilkins, including Tiffany Piper, Product Manager and Margie Orzech, Manufacturing Coordinator. Without the Lippincott Williams & Wilkins team's commitment to our readers and to the quality expected of Stedman's publications, this new edition would not have been possible.

Your Medical Word Resource Publisher

We strive to provide our readers of students, educators, and practitioners with the most up-to-date and accurate medical language references. We, as always, welcome any suggestions you may have for improvements, changes, corrections, and additions—whatever makes it possible for this Stedman's product to serve you better.

Julie K. Stegman   Eric Branger
Senior Publisher   Product Director

Stedman's Pocket Medical Dictionary, 1st Edition
Lippincott Williams & Wilkins
Baltimore, Maryland

Consultants to Stedman's Pocket Medical Dictionary

Tricia Berry, MATL, OTR/L
Assistant Dean of Clinical Placement, Kaplan University,
Ft. Lauderdale, FL, USA
Medical Assisting

Dolores Bertoti, MS, PT
Associate Professor and Department Chair, Alvernia College,
Reading, PA, USA
Physical Therapy

Mark Drnach, PT, DPT, MBA, PCS
Clinical Associate Professor, Department of Physical Therapy,
Wheeling Jesuit University, Wheeling, WV, USA
Physical Therapy

Kerri Hines, RN, BSN
San Jacinto College, Houston, TX, USA
Nursing

Nancy Hislop, RN, BSN
Online Instructor, Globe University/Minnesota School of Business,
Richfield, MN, USA
Medical Terminology

Laurie A. Milliken, PhD
Associate Professor, Department of Exercise and Health Sciences,
University of Massachusetts Boston, Boston, MA, USA
Exercise Science

Susan Polasek, MA, RD, LD
Austin, TX, USA
Nutrition

Georgina Sampson, RHIA
Professor, Rasmussen College, Brooklyn Park, MN, USA
Health Information Technology

Margaret M. Spieth, PhD, CMT
Faculty, Medical Transcription Program, Moraine Park Technical
College, West Bend, WI, USA
Medical Transcription

Nina Thierer, CMA (AAMA), BS, CPC, CCAT
Ivy Tech Community College Northeast, Fort Wayne, IN, USA
Medical Assisting

Bruce J. Walz, PhD
Professor and Chair, Department of Emergency Health Services,
University of Maryland, Baltimore County, Baltimore, MD, USA
Emergency Medical Services

Marsha Wamsley, RN, MS
Professor of Nursing, Sinclair Community College, Dayton, OH,
USA
Nursing

Barry M. Westling, MS, RRT-NPS, RPFT
Program Director, Respiratory Therapy, San Joaquin Valley
College, Visalia, CA, USA
Respiratory Therapy

Consultants to the Stedman's Dictionaries

Naomi Adams, RN, BN, CLNC
CEO, Adams Medical-Legal Consulting, Woodbridge, VA USA; Instructor, Practical Nursing Program MCI@ECPI College of Technology, Manassas, VA, USA

ESL

Steven Ades, MD, FRCPC
Associate Professor of Medicine and Oncology, McGill University Health Center, Montreal, Quebec, Canada

Oncology

Amy S. Alfriend, RN, MPH, COHN-S/CM
Assistant Director, Division of Occupational and Environmental Medicine, Johns Hopkins University School of Medicine, Baltimore, MD, USA

Nursing

R. Donald Allison, PhD
Associate Scientist, Department of Biochemistry and Molecular Biology, University of Florida College of Medicine, Gainesville, FL, USA

Biochemistry

Debra Kay Arver, RDH, BSDH, Masters Candidate
Dental Hygiene Instructor, Argosy University Health Sciences, Department of Dental Hygiene, Eagan, MN, USA

Dental Hygiene

Tricia Berry, OTR/L, MATL
Director of Clinical Placement, Kaplan University, Johnston, IA, USA

Medical Assisting

Dolores Bertoti, MS, PT
Associate Professor and Department Chair, Alvernia College, Reading, PA, USA

Physical Therapy

David A. Bloom, MD
The Jack Lapides Professor of Urology, University of Michigan, Ann Arbor, MI, USA

Genitourinary Surgery

Jane Bruner, PhD
Chair, Department of Biological Sciences, California State University, Stanislaus, Turlock, CA, USA

Bacteriology

Mary Ellen Camire, PhD
Professor, Department of Food Science and Human Nutrition, University of Maine, Orono, ME, USA

Nutrition

Kathleen E. Cavanagh, BSC, DVM
Fonthill, ON, Canada

Veterinary Medicine

Mitchell Charap, MD, FACP
The Abraham Sunshine Associate Professor of Clinical Medicine,
Associate Chair for Postgraduate Programs, Program Director,
Department of Medicine, NYU School of Medicine, New York,
NY, USA

Internal Medicine

George P. Chrousos, MD, FAAP, MACP, MACE
Professor and Chairman, First Department of Pediatrics, Athens
University Medical School, Aghia Sophia Children's Hospital,
Athens, Greece

Endocrinology

Mark B. Constantian, MD
St. Joseph Hospital, Southern New Hampshire Medical Center,
Nashua, NH, USA

Plastic/ Reconstructive Surgery

Arthur F. Dalley, II, PhD
Professor of Cell and Developmental Biology and Director, Gross
Anatomy Program, Department of Cell and Developmental
Biology, Vanderbilt University School of Medicine, Nashville,
TN, USA; Adjunct Professor for Anatomy, Belmont University
School of Physical Therapy, Nashville, TN, USA

Gross Anatomy

Ivan Damjanov, MD, PhD
Professor of Pathology, University of Kansas School of Medicine,
Kansas City, KS, USA

Pathology/ Anatomy

John A. Day, Jr., MD, FCCP
Assistant Professor of Medicine, University of Massachusetts
Medical School, Worcester, MA, USA

Pulmonary Diseases

John H. Dirckx, MD
Dayton, Ohio, USA

Etymologies and High Profile Terms

Philip Docking, EdD, MSc, Cert Ed, RN MFPHC
Associate Director, Education and Development, HMI Institute of
Health Sciences, Singapore

Nursing

Mark Drnach, PT, DPT, MBA, PCS
Clinical Associate Professor, Department of Physical Therapy,
Wheeling Jesuit University, Wheeling, WV, USA

Physical Therapy

Michelle R. Easton, PharmD
Assistant Dean, Professional and Student Affairs and Associate
Professor, School of Pharmacy, University of Charleston,
Charleston, WV, USA

Pharmacy

Nancy L. Evans, RN, MS
Professor of Nursing, Bristol Community College, Fall River,
MA, USA

Nursing

Thomas W. Filardo, MD
Physician-Consultant, Evendale, OH, USA

Chief Lexicographer and New Terms Editor

Benjamin K. Fisher, MD, FRCP(C)
Professor Emeritus, University of Toronto Medical School, Toronto, Ontario, Canada

Dermatology

Lee A. Fleisher, MD
Robert D. Dripps Professor and Chair of Anesthesiology and Critical Care, Professor of Medicine, University of Pennsylvania School of Medicine, Philadelphia, PA, USA

Anesthesiology

Robert J. Fontana, MD
Associate Professor of Medicine, University of Michigan, Ann Arbor, MI, USA

Gastroenterology

Paul J. Friedman, MD
Professor Emeritus, Department of Radiology, University of California, San Diego, CA, USA

Radiology

Leslie P. Gartner, PhD
Professor of Anatomy, Department of Biomedical Sciences, Dental School, University of Maryland at Baltimore, Baltimore, MD, USA

Histology

Douglas J. Gould, PhD
Associate Professor, University of Kentucky College of Medicine, Lexington, KY, USA

Gross Anatomy

Mary Kaye Griffin, BSH RT(R)(M)
Radiology Program Director, Spencerian College, Louisville, KY, USA

Radiology Technology

Joyce P. Griffin-Sobel, PhD, RN, AOCN, APRN.BC, CNE
Director, Undergraduate Programs, Bellevue School of Nursing, Hunter College, New York, NY, USA

Nursing Oncology

Steven Gutman, MD, MBA
Director, Office of In Vitro Diagnostics, Center for Devices and Radiological Health, Food and Drug Administration, Rockville, MD, USA

Stains/ Procedures

Duane E. Haines, PhD
Professor and Chairman of Anatomy, Professor of Neurosurgery and of Neurology, University of Mississippi Medical Center, Jackson, MS, USA

Neuroanatomy

Kerri Hines, RN, BSN   **Nursing**
San Jacinto College, Houston, TX, USA

Nicholas M. Hipskind, PhD, CCC-A   **Audiology**
Professor Emeritus, Department of Speech and Hearing Sciences,
Indiana University, Bloomington, IN, USA

Nancy Hislop, RN, BSN   **Medical**
Online Instructor, Globe University/Minnesota School of Business,   **Terminology**
Richfield, MN, USA

Nicola C. Y. Ho, MD   **Genetics**
Assistant Professor of Pediatrics and Active Staff of Johns
Hopkins Medical Institutions, Baltimore, MD, USA

Iain H. Kalfas MD, FACS   **Neurosurgery**
Chairman, Department of Neurosurgery, Cleveland Clinic
Foundation, Cleveland, OH, USA

John B. Kerrison, MD   **Ophthal-**
Assistant Professor of Ophthalmology, Neurology, and   **mology**
Neurosurgery, Wilmer Eye Institute, Johns Hopkins Hospital,
Baltimore, MD, USA

Jeffrey L. Kishiyama   **Immunology**
Associate Clinical Professor of Medicine, University of California,
San Francisco, CA, USA

Marian Kovatchitch, MS, RN   **Nursing**
Dean of Academic Affairs, St. Elizabeth College of Nursing,
Utica, NY, USA

John M. Last, MD, FRACP, FRCPC, FFPH(UK)   **Medical**
Professor Emeritus, Department of Epidemiology and Community   **Statistics/**
Medicine, University of Ottawa, Ottawa, Ontario, Canada   **Epidemiology**

James L. Lear, MD   **Nuclear**
Founder, Scientific Imaging, Inc., Larkspur, CO, USA; Professor   **Medicine**
and Director, Division of Nuclear Medicine, University of
Colorado Health Sciences Center, Denver, CO, USA

Joseph LoCicero, III, MD   **Thoracic**
Professor and Chair, Department of Surgery, University of South   **Surgery**
Alabama, Mobile, AL, USA

Kathy A. Locke, BA, CMA, RMA   **Medical**
Program Coordinator, School of Health Science, Northwestern   **Assisting**
Business College, Bridgeview, IL, USA

James M. Madsen, MD, MPH, FCAP, FACOEM COL, MC-FS, USA
Scientific Advisor, Chemical Casualty Care Division, U.S. Army Medical Research Institute of Chemical Defense (USAMRICD), APG-EA, MD; Associate Professor of Preventive Medicine and Biometrics; Assistant Professor of Pathology; Assistant Professor of Military and Emergency Medicine; Assistant Professor of Emerging Infectious Diseases, Uniformed Services University of the Health Sciences, Bethesda, MD, USA

Weapons of Mass Destruction/ Bioterrorism

Connie R. Mahon, MS, CLS
Microbiologist, Center for Drug Evaluation and Research, U.S. Food and Drug Administration, Rockville, MD, USA

Clinical Lab Sciences, Bacteriology and Mycology

Lisa Marcucci, MD
Fellow, Division of Critical Care, Department of Surgery, Johns Hopkins University, Baltimore, MD, USA

Biography/ Eponyms

Gail Metzger, MS, OTR/L
Assistant Professor, Department of Occupational Therapy, Alvernia College, Reading, PA, USA

Occupational Therapy

Laurie A. Milliken, PhD
Associate Professor, Department of Exercise and Health Sciences, University of Massachusetts Boston, Boston, MA, USA

Exercise Science

Keith L. Moore, MSc, PhD, FIAC, FRSM
Professor Emeritus, Division of Anatomy, Department of Surgery, Faculty of Medicine, University of Toronto, Toronto, Ontario, Canada; Recipient of the 2007 Henry Gray/Elsevier Distinguished Educator Award, awarded by the American Association of Anatomists

Embryology and British Medical Terminology

Marianna M. Newkirk, MSc, PhD
Associated Professor of Medicine, Physiology, Microbiology and Immunology, McGill University, Montreal, Quebec, Canada

Rheumatology

Marilyn H. Oermann, PhD, RN, FAAN
Professor and Division Chair, School of Nursing; Editor, Journal of Nursing Care Quality; The University of North Carolina at Chapel Hill, Chapel Hill, NC, USA

Nursing

J. Patrick O'Leary, MD
Associate Dean for Clinical Affairs, The Isidore Cohn, Jr. Professor and Chairman of Surgery, LSU Health Sciences Center, New Orleans, LA, USA

General Surgery

Kathleen M. O'Malley, CPhT
American Medical Careers, Flint, MI, USA

Pharm Tech

Stephen J. Peroutka, MD, PhD
Consultant, Hillsborough, CA, USA

Biotechnology

Sharon T. Phelan, MD, FACOG
Professor, Department of Obstetrics and Gynecology, University
of New Mexico, Albuquerque, NM, USA

Obstetrics/
Gynecology

Wanda Pierson, RN, MSN, PhD
Chair, Nursing Department, Langara College, Vancouver, BC,
Canada

Nursing

Susan Polasek, MA, RD, LD
Austin, TX, USA

Nutrition

Richard A. Prayson, MD
Section Head of Neuropathology, Department of Anatomic
Pathology, Cleveland Clinic Foundation, Cleveland, OH, USA

Neuropa-
thology

Lisa Radak, RT(R)(T)(CT)
Academic Clinical Coordinator, Radiation Therapy Program,
Baker College of Jackson, Jackson, MI, USA

Radiation
Therapy

Deneen Raysor, BS, CPT
Exercise Physiologist, Aquatic and Fitness Center, Philadelphia,
PA, USA

Physiology

William Reichel, MD
Affiliated Scholar, Center for Clinical Bioethics, Georgetown
University, School of Medicine, Washington, DC, USA

Geriatrics

Jo Ann Runewicz, RN.C, MSN, EdD
Drexel University, Philadelphia, PA, USA

Nursing

Georgina Sampson, RHIA
Professor, Rasmussen College, Brooklyn Park, MN, USA

Health
Information
Technology

George S. Schuster, DDS, MS, PhD
Ione and Arthur Merritt Professor, Chair, Department of Oral
Biology and Maxillofacial Pathology, Medical College of Georgia,
School of Dentistry, Augusta, GA, USA

Dentistry

Linda N. Sevier, MD
Pediatric Faculty, The Children's Hospital at Sinai, Baltimore,
MD, USA

Pediatrics

Susan Slajus, MBA, RHIA
Davenport University, Grand Rapids, MI, USA

Health
Information
Technology

James B. Snow, Jr., MD, FACS
Former Director, National Institute on Deafness and Other

Otorhinolaryn-
gology

Communication Disorders, National Institutes of Health, Bethesda, MD, USA; Professor Emeritus of Otorhinolaryngology, University of Pennsylvania, Philadelphia, PA, USA

Carlotta South, AAS, ADN, RN — Nursing
San Jacinto College North, Houston, TX, USA

Linda Spang, EMT-P, RMA, JD — Emergency Medical Services
Department Coordinator Allied Health, MA Program Director, Davenport University, Lansing, MI, USA

Margaret M. Spieth, PhD, CMT — Medical Transcription
Faculty, Medical Transcription Program, Moraine Park Technical College, West Bend, WI, USA

Scott Stanley, EdD, RRT, FAARC — Respiration Therapy
Assistant Dean for Undergraduate Affairs, Health and Liberal Arts Director of the Respiratory Care Programs School of Professional and Continuing Studies Northeastern University Boston, MA, USA

Erin K. Stauder, MS CCC/SLP — Speech-Language Pathology
Speech-Language Pathologist, Loyola College in Maryland, Baltimore, MD, USA

Nona K. Stinemetz, LPN — Medical Terminology
Vatterott College, Des Moines, IA, USA

Roger M. Stone, MD, MS, FAAEM, FACEP — Emergency Medicine
Clinical Assistant Professor, Emergency Medicine Residency, University of Maryland School of Medicine, Baltimore, MD, USA; EMS Medical Director, Montgomery and Caroline Counties, MD, USA

Janet L. Stringer, MD, PhD — Pharmacology/Toxicology
Associate Professor of Pharmacology and Neuroscience, Baylor College of Medicine, Houston, TX, USA

Deanna A. Sutton, PhD, MT, SM(ASCP), RM, SM(NRM) — Medical Mycology
Assistant Professor, Department of Pathology, Administrative Director, Fungus Testing Laboratory, University of Texas Health Science Center at San Antonio, San Antonio, TX, USA

Robin Sylvis, RDH, MS — Dental Hygiene
Director, International Business Development, The CoreMedical Group, Salem, NH, USA

Geoffrey Tabin, MD — Ophthalmology and Optometry
Professor of Ophthalmology and Visual Sciences, Moran Eye Center, University of Utah, Salt Lake City, UT, USA

Nina Thierer, CMA (AAMA), BS, CPC, CCAT — **Medical Assisting**
Ivy Tech Community College Northeast, Fort Wayne, IN, USA

Walter R. Thompson, PhD, FACSM, FAACVPR — **Exercise Science**
Professor, Department of Kinesiology and Health, College of
Education; Professor, Division of Nutrition, School of Health
Professions, College of Health and Human Sciences, Georgia
State University, Atlanta, GA, USA

Kelly S. Ullmer, ND, LDHS, OTR — **Alternative/Holistic Medicine**
Sheboygan, WI, USA

Alexandra Valsamakis, MD, PhD — **Virology**
Assistant Professor of Pathology, Johns Hopkins School of
Medicine, Baltimore, MD, USA

Amy Carson VonKadich, MEd, RTT — **Radiology Technology**
Radiation Therapy Program Director, New Hampshire Technical
Institute, Concord, NH, USA

Galen S. Wagner, MD — **Cardiology**
Duke University Medical Center, Durham, NC, USA

Bruce J. Walz, PhD — **Emergency Medical Services**
Professor and Chair, Department of Emergency Health Services,
University of Maryland, Baltimore County, Baltimore, MD, USA

Marsha Wamsley, RN, MS — **Nursing**
Professor of Nursing, Sinclair Community College, Dayton, OH,
USA

Dr. Brian J. Ward — **Parasitology/Tropical Medicine**
Chief, McGill University Division of Infectious Diseases,
Departments of Medicine & Microbiology, McGill University,
Montreal, Quebec, Canada

Ruth Werner, LMP, NCTMB — **Massage Therapy**
Faculty, Myotherapy College of Utah, Layton, UT, USA

Barry M. Westling, MS, RRT-NPS, RPFT — **Respiratory Therapy**
Program Director, Respiratory Therapy, San Joaquin Valley
College, Visalia, CA, USA

Asa J. Wilbourn, MD — **Neurology**
Director, EMG Laboratory, Cleveland Clinic; Clinical Professor of
Neurology, Case University School of Medicine, Cleveland, OH,
USA

Helaine R. Wolpert, MD
Anatomic and Clinical Pathologist, Newton, MA, USA

Clinical Pathology/ Hematology/ Laboratory Medicine

Douglas B. Woodruff, MD
Private Practice, Baltimore, MD, USA

Psychiatry/ Psychology

David B. Young, PhD
Professor, Physiology and Biophysics, University of Mississippi Medical Center, Jackson, MS, USA

Physiology

Joseph D. Zuckerman, MD
Professor & Chairman, Department of Orthopaedic Surgery, NYU – Hospital for Joint Diseases, New York, NY, USA

Orthopaedics

Å Abbreviation for angstrom.

AAPMR Abbreviation for American Academy of Physical Medicine and Rehabilitation.

ab-, abs- *Do not confuse words formed with this prefix and words formed with the prefix ad-.* **1.** From, away from, off. **2.** Prefix applied to electrical units in the CGS-electromagnetic system to distinguish them from units in the CGS-electrostatic system (prefix stat-) and those in the metric system or SI (no prefix).

Abad·ie sign of ta·bes dor·sa·lis (ah-bah-dē′ sīn tā′bēz dōr-sā′lis) Insensibility to pressure over the Achilles tendon.

A band (band) Muscle striation containing myosin filaments; appears dark under light microscope and light in polarized light.

a·ban·don·ment of care (ă-ban′dŏn-mĕnt kār) Situation in which a medical professional should have provided care for a patient but fails to do so.

a·bar·og·no·sis (ā-bar′ŏg-nō′sis) Loss of ability to appreciate the weight of objects held in the hand, or to differentiate objects of different weights.

a·ba·si·a (ă-bā′zē-ă) Inability to walk. SEE gait.

a·ba·si·a-a·sta·si·a (ă-bā′zē-ă-ă-stā′zē-ă) SEE astasia-abasia.

a·ba·si·a tre·pi·dans (ă-bā′zē-ă trep′i-danz) Gait defect due to trembling of the lower limbs.

a·bate·ment (ă-bāt′mĕnt) **1.** A diminution or easing. **2.** Reduction, ultimately elimination, of public-health nuisances such as smoke or loud noise.

ab·ax·i·al, ab·ax·ile (ab-ak′sē-ăl, -ak′sīl) **1.** Lying outside the axis of any body or part. **2.** Situated at the opposite extremity of the axis of a part.

ab·do·men (ab′dŏ-mĕn) [TA] The part of the trunk that lies between the thorax and the pelvis; considered by some anatomists to include the pelvis (abdominopelvic cavity). SYN venter (1).

ab·dom·i·nal (ab-dom′i-năl) Relating to the abdomen.

ab·dom·i·nal an·gi·na, an·gi·na ab·do·m·i·nis (ab-dom′i-năl an′ji-nă, an′ji-nă ab-dō′mi-nis) Intermittent abdominal pain, frequently occurring in a fixed time after eating, caused by inadequacy of the mesenteric circulation resulting from arteriosclerosis or other arterial disease, with associated significant weight loss. SYN intestinal angina.

ab·dom·i·nal ap·o·neu·ro·sis (ab-dom′i-năl ap′ō-nūr-ō′sis) Broad, flat, abdominal tendon.

ab·dom·i·nal au·ra (ab-dom′i-năl awr′ă) Epileptic aura characterized by abdominal discomfort, nausea, malaise, pain, and hunger. Some phenomena reflect ictal autonomic dysfunction. SEE ALSO aura (1).

ab·dom·i·nal cav·i·ty (ab-dom′i-năl kav′i-tē) [TA] Space bounded by the abdominal walls, the diaphragm, and the pelvis. SYN cavitas abdominalis [TA], cavum abdominis, enterocele (2).

ab·dom·i·nal fis·sure (ab-dom′i-năl fish′ŭr) Congenital failure of the ventral body wall to close. SEE ALSO celosomia, gastroschisis.

ab·dom·i·nal fis·tu·la (ab-dom′i-năl fis′tyū-lă) Fistulous passage connecting one of the abdominal viscera to the external surface.

ab·dom·i·nal guard·ing (ab-dom′i-năl gahrd′ing) A spasm of abdominal wall muscles, detected on palpation, to protect inflamed abdominal viscera from pressure.

ab·dom·i·nal her·ni·a (ab-dom′i-năl hĕr′nē-ă) A hernia protruding through or into any part of the abdominal wall. SYN laparocele.

ab·dom·i·nal hys·ter·ec·to·my (ab-dom′i-năl his′tĕr-ek′tŏ-mē) Removal of the uterus through an incision in the abdominal wall.

ab·dom·i·nal hysterotomy (ab-dom′i-năl his′tĕr-ot′ŏ-mē) Transabdominal incision into the uterus; also called abdominohysterotomy, celiohysterotomy, laparohysterotomy, and laparouterotomy.

ab·dom·i·nal mi·graine (ab-dom´i-năl mī´grăn) **1.** Migraine in children accompanied by paroxysmal abdominal pain. **2.** Disorder that causes intermittent abdominal pain and is believed to be related to migraine; has some features of migraine. The diagnosis depends on excluding other causes of abdominal pain.

ab·dom·i·nal mus·cle de·fi·cien·cy syn·drome (ab-dom´i-năl mŭs´ĕl dĕ-fish´ĕn-sē sin´drōm) Congenital absence (partial or complete) of abdominal muscles, in which the outline of the intestines is visible through the protruding abdominal wall; in men, genitourinary anomalies (urinary tract dilation and cryptorchidism) are also found.

ab·dom·i·nal ne·phrec·tomy (ab-dom´i-năl ne-frek´tŏ-mē) Transperitoneal removal of the kidney by an incision through the anterior abdominal wall.

ab·dom·i·nal pad (ab-dom´i-năl pad) SYN laparotomy pad.

ab·dom·i·nal re·flex·es (ab-dom´i-năl rē´fleks-ĕz) Contraction of the muscles of the abdominal wall on stimulation of the skin (superficial a. reflexes) or tapping on neighboring bony structures (deep a. reflexes). SYN supraumbilical reflex (2).

ab·dom·i·nal res·pi·ra·tion (ab-dom´i-năl res´pir-ā´shŭn) Breathing produced mainly by action of the diaphragm.

ab·dom·i·nal sal·pin·gec·to·my (ab-dom´i-năl sal-pin-jek´tŏ-mē) Removal of one or both uterine tubes through an abdominal incision.

ab·dom·i·nal sal·pin·got·o·my (ab-dom´i-năl sal-ping-got´ŏ-mē) Incision into the uterine tube through an opening in the abdominal wall.

ab·dom·i·nal sec·tion (ab-dom´i-năl sek´shŭn) SYN celiotomy.

ab·dom·i·no·car·di·ac re·flex (ab-dom´i-nō-kahr´dē-ak rē´fleks) Mechanical stimulation (usually distention) of abdominal viscera causing changes (usually a slowing) in the heart rate or the occurrence of extrasystoles.

ab·dom·i·no·cen·te·sis (ab-dom´i-nō-sen-tē´sis) *Avoid the incorrect form ab-dominal centesis.* Paracentesis of the abdomen.

ab·dom·i·no·cys·tic (ab-dom´i-nō-sis´tik) SYN abdominovesical.

ab·dom·i·no·gen·i·tal (ab-dom´i-nō-gen´i-tăl) Relating to the abdomen and the genital organs.

ab·dom·i·no·hys·ter·ot·o·my (ab-dom´i-nō-his-ter-ot´ŏ-mē) SYN abdominal hysterotomy.

ab·dom·i·no·pel·vic cav·i·ty (ab-dom´i-nō-pel´vik kav´i-tē) [TA] The combined and continuous abdominal and pelvic cavities. SEE ALSO abdominal cavity.

ab·dom·i·no·per·i·ne·al (ab-dom´i-nō-per-i-nē´ăl) Relating to both abdomen and perineum.

ab·dom·i·no·per·i·ne·al re·sec·tion (ab-dom´i-nō-per-i-nē´ăl rē-sek´shŭn) A surgical treatment for cancer involving resection of the lower sigmoid colon, rectum, anus, and surrounding skin, and formation of a sigmoid colostomy.

ab·dom·i·no·plas·ty (ab-dom´i-nō-plas-tē) An operation performed on the abdominal wall for cosmetic purposes.

ab·dom·i·nos·co·py (ab-dom´i-nos´kŏ-pē) SYN peritoneoscopy.

ab·dom·i·no·scro·tal (ab-dom´i-nō-skrō´tăl) Relating to the abdomen and the scrotum.

ab·dom·i·no·vag·i·nal (ab-dom´i-nō-vaj´i-năl) Relating to both the abdomen and the vagina.

ab·dom·i·no·ves·i·cal (ab-dom´i-nō-ves´i-kăl) Relating to the abdomen and urinary bladder, or to the abdomen and gallbladder. SYN abdominocystic.

ab·du·cens mus·cle (ab-dū´senz mŭs´ĕl) Small muscle that provides motion to the eyeball.

ab·du·cent (ab-dū´sĕnt) Abducting; drawing away, especially away from the median plane.

ab·du·cent nerve [CN VI] (ab-dū´sĕnt nĕrv) [TA] A small motor nerve supplying the lateral rectus muscle of the eye; its origin is in the facial colliculus of the tegmentum of the pons just below the surface of the rhomboid fossa. SYN nervus abducens [CN VI] [TA], sixth cranial nerve [CN VI].

ab·duct (ab-dŭkt′) *Do not confuse this word with adduct.* To move away from the median plane.

ab·duc·tion (ab-dŭk′shŭn) **1.** Movement of a body part away from the median plane (of the body, in the case of limbs; of the hand or foot, in the case of digits). **2.** Monocular rotation (duction) of the eye toward the temple. **3.** A position resulting from such movement. Cf. adduction.

ab·duc·tion boots (ab-dŭk′shŭn būts) Positioning device that maintains abduction of the hips.

ab·duc·tor di·gi·ti mi·ni·mi mus·cle of hand (ab-dŭk′tŏr dij′i-tī mi′ni-mī mŭs′ĕl hand) *Origin*, pisiform bone and pisohamate ligament; *insertion*, medial side of base of proximal phalanx of the little finger; *action*, abducts and flexes little finger; *nerve supply*, ulnar.

ab·duc·tor hal·lu·cis mus·cle (ab-dŭk′tŏr hal′ū-sis mŭs′ĕl) *Origin*, medial process of calcaneal tuberosity, flexor retinaculum, and plantar aponeurosis; *insertion*, medial side of proximal phalanx of great toe; *action*, abducts great toe; *nerve supply*, medial plantar. SYN musculus abductor hallucis [TA].

ab·duc·tor pol·li·cis brev·is mus·cle (ab-dŭk′tŏr pol′li-sis brev′is mŭs′ĕl) Superficial thenar muscle; *origin*, tubercle of trapezium and flexor retinaculum; *insertion*, lateral side of proximal phalanx of thumb; *action*, abducts thumb; *nerve supply*, median. SYN musculus abductor pollicis brevis, short abductor muscle of thumb.

ab·duc·tor pol·li·cis long·us mus·cle (ab-dŭk′tŏr pol′li-sis long′gŭs mŭs′ĕl) Outcropping muscle of posterior compartment of forearm; *origin*, interosseous membrane and posterior surfaces of radius and ulna; *insertion*, lateral side of base of first metacarpal bone; *action*, abducts and assists in extending thumb; *nerve supply*, radial. SYN long abductor muscle of thumb, musculus abductor pollicis longus,

musculus extensor ossis metacarpi pollicis.

ab·duc·tor spas·mo·dic dys·pho·nia (ab-dŭk′tŏr spaz-mod′ik dis-fō′nē-ă) A breathy form of spasmodic dysphonia caused by excessive and long vocal cord opening for voiceless phonemes extending into vowels.

A·bell-Ken·dall meth·od (ā′bel ken′dăl meth′ŏd) A methodology for determining total serum cholesterol that avoids interference by bilirubin, protein, and hemoglobin.

ab·er·rant (aber) (ab-er′ănt) **1.** Differing from the usual or norm. **2.** Wandering off; used to describe certain ducts, vessels, or nerves that deviate from the usual or normal course or pattern. **3.** SYN deviant (1).

ab·er·rant gan·gli·on (ab-er′ănt gang′glē-on) Collection of nerve cells sometimes found on a posterior spinal nerve root between the spinal ganglion and the spinal cord.

ab·er·rant goi·ter (ab-er′ănt goy′tĕr) Enlargement of a supernumerary thyroid gland. SYN struma aberrata.

aberrant goitre [Br.] SYN aberrant goiter.

ab·er·rant ven·tric·u·lar con·duc·tion (AVC) (ab-er′ănt ven-trik′yū-lăr kŏn-dŭk′shŭn) Abnormal intraventricular conduction of a supraventricular beat, especially where surrounding beats are normally conducted. SYN ventricular aberration.

ab·er·ra·tion (ab′ĕr-ā′shŭn) **1.** Deviation from the usual or normal course or pattern. **2.** Deviant development or growth. SEE ALSO chromosome aberration.

abetalipoproteinaemia [Br.] SYN abetalipoproteinemia.

a·be·ta·lip·o·pro·tein·e·mi·a (ā-bā′tă-lip′ō-prō′tē-nē′mē-ă) A disorder characterized by absence from plasma of low density lipoproteins that migrate electrophoretically as beta globulins, the presence of acanthocytes in the blood, retinal pigmentary degeneration, malabsorption, engorgement of upper intestinal absorptive cells with dietary triglycerides, and neuromuscular abnormalities. SYN abetalipoproteinaemia, Bassen-Kornzweig syndrome.

a·bey·ance (ă-bā'ăns) A state of temporary cessation of function.

ab·frac·tion (ab-frak'shŭn) To break away.

a·bi·ent (ab'ē-ĕnt) Characterized by avoidance or withdrawal.

a·bi·o·gen·e·sis (ā'bī-ō-jen'ĕ-sis) Spontaneous origination of living organ directly from lifeless matter. SEE ALSO spontaneous generation.

Ab·i·o·tro·phi·a (ab'ē-ō-trō'fē-a) A bacterial genus associated with various infections, particularly subacute bacterial endocarditis.

ab·la·tion (ab-lā'shŭn) Removing a body part or destroying its function, as by a surgical procedure, morbid process, or noxious substance.

ableph·ar·ia (ā-blef-ar'ē-ă) Congenital absence of the eyelids.

ab·lu·ent (ab'lū-ĕnt) *Avoid the mispronunciation ablu'ent.* 1. Cleansing. 2. Anything with cleansing properties.

ab·lu·ted (ă-blū'tĕd) Washed clean.

ab·nor·mal (A, AB, abn, ABN, abnor, abnorm, Abn) (ab-nōr'măl) *Negative and pejorative connotations of this word may render it offensive in some contexts.* 1. Not normal; differing in any way from the usual state, structure, condition, or rule. Cf. normal. 2. SYN deviant (1).

ab·nor·mal·i·ty (ab'nōr-mal'i-tē) 1. The state or quality of being abnormal; that which deviates from the norm. 2. An anomaly, deformity, malformation, impairment, or dysfunction.

ab·nor·mal oc·clu·sion (ab-nōr'măl ŏ-klū'zhŭn) An arrangement of the teeth that is not considered to be within the normal range of variation.

ABO blood group (blŭd grūp) The most significant and common blood group.

ABO haemolytic disease of the newborn [Br.] SYN ABO hemolytic disease of the newborn.

ABO he·mo·lyt·ic dis·ease of the new·born (HDN) (hē'mō-lit'ik di-zēz' nū'bŏrn) Erythroblastosis fetalis due to maternal-fetal incompatibility with respect to an antigen of the ABO blood group. SYN ABO haemolytic disease of the newborn.

ab·o·rad, ab·o·ral (ab-ōr'ad, -ăl) In a direction away from the mouth; opposite of orad.

a·bort (ă-bōrt') 1. The expulsion of an embryo or fetus before it is viable. SEE ALSO miscarry. 2. The removal of the products of conception prematurely. 3. To arrest a disease in its earliest stages. 4. To arrest any action or process before its normal completion.

a·bort·ed sys·to·le (ă-bōrt'ĕd sis'tŏ-lē) A loss of the systolic beat in the radial pulse through weakness of the ventricular contraction.

a·bor·ti·fa·cient (ă-bōr'ti-fā'shĕnt) *Avoid the misspelling abortefacient.* 1. Producing abortion. SYN abortive (3). 2. An agent that produces abortion.

a·bor·tion (ă-bōr'shŭn) Expulsion from the uterus of an embryo or fetus before the stage of viability (20 weeks' gestation or fetal weight less than 500 g); may be either spontaneous (occurring from natural causes) or induced (artificial or therapeutic).

a·bor·tion·ist (ă-bōr'shŭn-ist) One who interrupts a pregnancy.

a·bor·tion pill (ă-bōr'shŭn pil) A means of expelling an embryo or fetus during the first 7 weeks of pregnancy with a combination of a progesterone antagonist and prostaglandins.

a·bor·tive (ă-bōr'tiv) 1. Not reaching completion; e.g., said of an attack of a disease subsiding before it has fully developed or completed its course. 2. SYN rudimentary. 3. SYN abortifacient (1).

a·bor·tus (ă-bōr'tŭs) 1. An embryo or fetus and membranes. 2. Any product (or all products) of an abortion.

a·bove-el·bow am·pu·ta·tion (ă-bŭv' el'bŏ amp'yū-tā'shŭn) Surgical removal of the upper limb in a location proximal to the elbow.

a·bove-knee am·pu·ta·tion (ă-bŭv´ nē amp´yū-tā´shŭn) Surgical removal of the lower limb in a location proximal to the knee.

a·bra·chi·o·ceph·a·ly (ă-brā´kē-ō-sef´ă-lē) Congenital absence of upper limbs and head.

A·brams heart re·flex (ā´brămz hahrt rē´fleks) A contraction of the myocardium when the skin of the precordial region is irritated.

a·bra·sion (ă-brā´zhŭn) **1.** An excoriation or circumscribed removal of the superficial layers of skin or mucous membrane. **2.** A scraping away of a portion of the surface. **3.** In dentistry, the pathologic grinding or wearing away of tooth substance by incorrect tooth-brushing methods, the presence of foreign objects, bruxism, or similar causes. SYN grinding. SEE ALSO bruxism. Cf. attrition.

ab·re·ac·tion (ab-rē-ak´shŭn) Emotional release or catharsis associated with the recollection of previously repressed unpleasant experiences.

ab·ro·sia (ā-brō´zē-ă) Abstinence from food.

ab·rup·ti·o (ă-brŭp´shē-ō) Nonphysiologic separation of tissues that should normally adhere.

ab·rup·ti·o pla·cen·tae (ă-brŭp´shē-ō plă-sen´tē) Premature detachment of a normally situated placenta.

ab·scess (ab´ses) **1.** A circumscribed collection of purulent exudate appearing in an acute or chronic localized infection, caused by tissue destruction and frequently associated with swelling, pain, and other signs of inflammation. **2.** A cavity formed by liquefactive necrosis within solid tissue; healing may be promoted by excision and drainage.

ab·scon·si·o (ab-skon´sē-ō) A recess, cavity, or depression; used especially in osteology to denote a bony cavity that accommodates the head of another bone.

ab·sco·pal (ab-skō´păl) Denoting the effect that irradiation of a tissue has on remote nonirradiated tissue.

ab·sence seiz·ure (ab´sĕns sē´zhŭr) A brief seizure characterized by arrest of activity and occasionally clonic movements.

Ab·sid·i·a (ab-sid´ē-ă) A genus of fungi commonly found in nature (e.g., compost piles); may cause zygomycosis in humans.

ab·sinthe (ab´sinth) A liquor consisting of 60–75% ethanol flavored with absinthium, anise, fennel, and other herbs, long banned in the U.S. and some other countries because of its toxic effects and addictiveness.

ab·so·lute (abs, A) (ab-sō-lūt´) _Although the traditional pronunciation is as shown, the word is often stressed on the last syllable in the U.S._ Unconditional; unlimited; uncombined; undiluted (as in reference to alcohol); certain.

ab·so·lute al·co·hol (ab-sō-lūt´ al´kŏ-hol) **1.** 100% alcohol, water having been removed. SYN anhydrous alcohol. **2.** Alcohol with a minimum admixture of water, at most 1%. SYN dehydrated alcohol.

ab·so·lute glau·co·ma (ab-sō-lūt´ glaw-kō´mă) Final stage of blindness due to glaucoma.

ab·so·lute hem·i·a·no·pia (ab-sō-lūt´ hem-ē-ă-nō´pē-ă) Hemianopia in which the affected field is totally insensitive to all visual stimuli. SYN complete hemianopia.

ab·so·lute hy·per·o·pia (ab-sŏ-lūt´ hī´pĕr-ō´pē-ă) Manifest hyperopia that cannot be overcome by an effort of accommodation.

ab·so·lute rate ox·y·gen up·take (ab´sŏ-lūt´ rāt ok´si-jen ŭp´tāk) Rate of VO_2 conversion to energy expenditure or kilocalories.

ab·so·lute tem·per·a·ture (T) (ab-sŏ-lūt´ tem´pĕr-ă-chŭr) Temperature reckoned in the Kelvin scale from absolute zero.

ab·so·lute thresh·old (ab-sō-lūt´ thresh´ōld) Lowest limit of any perception. Cf. differential threshold. SYN stimulus threshold.

ab·so·lute ze·ro (ab-sŏ-lūt´ zēr´ō) The lowest possible temperature.

ab·sorb (ab-sōrb′) *Do not confuse this word with adsorb.* **1.** To take in by absorption. **2.** To reduce the intensity of transmitted light.

ab·sorb·a·ble gel·a·tin film (ab-sōr′bă-bĕl jel′ă-tin film) A sterile, nonantigenic, water-insoluble sheet of gelatin prepared by drying a gelatin-formaldehyde solution on plates.

ab·sorb·a·ble sur·gi·cal su·ture (ab-sōr′bĕnt sŭr′ji-kăl sū′chŭr) Suture material prepared from a substance that can be dissolved by body tissues and is therefore not permanent.

ab·sorbed dose (ab-sōrbd′ dōs) The amount of a substance that is absorbed by the body by penetrating an epithelial barrier such as the skin, eyes, respiratory tract, or gastrointestinal tract.

ab·sor·be·fa·cient (ab-sōr-bĕ-fā′shŭnt) **1.** Causing absorption. **2.** Any substance possessing such quality.

ab·sor·bent (ab-sōr′bĕnt) **1.** Having the power to soak up or take into itself a gas, liquid, light rays, or heat. **2.** Any substance possessing such power.

ab·sor·bent gauze (ab-sōr′bĕnt gawz) White cotton cloth in folds or rolls used for surgical or wound dressings.

ab·sorp·tion (ab-sōrp′shŭn) The taking in, incorporation, or reception of gases, liquids, light, or heat. Cf. adsorption.

ab·sorp·tion co·ef·fi·cient (ab-sōrp′shŭn kō-ĕ-fish′ĕnt) **1.** The milliliters of a gas at standard temperature and pressure that will saturate 100 mL of liquid. **2.** The amount of light absorbed in passing through 1 cm of a 1 molar solution of a given substance, expressed as a constant in Beer-Lambert law. **3.** RADIOLOGY a measure of the rate of decrease of intensity of a beam in its passage through matter, resulting from a combination of scattering and conversion to other forms of energy. SEE ALSO attenuation.

ab·sorp·tion lines (ab-sōrp′shŭn līnz) Dark lines in the solar spectrum due to absorption by the solar and the earth's atmosphere.

ab·sorp·tiv·i·ty (a) (ab-sōrp-tiv′i-tē) SYN specific absorption coefficient.

ab·sti·nence (ab′sti-nĕns) Refraining from the use of certain articles of diet, alcoholic beverages, illegal drugs, or sexual intercourse.

ab·sti·nence syn·drome (ab′sti-nĕns sin′drōm) Constellation of physiologic changes undergone by people or animals who have become physically dependent on a drug or chemical who are abruptly deprived of that substance. The intensity of the syndrome varies with the drug or chemical.

ab·stract (ab′strakt, ab-strakt′) **1.** A condensation, summary, or brief description of a scientific or literary article or the results of a study. **2.** A preparation made by evaporating a fluid extract to a powder and triturating it with milk sugar.

ab·strac·tion (ab-strak′shŭn) **1.** Distillation or separation of the volatile constituents of a substance. **2.** Malocclusion in which the teeth or associated structures are lower than their normal occlusal plane.

a·bu·li·a (ā-bū′lē-ă) Reduction in speech, movement, thought, and emotional reaction; a common result of bilateral frontal lobe disease.

a·buse (ă-byūs′) **1.** Misuse, wrong use, especially excessive use, of anything, intentionally or unintentionally. **2.** Injurious, harmful, or offensive treatment, as in child abuse or sexual abuse.

a·but·ment (ă-bŭt′mĕnt) A natural tooth or implanted tooth substitute.

Ac Abbreviation for actinium; acetyl.

a·cal·cu·li·a (ā-kal-kyū′lē-ă) A form of aphasia characterized by the inability to perform simple mathematical problems; often an early sign of dementia.

a·can·tha (ă-kan′thă) A spine or spinous process.

acanthaesthesia [Br.] SYN acanthesthesia.

a·can·tha·me·bi·a·sis (ă-kan′thă-mē-bī′ă-sis) Infection by free-living soil amebae of the genus *Acanthamoeba* that may result in a necrotizing dermal or tissue invasion. SYN acanthamoebiasis.

acanthamoebiasis [Br.] SYN acanthamebiasis.

a·can·thes·the·si·a (ă-kan'thes-thē'zē-ă) Paresthesia with the sensation of a pinprick. SYN acanthaesthesia.

a·can·thi·on (ă-kan'thē-on) The tip of the anterior nasal spine.

a·can·tho·cyte (ă-kan'thō-sīt) Erythrocytes characterized by spiny cytoplasmic projections.

a·can·thoid (ă-kan'thoyd) Spine shaped.

ac·an·thol·y·sis (ak'an-thol'i-sis) Separation of individual epidermal keratinocytes from their neighbors.

ac·an·tho·ma (ak'an-thō'mă) A tumor formed by proliferation of epithelial squamous cells. SEE ALSO keratoacanthoma.

ac·an·tho·me·a·tal line (ă-kan'thō-mē-ă'tăl līn) An imaginary line between the acanthion and the external auditory meatus; used for radiographic positioning of the skull.

ac·an·tho·sis (ak-an-thō'sis) An increase in the thickness of the stratum spinosum of the epidermis.

ac·an·tho·sis ni·gri·cans (ak-an-thō'sis nī'gri-kanz) An eruption of velvet warty benign growths and hyperpigmentation occurring in the skin of the axillae, neck, anogenital area, and groins.

a·cap·ni·a (ă-kap'nē-ă) Absence of carbon dioxide in the blood.

a·car·di·a (ā-kahr'dē-ă) Congenital absence of the heart.

a·car·di·us (ā-kahr'dē-ŭs) A twin without a heart that remains viable by using the placental circulation of its mate.

a·car·di·us a·ceph·a·lus (ā-kahr'dē-ŭs ā-sef'ă-lŭs) A cardiac conceptus in which the head and thoracic organs are absent.

a·car·di·us a·mor·phus (ā-kahr'dē-ŭs ă-mōr'fŭs) Shapeless product of conception covered by skin and hair.

ac·a·ri·a·sis (ak'ăr-ī'ă-sis) Any disease caused by mites, usually a skin infestation. SEE mange.

a·car·i·cide (ă-kar'i-sīd) An agent that kills acarines; commonly used to denote chemicals that kill ticks.

Ac·a·ri·na (ak-ă-rī'nă) An order of Arachnida that includes mites and ticks.

ac·a·ro·der·ma·ti·tis (ak'ă-rō-dĕr-mă-tī'tis) A skin inflammation or eruption produced by a mite.

a·cat·a·la·si·a (ā-kat'ă-lā'zē-ă) Absence or deficiency of catalase from blood and tissues, often manifested by recurrent infection or ulceration of the gingivae (gums) and related oral structures and caused by mutations in the catalase gene (*CAT*) on 11p. Homozygotes may have complete absence (Japanese variety) or very low levels (Swiss variety) of catalase; heterozygotes have reduced catalase levels (hypocatalasia), which overlap with the normal range. SYN Takahara disease.

a·cau·dal, a·cau·date (ā-kaw'dăl, ă-kaw'dāt) Having no tail.

ac·cel·er·ant (ak-sel'ĕr-ănt) SYN accelerator (3).

ac·cel·er·at·ed hy·per·ten·sion (ak-sel'ĕr-ā-tĕd hī'pĕr-ten'shŭn) Hypertension advancing rapidly with increasing blood pressure and associated with acute and rapidly worsening signs and symptoms.

ac·cel·er·at·ed id·i·o·ven·tri·cu·lar rhythm (ak-sel'ĕr-ā-tĕd id'ē-ō-ven-trik'yū-lăr ridh'ŭm) Tachycardia originating from a ventricular pacemaker.

ac·cel·er·at·ed res·pi·ra·tion (ak-sel'ĕr-āt-ĕd res'pir-ā'shŭn) Increased rate of breathing.

ac·cel·er·a·tion (ak-sel-er-ā'shŭn) *Avoid the mispronunciation uh-sel-er-ā'shŭn.* **1.** The act of accelerating. **2.** The rate of increase in velocity per unit of time; commonly expressed in *g* units; also expressed in centimeters or feet per second squared.

ac·cel·er·a·tor (ak-sel'ĕr-ā-tŏr) **1.** Anything that increases rapidity of action or function. **2.** PHYSIOLOGY a nerve, muscle, or substance that quickens movement or response. **3.** A catalytic agent used to hasten a chemical reaction.

ac·cel·er·a·tor fac·tor (ak-sel′ĕ-rā-tŏr fak′tŏr) SYN factor V.

ac·cel·er·a·tor fi·bers (ak-sel′ĕr-ā-tŏr fī′bĕrz) Postganglionic sympathetic nerve fibers originating in the superior, middle, and inferior cervical ganglia of the sympathetic trunk, conveying nervous impulses to the heart that increase the rapidity and force of the cardiac pulsations. SYN accelerator fibres.

accelerator fibres [Br.] SYN accelerator fibers.

ac·cen·tu·a·tor (ak-sen′chū-ā-tŏr) A substance (e.g., aniline) the presence of which allows a combination between a tissue or histologic element and a stain that might otherwise be impossible.

ac·cept·a·ble in·take (AI) (ak-sep′tă-bĕl in′tāk) Value for suggested daily intake of a nutrient in cases in which data are insufficient to determine an estimated average requirement (EAR) and thus a recommended dietary allowance (RDA). SEE ALSO Dietary Reference Intake.

ac·cept·a·ble mac·ro·nu·tri·ent dis·tri·bu·tion range (AMDR) (ak-sep′tă-bĕl mak′rō-nū′trē-ĕnt dis′tri-byū′shŭn rānj) A range of intakes for a particular energy source that is associated with reduced risk of chronic disease while providing adequate intakes of essential nutrients.

ac·cep·tor (ak-sept′ŏr) A compound that will take up a chemical group (e.g., an amine group, a methyl group, a carbamoyl group) from another compound (the donor).

ac·cess (ak′ses) *Do not confuse this word with assess or axis.* **1.** A way or means of approach or admittance. **2.** In dentistry, the space required for visualization and for manipulation of instruments to remove decay and prepare a tooth for restoration.

ac·ces·so·ry (ak-ses′ŏr-ē) ANATOMY denoting a muscle, nerve, gland, or similar, which is auxiliary or supernumerary to some other, generally more important structure.

ac·ces·so·ry ce·phal·ic vein (ak-ses′ŏr-ē sĕ-fal′ik vān) [TA] A variable vein that passes along the radial border of the forearm to join the cephalic vein near the elbow. SYN vena cephalicaaccessoria [TA].

ac·ces·so·ry chro·mo·some (ak-ses′ŏr-ē krō′mŏ-sōm) A supernumerary chromosome that is not an exact replica of any of the chromosomes in the normal cellular complement. SYN monosome (1), odd chromosome, unpaired allosome, unpaired chromosome.

ac·ces·so·ry gland (ak-ses′ŏr-ē gland) A small mass of glandular structure, detached from but lying near another and larger gland, to which it is similar in structure and probably in function.

ac·ces·so·ry hem·i·az·y·gos vein (ak-ses′ŏr-ē hem′ē-ā-zī′gos vān) [TA] Blood vessel formed by the union of the fourth to seventh left posterior intercostal veins. SYN vena hemiazygos accessoria [TA].

ac·ces·so·ry mus·cle (ak-ses′ŏr-ē mŭs′ĕl) A muscle that is not primarily responsible for but does provide assistance in initiating movement.

ac·ces·so·ry nerve [CN XI] (ak-ses′ŏr-ē nĕrv) [TA] Arises by two sets of roots: the presumed cranial, emerging from the side of the medulla, and spinal, emerging from the ventrolateral part of the first five cervical segments of the spinal cord; these roots unite to form the accessory nerve trunk, which divides into two branches, internal and external. SYN nervus accessorius [CN XI] [TA], eleventh cranial nerve [CN XI].

ac·ces·so·ry nip·ple (ak-ses′ŏr-ē nip′ĕl) A supernumerary nipple occurring on the mammary crest or line.

ac·ces·so·ry ob·tu·ra·tor ar·te·ry (ak-ses′ŏr-ē ob′tū-rā-tŏr ahr′tĕr-ē) [TA] Term applied to the anastomosis of the pubic branch of the inferior epigastric artery with the pubic branch of the obturator artery when it contributes a significant supply through the obturator canal. SYN arteria obturatoria accessoria [TA].

ac·ces·so·ry pan·cre·as (ak-ses′ŏr-ē pan′krē-ŭs) [TA] Detached portion of pancreatic tissue, usually the uncinate process (part of head of the pancreas), and hence most often found in the vicinity of the head, but which may occur within the gut wall (stomach or duodenum). SYN pancreas accessorium [TA].

ac·ces·so·ry pan·cre·at·ic duct (ak-ses'ŏr-ē pan-krē-at'ik dŭkt) [TA] The excretory duct of the head of the pancreas formed from the proximal part of the duct of the embryonic dorsal pancreatic bud. SYN ductus pancreaticus accessorius [TA], ductus dorsopancreaticus, Santorini canal, Santorini duct.

ac·ces·so·ry phren·ic nerves (ak-ses'ŏr-ē fren'ik nĕrvz) [TA] Accessory nerve strands that arise from the fifth cervical nerve. SYN nervi phrenici accessorii [TA].

ac·ces·so·ry pla·cen·ta (ak-ses'ŏr-ē plă-sen'tă) Mass of placental tissue distinct from the main placenta. SYN supernumerary placenta.

ac·ces·so·ry sign (ak-ses'ŏr-ē sīn) Finding frequently but not consistently present in a disease. SYN assident sign.

ac·ces·so·ry spleen (ak-ses'ŏr-ē splēn) [TA] One of the small globular masses of splenic tissue occasionally found in the region of the spleen, in one of the peritoneal folds, or elsewhere. SYN lien accessorius.

ac·ces·so·ry symp·tom (ak-ses'ŏr-ē simp'tŏm) A symptom that usually but not always accompanies a certain disease. SYN concomitant symptom.

ac·ces·so·ry ver·te·bral vein (ak-ses'ŏr-ē vĕr'tĕ-brăl vān) [TA] A vein that accompanies the vertebral vein but passes through the foramen of the transverse process of the seventh cervical vertebra and opens independently into the brachiocephalic vein. SYN vena vertebralis accessoria [TA].

ac·ci·den·tal host (ak-si-den'tăl hōst) Host that harbors an organism that usually does not infect it.

ac·ci·den·tal hy·po·ther·mi·a (ak-si-den'tăl hī'pō-thĕr'mē-ă) Unintentional decrease in body temperature, especially in the newborn, infants, and elderly, particularly during operations.

ac·ci·den·tal my·i·a·sis (ak-si-den'tăl mī-ī'ă-sis) Gastrointestinal myiasis due to ingestion of contaminated food.

ac·ci·den·tal par·a·site (ak-si-den'tăl par'ă-sīt) SYN incidental parasite.

ac·cli·mate (ak'li-māt) The process of becoming accustomed to something; may be either physiologic or psychological.

acclimatisation [Br.] SYN acclimatization.

ac·cli·ma·ti·za·tion, ac·cli·ma·tion (ă-klī'mă-tī-zā'shŭn, ak-li-mă'shŭn) Physiologic adaptation to a variation in environmental factors such as temperature, climate, or altitude.

ac·com·mo·dat·ing re·sis·tance (ă-kom'ŏ-dā-ting rĕ-zis'tăns) In isokinetic testing or training, application of a counterforce to muscle action to regulate the speed of contraction.

ac·com·mo·da·tion (ă-kom'ŏ-dā'shŭn) **1.** The act or state of adjustment or adaptation; especially change in the shape of the ocular lens for various focal distances. **2.** The ability of the ciliary muscle to adjust the curvature of the lens, increasing it for near vision and decreasing it for distant vision.

ac·com·mo·da·tive as·the·no·pi·a (ă-kom'ŏ-dā-tiv as'thĕ-nō'pē-ă) Ocular discomfort, headache, and other symptoms of eyestrain resulting from refractive error and excessive contraction of ciliary muscle.

ac·com·mo·da·tive in·suf·fi·cien·cy (ă-kom'ŏ-dā-tiv in'sŭ-fish'ĕn-sē) A lack of appropriate accommodation for near focus.

ac·com·mo·da·tive stra·bis·mus (ă-kom'ŏ-dā-tiv stră-biz'mŭs) Ocular condition in which the severity of deviation varies with accommodation.

ac·cor·di·on graft (ă-kōr'dē-ŏn graft) A skin graft in which multiple slits have been made, so it can be stretched to cover a large area.

ac·couche·ment (ak-kūsh-mawn[h]') Childbirth, particularly parturition.

ac·cou·cheur's hand (ah-kū-shurz' hand) Position of the hand in tetany or in muscular dystrophy; has resemblance to the position of the physician's hand in making a vaginal examination. SYN obstetric hand.

ac·cred·i·ta·tion (ă-kred′i-tā′shŭn) Approval, certification, or endorsement by an authority.

ac·cre·men·ti·tion (ak′rĕ-men-ti′shŭn) Reproduction by germination.

ac·cre·tion (ă-krē′shŭn) **1.** Increase by addition to the periphery of material of the same nature as that already present; e.g., the manner of growth of crystals. **2.** DENTISTRY foreign material (usually plaque or calculus) collecting on the surface of a tooth or in a cavity. **3.** A growing together of parts normally separate.

ac·cul·tur·a·tion (ă-kŭl′chŭr-ā′shŭn) Adaptation by a person or group to customs, values, beliefs, and behaviors of a new country or culture.

ac·cur·a·cy (ak′kyūr-ă-sē) *Do not confuse this word with precision.* The degree to which a measurement, or an estimate based on measurements, represents the true value of the attribute being measured.

a·cell·u·lar (ā-sel′yū-lăr) **1.** Devoid of cells. **2.** A term applied to unicellular organisms that do not become multicellular and are complete within a single cell unit.

a·ce·lo·mate, a·ce·lo·ma·tous (ā-sē′lŏ-māt, ā-sē-lō′mă-tŭs) Not having a celom or body cavity.

a·cen·tric (ā-sen′trik) Lacking a center.

a·ceph·al·gic mi·graine (ā-se-fal′jik mī′grān) A classic migraine episode in which the teichopsia is not followed by a headache.

a·ceph·a·lo·bra·chi·a (ā-sef′ă-lō-brā′kē-ă) SYN abrachiocephaly.

a·ceph·a·lous (ā-sef′ă-lŭs) Headless.

a·ceph·a·lus (ā-sef′ă-lŭs) A headless fetus.

a·ceph·a·ly (ā-sef′ă-lē) Congenital absence of the head.

ac·e·tab·u·lar (as′ĕ-tab′yū-lăr) Relating to the acetabulum.

ac·e·tab·u·lar la·brum (as′ĕ-tab′yū-lăr lā′brŭm) A fibrocartilaginous rim attached to the margin of the acetabulum of the hip bone. SYN cotyloid ligament.

ac·e·tab·u·lar notch (as′ĕ-tab′yū-lăr noch) [TA] A gap in the inferior margin of the acetabulum, bridged by the transverse acetabular ligament, giving passage to the acetabular branches of the obturator artery and vein. SYN incisura acetabuli [TA], cotyloid notch.

ac·e·tab·u·lec·to·my (as′ĕ-tab-yū-lek′tŏ-mē) Excision of the acetabulum.

ac·e·tab·u·lo·plas·ty (as′ĕ-tab′yū-lō-plas-tē) Any operation aimed at restoring the acetabulum to as near a normal state as possible.

ac·e·tab·u·lum, pl. **ac·e·tab·u·la** (as′ĕ-tab′yū-lŭm, -lă) [TA] A cup-shaped depression on the external surface of the hip bone, with which the head of the femur articulates. SYN cotyloid cavity.

ac·et·al·de·hyde (as′ĕ-tal′dĕ-hīd) An intermediary product in the metabolism of alcohol.

ac·et·a·min·o·phen (APAP) (ă-sē′tă-min′ō-fen) An antipyretic and analgesic, with potency similar to that of aspirin. SYN paracetamol.

ac·e·tate (as′ĕ-tāt) A salt or ester of acetic acid.

a·ce·tic (a-sē′tik, -set′ik) *Do not confuse this word with acidic or ascitic.* **1.** Denoting the presence of the two-carbon fragment of acetic acid. **2.** Relating to vinegar; sour.

a·ce·tic ac·id (HAc, AA) (a-sē′tik as′id) A product of the oxidation of ethanol and of the destructive distillation of wood; used locally as a counterirritant and occasionally internally, and also as a reagent. SYN ethanoic acid.

a·ce·tic fer·men·ta·tion, ac·e·tous fer·men·ta·tion (ă-sē′tik fĕr-men-tā′shŭn, as′ĕ-tŭs) Fermentation, as of wine or beer, whereby the alcohol is oxidized to acetic acid (vinegar).

ac·e·to·a·ce·tic ac·id (as′ĕ-tō-ă-sē′tik as′id) One of the ketone bodies, formed in excess and appearing in the urine in starvation or in diabetic acidosis. SYN diacetic acid.

acetonaemia [Br.] SYN acetonemia.

ac·e·tone (A) (as′ĕ-tōn) A colorless, volatile, flammable liquid; extremely small amounts are found in normal urine, but larger quantities occur in the urine and blood of people with diabetes. SYN dimethyl ketone.

ac·e·ton·e·mi·a (as′ĕ-tŏ-nē′mē-ă) The presence of acetone or acetone bodies in relatively large amounts in the blood. SYN acetonaemia.

ac·e·to·nu·ri·a (as′e-tō-nyūr′ē-ă) Excretion in the urine of large amounts of acetone.

ac·e·tous (as′ĕ-tŭs) Relating to vinegar; sour-tasting.

ac·e·to·whit·en·ing (ă-sē′tō-wīt′ĕn-ing) Blanching of skin or mucous membranes after application of 3–5% acetic acid solution, a sign of increased cellular protein and increased nuclear density. SYN cervicoscopy, visual inspection with acetic acid.

ac·e·tyl (Ac) (as′ĕ-til) An acetic acid molecule from which the hydroxyl group has been removed.

a·cet·y·la·tion (a-set′i-lā′shŭn) Formation of an acetyl derivative.

a·ce·tyl·cho·line (ACh) (as′ē-til-kō′lēn) A neurotransmitter that stimulates nicotinic receptors in autonomic ganglia, at the motor endplates of skeletal muscle, and in the central nervous system as well as muscarinic receptors in smooth muscle, in exocrine glands, and in the central nervous system.

a·ce·tyl·cys·te·ine, N-a·ce·tyl·cys·te·ine (AC) (as′ē-til-sis′tē-in) A mucolytic agent used to prevent liver injury due to acetaminophen toxicity.

N-ace·tyl·glu·co·sam·ine (as′ĕ-til-glū-cōs′ă-mēn) An acetylated amino sugar that is an important moiety of glycoproteins.

N-a·ce·tyl·neu·ra·min·ic ac·id (as′ĕ-til-nūr-ă-min′ik as′id) The most common form of sialic acid in mammals.

a·ce·tyl·sal·i·cyl·ic ac·id (ASA) (as′ĕ-til-sal-i-sil′ik as′id) Generic name of aspirin; this term is used in Canada and other countries where Aspirin remains a proprietary term.

a·ce·tyl·trans·fer·ase (as′ĕ-til-trans′fĕr-ās) Any enzyme transferring acetyl groups from one compound to another. SYN transacetylase.

a·cha·la·sia (ak-ă-lā′zē-ă) Failure to relax; referring especially to visceral openings such as the pylorus, cardia, or any other sphincter muscles.

a·cha·la·si·a of the car·di·a (ak-ă-lā′zē-ă kahr′dē-ă) SYN esophageal achalasia.

a·cha·la·si·a of the up·per sphinc·ter (ak-ă-lā′zē-ă ŭp′ĕr sfingk′tĕr) SYN cricopharyngeal achalasia.

ache (āk) A dull, poorly localized pain, usually of less than severe intensity.

a·chei·ri·a, a·chi·ri·a (ă-kī′rē-ă) **1.** Congenital absence of one or both hands. **2.** Anesthesia in one or both hands with loss of the sense of possession of the hand or hands. **3.** A sensibility disorder in which the patient is unable to identify which side of the body has received a stimulus.

a·chei·rop·o·dy, a·chi·rop·o·dy (ă-kī-rop′ŏ-dē) Congenital absence of the hands and feet; autosomal recessive inheritance.

a·chieve·ment age (ă-chēv′mĕnt āj) The relationship between the chronologic age and the age of achievement, as established by standard achievement tests.

Achil·les re·flex (ă-kil′ēz rē′fleks) A contraction of the calf muscles when the tendo calcaneus is sharply struck.

a·chil·lo·bur·si·tis (ă-kil′ō-bŭr-sī′tis) Inflammation of a bursa in proximity to the tendo calcaneus. SYN retrocalcaneobursitis.

a·chil·lo·dyn·i·a (ă-kil′ō-din′ē-ă) Pain due to inflammation of the bursa between the calcaneus and the tendo calcaneus (achillobursitis).

ach·il·lor·rha·phy (ak′il-ōr′ă-fē) Suture of the tendo calcaneus.

a·chil·lo·ten·ot·o·my (ă-kil'ō-ten-ot'ŏ-mē) Cutting of the tendo calcaneus.

a·chlor·hy·dri·a (ā-klōr-hī'drē-ă) Absence of hydrochloric acid from the gastric juice.

a·chlor·hy·dric ane·mi·a (ā-klōr-hī'drik ă-nē'mē-ă) A form of chronic hypochromic microcytic anemia associated with achlorhydria or achylia gastrica; observed most frequently in women in the third to fifth decades. SYN Faber syndrome.

a·cho·li·a (ā-kō'lē-ă) Suppressed or absent secretion of bile.

a·chol·ic (ā-kol'ik) Without bile, as in acholic (pale) stools.

a·chol·u·ric jaun·dice (ā-kō-lyūr'ik jawn'dis) Hepatic disorder with excessive amounts of unconjugated bilirubin in the plasma but without bile pigments in the urine.

a·chon·dro·gen·e·sis (ă-kon'drō-jen'ĕ-sis) Dwarfism accompanied by various bone aplasias of all four limbs, a normal or enlarged cranium, and a short trunk with delayed ossification of the lower vertebral column and pelvic bones.

achon·dro·gen·e·sis type IA (ă-kon'drō-jen'ĕ-sis tīp) The condition as seen with hypervascular cartilage and hypercellular bone; uncertain inheritance pattern. SYN Houston-Harris syndrome.

achon·dro·gen·e·sis type IB (ă-kon'drō-jen'ĕ-sis tīp) Disorder with severely disorganized intracartilaginous ossification.

achon·dro·gen·e·sis type II (ă-kon'drō-jen'ĕ-sis tīp) Genetic disorder with autosomal dominant inheritance, caused by mutation in the collagen type II gene (COL2A1) on chromosome 12q. SYN Langer-Saldino syndrome.

a·chon·dro·pla·si·a (ā-kon-drō-plā'zē-ă) This chondrodystrophy, characterized by an abnormality in conversion of cartilage to bone, is the most common form of short-limb dwarfism.

a·chon·dro·plas·tic dwarf (ā-kon'drō-plas'tik dwōrf) Most common form of dwarfism; related to defective abnormality of conversion of ligament to bone.

achrestic anaemia [Br.] SYN achrestic anemia.

a·chres·tic a·ne·mi·a (ă-kres'tik ă-nē'mē-ă) A potentially fatal form of the disorder chronic progressive macrocytic anemia in which the changes in bone marrow and circulating blood very closely resemble those found in pernicious anemia. SYN achrestic anaemia.

ach·ro·ma·si·a (ak'rō-mā'zē-ă) Pallor associated with hippocratic facies, emaciation, and weakness, often heralding a moribund state. SYN cachectic pallor.

ach·ro·mat (ăk-rō'măt) A person exhibiting achromatopsia.

ach·ro·mat·ic (ā'krō-mat'ik) 1. Without hue; of black, white, or gray color. 2. Not staining readily. 3. Refracting light without chromatic aberration.

ach·ro·mat·ic lens (ā-krō-mat'ik lenz) A compound lens made of two or more lenses having different indices of refraction.

ach·ro·ma·tin (ā-krō'mă-tin) The weakly staining components of the nucleus, such as the nuclear sap and euchromatin.

ach·ro·ma·tism (ā-krō'mă-tizm) 1. The quality of being achromatic. 2. The annulment of chromatic aberration by combining glasses of different refractive indices and different dispersion.

ach·ro·ma·tol·y·sis (ă-krō'mă-tol'i-sis) Dissolution of the achromatin of a cell or of its nucleus. SYN karyoplasmolysis.

ach·ro·mat·o·phil, ach·ro·mo·phil·ic, ach·ro·moph·i·lous (ă-krō-mat'ō-fil, -fil'ik, -mof'i-lŭs) 1. Not being colored by histologic or bacteriologic stains. 2. A cell or tissue that cannot be stained in the usual way. SYN achromophil.

ach·ro·ma·top·si·a, ach·ro·ma·top·sy (ă-krō-mă-top'sē-ă, ă-krō'mă-top-sē) A severe congenital deficiency in color perception, often associated with nystagmus and reduced visual acuity. SYN monochromatism (2).

ach·ro·ma·tous (ă-krō'mă-tŭs) Colorless.

ach·ro·ma·tu·ri·a (ă-krō-mă-tyūr′ē-ă) The passage of colorless or very pale urine.

ach·ro·mi·a (ă-krō′mē-ă) 1. Depigmentation (q.v.); absence or loss of natural pigmentation of the skin and iris. 2. Inability of a cell or tissue to be colored by one or more biologic stains

ach·y·li·a (ă-kī′lē-ă) 1. Absence of gastric juice or other digestive secretions. 2. Absence of chyle.

ac·ic·u·lar (ă-sik′yū-lar) Needle shaped.

ac·id (as′id) 1. A compound yielding a hydrogen ion in a polar solvent (e.g., in water); acids form salts by replacing all or part of the ionizable hydrogen with an electropositive element or radical. 2. In popular language, any sharp or sour tasting chemical compound. 3. Relating to acid; giving an acidic reaction.

acidaemia [Br.] SYN acidemia.

ac·id-ash di·et (as′id-ash dī′ĕt) SYN alkaline-ash diet.

ac·id-base ba·lance (as′id-bās bal′ăns) The normal balance between acid and base in the blood plasma.

ac·id-base man·age·ment: met·a·bol·ic ac·i·do·sis (asíd bās man′ăj-mĕnt met′ă-bol′ik as′i-dō′sis) Abnormal decrease in pH of the blood.

ac·id-base man·age·ment: met·a·bol·ic al·ka·lo·sis (as′id bās man′ăj-mĕnt met′ă-bol′ik al′ki-lō′sis) Abnormal increase in pH of the blood.

ac·id-base man·age·ment: res·pi·ra·to·ry ac·i·do·sis (as′id bās man′ăj-mĕnt res′pir-ă-tōr′ē as′i-dō′sis) Increase in carbon dioxide levels in blood that produces an abnormal decrease in pH.

ac·id-base man·age·ment: res·pir·a·to·ry al·ka·lo·sis (as′id bās man′ăj-mĕnt res′pir-ă-tōr′ē al′ki-lō′sis) Increase in carbon dioxide levels in the blood that produces an abnormal increase in pH.

ac·id-base reg·u·la·tion (as′id-bās reg-yū-lā′shŭn) The pH of body fluids ranges from a low of 1.0 to a high of 7.45. Regulation is by chemical buffers (bicarbon-

ate, phosphate, protein) and pulmonary excretion or retention of CO_2.

ac·i·de·mi·a (as-i-dē′mē-ă) An increase in the H^+ ion concentration of the blood or a fall below normal in pH, despite shifts in bicarbonate concentration. SYN acidaemia.

ac·id-fast (as′id-fast) Denoting bacteria that are not decolorized by acid-alcohol after having been stained with dyes such as basic fuchsin; e.g., the mycobacteria and nocardiae.

ac·id-fast ba·cil·lus (AFB) (as′id-fast bă-sil′ŭs) A type of bacterium that reacts in a given way when treated with an acid bath.

ac·id fuch·sin (as′id fūk′sin) Mixture of sodium salts, bi- and trisulfonic acids of rosanilin and pararosanilin; used as an indicator dye. SYN rubin S, rubine.

ac·id·ic (ă-sid′ik) Denotes something related to acid; forming acid.

ac·id·i·fied se·rum test (as-sid′i-fīd sēr′ŭm test) Lysis of the patient's red blood cells in acidified fresh serum, specific for paroxysmal nocturnal hemoglobinuria. SYN Ham test.

ac·id in·di·ges·tion (as′id in′di·jes′chŭn) Condition resulting from hyperchlorhydria; often used colloquially as a synonym for pyrosis.

ac·id·i·ty (ă-sid′i-tē) 1. The state of being acid. 2. The acid content of a fluid.

ac·i·do·phil, ac·i·do·phile (ă-sid′ŏ-fil, ă-sid′ŏ-fīl) 1. One of the acid-staining cells of the anterior pituitary. 2. A microorganism that grows well in a highly acid medium.

ac·i·do·phil ad·e·no·ma (ă-sid′ŏ-fil ad′ĕ-nō′mă) A tumor of the adenohypophysis in which cell cytoplasm stains with acid dyes. SYN eosinophil adenoma.

ac·i·do·phil·ic (A) (as′i-dŏ-fil′ik) Having an affinity for acid dyes; denoting a cell or tissue element that stains with an acid dye, such as eosin. SYN oxychromatic.

ac·i·doph·i·lus milk (as′i-dof′i-lŭs milk)

Milk inoculated with a culture of *Bacillus acidophilus*.

ac·i·do·sis (as'i-dō'sis) A pathologic state characterized by an increase in the concentration of hydrogen ions in the arterial blood below the normal range of pH 7.35 to 7.45.

ac·i·dot·ic (as'i-dot'ik) Pertaining to or indicating acidosis.

ac·id phos·pha·tase (AcP, ACP, ACPH, AP) (as'id fos'fā-tās) Phosphatase with an optimal pH of less than 7 (for several isozymes, it is 5.4), notably present in the prostate gland.

ac·id stain (as'id stān) A dye in which the anion is the colored component of the dye molecule, e.g., sodium eosinate (eosin).

ac·id tide (as'id tīd) A temporary increase in the acidity of the urine that occurs during fasting.

a·cid·u·lous (ă-sid'yŭ-lŭs) Acid or sour.

ac·i·du·ria (as'i-dyūr'ē-ă) 1. Excretion of acidic urine. 2. Excretion of an abnormal amount of any specified acid.

ac·i·du·ric (as'i-dyūr'ik) Pertaining to bacteria that tolerate an acid environment.

ac·i·nar (as'i-năr) Pertaining to the acinus. SYN acinic.

ac·i·nar car·ci·no·ma (as'i-năr kahr-si-nō'mă) SYN acinic cell adenocarcinoma.

ac·i·nar cell (as'i-năr sel) Any secreting cell lining an acinus, applied especially to the cells of the pancreas that furnish pancreatic enzymes. SYN acinous cell.

Ac·i·ne·to·bac·ter (as-i-nē'tō-bak'tĕr) A genus of nonmotile, aerobic bacteria (family Moraxellaceae), frequent cause of nosocomial infections; can also cause severe primary infections in immunocompromised patients. SYN *Lingelsheimia*.

ac·in·ic (ă-sin'ik) SYN acinar.

ac·in·i·form (ă-sin'i-fōrm) SYN acinous.

ac·i·ni·tis (as-in-ī'tis) Inflammation of an acinus.

ac·i·nous, ac·i·nose (as'i-nŭs) Resembling an acinus or grape-shaped structure. SYN aciniform.

ac·i·nous cell (as'i-nŭs sel) SYN acinar cell.

ac·i·nous gland (as'i-nŭs gland) A gland in which the secretory unit has a grapelike shape and a very small lumen.

ac·i·nus, gen. and pl. **ac·i·ni** (as'i-nŭs, as'i-nī) [TA] One of the minute grape-shaped secretory portions of an acinous gland.

ac·la·sis (ak'lă-sis) A state of continuity between normal and abnormal tissue. SYN aclasia.

ac·me (ak'mē) The period of greatest intensity of any symptom, sign, or process.

ac·mes·the·sia (ak'mes-thē'zē-ă) Sensitivity to pinprick.

ac·ne (ak'nē) Inflammatory disease of sebaceous follicles marked by papules and pustules. Typically begins during puberty; affects chest, back, and face, but sometimes other areas. Cause remains unknown.

ac·ne ca·chec·ti·co·rum (ak'nē kă-kek-ti-kōr'ŭm) Acne in persons who have a debilitating constitutional disease; characterized by large, soft, purulent, ulcerative, cystic, and scarred lesions.

ac·ne er·y·the·ma·to·sa (ak'nē ĕ-rith'ĕ-mă-tō'să) SYN rosacea.

ac·ne ful·mi·nans (ak'nē ful'mi-nanz) Severe scarring acne in male teenagers, which may be associated with fever, polyarthralgia, crusted ulcerative lesions, weight loss, and anemia.

ac·ne·ge·nic (ak'nē-jen'ik) Inducing acne or increasing its severity.

ac·ne in·du·ra·ta (ak'nē in-dū-rā'tă) Deeply seated acne, with large papules and pustules, large scars, and hypertrophic scars.

ac·ne ke·loid (ak'nē kē'loyd) A chronic

eruption of fibrous papules that develop at the site of follicular lesions, usually on the back of the neck at the hairline. SYN dermatitis papillaris capillitii, folliculitis keloidalis.

ac•ne ke•ra•to•sa (ak′nē ker-ă-tō′să) An eruption of papules consisting of horny plugs projecting from the hair follicles, accompanied by inflammation.

ac•ne ne•o•na•to•rum (AN) (ak′nē nē-ō-nā-tōr′ŭm) Condition of neonates, characterized by papules, pustules, and comedones on the forehead and cheeks, usually resolving in a few months.

ac•ne pa•pu•lo•sa (ak′nē pap-yū-lō′să) Dermatologic condition in which papular lesions predominate.

ac•ne punc•ta•ta (ak′nē pŭngk-tā′tă) Dermatologic condition with black comedones.

ac•ne vul•ga•ris (ak′nē vŭl-gā′ris) An eruption, predominantly of the face, upper back, and chest, composed of comedones, cysts, papules, and pustules on an inflammatory base.

ac•o•nite (ak′ō-nīt) The dried root of *Aconitum napellus,* commonly known as monkshood or wolfsbane; a powerful and rapid-acting poison used as an antipyretic, diuretic, diaphoretic, anodyne, cardiac and respiratory depressant, and externally as an analgesic. SYN fu tzu, monkshood.

a•co•re•a (ă-kōr′ē-ă) Congenital absence of the pupil of the eye.

a•corn-tip•ped cath•e•ter (ā′kōrn-tipt kath′ĕ-tĕr) Catheter used in ureteropyelography to occlude the ureteral orifice and prevent backflow from the ureter during and following the injection of an opaque medium.

a•cous•tic, a•cous•ti•cal (ă-kūs′tik, -tik-ăl) Pertaining to hearing and the perception of sound.

a•cous•tic im•ped•ance (ă-kū′stik im-pē′dăns) Resistance that a material offers to the passage of a sound wave (colloquial).

a•cou•stic me•a•tus (ă-kūs′tik mē-ā′tŭs) **1.** External: auditory canal; the passage leading inward through the tympanic portion of the temporal bone, from the auricle to the membrana tympani. **2.** Internal: a canal running through the petrous portion of the temporal bone, giving passage to the facial and vestibulocochlear nerves and to the labyrinthine artery and veins. SYN meatus acusticus.

a•cous•tic neu•ri•lem•o•ma (ă-kū′stik nūr′i-lē-mō′mă) Schwannoma arising from cranial nerve VIII.

a•cous•tic neu•ro•ma, a•cous•tic neu•ri•le•mo•ma (ă-kūs′tik nūr-ō′mă, ă-kūs′tik nūr′i-lē-mō′mă) A benign tumor arising from Schwann cells of the auditory nerve (CN VIII).

a•cous•tic ra•di•a•tion (ă-kūs′tik rā′dē-ā′shŭn) [TA] The fibers that pass from the medial geniculate body to the transverse temporal gyri of the cerebral cortex by way of the sublentiform part of the internal capsule. SYN radiatio acustica [TA].

a•cou•stic re•flex (ă-kūs′tik rē′fleks) Contraction of the stapedius muscle in response to intense sound, increasing impedance of the middle ear and thereby protecting the inner ear from the sound. SYN stapedial reflex.

a•cous•tics (ă-kūs′tiks) The science concerned with sounds and with their perception.

a•cou•stic stim•u•la•tion test (ă-kūs′tik stim′yū-lā′shŭn test) A test for fetal well-being through use of an acoustic device to stimulate the fetus and cause acceleration of fetal heart rate.

a•cous•tic trau•ma•tic hear•ing loss (ă-kūs′tik traw-mat′ik hēr′ing laws) Sensory hearing loss due to exposure to high-intensity noise.

ac•quired char•ac•ter (ă-kwīrd′ kar′ăk-tĕr) A character developed in a plant or animal as a result of environmental influences during the individual's life.

ac•quired ep•i•lep•tic a•pha•si•a (ă-kwīrd′ ep′i-lep′tik ă-fā′zē-ă) SYN Landau-Kleffner syndrome.

acquired hyperlipoproteinaemia [Br.] SYN acquired hyperlipoproteinemia.

ac•quired hy•per•lip•o•pro•tein•e•mi•a

(ă-kwīrd´ hĭ´pĕr-lip´ō-prō´tē-nē´mē-ă) Nonfamilial disorder that develops as a consequence of some primary disease, such as thyroid deficiency. SYN acquired hyperlipoproteinaemia.

ac·quired hy·po·gam·ma·glob·u·li·ne·mi·a (ă-kwīrd´ hī´pō-gam´ă-glob´yū-li-nē´mē-ă) SYN common variable immunodeficiency.

ac·quired im·mu·ni·ty (ă-kwīrd´ i-myū´ni-tē) Resistance resulting from previous exposure of the individual in question to an infectious agent or antigen.

ac·quired im·mu·no·de·fi·cien·cy syn·drome (AIDS) (ă-kwīrd´ im´yū-nō-dĕ-fish´ĕn-sē sin´drōm) Disorder of the immune system characterized by opportunistic diseases, including candidiasis, *Pneumocystis jiroveci* pneumonia, oral hairy leukoplakia, herpes zoster, Kaposi sarcoma, toxoplasmosis, isosporiasis, cryptococcosis, non-Hodgkin lymphoma, and tuberculosis.

ac·quired meg·a·co·lon (ă-kwīrd´ meg´ă-kō´lŏn) Megacolon occurring in association with an acquired disease.

acquired naevus [Br.] SYN acquired nevus.

ac·quired ne·vus (ă-kwīrd´ nē´vŭs) A melanocytic nevus that is not visible at birth, but appears in childhood or adult life. SYN acquired naevus.

ac·quired pel·li·cle (ă-kwīrd´ pel´i-kĕl) Thin film (about 1 mcm), derived mainly from salivary glycoproteins, which forms over the surface of a cleansed tooth crown when exposed to saliva. SYN acquired cuticle, acquired enamel cuticle, brown pellicle, posteruption cuticle.

ac·quired tox·o·plas·mo·sis in adults (ă-kwīrd´ tok´sō-plaz-mō´sis ă-dŭlts´) A form of toxoplasmosis that may result in fever, encephalomyelitis, chorioretinopathy, maculopapular rash, arthralgia, myalgia, myocarditis, and pneumonitis; frequently found in patients with AIDS.

ac·ral (ak´răl) Relating to or affecting the peripheral body parts.

Ac·re·mo·ni·um (ak´rĕ-mō´nē-ŭm) A genus of fungi that occurs in soil and decaying plant matter; causes onychomycosis, corneal ulcers, eumycotic mycetoma, and endophthalmitis.

ac·rid (ak´rid) Sharp, pungent, biting, or irritating.

ac·ro·ag·no·sis (ak´rō-ag-nō´sis) Loss or impairment of the sensory recognition of a limb.

acroanaesthesia [Br.] SYN acroanesthesia.

ac·ro·an·es·the·si·a (ak´rō-an-es-thē´zē-ă) Anesthesia of one or more of the extremities. SYN acroanaesthesia.

ac·ro·ar·thri·tis (ak´rō-ahr-thrī´tis) Inflammation of the joints of the hands or feet.

ac·ro·a·tax·i·a (ak´rō-ă-tak´sē-ă) Ataxia affecting the distal portion of the extremities. Cf. proximoataxia.

ac·ro·brach·y·ceph·a·ly (ak´rō-brak-i-sef´ă-lē) Type of craniosynostosis with premature closure of the coronal suture, resulting in an abnormally short anteroposterior diameter of the cranium.

ac·ro·ce·pha·li·a (ak´rō-se-fā´lē-ă) SYN oxycephaly.

ac·ro·ceph·a·lo·pol·y·syn·dac·ty·ly (ak´rō-sef´ă-lō-pol´ē-sin-dak´ti-lē) Rare autosomal disorder with mental retardation, syndactyly, oxycephaly, congenital heart defects, mild obesity, and hypogenitalism.

ac·ro·ceph·a·lo·syn·dac·tyly (ak´rō-sef´ă-lō-sin-dak´ti-lē) A group of congenital syndromes characterized by peaking of the cranium and fusion or webbing of fingers or digits.

ac·ro·ceph·a·ly, ac·ro·ce·pha·li·a (ak´rō-sef´ă-lē, -sĕ-fā´lē-ă) SYN oxycephaly.

ac·ro·chor·don (ak´rō-kōr´dŏn) SYN skin tag.

ac·ro·con·trac·ture (ak´rō-kŏn-trak´chŭr) Contracture of the joints of the hands or feet.

ac·ro·cy·a·no·sis (ak´rō-sī-ă-nō´sis) A circulatory disorder in which the hands, and less commonly the feet, are persistently cold and blue. SYN Crocq disease, Raynaud sign.

ac·ro·der·ma·ti·tis (ak′rō-dĕr-mă-tī′tis) *Do not confuse this word with acarodermatitis.* Inflammation of the skin of the extremities.

ac·ro·der·ma·ti·tis chron·i·ca a·tro·ph·i·cans (ACA) (ak′rō-dĕr-mă-tī′tis kron′i-kă ă-trō′fi-kanz) Gradually progressive late skin manifestation of Lyme disease, giving a tissue-paper appearance of the involved sites.

ac·ro·der·ma·ti·tis con·tin·u·a (ak′rō-dĕr-mă-tī′tis kon-tin′yū-ă) SYN pustulosis palmaris et plantaris.

ac·ro·der·ma·ti·tis en·ter·o·path·i·ca (ak′rō-dĕr′mă-tī′tis en′tĕr-ō-path′i-kă) A progressive hereditary defect of zinc metabolism in young children (onset, 3 weeks–18 months); often manifests first as a blistering, oozing, and crusting eruption on an extremity or around one of the orifices of the body, followed by loss of hair and by diarrhea or other gastrointestinal disturbances.

ac·ro·der·ma·ti·tis per·stans (ak′rō-dĕr′mă-tī′tis pĕr′stanz) SYN pustulosis palmaris et plantaris.

ac·ro·der·ma·to·sis (ak′rō-dĕr′mă-tō′sis) Any cutaneous affection involving the more distal portions of the extremities.

ac·ro·dyn·i·a (ak′rō-din′ē-ă) 1. Pain in peripheral or acral parts of the body. 2. A syndrome caused almost exclusively in the past by mercury poisoning: in children, characterized by erythema of the limbs, chest, and nose, gastrointestinal symptoms, behavioral changes, and polyneuritis; in adults, characterized by anorexia, photophobia, sweating, and tachycardia. SYN acrodynic erythema, dermatopolyneuritis, erythredema, Feer disease, pink disease.

ac·ro·es·the·si·a (ak′rō-es-thē′zē-ă) 1. An extreme degree of hyperesthesia. 2. Hyperesthesia of one or more of the extremities. SYN acroaesthesia.

ac·rog·no·sis (ak′rog-nō′sis) *In the diphthong gn, the g is silent only at the beginning of a word. Do not confuse this word with acroagnosis.* Normal sensory perception of the extremities.

ac·ro·ker·a·to·sis (ak′rō-ker-ă-tō′sis) Overgrowth of the horny layer of the skin, usually in nodular configurations, of the dorsum of the fingers and toes, and occasionally on the rim of the ear and tip of the nose.

ac·ro·ki·ne·si·a (ak′rō-ki-nē′zē-ă) SYN acrocinesia.

ac·ro·meg·a·ly (ak′rō-meg′ă-lē) A disorder marked by progressive enlargement of the head, face, hands, and feet.

ac·ro·mel·ic (ak′rō-mē′lik) Affecting the terminal part of a limb.

ac·ro·met·a·gen·e·sis (ak′rō-met-ă-jen′ĕ-sis) Abnormal growth of the limbs resulting in deformity.

ac·ro·mi·al (ă-krō′mē-ăl) Relating to the acromion.

ac·ro·mi·al an·gle (ă-krō′mē-ăl ang′gĕl) [TA] The prominent angle at the junction of the posterior and lateral borders of the acromion. SYN angulus acromii [TA].

ac·ro·mi·al pro·cess (ă-krō′mē-ăl pros′es) SYN acromion.

ac·ro·mic·ri·a (ak′rō-mik′rē-ă) Condition in which the bones of the face and limbs are overly small and delicate.

ac·ro·mi·o·cla·vic·u·lar (ă-krō′mē-ō-klă-vik′yū-lăr) Relating to the acromion and the clavicle. SYN scapuloclavicular (1).

ac·ro·mi·on (ă-krō′mē-on) [TA] The lateral end of the spine of the scapula, which projects as a broad flattened process overhanging the glenoid fossa. SYN acromial process.

ac·ro·mi·o·plas·ty (ă-krō′mē-ō-plas′tē) A surgical reshaping of the acromion.

ac·ro·mi·o·tho·rac·ic ar·te·ry (ă-krō′mē-ō-thōr-as′ik ahr′tĕr-ē) SYN thoracoacromial artery.

ac·rom·pha·lus (ak-rom′făl-ŭs) Abnormal projection of the umbilicus.

ac·ro·my·o·to·ni·a, ac·ro·my·ot·o·nus (ak′rō-mī-ō-tō′nē-ă, -mī-ot′ō-nŭs) Myotonia affecting the extremities only, resulting in spastic deformity of the hand or foot.

ac·ro·pach·y·der·ma (ak′rō-pak-i-dĕr′mă) SYN pachydermoperiostosis.

acroparesthaesia [Br.] SYN acroparesthesia.

ac·ro·par·es·the·si·a (ak′rō-par-es-thē′zē-ă) **1.** Paresthesia of one or more of the limbs. **2.** Nocturnal paresthesia involving the hands, most often of middle-aged women; formerly attributed to a lesion in the thoracic outlet but now known to be a classic symptom of carpal tunnel syndrome. SYN acroparaesthesia.

ac·rop·e·tal (ă-krop′ĕ-tăl) Developing from the base toward the apex.

ac·ro·pho·bi·a (ak′rŏ-fō′bē-ă) Morbid fear of heights.

ac·ro·pus·tu·lo·sis (ak′rō-pŭs-chū-lō′sis) Pustular eruptions of the hands and feet, often a form of psoriasis.

ac·ro·scle·ro·sis, ac·ro·scle·ro·der·ma (ak′rō-skler-ō′sis, -ō-dĕr′mă) Stiffness and tightness of the skin of the fingers, with atrophy of the soft tissue and osteoporosis of the distal phalanges of the hands and feet. SEE CREST syndrome. SYN sclerodactyly.

ac·ro·so·mal (ak′rō-sō′măl) Outer covering of a sperm; contains enzymes that allow it to penetrate an oocyte.

ac·ro·so·mal cap (ak′rō-sō′măl kap) SYN acrosome.

ac·ro·so·mal ves·i·cle (ak′rō-sō′măl ves′i-kĕl) A vesicle derived from the Golgi apparatus during spermiogenesis.

ac·ro·some (ak′rō-sōm) A caplike organelle or saccule derived from Golgi elements that surround the anterior two thirds of the nucleus of a sperm. SYN acrosomal cap, head cap.

ac·ro·spi·ro·ma (ak′rō-spī-rō′mă) A tumor of the distal dermal segment of a sweat gland.

ac·ro·tism (ak′rō-tizm) Absence or imperceptibility of the pulse.

a·cryl·a·mide (AM) (ă-kril′ă-mīd) A carcinogen that forms in starchy foods cooked at high temperature (e.g., fried potatoes, potato chips).

a·cryl·ate (ak′ri-lāt) A salt or ester of acrylic acid.

a·cryl·ic (Acr) (ă-kril′ik) Denoting certain synthetic plastic resins derived from acrylic acid.

ac·ti·gra·phy (ak-tig′ră-fē) Monitoring of movement, especially during testing to assess sleep disorders.

ac·tin (ak′tin) One of the protein components into which actomyosin can be split.

ac·tin fil·a·ment (ak′tin fil′ă-mĕnt) One of the contractile elements in muscular fibers and other cells.

act·ing out (akt′ing owt) An overt act or set of actions that provides an emotional outlet for the expression of emotional conflicts (usually unconscious).

ac·tin·ic (ak-tin′ik) Relating to the chemically active rays of the electromagnetic spectrum.

ac·tin·ic con·junc·ti·vi·tis (ak-tin′ik kŏn-jŭnk′ti-vī′tis) SYN ultraviolet keratoconjunctivitis.

ac·tin·ic der·ma·ti·tis (ak-tin′ik dĕr′mă-tī′tis) SYN photodermatitis.

ac·tin·ic gran·u·lo·ma (ak-tin′ik gran′yū-lō′mă) An anular eruption on sun-exposed skin. SYN Miescher granuloma.

ac·tin·ic ker·a·to·sis (ak-tin′ik ker′ă-tō′sis) A premalignant warty lesion occurring on the sun-exposed skin of the face or hands in aged light-skinned people.

actino- Combining form meaning a ray, as of light; applied to any form of radiation or to any structure with radiating parts. SEE ALSO radio-.

ac·ti·no·bac·il·lo·sis (ak′tin-ō-bas-i-lō′sis) A disease of cattle and swine, occasionally reported in humans, caused by the bacterium *Actinobacillus lignieresii*; primarily affects soft tissues.

Ac·ti·no·ba·cil·lus (ak′tin-ō-bă-sil′lŭs)

A genus of nonmotile, non-spore-forming, aerobic, facultatively anaerobic bacteria containing gram-negative rods interspersed with coccal elements.

ac·ti·no·der·ma·ti·tis (ak′ti-nō-dĕr′mă-tī′tis) SYN photodermatitis.

Ac·ti·no·ma·du·ra (ak′ti-nō-mă-dū′ră) A genus of aerobic, gram-positive, non-acid-fast fungi with filaments that fragment into spores.

Ac·ti·no·my·ces (ak′ti-nō-mī′sēz) A genus of slow-growing, nonmotile, non-spore-forming, anaerobic to facultatively anaerobic bacteria containing gram-positive, irregularly staining filaments; can cause chronic suppurative infection in humans. The type species is *A. bovis*.

Ac·ti·no·my·ces is·ra·eli·i (ak′ti-nō-mī′sēz iz-rā-el′ē-ī) A species of bacteria causing human actinomycosis and, occasionally, infections in cattle.

Ac·ti·no·my·ce·ta·ce·ae (ak′ti-nō-mī-sē-tā′shē-ē) A family of non-spore-forming, nonmotile, facultatively anaerobic bacteria containing gram-positive, non-acid-fast, predominantly diphtheroid cells that tend to form branched filaments.

Ac·ti·no·my·ce·ta·les (ak′ti-nō-mī-sē-tā′lēz) An order of bacteria consisting of moldlike, rod-shaped, clubbed, or filamentous forms with tendency to branching.

ac·ti·no·my·co·sis (ak′ti-nō-mī-kō′sis) A disease primarily of cattle and humans caused by *Actinomyces bovis* in cattle and by *Actinomyces israelii* and *Arachnia propionica* in humans. Part of the normal bacterial flora of the mouth and pharynx, but may produce chronic destructive abscesses or granulomas that eventually discharge a viscid pus. In humans, the disease commonly affects the cervicofacial area, abdomen, or thorax.

ac·ti·no·ther·a·py (ak′ti-nō-thār′ă-pē) DERMATOLOGY ultraviolet light therapy.

ac·tion cur·rent (ak′shŭn kŭr′rĕnt) An electrical current induced in muscle fibers when they are effectively stimulated; normally it is followed by contraction.

ac·tion po·ten·ti·al (ak′shŭn pŏ-ten′ shăl) The change in membrane potential occurring in nerve, muscle, or other excitable tissue when excitation occurs.

ac·tion tre·mor (ak′shŭn trem′ŏr) SYN intention tremor.

ac·ti·vate (ak′ti-vāt) **1.** To render active. **2.** To make radioactive.

ac·ti·vat·ed char·coal (AC) (ak′ti-vā-tĕd chahr′kōl) Residue from destructive distillation of various organic materials, treated to increase its adsorptive power; used to treat diarrhea, as an antidote to various poisons, and in purification processes in industry and research.

ac·ti·va·ted clot·ting time test (ak′ti-vāt-ĕd klot′ing tīm test) Diagnostic test that determines coagulation time of blood.

ac·ti·vat·ed par·tial throm·bo·plas·tin time (aPTT) (ak′ti-vā-tĕd pahr′ shăl throm-bō-plas′tin tīm) The time needed for plasma to form a fibrin clot following addition of calcium and a phospholipid reagent.

ac·ti·va·tion (ak′ti-vā′shŭn) **1.** The act of rendering active. **2.** An increase in the energy content of an atom or molecule, through the raising of temperature, absorption of light photons, or other means. **3.** Techniques of stimulating the brain by light, sound, electricity, or chemical agents, to elicit abnormal activity in the electroencephalogram. **4.** Stimulation of peripheral nerve fibers to the point that action potentials are initiated. **5.** The act of making radioactive.

ac·ti·va·tor (ak′ti-vā-tŏr) **1.** A substance that renders another substance active, or one that accelerates a process or reaction. **2.** The fragment, produced by chemical cleavage of a proactivator, that induces the enzymatic activity of another substance. **3.** An apparatus for making substances radioactive. **4.** A removable type of myofunctional orthodontic appliance that acts as a passive transmitter of force, which is produced by the function of the activated muscles, to the teeth and alveolar process that are in contact with it. **5.** A protein that binds to a DNA sequence before DNA polymerase transcription. **6.** Manually assisted thrust instrument that activates mechanoreceptors; used by many chiropractors.

ac·tive an·a·phy·lax·is (ak'tiv an'ă-fi-lak'sis) Reaction following inoculation of antigen in a subject previously sensitized to the specific antigen, in contrast to passive anaphylaxis.

ac·tive as·sist·ed ex·er·cise (ak'tiv ă-sist'ĕd ek'sĕr-sīz) Exercise that requires an individual to use as much personal movement as possible but also incorporates help from an outside source (either human or mechanical) to complete the movement.

ac·tive car·ri·er (ak'tiv kar'ē-ĕr) A living being (human or otherwise) that can transmit active forms of a disease to other living beings.

ac·tive chron·ic hep·a·ti·tis (ak'tiv kron'ik hep'ă-tī'tis) Liver disease with chronic portal inflammation and progressive hepatic degeneration. SYN posthepatitic cirrhosis.

ac·tive cool-down (ak'tiv kūl'down) SYN active recovery.

ac·tive e·lec·trode (ak'tiv ĕ-lek'trōd) Small electrode with an exciting effect used to stimulate or record potentials from a localized area. SYN exciting electrode, localizing electrode, therapeutic electrode.

ac·tive eu·tha·na·sia (ak'tiv yū'thă-nā'zē-ă) Mode of ending life in which the intent is to cause the patient's death in a single act (also called mercy killing).

ac·tive ex·er·cise (ak'tiv ek'sĕr-sīz) Exercise that requires someone to use one's own muscle power and does not require assistance from an outside source.

ac·tive ex·pi·ra·tion (ak'tiv eks'pĕr-ă'shŭn) Forceful exhalation of air from the lungs.

active hyperaemia [Br.] SYN active hyperemia.

ac·tive hy·per·e·mi·a (ak'tiv hī'pĕr-ē'mē-ă) Hyperemia due to an increased afflux of arterial blood into dilated capillaries. SYN active hyperaemia, fluxionary hyperemia.

ac·tive im·mu·ni·ty (ak'tiv i-myū'ni-tē) SEE acquired immunity.

ac·tive move·ment (ak'tiv mūv'mĕnt) **1.** Motion effected by the organism itself, unaided by external influences. **2.** In physical therapy, a movement that is effected entirely by the patient's muscles, often with the guidance of the therapist.

ac·tive play (ak'tiv plā) Refers to the type of play in which a child engages in an activity, rather than simply watching others passively.

ac·tive prin·ci·ple (ak'tiv prin'si-pĕl) A constituent of a drug, usually an alkaloid or glycoside, on which the characteristic therapeutic action of the substance largely depends.

ac·tive range of mo·tion (AROM) (ak' tiv rānj mō'shŭn) Amount of motion at a given joint when the subject moves the part voluntarily.

ac·tive re·cov·er·y (ak'tiv rĕ-kŭv'ĕr-ē) Exercising with gradually diminishing intensity immediately after a bout of vigorous exercise. SYN active cool-down, tapering-off.

ac·tive re·sist·ance ex·er·cise (ak'tiv rē-zis'tăns ek'sĕr-sīz) Exercise that incorporates weights of some type (e.g., provides resistance to a motion).

ac·tive splint (ak'tiv splint) SYN dynamic splint.

ac·tive trans·port (ak'tiv trans'pōrt) Passage of ions or molecules across a cell membrane, not by passive diffusion but by an energy-consuming process at the expense of catabolic processes proceeding within the cell.

ac·tive treat·ment (ak'tiv trēt'mĕnt) Therapeutic substance or course intended to ameliorate the basic disease, rather than supportive or palliative treatment. Cf. causal treatment.

ac·tiv·in (ak'ti-vin) Placental hormone that reaches maximum levels in maternal serum during labor.

ac·tiv·i·ties of daily liv·ing (ADL) (ak-tiv'i-tēz dā'lē liv'ing) Everyday routines generally involving functional mobility and personal care, such as bathing, dressing, toileting, and meal preparation. An inability to perform these renders one dependent on others, resulting in a self-care deficit.

ac·tiv·i·ties of dai·ly liv·ing scale (ak-tiv'i-tēz dā'lē liv'ing skāl) A measurement to score physical activity and its limitations, based on answers to simple questions about mobility, self-care, and grooming.

ac·tiv·i·ty (ak-tiv'i-tē) **1.** ELECTROENCE-PHALOGRAPHY the presence of neurogenic electrical energy. **2.** PHYSICAL CHEMISTRY an ideal concentration for which the law of mass action will apply perfectly; the ratio of the activity to the true concentration is the activity coefficient (γ), which becomes 1.00 at infinite dilution. **3.** For enzymes, the amount of substrate consumed (or product formed) in a given time under given conditions; turnover number. **4.** The number of nuclear transformations (disintegrations) in a given quantity of a material per unit time. Units: curie (Ci), millicurie (mCi), becquerel (Bq), megabecquerel (MBq). SEE ALSO radioactivity. **5.** Producing movement. **6.** A class of goal-directed human actions.

ac·tiv·i·ty grad·ing (ak-tiv'i-tē grād'ing) Incrementally changing the process, tools, materials, or environment of a given activity to increase or decrease performance demands gradually, and ultimately to ensure best performance. SYN sport-specific training.

ac·tiv·i·ty in·to·le·rance (ak-tiv'i-tē in-tol'ĕr-ăns) Inability to perform daily activities because of decreased energy for any reason.

ac·tiv·i·ty tol·er·ance (ak-tiv'i-tē tol'ĕr-ăns) A measure of a patient's ability to participate in daily required tasks.

ac·tu·al cau·te·ry (ak'chū-ăl kaw'tĕr-ē) A cautery acting directly through heat and not by chemical means.

a·cu·i·ty (ă-kyū'i-tē) **1.** Sharpness, clearness, distinctness. **2.** Severity.

a·cu·mi·nate (ă-kyū'mi-năt) Pointed; tapering to a point.

ac·u·pres·sure (ak'yū-presh-ŭr) Application of pressure in sites used for acupuncture with therapeutic intent.

ac·u·punc·ture (ak'yū-pŭngk'shŭr) An ancient Asian system of healing that uses long fine needles.

ac·u·punc·ture an·es·the·si·a (ak'yū-pŭngk'shŭr an'es-thē'zē-ă) Percutaneous insertion of, and stimulation by, needles placed in critical areas of the body to produce loss of sensation in another area.

ac·u·punc·ture points (ak'yū-pŭngk'shŭr poynts) Points on the body surface at which acupuncture is believed to correct disturbances of energy flow associated with disease.

a·cute (ă-kyūt') **1.** Referring to a disease of sudden onset and brief course, not chronic, sometimes loosely used to mean severe. **2.** Referring to treatment or exposure: brief, intense, short-term; sometimes specifically referring to brief exposure of high intensity.

a·cute ab·do·men (ă-kyūt' ab'dŏ-mĕn) Any serious sudden intraabdominal condition (e.g., appendicitis) attended by pain, tenderness, and muscular rigidity, and for which emergency surgery must be considered. SYN surgical abdomen.

a·cute a·dre·no·cor·ti·cal in·suf·fi·cien·cy (ă-kyūt' ă-drē'nō-kŏr'ti-kăl in'sŭ-fish'ĕn-sē) Sudden worsening of signs and symptoms of corticosteroid deficiency when trauma or illness causes increased demand in a patient with impaired adrenal insufficiency. SYN addisonian crisis, adrenal crisis.

a·cute al·co·hol·ism (ă-kyūt' al'kŏ-hol-izm) Temporary deterioration in mental function, accompanied by muscular incoordination and paresis, induced by the rapid ingestion of alcoholic beverages. SYN intoxication (2).

a·cute an·gle (ă-kyūt' ang'gĕl) Any angle measuring less than 90 degrees.

a·cute an·te·ri·or po·li·o·my·e·li·tis (ă-kyūt' an-tēr'ē-ŏr pō'lē-ō-mī-ĕ-lī'tis) Inflammation of the anterior cornua of the spinal cord; an acute infectious disease caused by the poliomyelitis virus marked by fever, pains, and gastroenteric disturbances, followed by a flaccid paralysis of one or more muscular groups, and later by atrophy.

a·cute ap·pen·di·ci·tis (AA, AAP) (ă-kyūt´ ă-pen´di-sī´tis) Sudden inflammation of the appendix, usually resulting from bacterial infection, which may be precipitated by obstruction of the lumen by a fecalith.

a•cute chor•e•a (ă-kyūt´ kōr-ē´ă) SYN Sydenham chorea.

a•cute com•pres•sion tri•ad (ă-kyūt´ kŏm-presh´ŭn trī´ad) The rising venous pressure, falling arterial pressure, and decreased heart sounds of pericardial tamponade. SYN Beck triad.

a•cute cor•o•nar•y syn•drome (ACS) (ă-kyūt´ kōr´ŏ-nār-ē sin´drōm) A general term for clinical syndromes due to reduction of blood flow in coronary arteries (e.g., unstable angina, acute myocardial infarction). SYN acute myocardial infarction, preinfarction angina, unstable angina.

a•cute dis•sem•i•nat•ed en•ceph•a•lo•my•e•li•tis (ă-kyūt´ di-sem´i-nā-tĕd en-sef´ă-lō-mī´ĕ-lī´tis) Demyelinating disorder of the central nervous system in which focal demyelination is present throughout the brain and spinal cord.

a•cute ep•i•dem•ic leu•ko•en•ceph•a•li•tis (ă-kyūt´ ep´i-dem´ik lū´kō-en-sef´ă-lī´tis) A disease characterized by acute onset of fever, followed by convulsions, delirium, and coma, and associated with perivascular demyelination and hemorrhagic foci in the central nervous system. SYN Strümpell disease (2).

a•cute fi•brin•ous per•i•car•di•tis (ă-kyūt´ fī´bri-nŭs per´i-kahr-dī´tis) Common lesion of acute pericarditis in which inflammation produces large quantities of fibrin.

a•cute ful•mi•nat•ing me•nin•go•coc•ce•mi•a (ă-kyūt´ ful´mi-nāt´ing mĕ-ning´gō-kok-sē´mē-ă) Rapidly systemic infection with *Neisseria meningitidis*, usually without meningitis, characterized by rash, usually petechial or purpuric, high fever, and hypotension. May lead to death within hours.

acute haemorrhagic conjunctivitis [Br.] SYN acute hemorrhagic conjunctivitis.

acute haemorrhagic pancreatitis [Br.] SYN acute hemorrhagic pancreatitis.

a•cute hal•lu•ci•na•to•ry pa•ra•noi•a (ă-kyūt´ hă-lū´si-nă-tōr-ē păr´ă-noy´ă) Mental disorder in which periods of hallucination occur in addition to the delusions.

a•cute hem•or•rhag•ic con•junc•ti•vi•tis (ă-kyūt´ hem´ŏr-aj´ik kŏn-jŭngk´ti-vī´tis) Specific acute endemic conjunctivitis with eyelid swelling, tearing, conjunctival hemorrhages, and follicles. SYN acute haemorrhagic conjunctivitis.

a•cute hem•or•rhag•ic pan•cre•a•ti•tis (ă-kyūt´ hem´ŏr-aj´ik pan´krē-ă-tī´tis) An acute inflammation of the pancreas accompanied by the formation of necrotic areas and hemorrhages into the substance of the gland; clinically marked by sudden severe abdominal pain, nausea, fever, and leukocytosis. SYN acute haemorrhagic pancreatitis.

a•cute id•i•o•path•ic pol•y•neu•ri•tis (ă-kyūt´ id´ē-ō-path´ik pol´ē-nūr-ī´tis) A neurologic syndrome, probably an immune-mediated disorder, often a sequela of certain virus infections, marked by paresthesia of the limbs and muscular weakness or a flaccid paralysis.

a•cute in•flam•ma•tion (AI) (ă-kyūt´ in´flă-mā´shŭn) Any inflammation that has a fairly rapid onset, quickly becomes severe, and is usually manifested for only a few days, but may persist for even a few weeks. SYN active inflammation.

a•cute in•flam•ma•to•ry de•my•e•li•na•ting pol•y•ra•di•cu•lo•neu•rop•a•thy (ă-kyūt´ in-flam´ă-tōr-ē dē-mī´ĕ-lin-āt-ing pol´ē-ră-dik´yū-lō-nūr-op´ă-thē) Classic Guillain-Barré syndrome (q.v.) in which the predominant type of underlying nerve fiber pathology is demyelination.

a•cute in•ter•mit•tent por•phy•ri•a, a•cute por•phy•ri•a (ă-kyūt´ in´tĕr-mit´ĕnt pōr-fir´ē-ă, ă-kyūt´ pōr-fir´ē-ă) SYN intermittent acute porphyria.

a•cute is•che•mic stroke (AIS) (ă-kyūt´ is-kē´mik strōk) Circulatory cerebral occlusion that produces varying degrees of neurologic deficits. Ischemic strokes account for 85% of all attacks; most are caused by thrombus formation or embolus due to atherosclerosis. Cardiogenic embolic stroke, usually caused by atrial fibrillation, is the second major cause of acute ischemic stroke. SYN brain attack, cerebral vascular attack.

a·cute i·so·lat·ed my·o·car·di·tis (ă-kyūt′ ī′sŏ-lā-tĕd mī′ō-kahr-dī′tis) An acute interstitial myocarditis of unknown cause, the endocardium and pericardium being unaffected. SYN Fiedler myocarditis.

a·cute liv·er ne·cro·sis (ă-kyūt′ liv′ĕr nĕ-krō′sis) Lesion with extensive and quick death of hepatic cells; may be due to infection or chemical poisoning.

acute lymphocytic leukaemia [Br.] SYN acute lymphocytic leukemia.

a·cute lym·pho·cy·tic leu·ke·mi·a (ALL) (ă-kyūt′ lim′fō-sit′ik lū-kē′mē-ă) SEE lymphocytic leukemia.

a·cute ma·la·ri·a (ă-kyūt′ mă-lar′ē-ă) A form of the disease consisting of a chill accompanied by and followed by fever with its attendant general symptoms and terminating in a sweating stage; the paroxysms, caused by release of merozoites from infected cells, recur after becoming synchronized every 48 hours in tertian (vivax or ovale) malaria, every 72 hours in quartan (malariae) malaria, and at indefinite but frequent intervals, usually about 48 hours, in malignant tertian (falciparum) malaria.

a·cute mas·sive liv·er ne·cro·sis (ă-kyūt′ mas′iv liv′ĕr nĕ-krō′sis) A lesion in which there is extensive and rapid death of parenchymal cells of the liver, sometimes with fatty degeneration.

a·cute my·e·lo·blas·tic leu·ke·mi·a (AML) (ă-kyūt′ mī′ĕ-lō-blas′tik lū-kē′mē-ă) SYN myeloblastic leukemia.

a·cute my·o·car·di·al in·farc·tion (AMI) (ă-kyūt′ mī′ō-kahr′dē-ăl in-fahrk′shŭn) SYN acute coronary syndrome.

a·cute nec·ro·tiz·ing en·ceph·a·li·tis (ă-kyūt′ nek′rō-tīz-ing en-sef′ă-lī′tis) Disorder characterized by destruction of brain parenchyma.

a·cute nec·ro·tiz·ing hem·or·rhag·ic en·ceph·a·lo·my·e·li·tis (ă-kyūt′ nek′rō-tīz-ing hem′or-aj′ik en-sef′ă-lō-mī′ĕ-lī′tis) A fulminating demyelinating

disorder of the central nervous system that affects mainly children and young adults.

a·cute phase re·ac·tion (ă-kyūt′ fāz rē-ak′shŭn) Host's response against microorganisms.

a·cute pos·te·rior mul·ti·fo·cal pla·coid pig·ment ep·i·the·li·op·a·thy (APMPPE) (ă-kyūt′ pos-tēr′ē-ŏr mŭl-tē-fō′kăl plak′oyd pig′mĕnt ep′i-thē-lē-op′ă-thē) An inflammatory, self-limited disease manifested by decreased vision and multifocal, cream-colored placoid lesions of the retinal pigment epithelium.

acute promyelocytic leukaemia [Br.] SYN acute promyelocytic leukemia.

a·cute pro·my·e·lo·cyt·ic leu·ke·mi·a (ă-kyūt′ prō′mī-ĕ-lō-sit′ik lū-kē′mē-ă) Disorder presenting with severe bleeding, with infiltration of bone marrow by abnormal promyelocytes and myelocytes, low plasma fibrinogen, and defective coagulation. SYN acute promyelocytic leukaemia.

a·cute pul·mo·na·ry al·ve·o·li·tis (ă-kyūt′ pul′mŏ-nār-ē al′vē-ō-lī′tis) Inflammation involving formation of exudate in pulmonary alveoli and impaired gas exchange.

a·cute ra·di·a·tion syn·drome (ARS) (ă-kyūt′ rā′dē-ā′shŭn sin′drōm) Syndrome caused by exposure of the body to large amounts of radiation (e.g., from certain forms of therapy, accidents, and nuclear explosions).

a·cute re·nal fail·ure (ARF) (ă-kyūt′ rē′năl fāl′yŭr) A rapid decline of kidney function due to tubular injury; commonly caused by ischemia or nephrotoxins.

a·cute res·pi·ra·to·ry dis·tress syn·drome (ARDS) (ă-kyūt′ res′pir-ă-tōr-ē dis-tres′ sin′drōm) SYN adult respiratory distress syndrome.

a·cute rhi·ni·tis (ă-kyūt′ rī-nī′tis) Sudden onset catarrhal inflammation of the mucous membrane of the nose, marked by sneezing, lacrimation, and a profuse secretion of watery mucus; usually associated with infection by one of the common cold viruses. SYN coryza.

a·cute sen·sor·y-mo·tor ax·o·nal neu·

rop·a·thy (ă-kyūt′ sen′sŏr-ē-mō′tŏr ak-sō′năl nūr-op′ă-thē) An acute axon-degenerating polyradiculoneuropathy that affects both motor and sensory fibers; a variant of Guillain-Barré syndrome.

a·cute sit·u·a·tion·al re·ac·tion (ă-kyūt′ sich′ū-ā′shŭn-ăl rē-ak′shŭn) SYN stress reaction.

a·cute stress dis·or·der (ASD) (ă-kyūt′ stres dis-ōr′dĕr) Development of characteristic symptoms within the first 4 weeks after a psychologically traumatic event that was outside the range of usual human experience.

a·cute tu·ber·cu·lo·sis (ă-kyūt′ tū-bĕr′ kyū-lō′sis) A rapidly fatal disease due to the general dissemination of acid-fast bacilli in the blood, resulting in the formation of miliary tubercles in various organs and tissues, and producing symptoms of profound toxemia. SYN disseminated tuberculosis.

a·cute vi·ral con·junc·ti·vi·tis (ă-kyūt′ vī′răl kŏn-jŭngk′ti-vī′tis) Disorder marked by intense hyperemia and a watery discharge; highly contagious. SYN pinkeye (1).

a·cy·a·not·ic (ā-sī′ă-not′ik) Characterized by absence of cyanosis.

a·cyc·lic com·pound (ā-sik′lik kom′ pownd) An organic compound in which the chain does not form a ring. SYN open chain compound.

ac·yl·a·tion (as′i-lā′shŭn) Introduction of an acyl radical into an organic compound or formation of such a radical within an organic compound.

ac·yl·trans·fer·ase (as′il-trans′fĕr-ās) An enzyme catalyzing the transfer of an acyl group from an acyl-CoA to any of various acceptors.

a·cys·ti·a (ā-sis′tē-ă) Congenital absence of urinary bladder.

a·dac·ty·ly, a·dac·tyl·i·a (ā-dak′ti-lē, -lē-ă) Congenital absence of digits (fingers or toes).

Ad·am's ap·ple (ad′ămz ap′ĕl) SYN laryngeal prominence.

Ad·ams-Stokes syn·drome (ad′ămz- stōks sin′drōm) A disorder characterized by slow or absent pulse, vertigo, syncope, convulsions, and sometimes Cheyne-Stokes respiration; usually as a result of advanced A-V block or sick sinus syndrome. SYN Spens syndrome, Stokes-Adams syndrome.

ad·ap·ta·tion (ad′ăp-tā′shŭn) **1.** Preferential survival of members of a species because of a phenotype that gives them an enhanced capacity to withstand the environment. **2.** An advantageous change in function or constitution of an organ or tissue to meet new conditions. **3.** Adjustment of the sensitivity of the retina to light intensity. **4.** A property of certain sensory receptors that modifies the response to repeated or continued stimuli at constant intensity. **5.** DENTISTRY The fitting, condensing, or contouring of a restorative material, foil, or shell to a tooth or cast so as to ensure close contact. **6.** The dynamic process wherein the thoughts, feelings, behavior, and biophysiologic mechanisms of a person continually change to adjust to a constantly changing environment. **7.** A homeostatic response. **8.** OCCUPATIONAL THERAPY The ability to anticipate, correct for, and benefit by learning from the consquences of errors that arise during task performances.

a·dap·ted cloth·ing (ă-dap′tĕd klōdh′ ing) Clothes that are modified so a person with a disability can dress without assistance.

a·dap·tive be·hav·ior scales (ă-dap′ tiv bē-hāv′yŏr skālz) A behavioral assessment device to quantify the levels of skills of mentally retarded and developmentally delayed people in interacting with the environment; consists of three developmentally related factors: 1) personal self-sufficiency, e.g., eating, dressing; 2) community self-sufficiency, e.g., shopping, communicating; 3) personal and social responsibility, e.g., use of leisure time, job performance. SEE intelligence.

a·dap·tive de·vice (ă-dap′tiv dĕ-vīs′) A tool that provides assistance in ADLs and IADLs to a person with a disability and allows a higher level of independence.

a·dap·tive ther·mo·gen·e·sis (ă-dap′ tiv thĕr′mō-jen′ĕ-sis) Regulated production of heat, which is influenced by environmental temperature and diet.

ad·ap·tom·e·ter (ad'ap-tom'ĕ-tĕr) A device for determining the course of retinal dark adaptation and for measuring the minimum light threshold.

ad·der (ad'ĕr) Common name for many members of the family Viperidae (the vipers), applied to several genera, although true adders are of the genus *Vipera*.

ad·dic·tion (ă-dik'shŭn) Habitual psychological and physiologic dependence on a substance or practice that is beyond voluntary control. Commonly abused substances include alcohol and drugs.

ad·dic·tion se·ver·i·ty in·dex (ASI) (ă-dik'shŭn sĕ-ver'i-tē in'deks) A measurement instrument used to assess a patient's level of substance abuse or dependency.

ad·dic·tive per·son·al·i·ty (ă-dik'tiv pĕr'sŏn-al'i-tē) Collective term indicating use of substances or behaviors to moderate effects of anxiety or neurosis.

Addison anaemia [Br.] SYN Addison anemia.

Ad·di·son a·ne·mi·a (ad'i-sŏn ă-nē'mē-ă) SYN pernicious anemia, Addison anaemia.

ad·di·so·ni·an cri·sis (ad'i-sŏn'ē-ăn krī'sis) SYN acute adrenocortical insufficiency.

ad·di·tive (ad'i-tiv) **1.** A substance not naturally part of a material (e.g., food) but deliberately added to fulfill some specific purpose (e.g., preservation). **2.** Tending to add or be added; denoting addition.

ad·du·cent (ă-dū'sĕnt) Bringing toward; adducting.

ad·duct (ă-dŭkt') *Do not confuse this word with abduct.* **1.** To draw toward the median plane. **2.** An addition product, or complex, or one part of the same.

ad·duc·tion (ă-dŭk'shŭn) **1.** Movement of a body part toward the median plane (of the body, in the case of limbs; of the hand or foot, in the case of digits) or midline of the body. **2.** Monocular rotation

(duction) of the eye toward the nose. **3.** A position resulting from such movement. Cf. abduction.

ad·duc·tor (ă-dŭk'tŏr) A muscle that draws a part toward the median plane; or, in the case of the digits, toward the normal axis of the middle finger or the second toe.

ad·duc·tor bre·vis (ă-dŭk'tŏr brev'is) One of a group of muscles that extends from the pubis to femur; serves to adduct the thigh.

ad·duc·tor ca·nal (ă-dŭk'tŏr kă-nal') [TA] The space in the middle third of the thigh between the vastus medialis and adductor muscles, converted into a canal by the overlying sartorius muscle. It gives passage to the femoral vessels and saphenous nerve, ending at the adductor hiatus. SYN canalis adductorius [TA], Hunter canal.

ad·duc·tor long·us (ă-dŭk'tŏr lawn'gŭs) One of a group of muscles that extends from the pubis to femur and serves to adduct the tight.

ad·duc·tor mag·nus (ă-dŭk'tŏr mag'nŭs) One of a group of muscles that extends from the pubis to femur and serves to adduct and extend the thigh.

ad·duc·tor spas·mod·ic dys·pho·ni·a (ă-dŭk'tŏr spaz-mod'ik dis-fō'nē-ă) A form of spasmodic dysphonia in which excessive closure of the vocal cords affects the initiation and maintenance of phonation.

a·del·o·mor·phous (ă-del'ō-mōr'fŭs) Of a not clearly defined form.

ad·e·nec·to·my (ad'ĕ-nek'tŏ-mē) Excision of a gland.

ad·e·nec·to·pia (ad'ĕ-nek-tō'pē-ă) Presence of a gland in other than its normal anatomic position.

ad·e·nine (A, Ade) (ad'ĕ-nēn) One of the two major purines (the other being guanine) found in both RNA and DNA, and also in various free nucleotides.

ad·e·ni·tis (ad'ĕ-nī'tis) Inflammation of a lymph node or of a gland.

ad·e·no·ac·an·tho·ma (ad'ĕ-nō-ak'an-thŏ′mă) A malignant neoplasm consisting chiefly of glandular epithelium (adenocarcinoma), usually well differentiated, with foci of squamous (or epidermoid) neoplastic cells.

ad·e·no·am·e·lo·blas·to·ma (ad′ĕ-nō-am′el-ō-blas-tō′mă) SYN adenomatoid odontogenic tumor.

ad·e·no·blast (ad′ĕ-nō-blast) A proliferating embryonic cell with the potential to form glandular parenchyma.

ad·e·no·car·ci·no·ma (ad′ĕ-nō-kahr′si-nō′mă) A malignant neoplasm of epithelial cells in a glandular or glandlike pattern.

ad·e·no·car·ci·no·ma in Bar·rett e·soph·a·gus (ad′ĕ-nō-kahr′si-nō′mă bar′ĕt ĕ-sof′ă-gŭs) Lesion arising in the esophagus, which has become lined with columnar cells (Barrett mucosa).

ad·e·no·car·ci·no·ma in si·tu (AIS, ACIS) (ad′ĕ-nō-kahr-si-nō′mă in si′tū) Noninvasive, abnormal proliferation of glands believed to precede the appearance of invasive adenocarcinoma.

ad·e·no·car·ci·no·ma·tous (ad′ĕ-nō-kahr′si-nō′mă-tŭs) Pertaining to a malignant tumor originating in glandular epithelium.

ad·e·no·cel·lu·li·tis (ad′ĕ-nō-sel′yū-lī′tis) Inflammation of a gland, usually a lymph node, and of the adjacent connective tissue.

ad·e·no·cys·to·ma (ad′ĕ-nō-sis-tō′mă) Adenoma in which the neoplastic glandular epithelium forms cysts.

ad·e·no·cyte (ad′ĕ-nō-sīt) A secretory cell of a gland.

ad·e·no·fi·bro·ma (ad′ĕ-nō-fī-brō′mă) A benign neoplasm composed of glandular and fibrous tissues, with a relatively large proportion of glands.

ad·e·no·fi·bro·my·o·ma (ad′ĕ-nō-fī′brō-mī-ō′mă) SYN adenomatoid tumor.

ad·e·no·fi·bro·sis (ad′ĕ-nō-fī-brō′sis) SYN sclerosing adenosis.

ad·e·nog·en·ous (ad′ĕ-noj′ĕn-ŭs) Having an origin in glandular tissue.

ad·e·no·hy·poph·y·sis (ad′ĕ-nō-hī-pof′i-sis) [TA] The anterior pituitary gland. SEE ALSO hypophysis. SYN lobus anterior hypophyseos [TA], anterior lobe of hypophysis.

ad·e·no·hy·poph·y·si·tis (ad′ĕ-nō-hī-pof-i-sī′tis) Inflammatory reaction or sepsis affecting the anterior pituitary gland, often related to pregnancy.

ad·e·noid (ad′ĕ-noyd) **1.** Glandlike; of glandular appearance. SYN adeniform, lymphoid (2). **2.** SEE adenoids.

ad·e·noi·dal-pha·ryn·ge·al-con·junc·ti·val vi·rus (A.P.C. virus) (ad-ĕ-noy′dăl-făr-in′jē-ăl-kŏn-jŭngk′ti-văl vī′rŭs) SYN adenovirus.

ad·e·noid cys·tic car·ci·no·ma (ad′ĕ-noyd sis′tik kahr′si-nō′mă) A histologic type of carcinoma characterized by round, glandlike spaces or cysts bordered by layers of epithelial cells without intervening stroma. SYN cylindromatous carcinoma.

ad·e·noid·ec·to·my (adn) (ad′ĕ-noyd-ek′tŏ-mē) Surgery to remove adenoid tissue from the nasopharynx.

ad·e·noid·i·tis (ad′ĕ-noyd-ī′tis) Inflammation of adenoid tissue caused by viral and bacterial infection and allergy.

ad·e·noids (ad′ĕ-noydz) A normal collection of unencapsulated lymphoid tissue in the nasopharynx. Also called pharyngeal tonsils.

ad·e·noid squa·mous cell car·cin·o·ma (ad′ĕ-noyd skwă′mŭs sel kahr′si-nō′mă) SYN adenoacanthoma.

ad·e·noid tis·sue (ad′ĕ-noyd tish′ū) SYN lymphatic tissue.

ad·e·no·li·po·ma (ad′ĕ-nō-li-pō′mă) A benign neoplasm of glandular and adipose tissues.

ad·e·no·lym·pho·ma (ad′ĕ-nō-lim-fō′mă) SYN Warthin tumor.

ad·e·no·ma, pl. **ad·e·no·mas,** pl. **ad·e·no·ma·ta** (ad′ĕ-nō′mă, -nō′măz, -nō′mă-tă) An ordinarily benign neoplasm of epithelial tissue in which the tumor cells form glands or glandlike structures in the stroma.

ad·e·no·ma·la·cia (ad'ĕ-nō-mă-lā'shē-ă) Abnormal softening of a gland.

ad·e·no·ma·toid (ad'ĕ-nō'mă-toyd) Resembling an adenoma.

ad·e·no·ma·toid odon·to·gen·ic tu·mor (ad'ĕ-nō'mă-toyd ō-don'tō-jen'ik tū'mŏr) A benign epithelial lesion surrounding the crown of an impacted tooth in an adolescent or young adult.

ad·e·no·ma·toid tu·mor (ad'ĕ-nō'mă-toyd tū'mŏr) A small benign neoplasm of the epididymis or female genital tract. SYN adenofibromyoma, Recklinghausen tumor.

ad·e·no·ma·to·sis (ad'ĕ-nō'mă-tō'sis) A condition characterized by numerous overgrowths of glandular tissue.

ad·e·nom·a·tous (ad'ĕ-nō'mă-tŭs) Relating to an adenoma.

ad·e·no·my·o·ma (ad'ĕ-nō-mī-ō'mă) A benign neoplasm of muscle (usually smooth muscle) with glandular elements; occurs most frequently in uterus and uterine ligaments.

ad·e·no·my·o·sis (ad'ĕ-nō-mī-ō'sis) The ectopic occurrence or diffuse implantation of adenomatous tissue in muscle.

ad·e·nop·a·thy, a·de·no·pa·li·a (ADP) (ad'ĕ-nop'ă-thē) Swelling or morbid enlargement of the lymph nodes.

ad·e·no·sar·co·ma (ad'ĕ-nō-sahr-kō'mă) A malignant neoplasm arising in mesodermal tissue and glandular epithelium of the same part.

a·den·o·sine (Ado) (ă-den'ō-sēn) A condensation product of adenine and D-ribose. SYN gamma (γ)-beta (β)-D-ribo-furanosyladenine.

a·den·o·sine 3′,5′-cy·clic mo·no·phos·phate, 5′-cyclic mo·no·phos·phate (cAMP) (ă-den'ō-sēn sik'lik mon' ō-fos'fāt) An activator of phosphorylase kinase and an effector of other enzymes, formed in muscle from ATP by adenylate cyclase and broken down to 5′-AMP by a phosphodiesterase; sometimes referred to as the "second messenger." SYN cyclic AMP.

a·den·o·sine de·am·i·nase (ADA, ADD, ADase) (ă-den'ō-sēn dē-am'ĭ-nās) Enzyme found in mammalian tissues, capable of catalyzing the deamination of adenosine, forming inosine and ammonia.

a·den·o·sine tri·phos·pha·tase (ATP ase) (ă-den'ō-sēn trī-fos'fă-tās) An enzyme that catalyzes the release of the terminal phosphate group of adenosine 5′-triphosphate.

a·den·o·sine 5′-tri·phos·phate (ATP) (ă-den'ō-sēn trī-fos'fāt) Adenosine (5) pyrophosphate; adenosine with triphosphoric acid esterfied at its 5′ position; immediate precursor of adenine nucleotides in RNA. The primary energy currency of a cell.

ad·e·no·squa·mous car·ci·no·ma (ad'ĕ-nō-skwā'mŭs kahr'si-nō'mă) Lung tumor exhibiting areas of clear-cut glandular and squamous cell differentiation.

Ad·e·no·vi·ri·dae (ad'ĕ-nō-vir'i-dē) A family of double-stranded DNA viruses, commonly known as adenoviruses, which develop in the nuclei of infected cells in mammals and birds.

ad·e·no·vi·rus (ad'ĕ-nō-vī'rŭs) Adenoidal-pharyngeal-conjunctival (A-P-C) virus; any virus of the family Adenoviridae. More than 40 types are known to infect humans, causing upper respiratory symptoms, acute respiratory disease, conjunctivitis, gastroenteritis, hemorrhagic cystitis, and serous infections in neonates. SYN adenoidal-pharyngeal-conjunctival virus.

a·den·y·late ki·nase (AK) (ă-den'i-lāt kī'nās) Adenylic acid kinase; a phosphotransferase that catalyzes the reversible phosphorylation of a molecule of ADP by MgADP.

ad·e·nyl cy·clase (ade'-nil sī'klās) An enzyme that converts adenosine monophosphate to 3′,5′-cyclic adenosine monophosphate.

ad·e·nyl·ic ac·id (ad'ĕ-nil'ik as'id) A condensation product of adenosine and phosphoric acid.

ad·e·quate stim·u·lus (ad'ĕ-kwăt stim' yū-lŭs) A stimulus to which a particular receptor responds effectively and that gives rise to a characteristic sensation

a·der·mo·gen·e·sis (ă-dĕr′mō-jen′ĕ-sis) Failure or imperfection in the regeneration of the skin.

ad·her·ence (ad-hēr′ĕns) The extent to which a patient continues a mode of treatment without close supervision.

ad·her·ent (ad-hēr′ĕnt) A substance that is stuck to, or assists something in sticking to, another structure or substance.

ad·he·sins (ad-hē′zins) Microbial surface antigens (usually of filamentous form) that bind to specific receptors on epithelial cell membranes.

ad·he·sion (ad-hē′zhŭn) The adhering or uniting of two surfaces or parts, especially the union of the opposing surfaces of a wound or adjacent layers of fascia. SYN conglutination (1).

ad·he·si·ot·o·my (ad-hē′zē-ot′ŏ-mē) Surgical section or lysis of adhesions.

ad·he·sive (ad-hē′siv) **1.** Relating to, or having the characteristics of, an adhesion. **2.** Any material that adheres to a surface or causes adherence between surfaces.

ad·he·sive in·flam·ma·tion (ad-hē′siv in′flă-mā′shŭn) Inflammation in which the amount of fibrin in the exudate is sufficient to result in a slight or moderate degree of adherence of adjacent tissues.

ad·he·sive o·ti·tis (ad-hē′siv ō-tī′tis) Inflammation of the middle ear caused by prolonged auditory tube dysfunction.

ad·he·sive pleu·ri·sy (ad-hē′siv plūr′i-sē) SYN dry pleurisy.

ad·he·sive vag·i·ni·tis (ad-hē′siv vaj′i-nī′tis) Inflammation of vaginal mucosa with adhesions of the vaginal walls to each other.

ad·i·ad·o·cho·ki·ne·si·a (ă-dī′ă-dō-kō-kin-ē′sē-ă) Inability to perform rapid alternating movements.

a·di·a·pho·ri·a (ă-dī′ă-fōr′ē-ă) Failure to respond to stimulation after a series of previously applied stimuli.

a·di·as·to·le (ă-dī-as′tō-lē) Absence or imperceptibility of the diastolic movement of the heart.

A·die syndrome, A·die pu·pil (a′dē sin′drŏm, pyū′pil) An idiopathic postganglionic denervation of the parasympathetically innervated intraocular muscles, usually complicated by signs of aberrant regeneration of these nerves. SYN Holmes-Adie pupil, Holmes-Adie syndrome, pupillotonic pseudostrabismus.

♻ **adip-, adipo-** Combining forms meaning fat, fatty.

ad·i·po·cel·lu·lar (ad′i-pō-sel′yū-lăr) Relating to both fatty and cellular tissues.

ad·i·po·cer·a·tous (ad′i-pō-ser′ă-tŭs) Relating to adipocere. SYN lipoceratous.

ad·i·po·cere (ad′i-pō-sēr) A fatty waxy substance into which dead animal tissues are sometimes converted when kept from the air under certain conditions of temperature. SYN lipocere.

ad·i·po·cyte (ad) (ad′i-pō-sīt) SYN fat cell.

ad·i·po·gen·ic, ad·i·pog·e·nous (ad′i-pō-jen′ik, ad′i-poj′ĕ-nŭs) SYN lipogenic.

ad·i·pom·e·ter (ad′i-pom′ĕ-tĕr) An instrument to determine skin thickness.

ad·i·pose (ad′i-pōs) Denoting fat.

ad·i·pose cap·sule (ad′i-pōs kap′sŭl) SYN paranephric fat.

ad·i·pose fos·sae (ad′i-pōs fos′ē) Subcutaneous spaces containing accumulations of fat in the breast.

ad·i·pose in·fil·tra·tion (ad′i-pōs in′fil-trā′shŭn) Growth of normal adult fat cells where not usually present.

ad·i·po·sis (ad′i-pō′sis) Excessive accumulation of body fat. SYN lipomatosis, liposis (1), steatosis (1).

ad·i·po·sis ce·re·bra·lis (ad′i-pō′sis ser′ĕ-brā′lis) Obesity due to intracranial disease, resulting in hyperphagia.

ad·i·po·sis do·lo·ro·sa (ad-i-pō′sis dō-lō-rō′să) Condition characterized by a deposit of symmetric nodular or pendulous masses of fat in various regions of the body, with discomfort or pain.

ad•i•pos•i•ty (ad′i-pos′i-tē) SYN obesity.

ad•i•po•su•ria (ad′i-pō-syūr′ē-ă) SYN lipuria.

a•dip•si•a, a•dip•sy (ă-dip′sē-ă, -dip′sē) Absence of thirst or desire to drink.

ad•just•able ax•is face-bow (ad-jŭs′tă-běl ak′sis fās′bō) A face-bow the caliper ends of which can be adjusted to permit location of the axis of rotation of the mandible. SYN kinematic face-bow.

ad•just•ment (adj) (ă-jŭst′měnt) 1. SYN spinal adjustment. 2. In health care accounting, any addition or deletion in a patient's record that will alter the balance due.

ad•just•ment dis•or•der (ă-jŭst′měnt dis-ōr′děr) A class of mental and behavioral disorders in which the development of symptoms is related to the presence of some environmental stressor or life event and is expected to remit when the stress ceases.

ad•ju•vant (ad′jū-vănt) 1. A substance added to a drug product formulation that affects the action of the active ingredient in a predictable way. 2. Additional therapy given to enhance or extend primary therapy's effect.

ad•ju•vant ra•di•o•ther•a•py (ad′jū-vănt rā′dē-ō-thār′ă-pē) Radiologic treatment used with another medical treatment to modify second's effects.

ad•neu•ral, ad•ner•val (ad-nūr′ăl, -něr′văl) 1. Lying near a nerve. 2. In the direction of a nerve.

ad•nex•al ad•e•no•ma (ad-nek′săl ad′ě-nō′mă) An adenoma arising in, or forming structures resembling, skin appendages.

ad•nex•ec•to•my (ad-nek-sek′tŏ-mē) 1. Excision of any adnexa. 2. In gynecology, excision of the uterine tube and ovary if unilateral, and excision of both tubes and ovaries (adnexa uteri) if bilateral.

ad•o•les•cence (ad′ŏ-les′ĕns) Life period beginning with puberty and ending with physical maturity.

ad•re•nal (ă-drē′năl) 1. Near or on the kidney; denoting the suprarenal (adrenal) gland. 2. A suprarenal gland or separate tissue or product thereof. SEE ALSO suprarenal.

ad•re•nal cri•sis (ă-drē′năl krī′sis) SYN acute adrenocortical insufficiency.

ad•re•nal gland (ă-drē′năl gland) SYN suprarenal gland.

ad•ren•a•line (A, Adr) (ă-dren′ă-lin) SYN epinephrine.

ad•re•nal•ism (ă-drē′năl-izm) SYN hypercorticoidism.

ad•re•nal•i•tis (ă-drē′năl-ī′tis) Inflammation of the suprarenal gland.

ad•re•na•lop•a•thy (ă-drē′nă-lop′ă-thē) Any pathologic condition of the suprarenal glands.

ad•ren•ar•che (ad-ren-ahr′kē) Growth of axillary and pubic hair induced by hyperactivity of the suprarenal cortex in early puberty.

ad•re•ner•gic (ad′rĕ-něr′jik) Relating to nerve cells or fibers of the autonomic nervous system that employ norepinephrine as their neurotransmitter. Cf. cholinergic.

ad•re•ner•gic block•ing a•gent (ad′rĕ-něr′jik blok′ing ā′jěnt) Drug that selectively blocks or inhibits responses to sympathetic adrenergic nerve activity and to epinephrine, norepinephrine, and other adrenergic amines.

ad•re•ner•gic bron•cho•di•la•tors (ad′rĕ-něr′jik brong′kō-dī′lā-tŏrz) Sympathomimetic drugs that stimulate receptors in the bronchi and other organs, producing smooth muscle relaxation.

ad•re•ner•gic neu•ro•nal block•ing agent (ad′rĕ-něr′jik nūr-ō′năl blok′ing ā′jěnt) A drug that prevents the release of norepinephrine from sympathetic nerve terminals.

adreno-, adrenal-, adren- Combining

forms meaning related to the suprarenal gland.

ad·re·no·cor·ti·cal (ă-drē′nō-kōr′ti-kăl) Pertaining to the cortex of the suprarenal gland.

ad·re·no·cor·ti·cal in·suf·fi·cien·cy (ă-drē′nō-kōr′ti-kăl in′sŭ-fish′ĕn-sē) Loss, to varying degrees, of adrenocortical function. SYN hypocorticoidism.

ad·re·no·cor·ti·coid (AC) (ă-drē′nō-kōr′ti-koyd) SYN corticosteroid.

ad·re·no·cor·ti·co·mi·met·ic (ă-drē′nō-kōr′ti-kō-mi-met′ik) Mimicking or producing effects similar to adrenocortical function.

ad·re·no·cor·ti·co·tro·pic, ad·re·no·cor·ti·co·tro·phic (ă-drē′nō-kōr′ti-kō-trō′pik, -trō′fik) Stimulating growth of the suprarenal cortex or secretion of its hormones. SYN adrenotropic, adrenotrophic.

ad·re·no·cor·ti·co·tro·pin (ă-drē′nō-kōr′ti-kō-trō′pin) Protein hormone of the anterior pituitary gland that stimulates the cortex of the suprarenal gland.

ad·re·no·med·ul·lar·y hor·mones (ă-drē′nō-med′ŭ-lar-ē hōr′mōnz) Those produced by the medulla of the suprarenal gland.

ad·re·no·meg·a·ly (ă-drē′nō-meg′ă-lē) Enlargement of the suprarenal gland.

ad·re·no·mi·met·ic (ă-drē′nō-mi-met′ik) Having an action similar to that of the compounds epinephrine and norepinephrine.

ad·re·no·my·e·lo·neu·rop·a·thy (ă-drē′nō-mī′ě-lō-nūr-op′ă-thē) Male disorder with adrenal insufficiency, hypogonadism, progressive myelopathy, peripheral neuropathy, and sphincter disturbances.

ad·re·no·tox·in (ă-drē-nō-tok′sin) A substance toxic to the suprarenal glands.

ad·re·no·tro·pic, a·dre·no·tro·phic (ă-drē-nō-trō′pik, -trō′fik) SYN adrenocorticotropic.

ad·sorb (ad-sōrb′) *Do not confuse this word with absorb.* To take up by adsorption.

ad·sorb·ent (ad-sōr′bĕnt) A solid substance with the property of attaching other substances to its surface without covalent bonding.

ad·sorp·tion (ad-sōrp′shŭn) Property of a solid to attract and hold to its surface a gas, liquid, or a substance.

ad·ul·ter·a·tion (ă-dŭl′tĕr-ā′shŭn) The alteration of any substance by the deliberate addition of a component not ordinarily part of that substance.

a·dult res·pi·ra·to·ry dis·tress syn·drome (ARDS) (ă-dŭlt′ res′pir-ă-tōr-ē dis-tres′ sin′drōm) Disorder with rapid onset of progressive malfunction of the lungs usually associated with malfunction of other organs attributable to inability to take in oxygen. SYN acute respiratory distress syndrome, white lung.

a·dult ric·kets (ă-dŭlt′ rik′ĕts) SYN osteomalacia.

ad·vanced car·di·ac life sup·port (ACLS) (ăd-vanst′ kahr′dē-ak līf sŭ-pōrt′) Definitive emergency medical care that includes defibrillation, airway management, and use of drugs and medications.

ad·vance·ment (ăd-vans′mĕnt) Surgical procedure in which an attachment (usually the point of origin) is partially severed or released so that tissue may be moved to a more distal point.

ad·ven·ti·ti·a (ad′vĕn-tish′ă) [TA] The outermost connective tissue covering of any organ, vessel, or other structure not covered by a serosa.

ad·ven·ti·tious (ad′vĕn-tish′ŭs) Arising from an external source or occurring in an unusual place or manner.

ad·verse side ef·fect (ad-vĕrs′ sīd ĕ-fekt′) Result of pharmacotherapy in addition to the desired therapeutic effect; usually considered detrimental.

a·dy·nam·i·a (ā-dī-nam′ē-ă) SYN asthenia.

A·e·des (ā-ē′dēz) A widespread genus of small mosquitoes found in tropic and subtropic regions.

aer-, aero- Combining forms meaning the air, a gas; aerial, gassy.

aer·obe (ār'ōb) **1.** An organism that lives and grows in oxygen. **2.** An organism that uses oxygen as a final electron acceptor in a respiratory chain.

aer·o·bic (ār-ō'bik) **1.** Living in air. **2.** Relating to an aerobe. **3.** Oxygen consumed to produce energy. SYN aerophilous.

aer·o·bi·ol·o·gy (ār'ō-bī-ol'ŏ-jē) The study of atmospheric constituents, living and nonliving, of biologic significance.

aer·o·bi·o·sis (ār'ō-bī-ō'sis) Existence in an atmosphere containing oxygen.

aer·o·cele (ār'ō-sēl) Distention of a small natural cavity with gas.

aer·o·don·tal·gi·a (ār'ō-don-tal'jē-ă) Dental pain caused by a change in atmospheric pressure.

aer·o·gen (ār'ō-jen) A gas-forming microorganism.

Aer·o·mo·nas (ār-ō-mō'năs) A genus of aerobic, facultatively anaerobic bacteria; found in water and sewage.

aer·o·pha·gi·a, aer·oph·a·gy (ār'ō-fā'jē-ă, -of'ă-jē) Excessive swallowing of air due to anxiety, hunger, or other causes.

aer·o·si·nus·i·tis (ār'ō-sī'nŭ-sī'tis) SYN barosinusitis.

aer·o·sol (ār'ŏ-sol) Liquid or particulate matter in the form of a stable suspension for therapeutic, insecticidal, or other purposes, including bioterrorism and bioweapons.

aer·o·ti·tis me·di·a (ār'ō-tī'tis mē'dē-ă) Inflammation of the middle ear caused by a reduction in pressure in the tympanic cavity relative to ambient pressure.

aer·o·tol·er·ant (ār'ō-tol'ĕr-ănt) Able to survive in the presence of oxygen; said of some anaerobic microorganisms.

aesthesodic [Br.] SYN esthesiodic.

aesthetics [Br.] SYN esthetics.

aetiology [Br.] SYN etiology.

afe·tal (ā-fē'tăl) Without relation to a fetus or intrauterine life.

af·fect (a'fekt) The emotional feeling, tone, and mood attached to a thought, including its external manifestations.

af·fec·tive (a-fek'tiv) Pertaining to mood, emotion, feeling, sensibility, or a mental state.

af·fer·ent (aff) (af'ĕr-ĕnt) Inflowing; conducting toward a center, denoting certain arteries, veins, lymphatics, and nerves. Opposite of efferent. SYN centripetal (1).

af·fer·ent lym·phat·ic (af'ĕr-ĕnt lim-fat'ik) A lymphatic vessel entering, or bringing lymph to, a node.

af·fer·ent nerves (af'ĕr-ĕnt nĕrvz) Nerves that carry impulses from the sensory organs to the central nervous system.

af·fer·ent ves·sel (af'ĕr-ĕnt ves'ĕl) Any artery conveying blood to a part.

af·fin·i·ty (ă-fin'i-tē) **1.** CHEMISTRY the force that impels certain atoms to unite with certain others. **2.** Selective staining of a tissue by a dye. **3.** The strength of binding between a Fab site of an antibody and an antigenic determinant. **4.** In a general sense, an attraction.

afibrinogenaemia [Br.] SYN afibrinogenemia.

a·fi·brin·o·gen·e·mi·a (ā-fī'brin-ō-jĕ-nē'mē-ă) The absence of fibrinogen in the plasma. SEE ALSO hypofibrinogenemia. SYN afibrinogenaemia.

af·la·tox·in (AF, AFT) (af'lă-tok'sin) Toxic metabolites of some *Aspergillus* strains including the fungi *A. flavus, A. parasiticus,* and *A. oryzae.*

af·ter·birth (af'tĕr-bĭrth) Placenta and fetal membranes extruded from the uterus after birth. SYN secundina, secundines.

af·ter·ef·fect (af'tĕr-ĕ-fekt') A physical, physiologic, psychological, or emotional effect that continues after removal of a stimulus.

af·ter·im·age (af'tĕr-im'ăj) Persistence

of a visual response after cessation of the stimulus.

af·ter·pains, af-ter-pains (af'tĕr-pānz) Painful cramplike contractions of the uterus occurring after childbirth.

af·ter·sen·sa·tion (af'tĕr-sen-sā'shŭn) Subjective persistence of sensation after cessation of stimulus.

af·ter·sound, af-ter-sound (af'tĕr-sownd) Subjective persistence of an auditory stimulus after cessation of the stimulus.

af·ter·taste, af-ter-taste (af'tĕr-tāst) Subjective persistence of a gustatory stimulus after contact with the stimulating substance has ceased.

a·func·tion·al oc·clu·sion (ā-fŭngk'shŭn-ăl ŏ-klŭ'zhŭn) A malocclusion that does not permit normal function of the dentition.

agammaglobulinaemia [Br.] SYN agammaglobulinemia.

a·gam·ma·glob·u·lin·e·mi·a (ā-gam'ă-glob'yū-li-nē'mē-ă) Absence of, or extremely low levels of, the gamma fraction of serum globulin. SYN agammaglobulinaemia.

ag·a·mo·gen·e·sis (ag'ă-mō-jen'ĕ-sis, ā-gam-ō-) SYN asexual reproduction.

a·gan·gli·on·ic (ā'gang-glē-on'ik) Without ganglia.

a·gan·gli·o·no·sis (ā-gang'glē-ŏ-nō'sis) The state of being without ganglia.

a·gar (a) (ā'gahr) Natural or synthetic complex polysaccharide (a sulfated galactan) derived from seaweed (various red algae); used as a solidifying agent in culture media.

ag·a·rose (AG) (ag'ă-rōs) The neutral linear polysaccharide fraction found in agar preparations; used in chromatography and electrophoresis.

a·gas·tric (ā-gas'trik) Without stomach or alimentary (digestive) tract.

age (āj) **1.** The period elapsed since birth. **2.** One of the periods into which human

life is divided, distinguished by physical evolution, equilibrium, and involution. **3.** To grow old.

a·gen·e·sis (ā-jen'ĕ-sis) Absence or failure of formation of any part.

a·gen·i·tal·ism (ā-jen'i-tăl-izm) **1.** Congenital absence of genitalia. **2.** Any condition caused by lack of sex hormones.

a·gen·o·so·mi·a (ā'jen-ō-sō'mē-ă) Markedly defective formation or absence of the genitalia.

a·gent (ā'jĕnt) **1.** An active force or substance capable of producing an effect. **2.** A factor such as a microorganism, chemical substance, or a form of radiation the presence or absence of which (as in deficiency diseases) results in disease or more advanced disease.

age-re·lat·ed mac·u·lar de·gen·er·a·tion (āj-rē-lāt'ĕd mak'yū-lăr dĕ-jen'ĕr-ā'shŭn) SYN macular degeneration.

a·geu·si·a (ă-gū'sē-ă) Loss of the sense of taste.

ag·ger, pl. **ag·ger·es** (aj'ĕr, -ēz) [TA] Any anatomic prominence.

ag·glu·ti·nant (ă-glū'ti-nănt) A substance that holds parts together or causes agglutination.

ag·glu·ti·na·tion (ă-glū'ti-nā'shŭn) **1.** The process by which suspended bacteria, cells, or other particles are caused to adhere and form clumps; similar to precipitation, but the particles are larger and are in suspension rather than being in solution. **2.** Adhesion of the surfaces of a wound.

ag·glu·ti·na·tive (ă-glū'ti-nă-tiv) Causing, or able to cause, agglutination.

ag·glu·ti·nin (ă-glū'ti-nin) **1.** An antibody that causes clumping or agglutination of the bacteria or other cells that either stimulated the formation of the agglutinin, or contain immunologically similar, reactive antigen. **2.** A substance, other than a specific agglutinating antibody, which causes organic particles to agglutinate.

ag·glu·tin·o·gen (ă-glū-tin'ō-jen) Antigenic substance that stimulates formation of specific agglutinin, which, under certain conditions, causes agglutination of affected cells. SYN agglutogen.

ag·glu·tin·o·phil·ic (ă-glū'tin-ō-fil'ik) Readily undergoing agglutination.

ag·glu·to·gen·ic (ă-glū'tō-jen'ik) SYN agglutinogenic.

ag·gre·gate (ag'rĕ-gāt, -ăt) **1.** To unite or come together in a mass or cluster. **2.** The total of individual units making up a mass or cluster.

ag·gre·gate a·na·phy·lax·is (ag'rĕ-gāt an'ă-fi-laks'is) Anaphylactic reaction initiated by the formation of antigen-antibody complexes that activate complement.

ag·gre·gat·ed fol·li·cle (ag'rĕ-gā-tĕd fol'i-kĕl) SEE Peyer patches.

ag·gre·ga·tion (ag'rĕ-gā'shŭn) A crowded mass of independent but similar units; a cluster.

ag·gres·sion (ă-gresh'ŭn) A domineering, forceful, or assaultive verbal or physical action toward another person as the motor component of anger, hostility, or rage.

ag·gres·sive an·gi·o·myx·o·ma (ă-gres'iv an'jē-ō-miks-ō'mă) Locally invasive, but nonmetastasizing, tumor of genital organs in young women.

ag·ing (ā'jing) The process of growing old, especially by failure of replacement of cells in sufficient number to maintain full functional capacity; particularly affects cells (e.g., neurons) incapable of mitotic division.

ag·no·gen·ic (ag'nō-jen'ik) SYN idiopathic.

ag·no·si·a (ag-nō'zē-ă) Impairment of ability to recognize, or comprehend the meaning of, various sensory stimuli, not attributable to disorders of the primary receptors or general intellect; receptive defects caused by lesions in various portions of the cerebrum.

-agogue, -agog Suffixes meaning leading, promoting, stimulating; a promoter or stimulant of.

a·go·nad·al (ā'gō-nad'ăl) Denoting the absence of gonads (testes or ovaries).

ag·o·nal (ag'ŏ-năl) Relating to struggles preceding death.

ag·o·nal res·pi·ra·tion (ag'ŏ-năl res'pir-ā'shŭn) Shallow breathing pattern that is often related to cardiac arrest and death.

ag·o·nal throm·bus (ag'ŏ-năl throm'bŭs) Cardiac clot formed when dying after prolonged heart failure.

ag·o·nist (ag'ŏn-ist) **1.** Denoting a muscle in a state of contraction, with reference to its opposing muscle, or antagonist. **2.** A drug capable of combining with receptors to initiate drug actions; it possesses affinity and intrinsic activity.

ag·o·nis·tic mus·cle (ag'ŏ-nis'tik mŭs'ĕl) Muscle that contracts in reaction to its opposing, or antagonistic, muscle.

ag·or·a·pho·bi·a (ag'ŏr-ă-fō'bē-ă) A mental disorder characterized by an irrational fear of leaving a familiar setting.

-agra Combining form denoting sudden onslaught of acute pain.

a·gram·ma·tism (ā-gram'ă-tizm) Aphasia characterized by reduced ability to understand or produce most grammatical markers.

ag·ran·u·lar (ā-gran'yū-lăr) Without granules.

a·gran·u·lo·cyte (ā-grăn'ŭ-lō-sīt) A nongranular leukocyte.

a·gran·u·lo·cy·to·sis (ā'gran'yŭ-lō-sī-tō'sis) Acute potentially lethal condition with pronounced leukopenia and great reduction in the number of polymorphonuclear leukocytes; infected ulcers develop in the throat, intestinal tract, and other mucous membranes, as well as in the skin. SYN agranulocytic angina, angina lymphomatosa, neutropenic angina.

a·gran·u·lo·plas·tic (ā'gran'yŭ-lō-plas'tik) Capable of forming nongranular cells, and incapable of forming granular cells.

a·graph·i·a (ă-graf'ē-ă) Inability to write properly in the absence of abnormalities of the limb.

a·gue (ā′gyū) An intermittent fever.

a·gyr·ia (ā-jī′rē-ă) Congenital lack or underdevelopment of the convolutional pattern of the cerebral cortex. SYN lissencephalia.

aid (ād) **1.** Help; assistance. **2.** A device that helps in the performance of an action.

AIDS (ādz) Acronym for acquired immune deficiency syndrome.

AIDS quack·er·y (ādz kwak′ĕr-ē) Unvalidated therapy that suggests—among other things—that HIV does not cause acquired immune deficiency syndrome (AIDS) and that antiretroviral drugs are poison; some believers assert that human immunodeficiency virus (HIV)/AIDS results from poverty, racism, or political policy.

AIDS-re·lat·ed com·plex (ARC) (ādz-rē-lāt′ĕd kom′pleks) Manifestations of acquired immune deficiency syndrome (AIDS) in patients who have not yet developed major deficient immune function, characterized by fever with generalized lymphadenopathy, diarrhea, weight loss, minor opportunistic infections, and cytopenias.

air (ār) A mixture of odorless gases found in the atmosphere in the following approximate percentages: oxygen, 20.95; nitrogen, 78.08; argon 0.93; carbon dioxide, 0.03; other gases, 0.01.

air-bone gap (ABG) (ār-bōn gap) An abnormal condition in which the auditory threshold for an air-conducted test tone is higher than that for a bone-conducted test tone of the same frequency. SEE ALSO conductive hearing loss.

air dose (E) (ār dōs) SYN exposure dose.

air em·bo·lism (ār em′bŏ-lizm) Blockage that occurs when air enters a blood vessel, usually a vein, as a result of trauma, surgery, or deliberate injection; can cause lethal derangement of cardiac function.

air·sick·ness (ār′sik-nĕs) A condition resembling seasickness occurring in airplane or space flight due to erratic, increased, reduced, or continuous stimulation of the inner ear.

air ther·mom·e·ter (ār thĕr-mom′ĕ-tĕr) SEE gas thermometer.

air·trap·ping (ār′trap-ing) Slow or incomplete emptying of air from all or part of a lung on expiration; implies obstruction of regional airways or emphysema.

air·way (ār′wā) Any part of the respiratory tract through which air passes during breathing.

air·way a·nat·o·my (ār′wā ă-nat′ŏ-mē) The tracheobronchial structure, similar in shape to that of an inverted tree, containing cartilaginous airways; membranous bronchioles, and respiratory bronchioles.

a·kar·y·o·cyte, a·kar·y·ote, a·car·y·ote (ā-kar′ē-ō-sīt, ā-kar′ē-ōt) A cell without a nucleus, such as the erythrocyte.

a·ka·thi·sia, a·ca·thi·sia (ak-ă-thiz′ē-ă) A syndrome characterized by inability to remain seated, with motor restlessness and a feeling of muscular quivering.

a·ki·ne·si·a al·ge·ra (ā-ki-nē′sē-ă al-jer′ă) Immobility due to pain caused by any movement; usually psychogenic.

a·kin·es·the·si·a (ā-kin′es-the′zē-ă) Inability to perceive movement or position. SYN akinaesthesia.

Al Symbol for aluminum.

a·la, gen. and pl. **a·lae** (ā′lă, ā′lē) [TA] SYN wing.

a·la na·si (ā′lă nā′sī) [TA] The lateral wall of each naris.

al·a·nine a·mi·no·trans·fer·ase (ALT) (al′ă-nēn ă-mē′nō-trans′fĕr-ās) An enzyme transferring amino groups from L-alanine to 2-ketoglutarate, or the reverse (from L-glutamate to pyruvate). SYN glutamic-pyruvic transaminase, serum glutamic-pyruvic transaminase.

Al·an·son am·pu·ta·tion (al′ăn-sŏn amp′ yū-tā′shŭn) A circular amputation, with the stump shaped like a cone.

a·lar (ā′lăr) **1.** Relating to a wing; winged. **2.** SYN axillary.

a·lar lig·a·ments (ā′lăr lig′ă-mĕnts) [TA] One of a pair of short stout bands that extends from the side of the dens of the axis to the tubercle on the medial aspect of the occipital condyle. SYN check ligaments of odontoid, ligamenta alaria [TA].

al·ba, pl. **al·bae** (al'bă) SYN white matter.

al·be·do (al-bē'dō) A white area of the retina resulting from edema or infarction.

al·bi·cans, pl. **al·bi·can·ti·a** (al'bi-kanz, -kan'shē-ă) **1.** SYN white. **2.** SYN corpus albicans.

al·bi·du·ria, al·bi·nu·ria (al-bi-dyūr'ē-ă, -nyūr'ē-a) The passing of pale or white urine of low specific gravity, as in chyluria.

al·bi·nism (al'bi-nizm) Inherited (usually autosomal recessive) disorders with deficiency or absence of pigment in the skin, hair, and eyes, or eyes only, due to an abnormality in production of melanin.

al·bi·no (al-bī'nō) An individual with albinism.

al·bi·not·ic (al-bi-not'ik) Pertaining to albinism.

Al·bright dis·ease (awl'brīt di-zēz') SYN McCune-Albright syndrome.

al·bu·gin·ea (al-bū-jin'ē-ă) A white fibrous tissue layer, such as the tunica albuginea (q.v.).

al·bu·min (al-bū'min) A simple protein, varieties of which are widely distributed throughout the tissues and fluids of plants and animals.

al·bu·mi·na·tu·ri·a (al-bū'mi-nā-tyūr'ē-ă) The presence of an abnormally large quantity of albuminates in the urine when voided.

al·bu·min:glob·u·lin ra·ti·o (al-bū'min-glob'yū-lin rā'shē-ō) The ratio of albumin to globulin in serum plasma or urine; the normal ratio in the serum is approximately 1.55.

al·bu·mi·noid (al-bū'min-oyd) **1.** Resembling albumin. **2.** Any protein. **3.** A simple type of protein, insoluble in neutral solvents, present in horny and cartilaginous tissues and in the lens of the eye; e.g., keratin, elastin, collagen.

al·bu·min·ur·i·a (al-bū'mi-nyūr'ē-ă) Presence of protein in urine. SYN proteinuria (2).

al·co·hol (al'kŏ-hol) **1.** One of a series of organic chemical compounds in which a hydrogen (H) attached to carbon is replaced by a hydroxyl (OH); alcohols react with acids to form esters and with alkali metals to form alcoholates. **2.** Ethanol, C_2H_5OH, made from carbohydrates by fermentation and synthetically from ethylene or acetylene. It has been used in beverages and as a solvent, vehicle, and preservative; medicinally, it is used externally as a rubefacient, coolant, and disinfectant, and internally as an analgesic, stomachic, and sedative. SYN ethanol, ethyl alcohol.

al·co·hol·ic (alc) (al'kŏ-hol'ik) **1.** Relating to, containing, or produced by alcohol. **2.** One who suffers from alcoholism.

al·co·hol·ism (al'kŏ-hol-ism) A chronic, progressive behavioral disorder characterized by a strong urge to consume ethanol and an inability to limit the amount of drinking despite adverse consequences, which may include social or occupational impairment and deterioration of physical health.

al·co·hol with·draw·al syn·drome (al'kŏ-hol with-draw'ăl sin'drōm) Cluster of symptoms found when someone who habitually consumed excessive amounts of ethanol ceases to do so.

al·co·hol·y·sis (al'kŏ-hol'i-sis) Splitting of a chemical bond with the addition of the elements of alcohol at the point of splitting.

al·dar·ic ac·id (al'dar-ik as'id) One of a group of sugar acids; e.g., glucaric acid.

al·dos·ter·one (al-dos'tĕr-ōn) A hormone produced by the cortex of the suprarenal gland; facilitates potassium exchange for sodium in the distal renal tubule.

al·dos·ter·on·ism (al-dos'tĕr-ŏn-izm) A disorder caused by excessive secretion of aldosterone. SYN hyperaldosteronism.

al·drin (al'drin) A volatile chlorinated hydrocarbon used as an insecticide; if absorbed through the skin, it causes toxic symptoms consisting of irritability followed by depression; now banned in many countries.

alert·ness (ă-lĕrt′nĕs) Condtion of being responsive to external and internal stimuli.

aleukaemia [Br.] SYN aleukemia.

aleukaemic [Br.] SYN aleukemic.

a·leu·ke·mi·a (ā-lū-kē′mē-ă) **1.** Literally, a lack of leukocytes in the blood. **2.** Leukemic changes in bone marrow associated with a subnormal number of leukocytes in the blood. SEE ALSO subleukemic leukemia. SYN aleukaemia.

a·leu·ke·mic (ā′lū-kē′mik) Pertaining to aleukemia. SYN aleukaemic.

a·leu·ko·cy·to·sis (ā′lū-kō-sī-tō′sis) Absence or great reduction of white blood cells in the circulating blood.

a·lex·i·a (ă-lek′sē-ă) An inability to comprehend the meaning of written or printed words and sentences, caused by a cerebral lesion. SYN word blindness, visual aphasia (1).

a·lex·ic (ă-lek′sik) Pertaining to alexia.

♻ **alge-, algesi-, algio-, algo-** Combining forms meaning pain; corresponds to L. dolor-.

al·ge·sim·e·ter (al′jē-sim′ĕ-ter) SYN algesiometer.

al·ge·si·o·gen·ic (al′jē-zē-ō-jen′ik) Pain-producing. SYN algogenic.

al·ge·si·om·e·ter (al′jē-zē-om′ĕ-tĕr) An instrument for measuring the degree of sensitivity to a painful stimulus. SYN algesimeter, odynometer.

♻ **-algia** Combining form meaning pain, painful condition.

al·gi·nate (al′ji-nāt) An irreversible hydrocolloid consisting of salts of alginic acid.

al·go·gen·ic (al′gō-jen′ik) SYN algesiogenic.

al·go·phil·i·a, al·go·phil·y (al′gō-fil′ē-ă, -fil′ē) **1.** Pleasure experienced in the thought of pain in others or in oneself. **2.** SYN algolagnia.

al·go·pho·bi·a (al′gō-fō′bē-ă) Abnormal fear of or sensitiveness to pain.

al·go·rithm (al′gŏr-idhm) In clinical medicine, a step-by-step protocol for management of a health care problem; in computed tomography, the formulas used to calculate the final image from the transmitted x-ray data.

al·go·spasm (al′gō-spazm) Spasm produced by pain.

al·go·vas·cu·lar (al′gō-vas′kyū-lăr) Relating to changes in the lumen of the blood vessels occurring under the influence of pain.

ali·as·ing (āl′ē-ăs-ing) Magnetic resonance imaging artifact produced when anatomy outside the field of view is mismapped inside it.

al·i·cy·clic (al-i-sik′lik) Denoting an alicyclic compound.

a·li·e·ni·a (ā′li-ē′nē-ă) Congenital absence of the spleen.

al·i·form (al′i-fŏrm) Wing-shaped.

al·i·men·ta·ry (al′i-men′tăr-ē) Relating to food or nutrition.

al·i·men·ta·tion (al′i-mĕn-tā′shŭn) Providing nourishment. SEE ALSO feeding.

al·i·na·sal (al′i-nā′zăl) Relating to the wings of the nose (alae nasi), or flaring portions of the nostrils.

al·i·phat·ic (al′i-fat′ik) Denoting the acyclic carbon compounds, most of which belong to the fatty acid series.

al·i·sphe·noid (al′i-sfē′noyd) Relating to the greater wing of the sphenoid bone.

alkalaemia [Br.] SYN alkalemia.

al·ka·le·mi·a (al′kă-lē′mē-ă) A decrease in H^+ ion concentration of the blood or a rise in pH.

al·ka·les·cent (al′kă-les′ĕnt) **1.** Slightly alkaline. **2.** Becoming alkaline.

al·ka·li, pl. **al·ka·lies**, pl. **al·ka·lis** (al′kă-lī, -līz, al′kă-līz) **1.** A strongly basic substance yielding hydroxide ions

(OH$^-$) in solution; e.g., sodium hydroxide, potassium hydroxide. **2.** SYN base (3).

al·ka·line (al′kă-lin) Relating to or having the reaction of an alkali.

al·ka·line-ash di·et (al′kă-lin-ash dī′ĕt) A diet consisting mainly of fruits, vegetables, and milk that, when catabolized, leaves an alkaline residue to be excreted in the urine. SYN acid-ash diet.

al·ka·lin·ur·i·a (al′kă-li-nyūr′ē-ă) The passage of alkaline urine. SYN alkaluria.

al·ka·liz·er (al′kă-līz-ĕr) An agent that neutralizes acids or renders a solution alkaline.

al·ka·loid (al′kă-loyd) Originally, any one of hundreds of plant products distinguished by alkaline (basic) reactions, but now restricted to heterocyclic nitrogen-containing and often complex structures possessing pharmacologic activity; synthesized by plants and are found in the leaf, bark, seed, or other parts.

al·ka·lo·sis (al-kă-lō′sis) A state characterized by a decrease in the hydrogen ion concentration of arterial blood below the normal level, 40 nmol/L, or pH over 7.4.

al·kane (al′kān) The general term for a saturated acyclic hydrocarbon (e.g., propane, butane).

al·kyl (al′kil) **1.** A hydrocarbon radical of the general formula C_nH_{2n+1}. **2.** A compound, such as tetraethyl lead, in which a metal is combined with alkyl radicals. SYN alkide.

al·kyl·a·mine (al-kil′ă-mēn) An alkane containing an $-NH_2$ group in place of one H atom; e.g., ethylamine.

al·kyl·a·tion (al′ki-lā′shŭn) Substitution of an alkyl radical for a hydrogen atom; e.g., introduction of a side chain into an aromatic compound.

allachaesthesia [Br.] SYN allachesthesia.

al·la·ches·the·si·a (al′ă-kes-thē′zē-ă) A condition in which a tactile sensation is referred to a point other than that to which the stimulus is applied. SYN allachaesthesia.

allanto-, allant-, allant- Combining forms meaning allantois; allantoid; sausagelike.

al·lan·to·ic (al′an-tō′ik) Relating to the allantois.

al·lan·to·ic di·ver·ti·cu·lum (al′an-tō′ik dī-vĕr-tik′yū-lŭm) An endoderm-lined outpouching of the hindgut representing the primordium of the allantois.

al·lan·toid (ă-lan′toyd) **1.** Sausage-shaped. **2.** Relating to, or resembling, the allantois.

al·lan·to·in (ă-lan′tō-in) A substance present in allantoic fluid, fetal urine and elsewhere. SYN 3-ureidohydantoin, cordianine, glyoxyldiureide.

al·lan·to·i·nu·ria (ă-lan′tō-i-nyūr′ē-ă) The urinary excretion of allantoin; normal in most other mammals, but abnormal in humans.

al·lan·to·is (ă-lan′tō-is) A fetal membrane developing from the hindgut (or umbilical vesicle, in humans). SYN allantoid membrane.

al·lele (ă-lēl′) Any one of a series of two or more different genes that may occupy the same locus on a specific chromosome.

al·le·lo·tax·is, al·le·lo·taxy (ă-lē′lō-taks′is, -taks′ē) Development of an organ from a number of embryonal structures or tissues.

al·ler·gen (al′ĕr-jĕn) An incitant of altered reactivity (allergy), an antigenic substance.

al·ler·gic con·junc·ti·vi·tis (ă-lĕr′jik kŏn-jŭngk′ti-vī′tis) Ocular disease characterized by itching and watery discharge.

al·ler·gic re·ac·tion (ă-lĕr′jik rē-ak′shŭn) A local or general reaction of an organism following contact with a specific allergen to which it has been previously exposed and sensitized.

al·ler·gy blood test (al′ĕr-jē blŭd test) Assessment used to diagnose an inappropriate immune response to a substance that does not normally trigger an immune reaction.

al·li·ga·tor for·ceps (al'i-gā-tŏr fōr' seps) A long forceps with a small hinged jaw on the end.

♻ **allo-** Prefix meaning other; differing from the normal or usual.

al·lo·an·ti·bod·y (al'ō-an'ti-bod-ē) An antibody specific for an alloantigen.

al·lo·an·ti·gen (al'ō-an'ti-jen) An antigen that occurs in some but not all members of the same species. Used by the immune system to distinguish self from nonself.

al·lo·chi·ri·a, al·lo·chei·ri·a (al'ō-kī'rē-ă) A form of allachesthesia in which the sensation of a stimulus in one limb is referred to the contralateral limb. SYN allesthesia, Bamberger sign (2).

al·lo·dyn·ia (al'ō-din'ē-ă) Condition in which ordinarily nonpainful stimuli evoke pain.

al·lo·er·o·tism (al'ō-ār'ō-tizm) Sexual attraction toward another person. Cf. autoerotism. SYN heteroerotism.

al·lo·ge·ne·ic graft (al'ō-jen'ik graft) SYN allograft.

al·lo·gen·ic, al·lo·ge·ne·ic (al'ō-jen' ik, -jě-nē'ik) Used in transplantation biology. It pertains to different gene constitutions within the same species; antigenically distinct.

al·lo·graft (al'ō-graft) A graft transplanted between genetically nonidentical individuals of the same species. SYN allogeneic graft, homologous graft, homoplastic graft.

al·lo·graft re·jec·tion (al'lō-graft rě-jek' shŭn) The rejection of tissue transplanted between two genetically different individuals of the same species.

al·lo·im·mu·ni·za·tion (al-lō'im-myū' nī-zā'shŭn) Immunization against a nonself protein, as occurs in patients receiving transfusions.

al·lo·mor·phism (al'ō-mōr'fizm) Change of shape in cells due to mechanical causes, such as flattening from pressure, or to progressive metaplasia, such as the change of bile duct cells into liver cells.

al·lop·a·thy (al-op'ă-thē) A therapeutic system in which a disease is treated by producing a second condition that is incompatible with or antagonistic to the first. Cf. homeopathy. SYN heteropathy (2).

al·lo·plast (al'ō-plast) An inert material used to construct, reconstruct, or augment tissue.

al·lo·plas·ty (al'ō-plas-tē) Repair of defects by allotransplantation.

al·lo·rhyth·mi·a (al'ō-ridh'mē-ă) An irregularity in the cardiac rhythm that repeats itself any number of times.

all-or-none law (awl nŭn law) Theory that when a muscle contracts it contracts completely or not at all. SEE Bowditch law.

al·lo·sen·si·ti·za·tion (al'ō-sen'si-ti-zā' shun) Exposure to an alloantigen that induces immunologic memory cells.

al·lo·ste·ric (al'ō-ster'ik) Pertaining to or characterized by allosterism.

al·lo·tope (al'ō-tōp) *Do not confuse this word with allotrope.* A polymorphic region constituting antigenic determinant on the constant region of an allotype.

al·lo·trans·plan·ta·tion (al'ō-trans'plan-tā'shŭn) Transplantation of an allograft.

al·lo·tro·pic (al'ō-trō'pik) Denoting a type of personality characterized by a preoccupation with the reactions of others.

al·lot·ro·pism, al·lot·ro·py (ă-lot'rō-pizm, -lot'rō-pē) The existence of certain elements, in several forms differing in physical properties; e.g., carbon black, graphite, and diamonds are all pure carbon.

al·lo·type (al'ō-tīp) Any one of the genetically determined antigenic differences within a given class of immunoglobulin that occur among members of the same species. SEE ALSO antibody.

alloxuraemia [Br.] SYN alloxuremia.

al·lox·u·re·mia (al'oks-yūr-ē'mē-ă) The presence of purine bases in the blood. SYN alloxuraemia.

al·lox·u·ria (al'oks-yūr'ē-ă) The presence of purine bodies in the urine.

al•oe (al′ō) The dried juice from the leaves of *Aloe perryi*, and *A. barbadensis* or of *A. capensis*; used as a purgative and topically in cosmetics where it has unproven value.

al•o•pe•ci•a (al-ō-pē′shē-ă) Complete or partial absence or loss of hair.

al•o•pe•ci•a ar•e•a•ta (al-ō-pē′shē-ă ā-rē-ā′tă) Circumscribed, nonscarring, usually asymmetric areas of baldness on the scalp, eyebrows, and beard area of unknown cause. SYN Cazenove vitiligo, Jonston alopecia.

al•o•pe•ci•a me•di•ca•men•to•sa (al-ō-pē′shē-ă med-i-kă-men-tō′să) Diffuse hair loss, most notably of the scalp, attributable to prescribed drugs.

alo•pe•ci•a se•ni•lis (al′ō-pē′shē-ă se-nil′is) Normal loss of scalp hair in old age.

alo•pe•ci•a to•ta•lis (al-ō-pē′shē-ă tō-tā′lis) Total loss of hair of the scalp either within a very short period of time or from progression of localized alopecia, especially alopecia areata. Cf. alopecia universalis.

alo•pe•ci•a tox•i•ca (al′ō-pē′shē-ă toks′i-kă) Hair loss attributed to febrile illness.

alo•pe•ci•a u•ni•ver•sa•lis (al-ō-pē′shē-ă yū′ni-věr-sā′lis) Total loss of hair from all parts of the body.

al•o•pe•cic (al′ō-pē′sik) Relating to alopecia.

al•pha (α) (al′fă) First letter of the Greek alphabet; used as a classifier in the nomenclature of many sciences.

al•pha (α)-ad•re•ner•gic block•ing agent (al′fă ad′rĕ-něr′jik blok′ing ā′jěnt) An agent that competitively blocks α-adrenergic receptors.

al•pha (α)-ad•re•ner•gic re•cep•tors (al′fă ad′rĕ-něr′jik rĕ-sep′tŏrz) Adrenergic receptors in effector tissues capable of selective activation by methoxamine and blockade by phenoxybenzamine. Their activation results in physiologic responses (e.g., increased peripheral vascular resistance, mydriasis, and contraction of pilomotor muscles).

al•pha (α) tha•las•se•mia (al′fă thal′ă-sē′mē-ă) Hematologic disorder due to one of two or more genes that depress synthesis of α-globin chains.

Al•pha•vi•rus (al′fă-vī′rŭs) One of the genera of the family Togaviridae that was formerly classified as part of the "group A" arboviruses and includes the viruses that cause eastern equine, western equine, and Venezuelan encephalitis.

Al•port syn•drome (AS) (al′pŏrt sin′drŏm) A genetically heterogeneous disorder characterized by nephritis associated with microscopic hematuria and slow progression of renal failure, sensorineural hearing loss, and ocular abnormalities such as lenticonus and maculopathy.

Als•tröm syn•drome (ahl′strem sin′drŏm) Retinal degeneration with nystagmus and loss of central vision, associated with obesity in childhood; sensorineural hearing loss and diabetes mellitus usually occur after age 10 years.

al•tered state of con•scious•ness (awl′těrd stāt kon′shŭs-něs) General term indicating that someone is failing to interact with environmental stimuli in a normal manner.

al•ter•e•go•ism (awl′ter-ē′gō-izm) Identification with people of similar personality to one's own.

Al•ter•nar•i•a (awl-tĕr-nā′rē-ă) A widespread rapidly growing dematiaceous fungal genus, associated with subcutaneous infections such as phaeohyphomycosis, sinusitis, erosion of the nasal septum, and infections of skin and nails.

al•ter•nat•ing trem•or (awl′tĕr-nāt-ing trem′ŏr) A form of hyperkinesia characterized by regular, symmetric, to-and-fro movements produced by patterned, alternating contraction of muscles and their antagonists.

al•ter•na•tion (awl′tĕr-nā′shŭn) The occurrence of two things or phases in succession and recurrently; used interchangeably with alternans.

al•ter•na•tive in•her•i•tance (awl-tĕr′nă-tiv in-her′i-tăns) 1. SYN mendelian inheritance. 2. Galtonian term for an assumed form in which all the characters are derived from one parent.

al·ter·na·tive med·i·cine (awl-tĕr′nă-tiv med′i-sin) A term used by some practitioners of Western medicine for methods of healing, some ancient and widely practiced, which may not be firmly based on accepted scientific principles and may thereby be of limited known effectiveness. SEE ALSO complementary and alternative medicine.

al·ter·na·tor (awl′ter-nā-tŏr) Mechanical apparatus with movable transparent racks to which a large number of radiographs can be attached, to enable selection and viewing in front of a stationary bank of lights.

al·ti·tude sick·ness (al′ti-tūd sik′nĕs) Syndrome caused by low inspired oxygen pressure (as at high altitude) and characterized by nausea, headache, dyspnea, and insomnia. SYN puna, soroche, aerial sickness, altitude disease.

alu·mi·no·sis (ă-lū′min-ō′sis) A pneumoconiosis caused by inhalation of aluminum particles into the lungs.

alu·mi·num (Al) (ă-lū′min-ŭm) A white silvery metal of very light weight; atomic no. 13, atomic wt. 26.981539. Many salts and compounds are used in medicine and dentistry.

alu·mi·num hy·drox·ide (ă-lū′mi-nŭm hī-drok′sīd) Astringent dusting powder; also used internally as a mild astringent antacid. SYN aluminum hydrate, hydrated alumina.

alu·mi·num ox·ide (ă-lū′mi-nŭm ok′sīd) Aluminum compound used as an abrasive, as a refractory, and in chromatography.

alu·mi·num phos·phate (ă-lū′mi-nŭm fos′fāt) Infusible powder used for dental cements with calcium sulfate and sodium silicate.

alu·mi·num sub·ac·e·tate (ă-lū′mi-nŭm sŭb-as′ĕ-tāt) Compound of aluminum used in solution as an astringent, as an ingredient in mouthwashes, and in embalming fluids. SYN aluminum diacetate.

al·ve·o·al·gi·a (al-vē′ō-al′jē-ă) A postoperative complication of tooth extraction in which the blood clot in the socket disintegrates, resulting in focal osteomyelitis and severe pain. SYN alveolalgia.

al·ve·o·lal·gia (al-vē′ō-lal′jē-ă) SYN alveoalgia.

al·ve·o·lar cell (al-vē′ŏ-lăr sel) Any of the cells lining the alveoli of the lung, including the squamous alveolar cells, the great alveolar cells, and the alveolar macrophages.

al·ve·o·lar mac·ro·phage (AM) (al-vē′ŏ-lăr mak′rō-fāj) A vigorously phagocytic macrophage on the epithelial surface of lung alveoli where it ingests inhaled particulate matter. SYN coniophage, dust cell.

al·ve·o·lar pores (al-vē′ō-lăr pōrz) Openings in the interalveolar septa of the lung that permit air flow between adjacent alveoli. SYN interalveolar pores, Kohn pores.

al·ve·o·lar pro·cess (al-vē′ŏ-lăr pros′es) That portion of bone in either the maxilla or the mandible that surrounds and supports the teeth.

al·ve·o·lar sac·cules (al-vē′ō-lăr sak′yūlz) Terminal dilations of the alveolar ducts that give rise to alveoli in the lungs.

al·ve·o·lar sep·tum (al-vē′ō-lăr sep′tŭm) SYN interalveolar septum.

al·ve·o·late (al-vē′ō-lāt) Pitted like a honeycomb.

al·ve·o·lec·to·my (al′vē-ō-lek′tŏ-mē) Surgical excision of a portion of the dentoalveolar process during tooth removal to facilitate dental prosthesis placement.

al·ve·o·li (al-vē′ō-lī) Plural of alveolus.

al·ve·o·li·tis (al-vē′ō-lī′tis) **1.** Inflammation of lung alveoli. **2.** Inflammation of a tooth socket.

alveolo- Combining form indicating an alveolus, the alveolar process; alveolar.

al·ve·o·lo·cla·si·a (al-vē′ŏ-lō-klā′zē-ă) Destruction of the alveolus.

al·ve·o·lo·den·tal (al-vē′ŏ-lō-den′tăl) Relating to the alveoli and the teeth.

al•ve•o•lo•plas•ty (al-vē′ŏ-lō-plas-tē) Surgical preparation of the alveolar ridges for the reception of dentures; shaping and smoothing of socket margins after extraction of teeth with subsequent suturing to ensure optimal healing.

al•ve•o•lus, gen. and pl. **al•ve•o•li** (al-vē′ō-lŭs, -lī) [TA] **1.** One of the terminal secretory portions of an alveolar or racemose gland. **2.** One of the honeycomb pits in the wall of the stomach. **3.** SYN tooth socket.

al•ve•us, pl. **al•ve•i** (al′vē-ŭs, -ī) A channel or trough.

a•lym•pho•cy•to•sis (ā-lim′fō-sī-tō′sis) Absence or great reduction of lymphocytes.

a•lym•pho•pla•si•a (ā-lim′fō-plā′zē-ă) Aplasia or hypoplasia of lymphoid tissue.

Alz•hei•mer dis•ease, Alz•heim•er de•men•ti•a (awlts′hī-měr di-zēz′, dě-men′shē-ă) Progressive mental deterioration manifested by loss of memory, ability to calculate, and visual-spatial orientation; confusion; and disorientation. Begins in late middle life and usually results in death in 5–10 years. SYN presenile dementia (2), dementia presenilis, primary senile dementia.

am•a•crine (am′ă-krēn) **1.** A cell or structure lacking a long, fibrous process. **2.** Denoting such a cell or structure. SEE ALSO amacrine cell.

am•a•crine cell (AM) (am′ă-krēn sel) Neural cell with short branching dendrites but believed to lack an axon.

a•mal•gam (ă-mal′găm) An alloy of an element or a metal with mercury. In dentistry, primarily of two types: silver-tin alloy, containing small amounts of copper, zinc, and perhaps other metals, and a second type containing more copper; they are used in restoring teeth.

a•mal•ga•ma•tion (ă-mal′gă-mā′shŭn) The process of combining mercury with a metal or an alloy to form a new alloy.

a•mal•gam car•ri•er (ă-mal′găm kar′ē-ěr) Dental instrument used to transport triturated amalgam to a cavity preparation and to deposit it therein.

Am•a•ni•ta (am′ă-nī′tă) A genus of fungi, many members of which are highly poisonous.

a•mas•ti•a (ā-mas′tē-ă) Absence of breasts.

a•mas•ti•gote (ă-mas′ti-gōt) SYN Leishman-Donovan body.

am•au•ro•sis (am′aw-rō′sis) Blindness, especially that occurring without apparent change in the eye itself, as from a brain lesion.

am•au•ro•sis con•gen•ita of Le•ber (am′aw-rō′sis kŏn-jen′i-tă lā′běr) A disorder of cone-rod abiotrophy causing blindness or severely reduced vision at birth.

am•au•rot•ic pu•pil (am′aw-rot′ik pyū′pil) Pupil in an eye that is blind because of ocular or optic nerve disease.

am•bi•dex•trous (am′bi-deks′trŭs) Having equal facility in the use of both hands.

am•bi•ent (amb) (am′bē-ěnt) Surrounding, encompassing; pertaining to the immediate environment in which an organism or apparatus functions.

am•big•u•ous (amb, ambig) (am-big′yū-ŭs) **1.** Having more than one interpretation. **2.** In anatomy, wandering; having more than one direction. **3.** In neuroanatomy, applied to a nucleus (nucleus ambiguus) supplying special visceral efferent fibers to the vagus and glossopharyngeal nerves.

am•bi•lat•er•al (am′bi-lat′ěr-ăl) Relating to both sides.

am•bi•le•vous (am′bi-lē′vŭs) Awkwardness in the use of both hands. SYN ambisinister, ambisinistrous.

am•bi•o•pia (am′bē-ō′pē-ă) Double vision.

am•bi•sex•u•al (am′bi-sek′shū-ăl) **1.** Denoting sexual characteristics found in both sexes (e.g., breasts, pubic hair). **2.** Bisexual.

am•biv•a•lence (am-biv′ă-lěns) The coexistence of antithetical attitudes or emotions toward a given person or thing, or idea, as in the simultaneous feeling and expression of love and hate toward the same person. SEE approach-avoidance conflict.

am·bly·a·phi·a (am′blē-ā′fē-ă) Diminution in tactile sensibility.

am·bly·geus·ti·a (am′blē-gū′stē-ă) A diminution in the sense of taste.

am·bly·o·gen·ic (am′blē-ō-jen′ik) Inducing amblyopia.

Am·bly·om·ma (am′blē-o′mă) A genus of male hard ticks characterized by eyes, festoons, and deeply imbedded ventral plates near these festoons.

am·bly·o·pi·a (am′blē-ō′pē-ă) Visual impairment not due to an ocular lesion and not fully correctable by an artificial lens.

am·bly·o·scope (am′blē-ō-skōp) A reflecting stereoscope used to evaluate or simulate binocular vision. SEE ALSO haploscope.

am·bu·la·to·ry, am·bu·lant (am′byū-lă-tōr-ē, am′byū-lănt) Walking about or able to walk about; denoting a patient who is not confined to bed or hospital as a result of disease or surgery.

Am·bu·la·to·ry Pay·ment Clas·sif·i·ca·tion (APC) (am′byū-lă-tōr-ē pā′ mĕnt klas′i-fi-kă′shŭn) In U.S. medical care, a system for grouping outpatient services provided by hospitals on the basis of similarity of costs and clinical indications.

a·me·ba, pl. **a·me·bae**, pl. **a·me·bas** (ă-mē′bă, -bē, -băz) Common name for *Amoeba* and similar naked, lobose, sarcodine protozoa. SYN amoeba.

a·me·bi·a·sis (am′ē-bī′ă-sis) Infection with *Entamoeba histolytica* or other pathogenic amebae.

a·me·bi·a·sis cu·tis (am′ē-bī′ă-sis kyū′ tis) Cutaneous amebiasis, usually appearing as an extension of underlying infection (e.g., perianal or at a colostomy site or over a liver abscess).

a·me·bic (ă-mē′bik) Relating to, resembling, or caused by amebas.

a·me·bic dys·en·te·ry (ă-mē′bik dis′ ĕn-ter′ē) Diarrhea resulting from ulcerative inflammation of the colon, caused chiefly by infection with *Entamoeba histolytica*.

a·me·bi·ci·dal (ă-mē′bi-sī′dăl) Destructive to amebae.

a·me·bi·cide (ă-mē′bi-sīd) Any agent that destroys amebae.

a·me·bi·form (ă-mē′bi-fōrm) Of the shape or appearance of an ameba.

a·me·boid (ă-mē′boyd) Resembling an ameba in appearance or characteristics.

a·me·boid cell (ă-mē′boyd sel) Cell (e.g., leukocyte), having ameboid movements, with a power of locomotion. SYN wandering cell, migratory cell.

am·e·bu·ria (am′ē-byūr′ē-ă) The presence of amebae in the urine.

a·mel·a·not·ic (ā-mel′ă-not′ik) Containing little to no melanin.

a·me·li·a (ă-mē′lē-ă) Congenital absence of a limb or limbs. Autosomal dominant, autosomal recessive, and X-linked forms have been reported, but most cases are sporadic.

a·me·li·o·ra·tion (ă-mē′lē-ō-rā′shŭn) Improvement; moderation in the severity of a disease or the intensity of its symptoms.

am·e·lo·blast (am′ĕl′ō-blast) One of the columnar epithelial cells of the inner layer of the enamel organ of a developing tooth, involved with the formation of enamel matrix. SYN enamel cell, enameloblast, ganoblast.

am·e·lo·blas·tic lay·er (am′el-ō-blas′ tik lā′ĕr) The internal layer of the enamel organ. SYN enamel layer.

am·e·lo·blas·to·ma (am′ĕ-lō-blas-tō′ mă) A benign odontogenic epithelial neoplasm; it behaves as a slowly growing expansile radiolucent tumor, occurs most commonly in the posterior regions of the mandible, and has a marked tendency to recur if inadequately excised.

am·e·lo·den·tin·al (am′ĕ-lō-den′ti-năl) SYN dentinoenamel.

am·e·lo·gen·e·sis (am′ē-lō-jen′ĕ-sis)

The deposition and maturation of enamel. SYN enamelogenesis.

am·e·lo·gen·e·sis im·per·fec·ta (am´ĕ-lŏ-jen´ĕ-sis im-pĕr-fek´tă) Hereditary ectodermal disorders in which the enamel is defective in structure or deficient in quantity. SYN enamel dysplasia, enamelogenesis imperfecta.

amel·o·gen·in (am´ĕ-lō-jen´in) Protein that forms much of the organic matrix during early development of tooth enamel.

a·men·or·rhea (ă-men-ŏr-ē´ă) Absence or abnormal cessation of the menses.

amenorrhoea [Br.] SYN amenorrhea.

a·men·ti·a (ă-men´shē-ă) SYN dementia.

A·mer·i·can A·cad·e·my of Nurs·ing (AAN) (ă-mer´i-kăn ă-kad´ĕ-mē nŭrs´ing) A professional group composed of about 1500 nursing leaders who address national and international issues of health care and policy; nursing leaders are selected as Fellows in recognition of their accomplishments within the nursing profession.

A·mer·i·can As·so·ci·a·tion for Med·i·cal Tran·scrip·tion (AAMT) (ă-mer´i-kăn ă-sŏ´sē-ā´shŭn med´i-kăl trans-krip´shŭn) Former name of Association for Healthcare Documentation Integrity (AHDI).

A·mer·i·can As·so·ci·a·tion of Med·i·cal Assistants (AAMA) (ă-mer´i-kăn ă-sŏ´sē-ā´shŭn med´i-kăl ă-sis´tănts) A professional organization comprising over 350 chapters nationally. The group awards a certificate verifying that the holder has met the standards of knowledge for the discipline and maintains them on a regular basis.

A·mer·i·can As·so·ci·a·tion of Oc·cu·pa·tion·al Health Nurs·es (AAOHN) (ă-mer´i-kăn ă-sŏ´sē-ā´shŭn ok´yū-pā´shŭn-ăl helth nŭr´sĕz) Professional organization founded in 1942 with headquarters in Georgia, whose members provide health care in the workplace.

A·mer·i·can Col·lege of Chest Phy·si·cians (ă-mer´i-kăn kol´ĕj chest fi-zish´ănz) Professional organization founded in 1935 with headquarters in Northbrook,

Illinois; multidisciplinary membership specializing in thoracic diseases.

A·mer·i·can Col·lege of Den·tists (ă-mer´i-kăn kol´ĕj den´tists) Honorary professional organization founded in 1920 with headquarters in Gaithersburg, Maryland; concerns include increasing professional knowledge and maintaining professional standards.

A·mer·i·can Col·lege of Phy·si·cians (ă-mer´i-kăn kol´ĕj fi-zish´ănz) Professional organization of health care specialists that was founded in 1915 in Philadelphia; its members specialize in all aspects of internal medicine.

A·mer·i·can Col·lege of Sur·geons (ACS) (ă-mer´i-kăn kol´ĕj sŭr´jŏnz) Professional organization based in Chicago that offers courses in continuing education, maintains professional standards, and is also involved in research.

A·mer·i·can Den·tal Hy·gien·ists As·so·ci·a·tion (ADHA) (ă-mer´i-kăn den´tăl hī-jen´ists ă-sŏ´sē-ā´shŭn) Professional organization in the United States; its mission is to promote the public's oral health and to advance the practice and techniques of dental hygiene.

Amer·i·can Man·u·al Al·pha·bet (ă-mer´i-kăn man´yū-ăl al´fă-bet) Specific hand and finger positions used to represent each letter of the alphabet, used in conjunction with American Sign Language and other sign languages. SEE ALSO fingerspelling, sign language.

A·mer·i·can Med·i·cal As·so·ci·a·tion (AMA) (ă-mer´i-kăn med´i-kăl ă-sŏ´sē-ā´shŭn) Professional organization for physicians.

A·mer·i·can Nurs·es As·so·ci·a·tion (ANA) (ă-mer´i-kăn nŭrs´ĕz ă-sŏ´sē-ā´shŭn) A full-service professional organization representing the U.S.'s 2.7 million registered nurses through its 54 constituent state associations. ANA advances the nursing profession by fostering high standards of nursing practice, promoting the economic and general welfare of nurses in the workplace, projecting a positive and realistic view of nursing, and by lobbying the U.S. Congress and regulatory agencies on health care issues affecting nurses and the public.

A·mer·i·can Oc·cu·pa·tion·al Ther·a·py Fel·lows (AOTF) (ă-mer′i-kăn ŏk′yū-pā′shŭn-ăl thār′ă-pē fel′ōz) Members of the professional organization representing occupational therapists.

A·mer·i·can Speech Lan·guage and Hear·ing As·so·ci·a·tion (ASHA) (ă-mer′i-kăn spēch lan′gwăj hēr′ing ă-sō′sē-ā′shŭn) U.S. national organization founded in 1958 with headquarters in Rockville, Maryland; its members include speech-language pathologists and other specialists concerned with the interplay of audition and the act of speaking.

Amer·i·cans with Dis·a·bil·i·ties Act (ADA) (ă-mer′i-kănz dis′ă-bil′i-tēz akt) U.S. federal legislation prohibiting discrimination against those with disabilities and ensuring equal access to employment, education, and other services.

Ames test (āmz test) A screening procedure for possible carcinogens using strains of *Salmonella typhimurium* that are unable to synthesize histidine.

am·e·tro·pi·a (am′ĕ-trō′pē-ă) Optic condition with an error of refraction so that with the eye at rest the retina is not in conjugate focus with light rays from distant objects.

am·e·tro·pic (am′ĕ-trō′pik) Relating to, or suffering from, ametropia.

♻ **-amic** Chemical suffix denoting the replacement of one COOH group of a dicarboxylic acid by a carboxamide group (—CONH$_2$); applied only to trivial names (e.g., succinamic acid).

a·mim·ia (ā-mim′ē-ă) Inability to express ideas by nonverbal communication, such as gestures or signs.

am·i·na·tion (am′i-nā′shŭn) The introduction of an amine moiety into a compound.

am·in·er·gic (a′mi-něr′jik) Relating to nerve cells or fibers.

♻ **amino-** Combining form denoting a compound containing the radical, —NH$_2$.

ami·no ac·id (AA, aa) (ă-mē′nō as′id) An organic acid in which one of the hydrogen atoms on a carbon atom have been replaced by NH$_2$. Usually refers to an aminocarboxylic acid. However, taurine is also an amino acid.

a·mi·no·ac·i·de·mi·a (ă-mē′nō-as′i-dē′mē-ă, am′i-nō-) The presence of excessive amounts of specific amino acids in the blood.

a·mi·no·ac·i·du·ri·a (ă-mē′nō-as′i-dyūr′ē-ă) Excretion of amino acids in the urine, especially in excessive amounts. SYN hyperaminoaciduria.

a·mi·no·ac·yl·ase (ă-mē′nō-as′i-lās) An enzyme catalyzing hydrolysis of a wide variety of *N*-acyl amino acids to the corresponding amino acid and an acid anion.

***p*-ami·no·ben·zo·ic acid (PABA)** (ă-mē′nō-ben-zō′ik as′id) A factor in the vitamin B complex, a part of all folic acids and required for its formation; neutralizes the bacteriostatic effects of the sulfonamides.

γ-a·mi·no·bu·tyr·ic ac·id (GABA, γ-Abu) (ă-mē′nō-byū-tēr′ik as′id) Constituent of the central nervous system; quantitatively, the principal inhibitory neurotransmitter. Used in the treatment of various neurologic disorders (e.g., epilepsy).

***p*-a·mi·no·hip·pur·ic acid (PAH)** (ă-mē′nō-hi-pyūr′ik as′id) Acid used in renal function tests to measure renal plasma flow; actively secreted (and filtered) by the kidney.

am·i·nol·y·sis (am′i-nol′i-sis) Replacement of a halogen in an alkyl or aryl molecule by an amine radical, with elimination of hydrogen halide.

***p*-a·mi·no·sal·i·cyl·ic ac·id (PAS, PASA)** (ă-mē′nō-sal-i-sil′ik as′id) A bacteriostatic agent against tubercle bacilli, used as a second-line agent; potassium, sodium, and calcium salts have the same use.

a·mi·no·trans·fer·ase (ă-mē′nō-trans′fĕr-ās) [EC sub-group 2.6.1] Enzyme transferring amino groups between an amino acid to (usually) a 2-keto acid.

am·i·nu·ri·a (am′i-nyūr′ē-ă) Excretion of amines in the urine.

am·i·to·sis (am′i-tō′sis) Direct division of the nucleus and cell, without the complicated changes in the nucleus that occur in the ordinary process of cell reproduction. SYN direct nuclear division, Remak nuclear division.

am·i·tot·ic (am′i-tot′ik) Relating to or marked by amitosis.

am·me·ter (am) (am′ē-tĕr) An instrument for measuring strength of electric current in amperes.

am·mo·nia (NH₃, amm, AMM, ammon.) (ă-mō′nē-ă) A colorless volatile gas, NH₃, highly soluble in water, capable of forming a weak base, which combines with acids to form ammonium compounds.

am·mo·ni·u·ri·a (ă-mō-nē-yūr′ē-ă) Excretion of urine that contains an excessive amount of ammonia.

am·mo·nol·y·sis (am′ō-nol′i-sis) The breaking of a chemical bond with the addition of the elements of ammonia (NH₂ and H) at the point of breakage.

am·ne·si·a (am-nē′zē-ă) A disturbance in the memory of information stored in long-term memory, in contrast to short-term memory, manifested by total or partial inability to recall past experiences.

am·ne·si·ac (am-nē′sē-ak) One suffering from amnesia.

am·ne·sic (am-nē′sik) Relating to or characterized by amnesia. SYN amnestic (1).

am·nes·tic (am-nes′tik) 1. SYN amnesic. 2. An agent causing amnesia.

am·nes·tic syn·drome (am-nes′tik sin′ drōm) 1. SYN Korsakoff syndrome. 2. An organic brain syndrome with short-term (but not immediate) memory disturbance, regardless of the etiology.

am·ni·o·cele (am′nē-ō-sēl) SYN omphalocele.

am·ni·o·cen·te·sis (am′nē-ō-sen-tē′sis) Transabdominal aspiration of fluid from the amniotic sac for diagnostic purposes.

am·ni·o·cho·ri·al, am·ni·o·cho·ri·on·

ic (am′nē-ō-kōr′ē-ăl, -kōr′ē-on′ik) Relating to both amnion and chorion.

am·ni·o·gen·e·sis (am′nē-ō-jen′ē-sis) Formation of the amnion.

am·ni·o·hook (am′nē-ō-huk) Instrument designed to tear a hole in the amnion without injuring the fetus.

am·ni·o·in·fu·sion (am′nē-ō-in-fyū′ zhŭn) Infusion of warmed saline through an intrauterine catheter during labor.

am·ni·on (Am) (am′nē-on) Innermost of the extraembryonic membranes enveloping the embryo in utero and containing the amniotic fluid.

am·ni·on·ic, am·ni·ot·ic (am′nē-on′ik, am′nē-ot′ik) Relating to the amnion.

am·ni·on·ic band, am·ni·ot·ic band (am′nē-on′ik band, am′nē-ot′ik) Strand of amnionic tissue adherent to the embryo or fetus, which constricts the embryonic limbs. SEE ALSO congenital amputation.

am·ni·o·ni·tis (am′nē-ō-nī′tis) Inflammation resulting from infection of the amnion, which, in turn, usually results from premature rupture of the membranes (a condition often associated with neonatal infection).

am·ni·or·rhe·a (am′nē-ōr-ē′ă) Escape of amniotic fluid.

am·ni·or·rhex·is (am′nē-ō-rek′sis) Rupture of the amniotic membrane.

am·ni·o·scope (am′nē-ō-skōp) An endoscope for studying amniotic fluid through the intact amnion.

am·ni·ot·ic band se·quence (ABS) (am-nē-on′ik band sē′kwĕns) Early rupture of the amnion with formation of bands that adhere to or compress parts of the fetus, resulting in a wide variety of anomalies.

am·ni·o·tome (am′nē-ō-tōm) An instrument for puncturing the fetal membranes.

am·ni·ot·o·my (am′nē-ot′ŏ-mē) Artificial rupture of the fetal membranes as a means of inducing or expediting labor.

Amoe·ba (ă-mē′bă) A genus of pseudo-pod-forming protozoa of the class Sarcodina (or Rhizopoda), which are abundant soil-dwellers, especially in rich organic debris, and are also commonly found as parasites.

amoeba [Br.] SYN ameba.

amoeboid [Br.] SYN ameboid.

a·mok, a·muck (ă-mŭk′) Colloquialism denoting maniacal, wild, or uncontrolled behavior threatening injury to others.

a·morph (ā′mōrf) An allele that has no phenotypically recognizable product and therefore its existence can be inferred on molecular evidence only.

a·mor·phi·a, a·mor·phism (ă-mōr′fē-ă, -fizm) Condition of being amorphous (1).

a·mor·pho·syn·the·sis (ă-mōr′fō-sin′thĕ-sis) Disorder of recognition of the right side of the body in spatial relationships, caused by a lesion of the left parietal lobe.

a·mor·phous (ā-mōr′fŭs) **1.** Without definite form or visible differentiation in structure. **2.** Not crystallized.

am·pere (A) (am′pēr) **1.** Legal definition: the current that, flowing for 1 second, will deposit 1.118 mg of silver from silver nitrate solution. **2.** Scientific (SI) definition: the current that, if maintained in two straight parallel conductors of infinite length and of negligible circular cross-sections and placed 1 m apart in a vacuum, produces between them a force of 2×10^{-7} N/m of length.

am·phet·a·mine (AMT, AMPH, A, AMP) (am-fet′ă-mēn) A chemical compound that is structurally a sympathomimetic amine, considered a psychostimulant, and approved by the U.S. Food and Drug Administration (FDA) to treat narcolepsy and attention deficit hyperactivity disorder. Because of its potential for abuse, it is scheduled by the FDA in the most restrictive classification for a drug with medical usefulness.

♻ **amphi-** Combining form meaning on both sides, surrounding, double; corresponds to L. *ambi-*.

am·phi·ar·thro·sis (am′fē-ahr-thrō′sis) SYN symphysis (1).

am·phi·bol·ic (am′fi-bol′ik) Referring to reactions or biologic pathways that serve in both biosynthesis and degradation (i.e., anabolism and catabolism).

am·phi·cen·tric (am′fi-sen′trik) Centering at both ends.

am·phi·di·ar·thro·di·al joint (am′fi-dī′ahrth-rō′dē-ăl joynt) SYN synovial joint.

am·phi·kar·y·on (am′fē-kar′ē-on) A diploid nucleus containing two haploid sets of chromosomes.

am·phi·mix·is (am′fi-mik′sis) **1.** Union of the paternal and maternal chromatin after impregnation of the oocyte. **2.** In psychoanalysis, a combination of genital and anal eroticism.

♻ **ampho-** Combining form meaning on both sides, surrounding, double.

am·pho·phil, am·pho·phile (am′fŏ-fil, -fīl) **1.** Having an affinity for both acid and basic dyes. SYN amphophilous. **2.** A cell that stains readily with either acidic or basic dyes. SYN amphochromatophil, amphochromatophile.

am·phor·ic (am-fōr′ik) Denoting the sound heard in auscultation (but not percussion) of the lungs; resembles the noise produced by blowing across the mouth of a bottle.

am·pho·ter·ic (am-fŏ-ter′ik) Having two opposite characteristics, especially having the capacity of reacting as either an acid or a base.

am·pho·tro·pic vi·rus (am′fŏ-trō′pik vī′rŭs) An oncornavirus that does not produce disease in its natural host but does replicate in tissue culture cells of the host species and also in cells from other species.

am·pli·fi·ca·tion (am′pli-fi-kā′shŭn) The process of making larger, as in increasing an auditory or visual stimulus to enhance its perception.

am·pli·tude (am.) (am′pli-tūd) Largeness; extent; breadth or range.

am·pli·tude of ac·com·mo·da·tion (AA) (am′pli-tūd ă-kom′ŏ-dā′shŭn) Difference in refractivity of the eye at rest and when fully accommodated.

am·pli·tude of con·ver·gence (am′pli-tūd kŏn-vĕr′jĕns) Distance between near and far points of convergence. SYN range of convergence.

ampoule [Br.] SYN ampule.

am·pule (am′pyūl) A hermetically sealed container, usually made of glass containing a sterile medicinal solution, or powder to be made up in solution, to be used for subcutaneous, intramuscular, or intravenous injection. SYN ampoule.

am·pul·la, gen. and pl. **am·pul·lae** (am-pul′ă, -ē) [TA] A saccular dilation of a canal or duct.

am·pul·la of u·ter·ine tube (am-pul′ă yū′tĕr-in tūb) [TA] The wide portion of the uterine (fallopian) tube near the fimbriated extremity.

am·pul·la rec·ti (am-pul′ă rek′tī) [TA] SYN rectal ampulla.

am·pul·lar preg·nan·cy (am-pul′ăr preg′năn-sē) Tubal pregnancy situated near the midportion of the oviduct.

am·pul·la·ry crest (am-pul′ă-rē krest) An elevation on the inner surface of the ampulla of each semicircular duct.

am·pul·li·tis (am′pul-ī′tis) Inflammation of any ampulla.

am·pul·lu·la (am-pul′ū-lă) A circumscribed dilation of any minute lymphatic or blood vessel or duct.

am·pu·ta·tion (amp′yū-tā′shŭn) The severing of a limb or part of a limb, the breast, or other projecting part. SEE ALSO congenital amputation.

am·pu·ta·tion neu·ro·ma (amp′yū-tā′shŭn nūr-ō′mă) SYN traumatic neuroma.

Am·sel cri·te·ria (am′sel krī-tēr′ē-ă) Findings necessary for clinical diagnosis of bacterial vaginosis.

amy·e·lous, a·my·e·lo·ic, a·mye·lon·ic (ă-mī′ē-lŭs, ă-mī′ē-lō′ik, ă-mī′ē-lon′ik) Without a spinal cord.

a·myg·da·la, gen. and pl. **a·myg·da·lae** (ă-mig′dă-lă, -lē) Denoting the cerebellar tonsil, as well as the lymphatic tonsils (pharyngeal, palatine, lingual, laryngeal, and tubal).

a·myg·da·loid bod·y (ă-mig′dă-loyd bod′ē) A rounded mass of gray matter in the temporal lobe internal to the cortex of the uncus and immediately anterior to the inferior horn of the lateral ventricle.

amyg·da·loid fos·sa (ă-mig′dă-loyd fos′ă) SYN tonsillar fossa.

am·yl (am′il) The radical formed from a pentane, C_5H_{12}, by removal of one H. Several isomeric forms exist. SYN pentyl (1).

am·y·la·ceous (am′i-lā′shē-ŭs) Starchy.

am·y·lase (AMS, AMY) (am′il-ās) One of a group of amylolytic enzymes that cleave starch, glycogen, and related 1,4-α-glucans.

am·y·la·su·ria (am′i-lă-syūr′ē-ă) The excretion of amylase in urine, especially increased amounts in acute pancreatitis. SYN diastasuria.

am·y·loid (am′i-loyd) **1.** Any of a group of chemically diverse proteins that appears microscopically homogeneous but is composed of linear nonbranching aggregated fibrils arranged in sheets when seen under the electron microscope. **2.** Resembling or containing starch.

am·y·loi·do·sis (am′i-loy-dō′sis) **1.** A disease characterized by extracellular accumulation of amyloid in various organs and tissues of the body; may be primary or secondary. **2.** The process of deposition of amyloid protein.

am·y·loid tu·mor (am′i-loyd tū′mŏr) SYN nodular amyloidosis.

am·y·lo·pec·tin (am′i-lō-pek′tin) A branched-chain polyglucose (glucan) in starch containing both 1,4 and 1,6 linkages. Cf. amylose.

am·y·lo·pha·gi·a (am′i-lō-fā′jē-ă) A morbid craving for starch. SYN starch-eating.

am·y·lop·sin (am-il-op′sin) The amylase of pancreatic juice.

am·y·lor·rhe·a (am′i-lō-rē′ă) Passage of undigested starch in the stools, implying a deficiency of amylase activity in the intestine. SYN amylorrhoea.

amylorrhoea [Br.] SYN amylorrhea.

am·y·lose (am′i-lōs) An unbranched polyglucose (glucan) in starch, similar to cellulose, containing α(1→4) linkages.

am·y·lo·su·ri·a, am·y·lu·ri·a (am′i-lō-syūr′ē-ă, -lyūr′ē-ă) Excretion of starch in the urine.

amyoaesthesia [Br.] SYN amyoesthesia.

am·y·o·es·the·si·a, a·my·o·es·the·sis (ă-mī′ō-es-thē′zē-ă, -thē′sis) Absence of muscle sensation. SYN amyoaesthesia.

am·y·o·pla·si·a (ă-mī′ō-plā′zē-ă) Deficient formation of muscle and muscle growth.

amy·o·sta·si·a (ă-mī′ō-stā′zē-ă) Difficulty in standing, due to muscular tremor or incoordination.

am·y·os·then·ic (ă-mī′os-then′ik) Relating to or causing muscular weakness.

a·my·o·tax·y, a·my·o·tax·i·a (ă-mī′ō-tak-sē, -tak′sē-ă) Muscular ataxia.

a·my·o·to·ni·a (ă-mī′ō-tō′nē-ă) Generalized absence of muscle tone.

am·y·o·to·nia con·gen·i·ta (ă-mī′ō-tō′nē-ă kon-jen′i-tă) Atonic pseudoparalysis of congenital origin (neither familial nor hereditary). SYN Thomsen disease.

amy·o·tro·phic lat·er·al scler·o·sis (ALS) (ă-mī′ō-trō′fik lat′ĕr-ăl sklĕr-ō′sis) A disease of the motor tracts of the lateral columns and anterior horns of the spinal cord, causing progressive muscular atrophy, increased reflexes, fibrillary twitching, and spastic irritability of muscles; associated with a defect in superoxide dismutase. SYN Aran-Duchenne disease, Charcot disease, Cruveilhier disease, Duchenne-Aran disease, Lou Gehrig disease, progressive muscular atrophy.

amy·ot·ro·phy, amy·o·tro·phi·a (ā′mī-ot′rō-fē, -ă) Muscular wasting or atrophy.

a·myx·or·rhea (ă-mik′sōr-ē′ă) Absence of the normal secretion of mucus.

ana- Prefix meaning up, toward, apart. USAGE NOTE not to be confused with *an-* (a form of the prefix *a-*, without, used before a vowel).

an·a·bi·o·sis (an′ă-bī-ō′sis) Resuscitation after apparent death.

an·a·bol·ic ster·oid (an′ă-bol′ik ster′oyd) Prescription drug abused by some athletes to increase muscle mass. SEE ALSO ergogenic aid.

a·nab·o·lism (ă-nab′ō-lizm) **1.** The building up in the body of complex chemical compounds from smaller simpler compounds (e.g., proteins from amino acids), usually with the use of energy. Cf. catabolism, metabolism. **2.** The sum of synthetic metabolic reactions.

a·nab·o·lite (ă-nab′ō-līt) Any substance formed as a result of anabolic processes.

an·ac·id·i·ty (an′ă-sid′i-tē) Absence of acidity; used especially to denote absence of hydrochloric acid in the gastric juice.

an·a·clit·ic (an′ă-klit′ik) Leaning or depending on; in psychoanalysis, relating to the dependence of the infant on the mother or mother substitute.

an·a·crot·ic, an·a·di·crot·ic (an′ă-krot′ik, -dī-krot′ik) Referring to the upstroke or ascending limb of the arterial pulse tracing.

an·a·crot·ic pulse, an·a·di·crot·ic pulse (an′ă-krot′ik pŭls, an′ă-dī-krot′ik) A pulse wave showing one or more notches or indentations on its rising limb that are sometimes detectable by palpation.

an·a·cu·sis, an·a·ku·sis (an′ă-kyū′sis) Absence of the ability to perceive sound.

an·ad·re·nal·ism (an′ă-drē′năl-izm) Complete lack of adrenal function.

anaemia [Br.] SYN anemia.

anaemic [Br.] SYN anemic.

an·aer·obe (an-ār′ōb) A microorganism

that can live and grow in the absence of dioxygen.

an·aer·o·bic, an·aer·o·bi·ot·ic (an'ār-ō'bik, ār-ō-bī-ot'ik) Relating to an anaerobe; living without oxygen.

an·ae·ro·bic ex·er·cise (an'ār-ō'bik ek'sĕr-sīz) Physical activity that alternates short bursts of energy with periods of rest.

an·aer·o·bic res·pi·ra·tion (an'ār-ō'bik res'pi-rā'shŭn) A form of respiration in which molecular oxygen is not consumed (e.g., nitrate respiration, sulfate respiration).

an·aer·o·bi·o·sis (an'ār-ō-bī-ō'sis) Existence in an oxygen-free atmosphere.

an·aer·o·gen·ic (an'ār-ō-jen'ik) Not producing gas.

anaesthekinesia [Br.] SYN anesthekinesia.

anaesthesia [Br.] SYN anesthesia.

anaesthesia dolorosa [Br.] SYN anesthesia dolorosa.

anaesthesiology [Br.] SYN anesthesiology.

anaesthetic [Br.] SYN anesthetic.

anaesthetist [Br.] SYN anesthetist.

an·a·gen (an'ă-jen) Growth phase of the hair cycle, lasting about 3–6 years in human scalp hair.

an·a·ku·sis (an'ă-kyū'sis) SYN anacusis.

a·nal (ā'năl) Relating to the anus.

a·nal a·tre·sia, a·tre·si·a a·ni (ā'năl ă-trē'zē-ă, ă-trē'zē-ă ā'nī) Congenital absence of an anal opening due to the persistence of epithelial plug or to complete absence of the anal canal. SYN imperforate anus, proctatresia.

analbuminaemia [Br.] SYN analbuminemia.

an·al·bu·mi·ne·mi·a (an-al-bū'mi-nē'mē-ă) Absence of albumin from the serum. SYN analbuminaemia.

a·nal ca·nal (ā'năl kă-nal') [TA] The terminal portion of the alimentary canal. SYN canalis analis [TA].

a·nal cleft (ā'năl kleft) SYN intergluteal cleft.

an·a·lep·tic (an'ă-lep'tik) 1. Strengthening, stimulating, or invigorating. 2. A central nervous system stimulant, particularly used to denote agents that reverse depressed central nervous system function.

a·nal fis·sure (ā'năl fish'ŭr) A crack or slit in the mucous membrane of the anus.

a·nal fis·tu·la (ā'năl fis'tyū-lă) A fistula opening at or near the anus; usually, but not always, opening into the rectum above the internal sphincter.

a·nal folds (ā'năl fōldz) Slightly elevated folds derived from the cloacal folds located just lateral to the anal membrane; form the anal margin.

an·al·ge·si·a (an'ăl-jē'zē-ă) A neurologic or pharmacologic state in which painful stimuli are moderated so that, although still perceptible, they are no longer painful. Cf. anesthesia.

an·al·ge·si·a do·lo·ro·sa (an'ăl-jē'zē-ă dō-lō-rō'să) Spontaneous pain in a body area that lacks sensation.

an·al·ge·sic (an'ăl-jē'zik) 1. A compound capable of producing analgesia, i.e., one that relieves pain by altering perception of nociceptive stimuli without producing anesthesia or loss of consciousness. 2. Characterized by reduced response to painful stimuli.

an·al·get·ic (an'ăl-jet'ik) Associated with decreased pain perception.

an·al·ler·gic (an'ă-ler'jik) Not allergic.

anal·o·gous (ă-nal'ō-gŭs) Possessing a functional resemblance, but having a different origin or structure.

an·a·logue (an'ă-lawg) 1. One of two organs or parts in different species of animals or plants that differ in structure or development but are similar in function. 2. A compound that resembles another in structure but is not necessarily an isomer; analogues are often used to block enzymatic reactions by combining with enzymes.

a·nal pec·ten (ā′năl pek′těn) [TA] The middle third of the anal canal. SYN pecten analis, pecten (2).

an·al·pha·li·po·pro·tein·e·mi·a (an-al′fă-lip′ō-prō′tēn-ē′mē-ă) Familial high density lipoprotein deficiency.

a·nal plug (ā′năl plŭg) A mass of anal epithelial cells that temporarily occludes the anal canal in the embryo.

a·nal re·flex (ā′năl rē′fleks) Contraction of the internal sphincter gripping the finger passed into the rectum.

a·nal si·nus·es (ā′năl sī′nŭs-ĕz) [TA] 1. The grooves between the anal columns. 2. Pockets or crypts in the columnar zone of the anal canal between the anocutaneous line and the anorectal line.

a·nal tri·an·gle (ā′năl trī′ang-gĕl) [TA] Posterior portion of the perineal region through which the anal canal opens; bounded by a line through both ischial tuberosities, the sacrotuberous ligaments, and the coccyx. SYN regio analis [TA].

a·nal verge (ā′năl věrj) The transitional zone between the moist, hairless, modified skin of the anal canal and the perianal skin.

a·nal·y·sand (ă-nal′i-sand) In psychoanalysis, the person being analyzed.

a·nal·y·sis, pl. **a·nal·y·ses** (ă-nal′i-sis, -sēz) 1. The disaggregation of a compound or mixture into simpler elements. 2. The study of a whole in terms of its parts. 3. SEE psychoanalysis.

a·nal·y·sis of var·i·ance (ANOVA) (ă-nal′i-sis var′ē-ăns) A statistical technique that isolates and assesses the contribution of categoric independent variables to variation in the mean of a continuous dependent variable.

an·a·lyte (an′ă-līt) Any material or chemical substance subjected to analysis.

an·a·lyt·ic chem·is·try (an′ă-lit′ik kem′is-trē) Using chemistry to determine and detect the composition and identification of specific substances.

an·a·lyz·er, an·a·lyz·or (an′ă-līz-ĕr, -ŏr) 1. Any instrument that performs an analysis. 2. The prism in a polariscope used to examine polarized light. 3. The neural basis of the conditioned reflex; includes all the sensory side of the reflex arc and its central connections. 4. A device that electronically determines the frequency and amplitude of a particular channel of an electroencephalogram.

an·am·ne·sis (an′am-nē′sis) 1. The act of remembering. 2. The medical or developmental history of a patient.

an·am·nes·tic (an′am-nes′tik) 1. Assisting the memory. 2. Relating to the medical history of a patient.

an·am·nes·tic re·ac·tion (an′am-nes′tik rē-ak′shŭn) Augmented production of an antibody due to previous response of the subject to stimulus by the same antigen.

an·a·phase (an′ă-fāz) The stage of mitosis or meiosis in which the chromosomes move from the equatorial plate toward the poles of the cell.

an·a·phi·a, an·ha·phi·a (an-ā′fē-ă, an-af′ē-ă) Absence of the sense of touch.

an·a·pho·re·sis (an′ă-fōr-ē′sis) Movement of negatively charged particles (anions) in a solution or suspension toward the anode in electrophoresis. Cf. cataphoresis.

an·aph·ro·di·si·ac (an′af-rō-diz′ē-ak) Repressing or destroying sexual desire.

an·a·phy·lac·tic (an′ă-fi-lak′tik) Relating to anaphylaxis; manifesting extremely great sensitivity to foreign protein or other material.

an·a·phy·lac·to·gen·e·sis (an′ă-fi-lak′tō-jen′ĕ-sis) The production of anaphylaxis.

an·a·phy·lac·toid (an′ă-fi-lak′toyd) Resembling anaphylaxis but not IgE-mediated. SYN pseudoanaphylactic.

an·a·phyl·a·tox·in (an′ă-fil′ă-tok′sin) A substance postulated to be the immediate cause of anaphylactic shock and assumed to result from in vivo combination of specific antibody and the specific sensitizing material.

an·a·phy·lax·is (an′ă-fi-lak′sis) The immediate, transient kind of immunologic (allergic) reaction characterized by contraction of smooth muscle and dilation of capillaries due to release of pharmacologically active substances (histamine, bradykinin, serotonin, and slow-reacting substance), classically initiated by the combination of antigen (allergen) with mast-cell–fixed, cytophilic antibody (chiefly IgE).

an·a·pla·si·a (an′ă-plā′zē-ă) Loss of structural differentiation, especially as seen in most, but not all, malignant neoplasms. SYN dedifferentiation (2).

an·a·plas·tic (an′ă-plas′tik) **1.** Relating to anaplasty. **2.** Characterized by or pertaining to anaplasia. **3.** Growing without form or structure, as in loss of cellular differentiation in association with malignancies.

an·a·poph·y·sis (an′ă-pof′i-sis) An accessory spinal process of a vertebra.

a·nap·tic (ă-nap′tik) Relating to anaphia.

an·ar·thri·a (an-ahrth′rē-ă) Loss of the power of articulate speech.

an·as·tig·mats (an′ă-stig′mats) Lenses with which astigmatism is corrected.

a·nas·to·mo·sis, pl. **a·nas·to·mo·ses** (ă-nas′tŏ-mō′sis, -mō′sēz) **1.** A natural communication, direct or indirect, between two blood vessels or other tubular structures. **2.** An opening created by surgery, trauma, or disease between two or more normally separate spaces or organs.

a·nas·to·mot·ic (ă-nas′tŏ-mot′ik) Pertaining to an anastomosis.

a·nas·to·mot·ic branch (ă-nas′tŏ-mot′ ik branch) [TA] A blood vessel that interconnects two neighboring vessels.

an·a·tom·ic, an·a·tom·ic·al (an′ă-tom′ ik, -tom′i-kăl) Relating to anatomy.

an·a·tom·ic age (an′ă-tom′ik āj) Age in terms of structure rather than of function or the passage of time. SYN physical age.

an·a·tom·ic im·po·tence (an′ă-tom′ik im′pŏ-těns) Inability of a male to achieve an erection or ejaculate due to physical defect. SEE erectile dysfunction.

an·a·tom·ic path·ol·o·gy (ATP) (an′ă-tom′ik pă-thol′ŏ-jē) Subspecialty of pathology that pertains to the gross and microscopic study of organs and tissues removed for biopsy or during postmortem examination, and also the interpretation of the results of such study.

an·a·tom·ic po·si·tion (an′ă-tŏm′ik pŏ-zish′ŏn) Standing erect, arms at the sides, with palms facing forward.

a·nat·o·my (ă-nat′ŏ-mē) [TA] **1.** The morphologic structure of an organism. **2.** The science of the morphology or structure of organisms. **3.** SYN dissection. **4.** A work describing the form and structure of an organism and its various parts.

an·a·tox·in (an′ă-toks′in) A weakened bacterial toxin.

an·chor·age (ang′kŏr-ăj) **1.** Operative fixation of loose or prolapsed abdominal or pelvic organs. **2.** DENTISTRY a tooth or an implanted tooth substitute with which a fixed or removable partial denture, crown, or restoration is retained.

an·chor splint (ang′kŏr splint) An apparatus used to support and immobilize a fractured jaw.

an·cip·i·tal, an·cip·i·tate, an·cip·i·tous (an-sip′i-tăl, -i-tāt, -i-tŭs) Two-headed; two-edged.

an·co·nad (an′kō-nad) Toward the elbow.

An·cy·los·to·ma, An·ky·lo·sto·ma (an′ki-lō-stō′mă) A genus of Nematoda, the Old World hookworm, the members of which are parasitic in the duodenum.

an·cy·lo·sto·mi·a·sis (an′ki-lō-stō-mī′ ă-sis) Hookworm disease caused by *Ancylostoma duodenale* and characterized by eosinophilia, anemia, emaciation, dyspepsia, and, in children with severe chronic infections, swelling of the abdomen and mental and physical maldevelopment.

an·cy·roid, an·ky·roid (an-kīr′oyd) Shaped like the fluke of an anchor.

An·der·son-Fab·ry dis·ease (an′dĕr-sŏn-fah′brē di-zēz′) SYN Fabry disease.

An·der·son splint (an'dĕr-sŏn splint) A skeletal traction splint with pins inserted into proximal and distal ends of a fracture.

andro- Combining form denoting masculine.

an·dro·blas·to·ma (an'drō-blas-tō'mă) A testicular tumor microscopically resembling fetal testis, with varying proportions of tubular and stromal elements; the tubules contain Sertoli cells, which may cause feminization.

an·dro·gen (an'drŏ-jen) Generic term for an agent, usually a hormone (e.g., androsterone, testosterone), which stimulates activity of the accessory male sex organs, promotes development of male sex characteristics, or prevents changes in the latter that follow castration.

an·dro·gen·e·sis (an'drō-jen'ĕ-sis) Development in the presence of paternal chromosomes only.

an·dro·gen·ic (an'drō-jen'ik) Relating to an androgen; having a masculinizing effect. SYN testoid (1).

an·dro·gen·ic al·o·pe·cia (an'drō-jen'ik al'ŏ-pē'shē-ă) Gradual decrease of scalp hair density in adults as a result of familial increased susceptibility of hair follicles to androgen secretion following puberty. SYN patterned alopecia.

an·drog·y·nous (an-droj'i-nŭs) Pertaining to androgyny.

an·drog·y·ny (an-droj'i-nē) Having both masculine and feminine characteristics, as in attitudes and behaviors that contain features of stereotyped, culturally sanctioned sexual roles of both male and female.

an·droid (an'droyd) SYN andromorphous.

an·droid pel·vis (an'droyd pel'vis) A masculine or funnel-shaped pelvis.

an·dro·mor·phous (an'drō-mōr'fŭs) Having a male form or habitus.

an·drop·a·thy (an-drop'ă-thē) A disease or disorder peculiar to males.

an·dro·pause (an'drō-pawz) A postulated decrease in function of male gonads with increasing age, analogous to menopause.

an·ec·dot·al (an'ek-dō'tăl) Report of clinical experiences based on individual experience, rather than an organized investigation with standard research features, such as appropriate controls.

an·e·cho·ic (an'ĕ-kō'ik) The property of appearing echo free on a sonographic image; a clear cyst appears anechoic.

a·ne·mi·a (ă-nē'mē-ă) Any condition in which the number of red blood cells per mm³, the amount of hemoglobin in 100 mL of blood, or the volume of packed red blood cells per 100 mL of blood is less than normal. SYN anaemia.

a·ne·mic (ă-nē'mik) Pertaining to or manifesting the various features of anemia. SYN anaemic.

an·en·ceph·a·ly (an'en-sef'ă-lē) SYN meroanencephaly.

an·er·ga·si·a (an'ĕr-gā'zē-ă) Absence of psychic activity as the result of organic brain disease.

an·er·gy (an'ĕr-jē) Lack of energy.

an·e·ryth·ro·pla·si·a (an'ĕ-rith'rō-plā'zē-ă) A condition in which red blood cells do not form.

an·es·the·ki·ne·si·a, an·es·the·ci·ne·si·a (an-es'thē-ki-nē'zē-ă, -si-nē'zē-ă) Combined sensory and motor paralysis. SYN anaesthekinesia.

an·es·the·si·a (an'es-thē'zē-ă) **1.** Loss of sensation resulting from pharmacologic depression of nerve function or from neurologic dysfunction. **2.** Broad term for anesthesiology as a clinical specialty. SYN anaesthesia.

an·es·the·si·a do·lo·ro·sa (an'es-thē'zē-ă dō-lō-rō'să) Severe spontaneous pain occurring in an anesthetized area. SYN anaesthesia dolorosa.

an·es·the·si·a ma·chine (an'es-thē'zē-ă mă-shēn') Equipment used for inhalation anesthesia.

an·es·the·si·ol·o·gy (an'es-thē'zē-ol'ŏ-jē) The medical specialty concerned with the pharmacologic, physiologic, and clinical basis of anesthesia and related fields, including resuscitation, intensive respiratory care, and the management of acute and chronic pain. SYN anaesthesiology.

an·es·thet·ic (an'es-thet'ik) **1.** A compound that depresses neuronal function, producing loss of ability to perceive pain and/or other sensations. **2.** Characterized by loss of sensation or capable of producing loss of sensation. SYN anaesthetic.

an·es·thet·ic depth (an'es-thet'ik depth) The degree of central nervous system depression produced by a general anesthetic agent.

a·nes·the·tist (ă-nes'thĕ-tist) One who administers an anesthetic, whether an anesthesiologist, a physician who is not an anesthesiologist, a nurse anesthetist, or an anesthesia assistant. SYN anaesthetist.

an·es·trus (an-es'trŭs) The period between two estrus (heat) cycles. SYN anoestrus.

an·eu·ploid (an'yū-ployd) Having an abnormal number of chromosomes not an exact multiple of the haploid number.

an·eu·rysm (an'yūr-izm) **1.** Circumscribed dilation of an artery in direct communication with the lumen, usually due to an acquired or congenital weakness of the wall of the artery. **2.** Circumscribed dilation of a cardiac chamber usually due to an acquired or congenital weakness of the wall of the heart.

an·eu·rys·mo·plas·ty (an'yūr-iz'mō-plas-tē) Repair of an aneurysm by opening the sac and suturing its walls to restore the normal dimension to the lumen of the artery. SEE ALSO aneurysmorrhaphy. SYN endoaneurysmoplasty, endoaneurysmorrhaphy.

an·eu·rys·mor·rha·phy (an'yūr-iz-mōr'ă-fē) Closure by suture of the sac of an aneurysm to restore the normal lumen dimensions.

an·eu·rys·mot·o·my (an'yūr-iz-mot'ŏ-mē) Incision into the sac of an aneurysm.

an·gel wing (ān'jĕl wing) A deformity in which both scapulae project conspicuously. SEE ALSO winged scapula.

♻ **angi-** (an'jē) SEE angio-.

an·gi·ec·ta·si·a, an·gi·ec·ta·sis (an'jē-ek-tā'zē-ă, -ek'tă-sis) Dilation of a lymphatic or blood vessel.

an·gi·ec·to·pi·a (an'jē-ek-tō'pē-ă) Abnormal location of a blood vessel.

an·gi·i·tis, an·gi·tis (an'jē-ī'tis, an-jī'tis) Inflammation of a blood vessel (arteritis, phlebitis) or lymphatic vessel (lymphangitis).

an·gi·na (an'ji-nă) A severe, often constricting pain; caused by reduced arterial blood to the myocardium, which reduces oxygen supplied to the myocardial cells; usually refers to angina pectoris.

an·gi·na cru·ris (an'ji-nă krū'ris) Intermittent claudication of the leg.

an·gi·na in·ver·sa (an'ji-nă in-vĕr'să) SYN Prinzmetal angina.

an·gi·na pec·to·ris (an'ji-nă pek'tŏ'ris) Paroxysmal severe constricting pain or pressure in the chest due to myocardial ischemia. SYN stenocardia.

an·gi·na scale (an'ji-nă skāl) A four-part measure used to describe the severity of angina (1 + = mild, to 4 + = severe).

♻ **angio-, angi-** Combining forms meaning blood or lymph vessels; a covering, an enclosure; corresponds to L. vas-, vaso-, vasculo-.

an·gi·o·blast (an'jē-ō-blast) **1.** A cell taking part in blood vessel formation. SYN vasoformative cell. **2.** Primordial mesenchymal tissue from which embryonic blood cells and vascular endothelium are differentiated.

an·gi·o·blas·to·ma (an'jē-ō-blas-tō'mă) SYN hemangioblastoma.

an·gi·o·car·di·og·ra·phy (an'jē-ō-kahr-dē-og'ră-fē) Diagnostic x-ray imaging of the heart and great vessels made visible by injection of a radiopaque solution. SEE coronary angiography.

an·gi·o·car·di·o·ki·net·ic, an·gi·o·car·di·o·ci·net·ic (an'jē-ō-kahr'dē-ō-ki-net'ik, -si-net'ik) Causing dilation or contraction in the heart and blood vessels.

an·gi·o·car·di·tis (an′jē-ō-kahr-dī′tis) Inflammation of the heart and blood vessels.

an·gi·o·cath·e·ter (an′jē-ō-kath′ĕ-tĕr) Hollow tube that allows for injection of contrast dye for imaging cadiac areas.

an·gi·o·dys·pla·sia (an′jē-ō-dis-plā′zē-ă) Degenerative or congenital structural abnormality of the normally distributed vasculature.

an·gi·o·e·de·ma (an′jē-ō-ĕ-dē′mă) Recurrent large circumscribed areas of subcutaneous or mucosal edema of sudden onset, usually disappearing within 24 hours. SYN giant hives, giant urticaria, periodic edema.

an·gi·o·en·do·the·li·oma (an′jē-ō-en-dō-thē-lē-ō′mă) A benign or malignant neoplasm arising from vascular endothelium.

an·gi·o·en·do·the·li·o·ma·to·sis (an′jē-ō-en-dō-thē′lē-ō-mă-tō′sis) Proliferation of endothelial cells within blood vessels.

an·gi·o·fi·bro·ma (an′jē-ō-fī-brō′mă) A benign but locally invasive neoplasm composed of dense fibrous tissue and thin-walled vascular spaces.

an·gi·o·fi·bro·sis (an′jē-ō-fī-brō′sis) Fibrosis of the walls of blood vessels.

an·gi·o·gen·e·sis (an′jē-ō-jen′ĕ-sis) Development of new blood vessels. SYN arteriogenesis.

an·gi·o·gen·ic (an′jē-ō-jen′ik) **1.** Relating to angiogenesis. **2.** Of vascular origin.

an·gi·og·ra·phy (an′jē-og′ră-fē) Radiography of vessels after the injection of a radiopaque contrast material; usually requires percutaneous insertion of a radiopaque catheter and positioning under fluoroscopic control.

an·gi·o·hy·a·li·no·sis (an′jē-ō-hī′ă-li-nō′sis) Hyaline degeneration of the walls of the blood vessels.

an·gi·oid (an′jē-oyd) Resembling blood vessels; in a branching pattern.

an·gi·oid streaks (an′jē-oyd strēks) Breaks in Bruch membrane visible in the peripapillary fundus oculi, and sometimes mistaken for choroidal vessels. SYN Knapp streaks, Knapp striae.

an·gi·o·ker·a·to·ma (an′jē-ō-ker-ă-tō′mă) A superficial capillary telangiectasis, over which wartlike hyperkeratosis and acanthosis appear. SYN telangiectatic wart.

an·gi·o·li·po·ma (an′jē-ō-li-pō′mă) A lipoma that contains an unusually large number or foci of proliferated, neoplasticlike, frequently dilated vascular channels. SYN lipoma cavernosum, telangiectatic lipoma.

an·gi·o·lu·poid (an′jē-ō-lū′poyd) A sarcoidlike eruption of the skin in which the granulomatous telangiectasic papules are distributed over the nose and cheeks.

an·gi·ol·y·sis (an′jē-ol′i-sis) Obliteration of a blood vessel, such as occurs in the newborn infant after tying of the umbilical cord.

an·gi·o·ma, gen. and pl. **an·gi·o·ma·ta** (an′jē-ō′mă, -tă) A swelling or benign tumor due to proliferation, with or without dilation, of the blood vessels (hemangioma) or lymphatics (lymphangioma).

an·gi·o·ma·toid (an′jē-ō′mă-toyd) Resembling a tumor of vascular origin.

an·gi·o·ma·to·sis (an′jē-ō-mă-tō′sis) A condition characterized by multiple angiomas.

an·gi·o·ma·tous (an′jē-ō′mă-tŭs) Relating to or resembling an angioma.

an·gi·o·my·o·li·po·ma (AML) (an′jē-ō-mī′ō-li-pō′mă) A benign neoplasm of adipose tissue (lipoma) in which muscle cells and vascular structures are fairly conspicuous.

an·gi·o·my·o·sar·co·ma (an′jē-ō-mī′ō-sahr-kō′mă) A myosarcoma that has an unusually large number of proliferated, frequently dilated vascular channels.

an·gi·o·myx·o·ma (an′jē-ō-miks-ō′mă) A myxoma in which there is an unusually large number of vascular structures.

an·gi·o·neu·rop·a·thy (an′jē-ō-nūr-op′ă-thē) A vascular disorder attributed to an abnormality of the autonomic nervous system fibers supplying the blood vessels (i.e., the vasomotor system).

an·gio-oedema [Br.] SYN angioedema.

an·gi·o·pa·ral·y·sis (an′jē-ō-pă-ral′i-sis) SYN vasoparalysis.

an·gi·op·a·thy (an′jē-op′ă-thē) Any disease of the blood vessels or lymphatics.

an·gi·o·plas·ty (an′jē-ō-plas-tē) Reconstitution or recanalization of a blood vessel.

an·gi·o·plas·ty bal·loon (an′jē-ō-plas-tē bă-lūn′) A balloon near the tip of an angiographic catheter, designed to distend narrowed vessels.

an·gi·o·poi·e·sis (an′jē-ō-poy-ē′sis) Formation of blood or lymphatic vessels. SYN vasifaction, vasoformation.

an·gi·o·poi·et·ic (an′jē-ō-poy-et′ik) Relating to angiopoiesis. SYN vasifactive, vasoformative.

an·gi·o·pres·sure (an′jē-ō-presh′ŭr) Forcing down on blood vessels or arteries to control bleeding.

an·gi·or·rha·phy (an′jē-ōr′ă-fē) Suture repair of any vessel, especially of a blood vessel.

an·gi·o·sar·co·ma (an′jē-ō-sahr-kō′mă) A rare malignant neoplasm occurring most often in the breast and skin, and believed to originate from the endothelial and fibroblastic cells of blood vessels.

an·gi·o·scler·o·sis (an′jē-ō-skler-ō′sis) Induration of the walls of blood vessels.

an·gi·o·scope (an′jē-ō-skōp) A modified microscope for studying the capillary vessels and a scope used for viewing larger vessels.

an·gi·os·co·py (an′jē-os′kŏ-pē) **1.** Visualization with a microscope of the passage of substances through capillaries after intravenous injection. **2.** Visualization of the interior of blood vessels, using a fiberoptic catheter inserted through a peripheral artery.

an·gi·o·sco·to·ma (an′jē-ō-skō-tō′mă) Ribbon-shaped defect of the visual fields caused by the retinal vessels overlying photoreceptors.

an·gi·o·sco·tom·e·try (an′jē-ō-skō-tom′ĕ-trē) The measurement or projection of the angioscotoma pattern.

an·gi·o·spasm (an′jē-ō-spazm) SYN vasospasm.

an·gi·o·ste·no·sis (an′jē-ō-stĕ-nō′sis) Narrowing of one or more blood vessels.

an·gi·o·te·lec·ta·sis, an·gi·o·tel·ec·ta·sia (an′jē-ō-tĕ-lek′tă-sis, -tel′ek-tā′zē-ă) SYN telangiectasia.

an·gi·o·ten·sin (an′jē-ō-ten′sin) A family of peptides with vasoconstrictive activity, produced by action of renin on angiotensinogen.

an·gi·o·ten·sin-con·vert·ing en·zyme (ACE) (an′jē-ō-ten′sin-kŏn-vĕrt′ing en′zīm) A hydrolase responsible for the conversion of angiotensin I to the vasoactive angiotensin II by removal of a dipeptide (histidylleucine) from angiotensin I.

an·gi·o·ten·sin·o·gen (an′jē-ō-ten-sin′ō-jen) The substrate for renin whereon through enzymatic action angiotensin I is liberated; an abundant α_2-globulin that circulates in the blood plasma. SYN angiotensin precursor.

an·gi·o·to·ni·a (an′jē-ō-tō′nē-ă) SYN vasotonia.

an·gle (ang′gĕl) [TA] The figure formed by the junction of two lines or planes; the space bounded on two sides by lines or planes that meet. SYN angulus [TA].

an·gle-clo·sure glau·co·ma (ang′gĕl-klō′zhŭr glaw-kō′mă) Primary glaucoma in which contact of the iris with the peripheral cornea excludes aqueous humor from the trabecular drainage meshwork. SYN narrow-angle glaucoma.

an·gle of re·frac·tion (r) (ang′gĕl rē-frak′shŭn) Angle that a ray leaving a refracting medium makes with a line drawn perpendicular to the surface of this medium.

an·gle of tor·sion (ang′gĕl tŏr′shŭn) The amount of rotation of a long bone along its axis or between two axes, measured in degrees.

an·gle re·ces·sion (ang′gĕl rĕ-sesh′ŭn) Tearing of the iris root between the longitudinal and circular ciliary muscles; often leading to glaucoma.

ang·strom (Å) (ang′strŏm) A unit of wavelength, 10^{-10} m, roughly the diameter of an atom; equivalent to 0.1 nm.

Ång·ström law (eng′strŏm law) A substance absorbs light of the same wavelength as it emits when luminous.

an·gu·lar ar·te·ry (ang′gyŭ-lăr ahr′tĕr-ē) [TA] The terminal branch of the facial artery. SYN arteria angularis [TA].

an·gu·lar chei·li·tis (ang′gyŭ-lăr kī-lī′tis) Inflammation and fissuring radiating from the commissures of the mouth. SYN commissural cheilitis, perlèche.

an·gu·lar cur·va·ture (ang′gyŭ-lăr kŭr′vă-chŭr) A gibbous deformity, i.e., a sharp angulation of the spine, occurring in Pott disease.

an·gu·lar gy·rus (ang′gyŭ-lăr jī′rŭs) [TA] A folded convolution in the inferior parietal lobule formed by the union of the posterior ends of the superior and middle temporal gyri.

an·gu·la·tion (ang′gyū-lā′shŭn) 1. Formation of an angle; an abnormal angle or bend in an organ. 2. In orthopaedics, a method of describing the alignment of long bones that have been affected by injury or disease.

an·gu·lus, gen. and pl. **an·gu·li** (ang′gyū-lŭs, -lī) [TA] SYN angle.

an·gu·lus pon·to·cer·e·bel·la·ris (ang′gyū-lŭs pon′tō-ser-ĕ-bel-ā′ris) [TA] SYN cerebellopontine angle.

an·he·do·nia (an′hē-dō′nē-ă) Absence of pleasure from the performance of acts that would ordinarily be pleasurable.

an·hi·dro·sis, an·i·dro·sis (an′hī-drō′sis, an′i-drō′sis) Absence of sweat glands or absence of sweating.

an·hi·drot·ic (an′hī-drot′ik) Relating to, or characterized by, anhidrosis. SYN adiaphoretic.

an·hy·dram·ni·os (an-hī-dram′nē-os) A lack of amniotic fluid.

an·hy·dra·tion (an′hī-drā′shŭn) SYN dehydration (1).

an·hy·dride (an-hī′drīd) An oxide that can combine with water to form an acid or is derived from an acid by the abstraction of water.

🔧 **anhydro-** Chemical prefix denoting the removal of water. Cf. pyro- (2).

an·ic·ter·ic (an′ik-ter′ik) Unrelated to jaundice.

an·id·e·an (an-id′ē-an) Shapeless; denoting a formless mass of tissue.

an·i·lide (an′i-līd) An *N*-acyl aniline, e.g., acetanilide.

an·il·ism (ani-lizm) Chronic aniline poisoning, characterized by nausea, vertigo, muscular weakness, cyanosis, and respiratory and circulatory failure.

an·i·ma (an′i-mă) The soul or spirit.

an·i·mal (an′i-măl) 1. A living, sentient organism that has membranous cell walls, requires oxygen and organic foods, and is capable of voluntary movement, as distinguished from a plant or mineral. 2. One of the lower animal organisms as distinguished from humans.

an·i·mus (an′i-mŭs) 1. An animating or energizing spirit. 2. Intention to do something; disposition. 3. PSYCHIATRY a spirit of active hostility or grudge. 4. The ideal image toward which a person strives.

an·i·on (A −) (an′ī-on) An ion that carries a negative charge.

an·i·on gap (an′ī-on gap) The arithmetic difference between the concentrations of routinely measured cations ($Na^+ + K^+$) and of routinely measured anions ($Cl^- + HCO_3^-$) in plasma or serum.

an·i·rid·i·a (an′i-rid′ē-ă) Absence of the iris. Cf. irideremia.

an·i·sa·ki·a·sis (an′i-să-kī′ă-sis) Infection of the intestinal wall by larvae of *Anisakis marina* and other genera of anisakid nematodes (*Phocanema*). SYN herring-worm disease.

an·is·ei·ko·ni·a (an'ĭ-sī-kō'nē-ă) An ocular condition in which the image of an object in one eye differs in size or shape from the image of the same object in the fellow eye.

aniso- Combining form meaning unequal, dissimilar, unlike.

an·i·so·chro·mat·ic (an-ī'sō-krō-mat'ik) Not uniformly of one color.

an·i·so·co·ri·a (an-ī'sō-kōr'ē-ă) A condition in which the two pupils are not of equal size.

an·i·so·cy·to·sis (ANIS, ANISO) (an-ī'sō-sī-tō'sis) Considerable variation in cell size that is normally uniform.

an·i·sog·a·my (an-ī-sog'ă-mē) Fusion of two gametes unequal in size or form.

an·i·so·kar·y·o·sis (an-ī'sō-kar-ē-ō'sis) Variation in size of nuclei, greater than the normal range for a tissue.

an·i·so·me·tro·pi·a (An, AN) (an-ī'sō-mĕ-trō'pē-ă) A difference in the refractive power of the two eyes.

an·i·so·pi·e·sis (an-ī'sō-pī-ē'sis) Unequal arterial blood pressure on the two sides of the body.

an·i·so·ton·ic (an-ī'sō-ton'ik) Not having equal tension; having unequal osmotic pressure.

an·i·so·tro·pic (an-ī'sō-trop'ik) Not having properties that are the same in all directions.

an·kle (ang'kĕl) **1.** SYN ankle joint. **2.** The region of the ankle joint. **3.** SYN talus.

an·kle bone (ang'kel bōn) SYN talus.

an·kle clo·nus (ang'kĕl klō'nŭs) Rhythmic contraction of the calf muscles following a sudden passive dorsiflexion of the foot, the leg being semiflexed.

an·kle-foot or·tho·tic (AFO) (ang'kĕl-fut ōr-thot'ik) A device that encompasses the ankle and foot to provide ankle stability and assist knee extension control during ambulation.

an·kle joint (ang'kĕl joynt) [TA] Hinged synovial articulation between the tibia and fibula above and the talus below.

an·kle re·flex (AR) (ang'kĕl rĕ'fleks) SYN Achilles reflex.

ankylo- Combining form meaning bent, crooked, stiff, fused, fixed, closed.

an·ky·lo·bleph·a·ron (ang'ki-lo-blef'ă-ron) Adhesion between upper and lower eyelids.

an·ky·lo·glos·sia (ang'ki-lō-glos'ē-ă) Partial or complete fusion of the tongue to the floor of the mouth.

an·ky·losed (ang'ki-lōst) Stiffened; bound by adhesions; denoting a joint in a state of ankylosis.

an·ky·los·ing spon·dy·li·tis (ang'ki-lōs-ing spon'di-lī'tis) Arthritis of the spine, resembling rheumatoid arthritis. SYN rheumatoid spondylitis.

an·ky·lo·sis (ang'ki-lō'sis) Stiffening or fixation of a joint as the result of a disease process, with fibrous or bony union across the joint.

an·ky·rin (ang'ki-rin) An erythrocyte membranal protein that binds spectrin.

an·la·ge, pl. **an·la·gen** (ahn'lah-ge, -gen) SYN primordium.

an·neal (ă-nēl') Process by which oligonucleotides affix to targeted DNA sequences.

an·nec·tent (ă-nek'tĕnt) Connected with; joined.

an·od·al (An, AN) (an'ōd-ăl) Of, pertaining to, or emanating from an anode.

an·o·don·ti·a (an'ō-don'shē-ă) Complete absence of teeth.

an·o·dyne (an'ō-dīn) A substance that soothes or relieves pain.

anoestrus [Br.] SYN anestrus.

a·no·gen·i·tal (ā'nō-jen'i-tăl) Relating to both the anal and the genital regions.

a·nom·a·lad (ă-nom'ă-lad) A malformation together with its subsequently derived structural changes. SEE anomaly.

a·nom·a·ly (ă-nom′ă-lē) A birth defect caused by a structural abnormality or a marked deviation from the average or normal standard; anything that is structurally unusual, irregular, or contrary to a general rule, especially a congenital defect.

an·o·mer (an′ō-měr) One of two sugar molecules that are epimeric at the hemiacetal or hemiketal carbon atom.

a·nom·ic a·pha·si·a (ă-nom′ik ă-fā′zē-ă) Aphasia in which the patient cannot name people and objects seen, heard, or felt.

an·o·nych·i·a, an·o·ny·cho·sis (an′ō-nik′ē-ă, -ni-kō′sis) Absence of the nails.

A·noph·e·les (ă-nof′ĕ-lēz) A genus of mosquitoes. The sporogenous cycle of the malarial parasite is passed in the body cavity of female mosquitoes of certain species of this genus.

an·oph·thal·mi·a (an′of-thal′mē-ă) Congenital absence of all tissues of the eyes.

a·no·plas·ty (ā′nō-plas-tē) Plastic surgery of the anus.

an·or·chism (an-ōr′kizm) Absence of the testes; may be congenital or acquired. SEE ALSO monorchia, monorchism.

an·o·rec·tic (an′ō-rek′tic) Relating to, characteristic of, or suffering from anorexia, especially anorexia nervosa.

an·o·rex·i·a (an′ō-rek′sē-ă) Diminished appetite; aversion to food.

an·o·re·xia ath·let·i·ca (an′ō-rek′sē-ă ath-let′i-kă) Continuum of subclinical eating behaviors of athletes who do not meet the criteria for a true eating disorder, but who practice at least one unhealthful method of weight control.

an·o·rex·ia ner·vo·sa (an′ō-rek′sē-ă něrvō′să) A personality disorder manifested by extreme fear of becoming obese and an aversion to eating, usually occurring in young women and often resulting in life-threatening weight loss, accompanied by a disturbance in body image, hyperactivity, and amenorrhea.

an·o·rex·i·gen·ic (an′ō-rek′si-jen′ik) Promoting or causing anorexia.

an·or·gas·mia (an′ōr-gaz′mē-ă) Failure to experience an orgasm.

a·no·sig·moid·os·co·py (ā′nō-sig′moy-dos′kŏ-pē) Endoscopy of the anus, rectum, and sigmoid colon.

an·os·mi·a (an-oz′mē-ă) Loss of the sense of smell.

an·os·mic (an-oz′mik) Relating to anosmia.

a·no·sog·no·si·a (ă-nō′sŏg-nō′sē-ă) *In the diphthong gn, the g is silent only at the beginning of a word.* Ignorance of the presence of disease, specifically of paralysis. Most often seen in patients with nondominant parietal lobe lesions, who deny presence of hemiparesis.

a·no·spi·nal (ā′nō-spī′năl) Relating to the anus and the spinal cord.

an·os·to·sis (an′os-tō′sis) Failure of ossification.

an·o·ti·a (an-ō′shē-ă) Congenital absence of one or both external ears.

ANOVA (ă-nō′vă) Acronym for analysis of variance.

a·no·ves·i·cal (ā′nō-ves′i-kăl) Relating in any way to both anus and urinary bladder.

an·ov·u·la·tion (an′ov-yū-lā′shŭn) Suspension or cessation of ovulation.

an·ov·u·la·to·ry (an-ov′yŭ-lă-tōr-ē) Absence of the development of a mature ovarian follicle and/or the discharge of the oocyte during a menstrual cycle.

an·ox·i·a (an-ok′sē-ă) Absence or almost complete absence of oxygen from inspired gases, arterial blood, or tissues; to be differentiated from hypoxia.

an·ox·ic an·ox·ia (an-ok′sik an-ok′sē-ă) Hypoxic hypoxia in which oxygen is almost completely lacking.

An·rep phe·nom·e·non (ahn′rep fĕ-nom′ĕ-non) Homeometric autoregulation of the heart whereby cardiac performance improves as the afterload (aortic pressure) is increased.

an·sa, gen. and pl. **an·sa·e** (an′să, -sē)

[TA] Any anatomic structure in the form of a loop or arc. SEE ALSO loop.

an·sae ner·vo·rum spi·na·li·um (an' sē nĕr-vō'rŭm spī-nā'lē-ŭm) SYN loops of spinal nerves.

an·sa len·tic·u·la·ris (an'să len-tik-yū-lā'ris) [TA] SYN lenticular loop.

an·ser·ine (an'sĕr-īn) Resembling or characteristic of a goose. SEE cutis anserina, pes anserinus. SYN N-methylcarnosine.

ant·ac·id (ant-as'id) **1.** Neutralizing an acid. **2.** Any agent that reduces or neutralizes acidity, as of the gastric juice or any other secretion.

an·tag·o·nism (an-tag'ŏ-nizm) Denoting mutual opposition in action among structures, agents, diseases, or physiologic processes.

an·tag·o·nist (an-tag'ŏ-nist) Something opposing or resisting the action of another; any structure, agent, disease, or physiologic process that tends to neutralize or impede some action or effect.

ant·al·gic gait (ant-al'jik gāt) Characteristic gait resulting from pain on weight-bearing in which the stance phase of gait is shortened on the affected side.

ante- Prefix meaning before, in front of (in time or place or order). SEE ALSO pre-, pro-(1).

an·te·bra·chi·um (an'tē-brā'kē-ŭm) [TA] SYN forearm.

an·te·flex·ion (an'tē-flek'shŭn) A bending forward; a sharp forward curve or angulation; denoting especially the normal forward bend in the uterus at the junction of corpus and cervix uteri.

an·te·grade (an'tĕ-grād) In the direction of normal movement, as in blood flow or peristalsis.

an·te·grade u·rog·ra·phy (an'tĕ-grād yūr-og'ră-fē) Radiography following percutaneous injection of contrast agent with a needle or catheter into the renal calyces or pelvis (antegrade pyelography), or into the urinary bladder (antegrade cystography).

an·te·mor·tem (an'tĕ-mōr'tĕm) Before death. Cf. postmortem.

an·te·par·tum (AP) (an'tĕ-pahr'tŭm) Before labor or childbirth.

an·te·py·ret·ic (an'tĕ-pī-ret'ik) Before the occurrence of fever; before the period of reaction following shock.

an·te·ri·or (an-tēr'ē-ŏr) HUMAN ANATOMY denoting the front surface of the body.

an·te·ri·or at·lan·to·oc·cip·i·tal mem·brane (an-tēr'ē-ŏr at-lan'tō-ok-sip'i-tăl mem'brān) [TA] Fibrous layer that extends from the anterior arch of the atlas to the anterior margin of the foramen magnum of the occipital bone. SYN membrana atlanto-occipitalis anterior [TA].

an·te·ri·or col·umn (an-tēr'ē-ŏr kol'ŭm) [TA] The pronounced, ventrally oriented ridge of gray matter in each half of the spinal cord. SEE ALSO gray columns.

an·te·ri·or com·mis·sure (an-tēr'ē-ŏr kŏ-mish'ŭr) [TA] A round bundle of nerve fibers that crosses the midline of the brain near the anterior limit of the third ventricle. SYN precommissure.

an·te·ri·or cor·ti·co·spi·nal tract (an-tēr'ē-ŏr kōr'ti-kō-spī'năl trakt) Uncrossed fibers forming a small bundle in the anterior funiculus of the spinal cord. SEE pyramidal tract, corticospinal tract. SYN tractus corticospinalis anterior [TA], anterior pyramidal fasciculus, anterior pyramidal tract, direct pyramidal tract, fasciculus corticospinalis anterior, fasciculus pyramidalis anterior, tractus pyramidalis anterior, Türck bundle, Türck column, Türck tract.

an·te·ri·or fo·cal point (an-tēr'ē-ŏr fō'kăl poynt) The point where parallel rays from the retina are focused.

an·te·ri·or fon·ta·nelle (an-tēr'ē-ŏr fon'tă-nel') [TA] Membrane-covered gap in the infant cranium where the parietal and frontal bones will meet after fusion occurs.

an·te·ri·or guide (an-tēr'ē-ŏr gīd) SYN incisal guide.

an·te·ri·or horn cell (an-tēr'ē-ŏr hōrn sel) SYN motor neuron.

an·te·ri·or lac·ri·mal crest (an-tēr'ē-ŏr lak'ri-măl krest) [TA] Vertical ridge on the lateral surface of the frontal process of the maxilla that forms part of the medial rim of the orbit. SYN crista lacrimalis anterior [TA].

an·te·ri·or pi·tu·i·ta·ry hor·mones (an-tēr'ē-ŏr pi-tū'i-tār-ē hōr'mōnz) The group of hormones produced by the front portion of the pituitary gland, including lutropin, thyrotropin, follitropin, somatotropin, prolactin, and adrenocorticotropic hormone.

an·te·ri·or staph·y·lo·ma (an-tēr'ē-ŏr staf'i-lō'mă) A bulging near the anterior pole of the eye. SYN corneal staphyloma.

an·te·ri·or tib·i·al com·part·ment syn·drome (an-tēr'ē-ŏr tib'ē-ăl kŏm-pahrt'mĕnt sin'drōm) Ischemic necrosis of the muscles of the anterior tibial compartment of the leg.

an·te·ri·or tooth (an-tēr'ē-ŏr tūth) Any of the incisor and canine teeth on the mandible or maxillae located at the front of the oral cavity.

🌣 **antero-** Prefix meaning anterior.

an·ter·o·grade (an'tĕr-ō-grād) 1. Moving forward. Cf. antegrade. 2. Extending forward from a particular timepoint.

an·ter·o·grade am·ne·sia (an'tĕr-ō-grād am-nē'zē-ă) Amnesia in reference to events occurring after the trauma or disease that caused the condition.

an·ter·o·grade block (an'tĕr-ō-grād blok) Conduction block of an impulse traveling in its ordinary direction, for example, from the sinuatrial node toward the ventricular myocardium.

an·ter·o·grade mem·o·ry (an'ter-ō-grād mem'ŏr-ē) Recollection of events and experiences after a given timepoint or sudden cerebral disturbance (e.g., stroke, trauma).

an·ter·o·in·fe·ri·or (an'tĕr-ō-in-fēr'ē-ŏr) In front and below.

an·ter·o·lat·er·al (an'tĕr-ō-lat'ĕr-ăl) In front and away from the middle line.

an·te·ro·lis·the·sis (an'tĕr-ō-lis'thē-sis) Forward displacement of a vertebral body with respect to the vertebral body immediately below it.

an·ter·o·me·di·al (an'tĕr-ō-mē'dē-ăl) In front and toward the middle line.

an·ter·o·pos·te·ri·or (AP, A/P) (an'tĕr-ō-pos-tēr'ē-ŏr) Relating to both front and rear.

an·te·ver·sion (an'tĕ-vĕr'zhŭn) Forward displacement or turning forward of a body segment.

ant·hel·min·tic, ant·hel·min·thic (ant'hĕl-min'tik, -min'thik) 1. An agent that destroys or expels intestinal worms. SYN helminthagogue. 2. Having the power to destroy or expel intestinal worms.

an·thra·coid (an'thră-koyd) Resembling a carbuncle or cutaneous anthrax.

an·thra·co·sil·i·co·sis (an'thră-kō-sil'i-kō'sis) Pneumoconiosis from accumulation of carbon and silica in the lungs from inhaled coal dust. SYN coal worker's pneumoconiosis.

an·thrax (an'thraks) Infection by the bacterium *Bacillus anthracis*, which in humans is caused by contact with infected animals or animal products, and ingestion or inhalation of spores of the bacterium. Worldwide concern is focused on the potential use of anthrax as a bioterrorist weapon, in particular as an inhalational agent. SYN charbon.

🌣 **anthropo-** Prefix meaning human.

an·thro·po·cen·tric (an'thrŏ-pō-sen'trik) With a human bias, under the assumption that humankind is the central fact of the universe.

an·thro·poid (an'thrŏ-poyd) 1. Resembling a human in structure and form. 2. One of the monkeys resembling humans.

an·thro·pol·o·gy (an'thrŏ-pol'ŏ-jē) The scientific study of human beings with respect to physical features, distribution, and social and cultural relationships.

an·thro·pom·e·try (an'thrŏ-pom'ĕ-trē) The branch of anthropology concerned with comparative measurements of the human body.

an·thro·po·mor·phism (an'thrŏ-pō-mōr'fizm) Ascription of human shape or qualities to nonhuman creatures or objects.

an·thro·po·phil·ic (an'thrŏ-pō-fil'ik) Human-seeking or human-preferring, especially with reference to bloodsucking arthropods.

an·thro·po·zo·o·no·sis (an'thrŏ-pō-zō'ō-nō'sis) A zoonosis maintained in nature by animals and transmissible to humans (e.g., rabies, brucellosis).

anti- 1. Combining form meaning against, opposing, or, in relation to symptoms and diseases, curative. 2. Combining form meaning an antibody (immunoglobulin) specific for the thing indicated (e.g., antitoxin, as in antibody specific for a toxin).

an·ti·ad·ren·er·gic (an'tē-ad-rĕ-nĕr'jik) Antagonistic to the action of sympathetic or other adrenergic nerve fibers. SEE ALSO sympatholytic.

an·ti·ag·glu·ti·nin (an'tē-ă-glū'ti-nin) A specific antibody that inhibits or destroys the action of an agglutinin.

antianaemic [Br.] SYN antianemic.

an·ti·an·a·phy·lax·is (an'tē-an'ă-fi-lak'sis) SYN desensitization (1).

an·ti·an·dro·gen (an'tē-an'drŏ-jĕn) Any substance capable of preventing full expression of the biologic effects of androgenic hormones on responsive tissues.

an·ti·a·ne·mic (an'tē-ă-nē'mik) Pertaining to factors or substances that prevent or correct anemic conditions. SYN antianaemic.

an·ti·an·ti·body (an'tē-an'tē-bod-ē) Antibody specific for another antibody.

an·ti·ar·rhyth·mic (an'tē-ă-ridh'mik) Combating an arrhythmia. SYN antidysrhythmic.

an·ti·ar·thrit·ic (an'tē-ahr-thrit'ik) 1. Relieving arthritis. 2. A remedy for arthritis.

an·ti·asth·mat·ic (an'tē-az-mat'ik) 1. Tending to relieve or prevent asthma. 2. An agent that prevents or halts an asthmatic attack. SYN antasthmatic.

an·ti·bac·te·ri·al (an'tē-bak-tēr'ē-ăl) Destructive to or preventing the growth of bacteria.

an·ti·bi·o·gram (an'tē-bī'ō-gram) A profile of the antimicrobial resistance and susceptibility of a particular microorganism.

an·ti·bi·o·sis (an'tē-bī-ō'sis) Production of an antibiotic by bacteria or other organisms inhibitory to other living things, especially among soil microbes.

an·ti·bi·ot·ic (an'tē-bī-ot'ik) 1. Relating to antibiosis. 2. Prejudicial to life. 3. Denotes any substance that acts against susceptible microorganisms. 4. Relating to such an action.

an·ti·bi·ot·ic-re·sis·tant (an'tē-bī-ot'ik rē-zis'tănt) Denotes those pathogens that do not respond to antibiotic pharmacotherapy.

an·ti·bi·ot·ic sen·si·tiv·i·ty test (an'tē-bī-ot'ik sen'si-tiv'i-tē test) In vitro testing of bacterial cultures with antibiotics to determine susceptibility of bacteria to antibiotic therapy. SEE ALSO Bauer-Kirby test.

an·ti·bod·y (Ab) (an'tē-bod-ē) An immunoglobulin molecule with a specific amino acid sequence evoked in humans or other animals by an antigen and characterized by reacting specifically with the antigen in some demonstrable way, produced by B lymphocytes in response to an antigen. SEE ALSO immunoglobulin.

an·ti·body ti·ter (an'tē-bod'ē tī'tĕr) A diagnostic blood test that assesses the levels of specific antibodies.

an·ti·cho·lin·er·gic (an'tē-kō'li-nĕr'jik) 1. Antagonistic to the action of parasympathetic or other cholinergic nerve fibers (e.g., atropine). 2. Any of a class of compounds exerting anticholinergic effects.

an·ti·cho·lin·es·ter·ase (AChe) (an'tē-kō-lin-es'tĕr-ās) One of the drugs that inhibit or inactivate acetylcholinesterase.

an·ti·cli·nal (an'tē-klī'năl) Inclined in opposite directions, as two sides of a pyramid.

an·ti·co·ag·u·lant (an'tē-kō-ag'yŭ-lănt) 1. Preventing coagulation. 2. An agent having such action (e.g., warfarin ethylenediaminetetraacetic acid).

an·ti·co·ag·u·lant ther·a·py (ACT) (an′tē-kō-ag′yŭ-lănt thār′ă-pē) Use of anticoagulant drugs to reduce or prevent intravascular or intracardiac clotting.

an·ti·co·don (an′tē-kō′don) The trinucleotide sequence complementary to a codon found in one loop of a tRNA molecule.

an·ti·com·ple·ment (an′tē-kom′plĕ-mĕnt) A substance that combines with a complement and neutralizes its action by preventing its union with an antibody.

an·ti·con·vul·sant (AC) (an′tē-kŏn-vŭl′sănt) 1. Preventing or arresting seizures. 2. An agent having such action. SYN anticonvulsive.

an·ti·de·pres·sant (AD) (an′tē-dĕ-pres′ănt) 1. Counteracting depression. 2. A pharmacologic agent used in treating depression.

an·ti·di·a·bet·ic (an′tē-dī-ă-bet′ik) Counteracting diabetes; denoting an agent that reduces blood sugar (e.g., insulin).

an·ti·di·ar·rhe·al (an′tē-dī-ă-rē′ăl) Counteracting diarrhea. SYN antidiarrhoeal.

antidiarrhoeal [Br.] SYN antidiarrheal.

an·ti·di·u·re·sis (an′tē-dī-yŭr-ē′sis) Reduction of urinary volume.

an·ti·di·u·ret·ic (an′tē-dī-yŭr-et′ik) An agent that reduces output of urine.

an·ti·dot·al (an′ti-dō′tăl) Relating to or acting as an antidote.

an·ti·dote (an′ti-dōt) An agent that neutralizes a poison or counteracts its effects.

an·ti·drom·ic (an′tē-drom′ik) Denoting the propagation of an impulse along a conduction system (e.g., nerve fiber) in the direction opposite to that which it normally travels.

an·ti·dump·ing law (an′tē-dŭmp′ing law) Governmental regulation that may vary by jurisdiction, but which, in general, mandates that a hospital or care fa-

cility must either provide therapy regardless of ability to pay or transfer the penurious or destitute patient to another facility; such laws generally forbid health care facilities from refusing care to such patients or 'dumping' them on another care provider (or city street).

an·ti·em·bo·lism stock·ings (an′tē-ĕm′bŏ-lizm stok′ingz) Specially fitted elastic stockings used to compress lower extremities.

an·ti·e·met·ic (an′tē-ĕ-met′ik) 1. Preventing or arresting vomiting. 2. A remedy that tends to control nausea and vomiting.

an·ti·es·tro·gen (an′tē-es′trō-jĕn) Any substance capable of preventing full expression of the biologic effects of estrogenic hormones on responsive tissues. SYN antioestrogen.

an·ti·fi·bril·la·tory (an′tē-fi′bri-lă-tōr-ē) Any measure or medication that tends to suppress fibrillary arrhythmias (atrial fibrillation, ventricular fibrillation).

an·ti·fi·bri·no·lyt·ic (an′tē-fī-brin-ō-lit′ik) Denoting a substance that decreases the breakdown of fibrin (e.g., aminocaproic acid).

an·ti·flux (an′tē-flŭks) In dentistry, a material that prevents flow of solder.

an·ti·fun·gal (AF) (an′tē-fŭng′ăl) SYN antimycotic.

an·ti·gen (Ag) (an′ti-jen) Any substance that, as a result of coming in contact with target cells, induces a state of sensitivity or immune responsiveness after a latent period (days to weeks) and reacts in a demonstrable way with antibodies or immune cells of the sensitized subject in vivo or in vitro. SEE ALSO hapten. SYN immunogen.

antigenaemia [Br.] SYN antigenemia.

an·ti·gen-bind·ing site (an′ti-jen-bīnd′ing sīt) SYN paratope.

an·ti·ge·ne·mi·a (an′ti-jĕ-nē′mē-ă) Persistence of antigen in circulating blood.

an·ti·gen·ic (an′ti-jen′ik) Having the properties of an antigen (allergen). SYN allergenic, immunogenic.

an·ti·gen·ic com·pe·ti·tion (an'ti-jen´ik kom'pĕ-tish'ŏn) Competition that occurs when two different antigens, each of which can evoke an immunologic response when inoculated alone, are mixed and inoculated together.

an·ti·gen·ic de·ter·mi·nant (AD) (an'ti-jen'ik dĕ-tĕr'mi-nănt) The particular chemical group of a molecule that determines immunologic specificity. SYN determinant group.

an·ti·ge·nic·i·ty (an'ti-jĕ-nis'i-tē) The state or property of being antigenic. SYN immunogenicity.

an·ti·glob·u·lin (an'tē-glob'yū-lin) Antibody that combines with and precipitates globulin.

an·ti·glob·u·lin test (an'tē-glob'yū-lin test) Laboratory assessment to detect red blood cell antibodies in patient serum (indirect) or immunoglobulin bound to the surface of the red blood cell (direct).

an·ti·grav·i·ty mus·cles (an'tē-grav´i-tē mus'ĕlz) Muscles that maintain the posture characteristic of a given animal species. In most mammals and especially in bipeds, they are the extensor muscles. SYN postural muscles.

antihaemolysin [Br.] SYN antihemolysin.

antihaemophilic [Br.] SYN antihemophilic.

antihaemophilic factor a [Br.] SYN antihemophilic factor A.

antihaemorrhagic [Br.] SYN antihemorrhagic.

an·ti·he·mo·ly·sin (an'tē-hē-mol'i-sin) A substance (including antibody) that inhibits or prevents the effects of hemolysin. SYN antihaemolysin.

an·ti·he·mo·phil·ic (an'tē-hē-mō-fil'ik) Correcting or counteracting the hemorrhagic tendency in hemophilia. SYN antihaemophilic.

an·ti·he·mo·phil·ic factor A (AHF) (an'tē-hē-mō-fil'ik fak'tŏr) SYN factor VIII, antihaemophilic factor A.

an·ti·he·mo·phil·ic factor B (an'tē-hē´mō-fil'ik fak'tŏr) SYN factor IX.

an·ti·he·mo·phil·ic glob·u·lin (AHG) (an'tē-hē´mō-fil'ik glob'yū-lin) 1. SYN factor VIII. 2. SYN human antihemophilic factor.

an·ti·hem·or·rhag·ic (an'tē-hem-ō-raj´ik) Arresting hemorrhage. SYN antihaemorrhagic, hemostatic (2).

an·ti·his·ta·mine (an'tē-his'tă-mēn) Medication that suppresses histamine production in the body.

an·ti·his·ta·min·ic (an'tē-his-tă-min'ik) 1. Tending to neutralize or antagonize the action of histamine or to inhibit its production in the body. 2. An agent having such an effect, used to relieve allergy symptoms.

an·ti·hy·per·lip·i·de·mic (an'tē-hī'pĕr-lip'i-dē'mik) Acting to prevent or counteract the buildup of lipids in the blood.

an·ti·hy·per·ten·sive (an'tē-hī-pĕr-ten'siv) Indicating a drug or mode of treatment that reduces the blood pressure of people with hypertension.

an·ti·hy·po·ten·sive (an'tē-hī'pō-ten'siv) Any measure or medication that tends to raise reduced blood pressure.

an·ti·in·flam·ma·to·ry (an'tē-in-flam'ă-tōr-ē) Reducing inflammation by acting on body responses, without directly antagonizing the causative agent.

an·ti·lith·ic (an'tē-lith'ik) 1. Preventing the formation of calculi or promoting their dissolution. 2. An agent so acting.

an·ti·lym·pho·cyte glob·u·lin (ALG) (an'tē-lim'fō-sīt glob'yū-lin) SYN antilymphocyte serum.

an·ti·lym·pho·cyte se·rum (ALS) (an'tē-lim'fō-sīt sēr'ŭm) Antiserum against lymphocytes.

an·ti·ma·lar·i·al (an'tē-mă-lār'ē-ăl) 1. Preventing or curing malaria. 2. A chemotherapeutic agent that inhibits or destroys malarial parasites.

an·ti·mere (an'ti-mēr) 1. A segment of an animal body formed by planes cutting the axis of the body at right angles. 2. One of the symmetric parts of a bilateral organism. 3. The right or left half of the body.

an·ti·me·tab·o·lite (an'tē-mĕ-tab'ō-līt) A substance that competes with, replaces, or antagonizes a particular metabolite.

an·ti·me·tro·pi·a (an'tē-mĕ-trō'pē-ă) A form of anisometropia in which one eye is myopic and the other hypermetropic.

an·ti·mi·cro·bi·al (an'tē-mī-krō'bē-ăl) Tending to destroy microbes, to prevent their multiplication or growth, or to prevent their pathogenic action.

an·ti·mi·cro·bi·al break·point (an'tē-mī-krō'bē-ăl brāk'poynt) The concentration of an antimicrobial agent that can be achieved in the body fluids or target site(s) during optimal therapy.

an·ti·mi·cro·bi·al drugs (an'tē-mī-krō'bē-ăl drŭgz) Substances that kill or inhibit growth of microscopic pathogens such as bacteria and viruses.

an·ti·mus·ca·rin·ic (an'tē-mŭs'kă-rin'ik) Inhibiting or preventing the actions of muscarine and muscarinelike agents, or the effects of parasympathetic stimulation at the neuroeffector junction (e.g., atropine).

an·ti·my·as·then·ic (an'tē-mī'as-then'ik) Tending toward the correction of the symptoms of myasthenia gravis, (e.g., as in the action of neostigmine).

an·ti·my·cot·ic (an'tē-mī-kot'ik) Antagonistic to fungi.

an·ti·nau·se·ant (an'tē-naw'zē-ănt) Having an action to prevent nausea.

an·ti·ne·o·plas·tic (an'tē-nē'ō-plas'tik) Preventing the development, maturation, or spread of neoplastic cells.

an·tin·i·on (an-tin'ē-on) The space between the eyebrows; the point on the cranium opposite the inion.

an·ti·nu·cle·ar (an'tē-nū'klē-ĕr) Having an affinity for or reacting with the cell nucleus.

an·ti·nu·cle·ar an·ti·body, an·ti·nu·cle·ar fac·tor (ANF, ANA) (an'tē-nū'klē-ăr an'ti-bod-ē, fak'tŏr) An antibody showing an affinity for cell nuclei, demonstrated by exposing a cell substrate to the serum to be tested, followed by exposure to an antihuman-globulin serum.

antioestrogen [Br.] SYN antiestrogen.

an·ti·ox·i·dant (an'tē-ŏks-i-dănt) Any substance that may prevent organ damage by scavenging free radicals, including catalase, glutathione, peroxidase, superoxide dismutase, and vitamins A, C, and E. SEE ALSO angina, free radical.

an·ti·par·al·lel (an'tē-par'ă-lel) Denoting molecules that are parallel but have opposite directional polarity, e.g., the two strands of a DNA double helix.

an·ti·par·a·sit·ic (an'tē-par-ă-sit'ik) Destructive to parasites.

an·ti·pe·dic·u·lot·ic (an'tē-pe-dik'yū-lot'ik) Effective in the treatment of pediculosis, especially denoting such an agent.

an·ti·per·i·stal·sis (an'tē-per-i-stal'sis) SYN reversed peristalsis.

an·ti·per·spi·rant (an'tē-pĕr'spir-ănt) An agent that inhibits the secretion of sweat (e.g., aluminum chloride).

an·ti·plas·min (AP) (an'tē-plaz'min) A substance that inhibits or prevents the effects of plasmin; found in plasma and some tissues, especially the spleen and liver.

an·ti·port (an'ti-pōrt) The coupled transport of two different molecules or ions through a membrane in opposite directions by a common carrier mechanism.

an·ti·pro·ges·tin (an'tē-prō-jes'tin) A substance that inhibits progesterone formation.

an·ti·pro·throm·bin (an'tē-prō-throm'bin) An anticoagulant that inhibits or prevents the conversion of prothrombin into thrombin.

an·ti·pru·rit·ic (an'tē-prūr-it'ik) 1. Preventing or relieving itching. 2. An agent that relieves itching.

an·ti·psy·chot·ic agent (an'tē-sī-kot'ik ā'jĕnt) Functional category of neuroleptic drugs helpful in treatment of psychosis; have a capacity to decrease symptoms of thought disorders.

an·ti·py·re·sis (an'tē-pī-rē'sis) Symptomatic treatment of fever itself rather than of the underlying disease.

an·ti·py·ret·ic (an'tē-pī-ret'ik) 1. Reducing fever. 2. A drug that reduces fever.

an·ti·py·rot·ic (an'tē-pī-rot'ik) 1. Relieving the pain and promoting the healing of superficial burns. 2. A topical application for burns.

an·ti·ra·chit·ic (an'tē-ră-kit'ik) Agent used to prevent the development of rickets.

an·ti·rheu·mat·ic (an'tē-rū-mat'ik) *Although the digraph rh occurring at the beginning of a syllable in a word of Greek origin is ordinarily changed to rrh when a prefix or other lexical element is placed before it, the r is not doubled in this word.* 1. Denoting an agent that suppresses manifestations of rheumatic disease; usually applied to antiinflammatory agents or agents that are capable of delaying progression of the basic disease process in inflammatory arthritis. 2. An agent possessing such properties (e.g., gold compounds).

an·ti·schis·to·so·mal (an'tē-shis'tō-sō'mal) 1. Destructive or harmful to schistosomes. 2. An agent capable of affecting the viability of schistosomes.

an·ti·scor·bu·tic (an'tē-skōr-byū'tik) 1. Preventive or curative of scurvy. 2. A treatment for scurvy (e.g., vitamin C).

an·ti·seb·or·rhe·ic (an'tē-seb'ŏr-ē'ik) 1. Preventing or relieving excessive secretion of sebum; preventing or relieving seborrheic dermatitis. 2. An agent having such actions.

an·ti·se·cre·to·ry (an'tē-sĕ-krē'tŏr-ē) Inhibitory to secretion, said of certain drugs that reduce or suppress gastric secretion (e.g., ranitidine, omeprazole).

an·ti·sense (an'tē-sens) Pertaining to the strand of a double-stranded DNA or RNA molecule that is complementary to the sense strand.

an·ti·sep·sis (an'ti-sep'sis) Prevention of infection by inhibiting the growth of infectious agents. SEE ALSO disinfection.

an·ti·sep·tic (an'ti-sep'tik) 1. Relating to antisepsis. 2. An agent or substance capable of effecting antisepsis.

an·ti·sep·tic dress·ing (an'ti-sep'tik dres'ing) A sterile dressing of gauze impregnated with an antiseptic.

an·ti·se·rum (an'tē-sēr'ŭm) Serum that contains demonstrable antibody or antibodies specific for one or more antigens. SYN immune serum.

an·ti·se·rum an·a·phy·lax·is (an'tē-sēr'ŭm an'ă-fī-lak'sis) SYN passive anaphylaxis.

an·ti·si·al·a·gogue (an'tē-sī-al'ă-gog) An agent that diminishes or stops saliva flow.

an·ti·so·cial (AS) (an'tē-sō'shăl) Manifesting at least some of the traits of an antisocial personality disorder; disregard for social or legal norms, lying, aggressiveness, indifference to others' rights or safety, irresponsibility, blaming others, and showing minimal or no remorse. SEE antisocial personality disorder.

an·ti·so·cial per·son·al·i·ty dis·or·der (an'tē-sō'shăl pĕr-sōn-al'i-tē dis-ōr'dĕr) Mental state characterized by continuous and chronic antisocial behavior with disregard and violation of the rights of others, beginning before age 15; early childhood signs include chronic lying, stealing, fighting, and truancy.

an·ti·spas·mod·ic (an'tē-spaz-mod'ik) 1. Preventing or alleviating muscle spasms (cramps). 2. An agent that quiets spasm.

an·ti·throm·bin (AT, At) (an'tē-throm'bin) Substance that inhibits or prevents effects of thrombin so blood does not coagulate.

an·ti·thy·roid (an'tē-thī'royd) Relating to an agent that suppresses thyroid function.

an·ti·tox·in (an'tē-tok'sin) Antibody formed in response to antigenic poisonous substances of biologic origin (e.g., bacterial exotoxins, phytotoxins, and zootoxins).

an·ti·tra·gus (an'tē-tră'gŭs) [TA] A projection of the cartilage of the auricle.

an·ti·tris·mus (an'tē-triz'mŭs) A condition of tonic muscular spasm that prevents closing of the mouth.

an·ti·tryp·sin (an'tē-trip'sin) A substance that blocks the action of trypsin.

an·ti·tus·sive (an'tē-tŭs'iv) **1.** Relieving cough. **2.** A cough remedy (e.g., codeine).

an·ti·ven·in (an'tē-ven'in) An antitoxin specific for an animal or insect venom.

an·ti·vi·ral (an'tē-vī'răl) Opposing a virus; interfering with its replication; weakening or abolishing its action.

an·ti·xe·rot·ic (an'tē-zē-rot'ik) Preventing dryness.

♻ **antro-** Prefix meaning an antrum.

an·tro·na·sal (an'trō-nā'zăl) Relating to a maxillary sinus and the corresponding nasal cavity.

an·tro·scope (an'trō-skōp) An instrument to aid in the visual examination of any cavity, particularly the maxillary sinus.

an·tros·to·my (an-tros'tŏ-mē) Formation of a permanent opening into any antrum.

an·trot·o·my (an-trot'ŏ-mē) Incision through the wall of any antrum.

an·trum, gen. **an·tri,** pl. **an·tra** (an'trŭm, -trī, -tră) [TA] Any nearly closed cavity, particularly one with bony walls.

an·trum car·di·a·cum (an'trŭm kahr-dē-ā'kŭm) SYN cardiac antrum.

An·tyl·lus method (an-til'ŭs meth'ŏd) Ligation of the artery above and below an aneurysm, followed by incision into and emptying of the sac.

an·u·lar, an·nu·lar (an'yŭ-lăr) Ring-shaped.

an·u·lar cat·a·ract (an'yŭ-lăr kat'ăr-akt) Congenital cataract in which a central white membrane replaces the nucleus.

an·u·lar lig·a·ment (an'yŭ-lăr lig'ă-měnt) [TA] A ligament that encircles a body part. SYN ligamentum anulare [TA], orbicular ligament.

an·u·lar pla·cen·ta (an'yŭ-lăr plă-sen'tă) A placenta in the form of a band encircling the interior of the uterus.

an·u·lar scle·ri·tis (an'yŭ-lăr skler-ī'tis) An often protracted inflammation of the anterior portion of the sclera, forming a ring around the corneoscleral limbus.

an·u·lar sco·to·ma (an'yŭ-lăr skō-tō'mă) A circular scotoma surrounding the center of the field of vision.

an·u·lar staph·y·lo·ma (an'yŭ-lăr staf'i-lō'mă) A staphyloma extending around the periphery of the cornea.

an·u·lo·a·or·tic ec·ta·si·a (AAE) (an'yū-lō-ā-ōr'tik ek-tā'zē-ă) Supravalvular dilation of the aorta involving both its wall and the valve ring, which, however, remains of smaller diameter than the more distal ectatic wall. SYN aortoanular ectasia.

an·u·lo·plast·y (an'yū-lō-plas'tē) Reconstruction of the ring (or anulus) of a cardiac valve.

an·u·lor·rha·phy (an-yū-lōr'ă-fē) Closure of a hernial ring by suture.

an·u·lus, an·nu·lus, gen. and pl. **an·u·li** (an'yū-lŭs, -li) [TA] SYN ring (1).

an·u·lus fi·bro·sus (an'yū-lŭs fī-brō'sŭs) [TA] **1.** SYN right and left fibrous rings of heart. **2.** SYN anulus fibrosus of intervertebral disc.

an·u·lus fi·bro·sus of in·ver·te·bral disc (an'yū-lŭs fī-brō'sŭs in-vĕr'tĕ-brăl disk) Ring of cartilage and fibrous tissue forming the circumference of the intervertebral disc. SYN annulus fibrosis.

an·u·re·sis (an'yūr-ē'sis) Inability to urinate.

an·u·ri·a (ă-nyūr'ē-ă) Absence of urine formation.

a·nus, gen. and pl. **a·ni** (ā'nŭs, ā'nī) [TA] The lower opening of the alimentary (digestive) tract, lying in the intergluteal cleft between the buttocks, through which feces or excrement is discharged.

an·vil (an'vil) SYN incus.

anx·i·e·ty (ang-zī'ĕ-tē) **1.** Apprehension

of danger and dread accompanied by restlessness, tension, tachycardia, and dyspnea unattached to a clearly identifiable stimulus. **2.** EXPERIMENTAL PSYCHOLOGY a drive or motivational state learned from and thereafter associated with previously neutral cues.

an·xi·e·ty at·tack (ang-zī′ĕ-tē ă-tak′) Acute episode of anxiety.

anx·i·e·ty dis·or·ders (ang-zī′ĕ-tē dis-ōr′dĕrz) A category of interrelated mental illnesses involving anxiety reactions in response to stress.

anx·i·e·ty re·ac·tion (anx react) (ang-zī′ĕ-tē rē-ak′shŭn) Psychological state involving apprehension of danger accompanied by dread and attendant physical symptoms.

anx·i·o·lyt·ic (ang′zē-ō-lit′ik) Something that diminishes anxiety (e.g., a drug).

a·or·ta, gen. and pl. **a·or·tae** (ā-ōr′tă, -tē) [TA] A large artery that is the main trunk of the systemic arterial system, arising from the left ventricle and ending at the left side of the body of the fourth lumbar vertebra.

a·or·tic an·eu·rysm (AA) (ā-ōr′tik an′yūr-izm) Diffuse or circumscribed dilation of a portion of the aorta.

a·or·tic an·gi·o·gram (ā-ōr′tik an′jē-ō-gram) A radiographic procedure that produces an image of the aorta after injection of a radiopaque substance.

a·or·tic arch (ā-ōr′tik ahrch) **1.** The curved portion of the aorta between its ascending and descending parts. **2.** One of several pairs of arterial channels encircling the embryonic pharynx in the branchial arches, mesenchyme.

a·or·tic a·tre·si·a (ā-ōr′tik ă-trē′zē-ă) Congenital absence of the normal valvular orifice into the aorta.

a·or·tic for·a·men (ā-ōr′tik fōr-ā′men) SYN aortic hiatus.

a·or·tic hi·a·tus (ā-ōr′tik hī-ā′tŭs) [TA] The opening in the diaphragm bounded by the two crura, the vertebral column, and the median arcuate ligament, through which pass the aorta and thoracic duct; also called aortic opening.

a·or·tic mur·mur (ā-ōr′tik mŭr′mŭr) Bruit at the aortic orifice, either obstructive or regurgitant.

a·or·tic notch (ā-ōr′tik noch) The notch in a sphygmographic tracing caused by rebound following closure of the aortic valves.

a·or·ti·co·pul·mo·nary sep·tum (ā-ōr′ti-kō-pul′mŏ-nār-ē sep′tŭm) This wall dividing the embryonic bulbus cordis and truncus arteriosus into pulmonary and aortic outflow tracts from the developing heart. SYN spiral bulbar septum, spiral septum.

a·or·tic or·i·fice (ā-ōr′tik ōr′i-fis) [TA] Opening from the left ventricle into the ascending aorta; it is guarded by the aortic valve. SYN ostium aortae [TA], aortic ostium.

a·or·tic re·gur·gi·ta·tion (ā-ōr′tik rē-gŭr′ji-tā′shŭn) Reflux of blood through an incompetent aortic valve into the left ventricle during ventricular diastole; also called aortic insufficiency.

a·or·tic sep·tal de·fect, a·or·ti·co·pul·mo·nary sep·tal defect (ā-ōr′tik sep′tăl dē′fekt, ā-ōr′ti-kō-pul′mŏ-nār-ē) Small congenital opening between the aorta and pulmonary artery 1 cm above the semilunar valves.

a·or·tic si·nus (ā-ōr′tik sī′nŭs) [TA] Space between the superior aspect of each cusp of the aortic valve and the dilated portion of the wall of the ascending aorta. SYN sinus aortae [TA], Petit sinus, Valsalva sinus.

a·or·tic valve (ā-ōr′tik valv) [TA] The valve between the left ventricle and the ascending aorta, consisting of three fibrous semilunar cusps (valvules).

a·or·ti·tis (ā-ōr-tī′tis) Inflammation of the aorta.

a·or·tog·ra·phy (ā-ōr-tog′ră-fē) Radiographic imaging of the aorta and its branches, or a portion of the aorta, by injection of contrast medium.

a·or·to·il·i·ac by·pass (ā-ōr′tō-il′ē-ak bī′pas) An operation in which a vascular prosthesis is united with the aorta and iliac artery to relieve obstruction of the lower abdominal aorta, its bifurcation, and the proximal iliac branches.

a·or·to·plas·ty (ā-ōr'tō-plas'tē) A procedure for surgical repair of the aorta.

a·or·to·re·nal by·pass (ā-ōr'tō-rē'năl bī'pas) Insertion of a graft of autogenous artery, saphenous vein, or synthetic material between the aorta and the distal renal artery.

a·or·tor·rha·phy (ā-ōr-tōr'ă-fē) Suture of the aorta.

a·or·to·scle·ro·sis (ā-ōr'tō-skler-ō'sis) Arteriosclerosis of the aorta.

a·or·tot·o·my (ā-ōr-tot'ŏ-mē) Incision of the aorta.

a·par·eu·ni·a (ă-păr-yū'nē-ă) Absence or impossibility of coitus.

ap·a·thy (ap'ă-thē) Indifference; absence of interest in the environment.

A-pat·tern eso·tro·pi·a (pat'ĕrn es'ō-trō'pē-ă) Convergent strabismus greater in upward than in downward gaze.

A-pat·tern exo·tro·pi·a (pat'ĕrn ek'sō-trō'pē-ă) Divergent strabismus greater in downward than in upward gaze.

a·pel·lous (ă-pel'ŭs) 1. Without skin. 2. Without foreskin; circumcised.

a·per·i·stal·sis (ā'per-i-stal'sis) Absence of peristalsis.

ap·er·to·gna·thi·a (ă-per-tōg-nath'ē-ă) An open bite deformity, a type of malocclusion characterized by premature posterior occlusion and absence of anterior occlusion.

A·pert syn·drome (ah-pār' sin'drōm) Disorder characterized by craniosynostosis and syndactyly of all the fingers and usually the toes as well.

ap·er·ture (ap'ĕr-chŭr) [TA] 1. An inlet or entrance to a cavity or channel; in anatomy, an open gap or hole; also called apertura. 2. The diameter of the objective of a microscope.

a·pex, gen. **ap·i·cis,** pl. **ap·i·ces** (ā'peks, ap'i-sis, -i-sēz) [TA] Extremity of a conic or pyramidal structure.

a·pex beat (ā'peks bēt) The visible and/or palpable pulsation made by the apex of the left ventricle as it strikes the chest wall in systole. SYN ictus cordis.

a·pex·car·di·o·gram (ACG, APCG) (ā'peks-kahr'dē-ō-gram) Graphic recording of the movements of the chest wall produced by the apex beat of the heart.

a·pex·car·di·og·ra·phy (ā'peks-kahr' dē-og'ră-fē) Noninvasive graphic recording of cardiac pulsations from the region of the apex, usually of the left ventricle, and resembling the ventricular pressure curve.

Ap·gar score (ap'gahr skōr) Evaluation of a newborn infant's physical status by assigning numeric values (0–2) to each of 5 criteria: 1) heart rate, 2) respiratory effort, 3) muscle tone, 4) response to stimulation, and 5) skin color; a score of 8–10 indicates the best possible condition.

a·pha·gi·a (ă-fā'jē-ă) Inability to eat.

a·pha·ki·a (ă-fā'kē-ă) Absence of the lens of the eye.

a·pha·lan·gi·a (ă-fă-lan'jē-ă) Congenital absence of a digit, or more specifically, absence of one or more of the long bones (phalanges) of a finger or toe.

a·pha·si·a (aph) (ă-fā'zē-ă) Impaired or absent comprehension or production of, or communication by, speech, reading, writing, or signs, caused by an acquired lesion of the dominant cerebral hemisphere.

a·pha·si·ol·o·gy (ă-fā'zē-ol'ŏ-jē) The science of language disorders caused by dysfunction of the cerebral language areas.

a·pher·e·sis (ā-fĕr-ē'sis) Extraction of certain fluid or cellular elements from withdrawn blood, which is then reinfused into the donor or patient.

a·pho·ni·a (ă-fō'nē-ă) Loss of the voice.

a·phra·si·a (ă-frā'zē-ă) Inability to speak.

aph·ro·di·si·ac (af-rō-diz'ē-ak) 1. Increasing sexual desire. 2. Anything that arouses or increases sexual desire.

aph·tha, pl. **aph·thae** (af′thă, -thē) **1.** In the singular, a small ulcer on a mucous membrane. **2.** In the plural, stomatitis characterized by episodes of painful oral ulcers of unknown etiology that are covered by gray exudate. SYN canker sores, recurrent aphthous ulcers, recurrent ulcerative stomatitis, ulcerative stomatitis.

aph·thae ma·jor (af′thē mā′jŏr) A severe form of aphthae characterized by unusually numerous, large, deep, and frequent ulcers.

aph·tho·sis (af-thō′sis) Any condition characterized by the presence of aphthae.

aph·thous (af′thŭs) Characterized by or relating to aphthae or aphthosis.

ap·i·cal (ap′i-kăl) [TA] **1.** Relating to the apex or tip of a pyramidal or pointed structure. **2.** Situated nearer to the apex of a structure in relation to a specific reference point; opposite of basal.

ap·i·cal gran·u·lo·ma (ap′i-kăl gran′yū-lō′mă) SYN periapical granuloma.

ap·i·cal mem·brane (ap′i-kăl mem′brăn) The microvilli-bearing portion of the epithelial cell membrane at the secretory pole.

ap·i·cal space (ap′i-kăl spās) Area between the alveolar wall and the apex of the root of a tooth.

ap·i·ci·tis (ap-i-sī′tis) Inflammation of the apex of a structure or organ.

apico- Prefix meaning an apex; apical.

ap·i·co·ec·to·my (ap′i-kō-ek′tŏ-mē) Surgical removal of a tooth root apex.

a·pi·tu·i·tar·ism (ā′pi-tū′i-tăr-izm) Total lack of functional pituitary tissue.

ap·la·nat·ic (ap-lă-nat′ik) Pertaining to aplanatism, or to an aplanatic lens.

ap·la·nat·ic lens (ap-lă-nat′ik lenz) Spectacle lens designed to correct spheric aberration and coma.

a·pla·si·a (ă-plā′zē-ă) **1.** Defective development or congenital absence of an organ or tissue. **2.** In hematology, incomplete, retarded, or defective development, or cessation of the usual regenerative process.

a·plas·tic (ā-plas′tik) Pertaining to aplasia, or conditions characterized by defective regeneration, as in aplastic anemia.

a·plas·tic a·ne·mia (ā-plas′tik ă-nē′mē-ă) Disorder characterized by a greatly decreased formation of erythrocytes and hemoglobin. SYN Ehrlich anemia.

a·plas·tic lymph (ā-plas′tik limf) Fluid containing a relatively large number of leukocytes, but comparatively little fibrinogen.

ap·ne·a (ap′nē-ă) *Although the correct pronunciation of this word is with stress on the second-last syllable, the pronunciation shown is usually heard in the U.S.* Absence of breathing.

ap·nea mon·i·tor (ap′nē-ă mon′i-tŏr) A portable machine used by patients with apnea to monitor breathing in at-risk situations; typically used at night.

ap·ne·ic (ap′nē-ik) Related to or suffering from apnea. SYN apnoeic.

ap·neu·sis (ap-nū′sis) An abnormal respiratory pattern consisting of a pause at full inspiration.

apnoea [Br.] SYN apnea.

apnoeic [Br.] SYN apneic.

apo- Combining form meaning, usually, separated from or derived from.

ap·o·crine (ap′ō-krin) Denoting a mechanism of glandular secretion in which the apical portion of secretory cells is shed and secreted. SEE ALSO apocrine sweat gland.

ap·o·crine car·ci·no·ma (ap′ō-krin kahr′si-nō′mă) Carcinoma composed predominantly of cells with abundant eosinophilic granular cytoplasm, occurring in the apocrine glands.

ap·o·crine sweat gland (ap′ō-krin swet gland) Specialized sudoriferous gland located primarily in the armpits, groin, breasts, ears, and eyelids.

ap·o·en·zyme (apo, AE) (ap′ō-en-zīm)
The protein portion of an enzyme as contrasted with the nonprotein portion, coenzyme, or prosthetic portion (if present in
the intact protein).

ap·o·fer·ri·tin (ap-ō-fer′i-tin) A protein
in the intestinal wall that combines with
a ferric hydroxide-phosphate compound
to form ferritin, the first stage in the absorption of iron.

a·po·gee (ap′ō-jē) The peak of severity of
the clinical manifestations of an illness.

a·po·lar (ā-pō′lăr) **1.** Without poles; specifically denoting embryonic nerve cells
(neuroblasts) that have not yet begun to
sprout processes. **2.** SYN hydrophobic
(2).

ap·o·lip·o·pro·tein (ap′ō-lip-ō-prō′tēn)
The protein component of lipoprotein
complexes that is a normal constituent of
plasma chylomicrons.

ap·o·neu·rec·to·my (ap′ō-nūr-ek′tŏ-mē)
Excision of an aponeurosis.

ap·o·neu·ror·rha·phy (ap′ō-nūr-ōr′ă-
fē) SYN fasciorrhaphy.

ap·o·neu·ro·sis, pl. **ap·o·neu·ro·ses**
(ap′ō-nūr-ō′sis, -sēz) [TA] A fibrous
sheet or flat, expanded tendon, giving attachment to muscular fibers and serving
as the means of proximal or distal attachment (origin or insertion) of a flat
muscle.

ap·o·neu·ro·si·tis (ap′ō-nūr′ō-sī′tis) Inflammation of an aponeurosis.

ap·o·neu·rot·ic pto·sis (ap′ō-nūr-ot′ĭk
tō′sis) Drooping eyelid caused by dehiscence of the levator muscle tendon.
SYN involutional ptosis.

ap·o·neu·rot·o·my (ap′ō-nūr-ot′ŏ-mē)
Incision of an aponeurosis.

a·poph·y·sis, pl. **a·poph·y·ses** (ă-pof′
i-sis, -sēz) [TA] An outgrowth or projection, especially one from a bone.

a·poph·y·si·tis (ă-pof-i-sī′tis) Inflammation of any apophysis.

ap·o·plec·ti·form (ap′ō-plek′ti-fōrm) Resembling apoplexy.

ap·o·plexy (ap′ō-pleks-ē) SYN stroke.

ap·o·pro·tein (ap′ō-prō′tēn) A polypeptide chain (protein) not yet complexed
with the prosthetic group that is necessary to form the active holoprotein.

ap·o·pto·sis (ap-ō-tō′sis) Programmed
cell death.

ap·o·re·pres·sor (ap′ō-rĕ-pres′ŏr) A
regulatory protein that, when combined
with another corepressor, undergoes allosteric transformation, which allows it
to combine with an operator locus and
inhibit transcription of certain genes.

ap·pa·ra·tus, pl. **ap·pa·ra·tus** (ap′ă-
rat′ŭs) [TA] A group or system of glands,
ducts, blood vessels, muscles, or other
anatomic structures involved in the performance of some function. SEE ALSO
system.

ap·pa·ra·tus la·cri·ma·lis (ap′ă-rā′tŭs
lak-ri-mā′lis) [TA] SYN lacrimal apparatus.

ap·pend·age (ă-pen′dăj) Any part, subordinate in function or size, attached to
a main structure. SYN appendix (1).

ap·pend·ages of skin (ă-pend′dăj-ĕz
skin) Hair, fingernails, toenails, and the
sweat, sebaceous, and mammary glands.

**ap·pen·dec·to·my, ap·pen·di·cec·to·
my** (ap′pĕn-dek′tŏ-mē, ă-pen′di-sek′tŏ-
mē) Surgical removal of the vermiform
appendix. SYN appendicectomy.

ap·pen·dic·e·al, ap·pen·di·cal (ap′ĕn-
dis′ē-ăl, ă-pen′di-kăl) Relating to an appendix.

ap·pen·di·ci·tis (ă-pen′di-sī′tis) Inflammation of the vermiform appendix.

appendico- Combining form meaning
an appendix, usually the vermiform appendix.

ap·pen·di·cos·to·my (ă-pen′di-kos′tŏ-
mē) An operation to open the intestine
through the tip of the vermiform appendix.

ap·pen·di·co·ves·i·cos·to·my (ă-pen′
di-ko-ves′i-kos′tŏ-mē) Use of an isolated
appendix on a vascularized pedicle as a

catheterizable route of access to the bladder from the skin.

ap·pen·dic·u·lar (ap′ĕn-dik′yŭ-lăr) **1.** Relating to an appendix or appendage. **2.** Relating to the limbs, as opposed to axial, which refers to the trunk and head.

ap·pen·dix, pl. **ap·pen·dix·es**, gen. **ap·pen·di·cis**, pl. **ap·pen·di·ces** (ă-pen′diks, -diks-ĕz, -di-sis, -di-sēz) [TA] **1.** SYN appendage. **2.** A wormlike intestinal diverticulum extending from the blind end of the cecum; it varies in length and ends in a blind extremity.

ap·per·cep·tion (ap′ĕr-sep′shŭn) The final stage of attentive perception in which something is clearly apprehended and thus is relatively prominent in awareness.

ap·pe·stat (ap′ĕ-stat) Cerebral mechanism concerned with the appetite and control of food intake.

ap·pla·na·tion (ap′lă-nā′shŭn) Flattening of the cornea by pressure from a tonometer. SEE ALSO applanation tonometer.

ap·pla·na·tion to·nom·e·ter (ap′lă-nā′shŭn tō-nom′ĕ-tĕr) Device used to gauge ocular tension by application of a small, flat disc to the cornea.

ap·ple jel·ly no·dules (ap′ĕl jel′ē nod′yūlz) Descriptive term for the papular lesions of lupus vulgaris, as they appear on diascopy.

ap·pli·ance (ă-plī′ăns) A device used to provide function to a part, or for therapeutic purposes.

ap·plied a·nat·o·my (ă-plīd′ ă-nat′ŏ-mē) **1.** SYN clinical anatomy. **2.** Any practical application related to human structure or a structural feature.

ap·po·si·tion (ap′ŏ-zish′ŭn) **1.** Putting two substances in contact. **2.** The relationship of fracture fragments to one another. **3.** The process of thickening of the cell wall. **4.** The deposition of the matrix of the hard dental structures; enamel, dentin, and cementum.

ap·po·si·tion su·ture (ap′ŏ-zish′ŭn sū′chŭr) A suture that holds together dermatologic margins.

ap·proach (ă-prōch′) **1.** PSYCHIATRY a term used to describe how interpersonal relationships are negotiated. **2.** The path or method used to expose the operative field during an operation.

AP pro·jec·tion (prŏ-jek′shŭn) A radiographic study in which x-rays travel from anterior to posterior. SYN anteroposterior projection.

ap·pro·pri·ate for ges·ta·tion·al age in·fant (ă-prō′prē-ăt jes-tā′shŭn-ăl ăj in′fănt) Infant who has met the appropriate developmental milestones.

ap·prox·i·ma·tion (ă-prok′si-mā′shŭn) In surgery, bringing tissue edges into desired apposition for suturing.

ap·prox·i·ma·tion su·ture (ă-prok′si-mā′shŭn sū′chŭr) Suture that pulls together the deep tissues.

a·prax·i·a (ă-prak′sē-ă) A disorder of voluntary movement, consisting of impairment in the performance of skilled or purposeful movements.

a·prax·ic, a·prac·tic (ă-prak′sik, -prak′tik) Marked by or pertaining to apraxia.

a·proc·ti·a (ă-prok′shē-ă) Congenital absence or imperforation of the anus.

ap·ron·ec·to·my (ap′rō-nek′tŏ-mē) Surgical excision of a redundant and dependent panniculus adiposus of the abdominal wall, which is commonly called an apron.

ap·ti·tude test (ap′ti-tūd test) An occupation-oriented intelligence test used to evaluate a person's abilities, talents, and skills; particularly valuable in vocational counseling.

APUD, APUD cells (ap′ŭd, selz) Designation for cells in various organs secreting polypeptide hormones.

a·py·ret·ic (ā-pī-ret′ik) Without fever, denoting apyrexia; having a normal body temperature.

a·py·rex·i·a (ā-pī-rek′sē-ă) Absence of fever.

aq·ua, gen. and pl. **aq·uae** (ah′kwäh) H_2O. Pharmaceutical waters, aquae, are aqueous solutions of volatile substances (e.g., rose water). Pharmaceutical solutions, liquors, are aqueous solutions of nonvolatile substances.

aq·ua·gen·ic pru·ri·tus (ahk'wă-jen'ik prū-rī'tŭs) Intense itching produced by brief contact with water at any temperature without visible changes in the skin.

aq·ue·duct (ahk'wă-dŭkt) [TA] A conduit or canal. SYN aqueductus [TA].

aq·ue·duc·tus, pl. **aq·ue·duc·tus** (ahk'wĕ-dŭk'tŭs) [TA] SYN aqueduct.

a·que·ous (ā'kwē-ŭs) Watery; of, like, or containing water.

a·que·ous hu·mor (ā'kwē-ŭs hyū'mŏr) [TA] The watery fluid that fills the anterior chamber of the eye.

a·que·ous so·lu·tion (AS, A.S.) (ā'kwē-ŭs sŏ-lū'shŭn) Liquid containing water as solvent (e.g., lime water, rose water, saline solution), and many solutions intended for intravenous administration.

♻ **arab-** Combining form meaning gum arabic or similar gummy substances.

ar·a·chid·ic ac·id (ar'ă-kid'ik as'id) A saturated fatty acid in peanut oil, butter, and other fats. SYN *N*-eicosanoic acid, *N*-icosanoic acid.

ar·a·chi·don·ic ac·id (AA) (ar'ă-ki-don'ik as'id) An unsaturated fatty acid, usually essential in nutrition; the biologic precursor of the prostaglandins, the thromboxanes, and the leukotrienes (collectively known as eicosanoids).

a·rach·no·dac·ty·ly, a·rach·no·dac·ty·li·a (ă-rak'nō-dak'ti-lē, -dak-til'ē-ă) A condition in which the hands and fingers, and often the feet and toes, are abnormally long and slender; a characteristic of Marfan and other hereditary syndromes. SYN spider finger.

a·rach·noid (ă-rak'noyd) A delicate fibrous membrane forming the middle of the three coverings (i.e., meninges) of the central nervous system.

ar·ach·noi·dal (ar'ak-noy'dăl) Relating to the arachnoid membrane, or arachnoidea.

a·rach·noid cyst (ă-rak'noyd sist) A fluid-filled cyst lined with arachnoid mater, frequently situated near the lateral aspect of the lateral sulcus; usually congenital in origin.

a·rach·noid gran·u·la·tions (ă-rak'noyd gran-yū-lā'shŭnz) [TA] Tufted prolongations of pia-arachnoid, composed of numerous arachnoid villi that penetrate the dural sinuses and effect transfer of cerebrospinal fluid to the venous system. SYN granulationes arachnoideales [TA], pacchionian bodies.

a·rach·noid·i·tis (ă-rak'noy-dī'tis) Inflammation of the arachnoid membrane.

a·rach·noid vil·li (ă-rak'noyd vil'ī) Tufted prolongations of pia-arachnoid that protrude through the meningeal layer of the dura mater and have a thin limiting membrane. SEE ALSO arachnoid granulations.

Aran-Du·chenne dis·ease (ah-rahn' dū-shen' di-zēz') SYN amyotrophic lateral sclerosis.

ar·bor, pl. **ar·bo·res** (ahr'bŏr) ANATOMY Any treelike structure with branchings.

ar·bo·ri·za·tion (ahr'bŏr-ī-zā'shŭn) The terminal branching of nerve fibers or blood vessels in a treelike pattern.

ar·bor vi·tae (ahr'bŏr vī'tē) [TA] Arborescent appearance of gray and white matter in sagittal sections of the cerebellum.

ar·bo·vi·rus (ahr'bō-vī'rŭs) A name for a large, heterogeneous group of RNA viruses. There are more than 500 species and cause yellow fever and other diseases.

arc (ahrk) **1.** A curved line or segment of a circle. **2.** Continuous luminous passage of an electric current in a gas or vacuum between two or more separated carbon or other electrodes.

Ar·can·o·bac·te·ri·um (ahr-kā'nō-bak-tēr'ē-ŭm) A genus of nonmotile, facultatively anaerobic bacteria containing gram-positive slender irregular rods, sometimes showing clubbed ends; obligate parasites of the pharynx in farm animals and humans.

arch (ahrch) [TA] Any structure resembling a bent bow or an arch; an arc. ANATOMY any vaulted or archlike structure. SYN arcus [TA].

arch-, arche-, archi-, archo- 1. Combining forms meaning primordial, ancestral, first, chief, or extreme. 2. DENTISTRY denoting the maxillary or mandibular arch.

arch•en•ter•on (arhk-en′ter-on) SYN primordial gut.

ar•che•type (ahr′kĕ-tīp) 1. A primordial structural plan from which various modifications have evolved. 2. PSYCHOLOGY C.G. Jung's term for structural manifestation of the collective unconscious. SYN imago (2).

ar•chi•cer•e•bel•lum (ahr′ki-ser′ĕ-bel′ŭm) [TA] The small, phylogenetically oldest portion of the cerebellum.

ar•chi•cor•tex (ahr′ki-kōr′teks) [TA] 1. Typically, the phylogenetically older parts of the cerebral cortex. 2. More specifically, the cortex forming the hippocampus. SEE ALSO cerebral cortex.

Ar•chi•me•des prin•ci•ple (ahr-ki-mē′dēz prin′si-pĕl) Tenet that a body placed in liquid is buoyed up by a force equal to the weight of the liquid displaced.

arch•wire (ahrch′wīr) A device consisting of various types of wires from which the dental arch will take its shape, conforming to the alveolar or dental arch, used as an anchorage in correcting irregularities in the position of the teeth.

ar•ci•form (ahr′si-fōrm) SYN arcuate.

ar•cu•ate ar•ci•form (ahr′kyū-ăt ahr′si-fōrm) Denoting a form that is arched or has the shape of a bow. SYN arciform.

ar•cu•ate fi•bers (ahrk′yū-ăt fī′bĕrz) Nervous or tendinous fibers passing in the form of an arch from one part to another.

ar•cu•ate line (ahr′kyū-ăt līn) An arching or bow-shaped line. SYN linea arcuata [TA].

ar•cu•ate sco•to•ma (ahr′kyū-ăt skō-tō′mă) Ocular area extending from the blind spot and arching into the nasal field following the lines of retinal nerve fibers.

ar•cu•ate zone (ahr′kyū-ăt zōn) The inner third of the basilar membrane of the cochlear duct extending from the tympanic lip of the osseous spiral lamina to the outer pillar cell of the spiral organ (organ of Corti). SYN zona arcuata.

ar•cu•a•tion (ahr′kyū-ā′shŭn) A bending or curvature.

ar•cus se•ni•lis (ahr′kŭs sĕ-nil′is) An opaque, grayish ring at the periphery of the cornea just within the sclerocorneal junction; frequent finding in old people. SYN gerontoxon.

ar•e•a (a), pl. **ar•e•ae** (ār′ē-ă, -ē) [TA] 1. Any circumscribed surface or space. 2. All of the part supplied by a given artery or nerve. 3. A part of an organ having a special function, as the motor area of the brain. SEE ALSO regio, region, space, spatium, zone.

a•re•flex•i•a (ā-rĕ-flek′sē-ă) Absence of reflexes.

A•re•na•vi•ri•dae (ă-rē-nă-vir′i-dē) A family of more than 15 RNA viruses, many of which are natural parasites of rodents.

A•re•na•vi•rus (ă-rē′nă-vī′rŭs) A genus in the family Arenaviridae that is associated with lymphocytic choriomeningitis and a number of hemorrhagic fevers.

a•re•o•la, pl. **a•re•o•lae** (ă-rē′ō-lă, -lē)- 1. Any small area. 2. One of the spaces or interstices in areolar tissue. 3. A pigmented, depigmented, or erythematous zone surrounding a papule, pustule, wheal, or cutaneous neoplasm. SYN halo (3).

a•re•o•lar glands (ă-rē′ō-lăr glandz) A number of small mammary glands forming small rounded projections from the surface of the areola of the breast; they enlarge with pregnancy and during lactation secrete a substance presumed to resist chapping.

ar•ga•sid (ahr′gă-sid) Common name for members of the family Argasidae.

Ar·gas·i·dae (ahr-gas′i-dē) Family of soft ticks; so-called because of their wrinkled, leathery, tuberculated appearance that fills out when the tick is engorged with blood.

ar·gen·taf·fin, ar·gen·taf·fine (ahr-jen′tă-fin, -fēn) Pertaining to cells or tissue elements that reduce silver ions in solution, thereby becoming stained brown or black.

ar·gi·nase (ahr′ji-nās) Liver enzyme that catalyzes hydrolysis of L-arginine to L-ornithine and urea; key enzyme of the urea cycle.

ar·gi·nine (ahr′ji-nēn) An amino acid occurring among the hydrolysis products of proteins, particularly abundant in the basic proteins such as histones and protamines.

ar·gon la·ser (ahr′gon lā′zĕr) Laser used for ophthalmic procedures, consisting of photons in the blue (488 nm) or green (514 nm) spectrum.

Ar·gyll Ro·bert·son pu·pil (ahr′gĭl rob′ĕrt-sŏn pyū′pil) A form of reflex iridoplegia characterized by miosis, irregular shape, and a loss of the direct and consensual pupillary reflex to light, with normal pupillary constriction to a near vision effort (light-near dissociation).

ar·gyr·ia, ar·gy·rism, ar·gy·ro·sis (ahr-jir′ē-a, ahr′jir-izm, -jir-ō′sis) A slate-gray or bluish discoloration of the skin and deep tissues due to the deposit of silver, occurring after medicinal administration of a soluble silver salt.

ar·ith·me·tic mean (ar′ith-met′ik mēn) The mean calculated by adding a set of values and then dividing the sum by the number of values. SYN average (2).

arm (ahrm) [TA] **1.** The segment of the upper limb between the shoulder and the elbow; colloquially, the whole upper limb. SYN brachium (1) [TA], brachio- (1). **2.** An anatomic extension resembling an arm. **3.** A specifically shaped and positioned extension of a removable partial denture framework.

arm cyl·in·der cast (ahrm sil′in-dĕr kast) A plaster cast that encases the upper limb to provide stabilization.

ar·ni·ca (ahr′ni-kă) (*A. montana*) Herbal agent of purported value in therapy for muscular pain and in wound healing. Serious reactions in children reported after overingestion. SYN leopard bane, mountain daisy, wolf bane.

Ar·nold re·flex (ahr′nŏld rē′fleks) Coughing or discomfort resulting from touching the external auditory meatus during cerumen extraction or the insertion of earplugs, earmolds, or hearing aids.

aro·ma·ther·a·py (ă-rō′mă-thār′ă-pē) Use of essential oils through inhalation or direct application to promote healing and well-being.

ar·o·mat·ic (ār′ō-mat′ik) **1.** Having an agreeable, somewhat pungent, spicy odor. **2.** One of a group of vegetable drugs having a fragrant odor and slightly stimulant properties.

a·rou·sal (ă-row′zăl) State of heightened level of consciousness or awareness.

a·rou·sal in·dex (ă-row′zăl in′deks) A measurement calculated from sleep disruptions observed during a sleep study.

ar·rec·tor, pl. **ar·rec·to·res** (ă-rek′tōr, ă-rek-tō′rēz) SYN erector.

ar·rest (ă-rest′) **1.** To stop, check, or restrain. **2.** A stoppage; interference with, or checking of, the regular course of a disease, a symptom, or the performance of a function.

ar·rest of la·bor (ă-rest′ lā′bŏr) Absence of progress of active labor (as defined by cervical dilation and descent of the presenting part) for 2 hours or longer.

ar·rhyth·mi·a (arry) (ā-ridh′mē-ă) Loss or abnormality of rhythm; denoting especially an irregularity of the heartbeat. Cf. dysrhythmia.

ar·rhyth·mo·gen·ic (ă-ridh′mō-jen′ik) Capable of inducing cardiac arrhythmias. SYN dysrhythmogenic.

ar·se·nic (As) (ahr′sĕ-nik) A metallic element, atomic no. 33, atomic wt. 74.92159; forms a number of poisonous compounds, some of which are used in medicine.

ar·sine (ahr′sēn) A cell and blood poison,

many organic derivatives of which have been used in chemical warfare. SYN arsenic trihydride, arseniureted hydrogen, arsenous hydride.

arteri- (ar-tēr'ē) SEE arterio-.

ar·te·ri·a, gen. and pl. **ar·te·ri·ae (aa)** (ahr-tēr'ē-ă, -ē) [TA] SYN artery.

ar·te·ri·al (ahr-tēr'ē-ăl) Relating to one or more arteries or to the entire system of arteries.

ar·te·ri·al bleed·ing (ahr-tēr'ē-ăl blēd' ing) Loss of blood from a vessel that is carrying oxygenated blood away from the heart.

ar·te·ri·al blood (a) (ahr-tēr'ē-ăl blŭd) Blood that is oxygenated in the lungs, found in the left chambers of the heart and in the arteries.

ar·te·ri·al blood gas test (ahr-tēr'ē-ăl blŭd gas test) Measurement of levels of oxygen and carbon dioxide in blood that is moving away from the heart.

ar·te·ri·al blood pres·sure (ahr-tēr'ē-ăl blŭd presh'ŭr) Measurement of the force of the movement of blood against the vessels that carry blood away from the heart.

ar·te·ri·al cap·il·la·ry (ahr-tēr'ē-ăl kap' i-lar-ē) A capillary opening from an arteriole or metarteriole.

ar·te·ri·al for·ceps (ahr-tēr'ē-ăl fōr' seps) A locking forceps with sloping blades for grasping the end of a blood vessel until a ligature is applied.

ar·te·ri·al in·suf·fi·cien·cy (ahr-tēr'ē-ăl in'sŭ-fish'ĕn-sē) Inadequate action of the vessels carrying blood away from the heart.

ar·te·ri·al mur·mur (ahr-tēr'ē-ăl mŭr' mŭr) Bruit heard on arterial auscultation.

ar·te·ri·al oc·clu·sive dis·ease (ahr-tēr'ē-ăl ŏ-klū'siv di-zēz') Obstruction of a major artery, resulting in ischemia distal to the obstruction; causes include atherosclerosis, emboli, thrombosis, trauma, and fracture.

ar·te·ri·al pH (ahr-tēr'ē-ăl) Measurement of the acidity and alkalinity of the blood in the arteries carrying blood away from the heart.

ar·te·ri·al ten·sion (ahr-tēr'ē-ăl ten' shŭn) The blood pressure within an artery.

ar·te·ri·ec·to·my (ahr-tēr'ē-ek'tō-mē) Excision of part of an artery.

arterio-, arteri- Combining forms denoting artery.

ar·te·ri·og·ra·phy (ahr-tēr'ē-og'ră-fē) X-ray view of an artery after injection of a radiopaque contrast medium.

ar·te·ri·o·la, pl. **ar·te·ri·o·lae** (ahr-tēr-ē-ō'lă, ahr-tēr-ē-ō'lē) [TA] SYN arteriole.

ar·te·ri·o·lar neph·ro·scler·o·sis (ahr-tēr'ē-ō'lăr nef'rō-skler-ō'sis) Renal scarring due to arteriolar sclerosis resulting from long-standing hypertension.

ar·te·ri·o·lar scle·ro·sis (ahr-tēr'ē-ō' lăr skler-ō'sis) SYN arteriolosclerosis.

ar·te·ri·ole (ahr-tēr'ē-ōl) [TA] A minute artery with a tunica media comprising only one or two layers of smooth muscle cells. SYN arteriola [TA].

ar·te·ri·o·lith (ahr-tēr'ē-ō-lith) A calcareous deposit in an arterial wall or thrombus.

ar·ter·i·o·li·tis (ahr-tēr'ē-ō-lī'tis) Inflammation of the wall of the arterioles.

arteriolo- Combining form indicating the arterioles.

ar·te·ri·o·lo·ne·cro·sis (ahr-tēr'ē-ō'lō-nĕ-krō'sis) SYN necrotizing arteriolitis.

ar·te·ri·o·lo·scle·ro·sis (ahr-tēr'ē-ō'lō-skler-ō'sis) Arteriosclerosis affecting mainly the arterioles, seen especially in chronic hypertension.

ar·te·ri·o·mo·tor (ahr-tēr'ē-ō-mō'tŏr) Causing changes in the caliber of an artery.

ar·te·ri·op·a·thy (ahr-tēr'ē-op'ă-thē) Any disease of the arteries.

ar·te·ri·o·plas·ty (ahr-tēr'ē-ō-plas-tē)

Any operation for the reconstruction of the wall of an artery.

ar·te·ri·o·pres·sor (ahr-tēr′ē-ō-pres′ŏr) Something that increases arterial blood pressure.

ar·te·ri·or·rha·phy (ahr-tēr′ē-ōr′ă-fē) Suture of an artery.

ar·te·ri·or·rhex·is (ahr-tēr′ē-ō-rek′sis) Rupture of an artery.

ar·te·ri·o·scle·ro·sis (ahr-tēr′ē-ō-skler-ō′sis) Hardening of the arteries.

ar·te·ri·o·scle·ro·sis ob·li·te·rans (ahr-tēr′ē-ō-skler-ō′sis ob-lit′ĕr-anz) Arteriosclerosis producing narrowing and occlusion of the arterial lumen.

ar·te·ri·o·ste·no·sis (ahr-tēr′ē-ō-stĕ-nō′sis) Narrowing of the caliber of an artery, either temporary, through vasoconstriction, or permanent, through arteriosclerosis.

ar·te·ri·o·ve·nous (A-V, AV) (ahr-tēr′ē-ō-vē′nŭs) Relating to both an artery and a vein or to both arteries and veins in general.

ar·te·ri·o·ve·nous an·as·to·mo·sis (ava) (ahr-tēr′ē-ō-vē′nŭs ă-nas′tŏ-mō′sis) Vessels through which blood is shunted from arterioles to venules without passing through the capillaries.

ar·te·ri·o·ve·nous an·eur·ysm (ahr-tēr′ē-ō-vē′nŭs an′yūr-izm) **1.** A dilated arteriovenous shunt. **2.** Communication between an artery and a vein, sometimes congenital.

ar·te·ri·o·ve·nous fis·tu·la (ahr-tēr′ē-ō-vē′nŭs fis′tyū-lă) An abnormal communication between an artery and a vein, usually resulting in the formation of an arteriovenous aneurysm.

ar·te·ri·o·ve·nous graft (ahr-tēr′ē-ō-vē′nŭs graft) A synthetic tube that connects an artery to a vein.

ar·te·ri·o·ve·nous shunt (ahr-tēr′ē-ō-vē′nŭs shŭnt) The passage of blood directly from arteries to veins, without going through the capillary network.

ar·te·ri·tis (ahr′tĕr-ī′tis) Inflammation or infection involving an artery or arteries.

ar·te·ry (ahr′tĕr-ē) [TA] Thick-walled, muscular blood vessel conveying blood away from the heart and pulsating with each heartbeat. With the exception of the pulmonary and umbilical arteries, the arteries convey red or oxygenated blood. SYN arteria [TA].

ar·thral·gia (ahr-thral′jē-ă) Pain in a joint, especially one not inflammatory in character. SYN arthrodynia.

ar·thral·gic (ahr-thral′jik) Relating to or affected with arthralgia. SYN arthrodynic.

ar·threc·to·my (ahr-threk′tŏ-mē) Excision of a joint.

ar·thres·the·si·a (ahr-thres-thē′zē-ă) SYN articular sensibility.

ar·thrit·ic (ahr-thrit′ik) Relating to arthritis.

ar·thri·tis, pl. **ar·thrit·i·des** (ahr-thrī′tis, ahr-thrit′i-dēz) Inflammation of a joint or a state characterized by inflammation of joints. SYN articular rheumatism.

ar·thri·tis mu·ti·lans (ahr-thrī′tis myū′ti-lanz) Chronic rheumatoid arthritis in which osteolysis occurs with extensive destruction of the joint cartilages and bony surfaces with pronounced deformities, chiefly of the hands and feet. SYN chronic absorptive arthritis.

ar·thro·cele (ahr′thrō-sēl) **1.** Hernia of the synovial membrane through the capsule of a joint. **2.** Any swelling of a joint.

ar·thro·cen·te·sis (ahr′thrō-sen-tē′sis) Aspiration of fluid from a joint performed by needle puncture.

ar·thro·chon·dri·tis (ahr′thrō-kon-drī′tis) Inflammation of an articular cartilage.

ar·thro·cla·si·a (ahr′thrō-klā′zē-ă) The forcible breaking up of the adhesions in ankylosis.

ar·throd·e·sis (ahr-throd′ĕ-sis) The stiffening of a joint by operative means. SYN syndesis.

ar·thro·di·al joint (ahr-thrō′dē-ăl joynt) SYN plane joint.

ar•thro•dys•pla•si•a (ahr′thrō-dis-plā′zē-ă) Hereditary congenital defect of joint development.

ar•thro•en•dos•co•py (ahr′thrō-en-dos′kŏ-pē) SYN arthroscopy.

ar•throg•ra•phy (ahr-throg′ră-fē) Radiography of a joint after injecting one or more contrast media into the joint.

ar•thro•gry•po•sis (ahr′thrō-gri-pō′sis) Congenital defect of the limbs characterized by contractures of multiple joints.

ar•thro•lith (ahr′thrō-lith) A loose body in a joint.

ar•throl•o•gy (ahr-throl′ŏ-jē) The branch of anatomy concerned with the joints. SYN syndesmologia, synosteology.

ar•thro•oph•thal•mop•a•thy (ahr′thrō-of′thal-mop′ă-thē) Disease affecting joints and eyes.

ar•throp•a•thy (ahr-throp′ă-thē) Any disease affecting a joint.

ar•thro•plas•ty (ahr′thrō-plas-tē) 1. Creation of an artificial joint to correct ankylosis. 2. An operation to restore as far as possible the integrity and functional power of a joint.

ar•thro•pod (ahr′thrō-pod) A member of the phylum Arthropoda.

Ar•throp•o•da (ahr-throp′ŏ-dă) A phylum of the Metazoa that includes the classes Crustacea (crabs, shrimp, crayfish, lobsters), Insecta, Arachnida (spiders, scorpions, mites, ticks), Chilopoda (centipedes), Diplopoda (millipedes), Merostomata (horseshoe crabs), and various other extinct or lesser known groups.

ar•thro•py•o•sis (ahr′thrō-pī-ō′sis) Suppuration in a joint.

ar•thro•scle•ro•sis (ahr′thrō-skler-ō′sis) Stiffness of the joints.

ar•thro•scope (ahr′thrō-skōp) An endoscope for examining the internal anatomy of a joint.

ar•thros•co•py (ahr-thros′kŏ-pē) Endoscopic examination of the interior of a joint. SYN arthroendoscopy.

ar•thro•sis, pl. **ar•thro•ses** (ahr-thrō′sis, -sēz) 1. SYN joint. 2. A degenerative disorder of a joint.

ar•thros•to•my (ahr-thros′tŏ-mē) Establishment of a temporary opening into a joint cavity.

ar•thro•sy•no•vi•tis (ahr′thrō-sin-ō-vī′tis) Inflammation of the synovial membrane of a joint.

ar•throx•e•sis (ahr-throk′sĕ-sis) Removal of diseased tissue from a joint by means of a sharp spoon or other scraping instrument.

ar•tic•u•lar (ahr-tik′yū-lăr) Relating to a joint.

ar•tic•u•lar cap•sule (ahr-tik′yū-lăr kap′sŭl) SYN joint capsule.

ar•tic•u•lar disc (ahr-tik′yū-lăr disk) [TA] A plate or ring of fibrocartilage attached to the joint capsule and separating the articular surfaces of the bones for a varying distance.

ar•tic•u•lar frac•ture (ahr-tik′yū-lăr frak′shŭr) Breakage involving the joint surface of a bone.

ar•tic•u•lar head (ahr-tik′yū-lăr hed) [TA] Generic term for the rounded articulating surface of a long bone or process received by an articular fossa. SYN caput articulare [TA].

ar•tic•u•lar mus•cle (ahr-tik′yū-lăr mŭs′ĕl) A muscle that inserts directly onto the capsule of a joint, acting to retract the capsule in certain movements.

ar•tic•u•lar nerve (ahr-tik′yū-lăr nĕrv) A branch of a nerve supplying a joint.

ar•tic•u•lar sen•si•bil•i•ty (ahr-tik′yū-lăr sen′si-bil′i-tē) Appreciation of sensation in joint surfaces. SYN arthresthesia, joint sense.

ar•tic•u•late (ahr-tik′yū-lăt, -lāt) 1. Capable of distinct and connected speech. 2. To join or connect together loosely to allow motion between the parts. 3. To speak distinctly and connectedly.

ar•tic•u•la•ti•o, pl. **ar•tic•u•la•ti•o•nes** (ahr-tik-ū-lā′shē-ō, -nēz) [TA] SYN synovial joint.

ar·tic·u·la·tion (ahr-tik´yū-lā´shŭn) **1.** SYN joint. **2.** A loose juncture or connection that permits motion between parts. **3.** The process of moving and coordinating oral, laryngeal, and pharyngeal structures to produce speech.

ar·tic·u·la·tion dis·or·der (ahr-tik´yū-lā´shŭn dis-ōr´dĕr) Any error in pronunciation including phoneme omissions, substitutions, distortions, and additions.

ar·ti·fact, ar·te·fact (ahr´ti-fakt) **1.** Anything (especially in a histologic specimen or a graphic record) that is caused by the technique used or is not a natural occurrence but is merely incidental. **2.** A skin lesion produced or perpetuated by self-inflicted action, such as scratching in dermatitis artefacta.

ar·ti·fi·cial an·ky·lo·sis (ahr´ti-fish´ăl ang´ki-lō´sis) SYN arthrodesis.

ar·ti·fi·cial crown (ahr´ti-fish´ăl krown) Restoration and covering of the major part of the entire coronal part of a natural tooth.

ar·ti·fi·cial fe·ver (ahr´ti-fish´ăl fē´vĕr) SYN pyretotherapy.

ar·ti·fi·cial heart (ahr´ti-fish´ăl hahrt) A mechanical pump used to replace the function of a damaged heart, either temporarily or as a permanent prosthesis.

ar·ti·fi·cial in·sem·i·na·tion (AI) (ahr´ti-fish´ăl in-sem´i-nā´shŭn) Introduction of semen into the vagina other than by coitus.

ar·ti·fi·cial in·sem·i·na·tion do·nor (AID) (ahr´ti-fish´ăl in-sem´i-nā´shŭn dō´nŏr) A man who provides semen used to impregnate a woman whose spouse is incapable of providing viable sperms.

ar·ti·fi·cial in·tel·li·gence (AI) (ahr´ti-fish´ăl in-tel´i-jĕns) Branch of computer science in which attempts are made to replicate human intellectual functions.

ar·ti·fi·cial kid·ney (ahr´ti-fish´ăl kid´nē) SYN hemodialyzer.

ar·ti·fi·cial la·bor (ahr´ti-fish´ăl lā´bŏr) Induced labor.

ar·ti·fi·cial lar·ynx (ahr´ti-fish´ăl lar´-

ingks) Mechanical device used to create alaryngeal speech.

ar·ti·fi·cial ra·di·o·ac·tiv·i·ty (ahr´ti-fish´ăl rā´dē-ō-ak-tiv´i-tē) The radioactivity of isotopes created by the bombardment of naturally occurring isotopes by subatomic particles, or high levels of x- or gamma radiation.

ar·ti·fi·cial tears (AT) (ahr´ti-fish´ăl tērz) Mixtures of fluid compounds used to substitute for naturally produced tears.

ar·y·ep·i·glot·tic (AE) (ar´ē-ep-i-glot´ik) Relating to the arytenoid cartilage and the epiglottis.

ar·y·ep·i·glot·tic fold, ar·y·te·no·ep·i·glot·tid·e·an fold (ar´ē-ep-i-glot´ik fōld, ar-it´ē-nō-ep´i-glot-id´ē-ăn fōld) [TA] A prominent fold of mucous membrane stretching between the lateral margin of the epiglottis and the arytenoid cartilage on either side. SYN plica aryepiglottica [TA].

ar·yl·sul·fat·ase (ar´il-sŭl´fă-tās) An enzyme that cleaves phenol sulfates, including cerebroside sulfates (i.e., a phenol sulfate + H_2O → a phenol + sulfate anion). Some arylsulfatases are inhibited by sulfate (type II) and some are not (type I). SYN sulfatase (2).

ar·y·te·noid (ar-i-tē´noyd) [TA] Denoting a cartilage (arytenoid cartilage) and muscles (oblique and transverse arytenoid muscles) of the larynx.

ar·y·te·noid car·ti·lage (ar-i-tē´noyd kahr´ti-lăj) [TA] One of a pair of small triangular pyramidal laryngeal cartilages that articulate with the lamina of the cricoid cartilage. SYN cartilago arytenoidea [TA], triquetrous cartilage (2).

ar·y·te·noi·do·pex·y (ar´i-tē-noy´dō-pek´sē) Excision of an arytenoid cartilage, usually in bilateral vocal fold paralysis, to improve breathing.

ASA Abbreviation for acetylsalicylic acid; American Society of Anesthesiologists.

ASA class·i·fi·ca·tion (klas´i-fi-kā´shŭn) SYN Dripps classification.

as·bes·tos (as-bes´tŏs) Product obtained from fibrous hydrated silicates divided into amphiboles and serpentines; inhalation of asbestos particles can cause asbestosis and cancer of the lung and pleura.

as·bes·tos bo·dies (as-bes´tŏs bod´ēz) Ferruginous bodies with core asbestos fibers; hallmark of exposure to asbestos.

as·bes·to·sis (as-bes-tō´sis) Pneumoconiosis due to inhalation of asbestos fibers suspended in the ambient air; sometimes complicated by pleural mesothelioma or bronchogenic carcinoma.

As·ca·ris (as´kă-ris) A genus of large, heavy-bodied roundworms parasitic in the small intestine; abundant in humans and many other vertebrates.

as·cend·ing (ă-send´ing) Moving in an upward direction.

as·cend·ing de·gen·er·a·tion (ă-send´ing dĕ-jen´ĕr-ā´shŭn) Retrograde degeneration of an injured nerve fiber.

as·cend·ing neu·ri·tis (ă-send´ing nūr-ī´tis) Inflammation progressing upward along a nerve trunk in a direction away from the periphery.

as·cer·tain·ment (as´sĕr-tān´mĕnt) In epidemiologic and genetic research, the method by which a person, pedigree, or cluster is brought to the attention of an investigator.

Asch·er syn·drome (ahsh´ĕr sin´drōm) A condition in which a congenital double lip is associated with blepharochalasis and nontoxic thyroid gland enlargement.

as·ci·tes (ă-sī´tēz) Accumulation of serous fluid in the peritoneal cavity. SYN hydroperitoneum, hydroperitonia.

As·co·li test (as-kō´ē test) Method to detect anthrax that uses a precipitin test with antiserum and tissue extract.

As·co·my·ce·tes (as´kō-mī-sē´tēz) A class of fungi characterized by the presence of asci and ascospores. Such fungi have generally two distinct reproductive phases, the sexual or perfect stage and the asexual or imperfect stage.

as·cor·bic ac·id (ă-skōr´bik as´id) Used in preventing scurvy, as a strong reducing agent, and as an antioxidant. SYN vitamin C.

-ase A suffix denoting an enzyme; attached to the end of the name of the substance (substrate) on which the enzyme acts; e.g., phosphatase, lipase, proteinase. May also indicate the reaction catalyzed, e.g., decarboxylase, oxidase.

a·sep·sis (ā-sep´sis) A condition in which living pathogenic organisms are absent; a state of sterility (q.v.).

a·sep·tic (ā-sep´tik) *Do not confuse this word with antiseptic.* Marked by or relating to asepsis.

a·sep·tic fe·ver (ā-sep´tik fē´vĕr) Fever accompanied by malaise caused by absorption of dead but noninfected tissue following an injury.

a·sep·tic gauze (ā-sep´tik gawz) Sterilized gauze.

a·sep·tic ne·cro·sis (ā-sep´tik nĕ-krō´sis) Death or decay of tissue due to local ischemia in the absence of infection. SYN avascular necrosis.

a·sep·tic sur·ge·ry (ā-sep´tik sŭr´jĕr-ē) The performance of an operation with sterilized hands, instruments, and environment, taking precautions against the introduction of infectious microorganisms from without.

a·sep·tic tech·nique (ā-sep´tik tek-nēk´) Health care procedures designed to reduce the risk of transmission of pathogenic microorganisms to patients.

a·sex·u·al (ā-sek´shū-ăl) **1.** Referring to reproduction without nuclear fusion in an organism. **2.** Having no sexual desire or interest.

a·sex·u·al gen·er·a·tion (ā-sek´shū-ăl jen-ĕr-ā´shŭn) Reproduction by fission, gemmation, or in any other way without union of the male and female cells, or conjugation. SEE ALSO parthenogenesis. SYN heterogenesis (2), nonsexual generation.

Ash·er·man syn·drome (ash´ĕr-măn sin´drōm) SYN traumatic amenorrhea.

Ash·worth scale (ash´wŏrth skāl) An

0–4 ordinal scale used to apply a grade to increased muscle tone.

a·si·al·ism (ā-sī′ă-lizm) Absence of saliva.

A·si·an flu (ā′zhăn flū) Influenza caused by H_2N_2 influenza A that was responsible for over 60,000 deaths in the United States during the 1957 to 1958 influenza pandemic.

a·so·cial (ā-sō′shăl) Not social; withdrawn from society.

a·so·ma, pl. **a·so·ma·ta** (ā-sō′mă, -sō′ mă-tă) A fetus with only a rudimentary body.

as·par·a·gi·nase (as-par′ă-ji-nās) An enzyme catalyzing the hydrolysis of L-asparagine to L-aspartate and ammonia.

as·par·tate ki·nase (as-pahr′tāt kī′nās) An enzyme catalyzing phosphorylation by ATP of L-aspartate to form 4-phospho-L-aspartate (β-aspartyl phosphate) and ADP.

as·pect (as′pekt) **1.** The manner of appearance; looks. **2.** The side of an object that is exposed to a view from a designated direction.

As·per·ger syn·drome (ahs′bĕr-gĕr sin′ drŏm) Developmental disorder that is a part of the continuum of autism symptoms typically including the need to adhere to strict routines and rituals as well as impaired abilities with social interactions.

as·per·gil·lo·ma (as′pĕr-ji-lō′mă) **1.** An infectious granuloma caused by the fungus *Aspergillus*. **2.** A variety of bronchopulmonary aspergillosis; a ball-like mass of *Aspergillus fumigatus* colonizing an existing cavity in the lung.

a·sper·mi·a (ā-spĕr′mē-ă) Inability to produce or ejaculate semen.

as·phyx·i·a (as-fik′sē-ă) Impaired or absent exchange of oxygen and carbon dioxide on a ventilatory basis; combined hypercapnia and hypoxia or anoxia.

as·phyx·i·a·ting thor·a·cic dys·tro·phy (as-fik′sē-āt-ing thŏr-as′ik dis′trŏ-fē) Hereditary hypoplasia of the thorax, associated with pelvic skeletal abnormality.

as·phyx·i·a·tion (as-fik′sē-ā′shŭn) The production of, or the state of, asphyxia.

as·pi·rate (asp.) (as′pir-āt, -ăt) **1.** To remove by aspiration. **2.** To inhale into the airways foreign particulate material, such as vomitus. **3.** Foreign body, food, gastric contents, or fluid, including saliva, which is inhaled.

as·pi·rat·ing needle (as′pir-āt-ing nē′ dĕl) Hollow needle used to withdraw fluid from a cavity, when combined with an aspirator tube attached to one end.

as·pi·ra·tion (as-pir-ā′shŭn) **1.** Removal, by suction, of a gas or fluid from a body cavity, from unusual accumulations, or from a container. **2.** Inhalation into the airways of fluid or foreign body (e.g., vomitus, food, fluid).

as·pi·ra·tion bi·op·sy (as-pir-ā′shŭn bī′op-sē) SYN needle biopsy.

as·pi·ra·tion pneu·mo·ni·a (as-pir-ā′ shŭn nū-mō′nē-ă) Bronchopneumonia due to the inhalation of foreign material, usually food particles or vomitus, into the bronchi.

as·pi·ra·tor (as′pir-ā-tŏr) An apparatus for removing fluid by aspiration from any of the body cavities.

as·pi·rin (ASA) (as′pĭr-in) A widely used analgesic, antipyretic, and antiinflammatory agent; also used as an antiplatelet agent. Although a generic in the U.S., aspirin remains a proprietary name in other countries. SYN acetylsalicylic acid.

a·sple·ni·a (ā-splē′nē-ă) Congenital or surgical absence of the spleen (e.g., after surgical removal).

as·sault (ă-sawlt′) Any sort of physical or psychological attack on another person.

as·say (as′ā) **1.** Test of purity; trial. **2.** To examine; to subject to analysis. **3.** The quantitative or qualitative evaluation of a substance for impurities, toxicity, or other attributes; the results of such an evaluation.

as·ser·tive train·ing (ă-sĕr′tiv trăn′ing) Behavior modification therapy in which

as·si·mi·late (ă-sim´ĭ-lāt) **1.** Gradual personal adaptation to a specific situation; either physiologic or psychological. **2.** Incorporating digested materials from food into the tissues.

as·sist·ed cir·cu·la·tion (ă-sis´tĕd sĭr´kyū-lā´shŭn) Application of external devices to improve pressure, flow, or both in the heart or arteries.

as·sist·ed con·cep·tion (ă-sis´tĕd kŏn-sep´shŭn) Creation of an embryo through the use of medical procedures.

as·sist·ed re·pro·duc·tive tech·nol·o·gy (ART) (ă-sis´tĕd rē-prō-duk´tiv tek-nol´ŏ-jē) Techniques for manipulating oocytes and sperms to overcome infertility.

as·sist·ed su·i·cide (ă-sis´tĕd sū´i-sīd) A process in which a patient dies with compliance from a health care professional.

as·so·ci·at·ed an·tag·o·nist (ă-sō´sē-āt-ĕd an-tag´ŏ-nist) A muscle or muscle group that pulls in nearly opposite directions but that, when acting together, move the part in a path between their diverging lines of action.

as·so·ci·a·ted move·ment (ă-sō´sē-āt-ĕd mūv´mĕnt) A motion seen in the contralateral limb when increased concentration, muscle tone, or effort is exerted.

as·so·ci·a·tion (ă-sō´sē-ā´shŭn) **1.** A connection of people, things, or ideas by some common factor. **2.** A movement seen in the opposite limb when increased concentration, tone, or effort is exerted (e.g., increased elbow flexion in one arm while the other moves).

as·so·ci·a·tion test (ă-sō´sē-ā´shŭn test) A word (i.e., stimulus word) is spoken to the subject, who is to reply immediately with another word (reaction word) suggested by the first; used as a diagnostic aid in psychiatry and psychology.

as·so·ci·a·tive a·pha·si·a (ă-sō´sē-ă-tiv ă-fā´zē-ă) SYN conduction aphasia.

as·so·ci·a·tive play (ă-sō´sē-ă-tiv plā) Play in which each child participates in a separate activity, but with the cooperation and assistance of the others.

as·sort·a·tive mat·ing (ă-sŏrt´ă-tiv māt´ing) Selection of a mate with preference for (or aversion to) a particular genotype, i.e., nonrandom mating.

as·sort·ment (ă-sŏrt´mĕnt) In genetics, the relationship between nonallelic genetic traits that are transmitted from parent to child more or less independently in accordance with the degree of linkage between the respective loci.

a·sta·si·a (ă-stā´zē-ă) Inability, through muscular incoordination, to stand.

a·sta·si·a·a·ba·si·a (ă-stā´zē-ă-ă-bā´zē-ă) Inability to stand or walk in a normal manner. SYN Blocq disease.

a·stat·ic sei·zure (ā-stat´ik sē´zhŭr) Seizure causing loss of erect posture.

as·te·a·to·sis (as´tē-ă-tō´sis) Diminished or arrested secretion of the sebaceous glands.

as·ter (as´tĕr) SYN astrosphere.

as·te·ri·on (as-tē´rē-on) [TA] A craniometric point at the junction of the lambdoid, occipitomastoid, and parietomastoid sutures.

as·ter·ix·is (as-tĕr-ik´sis) Involuntary jerking movements, especially in the hands, due to arrhythmic lapses of sustained posture. SYN flapping tremor.

a·ster·nal (ā-stĕr´năl) **1.** Not related to or connected with the sternum. **2.** Without a sternum.

a·ster·ni·a (ā-stĕr´nē-ă) Congenital absence of the sternum.

as·ter·oid body (as´tĕr-oyd bod´ē) **1.** An eosinophilic inclusion resembling a star with delicate radiating lines, occurring in a vacuolated area of cytoplasm of a multinucleated giant cell. **2.** A structure that is characteristic of sporotrichosis when found in the skin or secondary lesions of this mycosis; in tissue, it surrounds the 3- to 5-mcm (diameter) ovoid yeast of *Sporothrix schenkii*.

as·ter·oid hy·a·lo·sis (as´tĕr-oyd hī´ă-lō´sis) Small refractive spheric bodies in the vitreous (composed of calcium soaps), visible ophthalmoscopically.

as·the·ni·a (as-thē′nē-ă) Weakness or debility. SYN adynamia (1).

as·the·no·zo·o·sper·mi·a (as′thē-nō-zō-ō-spĕrm′ē-ă) Loss or reduction of mobility of sperms, frequently associated with infertility.

asth·ma (az′mă) An inflammatory disease of the lungs characterized by reversible (in most cases) inflammation and narrowing of the airway.

asth·mat·ic breath·ing (az-mat′ik brēdh′ing) Difficulty with breathing typically characterized by wheezing; most generally triggered by an allergic reaction.

asth·mat·ic bron·chi·tis (AB) (az-mat′ik brong-kī′tis) Disorder that causes or aggravates bronchospasm.

as·tig·mat·ic (as′tig-mat′ik) Relating to or suffering from astigmatism.

as·tig·mat·ic lens (as′tig-mat′ik lenz) SYN cylindric lens.

a·stig·ma·tism (ă-stig′mă-tizm) **1.** A lens or optic system having different refractivity in different meridians. **2.** A condition of unequal curvatures along the different meridians in one or more of the refractive surfaces (cornea, anterior or posterior surface of the lens) of the eye, in consequence of which the rays from a luminous point are not focused at a single point on the retina. SYN astigmia.

a·sto·mi·a (ă-stō′mē-ă) Congenital absence of the mouth.

as·trag·a·lec·to·my (as-trag′ă-lek′tŏ-mē) Removal of the astragalus or talus.

as·trag·a·lus (ă-strag′ă-lŭs) SYN talus.

as·tral (as′trăl) Relating to an astrosphere.

as·trin·gent (ă-strin′jĕnt) **1.** Causing contraction of the tissues, arrest of secretion, or control of bleeding. **2.** An agent having these effects.

as·tro·blast (as′trō-blast) A primordial cell developing into an astrocyte.

as·tro·blas·to·ma (as′trō-blas-tō′mă) A relatively poorly differentiated glioma composed of young, immature, neoplastic cells of the astrocytic series.

as·tro·cyte (as′trō-sīt) One of the large neuroglia cells of nervous tissue. SYN astroglia, macroglia.

as·tro·cy·to·ma (as′trō-sī-tō′mă) A glioma derived from astrocytes.

as·trog·li·a (as-trog′lē-ă) SYN astrocyte.

As·tro·vi·rus (as′trō-vī′rŭs) A small RNA virus and the only genus in the family Astroviridae; it is associated with diarrhea and is detected in the feces of numerous animals.

a·sym·bo·li·a (ă-sim-bō′lē-ă) Aphasia in which the significance of signs and symbols is not appreciated.

a·sym·met·ric, a·sym·met·ric·al (a) (ă-si-met′rik, -rik-ăl) Not symmetric; denoting a lack of symmetry between two or more like parts.

a·sym·met·ric fe·tal growth re·stric·tion (ă-si-met′rik fē′tăl grōth rĕ-strik′shŭn) Normal fetal head size due to preferential shunting of blood to brain, and decreased abdominal circumference from decreased adipose tissue and liver size.

a·sym·me·try (ă-sim′ĕ-trē) Lack of symmetry; disproportion between two parts normally alike.

a·symp·tom·at·ic neu·ro·sy·phil·is (ă-simp-tŏ-mat′ik nūr′ō-sif′i-lis) Clinically nonapparent (except, possibly, for abnormal pupils) syphilitic meningeal infection, diagnosed by examination of the cerebrospinal fluid.

a·syn·cli·tism (ă-sin′kli-tizm) Absence of synclitism or parallelism.

a·syn·ech·i·a (ă-si-nek′ē-ă) Discontinuity of structure.

a·syn·er·gy, a·syn·er·gi·a (ă-sin′ĕr-jē, ā-sin-ĕr′jē-ă) Lack of coordination among various muscle groups during the performance of complex movements, resulting in loss of skill and speed.

a·sys·to·le, a·sys·to·li·a (ă-sis′tō-lē, -sis-tō′lē-ă) Absence of contractions of the heart.

a•tac•tic a•ba•si•a, a•tax•ic a•ba•si•a (ă-tak´tik ă-bā´zē-ă, ă-tak´sik) Difficulty in walking due to ataxia of the legs.

at•a•rac•tic (at´ăr-ak´tik) Tending to tranquilize.

at•a•rax•i•a, at•a•rax•y (at-ă-rak´sē-ă, -sē) Calmness and peace of mind; tranquility.

at•a•vism (at´ă-vizm) The appearance in an individual of characteristics presumed to have been present in some remote ancestor; a throwback.

a•tax•ia tel•an•gi•ec•ta•si•a (ă-tak´sē-ă tel-an´jē-ek-tā´zē-ă) A slowly progressive multisystem disorder with ataxia appearing with the onset of walking.

a•tax•ic breath•ing (ă-tak´sik brēdh´ing) SYN Biot respiration.

a•tax•i•o•phe•mi•a, a•tax•o•phe•mi•a (ă-tak´sē-ō-fē´mē-ă, -tak´sō-fē´mē-ă) Incoordination of the muscles concerned in speech production.

-ate Suffix used as a replacement for ''-ic acid'' when the acid is neutralized (e.g., sodium acetate) or esterified (e.g., ethyl acetate).

at•el•ec•ta•sis (at-ĕ-lek´tă-sis) Reduction or absence of air in part or all of a lung, with resulting loss of lung volume. SEE ALSO pulmonary collapse.

at•e•lec•tat•ic (at-ĕ-lek-tat´ik) Relating to atelectasis.

a•the•li•a (ă-thē´lē-ă) Congenital absence of the nipples.

ath•er•ec•to•my (ath-ĕr-ek´tŏ-mē) Invasive removal of an atheroma or plaque from an artery.

a•ther•mo•sys•tal•tic (ă-thĕr´mō-sis-tal´tik) Not contracted or constricted by ordinary variations of temperature; said of certain tissues.

athero- Combining form meaning gruellike, soft, pasty materials; atheroma, atheromatous.

ath•er•o•gen•e•sis (ath´ĕr-ō-jen´ĕ-sis) Formation of atheroma, important in the pathogenesis of arteriosclerosis.

ath•er•o•ma (ath´ĕr-ō´mă) The lipid deposits in the intima of arteries, producing a yellow swelling on the endothelial surface.

ath•er•o•ma•to•sis (ath´ĕr-ō-mă-tō´sis) Disease characterized by atheromatous degeneration of the arteries.

ath•er•om•a•tous de•gen•er•a•tion (ath´ĕr-ō´mă-tŭs dĕ-jen´ĕr-ā´shŭn) Focal accumulation of lipid material (atheroma) in the intima and subintimal portion of arteries, eventually resulting in fibrous thickening or calcification.

ath•er•om•a•tous plaque (ath-ĕr-ō´mă-tŭs plak) A well-demarcated yellow area or swelling on the intimal surface of an artery.

ath•er•o•scle•ro•sis (ath´ĕr-ō-skler-ō´sis) Arteriosclerosis characterized by irregularly distributed lipid deposits in the intima of large and medium arteries; such deposits provoke fibrosis and calcification.

ath•er•o•scle•rot•ic an•eu•rysm (ath´ĕr-ō-sler-ot´ik an´yūr-izm) Most common type of aneurysm, occurring in the abdominal aorta and other large arteries, primarily in old people.

ath•er•o•throm•bo•sis (ath´ĕr-ō-throm-bō´sis) Thrombus formation in an atheromatous vessel.

ath•e•to•sis (ath´ĕ-tō´sis) A condition in which there is a constant succession of slow, writhing, involuntary movements of flexion, extension, pronation, and supination of the fingers and hands, and sometimes of the toes and feet. SYN extrapyramidal cerebral palsy, Hammond disease.

ath•lete's foot (ath´lēts fut) SYN tinea pedis.

ath•lete's heart (ath´lēts hahrt) Nonpathologic enlarged heart in athletes reflecting specific adaptation to prolonged training. SEE hypertrophy.

ath•let•ic a•men•or•rhe•a (ath-let´ik ā-men´ŏr-ē´ă) Irregularities in the menstrual cycle presenting as either oligomenorrhea (35–90 days between menses) or secondary amenorrhea (cessation of menstrual cycles for at least 3 months) caused by intense athletic training or disordered eating behavior.

ath·le·tic train·er, ath·le·tic ther·a·pist (ath-let′ik trān′ẽr, thār′ă-pist) One who is skilled in the prevention, evaluation, treatment, and rehabilitation of athletic injuries.

a·thy·mi·a (ā-thī′mē-ă) **1.** PSYCHOLOGY absence of affect or emotion; morbid impassivity. **2.** Congenital absence of the thymus, often with associated immunodeficiency.

a·thy·re·a (ă-thī′rē-ă) **1.** SYN hypothyroidism. **2.** SYN athyroidism.

athy·roid·ism (ā-thī′royd-izm) Congenital absence of the thyroid gland or suppression or absence of its hormonal secretion.

at·lan·tad (at-lan′tad) In a direction toward the atlas.

at·lan·tal (at-lan′tăl) Relating to the atlas.

atlanto-, atlo- Combining forms denoting the atlas (the bone that supports the head).

at·lan·to·ax·i·al, at·lo·ax·oid (at-lan′tō-ak′sē-ăl, -ak′soyd) Pertaining to the atlas and the axis; denoting the joint between the first two cervical vertebrae.

at·las (at′lăs) [TA] First cervical vertebra, articulating with the occipital bone and rotating around the dens of the axis. SYN vertebra C1.

atlo- SEE atlanto-.

atm Abbreviation for standard atmosphere.

atmo- Prefix denoting steam or vapor; or derived by action of steam or vapor.

at·mos·phere (at′mŏs-fēr) **1.** Any gas surrounding a given body; a gaseous medium. **2.** A unit of air pressure equal to 101.325 kPa. SEE ALSO standard atmosphere.

at·mo·spher·ic press·ure (Patm) (at-mŏs-fēr′ik presh′ŭr) SYN barometric pressure.

at·om (at′ŏm) Formerly considered the ultimate particle of an element, believed to be as indivisible as its name indicates.

Discovery of radioactivity demonstrated the existence of subatomic particles, notably protons, neutrons, and electrons, the first two comprising most of the mass of the atomic nucleus. We now know that subatomic particles are further divisible into hadrons, leptons, and quarks.

a·tom·ic mass (ă-tom′ik mas) Total number of protons, neutrons, and electrons in an atom.

a·tom·ic nu·cle·us (ă-tom′ik nū′klē-ŭs) Centralized portion of the atom; composed of protons and neutrons.

a·tom·ic num·ber (Z, at. no.) (ă-tom′ik nŭm′bĕr) Number of protons in the atomic nucleus.

a·tom·ic weight (AW, at. wt.) (ă-tom′ik wāt) The mass in grams of 1 mol (6.02×10^{23}, atoms) of an atomic species. SEE ALSO molecular weight.

at·om·i·za·tion (at′ŏm-ī-zā′-shŭn) Spray production; reduction of a fluid to small-droplets.

at·om·iz·er (at′ŏm-ī-zĕr) A device used to reduce liquid medication to fine particles in the form of a spray or aerosol.

a·ton·ic im·po·tence (ā-ton′ik im′pŏ-tĕns) Physiologic dysfunction that makes penile erection impossible due to neurologic or muscular conditions, rather than psychological factors.

at·o·nic·i·ty (ā′tō-nis′i-tē) SYN atony.

a·ton·ic sei·zure (ā-ton′ik sē′zhŭr) Seizure characterized by sudden, brief (1–2 second) loss of muscle tone, involving postural muscles.

at·o·ny, ato·ni·a (at′ŏ-nē, ă-tō′nē-ă) Relaxation, flaccidity, or lack of tone or tension. SYN atonia, atonicity.

a·top·ic (ā-top′ik) Relating to or marked by atopy; allergic.

a·top·ic cat·a·ract (ā-top′ik kat′ăr-akt) A cataract associated with atopic dermatitis.

a·top·ic der·ma·ti·tis (ā-top′ik dĕr′mă-tī′tis) Skin disorder characterized by the distinctive phenomena of atopy, including infantile and flexural eczema.

a·top·og·no·si·a, a·top·og·no·sis (ă-top-og-nō′zē-ă, -og-nō′sis) Inability to locate a sensation properly.

at·o·py (at′ŏ-pē) A genetically determined state of hypersensitivity to environmental allergens.

ATPS Symbol indicating that a gas volume has been expressed as if it were saturated with water vapor at the ambient temperature and barometric pressure; the condition of an expired gas equilibrated in a spirometer.

a·tre·si·a (ă-trē′zē-ă′) Congenital absence of a normal opening or normally patent lumen.

atret·ic (ă-tret′ik) Relating to atresia. SYN imperforate.

atreto- Prefix meaning lack of an opening.

a·tri·al (ā′trē-ăl) Relating to an atrium.

a·tri·al bi·gem·i·ny (ā′trē-ăl bī-jem′i-nē) Pairing of atrial beats, as when an atrial extrasystole is coupled to each sinus beat.

a·tri·al cap·ture (ā′trē-ăl kap′shŭr) Control of the atria for one or more beats after a period of independent beating.

a·tri·al cha·ot·ic tach·y·car·di·a (ā′trē-ăl kā-ot′ik tak′i-kahr′dē-ă) Multifocal origin of tachycardia within the atrium. SYN multifocal atrial tachycardia.

a·tri·al com·plex (ā′trē-ăl kom′pleks) P wave in the electrocardiogram.

a·tri·al dis·so·ci·a·tion (ā′trē-ăl di-sō′sē-ā′shŭn) Mutually independent beating of the two atria or of parts of the atria.

a·tri·al ex·tra·sys·to·le (ā′trē-ăl eks′tră-sis′tŏ-lē) A premature contraction of the heart arising from an ectopic atrial focus.

a·tri·al fi·bril·la·tion, au·ric·u·lar fi·bril·la·tion (ā′trē-ăl fib′ri-lā′shŭn, awr-ik′yū-lăr fib′ri-lā′shŭn) Fibrillation in which the normal rhythmic contractions of the cardiac atria are replaced by rapid irregular twitchings of the muscular wall.

a·tri·al flut·ter, au·ric·u·lar flut·ter (ā′trē-ăl flŭt′ĕr, awr-ik′yū-lăr flŭt′ĕr) Rapid regular atrial contractions occurring usually at rates between 250 and 350 per minute and often producing "saw-tooth" waves in the electrocardiogram.

a·tri·al myx·o·ma (AM) (ā′trē-ăl miks-ō′mă) Primary cardiac neoplasm arising most commonly in the left atrium as a soft polypoid mucinous mass attached by a stalk to the atrial septum.

a·tri·al na·tri·u·ret·ic fac·tor (ANDF, ANF) (ā′trē-ăl nā′trē-yūr-et′ik fak′tŏr) A hormone produced by cardiac atria in response to increased fluid volume or pressure.

a·tri·al na·tri·u·ret·ic pep·tide (ANP) (ā′trē-ăl nā′trē-ūr-et′ik pep′tīd) 28–amino acid peptide (α-ANP) derived from cardiac atria, several smaller fragments of α-ANP, and a dimer of α-ANP with 56 amino acids (β-ANP) that are present in plasma in heart failure. SYN cardionatrin, natriuretic peptide.

a·tri·al pres·sure test (ā′trē-ăl presh′ŭr test) Measurement of the force of blood moving against the walls of the smaller, upper chambers of the heart.

a·tri·al sep·tum (ā′trē-ăl sep′tŭm) Thin wall between the two smaller, upper chambers of the heart.

a·tri·al sys·to·le (ā′trē-ăl sis′tō-lē) Contraction of the atria.

a·tri·al tach·y·car·di·a (AT) (ā′trē-ăl tak-i-kahr′dē-ă) Paroxysmal tachycardia originating in an ectopic focus in the atrium.

a·trich·ous (ă-trik′ŭs) Without hair.

atrio- Combining form meaning the atrium; atrial.

a·tri·o·meg·a·ly (ā′trē-ō-meg′ă-lē) Enlargement of the atrium.

a·tri·o·sep·to·plas·ty (ā′trē-ō-sep′tō-plas-tē) Surgical repair of an atrial septal defect.

a·tri·o·ven·tric·u·lar, au·ri·cu·lo·ven·tric·u·lar (A-V, AV) (ā′trē-ō-ven-trik′yū-lăr, aw-rik′yū-lō-ven-trik′yū-lăr) Relating to both the atria and the ventricles of the heart, especially to the ordinary, orthograde transmission of conduction or blood flow.

a·tri·o·ven·tric·u·lar (AV) con·duc·tion (ā′trē-ō-ven-trik′yū-lăr kŏn-dŭk′shŭn) Forward conduction of the cardiac impulse from atria to ventricles via the AV node or any bypass tract, represented in the electrocardiogram by the P-R interval.

a·tri·o·ven·tric·u·lar (AV) ex·tra·sys·to·le (ā′trē-ō-ven-trik′yū-lăr eks′tră-sis′tŏ-lē) An extrasystole arising from the ''junctional'' tissues, either the AV node or AV bundle.

a·tri·o·ven·tric·u·lar (AV) no·dal ex·tra·sys·to·le (ā′trē-ō-ven-trik′yū-lăr nō′dăl eks′tră-sis′tŏ-lē) A premature beat arising from the AV junction and leading to a simultaneous or almost simultaneous contraction of atria and ventricles.

a·tri·o·ven·tric·u·lar junc·tion·al rhythm (ā′trē-ō-ven-trik′yū-lăr jungk′shŭn-ăl ridh′ŭm) The cardiac rhythm when the heart is controlled by the A-V junction (including node); arising in the A-V junction, the impulse ascends to the atria and descends to the ventricles, each at varying speeds depending on site of the pacemaker. SYN AV junctional rhythm.

a·tri·o·ven·tric·u·lar node (ā′trē-ō-ven-trik′yū-lăr nōd) [TA] A small node of modified cardiac muscle fibers located near the ostium of the coronary sinus; it gives rise to the atrioventricular bundle of the conduction system of the heart.

a·tri·o·ven·tric·u·lar valves (ā′trē-ō-ven-trik′yū-lăr valvz) SEE tricuspid valve, mitral valve.

a·tri·um, pl. **a·tri·a** (ā′trē-ŭm, ā′trē-ă) [TA] **1.** A chamber or cavity to which are connected several chambers or passageways. **2.** SYN atrium of heart. **3.** That part of the tympanic cavity that lies immediately deep to the tympanic membrane (eardrum). **4.** In the lung, a subdivision of the alveolar duct from which alveolar sacs open.

a·tri·um cor·dis dex·trum (ā′trē-ŭm kōr′dis deks′trŭm) [TA] SYN right atrium of heart.

a·tri·um of heart (ā′trē-ŭm hahrt) [TA] The upper chamber of each half of the heart. SYN atrium cordis [TA], atrium (2) [TA].

a·troph·ic (ā-trō′fik) Denoting atrophy.

a·troph·ic gas·tri·tis (ā-trō′fik gas-trī′tis) Chronic gastritis with atrophy of the mucous membrane and destruction of the peptic glands, sometimes associated with pernicious anemia or gastric carcinoma; also applied to gastric atrophy without inflammatory changes.

a·troph·ic glos·si·tis (ā-trō′fik glos-ī′tis) An erythematous, edematous, and painful tongue that appears smooth because of loss of the filiform and sometimes the fungiform papillae secondary to certain nutritional deficiencies, especially B-vitamin deficiencies. SYN bald tongue, bald tongue.

a·troph·ic rhi·ni·tis (ā-trō′fik rī-nī′tis) Chronic disorder with thinning of the mucous membrane; often associated with crusts and foul-smelling discharge.

a·troph·ic vag·i·ni·tis (ā-trō′fik vaj′i-nī′tis) Thinned atrophic vaginal epithelium usually due to diminished estrogen stimulation; common in postmenopausal women.

at·ro·pho·der·ma (at′rŏ-fō-dĕr′mă) Atrophy of the skin that may occur either in discrete localized or widespread areas.

at·ro·pho·der·ma·to·sis (at′rŏ-fō-dĕr′mă-tō′sis) Any cutaneous disorder in which a prominent symptom is skin atrophy.

at·ro·phy (at′rŏ-fē) A wasting of tissues, organs, or the entire body, as from death and reabsorption of cells, diminished cellular proliferation, decreased cellular volume, pressure, ischemia, malnutrition, lessened function, or hormonal changes.

at·tached gin·gi·va (ă-tacht′ jin′ji-vă) That part of the oral mucosa that is firmly bound to the tooth and alveolar process.

at·tack (ă-tak′) A sudden illness or an episode or exacerbation of chronic or recurrent illness.

at·tend·ing (att) (ă-tend′ing) Colloquial for attending physician.

at·tend·ing staff (ă-tend′ing staf) Physicians and surgeons who are members of a hospital staff and regularly see their patients at the hospital; may also supervise and teach house staff, fellows, and medical students.

at·ten·tion def·i·cit dis·or·der (ADD)

(ă-ten′shŭn def′i-sit dis-ōr′dĕr) A disorder of attention and impulse control with specific criteria, appearing in childhood and sometimes persisting to adulthood. SEE ALSO attention deficit hyperactivity disorder.

at·ten·tion def·i·cit hy·per·ac·tiv·i·ty dis·or·der (ADHD) (ă-ten′shŭn def′i-sit hī′pĕr-ak-tiv′i-tē dis-ōr′dĕr) A disorder of childhood and adolescence manifested at home, in school, and in social situations by developmentally inappropriate degrees of inattention, impulsiveness, and hyperactivity; also called hyperactivity or hyperactive child syndrome. SEE ALSO attention deficit disorder.

at·ten·u·ate (AT) (ă-ten′yū-āt) To dilute, thin, reduce, weaken, diminish.

at·ten·u·at·ed vac·cine (ă-ten′yū-āt-ĕd vak-sēn′) Live pathogens that have lost their virulence but are still capable of inducing a protective immune response to the virulent forms of the pathogen.

at·ten·u·a·tion (ă-ten′yū-ā′shŭn) 1. The act of attenuating. 2. Diminution of virulence in a strain of an organism, obtained through selection of variants that occur naturally or through experimental means.

at·tic (at′ik) SYN epitympanum.

at·ti·tude (at′i-tūd) 1. Position of the body and limbs. 2. Manner of acting. 3. PSYCHOLOGY a predisposition to behave or react in a certain way toward people, objects, institutions, or issues.

atto- (a) Prefix used in the SI and metric system to signify one quintillionth (10^{-18}).

a·typ·i·cal li·po·ma (ā-tip′i-kăl li-pō′mă) Skin eruption, occurring primarily in older men on the posterior neck, shoulders, and back, which is benign but microscopically atypical, containing giant cells with multiple overlapping nuclei forming a circle. SYN pleomorphic lipoma.

a·typ·i·cal mea·sles (ā-tip′i-kăl mē′zĕlz) Unusual clinical manifestation of natural measles infection in people with waning vaccination immunity, particularly in those who had received formaldehyde-inactivated vaccine.

a·typ·i·cal my·co·bac·te·ri·a (ā-tip′i-kăl mī′kō-bak-tēr′ē-ă) Species of mycobacteria other than *M. tuberculosis* or *M. bovis* that can cause disease in immunocompromised humans.

a·typ·i·cal pneu·mo·ni·a (ā-tip′i-kăl nū-mō′nē-ă) SYN primary atypical pneumonia.

a·typ·i·cal ver·ru·cous en·do·car·di·tis (ā-tip′i-kăl vĕ-rū′kŭs en′dō-kahr-dī′tis) SYN Libman-Sacks endocarditis.

audio- Combining form meaning the sense of hearing.

au·di·o·gen·ic (aw′dē-ō-jen′ik) 1. Caused by sound, especially a loud noise. 2. Sound-producing.

au·di·ol·o·gy (aw′dē-ol′ŏ-jē) The study of hearing disorders through the identification and measurement of hearing impairment.

au·di·om·e·trist (aw′dē-om′ĕ-trist) A person trained in the use of an audiometer in hearing testing.

au·di·om·e·try (aw′dē-om′ĕ-trē) Rapid measurement of the hearing of an individual or a group against a predetermined limit of normality; auditory responses to different frequencies presented at a constant intensity level are tested.

au·di·tion (aw-dish′ŭn) SYN hearing.

au·di·to·ry (aw′di-tōr-ē) Pertaining to the sense of hearing or to the organs of hearing.

au·di·to·ry ag·no·si·a (aw′di-tōr-ē ag-nō′zē-ă) Inability to recognize sounds, words, or music; caused by a lesion of the auditory cortex of the temporal lobe.

au·di·to·ry a·pha·si·a (aw′di-tōr-ē ă-fā′zē-ă) An impairment in comprehension of the auditory forms of language and communication, including the ability to write from dictation in the presence of normal hearing.

au·di·to·ry ar·e·a (aw′di-tōr-ē ăr′ē-ă) SYN auditory cortex.

au·di·to·ry cap·sule (aw′di-tōr-ē kap′sŭl) SYN otic capsule.

au·di·to·ry cor·tex (aw′di-tōr-ē kōr′teks) The region of the cerebral cortex that receives the auditory radiation from the medial geniculate body, a thalamic cell group receiving auditory input from the cochlear nuclei in the rhombencephalon. SYN auditory area.

au·di·to·ry de·fen·sive·ness (aw′di-tōr-ē dĕ-fen′siv-nĕs) Excessive reaction to sound (e.g., because of its volume or novelty).

au·di·to·ry field (aw′di-tōr-ē fēld) The space included within the limits of hearing of a definite sound, as of a tuning fork.

au·di·to·ry hal·lu·ci·na·tion (AH) (aw′di-tōr-ē hă-lū′si-nā′shŭn) Symptom commonly seen in a schizophrenic or psychotic mood disorder that, in the absence of an external source, consists of hearing a voice or other auditory stimulus that other people do not perceive.

au·di·to·ry hy·per·es·the·si·a (aw′di-tōr-ē hī′pĕr-es-thē′zē-ă) Abnormal hearing sensitivity.

au·di·to·ry neu·rop·a·thy (aw′di-tōr-ē nūr-op′ă-thē) A distinctive type of hearing deficit that seemingly is due to a malfunction of the eighth cranial nerve.

au·di·to·ry re·flex (aw′di-tōr-ē rē′fleks) Any reflex occurring in response to a sound (e.g., cochleopalpebral reflex).

au·di·to·ry thresh·old (aw′di-tōr-ē thresh′ōld) Level at which sound becomes audible.

au·di·to·ry ves·i·cle (aw′di-tōr-ē ves′i-kĕl) SYN otic vesicle.

aug·men·ta·tive and al·ter·na·tive com·mu·ni·ca·tion (awg-men′tă-tiv awl-tĕr′nă-tiv kŏ-myū′ni-kā′shŭn) The clinical practice of determining appropriate compensatory techniques for inadequate verbal communication and providing training in the use of those techniques. SYN nonoral communication, nonverbal communication.

aug·ment·ed la·bor (awg-men′tĕd lā′bŏr) Induced labor.

au·ra (awr′ă) **1.** Subjective symptoms occurring at the onset of a partial epileptic seizure; often characteristic for the brain region involved in the seizure, e.g., visual aura, occipital lobe auditory aura, temporal lobe. **2.** Subjective symptoms at the onset of a migraine headache.

au·ral, au·ric·u·lar (awr′ăl, aw-rik′yū-lăr) **1.** Relating to the ear (auris). **2.** Relating to an aura.

au·ral·ly (awr′ă-lē) Related to the ear or sense of hearing.

♻ **auri-** Combining form denoting the ear. SEE ALSO ot-, oto-.

au·ri·cle, au·ric·u·la (awr′i-kĕl, aw-rik′yū-lă) [TA] **1.** The projecting shell-like structure on the side of the head, constituting, with the external acoustic meatus, the external ear. SYN pinna (1). **2.** SYN auricle of atrium.

au·ri·cle of a·tri·um (awr′i-kĕl ā′trē-ŭm) A small conic (''ear-shaped'') pouch projecting from the upper anterior portion of each atrium of the heart, increasing slightly the atrial volume. SYN atrial auricle, auricle (2).

au·ric·u·lar (aur) (awr-ik′yū-lăr) Relating to the ear, or to an auricle in any sense.

au·ric·u·lar tu·ber·cle (awr-ik′yū-lăr tū′bĕr-kĕl) [TA] A small projection from the upper end of the posterior portion of the incurved free margin of the helix. SYN darwinian tubercle.

au·ric·u·lo·cra·ni·al (aw-rik′yū-lō-krā′nē-ăl) Relating to the auricle or pinna of the ear and the cranium.

au·ric·u·lo·pres·sor re·flex (awr-ik′yū-lō-pres′ŏr rē′fleks) Peripheral vasoconstriction and a rise in blood pressure in response to a fall in pressure in the great veins.

au·ric·u·lo·tem·po·ral (awr-ik′yū-lō-tem′pŏr-ăl) Relating to the auricle or pinna of the ear and the temporal region.

au·ris, pl. **au·res** (awr′is, awr′ēz) [TA] SYN ear.

aus·cul·ta·tion (aws′kŭl-tā′shŭn) Listening to the sounds made by various body structures and functions as a diagnostic method, usually with a stethoscope.

aus·cul·ta·to·ry al·ter·nans (aws-kŭl′tă-tōr-ē awl-tĕr′nanz) Alternation in the intensity of heart sounds or murmurs in the presence of a regular cardiac rhythm.

aus·cul·ta·to·ry per·cus·sion (aws-kŭl′tă-tōr-ē pĕr-kŭsh′ŭn) Auscultation of the chest or other part at the same time that percussion is made, to facilitate hearing the sound made by percussion.

Au•spitz sign (ow′spits sīn) A finding typical of psoriasis, in which removal of a scale leads to pinpoint bleeding.

au•tism (aw′tizm) A mental disorder characterized by severely abnormal development of social interaction and of verbal and nonverbal communication skills. Affected people may adhere to inflexible, nonfunctional rituals or routines.

au•tis•tic (aw-tis′tik) Pertaining to or characterized by autism.

au•tis•tic spec•trum dis•or•der (aw-tis′tik spek′trŭm dis-ōr′dĕr) A nonspecific diagnosis of any developmental disorder characterized by poor social abilities and impaired communication.

au•to•ag•glu•ti•na•tion (aw′tō-ă-glū′ti-nā′shŭn) Nonspecific agglutination or clumping together of cells (e.g., bacteria, erythrocytes) due to physical-chemical factors.

au•to•ag•glu•ti•nin (aw′tō-ă-glū′ti-nin) An agglutinating autoantibody.

au•to•an•ti•body (autoAB) (aw′tō-an′ti-bod-ē) An antibody that occurs in response to antigenic constituents of the host's tissue (or ''self antigen'') and reacts with the inciting target tissue.

au•to•an•ti•gen (aw′to-an′ti-jĕn) A ''self'' antigen; any tissue constituent that evokes an immune response by the host.

au•to•ca•tal•y•sis (aw′tō-kă-tal′i-sis) A reaction in which one or more of the products formed acts to catalyze the reaction; beginning slowly, the rate of such a reaction rapidly increases.

au•toch•thon•ous (aw-tok′thŏn-ŭs) Originating in the place where found.

au•toc•la•sis, au•to•cla•sia (aw-tok′lă-sis, aw′tō-klā′zē-ă) **1.** A breaking up or rupturing from intrinsic or internal causes. **2.** Progressive immunologically induced tissue destruction.

au•to•clave (aw′tō-klāv) An apparatus for sterilization by steam under pressure; also used as a verb.

au•to•crine (aw′tō-krin) Denoting self-stimulation through cellular production of a factor and a specific receptor for it.

au•to•cy•to•tox•in (aw′tō-sī-tō-toks′in) A cytotoxic autoantibody.

au•to•der•mic graft (aw′tō-dĕr′mik graft) A skin autograft.

au•to•e•rot•i•cism (aw′tō-ĕ-rot′i-sizm) Sexual arousal or gratification using one's own body, as in masturbation.

au•to•e•ryth•ro•cyte sen•si•ti•za•tion syn•drome (aw′tō-ĕ-rith′rō-sīt sen′si-tī-zā′shŭn sin′drōm) A condition that usually occurs primarily in women, in which the person bruises easily (purpura simplex).

au•to•gen•e•sis (aw′tō-jen′ĕ-sis) **1.** The origin of living matter within the organism itself. **2.** In bacteriology, the process by which vaccine is made from bacteria obtained from the patient's own body.

au•tog•e•nous (aw-toj′ĕ-nŭs) Originating within the body.

au•to•graft (aw′tō-graft) A tissue or an organ transferred by grafting into a new position in the body of the same individual.

au•to•hem•ag•glu•ti•na•tion (aw′tō-hē′mă-glū-ti-nā′shŭn) Autoagglutination of erythrocytes. SYN autohaemagglutination.

au•to•he•mo•ly•sin (aw′tō-hē-mol′i-sin) An autoantibody that causes lysis of erythrocytes in the same person in whose body the lysin is formed. SYN autohaemolysin.

au•to•he•mol•y•sis (aw′tō-hē-mol′i-sis) Hemolysis occurring in certain diseases as a result of an autohemolysin. SYN autohaemolysis.

au•to•he•mo•ther•a•py (aw-tō-hē′mō-thār′ă-pē) An unproven mode of alternative therapy in which a quantity of the patient's blood is withdrawn and either reinjected intramuscularly at once or reinfused intravenously after being treated with ultraviolet radiation, ozone, or some other agent.

au•to•hyp•no•sis (aw′tō-hip-nō′sis) Self-induced hypnosis, accomplished by concentrating on self-absorbing thought or on the idea of being hypnotized. SYN idiohypnotism.

au·to·im·mune (AI) (aw'tō-i-myūn') Term describing cells and antibodies arising from and directed against the individual's own tissues, as in autoimmune disease.

au·to·im·mune dis·ease (aw'tō-i-myūn' di-zēz') Any disorder in which loss of function or destruction of normal tissue arises from humoral or cellular immune responses of the person to her or his own tissue constituents.

au·to·im·mu·ni·ty (aw'tō-i-myū'ni-tē) Immune response against the body's own tissues. SYN autoallergy.

au·to·im·mu·no·cy·to·pe·ni·a (aw'tō-im'yū-nō-sī-tō-pē'nē-ă) Anemia, thrombocytopenia, and leukopenia resulting from cytotoxic autoimmune reactions.

au·to·in·oc·u·la·tion (aw'tō-in-ok-yū-lā'shŭn) A secondary infection originating from a focus of infection already present in the body.

au·to·i·sol·y·sin (aw'tō-ī-sol'i-sin) An antibody that in the presence of complement causes lysis of cells in the person in whose body the lysin is formed, as well as in others of the same species.

au·to·ker·a·to·plas·ty (aw'tō-ker'ă-tō-plas-tē) Grafting of corneal tissue from one eye of a patient to the fellow eye.

au·to·le·sion (aw'tō-lē'zhŭn) A self-inflicted injury.

au·tol·o·gous do·na·tion (aw-tol'ŏ-gŭs dō-nā'shŭn) A blood transfusion or tissue graft involving one person as both donor and recipient.

au·tol·y·sin (aw-tol'i-sin) An antibody that causes lysis of the cells and tissues in the body of the individual in whom the lysin is formed. SYN autocytolysin.

au·tol·y·sis (aw-tol'i-sis) **1.** Enzymatic digestion of cells (especially dead or degenerated) by enzymes present within them (autogenous). **2.** Destruction of cells as a result of a lysin formed in those cells or others in the same organism. SYN isophagy.

au·to·mo·tor sei·zure (aw'tō-mō'tŏr sē'zhŭr) Seizure characterized by an auto-matism predominantly involving the distal limbs.

au·to·nom·ic ep·i·lep·sy (aw'tō-nom'ik ep'i-lep-sē) Episodes of autonomic dysfunction presumably resulting from diencephalic irritation.

au·to·nom·ic nerve (aw'to-nom'ik něrv) A bundle of autonomic nerve fibers outside the central nervous system belonging or relating to the autonomic (visceral motor) nervous system. SYN nervus autonomicus [TA].

au·to·nom·ic neu·ro·gen·ic blad·der (aw'tō-nom'ik nūr-ō-jen'ik blad'ĕr) Malfunctioning urinary bladder, secondary to low spinal cord lesions.

au·to·no·mic sei·zure (aw'tō-nom'ik sē'zhŭr) Seizure characterized by objectively documented dysfunction of the autonomic nervous system, usually involving cardiovascular, gastrointestinal, or sudomotor functions.

au·to·nom·o·tro·pic (aw'tō-nom-ō-trō'pik) Acting on the autonomic nervous system.

au·to·pha·go·ly·so·some (aw'tō-fā'gō-lī'sō-sōm) The digestive vacuole of autophagy that results from the fusion of a lysosome with an autophagic vacuole.

au·to·plas·ty (aw'tō-plas-tē) Repair of defects by autotransplantation.

au·to·po·di·um, pl. **au·to·po·di·a** (aw'tō-pō'dē-ŭm, -dē-ă) The distal major subdivision of a limb (hand or foot). SYN autopod.

au·to·pol·y·mer res·in (aw'to-pol'i-měr rez'in) Any resin that can be polymerized by chemical catalysis rather than by the application of heat; in dentistry used in making dental restorations, denture repairs, and impression trays.

au·top·sy (aw'top-sē) An examination of a corpse and the organs of a dead body to determine the cause of death or to study the pathologic changes present. (Colloquially called postmortem or post.) SYN necropsy.

au·to·ra·di·og·ra·phy (aw'tō-rā-dē-og'ră-fē) The process of producing an autoradiograph.

au·to·reg·u·la·tion (aw′tō-reg-yū-lā′ shŭn) The tendency of the blood flow to an organ or part to remain at or return to the same level despite changes in the pressure in the artery which conveys blood to it.

au·to·sep·ti·ce·mia (aw′tō-sep′ti-sē′ mē-ă) Septicemia apparently originating from microorganisms existing within the individual and not introduced from without.

au·to·so·ma·tog·no·sis (aw′tō-sō′mă-tog-nō′sis) The sensation that an amputated portion of the body is still present. SEE phantom limb.

au·to·some (aw′tō-sōm) Any chromosome other than a sex chromosome; autosomes normally occur in pairs in somatic cells and singly in gametes.

au·to·sug·ges·tion (aw′tō-sŭg-jes′ chŭn) Constant dwelling on an idea or concept, thereby inducing some change in the mental or bodily functions.

au·to·top·ag·no·sia (aw′tō-top′ag-nō′ zē-ă) *In the diphthong gn, the g is silent only at the beginning of a word.* Inability to recognize or to orient any part of one's own body; caused by a parietal lobe lesion. Cf. somatotopagnosis.

au·to·tox·e·mia (aw′tō-tok-sē′mē-ă) The presence of autointoxicants in the blood.

au·to·tox·ic (aw′tō-toks′ik) Relating to autointoxication.

au·to·trans·fu·sion (aw′tō-trans-fyū′ zhŭn) Withdrawal and reinjection-transfusion of the patient's own blood.

au·to·trans·plan·ta·tion (aw′tō-trans-plan-tā′shŭn) The performance of an autograft.

au·to·vac·ci·na·tion (aw′tō-vak′si-nā′ shŭn) A second vaccination with virus from a vaccine sore or liberation of antigenic products from invading microorganisms on the same patient.

au·to·zy·gous (aw′tō-zī′gŭs) Denoting genes in a homozygote that are copies of the identical ancestral gene as a result of a consanguineous mating.

auxano-, auxo-, aux- Combining forms meaning increase (e.g., in size, intensity, speed).

aux·e·sis (awk-sē′sis) Increase in size, especially as in hypertrophy.

aux·i·lyt·ic (awk′si-lit′ik) Increasing the destructive power of a lysin, or favoring lysis.

a·ver·sive (ă-věr′siv) Denotes type of therapy using unpleasant stimuli that seeks to cause a patient to avoid one or more transgressive behaviors.

A·vo·gad·ro number (NA, lambda) (ah-vō-gahd′rō nŭm′běr) The number of molecules in 1 gram-molecular weight (1 mol) of any compound; defined as the number of atoms in 0.0120 kg of pure carbon-12; equivalent to 6.0221367×10^{23}. SYN Avogadro constant.

a·void·ance (a-voyd′-ăns) In psychiatry, a term describing a decrease in strength of relationships or fear and withdrawal when conflict emerges. SEE attachment.

a·vulsed wound (ă-vŭlst′ wūnd) A wound caused by or resulting from forcible shearing.

a·vul·sion frac·ture (ă-vŭl′shŭn frak′ shŭr) Break that occurs when a joint capsule, ligament, or muscle insertion of origin is pulled from the bone as a result of a sprain, dislocation, or strong contracture of the muscle against resistance.

a·xen·ic (ă-zen′ik) Sterile, denoting especially a pure culture; also used to denote ''germ-free'' animals born and raised in a sterile environment.

ax·i·al (ak′sē-ăl) [TA] **1.** Relating to or situated in the central part of the body, in the head and trunk as distinguished from the limbs, e.g., axial skeleton. **2.** DENTISTRY relating to or parallel with the long axis of a tooth.

ax·i·al an·gle (ak′sē-ăl ang′gĕl) An angle formed by two surfaces of a body, the line of union of which is parallel with its axis; the axial angles of a tooth are the distobuccal, distolabial, distolingual, mesiobuccal, mesiolabial, and mesiolingual.

ax·i·al plane (aks′ē-ăl plăn) Transverse plane at right angles to the long axis of the body, as in computed tomographic scanning. SYN transaxial plane.

ax·i·al skel·e·ton (ak'sē-ăl skel'ĕ-tŏn) [TA] Articulated bones of head and vertebral column, i.e., head and trunk, as opposed to the appendicular skeleton, the articulated bones of the upper and lower limbs.

ax·il·la, gen. and pl. **ax·il·lae** (ak-sil'ă, -sil'ē) [TA] The space below the shoulder joint, bounded by the pectoralis major anteriorly, the latissimus dorsi posteriorly, the serratus anterior medially, and the humerus laterally; commonly, the armpit.

ax·il·lar·y (ak'si-lar-ē) Relating to the axilla. SYN alar (2).

ax·il·la·ry fos·sa (ak'si-lar-ē fos'ă) [TA] Depression between the anterior and posterior axillary folds forming the floor of the axilla. SYN fossa axillaris [TA], armpit.

ax·il·la·ry glands (ak'si-lar-ē glandz) SYN axillary lymph nodes.

ax·il·lar·y lymph nodes (ak'si-lar-ē limf nōdz) Numerous nodes around the axillary veins that receive the lymphatic drainage from the upper limb, scapular region, and pectoral region (including mammary glands); they drain into the subclavian trunk.

axio- Prefix meaning an axis. SEE ALSO axo-.

ax·i·on (ak'sē-on) The brain and spinal cord (cerebrospinal axis).

ax·ip·e·tal (ak-sip'ĕ-tăl) SYN centripetal (2).

ax·is (ax) (ak'sis, ak'sēz) [TA] **1.** A straight line joining two opposing poles of a spheric body, about which the body may revolve. **2.** The central line of the body or any of its parts. **3.** The vertebral column. **4.** The central nervous system. **5.** The second cervical vertebra. SYN epistropheus, vertebra C2, vertebra dentata. **6.** An artery that divides, immediately on its origin, into a number of branches, e.g., celiac axis. SEE trunk.

axo- Prefix meaning axis; axion.

ax·o·ax·on·ic (ak'sō-ak-son'ik) Relating to synaptic contact between the axon of one nerve cell and that of another. SEE synapse.

ax·o·den·drit·ic syn·apse (aks'ō-den-drit'ik sin'aps) Synaptic contact between an axon terminal of one nerve cell and a dendrite of another.

ax·o·lem·ma (ak'sō-lem'ă) The plasma membrane of the axon. SYN Mauthner sheath.

ax·on (ak'son) The single process of a nerve cell that normally conducts nervous impulses away from the cell body and its remaining processes (dendrites).

ax·o·neme (ak'sō-nēm) The central thread running in the axis of the chromosome.

ax·o·plasm (ak'sō-plazm) Neuroplasm of the axon.

ax·o·so·mat·ic (ak'sō-sō-mat'ik) Relating to the synaptic relationship of an axon with a nerve cell body. SEE synapse.

A·yer·za syn·drome (ah-yer'sah sin'drōm) Sclerosis of the pulmonary arteries in chronic cor pulmonale.

Ayur·ve·dic med·i·cine (ī'yŭr-vā'dik med'i-sin) A system of alternative medicine that uses herbs, aromatherapy, music therapy, massage, yoga, and other measures; places equal emphasis on mind, body, and spirit.

azo- Prefix denoting the presence in a molecule of the group ≡C–N=N–C≡. Cf. diazo-.

azo·ic (ă-zō'ik, ā-) Containing no living things; without organic life.

azo·o·sper·mi·a (ā'zō-ō-spĕrmē-ă) Absence of living sperms in the semen; failure of spermatogenesis.

azotaemia [Br.] SYN azotemia.

az·o·te·mi·a (ā'zō-tē'mē-ă) SYN uremia, azotaemia.

a·zo·tu·ri·a (az'ō-tyūr'ē-ă) An increased elimination of urea in the urine.

az·u·ro·phil, az·u·ro·phile (azh'ŭr-ō-fil, -fīl) Staining readily with an azure dye.

az·u·ro·phil·ia (azh-ū'rō-fil'ē-ă) A condition in which the blood contains cells having azurophil granulations.

B

B$_e$ Symbol for beryllium.

Ba Symbol for barium.

Ba·be·si·a (bă-bē'zē-ă) The most important genus of the family Babesiidae; characterized by multiplication in host red blood cells to form pairs and tetrads. It causes babesiosis (piroplasmosis) in domestic animals; two species cause disease in splenectomized or normal people. Vectors are ixodid or argasid ticks.

Ba·bin·ski sign (bă-bin'skē sīn) **1.** Extension of the great toe and abduction of the other toes instead of the normal flexion reflex to plantar stimulation, considered indicative of pyramidal tract involvement (''positive'' Babinski). SYN Babinski phenomenon, paradoxic extensor reflex. **2.** In hemiplegia, weakness of the platysma muscle on the affected side, as evident in such actions as blowing or opening the mouth. **3.** When the patient is lying supine with arms crossed on the front of the chest, and attempts to assume the sitting posture, the thigh on the side of an *organic* paralysis is flexed and the heel raised, whereas the limb on the sound side remains flat. **4.** In hemiplegia, the forearm on the affected side turns to a pronated position when placed in a position of supination.

Ba·bin·ski syn·drome (bă-bin'skē sin'drōm) The combination of cardiac, arterial, and central nervous system manifestations of late-stage syphilis.

Bach·e·lor of Phar·ma·cy (Phar.B.) (bach'ĕ-lŏr fahr'mă-sē) An undergraduate academic degree in the field of pharmacy that has now largely been supplanted in the U.S. by the Pharm.D.

Ba·cil·la·ce·ae (ă-si-lā'sē-ē) A family of aerobic or facultatively anaerobic, spore-forming, ordinarily motile bacteria containing gram-positive rods. Some species are pathogenic. Ordinarily two genera, *Bacillus* and *Clostridium*, are included.

ba·cil·lar, bac·il·la·ry (bas'i-lăr, bas'i-lăr-ē) Shaped like a rod; consisting of rods or rodlike elements.

bac·il·la·ry an·gi·o·ma·to·sis (bas'i-lăr-ē an'jē-ō-mă-tō'sis) An infection of immunocompromised patients by the rickettsial species *Bartonella henselae*, characterized by fever and granuloma-tous cutaneous nodules, and peliosis hepatis in some cases.

bac·il·la·ry dys·en·ter·y (bas'i-lār-ē dis'en-ter'ē) Infection with *Shigella dysenteriae, S. flexneri,* or other organisms.

ba·cil·le Cal·mette-Gué·rin (BCG) (bah-sēl' kahl-met'gā-rin[h]') An attenuated strain of *Mycobacterium bovis* used in BCG vaccine for immunization against tuberculosis and in cancer chemotherapy. SYN Calmette-Guérin bacillus.

ba·cil·lin (ba-sil'in) An antibiotic substance produced by *Bacillus subtilis.*

bac·il·lu·ri·a (bas-il-yūr'ē-ă) The presence of bacilli in the urine.

Ba·cil·lus (bă-sil'ŭs) A genus of aerobic or facultatively anaerobic, spore-forming, ordinarily motile bacteria containing gram-positive rods.

ba·cil·lus, pl. **ba·cil·li** (bă-sil'ŭs, bă-sil'ī) **1.** A term used to refer to any member of the genus *Bacillus.* **2.** Term used to refer to any rod-shaped bacterium.

bac·i·tra·cin (bas'i-trā'sin) An antibacterial antibiotic polypeptide of known chemical structure isolated from cultures of an aerobic, gram-positive, spore-bearing bacillus; active against hemolytic streptococci, staphylococci, and several types of gram-positive, aerobic, rod-shaped organisms; usually applied locally.

back (bk) (bak) [TA] **1.** Posterior aspect of trunk, below neck and above buttocks. **2.** Vertebral column with associated muscles (erector spinae and transversospinalis) and overlying integument. SEE dorsum.

back·cross (bak'kraws) Mating of an individual heterozygous at one or more loci to an individual homozygous at the same loci.

back·flow (bak'flō) The reversal of the normal flow of a current.

back·ing (bak'ing) In dentistry, a metal support that serves to attach a facing to a prosthesis.

bacteraemia [Br.] SYN bacteremia.

bac•te•re•mi•a (bak'tĕr-ē'mē-ă) Having viable bacteria in circulating blood; may be transient after trauma such as dental or other iatrogenic manipulation or persistent or recurrent due to infection. SYN bacteraemia.

bacteri- SEE bacterio-.

bac•te•ri•al (bak-tēr'ē-ăl) Relating to bacteria.

bac•te•ri•al cap•sule (bak-tēr'ē-ăl kap' sŭl) Layer of slime of variable composition on surface of some bacteria; capsulated cells of pathogenic bacteria are usually more virulent than unencapsulated because capsulated bacteria are more resistant to phagocytic (q.v.) action.

bac•te•ri•al end•ar•ter•i•tis (bak-tēr' ē-ăl end'ahr-tĕr-ī'tis) Implantation and growth of bacteria on the arterial wall.

bac•te•ri•al en•do•car•di•tis (bak-tēr' ē-ăl en'dō-kahr-dī'tis) Disorder due to direct invasion of bacteria leading to deformity and destruction of the valve leaflets.

bac•te•ri•al plaque (bak-tēr'ē-ăl plak) DENTISTRY filamentous microorganisms and diverse smaller forms attached to tooth surface; may give rise to caries, calculus, or inflammatory changes in adjacent tissue. SYN dental plaque (2).

bac•te•ri•al pneu•mo•ni•a (bak-tēr'ē-ăl nū-mō'nē-ă) Lung infection with any of a large variety of bacteria, especially *Streptococcus pneumoniae*.

bac•te•ri•al tox•in (bak-tēr'ē-ăl tok'sin) Any intracellular or extracellular toxin formed in or elaborated by bacterial cells.

bac•te•ri•cid•al, bac•te•ri•o•ci•dal (bak-tēr'i-sī'dăl, -ēr'ē-ō-sī'dăl) Causing the death of bacteria. Cf. bacteriostatic.

bac•te•ri•ci•din (bak-tēr'i-sī'din) An antibody that kills bacteria in the presence of complement.

bac•ter•id (bak'tĕr-id) A recurrent or persistent eruption of discrete sterile pustules of the palms and soles, thought to be an allergic response to bacterial infection at a remote site.

bacterio-, bacteri- Combining forms meaning bacteria. SEE bacterium.

bac•te•ri•o•cid•in (bak-tēr-ē-ō-sī'din) Antibody having bactericidal activity.

bac•ter•i•o•cin (bak-tēr-ē-ō'sin) A protein toxin produced and released by bacteria to inhibit the growth of similar bacteria.

bac•te•ri•o•cin•o•gens (bak-tēr'ē-ō-sin' ō-jĕnz) SYN bacteriocinogenic plasmids.

bac•te•ri•ol•o•gy (bact) (bak-tēr'ē-ol' ō-jē) The branch of science concerned with the study of bacteria.

bac•te•ri•o•ly•sin (bak-tēr'ē-ol'i-sin) Specific antibody that combines with bacterial cells (i.e., antigen) and, in the presence of complement, causes lysis or dissolution of the cells.

bac•te•ri•o•phage (bak-tēr'ē-ō-fāj) *Avoid the mispronunciation bak-te′rē-ō-fahzh.* A virus with specific affinity for bacteria, found in association with nearly all groups of bacteria. SYN phage.

bac•te•ri•o•phage typ•ing (bak-tēr'ē-ō-fāj tīp'ing) Microbiologic typing procedure, of epidemiologic importance, for distinguishing types within a seemingly homogeneous bacterial species or strain.

bac•te•ri•op•so•nin (bak-tēr'ē-op'sō-nin) An opsonin that acts on bacteria.

bac•te•ri•o•sper•mi•a (bak-tēr'ē-ō-spĕr' mē-ă) Bacteria in the semen or ejaculate.

bac•te•ri•o•sta•sis (bak-tēr'ē-os'tă-sis) An arrest or retardation of growth of bacteria.

bac•te•ri•o•stat•ic (bak-tēr'ē-ō-stat'ik) Inhibiting or retarding the multiplication of bacteria.

bac•te•ri•um, pl. **bac•te•ria** (bak-tēr'ē-ŭm, -ă) A unicellular prokaryotic microorganism that usually multiplies by cell division and has a cell wall that provides a constancy of form; may be aerobic or anaerobic, motile or nonmotile, and free-living, saprophytic, parasitic, or pathogenic.

bac•te•ri•u•ri•a (bak-tēr'ē-yūr'ē-ă) The presence of bacteria in the urine.

Bac·te·roi·des (bak-ter-oy′dēz) A genus that includes species of obligate anaerobic, non-spore-forming bacteria containing gram-negative rods. The type species is *B. fragilis*.

bag of wa·ters (BOW) (bag waw′tĕrs) Colloquialism for the amnionic sac containing amnionic fluid.

Ba·ker cyst (bā′kĕr sist) Synovial fluid that has escaped from the knee joint or a bursa to form a new synovial-fluid-lined sac in the popliteal space.

bak·ing soda (bāk′ing sō′dă) SYN sodium bicarbonate.

bal·ance (bal′ăns) **1.** An apparatus for weighing (e.g., scales). **2.** The normal state of action and reaction between two or more parts or organs of the body. **3.** Quantities, concentrations, and proportionate amounts of bodily constituents. **4.** The difference between intake and use, storage, or excretion of a substance by the body. **5.** The system that depends on vestibular function, vision, and proprioception to maintain posture, navigate in one's surroundings, coordinate motion of body parts, modulate fine motor control, and initiate the vestibulooculomotor reflexes.

bal·anced di·et (bal′ănst dī′ĕt) One containing the essential nutrients with a reasonable ration of all the major food groups.

bal·anced oc·clu·sion (bal′ănst ŏ-klū′zhŭn) The simultaneous contacting of the upper and lower teeth on the right and left and in the anterior and posterior occlusal areas in centric and eccentric positions within the functional range.

bal·anced pol·y·mor·phism (bal′ănst pol′ē-mōr′fizm) A unilocal trait in which two alleles are maintained at stable frequencies because the heterozygote is more fit than either of the homozygotes.

bal·anc·ing con·tact (bal′ăns-ing kon′ takt) **1.** Contacts between upper and lower dentures on the balancing or mediotrusive side for the purpose of stabilizing the dentures. **2.** Contacts between upper and lower dentures at the opposite side from the working or laterotrusive side (anteroposteriorly or laterally) to purpose stabilize dentures. **3.** Contacts between upper

and lower natural or artificial teeth at the opposite side from the working or laterotrusive side. SYN balancing occlusal surface.

ba·lan·ic (bă-lan′ik) Relating to the glans penis or glans clitoridis.

bal·a·ni·tis (bal′ă-nī′tis) Inflammation of the glans penis or clitoris.

bal·a·ni·tis di·a·be·ti·ca (bal′ă-nī′tis dī-ă-bet′i-kă) Glandular inflammation in diabetic patients related to urinary infection or concomitant posthitis.

bal·a·ni·tis xe·ro·ti·ca ob·li·te·rans (BXO) (bal′ă-nī′tis zē-rot′i-kă ob-lit′ĕranz) Infection with lichen sclerosus et atrophicus of the glans penis, may result in meatal stenosis.

balano-, balan- Combining forms denoting glans penis.

bal·a·no·pos·thi·tis (bal′ă-nō-pos-thī′ tis) Inflammation of the glans penis and overlying prepuce.

bal·an·ti·di·a·sis (bal′an-ti-dī′ă-sis) A disease due to *Balantidium coli* in the large intestine.

Ba·lan·ti·di·um (bal-an-tid′ē-ŭm) A genus of ciliates (family Balantidiidae) found in the digestive tract of vertebrates and invertebrates.

Bal·kan frame, Bal·kan splint (bawl′ kăn frām, splint) An overhead frame, supported on uprights attached to the bedposts or to a separate stand, from which a splinted limb is slung in the treatment of fracture or joint disease.

Balke-Ware tread·mill pro·to·col (bawlk-wār tred′mil prō′tŏ-kawl) A submaximal exercise test performed on a treadmill to evaluate patients with acute myocardial infarction and high risk dysrhythmias.

ball (bawl) **1.** Any round mass. **2.** In veterinary medicine, a large pill or bolus.

ball-and-sock·et joint (bawl-and-sok′ ĕt joynt) A multiaxial synovial joint in which a more or less extensive sphere on the head of one bone fits into a rounded cavity in the other bone. SYN cotyloid joint, enarthrodial joint, enarthrosis, spheroid joint.

Bal·lan·tyne dis·ease (bal′ăn-tīn di-zēz′) Neonatal disorder marked by prolonged gestation (i.e., longer than 39 weeks), decreased alertness, low birth weight, and increased respiratory distress. SYN Clifford disease, dysmaturity syndrome, Runge disease.

bal·lis·mus (bă-liz′mŭs) Involuntary movement affecting the proximal limb musculature, manifested as jerking, flinging movements of the extremity; caused by a lesion of or near the contralateral subthalamic nucleus.

bal·loon ang·i·o·plas·ty (bă-lūn′ an′jē-ō-plas′tē) Dilation of an obstructed atherosclerotic artery by passage of a balloon catheter through the vessel to the area of disease where the plaque is compressed against the vessel wall.

bal·loon cath·e·ter (bă-lūn′ kath′ĕ-tĕr) Catheter used in arterial embolectomy or to float into the pulmonary artery.

bal·loon cell ne·vus (bă-lūn′ sel nē′vŭs) Nevus in which many of the cells are large, with clear cytoplasm.

balm (bawlm) **1.** SYN balsam. **2.** An ointment, especially a fragrant one. **3.** A soothing application.

bal·sam (bal, bals) (bawl′săm) A fragrant, resinous or thick, oily exudate from various trees and plants. SYN balm (1), oleoresin (3).

bam·boo hair (bam-bū′ hār) Hair with regularly spaced nodules along the shaft caused by intermittent fractures with invagination of the distal hair into the proximal portion, with intervening lengths of normal hair, giving the appearance of bamboo. SYN trichorrhexis invaginata.

bam·boo spine (bam-bū′ spīn) RADIOLOGY the appearance of the thoracic or lumbar spine with ankylosing spondylitis.

band (band) **1.** Any appliance or part of an apparatus that encircles or binds a part of the body. **2.** Any ribbon-shaped or cordlike anatomic structure that encircles or binds another structure or that connects two or more parts. **3.** DENTISTRY a strip of metal that fits around a tooth and serves as an attachment for orthodontic components. **4.** A nonfilamentous neutrophil.

ban·dage (ban′dăj) **1.** A piece of cloth or other material, of varying shape and size, applied to a body part to provide compression, protect from external contamination, prevent drying, absorb drainage, prevent motion, and retain surgical dressings. **2.** To cover a body part by application of a bandage.

band cell (band sel) Any cell of the granulocytic (leukocytic) series that has a nucleus that could be described as a curved or coiled band, no matter how marked the indentation, if it does not completely segment the nucleus into lobes connected by a filament. SYN staff cell.

band·ing (band′ing) The process of differential staining of chromosomes to reveal characteristic patterns of bands that permit identification of individual chromosomes and recognition of missing segments.

Bandl ring (bahn′dĕl ring) SYN pathologic retraction ring.

band-shap·ed ker·a·top·a·thy (band′ shāpt ker′ă-top′ă-thē) A horizontal, gray, interpalpebral opacity of the cornea from calcium deposits at the Bowman layer.

bank (bangk) Any facility for storage of viable preserved tissue, blood, or medical supplies for future study or use.

Ban·kart le·sion (bangk′ărt lē′zhŭn) Avulsion or damage to the anterior lip of the glenoid fossa when the humerus slides forward in an anterior dislocation.

Ban·nis·ter dis·ease (ban′is-tĕr di-zēz′) SYN angioedema.

Bann·warth syn·drome (bahn′vahrt sin′drŏm) Neurologic manifestations of Lyme disease, also called chronic lymphocytic meningitis and tick-borne meningopolyneuritis.

bar (bahr) **1.** A unit of pressure equal to 1 megadyne (10^6 dyne) per cm^2 in the CGS system, 0.9869233 atmosphere, or 10^5 Pa (N/m^2) in the SI system. **2.** A metal segment of greater length than width that serves to connect two or more parts of a removable partial denture. **3.** A segment of tissue or bone that unites two or more similar structures.

baraesthesiometer [Br.] SYN baresthesiometer.

bar·ag·no·sis (bar-ag-nō'sis) *In the diphthong gn, the g is silent only at the beginning of a word.* Loss of ability to appreciate the weight of objects held in the hand. When the primary senses are intact, caused by contralateral parietal lobe lesion.

bar·ber's pi·lo·ni·dal si·nus (bahr' bĕrz pī'lō-nī'dăl sī'nŭs) Pilonidal abscess occurring in barbers, usually in the web between the fingers, due to the burying of exogenous hairs by alternate loosening and tightening of hand tissues by using scissors.

bar·bi·tu·rate (bahr-bich'ŭr-ăt) Any of various derivatives of barbituric acid used as sedatives, hypnotics, and anticonvulsants.

bar·bo·tage (bahr-bō-tahzh') Spinal anesthesia in which some anesthetic solution is injected into the cerebrospinal fluid, which is then aspirated back into the syringe and reinjected.

bar clasp arm (bahr klasp ahrm) Device with its origin in the denture base or major connector; consists of the arm that traverses but does not contact the gingival structures, and a terminal end that approaches its contact with the tooth gingivoocclusally.

Bard-Pic dis·ease (bahrd-pik di-zēz') SYN Courvoisier gallbladder.

bar·es·the·si·om·e·ter (bar'es-thē'zē-om'ĕ-tĕr) An instrument for measuring the pressure sense.

bar·i·at·rics (bar'ē-at'riks) That branch of medicine concerned with the management of obesity.

bar·i·at·ric sur·ger·y (bar'ē-at'rik sŭr'jĕr-ē) Operation performed for the management of obesity.

bar·i·to·sis (bar'i-tō'sis) Pneumoconiosis caused by barite or barium dust.

bar·i·um (Ba) (bar'ē-ŭm) A metallic, alkaline, divalent earth element; atomic no.

56, atomic wt. 137.327. Salts are often used in diagnosis.

bar·i·um en·e·ma (BE) (bar'ē-ŭm en'ĕ-mă) A type of contrast enema; administration of barium, a radiopaque medium, for radiographic and fluoroscopic study of the lower intestinal tract.

bar·i·um meal (BaM) (bār'ē-ŭm mēl) Oral administration of barium sulfate suspension for radiographic study of the upper gastrointestinal tract (British usage). SEE ALSO barium sulfate, barium swallow.

bar·i·um sul·fate (BaSO₄) (bār'ē-ŭm sŭl'fāt) Suspension given orally, rectally, or through a tube, for radiographic demonstration of a part of the gastrointestinal tract.

bar·i·um swal·low (bar'ē-ŭm swahl'ō) Oral administration of barium sulfate suspension for radiographic investigation of the hypopharynx and esophagus.

bark (bahrk) The envelope or covering of the roots, trunk, and branches of plants.

Bark·man re·flex (bahrk'mahn rē'fleks) Contraction of the ipsilateral rectus muscle in response to a stimulus applied to the skin below a nipple.

Bar·low ma·neu·ver (bahr'lō mă-nū'vĕr) Test for hip instability, with dislocation occurring with flexion, adduction, and posterior force.

Bar·mah For·est vi·rus (bahr'mă fōr'ĕst vī'rus) A mosquito-borne alphavirus that caused outbreaks of polyarthritis in humans in Australia.

baro- Prefix meaning weight, pressure.

bar·o·cep·tor (bar'ō-sep-tŏr) SYN baroreceptor.

bar·og·no·sis (bar'og-nō'sis) Ability to appreciate the weight of objects, or to differentiate objects of different weights.

bar·o·graph (bar'ō-graf) A device that gives a continuous record of barometric pressure. SYN barometrograph.

bar·o·phil·ic (bar'ō-fil'ik) Thriving under high environmental pressure; applied to microorganisms.

bar•o•re•cep•tor (băr′ō-rĕ-sep′tŏr) In general, any sensor of pressure changes. SYN baroceptor.

bar•o•re•flex (BR) (băr′ō-rē′fleks) A reflex triggered by stimulation of a baroreceptor.

bar•o•si•nus•i•tis (băr′ō-sī-nŭs-ī′tis) Inflammation of the mucous membrane of the paranasal sinuses caused by pressure difference within the sinus relative to ambient pressure. SYN aerosinusitis.

bar•o•ti•tis me•di•a (băr′ō-tī′tis mē′dē-ă) Inflammation of the mucous membrane of the middle ear caused by pressure difference within the middle ear relative to ambient pressure. SYN aerotitis media.

bar•o•trau•ma (băr′ō-traw′mă) **1.** Injury to the middle ear or paranasal sinuses, resulting from imbalance between ambient pressure and that within the affected cavity. **2.** Lung injury that occurs when a ventilated patient is subjected to excessive airway pressure.

bar•rel dis•tor•tion (băr′ĕl dis-tŏr′shŭn) Irregular image produced when peripheral magnification is greater than axial magnification. SEE Petzval surface.

Bar•ré sign (bah-rā′ sīn) When a patient with a pyramidal tract lesion is lying prone, and the affected leg is passively flexed 90° at the knee, the patient cannot maintain the lower leg in a vertical position; instead, it drops into full extension.

Bar•rett syn•drome, Bar•rett esoph•a•gus, Bar•rett met•a•pla•sia (băr′ĕt sin′drōm, ĕ-sof′ă-gŭs, met-ă-plā′zē-ă) Chronic peptic ulceration of the lower esophagus, which is lined by columnar epithelium, resembling the mucosa of the gastric cardia, acquired as a result of long-standing chronic esophagitis.

bar•ri•er (băr′ē-ĕr) PSYCHIATRY a conflictual agent that blocks behavior that could help resolve a personal struggle.

bar•ri•er con•tra•cep•tive (băr′ē-ĕr kon-tră-sep′tiv) Mechanical device designed to prevent sperms from penetrating the cervical os; usually used with a spermicide.

Bar•thel Self-Care In•dex (bahr′tel self-kār in′deks) A screening scale used in geriatric patients to measure ten self-care tasks (e.g., activities of daily living, instrumental activities of daily living) on a scale from 1–10.

Barth her•ni•a (bahrt hĕr-nē′ă) A loop of intestine between a persistent vitelline duct and the abdominal wall.

Bar•tho•lin duct (bahr′tō-lin dŭkt) Large duct draining the sublingual gland and opening into the Wharton duct or near it.

Bar•ton ban•dage (bahr′tŏn ban′dăj) A figure-of-8 bandage supporting the mandible below and anteriorly.

Bar•ton•el•la (bahr-tō-nel′ă) A genus of bacteria closely resembling *Rickettsia* in staining properties, morphology, and mode of transmission between hosts.

Bar•ton•el•la•ce•ae (bahr-ton-el-ā′sē-ē) A family of bacteria that currently includes the genus *Bartonella*. On the basis of S16 rRNA studies, the former genera of *Rochalimaea* and *Grahamella* have been merged with the genus *Bartonella*, retaining their species names.

Bar•ton frac•ture (bahr′tŏn frak′shŭr) Break in the distal radius with volar subluxation or dislocation of the radiocarpal joint.

Bart•ter syn•drome (bahr′tĕr sin′drōm) A disorder due to a defect in active chloride reabsorption in the loop of Henle.

ba•sad (bā′sad) In a direction toward the base of any object or structure.

ba•sal, ba•si•lar (bā′săl, bas′ĭ-lăr) [TA] **1.** Situated nearer the base of a pyramidal organ in relation to a specific reference point; opposite of apical. **2.** In dentistry, denoting the floor of a cavity in the grinding surface of a tooth. **3.** Denoting a standard or reference state of a function for comparison.

ba•sal an•es•the•si•a (bā′săl an′es-thē′zē-ă) Parenteral administration of one or more sedatives to produce a state of depressed consciousness short of a general anesthesia.

ba•sal bod•y (bā′săl bod′ē) An elongated centriolar structure situated at the base of each cilium at the apical margin of a cell.

ba·sal bod·y tem·per·a·ture (BBT) (bā'săl bod'ē tem'pĕr-ă-chŭr) Temperature at rest, usually obtained on arising in the morning, without any influences that might increase it; can give indirect evidence of ovulation.

ba·sal bone (bā'săl bōn) Osseous tissue of the mandible and maxillae except the alveolar processes.

ba·sal cell (bā'săl sel) A cell of the deepest layer of stratified epithelium.

ba·sal cell ad·e·no·ma (bā'săl sel ad-ĕ-nō'mă) Benign tumor of major or minor salivary glands or other organs composed of small cells showing peripheral palisading.

ba·sal cell car·ci·no·ma, ba·sal cell ep·i·the·li·o·ma (bā'săl sel kahr'si-nō'mă, ep'i-thē-lē-ō'mă) A slow-growing, malignant, but usually nonmetastasizing epithelial neoplasm of the epidermis or hair follicles, most commonly arising in sun-damaged skin of the elderly and fair-skinned.

ba·sal cell ne·vus syn·drome (bā'săl sel nē'vŭs sin'drōm) A syndrome of myriad basal cell nevi with development of basal cell carcinomas in adult life, odontogenic keratocysts, erythematous pitting of the palms and soles, calcification of the cerebral falx, and frequently skeletal anomalies, particularly ribs that are bifid or broadened anteriorly. SYN Gorlin syndrome.

ba·sal gan·glia (bā'săl gang'glē-ă) Large masses of gray matter at the base of the cerebral hemisphere.

ba·sal lam·i·na (BL) (bā'săl lam'i-nă) Amorphous extracellular layer applied to the basal surface of epithelium and also investing muscle cells, fat cells, and Schwann cells.

ba·sal met·a·bol·ic rate (BMR) (bā'săl met'ă-bol'ik rāt) The minimal amount of energy required to sustain life in the waking state. SEE ALSO resting energy expenditure.

ba·sal seat a·re·a (bā'săl sēt ār'ē-ă) Part of the oral structures available to support

a denture. SEE ALSO denture foundation.

base, ba·sis (bās, bā'sis) [TA] **1.** The lower part or bottom; the part of a pyramidal or conic structure opposite the apex; the foundation. [TA]. **2.** PHARMACY the chief ingredient of a mixture. **3.** CHEMISTRY an electropositive element (cation) that unites with an anion to form a salt; a compound ionizing to yield hydroxyl ion. SYN alkali (2). **4.** A substance with a pH over 7.0, in contrast to an acid. SEE ALSO Lewis base.

base·ball fin·ger (bās'bawl fing'gĕr) An avulsion, partial or complete, of the long finger extensor from the base of the distal phalanx. SYN mallet finger (2).

base·line (bās'līn) A line approximating the base of the skull, passing from the infraorbital ridge to the midline of the occiput, intersecting the superior margin of the external auditory meatus; the skull is in the anatomic position when the baseline lies in the horizontal plane. SYN orbitomeatal line.

base·line fe·tal heart rate (bās'līn fē'tăl hahrt rāt) Average cardiac rate for a particular fetus during diastolic phase of uterine contractions.

base·line pain (bās'līn pān) Long-term discomfort at a persistent level.

base·ment mem·brane (bās'mĕnt mem'brān) An amorphous extracellular layer closely applied to the basal surface of epithelium and also investing muscle cells, fat cells, and Schwann cells. SYN basilemma.

base of sta·pes (bās stā'pēz) [TA] Flat portion of the stapes to which the limbs attach that fits in the oval window. SYN basis stapedis [TA], footplate (1).

base·plate (bās'plāt) A temporary form representing the base of a denture; used for making maxillomandibular (jaw) relation records or for arranging artificial trial placement in the mouth to ensure exact fit of a denture.

basi-, basio-, baso- Combining forms meaning base; basis.

ba·si·breg·mat·ic ax·is (bā'si-breg-mat'

ik ak′sis) A line extending from the basion to the bregma.

ba·sic (bā′sik) Relating to a base.

ba·sic ami·no ac·id (bā′sik ă-mē′nō as′id) One containing a second basic group (e.g., lysine, arginine, ornithine). SYN dibasic amino acid.

ba·sic fuch·sin (bā′sik fūk′sin) [CI 42500] A triphenylmethane dye the dominant component of which is pararosanilin; an important stain in histology, histochemistry, and bacteriology.

ba·sic·i·ty (bā-sis′i-tē) **1.** The valence or combining power of an acid, or the number of replaceable atoms of hydrogen in its molecule. **2.** The characteristic(s) of being a chemical base.

ba·si·cra·ni·al ax·is (bā′si-krā′nē-ăl ak′sis) A line drawn from the basion to the midpoint of the sphenoethmoidal suture.

ba·sic salt (bā′sik sawlt) One in which one or more hydroxyl ions not replaced by the electronegative element of an acid.

ba·sid·i·um, pl. **ba·sid·i·a** (bă-sid′ē-ŭm, -ă) A cell or spore-bearing organ, usually club-shaped, characteristic of the Basidiomycota.

ba·si·fa·cial (bā′si-fā′shăl) Relating to the lower portion of the face.

ba·si·fa·cial ax·is (bā′si-fā′shăl ak′sis) A line drawn from the subnasal point to the midpoint of the sphenoethmoidal suture. SYN facial axis.

bas·i·lar, bas·i·la·ris (bas′i-lăr, bas-i-lā′ris) [TA] Relating to the base of a pyramidal or broad structure.

bas·i·lar ar·te·ry (bas′i-lăr ahr′tĕr-ē) [TA] Formed by union of the intracranial portions of the two vertebral arteries. SYN arteria basilaris [TA].

bas·i·lar im·pres·sion (BI) (bas′i-lăr im-presh′ŭn) Invagination of the base of the skull into the posterior fossa with compression of the brainstem and cerebellar structures into the foramen magnum. Cf. platybasia.

bas·i·lar in·dex (bas′i-lăr in′deks) Ratio between the basialveolar line and the maximum length of the cranium, according to the formula: (basialveolar line × 100)/length of cranium.

bas·i·lar in·vag·i·na·tion (bas′i-lăr in-vaj′i-nā′shŭn) SYN platybasia.

bas·i·lar men·in·gi·tis (bas′i-lăr men′in-jī′tis) Meningitis at the base of the brain; may result in an internal hydrocephalus.

bas·i·lar mi·graine (bas′i-lăr mī′grān) Headache accompanied by transient brainstem signs (e.g., vertigo, tinnitus, perioral numbness, diplopia). SYN Bickerstaff migraine.

bas·i·lar pon·tine sul·cus (bas′i-lăr pon′tēn sŭl′kŭs) A median groove on the ventral surface of the pons varolii in which lies the basilar artery.

bas·i·lar ver·te·bra (bas′i-lăr vĕr′tĕ-bră) The lowest lumbar vertebra.

ba·si·lem·ma (bā′si-lem′ă) SYN basement membrane.

ba·sin (bā′sin) A receptacle for fluids.

ba·si·na·sal line (bā′si-nā′zăl līn) A line connecting the basion and the nasion. SYN nasobasilar line.

basio- SEE basi-.

ba·si·oc·cip·i·tal (bā′sē-ok-sip′i-tăl) Relating to the basilar process of the occipital bone.

ba·si·on (bā′sē-on) [TA] The middle point on the anterior margin of the foramen magnum, opposite the opisthion.

ba·sip·e·tal (bā′sip-ĕ-tăl) In a direction toward the base.

ba·sis (bā′sis) [TA] SYN base (1).

ba·si·sphe·noid (bā′si-sfē′noyd) Relating to the base or body of the sphenoid bone.

bas·ket (bas′kĕt) A basketlike arborization of the axon of cells in the cerebellar cortex, surrounding the cell body of Purkinje cells.

bas·ket cell (bas′kĕt sel) A neuron enmeshing the cell body of another neuron with its terminal axon ramifications.

baso- SEE basi-.

ba·so·e·ryth·ro·cy·to·sis (bā'sō-ĕ-rith'rō-sī-tō'sis) An increase of red blood cells with basophilic degenerative changes, frequently observed in hypochromic anemia.

ba·so·phil, ba·so·phile (bā'sō-fil, -fīl) **1.** A cell with granules that stain specifically with basic dyes. **2.** A phagocytic leukocyte of the blood characterized by basophilic granules containing heparin and histamine.

ba·so·phil a·de·no·ma (bā'sō-fil ad'ĕ-nō'mă) Adenohypophysial lesion in which the cell cytoplasm stains with basic dyes.

ba·so·phil gran·ule (bā'sō-fil gran'yūl) One that stains readily with a basic dye.

ba·so·phil·i·a (bā'sō-fil'ē-ă) A condition in which there are more than the usual number of basophilic leukocytes in the circulating blood (basophilic leukocytosis) or an increase in the proportion of parenchymatous basophilic cells in an organ (in the bone marrow, basophilic hyperplasia).

basophilic leukaemia [Br.] SYN basophilic leukemia.

ba·so·phil·ic leu·ke·mi·a, ba·so·phil·o·cyt·ic leu·ke·mi·a (bā'sō-fil'ik lū-kē'mē-ă, bā'sō-fil-ō-sit'ik) Granulocytic leukemia with unusually high numbers of basophilic granulocytes in tissues and circulating blood. SYN basophilic leukaemia, mast cell leukemia.

ba·so·phil·ic leu·ko·cyte (bā'sō-fil'ik lū'kō-sīt) A polymorphonuclear leukocyte characterized by many large, coarse, metachromatic granules that usually fill the cytoplasm and may almost mask the nucleus; they usually do not occur in increased numbers as the result of acute infectious disease. SYN mast leukocyte.

ba·so·phil·ic leu·ko·cy·to·sis (bā-sō-fil'ik lū'kō-sī-tō'sis) Presence of an abnormally high number of basophilic granulocytes in the blood. SYN basocytosis.

ba·so·phil·ic leu·ko·pe·ni·a (bā'sō-fil'ik lū-kō-pē'nē-ă) A decrease in the number of basophilic granulocytes in the circulating blood.

Bas·sen-Korn·zweig syn·drome (bas'en kōrn'zwīg sin'drōm) SYN abetalipoproteinemia.

Bas·si·ni her·ni·or·rha·phy (bă-sē'nē hĕr'nē-ōr'ă-fē) An operation for indirect inguinal hernia repair.

bath (bath) **1.** Immersion of the body or any of its parts in water or any other yielding or fluid medium, or application of such medium in any form to the body or any of its parts. May be used for cleansing or therapy. **2.** Apparatus used in giving a bath of any form. **3.** Fluid used for maintenance of metabolic activities or growth of living organisms, e.g., cells derived from body tissue.

bath·ing trunk ne·vus (bādh'ing trŭngk nē'vŭs) A large hairy congenital pigmented nevus with a predilection for the entire lower trunk.

batho-, bathy- Combining forms meaning depth.

bathyaesthesia [Br.] SYN bathyesthesia.

bath·y·car·di·a (bath'ē-kahr'dē-ă) A condition in which the heart occupies a lower position than normal.

bath·y·es·the·si·a (bath'ē-es-thē'zē-ă) General term for all sensation coming from tissues beneath the skin. SYN bathyaesthesia.

bathyhypaesthesia [Br.] SYN bathyhypesthesia.

bathyhyperaesthesia [Br.] SYN bathyhyperesthesia.

bath·y·hy·per·es·the·si·a (bath'ē-hī'pĕr-es-thē'zē-ă) Exaggerated sensitiveness of deep body structures, e.g., muscular tissue. SYN bathyhyperaesthesia.

bath·y·hyp·es·the·si·a (bath'ē-hip'es-thē'zē-ă) Impairment of sensation in the structures beneath the skin, e.g., muscle tissue. SYN bathyhypaesthesia.

bat·ter·y (bat'ĕr-ē) **1.** A group or series of tests administered for analytic or diagnostic purposes. **2.** Device that turns chemical energy into electrical. **3.** Unlawful touching of another person. **4.** Any form of physical violence against another person.

bat·tle·dore pla·cen·ta (bat′ĕl-dōr plă-sen′tă) Placenta with the umbilical cord attached at the placental margin.

Bat·tle sign (bat′ĕl sīn) Postauricular ecchymosis in cases of fracture of the base of the skull.

Bau·mé scale (bō-mā′ skāl) Measurement allowing calculation of specific gravity of fluids at a baseline temperature of 60°F.

Bayle dis·ease (bāl di-zēz′) SYN paresis (2).

bay·o·net for·ceps (bā-ŏ-net′ fōr′seps) Device with offset blades, such as those for use through an otoscope.

***Ba·you vi·rus* (BAYV)** (bī′yū vī′rŭs) U.S. species of hantavirus that causes hantavirus pulmonary syndrome; transmitted by rice rats.

Ba·zin dis·ease (bah-zin[h]′ di-zēz′) SYN erythema induratum.

B cell-me·di·a·ted im·mu·ni·ty (sel mē′dē-āt-ĕd i-myū′ni-tē) The body's ability to defend itself from diseases through the production of antibodies.

B cells (selz) SYN beta (β) cells (1).

B com·plex vi·ta·mins (kom′pleks vī′tă-minz) A group of water-soluble vitamins that support many physiologic functions (e.g., metabolism, immunity, cellular reproduction).

bead·ed (bēd′ĕd) Marked by numerous small rounded projections, often arranged in a row like a string of beads.

bead·ed hair (bēd′ĕd hār) SYN monilethrix.

beak (bēk) **1.** The nose of dental pliers to contour and adjust wrought or cast metal dental appliances. **2.** Denotes a beak-shaped anatomic structure. SEE rostrum.

beak·ed pel·vis (bēkt pel′vis) SYN osteomalacic pelvis.

beak·er (bē′kĕr) A thin glass vessel, with a lip (beak) for pouring, used as containers for liquids.

beak·er cell (bē′kĕr sel) SYN goblet cell.

beak sign (bēk sīn) Appearance of the distal esophagus, on a contrast esophagram, in achalasia; also used to describe the proximal pyloric canal on upper GI series in congenital pyloric stenosis.

bean (bēn) The flattened seed, contained in a pod, of various leguminous plants.

bear·ber·ry (bār′ber-ē) Dried shrub leaves; purported value as a diuretic; use has been known to discolor urine.

bear·ing-down pain (bār′ing-down pān) Second-stage uterine contraction accompanied by straining and tenesmus.

beat (bēt) **1.** To strike; to throb or pulsate. **2.** A stroke, impulse, or pulsation, as of the heart or pulse. **3.** Mechanical activity of a cardiac chamber produced by catching a stimulus generated elsewhere in the heart.

Beau lines (bō līnz) Transverse grooves on the fingernails following fever, malnutrition, trauma, or other severe illness.

Bech·te·rew dis·ease (bek-ter′yev di-zēz′) SYN spondylitis deformans.

Bech·te·rew-Men·del re·flex (bek-ter′ yev men′dĕl rē′fleks) Percussion of the dorsum of the foot causes flexion of the toes; present in a pyramidal lesion. SYN Mendel-Bechterew reflex.

Bech·te·rew sign (bek-ter′yev sīn) Paralysis of automatic facial movements, the power of voluntary movement being retained.

Beck·er mus·cu·lar dys·tro·phy, (BMD) (bek′er mŭs′kyū-lăr dis′trō-fē) Hereditary late-onset muscle disorder, usually in the second or third decade, affecting the proximal muscles with characteristic pseudohypertrophy of the calves.

Beck·er ne·vus (bek′ĕr nē′vŭs) A nevus first seen as an irregular pigmentation of the shoulders, upper chest, or scapular area, gradually enlarging irregularly and becoming thickened and hairy.

Beck tri·ad (bek trī′ad) SYN acute compression triad.

Beck·with-Wie·de·mann syn·drome (bek′with vē′de-mahn sin′drōm) Exomphalos, macroglossia, and gigantism, often with neonatal hypoglycemia.

Bé·clard her·ni·a (bā-klahr′ hĕr′nē-a) One through the opening for the saphenous vein.

bec·que·rel (bek-ă-rel′) The SI unit of measurement of radioactivity, equal to 1 disintegration per second; 1 Bq = 0.027 × 10^{-9} Ci. SEE ALSO absorption.

bed (bed) **1.** ANATOMY a base or structure that supports another structure. **2.** A piece of furniture used for rest, recuperation, or treatment.

bed·bug (bed′bŭg) SEE *Cimex.*

Bed·nar aph·thae (bed′nahr af′thē) Traumatic ulcers located on the posterior portion of the hard palate in infants who place infected objects in the mouth.

Beer law (bēr law) Color intensity is inversely proportional to the depth of liquid through which it is transmitted; absorption thus depends on the number of molecules in the path of the ray.

bees·wax (bēz′waks) SYN wax (1).

beet su·gar (bēt shug′ăr) SEE sucrose.

be·hav·ior (bē-hāv′yŏr) **1.** Any response emitted by or elicited from an organism. **2.** Any mental or motor act or activity. **3.** Parts of a total response pattern. SYN behaviour.

be·hav·ior·al med·i·cine (bē-hāv′yŏr-ăl med′ĭ-sin) Interdisciplinary field concerned with development and integration of behavioral and biomedical science knowledge and techniques relevant to health and illness.

be·hav·ior·ism (bē-hāv′yŏr-izm) A branch of psychology that formulates, through systematic observation and experimentation, the laws and principles that underlie the behavior of humans and animals. SYN behavioral psychology, behaviourism.

be·hav·ior ther·a·py (bē-hāv′yŏr thār′ ă-pē) An offshoot of psychotherapy that uses procedures and techniques associated with conditioning and learning to treat psychological conditions.

behaviour [Br.] SYN behavior.

behaviourism [Br.] SYN behaviorism.

Beh·çet syn·drome (beh-chet′ sin′drōm) Disorder characterized by simultaneously or successively occurring recurrent attacks of genital and oral ulcerations (aphthae) and uveitis or iridocyclitis with hypopyon, often with arthritis.

bej·el (bej′el) Nonvenereal endemic syphilis, now found chiefly among Arab children; apparently due to *Treponema pallidum.* SEE ALSO nonvenereal syphilis.

Bé·ké·sy au·di·om·e·try (bā′kā-shē aw′dē-om′ĕ-trē) Hearing test where the subject controls increases and decreases in intensity at a fixed frequency or, more unusually, as the frequency of the stimulus is gradually changed so that the subject traces back and forth across the threshold of hearing. SYN automatic audiometry.

bel (B) (bel) Unit expressing the relative intensity of a sound. The intensity in bels is the logarithm (to a base 10) of the ratio of the power of the sound to that of a reference sound.

bel·la·don·na (bel′ă-don′ă) Perennial herb with dark purple flowers and berries; originally used as a source of atropine. SYN deadly nightshade.

Bell pal·sy (bel pawl′zē) Paresis or paralysis, usually unilateral, of the facial muscles, caused by dysfunction of the seventh cranial nerve; probably due to viral infection; usually demyelinating.

bel·ly (bel′ē) **1.** The abdomen. **2.** The wide fleshy part of a muscle. SYN venter (2) [TA]. **3.** Popularly, the stomach or womb.

bench sur·ger·y (bench sŭr′jĕr-ē) A surgical procedure carried on outside the patient's body (e.g., removal of cardiac tumors from the heart while that organ is itself extracorporeal).

bend frac·ture (bend frak′shŭr) An injury in which a long bone or bones, usually the radius and ulna, are bent (i.e., angulated) due to multiple microfractures, invisible on x-ray imaging.

bends (bendz) Colloquialism for caisson disease or decompression sickness.

Ben·e·dict test (ben′ĕ-dikt test) A copper-reduction test for glucose in urine; a red or orange precipitate indicates a sugar content exceeding 2%.

Ben·e·dikt syn·drome (ben′ĕ-dikt sin′drōm) Hemiplegia with clonic spasm or tremor and oculomotor paralysis on the opposite side.

be·nign (bĕ-nīn′) Denoting the mild character of an illness or the nonmalignant character of a neoplasm.

be·nign con·gen·it·al hy·po·to·ni·a (bĕ-nīn′ kŏn-jen′i-tăl hī′pō-tō′nē-ă) Nonprogressive hypotonia of unknown etiology in infants and children; other known causes of hypotonia must be excluded.

be·nign fa·mil·ial chron·ic pem·phi·gus (bĕ-nīn′ fă-mil′ē-ăl kron′ik pem′fĭ-gŭs) Recurrent eruption of vesicles and bullae that become scaling and crusted lesions with vesicular borders, predominantly of the neck, groin, and axillary regions.

be·nign gi·ant lymph node hy·per·pla·si·a (bĕ-nīn′ jī′ănt limf nōd hī′pĕr-plā′zhă) Solitary masses of lymphoid tissue containing concentric perivascular aggregates of lymphocytes, occurring usually in the mediastinum or hilar region of young adults.

be·nign in·fan·tile my·o·clo·nus (bĕ-nīn′ in′făn-tīl mī-ok′lō-nŭs) A seizure disorder of infancy in which myoclonic movements occur in the neck, trunk, and extremities.

be·nign lym·pho·ep·i·the·li·al le·sion (BLL, BLEL) (bĕ-nīn′ lim′fō-ep-i-thē′lē-ăl lē′zhŭn) Tumorlike masses of lymphoid tissue in the parotid gland, containing scattered small islands of epithelial cells. SYN Godwin tumor.

be·nign mi·gra·to·ry glos·si·tis (bĕ-nīn′ mī′gră-tōr-ē glos-ī′tis) SYN geographic tongue.

be·nign neph·ro·scler·o·sis (BNS) (bĕ-nīn′ nef′rō-sker-ō′sis) SYN arteriolar nephrosclerosis.

be·nign po·si·tion·al ver·ti·go (bĕ-nīn′ pŏ-zish′ŭn-ăl vĕr′ti-gō) Brief attacks of paroxysmal vertigo and nystagmus that occur solely with certain head movements or positions. SYN postural vertigo (1).

be·nign pros·tatic hy·per·pla·si·a (BPH) (bĕ-nīn′ pros-tat′ik hī′pĕr-plā′zē-ă) Progressive enlargement of the prostate due to hyperplasia of both glandular and stromal components.

be·nign pros·tat·ic hy·per·tro·phy (BPH) (bĕ-nīn′ pros-tat′ik hī-pĕr′trō-fē) Erroneous term; mistakenly used as a synonym of nodular hyperplasia of prostate.

be·nign stu·por (bĕ-nīn′ stū′pŏr) A syndrome from which recovery is the rule, as opposed to malignant stupor. SYN depressive stupor.

Ben·nett move·ment (ben′ĕt mūv′mĕnt) A lateral, bodily shift of the condyles of the lower jaw during lateral excursions.

Ben·son dis·ease (bens′ŏn di-zēz′) Disorder marked by presence of crystals of calcium stearate or polynitrile precipitating as irregularly shaped bodies in the vitreous of the eye; negligible impairment of vision.

ben·tir·o·mide test (bĕn-tēr′ō-mīd test) A measurement of pancreatic exocrine function that does not require duodenal intubation.

benz- Combining form denoting benzene.

benz·al·de·hyde (ben-zal′dĕ-hīd) Aldehyde produced artificially or obtained from oil of bitter almond, containing not less than 80% of benzaldehyde; a flavoring agent used in medicines. SYN benzoic aldehyde.

ben·zal·ko·ni·um chlo·ride (BAC, BZK, BAK) (ben′zal-kō′nē-ŭm klōr′īd) Aqueous solutions of this agent have a low surface tension, and possess detergent, keratolytic, and emulsifying properties that aid penetration and wetting of tissue surfaces.

ben·zene (ben′zēn) *Do not confuse this*

word with benzine. The basic six-carbon ring structure in most aromatic compounds; a highly toxic hydrocarbon from light coal tar oil; used as a solvent. SYN benzol, coal tar naphtha.

ben·zene ring (ben'zēn ring) The closed-chain arrangement of the carbon and hydrogen atoms in the benzene molecule. SEE ALSO cyclic compound.

benz·e·tho·ni·um chlo·ride (benz'ĕ-thō'nē-ŭm klōr'ĭd) A synthetic quaternary ammonium compound, one of the cationic class of detergents; germicidal and bacteriostatic.

ben·zo·ate (benz., B) (ben'zō-āt) A salt or ester of benzoic acid. The salts are often used as pharmaceutical or food preservatives.

ben·zo·caine (ben'zō-kān) The ethyl ester of *p*-aminobenzoic acid; a topical anesthetic agent. SYN ethyl aminobenzoate.

ben·zo·di·az·e·pine (BD, BDP, BZ, BZD, BZDZ, bz) (ben'zō-dī-az'ĕ-pēn) **1.** Parent compound for the synthesis of a number of psychoactive compounds (e.g., diazepam, chlordiazepoxide). **2.** A class of compounds with antianxiety, hypnotic, anticonvulsant, and skeletal muscle relaxant properties.

ben·zo·ic ac·id (ben-zō'ik as'id) Used as a food preservative, locally as a fungistatic, and orally as an antiseptic. SYN benzoyl hydrate, flowers of benzoin.

ben·zo·na·tate (ben-zō'nă-tāt) An antitussive agent related chemically to tetracaine; thought to act by depressing mechanoreceptors in the lungs.

ben·zo·yl·ec·gon·ine (ben'zō-il-ek'gō-nēn) Cocaine metabolite produced by hydrolysis; detectable in urine. SYN ecgonine benzoate.

ben·zo·yl per·ox·ide (BP, Oxy-5, BPO) (ben'zoyl pĕr-ok'sīd) Agent used in oil as an application to ulcers and to burns and scalds, in promoting the polymerization of dental resins, and as a keratolytic in the treatment of acne.

benz·thi·a·zide (benz-thī'ă-zīd) A diuretic and antihypertensive agent.

ben·zyl al·co·hol (BA) (ben'zil al'kŏ-hawl) Therapeutic liquid that possesses local anesthetic and bacteriostatic properties. SYN phenmethylol, phenylcarbinol.

ben·zyl ben·zo·ate (ben'zil ben'zō-āt) Agent that reduces the contractility of smooth muscular tissue, possessing marked antispasmodic properties; used now as a pediculicide and scabicide.

ber·ber·ine (bĕr'bĕr-ēn) An alkaloid from *Hydrastis canadensis*; has been used as an antimalarial, antipyretic, and carminative, and externally for indolent ulcers.

Berg Bal·ance Scale (BBS) (bĕrg bal'ăns skāl) An assessment of balance to determine risk of falling in older and neurologically impaired patients; comprises 14 tasks that are rated from 0 (cannot perform) to 4 (normal performance) for a total of 56 points.

Ber·gey clas·si·fi·ca·tion (bĕr'gē klas'i-fi-kā'shŭn) System for categorization of bacteria based on findings on Gram stain, morphology, order, family, genus, and species.

ber·i·ber·i (ber'ē-ber'ē) A nutritional (thiamine) deficiency syndrome occurring in endemic form in eastern and southern Asia; characterized by painful polyneuritis, diarrhea, weight loss, fatigue, poor memory, and edema. SYN endemic neuritis.

Ber·nard-Can·non ho·me·o·sta·sis (bār-nahr' kan'ŏn hō'mē-ō-stā'sis) The set of mechanisms responsible for the cybernetic adjustment of physiologic and biochemical states in postnatal life. SYN physiologic homeostasis.

Bern·hardt dis·ease (bern'hahrt di-zēz') SYN meralgia paraesthetica.

Bern·hardt sign (bern'harht' sīn) Pain on anterior lateral thigh; caused by injury to external cutaneous nerve. SYN Roth sign.

ber·ry an·eu·rysm (ber'ē an'yūr-izm) A small saccular aneurysm of a cerebral artery that resembles a berry.

ber·yl·li·o·sis (bĕ-ril'ē-ō'sis) Beryllium poisoning characterized by granulomatous fibrosis of the lungs from chronic inhalation of beryllium; toxic white metal element belonging to the alkaline earths.

Best dis·ease (best di-zēz′) Autosomal dominant macular degeneration beginning during the first years of life. SYN vitelliform retinal dystrophy.

bes·ti·al·i·ty (bes-tē-al′i-tē) Sexual relations between a human and an animal. SYN zooerastia.

be·ta (β) (bā′tă) **1.** Second letter of the Greek alphabet. **2.** CHEMISTRY denotes the second in a series, the second carbon from a functional (e.g., carboxylic) group, or the direction of a chemical bond toward the viewer.

be·ta (β)-**ad·re·ner·gic block·ing agent** (bā′tă ad′rĕ-nĕr′jik blok′ing ā′jĕnt) A class of drugs that competes with β-adrenergic agonists for available receptor sites; used to treat cardiovascular diseases and related conditions. Also called beta (β)-blocker.

be·ta (β)-**ad·re·ner·gic re·cep·tors** (bā′tă ad′rĕ-nĕr′jik rĕ-sep′tŏrz) Adrenergic receptors in effector tissues capable of selective activation by isoproterenol and blockade by propranolol.

be·ta (β) **car·o·tene** (bā′tă kar′ŏ-tēn) Isomer of carotene found in dark green and yellow vegetables and fruits.

be·ta (β) **cells** (bā′tă selz) **1.** Basophil cells of the anterior lobe of the hypophysis that contain basophil granules and are believed to produce gonadotropic hormones. SYN B cells. **2.** The predominant cells of the islets of Langerhans, which produce insulin.

be·ta fi·bers (bā′tă fī′berz) Nerve fibers that have conduction velocities of 40–70 m/sec.

be·ta (β)-ᴅ-**ga·lac·to·sid·ase** (bā′tă gă-lak-tō′si-dās) A sugar-splitting enzyme that catalyzes the hydrolysis of lactose into ᴅ-glucose and ᴅ-galactose, and that of other β-ᴅ-galactosides.

be·ta (β)-ᴅ-**glu·cu·ron·i·dase** (bā′tă glū-kyū-ron′i-dās) An enzyme catalyzing the hydrolysis of various β-ᴅ-glucuronides, liberating free ᴅ-glucuronic acid and an alcohol.

Be·ta·her·pes·vir·i·nae (bā′tă-hĕr′pĕz-vir′ĭ-nē) A subfamily of herpesviridiae containing cytomegalovirus and roseolavirus.

be·ta·ine (bā′tă-ēn) An oxidation product of choline and a transmethylating intermediate in metabolism.

β-lac·ta·mase (bā′tă lak′tă-mās) An enzyme that elicits hydrolysis of a beta lactam; found in most staphylococcal strains resistant to penicillin.

beta (β) **ox·i·da·tion** (bā′tă oks-i-dā′shŭn) Oxidation of the β-carbon (carbon 3) of a fatty acid, forming the β-keto (β-oxo) acid analogue; of importance in fatty acid catabolism.

be·ta par·ti·cle (bā′tă pahr′ti-kĕl) Electron, either positively (positron, β^+) or negatively (negatron, β^-) charged, emitted during beta decay of a radionuclide.

be·ta rhythm (bā′tă ridh′ŭm) Wave pattern in the electroencephalogram in the frequency band of 18–30 Hz. SYN beta wave.

be·ta test·ing (bā′tă test′ing) In health care, assessment of a product (e.g., software) in the manner it will, in fact, be used in clinical practice, so as to discover and remove any difficulties before such product is put onto the general market.

beta (β) **thalassaemia** [Br.] SYN beta (β) thalassemia.

be·ta (β) **thal·as·se·mi·a** (bā′tă thal′ă-sē′mē-ă) Hematologic disorder due to one of two or more genes that depress (partially or completely) synthesis of β-globin chains. SYN beta-thalassaemia.

be·ta wave (bā′tă wāv) SYN beta rhythm.

Be·thes·da system, Be·thes·da class·i·fi·ca·tion (bĕ-thez′dă sis′tĕm, klas′i-fi-kā′shŭn) A comprehensive system for reporting findings on cervical Papanicolaou smears.

Be·thes·da u·nit (bĕ-thez′dă yū′nit) A measure of inhibitor activity: the amount of inhibitor that will inactivate 50% or 0.5 unit of a coagulation factor during the incubation period.

Bet·ke-Klei·hau·er test (bet′kĕ klī′

how•ěr test) A slide-based procedure for the presence of fetal red blood cells among maternal cells.

bet•o•ny (bet′ŏ-nē) Herbal medicine suggested useful in lowering blood pressure levels. Other claims remain untested.

Betz cells (bets selz) Large pyramidal cells in the motor area of the precentral gyrus of the cerebral cortex.

be•zoar (bē′zōr) A concretion (hair, food, fiber) formed in the alimentary canal of animals, and occasionally humans.

Bi Symbol for bismuth.

bi- 1. Prefix meaning twice or double, referring to double structures, dual actions, for example. 2. CHEMISTRY used to denote a partially neutralized acid (an acid salt); e.g., bisulfate. Cf. bis-, di-.

bi•as (bī′ăs) Any trend in the collection, analysis, interpretation, publication, or review of data that can lead to conclusions that differ systematically from the truth.

bi•au•ric•u•lar (bī′awr-ik′yū-lăr) Relating to both auricles, in any sense.

bi•ax•i•al joint (bī-ak′sē-ăl joynt) Articulation with two principal axes of movement situated at right angles to each other; e.g., saddle joints.

bib•li•o•ther•a•py (bib′lē-ō-thār′ă-pē) Use of specific reading materials as therapy in psychiatry.

bi•cam•er•al (bī-kam′ěr-ăl) Having two chambers; denoting especially an abscess divided by a more or less complete septum.

bi•cam•er•al ab•scess (bī-kam′ěr-ăl ab′ ses) Lesion with two separate chambers.

bi•car•bon•ate (bī-kahr′bŏn-āt) The ion remaining after the first dissociation of carbonic acid; a central buffering agent in blood.

bi•ceps, pl. **bi•cep•ses** (bī′seps, -ěz) A muscle with two origins or heads. Commonly used to refer to the biceps brachii muscle.

bi•ceps bra•chi•i mus•cle (bī′seps brā′ kē-ī mŭs′ěl) *Origin*, long head from supraglenoidal tuberosity of scapula, short head from coracoid process; *insertion*, tuberosity of radius; *action*, flexes and supinates forearm (it is the primary supinator of the forearm); *nerve supply*, musculocutaneous. SYN musculus biceps brachii [TA].

bi•ceps fe•mo•ris mus•cle (bī′seps fem′ ōr-is mŭs′ěl) *Origin*, long head (caput longum) from tuberosity of ischium, short head (caput breve) from lower half of lateral lip of linea aspera; *insertion*, head of fibula; *action*, flexes knee and rotates leg laterally; *nerve supply*, long head, tibial, short head, peroneal. SYN musculus biceps femoris [TA].

bi•ceps re•flex (bī′seps rē′fleks) Contraction of the biceps brachii muscle when its tendon of insertion is struck.

Bi•chat mem•brane (bē-shah′ mem′ brăn) The inner elastic membrane of arteries.

bi•cip•i•tal (bī-sip′i-tăl) 1. Two-headed. 2. Relating to a biceps muscle.

bi•cip•i•tal groove (bī-sip′i-tăl grūv) SYN intertubercular sulcus.

bi•con•cave (bī-kon′kāv) Concave on two sides. SYN concavoconcave.

bi•con•dy•lar joint (bī-kon′di-lăr joynt) [TA] A synovial joint in which two distinct rounded surfaces of one bone articulate with shallow depressions on another bone.

bi•con•vex (bī-kon′veks) Convex on two sides. SYN convexoconvex.

bi•cor•nate, bi•cor•nous (bī-kōr′nāt, -nŭs) SYN bicornuate.

bi•cor•nu•ate (bī-kōrn′yū-āt) Two-horned; having two processes or projections.

bicro- SYN pico (2).

bi•cus•pid (bī-kŭs′pid) Having two points, prongs, or cusps.

bi•cus•pid mur•mur (bī-kŭs′pid mŭr′ mŭr) SYN Flint murmur.

bi•cus•pid tooth (bī-kŭs′pid tūth) SYN premolar tooth.

bi·cus·pid valve (bī-kŭs'pid valv) SYN mitral valve.

bi·di·rec·tion·al ven·tric·u·lar tach·y·car·di·a (bī-dir-ek'shŭn-ăl ven-trik' yū-lăr tak'i-kahr'dē-ă) Ventricular tachycardia in which the QRS complexes in the electrocardiogram are alternately mainly positive and mainly negative.

bi·dis·coi·dal pla·cen·ta (bī-dis-koy' dăl plă-sen'tă) A placenta with two separate disc-shaped portions attached to opposite uterine walls, occasionally found in humans.

Bi·el·schow·sky sign (byels-chov'skē sīn) In paralysis of a superior oblique muscle, tilting the head to the side of the involved eye causes that eye to rotate upward.

Bier am·pu·ta·tion (bēr amp'yū-tā'shŭn) Osteoplastic amputation of tibia and fibula.

Bier·nac·ki sign (byer-naht'skē sīn) Lack of feeling in the ulnar nerve in tabes dorsalis and dementia paralytica.

bi·fas·cic·u·lar (bī'fă-sik'yū-lăr) Involving two of the presumed three major fascicles of the ventricular conduction system of the heart.

bi·fid (bī'fid) Split or cleft; separated into two parts.

Bi·fi·do·bac·te·ri·um (bī'fĭ-dō-bak-tēr' ē-ŭm) A genus of anaerobic bacteria containing gram-positive rods of highly variable appearance.

bi·fid tongue (bī'fid tŭng) A congenital structural defect of the tongue in which its anterior part is divided longitudinally for a greater or lesser distance. SEE ALSO diglossia. SYN cleft tongue.

bi·fid uvu·la (bī'fid yū'vyū-lă) Bifurcation of the uvula, constituting a partially cleft soft palate.

bi·fo·cal (BI, bif, BIF) (bī-fō'kăl) Having two foci.

bi·fo·cal lens (bī-fō'kăl lenz) A lens used in cases of presbyopia, in which one portion is suited for distant vision, the other for reading and close work in general.

bi·fo·rate (bī-fōr'ăt) Having two openings.

bi·fur·ca·tion (bī'fŭr-kā'shŭn) [TA] A forking; a division into two branches.

bi·gem·i·nal bod·ies (bī-jem'i-năl bod' ēz) A bilateral single swelling of the roofplate of the embryonic midbrain that later in development becomes subdivided into a superior and an inferior colliculus. SYN corpora bigemina.

bi·gem·i·nal pulse (bī-jem'i-năl pŭls) A pulse in which the beats occur in pairs. SYN coupled pulse, pulsus bigeminus.

bi·gem·i·ny (bī-jem'i-nē) Pairing; especially, the occurrence of heartbeats in pairs.

bi·labe (bī'lāb) Forceps for seizing and removing urethral or small vesical calculi.

bi·lat·er·al (bī-lat'ĕr-ăl) Relating to, or having, two sides.

bi·lat·er·al left-sid·ed·ness (bī-lat'ĕr-ăl left-sī'dĕd-nĕs) A syndrome in which normally unpaired organs develop more symmetrically in mirror image; two spleens, one on each side, are usually present, and cardiovascular anomalies are common.

bi·lat·er·al syn·chro·ny (bī-lat'ĕr-ăl sin'krō-nē) Electroencephalographic activity recorded over both hemispheres simultaneously; usually used in reference to spike-and-wave activity.

bil·berry (bil'ber-ē) Agent derived from dried fruit of *Vaccinum myrtillus;* studies suggest value in cardiovascular disease; also used to treat optic disorders. SYN European blueberry, huckleberry, whortleberry.

bile (bīl) The yellowish-brown or greenish fluid secreted by the liver and discharged into the duodenum, where it aids in the emulsification of fats, increases peristalsis, and retards putrefaction.

bi·leaf·let valve (bī-lēf'lĕt valv) Low profile mechanical heart valve that is less obstructive to outflow, especially in small size.

bile duct (bīl dŭkt) Any of the ducts conveying bile between the liver and the intestine, including hepatic, cystic, and common bile duct. SYN biliary duct.

bile salts (bīl sawlts) Salt forms of bile acids; e.g., taurocholate, glycocholate.

bile sol·u·bil·i·ty test (bīl sol-yū-bil´i-tē test) Procedure that differentiates *Streptococcus pneumoniae* from other α-hemolytic streptococci by demonstrating its susceptibility to lysis in the presence of bile.

bil·har·zi·a·sis, bil·har·zi·o·sis (bil´hahr-zī´ă-sis, bil-hahr-zē-ō´sis) SYN schistosomiasis.

bili- Combining form denoting bile.

bil·i·ar·y (bil´ē-ār-ē) Relating to bile or the biliary tract.

bil·i·ar·y a·tre·sia (bil´ē-ār-ē ă-trē´zē-ă) Atresia of the major bile ducts.

bil·i·ar·y cal·cu·lus (bil´ē-ār-ē kal´kyū-lŭs) SYN gallstone.

bil·i·ar·y cir·rho·sis (bil´ē-ār-ē sir-ō´sis) Hepatic disorder due to biliary obstruction.

bil·i·ar·y col·ic (bil´ē-ār-ē kol´ik) Steady, ill-defined epigastric or right upper quadrant pain.

bil·i·ar·y duct (bil´ē-ār-ē dŭkt) SYN bile duct.

bil·i·ar·y dys·ki·ne·si·a (bil´ē-ār-ē dis-ki-nē´zē-ă) SYN sphincter of Oddi dysfunction.

bil·i·ar·y fis·tu·la (bil´ē-ār-ē fis´tyū-lă) Passage leading to the biliary tract.

bil·i·ra·chi·a (bil´i-rā´kē-ă) Occurrence of bile pigments in the spinal fluid.

bil·i·ru·bin (bil´i-rū´bin) A yellow bile pigment found as sodium bilirubinate (soluble), or as an insoluble calcium salt in gallstones.

bilirubinaemia [Br.] SYN bilirubinemia.

bil·i·ru·bi·ne·mi·a (bil´i-rū-bin-ē´mē-ă) The presence of increased amounts of bilirubin in the blood, where it is normally present in only relatively small amounts. SYN bilirubinaemia.

bil·i·ru·bin en·ceph·a·lop·a·thy (bil´i-rū´bin en-sef´ă-lop´ă-thē) SYN kernicterus.

bil·i·u·ri·a (bil´ē-yūr´ē-ă) The presence of various bile salts, or bile, in the urine. SYN choleuria, choluria.

bil·i·ver·din, bil·i·ver·dine (bil´i-vĕr-din, -ēn) Green pigment that occurs in bile.

Bill·roth dis·ease (bil´rōt di-zēz´) **1.** Bladder cancer caused by chronic infection by *Schistosoma haematobium*. **2.** Fluid accumulation under scalp caused by skull fracture and arachnoid tear.

Bill·roth-von Wi·ni·war·ter dis·ease (bil´rōt-fŏn vē-nē´vahr-ter di-zēz´) SYN Buerger disease.

bi·lobed (bī´lōbd) Having two lobes.

bi·lo·bate pla·cen·ta (bī-lō´bāt plă-sen´tă) Placenta divided into two lobes.

bi·loc·u·lar, bi·loc·u·late (bī-lok´yū-lăr, -yū-lăt) Having two compartments or spaces.

bi·loc·u·lar joint (bī-lok´yū-lăr joynt) One in which the intraarticular disc is complete, dividing the joint into two distinct cavities.

bi·man·u·al (bī-man´yū-ăl) Relating to, or performed by, both hands.

bi·man·u·al pal·pa·tion (bī-man´yū-ăl pal-pā´shŭn) Use of both hands to feel organs or masses, especially in the abdomen or pelvis.

bi·man·u·al per·cus·sion (bī-man´yū-ăl pĕr-kŭsh´ŭn) Percussion in which the finger of one hand taps the other hand; a form of mediate percussion.

bi·man·u·al ver·sion (bī-man´yū-ăl vĕr´zhŭn) Turning the baby in utero, performed by the hands acting on both extremities of the fetus; may be external or combined version. SYN bipolar version.

bin·an·gle (bin-ang´gĕl) The second angle given the shank of an angled instrument to bring its working end close to the axis of the handle to prevent it from turning about the axis.

bi·na·ry (bī´nar-ē) Comprising two components, elements, molecules, or other.

bi·na·ry digit (bī′nar-ē dij′it) **1.** The smallest unit of digital information expressed in the binary system of notation (either 0 or 1). **2.** The signal in computing.

bi·na·sal hem·i·a·no·pi·a (bī-nā′zăl hem′ē-ă-nō′pē-ă) Blindness in the nasal field of vision of both eyes.

bin·au·ral (bī-naw′răl) Relating to both ears. SYN binotic.

bi·nau·ral dip·la·cu·sis (bī-naw′răl dip′ lă-kyū′sis) A diplacusis in which the same sound is heard differently by the two ears.

bind (bīnd) **1.** To confine or encircle with a band or bandage. **2.** To join together with a band or ligature. **3.** To combine or unite molecules by means of reactive groups.

bind·er (bīnd′ĕr) **1.** A broad bandage, especially one encircling the abdomen. **2.** Anything that binds.

Bing re·flex (bing rē′fleks) When the foot is passively dorsiflexed, plantar flexion occurs if any point on the ankle between the two malleoli is tapped.

bin·oc·u·lar (bin-ok′yū-lăr) Adapted to the use of both eyes; said of an optic instrument.

bin·oc·u·lar fix·a·tion (bin-ok′yū-lăr fik-sā′shŭn) Condition in which both eyes are simultaneously directed to the same target. SYN bifoveal fixation.

bin·oc·u·lar mi·cro·scope (bin-ok′yū-lăr mī′krŏ-skōp) A microscope with two eyepieces.

bin·oc·u·lar oph·thal·mo·scope (bin-ok′yū-lăr of-thal′mŏ-skōp) Optic device that provides a stereoscopic view of the fundus.

bin·oc·u·lar pa·ral·lax (bin-ok′yū-lăr par′ă-laks) Difference in the angles formed by the lines of sight to two objects situated at different distances from the eyes; a factor in the visual perception of depth. SYN stereoscopic parallax.

bin·oc·u·lar per·cep·tion (bin-ok′yū-lăr pĕr-sep′shŭn) Ability of the brain to incorporate images received from each eye and integrate them.

bin·oc·u·lar vi·sion (bin-ok′yū-lăr vizh′ ŭn) Vision with a single image, by both eyes simultaneously.

bi·no·mi·al (bī-nō′mē-ăl) A set of two terms or names; in the probabilistic or statistical sense it corresponds to a Bernoulli trial.

bi·no·mi·al no·men·cla·ture (bī-nō′ mē-ăl nō′mĕn-klā′chŭr) Naming system in which each species of animal or plant has a name composed of two terms, one identifying the genus to which it belongs and the second the species.

bin·ov·u·lar (bin-ov′yū-lăr) Derived from two ova; of fraternal twins.

Bin·swan·ger dis·ease (bin′swahng-er di-zēz′) Form of dementia, with many infarcts and lacunae in the white matter.

bi·nu·cle·ate (bī-nū′klē-ăt) Having two nuclei.

bi·o·ac·tive (BA) (bī′ō-ak′tiv) Referring to a substance that can be acted on by a living organism or by an extract from a living organism.

bi·o·ac·ti·vi·ty (bī′ō-ak-tiv′i-tē) Having an effect on a living organism.

bi·o·as·say (bī′ō-as′ā) Determination of the potency or concentration of a compound by its effect on animals, isolated tissues, or microorganisms.

bi·o·as·tro·nau·tics (bī′ō-as-trŏ-naw′ tiks) The study of the effects of space travel and space habitation on living organisms.

bi·o·a·vail·a·bil·i·ty (bī′ō-ă-vāl′ă-bil′i-tē) Physiologic availability of a given amount of a drug, as distinct from its chemical potency; part of administered dose absorbed into bloodstream.

bi·o·ce·no·sis (bī′ō-se-nō′sis) An assemblage of species living in a particular biotope. SYN biotic community.

bi·o·chem·i·cal ge·net·ics (bī′ō-kem′ i-kăl jĕ-net′iks) Study of genetics in terms of the chemical (biochemical) events involved.

bi·o·chem·i·cal mod·u·la·tion (bī′ō-kem′ĭ-kăl mod-yū-lā′shŭn) Modification of a chemotherapeutic agent by another agent, which may or may not have antineoplastic activity of its own.

bi·o·chem·is·try (bī′ō-kem′is-trē) The chemistry of living organisms and of the chemical, molecular, and physical changes occurring therein. SYN biologic chemistry, physiologic chemistry.

bi·o·cli·ma·tol·o·gy (bī′ō-klī′mă-tol′ō-jē) The science of the relationship of climatic factors to the distribution, numbers, and types of living organisms; an aspect of ecology.

bi·o·de·grad·a·ble (bī′ō-dĕ-grād′ă-bĕl) Denoting a substance that can be chemically degraded or decomposed by natural effectors (e.g., weather, soil bacteria, plants, animals).

bi·o·de·gra·da·tion (bī′ō-deg-rĕ-dā′shŭn) SYN biotransformation.

bi·o·eth·ics (bī′ō-eth′iks) Discipline dealing with the use of the human body or body tissue in medical procedures (i.e., organ and fetal tissue transplants).

bi·o·feed·back (bī′ō-fēd′bak) A training technique that enables a person to gain some element of voluntary control over autonomic body functions.

bi·o·gen·e·sis (bī′ō-jen′ĕ-sis) **1.** Idea that life originates from only preexisting life and never from nonliving material. SEE spontaneous generation, recapitulation theory. **2.** SYN biosynthesis.

bi·o·gen·ic (bī′ō-jen′ik) Produced by a living organism.

bi·o·grav·ics (bī′ō-grav′iks) That field of study dealing with the effect on living organisms (particularly humans) of abnormal gravitational effects produced, e.g., by acceleration or by free fall; in the former case, heavier than normal weight is induced, and in the latter weightlessness.

bi·o·haz·ard (bī′ō-haz′ărd) Contaminated or infective waste such as blood, body fluids, sharps.

bi·o·ki·net·ics (bī′ō-ki-net′iks) The study of the growth changes and movements that developing organisms undergo.

bi·o·log·ic, bi·o·log·i·cal (bī′ŏ-loj′ik, -loj′i-kăl) Relating to biology.

bi·o·log·ic res·ponse mod·i·fi·er (bī′ŏ-loj′ik rĕ-spons′ mod′i-fī-ĕr) Agent that modifies host responses to neoplasms by enhancing immune systems or reconstituting impaired immune mechanisms.

bi·o·log·ic-war·fare (BW) agent (bī′ŏ-loj′ik wŏr′fār ā′jĕnt) Living organisms (e.g., bacteria, viruses, fungi) used for military purposes.

bi·ol·o·gy (bī-ol′ō-jē) The science concerned with the phenomena of life and living organisms.

bi·o·mark·er (bī-ō-mahrk′ĕr) A detectable cellular or molecular indicator of exposure, health effects, or susceptibility.

bi·o·mass (bī′ō-mas) The total weight of all living things in a given area, biotic community, species population, or habitat; a measure of total biotic productivity.

bi·o·ma·ter·i·al (bī′ō-mă-tēr′ē-ăl) A synthetic or semisynthetic material chosen for its biocompatibility and used in a biologic system to construct an implantable prosthesis.

bi·o·med·i·cal (bī′ō-med′i-kăl) Pertaining to aspects of the biologic sciences that relate to or underlie medicine and medical technology.

bi·o·mem·brane (bī′ō-mem′brān) A structure bounding a cell or cell organelle; it contains lipids, proteins, glycolipids, and steroids. SYN membrana [TA], membrane (2).

bi·om·e·try (bī-om′ĕ-trē) The application of statistical methods to the study of numeric data based on biologic observations and phenomena.

bi·o·mi·cro·scope (bī′ō-mī′krŏ-skōp) SYN slitlamp.

bi·on·ics (bī-on′iks) **1.** The science of biologic functions and mechanisms as applied to electronic chemistry. **2.** The science of applying the knowledge gained by studying the characteristics of living organisms to the formulation of nonorganic devices and techniques.

B

bi·o·phys·ics (bī′ō-fiz′iks) **1.** The study of biologic processes and materials by means of the theories and tools of physics. **2.** The study of physical processes (e.g., electricity, luminescence) occurring in organisms.

bi·op·sy (bī′op-sē) **1.** Process of removing tissue from living patients for macroscopic diagnostic examination. **2.** A specimen obtained by brush or needle and syringe aspiration for biopsy.

bi·o·psy·chol·o·gy (bī′ō-sī-kol′ŏ-jē) An interdisciplinary area of study involving psychology, biology, physiology, biochemistry, the neural sciences, and related fields.

bi·o·psy·cho·so·cial (bī′ō-sī′kō-sō′shăl) Involving interplay of biologic, psychological, and social influences.

bi·op·tome (bī′ō-tōm) A biopsy instrument passed through a catheter into the heart to obtain tissue for diagnosis.

bi·o·reg·u·la·tor (bī′ō-reg-yŭ′lā-tŏr) Any endogenous substance that modifies the rate or intensity of a biologic process so as to maintain homeostasis or meet changing needs of the organism.

bi·o·rhythm (bī′ō-ridh-ĕm) A biologically inherent cyclic variation or recurrence of an event or state, such as the sleep cycle, circadian rhythms, or periodic diseases.

bi·o·safe·ty (bī′ō-sāf′tē) Safety measures applied to the handling of biologic materials or organisms with a known potential to cause disease in humans.

bi·o·sta·tis·tics (bī′ō-stă-tis′tiks) The science of statistics applied to biologic or medical data.

bi·o·syn·the·sis (bī′ō-sin′thĕ-sis) Formation of a chemical compound by enzymes, either in the organism (in vivo) or by fragments or extracts of cells (in vitro). SYN biogenesis (2).

bi·o·ta (bī-ō′tă) The collective flora and fauna of a region.

Bi·ot breath·ing sign (bē-ō′ brēdh′ing sīn) Irregular periods of apnea alternating with four or five deep breaths; seen with increased intracranial pressure.

bi·o·tech·nol·o·gy (bī′ō-tek-nol′ŏ-jē) Science of applying techniques of biochemistry, cellular biology, biophysics, and molecular biology to addressing practical issues related to human beings and the environment.

bi·o·te·lem·e·try (bī′ō-tĕ-lem′ĕ-trē) The technique of monitoring vital processes and transmitting data without wires to a point remote from the subject.

bi·ot·ic (bī-ot′ik) Pertaining to life.

bi·ot·ic com·mu·ni·ty (bī-ot′ik kŏ-myū′ni-tē) SYN biocenosis.

bi·ot·ic po·ten·ti·al (BP) (bī-ot′ik pŏ-ten′shăl) Theoretic measurement of the capacity of a species to survive or to compete successfully.

bi·o·tin (bī′ō-tin) The D-isomer component of the vitamin B2 complex occurring in or required by most organisms and inactivated by avidin; participates in biologic carboxylations. SEE ALSO avidin. SYN coenzyme R, vitamin H, W factor.

bi·o·tox·i·col·o·gy (bī′ō-tok′si-kol′ŏ-jē) The study of poisons produced by living organisms.

bi·o·trans·for·ma·tion (bī′ō-trans′fŏr-mā′shŭn) The conversion of molecules from one form to another within an organism. SYN biodegradation.

Bi·ot res·pi·ra·tion (bē-ō′ res-pir-ā′ shŭn) Completely irregular breathing pattern, with continually variable rate and depth of breathing; results from lesions in the respiratory centers in the brainstem, extending from the dorsomedial medulla caudally to the obex.

bi·o·type (bī′ō-tīp) **1.** A population or group of individuals composed of the same genotype. **2.** SYN biovar (2).

bi·o·var (bī′ō-vahr) **1.** A group of bacterial strains distinguishable from other strains of the same species on the basis of physiologic characters. **2.** SYN biotype (2).

bi·ov·u·lar (bī-ov′yū-lăr) SYN diovular.

bip·a·rous (bip′ă-rŭs) Bearing two offspring or children.

bi·ped (bī'ped) **1.** Two-footed. **2.** Any animal with only two feet.

bip·e·dal (bip'ĕ-dal) **1.** Relating to a biped. **2.** Capable of locomotion on two feet.

bi·per·fo·rate (bī-per'fŏ-răt) Having two foramina or perforations.

bi·pha·sic (bī-fā'zik) Cellular structure with two histomorphologic patterns.

bi·phen·yl (bī-fen'il) SYN diphenyl.

bi·po·lar (bī-pō'lăr) **1.** Having two poles, ends, or extremes. **2.** Pertaining to a mood disorder involving alternating mania and depression.

bi·po·lar cell (bī-pō'lăr sel) A neuron with two processes (e.g., retina spiral and vestibular ganglia of the eighth cranial nerve).

bi·po·lar lead (bī-pō'lăr lēd) A record obtained with two electrodes placed on different regions of the body, each electrode contributing significantly to the record.

bi·po·lar ver·sion (bī-pō'lăr vĕr'zhŭn) SYN bimanual version.

bi·po·ten·ti·al·i·ty (bī'pŏ-ten'shē-al'i-tē) Capability of differentiating along either of two developmental pathways.

bi·ra·mous (bī-rā'mŭs) Having two branches.

bird-breed·er's lung, bird-fan·ci·er's lung (bĭrd'brēd-ĕrz lŭng, bĭrd'fan'sē-ĕrz lŭng) Extrinsic allergic alveolitis caused by inhalation of particulate avian emanations.

bird shot ret·in·o·chor·oid·i·tis (bĭrd shot ret'i-nō-kōr'oyd-ī'tis) Bilateral diffuse retinal vasculitis with depigmentation of multiple areas of the choroid and retinal pigment epithelium. SYN vitiliginous choroiditis.

bi·re·frin·gence (bī-rĕ-frin'jĕns) SYN double refraction.

birth (bĭrth) **1.** Passage of the fetus from the uterus to the outside world; the act of being born. **2.** Specifically, complete expulsion or extraction of a fetus from its mother.

birth ca·nal (bĭrth kă-nal') Cavity of the uterus and vagina through which the fetus passes. SYN parturient canal.

birth control (bĭrth kŏn-trōl') Restriction of conception by contraceptive measures.

birth de·fect (bĭrth dē-fekt') Any structural or biochemical abnormality present at birth.

birth·ing (bĭrth'ing) Parturition; the act of giving birth.

birth in·ju·ry (bĭrth in'jŭr-ē) SYN birth trauma.

birth·mark (BMK) (bĭrth'mahrk) A persistent visible lesion, usually on the skin, identified at or near birth; commonly a nevus or hemangioma. SEE nevus (1).

birth pal·sy (bĭrth pawl'zē) Any motor abnormality in the infant caused by or attributed to the birthing process.

birth rate (bĭrth rāt) Summation based on the number of live births in a population over a given period, usually 1 year.

birth trau·ma (bĭrth traw'mă) Physical injury to an infant during its delivery.

bis- 1. Prefix signifying two or twice. **2.** CHEMISTRY used to denote the presence of two identical but separated complex groups in one molecule. Cf. bi-, di-.

bis·a·cro·mi·al (bis'ă-krō'mē-ăl) Relating to both acromions of the scapular processes.

bi·sex·u·al (bī-sek'shū-ăl) **1.** Having gonads of both sexes. SEE ALSO hermaphroditism. **2.** Denoting a person who engages in both heterosexual and homosexual activities.

bis·fer·i·ous, bi·fer·i·ous (bis-fēr'ē-ŭs, bī-) Striking twice. SYN bisferient.

bis·fer·i·ous pulse (bis-fēr'ē-ŭs pŭls) Having two beats; an arterial pulse with peaks that may be palpable. SYN pulsus bisferiens.

Bish·op score (bish'ŏp skōr) System to determine the inducibility of the cervix in a pregnant patient, based on dilation, effacement, and cervical consistency and position.

bis·il·i·ac (bis-il′ē-ak) Relating to any two corresponding iliac parts or structures, as the iliac bones or iliac fossae.

bis in die, bid (bis in dē′ā) Twice a day.

bis·muth (Bi) (biz′mŭth) A trivalent metallic element; atomic no. 83, atomic wt. 20.98037. Several of its salts are used in medicine.

bis·muth line (biz′mŭth līn) A black zone on the free marginal gingiva, often the first sign of poisoning from prolonged parenteral administration of bismuth.

bis·mu·tho·sis (biz′mŭ-thō′sis) Chronic bismuth poisoning.

bis·phos·pho·nate (bĭs-fos′fō-nāt) Member of a class of drugs used for treatment of osteoporosis; works by inhibiting osteoclast-mediate resorption of bone.

bis·tou·ry (bis′tū-rē) A long, narrow-bladed knife, with a straight or curved edge and sharp or blunt point (probe-point); used for opening or slitting cavities or hollow structures.

bi·sul·fate (bī-sŭl′fāt) A salt containing HSO_{4-}. SYN acid sulfate, bisulphate.

bisulphate [Br.] SYN bisulfate.

bi·tar·trate (bī-tahr′trāt) A salt or anion resulting from the neutralization of one of tartaric acid's two acid groups.

bite (bīt) 1. To incise or seize with the teeth. 2. Term used to denote the amount of pressure developed in closing the jaws. 3. Undesirable jargon for terms such as interocclusal record, maxillo-mandibular registration, denture space, and interarch distance.

bite an·al·y·sis (bīt ă-nal′i-sis) SYN occlusal analysis.

bi·tem·po·ral (bī-tem′pŏr′ăl) Relating to both temporal bones, especially to the greatest diameter measured externally from one temporal bone to the other.

bi·tem·po·ral hem·i·a·no·pi·a (bī-tem′pŏr-ăl hem′ē-ă-nō′pē-ă) Blindness in the temporal field of vision of both eyes.

bite·plate (bīt′plāt) A removable appliance that incorporates a plane of acrylic designed to occlude with the opposing teeth.

bite rim (bīt rim) SYN occlusion rim.

bi·ther·mal ca·lor·ic test (bī-thĕr′măl kă-lōr′ik test) Assessment of vestibular function in which each ear canal is alternately or simultaneously irrigated with water at 7°C above or below body temperature. SEE ALSO Bárány sign.

Bi·tot spots (bē-tō′ spots) Small, circumscribed, grayish white, foamy, triangular deposits on the bulbar conjunctiva adjacent to the cornea in the area of the palpebral fissure of both eyes.

bi·tro·chan·ter·ic (bī′trō-kan-ter′ik) Relating to two trochanters, either to the two trochanters of one femur or to both greater trochanters.

bi·u·ret (bī′yŭr-et′) Agent obtained by eliminating one NH_3 between two urea molecules; used in protein determinations. SYN carbamoyl urea.

bi·va·lent (bī-vā′lĕnt) 1. Having a combining power (valence) of two. SYN divalent. 2. CYTOLOGY a structure consisting of two paired homologous chromosomes, each split into two sister chromatids.

bi·va·lent an·ti·bod·y (bī-vā′lĕnt an′ti-bod-ē) Antibody that causes a visible reaction with a specific antigen as in agglutination, precipitation, and other processes.

bi·va·lent chro·mo·some (bī-vā′lĕnt krō′mŏ-sōm) A pair of chromosomes temporarily united.

bi·val·i·ru·din (bī-val′i-rū-din) SYN hirulog.

bi·valve spec·u·lum (bī′valv spek′yū-lŭm) Probe with two adjustable blades.

bi·ven·tric·u·lar (bī′ven-trik′yū-lăr) Pertaining to both right and left ventricles.

bi·zy·go·mat·ic (bī′zī-gō-mat′ik) Relating to both zygomatic bones or arches.

Bk Symbol for berkelium.

black cat·a·ract (blak kat′ăr-akt) SYN brunnescent cataract.

Black clas·si·fi·ca·tion (blak klas′i-fi-kā′shŭn) A classification of cavities of the teeth based on the tooth surface(s) involved.

black co·hosh (blak kō′hosh) A herbal made from *Cimifuga racemosa*; widely used for purported value in treating disorders of the female reproductive system, and other uses. SYN baneberry, black snake root, rattleweed, squaw root (1).

black death (blak deth) Term applied to the worldwide epidemic of the 14th century, during which some 60 million people are said to have died. SEE ALSO plague (2).

black eye (blak ī) Ecchymosis of the eyelids and surroundings.

black·head (blak′hed) **1.** SYN open comedo. **2.** SYN histomoniasis.

black lung (blak lŭng) A form of pneumoconiosis, common in coal miners, characterized by deposit of carbon particles in the lung. SYN miner's lung (2).

black mea·sles (blak mē′zĕlz) **1.** SYN hemorrhagic measles. **2.** SYN Rocky Mountain spotted fever.

black·out (blak′owt) **1.** Temporary loss of consciousness. **2.** Temporary loss of vision, without alteration of consciousness, due to positive gravity forces.

black tongue (blak tŭng) Black to yellowish-brown discoloration of the dorsum of the tongue due to staining by exogenous material such as the components of tobacco or the use of broad spectrum antibiotics. Also called black hairy tongue.

black vom·it (blak vom′it) Vomitus with the consistency of coffee-grounds. SEE ALSO coffee-grounds vomit. SYN vomitus niger.

black·wa·ter fe·ver (blak′waw′tĕr fē′vĕr) Hemoglobinuria resulting from severe hemolysis occurring in falciparum malaria.

black widow spi·der (blak wid′ō spī′dĕr) A venomous arachnid, attacks always come from female (*Latrodectus mactans*); reported throughout the U. S., but more common in the South; marked on underside with a white 'hourglass' shape.

blad·der (blad′ĕr) [TA] **1.** A distensible musculomembranous organ serving as a receptacle for fluid. SEE detrusor. **2.** SYN vesica (1).

blad·der ear (blad′ĕr ēr) Protrusion of a portion of the bladder into proximal inguinal canal; rarely of clinical significance.

blad·der sphinc·ter (blad′ĕr sfingk′tĕr) Circular muscle that controls the release of urine from the bladder.

blad·der train·ing (blad′ĕr trān′ing) A predetermined schedule of voiding and toileting to maintain or improve bladder functioning.

Blain·ville ears (blăn-vēl′ ērz) Asymmetry in size or shape of the auricles.

Blair-Brown graft (blār-brown graft) A split-thickness graft of intermediate thickness.

Bla·lock-Taus·sig op·er·a·tion (blā′lok taw′sig o-ĕr-ā′shŭn) Surgery for congenital malformations of the heart.

Bla·lock-Taus·sig shunt (blă′lok taw′sig shŭnt) Palliative anastomosis of subclavian artery to pulmonary artery.

bland di·et (bland dī′ĕt) A regular diet omitting foods that mechanically or chemically irritate the gastrointestinal tract.

blan·ket su·ture (blangk′ĕt sū′chŭr) A continuous lock-stitch used to approximate the skin of a wound.

-blast A suffix meaning an immature precursor cell of the type indicated by the preceding word.

blast cell, blast (blast sel) An immature precursor cell.

blast cri·sis (BC) (blast krī′sis) Sudden alteration in the status of a patient with leukemia in which the peripheral blood cells are almost exclusively blast cells of the type characteristic of leukemia.

blas·te·ma (blas-tē'mă) **1.** The primordial cellular mass (precursor) from which an organ or part is formed. **2.** A cluster of cells competent to initiate the regeneration of a damaged or ablated structure.

♻ **blasto-** Prefix pertaining to the process of budding by cells or tissue.

blas·to·cele (blas'tō-sēl) The cavity in the blastula of a developing embryo. SYN blastocoele, cleavage cavity, segmentation cavity.

blas·to·coele [Br.] SYN blastocele.

blas·to·cyst (blas'tō-sist) The modified blastula stage of mammalian embryos (including human), consisting of the embryoblast (inner cell mass) and a thin trophoblast layer enclosing the blastocystic cavity. Also called blastodermic vesicle.

blas·to·cyte (blas'tō-sīt) An undifferentiated blastomere of the morula, blastula, or blastocyst stage of an embryo.

blas·to·derm, blas·to·der·ma (blas'tō-děrm, -děr'mă) The thin, disc-shaped cell mass of a young embryo and its extraembryonic extensions over the surface of the yolk. SYN germ membrane, germinal membrane, membrana germinativa.

blas·to·gen·e·sis (blas'tō-jen'ĕ-sis) **1.** Reproduction of unicellular organisms by budding. **2.** Development of an embryo during cleavage and germ layer formation. **3.** Transformation of small lymphocytes of human peripheral blood in tissue culture into large, morphologically primordial blastlike cells capable of undergoing mitosis.

blas·to·kin·in (blas-tō-kin'in) SYN uteroglobin.

blas·tol·y·sis (blas-tol'i-sis) Dissolution or destruction of the blastocyst or blast cells and subsequent death.

blas·to·ma (blas-tō'mă) A neoplasm composed chiefly or entirely of immature undifferentiated cells (i.e., blast forms), with little or virtually no stroma. SYN blastocytoma.

blas·to·mere (blas'tō-mēr) Cells into which the oocyte divides after its fertilization. SYN cleavage cell, embryonic cell.

blas·to·mer·ot·o·my (blas'tō-mēr-ot'ŏ-mē) SYN blastotomy.

Blas·to·my·ces der·ma·tit·i·dis (blas'tō-mī'sēz děr-mă-tit'i-dis) A dimorphic soil fungus that causes blastomycosis.

blas·to·my·co·sis (blas'tō-mī-kō'sis) A chronic respiratory granulomatous and suppurative disease caused by *Blastomyces dermatitidis*. SYN Gilchrist disease.

blas·tot·o·my (blas-tot'ŏ-mē) Experimental destruction of one or more blastomeres. SYN blastomerotomy.

blas·tu·la (blas'chŭ-lă) An early stage of an embryo formed by the rearrangement of the blastomeres of the morula to form a hollow sphere.

Bla·tin syn·drome (blă-tahn[h]' sin' drōm) SYN hydatid thrill.

bleb (bleb) **1.** A large, flaccid vesicle. **2.** An acquired lung cyst, usually smaller than 1 cm in diameter, similar to but smaller than a bulla; occurs mainly in lung apex.

bleed·er (blē'dĕr) **1.** A person with a hemorrhagic disease. **2.** A blood vessel severed during surgery.

bleed·ing (bl, BL, bldg) (blēd'ing) **1.** Losing blood as a result of the rupture or severance of blood vessels. **2.** Phlebotomy; the letting of blood.

bleed·ing time (blēd'ing tīm) A screening procedure to detect congenital and acquired platelet disorders.

blen·nad·e·ni·tis (blen'ad-ě-nī'tis) Inflammation of the mucous glands.

♻ **blenno-, blenn-** Combining forms indicating mucus.

blen·noid (blen'oyd) SYN muciform.

ble·o·my·cin sul·fate (blē-ō-mī'sin sŭl'fāt) An antineoplastic antibiotic obtained from *Streptomyces verticillus;* often induces pulmonary fibrosis.

blephar- Combining form denoting eyelid.

bleph·ar·ad·e·ni·tis, bleph·a·ro·ad·e·ni·tis (blef′ăr-ad′ĕ-nī′tis, blef′ă-rō-ad′ĕ-nī′tis) Inflammation of the meibomian glands or the marginal glands of Moll or Zeis. SYN blepharoadenitis.

bleph·ar·e·de·ma (blef′ăr-ĕ-dē′mă) Edema of the eyelids. SYN blepharoedema.

bleph·a·ri·tis (blef′ă-rī′tis) Inflammation of the eyelids.

bleph·a·ri·tis an·gu·la·ris (blef-ă-rī′tis ang-gyū-lā′ris) Inflammation of the lid margins at the angles of the commissure.

bleph·a·ri·tis mar·gi·na·lis (blef′ăr-ī′tis mahr-ji-nā′lis) Inflammation of the margins of the eyelids. SYN marginal blepharitis.

blepharo-, blephar- Combining forms meaning eyelid.

bleph·a·ro·chal·a·sis (blef′ă-rō-kal′ă-sis) A condition with redundancy of eyelid skin. SYN ptosis adiposa.

bleph·a·roc·lo·nus (blef′ăr-ok′lō-nŭs) Clonic spasm of the eyelids.

blepharoedema [Br.] SYN blepharedema.

bleph·a·ro·phi·mo·sis (blef′ă-rō-fi-mō′sis) Decrease in the width of the palpebral aperture without fusion of lid margins. SYN blepharostenosis.

bleph·a·ro·plas·ty (blef′ă-rō-plast-tē) Any operation to correct eyelid defects.

bleph·a·ro·ple·gi·a (blef′ă-rō-plē′jē-ă) Paralysis of an eyelid.

bleph·a·rop·to·sis, bleph·a·rop·to·si·a (blef-ăr-op-tō′sis, -tō′sē-ă) Drooping of the upper eyelid. SYN ptosis (2).

bleph·a·ror·rha·phy (blef-ăr-ōr′ă-fē) Reconstructive repair of an eyelid.

bleph·a·ro·spasm, bleph·a·ro·spas·mus (blef′ă-rō-spazm, -spaz′mŭs) Involuntary spasmodic contraction of the orbicularis oculi muscle.

bleph·a·ro·syn·ech·i·a (blef′ă-rō-si-nek′ē-ă) Adhesion of the eyelids to each other or to the eyeball.

bleph·a·rot·o·my (blef-ă-rot′ŏ-mē) A cutting operation on an eyelid.

bless·ed this·tle (bles′ĕd this′ĕl) An herbal made from the leaves and flowers of *Cnicus benedictus*; purported therapeutic effect on many internal organs. SYN cardo santo, holy thistle, spotted thistle, St. Benedict thistle.

blind (blīnd) Unable to see; without useful sight. SEE blindness.

blind fis·tu·la (blīnd fis′tyū-lă) Passage that ends in a cul-de-sac, thus open at only one extremity.

blind gut (blīnd gŭt) SYN cecum (1).

blind·ing glare (blīnd′ing glār) Glare resulting from excessive illumination.

blind loop syn·drome (blīnd lūp sin′drŏm) Symptoms that result from bacterial overgrowth in a surgically bypassed or disconnected segment of intestine.

blind·ness (blīnd′nĕs) 1. Loss of the sense of sight; absolute blindness connotes no light perception. 2. Loss of visual appreciation of objects although visual acuity is normal. 3. Absence of the appreciation of sensation, e.g., taste blindness. SYN typhlosis.

blind spot (blīnd spot) 1. SYN physiologic scotoma. 2. SYN optic disc.

blink re·sponse, blink re·flex (blingk rĕ-spons′, rĕ′fleks) A response elicited during nerve conduction studies, consisting of muscle action potentials evoked from orbicularis oculi muscles after brief electric or mechanical stimuli.

blis·ter (blis′tĕr) 1. A fluid-filled thin-walled structure under the epidermis or within the epidermis (subepidermal or intradermal). 2. To form a blister with heat or some other vesiculating agent.

bloat, bloat·ing (blōt, blōt′ing) Abdominal distention from swallowed air or intestinal gas from fermentation.

Bloch-Sulz·ber·ger disease (blok-sŭlts′ber-ger di-zēz′) Variously colored hyperpigmented lesions after development of bullous skin lesions; disorder usually causes death of pediatric patients.

block (blok) 1. To obstruct; to arrest passage. 2. A condition in which the passage of an electrical impulse is arrested, wholly or in part, temporarily or permanently. 3. Regional anesthesia. 4. SYN atrioventricular block.

block·ade (blok-ād′) Isolation of an organ, tissue, or system from communication with or influence by external forces or events.

block·er (blok′ĕr) 1. An instrument used to obstruct a passage. 2. SEE blocking agent.

block·ing (blok′ing) 1. Obstructing; arresting passage, conduction, or transmission. 2. In psychoanalysis, a sudden break in free association occurring when a painful subject or repressed complex is touched. 3. Sudden cessation of thoughts and speech, which may indicate the presence of a severe thought disorder or a psychosis.

block·ing a·gent (blok′ing ā′jĕnt) Drugs that inhibit a biologic activity or process; frequently called ''blockers.''

Blocq dis·ease (blawk di-zēz′) SYN astasia-abasia.

blood (blŭd) The fluid and its suspended formed elements that are circulated through the heart, arteries, capillaries, and veins; the means by which oxygen and nutritive materials are transported to the tissues, and carbon dioxide and various metabolic products are removed for excretion. The blood consists of a pale yellow or gray-yellow fluid, plasma, in which red blood cells (erythrocytes), white blood cells (leukocytes), and platelets are suspended. SEE ALSO arterial blood, venous blood.

blood a·gar (BA) (blŭd ah′gahr) Mixture of animal blood and an agar-based medium used to cultivate many medically important microorganisms.

blood-air bar·ri·er (blŭd-ār bar′ē-ĕr) Matter formed between alveolar air and blood; consists of a nonstructural film or surfactant, alveolar epithelium, basal lamina, and endothelium.

blood al·bu·min (blŭd al-bū′min) SYN serum albumin.

blood-a·que·ous bar·ri·er (blŭd-ā′kwē-ŭs bar′ē-ĕr) A selectively permeable barrier between the capillary bed in the ciliary body and the aqueous humor.

blood bank (blŭd bank) A place, usually a separate part or division of a hospital laboratory or a free-standing facility, in which blood is collected from donors, typed, tested, separated into several components, stored, and/or prepared for transfusion to recipients.

blood blis·ter (blŭd blis′tĕr) A sac resulting from a pinch or crushing injury.

blood-borne in·fec·tion (blŭd′bōrn in-fek′shŭn) Infection transmitted through blood or blood products (e.g., hepatitis virus, HIV-1).

blood-borne path·o·gens (BBP) (blŭd′bōrn path′ŏ-jĕnz) Disease-producing microorganisms transmitted by means of blood, tissue, and body fluids containing blood.

blood-brain bar·ri·er (BBB) (blŭd-brān bar′ē-ĕr) A selective mechanism opposing the passage of most ions and large-molecular weight compounds from the blood to brain tissue.

blood cap·il·la·ries (blŭd kap′i-lār-ēz) Smallest vessels in the circulatory system.

blood-ce·re·bro·spi·nal flu·id bar·rier, blood-CSF barrier (CSF) (blŭd-ser′ă-brō-spī′năl flū′id bar′ē-ĕr, blŭd bar′ē-ĕr) A barrier located at the tight junctions that surround and connect the cuboidal epithelial cells on the surface of the choroid plexus.

blood cir·cu·la·tion (blŭd sĭr-kyū-lā′shŭn) Course of blood from the heart through arteries, capillaries, and veins back again to the heart.

blood clot (blŭd klot) SYN thrombus.

blood clot·ting (blŭd klot′ing) Process in which platelets, in conjunction with clotting factors, transform blood from a liquid into a semisolid mass. Also called blood coagulation.

blood count (blŭd kownt) A determination of the number of red blood cells (RBCs) or white blood cells (WBCs) in a cubic millimeter of blood; calculated by counting the cells in an accurate volume of diluted blood.

blood crys·tals (blŭd kris′tălz) SYN hematoidin.

blood dop·ing (blŭd dōp′ing) Infusion of red blood cells, usually freeze-preserved autologous packed red blood cells, to increase hematocrit and hemoglobin levels; used by endurance athletes to increase blood's oxygen-carrying capacity and thus enhance endurance performance. SYN blood boosting, induced erythrocythemia.

blood gas a·nal·y·sis (blŭd gas ă-nal′i-sis) The direct electrode measurement of the partial pressure of oxygen and carbon dioxide in the blood.

blood group (blŭd grūp) A system of classifying genetically determined antigens or agglutinogens located on the surface of the erythrocyte; significant in blood transfusions, maternal-fetal incompatibilities (erythroblastosis fetalis), tissue and organ transplantation, disputed paternity cases, and in genetic and anthropologic studies. Often used as synonymous with blood type. SEE ALSO blood type.

blood is·land (blŭd ī′lănd) Aggregation of splanchnic mesodermal cells on the embryonic yolk sac, with the potentiality of forming vascular endothelium and primordial blood cells.

blood pH (blŭd) pH of arterial blood; normal is 7.4 (range, 7.36–7.44).

blood plas·ma (blŭd plaz′mă) SYN plasma (1).

blood poi·son·ing (blŭd poy′zŏn-ing) SEE septicemia, pyemia.

blood pres·sure (blŭd presh′ŭr) Tension of blood within the systemic arteries, maintained by the contraction of the left ventricle, the resistance of the arterioles and capillaries, the elasticity of the arterial walls, as well as the viscosity and volume of the blood.

blood rel·a·tive (blŭd rel′ă-tiv) A popular term describing a relative of a person sharing a common ancestor.

blood se·rum (blŭd sēr′ŭm) SEE serum (2).

blood sub·sti·tute (blŭd sŭb′sti-tūt) Material (e.g., human plasma, serum albumin, a solution of substances such as dextran) used for transfusion in hemorrhage and shock.

blood sug·ar (blŭd shug′ăr) Amount of glucose in blood; measured regularly by patients with diabetes. SEE ALSO glucose.

blood-thy·mus bar·ri·er (blŭd-thī′mŭs bar′ē-ĕr) A sheath of pericytes and epithelial reticular cells around thymic capillaries that prevents the developing T lymphocytes of the thymus from being exposed to circulating antigens.

blood trans·fu·sion (blŭd tranz-fyū′zhŭn) Process whereby a donor's blood cells or whole blood is infused into a recipient.

blood type (BT, BLT) (blŭd tīp) The specific agglutination pattern of erythrocytes of an individual to the antisera of one blood group.

blood typ·ing (blŭd tīp′ing) Process of testing a sample of blood to determine antigen and antibody factors to determine whether the patient has Type A, Type B, Type AB, or Type O blood.

blood u·re·a ni·tro·gen (BUN) (blŭd yūr-ē′ă nī′trŏ-jĕn) Nitrogen, in the form of urea, in the blood; the most prevalent of the nonprotein nitrogenous compounds in blood, which normally contains 10–15 mg of urea/100 mL. SEE ALSO urea nitrogen.

blood ves·sel (blŭd ves′ĕl) [TA] Any vessel conveying blood: arteries, arterioles, capillaries, venules, veins.

blot (blot) SEE Northern blot analysis, Southern blot analysis, Western blot analysis, zoo blot analysis.

blow-out frac·ture (blō′owt frak′shŭr) Trauma to the floor or medial wall of the ocular orbit, without break of the rim.

blue (blū) A range of hues in the visible

spectrum lying between green and indigo.

blue di·a·per syn·drome (blū dī´ă-pĕr sin´drōm) Disorder of tryptophan absorption manifest in indigo urine.

blue fe·ver (blū fē´vĕr) SYN Rocky Mountain spotted fever.

blue line (blū līn) A bluish striation along the free border of the gingiva, occurring in chronic heavy metal poisoning. SEE ALSO Burton line.

blue ne·vus (blū nē´vŭs) Dark blue or blue-black nevus covered by smooth skin and formed by heavily pigmented spindle-shaped or dendritic melanocytes in the reticular dermis.

blue pus (blū pŭs) An inflammatory fluid tinged with pyocyanin, a product of *Pseudomonas aeruginosa*.

blue spot (blū spot) 1. SYN macula cerulea. 2. SYN mongolian spot.

Blum·berg sign (blŭm´berg sīn) Pain felt on sudden release of steadily applied pressure on a suspected area of the abdomen, indicative of peritonitis. SYN rebound tenderness.

blunt dis·sec·tion (blŭnt di-sek´shŭn) Separating or incising tissue using a dull object, such as one's fingers or the opening action of a pair of scissors.

blush (blŭsh) 1. A sudden and brief redness of the face and neck due to emotion. 2. In angiography, used metaphorically to describe neovascularity or, in some cases, extravasation.

BMI Abbreviation for body mass index.

bob·bing (bob´ing) An up-and-down movement.

Boch·da·lek her·ni·a (bok´di-lĕk hĕr´nē-ă) SYN congenital diaphragmatic hernia.

Bo·dan·sky u·nit (bō-dan´skē yū´nit) The amount of phosphatase that liberates 1 mg of phosphorus as inorganic phosphate during the first hour of incubation with a buffered substrate containing sodium β-glycerophosphate.

bod·y (bod´ē) 1. The head, neck, trunk, and limbs; the human body, consisting of head (caput), neck (collum), trunk (truncus), and limbs (membra). 2. The material part of a human, as distinguished from the mind and spirit. 3. The principal mass of any structure. 4. A thing; a substance. SEE ALSO soma. SYN corpus (1) [TA].

bod·y cav·i·ty (bod´ē kav´i-tē) The collective visceral cavity of the trunk (thoracic cavity plus abdominopelvic cavity), bounded by the superior thoracic aperture above, the pelvic floor below, and the body walls (parietes) in between. SYN celom (3), celoma.

bod·y com·po·si·tion (bod´ē kom-pŏ-zish´ŭn) An estimate of the proportions of major components of a living body, as water, nitrogen, sodium; more specifically, the proportion of lean body mass to fat.

bod·y dys·mor·phic dis·or·der (bod´ē dis-mōr´fik dis-ōr´dĕr) A psychosomatic (somatoform) disorder characterized by preoccupation with some imagined defect in appearance in a person who looks normal.

bod·y im·age (bod´ē im´ăj) 1. The cerebral representation of all body sensation organized in the parietal cortex. 2. Personal conception of one's own body as distinct from one's actual body or the conception other people have of it.

bod·y im·age dis·tur·bance (bod´ē im´ăj dis-tŭr´băns) Distortion of one's mental picture of oneself. NANDA-approved diagnosis.

bod·y in·teg·ri·ty dis·or·der (bod´ē in-teg´ri-tē dis-ōr´dĕr) Mental state in which the person requests an elective amputation.

bod·y mass in·dex (BMI) (bod´ē mas in´deks) A rough method of assessing weight status; correlates with risk of disease and death due to causes associated with obesity. BMI = weight (kg) ÷ height (m²).

bod·y me·chan·ics (bod´ē mĕ-kan´iks) The application of physical principles to achieve maximum efficiency and to limit risk of physical stress or injury to the practitioner of physical therapy, massage therapy, or chiropractic or osteopathic manipulation. SEE ALSO ergonomics.

bod·y of ster·num (bod′ē stĕr′nŭm) [TA] Middle and largest portion of the sternum, lying between the manubrium superiorly and the xiphoid process inferiorly. SYN corpus sterni [TA], gladiolus, midsternum.

bod·y of uter·us (bod′ē yū′tĕr-ŭs) The part of the uterus above the isthmus, comprising about two thirds of the nonpregnant organ. SYN corpus uteri [TA].

bod·y pleth·ys·mo·graph (bod′ē plĕthiz′mō-graf) A testing device surrounding the entire body, commonly used in studies of respiratory function.

bod·y stalk (bod′ē stawk) SYN connecting stalk.

bod·y sur·face ar·e·a (BSA) (bod′ē sŭr′făs ăr′ē-ă) The entire external surface of the body, expressed in square meters (m²); used to calculate metabolic, electrolyte, nutritional requirements, drug dosage, and expected pulmonary function measurements.

bod·y:weight ra·ti·o (bod′ē-wāt′ rā′shē-ō) Body weight (in grams) divided by stature (in centimeters).

bod·y·work (bod′ē-wŏrk) Any technique involving touch, massage, manipulation, and/or energetic principles for the improvement or restoration of health. SEE ALSO massage therapy.

Boeck dis·ease (bĕrk di-zēz′) SYN sarcoidosis.

Boer·haa·ve syn·drome (būr′hah-vē sin′drōm) Esophageal rupture caused by increased intraluminal pressure and distention during retching or vomiting.

bohr·i·um (bōr′ē-ŭm) An artificial transplutonium element; atomic number 107; atomic weight 262 [Formerly called Unnilseptium, Uns 262.]

boil (boyl) SYN furuncle.

boil·ing point (BP, b.p., bp) (boyl′ing poynt) Temperature at which the vapor pressure of a liquid equals the ambient atmospheric pressure.

bo·lus (bō′lŭs) **1.** A single, relatively large quantity of a substance, usually one intended for therapeutic use (e.g., bolus dose of an intravenously injected drug) generally followed by smaller doses. **2.** A masticated morsel of food or another substance ready to be swallowed (e.g., a bolus of barium for x-ray studies).

bom·bard (bom-bahrd′) To expose a substance to particulate or electromagnetic radiations to make it radioactive.

bom·be·sin (BBS) (bomb′ĕ-sin) Pharmacologically active tetradecapeptide found in skins of European amphibians of the family Discoglossidae. A potent stimulant of gastric and pancreatic secretions; a bombesinlike immunoreactive peptide is found in both brain and gut.

bond (bond) CHEMISTRY the force holding two neighboring atoms in place and resisting their separation; a bond is electrovalent if it consists of the attraction between oppositely charged groups, or covalent if it results from the sharing of one, two, or three pairs of electrons by the bonded atoms.

bone (bōn) [TA] Osseous tissue of definite shape and size, forming a part of the animal skeleton; in human adults there are approximately 200 distinct bones in the skeleton, not including the auditory ossicles of the tympanic cavity or the sesamoid bones other than the two patellae. The core of a long bone is filled with marrow. SYN os [TA].

bone age (BA) (bōn āj) Stage of osseous development (in years) as adjudged by radiography, in contrast to chronologic age.

bone and mar·row trans·plan·ta·tion (BMT) (bōn mar′ō trans′plan-tā′shŭn) Grafting of bone marrow tissue.

bone cell (bōn sel) SYN osteocyte.

bone con·duc·tion (BC) (bōn kŏn-dŭk′shŭn) In relation to hearing, the transmission of sound to the inner ear through vibrations applied to the bones of the skull. SYN osteophony.

bone cyst (bōn sist) SEE solitary bone cyst.

bone den·si·ty (bōn den′si-tē) Quantitative measurement of the mineral content of bone, used as an indicator of the structural strength of the bone and as a screen for osteoporosis.

bone flap (bōn flap) Portion of cranium removed but left attached to overlying muscle-fascial blood supply.

bone graft (BG) (bōn graft) Osseous matter transplanted from a donor site to a recipient site, without anastomosis of nutrient vessels. SEE ALSO osteoplasty.

bone island (bōn ī'lănd) Macroscopic focus of cortical bone within medullary bone, commonly seen as a dense round or oval opacity on radiographs of the pelvis, femoral head, humerus, or ribs.

bone mar·row (bōn mar'ō) [TA] The tissue filling the cavities of bones, having a stroma of reticular fibers and cells.

bone mar·row bi·op·sy (bōn mar'ō bī'op-sē) Process whereby bone marrow is aspirated with a needle or trocar for microscopic examination.

bone ma·trix (bōn mā'triks) The intercellular substance of bone tissue consisting of collagen fibers, ground substance, and inorganic bone salts.

bone min·er·al den·si·ty (BMD) (bōn min'ĕr-ăl den'si-tē) Measurement of the amount of calcium in bone. Most methods for measuring BMD (also called bone densitometry) are fast, noninvasive, painless, and available on an outpatient basis.

bone plate (bōn plāt) Metal bar with perforations for the insertion of screws; used to immobilize fractured segments.

bone scan (bōn skan) Examination involving nuclear medicine of bone after injection of radioactive material, to identify areas of injury, disease, or regeneration, using a gamma camera.

bones of cra·ni·um (bōnz krā'nē-ŭm) The paired inferior nasal concha, lacrimal, maxilla, nasal, palatine, parietal, temporal, and zygomatic; and the unpaired ethmoid, frontal, occipital, sphenoid, and vomer.

Bon·fer·ro·ni meth·od (bōn-fer-rō'nē meth'ŏd) Multiple comparison method used in studies involving analysis of variants.

Bon·hoef·fer sign (bon'hĕrf-ĕr sīn) Loss of normal muscle tone in chorea.

Bon·nier syn·drome (bōn-yā' sin'drōm) A disorder due to a lesion of vestibular nuclei and connection; the symptoms include ocular disturbances (e.g., paralysis of accommodation, nystagmus, diplopia), as well as deafness, nausea, thirst, anorexia, and other symptoms.

bony (bō'nē) Pertaining to or characteristic of bone.

bon·y an·ky·lo·sis (bō'nē ang'ki-lō'sis) SYN synostosis.

bon·y lab·y·rinth (bō'nē lab'i-rinth) [TA] A series of cavities (cochlea, vestibule, semicircular canals) contained within the otic capsule of the petrous portion of the temporal bone; filled with perilymph, in which the delicate, endolymph-filled membranous labyrinth is suspended.

boost·er, boost·er dose (būs'tĕr, dōs) A dose given at some time after an initial dose to enhance the effect.

boot (būt) A boot-shaped appliance.

bor·age (bōr'ăj) A herbal prepared from the plant parts and seeds of *Borago officinalis*. Value as antiinflammatory and tonic. Plant contains toxic pyrrolizidine alkaloids. SYN beebread, ox's tongue, starflower.

bo·rate (bōr'āt) A salt of boric acid.

bo·rax (bōr'aks) SYN sodium borate.

bor·bo·ryg·mus, gen. and pl. **bor·bo·ryg·mi** (bōr-bō-rig'mŭs, -rig'mī) Audible sounds produced by gas or fluid moving through the gastrointestinal tract.

bor·der (bōr'dĕr) [TA] The part of a surface that forms its outer boundary. SEE ALSO margin. SYN margo [TA].

bor·der·line hy·per·ten·sion (BHT) (bōr'dĕr-līn hī'pĕr-ten'shŭn) By consensus, that blood pressure zone between highest acceptable "normal" blood pressure and hypertensive blood pressure. The Framingham Heart Study defines this as pressures between 140–160 mm/ Hg systolic and 90–95 mm/Hg diastolic.

Bor·de·tel·la (bor-dĕ-tel'ă) A genus of strictly aerobic bacteria containing minute gram-negative coccobacilli.

bo·ric ac·id (BA) (bōr'ik as'id) A weak acid, used as an antiseptic dusting powder, in saturated solution as a collyrium, and with glycerin in aphthae and stomatitis. Also called boracic acid.

bo·ron (B) (bōr'on) A nonmetallic trivalent element, atomic no. 5, atomic wt. 10.811; occurs as a hard crystalline mass or as a brown powder, and forms borates and boric acid.

Bor·rel·i·a (bŏ-rel'ē-ă) A genus of bacteria containing cells 8– 16 mcm in length, with coarse, shallow, irregular spirals and tapered, finely filamented ends; most are transmitted to animals or humans by the bites of arthropods. *B. burgdorferi* causes Lyme disease.

bor·re·li·o·sis (bōr-el'ē-ō'sis) Disease caused by bacteria of the genus *Borrelia*.

boss (baws) **1.** A protuberance; a circumscribed rounded swelling. **2.** The prominence of a kyphosis.

bos·se·lat·ed (baws'ĕ-lā-ted) Marked by numerous rounded protuberances.

bot·ry·oid (bot'rē-oyd) Having numerous rounded protuberances resembling a bunch of grapes. SYN uviform.

bot·ry·oid sar·co·ma (bot'rē-oyd sahr-kō'mă) A polypoid form of embryonal rhabdomyosarcoma that occurs in children, most frequently in the urogenital tract, characterized by the formation of grossly apparent grapelike clusters of neoplastic tissue; highly malignant.

bot·u·li·num tox·in (bot-yū-lī'nŭm tok'sin) An extremely potent neurotoxin produced by *Clostridium botulinum*, a gram-positive, strictly anaerobic bacillus; causes botulism when the preformed toxin is ingested in previously contaminated food products.

bot·u·lism (boch'ŭ-lizm) Food poisoning caused by the ingestion of the neurotoxin produced by *Clostridium botulinum* and

related bacteria, usually in improperly canned or preserved food.

bot·u·lism an·ti·tox·in (boch'ŭ-lizm an'tē-toks'in) Antitoxin specific for a toxin of one or more strains of *Clostridium botulinum*.

Bou·chard dis·ease (bū-shahr' di-zēz') Myopathic dilation of the stomach.

bou·gie (bū-zhē') A cylindric instrument, usually somewhat flexible and yielding, used for calibrating, examining, measuring, or dilating constricted areas in tubular organs.

bound (B, BD) (bownd) **1.** Limited; circumscribed; attached; enclosed. **2.** Denoting a substance, such as iodine, phosphorus, calcium, morphine, or some other drug, which is not in readily diffusible form but exists in combination with a high molecular weight substance, especially protein.

bound wa·ter (bownd waw'tĕr) Water held to colloids and other substances and not removed by simple filtration.

bou·ton (bū-tōn[h]') A button, pustule, or knoblike swelling.

bou·ton·neuse fe·ver (bu-tō-nuz' fē'vĕr) Tick-borne infection with *Rickettsia conorii* seen in Africa, Europe, the Middle East, and India. SYN tick typhus.

bo·vine (bō'vīn) Relating to cattle.

bo·vine ba·be·si·o·sis (bō'vīn ba-bē-sē-ō'sis) An infectious disease of cattle caused by *Babesia* species and transmitted by ticks.

bo·vine spon·gi·form en·ceph·a·lop·a·thy (bō'vīn spŭn'ji-fōrm en-sef'a-lop'ă-thē) Cattle disease first reported in 1986 in Great Britain; characterized by apprehensive behavior, hyperesthesia, and ataxia, with spongiform changes in the gray matter of the brainstem; caused by a prion.

bow (bō) Any flexible device bent in a simple curve.

Bow·ditch law (bō'dich law) Consistently total response to any effective stimulus. SYN all or none law.

bow·el (bow'ĕl) SYN intestine.

bow·el by·pass syn·drome (bow'ĕl bī'pas sin'drōm) Recurrent fever, chills, malaise, and inflammatory cutaneous papules and pustules on the extremities and upper trunk with diffuse neutrophil infiltration due to bowel bypass surgery.

bowel train·ing (bow'ĕl trān'ing) A method of establishing or reestablishing regularity of defecation.

Bow·en dis·ease (bō'ĕn di-zēz') A form of intraepidermal carcinoma characterized by the development of slowly enlarging pinkish or brownish papules or eroded plaques covered with a thickened horny layer.

bow·en·oid pap·u·lo·sis (bō'ĕn-oyd pap'yū-lō'sis) Condition associated with variant of the human papillomavirus; characterized by pigmented anogenital papules that are typically benign.

bow·ing frac·ture (bō'ing frak'shŭr) Osseous breakage due to impact that ruptures a bone along the longitudinal axis.

bow·leg, bow-leg (bō'leg) SYN genu varum.

bowl·er's thumb (bō'lĕrz thŭmb) Compression of the digital nerve on the medial aspect of the thumb, causing paresthesia.

box·er's de·men·tia (boks'ĕrz dĕ-men'shē-ă) Mental disorder due to cumulative damage sustained over some years in boxing, with slowed thought, memory loss, dysarthria, and other movement disorders. SYN dementia pugilistica.

box·ing (boks'ing) In dentistry, the building up of vertical walls, usually in wax, around a dental impression after beading, to produce the desired size and form of the dental cast, and to preserve certain landmarks of the impression.

Boy·er cyst (bwah-yā' sist) A subhyoid cyst.

Boyle law (boyl law) At constant temperature, the volume of a given quantity of gas varies inversely with its absolute pressure. SYN Mariotte law.

Boze·man pos·i·tion (bōz'măn pŏ-zish'ŏn) Knee-elbow position, the patient being strapped to supports.

Boz·zo·lo sign (bōts'sō-lō sīn) Pulsating vessels in the nasal mucous membrane, noted occasionally in thoracic aneurysm.

Br Symbol for bromine.

brace (brās) An orthosis or orthopedic appliance that supports or holds in correct position any movable part of the body and that allows motion of the part, in contrast to a splint, which prevents motion of the part.

brach·i·al (brā'kē-ăl) Relating to the arm.

bra·chi·al·gi·a (brā'kē-al'jē-ă) Pain in the arm.

brach·i·al plex·us (brā'kē-ăl plek'sŭs) [TA] Major nerve plexus formed of the ventral primary rami of the fifth cervical to first thoracic spinal nerves for innervation of the upper limb. SYN plexus brachialis [TA].

bra·chi·al plex·us in·ju·ry (brā'kē-ăl plek'sŭs in'jŭr-ē) Damage to the brachial plexus related to delivery; associated with excessive lateral stretching of the head, typically in cases of shoulder dystocia or breech deliveries.

bra·chi·al pulse (brā'kē-ăl pŭls) A palpable rhythmic expansion of the brachial artery in the antecubital space.

bra·chi·al re·gion (brā'kē-ăl rē'jŭn) [TA] Area of the arm, between deltoid and axillary regions proximally and cubital region distally. SYN arm region.

bra·chi·al vein (brā'kē-ăl vān) The vein that transports blood from the elbow upward to the shoulder.

brachio- Combining form denoting **1.** SYN arm (1). **2.** SYN radial.

bra·chi·o·ce·phal·ic (BC) (brā'kē-ō-se-fal'ik) Relating to both arm and head.

bra·chi·o·cu·bi·tal (brā'kē-ō-kyū'bi-tăl) Relating to both arm and elbow or to both arm and forearm.

bra·chi·o·plas·ty (brā'kē-ō-plas'tē) Surgical repair of the arm to restore form or function.

bra·chi·o·ra·di·a·lis (brā′kē-ō-rā′dē-ā′lis) Forearm muscle that allows elbow flexion.

bra·chi·um, pl. **bra·chi·a** (brā′kē-ŭm, brā′kē-ă) [TA] **1.** SYN arm (1). **2.** An anatomic structure resembling an arm.

bra·chi·um col·lic·u·li in·fe·ri·o·ris (brā′kē-ŭm kol-ik′yū-lī in-fēr-ē-ōr′is) [TA] SYN brachium of inferior colliculus.

bra·chi·um col·lic·u·li su·pe·ri·o·ris (brā′kē-ŭm kol-ik′yū-lī sū-pēr-ē-ōr′is) [TA] SYN brachium of superior colliculus.

bra·chi·um of in·fe·ri·or col·lic·u·lus (brā′kē-ŭm in-fēr′ē-ŏr kŏ-lik′yū-lŭs) [TA] A fiber bundle passing from the inferior colliculus on either side of the brainstem along the lateral border of the superior colliculus.

bra·chi·um of su·pe·ri·or col·lic·u·lus (brā′kē-ŭm sū-pēr′ē-ŏr kŏ-lik′yū-lŭs) [TA] A band of fibers of the optic tract bypassing the lateral geniculate body to terminate in the superior colliculus and pretectal region.

brachy- Combining form meaning short.

brach·y·ba·si·a (brak′ē-bā′sē-ă) The shuffling gait of pyramidal tract disease.

brach·y·ceph·a·ly, brach·y·ceph·a·li·a, brach·y·ceph·al·ism (brak′ē-sef′ă-lē, -sē-fā′lē-ă, -sef′ă-lizm) Shortness or broadness of the head.

brach·y·dac·ty·ly (brak′ē-dak′ti-lē) Abnormal shortness of the fingers.

bra·chyg·na·thi·a (brak′ig-nā′thē-ă) *In the diphthong gn, the g is silent only at the beginning of a word.* Abnormal shortness or recession of the mandible. SEE ALSO micrognathia. SYN bird face.

brach·y·me·li·a (brak′ē-mē′lē-ă) Disproportionate shortness of the limbs.

brach·y·me·so·pha·lan·gi·a (brak′ē-mez′ō-fă-lan′jē-ă) Abnormal shortness of the middle phalanges.

brach·y·met·a·car·pi·a, brach·y·met·

a·car·pa·li·a (brak′ē-met-ă-kahr′pē-ă, kahr-pā′lē-ă) Abnormal shortness of the metacarpals, especially the fourth and fifth; also called brachymetatarsia.

brach·y·o·dont (brak′ē-ō-dont) A tooth in which the root length exceeds that of the crown.

brach·y·o·nych·i·a (brak′ē-ō-nik′ē-ă) Short nails, in which the width of the nail plate and nail bed is greater than the length.

brach·y·pel·lic pel·vis (brak′ē-pel′ik pel′vis) A pelvis in which the transverse diameter is more than 1 cm longer but less than 3 cm longer than the anteroposterior diameter.

brach·y·pha·lan·gi·a (brak′ē-fă-lan′jē-ă) Abnormal shortness of the phalanges.

brach·y·syn·dac·ty·ly (brak′ē-sin-dak′ti-lē) Abnormal shortness of the digits (i.e., fingers, toes) combined with a webbing between the adjacent digits.

brach·y·te·le·pha·lan·gi·a (brak′ē-tel′ĕ-fă-lan′jē-ă) Abnormal shortness of the distal phalanges.

brach·y·ther·a·py (brak′ē-thār′ă-pē) Radiotherapy in which the source of irradiation is placed close to the surface of the body or implanted in the tissues to be treated.

brack·et (brak′ĕt) In dentistry, a small metal attachment that is soldered or welded to an orthodontic band or bonded directly to the teeth, serving to fasten the arch wire to the band or tooth.

Brad·bur·y-Eg·gle·ston syn·drome (brad′bŭr-ē eg′ĕl-stŏn sin′drōm) SYN pure autonomic failure.

brady- Combining form meaning slow.

bradyaesthesia [Br.] SYN bradyesthesia.

bra·dy·ar·rhyth·mi·a (brad′ē-ă-ridh′mē-ă) Any disturbance of the heart's rhythm resulting in a rate less than 60 beats per minute.

bra·dy·arth·ri·a (brad′ē-ahrth′rē-ă) A form of dysarthria characterized by an abnormal slowness or deliberateness of speech.

bra·dy·car·di·a (brad'ē-kahr'dē-ă) Slowness of the heartbeat, usually a rate less than 60 beats per minute.

brad·y·car·di·ac, bra·dy·car·dic (brad'ē-kahr'dē-ak, brad'ē-kahr'dik) Relating to or characterized by bradycardia.

bra·dy·di·as·to·le (brad'ē-dī-as'tŏ-lē) Prolongation of the diastole of the heart.

bra·dy·es·the·si·a (brad'ē-es-thē'zē-ă) Slow sensory perception. SYN bradyaesthesia.

bra·dy·ki·ne·si·a (brad'ē-kin-ē'sē-ă) A decrease in spontaneity and movement. One of the features of extrapyramidal disorders (e.g., parkinsonism).

bra·dy·ki·net·ic (brad'ē-ki-net'ik) Characterized by or pertaining to slow movement.

bra·dy·ki·nin (brad'ē-kī'nin) The vasodilatory nonapeptide normally present in blood in an inactive form; one of the plasma kinins.

bra·dy·pha·gi·a (brad'ē-fā'jē-ă) Slowness in eating.

bra·dy·pha·si·a (brad'ē-fā'zē-ă) A form of aphasia characterized by abnormal slowness of speech. SYN bradyphemia.

bra·dyp·ne·a (brad'ip-nē'ă) *In the diphthong pn, the p is silent only at the beginning of a word.* Abnormal slowness of respiration, specifically a low respiratory frequency.

bra·dy·sper·ma·tism (brad'ē-spěr'mă-tizm) Absence of ejaculatory force, so that the semen trickles out slowly.

bra·dy·sphyg·mi·a (brad'ē-sfig'mē-ă) Slowness of pulse.

bra·dy·stal·sis (brad'ē-stal'sis) Slow bowel motion.

bra·dy·tach·y·car·dia (brad'ē-tak'ĭ-kahr'dē-ă) Alternating episodes of slow heart beat (bradycardia) and rapid heart beat (tachycardia).

bra·dy·to·ci·a (brad'ē-tō'sē-ă) Tedious labor; slow delivery.

bra·dy·u·ri·a (brad'ē-yūr'ē-ă) Slow micturition.

brain (brān) [TA] That part of the central nervous system contained within the cranium. SEE ALSO encephalon.

brain ab·scess (brān ab'ses) Cranial infection, frequently confined to a specific cerebral region.

brain at·tack (brān ă-tak') SYN stroke (1).

brain death (brān deth) Loss of brain function.

brain·stem (brān'stem) [TA] Originally, the entire unpaired subdivision of the brain, composed of the rhombencephalon, mesencephalon, and diencephalon as distinguished from the brain's only paired subdivision, the telencephalon.

brain·stem aud·i·to·ry evoked po·ten·tial (brān'stem aw'di-tōr-ē ē-vōkt' pŏ-ten'shăl) Responses triggered by click stimuli, which are generated in the acoustic nerve and brainstem auditory pathways; recorded over the scalp.

brain·stem au·di·to·ry e·voked res·ponse (BAER, BSAER) (brān'stem aw'di-tōr-ē ē-vōkt' rē-spons') SEE auditory brainstem response.

brain·stem im·plant (brān'stem im'plant) A nonphysiologic structure used to improve or restore audition by stimulation of the cochlear area.

brain tu·mor (brān tū'mŏr) Cerebral neoplasm that can be either benign or malignant; often produced by metastasis.

brain·wash·ing (brān'wawsh'ing) Inducing a person to modify his attitudes and behavior in certain directions using psychological pressure or torture.

bran (bran) The outer coatings of grains, which are rich in nutrients and fiber.

branch (branch) [TA] An offshoot; in anatomy, one of the primary divisions of a nerve or blood vessel. SEE ramus, artery, nerve, vein. SYN ramus (1).

branch·er gly·co·gen stor·age dis·ease (branch'ĕr glī'kō-jen stōr'ăj di-zēz') Disorder due to deficiency of amylo-

1,4-1,6-transglucosidase (brancher enzyme).

bran·chi·al (BR) (brang′kē-ăl) **1.** Relating to branchiae or gills (e.g., in fish). **2.** In human embryology, denoting the various structures constituting the pharyngeal apparatus.

bran·chi·al arch·es (brang′kē-ăl ahr′chĕz) Typically, six arches in vertebrates; in lower vertebrates, they bear gills; called pharyngeal arches (q.v.) in human embryos.

bran·chi·al cleft (brang′kē-ăl kleft) SYN pharyngeal groove.

bran·chi·al cyst (brang′kē-ăl sist) Cervical lesion arising from developmental persistence of an ectodermal pharyngeal groove, usually the second.

bran·chi·al fis·sure (brang′kē-ăl fish′ŭr) Persistent pharyngeal groove or cleft.

bran·chi·al si·nus (brang′kē-ăl sī′nŭs) Abnormal cavity or space that opens on the lower third of the neck, usually results from failure of the second pharyngeal groove and cervical sinus to obliterate themselves.

branch·ing (branch′ing) Dividing into parts; sending out offshoots; bifurcating.

branch·ing en·zyme (branch′ing en′zīm) SYN 1, 4-α-d-glucan-branching enzyme.

bran·chi·o·gen·ic, bran·chi·og·en·ous (brang′kē-ō-jen′ik, -kē-ō-oj′ĕn-ŭs) Originating from the pharyngeal arches.

bran·chi·o·ot·o·re·nal syn·drome (brang′kē-ō-ō′tō-rē′năl sin′drōm) An autosomal dominant disorder characterized by anomalies of the pharyngeal arch derivatives, sensory hearing impairment, and renal abnormalities.

Brandt-An·drews ma·neu·ver (brahnt an′drūz mă-nū′vĕr) The expression of the placenta by grasping the umbilical cord with one hand and placing the other hand on the abdomen. SYN Andrews maneuver.

Bran·ha·mel·la (bran-hă-mel′ă) A subgenus of aerobic, nonmotile, non-spore-forming bacteria containing gram-negative cocci that occur in pairs with adjacent sides flattened. Found in the mucous membranes of the upper respiratory tract.

Bran·ham sign (bran′ăm sīn) Bradycardia following compression or excision of an arteriovenous fistula.

brass found·er's fe·ver (bras fown′dĕrz fē′vĕr) An occupational disease, characterized by influenzalike symptoms, due to inhalation of particles and fumes of metallic oxides.

brawn·y arm (braw′nē ahrm) Swollen upper limb caused by lymphedema; can be seen after ipsilateral radical mastectomy.

brawn·y e·de·ma (brawn′ē ĕ-dē′mă) SYN nonpitting edema.

Brax·ton Hicks sign (braks′tŏn hiks sīn) Irregular uterine contractions occurring after the third month of pregnancy.

break test (brāk test) A form of manual muscle procedure in which the therapist opposes the force exerted by a muscle that is isometrically contracted at its greatest mechanical advantage, so as to grade its strength.

break·through (brāk′thrū) A sudden manifestation of new insights and more constructive attitudes following a period of resistance during psychotherapy.

break·through dose (brāk′thrū dōs) As needed dosage of medication for sporadic worsening of pain; given to palliate breakthrough pain. SEE ALSO prn.

break·through pain (brāk′thrū pān) Discomfort, usually acute and severe, which is experienced by patients between the normal doses of a medication that generally controls or palliates such pain.

breast (brest) [TA] **1.** The pectoral surface of the thorax. **2.** The organ of milk secretion; one of two hemispheric projections situated in the subcutaneous tissue anterior to the pectoralis major muscle on either side of the thorax or chest of the mature female. SYN mamma [TA], teat (2).

breast im·plant (brest im′plant) Insertion of a nonphysiologic substance to enlarge the female breast for cosmetic purposes or in reconstruction of a breast that suffered surgical scarring during mastectomy or trauma.

breast pump (brest pŭmp) A suction instrument for withdrawing milk from the breast.

breath (breth) **1.** The respired air. **2.** An inspiration. **3.** A single cycle of inhalation followed by exhalation.

breath-hold•ing (breth′hōld-ing) Voluntary or involuntary cessation of breathing; often seen in young children as a response to frustration.

breath-hold•ing test (breth-hōld′ing test) A rough index of cardiopulmonary reserve measured by the length of time that a person can voluntarily stop breathing; normal duration is 30 seconds or longer; diminished cardiac or pulmonary reserve is indicated by a duration of 20 seconds or less.

breath•ing (brēdh′ing) Inhalation and exhalation of air or gaseous mixtures. SEE ALSO respiration.

breath•ing bag (brēdh′ing bag) A collapsible reservoir from which gases are inhaled and into which gases may be exhaled during general anesthesia or artificial ventilation.

breath•ing re•serve (brēdh′ing rē-zěrv′) The difference between the pulmonary ventilation (i.e., the volume of air breathed under ordinary resting conditions) and the maximum breathing capacity.

breath sounds (BR S, bs, BS) (breth sowndz) A murmur, bruit, fremitus, rhonchus, or rale heard on auscultation over the lungs or any part of the respiratory tract. SYN respiratory sounds.

breath test (breth test) **1.** Any diagnostic procedure in which endogenous or exogenous materials are measured in samples of breath as a means of identifying pathologic processes. **2.** A test to measure alcohol consumption.

breech (brēch) SYN buttocks.

breech pres•en•ta•tion (brēch prez′ěn-tā′shŭn) Presentation of any part of the pelvic extremity of the fetus, the nates,

knees, or feet; more properly only of the nates.

breg•ma (breg′mă) [TA] Cranial point corresponding to junction of the coronal and sagittal sutures.

Bren•ner tu•mor (bren′er tū′mŏr) A relatively infrequent benign neoplasm of the ovary, consisting chiefly of fibrous tissue that contains nests of cells resembling transitional type epithelium, as well as glandlike structures that contain mucin.

bre•tyl•i•um (bre-til′ē-ŭm) An antiarrhythmic used to treat life-threatening ventricular arrhythmias. Initially releases norepinephrine, then blocks its reuptake, thus depressing excitability of sympathetic nerve terminals.

brev•i•col•lis (brev-ē-kol′is) Abnormal shortness of the neck.

brew•er's yeast (brū′ěrz yēst) Agent used in gastrointestinal disorders; purported value against acne and dermatitis; dermatologic adverse reactions, however, have been reported.

bridge (brij) **1.** The upper part of the ridge of the nose formed by the nasal bones. **2.** One of the threads of protoplasm that appear to pass from one cell to another.

bridge•work (brij′wŏrk) SYN partial denture.

Brill dis•ease (bril di-zēz′) SYN Brill-Zinsser disease.

Brill-Zins•ser dis•ease (bril-zin′sĕr di-zēz′) An endogenous reinfection in people who previously had epidemic typhus fever; it is mild and may be mistaken for endemic (murine) typhus. SYN Brill disease, recrudescent typhus.

brim (brim) The upper edge or rim of a hollow structure.

Bri•quet a•tax•i•a (brē-kā′ ă-tak′sē-ă) Weakening of the muscle sense and increased sensibility of the skin, in hysteria.

Bri•quet syn•drome (brē-kā′ sin′drōm) A chronic but fluctuating mental disorder, usually of young women, characterized by frequent complaints of physical illness involving multiple organ systems simultaneously.

brise·ment for·cé (brēs-mŏn[h]′ fŏr-sā′) Procedure to treat frozen shoulder in which a forceful manipulation is performed to restore range of motion.

Bris·saud re·flex (brē-sō′ rē′fleks) Tickling the sole causes a contraction of the tensor fasciae latae muscle, even without responsive toe movement.

Brit·ish ther·mal u·nit (BTU) (brit′ish thĕr′măl yū′nit) The quantity of heat required to raise 1 pound of water from 3.9–4.4°C; equal to 251.996 calories or to 1055.056 joules.

brit·tle bones (brit′ĕl bōnz) SYN osteogenesis imperfecta.

brit·tle di·a·be·tes (brit′ĕl dī-ă-bē′tēz) Diabetes mellitus in which there are marked fluctuations in blood glucose concentrations that are difficult to control.

broach (brōch) A dental instrument for removing the pulp of a tooth or exploring the dentinal canal.

Broad·bent sign (brawd′bent sīn) Retraction of the thoracic wall, synchronous with cardiac systole, visible anywhere, but particularly in the left posterior axillary line; a sign of adherent pericardium.

broad be·ta dis·ease (brawd bā′tă di-zēz′) SYN Type III familial hyperlipoproteinemia.

broad-spec·trum an·ti·bi·ot·ic (brawd-spek′trŭm an′tē-bī-ot′ik) An antibiotic having a wide range of activity against both gram-positive and gram-negative organisms.

Bro·ca a·pha·si·a (brō′kă ă-fā′zē-ă) 1. SYN motor aphasia. 2. SYN expressive aphasia.

Bro·ca cen·ter (brō′kă sen′tĕr) The posterior part of the inferior frontal gyrus of the left or dominant hemisphere, corresponding approximately to Brodmann area 44; Broca identified this region as an essential component of the motor mechanisms governing articulated speech. SYN motor speech center.

Bro·die ab·scess (brō′dē ab′ses) A chronic bone lesion surrounded by dense fibrous tissue and sclerotic bone.

Bro·die dis·ease (brō′dē di-zēz′) 1. SYN Brodie knee. 2. Hysteric spinal neuralgia, simulating Pott disease, following a trauma.

Bro·die knee (brō′dē nē) Chronic hypertrophic synovitis of the knee. SYN Brodie disease (1).

Brod·mann ar·e·as (brod′mahn ār′ē-ăz) Regions of the cerebral cortex distinguished on the basis of histologic differences and presumed differences in function.

brom-, bromo- Prefixes that indicate bromine or a foul odor.

bro·mate (brō′māt) Salt or anion of bromic acid.

bro·me·lain, bro·me·lin (brō′mĕ-lān, -lin) One of a group of peptide hydrolases, all thiol proteinases, obtained from pineapple stems and fruit; used in tenderizing meats and in producing hydrolysates of proteins; orally administered in the treatment of inflammation and edema of soft tissues associated with traumatic injury.

brom·hi·dro·sis, brom·i·dro·sis (brom′hi-drō′sis, -i-drō′sis) Fetid or foul-smelling perspiration. Apocrine bromhidrosis affects the axillae after puberty, and eccrine bromhidrosis is generalized, with excessive sweating.

bro·mide (brom) (brō′mīd) The anion Br$^-$; salt of hydrogen bromide (HBr); several salts formerly used as sedatives, hypnotics, and anticonvulsants.

bro·mine (Br) (brō′mēn) A nonmetallic, reddish, volatile, liquid element; atomic no. 35, atomic wt. 79.904; valences 1–7, inclusive; reacts with many metals to form bromides, some of which are used in medicine.

brom·phe·nol test (brōm-fē′nol test) A colorimetric measurement of protein, albumin, and globulin in the urine by use of reagent strips.

bron·chi (bron) (brong′kī) Plural of bronchus.

bron·chi·al (brong′kē-ăl) Relating to the bronchi.

bron·chi·al asth·ma (brong′kē-ăl az′

mă) Pulmonary disorder with extensive airway narrowing, varying over short periods either spontaneously or as a result of treatment, due to contraction (spasm) of smooth muscle, edema of the mucosa, chronic or recurrent local inflammation of the submucosa with eventual fibrosis, and presence of excessive mucus.

bron·chi·al a·tre·si·a (brong′kē-ăl ă-trē′zē-ă) Severe focal narrowing or obliteration of a segmental, subsegmental, or lobar bronchus, usually associated with distal air trapping and bronchial mucoid impaction distal to the obstruction.

bron·chi·al cast (brong′kē-ăl kast) A fragment of thick, tenacious mucus in the shape of a small bronchus; often coughed up as an acute asthma attack resolves. SEE ALSO mucous plug.

bron·chi·al frem·i·tus (brong′kē-ăl frem′i-tŭs) Adventitious pulmonary sounds or voice sounds perceptible to the hand resting on the chest, as well as by the ear.

bron·chi·al glands (brong′kē-ăl glandz) [TA] 1. SYN bronchopulmonary lymph nodes. 2. Mucous and seromucous glands with secretory units that lie outside the muscle of the bronchi.

bron·chi·al hy·giene (brong′kē-ăl hī′jēn) Those activities contributing to the removal of bronchial secretions and the maintenance of open airways.

bron·chi·al pneu·mo·ni·a (brong′kē-ăl nū-mō′nē-ă) SYN bronchopneumonia.

bron·chi·al spasm (brong′kē-ăl spazm) Acute constriction of the bronchi and bronchioles resulting in decreased pulmonary function; also known as bronchospasm.

bron·chi·al sten·o·sis (brong′kē-ăl stĕ-nō′sis) Narrowing of the lumen of a bronchial tube.

bron·chi·ec·ta·sis (BE) (brong′kē-ek′tă-sis) Chronic dilation of bronchi or bronchioles as a sequel of inflammatory disease or obstruction often associated with heavy sputum production. SYN bronchiectasia.

bron·chi·o·gen·ic (brong′kē-ō-jen′ik) SYN bronchogenic.

bron·chi·o·lar car·ci·no·ma (brong′kē-ō′lăr kahr′si-nō′mă) Malignancy thought to be derived from epithelium of terminal bronchioles, in which the neoplastic tissue extends along the alveolar walls and grows in small masses within the alveoli. SYN bronchiolar adenocarcinoma.

bron·chi·ole (brong′kē-ōl) [TA] One of approximately six generations of increasingly finer subdivisions of the bronchi, each smaller than 1 mm in diameter, and having no cartilage in its wall, but relatively abundant smooth muscle and elastic fibers. SYN bronchiolus [TA].

bron·chi·o·lec·ta·sis, bron·chi·o·lec·ta·si·a (brong′kē-ō-lek′tă-sis, -lek-tā′zē-ă) Bronchiectasis involving the bronchioles.

bron·chi·o·li·i·tis (brong′kē-ō-lī′tis) Inflammation of the bronchioles, often associated with bronchopneumonia.

bron·chi·o·li·tis fi·bro·sa ob·li·te·rans (brong′kē-ō-lī′tis fī-brō′să ob-lit′ĕr-anz) Obstruction of bronchioles and alveolar ducts by fibrous granulation tissue induced by mucosal ulceration.

♻ **bronchiolo-** Combining form meaning bronchiole.

bron·chi·o·lus (brong-kī′ō-lŭs) [TA] SYN bronchiole.

bron·chi·o·ste·no·sis (brong′kē-ō-stĕ-nō′sis) Narrowing of the lumen of a bronchial tube.

bron·chit·ic (brong-kit′ik) Relating to bronchitis.

bron·chi·tis (brong-kī′tis) Acute (e.g., caused by recent infection) or chronic (e.g., long-term infection, smoking, cystic fibrosis) inflammation of the mucous membrane of the bronchial tubes.

♻ **broncho-, bronch-, bronchi-** Combining forms meaning bronchus.

bron·cho·al·ve·o·lar (brong′kō-al-vē′ō-lăr) SYN bronchovesicular.

bron·cho·al·ve·o·lar car·ci·no·ma (brong′kō-al-vē′ō-lăr kahr′si-nō′mă) SYN bronchiolar carcinoma.

bron·cho·al·ve·o·lar flu·id (brong'kō-al-vē'ŏ-lăr flū'id) A liquid (containing several lytic enzymes) that serves to remove inspired particulates from the pulmonary airways.

bron·cho·cele (brong'kō-sēl) A circumscribed dilation of a bronchus.

bron·cho·con·stric·tion (brong'kō-kŏn-strik'shŭn) Constriction of the bronchi.

bron·cho·con·stric·tor (brong'kō-kŏn-strik'tŏr) **1.** Causing a reduction in caliber of a bronchus or bronchial tube. **2.** An agent that possesses this action (e.g., histamine).

bron·cho·di·la·tor (brong'kō-dī'lā-tŏr) **1.** Causing an increase in caliber of a bronchus. **2.** An agent that possesses this power (e.g., epinephrine).

bron·cho·e·soph·a·ge·al (brong'kō-ĕ-sof'ă-jē'ăl) Pertaining to the bronchial tubes and esophagus.

bron·cho·e·soph·a·gos·co·py (brong'kō-ē-sof-ă-gos'kŏ-pē) Examination of the tracheobronchial tree and esophagus with appropriate endoscopes. SYN bronchooesophagoscopy.

bron·cho·fi·ber·scope (brong'kō-fī'bĕr-skōp) A fiberoptic endoscope adapted for visualization of the trachea and bronchi. SYN bronchofibrescope.

bronchofibrescope [Br.] SYN bronchofiberscope.

bron·cho·gen·ic (brong'kō-jen'ik) Of bronchial origin; emanating from the bronchi. SYN bronchiogenic.

bron·cho·gen·ic car·ci·no·ma (brong'kō-jen'ik kahr'si-nō'mă) Squamous cell or oat cell carcinoma that arises in the mucosa of the large bronchi.

bron·cho·gen·ic cyst (brong'kō-jen'ik sist) A cyst lined by ciliated columnar epithelium believed to represent bronchial differentiation; smooth muscle and mucous glands may be present.

bron·cho·gram (brong'kō-gram) A radiograph obtained by bronchography.

bron·chog·ra·phy (brong-kog'ră-fē) Radiographic examination of the tracheobronchial tree following introduction of a radiopaque material, usually an iodinated compound in a viscous suspension; has been superseded by high resolution computed tomography.

bron·cho·li·thi·a·sis (brong'kō-li-thī'ă-sis) Bronchial inflammation or obstruction caused by broncholiths.

bron·cho·ma·la·ci·a (brong'kō-mă-lā'shē-ă) Degeneration of elastic and connective tissue of bronchi and trachea.

bron·cho·mo·tor (brong'kō-mō'tŏr) **1.** Relating to a change in caliber, dilation, or contraction of a bronchus or bronchiole. **2.** An agent possessing this action.

broncho-oesophagoscopy [Br.] SYN bronchoesophagoscopy.

bron·chop·a·thy (brong-kop'ă-thē) Any disease or condition involving the major air passages of the lungs.

bron·choph·o·ny (Brph) (brong-kof'ŏ-nē) Increased intensity and clarity of voice sounds heard over a bronchus surrounded by consolidated lung tissue. SEE ALSO tracheophony. SYN bronchial voice.

bron·cho·plas·ty (brong'kō-plas-tē) Surgical repair of the configuration of a bronchus.

bron·cho·pleu·ral (brong'kō-plūr'ăl) Pertaining to the bronchial tubes and pleura (the double-folded membrane surrounding each lung or the pulmonary cavity).

bron·cho·pneu·mo·ni·a (brong'kō-nū-mō'nē-ă) Acute inflammation of the walls of the smaller bronchial tubes, with varying amounts of pulmonary consolidation due to the spread of the inflammation into peribronchiolar alveoli and the alveolar ducts; may become confluent or may be hemorrhagic. SYN bronchial pneumonia.

bron·cho·pul·mo·nar·y (BP) (brong'kō-pul'mŏ-nār-ē) Relating to the bronchial tubes and the lungs.

bron·cho·pul·mo·nar·y dys·pla·si·a (brong'kō-pul'mŏ-nār-ē dis-plā'zē-ă) Chronic pulmonary insufficiency arising from long-term artificial pulmonary ventilation; seen more frequently in premature than in mature infants.

bron·cho·pul·mo·na·ry lymph glands (brong′kō-pul′mŏ-nar-ē limf glandz) Lymph nodes located in the hilum of the lung.

bron·chor·rha·phy (brong-kōr′ă-fē) Suture of a wound of the bronchus.

bron·cho·scope (brong′kō-skōp) An endoscope for inspecting the interior of the tracheobronchial tree.

bron·chos·co·py (brong-kos′kŏ-pē) Inspection of the interior of the tracheobronchial tree through a bronchoscope.

bron·cho·spasm (BSp) (brong′kō-spazm) Contraction of smooth muscle in the walls of the bronchi and bronchioles, causing narrowing of the lumen. Cf. bronchoconstriction.

bron·cho·spi·rom·e·ter (brong′kō-spī-rom′ĕ-tĕr) A device for measurement of rates and volumes of airflow into each lung separately, using a double-lumen endobronchial tube.

bron·cho·spi·rom·e·try (brong′kō-spī-rom′ĕ-trē) Use of a bronchospirometer to measure ventilatory function of each lung separately.

bron·cho·ste·no·sis (brong′kō-stĕ-nō′sis) Chronic narrowing of a bronchus.

bron·chos·to·my (brong-kos′tŏ-mē) Surgical formation of a new opening into a bronchus.

bron·cho·tra·che·al (brong′kō-trā′kē-ăl) Relating to the trachea and bronchi.

bron·cho·ve·sic·u·lar (brong′kō-vĕ-sik′yū-lăr) Relating to the bronchioles and alveoli in the lungs. SYN bronchoalveolar.

bron·chus (brong′kŭs) [TA] One of the two subdivisions of the trachea serving to convey air to and from the lungs.

bronze di·a·be·tes, bron·zed di·a·be·tes (bronz dī-ă-bē′tēz, bronzd) Diabetes mellitus associated with hemochromatosis, with iron deposits in the skin, liver, pancreas, and other viscera, often with severe liver damage and glycosuria. SEE ALSO hemochromatosis.

Brooke tu·mor (bruk tū′mŏr) SYN trichoepithelioma.

brow (brow) **1.** The eyebrow (q.v.). **2.** SYN forehead.

brown·i·an move·ment, brown·i·an mo·tion (brown′ē-ăn mūv′mĕnt, mō′shŭn) Erratic, nondirectional, zigzag movement observed by microscope in suspensions of particles in fluid, resulting from the jostling or bumping of the larger particles by the molecules in the suspending medium. SYN molecular movement, pedesis.

brown lung (brown lŭng) Obstructive airway disease with asthma produced by exposure to cotton dust, flax, or hemp. SEE ALSO byssinosis.

Brown-Sé·quard syn·drome (brūn′ sā-kahr′ sin′drōm) Syndrome with unilateral spinal cord lesions, proprioception loss and weakness occur ipsilateral to the lesion, while pain and temperature loss occur contralateral. SYN Brown-Séquard paralysis.

brow pre·sen·ta·tion (brow prez′ĕn-tā′shŭn) SEE cephalic presentation.

Bru·cel·la (brū-sel′ă) A genus of encapsulated, nonmotile bacteria containing short, rod-shaped to coccoid, gram-negative cells. These organisms are parasitic, invading all animal tissues and causing infection of the genital organs, the mammary gland, and the respiratory and intestinal tracts, and are pathogenic for humans and various species of domestic animals.

bru·cel·lo·sis (brū-sel-ō′sis) An infectious disease caused by *Brucella*, characterized by fever, sweating, weakness, and aching; transmitted to humans by direct contact with diseased animals or through ingestion of infected meat or milk. SYN undulant fever.

Bruck dis·ease (bruk di-zēz′) A disorder marked by osteogenesis imperfecta, ankylosis of the joints, and muscular atrophy.

bruise (brūz) **1.** An injury producing a hematoma or diffuse extravasation of blood without rupture of the skin. **2.** SYN contuse.

bru·it (brū-ē′) An abnormal swishing, blowing, or murmuring sound.

bru·it de tam·bour (brū-ē′ dĕ tam-būr′) Reverberating drumlike tone heard as the second heart sound over the aortic area, associated with syphilitic aortic valvular disease. .

brun·nes·cent cat·a·ract (brŭn′ĕ-sĕnt kat′ă-rakt) A cataract in which the lens is hardened and of a dark brown color. SYN black cataract.

Brunn mem·brane (brŭn mem′brăn) Epithelium of the olfactory region of the nose.

Bruns a·tax·i·a (brŭnz ă-taks′ē-ă) Neuromuscular disorder involving difficulty in initiation of walking forward, although leg strength, coordination, and forward movement are normal. SYN glue-footed gait, magnetic gait (1), magnetic gait (2).

Bruns ny·stag·mus (brŭnz nis-tag′mŭs) A fine, jerking (vestibular) nystagmus on horizontal gaze in one direction, together with a slower, larger amplitude (gaze, paretic) nystagmus on looking in the opposite direction.

brush bi·op·sy (brŭsh bī′op-sē) Obtained by abrading the surface of a lesion with a brush to obtain cells and tissue for microscopic examination.

brush cath·e·ter (brŭsh kath′ĕ-tĕr) A ureteral catheter with a finely bristled brush tip that is endoscopically passed into the ureter or renal pelvis.

brux·ism (brŭk′sizm) A clenching of the teeth, associated with forceful lateral or protrusive jaw movements, resulting in rubbing, gritting, or grinding together of the teeth, usually during sleep; sometimes a pathologic condition. SEE ALSO parafunction.

Bryant line (brī′ănt līn) Vertical border of the iliofemoral triangle.

Bryant sign (brī′ănt sīn) Lowering of axillary skin folds; seen in association with dislocation of shoulder.

BTPS Abbreviation that indicates a gas volume has been expressed as if it were saturated with water vapor at body temperature (37°C) and at the ambient barometric pressure; used for measurements of lung volumes.

bub·ble gum der·ma·ti·tis (bŭb′ĕl gŭm dĕr′mă-tī′tis) Allergic contact dermatitis developing about the lips in children who chew bubble gum; caused by plastics in the gum.

bu·bo (bū′bō) Inflammatory swelling of one or more lymph nodes, usually in the groin; the confluent mass of nodes usually suppurates and drains pus.

bu·bon·ic plague (bū-bon′ik plāg) The most common form of plague (infection by *Yersinia pestis*), characterized by fever, cutaneous and visceral hemorrhages, and enlarged lymph nodes.

buc·ca, gen. and pl. **buc·cae** (bŭk′ă, bŭk′ē) SYN cheek.

buc·cal (bŭk′ăl) Pertaining to, adjacent to, or in the direction of the cheek.

buc·cal fat pad (bŭk′ăl fat pad) Encapsuled mass of fat in the cheek on the outer side of the buccinator muscle, especially marked in the infant. SYN corpus adiposum buccae.

buc·cal flange (bŭk′ăl flanj) Portion of the flange of a denture that occupies the buccal vestibule of the mouth.

buc·cal mu·co·sa (bŭk′ăl myū-kō′ză) Membrane the forms the inner lining of the cheeks.

buc·cal smear (bŭk′ăl smēr) Cytologic smear containing material obtained by scraping the lateral buccal mucosa above the dentate line, smearing, and fixing immediately.

buc·cal speech (buk′ăl spēch) A way to produce a sound source for speech by trapping air between the cheek and teeth and squeezing it out while articulating.

buc·cal tab·let (bŭk′ăl tab′lĕt) A small, flat lozenge intended to be inserted between cheek and gum, where the active ingredient is absorbed directly through the oral mucosa.

buc·co·ver·sion (bŭk′ō-vĕr-zhŭn) Malposition of a posterior tooth from the normal line of occlusion toward the cheek.

Buch·wald at·ro·phy (būk'vold at'rŏ-fē) A progressive form of cutaneous atrophy.

buck·le frac·ture (bŭk'ĕl frak'shŭr) SYN torus fracture.

bud (bŭd) **1.** An outgrowth that resembles the bud of a plant, usually pluripotential, and capable of differentiating and growing into a definitive structure. **2.** To give rise to such an outgrowth. SEE ALSO gemmation. **3.** A small outgrowth from a parent cell; a form of asexual reproduction.

Budd-Chi·a·ri syn·drome (bŭd kē-ahr'ē sin'drōm) Hepatic vein obstruction; most often associated with hepatomegaly and ascites. SYN Rokitansky syndrome.

bud·dy splint (bŭd'ē splint) Brace that anchors an injured digit to its neighbor for protection and support during the healing process.

Buer·ger dis·ease (bĕr'gĕr di-zēz') Pain in extremities similar to those caused by intermittent claudication in association with medial arterial sclerosis. SYN Billroth-von Winiwarter disease, endoarteritis obliterans, Winiwarter-Manteuffel-Buerger disease.

buf·fa·lo neck (bŭf'ă-lō nek) Combination of moderate kyphosis with a thick heavy fat pad on the neck, seen especially in people with Cushing disease or syndrome. Also called buffalo hump.

buff·er (bŭf'ĕr) A mixture of an acid and its conjugate base (salt), such as H_2CO_3 or HCO_3^-; $H_2PO_4^-/HPO_4^{2-}$, that, when present in a solution, reduces any changes in pH that would otherwise occur in the solution when acid or alkali is added to it.

buff·y coat (BC) (bŭf'ē kōt) Upper lighter portion of the blood clot (coagulated plasma and white blood cells), occurring when coagulation is delayed so that the red blood cells have had time to settle; the portion of centrifuged, anticoagulated blood that contains leukocytes and platelets. SYN crusta inflammatoria, crusta phlogistica, leukocyte cream.

bulb (bŭlb) [TA] **1.** Any rounded, globular, or fusiform structure. SYN bulbus [TA]. **2.** A short, vertical, underground stem of plants, such as onions and garlic.

bul·bar (bŭl'bahr) **1.** Relating to a bulb. **2.** Relating to the rhombencephalon (hindbrain). **3.** Bulb-shaped; resembling a bulb.

bul·bar pa·ral·y·sis (bŭl'bahr păr-al'i-sis) SYN progressive bulbar palsy.

bul·bi·form (bŭl'bi-fōrm) Resembling a bulb or in the shape of a bulb; bulbous.

bul·bi·tis (bŭl-bī'tis) Inflammation of the bulbous portion of the urethra.

bulbo- Combining form denoting a bulb; bulbus

bul·bo·cav·er·no·sus (bŭl'bō-kav'ĕr-nō'sŭs) SEE bulbospongiosus muscle.

bul·bo·cav·er·no·sus re·flex (BCR) (bŭl'bō-kav'ĕr-nō'sŭs rē'fleks) Sharp contraction of the bulbocavernosus and ischiocavernosus muscles when the glans penis is suddenly compressed or tapped.

bulb of cor·pus spon·gi·o·sum (bŭlb kōr'pŭs spŏn-jē-ō'sŭm) SYN bulb of penis.

bulb of hair, hair bulb (bŭlb hār) Lower expanded end of the hair follicle that caps the papilla pili.

bulb of pe·nis (bŭlb pē'nis) [TA] The expanded posterior part of the corpus spongiosum of the penis lying in the interval between the crura of the penis. SYN bulbus penis [TA], bulb of corpus spongiosum.

bul·bo·spi·nal (bŭl'bō-spī'năl) Relating to the medulla oblongata and spinal cord, particularly to nerve fibers interconnecting the two. SYN spinobulbar.

bul·bo·u·re·thral (bŭl'bō-yūr-ē'thrăl) Relating to the bulbus penis and the urethra.

bul·bo·u·re·thral gland (bŭl'bō-yūr-ē'thrăl gland) [TA] One of two small compound racemose glands, which produce a mucoid secretion, lying side by side along the membranous urethra just above the bulb of the corpus spongiosum; they discharge through a small duct into the spongy portion of the urethra. SYN Cowper gland.

bul·bous (bŭl′bŭs) Resembling a bulb or in the shape of a bulb. SYN bulbiform.

bul·bous bou·gie (bŭl′bŭs bū-zhē′) Cylindric probe with a bulb-shaped tip; some are shaped like an acorn or an olive.

bul·bus, gen. and pl. **bul·bi** (bŭl′bŭs, -bī) [TA] SYN bulb (1).

bu·li·mi·a ner·vo·sa (bŭ-lē′mē-ă nĕr-vō′să) A chronic morbid disorder involving repeated and secretive episodic bouts of eating characterized by uncontrolled rapid ingestion of large quantities of food over a short period of time (binge eating), followed by self-induced vomiting, use of laxatives or diuretics, fasting, or vigorous exercise to prevent weight gain; often accompanied by feelings of guilt, depression, or self-disgust.

bul·la, gen. and pl. **bul·lae** (bul′ă, -ē) **1.** A large blister appearing as a circumscribed area of separation of the epidermis from subepidermal structures or as a circumscribed area of separation of epidermal cells caused by the presence of serum, or an injected substance. **2.** A bubblelike structure.

bul·lec·to·my (bul-ek′tŏ-mē) Resection of a bulla; helpful in treating some forms of bullous emphysema, in which giant bullae compress functioning lung tissue.

bul·lous (bul′ŭs) Relating to, of the nature of, or marked by, bullae.

bul·lous con·gen·i·tal ich·thy·o·si·form e·ryth·ro·der·ma (bul′ŭs kŏn-jen′i-tăl ik-thē-os′i-fōrm ĕ-rith′rō-dĕr′mă) Diffusely red, eroded skin at birth, with subsequent scaling, tending to improve in later life, characterized by generalized epidermolytic hyperkeratosis.

bul·lous em·phy·se·ma (bul′ŭs em′fi-sē′mă) Lung disorder in which the enlarged airspaces are 1 to several cm in diameter, often visible on chest radiographs. Thin-walled air sacs, under tension, compress pulmonary tissue, either single or multiple.

bul·lous im·pe·ti·go of new·born (bul′ŭs im-pē-tī′gō nū′bōrn) Disseminated bullous lesions appearing soon after birth, caused by infection with *Staphylococcus aureus*. SYN impetigo neonatorum (2), pemphigus gangrenosus (2).

bul·lous ker·a·top·a·thy (bul′ŭs ker′ă-top′ă-thē) Edema of the corneal stroma and epithelium resulting in formation of bullae on the corneal surface. It occurs in Fuchs epithelial dystrophy, advanced glaucoma and iridocyclitis, endothelial failure, and sometimes after intraocular lens implantation.

bul·lous myr·in·gi·tis (BM) (bul′ŭs mir-in-jī′tis) Painful inflammation of the tympanic membrane accompanied by bullae.

bull's eye rash (bulz ī rash) A cutaneous eruption consisting of two or more concentric erythematous rings.

Bum·ke pu·pil (bum′ke pyū′pil) Dilation of the pupil in response to anxiety or other psychic stimuli.

bun·dle (bŭn′dĕl) [TA] A structure composed of a group of fibers, muscular or nervous. SYN fasciculus (3) [TA].

bun·dle-branch block (bŭn′dĕl-branch blok) Intraventricular block due to interruption of conduction in one of the two main branches of the bundle of His and manifested in the electrocardiogram by marked prolongation of the QRS complex. Block to each branch has distinctive QRS morphology.

bun·ion (bŭn′yŏn) A localized swelling at either the medial or dorsal aspect of the first metatarsophalangeal joint, caused by bursal inflammation and fibrosis; a medial bunion is usually associated with hallux valgus.

bun·ion·ec·to·my (bŭn-yŏn-ek′tŏ-mē) Excision of swelling of the first metatarsophalangeal joint.

bun·i·on·ette (bŭn-yŏ-net′) Enlargement of the fifth metatarsophalangeal joint.

Bun·sen burn·er (bŭn′sĕn bŭr′nĕr) A gas lamp supplied with openings admitting sufficient air that carbon is completely burned, giving a hot but only slightly luminous flame.

Bun·ya·vi·rus en·ceph·a·li·tis (bŭn′ yă-vī-rŭs en-sef′ă-lī′tis) Encephalitis of abrupt onset, with severe frontal headache and low-grade to moderate fever, caused by members of the genus *Bunyavirus*.

buoy·ant den·si·ty (Bd) (bwoy′ănt den′si-tē) Density that allows a substance to float in some standard fluid.

buph·thal·mi·a (bŭf-thal′mē-ă) Enlargement of the eyeball as a result of congenital glaucoma.

bur, burr (bŭr) *This first spelling is preferred.* 1. A rotary cutting instrument. 2. In ophthalmology, a device used to remove rust rings embedded in the cornea.

bur holes (bŭr hōlz) Small openings in the skull made with a surgical drill during operations.

bur·ied su·ture (ber′ēd sū′chŭr) Any suture placed entirely below the surface of the skin.

Burk·hol·der·i·a (bŭrk-hol-der′ē-ă) A genus of motile, nonfermentative, non-spore-forming gram-negative rods, containing significant species of human pathogens; formerly classified as in the genus *Pseudomonas*.

Bur·kitt lymph·o·ma (bŭr′kit lim-fō′ mă) A form of malignant lymphoma reported in African children, frequently involving the jaw and abdominal lymph nodes. Geographic distribution of Burkitt lymphoma suggests that it is found in areas with endemic malaria.

burn (bŭrn) 1. To cause a lesion by means of heat or a similar lesion by other means. 2. A sensation of pain caused by excessive heat, or similar pain from another cause. 3. A lesion caused by heat or any cauterizing agent, including friction, caustic agents, electricity, or electromagnetic energy. Types of burns resulting from different agents are relatively specific and diagnostic. Burns are divided into three types: superficial (formerly first-degree), partial thickness (second-degree), and full thickness (third-degree) depending on dermatologic severity (ery-

thema, blisters, charring), respectively. SEE ALSO rule of nines.

burn·er syn·drome (bŭr′nĕr sin′drōm) Multiple episodes of upper extremity burning pain, sometimes accompanied by shoulder girdle weakness, experienced during contact sports, especially U.S.-rules football.

Bur·nett syn·drome (bŭr-net′ sin′drōm) SYN milk-alkali syndrome.

burn·ing drops sign (bŭrn′ing drops sīn) In some cases of perforated gastric ulcer, a sensation of drops of hot liquid falling into the abdominal cavity or as of a stream of intensely hot liquid being poured into the cavity.

burn·ing tongue (bŭrn′ing tŭng) SYN glossodynia.

bur·nish·ing (bŭr′nish-ing) Smoothing the surface of a dental amalgam after initial carving, or adapting margins of gold restorations by rubbing with a broad-surfaced metal instrument. This term also refers to the rubbing of a medication into the dentinal tubules.

burr cell (bŭr sel) A crenated red blood cell.

bur·sa, pl. **bur·sae** (bŭr′să, -sē) [TA] A closed sac or envelope lined with synovial membrane and containing synovial fluid, usually located or formed in areas subject to friction (e.g., over an exposed or prominent part or where a tendon passes over a bone).

bur·sal ab·scess (bŭr′săl ab′ses) Suppuration within a bursa.

bur·si·tis (bŭr-sī′tis) Inflammation of a bursa. SYN bursal synovitis.

bur·sot·o·my (bŭr-sot′ŏ-mē) Incision through the wall of a bursa.

Bus·quet dis·ease (būs-kā′ di-zēz′) An osteoperiostitis of the metatarsal bones, leading to exostoses on the dorsum of the foot.

Bus·se-Busch·ke dis·ease (bus′e-būsh′ke di-zēz′) SYN cryptococcosis.

bu·tane (byū′tān) A gaseous hydrocarbon present in natural gas.

butt (bŭt) **1.** To bring any two square-ended surfaces in contact so as to form a joint. **2.** In dentistry, to place a restoration directly against the tissues covering the alveolar ridge.

but·ter (bŭt′ĕr) **1.** A coherent mass of milk fat, obtained by churning or shaking cream until the separate fat globules run together, leaving a liquid residue, buttermilk. **2.** A soft solid having the consistency of butter.

but·ter·fly (bŭt′ĕr-flī) **1.** Any structure or apparatus resembling in shape a butterfly with outstretched wings. **2.** A scaling erythematous lesion on each cheek, joined by a narrow band across the nose; seen in lupus erythematosus and seborrheic dermatitis.

but·ter·fly pat·tern (bŭt′ĕr-flī pat′ĕrn) Bilateral, symmetric, pulmonary alveolar opacities sparing the periphery, on chest radiographs; usually caused by pulmonary edema.

but·ter·fly rash (bŭt′ĕr-flī rash) SYN butterfly (2).

but·ter stools (bŭt′ĕr stūlz) Fatty excrement, occurring especially in steatorrhea.

but·tocks (bŭt′ŏks) [TA] *This word is grammatically plural.* The prominence formed by the gluteal muscles of either side. SYN nates [TA], clunes, breech.

but·ton (bŭt′ŏn) A knob-shaped structure, lesion, or device.

bu·tyl (byū′til) A radical of *N*-butane.

bu·ty·rate (byū′ti-rāt) A salt or ester of butyric acid.

bu·tyr·ic ac·id (byū-tir′ik as′id) Foul-smelling acid found in butter, cod liver oil, sweat, and other substances.

bu·ty·ro·cho·lin·es·ter·ase (byū′tir-ō-kō′lin-es′tĕr-ās) Pseudocholinesterase or plasma cholinesterase.

bu·ty·roid (byū′ti-royd) **1.** Buttery. **2.** Resembling butter.

by·pass (bī′pas) **1.** A shunt or auxiliary flow. **2.** To create new flow from one structure to another through a diversionary channel. SEE ALSO shunt.

by·prod·uct ma·te·ri·al (bī′pro-dŭkt mă-tēr′ē-ăl) Radioactive material produced by nuclear fission or in a nuclear reactor or similar device.

bys·si·no·sis (bis′i-nō′sis) Obstructive airway disease in people who work with unprocessed cotton, flax, or hemp.

C

CA-125 an•ti•gen (an'ti-jen) Tumor marker elevated in 85% of women with advanced ovarian cancer.

ca•ble graft (kā'bĕl graft) A multiple strand nerve graft arranged as a pathway for regeneration of axons.

Cab•ot ring bodies (kab'ŏt ring bod'ēz) Ring-shaped or figure-8-shaped structures that stain red with Wright stain, found in red blood cells in severe anemias.

♻ **cac-** SEE caco-.

ca•cao (kă-kah'ū) Prepared cacao, or cocoa, a powder prepared from the roasted cured kernels of the ripe seed of *Theobroma cacao Linné.* SYN theobroma.

ca•chec•tic (kă-kek'tik) Relating to or suffering from cachexia.

ca•chec•tin (ka-kek'tin) A polypeptide cytokine, produced by endotoxin-activated macrophages, which has the ability to modulate adipocyte metabolism, lyse tumor cells in vitro, and induce hemorrhagic necrosis of certain transplantable tumors in vivo.

ca•chet (kash'ā) Discoid capsule or wafer made of flour for enclosing medicinal powders of disagreeable taste.

ca•chex•ia (kă-kek'sē-ă) A general weight loss and wasting due to chronic disease or emotional disturbance.

cach•in•na•tion (kak'i-nā'shŭn) Laughter without apparent cause, often observed in schizophrenia.

♻ **caco-, caci-, cac-** Combining forms meaning bad; ill. Cf. mal-.

cac•o•dyl•ic ac•id (kak'ō-dil'ik as'id) Arsenical contact herbicide that defoliates or desiccates a wide variety of plant species. SYN dimethylarsinic acid.

cac•o•geu•sia (kak'ō-gū'sē-ă) A bad taste.

cac•o•me•lia (kak'ō-mē'lē-ă) Congenital deformity of one or more limbs.

ca•coph•o•ny (kă-kof'ŏ-nē) Din; noise; collection of loud harsh sounds.

cac•o•plas•tic (kak'ō-plas'tik) **1.** Relating to or causing abnormal growth. **2.** Incapable of normal or perfect formation.

cac•u•men, pl. **cac•u•mi•na** (kak-ū'men, -mi-nă) The top or apex of a plant or an anatomic structure.

ca•dav•er (CAD) (kă-dav'ĕr) A dead body.

ca•dav•er•ine (kă-dav'ĕr-in) A foul-smelling poisonous diamine formed by bacterial decarboxylation of lysine.

cad•mi•um (Cd) (kad'mē-ŭm) A metallic element, atomic no. 48, atomic wt. 112.411; its salts are poisonous and little used in medicine.

ca•du•ce•us (kă-dū'sē-ŭs) A staff with two oppositely twined serpents and surmounted by two wings; emblem of the U.S. Army Medical Corps.

♻ **cae-** For words beginning with this, see under ce-.

caec- [Br.] SYN cec-.

caecal [Br.] SYN cecal.

caecectomy [Br.] SYN cecectomy.

caecitis [Br.] SYN cecitis.

caeco- [Br.] SYN ceco-.

caecocolostomy [Br.] SYN cecocolostomy.

caecoileostomy [Br.] SYN -stomy.

caecoplication [Br.] SYN cecoplication.

caecorrhaphy [Br.] SYN cecorrhaphy.

caecosigmoidostomy [Br.] SYN cecosigmoidostomy.

caecostomy [Br.] SYN cecostomy.

caecotomy [Br.] SYN cecotomy.

caecoureterocele [Br.] SYN cecoureterocele.

caecum [Br.] SYN cecum.

Caesarean hysterectomy [Br.] SYN cesarean hysterectomy.

Caesarean section [Br.] SYN cesarean section.

caesium [Br.] SYN cesium.

ca·fé au lait spots (ka-fā′ ō lā spots) Pigmented cutaneous lesions, ranging from light to dark brown; due to an excess of melanosomes in the malpighian cells.

ca·fe cor·o·nary (ka-fā′ kōr′ŏ-nar-ē) Sudden collapse while eating that results from food impaction closing the glottis.

caf·feine (kaf′ēn) Stimulant alkaloid obtained from the dried leaves of *Thea sinensis*, tea, or the dried seeds of *Coffea arabica*, coffee.

caf·fein·ism (kaf′ēn-izm) Caffeine intoxication characterized by restlessness, tachycardia, and other symptoms.

cage (kāj) [TA] An inert network surrounding an active molecule to be delivered to a chosen locus in its active state. SYN cavea.

Ca·got ear (kah′zhō ēr) An auricle having no lobulus.

cais·son dis·ease (kā′son di-zēz′) SYN decompression sickness.

caj·e·put oil, caj·u·put oil (kaj′ĕ-pŭt oyl, -ū-pŭt) A volatile oil distilled from the fresh leaves of *Melaleuca leucodendra*; a stimulant, counterirritant, and expectorant.

cake kid·ney (kāk kid′nē) A solid, irregularly lobed organ of peculiar shape, usually situated in the pelvis toward the midline, produced by fusion of the renal primordia.

cal·a·mine (kal′ă-mīn) Zinc oxide with a small amount of ferric oxide or basic zinc carbonate colored with ferric oxide; used for skin disorders.

cal·a·mus (kal′ă-mŭs) Any reed-shaped structure.

cal·a·mus scrip·to·ri·us (kal′ă-mŭs skrip-tō′rē-ŭs) Inferior part of the rhomboid fossa; the narrow lower end of the fourth ventricle between the two clavae.

calcaemia [Br.] SYN calcemia.

cal·ca·ne·al, cal·ca·ne·an (kal-kā′nē-ăl, -ăn) Relating to the calcaneus or heel bone.

cal·ca·ne·al spur (kal-kā′nē-ăl spŭr) SYN heel spur.

cal·ca·ne·al tu·ber·os·i·ty (kal-kā′nē-ăl tū′bĕr-os′i-tē) [TA] The posterior extremity of the calcaneus, or os calcis, forming the projection of the heel.

calcaneo- Combining form denoting the calcaneus.

cal·ca·ne·o·a·poph·y·si·tis (kal-kā′nē-ō-ă-pof′i-sī′tis) Inflammation at the posterior part of the os calcis, at the insertion of the Achilles tendon.

cal·ca·ne·o·as·trag·a·loid (kal-kā′nē-ō-as-trag′ă-loyd) Relating to the calcaneus and astragalus.

cal·ca·ne·o·dyn·i·a (kal-kā′nē-ō-din′ē-ă) SYN painful heel.

cal·ca·ne·us (kal-kā′nē-ŭs) **1.** [TA] The largest of the tarsal bones; it forms the heel and articulates with the cuboid anteriorly and the talus superiorly. SYN calcaneal bone, heel bone, os calcis. **2.** SYN talipes calcaneus.

cal·car (kal′kahr) [TA] A small projection from any structure; a spur.

cal·car·e·ous (kal-kār′ē-ŭs) Chalky; relating to or containing lime or calcium.

cal·car·e·ous de·gen·er·a·tion (kal-kār′ē-ŭs dĕ-jen′ĕr-ā′shŭn) Not a true degenerative process, rather a deposition of insoluble calcium salts in degenerated tissue.

cal·ca·rine (kal′kă-rēn) **1.** Relating to a calcar. **2.** Spur-shaped.

cal·ca·rine sul·cus (kal′kă-rēn sŭl′kŭs) [TA] A deep fissure on the medial aspect of the cerebral cortex, marking the border between the lingual gyrus below and the cuneus above it.

cal·car·i·u·ria (kal-kar-ē-yūr′ē-ă) Excretion of calcium (lime) salts in the urine.

cal·ce·mi·a (kal-sē′mē-ă) SYN hypercalcemia, calcaemia.

cal·ci·co·sis (kal-si-kō'sis) Pneumoconiosis due to the inhalation of limestone dust.

cal·ci·di·ol, cal·ci·fe·di·ol (kal-si-dī'ol, kal-sĭ-fē-dī'ol) The first step in the biologic conversion of vitamin D3 to the more active form, calcitriol; it is more potent than vitamin D3.

cal·cif·er·ol (kal-sif'ĕr-ol) SYN ergocalciferol.

cal·cif·ic (kal-sif'ik) Involving or caused by calcification.

cal·ci·fi·ca·tion (kal'si-fi-kā'shŭn) 1. Deposition of lime or other insoluble calcium salts. 2. A process in which tissue or noncellular material in the body hardens due to precipitates or larger deposits of insoluble salts of calcium (and also magnesium), normally found only in bones and teeth.

cal·ci·fic bur·si·tis (kal-sif'ik bŭr-sī'tis) Inflammation of a bursa that results in the deposition of calcium salts.

cal·cif·ic ten·din·i·tis (kal-sif'ik ten'din-ī'tis) Chronic tendinitis with formation of mineral deposits in and around the tendon.

cal·ci·no·sis (kal-si-nō'sis) A disorder of deposition of calcium salts in nodular foci in various tissues.

cal·ci·no·sis cir·cum·scrip·ta (kal-si-nō'sis sĭr-kŭm-skrip'tă) Localized deposits of calcium salts in skin and subcutaneous tissues.

cal·ci·no·sis u·ni·ver·sa·lis (kal-si-nō'sis yū-ni-vĕr-sā'lis) Diffuse deposits of calcium salts in skin and subcutaneous tissues, connective tissue, and other sites.

cal·ci·pex·is, cal·ci·pex·y (kal'si-pek'sis, -sē) Fixation of calcium in the tissues, an occasional cause of tetany in infants.

cal·ci·phy·lax·is (kal-si-fī-lak'sis) A condition of induced systemic hypersensitivity in which tissues respond to appropriate challenging agents with a sudden, but sometimes transient, local calcification.

cal·ci·priv·ia (kal-si-priv'ē-ă) Lack of dietary calcium.

cal·ci·to·nin (kal-si-tō'nin) A peptide hormone, produced by the parathyroid, thyroid, and thymus glands; increases osseous deposition of calcium and phosphate and lowers hematologic calcium.

cal·ci·tri·ol (CCT) (kal'si-trī'ol) Part of the biologic conversion of vitamin D3 to its active form.

cal·ci·um (Ca), gen. **cal·ci·i** (kal'sē-ŭm, -sē-ī) A metallic bivalent element; salts have crucial uses in metabolism and in medicine and are responsible for the radiopacity of bone, calcified cartilage, and arteriosclerotic plaques in arteries.

cal·ci·um car·bide (kal'sē-ŭm kahr'bīd) Blackish crystalline lumps that yield acetylene gas when in contact with water.

cal·ci·um car·bon·ate ($CaCO_3$) (kal'sē-ŭm kahr'bŏ-nāt) An antacid and a dietary supplement. SYN chalk, creta.

cal·ci·um chan·nel block·ing agent (kal'sē-ŭm chan'ĕl blok'ing ā'jĕnt) Drug group that inhibits calcium movement; used to treat hypertension, angina pectoris, and cardiac arrhythmias. SYN slow channel-blocking agent.

cal·ci·um chlo·ride ($CaCl_2$) (kal'sē-ŭm klōr'īd) Agent used to correct calcium deficiencies and in the treatment of hypocalcemia, magnesium intoxication, hyperkalemia, cardiac failure, and in some cases of drug overdose.

cal·ci·um glu·bi·o·nate (kal'sē-ŭm glū-bī'ŏ-nāt) A calcium replenisher.

cal·ci·um glu·cep·tate (kal'sē-ŭm glū-sep'tāt) A nutrient or dietary supplement. SYN calcium glucoheptonate.

cal·ci·um glu·co·nate (CaG, CG) (kal'sē-ŭm glū'kŏ-nāt) A salt of calcium more palatable than the chloride, sometimes used as a calcium supplement.

cal·ci·um glyc·er·o·phos·phate (kal'sē-ŭm glis'ĕr-ō-fos'fāt) A calcium and phosphorus dietary supplement.

cal·ci·um hy·drox·ide (CH) (kal'sē-ŭm

hī-drok′sīd) Agent used as a carbon dioxide absorbent.

cal·ci·um ox·a·late (CO) (kal′sē-ŭm ok′să-lāt) Substance found as sediment in urine and in urinary calculi. Toxic end product of ethylene glycol consumption.

cal·ci·um ox·ide (kal′sē-ŭm ok′sīd) SYN lime (1).

cal·ci·um pump (kal′sē-ŭm pŭmp) A membranal protein that can transport calcium ions across the membrane using energy from adenosine triphosphate.

cal·ci·um py·ro·phos·phate dep·o·si·tion dis·ease (CPPD, CPDD, CPPDD) (kal′sē-ŭm pīr′ō-fos′fāt dep-ō-zish′ŭn di-zēz′) A crystal deposition arthritis that may simulate gout.

cal·ci·um sul·fate (kal′sē-ŭm sŭl′fāt) Ingredient of plaster of Paris. SEE ALSO gypsum.

cal·co·dyn·ia (kal-kō-din′ē-ă) SYN painful heel.

cal·co·sphe·rite (kal-kō-sfēr′īt) A tiny, spheroidal, concentrically laminated body containing accretive deposits of calcium salts. SYN psammoma bodies (3).

cal·cu·lo·sis (kal-kyū-lō′sis) The tendency or disposition to form calculi or stones.

cal·cu·lus, gen. and pl. **cal·cu·li** (kal′kyū-lŭs, -lī) A concretion found in any body part, most commonly in the passages of the biliary and urinary tracts. SEE ALSO dental calculus. SYN stone (1).

Cald·well-Luc op·er·a·tion (kawld′wel lŭk op-ĕr-ā′shŭn) Intraoral procedure for opening into the maxillary antrum through the supradental (canine) fossa above the maxillary premolar teeth. SYN intraoral antrostomy, Luc operation.

Cald·well-Mo·loy clas·si·fi·ca·tion (kawld′wel mŏl-oy′ klas′i-fi-kā′shŭn) Classification of female pelvic types.

cal·e·fa·cient (kal-ĕ-fā′shĕnt) 1. Making warm or hot. 2. An agent causing this.

calf, pl. **calves** (kaf, kavz) 1. A young bovine animal, male or female. 2. The posterior prominence of the leg, caused by the underlying triceps surae muscles. SYN sura.

cal·i·ber (kal′i-bĕr) The diameter of a hollow tubular structure.

cal·i·bra·tion (kal′i-brā′shŭn) The act of standardizing or calibrating an instrument or laboratory procedure.

cal·i·cot·o·my, cal·i·cec·to·my, cal·i·ot·o·my (kal′i-sot′ŏ-mē, -sek′tŏ-mē, -ē-ot′ŏ-mē) Incision into a calyx, usually for removal of a calculus.

ca·lic·u·lus, pl. **ca·lic·u·li** (kă-lik′yŭ-lŭs, -lī) A bud-shaped or cup-shaped structure, resembling the closed calyx of a flower. SYN calycle, calyculus.

ca·li·ec·ta·sis (kā-lē-ek′tă-sis) Dilation of the calyces, usually due to obstruction or infection.

cal·i·for·ni·um (Cf) (kal-i-fōr′nē-ŭm) An artificial transuranium element, atomic no. 98, atomic wt. 251.08.

cal·i·pers (kal′i-pĕrz) Two-handled hinged instrument used for measuring diameters.

ca·lix (kā′liks) [TA] SYN calyx.

cal·los·al agen·e·sis (kal-ō′săl ā-jen′ĕ-sis) Congenital absence of the corpus collosum.

cal·los·i·ty (kă-los′i-tē) A circumscribed thickening of the keratin layer of the epidermis. SYN callus (1), keratoma (1), poroma (1), tyloma.

cal·lo·so·mar·gin·al fis·sure (ka-lō′sō-mahr′ji-năl fish′ŭr) SYN cingulate sulcus.

cal·lus (kal′ŭs) 1. SYN callosity. 2. A composite mass of tissue that forms at a fracture site to establish continuity between the bone ends.

Cal·mette-Guérin ba·cil·lus (kahl-mĕt′ gār-rin[h]′ bă-sil′ŭs) SYN bacille Calmette-Guérin.

cal·mod·u·lin (CM, CaM) (kal-mod′yū-lin) A small, ubiquitous eukaryotic protein that binds calcium ions.

cal·o·mel e·lec·trode (kal´ō-mel ĕ-lek´trōd) One in which the wire is connected through a pool of mercury to a paste of mercurous chloride in a potassium chloride solution covered by additional potassium chloride solution.

ca·lor (kā´lōr) Heat, as one of the four signs of inflammation (the others are rubor, tumor, dolor) enunciated by Celsus.

Ca·lo·ri bur·sa (kah-lō´rē bŭr´să) Cavity between aortic arch and trachea.

ca·lor·ic (kă-lōr´ik) 1. Relating to a calorie. 2. Relating to heat.

ca·lor·ic ny·stag·mus (kă-lōr´ik nis-tag´mŭs) Jerky nystagmus induced by labyrinthine stimulation with hot or cold water in the ear.

ca·lor·ic stim·u·la·tion (kă-lōr´ik stim´yŭ-lā´shŭn) To treat swallowing disorders, use of cold or hot temperatures to increase awareness of the bolus in the mouth and pharynx. SYN thermal stimulation.

cal·o·rie (kal´ŏr-ē) A unit of heat content or energy. The amount of heat necessary to raise 1 g of water from 14.5–15.5°C (small calorie). Calorie is being replaced by joule, the SI unit equal to 0.239 calorie. SEE ALSO British thermal unit.

ca·lor·i·gen·ic (kă-lōr-i-jen´ik) 1. Capable of generating heat. 2. Stimulating metabolic production of heat. SYN thermogenetic (2), thermogenic.

cal·o·rim·e·ter (kal-ŏr-im´ĕ-tĕr) An apparatus to measure the amount of heat liberated in a chemical reaction.

cal·re·tic·u·lin (kal-re-tik´yū-lin) Intracellular calcium-binding protein, with cell adhesion and vascular regulatory actions.

cal·se·ques·trin (CASQ) (kal´sē-kwes´trin) A calcium-binding protein found in the interior of sarcoplasmic reticulum of muscles.

cal·var·i·a, pl. **cal·var·i·ae** (kal-vār´ē-ă, -ē) [TA] The upper domelike portion of the skull.

calx, gen. **cal·cis,** pl. **cal·ces** (kalks, kal´sis, -sēz) 1. SYN lime (1). 2. The posterior rounded extremity of the foot. SYN heel (1).

Ca·lym·ma·to·bac·te·ri·um (kă-lim´mă-tō-bak-tēr´ē-ŭm) A genus of nonmotile bacteria containing gram-negative, pleomorphic rods with single or bipolar condensations of chromatin; pathogenic only for humans.

ca·lyx, pl. **ca·ly·ces** (kā´liks, -li-sēz) [TA] A flower-shaped or funnel-shaped structure; specifically one of the branches or recesses of the pelvis of the kidney into which the orifices of the malpighian renal pyramids project. Also spelled calix.

cam·era, pl. **cam·er·as,** pl. **cam·er·ae** (kam´ĕr-ă, -ăz, -ē) [TA] 1. A closed box; one containing a lens, shutter, and light-sensitive film or digital medium for photography. 2. ANATOMY any chamber or cavity.

cam·era oc·u·li (kam´ĕr-ă ok´yū-lī) SEE anterior chamber of eyeball, posterior chamber of eyeball.

cam·i·sole (kam´i-sōl) SYN straitjacket.

cam·phor (kam´fŏr) A ketone distilled from the bark and wood of *Cinnamonum camphora*; also prepared synthetically from oil of turpentine; used as a topical antiinfective and antipruritic agent.

cam·pim·e·ter (kam-pim´ĕ-tĕr) A small tangent screen used to measure the central visual field.

cam·pot·o·my (kam-pot´ŏ-mē) Subthalamic incision used to palliate parkinsonian tremor.

camp·to·cor·mi·a, camp·to·cor·my (kamp-tō-kōr´mē-ă, -kōr´mē) Static, often marked forward flexion of the trunk.

camp·to·dac·ty·ly, camp·to·dac·tyl·i·a, camp·to·dac·tyl·ism, streb·lo·dac·ty·ly (kamp-tō-dak´ti-lē, -dak-til´ē-ă, -til-izm, streb´lō-dak´ti-lē) Permanent flexion of one or both interphalangeal joints of one or more fingers.

camp·to·me·li·a (kamp-tō-mē´lē-ă) A skeletal dysplasia characterized by bending long bones of the limbs, resulting in permanent bowing or curvature of affected part.

camp·to·mel·ic dwarf·ism (kamp-tō-mel'ik dwōrf'izm) Dwarfism with shortening of the lower limbs due to anterior bending of the femur and tibia.

camp·to·mel·ic syn·drome (kamp'tō-mel'ik sin'drōm) Disorder associated with flat facies, short vertebrae, hypoplastic scapula, and bowed tibia.

Cam·py·lo·bac·ter (kam'pi-lō-bak'tĕr) A genus of bacteria containing gramnegative, non-spore-forming, curved spiral rods with a single polar flagellum at one or both ends of the cell; they are motile with a characteristic corkscrewlike motion.

Cam·py·lo·bac·ter fe·tus (kam'pi-lō-bak'tĕr fē'tŭs) A species that contains various subspecies, particularly *C. jejuni*, which can cause acute bacterial gastroenteritis in humans.

ca·nal (kă-nal') [TA] A duct or channel; a tubular structure. SYN canalis [TA].

can·a·lic·u·li den·ta·les (kan-ă-lik'yū-lī den-tā'lēz) [TA] Minute, wavy, branching tubes or canals in the dentin. SYN dentinal tubules.

can·a·lic·u·lus, pl. **can·a·lic·u·li** (kan-ă-lik'yū-lŭs, -lī) [TA] A small canal or channel. SEE ALSO iter.

ca·na·lis, pl. **ca·na·les** (kă-nā'lis, -lēz) [TA] SYN canal.

can·a·li·za·tion (kan-ă-lī-zā'shŭn) The formation of canals or channels in a tissue.

Can·a·van dis·ease (kan'ă-van di-zēz') Progressive pediatric degenerative disease of central nervous system. SYN Canavan sclerosis, Canavan-van Bogaert-Bertrand disease, spongy degeneration of infancy.

can·cel·lous (kan'sĕ-lŭs) *Do not confuse this word with the noun cancellus.* Denoting bone that has a latticelike or spongy structure. SYN cancelled.

can·cel·lous bone (kan'sĕ-lŭs bōn) SYN substantia spongiosa.

can·cel·lous tis·sue (kan'sĕ-lŭs tish'ū) Latticelike or spongy osseous tissue.

can·cel·lus, pl. **can·cel·li** (kan-sel'ŭs, -ī) A latticelike structure, as in spongy bone.

can·cer (CA, Ca) (kan'sĕr) General term for malignant neoplasms; carcinoma or sarcoma, especially the former.

can·cer cord (kan'sĕr kōrd) A specific pattern of cells found in bronchial carcinoma.

can·cer·i·gen·ic (kan'sĕr-i-jen'ik) Pertaining to producing cancer; carcinogenic.

can·cer·o·pho·bi·a (kan'sĕr-ō-fō'bē-ă) A morbid fear of acquiring a malignant growth.

can·cer stag·ing (kan'sĕr stāj'ing) Assessment of spread of cancerous tumors (e.g., TNM staging, with T referring to tumor size and extension, N lymph node involvement, and M the presence or absence of metastasis).

can·cri·form (kang'kri-fōrm) Resembling cancer.

can·crum, pl. **can·cra** (kang'krŭm, -kră) A gangrenous, ulcerative, inflammatory lesion.

can·crum o·ris (kang'krŭm ō'ris) SYN noma.

can·de·la (cd) (kan-dē'lă) The SI unit of luminous intensity, 1 lumen per m²; the luminous intensity, in a given direction. SYN candle.

Can·di·da (kan'di-dă) A genus of yeast fungi found in nature; a few species are isolated from the skin, feces, and vaginal and pharyngeal tissue, but the gastrointestinal tract is the primary source of the single most important species, *C. albicans*, which causes infection and sepsis.

can·di·di·a·sis, can·di·do·sis (kan-di-dī'ă-sis, -di-dō'sis) Infection with, or disease caused by, *Candida*, especially *C. albicans*. This disease usually results from debilitation (as in immunosuppression and especially AIDS), physiologic change, prolonged administration of antibiotics, and iatrogenic and barrier breakage.

can·dle (c, ca) (kan'dĕl) SYN candela.

cane sug·ar (kān shu´găr) D-sucrose.

ca·nine (kā´nīn) **1.** Relating to the dog. **2.** Relating to the canine teeth.

ca·nine fos·sa (kā´nīn fos´ă) [TA] Depression on anterior maxillary surface below the infraorbital foramen and on the lateral side of the canine eminence. SYN fossa canina [TA].

ca·nine tooth (kā´nīn tūth) [TA] A tooth with a crown of thick conic shape and a long, slightly flattened conic root; there are two canine teeth in each jaw, one on either side adjacent to the distal surface of the lateral incisors, in both deciduous and permanent dentition. SYN dens caninus [TA], canine (3), cuspid (2), eye tooth.

ca·nit·i·es (kă-nish´ē-ēz) Graying of hair.

can·ker (kang´kĕr) *Do not confuse this word with cancer or chancre.* In cats and dogs, acute inflammation of the external ear and auditory canal. SEE aphtha.

can·ker sore (kangk´ĕr sōr) SYN aphtha (2).

can·nab·i·noids (kă-nab´i-noydz) Organic substances present in *Cannabis sativa*, with many pharmacologic properties.

can·na·bis, mar·i·juan·a (kan´ă-bis, mahr´i-hwah´nă) The dried flowering tops of the pistillate plants of *Cannabis sativa* containing isomeric tetrahydrocannabinols, cannabinol, and cannabidiol. Preparations are smoked or ingested to induce psychotomimetic effects such as euphoria, hallucinations, drowsiness, and other mental changes; formerly used as a sedative and analgesic; now available in some jurisdictions for restricted use in management of iatrogenic anorexia, especially that associated with oncologic chemotherapy and radiation therapy.

can·non·ball pulse (kan´ŏn-bawl pŭls) SYN water-hammer pulse.

can·nu·la, can·u·la, pl. **can·nu·las,** pl. **can·nu·lae** (kan´yū-lă, -lăz, -lē) A tube that can be inserted into a cavity or vein, usually by means of a trocar filling its lumen; after insertion of the cannula,

the trocar is withdrawn, the cannula remains as a channel for the transport of fluid.

Can·tel·li sign (kahn-tel´lē sīn) SEE doll's eye sign.

can·ter·ing rhythm (kan´tĕr-ing ridh´ŭm) SYN gallop.

can·tha·ris, gen. **can·thar·i·dis,** pl. **can·thar·i·des** (kan´thăr-is, -i-dis, -i-dēz) A dried beetle, *Lytta (Cantharis) vesicatoria,* used as a counterirritant and vesicant. SYN Russian fly, Spanish fly.

can·thi·tis (kan-thī´tis) Inflammation of a canthus.

can·tho·plas·ty (kan´thō-plas-tē) **1.** Disruption of canthal tendon insertion; often performed surgically. SYN cantholysis. **2.** An operation to restore the canthus.

can·thot·o·my (kan-thot´ŏ-mē) Slitting of the canthus.

can·thus, pl. **can·thi** (kan´thŭs, -thī) The angle of the eye.

can·ti·le·ver bridge (kan´ti-lē-vĕr brij) Fixed partial denture in which the pontic is retained only on one side by an abutment tooth. SYN extension bridge.

ca·pac·i·tance (C) (kă-pas´i-tăns) The quantity of electric charge that may be stored upon a body per unit of electric potential; expressed in farads, abfarads, or statfarads.

ca·pac·i·ta·tion (kă-pas´i-tā´shŭn) Conditioning whereby the glycoprotein coat and seminal proteins are removed from the acrosome of a sperm.

ca·pac·i·tor (kă-pas´i-tŏr) A device for holding a charge of electricity. SYN condenser (4).

ca·pac·i·ty (kă-pas´i-tē) **1.** The potential cubic contents of a cavity or receptacle. **2.** Ability to do. SEE ALSO volume.

ca·pe·cit·a·bine (kap-ē-sit´ă-bēn) A prodrug converted to 5-fluorouracil.

ca·pil·la·ri·a·sis (kap´i-lar-ī´ă-sis) A disease caused by infection with nematodes of the genus *Capillaria*.

cap·il·lar·i·ty (kap'i-lar'i-tē) The rise of liquids in narrow tubes or through the pores of a loose material.

cap·il·la·rop·a·thy (kap'i-lă-rop'ă-thē) Any disease of the capillaries, often applied to vascular changes in diabetes mellitus. SYN microangiopathy.

cap·il·lar·y (kap'i-lār-ē) [TA] **1.** Resembling a hair; fine; minute. **2.** A capillary vessel. **3.** Relating to a blood or lymphatic capillary vessel.

cap·il·lar·y at·trac·tion (kap'i-lār-ē ă-trak'shŭn) The force that causes fluids to rise up very fine tubes or pass through the pores of a loose material.

cap·il·lar·y bed (kap'i-lār-ē bed) The capillaries considered collectively and their volume capacity for blood.

cap·il·lar·y drain·age (kap'i-lār-ē drān'ăj) Drainage by means of a wick of gauze or other material.

cap·il·lar·y fra·gil·i·ty (kap'i-lār-ē fră-jil'i-tē) The susceptibility of capillaries to breakage and extravasation of red blood cells under conditions of increased stress.

cap·il·lar·y he·man·gi·o·ma (kap'i-lār-ē hē-man'jē-ō'mă) An overgrowth of capillary blood vessels, seen most commonly in the skin, at or soon after birth, as a soft bright red to purple nodule or plaque that usually disappears by the fifth year. SYN nevus vascularis, nevus vasculosus.

ca·pil·lus (kă-pil'ŭs) A hair.

cap·i·tate (kap'i-tāt) [TA] **1.** The largest of the carpal bones; located in the distal row. SYN os capitatum [TA], magnum, os magnum. **2.** Head-shaped; having a rounded extremity.

cap·i·ta·tion (kap'i-tā'shŭn) A system of medical reimbursement wherein the provider is paid an annual fee per covered patient by an insurer or other financial source.

cap·i·tel·lum (kap-i-tel'ŭm) SYN capitulum.

ca·pit·u·lum, pl. **ca·pit·u·la** (kă-pit'yū-lŭm, -lă) [TA] A small head or rounded articular extremity of a bone. SYN capitellum.

Cap·no·cy·toph·a·ga (kap'nō-sī-tof'ă-gă) A genus of gram-negative, fusiform bacteria associated with human periodontal disease.

cap·no·gram (kap'nō-gram) A continuous record of the carbon dioxide content of expired air.

cap·no·graph (kap'nō-graf) Instrument by which a continuous graph of the carbon dioxide content of expired air is obtained.

cap·nom·e·ter (kap-nom'ĕ-tĕr) An instrument that measures the carbon dioxide concentration of exhaled air. SYN CO_2 analyzer.

cap·nom·e·try (kap nom'ĕ-trē) The process of measuring and recording the carbon dioxide concentration of exhaled air at the patient's airway using a capnometer.

cap·ping (kap'ing) **1.** Covering. **2.** The aggregation at one end of a cell of surface antigens that have been bound and cross linked by antibodies; this cap is then endocytosed by the cell.

cap pol·y·po·sis (kap pol-i-pō'sis) Disorder characterized by hundreds to thousands of precancerous colonic polyps beginning at about age 16 years. Colon cancer predisposition syndrome (i.e., familial polyposis coli, Peutz-Jeghers syndrome, juvenile polyposis syndrome).

cap·ro·ate (kap'rō-āt) A salt or ester of *N*-caproic acid.

cap·ry·late (kap'ri-lāt) A salt or ester of caprylic acid.

cap·ryl·ic ac·id (kă-pril'ik as'id) Acid found among the hydrolysis products of fat in butter and other substances.

cap·si·cum (kap'si-kŭm) Dried herbal remedy (and spice) made from *Capsicum frutescens*; internal and external medicinal uses have been described. SYN cayenne, hot pepper, red pepper.

cap·sid (CA) (kap'sid) Protein coat of a virus. SEE virion.

cap·so·mer, cap·so·mere (kap′sō-měr, -mēr) A subunit of the protein coat or capsid of a virus particle. SEE ALSO virion.

cap·su·la, gen. and pl. **cap·su·lae** (kap′sū-lă, -lē) [TA] **1.** A membranous structure, usually dense collagenous connective tissue, which envelops an organ, a joint, or any other part. **2.** An anatomic structure resembling a capsule or envelope. SYN capsule (1).

cap·su·lar an·ti·gen (kap′sū-lăr an′ti-jen) That found only in the capsules of certain microorganisms.

cap·su·lar cat·a·ract (kap′sū-lăr kat′ărakt) A cataract in which the opacity affects the capsule.

cap·su·lar space (kap′sū-lăr spās) The area between the visceral and parietal layers of the capsule of the renal corpuscle. SYN Bowman space, filtration space, urinary space.

cap·su·la·tion (kap′sū-lā′shŭn) Enclosure in a capsule.

cap·sule (kap′sŭl) [TA] **1.** SYN capsula. **2.** A fibrous tissue layer enveloping an organ, joint, or a neoplasm. **3.** A solid dosage form in which a drug is enclosed in either a hard or soft shell of soluble material. **4.** A hyaline polysaccharide coating around a fungal or bacterial wall of a cell.

cap·sul·ec·to·my (kap′sū-lek′tō-mē) Removal of a capsule.

cap·sule of lens (kap′sŭl lenz) [TA] The covering enclosing the lens of the eye.

cap·su·li·tis (kap′sū-lī′tis) Inflammation of the capsule of an organ or part, as of the liver, the lens of the eye, or surrounding a joint.

cap·su·lo·plas·ty (kap′sū-lō-plas-tē) Rearrangement or reshaping of a capsule; often the capsule of a joint.

cap·su·lor·rhex·is (kap′sū-lō-reks′sis) Technique used in cataract surgery by which a continuous circular tear is made in the anterior lens capsule.

cap·su·lot·o·my (kap′sū-lot′ŏ-mē) **1.** Division of a capsule. **2.** Creation of an opening through a capsule. **3.** Incision of the capsule of the lens in the extracapsular cataract operation.

cap·ture (kap′shŭr) Catching and holding a particle or an electrical impulse originating elsewhere.

ca·put, gen. and pl. **ca·pi·tis,** pl. **ca·pi·ta** (kah′put, pī-tis, -tă) [TA] **1.** Head: the superior extremity of the human body, comprising the cranium and face, and containing the brain and organs of sight, hearing, taste, and smell. **2.** The superior, anterior, or larger extremity, expanded or rounded, of any body, organ, or other anatomic structure. **3.** The rounded extremity of a bone. **4.** The end of a muscle that is attached to the less movable part of the skeleton.

ca·put me·du·sae (kah′put me-dū′sē) **1.** Varicose veins radiating from the umbilicus. **2.** Dilated ciliary arteries girdling the corneoscleral limbus in rubeosis iridis. SYN Medusa head.

ca·put suc·ce·da·ne·um (kah′pŭt sŭk-sĕ-dā′nē-ŭm) An edematous swelling formed on the presenting portion of the scalp of an infant during birth.

carb-, carbo- Combining forms indicating carbon.

car·ba·mate (kahr′bă-māt) A salt or ester of carbamic acid forming the basis of urethane hypnotics. SYN carbamoate.

car·bam·ic ac·id (kahr-bam′ik as′id) Hypothetical acid, NH_2-COOH, forming carbamates; acyl radical is carbamoyl.

carbaminohaemoglobin [Br.] SYN carbaminohemoglobin.

car·bam·i·no·he·mo·glo·bin (HbCO₂) (kahr-bam′i-nō-hē′mŏ-glō′bin) Carbon dioxide bound to hemoglobin by means of a reactive amino group on the hemoglobin. SYN carbhemoglobin, carbohemoglobin.

car·ba·mo·yl (kahr′bă-mō-il) The acyl radical, NH_2-CO-, the transfer of which plays an important role in certain biochemical reactions. SYN carbamyl.

car·ben·i·cil·lin (CB, CBC, CBCN) (kahr-ben′i-sil′in) A semisynthetic extended-spectrum penicillin active against a wide variety of gram-positive and gram-negative bacteria.

car·bi·do·pa (kahr′bi-dō′pă) A dopa decarboxylase inhibitor that does not enter the brain used in conjunction with levodopa in the treatment of parkinsonism to reduce L-dopa dosage and mitigate side effects.

car·bi·nol (kahr′bi-nol) SYN methyl alcohol.

carbo- SEE carb-.

car·bo·hy·drate (kahr′bō-hī′drāt) Organic compound of carbon, hydrogen, and oxygen.

car·bo·hy·drate-in·duced hy·per·li·pe·mi·a (kahr-bō-hī′drāt-in-dūst′ hī′pĕr-li-pē′mē-ă) SYN familial hyperlipoproteinemia type IV.

car·bol·ic ac·id (kahr-bol′ik as′id) SYN phenol.

car·bon (C) (kahr′bŏn) A nonmetallic tetravalent element, atomic no. 6, atomic wt. 12.011; the major bioelement. Its compounds are found in all living tissues, and the study of its vast number of compounds constitutes most of organic chemistry.

car·bon·ate (kahr′bŏn-āt) **1.** A salt of carbonic acid. **2.** The ion $CO_3^=$.

car·bon di·ox·ide (CO_2, CD, bicarb) (kahr′bŏn dī-oks′īd) The product of the combustion of carbon with an excess of air; used as a respiratory stimulant.

car·bon di·ox·ide cycle, car·bon cy·cle (kahr′bŏn dī-oks′īd sī′kĕl, kahr′bŏn sī′kĕl) The circulation of carbon as CO_2 from the expired air of animals and decaying organic matter to plant life where it is synthesized (through photosynthesis) to carbohydrate material, from which, as a result of catabolic processes in all life, it is again ultimately released to the atmosphere as carbon dioxide.

car·bon di·ox·ide snow (kahr′bŏn dī-ok′sīd snō) Solid carbon dioxide used to treat skin disease. SYN dry ice.

car·bon·ic ac·id (kahr-bon′ik as′id) Abbreviated H_2CO_3; formed from water and carbon dioxide.

car·bon·ic an·hy·drase (CA) (kahr-bon′ik an-hī′drās) A zinc-containing enzyme that catalyzes the interconversion of carbon dioxide with bicarbonate and a hydrogen ion. A deficiency can result in osteopetrosis and metabolic acidosis. SYN carbonate dehydratase, carbonate hydrolyase.

car·bon mon·ox·ide (CO) (kahr′bŏn mŏ-noks′īd) A colorless, practically odorless, poisonous gas formed by incomplete combustion of carbon; toxicity due to its strong affinity for hemoglobin, myoglobin, and cytochromes, which inhibit oxygen activity.

car·bon mon·ox·ide he·mo·glob·in (kahr′bŏn mŏ-noks′īd hē′mŏ-glō-bin) SYN carboxyhemoglobin.

car·bon tet·ra·chlo·ride (CCl_4) (kahr′bŏn tet-ră-klōr′īd) A colorless, mobile liquid having a characteristic ethereal odor resembling that of chloroform. SYN tetrachloromethane.

car·bon·yl (kahr′bŏn-il) The characteristic group, —CO—, of the ketones, aldehydes, and organic acids.

car·bo·plat·in (C, Cb) (kahr′bō-pla-tin) A platinum-containing anticancer agent used in the chemotherapy of solid tumors.

carboxy- Combining form indicating addition of carbon monoxide or carbon dioxide.

carboxyhaemoglobin [Br.] SYN carboxyhemoglobin.

carboxyhaemoglobinaemia [Br.] SYN carboxyhemoglobinemia.

car·box·y·he·mo·glo·bin (kahr-bok′sē-hē′mŏ-glō′bin) A stable union of carbon monoxide with hemoglobin. SYN carbon monoxide hemoglobin, carboxyhaemoglobin.

car·box·y·he·mo·glo·bi·ne·mi·a (kahr-bok′sē-hēmŏ-glō-bi-nē′mē-ă) Presence of carboxyhemoglobin in the blood. SYN carboxyhaemoglobinaemia.

car·box·yl (kahr-bok′sil) The characterizing group (–COOH) of certain organic acids, e.g., HCOOH (formic acid),

CH_3COOH (acetic acid), $CH_3CH(NH_2)$ COOH (alanine).

car·box·yl·ase (kahr-bok'sil-ās) One of several carboxylyases catalyzing addition of CO_2 to another molecule to create an additional —COOH group.

car·box·yl·a·tion (kahr-bok'si-lā'shŭn) Addition of CO_2 to an organic acceptor, as in formation of malonyl-CoA or in photosynthesis, to yield a —COOH group; catalyzed by carboxylases.

car·box·yl·ic ac·id (kahr-bok'sil-ik as' id) An organic acid with a carboxyl group. Cf. carboxyl.

car·box·y·meth·yl·cel·lu·lose (CM, CMC, CM-cellulose) (kahr-bok'sē-meth'il-sel'yū-lōs) A cellulose derivative that forms a colloidal dispersion in water; absorbs water and is used as a bulk laxative.

car·box·y·pep·ti·dase (kahr-bok'sē-pep'ti-dās) A hydrolase that removes the amino acid at the free carboxyl end of a polypeptide chain; an exopeptidase.

car·bun·cle (kahr'bŭng-kĕl) Deep-seated pyogenic infection of the skin and subcutaneous tissues, usually arising in several contiguous hair follicles, with formation of connecting sinuses.

car·ci·no·em·bry·on·ic (kahr'si-nō-em-brē-on'ik) Pertaining to a substance found in embryonic tissue but absent from adult tissue except in certain carcinomas of the lung, digestive tract, and pancreas.

car·ci·no·em·bry·on·ic an·ti·gen (CEA) (kahr'si-nō-em-brē-on'ik an'ti-jen) A glycoprotein constituent of the glycocalyx of embryonic endodermal epithelium, generally absent from adult cells with the exception of some carcinomas.

car·cin·o·gen (kahr-sin'ŏ-jen) Any cancer-producing substance or organism.

car·ci·no·gen·i·ci·ty (kahr'sin-ō-jen-is' i-tē) Ability to cause cancer.

car·ci·noid syn·drome (kahr'si-noyd sin'drōm) A combination of symptoms and lesions usually produced by the release of serotonin from carcinoid tumors

of the gastrointestinal tract that have metastasized to the liver.

car·ci·noid tu·mor (kahr'si-noyd tū'mŏr) A neoplasm composed of cells of medium size, with moderately small vesicular nuclei; present in the gastrointestinal tract, lungs, and other sites, with approximately 90% in the appendix. SEE ALSO carcinoid syndrome. SYN argentaffinoma.

car·ci·no·lyt·ic (kahr'si-nō-lit'ik) Destructive to the cells of carcinoma.

car·ci·no·ma (CA, Ca), pl. **car·ci·no·ma·ta, car·ci·no·mas** (kahr'si-nō'mă, -mă-tă, -măz) Any of the various types of malignant neoplasm derived from epithelial tissue, occurring more frequently in the skin and large intestine in both sexes, the lung and prostate gland in men, and the lung and breast in women.

car·ci·no·ma ex ple·o·mor·phic ad·e·no·ma (kar'si-nō'mă eks plē-ō-mōr'fik ad'ĕ-nō'mă) That arising in a benign mixed tumor of a salivary gland, characterized by fast growth and pain.

car·ci·no·ma in si·tu (CIS) (kahr'si-nō'mă in sit'ū) A lesion characterized by cytologic changes of the type associated with invasive carcinoma, but with the pathologic process limited to the lining epithelium and without histologic evidence of extension to adjacent structures.

car·ci·no·ma of the breast (kahr'si-nō'mă brest) A malignant tumor arising from epithelial cells of the female (and occasionally the male) breast.

car·ci·no·ma sim·plex (kahr'si-nō'mă sim'pleks) Any poorly differentiated malignant lesion.

car·ci·no·ma·to·sis, car·ci·no·sis (kahr'si-nō-mă-tō'sis, -si-nō'sis) Widespread dissemination of carcinoma in various organs or tissues of the body.

car·ci·nom·a·tous (kahr'si-nō'mă-tŭs) Pertaining to or manifesting the characteristic properties of carcinoma.

car·ci·nom·a·tous my·e·lop·a·thy (kahr'si-nō'mă-tŭs mī-ĕ-lop'ă-thē) Degeneration or necrosis of the spinal cord associated with a carcinoma.

car·ci·no·sar·co·ma (kahr'si-nō-sahr-kō'mă) A malignant neoplasm that contains elements of carcinoma and sarcoma.

car·da·mom (kahr'dă-mŏm) Herbal agent derived from *Elettaria cardamomum;* purportedly useful against flatulence. SYN Alpinia cardamom, Malabar cardamom.

cardi- SEE cardio-.

car·dia (kahr'dē-ă) [TA] The area of the stomach close to the esophageal opening (cardiac orifice or cardia) that contains the cardiac glands. SYN pars cardiaca gastricae [TA], cardiac part of stomach, cardial part of stomach, gastric cardia, pars cardiaca ventriculi.

car·di·ac an·trum (kahr'dē-ak an'trŭm) Dilation in the abdominal part of the esophagus. SYN antrum cardiacum, forestomach.

car·di·ac ar·rest (CA) (kahr'dē-ak ă-rest') Complete cessation of cardiac activity; either electric, mechanical, or both.

car·di·ac cath·e·ter (kahr'dē-ak kath'ĕ-tĕr) SYN intracardiac catheter.

car·di·ac cath·e·ter·i·za·tion (kahr'dē-ak kath'ĕ-tĕr-ī-zā'shŭn) Process whereby a thin flexible catheter is introduced into an artery and advanced into the heart for diagnosis or therapy.

car·di·ac cir·rho·sis (kahr'dē-ak sir-ō'sis) An extensive fibrotic reaction within the liver as a result of chronic constrictive pericarditis or prolonged congestive heart failure.

car·di·ac cy·cle (CC) (kahr'dē-ak sī'kĕl) Complete round of cardiac systole and diastole with the intervals between, or commencing with, any event in the heart's action to the moment when that same event is repeated.

car·di·ac de·com·pres·sion (kahr'dē-ak dē-kŏm-presh'ŭn) Incision into the pericardium or aspiration of fluid from the pericardium to relieve pressure. SYN pericardial decompression.

car·di·ac e·de·ma (kahr'dē-ak ĕ-dē'mă) Swelling resulting from congestive heart failure. SYN cardiac oedema.

car·di·ac gan·gli·a (kahr'dē-ak gang'glē-ă) [TA] Parasympathetic ganglia of the cardiac plexus.

car·di·ac im·pulse (kahr'dē-ak im'pŭls) Movement of the chest wall produced by cardiac contraction.

car·di·ac index (kahr'dē-ak in'deks) The amount of blood ejected by the heart in a unit of time divided by the body surface area.

car·di·ac in·farc·tion (kahr'dē-ak in-fahrk'shŭn) SYN myocardial infarction.

car·di·ac in·suf·fi·cien·cy (kahr'dē-ak in'sŭ-fish'ĕn-sē) SYN heart failure (1).

car·di·ac jelly (kahr'dē-ak jel'ē) The gelatinous, noncellular material between the endothelial lining and the myocardial layer of the heart in very early embryos; later in development it serves as a substratum for cardiac mesenchyme (i.e., embryonic connective tissue).

car·di·ac mas·sage (kahr'dē-ak mă-sahzh') SYN heart massage.

car·di·ac mur·mur (m, M, CM) (kahr'dē-ak mŭr'mŭr) Sound produced within the heart, at one of its valvular orifices or across ventricular septal defects.

car·di·ac mus·cle (kahr'dē-ak mŭs'ĕl) The muscle forming the myocardium, consisting of anastomosing transversely striated muscle fibers formed of cells united at intercalated discs. SYN muscle of heart.

car·di·ac notch (kahr'dē-ak noch) A deep notch between the esophagus and fundus of the stomach.

cardiacoedema [Br.] SYN cardiac edema.

car·di·ac or·i·fice (kahr'dē-ak ōr'i-fis) The trumpet-shaped opening of the esophagus into the stomach.

car·di·ac out·put (CO) (kahr'dē-ak owt'put) The product of heart rate and stroke volume, measured in liters per minute.

car·di·ac pace·ma·ker (kahr′dē-ak pās′māk-ĕr) Surgically implanted electronic device to regulate the heartbeat.

car·di·ac plex·us (kahr′dē-ak pleks′ŭs) A wide-meshed network of cardiopulmonary and splanchnic nerves arising from the afferent and autonomic nerve fibers (sympathetic) and vagus (parasympathetic) nerves, surrounding the arch of the aorta, the pulmonary artery, and continuing to the atria, ventricles, and coronary vessels.

car·di·ac re·serve (kahr′dē-ak rē-zĕrv′) The work the heart is able to perform beyond that required under the ordinary circumstances of daily life.

car·di·ac souf·fle (kahr′dē-ak sū′fĕl) A soft, puffing heart murmur.

car·di·ac sphinc·ter (kahr′dē-ak sfingk′tĕr) A physiologic sphincter at the esophagogastric junction.

car·di·ac syn·co·pe (kahr′dē-ak sin′kŏ-pē) Fainting with unconsciousness of any cardiac cause.

car·di·ac tam·po·nade (kahr′dē-ak tam′pŏ-nahd′) Compression of the heart due to critically increased volume of fluid in the pericardium.

car·di·al or·i·fice (kahr′dē-ăl ōr′i-fis) [TA] Trumpet-shaped opening of the esophagus into the stomach. SYN ostium cardiacum [TA], esophagogastric orifice.

car·di·nal (kahr′di-năl) Chief or principal; in embryology, relating to the main venous drainage.

car·di·nal lig·a·ment (kahr′di-năl lig′ă-mĕnt) [TA] A fibrous band attached to the uterine cervix and the vault of the lateral fornix of the vagina.

car·di·nal points (kahr′di-năl poynts) The four points in the pelvic inlet toward one of which the occiput of the baby is usually directed in case of head presentation: two sacroiliac articulations and the two iliopectineal eminences corresponding to the acetabula.

car·di·nal veins, pos·te·ri·or car·di·nal veins, com·mon car·di·nal veins, an·te·ri·or car·di·nal veins (kahr′di-năl vānz, pos-tēr′ē-ŏr, kom′ŏn, an-tēr′ē-ŏr) The major systemic venous channels in adult primitive vertebrates and in the embryos of higher vertebrates.

cardio-, cardi- Combining forms indicating the heart.

car·di·o·ac·cel·er·a·tor (kahr′dē-ō-ak-sel′ĕr-ā-tŏr) Accelerator of the heart beat.

car·di·o·ar·te·ri·al (kahr′dē-ō-ahr-tēr′ē-ăl) Relating to the heart and the arteries.

car·di·o·ar·te·ri·al (c-a) in·ter·val (kahr′dē-ō-ahr-tēr′ē-ăl in′tĕr-văl) Duration between the apex beat of the heart and the radial pulse beat.

Car·di·o·bac·te·ri·um (kahr′dē-ō-bak-tē′rē-ŭm) A genus of nonmotile, pleomorphic, gram-negative, facultatively anaerobic, rod-shaped bacteria found in the nasal flora and associated with endocarditis in humans.

Car·di·o·bac·te·ri·um hom·i·nis (kahr′dē-ō-bak-tē′rē-ŭm hom′i-nis) A species found as normal flora of the human upper respiratory tract that causes endocarditis. The type species of *Cardiobacterium*. SEE HACEK group.

car·di·o·cele (kahr′dē-ō-sēl) A herniation or protrusion of the heart through an opening in the diaphragm, or through a wound.

car·di·o·cen·te·sis (kahr′dē-ō-sen-tē′sis) Surgical puncture to withdraw fluid from the pericardial space.

car·di·o·cha·la·sia (kahr′dē-ō-kă-lā′zē-ă) **1.** Achalasia of the cardia. **2.** Relaxation or incompetence of the cardiac orifice of the stomach.

car·di·o·dy·nam·ics (kahr′dē-ō-dī-nam′iks) The mechanics of the heart's action.

car·di·o·dyn·i·a (kahr′dē-ō-din′ē-ă) Pain in the heart.

car·di·o·e·soph·a·ge·al (kahr′dē-ō-ē-sō-fā′jē-ăl) Denoting the junction of the esophagus and cardiac part of the stomach. SYN cardio-oesophageal.

car·di·o·gen·e·sis (kahr′dē-ō-gen′ĕ-sis) Formation of the heart in the embryo.

car·di·o·gen·ic (kahr′dē-ō-jen′ik) Of cardiac origin.

car·di·o·gen·ic shock (kahr′dē-ō-jen′ik shok) Condition resulting from decline in cardiac output secondary to serious heart disease, usually myocardial infarction.

car·di·o·gram (kahr′dē-ō-gram) 1. The graphic tracing made by the stylet of a cardiograph. 2. Any recording derived from the heart, with such prefixes as apex-, echo-, electro-, phono-, or vector-being understood.

car·di·og·ra·phy (kahr′dē-og′ră-fē) The use of the cardiograph.

car·di·o·in·hib·i·to·ry (kar′dē-ō-in-hib′i-tōr-ē) Arresting or slowing the action of the heart, either through effects on rate or muscle contraction.

car·di·o·ky·mog·ra·phy (kahr′dē-ō-kī-mog′ră-fē) Use of a cardiokymograph.

car·di·o·lip·in (CL) (kahr′dē-ō-lip′in) A glycerol found in many biomembranes with immunologic properties; used in serologic diagnosis of syphilis. SYN acetone-insoluble antigen, heart antigen.

car·di·ol·o·gy (kahr′dē-ol′ŏ-jē) The medical specialty concerned with the diagnosis and treatment of heart disease.

car·di·o·ma·la·cia (kahr′dē-ō-mă-lā′shē-ă) Softening of the walls of the heart.

car·di·o·meg·a·ly (kahr′dē-ō-meg′ă-lē) Enlargement of the heart. SYN macrocardia, megacardia, megalocardia.

car·di·o·mo·til·i·ty (kahr′dē-ō-mō-til′i-tē) Movements of the heart.

car·di·o·my·o·li·po·sis (kahr′dē-ō-mī′ō-li-pō′sis) Fatty degeneration of the myocardium.

car·di·o·my·op·a·thy (kahr′dē-ō-mī-op′ă-thē) Disease of the myocardium; a primary disease of heart muscle in the absence of a known underlying etiology. SYN myocardiopathy.

cardio-oesophageal [Br.] SYN cardio-oesophageal.

car·di·op·a·thy (kahr′dē-ō-op′ă-thē) Any disease of the heart.

car·di·o·pho·bia (kahr′dē-ō-fō′bē-ă) Morbid fear of heart disease.

car·di·o·plas·ty (kahr′dē-ō-plas-tē) An operation on the cardia of the stomach. SYN esophagogastroplasty.

car·di·o·ple·gia (kahr′dē-ō-plē′jē-ă) 1. Paralysis of the heart. 2. An elective stopping of cardiac activity temporarily by injection of chemicals, selective hypothermia, or electrical stimuli.

car·di·op·to·si·a, car·di·op·to·sis (kahr′dē-op-tō′sē-ă, -op′tŏ-sis) A condition in which the heart is unduly movable and displaced downward.

car·di·o·pul·mo·nar·y (CP) (kahr′dē-ō-pul′mŏ-nār-ē) Relating to the heart and lungs. SYN pneumocardial.

car·di·o·pul·mo·nar·y by·pass (CPB) (kahr′dē-ō-pul′mŏ-nār-ē bī′pas) Diversion of the blood flow returning to the heart through a pump oxygenator (heart-lung machine) and then returning it to the arterial side of the circulation.

car·di·o·pul·mo·nar·y re·sus·ci·ta·tion (CPR) (kahr′dē-ō-pul′mŏ-nār-ē rĕ-sŭs′i-tā′shŭn) Restoration of cardiac output and pulmonary ventilation following cardiac arrest and apnea, using artificial respiration and manual or mechanical closed chest compression or open chest cardiac massage.

car·di·or·rha·phy (kahr′dē-ōr′ă-fē) Suture of the heart wall.

car·di·or·rhex·is (kahr′dē-ō-rek′sis) Rupture of the heart wall.

car·di·o·se·lec·tive (kahr′dē-ō-sĕ-lek′tiv) Denoting or having the properties of cardioselectivity.

car·di·o·spasm (kahr′dē-ō-spazm) SYN esophageal achalasia.

car·di·o·ta·chom·e·ter (CTM) (kahr′dē-ō-tă-kom′ĕ-tĕr) An instrument for measuring the heart rate.

car·di·o·tho·rac·ic (kahr′dē-ō-thōr-as′ik) Pertaining to the heart and chest.

car·di·o·tho·rac·ic ra·tio (CT, CTR) (kahr′dē-ō-thōr-as′ik rā′shē-ō) Ratio of the horizontal diameter of the heart to the

car·di·o·to·cog·ra·phy (CTG) (kahr′de-ō-tō-kog′ră-fē) Method of monitoring and recording fetal heart rate and uterine contractions during pregnancy and labor.

car·di·ot·o·my (kahr′dē-ot′ō-mē) **1.** Incision of a heart wall. **2.** Incision of the cardiac part of the stomach.

car·di·o·ton·ic (kahr′dē-ō-ton′ik) Exerting a favorable, so-called tonic effect on the action of the heart.

car·di·o·tox·ic (kahr′dē-ō-tok′sik) Having a deleterious effect on the action of the heart.

car·di·o·val·vu·li·tis (kahr′dē-ō-val-vyū-lī′tis) Heart valve inflammation.

car·di·o·vas·cu·lar (kahr′dē-ō-vas′kyū-lăr) [TA] Relating to the heart and the blood vessels or the circulation. SYN cardiovasculare.

car·di·o·vas·cu·lar sys·tem (CVS) (kahr′dē-ō-vas′kyū-lăr sis′tĕm) [TA] The heart and blood vessels considered as one entity. SYN systema cardiovasculare [TA], blood-vascular system.

car·di·o·ver·sion (kahr′dē-ō-vĕr′zhŭn) Restoration of the heart's rhythm to normal by electrical countershock.

car·di·o·ver·ter (kahr′dē-ō-vĕr′tĕr) A machine used to perform cardioversion.

car·di·tis (kahr-dī′tis) Inflammation of the heart.

care (kār) In medicine and public health, a general term for the application of knowledge to the benefit of a community or individual patient.

Car·ey Coombs mur·mur (kār′ē kŭmz mŭr′mŭr) *Do not hyphenate Carey Coombs.* A blubbering apical middiastolic murmur occurring in the acute stage of rheumatic mitral valvulitis and disappearing as the valvulitis subsides. SYN Coombs murmur.

ca·ri·na, gen. and pl. **ca·ri·nae** (kă-rī′nă, -nē) In humans, a term applied or applicable to several anatomic structures forming a projecting central ridge.

ca·ri·na of tra·che·a (kă-rī′nă trā′kē-ă) [TA] The ridge separating the openings of the right and left main bronchi at their junction with the trachea. SYN tracheal carina.

car·i·nate (kar′i-nāt) Shaped like a keel; relating to or resembling a carina.

car·i·nate ab·do·men (kar′i-nāt ab′dŏ-mĕn) A sloping of the sides with prominence of the central line of the abdomen.

cario- Prefix meaning caries.

car·i·o·gen·e·sis (kar′ē-ō-jen′ĕ-sis) The process of producing caries; the mechanism of caries production.

car·min·a·tive (kahr-min′ă-tiv) An agent such as peppermint oil that is taken after a meal to facilitate belching through relaxation of the lower esophageal sphincter, thereby averting passage of swallowed air into the intestine as flatus.

car·mine (kahr′mĕn) [CI 75470] Red coloring matter used as a histology stain.

car·min·o·phil, car·min·o·phile, car·mi·noph·i·lous (kahr-min′ō-fil, -fīl, -mi-nof′ŏ-lŭs) Staining readily with carmine dyes.

car·mus·tine (kahr-mŭs′tēn) An antineoplastic agent. SYN BCNU.

car·ni·tine (kahr′ni-tēn) A trimethylammonium (betaine) derivative of gamma-amino-beta-hydroxybutyric acid.

car·ni·vore (kahr′ni-vōr) One of the Carnivora; any animal that consumes meat.

car·nos·in·ase (kahr′nō-si-nās) Mammalian enzyme that catalyzes the hydrolysis of carnosine.

car·no·sine (kahr′nō-sēn) The dominant nonprotein nitrogenous component of brain tissue, first found in high amounts in muscle. SYN ignotine, inhibitine.

car·no·si·ne·mia (kahr′nō-si-nē′mē-ă) An autosomal recessive congenital disease, characterized by the presence of excess amounts of carnosine in blood and urine; caused by a genetic deficiency of the enzyme carnosinase.

carotenaemia [Br.] SYN carotenemia.

car•o•tene (kar'ŏ-tēn) Yellow-red pigments (lipochromes) widely distributed in plants and animals closely related in structure to the xanthophylls and lycopenes and to the open-chain squalene.

car•o•ten•e•mia (kar'ŏ-tĕ-nē'mē-ă) Carotene in the blood that sometimes causes a pale yellow-red skin pigmentation that may resemble icterus. SYN carotenaemia, xanthemia.

ca•rot•e•noid (kă-rot'ĕ-noyd) 1. Resembling carotene; having a yellow color. 2. One of the carotenoids.

car•ot•i•co•tym•pan•ic (kă-rot'i-kō-tim-pan'ik) Relating to the carotid canal and the tympanum.

ca•rot•id (kă-rot'id) Pertaining to any carotid structure.

ca•rot•id bod•y (kă-rot'id bod'ē) [TA] A small epithelioid structure located just above the bifurcation of the common carotid artery on each side. SYN intercarotid body.

ca•rot•id can•al (kă-rot'id kă-nal') [TA] A pathway through the petrous part of the temporal bone from its inferior surface upward, medially, and forward to the apex where it opens into the foramen lacerum. SYN canalis caroticus [TA].

ca•rot•id sheath (kă-rot'id shēth) [TA] The dense fibrous investment of the carotid artery, internal jugular vein, and vagus nerve on each side of the neck. SYN vagina carotica [TA].

ca•rot•id si•nus (kă-rot'id sī'nŭs) [TA] A slight dilation of the common carotid artery at its bifurcation into external and internal carotids.

ca•rot•id si•nus re•flex (kă-rot'id sī'nŭs rē'fleks) A normal reflex relating to the carotid sinus syndrome, which results from hypersensitivity or hyperactivation of the carotid sinus.

ca•rot•id si•nus syn•drome (kă-rot'id sī'nŭs sin'drōm) Stimulation of a hyperactive carotid sinus, causing a marked fall in blood pressure due to vasodilation, cardiac slowing, or both.

ca•rot•o•dyn•i•a, ca•rot•i•dyn•i•a (kă-rot'ō-din'ē-ă, -i-din'ē-ă) Pain caused by pressure on the carotid artery.

car•pal (kahr'păl) Relating to the carpus.

car•pal bones (kahr'păl bōnz) [TA] Eight bones arranged in two rows that articulate proximally with the radius and indirectly with the ulna, and distally with the five metacarpal bones. SYN carpus (2) [TA].

car•pal joints (kahr'păl joynts) Synovial joints between the carpal bones.

car•pal tun•nel (kahr'păl tŭn'ĕl) [TA] Passageway deep to the transverse carpal ligament between tubercles of the scaphoid and trapezoid bones on the radial side and the pisiform and hook of the hamate on the ulnar side. SYN canalis carpi [TA].

car•pal tun•nel syn•drome (kahr'păl tŭn'ĕl sin'drōm) A common median nerve entrapment syndrome, characterized by hand paresthesia and pain.

car•pec•to•my (kahr-pek'tŏ-mē) Partial or total carpal excision.

car•po•ped•al (kahr'pō-ped'ăl) Relating to the wrist and the foot, or the hands and feet.

car•po•ped•al spasm (kahr'pō-ped'ăl spazm) Contraction of the feet and hands observed in hyperventilation, calcium deprivation, and tetany. Also called carpopedal contraction.

car•pop•to•sis, car•pop•to•si•a (kahr'pop-tō'sis, -tō'zē-ă) SYN wrist-drop.

car•pus, gen. and pl. **car•pi** (kahr'pŭs, -pī) [TA] 1. SYN wrist. 2. SYN carpal bones.

Car•rel-Lind•bergh pump (kar'ĕl-lind'bĕrg pŭmp) A device used to keep transplantation organs healthy during transport.

car•ri•er (kar'ē-ĕr) 1. A person or animal harboring a specific infectious agent in the absence of clinical disease symptoms and serving as a potential source of infection. **2.** Any chemical capable of accepting an atom, radical, or subatomic particle from one compound, then passing it to another. **3.** A large immunogen that when coupled to a hapten facilitates an immune response to the hapten.

car·ri·er-free (CF) (kar′ē-ĕr frē) Said of a substance in which a radioactive or other tagged atom is found in every molecule; the highest possible specific activity.

car·ri·er screen·ing (kar′ē-ĕr skrēn′ing) Indiscriminate examination of members of a population to detect heterozygotes for serious disorders and provide subsequent counsel about the risks of marriages to other carriers, and by prenatal diagnosis when both spouses in a married couple are both carriers.

car·ry·ing ca·pac·i·ty (kar′ē-ing kă-pas′i-tē) Estimate of the population a region, nation, or planet can sustain.

car sick·ness (kahr sik′nĕs) Motion sickness caused by riding in a car, bus, or train.

car·ti·lage bone (kahr′ti-lăj bōn) SYN endochondral bone.

car·ti·lage cap·sule (kahr′ti-lăj kap′sŭl) The more intensely basophilic matrix in hyaline cartilage surrounding the lacunae in which the cartilage cells lie.

car·ti·lage cell (kahr′ti-lăj sel) SYN chondrocyte.

car·ti·lage la·cu·na (kahr′ti-lăj lă-kū′nă) A cavity within the matrix of cartilage. SYN cartilage space.

car·ti·lage ma·trix (kahr′ti-lăj mā′triks) Intercellular substance composed of cartilaginous fibers and ground substance.

car·ti·lag·i·nous (kahr-ti-laj′i-nŭs) Relating to or consisting of cartilage.

car·ti·lag·i·nous joint (kahr-ti-laj′i-nŭs joynt) [TA] Articulation in which the apposed bony surfaces are united by cartilage. SYN junctura cartilaginea [TA], articulatio cartilaginis, cartilaginous articulation, synarthrodial joint (2).

ca·run·cu·la, pl. **ca·run·cu·lae** (kă-rŭng′kyū-lă, -lē) [TA] A small, fleshy

protuberance, or similarly shaped structure.

car·ve·di·lol (CAR) (kahr-vē′dil-ol) An antihypertensive and antianginal agent.

carve-out (kahrv′owt) Portion of a health care provider charge denied for payment.

car·ver (kahr′vĕr) A dental hand instrument, available in a wide variety of end shapes, used for forming and contouring.

caryo- Combining form meaning nucleus. SEE karyo-.

cas·cade (kas-kād′) A series of sequential interactions which after being initiated continues to the final one.

cas·cade stom·ach (kas-kād′ stŏm′ăk) Radiographic description: when contrast material is swallowed while the patient is upright, the gastric fundus acts as a reservoir until contrast overflows (cascades) into the antrum.

cas·ca·ra sa·gra·da (kas-kar′ă să-grä′dă) An herbal laxative made from the bark of *Rhamnus purshiana*.

case (kās) An instance of disease.

ca·se·a·tion (kā-sē-ā′shŭn) A form of necrotic coagulation in which the tissue resembles cheese.

case fa·tal·i·ty rate (kās fă-tal′i-tē rāt) Proportion of people contracting a disease who die as a result.

case his·to·ry (kās his′tŏr-ē) Detailed synopsis, generally written, of all particulars of a patient's familial, medical, and social involvements related to a condition or disease.

ca·sein (kā′sēn) The principal protein of cow's milk and the chief constituent of cheese.

ca·se·ous (kā′sē-ŭs) Cheeselike; showing features of caseation in tissue.

ca·se·ous ab·scess (kā′sē-ŭs ab′ses) An abscess containing white solid or semisolid material of cheeselike consistency. SYN cheesy abscess.

ca·se·ous ne·cro·sis (kā′sē-ŭs nĕ-krŏ′sis) Regional cell death characteristic of certain inflammations.

case study (kās stud′ē) In-depth study of an individual patient.

cas•sette (kă-set′) A plate, film, or tape holder for use in photography or radiography. A radiographic cassette contains one or two intensifying screens and a sheet of x-ray film.

cast (kast) **1.** An object formed by solidification of a liquid poured into a mold. **2.** Rigid encasement of a body part, with plaster, fiberglass, or plastic, to immobilize it after fracture (e.g., long-leg cast, short-leg cast). **3.** An elongated or cylindric mold formed in a tubular structure that may be observed in histologic sections or in material such as urine or sputum; results from inspissation of fluid material secreted or excreted in the tubular structures.

cast•ing (kast′ing) **1.** A metallic object formed in a mold. **2.** The act of forming a casting in a mold.

cas•tor oil (kas′tŏr oyl) Fatty oil from castor beans used as a cathartic or lubricant.

cas•trate (kas′trāt) To remove the testicles or the ovaries.

cas•tra•tion com•plex (kas-trā′shŭn kom′pleks) A child's fear of injury to the genitals by the parent of the same sex as punishment for unconscious guilt over oedipal feelings. Also called castration anxiety.

cata- Down; opposite of ana-. SEE ALSO kata-, de-.

ca•tab•o•lism (kă-tab′ō-lizm) **1.** The breaking down in the body of complex chemical compounds into simpler ones often accompanied by the liberation of energy. **2.** The sum of all degradative processes. SYN dissimilation (2).

ca•tac•ro•tism (kă-tak′rō-tizm) An anomaly of the pulse with one or more secondary expansions of the artery following the main beat.

cat•a•di•cro•tism (kat′ă-dī′krō-tizm) A condition of the pulse marked by two minor expansions of the artery following the main beat.

cat•a•gen (kat′ă-jen) A regressing phase of the hair growth cycle during which cell proliferation ceases, the hair follicle shortens, and an anchored club hair is produced.

cat•a•lase (kat′ă-lās) A hemoprotein catalyzing the decomposition of hydrogen peroxide to water and oxygen.

cat•a•lep•sy (kat′ă-lep-sē) A morbid condition characterized by waxy rigidity of the limbs, lack of response to stimuli, mutism, and inactivity.

ca•tal•y•sis (kă-tal′i-sis) The effect that a catalyst exerts on a chemical reaction.

cat•a•pla•si•a, cat•a•pla•sis (kat′ă-plā′zē-ă, -plā′sis) A degenerative change in cells or tissues that is the reverse of constructive or developmental change.

cat•a•plex•y, cat•a•plex•is (kat′ă-plek-sē, -sis) A transient attack of extreme generalized muscular weakness, often precipitated by an emotional state such as laughing, surprise, fear, or anger.

cat•a•ract (kat′ă-rakt) Complete or partial opacity of the ocular lens. Also called cataracta.

cat•a•ra•cta bru•nes•cens (kat-ă-rak′tă brū-nes′enz) SYN black cataract.

cat•a•ract nee•dle (kat′ăr-akt nē′dĕl) SYN knife needle.

ca•tarrh (kă-tahr′) Inflammation of a mucous membrane that increases flow of mucus.

ca•tar•rhal gas•tri•tis (kă-tahr′ăl gas-trī′tis) Stomach inflammation with excessive secretion of mucus.

ca•tar•rhal in•flam•ma•tion (kă-tahr′ăl in′flă-mā′shŭn) Inflammatory process most frequently seen in the respiratory tract.

ca•tar•rhal oph•thal•mi•a (kă-tahr′ăl of-thal′mē-ă) Mild conjunctivitis with mucopurulent secretion.

cat•a•to•ni•a (kat′ă-tō′nē-ă) A syndrome of psychomotor disturbances characterized by periods of physical rigidity, negativism, or stupor; may occur in schizophrenia or other mental disorders.

cat·a·ton·ic ex·cite·ment (kat-ă-ton´ik ek-sīt´mĕnt) Agitated catatonic state seen in one of the schizophrenic disorders. SEE catatonia.

cat·a·ton·ic ri·gi·di·ty (kat´ă-ton´ik ri-jid´i-tē) Rigidity associated with catatonic psychotic states in which all muscles exhibit flexibilitas cerea (q.v.).

cat·a·ton·ic schiz·o·phre·nia (kat´ă-ton´ik skits´ō-frē´nē-ă) Mental disorder characterized by marked disturbance, which may involve stupor, negativism, rigidity, excitement, or posturing.

catch·ment ar·ea (kach´mĕnt ār´ē-ă) Geographic jurisdiction of a community mental health center.

cat·e·chol (kat´ĕ-kol) SYN pyrocatechol.

ca·te·chol·a·mine (kat´ĕ-kō´lă-mēn) Hormone secreted by the suprarenal gland in response to stress.

cat·gut (kat´gŭt) An absorbable surgical suture material made from the collagenous fibers of the submucosa of certain animals, usually sheep or cows.

ca·thar·sis (kă-thahr´sis) **1.** The release or discharge of emotional tension or anxiety by psychoanalytically guided emotional reliving of past, especially repressed, events.

ca·thar·tic (kă-thahr´tik) **1.** Relating to catharsis. **2.** An agent having purgative action (i.e., of the bowel).

cath·e·ter (kath´ĕ-tĕr) **1.** A flexible tube that enables passage of fluid from or into a body cavity or blood vessel. SEE ALSO line (3). **2.** A tube designed to be passed through the urethra into the bladder to drain it of urine; usually composed of latex, silicone, or soft plastic.

cath·e·ter em·bo·lus (kath´ĕ-tĕr em´bō-lŭs) Coiled worm-shaped platelet and fibrin aggregates produced during vascular catheterization, originating on the catheter or its guide wire; embolization of the catheter itself.

catheterisation [Br.] SYN catheterization.

cath·e·ter·i·za·tion (kath´ĕ-tĕr-ī-zā´shŭn) Passage of a catheter. SYN catheterisation.

cath·e·ter spe·ci·men of u·rine (CSU) (kath´ĕ-tĕr spes´i-mĕn yūr´in) Specimen collected from an indwelling urinary catheter under clean conditions for testing.

ca·thex·is (kă-thek´sis) A conscious or unconscious attachment of psychic energy to an idea, object, or person.

cath·ode (C) (kath´ōd) The negative pole of a galvanic battery or the electrode connected with it.

cath·ode ray tube (CRT) (kath´ōd rā tūb) An evacuated tube containing a beam of electrons that can be deflected to various parts of a fluorescent screen.

cat·i·on (kat´ī-on) An ion carrying a charge of positive electricity, therefore going to the negatively charged cathode.

cat·i·on ex·change (kat´ī-on eks-chānj´) The process by which a cation in a liquid phase exchanges with another cation present as the counter-ion of a negatively charged solid polymer.

ca·top·tric (ka-top´trik) Relating to reflected light.

cat·scratch dis·ease, cat·scratch fe·ver (CSD) (kat´skrach di-zēz´, fē´vĕr) An infection that causes chronic benign adenopathy in most cases, especially in children and young adults, usually associated with a cat scratch or bite. SYN benign inoculation lymphoreticulosis, benign inoculation reticulosis, regional granulomatous lymphadenitis.

cau·dad (CD) (kaw´dad) In a direction toward the tail.

cau·da e·qui·na (kaw´dă ē-kwī´nă) [TA] The bundle of spinal nerve roots arising from the lumbosacral enlargement and medullary cone and running through the lumbar cistern.

cau·da e·qui·na syn·drome (kaw´dă ē-kwī´nă sin´drōm) Dull pain in upper sacral region, with anesthesia or analgesia in buttocks, genitalia, or thigh.

cau·dal (kaw´dăl) [TA] **1.** Pertaining to

the tail. **2.** VETERINARY ANATOMY denoting a position nearer to the tail.

cau·dal an·es·the·sia (kaw´dăl an´es-thē´zē-ă) Regional anesthesia by injection of local anesthetic solution into the epidural space through the sacral hiatus.

cau·dal em·i·nence (kaw´dăl em´i-nĕns) Rapidly proliferating mass of cells in the form of a taillike prominence found at the caudal extremity of the embryo. SYN end bud.

cau·dal flex·ure (kaw´dăl flek´shŭr) The bend in the lumbosacral region of the embryo.

cau·date (kaw´dāt) Tailed; possessing a tail.

cau·date pro·cess (kaw´dāt pros´es) A narrow band of hepatic tissue connecting the caudate and right lobes of the liver posterior to the porta hepatis.

caul, cowl (kawl, kowl) **1.** The amnion, either as a piece of membrane capping the baby's head at birth or the whole membrane when delivered unruptured with the baby. SYN galea (4), velum (2). **2.** SYN greater omentum.

caumaesthesia [Br.] SYN caumesthesia.

cau·sal·gi·a (kaw-zal´jē-ă) Persistent severe burning sensation, usually following partial injury of a peripheral nerve.

cau·sal·i·ty (kaw-zal´i-tē) The relating of causes to the effects they produce; the pathogenesis of disease and epidemiology are largely concerned with causality.

caus·al treat·ment (kaw´zăl trēt´mĕnt) Therapy aimed at reversing the causal factor in a disease.

cause (kawz) That which produces an effect or condition; that by which a morbid change or disease is brought about.

caus·tic (kaws´tik) **1.** Exerting an effect resembling a burn. **2.** An agent producing this effect. **3.** Denoting a solution of a strong alkali (e.g., caustic soda).

cau·ter·ant (kaw´tĕr-ănt) **1.** Cauterizing. **2.** A cauterizing agent.

cauterisation [Br.] SYN cauterization.

cauterise [Br.] SYN cauterize.

cau·ter·i·za·tion (kaw-tĕr-ī-zā´shŭn) The act of cauterizing. SEE ALSO cautery. SYN cauterisation.

cau·ter·ize (kaw´tĕr-īz) To apply a cautery; to burn with a cautery. SYN cauterise.

cau·tery (kaw´tĕr-ē) **1.** An agent or device used for scarring, burning, or cutting the skin or other tissues by means of heat, cold, electric current, or caustic chemicals. **2.** Use of a cautery.

cau·tery knife (kaw´tĕr-ē nīf) Knife that sears while cutting, to staunch bleeding.

cave (kāv) Any hollow or enclosed space or cavity. SYN cavum.

cav·e·o·la, pl. **ca·ve·o·lae** (kā-vē-ō´lă, -lē) A small pocket, vesicle, cave, or recess communicating with the outside of a cell and extending inward, indenting the cytoplasm and the cell membrane.

ca·ver·na, pl. **ca·ver·nae** (kă-ver´nă, -nē) [TA] SYN cavernous space.

cav·er·ni·tis, cav·er·no·si·tis (kav´ĕr-nī´tis, kav´ĕr-nō-sī´tis) Inflammation of the penile corpus cavernosum.

cav·ern·ous (kav´ĕr-nŭs) Relating to a cavern or a cavity; containing many cavities.

cav·ern·ous an·gi·o·ma (kav´ĕr-nŭs an´jē-ō´mă) Vascular malformation composed of sinusoidal vessels without a large feeding artery.

cav·ern·ous he·man·gi·o·ma (kav´ĕr-nŭs hē-man´jē-ō´mă) Deep cutaneous hemangioma with dilated vessels on gross and microscopic examination. Also used incorrectly for venous malformation.

cav·ern·ous lymph·an·gi·o·ma (kav´ĕr-nŭs lim-fan´jē-ō´mă) Extensive lymphangioma that has not only superficial and deep skin involvement but also subcutaneous and sometimes musculofascial components.

cav·ern·ous rale (kav´ĕr-nŭs rahl) A

resonating, bubbling sound caused by air entering a cavity partly filled with fluid.

cav·ern·ous si·nus (kav´ĕr-nŭs sī´nŭs) [TA] A paired dural venous sinus on either side of the sella turcica. SYN sinus cavernosus [TA].

cav·ern·ous si·nus syn·drome (CSS) (kav´ĕr-nŭs sī´nŭs sin´drŏm) Partial or complete external ophthalmoplegia.

cav·er·nous space (kav´ĕr-nŭs spās) [TA] An anatomic cavity with many interconnecting chambers.

cav·i·tar·y (kav´i-tār-ē) Relating to or having a cavity.

cav·i·tas, pl. **cav·i·ta·tes** (kav´i-tahs, -tā´tēz) SYN cavity.

ca·vi·tis (kā-vī´tis) SYN celophlebitis.

cav·i·ty (kav´i-tē) 1. A hollow space; hole. SEE cavernous space. 2. Common term for the loss of tooth structure due to dental caries. SYN cavitas.

cav·i·ty prep·a·ration (kav´i-tē prep´ăr-ā´shŭn) 1. Removal of dental caries and surgical preparation of the remaining tooth structure to receive a dental restoration. 2. Final form of an excavation in a tooth resulting from such preparation.

ca·vo·pul·mo·nar·y an·as·to·mo·sis (kā-vō-pul´mŏ-nār-ē ă-nas´tŏ-mō´sis) A means of palliating cyanotic heart disease by anastomosing the right pulmonary artery to the superior vena cava.

ca·vo·sur·face be·vel (kā´vō-sŭr´făs bev´ĕl) Incline of the cavosurface angle of a prepared cavity wall in relation to the plane of the enamel wall.

ca·vum (kā´vŭm) [TA] SYN cave.

cay·enne (kī-en´) SYN capsicum.

Cd Symbol for cadmium.

cd Symbol for candela.

Ce Symbol for cerium.

♻ **cec-** (sēk) SEE ceco-.

ce·cal (sē´kăl) 1. Relating to the cecum.

2. Ending blindly or in a cul-de-sac. SYN caecal.

ce·cec·to·my (sē-sek´tŏ-mē) Excision of the cecum. SYN caecectomy, typhlectomy.

ce·ci·tis (sē-sī´tis) Inflammation of the cecum. SYN caecitis, typhlenteritis, typhlitis, typhloenteritis.

♻ **ceco-, cec-** Combining forms denoting the cecum. SEE ALSO typhlo- (1). SYN caeco-.

ce·co·cele (sē´kō-sēl) Herniation of the cecum.

ce·co·co·los·to·my (sē´kō-kō-los´tŏ-mē) Formation of an anastomosis between cecum and colon. SYN caecocolostomy.

ce·co·cys·to·plas·ty (sē´kō-sis´tō-plas´ tē) Surgical repair of the bladder using a portion of the cecum.

ce·co·il·e·os·to·my (sē´kō-il-ē-os´tŏ-mē) SYN ileocecostomy.

ce·co·pli·ca·tion (sē´kō-pli-kā´shŭn) Operative reduction in size of a dilated cecum by the formation of folds or tucks in its wall. SYN caecoplication.

ce·cor·rha·phy (sē-kōr´ă-fē) Suture of the cecum. SYN typhlorrhaphy.

ce·co·sig·moid·os·to·my (sē´kō-sig-moy-dos´tŏ-mē) Formation of a communication between the cecum and the sigmoid colon. SYN caecosigmoidostomy.

ce·cos·to·my (sē-kos´tŏ-mē) Operative formation of a cecal fistula. SYN caecostomy, typhlostomy.

ce·cot·o·my (sē-kot´ŏ-mē) Incision into the cecum. SYN caecotomy, typhlotomy.

ce·co·u·re·ter·o·cele (sē´kō-yūr-ē´tĕr-ō-sēl) A ureterocele that extends far along the urethra, sometimes even out the urethral meatus.

ce·cum, pl. **ce·ca** (sē´kŭm, -kă) [TA] 1. The cul-de-sac, about 6 cm in depth, lying below the terminal ileum forming the first part of the large intestine. 2. Any similar structure ending in a cul-de-sac. SYN blind gut

ce·li·ac (sē′lē-ak) Relating to the abdominal cavity.

ce·li·ac (ar·te·ri·al) trunk (sē′lē-ak ahr-tēr′ē-ăl trŭngk) *Origin*, abdominal aorta just below diaphragm; *branches*, left gastric, common hepatic, splenic. SYN celiac axis.

ce·li·ac ax·is (CA) (sē′lē-ak ak′sis) SYN celiac (arterial) trunk.

ce·li·ac dis·ease (sē′lē-ak di-zēz′) A disease characterized by sensitivity to gluten, with chronic inflammation and atrophy of the mucosa of the upper small intestine. SYN coeliac disease, gluten enteropathy.

ce·li·ac gan·glia (sē′lē-ak gang′glē-ă) [TA] Largest and highest group of prevertebral sympathetic ganglia, located on the superior part of the abdominal aorta. SYN ganglia coeliaca [TA], solar ganglia, Vieussens ganglia, Willis centrum nervosum.

ce·li·ac trunk (sē′lē-ak trŭngk) *Origin*, abdominal aorta just below diaphragm; *branches*, left gastric, common hepatic, splenic. SYN truncus celiacus [TA], arteria celiaca, coeliac trunk.

celio- Prefix meaning the abdomen. SYN coelio-.

ce·li·o·gas·trot·o·my, ce·li·o·gas·tros·to·my (sē′lē-ō-gas-trot′ŏ-mē, -tros′tŏ-mē) Surgical incision of the abdomen and stomach.

ce·li·o·my·o·si·tis (sē′lē-ō-mī′ō-sī′tis) Inflammation of the abdominal muscles.

ce·li·os·co·py (sē′lē-os′kŏ-pē) SYN peritoneoscopy, coelioscopy.

ce·li·ot·o·my (sē′lē-ot′ŏ-mē) Transabdominal incision into the peritoneal cavity. SYN coeliotomy, abdominal section, laparotomy (2), ventrotomy.

ce·li·tis (sē-lī′tis) Any inflammation of the abdomen. SYN coelitis.

cell (sel) The smallest unit of living structure capable of independent existence.

cel·la, gen. and pl. **cel·lae** (sel′ă, -lē) A room or cell.

cell body (sel bod′ē) The part of the cell containing the nucleus.

cell cul·ture (sel kŭl′chŭr) The maintenance or growth of dispersed cells after removal from the body, commonly on a glass surface immersed in nutrient fluid.

cell cy·cle (sel sī′kĕl) The periodic biochemical and structural events occurring during proliferation of cells such as in tissue culture.

cell death (sel deth) The cessation of respiration within the cell that stops the production of energy, nutrients, active molecular transport, and the like.

cell de·ter·min·a·tion (sel dĕ-tĕr′mi-nā′shŭn) The process by which embryonic cells, previously undifferentiated, take on a specific developmental character. SEE morphogenesis, induction, evocator.

cell in·clu·sions (sel in-klū′zhŭnz) The residual elements of the cytoplasm that are metabolic products of the cell (e.g., pigment granules or crystals). SYN metaplasm.

cell-me·di·at·ed im·mu·ni·ty, cel·lu·lar im·mu·ni·ty (CMI) (sel′mē′dē-āt-ĕd i-myū′ni-tē, sel′yū-lăr) Immune responses that are initiated and mediated by T lymphocytes, macrophages, or both.

cell mem·brane (sel mem′brān) The protoplasmic boundary of all cells that controls permeability and may serve other functions through surface specializations.

cell or·gan·elle (sel ōr′gă-nel′) SYN organelle.

cel·lu·la, gen. and pl. **cel·lu·lae** (sel′yū-lă, -lē) 1. GROSS ANATOMY a small but macroscopic compartment. SYN cellule. 2. IN HISTOLOGY a cell.

cel·lu·lar (sel′yū-lăr) 1. Relating to, derived from, or composed of cells. 2. Having numerous compartments or interstices.

cel·lu·lar in·fil·tra·tion (sel′yū-lăr in′fil-trā′shŭn) Migration of cells from their sources of origin.

cel·lu·lar path·ol·o·gy (sel'yū-lăr pă-thol'ŏ-jē) **1.** The interpretation of diseases in terms of cellular alterations. **2.** Sometimes used as a synonym for cytopathology (1).

cel·lule (sel'yūl) SYN cellula (1).

cel·lu·lif·u·gal (sel'yū-lif'ŭ-găl) Moving from, or extending in a direction away from, a cell or cell body.

cel·lu·lip·e·tal (sel'yū-lip'ĕ-tăl) Moving toward, or extending in a direction toward, a cell or cell body.

cel·lu·lite (sel'yū-līt) **1.** Colloquial term for deposits of fat and fibrous tissue causing dimpling of the overlying skin. **2.** SYN lipoedema.

cel·lu·li·tis (sel'yū-lī'tis) Inflammation of subcutaneous, loose connective tissue (formerly called cellular tissue).

cel·lu·lose (sel'yū-lōs) A linear B1→4 glucan, composed of cellobiose residues, differing in this respect from starch, which is composed of maltose residues; it forms the basis of vegetable and wood fiber and is the most abundant organic compound. SYN cellulin.

cell wall (CW, cw) (sel wawl) **1.** The outer layer or membrane of some animal and plant cells.

♻ **celo-, coelo-** Combining forms denoting (1) the celom; (2) hernia. SEE ALSO celio-.

ce·lom, ce·lo·ma (sē'lŏm, sē-lō'mă) **1.** The cavity between the splanchnic and somatic mesoderm in the embryo. SYN coelom. **2.** SYN body cavity.

ce·lo·phle·bi·tis (sē'lō-flĕ-bī'tis) Inflammation of a vena cava. SYN cavitis.

Cel·si·us scale (sel'sē-ŭs skāl) A temperature scale that is based on the triple point of water (defined to be 273.16°K) and assigned the value of 0.01°C; has replaced the centigrade scale because the triple point of water can be more accurately measured than the ice point; for most practical purposes, however, the two scales are equivalent.

ce·ment (sĕ-ment') [TA] DENTISTRY a nonmetallic material used for luting, fill-

ing, or permanent or temporary restoration, or as an adherent sealer in attaching various dental restorations in or on the tooth made by mixing components into a plastic mass that sets.

ce·men·ta·tion (sē'men-tā'shŭn) **1.** The process of attaching parts by means of a cement. **2.** In dentistry, attaching a restoration to natural teeth by means of a cement.

ce·ment base (sĕ-ment' bās) In dentistry, a layer of dental cement, sometimes medicated, which is placed in the deep portion of a cavity preparation to protect the pulp, reduce the bulk of a metallic restoration, or eliminate undercuts. SYN cavity preparation base.

ce·ment dis·ease (sĕ-ment' di-zēz') The osteolysis that frequently occurs in association with loosening of cemented total hip replacements.

ce·ment·i·fi·ca·tion (sĕ-men'ti-fi-kā'shŭn) Metaplastic production of cementum or cementoid within a less differentiated connective tissue, e.g., cementification of a fibroma.

ce·ment·o·blast (sĕ-men'tō-blast) One of the cells concerned with the formation of the layer of cementum on the roots of teeth.

ce·ment·o·cyte (sĕ-men'tō-sīt) An osteocytelike cell with numerous processes, trapped in a lacuna in the cementum of the tooth.

ce·men·to·den·ti·nal junc·tion (sĕ-men'tō-den'ti-năl jŭngk'shŭn) The surface at which the cementum and dentin of the root of a tooth are joined.

ce·men·to·e·nam·el junction (CEJ) (sĕ-men'tō-ĕ-nam'ĕl jŭngk'shŭn) The surface at which the enamel of the crown and the cementum of the root of a tooth are joined. SEE ALSO cervical line.

ce·men·tum (sĕ-men'tŭm) [TA] A layer of bonelike mineralized tissue covering the dentin of the root and neck of a tooth that blends with the fibers of the periodontal ligament.

♻ **ceno-** Combining form denoting (1) shared in common [G. *koinos,* common];

(2) [G. *kainos*, new]. [G. *kenos*, empty].
SEE ALSO coeno-.

cen•o•site (sē'nō-sīt) A facultative commensal organism that can sustain itself apart from its usual host. SYN coinosite.

cen•sor (sen'sŏr) PSYCHOANALYTIC THEORY the psychic barrier that prevents certain unconscious thoughts and wishes from coming to consciousness.

cen•ter (sen'tĕr) [TA] **1.** The middle point of a body; loosely, the interior of a body. A center of any kind, especially an anatomic center. SYN centrum [TA]. **2.** A group of nerve cells governing a specific function. **3.** A health care or therapeutic facility performing a particular function or service for people in the surrounding area. SYN centre.

cen•ter of ex•cel•lence (sen'tĕr ek'sĕ-lĕns) A colloquial, jargonistic, and vastly overused term for any health care facility that is reputed, by means of public survey or in the opinion of the facility itself, to be superior in one or more ways to other such care facilities.

cen•ter of gra•vi•ty (COG) (sen'tĕr grav'i-tē) The point on a body or system where, if pressure equal to the weight of the object is applied, forces acting on the object will be in equilibrium; the point around which the mass is centered; the location of the COG in an adult human being in the anatomic position is just anterior to the second sacral vertebra. SYN centre of gravity.

Cen•ters for Dis•ease Con•trol and Pre•ven•tion (CDC) (sen'tĕrz di-zēz' kŏn-trōl' prĕ-ven'shŭn) The U.S. federal facility for disease eradication, epidemiology, and education headquartered in Atlanta, Georgia, which encompasses the Center for Infectious Diseases, Center for Environmental Health, Center for Health Promotion and Education, Center for Prevention Services, Center for Professional Development and Training, and Center for Occupational Safety and Health. It maintains several coding sets included in HIPAA standards (e.g., ICD-9-CM codes). Formerly named the Center for Disease Control (1970) and the Communicable Disease Center (1946).

Cen•ters for Med•i•care and Med•i•caid Ser•vices (CMS) (sen'tĕrz med'i-kār med'i-kād sĕr'vi-sĕz) An agency of the U.S. Department of Health and Human Services that manages the federal health care programs of Medicare and Medicaid; before July 2001, known as the Health Care Financing Administration (HCFA).

cen•te•sis (sen-tē'sis) Puncture, especially when used as a suffix, as in paracentesis.

centi- (c) Prefix used in the SI and metric system to signify one hundredth (10^{-2}).

cen•ti•grade (sen'ti-grād) Older term for metric measure of temperature (normal human body temperature is 36.7 degrees); usually replaced by Celsius. SYN Celsius.

cen•ti•me•ter (cm) (sen'ti-mē-tĕr) One hundredth of a meter; 0.3937008 inch. SYN centimetre.

cen•ti•me•ter-gram-sec•ond sys•tem (CGS, cgs) (sen'ti-mē-tĕr-gram-sek'ŏnd sis'tĕm) The scientific system of expressing the fundamental physical units of length, mass, and time, and those units derived from them, in centimeters, grams, and seconds; is being replaced by the International System of Units based on the meter, kilogram, and second.

centimetre [Br.] SYN centimeter.

cen•trad (sen'trad) **1.** Toward the center. **2.** A unit of measurement of the refracting strength of a prism; it corresponds to the deviation of a ray of light, the arc of which is 1/100 of the radius of the circle, or 0.57°.

cen•tral ap•ne•a (sen'trăl ap'nē-ă) Apnea as the result of medullary depression, which inhibits respiratory movement.

cen•tral cloud•y cor•ne•al dys•tro•phy of Fran•cois (sen'trăl klow'dē kōr'nē-ăl dis'trŏ-fē frahn-swah') An autosomal dominant opacification of the central corneal stroma consisting of cloudy polygonal areas.

cen•tral deaf•ness (sen'trăl def'nĕs) Deafness due to disorder of the auditory system of the brainstem or cerebral cortex.

cen•tral gan•gli•o•neu•ro•ma (sen'trăl

gang´glē-ō-nūr-ō´mă) SYN gangliocytoma.

cen·tral im·plan·ta·tion (sen´trăl im´plan-tā´shŭn) Implantation in which the blastocyst remains in the uterine cavity, as in carnivores, rhesus monkeys, and rabbits.

cen·tral in·ci·sor (sen´trăl in-sī´zŏr) The first tooth in the maxilla and mandible on either side of the midsagittal plane of the head.

cen·tral line (sen´trăl līn) Catheter placed into the femoral, subclavian, or jugular vein used for patient monitoring and administration of medication.

cen·tral nec·ro·sis (sen´trăl nĕ-krō´sis) Necrosis involving the deeper or inner portions of a tissue, or an organ or its units.

cen·tral ner·vous sys·tem (CNS) (sen´trăl nĕr´vŭs sis´tĕm) [TA] The brain and the spinal cord.

cen·tral ner·vous sys·tem de·pres·sant (sen´trăl nĕr´vŭs sis´tĕm dĕ-pres´ănt) Medication used to slow down neuronal activity.

cen·tral ner·vous sys·tem stim·u·lant (sen´trăl nĕr´vŭs sis´tĕm stim´yū-lănt) Medication used to speed up neuronal activity.

cen·tral os·si·fy·ing fi·bro·ma (sen´trăl os´i-fī-ing fī-brō´mă) A painless, slowly expansile, sharply circumscribed benign fibroosseous tumor of the jaws that is derived from cells of the periodontal ligament; presents initially as a radiolucency that becomes progressively more opaque as it matures.

cen·tral os·te·it·is (sen´trăl os-tē-ī´tis) 1. SYN osteomyelitis. 2. SYN endosteitis.

cen·tral sco·to·ma (sen´trăl skō-tō´mă) A scotoma involving the fixation point.

cen·tral sleep ap·ne·a (CSA) (sen´trăl slēp ap´nē-ă) Cessation of breathing during sleep secondary to blunted drive to the respiratory muscles. This is not a single disease but comprises several disorders that manifest as apneic episodes during sleep.

cen·tral ve·nous cath·e·ter (sen´trăl vē´nŭs kath´ĕ-tĕr) Tube surgically inserted into a vein in the central circulation (usually the superior vena cava). Commonly used for long-term intravenous therapy, nutritional support, or chemotherapy.

cen·tral ve·nous pres·sure (CVP) (sen´trăl vē´nŭs presh´ŭr) The pressure of the blood within the venous system in the superior and inferior vena cava cephalad to the diaphragm.

cen·tral vi·sion (sen´trăl vizh´ŭn) Vision stimulated by an object imaged on the fovea centralis. SYN direct vision.

centre [Br.] SYN center.

cen·tren·ce·phal·ic (sen´tren-sĕ-fal´ik) Relating to the center of the encephalon.

centre of gravity [Br.] SYN center of gravity.

centri- *Do not confuse this combining form with the prefix centi-.* Combining form denoting center.

-centric Combining form meaning having a center (of a specific kind or number) or having a specific thing as its center (of interest, focus).

cen·tric (sen´trik) Having a center (of a specific kind or number) or having a specific thing as its center (e.g., of interest, focus).

cen·tric·i·put (sen-tris´i-put) The central portion of the upper surface of the skull, between the occiput and the sinciput.

cen·trif·u·gal (sen-trif´ŭ-găl) 1. Denoting the direction of the force pulling an object outward (away) from an axis of rotation. 2. Sometimes, by analogy, extended to describe any movement away from a center. Cf. eccentric (2).

cen·trif·u·gal nerve (sen-trif´ŭ-găl nĕrv) SYN efferent nerve.

cen·trif·u·ga·tion (sen-trif´ŭ-gā´shŭn) Subjection to sedimentation, by means of a centrifuge, of solids suspended in a fluid. SYN centrifugalization.

cen·tri·fuge (sen´tri-fyūzh) 1. An apparatus by means of which particles in suspension in a fluid are separated by spinning the fluid, the centrifugal force throwing the particles to the periphery of the rotated vessel. **2.** To submit to rapid rotary action, as in a centrifuge.

cen·tri·lob·u·lar (sen'tri-lob'yū-lăr) At or near the center of a lobule, e.g., of the liver.

cen·tri·ole (sen'trē-ōl) Tubular structures, 150 nm by 300–500 nm, with a wall having nine triple microtubules, usually seen as paired organelles lying in the cytocentrum.

cen·trip·e·tal (sĕn-trip'ĕ-tăl) **1.** SYN afferent. **2.** Denoting the direction of the force pulling an object toward an axis of rotation. SYN axipetal.

cen·trip·e·tal nerve (sĕn-trip'ĕ-tăl nĕrv) SYN afferent nerve.

centro- Combining form denoting center.

cen·tro·blast (sen'trō-blast) A lymphocyte with a large noncleaved nucleus.

cen·tro·cyte (sen'trō-sīt) **1.** A cell with a protoplasm that contains single and double granules of varying size stainable with hematoxylin; seen in lesions of lichen planus. SYN Lipschütz cell. **2.** A lymphocyte with a cleaved nucleus. **3.** A nondividing, activated B cell that expresses membrane immunoglobulin.

cen·tro·mere (cen) (sen'trō-mēr) The nonstaining primary constriction of a chromosome that is the point of attachment of the spindle fiber; provides the mechanism of chromosome movement during cell division; the centromere divides the chromosome into two arms, and its position is constant for a specific chromosome: near one end (acrocentric), near the center (metacentric), or between (submetacentric).

cen·tro·some (sen'trō-sōm) SYN cytocentrum.

cen·trum, pl. **cen·tra** (sen'trŭm, -tră) [TA] SYN center (1).

cephal- SEE cephalo-.

ceph·a·lad (sef'ă-lad) In a direction toward the head. SEE ALSO cranial (1).

ceph·al·hy·dro·cele (sef-ăl-hī'drō-sēl) An accumulation of serous or watery fluid under the pericranium.

ce·phal·ic (sĕ-fal'ik) SYN cranial (1).

ce·phal·ic curve (sĕ-fal'ik kŭrv) Curve conforming to that of the fetal head, used in reference to the shape of obstetric forceps.

ce·phal·ic flex·ure (sĕ-fal'ik flek'shŭr) The sharp, ventrally concave bend in the developing midbrain of the embryo. SYN cranial flexure, mesencephalic flexure.

ce·phal·ic in·dex (se-fal'ik in'deks) The ratio of the maximal breadth to the maximal length of the head, obtained by the formula: (breadth $\times$ 100)/length. SYN length-breadth index.

ce·phal·ic pole (sĕ-fal'ik pōl) The head end of the embryo or fetus.

ce·phal·ic pre·sen·ta·tion (sĕ-fal'ik prez'ĕn-tā'shŭn) Presentation of any part of the fetal head, usually the upper and back part as a result of flexion such that the chin is in contact with the thorax in vertex presentation.

ce·phal·ic tet·a·nus (sĕ-fal'ik tet'ă-nŭs) A type of local tetanus that follows wounds to the face and head.

ce·phal·ic ver·sion (sĕ-fal'ik vĕr'zhŭn) Placement in which the fetus is turned so that the head presents; can be external cephalic version (q.v.) or internal cephalic version (q.v.).

cephalo-, cephal- Combining forms meaning the head.

ceph·a·lo·cau·dal, ceph·a·lo·cau·dad (sef'ă-lō-kaw'dăl, -kaw'dad) Relating to both head and tail, i.e., to the long axis of the body.

ceph·a·lo·cau·dal ax·is (sef'ă-lō-kaw'dăl ak'sis) Long axis of the body.

ceph·a·lo·cele (sef'ă-lō-sēl) Protrusion of part of the cranial contents. SEE ALSO encephalocele.

ceph·a·lo·cen·te·sis (sef'ă-lō-sen-tē'sis) Passage of a hollow needle or trocar into the brain to drain an abscess or hydrocephalic fluid.

ceph·a·lo·dyn·i·a (sef′ă-lō-din′ē-ă) Headache.

ceph·a·lo·gy·ric (sef′ă-lō-jī′rik) Relating to rotation of the head.

ceph·a·lo·meg·a·ly (sef′ă-lō-meg′ă-lē) Enlargement of the head.

ceph·a·lom·e·lus (sef′ă-lom′ĕ-lŭs) Malformed person with an accessory limb, resembling a leg or arm, growing from the head.

ceph·a·lom·e·ter (sef′ă-lom′ĕ-tĕr) An instrument used to position the head to produce oriented, reproducible lateral and posterior-anterior head films. SYN cephalostat.

ceph·a·lo·met·rics (sef′ă-lō-met′riks) ORAL SURGERY, ORTHODONTICS the scientific measurement of the bones of the cranium and face, using a fixed, reproducible position for lateral radiographic exposure of skull and facial bones.

ceph·a·lom·e·try (sef′ă-lom′ĕ-trē) Measurements on the living head, or head without removal of the soft parts. SEE ALSO cephalometrics.

ceph·a·lo·mo·tor (sef′ă-lō-mō′tŏr) Relating to movements of the head.

ceph·a·lop·a·thy (sef′ă-lop′ă-thē) SYN encephalopathy.

ceph·a·lo·pel·vic (sef′ă-lō-pel′vik) Pertaining to the size of the fetal head in relation to the maternal pelvis.

ceph·a·lo·pel·vic dis·pro·por·tion (CPT) (sef′ă-lō-pel′vik dis′prŏ-pōr′shŭn) A condition in which the fetal head is too large to traverse the maternal pelvis, causing arrest of labor.

ceph·a·lo·spo·rin (CEPH) (sef′ă-lō-spōr′in) Antibiotic produced by a *Cephalosporium.*

Ceph·a·lo·spo·ri·um (sef′ă-lō-spō′rē-ŭm) Former name of *Acremonium.*

ceph·a·lo·stat (sef′ă-lō-stat) SYN cephalometer.

ceph·a·lo·tho·rac·ic (sef′ă-lō-thōr-as′ik) Relating to the head and the chest.

ceph·a·lot·o·my (sef′ă-lot′ŏ-mē) Formerly used operation of cutting into the head of the fetus.

-cephaly Suffix indicating an anomalous condition of the head.

-ceptor Combining form denoting taker, receiver.

ce·ra (sē′ră) SYN wax (1).

cerat- SEE kerat-.

cerato- SEE kerato-.

cer·car·i·a, pl. **cer·car·i·ae** (sĕr-kar′ē-ă, -ē) The free-swimming trematode larva that emerges from its host snail.

cer·clage (ser-klazh′) Bringing into close opposition and binding together the ends of an obliquely fractured bone or the fragments of a broken patella by a ring or by an encircling, tightly drawn wire loop.

cer·co·cys·tis (ser′kō-sis′tis) Tapeworm larva that develops within a vertebrate host villus rather than in an invertebrate host's. SEE ALSO *Cysticercus.*

cer·e·bel·lar (ser-ĕ-bel′ăr) Relating to the cerebellum.

cer·e·bel·lar atax·ia (CLA) (ser-ă-bel′ăr ă-tak′sē-ă) Loss of muscle coordination caused by disorders of the cerebellum.

cer·e·bel·lar at·ro·phy (ser-ă-bel′ăr at′rō-fē) Degeneration of the cerebellum, particularly the Purkinje cells, as the result of abiotrophy or exposure to toxic agents, as in alcoholism.

cer·e·bel·lar cyst (ser-ă-bel′ăr sist) Lesion usually in the lateral cerebellar white matter.

cer·e·bel·lar hem·i·sphere (ser-ĕ-bel′ăr hem′is-fēr) The large part of the cerebellum lateral to the vermis cerebelli.

cerebello- Prefix meaning the cerebellum.

cer·e·bel·lo·pon·tine, cer·e·bel·lo·pon·tile (CP) (ser′e-bel′ō-pon′tēn, -tīl) Relating to the cerebellum and the pons.

cer·e·bel·lo·pon·tine an·gle (ser′ĕ-bel-ō-pon′tēn ang′gĕl) The recess at the junction of the cerebellum, pons, and medulla. SYN angulus pontocerebellaris [TA].

cer·e·bel·lo·spi·nal (ser′ĕ-bel′ō-spī′năl) Pertaining to the cerebellum and spinal cord.

cer·e·bel·lum, pl. **cer·e·bel·la** (ser-ĕ-bel′ŭm, -lă) [TA] Large posterior brain mass lying dorsal to the pons and medulla and ventral to the posterior portion of the cerebrum.

cerebr- SEE cerebro-.

ce·re·bral (ser′ĕ-brăl) Relating to the cerebrum.

cer·e·bral an·eur·ysm (ser′ĕ-brăl an′yūr-izm) Local widening or bulging in an artery in the brain.

ce·re·bral an·gi·og·ra·phy (ser′ĕ-brăl an-jē-og′ră-fē) Radiographic visualization of the blood vessels supplying the brain, including their extracranial portions. SYN cerebral arteriography.

ce·re·bral com·pres·sion (ser′ĕ-brăl kŏm-presh′ŏn) Pressure on intracranial tissues by an effusion of blood or cerebrospinal fluid, an abscess, a neoplasm, a depressed fracture of the skull, or an edema of the brain. SYN compression of brain.

cer·e·bral cor·tex (ser′ĕ-brăl kōr′teks) [TA] The gray cellular mantle (1–4 mm thick) covering the entire surface of the cerebral hemisphere of mammals. SEE ALSO Brodmann areas.

ce·re·bral death (ser′ĕ-brăl deth) A clinical syndrome characterized by the permanent loss of cerebral and brainstem function, manifested by absence of responsiveness to external stimuli, absence of cephalic reflexes, and apnea.

ce·re·bral de·com·pres·sion (ser′ĕ-brăl dē-kŏm-presh′ŭn) Removal of a piece of the cranium, usually in the subtemporal region, with incision of the dura, to relieve intracranial pressure.

ce·re·bral di·a·tax·i·a (ser′ĕ-brăl dī-ă-tak′sē-ă) Ataxic type of cerebral birth palsy.

ce·re·bral dys·pla·si·a (ser′ĕ-brăl dis-plā′zē-ă) Abnormal development of the telencephalon.

ce·re·bral gi·gan·tism (ser′ĕ-brăl jī-gant′izm) A syndrome characterized by increased birth weight and length (above the 90th percentile), an accelerated growth rate for the first 4 or 5 years without elevation of serum growth hormone levels, then reversion to normal growth rate.

ce·re·bral hem·is·phere (ser′ĕ-brăl hem′is-fēr) [TA] SYN hemisphere.

ce·re·bral hem·or·rhage (ser′ĕ-brăl hem′ŏr-ăj) Hemorrhage into the substance of the cerebrum. SYN hematencephalon, intracerebral hemorrhage.

ce·re·bral in·dex (ser′ĕ-brăl in′deks) The ratio of the transverse to the anteroposterior diameter of the cranial cavity multiplied by 100.

ce·re·bral in·farc·tion (ser′ĕ-brăl in-fahrk′shŭn) Localized necrosis of brain tissue caused by impaired blood flow.

ce·re·bral lo·cal·i·za·tion (ser′ĕ-brăl lō′kăl-ī-zā′shŭn) 1. Mapping of the cerebral cortex into areas and the correlation of the various areas with cerebral function. 2. Determination of the site of a brain lesion based on signs and symptoms or neuroimaging.

ce·re·bral pal·sy (ser′ĕ-brăl pawl′zē) Defect of motor power and coordination related to damage to the brain that occurred prenatally, perinatally, or in the first 3 years of life.

cer·e·bral re·vas·cu·lar·i·za·tion (ser′ĕ-brăl rē-vas′kyū-lăr-ī-zā′shŭn) Restoration of blood flow to the brain by surgical intervention.

ce·re·bral sul·ci (ser′ĕ-brăl sŭl′sī) [TA] Grooves between the cerebral gyri or convolutions. SYN sulci cerebri [TA].

ce·re·bral throm·bo·sis (CT) (ser′ĕ-brăl throm-bō′sis) Clotting of blood in a cerebral vessel.

cer·e·bral vas·cu·lar at·tack (CVA) (ser'ĕ-brăl vas'kyū-lăr ă-tak') SYN acute ischemic stroke.

cer·e·bra·tion (ser'ĕ-brā'shŭn) Activity of the mental processes; thinking.

cerebri- SEE cerebro-.

cer·e·bri·form (se-rē'bri-fōrm) Resembling the external fissures and convolutions of the brain.

cer·e·bri·tis (ser'ĕ-brī'tis) Focal inflammatory infiltrates in the brain parenchyma.

cerebro-, cerebr-, cerebri- Combining forms meaning the cerebrum. SEE ALSO encephalo-.

cer·e·bro·ma·la·ci·a (ser'ĕ-brō-mă-lā'shē-ă) SYN encephalomalacia.

cer·e·bro·men·in·gi·tis (ser'ĕ-brō-men-in-jī'tis) SYN meningoencephalitis.

cer·e·bron·ic ac·id (ser'ĕ-bron'ik as'id) A constituent of brain cerebrosides and other glycolipids. SYN phrenosinic acid.

cer·e·bro·path·i·a, cer·e·brop·a·thy (ser'ĕ-brō-path'ē-ă, ser'ĕ-brop'ă-thē) SYN encephalopathy.

cer·e·bro·phys·i·ol·o·gy (ser'ĕ-brō-fiz'ē-ol'ŏ-jē) The physiology of the cerebrum.

cer·e·bro·ret·i·nal an·gi·o·ma·to·sis (ser'ĕ-brō-ret'i-năl an'jē-ō-mă-tō'sis) SYN von Hippel-Lindau syndrome.

cer·e·bro·scle·ro·sis (ser'ĕ-brō-skler-ō'sis) Hardening of the cerebral hemispheres.

cer·e·bro·spi·nal (CS) (ser'ĕ-brō-spī'năl) Relating to the brain and the spinal cord.

cer·e·bro·spi·nal flu·id (CSF) (ser'ĕ-brō-spī'năl flū'id) [TA] A fluid largely secreted by the choroid plexuses of the ventricles of the brain, filling the ventricles and the subarachnoid cavities of the brain and spinal cord.

cer·e·bro·spi·nal flu·id rhi·nor·rhea (ser'ĕ-brō-spī'năl flū'id rī-nōr-ē'ă) Discharge of cerebrospinal fluid from the nose.

cer·e·bro·spi·nal men·in·gi·tis (ser'ĕ-brō-spī'năl men-in-jī'tis) SYN meningitis.

cer·e·bro·spi·nal pres·sure (ser'ĕ-brō-spī'năl presh'ŭr) Pressure of the cerebrospinal fluid, normally 100–150 mm of water, relative to the ambient atmospheric pressure.

cer·e·brot·o·my (ser'ĕ-brot'ŏ-mē) Incision of the brain.

cer·e·bro·vas·cu·lar (ser'ĕ-brō-vas'kyū-lăr) Relating to the blood supply to the brain, particularly with reference to pathologic changes.

cer·e·bro·vas·cu·lar ac·ci·dent (CVA) (ser'ĕ-brō-vas'kyū-lăr ak'si-dĕnt) An imprecise but common term for cerebral stroke.

cer·e·brum, pl. **cer·e·bra,** pl. **cer·e·brums** (ser'ĕ-brŭm, -bră, -brŭmz) [TA] Those parts of the brain derived from the telencephalon; includes mainly the cerebral hemispheres.

ce·ro·plas·ty (sē'rō-plas'tē) Wax models of anatomic and pathologic specimens or skin lesions.

cer·ti·fied mas·sage ther·a·pist (CMT) (sĕr'ti-fīd mă-sazh' thār'ă-pist) Health care professional who has passed examinations to verify that professional standards and necessary knowledge of the human body have been attained. SEE ALSO massage therapy.

cer·ti·fied med·i·cal as·sis·tant (CMA) (sĕr'ti-fīd med'i-kăl ă-sis'tănt) A health care professional whose skills have been verified by meeting examination standards set by a national board.

cer·ti·fied med·i·cal trans·crip·tion·ist (CMT) (sĕr'ti-fīd med'i-kăl tran-skrip'shŭn-ist) A health care professional who has passed board-administered examinations that confirm that standards of knowledge and accuracy have been met. SEE ALSO medical transcriptionist.

cer·ti·fied milk (sĕr'ti-fīd milk) Cow's milk that does not have more than the maximal permissible limit of 10,000 bacteria per mL at any time prior to delivery to the consumer.

Cer·ti·fied Oc·cu·pa·tion·al Health Nurse (COHN) (sĕr′ti-fīd ok-yū-pā′shŭn-ăl helth nŭrs) Specialty designation signifying the successful completion of an examination.

Cer·ti·fied Phar·ma·cy Tech·ni·cian (CPhT) (sĕr′ti-fīd fahr′mă-sē tek-ni′shŭn) A pharmacy technician who has successfully passed the Pharmacy Technician Certification Board (PTCB) examination.

Cer·ti·fied Res·pi·ra·to·ry Ther·a·pist (CRT) (sĕr′tĭ-fīd res′pir-ă-tōr-ē thār′ă-pist) A health care professional, generally holding an associate's degree, licensed at the state level to treat patients with various lung disorders.

cer·ti·fy (ser′ti-fī) To commit a patient to a mental hospital in accordance with state laws.

ce·ru·le·an (sĕ-rū′lē-ăn) SYN blue.

ce·ru·men (sĕ-rū′mĕn) The soft, brownish yellow, waxy secretion in the external auditory canal. SYN ear wax, earwax.

ce·ru·mi·no·ma (sĕ-rū′mi-nō′mă) A usually benign adenomatous tumor of ceruminous glands of the external auditory canal.

ce·ru·mi·nous glands (sĕ-rū′mi-nŭs glandz) Apocrine sudoriferous glands in the external acoustic meatus. SYN glandulae ceruminosae (1) [TA].

cer·vi·cal (sĕr′vi-kăl) Relating to a neck, or cervix, in any sense.

cer·vi·cal ad·e·ni·tis (sĕr′vi-kăl ad′ĕ-nī′tis) Inflammation of lymph nodes of the neck.

cer·vi·cal am·pu·ta·tion (sĕr′vi-kăl am-pyū-tā′shŭn) Surgical removal of the uterine cervix.

cer·vi·cal cap (sĕr′vi-kăl kap) Contraceptive diaphragm that fits over the uterine cervix.

cer·vi·cal col·lar (sĕr′vi-kăl kol′ăr) Splinting device used to stabilize the neck.

cer·vi·cal com·pres·sion test (sĕr′vi-kăl kŏm-presh′ŭn test) Maneuver in which the examiner exerts downward pressure on the subject's head. Increased pain or altered sensation indicates pressure on a nerve root.

cer·vi·cal dys·pla·sia (sĕr′vi-kăl dis-plā′zē-ă) Dysplasia of the uterine cervix, epithelial atypia involving part or all of the thickness of cervical squamous epithelium, occurring most often in young women.

cer·vi·cal flex·ure (sĕr′vi-kăl flek′shŭr) Ventrally concave bend at the juncture of the brainstem and spinal cord in the embryo.

cer·vi·cal in·tra·ep·i·the·li·al ne·o·pla·sia (CIN) (sĕr′vi-kăl in′tră-ep-i-thē′lē-ăl nē-ō-plā′zē-ă) Dysplastic changes beginning at the squamocolumnar junction in the uterine cervix that may be precursors of squamous cell carcinoma.

cer·vi·cal line (sĕr′vi-kăl līn) A continuous anatomic irregular curved line marking the junction of the crown and the root of a tooth. SEE ALSO cementoenamel junction.

cer·vi·cal or·tho·sis (sĕr′vi-kăl ōr-thō′sis) An orthosis designed to limit cervical spine motion to varying degrees.

cer·vi·cal plex·us (sĕr′vi-kăl pleks′ŭs) Formed by loops joining the adjacent ventral primary rami of the first four cervical nerves and receiving gray communicating rami from the superior cervical ganglion; it lies deep to the sternocleidomastoid muscle, and sends out numerous cutaneous, muscular, and communicating rami.

cer·vi·cal preg·nan·cy (sĕr′vi-kăl preg′năn-sē) Implantation and development of a blastocyst in the mucosal lining of the cervix.

cer·vi·cal si·nus (sĕr′vi-kăl sī′nŭs) In young mammalian embryos, depression in the nuchal region caudal to the second pharyngeal arch, with the third and fourth pharyngeal arches and ectodermal grooves in its floor. SYN precervical sinus.

cer·vi·cal smear (sĕr'vi-kăl smēr) Generic name for various types of smears of the cervix uteri.

cer·vi·cal spine (sĕr'vi-kăl spīn) A unit comprising the first seven bones of the spinal column. SYN cervical vertebrae, C-spine.

cer·vi·cal spon·dy·lo·sis (sĕr'vi-kăl spon-di-lō'sis) Ankylosis affecting the cervical vertebrae, intervertebral discs, and surrounding soft tissue.

cer·vi·cal tri·an·gle (sĕr'vi-kăl trī'ang-gĕl) Any triangular areas of the neck.

cer·vi·cal ver·te·brae (sĕr'vi-kăl vĕr'ti-brē) The first seven bones of the spinal column, the neck bones. SYN cervical spine, C-spine.

cer·vi·cec·to·my (sĕr'vi-sek'tŏ-mē) Excision of the cervix uteri.

cer·vi·ci·tis (sĕr'vi-sī'tis) Inflammation of the mucous membrane, frequently involving also the deeper structures of the cervix uteri. SYN trachelitis.

♻ **cervico-** Prefix meaning a cervix, or neck, in any sense.

cer·vi·co·la·bi·al (ser'vi-kō-lā'bē-ăl) Relating to the labial region of the neck of an incisor or canine tooth.

cer·vi·co·tho·rac·ic (sĕr'vi-kō-thōr-as'ik) Term describing: 1) the neck and thorax; 2) the transition between the neck and thorax; 3) the fusion of the cervical and thoracic vertebrae.

cer·vi·cot·o·my (sĕr-vi-kot'ŏ-mē) Incision into the cervix uteri.

cer·vi·co·u·te·rine (sĕr'vi-kō-yū'tĕr-in) Pertaining to the cervical os and uterus.

cer·vi·co·vag·i·ni·tis (sĕr'vi-kō-vaj'i-nī'tis) Inflammation of the cervical os and vagina.

cer·vi·co·ves·i·cal (sĕr'vi-kō-ves'i-kăl) Relating to the cervix of the uterus and the bladder.

cer·vix, gen. **cer·vi·cis,** pl. **cer·vi·ces** (sĕr'viks, -vi-sis, -sēz) [TA] **1.** SYN neck. **2.** Any necklike structure.

ce·sar·e·an (se-zār'ē-ăn) Denoting a cesarean section, which was included under *lex cesarea*, Roman law (715 BCE); not because performed at the birth of Julius Caesar (100 BCE).

ce·sar·e·an hys·ter·ec·to·my (se-zār'ē-ăn his'tĕr-ek'tŏ-mē) Cesarean section followed by hysterectomy.

ce·sar·e·an sec·tion (se-zār'ē-ăn sek'shŭn) Incision through the abdominal wall and the uterus (abdominal hysterotomy) for extraction of the fetus.

ce·si·um (Cs) (sē'zē-ŭm) A metallic element, atomic no. 55, atomic wt. 132.90543; a member of the alkali metal group. ^{137}Cs (half-life equal to 30.1 years) used in treatment of certain malignancies. SYN caesium.

Ces·to·da (ses-tō'dă) A subclass of tapeworms, containing the typical members of this group, including the segmented tapeworms that parasitize humans and domestic animals. SYN Eucestoda.

Ces·toi·de·a (ses-toy'dē-ă) The tapeworms, a class of platyhelminth flatworms characterized by lack of an alimentary canal and a segmented body with a scolex or holdfast organ at one end.

ce·tyl al·co·hol (sē'tăl al'kŏ-hol) The 16-carbon alcohol corresponding to palmitic acid used as an emulsifying aid and in the preparation of ''washable'' (oil in water emulsions) ointment bases. SYN 1-hexadecanol, palmityl alcohol.

ce·tyl pal·mi·tate (sē'tăl pal'mi-tāt) A wax; the chief constituent of spermaceti.

ce·tyl·pyr·i·din·i·um chlor·ide (CPC) (sē'til-pī'ri-din'ē-ŭm klōr'īd) The monohydrate of the quaternary salt of pyridine and cetyl chloride; a cationic detergent with antiseptic action against nonsporulating bacteria.

Cf Symbol for californium.

C fi·bers (fī'bĕrz) Unmyelinated fibers, 0.4–1.2 mcm in diameter, conducting nerve impulses at a velocity of 0.7–2.3 m/sec. SYN C fibres.

C fibres [Br.] SYN C fibers.

Chad·wick sign (chad′wik sīn) A bluish discoloration of the cervix and vagina; a sign of pregnancy.

chafe (chāf) To cause irritation of the skin by friction.

chain (chān) **1.** CHEMISTRY a series of atoms held together by one or more covalent bonds. **2.** BACTERIOLOGY a linear arrangement of living cells that have divided in one plane and remain attached to each other. **3.** A series of reactions. **4.** ANATOMY a linked series of structures, e.g., ossicular chain, chain ganglia. SEE ALSO sympathetic trunk.

chain·ing (chān′ing) Learning related behaviors in a series in which each response serves as a stimulus for the next response.

chain of sur·vi·val (chān sŭr-vī′văl) The American Heart Association's term for four major interventions designed to reduce sudden cardiac death—early access, early cardiopulmonary resuscitation (CPR), early defibrillation, and early advanced life support (ALS).

chain re·flex (chān rē′fleks) A series of reflexes, each serving as a stimulus for the next.

cha·la·sia, cha·la·sis (kă-lā′zē-ă, -lā′sis) Inhibition and relaxation of any previously sustained contraction of muscle, usually of a synergic group of muscles.

cha·la·zi·on, cha·la·za, gen. and pl. **cha·la·zi·a** (kă-lā′zē-on, -ză, -zē-ă) Chronic inflammatory granuloma of a meibomian gland. SYN meibomian cyst, tarsal cyst.

chal·co·sis (kal-kō′sis) Chronic copper poisoning.

chal·i·co·sis (kal-i-kō′sis) Pneumoconiosis caused by inhalation of dust due to stone cutting or masonry. SYN flint disease.

cham·ber (chām′bĕr) [TA] A compartment or enclosed space. SEE ALSO camera.

Cham·ber·len for·ceps (chām′bĕr-lĕn fōr′seps) The original obstetric forceps, without a curvature.

cham·fer (sham′fer) A marginal finish on an extracoronal cavity preparation of a tooth; describes a curve from an axial wall to the cavosurface.

chan·cre (shang′kĕr) The dull red primary lesion of syphilis. SYN hard chancre, hard ulcer.

chan·cre re·dux (shang′kĕr rē′duks) Second chancre occurring in a patient with syphilis.

chan·croid (shang′kroyd) An infectious, painful venereal ulcer at the site of infection by *Haemophilus ducreyi*.

chan·de·lier sign (shan′dĕ-lēr′ sīn) Colloquial term referring to severe pain elicited during pelvic examination of patients with pelvic inflammatory disease, in which the patient responds by reaching upward toward the ceiling for relief.

change (chānj) An alteration; in pathology, structural alteration of which the cause and significance is uncertain.

change blind·ness (chānj blīnd′nĕs) Failure to observe large changes in the vision field that occur simultaneously with brief disturbances.

chan·nel (chan′ĕl) A furrow, gutter, or groovelike passageway. SEE ALSO canal.

cha·ot·ic rhythm (kā-ot′ik ridh′ŭm) Completely irregular cardiac rhythm at varying rates. SEE ALSO arrhythmia.

chap·e·rone (shap′ĕ-rōn) One who accompanies a physician during physical examination of a patient of the opposite gender (from the physician).

chap·e·ro·nin (shap-ĕr-ō′nin) Molecular complex composed of multiple heat shock protein subunits that assemble into double ring structures.

char·ac·ter·is·tic curve (kar′ăk-tĕr-is′tik kŭrv) Sensitometric curve of radiographic film, a plot of the film density versus the logarithm of the relative exposure. SYN H and D curve, Hunter and Driffield curve.

char·coal (chahr′kōl) Carbon obtained by heating or burning wood with restricted access of air. SYN carbo.

Char·cot an·gi·na (shahr-kō′ an′ji-nă) Global insufficiency of blood flow to supply metabolic tissue demand during exertion; marked by cold extremities, weakness, cramps, and pain.

Char·cot dis·ease (shahr-kō′ di-zēz′) SYN amyotrophic lateral sclerosis.

Char·cot joint (shahr-kō′ joynt) SYN neuropathic joint.

Char·cot-Ley·den crys·tals (shahr-kō′ lī′děn kris′tălz) Crystals in the shape of elongated double pyramids, formed from eosinophils, found in the sputum in bronchial asthma.

Char·cot-Ma·rie-Tooth dis·ease (shahr-kō′ mah-rē′ tūth di-zēz′) SYN peroneal muscular atrophy.

Char·cot syn·drome (shahr-kō′ sin′ drōm) SYN intermittent claudication.

Char·cot ver·ti·go (shahr-kō′ věr′ti-gō) SYN tussive syncope.

charge nurse (chahrj nŭrs) The nurse who supervises patient care during a shift in a hospital unit.

char·la·tan (shahr′lă-tăn) A medical fraud claiming to cure disease by useless procedures, secret remedies, and worthless diagnostic and therapeutic machines. SYN quack.

char·la·tan·ism (shahr′lă-tăn-izm) A fraudulent claim to medical knowledge; treating the sick without knowledge of medicine or authority to practice medicine.

chart (chahrt) **1.** A record, handwritten or on computer, of clinical data relating to a patient's case. **2.** SYN curve (2). **3.** OPHTHALMOLOGY symbols of graduated size for measuring visual acuity, or test types for determining far or near vision. SEE ALSO Snellen test type.

chart·ing (chahrt′ing) Making a record in tabular or graph form of the progress of a patient's condition. SYN clinical recording.

Chaus·si·er sign (shō-sē-ā′ sīn) Severe pain in the epigastrium, a prodrome of eclampsia; may be of central origin or caused by distention of the capsule of liver by hemorrhage.

cheek (chēk) The side of the face forming the lateral wall of the mouth. SYN bucca, gena, mala (1).

cheek tooth (chēk tūth) Colloquialism for a posterior tooth, specifically a premolar or molar.

cheese work·er's lung (chēz wŏrk′ěrz lŭng) Extrinsic allergic alveolitis caused by inhalation of spores of *Penicillium casei* from moldy cheese.

cheesy ab·scess (chē′zē ab′ses) SYN caseous abscess.

cheil- SEE cheilo-.

chei·lec·to·my, chi·lec·to·my (kī-lek′ tŏ-mē) **1.** Excision of a portion of the lip. **2.** Chiseling away bony irregularities at osteochondral margin of a joint cavity that interfere with movements of the joint.

chei·lec·tro·pi·on, chil·ec·tro·pi·on (kī-lek-trō′pē-on) Eversion of the lips or a lip.

chei·li·tis, chi·li·tis (kī-lī′tis) Inflammation of the lips or lip.

cheilo-, cheil- Combining forms meaning lips. SEE ALSO chilo-, labio-.

chei·lo·car·ci·no·ma (kī′lō-kahr-si-nō′ mă) Cancerous tumor of the lip.

chei·lo·plas·ty, chi·lo·plas·ty (kī′lō-plas-tē) Surgical repair of the lips.

chei·lor·rha·phy, chi·lor·rha·phy (kī-lōr′ă-fē) Suturing of the lip.

chei·lo·schis·is (kī-los′ki-sis) Congenital defect in which the mid upper lip is split (cleft). SYN cleft lip.

chei·lo·sis, chi·lo·sis (kī-lō′sis) A condition characterized by dry scaling and fissuring of the lips.

chei·lot·o·my, chi·lot·o·my (kī-lot′ŏ-mē) Incision into the lip.

cheir- SEE cheiro-.

cheiro-, cheir- Combining forms meaning hand. SEE ALSO chiro-.

chei·ro·kin·aes·the·sia [Br.] SYN cheirokinesthesia.

chei·ro·kin·aes·thet·ic [Br.] SYN cheirokinesthetic.

chei·ro·kin·es·the·si·a, chi·ro·kin·es·the·si·a (kī′rō-kin-es-thē′zē-ă) Subjective sensation of hand movement. SYN chirokinesthesia.

chei·ro·kin·es·thet·ic (kī′rō-kin-ĕs-thet′ik) Relating to cheirokinesthesia. SYN cheirokinesthetic.

chei·ro·pom·pho·lyx, chi·ro·pom·pho·lyx (kī′rō-pom′fō-liks) SYN dyshidrosis.

che·late (kē′lāt) 1. To effect chelation. 2. Pertaining to chelation. 3. A complex formed through chelation.

chem- SEE chemo-.

chem·ex·fo·li·a·tion (kem′eks-fō-lē-ā′shŭn) Chemosurgery to remove acne scars or treat chronic skin changes caused by sun exposure. SYN chemical peeling.

chem·i·cal (kem′i-kăl) Relating to chemistry.

chem·i·cal an·ti·dote (kem′i-kăl an′ti-dōt) A substance that unites with a poison to form an innocuous chemical compound.

chem·i·cal burn (kem′i-kăl bŭrn) One due to a caustic chemical.

chem·i·cal der·ma·ti·tis (kem′i-kăl dĕr′mă-tī′tis) Allergic contact dermatitis or primary irritation dermatitis due to application of chemicals; usually characterized by erythema, edema, and vesiculation.

chem·i·cal for·mu·la (kem′i-kăl fōr′myū-lă) Statement of the structure of a molecule expressed in chemical symbols.

chem·i·cal hy·giene plan (kem′i-kăl hī′jēn plan) All safety procedures, special precautions, and emergency procedures used when working with chemicals.

chem·i·cal kin·et·ics (kem′i-kăl ki-net′iks) Study of chemical reaction rates.

chem·i·cal per·i·to·ni·tis (kem′i-kăl per′i-tŏ-nī′tis) Peritonitis due to the escape of bile, contents of the gastrointestinal tract, or pancreatic juice into the peritoneal cavity.

chem·ic·al preg·nan·cy (kem′i-kăl preg′năn-sē) Slight, unsustained rise in levels of human chorionic gonadotropin.

chem·i·cal shift (kem′i-kăl shift) Magnetic resonance artifact along the frequency axis caused by the difference in frequency between fat and water.

chem·i·cal sym·pa·thec·to·my (CS) (kem′i-kăl sim-pă-thek′tŏ-mē) SYN Doppler operation.

chem·i·cal-war·fare (CW) a·gent (kem′i-kăl-wōr′făr ā′jĕnt) In U.S. military parlance, any chemical compound developed for battlefield use either to kill or seriously injure or else to incapacitate humans or animals by means of its toxicologic effects.

chem·i·lu·mi·nes·cence, chem·o·lu·mi·nes·cence (kem′ē-lū-mi-nes′ĕns, kē′mō-) Light produced by chemical action usually at, or below, room temperature.

chem·ist (kem′ist) 1. A specialist or expert in chemistry. 2. Pharmacist (U.K. and some areas of Canada).

chem·is·try (chem) (kem′is-trē) 1. The science concerned with the atomic composition of substances, the elements, and their interrelations, as well as the formation, decomposition, and properties of molecules. 2. The chemical properties of a substance. 3. Chemical processes.

chemo-, chem- Combining forms denoting chemistry.

che·mo·at·tract·ant (kē′mō-ă-trak′tănt) A chemical substance that influences the migration of cells.

che·mo·cau·tery (kē′mō-kaw′tĕr-ē) Destruction of tissue by application of a chemical substance.

che·mo·dif·fer·en·ti·a·tion (kē′mō-dif′ĕr-en-shē-ā′shŭn) Differentiation of the cellular chemical constituents in the embryo before cytodifferentiation; sometimes recognizable histochemically.

che·mo·ki·ne·sis (kē′mō-ki-nē′sis) Stimulation of an organism by a chemical.

che·mo·ki·net·ic (kē′mō-ki-net′ik) Referring to chemokinesis.

che·mo·or·ga·no·troph (kē′mō-ōr′gă-nō-trōf) An organism that depends on organic chemicals for its energy and carbon.

che·mo·pro·phy·lax·is (kē′mō-prō′fi-lak′sis) Prevention of disease by the use of chemicals or drugs.

che·mo·ra·di·o·ther·a·py (kē′mō-rā′dē-ō-thār′ă-pē) A treatment plan that combines chemotherapy and radiotherapy.

che·mo·re·cep·tion (kē′mō-rĕ-sep′shŭn) The ability to perceive chemicals in the environment that are odorants or tastants. SYN chemosensation.

che·mo·re·cep·tor, che·mo·ceptor (kē′mō-rĕ-sep′tŏr, kē′mō-sep′tŏr) Any cell that when activated by a change in its chemical milieu produces a nerve impulse. SYN chemoceptor.

che·mo·re·flex (kē′mō-rē′fleks) A reflex initiated by the stimulation of chemoreceptors, e.g., of a carotid body.

che·mo·re·sis·tance (kē′mō-rē-zis′tăns) The state of being resistant to a chemical's action.

che·mo·re·sponse (kē′mō-rĕ-spons′) A reaction to chemical stimulation.

che·mo·sen·sa·tion (kē′mō-sen-sā′shŭn) SYN chemoreception.

che·mo·sen·si·tive (kē′mō-sen′si-tiv) Capable of perceiving changes in the chemical composition of the environment.

che·mo·sis (kē-mō′sis) Edema of the bulbar conjunctiva, forming a swelling around the cornea.

che·mo·stat (kē′mō-stat) A fermenter for microbial growth in which the ratio of growth to synthesis of secondary products is controlled by the rate at which new medium is added to the culture.

che·mo·sur·ger·y (kē′mō-sŭr′jĕr-ē) Ex-

cision of diseased tissue after it has been fixed in situ by chemical means.

che·mo·syn·the·sis (kē′mō-sin′thĕ-sis) **1.** Chemical synthesis. **2.** Chemolithotrophy.

che·mo·tac·tic (kē′mō-tak′tik) Relating to chemotaxis.

che·mo·ther·a·py (kē′mō-thār′ă-pē) Treatment of disease by means of chemical substances or drugs; usually used in reference to neoplastic disease. SEE ALSO pharmacotherapy.

che·mot·ic (kē-mot′ik) Relating to chemosis.

cher·ry-red spot my·oc·lo·nus syn·drome (cher′ē-red spot mī-ok′lō-nŭs sin′drōm) A neuronal storage disorder in children characterized by a cherry-red spot at the macula, progressive myoclonus, and easily controlled seizures.

chest (chest) The anterior wall of the thorax. SEE ALSO thorax. SYN pectus [TA].

chest lead (chest lēd) Electrocardiographic connector placed in one of six positions on the chest; used to record cardiac electricity. SYN precordial lead.

chest phys·ic·al ther·a·py (chest fiz′i-kăl thār′ă-pē) A type of respiratory care performed to promote coughing and the removal of lung secretions through percussion (clapping) and vibration on the affected areas, postural drainage, and breathing exercises. SYN chest physiotherapy, pulmonary rehabilitation, pulmonary toileting.

chest wall (chest wawl) RESPIRATORY PHYSIOLOGY All the structures outside the lungs that move as a part of breathing; comprises the rib cage, diaphragm, abdominal wall and contents. SYN thoracic wall.

chest wall com·pli·ance (chest wawl kŏm-plī′ăns) The change in chest wall volume per unit change in transmural pressure; may be static or dynamic.

chest x-ray (CXR) (chest eks′rā) SEE radiograph.

chi (kī) **1.** The 22nd letter of the Greek

alphabet, χ. **2.** In Asian medical traditions, the force of energy existing in all life forms. Chi manifests as five different elements; these are labeled according to either the Asian or Ayurvedic tradition. SYN qi, ki.

chi·asm, chi·as·ma (kī′azm, kī-az′mă) **1.** An intersection or crossing of two lines. **2.** ANATOMY a decussation or crossing of two fibrous bundles, such as tendons, nerves, or tracts.

chi·as·ma·pexy (kī-as′mă-pek′sē) Surgical fixation of the optic chiasm.

chick·en·pox (chik′ĕn-poks) SYN varicella.

chick·en·pox vi·rus (chik′ĕn-poks vī′rŭs) SYN varicella-zoster virus.

chief ag·glu·ti·nin (chēf ă-glū′ti-nin) SYN major agglutinin.

chief com·plaint (cc, c.c., CC) (chēf kŏm-plānt′) The primary symptom that a patient states as the reason for seeking medical care.

chig·ger (chig′ĕr) The six-legged larva of *Trombicula* species; a bloodsucking stage of mites that includes the vectors of scrub typhus.

chil- SEE chilo-.

Chi·lai·di·ti syn·drome (kī-lā′dē-tē sin′drōm) Interposition of the colon between the liver and the diaphragm.

chil·blain (chil′blān) Erythema, itching, and burning, especially of the dorsa of the fingers and toes, and of the heels, nose, and ears caused by vascular constriction on exposure to extreme cold. SYN erythema pernio, perniosis.

child·bed fe·ver (chīld′bed fē′vĕr) SYN puerperal fever.

child·birth (chīld′birth) The process of labor and delivery in the birth of a child. SEE ALSO birth. SYN parturition.

child·hood ab·sence ep·i·lep·sy (chīld′hud ab′sĕns ep′i-lep-sē) A generalized epilepsy syndrome characterized by the onset of absence seizures in childhood, typically at age 6 or 7 years. There

is a strong genetic predisposition and girls are affected more often than boys.

child·hood aprax·ia (chīld′hud ă-prak′sē-ă) SYN developmental apraxia of speech.

child·hood dis·in·te·gra·tive dis·or·der (CDD) (chīld′hud dis-in′tĕ-grā-tiv dis-ōr′dĕr) Severe regression including loss of bowel and bladder control in a previously normal child aged 2–10 years old.

child·hood schiz·o·phre·nia (chīld′hud skit′sō-frē′nē-ă) SYN infantile autism.

child psy·chol·o·gy (CP) (chīld sī-kol′ŏ-jē) Branch of psychology the theories and applications of which focus on the cognitive and intellectual development of the child in contrast to the adult; subspecialties include developmental psychology, clinical child psychology, pediatric psychology, and pediatric neuropsychology.

chill (chil) A sensation of cold.

chilo-, chil- Combining forms meaning lips. SEE ALSO cheilo-.

chi·me·ra (kī-mēr′ă) The individual produced by grafting an embryonic part of one animal onto the embryo of another, either of the same or of another species.

chin (chin) [TA] The prominence formed by the anterior projection of the mandible, or lower jaw. SYN mentum.

Chi·nese res·tau·rant syn·drome (chī-nēz′ rest′ă-rahnt sin′drōm) Colloquial usage for development of chest pain, feelings of facial pressure, and a sensation of burning over variable portions of the body surface after ingestion of food that contains monosodium L-glutamate (MSG) by people sensitive to this food additive.

chip (chip) A small fragment resulting from breakage, cutting, or avulsion.

chi·ral·gi·a (kī-ral′jē-ă) A traumatic pain in the hand.

chi·ral·i·ty (kī-ral′i-tē) The property of nonidentity of an object with its mirror image; used in chemistry with respect to stereochemical isomers.

chiro-, chir- Combining forms meaning the hand. SEE ALSO cheiro-.

chi·ro·kin·es·the·si·a (kī′rō-kin-es-thē′zē-ă) SYN cheirokinesthesia.

chi·ro·po·dal·gi·a (kī′rō-pō-dal′jē-ă) SYN cheiropodalgia.

chi·rop·o·dy (kī-rop′ŏ-dē) SYN podiatry.

chi·ro·prac·tic (kī′rō-prak′tik) A system that, in theory, uses the recuperative powers of the body and the relationship between the musculoskeletal structures and functions of the body, particularly of the spinal column and the nervous system, in the restoration and maintenance of health.

chi·ro·spasm (kī′rō-spazm) SYN cheirospasm.

chi-square (χ^2) (kī′skwār) A statistical technique whereby variables are categorized to determine whether a distribution of scores is due to chance or experimental factors.

chi-square (χ^2) **dis·tri·bu·tion** (kī′skwār dis-tri-byū′shŭn) Variable is said to have a chi-square distribution with K degrees of freedom if it is distributed like the sum of the squares of K independent random variables, each of which has a normal (gaussian) distribution with mean zero and variance one. The chi-square distribution is the basis for many variations of the chi-square(d) test, perhaps the most widely used test for statistical significance in biology and medicine.

Chla·myd·i·a (klă-mid′ē-ă) Bacterium that causes more sexually transmitted infections than any other; largely asymptomatic.

chla·myd·i·al (klă-mid′ē-ăl) Relating to or caused by any bacterium of the genus *Chlamydia*.

chlo·as·ma (klō-az′mă) Melanoderma or melasma characterized by brown patches of irregular shape and size on the face and elsewhere; associated most commonly with pregnancy or use of oral contraceptives.

chlor-, chloro- Combining forms meaning (1) green, (2) chlorine.

chlor·ac·ne, chlo·rine ac·ne (klōr-ak′nē, klōr′ĕn ak′nē) An occupational acnelike eruption due to prolonged contact with certain chlorinated compounds.

chlor·al hy·drate (CH) (klōr′ăl hī′drāt) Hypnotic and sedative; it is also used externally as a rubefacient, anesthetic, and antiseptic.

chlor·am·phen·i·col, chlor·o·my·ce·tin (klōr′am-fen′i-kol, klōr′ō-mī-sē′tin) An antibiotic effective against a number of pathogenic microorganisms, including *Staphylococcus aureus*, *Brucella abortus*, and others.

chlor·dane (klōr′dān) A chlorinated hydrocarbon used as an insecticide; may be absorbed dermally with resultant severe toxic effects.

chlor·e·mia (klōr-ē′mē-ă) **1.** SYN chlorosis. **2.** SYN hyperchloremia.

chlor·hy·dria (klōr-hī′drē-ă) SYN hyperchlorhydria.

chlo·ride (klōr′īd) A compound containing chlorine, at a valence of -1, as in the salts of hydrochloric acid.

chlor·i·dom·e·ter (klōr′i-dom′ĕ-ter) An apparatus for determining the amount of chlorides in blood, or other fluids.

chlor·i·dor·rhea (klō-rid-ō-rē′ă) A congenital autosomal recessive condition of intestinal chloride malabsorption, with intrauterine and life-long diarrhea.

chlo·ri·nat·ed (klōr′in-āt-ĕd) Having been treated with chlorine.

chlo·rine (Cl) (klōr′ēn) A greenish, toxic gas; a halogen used as a disinfectant and bleaching agent in the form of hypochlorite or chlorine water, because of its oxidizing power; also used as a chemical warfare agent.

chlo·rite (klōr′īt) A salt of chlorous acid; the radical ClO_2-.

o-**chlor·o·ben·zyl·i·dene mal·o·no·ni·trile** (klōr-ō-bĕn-zil′i-dēn măl-ō′nō-nī′tril) A compound (NATO code CS) widely used as a lacrimator on the battlefield and as a riot-control agent in law enforcement.

chlor·o·form (chl, chlor) (klōr′ŏ-fōrm) Formerly used by inhalation to produce general anesthesia; also used as a solvent. SYN trichloromethane.

chlo·ro·ma, chlo·ro·leu·ke·mia (klōr-ō′mă, klōr′ŏ-lū-kē′mē-ă) A condition characterized by the development of multiple localized green masses of abnormal cells (in most instances, myeloblasts), especially in relation to the periosteum of the skull, spine, and ribs.

chlo·ro·my·e·lo·ma (klōr′ŏ-mī-ĕ-lō′mă) SYN chloroma.

chlor·o·phyll (klōr′ŏ-fil) A complex of light-absorbing green pigments that, in living plants, convert light energy into oxidizing and reducing power.

chlor·o·plast (klōr′ŏ-plast) A plant cell inclusion body containing chlorophyll; site of photosynthesis in higher plants.

chlor·o·pri·vic (klōr′ŏ-priv′ik) Pertaining to loss of chlorides.

chlo·rop·si·a (klōr-op′sē-ă) A condition in which objects appear to be colored green.

chlor·o·quine (CQ) (klōr′ŏ-kwīn) An antimalarial agent; also used for hepatic amebiasis and skin diseases.

chlor·o·thi·a·zide (CTZ, CT) (klōr′ŏ-thī′ă-zīd) An orally effective diuretic inhibiting renal tubular reabsorption of sodium.

chlor·u·re·sis, chlor·u·ri·a (klōr-yū-rē′sis, -yūr′ē-ă) The excretion of chloride in the urine.

cho·a·na, gen. and pl. **cho·a·nae** (kō′ă-nă, -nē) The opening into the nasopharynx of the nasal cavity on either side.

cho·a·noid (kō′ă-noyd) Funnel-shaped. SYN infundibuliform.

choke (chōk) To prevent respiration by compression or obstruction of the larynx or trachea.

choked disc (chōkt disk) SYN papilledema.

cholaemia [Br.] SYN cholemia.

cho·la·gogue, cho·la·gog·ic (kō′lă-gog, -goj′ik) **1.** An agent that promotes the flow of bile into the intestine, especially as a result of contraction of the gallbladder. **2.** Relating to such an agent or effect. SYN cholagogic.

cho·lan·ge·i·tis (kō′lan-jē-ī′tis) SYN cholangitis.

chol·an·gi·ec·ta·sis (kō-lan′jē-ek′tă-sis) Dilation of the bile ducts, usually as a sequel to obstruction.

chol·an·gi·o·car·ci·no·ma (kō-lan′jē-ō-kahr-si-nō′mă) An adenocarcinoma, primarily in intrahepatic bile ducts, composed of ducts lined by cuboidal or columnar cells that do not contain bile, with abundant fibrous stroma.

chol·an·gi·o·en·ter·os·to·my (kō-lan′jē-ō-en-tĕr-os′tŏ-mē) Surgical anastomosis of bile duct to intestine.

chol·an·gi·o·fi·bro·sis (kō-lan′jē-ō-fī-brō′sis) Fibrosis of the bile ducts.

chol·an·gi·og·ra·phy (CAG) (kō-lan′jē-og′ră-fē) Radiographic examination of the bile ducts with contrast medium.

cho·lan·gi·o·hep·a·ti·tis (kō-lan′jē-ō-hep′ă-tī′tis) Inflammation of the bile ducts and liver.

cho·lan·gi·o·hep·a·to·ma (kō-lan′jē-ō-hep′ă-tō′mă) Carcinoma of the bile duct and liver.

chol·an·gi·ole (kō-lan′jē-ōl) A ductule occurring between a bile canaliculus and an interlobular bile duct.

chol·an·gi·o·li·tis (kō-lan′jē-ō-lī′tis) Inflammation of the small bile radicles or cholangioles.

chol·an·gi·o·ma (kō-lan′jē-ō′mă) A neoplasm of bile duct origin, especially within the liver; may be either benign or malignant (cholangiocarcinoma).

chol·an·gi·o·pan·cre·a·tog·ra·phy (kō-lan′jē-ō-pan′krē-ă-tog′ră-fē) Radiographic examination of the bile and pancreatic ducts with contrast medium.

chol·an·gi·os·to·my (kō-lan′jē-os′tŏ-mē) Formation of a fistula into a bile duct.

chol·an·gi·ot·o·my (kō-lan'jē-ot'ŏ-mē) Incision into a bile duct.

chol·an·gi·tis, cho·lan·ge·i·tis (kō'lan-jī'tis, -jē-ī'tis) Inflammation of a bile duct or the entire biliary tree.

cho·lan·o·poi·e·sis (kō'lă-nō-poy-ē'sis) Synthesis by the liver of cholic acid or its conjugates, or of natural bile salts.

cho·lan·o·poi·et·ic (kō'lă-nō-poy-et'ik) Pertaining to or promoting cholanopoiesis.

cho·late (kō'lāt) A salt or ester of a cholic acid.

♻ **chole-, chol-, cholo-** *Do not confuse these combining forms with coleo- or colo-.* Bile. SEE ALSO bili-.

cho·le·cal·cif·er·ol (kō'lĕ-kal-sif'ĕr-ol) The vitamin D of animal origin found in the skin, fur, and feathers of animals and birds exposed to sunlight, and also in butter, brain, fish oils, and egg yolk. SYN vitamin D3.

cho·le·cys·ta·gogue (kō'lĕ-sis'tă-gog) A substance that stimulates activity of the gallbladder.

cho·le·cys·tec·to·my (kō'lĕ-sis-tek'tŏ-mē) Surgical removal of the gallbladder.

cho·le·cyst·en·ter·os·to·my (kō'lĕ-sist-en'tĕr-os'tŏ-mē) Formation of a direct communication between the gallbladder and the intestine.

cho·le·cys·ti·tis (kō'lĕ-sis-tī'tis) Inflammation of the gallbladder.

cho·le·cys·to·co·los·to·my (kō'lĕ-sis'tō-kō-los'tŏ-mē) Establishment of a communication between the gallbladder and the colon. SYN colocholecystostomy.

cho·le·cys·to·du·o·de·nos·to·my (kō'lĕ-sis'tō-dū'ō-dē-nos'tŏ-mē) Establishment of a direct communication between the gallbladder and the duodenum. SYN duodenocholecystostomy, duodenocystostomy (1).

cho·le·cys·to·gas·tros·to·my (kō'lĕ-sis'tō-gas-tros'tŏ-mē) Establishment of a communication between the gallbladder and the stomach.

cho·le·cys·tog·ra·phy (CG, CCG) (kō'lĕ-sis-tog'ră-fē) Radiographic study of the gallbladder after oral administration of a cholecystopaque.

cho·le·cys·to·je·ju·nos·to·my (kō'lĕ-sis'tō-jĕ-jū-nos'tŏ-mē) Establishment of a communication between the gallbladder and the jejunum.

cho·le·cys·to·ki·net·ic (kō'lĕ-sis'tō-ki-net'ik) Promoting emptying of the gallbladder.

cho·le·cys·to·ki·nin (CCK) (kō'lĕ-sis'tō-kī'nin) A polypeptide hormone liberated by the upper intestinal mucosa on contact with gastric contents.

cho·le·cys·to·li·thi·a·sis (kō'lĕ-sis'tō-li-thī'ă-sis) Presence of one or more gallstones in the gallbladder.

cho·le·cys·to·lith·o·trip·sy (kō'lĕ-sis'tō-lith'ŏ-trip-sē) Fragmentation of a gallstone most commonly by the application of transcutaneously applied sonic energy.

cho·le·cys·top·a·thy (kō'lĕ-sis-top'ă-thē) Disease of the gallbladder.

cho·le·cys·to·pex·y (kō'lĕ-sis'tō-pek-sē) Suture of the gallbladder to the abdominal wall.

cho·le·cys·tor·rha·phy (kō'lĕ-sis-tōr'ă-fē) Suture of an incised or ruptured gallbladder.

cho·le·cys·to·so·nog·ra·phy (kō'lĕ-sis'tō-sŏ-nog'ră-fē) Ultrasonic examination of the gallbladder.

cho·le·cys·tot·o·my, cho·le·cys·to·my (kō'lĕ-sis-tot'ŏ-mē, -sis'tŏ-mē) Incision into the gallbladder. SYN cholecystomy.

cho·le·doch·al (kō-led'ŏ-kăl) Relating to the common bile duct.

cho·le·doch·al cyst (kō-led'ŏ-kăl sist) Lesion originating in common bile duct.

cho·le·doch·ec·to·my (kō'lĕ-dō-kek'tŏ-mē) Surgical removal of a portion of the common bile duct.

cho·led·o·chi·tis (kō'lĕ-dō-kī'tis) Inflammation of the common bile duct.

choledocho-, choledoch- Combining forms meaning the ductus choledochus (the common bile duct).

cho·led·o·cho·lith (kō′lĕ-dō-kō-lith) Stone in the common bile duct.

cho·led·o·cho·li·thi·a·sis (kō′lĕ-dō-kō-lith-ī′ă-sis) Presence of a gallstone in the common bile duct.

cho·led·o·cho·li·thot·o·my (kō′lĕ-dō-kō-li-thot′ŏ-mē) Incision of the common bile duct for the extraction of an impacted gallstone.

cho·led·o·cho·lith·o·trip·sy (kō′lĕ-dō-kō-lith′ŏ-trip-sē) Fragmentation of a gallstone in the common bile duct.

cho·led·o·cho·plas·ty (kō′lĕ-dō-kō-plas-tē) Plastic surgery of the common bile duct.

cho·led·o·chor·rha·phy (kō′lĕ-dō-kōr′ră-fē) Suturing together the divided ends of the common bile duct.

cho·led·o·chos·to·my (kō′lĕ-dō-kos′tŏ-mē) Establishment of a fistula into the common bile duct.

cho·led·o·chot·o·my (kō′lĕ-dō-kot′ŏ-mē) Incision into the common bile duct.

cho·led·o·chous (kō′lĕ-dō-kŭs) Containing or conveying bile.

cho·led·o·chus (kō′lĕ-dō-kŭs) SYN common bile duct.

cho·le·ic (kō-lē′ik) SYN cholic.

cho·le·lith, cho·lo·lith (kō′lĕ-lith, -lō-lith) SYN gallstone.

cho·le·li·thi·a·sis, cho·lo·li·thi·a·sis (CL) (kō′lĕ-li-thī′ă-sis, -lō-li-thī′ă-sis) Presence of concretions in the gallbladder or bile ducts. SYN chololithiasis.

cho·le·li·thot·o·my (kō′lĕ-li-thot′ŏ-mē) Operative removal of a gallstone.

cho·lem·e·sis (kō-lem′ĕ-sis) Vomiting bile.

cho·le·mia (kō-lē′mē-ă) The presence of bile salts in the circulating blood. SYN cholaemia.

cho·le·per·i·to·ne·um (kō′lĕ-per′i-tŏ-nē′ŭm) Bile in the peritoneum, which may lead to bile peritonitis.

cho·le·poi·e·sis, cho·lo·poi·e·sis (kō′lĕ-poy-ē′sis, -lō-poy-ē′sis) Formation of bile.

cho·le·poi·et·ic (kō′lĕ-poy-et′ik) Relating to the formation of bile.

chol·er·a (kol′ĕr-ă) An acute epidemic infectious disease caused by the bacterium *Vibrio cholerae*, occurring primarily in Asia.

chol·er·a·gen (kol′ĕr-ă-jen) The exotoxin produced during growth in vitro of *Cholera vibrio* and responsible for the diarrhea seen in association with this infection.

chol·er·a·ic (kol′ĕr-ā′ik) Relating to cholera.

chol·er·a·ic diar·rhea (kol′ĕr-ā′ik dī′ă-rē′ă) SYN summer diarrhea.

cho·le·re·sis (kō′lĕ-rē′sis) The secretion, as opposed to the expulsion, of bile by the gallbladder.

cho·le·ret·ic (kō′lĕr-et′ik) **1.** Relating to choleresis. **2.** An agent, usually a drug, which stimulates the liver to increase bile output.

chol·er·i·form, chol·er·oid (kol-ler′i-fōrm, kol′ĕr-i-fōrm, -ĕr-oyd) Resembling cholera.

cho·ler·rha·gic (kol′ĕr-aj′ik) Referring to the flow of bile.

chol·e·scin·tig·ra·phy, cho·le·scin·to·gra·phy (kō′lĕ-sin-tig′ră-fē, -tog′ră-fē) Examination of the gallbladder and bile ducts by nuclear medicine scanning.

cho·le·sta·sia, cho·le·sta·sis (kō-lĕ-stā′sē-ă, -sis) An arrest in the flow of bile.

cho·le·stat·ic hep·a·ti·tis (kō-les-tat′ik hep′ă-tī′tis) Jaundice with bile stasis in inflamed intrahepatic bile ducts; usually due to toxic effects of a drug.

cho·le·stat·ic jaun·dice (kō′lĕ-stat′ik jawn′dis) Liver disorder produced by inspissated bile or bile plugs in small biliary passages in the liver.

cho·les·te·a·to·ma (kŏ′lĕ-stē′ă-tō′mă) Squamous metaplasia that may involve the middle ear or mastoid, erode surrounding bone, and become filled with a mass of keratinized squamous cell epithelial debris.

cholesteraemia [Br.] SYN cholesteremia.

cho·les·ter·e·mi·a, cho·les·ter·ol·e· mi·a, cho·les·ter·i·ne·mi·a (kŏ-les′ tĕr-ē′mē-ă, kŏ-les′tĕr-ol-ē′mē-ă, -ĕr-i-nē′ mē-ă) The presence of excessive cholesterol in the blood. SYN cholesteraemia.

cho·les·ter·in·o·sis (kŏ-les′tĕr-in-ō′sis) SYN cholesterolosis.

cho·les·ter·ol (kŏ-les′tĕr-ol) The most abundant steroid in animal tissues.

cholesterolaemia [Br.] SYN cholesterolemia.

cho·les·ter·ol·e·mi·a (kŏ-les′tĕr-ol-ē′ mē-ă) The presence of excessive cholesterol in the blood. SYN cholesterolaemia.

cho·les·ter·ol·o·poi·e·sis (kŏ-les′tĕr- ŏ-lō-poy-ē′sis) Formation of cholesterol.

cho·les·ter·ol·o·sis, cho·les·ter·i·no· sis, cho·les·ter·o·sis (kŏ-les′tĕr-ol-ō′sis, -ĕr-i-nō′sis, -tĕr-ō′sis) A condition resulting from a disturbance in metabolism of lipids, characterized by deposits of cholesterol in tissue.

cho·les·ter·o·lu·ri·a (kŏ-les′tĕr-ol-yūr′ ē-ă) The excretion of cholesterol in the urine.

cho·le·u·ri·a (kŏ′lē-yūr′ē-ă) SYN biliuria.

cho·line (kŏ′lēn) An amine found in most animal tissues; part of vitamin B complex.

cho·line chlo·ride (kŏ′lēn klŏr′ĭd) A lipotropic agent.

cho·lin·er·gic (kŏ′lin-ĕr′jik) Relating to nerve cells or fibers that employ acetylcholine as their neurotransmitter. Cf. adrenergic.

cho·lin·er·gic re·cep·tors (kŏ′lin-ĕr′ jik rē-sep′tŏrz) Chemical sites in effector cells or at synapses through which acetylcholine exerts its action.

cho·line sal·i·cyl·ate (kŏ′lēn să-lis′i-lāt) Choline salt of salicyclic acid, an analgesic and antipyretic (because of the salicylate moiety).

cho·lin·es·ter·ase (ChE) (kŏ′lin-es′tĕr-ās) An enzyme capable of catalyzing hydrolysis of acylcholines and other compounds.

cho·lin·es·ter·ase in·hib·i·tor (kŏ′ lin-es′tĕr-ās in-hib′i-tŏr) A drug, such as neostigmine, which, by inhibiting biodegradation of acetylcholine, restores myoneural function in myasthenia gravis or after nondepolarizing neuromuscular relaxants have been administered.

cho·li·no·lyt·ic (kŏ′lin-ō-lit′ik) Impeding acetylcholine action.

chol·i·no·mi·met·ic (kŏ′lin-ō-mi-met′ ik) Having action similar to acetylcholine; replaces the less specific term parasympathomimetic. Cf. adrenomimetic.

cholo- SEE chole-.

chol·o·li·thi·a·sis (kŏ′lŏ-li-thī′ă-sis) SYN cholelithiasis.

chol·o·poi·e·sis (kŏ′lŏ-poy-ē′sis) SYN cholepoiesis.

cho·lu·ri·a (kŏ-lyūr′ē-ă) SYN biliuria.

chon·dral frac·ture (kon′drăl frak′shŭr) Breakage involving the articular cartilage of a joint. SEE ALSO articular cartilage.

chon·dral·gi·a (kon-dral′jē-ă) SYN chondrodynia.

chon·drec·to·my (kon-drek′tŏ-mē) Excision of cartilage.

chon·dri·fi·ca·tion (kon′dri-fi-kā′shŭn) Conversion into cartilage.

chon·dri·fi·ca·tion cen·ter (kon′dri-fi-kā′shŭn sen′tĕr) Site of earliest cartilage formation in the fetus.

chon·dri·tis (kon-drī′tis) Inflammation of cartilage.

chondro-, chondrio- Combining forms meaning (1) cartilage or cartilaginous, (2) granular or gritty substance.

chon·dro·blast (kon′drō-blast) A dividing cell of growing cartilage tissue. SYN chondroplast.

chon·dro·blas·to·ma (kon′drō-blas-tō′mă) A benign tumor arising in the epiphyses of long bones, consisting of highly cellular tissue resembling fetal cartilage.

chon·dro·cal·ci·no·sis (CC) (kon′drō-kal-si-nō′sis) Calcification of cartilage.

chon·dro·car·ci·no·ma (kon′drō-kahr′si-nō′mă) Malignant, cartilaginous epithelial tumor.

chon·dro·cos·tal (kon′drō-kos′tăl) SYN costochondral.

chon·dro·cra·ni·um (kon′drō-krā′nē-ŭm) A cartilaginous cranium; the cartilaginous parts of the developing cranium.

chon·dro·cyte (kon′drō-sīt) A nondividing cartilage cell; occupies a lacuna within the cartilage matrix.

chon·dro·dyn·i·a (kon′drō-din′ē-ă) Pain in cartilage. SYN chondralgia.

chon·dro·dys·pla·si·a (kon′drō-dis-plā′zē-ă) SYN chondrodystrophy.

chon·dro·dys·pla·si·a cal·ci·fi·cans con·gen·i·ta (kon′drō-dis-plā′zē-ă kal-sif′i-kanz kon-jen′i-tă) A form of hereditary chondrodysplasia characterized by asymmetric calcifications, dysplastic skeletal changes, but relatively good prognosis.

chon·dro·dys·tro·phic dwarf·ism (kon′drō-dis-trō′fik dwōrf′izm) SEE chondrodystrophy.

chon·dro·dys·tro·phy, chon·dro·dys·tro·phi·a (kon′drō-dis-trō′fē, -dis-trō′fē-ă) A disturbance in the development of the cartilage of the long bones, especially of the epiphysial plates, resulting in arrested growth and short-limb dwarfism but the head and trunk are normal. SYN chondrodysplasia.

chon·dro·dys·tro·phy with sen·sor·i·neu·ral deaf·ness (kon′drō-dis′trō-fē sen′sŏr-ē-nūr′ăl def′něs) A skeletal dysplasia characterized by dwarfism, flat nasal bridge, cleft palate, sensorineural deafness, large epiphyses, and flattening of the vertebral bodies. SYN Nance-Sweeney chondrodysplasia, otospondylomegaepiphysial dysplasia.

chon·dro·ec·to·der·mal (kon′drō-ek-tō-děr′măl) Relating to ectodermally derived cartilage.

chon·dro·ec·to·der·mal dys·pla·si·a (kon′drō-ek-tō-děr′măl dis-plā′zē-ă) Triad of chondrodysplasia, ectodermal dysplasia, and polydactyly, with congenital heart defects in over half of affected patients.

chon·dro·gen·e·sis (kon′drō-jen′ě-sis) Formation of cartilage. SYN chondrosis.

chon·droid (kon′droyd) **1.** Resembling cartilage. SYN cartilaginoid. **2.** Uncharacteristically developed cartilage, primarily cellular with a basophilic matrix and thin or nonexistent capsules.

chon·dro·ma (kon-drō′mă) A benign neoplasm derived from mesodermal cells that form cartilage.

chon·dro·ma·la·ci·a (kon′drō-mă-lā′shē-ă) Softening of any cartilage.

chon·dro·ma·to·sis (kon′drō-mă-tō′sis) Presence of multiple tumorlike foci of cartilage.

chon·dro·mere (kon′drō-mēr) A cartilage unit of the fetal axial skeleton developing within a single metamere of the body.

chon·dro·os·se·ous (kon′drō-os′ē-ŭs) Relating to cartilage and bone.

chon·dro·os·te·o·dys·tro·phy (kon′drō-os′tē-ō-dis′trŏ-fē) Term used for a group of disorders of bone and cartilage.

chon·drop·a·thy (kon-drop′ă-thē) Any disease of cartilage.

chon·dro·phyte (kon′drō-fīt) An abnormal cartilaginous mass that develops at the articular surface of a bone.

chon·dro·plast (kon′drō-plast) SYN chondroblast.

chon·dro·plas·ty (kon′drō-plas-tē) Reparative or plastic surgery of cartilage.

chon·dro·po·ro·sis (kon′drō-pōr-ō′sis) Condition of cartilage in which spaces appear, either normal (in the process of ossification) or pathologic.

chon·dro·sar·co·ma (kon′drō-sahr-kō′mă) Malignant tumor of flesh or connective tissue.

chon·dro·sis (kon-drō′sis) SYN chondrogenesis.

chon·dro·ster·nal (kon′drō-stěr′năl) **1.** Relating to a sternal cartilage. **2.** Relating to the costal cartilages and the sternum.

chon·dro·ster·no·plas·ty (kon′drō-stěr′nō-plas-tē) Surgical correction of malformations of the sternum.

chon·drot·o·my (kon-drot′ŏ-mē) Division of cartilage.

chon·dro·xi·phoid (kon′drō-zī′foyd) Relating to the xiphoid or ensiform cartilage.

♻ **chord-** Combining form for cord.

chor·da, pl. **chor·dae** (kōr′dă, -dē) [TA] A tendinous or a cordlike structure. SEE ALSO cord.

Chor·da·ta (kor-dā′tă) The phylum that includes the vertebrates.

chor·date (kōr′dāt) *Do not confuse this word with cordate.* An animal of the phylum Chordata.

chor·dee (kor-dē′) Painful erection of the penis in association with gonorrhea or Peyronie disease, with curvature resulting from lack of distensibility of the corpora cavernosa of the urethra.

chor·di·tis (kōr-dī′tis) Inflammation of a cord; usually a vocal cord.

chor·do·skel·e·ton (kōr′dō-skel′ĕ-tŏn) The part of the embryonic skeleton that develops in conjunction with the notochord.

chor·dot·o·my (kōr-dot′ŏ-mē) SYN cordotomy.

cho·rea (kōr-ē′ă) Irregular, spasmodic, involuntary movements of the limbs or facial muscles, often accompanied by hy-

potonia. The location of the responsible cerebral lesion is not known. SEE ALSO Huntington chorea, Sydenham chorea.

cho·re·a grav·i·dar·um (kōr-ē′ă grav-i-dā′rŭm) Sydenham chorea occurring during pregnancy.

cho·re·al (kōr-ē′ăl) Relating to involuntary writhing of the limbs or facial muscles.

cho·re·ic a·ba·si·a (kōr-ē′ik ă-bā′zē-ă) Abasia related to choreiform movements of the legs.

cho·re·ic move·ment (kōr-ē′ik mūv′mĕnt) An involuntary spasmodic twitching or jerking in groups of muscles not associated in the production of definite purposeful movements.

cho·re·i·form (kōr-ē′i-fŏrm) SYN choreoid.

♻ **choreo-** Combining form denoting chorea.

cho·re·o·ath·e·toid (kōr′ē-ō-ath′ĕ-toyd) Pertaining to or characterized by choreoathetosis.

cho·re·o·ath·e·to·sis (kōr′ē-ō-ath-ĕ-tō′sis) Abnormal movements of body of combined choreic and athetoid pattern.

cho·re·oid (kōr′ē-oyd) Resembling chorea. SYN choreiform.

cho·re·o·phra·si·a (kōr′ē-ō-frā′zē-ă) Continual repetition of meaningless phrases.

♻ **chorio-** Combining form denoting any membrane, but especially that enclosing the embryo, and later, fetus.

cho·ri·o·ad·e·no·ma (kōr′ē-ō-ad-ĕ-nō′mă) A benign neoplasm of chorion, especially with hydatidiform mole formation.

cho·ri·o·am·ni·o·ni·tis (kōr′ē-ō-am′nē-ō-nī′tis) Infection involving the chorion, amnion, and amniotic fluid; usually the placental villi and decidua are also involved.

cho·ri·o·an·gi·o·ma (kōr′ē-ō-an-jē-ō′mă) Benign tumor of placental blood vessels, usually of no clinical significance. SEE ALSO chorioangiosis.

cho·ri·o·an·gi·o·sis (kōr′ē-ō-an-jē-ō′sis) An abnormal increase in the number of vascular channels in placental villi; severe chorioangiosis is associated with a high incidence of neonatal death and major congenital malformations.

cho·ri·o·cap·il·la·ry lay·er (kōr′ē-ō-kap′i-lar-ē lā′ĕr) The internal layer of the choroidea of the eye, composed of a very close capillary network. SYN entochoroidea, Ruysch membrane.

cho·ri·o·car·ci·no·ma (kō′rē-ō-kahr-si-nō′mă) A highly malignant neoplasm derived from placental syncytial trophoblasts and cytotrophoblasts.

cho·ri·o·cele (kō′rē-ō-sēl) A hernia of the choroid coat of the eye through a defect in the sclera.

cho·ri·o·gen·e·sis (kōr′ē-ō-jen′ē-sis) Formation of the chorion.

cho·ri·o·go·nad·o·tro·pin (kō′rē-ō-go-nad′ō-trō′pin) SYN chorionic gonadotropin.

cho·ri·o·ma (kōr′ē-ō′mă) Neoplasm of chorionic tissue that can be either benign or malignant.

cho·ri·o·men·in·gi·tis (kōr′ē-ō-men-in-jī′tis) A cerebral meningitis in which there is a more or less marked cellular infiltration of the meninges, often with a lymphocytic infiltration of the choroid plexuses, particularly of the third and fourth ventricles.

cho·ri·on (kōr′ē-on) The multilayered, outermost fetal membrane consisting of extraembryonic somatic mesoderm, trophoblast, and, on the maternal surface, its villi are bathed by maternal blood; as pregnancy progresses, part of the villous chorion becomes the fetal part of placenta. SYN membrana serosa (1).

cho·ri·on fron·do·sum (kōr′ē-on fron-dō′sŭm) SYN villous chorion.

cho·ri·on·ic go·nad·o·tro·pin (kōr′ē-on′ik gō-nad′ō-trō′pin) A glycoprotein; its most important role appears to be stimulation (during the first trimester) of ovarian secretion of the estrogen and progesterone required for the integrity of the conceptus. SYN anterior pituitary-like hormone.

cho·ri·on·ic vil·lus sam·pling (CVS) (kōr′ē-on′ik vil′ŭs samp′ling) Biopsy of the villous chorion through the abdominal wall or through the endocervical canal at 6–12 weeks' gestation to obtain fetal cells for diagnosis of chromosomal abnormalities.

cho·ri·on lae·ve (kōr′ē-on lē′vē) SYN smooth chorion.

♻ **cho·ri·o·ret·i·ni·tis** (kōr′ē-ō-ret′i-nī′tis) Inflammation in the choroid and retina with its origin in the choroid.

cho·ri·o·ret·i·nop·a·thy (kōr′ē-ō-ret′i-nop′ă-thē) A primary abnormality of the choroid with extension to the retina. SEE ALSO choroidopathy.

cho·ris·to·ma (kor′is-tō′mă) A mass formed by maldevelopment of tissue of a type not normally found at that site.

cho·roid (kōr′oyd) [TA] The middle vascular tunic of the eye lying between the retina and the sclera. SYN choroidea [TA].

cho·roi·de·a (kōr-oyd′ē-ă) [TA] SYN choroid.

cho·roid en·large·ment (kōr′oyd en-lahrg′mĕnt) The enlarged portion of the choroid plexus located in the atrium of the lateral ventricle; may become partially calcified with age and appear white in computed tomography scan. SYN glomus choroideum [TA]

choroideraemia [Br.] SYN choroideremia.

cho·roi·der·e·mi·a (kōr′oyd-ĕr-ē′mē-ă) Progressive degeneration of the ocular choroid. SYN choroideraemia, progressive choroidal atrophy, progressive tapetochoroidal dystrophy.

cho·roid·i·tis (kōr′oyd-ī′tis) Inflammation of the choroid.

♻ **choroido-** Combining form meaning the choroid.

cho·roid·o·cy·cli·tis (kōr-oyd′ō-sik-lī′tis) Inflammation of the choroid coat and the ciliary body.

cho·roid·o·ret·i·ni·tis (kōr-oyd′ō-ret-i-nī′tis) Inflammation of the choroid and retina with the primary process in the choroid.

Christ·mas dis·ease (kris′măs di-zēz′) SYN hemophilia B.

Christ·mas fac·tor (CF) (kris′măs fak′tŏr) SYN factor IX.

♻ **chrom-, chromat-, chromato-, chromo-** Combining forms denoting color.

chromaesthesia [Br.] SYN chromesthesia.

chro·maf·fin (krō-maf′in) Giving a brownish yellow reaction with chromic salts; denoting certain cells in the medulla of the suprarenal glands and paraganglia. SYN chromatophil (3), chromophil (3), chromophile, pheochrome (1).

chro·maf·fin·o·ma (krō-maf′in-ō′mă) A neoplasm composed of chromaffin cells. SYN chromaffin tumor.

chro·maf·fin sys·tem (krō′maf-in sis′těm) Body cells that stain with chromium salts and occur in the medullary portion of the suprarenal gland and paraganglia.

chro·maf·fin tis·sue (krō-maf′in tish′ū) A cellular tissue, vascular and well supplied with nerves, made up chiefly of chromaffin cells; found in the medulla of the suprarenal glands and, in smaller collections, in the paraganglia.

♻ **chromat-** SEE chrom-.

chro·mate (krō′māt) A salt of chromic acid.

chro·mat·ic (krō-mat′ik) Of or pertaining to color or colors; produced by, or made in, a color or colors.

chro·mat·ic chart (krō-mat′ik chahrt) SYN color chart.

chro·mat·ic vi·sion (krō-mat′ik vizh′ŭn) SYN chromatopsia.

chro·ma·tin (krō′mă-tin) The genetic material of the nucleus, consisting of deoxyribonucleoprotein. During mitotic division the chromatin condenses into chromosomes.

chro·ma·tin body (krō′mă-tin bod′ē)

The genetic apparatus of bacteria. SEE nucleus (2).

chro·ma·ti·nol·y·sis (krō′mă-ti-nol′i-sis) SYN chromatolysis.

chro·ma·tism (krō′mă-tizm) Abnormal pigmentation.

♻ **chromato-** SEE chrom-.

chro·ma·tog·e·nous (krō′mă-toj′ĕ-nŭs) Producing color; causing pigmentation.

chro·mat·o·gram (krō-mat′ō-gram) A graphic record produced by chromatography.

chro·mat·o·graph (krō-mat′ō-graf) To perform chromatography.

chro·ma·tog·ra·phy (krō′mă-tog′ră-fē) The separation of chemical substances and particles by differential movement through a two-phase system. SYN absorption chromatography.

chro·ma·tol·y·sis, chro·ma·ti·nol·y·sis (krō′mă-tol′i-sis, -ti-nol′i-sis) The disintegration of the granules of chromophil substance (Nissl bodies) in a nerve cell body that may occur after exhaustion of the cell or damage to its peripheral process. SYN chromatinolysis, chromolysis, tigrolysis.

chro·mat·o·lyt·ic (krō-mat′ō-lit′ik) Relating to chromatolysis.

chro·mat·o·phil (krō-mat′ō-fil) **1.** SYN chromophil (2). **2.** SYN chromaffin.

chro·mat·o·pho·bi·a (krō′mă-tō-fō′bē-ă) SYN chromophobia.

chro·ma·top·si·a (krō′mă-top′sē-ă) A condition in which objects appear to be abnormally colored or tinged with color. SYN chromatic vision, colored vision.

chro·ma·tu·ri·a (krō′mă-tyūr′ē-ă) Abnormal coloration of the urine.

♻ **-chrome** A suffix indicating relationship to color.

chro·mes·the·sia (krō′mes-thē′zē-ă) **1.** The color sense. **2.** A condition in which nonvisual stimuli, such as taste or smell, cause the perception of color. SYN chromaesthesia.

chrom·hi·dro·sis, chrom·i·dro·sis (krōm′hī-drō′sis, krō′mi-drō′sis) A condition characterized by the excretion of sweat containing pigment.

chro·mic ac·id (krō′mik as′id) A strong oxidizing agent formed by dissolving chromium trioxide (CrO_3) in water. Has been used in solution as a topical antiseptic.

chro·mic cat·gut, chro·mic gut (krō′mik kat′gŭt) Catgut impregnated with chromium salts to prolong its tensile strength and retard its absorption.

chro·mi·um (Cr) (krō′mē-ŭm) A dietary essential bioelement;[51] used as a diagnostic aid in many disorders (e.g., gastrointestinal protein loss).

chro·mi·um pic·o·lin·ate (krō′mē-ŭm pik-ō′lin-āt) A chromium salt taken by many athletes with the unsubstantiated belief that additional chromium promotes muscle growth, curbs appetite, and fosters body fat loss.

chromium tri·ox·ide (krō′mē-ŭm trī-oks′īd) Chromic acid, a strong oxidizing agent used as a caustic to remove warts and other small growths from the skin and genitals.

chromo- SEE chrom-.

chro·mo·cyte (krō′mō-sīt) Any pigmented cell, such as a red blood corpuscle.

chro·mo·dac·ry·or·rhe·a (krō′mō-dak′rē-ōr-ē′ă) Flow of bloody tears.

chro·mo·gen (krō′mō-jen) 1. A substance, itself without definite color, that may be transformed into a pigment. 2. A microorganism that produces pigment.

chro·mo·gen·e·sis (krō′mō-jen′ĕ-sis) Production of coloring matter or pigment, often through an enzyme-catalyzed reaction.

chro·mol·y·sis (krō-mol′i-sis) SYN chromatolysis.

chro·mo·mere (krō′mō-mēr) 1. A condensed segment of a chromonema; densely staining bands visible in chromosomes under certain conditions. 2. SYN granulomere.

chro·mo·ne·ma, pl. **chro·mo·ne·ma·ta** (krō′mō-nē′mă, -tă) The coiled filament in which the genes are located, which extends the entire length of a chromosome.

chro·mo·phil, chro·mo·phile (krō′mō-fil, -fīl) 1. A cell or any histologic element that stains readily. SYN chromatophil (2). 2. SYN chromaffin.

chro·mo·phil ad·e·no·ma (krō′mō-fil ad′ĕ-nō′mă) Any adenoma composed of cells that stain readily.

chro·mo·phil·i·a (krō′mō-fil′ē-ă) The property possessed by most cells of staining readily with appropriate dyes. SYN chromatophilia.

chro·mo·phobe (krō′mō-fōb) Resistant to stains, staining with difficulty or not at all; denoting certain degranulated cells in the anterior lobe of the pituitary gland.

chro·mo·pho·bi·a (krō′mō-fō′bē-ă) 1. Resistance to stains on the part of cells and tissues. 2. A morbid dislike of color. SYN chromatophobia.

chro·mo·phore (krō′mō-fōr) The atomic grouping on which the color of a substance depends.

chro·mo·phor·ic, chro·moph·o·rous (krō′mō-fōr′ik, -mof′ŏr-ŭs) 1. Relating to a chromophore. 2. Producing or carrying color; denoting certain microorganisms.

chro·mo·som·al de·le·tion (krō′mŏ-sō′măl dĕ-lē′shŭn) A microscopically evident loss of part of a chromosome. SEE ALSO monosomy.

chro·mo·som·al map (krō′mŏ-sō′măl map) A formal, stylized representation of the karyotype and of the positioning and ordering on it of those loci localized by any of several mapping methods.

chro·mo·som·al re·gion (krō′mŏ-sō′măl rē′jŭn) That part of a chromosome defined either by anatomic details, notably banding, or by its linkages (linkage group).

chro·mo·som·al syn·drome (krō′mŏ-sō′măl sin′drōm) General designation for syndromes due to chromosomal aberrations; typically associated with mental retardation and multiple congenital anomalies.

chro•mo•som•al trait (krō′mŏ-sŏ′măl trāt) A trait dependent on a recurrent chromosomal aberration.

chro•mo•some (krō′mŏ-sŏm) A body in the cell nucleus (of which there are normally 46 in humans) that is a bearer of genes, has the form of a delicate chromatin filament during interphase, contracts to form a compact cylinder segmented into two arms by the centromere during metaphase and anaphase stages of cell divison, and is capable of reproducing its physical and chemical structure through successive cell divisons.

chro•mo•some ab•er•ra•tion (krō′mŏ-sŏm ab-ĕr-ā′shŭn) Any deviation from the normal number or morphology of chromosomes; also the phenotypic consequences thereof.

chro•mo•some band (krō′mŏ-sŏm band) A region of darker or contrasting staining across the width of a chromosome; the pattern of bands is characteristic for most chromosomes. SEE banding.

chro•mo•some map•ping (krō′mŏ-sŏm map′ing) The process of determining the position of loci on specific chromosomes and constructing a diagram of each chromosome showing the relative positions of loci; techniques include family studies with linkage analysis, somatic cell hybridization, and chromosome deletion mapping.

chro•mo•some sat•el•lite (krō′mŏ-sŏm sat′ĕ-līt) A small chromosomal segment separated from the main body of the chromosome by a secondary constriction.

chro•mo•trope (krō′mŏ-trōp) Any of several dyes containing chromotropic acid that have the property of changing from red to blue on afterchroming stain.

chro•nax•ie, chro•nax•ia, chro•nax•y, chro•nax•is (krō′nak-sē, -sē-ă, -sē, -sis) A measurement of excitability of nervous or muscular tissue; the shortest duration of an effective electrical stimulus having a strength equal to twice the minimum strength required for excitation. SYN chronaxia, chronaxis, chronaxy.

chron•ic (kron′ik) Term used to describe persistent disease or illness.

chron•ic ab•scess (kron′ik ab′ses) Long-standing mass of pus surrounded by fibrous tissue.

chron•ic act•ive hep•a•ti•tis (CAH) (kron′ik ak′tiv hep-ă-tī′tis) Liver disease with long-term portal inflammation. SYN juvenile cirrhosis, posthepatitic cirrhosis, subacute hepatitis.

chron•ic al•co•hol•ism (kron′ik al′kŏ-hol-izm) Pathologic condition, affecting chiefly the nervous and gastroenteric systems, associated with impairment in social and occupational functioning, caused by the habitual use of alcoholic beverages in toxic amounts.

chron•ic ap•pen•di•cit•is (kron′ik ă-pend-di-sī′tis) Fibrous adhesions, scarring, or deformity of the appendix following subsidence of acute appendicitis; term frequently signifying repeated mild attacks of acute appendicitis.

chron•ic a•troph•ic pol•y•chon•dri•tis (kron′ik ă-trō′fik pol′ē-kon-drī′tis) SYN relapsing polychondritis.

chron•ic a•troph•ic thy•roi•di•tis (kron′ik ă-trō′fik thī-roy-dī′tis) Replacement of the thyroid gland by fibrous tissue, the commonest cause of myxedema in older people.

chron•ic bron•chi•tis (kron′ik brong-kī′tis) A condition of the bronchial tree characterized by cough, hypersecretion of mucus, and expectoration of sputum over a long period, associated with frequent bronchial infections; usually due to smoking.

chron•ic des•qua•ma•tive gin•gi•vi•tis (kron′ik des-kwahm′ă-tiv jin′ji-vī′tis) A gingival condition of unknown etiology in middle-aged and older women.

chron•ic er•y•thre•mic my•e•lo•sis (kron′ik er′i-thrē′mik mī-ĕ-lō′sis) SYN myelodysplastic syndrome.

chron•ic fa•tigue syn•drome (kron′ik fă-tēg′ sin′drōm) Clinically evaluated new onset debilitating exhaustion not substantially relieved by rest and concurrent four of eight symptoms persisting or occurring during 6 or more consecutive months and not predating the fatigue: substantial short-term memory impairment or concentration; sore throat; tender lymph nodes; muscle and multijoint pain; unusual headache; unrefreshing sleep; postexertional malaise lasting more than 24 hours; of unknown etiology. Also called chronic fatigue and immune dysfunction syndrome.

chron·ic ill·ness (kron´ik il´nĕs) An ongoing, long-term medical condition.

chron·ic lymph·o·cyt·ic leu·ke·mi·a (CLL) (kron´ik lim´fō-sit´ik lū-kē´mē-ă) SEE lymphocytic leukemia.

chron·ic ma·lar·i·a (kron´ik mă-lar´ē-ă) Form of the disease that develops after frequently repeated attacks of one of the acute forms, usually falciparum malaria; characterized by profound anemia, enlarged spleen, emaciation, mental depression, sallow complexion, edema of the ankles, feeble digestion, and muscular weakness.

chron·ic my·e·lo·cyt·ic leu·ke·mi·a (kron´ik mī´ĕ-lō-sit´ik lū-kē´mē-ă) A heterogeneous group of myeloproliferative disorders that may evolve into acute leukemia in late stages (i.e., blast crisis). Slow onset, usually in older adults. SYN chronic myelogenous leukemia, chronic myeloid leukemia.

chron·ic my·e·log·e·nous leu·ke·mi·a (kron´ik mī´ĕ-loj´ĕ-nŭs lū-kē´mē-ă) SYN chronic myelocytic leukemia.

chron·ic my·e·loid leu·ke·mi·a (kron´ik mī´ĕ-loyd lū-kē´mē-ă) SYN chronic myelocytic leukemia.

chron·ic ob·struc·tive pul·mo·nar·y dis·ease (COPD) (kron´ik ŏb-strŭk´tiv pul´mŏ-nar-ē di-zēz´) General term used for those diseases with permanent or temporary narrowing of small bronchi, in which forced expiratory flow is slowed, especially when no etiologic or other more specific term can be applied.

chron·ic pan·cre·a·ti·tis (CP) (kron´ik pan-krē-ă-tī´tis) Recurrent bouts of inflammatory disease of the pancreas characterized by fibrosis and varying degrees of irreversible loss of exocrine and ultimately endocrine function.

chron·ic pos·te·ri·or lar·yn·gi·tis

(kron´ik pos-tēr´ē-ŏr lar-in-jī´tis) A form of laryngitis involving principally the interarytenoid area; thought to be caused by regurgitation of gastric contents.

chron·ic re·jec·tion (CR) (kron´ik rē-jek´shŭn) Rejection of surgical transplant occurring gradually, sometimes months later.

chrono- Combining form referring to time.

chron·o·bi·ol·o·gy (kron´ō-bī-ol´ō-jē) That aspect of biology concerned with the timing of biologic events, especially repetitive or cyclic phenomena.

chron·og·no·sis (kron´og-nō´sis) Perception of the passage of time.

chro·no·graph (kron´ō-graf) An instrument for graphic measurement and recording brief time periods.

chron·o·log·ic (kron´ŏ-loj´ik) Pertaining to time sequence.

chron·o·on·col·o·gy (kron´ō-on-kol´ō-jē) The study of the influence of biologic rhythms on cancer.

chron·o·ta·rax·is (kron´ō-tă-rak´sis) Distortion or confusion in the perception of time.

chron·o·ther·a·peu·tics (kron´ō-thār-ă-pyū´tiks) Timing of dosage of medication according to the circadian rhythms attached to the given disease.

chron·o·tro·pic (kron´ō-trō´pik) Affecting the rate of rhythmic movements such as the heartbeat.

chro·not·ro·pism (krō-not´rō-pizm) Modification of the rate of a periodic movement, e.g., the heartbeat, through some external influence.

chrys-, chryso- Combining forms denoting gold; corresponds to L. *auro-*.

chrys·a·ro·bin (kris´ă-rō´bin) An extract of a complex mixure of reduction products of chrysophanic acid, emodin, and emodin monomethyl ether; used as a topical dermatologic agent.

chry·si·a·sis (kris-ī´ă-sis) A permanent

slate-gray discoloration of the skin and sclera resulting from deposition of gold in macrophages. SYN auriasis, aurochromoderma.

chrys·o·der·ma (kris-ō-dĕr'mă) SYN chrysiasis.

Chrys·o·my·ia (kris'ō-mī'yă) A genus of myiasis-producing fleshflies with medium-sized metallic-colored adults.

Chrys·ops (kris'ops) The deerfly, a genus of biting flies with about 80 North American species, characterized by a splotched wing pattern; *Chrysops discalis* is a vector of *Francisella tularensis* in the U.S.

Churg-Strauss dis·ease (chŭrg-strows di-zēz') Allergic vasculitis marked by involvement of small and medium-sized arteries (e.g., in lungs), fever, weight loss, myalgia, headache, and respiratory distress. Usually determined by cutaneous biopsy revealing eosinophilic vasculitis.

Chvos·tek sign (kvos'tek sīn) Facial irritability in tetany, unilateral spasm of the orbicularis oculi or oris muscle being excited by a slight tap over the facial nerve just anterior to the external auditory meatus. SYN Weiss sign.

♻ **chyl-** SEE chylo-, chyle.

chylaemia [Br.] SYN chylemia.

chy·lan·gi·o·ma (kī-lan'jē-ō'mă) A mass of prominent, dilated lacteals and larger intestinal lymphatic vessels.

chyle (kīl) A turbid white or pale yellow fluid taken up by the lacteals from the intestine during digestion and carried by the lymphatic system through the thoracic duct into the circulation.

chyle fis·tu·la (kīl fis'tyū-lă) A leak of chyle from a lymph vessel to the skin surface; a complication of radical neck dissection when the thoracic duct is injured.

chy·le·mi·a (kī-lē'mē-ă) The presence of chyle in the circulating blood. SYN chylaemia.

♻ **chyli-** SEE chyl.

chy·lif·er·ous (kī-lif'ĕr-ŭs) Conveying chyle. SYN chylophoric.

chy·li·form (kī'li-fōrm) Resembling chyle.

chy·li·form as·ci·tes (kī'li-fōrm ă-sī'tēz) SYN chylous ascites.

♻ **chylo-, chyl-** Prefix meaning chyle.

chy·lo·cyst (kī'lō-sist) SYN cisterna chyli.

chy·lo·me·di·as·ti·num (kī'lō-mē-dē-as-tī'nŭm) Abnormal presence of chyle in the mediastinum.

chy·lo·mi·cron (kī'lō-mī'kron) A droplet of reprocessed lipid synthesized in epithelial cells of the small intestine; the least dense of the plasma lipoproteins.

chy·lo·per·i·car·di·um (kī'lō-per'i-kahr'dē-ŭm) A milky pericardial effusion resulting from obstruction of the thoracic duct, from trauma, or of idiopathic origin.

chy·lo·per·i·to·ne·um (kī'lō-per'i-tō-nē'ŭm) SYN chylous ascites.

chy·lo·phor·ic (kī'lō-fōr'ik) SYN chyliferous.

chy·lo·pneu·mo·tho·rax (kī'lō-nū-mō-thōr'aks) Free chyle and air in the pleural space.

chy·lo·poi·e·sis (kī'lō-poy-ē'sis) Formation of chyle in the intestine. SYN chylifaction.

chy·lo·tho·rax (kī'lō-thōr'aks) An accumulation of milky chylous fluid in the pleural space, usually on the left.

chy·lous (kī'lŭs) Relating to chyle.

chy·lous as·ci·tes, as·ci·tes chy·lo·sus (kī'lŭs ă-sī'tēz, kī-lō'sŭs) Presence in the peritoneal cavity of a milky fluid containing suspended fat, ordinarily caused by an obstruction or injury of the thoracic duct or cisterna. SYN chyloperitoneum.

chy·lu·ri·a (kī-lyūr'ē-ă) The passage of chyle in the urine; a form of albiduria.

chy·mase (kī'mās) SYN chymosin.

chyme, chy·mus (kīm, kī′mŭs) The semifluid mass of partly digested food passed from the stomach into the duodenum. SYN pulp (3).

chy·mi·fi·ca·tion (kī′mi-fi-kā′shŭn) SYN chymopoiesis.

chy·mo·poi·e·sis (kī′mō-poy-ē′sis) The production of chyme; the physical state of food (semifluid) brought about by digestion in the stomach. SYN chymification.

chy·mo·sin (kī′mō-sin) A proteinase structurally homologous with pepsin; the milk-curdling enzyme obtained from the stomach of the calf.

chy·mo·tryp·sin·o·gen (kī′mō-trip-sin′ŏ-jen) The precursor of chymotrypsin. Converted to π-chymotrypsin by the action of trypsin.

Ci·an·ca syn·drome (chē-ahn′kă sin′drōm) A severe form of infantile esotropia, an optic disease, characterized by cross-fixation, tight medial rectus muscles, and nystagmus with abduction of the fixating eye.

cib. Abbreviation for L. cibus, food.

cic·a·trec·to·my (sik′ă-trek′tŏ-mē) Excision of a scar.

cic·a·tri·cial (sik′ă-trish′ăl) Relating to a scar.

cic·a·tri·cial al·o·pe·ci·a (sik′ă-trish′ăl al-ō-pē′shē-ă) SYN scarring alopecia.

cic·a·tri·cial horn (sik′ă-trish′ăl hōrn) Keratinous horn projecting out from a scar.

cic·a·trix, gen. and pl. **cic·a·tri·ces** (sik′ă-triks, -tri-sēz) A scar.

cic·a·tri·za·tion (sik′ă-trī-zā′shŭn) **1.** The process of scar formation. **2.** The healing of a wound otherwise than by first intention.

-cidal SEE -cide.

-cide, -cido Combining forms denoting an agent that kills (e.g., insecticide), or the act of killing (e.g., suicide).

ci·gua·tox·in (sē′gwă-tok′sin) Toxic substance that causes ciguatera.

cili- SEE cilio-.

cil·i·ar·ot·o·my (sil-ē-ăr-ot′ŏ-mē) Surgical dissection of the ciliary region of the iris.

cil·i·ar·y (sil′ē-ar-ē) **1.** Relating to cilia found widely in the animal kingdom from single-cell to more complex organisms and serving various motile and sensory functions. **2.** Relating to any cilia or hairlike process, specifically the eyelashes. **3.** Relating to certain structures of the eyeball (e.g., ciliary body, ciliary muscle, ciliary process, anterior ciliary vein). **4.** Relating to the cilia of the pseudostratified columnar cells of the respiratory tract from the nose to the alveoli. **5.** Relating to cilia of the uterine tubes. **6.** Relating to the cilia of the olfactory receptor cells that contain the olfactory receptors. **7.** Relating to motile protoplasmic extensions of some cells. SEE ALSO cilium.

cil·i·ar·y bod·y (sil′ē-ar-ē bod′ē) [TA] Three-part thickened portion of the vascular tunic of the eye between the choroid and the iris. SYN corpus ciliare [TA].

cil·i·ar·y glands (sil′ē-ar-ē glandz) [TA] Modified apocrine sudoriferous glands in the eyelids, with ducts that usually open into the follicles of the eyelashes.

cil·i·ar·y zone (sil′ē-ar-ē zōn) Outer wider zone of the anterior surface of the iris, separated from the pupillary zone by the collarette. SYN zona ciliaris.

cil·i·ar·y zo·nule (sil′ē-ar-ē zōn′yūl) [TA] A series of delicate meridional fibers arising from the inner surface of the orbiculus ciliaris that run in bundles between, and in a very thin layer over, the ciliary processes. SYN zonula ciliaris [TA], suspensory ligament of lens, Zinn zonule.

Cil·i·a·ta (sil-ē-ā′tă) Pathogens; typical members, such as *Paramecium* or *Balantidium coli* (a parasite of humans, swine, nonhuman primates, rats and rarely, in dogs) possess two distinctive nuclei, a macronucleus and a micronucleus. SYN Ciliophora.

cil·i·ec·to·my (sil′ē-ek′tŏ-mē) SYN cyclectomy.

cilio-, cili- Combining forms meaning cilia or ciliary, in any sense; eyelashes.

Ci·li·oph·o·ra (sil'ē-of'ŏ-ră) A phylum of protozoa that includes the abundant free-living ciliates and the sessile suctorians. SYN ciliates, Ciliata.

cil·i·o·spi·nal (sil'ē-ō-spī'năl) Relating to the ciliary body and the spinal cord; denoting in particular the ciliospinal center.

cil·i·o·spi·nal cen·ter (sil'ē-ō-spī'năl sen'tĕr) Preganglionic motor neurons in the first thoracic segment of the spinal cord that give rise to the sympathetic innervation of the dilator muscle of the pupil.

cil·i·o·spi·nal re·flex (sil'ē-ō-spī'năl rē'fleks) SYN pupillary-skin reflex.

cil·i·um, pl. **cil·i·a** (sil'ē-ŭm, -ă) **1.** SYN eyelash. **2.** A motile extension of a cell surface.

ci·met·i·dine (CIM) (si-met'i-dēn) A histamine analogue and antagonist used to treat peptic ulcer and hypersecretory conditions by blocking histamine H_2 receptor sites, thus inhibiting gastric acid secretion.

Ci·mex (sī'meks) A genus of bedbugs with flat, reddish-brown, wingless bodies, prominent lateral eyes, a three-jointed beak, and a characteristic odor from thoracic stink glands; an abundant pest in human abodes. SYN bedbug.

cin·cho·na (sin-kō'nă) The dried bark of the root and stem of various species of *Cinchona* that produce quinine and quinidine. SYN bark (2), Jesuits' bark, Peruvian bark, quina, quinaquina, quinquina.

cin·cho·nism (sin'kō-nizm) Poisoning by cinchona, quinine, or quinidine; characterized by tinnitus, headache, deafness, and occasionally, anaphylactoid shock.

cine-, cin- Combining forms denoting movement, usually relating to motion pictures.

cin·e·an·gi·o·car·di·og·ra·phy (sin'ē-an'jē-ō-kahr-dē-og'ră-fē) Motion pictures of the passage of a contrast medium through chambers of the heart and great vessels.

cin·e·an·gi·o·gram (sin'ē-an'jē-ō-gram) Radiographic imaging of the cardiac vessels after injection of contrast material.

cin·e·an·gi·o·graph (sin'ē-an'jē-ō-graf) Instrument to record radiographic imaging of the cardiac vessels after injection of contrast material.

cin·e·an·gi·og·ra·phy (sin'ē-an'jē-og'ră-fē) Modality of radiographic imaging of the cardiac vessels after injection of contrast material.

cin·e·ole (sin'ē-ōl, -ol) A stimulant expectorant obtained from the volatile oil of *Eucalyptus globulus* and other species of *Eucalyptus*. SYN eucalyptol.

cin·e·ra·di·og·ra·phy (sin'ē-rā-dē-og'ră-fē) Radiography of an organ in motion, e.g., the heart, the gastrointestinal tract. SYN cinefluorography, cinefluoroscopy, cineroentgenography.

cin·gu·late (sing'gyū-lāt) Relating to a cingulum.

cin·gu·late gy·rus (sing'gyū-lāt jī'rŭs) [TA] Long, curved convolution of the medial surface of the cortical hemisphere, arched over the corpus callosum from which it is separated by the deep sulcus of the corpus callosum.

cin·gu·late sul·cus (sing'gyū-lāt sŭl'kŭs) [TA] A fissure on the mesial surface of the cerebral hemisphere, bounding the upper surface of the cingulate gyrus (callosal convolution).

cin·gu·lot·o·my, cin·gu·lec·to·my, cin·gu·lu·mot·o·my (sing'gyū-lot'ŏ-mē, -lek'tŏ-mē, -lŭ-mot'ŏ-mē) Electrolytic destruction of the anterior cingulate gyrus and callosum.

cin·gu·lum, gen. **cin·gu·li,** pl. **cin·gu·la** (sing'gyū-lŭm, -lī, -lă) [TA] **1.** SYN girdle. **2.** A well-marked fiber bundle passing longitudinally in the white matter of the cingulate gyrus. **3.** The lingual portion of an incisor or canine tooth, which forms a convexity on the cervical third of the crown. **4.** The cervical third of the crown of a molar, which is the source of the developing cusps.

cir·ca·di·an (sĭr-kā'dē-ăn) Relating to biologic variations or rhythms with a cycle of about 24 hours. Cf. infradian, ultradian.

cir·ca·di·an rhythm (sĭr-kā´dē-ăn ridh´ĕm) SEE circadian.

cir·ci·nate (sĭr´si-nāt) Circular; ring-shaped, anular.

cir·cle (sĭr´kĕl) **1.** A ring-shaped structure or group of structures. SYN circulus (1) [TA]. **2.** A line or process with every point equidistant from the center.

cir·cle of Wil·lis (sĭr´kĕl wil´is) A ring of arteries at the base of the brain formed by anastomoses of the internal carotid arteries and the basilar artery.

cir·cuit (sĭr´kŭt) The path or course of flow of electric or other currents.

cir·cuit re·sis·tance train·ing (CRT), cir·cuit train·ing, cir·cuit weight train·ing (sĭr´kŭt rĕ-zis´tăns trān´ing, sĭr´kŭt trān´ing, sĭr´kŭt wāt trān´ing) Modification of standard strength training emphasizing relatively light load (40–60% of maximum strength) and continuous exercise to provide a more general conditioning to improve body composition, muscular strength and endurance, and cardiovascular fitness.

cir·cu·lar am·pu·ta·tion (sĭr´kyū-lăr amp-yū-tā´shŭn) Surgical removal performed by a circular incision through the skin, the muscles being similarly divided higher up, and the bone higher still.

cir·cu·lar ban·dage (sĭr´kyū-lăr ban´dăj) Dressing encircling a limb, or a portion of it, or the trunk of the body.

cir·cu·lar si·nus (sĭr´kyū-lăr sī´nŭs) **1.** Dural venous formation that surrounds the hypophysis, composed of right and left cavernous sinuses and the intercavernous sinuses. SYN circulus venosus ridleyi, Ridley circle. **2.** Venous sinus at the periphery of the placenta.

cir·cu·la·tion time (CT) (sĭr´kyū-lă´shŭn tīm) Duration elapsed for blood to pass through a given circuit of the vascular system.

cir·cu·la·to·ry (sĭr´kyū-lă-tōr-ē) **1.** Relating to the circulation. **2.** SYN sanguiferous.

cir·cu·la·to·ry col·lapse (CC) (sĭr´kyū-lă-tōr-ē kŏ-laps´) Failure of circulation, either cardiac or peripheral.

cir·cu·la·to·ry sys·tem (sĭr´kyū-lă-tōr-ē sis´tĕm) SYN vascular system.

cir·cu·lus, gen. and pl. **cir·cu·li** (sĭr´kū-lŭs, -lī) [TA] A circle formed by connecting arteries, veins, or nerves. SYN circle.

circum- Combining form indicating a circular movement, or a position surrounding the part indicated by the word to which it is joined. SEE ALSO peri-.

cir·cum·a·nal (sĭr´kŭm-ā´năl) Surrounding the anus. SYN perianal, periproctic.

cir·cum·a·nal glands (sĭr´kŭm-ā´năl glandz) Large apocrine sweat glands surrounding the anus.

cir·cum·ar·tic·u·lar (sĭr´kŭm-ahr-tik´yū-lăr) Surrounding a joint.

cir·cum·cise (sĭr´kŭm-sīz) To perform circumcision, especially of the prepuce of the penis.

cir·cum·ci·sion (sĭr´kŭm-sizh´ŭn) **1.** Operation to remove part or all of the prepuce. SYN peritomy (2). **2.** Cutting around an anatomic part (e.g., the areola of the breast). SYN peritectomy (2).

cir·cum·cor·ne·al (sĭr´kŭm-kōr´nē-ăl) SYN pericorneal.

cir·cum·duc·ti·o (sĭr´kŭm-dŭk´shē-ō) Circular movement of a body part (i.e., a limb). SYN circumduction.

cir·cum·duc·tion (sĭr´kŭm-dŭk´shŭn) [TA] **1.** Movement of a body part, e.g., a limb, in a circular direction. **2.** SYN circumductio [TA].

cir·cum·fer·en·tial la·mel·la (sĭr´kŭm-fĕr-en´shăl lă-mel´ă) A bony thin layer that encircles the outer or inner surface of a bone.

cir·cum·flex (sĭr´kŭm-fleks) Describing an arc of a circle or that which winds around something else.

cir·cum·len·tal (sĭr´kŭm-len´tăl) SYN perilenticular.

cir·cum·oc·u·lar (sĭr´kŭm-ok´yū-lăr) Around the eye.

cir·cum·o·ral (sĭr'kŭm-ōr'ăl) SYN perioral.

cir·cum·or·bit·al (sĭr'kŭm-ōr'bi-tăl) Around the orbit. SYN periorbital (2).

cir·cum·pul·pal (sĭr'kŭm-pŭl'păl) Pertaining to areas adjacent to pulp.

cir·cum·scribed (sĭr'kŭm-skrībd) Bounded by a line; limited or confined. SYN circumscriptus.

cir·cum·val·late (sĭr'kŭm-val'āt) Denotes something surrounded by an elevated border.

cir·cum·val·late pa·pil·lae (sĭr'kŭm-val'ăt pă-pil'ē) SYN vallate papilla.

cir·cus move·ment (sĭr'kŭs mūv'mĕnt) Contraction or excitation wave traveling continuously in circular fashion around a ring of muscle or through the wall of the heart. SYN circus rhythm.

cir·rho·sis (sĭr-ō'sis) Liver disease characterized by diffuse damage to hepatic parenchymal cells, with nodular regeneration, fibrosis, and disturbance of normal architecture.

cir·rhot·ic (sĭr-rot'ik) Relating to or affected with cirrhosis or advanced fibrosis.

cir·soid (sĭr'soyd) SYN variciform.

cir·soid an·eu·rysm (sĭr'soyd an'yūrizm) Dilation of a group of blood vessels owing to congenital malformation with arteriovenous shunting. SYN racemose aneurysm.

cis- Prefix meaning on this side, on the near side; opposite of trans-.

cis con·fig·u·rat·ion (sis kŏn-fig'yŭrā'shŭn) SEE cis- (3).

cis·plat·in, meth·o·trex·ate, vin·blas·tine (CMV) (sis-plat'in meth'ō-treks'āt vin-blas'tēn) A drug combination used in the treatment of bladder cancer as well as malignancies in other sites.

cis·tern (sis'tĕrn) [TA] Any cavity or enclosed space serving as a reservoir, especially for chyle, lymph, or cerebrospinal fluid.

cis·ter·na chy·li (sis-tĕr'nă kī'lī) Dilated sac at the lower end of the thoracic duct into which the intestinal trunk and two lumbar lymphatic trunks open. SYN chyle cistern, ampulla chyli, chylocyst, Pecquet cistern, Pecquet reservoir, receptaculum chyli, receptaculum pecqueti.

cis·ter·nal punc·ture (sis-tĕr'năl pŭngk'shŭr) Passage of a hollow needle through the posterior atlantooccipital membrane into the cisterna cerebellomedullaris.

cis·tern·og·ra·phy (sis'tĕrn-og'ră-fē) Radiographic study of the basal cisterns of the brain after the subarachnoid introduction of contrast medium.

cis·tron (sis'tron) **1.** The smallest functional unit of heritability; a length of chromosomal DNA associated with a single biochemical function. **2.** The genetic unit defined by the cis/trans test.

cit·rate (sit'rāt) A salt or ester of citric acid; used as an anticoagulant because it binds calcium ions.

cit·ric ac·id (sit'rik as'id) The acid of citrus fruits, widely distributed in nature and a key intermediate in intermediary metabolism.

cit·ric ac·id cy·cle (sit'rik as'id sī'kĕl) SYN tricarboxylic acid cycle.

cit·ro·nel·la (sit'rō-nel'ă) *Cymbopogon (Andropogon) nardus*; a fragrant grass (Sri Lanka), from which comes a volatile oil (c. oil) used as a perfume and insect repellent.

clad·o·spo·ri·o·sis (klad'ō-spō'rē-ō'sis) Infection with a fungus of the genus *Cladosporium*.

Clad·o·spo·ri·um (klad-ō-spō'rē-ŭm) A genus of fungi having dematiaceous or dark-colored conidiophores with long chains of oval or round spores; commonly isolated in soil or plant residues.

clair·voy·ance (klār-voy'ăns) Perception of objective events (past, present, or future) not ordinarily discernible by the senses; a type of extrasensory perception.

clamp (klamp) An instrument for compression of a structure. Cf. forceps.

clamp for·ceps (klamp fōr′seps) Instrument with pronged jaws designed to engage the jaws of a rubber dam clamp so that they may be separated to pass over the widest buccolingual contour of a tooth. SYN rubber dam clamp forceps.

clam-shell brace (klam′shel brās) An orthopedic cast that encloses the trunk between anterior and posterior foam-lined rigid plastic components; permits ambulation of patients with injuries of the vertebral column and neck. SYN Risser cast.

cla·rif·i·cant (klar-if′i-kănt) An agent that makes a turbid liquid clear.

clar·i·fi·ca·tion (klar′i-fi-kā′shŭn) The process of making a turbid liquid clear. SYN lucidification.

Clark lev·el (klahrk lev′ĕl) The progressive depth of invasion of primary malignant melanoma of the skin.

Clark ne·vus (klahrk nē′vŭs) Dysplastic melanotic nevi with notched, irregular borders on lesions; considered premalignant and marker for increased risk of melanoma.

clasp (klasp) **1.** A part of a removable partial denture that acts as a direct retainer or stabilizer for the denture by partially surrounding or contacting an abutment tooth. **2.** A direct retainer of a removable partial denture, usually consisting of two arms joined by a body that connects with an occlusal rest; at least one arm of a clasp usually terminates in the infrabulge (gingival convergence) area of the tooth enclosed. **3.** Any device for holding tissues together.

class (klas) In biologic classification, the next division below the phylum (or subphylum) and above the order.

clas·sic (klas′ik) Common, prototypical.

classic haemophilia [Br.] SYN classic hemophilia.

clas·sic he·mo·phil·i·a (klas′ik hē′mō-fil′ē-ă) SYN hemophilia A, classic haemophilia.

clas·sic mi·graine (klas′ik mī′grān) A form of hemicrania migraine preceded by a scintillating scotoma (teichopsia).

class I an·ti·gens (klas an′ti-jenz) Cell-membrane-bound glycoproteins coded by genes of the major histocompatibility complex.

class II an·ti·gens (klas an′ti-jenz) A cell-membrane glycoprotein encoded by genes of the major histocompatibility complex. These antigens are distributed on antigen-presenting cells such as macrophages, B cells, and dendritic cells.

class III an·ti·gens (klas an′ti-jenz) Non-cell-membrane molecules that are encoded by the S region of the major histocompatibility complex. These antigens are not involved in determining histocompatibility and include the complement proteins.

clas·tic (klas′tik) Breaking up into pieces, or exhibiting a tendency so to break or divide.

clas·to·gen·ic (klas-tō-jen′ik) Relating to the action of a clastogen.

clas·to·thrix (klas′tō-thriks) SYN trichorrhexis nodosa.

Claude syn·drome (klōd sin′drōm) Midbrain disorder with oculomotor palsy on the side of the lesion and incoordination on the opposite side.

clau·di·ca·tion (klaw′di-kā′shŭn) *This word means 'limping' or 'walking with difficulty'. Avoid nonsense phrases such as jaw claudication and claudication at rest.* Limping, usually referring to intermittent claudication.

clau·di·ca·tor·y (klaw′di-kă-tōr-ē) Relating to claudication, especially intermittent claudication.

Clau·di·us cells (klaw′dē-ŭs selz) Columnar cells on the floor of the ductus cochlearis external to the organ of Corti.

claus·tral (klaws′trăl) Relating to the claustrum.

claus·tro·pho·bi·a (klaw′strō-fō′bē-ă) A morbid fear of being in a confined place.

claus·trum, pl. **claus·tra** (klaws′trŭm, -tră) [TA] **1.** One of several anatomic structures bearing a resemblance to a barrier. **2.** [TA] A thin, vertically placed lamina of gray matter lying close to the putamen, from which it is separated by the external capsule.

clav·i·cle (klav′i-kĕl) [TA] A doubly curved long bone that forms part of the shoulder girdle. SYN clavicula [TA], collar bone.

cla·vi·cot·o·my (klav′i-kot′ŏ-mē) Surgical separation of the clavicle.

cla·vic·u·la, pl. **cla·vic·u·lae** (klă-vik′yū-lă, -lē) [TA] SYN clavicle.

cla·vus, pl. **cla·vi** (klā′vŭs, -vī) A small conic callosity caused by pressure over a bony prominence, usually on a toe. SYN corn.

claw (klaw) A sharp, slender, usually curved nail on the toe of an animal.

claw·foot, claw foot (klaw′fut) SYN pes cavus.

claw·hand, claw hand (klaw′hand) Atrophy of the interosseous muscles of the hand with hyperextension of the metacarpophalangeal joints and flexion of the interphalangeal joints; develops as a result of nerve injury either at the spinal cord or peripheral nerve level.

claw toe (klaw tō) Hyperextension and subluxation of a metatarsophalangeal joint, with flexion deformity of the interphalangeal joints and transfer of weight-bearing to the metatarsal head.

clay shov·el·er's frac·ture (klā-shŏv′ĕl-ĕrz frak′shŭr) An avulsion fracture of the base of spinous processes of C-7, C-6, or T-1 (in order of prevalence).

clear·ance (klēr′ăns) **1.** Indicated as *C* with a subscript to show the substance removed. **2.** A condition in which bodies may pass each other without hindrance, or the distance between bodies. **3.** Removal of something from some place; e.g., "esophageal acid clearance" refers to removal from the esophagus of acid refluxed into it from the stomach, evaluated by the time taken for restoration of a normal pH in the esophagus.

clear cell car·ci·no·ma (klēr sel kahr′si-nō′mă) SYN mesonephroma.

clear·ing me·di·um (klēr′ing mē′dē-ŭm) Medium used in histology for making specimens translucent or transparent.

cleav·age (klēv′ăj) **1.** Series of mitotic cell divisions occurring in the oocyte immediately after its fertilization. **2.** Splitting of a complex molecule into two or more simpler molecules. SYN scission (2). **3.** Linear clefts in the skin indicating the direction of the fibers in the dermis. SEE ALSO cleavage lines.

cleav·age ca·vi·ty (klēv′ăj kav′i-tē) SYN blastocele.

cleav·age prod·uct (klēv′ăj prod′ŭkt) Substance resulting from splitting a molecule into two or more simpler molecules.

cleave (klēv) To incise, cut apart.

cleft (kleft) [TA] A fissure or groove.

cleft hand (kleft hand) A congenital deformity in which the division between the fingers, especially between the third and fourth, extends into the metacarpal region. SYN split hand.

cleft jaw (kleft jaw) Congenital anomaly of the jaw due to failure of fusion of the mandibular prominences. SYN gnathoschisis.

cleft lip (kleft lip) A congenital facial defect of the lip (usually the upper) due to failure of fusion of the medial and lateral nasal prominences and maxillary prominence. SYN harelip.

cleft pal·ate (kleft pal′ăt) A congenital fissure in the median line of the palate, often associated with cleft lip; often occurs as a feature of a syndrome or generalized condition (e.g., diastrophic dwarfism or spondyloepiphysial dysplasia congenita). Care of the affected child requires a team approach involving a plastic surgeon, orthodontist, dentist, nurse, speech and hearing specialists, and social workers. SYN palatoschisis.

cleft spine (kleft spīn) SEE spina bifida.

cleft tongue (kleft tŭng) SYN bifid tongue.

cleido-, cleid- Combining forms indicating the clavicle; also spelled clido-, clid-.

clei·do·cra·ni·al (klī′dō-krā′nē-ăl) Relating to the clavicle and the cranium. SYN clidocranial.

clei·dot·o·my (klī-dot′ŏ-mē) Cutting the clavicle of a dead fetus to effect a vaginal delivery.

-cleisis Suffix indicating closure.

clench·ed fist sign (klencht fist sīn) In angina pectoris, pressing of the clenched fist against the chest to indicate the constricting, pressing quality of the pain.

clench·ing (klench′ing) Constricting or tightening (e.g., teeth, jaws).

cle·oid (klē′oyd) A dental instrument with a pointed elliptic cutting end, used in excavating cavities or carving fillings and waxes.

click (klik) A slight, sharp sound.

click·ing (klik′ing) A snapping, crepitant noise noted on excursions of the temporomandibular articulation, due to an asynchronous movement of the disc and condyle.

click·ing rale (klik′ing rahl) Short, sticking sound usually associated with opening of small bronchi on deep breathing; sometimes heard in early pulmonary tuberculosis.

clido-, clid- Combining forms denoting the clavicle. SEE ALSO cleido-.

Cliff·ord dis·ease (klif′ŏrd di-zēz′) SYN Ballantyne disease.

cli·mac·ter·ic, cli·mac·te·ri·um (klī-mak′tĕr-ik, -mak-tē′rē-ŭm) 1. The period of endocrinal, somatic, and transitory psychological changes occurring in the transition to menopause. 2. A critical period of life. SYN climacterium.

cli·max (klī′maks) 1. The height or acme of a disease; its stage of greatest severity. 2. SYN orgasm.

clin·ic (cl, clin) (klin′ik) 1. An institution, building, or part of a building where ambulatory patients receive health care. 2. An institution, building, or part of a building in which medical instruction is given to students by means of demonstrations in the presence of the sick. 3. A lecture or symposium on a subject relating to disease.

clin·i·cal (klin′i-kăl) 1. Relating to the bedside of a patient. 2. Denoting the symptoms and course of a disease, as distinguished from the laboratory findings of anatomic changes. 3. Relating to a clinic.

clin·i·cal a·nat·o·my (klin′i-kăl ă-nat′ŏ-mē) The practical application of anatomic knowledge to diagnosis and treatment.

clin·i·cal a·ttach·ment lev·el (klin′i-kăl ă-tach′měnt lev′ĕl) The estimated position of structures that support the tooth as measured with a periodontal probe to provide an estimate of a tooth's stability and loss of bone support.

clin·i·cal a·ttach·ment loss (klin′i-kăl ă-tach′měnt laws) The extent of periodontal support that has been destroyed around a tooth.

clin·i·cal crown (klin′i-kăl krown) Part of the crown of a tooth visible in the oral cavity. SYN corona clinica.

clin·i·cal di·ag·no·sis (klin′i-kăl dī-ăg-nō′sis) A diagnosis made from a study of the signs and symptoms of a disease.

clin·i·cal drug tri·al (klin′i-kăl drŭg trī′ăl) SYN drug use review.

clin·i·cal end point (klin′i-kăl end poynt) Traditional medical measures of a diagnostic or therapeutic impact that may or may not be perceived by the patient.

clin·i·cal ep·i·de·mi·ol·o·gy (klin′i-kăl ep′i-dē-mē-ol′ŏ-jē) Field concerned with applying epidemiologic principles in a clinical setting.

clin·i·cal fit·ness (klin′i-kăl fit′něs) Absence of frank disease or of subclinical precursors.

clin·i·cal ge·net·ics (klin′i-kăl jĕ-net′iks) Genetics applied to the diagnosis, prognosis, management, and prevention of genetic diseases. Cf. medical genetics.

clin·i·cal in·di·ca·tor (klin′i-kăl in′di-kā-tŏr) A measure, process, or outcome used to judge a particular clinical situation and indicate whether the therapy delivered was appropriate.

clin·i·cal le·thal (klin'i-kăl lē'thăl) A term describing a disorder that culminates in premature death.

clin·i·cal med·i·cine (CM) (klin'i-kăl med'i-sin) Study and practice of medicine in relation to the care of patients; the art of medicine as distinguished from laboratory science.

clin·i·cal nurse spe·cial·ist (klin'i-kăl nŭrs spesh'ăl-ist) A registered nurse with at least a master's degree in nursing who has advanced education in a particular area of clinical practice, such as oncology or psychiatry.

clin·i·cal pa·thol·o·gy (clin path, CP, CLP) (klin'i-kăl pă-thol'ŏ-jē) 1. Any part of the medical practice of pathology as it pertains to the care of patients. 2. Subspecialty in pathology concerned with the theoretical and technical aspects (i.e., the methods or procedures) of chemistry, immunohematology, microbiology, parasitology, immunology, hematology, and other fields as they pertain to diagnosis and the care of patients, as well as to the prevention of disease.

clin·i·cal prac·tice guide·lines (klin'i-kăl prak'tis gīd'līnz) A formal statement about a defined task or function in clinical practice, such as desirable diagnostic tests or the optimal treatment regimen for a specific diagnosis.

clin·i·cal psy·chol·o·gy (klin'i-kăl sī-kol'ŏ-jē) A branch of psychology that specializes in both discovering new knowledge and in applying the art and science of psychology to those with emotional or behavioral disorders.

clin·i·cal spec·i·fic·i·ty (klin'i-kăl spes'i-fis'i-tē) The frequency of negative results in patients without the disease (true-negative results).

clin·i·cal sus·pi·cion (klin'i-kăl sŭs-pi'shŭn) A strong presumption that, absent a diagnostic or algorithmic certainty, a patient is suffering from a given disorder or state.

clin·i·cal ther·mom·e·ter (klin'i-kăl thĕr-mom'ĕ-tĕr) A device for measuring the temperature of the human body.

clin·i·cal trial (klin'i-kăl trī'ăl) A controlled experiment involving a defined set of human subjects, having a clinical event as an outcome measure, and intended to yield scientifically valid information about the efficacy or safety of a drug, vaccine, diagnostic test, surgical procedure, or other form of medical intervention.

cli·ni·cian (klin-ish'ŭn) A health care professional engaged in the care of patients, as distinguished from one working in other areas.

clin·i·co·path·o·log·ic, clin·i·co·path·o·log·ic·al (klin'i-kō-path-ŏ-loj'ik, -i-kăl) Pertaining to the signs and symptoms manifested by a patient, and also the results of laboratory studies.

clino- Prefix meaning a slope (inclination or declination) or bend.

cli·no·ceph·a·ly (klī'nō-sef'ă-lē) Craniosynostosis in which the superior surface of the cranium is concave, presenting a saddle-shaped appearance in profile. SYN saddle head.

cli·no·dac·ty·ly (klī'nō-dak'ti-lē) Permanent deflection of one or more fingers.

cli·noid (klī'noyd) 1. Resembling a four-poster bed. 2. SYN clinoid process.

cli·noid pro·cess (klin'ōyd pros'es) [TA] One of three pairs of bony projections from the sphenoid bone.

cli·no·me·ter (klī-nom'ĕ-tĕr) Device used to measure slope and angle of elevation.

clip (klip) 1. A fastener used to hold a part or thing together with another. 2. A fastener used to close off a small vessel.

clith·ro·pho·bi·a (klīth'rō-fō'bē-ă) Morbid fear of being locked in.

clit·i·on (klit'ē-on) A craniometric point in the middle of the highest part of the clivus on the sphenoid bone.

clit·o·ri·dec·to·my (klit'ōr-i-dek'tŏ-mē) Surgical removal of the clitoris.

clit·o·ri·di·tis, clit·o·ri·tis (klit'ōr-i-dī'tis, -ōr-ī'tis) Inflammation of the clitoris.

clit·or·i·meg·a·ly, clit·o·ro·meg·a·ly (klit′ŏr-i-meg′ă-lē, -ŏr-ō-meg′ă-lē) Abnormally enlarged clitoris.

clit·o·ris, gen. **cli·to·ri·dis,** pl. **cli·to·ri·des** (klit′ŏr-is, klit-ōr′i-dis, -dēz) [TA] A cylindric, erectile body, rarely exceeding 2 cm in length, situated at the most anterior portion of the vulva and projecting between the branched limbs or laminae of the labia minora, which form its prepuce and frenulum. It consists of a glans, a corpus, and two crura.

clit·o·rism (klit′ŏr-ism) Prolonged and usually painful erection of the clitoris; the female analogue of priapism.

clit·or·o·plas·ty (klit′ŏr-ō-plas′tē) Any plastic surgery procedure on the clitoris.

cli·vog·ra·phy (klīv-og′ră-fē) Process of recording a radiographic image of the clivus.

cli·vus, pl. **cli·vi** (klī′vŭs, -vī) [TA] A downward sloping surface.

clo·a·ca, pl. **clo·a·cae** (klō-ā′kă, -kē) In early embryos, the endodermally lined chamber into which the hindgut and allantois empty.

clo·nal de·le·tion the·o·ry (klō′năl dĕ-plē′shŭn thē′ŏr-ē) Elimination of certain T-cell populations in the thymus that have specificity for self-antigens (forbidden clones). SEE immunologic tolerance.

clo·nal ex·pan·sion (klō′năl ek-span′shŭn) Production of daughter cells all arising originally from a single cell.

clo·nal·i·ty (klōn-al′i-tē) The capacity to be cloned.

clo·nal se·lec·tion the·or·y (klō′năl sĕ-lek′shŭn thē′ŏr-ē) A theory that states that each lymphocyte has membrane-bound immunoglobulin receptors specific for a particular antigen and after the receptor is engaged, proliferation of the cell occurs such that a clone of antibody producing cells (plasma cell) is produced.

clone (klōn) **1.** A colony of organisms or cells derived from a single organism or cell by asexual reproduction, all having identical genetic constitutions. **2.** To produce such a colony or individual. **3.** A short section of DNA that has been copied by means of gene cloning. SEE cloning.

clo·nic (klon′ik) Relating to or characterized by clonus.

clo·nic con·vul·sion (klon′ik kŏn-vŭl′shŭn) A convulsion in which the contractions are intermittent, the muscles alternately contracting and relaxing.

clon·i·co·ton·ic (klon′i-kō-ton′ik) Both clonic and tonic; said of certain forms of muscular spasm.

clo·nic sei·zure (klon′ik sē′zhŭr) One characterized by repetitive rhythmic jerking of all or part of the body.

clo·nic spasm (klon′ik spazm) Alternate involuntary contraction and relaxation of a muscle.

clo·nic state (klon′ik stāt) Movement marked by repetitive muscle contractions and relaxations in rapid succession.

clon·ing (klōn′ing) **1.** Growing a colony of genetically identical cells or organisms in vitro. **2.** Transplantation of a nucleus from a somatic cell to an oocyte or ovum, which then develops into an embryo; many identical embryos can thus be generated by asexual reproduction.

clon·ism (klō′nizm) A long continued state of clonic spasms.

clo·no·gen·ic (klō-nō-jen′ik) Arising from or consisting of a clone.

clo·nus, clon·o·spasm (klō′nŭs, klon′ō-spazm) A form of movement marked by contractions and relaxations of a muscle, occurring in rapid succession seen with, among other conditions, spasticity, and some seizure disorders. SEE ALSO contraction.

closed an·est·he·si·a (klōzd an′es-thē′zē-ă) Inhalation anesthesia in which there is total rebreathing of all exhaled gases, except carbon dioxide, which is absorbed.

closed bite (klōzd bīt) Reduced vertical interarch distance with excessive vertical overlap of the anterior teeth.

closed chest mas·sage (klōzd chest mă-sahzh′) Rhythmic compression of the heart between sternum and spine by depressing the lower sternum with the heels of the hands with the patient lying supine.

closed co·me·do (klōzd kom′ĕ-dō) An acne lesion with a narrow or obstructed opening on the skin surface; may rupture, producing a low-grade dermal inflammatory reaction. SYN whitehead (2).

closed drain·age (klōzd drān′ăj) Drainage of a body cavity through a water- or air-tight system.

closed frac·ture (klōzd frak′shŭr) Breakage in which skin is intact at site of fracture.

closed head in·jury (klōzd hed in′jŭr-ē) Head trauma in which continuity of the scalp and mucous membranes is maintained.

closed re·duc·tion (klōzd rĕ-duk′shŭn) Therapeutic intervention whereby fractured bone is restored to normal alignment without surgical incision.

closed sys·tem (klōzd sis′tĕm) Process in which there is no exchange of material, energy, or information with the environment.

close-packed po·si·tion (klōs′pakt pŏ-zish′ŭn) Joint position in which contact between the articulation structures is maximal. SYN joint extension.

clos·ing plug (klōz′ing plŭg) Fibrinous coagulum of blood that fills the defect in the endometrial epithelium created by the implanting blastocyst.

***Clos·trid·i·um* (C, Cl)** (klos-trid′ē-ŭm) A genus of anaerobic (or anaerobic, aerotolerant), spore-forming, motile (occasionally nonmotile) bacteria containing gram-positive rods; generally found in soil and in the mammalian intestinal tract, where they may cause disease.

Clos·trid·i·um bi·fer·men·tans (klos-trid′ē-ŭm bī-fĕr-men′tanz) Bacterial species found in putrid meat and gaseous gangrene; also commonly found in soil, feces, and sewage.

Clos·trid·i·um bot·u·li·num (klos-trid′ē-ŭm boch-ū-lī′nŭm) A bacterial species that occurs widely in nature and is a frequent cause of food poisoning (botulism) from preserved meats, fruits, or vegetables that have not been properly sterilized before canning.

Clos·trid·i·um dif·fi·ci·le (klos-trid′ē-ŭm dif-ē-sē′lē) Gram-positive obligate anaerobic or microaerophilic, rod-shaped bacterium; causes antibiotic-associated colitis. SYN C-Diff, CDT.

Clos·trid·i·um his·to·ly·t·i·cum (klos-trid′ē-ŭm his-tō-lit′i-kŭm) A bacterial species found in war wounds, where it induces necrosis of tissue.

Clos·trid·i·um per·frin·gens (klos-trid′ē-ŭm pĕr-frin′jenz) Bacterial species that is the chief causative agent of food poisoning and gas gangrene in humans. This organism is found in soil, water, milk, dust, sewage, and the intestinal tract of humans and other animals. Also called *Clostridium welchii*, gas bacillus, Welch bacillus.

Clos·trid·i·um spo·ro·ge·nes (klos-trid′ē-ŭm spō-roj′ĕ-nēz) Bacterial species found in intestinal contents, gaseous gangrene, and soil.

Clos·trid·i·um te·ta·ni (klos-trid′ē-ŭm tet′ă-nī) Bacterial species that causes tetanus.

clo·sy·late (klō′si-lāt) USAN-approved contraction for *p*-chlorobenzene sulfonate.

clot (klot) 1. To coagulate, said especially of blood. 2. A soft, nonrigid, insoluble mass formed when a liquid (e.g., blood or lymph) gels.

clot·ting (klot′ing) Process of coagulation, the transformation of blood from a liquid into a semisolid mass.

clot·ting fac·tor (klot′ing fak′tŏr) Any of the various plasma components involved in the clotting process.

clot·ting time (CT, CLT) (klot′ing tīm) SYN coagulation time.

cloud·y swell·ing (klow′dē swel′ing) Swelling of cells due to injury to the membranes affecting ionic transfer; causes an accumulation of intracellular water. SYN hydropic degeneration, parenchymatous degeneration.

clove oil (klōv oyl) SYN oil of clove.

club·bed pe·nis (klŭbd pē´nis) Deformity of the erect penis marked by a curve to one side or toward the scrotum.

club·bing (klŭb´ing) A condition affecting the fingers and toes in which proliferation of distal tissues, especially the nail beds, results in thickening and widening of the extremities of the digits; the nails are abnormally curved and shiny; the nail beds excessively compressible; overlying skin is red and shiny.

club drug (klŭb drŭg) A drug of abuse (e.g., ecstasy) that is typically used by most or all members of a social gathering rather than in solitude.

club hair (klŭb hār) A hair in resting state, before shedding, in which the bulb has become a club-shaped mass.

club·hand, club hand (klŭb´hand) Congenital or acquired angulation deformity of the hand associated with partial or complete absence of the radius or ulna; usually with intrinsic deformities in the hand in congenital variants.

clue cell (klū sel) A type of vaginal epithelial cell that appears granular and is coated with coccobacillary organisms; seen in bacterial vaginosis.

clump·ing (klŭmp´ing) The massing together of bacteria or other cells suspended in a fluid.

clus·ter anal·y·sis (klŭs´tĕr ă-nal´i-sis) Set of statistical methods used to group variables or observations into strongly interrelated subgroups.

clus·ter head·ache, Hor·ton syn·drome (klŭs´tĕr hed´āk, hōr´tŏn sin´drŏm) Possibly due to a hypersensitivity to histamine; usually characterized by recurrent, severe, unilateral orbitotemporal headaches associated with ipsilateral photophobia, lacrimation, and nasal congestion. SYN histaminic headache, Horton headache.

clus·ter of dif·fer·en·ti·a·tion (CD) (klŭs´tĕr dif´ĕr-en-shē-ā´shŭn) Cell membrane molecules that are used to classify leukocytes into subsets. CD molecules are classified by monoclonal antibodies.

cly·sis (klī´sis) An infusion of fluid, usually subcutaneously, for therapeutic purposes.

Cm Symbol for curium.

CNS Symbol for the thiocyanate radical, CNS− or —CNS; abbreviation for central nervous system.

Co Symbol for cobalt.

co·ad·ap·ta·tion (kō´ad-ap-tā´shŭn) The operation of selection jointly on two or more loci.

co·ag·glu·ti·na·tion (COA) (kō´ă-glū´tin-a´shŭn) Aggregation of particulate antigens bound with agglutinins of more than one specificity.

co·ag·u·la·ble (kō-ag´yū-lă-bĕl) Capable of being coagulated or clotted.

co·ag·u·lant (kō-ag´yū-lănt) **1.** An agent that causes, stimulates, or accelerates coagulation, especially with reference to blood. **2.** SYN coagulative.

co·ag·u·lase-neg·a·tive *Staph·y·lo·coc·cus* **spe·cies** (kō-ag´yū-lās neg´ă-tiv staf´i-lō-kok´ŭs spē´shēz) A group of bacterial species that includes a group of those present as normal flora of human skin, respiratory, and mucous membrane surfaces; prominent cause of nosocomial infections. Some strains form abscesses and cause diverse pathologic processes, such as sinusitis, wound infections, and osteomyelitis.

co·ag·u·late (kō-ag´yū-lāt) **1.** To convert a fluid or a substance in solution into a solid or gel. **2.** To clot; to curdle; to change from a liquid to a solid or gel.

co·ag·u·la·ted (kō-ag´yū-lāt-ĕd) Condition whereby blood is transformed from a liquid into a semisolid mass. SYN clotted.

co·ag·u·la·tion (kō-ag´yū-lā´shŭn) **1.** Clotting; the process by which a liquid, especially blood, changes from a liquid to a solid. **2.** A clot or coagulum. **3.** Transformation of a solution into a gel or semisolid mass.

co·ag·u·la·tion fac·tor (kō-ag'yū-lā' shŭn fak'tŏr) SYN clotting factor.

co·ag·u·la·tion time (CT, coag T) (kō-ag'yū-lā'shŭn tīm) Temporal duration required for blood to coagulate. SYN clotting time.

co·ag·u·la·tive (kō-ag'yū-lă-tiv) Causing coagulation. SYN coagulant (2).

co·ag·u·lop·a·thy (kō-ag'yū-lop'ă-thē) A disease affecting the coagulability of the blood.

co·ag·u·lum, pl. **co·ag·u·la** (kō-ag'yū-lŭm, -lă) A clot or a curd; a soft, nonrigid, insoluble mass formed when a solution undergoes coagulation.

co·al·co·hol·ic (kō-al'kŏ-hol'ik) **1.** The person who enables an alcoholic person by assuming responsibilities on the alcoholic's behalf, minimizing or denying the problem drinking, or making amends for the alcoholic's behavior. SEE ALSO codependent. **2.** Pertaining to the coalcoholic or to coalcoholism.

co·a·lesce (kō'ă-les') To fuse together, meld.

co·a·les·cence (kō'ă-les'ĕns) Fusion of originally separate parts. SYN concrescence (1).

coal tar (kōl tahr) Agent used to treat skin diseases.

coal work·er's pneu·mo·co·ni·o·sis (kōl wŏrk'ĕrz nū'mō-kō-nē-ō'sis) SYN anthracosilicosis.

co·apt (kō'apt) To join or fit together.

co·ap·ta·tion (kō'ap-tā'shŭn) Joining or fitting together of two surfaces.

co·ap·ta·tion su·ture (kō'ap-tā'shŭn sū' chŭr) SYN apposition suture.

co·arc·tate (kō-ahrk'tāt) Pressed together.

co·arc·ta·tion (kō'ahrk-tā'shŭn) A constriction, stricture, or stenosis, particularly of the aorta.

coarse (kōrs) Not smooth; rough; not fine.

coarse trem·or (kōrs trem'ŏr) One in with large amplitude and irregular and slow oscillations.

coat (kōt) The outer covering or envelope of an organ or part. SEE tunic.

coat·ed tongue (kōt'ĕd tŭng) One with a whitish layer on its upper surface, composed of epithelial debris, food particles, and bacteria; often an indication of indigestion or of fever. SYN furred tongue.

co·balt (Co) (kō'bawlt) A steel-gray metallic element, and a constituent of vitamin B12; certain of its compounds are pigments.

cob·bler's su·ture (kob'lĕrz sū'chŭr) SYN doubly armed suture.

co·ca (kō'kă) The dried leaves of *Erythroxylon coca*, yielding not less than 0.5% of ether-soluble alkaloids; source of cocaine and several other alkaloids.

co·caine (kō-kān') A crystalline alkaloid obtained from the leaves of *Erythroxylon coca* and other species, or by synthesis from ecgonine or its derivatives; a potent central nervous system stimulant, vasoconstrictor, and topical anesthetic, widely abused as a euphoriant and associated with the risk of severe adverse physical and mental effects.

co·caine nose (kō-kān' nōz) A constellation of findings in chronic intranasal abusers of cocaine, including damage to the mucous membrane of the nose, nasal collapse with saddle-nose deformity, palatal retraction and perforation, pharyngeal wall ulceration, sinusitis, and turbinate necrosis.

co·car·cin·o·gen (kō'kahr-sin'ŏ-jen) A substance that works symbiotically with a carcinogen in the production of cancer.

Coc·cid·i·a (kok-sid'ē-ă) A subclass of protozoa in which mature trophozoites are small and typically intracellular.

Coc·cid·i·oi·des (kok-sid'ē-oy'dēz) A genus of fungi found in the soil of the semiarid areas of the southwestern U.S. and smaller areas throughout Central and South America. The only pathogenic species, *Coccidioides immitis*, causes coccidioidomycosis.

coc·cid·i·oi·do·ma (kok-sid′ē-oy-dō′mă) Benign localized residual granulomatous lung lesion or scar following primary coccidioidomycosis.

coc·cid·i·o·sis (kok-sid′ē-ō′sis) Group name for diseases due to any species of coccidia; both intestinal and pulmonary coccidiosis have been reported in humans with AIDS.

coc·cid·i·um, gen. and pl. **coc·cid·ia** (kok-sid′ē-ŭm, -ă) Common name given to protozoan parasites in which schizogony occurs within epithelial cells, generally in the intestine; parasitic species occasionally in humans; most are nonpathogenic. SEE Isospora.

coc·co·ba·cil·lus (kok′ō-bă-sil′ŭs) A short, thick bacterial rod of the shape of an oval or slightly elongated coccus.

coc·cus, pl. **coc·ci** (kok′ŭs, -sī) A bacterium of round, spheroid, or ovoid form.

coc·cy·al·gi·a (kok′sē-al′jē-ă) SYN coccygodynia.

coc·cyg·e·al (Co) (kok-sij′ē-ăl) Relating to the coccyx.

coc·cyg·e·al gland (kok-sij′ē-ăl gland) [TA] An arteriovenous anastomosis supplied by the middle sacral artery and located on the pelvic surface of the coccyx.

coc·cyg·e·al plex·us (kok-sij′ē-ăl plek′sŭs) [TA] A small plexus formed by the fifth sacral and the coccygeal nerves.

coc·cy·gec·to·my (kok′si-jek′tŏ-mē) Removal of the coccyx.

coc·cyg·e·us (kok-sij′ē-ŭs) SEE coccygeus muscle.

coc·cyg·e·us mus·cle (kok-sij′ē-ŭs mŭs′ĕl) *Origin*, spine of ischium and sacrospinous ligament; *insertion*, sides of lower part of sacrum and upper part of coccyx; *action*, assists in support of pelvic floor, especially when intraabdominal pressures increase; *nerve supply*, third and fourth sacral. SYN ischiococcygeus.

coc·cy·go·dyn·i·a (kok′si-gō-din′ē-ă) Pain in the coccygeal region. SYN coccyalgia, coccydynia, coccyodynia.

coc·cy·got·o·my (kok′si-got′ŏ-mē) Operation for freeing the coccyx from its attachments.

coc·cyx, gen. **coc·cy·gis,** pl. **coc·cy·ges** (kok′siks, -si-jis, -jēz) [TA] *Avoid the mispronunciations kok′iks and kos′iks.* The small bone at the end of the vertebral column in humans, formed by the fusion of four rudimentary vertebrae; it articulates above with the sacrum. SYN os coccygis [TA], coccygeal bone, tail bone.

coch·le·a, pl. **coch·le·ae** (kok′lē-ă, -ē) [TA] The snail-shell-shaped dense bone in the petrous portion of the temporal bone, forming the anterior division of the labyrinth or internal ear (bony cochlea).

coch·le·ar ca·nal (kok′lē-ăr kă-nal′) The winding tube of the bony labyrinth that makes two-and-a-half turns about the modiolus of the cochlea; divided incompletely into two compartments by a winding shelf of bone. SYN canalis spiralis cochleae [TA].

coch·le·ar duct (kok′lē-ăr dŭkt) [TA] A spirally arranged membranous tube suspended within the cochlea, occupying the lower portion of the scala vestibuli.

coch·le·ar dys·pla·si·a (kok′lē-ăr dis-plāz′ē-ă) Failure of the bony cochlea to develop completely.

coch·le·ar·i·form (kok′lē-ar′i-fōrm) Spoon-shaped.

coch·le·ar im·plant (kok′lē-ăr im′plant) Auditory amplification device surgically implanted with its stimulating electrodes inserted directly into the nonfunctioning cochlea. SEE hearing aid. SEE ALSO amplification.

coch·le·ar joint (kok′lē-ăr joynt) A hinge articulation in which the elevation and depression, respectively, on the opposing articular surfaces form part of a spiral, flexion being accompanied by a certain amount of lateral deviation.

coch·le·ar lab·y·rinth (kok′lē-ăr lab′i-rinth) [TA] Part of the membranous labyrinth concerned with the sense of hearing (vs. the vestibular labyrinth, which is concerned with the sense of equilibration) and innervated by the cochlear nerve. SYN labyrinthus cochlearis [TA], organ of hearing.

coch·le·ar nerve (kok'lē-ăr nĕrv) [TA] Part of the vestibulocochlear nerve [CN VIII] peripheral to the cochlear root. SYN nervus cochlearis [TA], auditory nerve, cochlear part of vestibulocochlear nerve, inferior part of vestibulocochlear nerve, pars cochlearis nervi vestibulocochlearis.

coch·le·i·tis (kok'lē-ī'tis) Inflammation of the cochlea.

coch·le·o·pal·pe·bral re·flex (kok'lē-ō-pal'pĕ-brăl rē'fleks) A form of the wink reflex in which there is a contraction, sometimes very slight, of the orbicularis palpebrarum muscle when a sudden noise is made close to the ear. It is absent in labyrinthine disease with total deafness. SYN startle reflex (2).

coch·le·o·top·ic (kok'lē-ō-top'ik) Referring to the frequency-responsive organization of the central auditory pathways in the brain.

Coch·rane col·lab·o·ra·tion (kok'răn kŏ-lab'ŏr-ā'shŭn) A worldwide network of clinical epidemiologists who review and publish results of randomized controlled trials. The aim is to provide improved data for use in evidence-based medicine and for setting clinical practice guidelines. SEE ALSO evidence-based medicine.

cock·tail (kok'tāl) A mixture that includes several ingredients or drugs.

co·con·scious·ness (kō-kon'shŭs-nes) 1. A splitting of consciousness into two streams. 2. Awareness by one personality of the thoughts of another personality in dissociative disorder.

coc·to·la·bile (kok'tō-lā'bil) Subject to alteration or destruction when exposed to the temperature of boiling water.

coc·to·sta·bile, coc·to·sta·ble (kok'tō-stā'bil, -bĕl) Resisting the temperature of boiling water without alteration or destruction.

code (kōd) 1. A set of rules, principles, or ethics. 2. Any system devised to convey information or facilitate communication. 3. Term used in hospitals to describe an

emergency requiring situation-trained members of the staff, such as a cardiopulmonary resuscitation team, or the signal to summon such a team. 4. A numeric system for ordering and classifying information, e.g., about diagnostic categories.

co·deine (COD, cod.) (kō'dēn) Alkaloid obtained from opium, which contains 0.7–2.5%, but usually made from morphine. Used as an analgesic and antitussive; drug dependence (physical and psychic) may develop, but codeine is less liable to produce addiction than morphine. SYN methylmorphine.

co·deine phos·phate (kō'dēn fos'fāt) Water-soluble salt of codeine often used in the pharmaceutical preparation of liquid medications containing codeine.

co·deine sul·fate (kō'dēn sŭl'fāt) Water-soluble salt of codeine, often used in solid pharmaceutical dosage forms. Also used in preparations in which the drug suppresses the cough reflex.

code link·age (kōd lingk'ăj) In health care accounting, verification that the diagnosis code and procedure code match up to support medical necessity for therapy.

cod·ing (kōd'ing) Assigning a number to a disease process, surgical procedure, or other type of health care service for the purpose of reimbursement, health care planning, and research.

cod liv·er oil (CLO) (kod liv'ĕr oyl) The partially destearinated fixed oil extracted from the fresh livers of the codfish (*Gadus morrhuae*) and other species of the family Gadidae, containing vitamins A and D; used as a supplementary source of vitamins A and D.

co·don (kō'don) A set of three consecutive nucleotides in a strand of DNA or RNA that provides the genetic information to code for a specific amino acid that will be incorporated into a protein chain or serve as a termination signal. SEE ALSO genetic code. SYN triplet (3).

coe- For words so beginning, and not found here, see ce-.

co·ef·fi·cient (kō'ĕ-fish'ĕnt) 1. The expression of the amount or degree of any quality possessed by a substance, or of the degree of physical or chemical change normally occurring in that substance under stated conditions. **2.** The ratio or factor that relates a quantity observed under one set of conditions to that observed under standard conditions, usually when all variables are either 1 or a simple power of 10.

co•ef•fi•cient of var•i•a•tion (CV) (kō'ĕ-fish'ĕnt var'ē-ā'shŭn) A unitless number used to describe dispersion of data. It allows comparison of standard deviations of test results expressed in different units. It is calculated from the standard deviation (s) and mean (x). $CV = 100s \div x$.

Coe•len•ter•a•ta (sē-len-tĕ-rā'tă) One of the major phyla of invertebrates, to which forms such as jellyfish belong; members called coelenterates.

coeliac [Br.] SYN celiac.

coeliac disease [Br.] SYN celiac disease.

coeliac ganglia [Br.] SYN celiac ganglia.

coeliac trunk [Br.] SYN celiac trunk.

coelio- [Br.] SYN celio-.

coelioscopy [Br.] SYN celios copy.

coeliotomy [Br.] SYN celiotomy.

coelitis [Br.] SYN celitis.

coelo- [Br.] SYN celo-.

coelom [Br.] SYN celom.

coeno- Combining form meaning shared in common. SEE ALSO ceno-.

co•en•zyme (kō-en'zīm) A substance (excluding solo metal ions) that enhances or is necessary for the action of enzymes; smaller molecular size than the enzymes themselves. SYN cofactor (1).

co•en•zyme A (CoA) (kō-en'zīm) A coenzyme containing pantothenic acid, adenosine 3'-phosphate 5'-pyrophosphate, and cysteamine; involved in the transfer of acyl groups, notably in transacetylations.

co•en•zyme Q (Q) (kō-en'zīm) Quinones with isoprenoid side chains (specifically, ubiquinones) that mediate electron transfer between cytochrome b and cytochrome c.

coeur (kur) SYN heart.

co•fac•tor (kō'fak'tŏr) **1.** SYN coenzyme. **2.** An atom or molecule essential for the action of a large molecule.

cof•fee-ground vom•i•tus (kaw'fē grownd vom'i-tŭs) Emesis with small pebbled lumps (e.g., having the appearance of ground coffee) due to bleeding in upper gastrointestinal tract.

Co•gan-Reese syn•drome (kō'găn rēs sin'drōm) SYN iridocorneal endothelial syndrome.

cog•ni•tion (COGN) (kog-ni'shŭn) Generic term embracing the mental activities associated with thinking, learning, and memory.

cog•ni•tive-be•ha•vior•al ther•a•py (CBT) (kog'ni-tiv-bē-hāv'yŭr-ăl thār'ă-pē) Broadening of behavior therapy to include consideration of cognitive processes and use specific techniques for teaching cognitive skills that help the patient adaptively perceive, interpret, and respond to the environment. SEE ALSO cognitive therapy, psychotherapy.

cog•ni•tive de•vel•op•ment (kog'ni-tiv dĕ-vel'ŏp-mĕnt) Process of acquiring more complex ways of thinking as a person grows from infancy through adulthood.

cog•ni•tive func•tion (kog'ni-tiv fŭngk'shŭn) Denotes the brain's ability to process information.

cog•ni•tive psy•chol•o•gy (kog'ni-tiv sī-kol'ŏ-jē) Branch of psychology that attempts to integrate into a whole the disparate knowledge from the subfields of perception, learning, memory, intelligence, and thinking.

cog•ni•tive ther•a•py (kog'ni-tiv thār'ă-pē) Any one of a variety of techniques in psychotherapy that uses guided self-discovery, imaging, self-instruction, symbolic modeling, and related forms of explicitly elicited cognitions as the principal mode of treatment.

cog·wheel res·pi·ra·tion (kog′wēl res′ pir-ā′shŭn) Inspiratory sound interrupted by one or two by silent intervals. SYN interrupted respiration, jerky respiration.

cog·wheel ri·gid·i·ty (kog′wēl ri-jid′i-tē) A type of inflexibility seen in parkinsonism in which the muscles respond with cogwheellike jerks to the use of constant force in bending the limb.

co·he·rence (kō-hēr′ĕns) A characteristic of laser light, in which all light waves are aligned and move in phase.

co·he·rin (kō-hēr′in) A posterior pituitary hormone that regulates peristaltic activity in intestinal smooth muscle.

co·he·sion (kō-hē′zhŭn) The attraction between molecules or masses that holds them together.

co·hort (kō′hōrt) **1.** Component of the population born during a particular period and identified by period of birth so that its characteristics can be ascertained as it enters successive time and age periods. **2.** Any designated group followed or traced over a period, as in an epidemiologic or research cohort study.

coil (koyl) **1.** A spiral or series of loops. **2.** An object made of wire wound in a spiral configuration, used in electronic applications.

co·in·fec·tion (kō′in-fek′shŭn) Concurrent infection by two or more pathogens.

coin·o·site (koyn′ō-sīt) SYN cenosite.

co·i·to·pho·bi·a (kō′i-tō-fō′bē-ă) Morbid fear of sexual intercourse.

co·i·tus (kō′i-tŭs) Sexual union. SYN coition, copulation (1), pareunia, sexual intercourse.

co·i·tus in·ter·rup·tus (kō′i-tŭs in-tĕr-rŭp′tŭs) Sexual intercourse that is interrupted before the male ejaculates.

co·i·tus re·ser·va·tus (kō′i-tŭs rez-ĕr-vā′tŭs) Sexual intercourse in which ejaculation is postponed or suppressed.

Co·ker·o·my·ces (kō′ker-ō-mī′sēz) A fungal genus in the order Mucorales.

col (kol) A craterlike area of the interproximal oral mucosa joining the lingual and buccal interdental papillae.

col·chi·cine (kol′chi-sin) An alkaloid obtained from *Colchicum autumnale* used to treat chronic gout.

cold (kōld) **1.** A low temperature; the sensation produced by a temperature notably below an accustomed norm or a comfortable level. **2.** Popular term for a virus infection involving the upper respiratory tract and characterized by congestion of the mucosa, watery nasal discharge, and general malaise, with a duration of 3–5 days. SEE ALSO rhinitis. SYN common cold, frigid (1), upper respiratory infection, upper respiratory tract infection.

cold ab·scess (kōld ab′ses) **1.** An abscess without heat or other usual signs of inflammation. **2.** SYN tuberculous abscess.

cold ag·glu·ti·nin (kōld ă-glū′ti-nin) An antibody that reacts more efficiently at temperatures below 37°C.

cold al·ler·gy (kōld al′ĕr-jē) Physical symptoms produced by hypersensitivity to cold.

cold-blood·ed (kōld-blŭd′ed) SYN poikilothermic.

cold cau·ter·y (kōld kaw′tĕr-ē) SYN cryocautery.

cold er·y·the·ma (kōld er-i-thē′mă) Rash characterized by redness and itching, brought on by exposure to cold.

cold-in·duced ur·ti·ca·ri·a (kōld′in-dūst′ ŭr′ti-kar′ē-ă) Hives resulting from exposure to cold.

cold knife co·ni·za·tion (kōld nīf kon′i-zā′shŭn) Obtaining a cone of endocervical tissue with a cold knife blade so as to preserve histologic characteristics and avoid desiccating tissue.

cold sore (kōld sōr) Colloquialism for blister caused by herpes simplex.

cold stage (kōld stāj) The stage of chill in a malarial paroxysm.

cold ther·a·py (kōld thār′ă-pē) A type of care in which ice or cold water is applied to a body part. SYN cryotherapy.

cold ur·ti·ca·ria (kōld ŭr′ti-kar′ē-ă) Hypersensitivity to cold leading to superficial vascular reaction manifested by transient itching, erythema, and hives. SEE ALSO hypothermia.

col·ec·to·my (kŏ-lek′tŏ-mē) Excision of a segment or of the entire colon.

co·le·ot·o·my (kō′lē-ot′ŏ-mē) SYN colpotomy.

co·li·bac·il·lo·sis (kō′li-bas-i-lō′sis) Diarrheal disease caused by the bacterium *Escherichia coli*; often called enteric colibacillosis.

col·ic (kol′ik) 1. Relating to the colon. 2. Spasmodic pains in the abdomen. 3. In young infants, paroxysms of gastrointestinal pain, with crying and irritability, due to a variety of causes, such as swallowing of air, emotional upset, or overfeeding.

col·i·cin (kol′i-sin) Bacteriocin produced by strains of *Escherichia coli* and other enterobacteria.

col·ick·y (kol′ik-ē) Denoting or resembling the pain of colic (q.v.).

col·i·co·ple·gi·a (kol′i-kō-plē′jē-ă) Lead poisoning marked by both colic and palsy.

col·i·form ba·cil·li (kō′li-fōrm bă-sil′ī) Common name for *Escherichia coli* that is used as an indicator of fecal contamination of water, measured in terms of coliform count. Occasionally used to refer to all lactose-fermenting enteric bacteria.

co·li·phage (kol′i-fāj) A bacteriophage with an affinity for one or another strain of *Escherichia coli*.

co·li·punc·ture (kō′li-pŭngk-shŭr) SYN colocentesis.

co·li·tis, pl. **co·lit·i·des** (kō-lī′tis, -ti-dēz) Inflammation of the colon.

col·i·tox·in (kō′li-toks′in) A toxin of *Escherichia coli*.

col·la·gen (kol′ă-jen) The major protein of the white fibers of connective tissue, cartilage, and bone; insoluble in water but can be altered to easily digestible, soluble gelatins by boiling in water, dilute acids, or alkalies. SYN ossein, osseine, ostein, osteine.

col·la·gen·ase (kŏ-laj′ĕ-nās) A proteolytic enzyme that acts on one or more of the collagens.

col·la·gen disease, col·la·gen-vas·cu·lar dis·ease (kol′ă-jen di-zēz′, kol′ă-jen-vas′kyū-lăr) A group of generalized diseases affecting connective tissue and frequently characterized by fibrinoid necrosis or vasculitis.

col·la·gen fi·brils (kol′ă-jen fī′brilz) SYN unit fibrils.

col·lag·e·ni·tis (kol′ă-jĕ-nī′tis) Inflammation of collagen fibers of connective tissue.

col·lag·e·ni·za·tion (kŏ-laj′ĕ-nī-zā′shŭn) 1. Replacement of tissues or fibrin by collagen. 2. Synthesis of collagen by fibroblasts.

col·lag·e·no·lyt·ic (kŏ-laj′ĕ-nō-lit′ik) Causing the lysis of collagen, gelatin, and other proteins containing proline.

col·lag·e·nous (kŏ-laj′ĕ-nŭs) Producing or containing collagen. SYN collagenic.

col·lapse (kŏ-laps′) 1. A condition of extreme prostration. 2. A state of profound physical depression. 3. A falling together of the walls of a structure or the failure of a physiologic system.

col·lar (kol′ăr) 1. A garment or part of a garment surrounding the neck. 2. Any encircling band.

col·lar bone (kol′ăr bōn) SYN clavicle.

col·lar-but·ton ab·scess (kol′ăr-bŭt′ŏn ab′ses) An abscess consisting of two cavities connected by a narrow channel, usually formed by rupture of an abscess through an overlying fascia. SYN shirt-stud abscess.

col·lar·ette (kol′ăr-et′) 1. The sinuous, scalloped line in the iris that divides the central pupillary zone from the peripheral ciliary zone and marks the embryonic site of the atrophied minor vascular circle of the iris. 2. Brittle scales encircling eyelashes in staphylococcal blepharitis. SYN iris frill.

col·lat·er·al (kŏ-lat′ĕr-ăl) **1.** Indirect, subsidiary, or accessory to the main thing; side by side. **2.** A side branch of a nerve axon or blood vessel.

col·lat·er·al cir·cu·la·tion (kŏ-lat′ĕr-ăl sĭr′kyū-lā′shŭn) Circulation maintained in small anastomosing vessels when the main vessel is obstructed.

col·lat·er·al hy·per·e·mia (kŏ-lat′ĕr-ăl hī′pĕr-ē′mē-ă) Increased blood flow through abundant collateral channels when circulation through the main artery to a part is arrested.

col·lat·er·al in·her·i·tance (kŏ-lat′ĕr-ăl in-her′i-tăns) Appearance of characters in collateral members of a family group, as when an uncle and a niece show the same character inherited from a common ancestor; in recessive characters it may appear irregularly, in contrast to dominant characters transmitted directly from one generation to the next.

col·lat·er·al ven·til·a·tion (kŏ-lat′ĕr-ăl ven-ti-lā′shŭn) Process by which gas passes from one lung unit to a contiguous unit through alveolar pores or direct airway anastomoses; sometimes also called collateral air drift.

col·lat·er·al ves·sel (kŏ-lat′ĕr-ăl ves′ĕl) [TA] **1.** A branch of an artery running parallel with the parent trunk. **2.** A vessel that runs in parallel with another vessel, nerve, or other long structure.

col·lec·tive un·con·scious (kŏ-lek′tiv ŭn-kon′shŭs) PSYCHOLOGY Combined engrams or memory potentials inherited from a person's phylogenetic past in Jung's theory.

col·lic·u·lec·to·my (kŏ-lik′yū-lek′tŏ-mē) Excision of the colliculus seminalis.

col·lic·u·li·tis (kŏ-lik′yū-lī′tis) Inflammation of the urethra in the region of the colliculus seminalis.

col·lic·u·lus, gen. and pl. **col·lic·u·li** (kŏ-lik′yū-lŭs, -lī) [TA] A small elevation above the surrounding parts.

col·lic·u·lus se·mi·na·lis (ko-lik′yū-lŭs sem-i-nā′lis) [TA] SYN seminal colliculus.

Col·lier sign (kol′yĕr sīn) Unilateral or bilateral lid retraction due to midbrain lesion; occurring at any age. SEE setting sun sign, Epstein sign. SYN Collier tucked lid sign.

col·li·ga·tive (ko-lig′ă-tiv) **1.** Depending on numbers of particles. **2.** Referring to properties of solutions that depend only on the concentration of dissolved substances and not on their nature (e.g., osmotic pressure, elevation of boiling point, vapor pressure lowering, freezing point depression).

col·li·ma·tion (kol′i-mā′shŭn) **1.** RADIOLOGY the process of restricting and confining the x-ray beam to a given area. **2.** NUCLEAR MEDICINE restricting the detection of emitted radiations from a given area of interest.

col·liq·ua·tive (kŏ-lik′wă-tiv) Denoting or characteristic of colliquation.

col·lo·di·on, col·lo·di·um (ko-lō′dē-on, -dē-ŭm) A liquid made by dissolving pyroxylin or gun cotton in ether and alcohol; on evaporation it leaves a glossy contractile film; used as a protective for cuts or as a vehicle for the local application of medicinal substances.

col·loid (kol′oyd) **1.** Aggregates of atoms or molecules in a finely divided state (submicroscopic), dispersed in a gaseous, liquid, or solid medium, and resisting sedimentation, diffusion, and filtration, thus differing from precipitates. SEE ALSO hydrocolloid. **2.** Gluelike. **3.** A translucent, yellowish, homogeneous material of the consistency of glue, less fluid than mucoid or mucinoid, found in the cells and tissues in a state of colloid degeneration. SYN colloidin. **4.** The stored secretion within follicles of the thyroid gland.

col·loid ad·e·no·ma (kol′oyd ad′ĕ-nō′mă) A follicular adenoma of the thyroid, composed of large follicles containing colloid. SYN macrofollicular adenoma.

col·loi·dal so·lu·tion (kol-oyd′ăl sŏ-lū′shŭn) A dispersoid, emulsoid, or suspensoid.

col·loid bath (kol′oyd bath) A therapeutic bath prepared by adding soothing agents such as sodium bicarbonate or oatmeal to the bath water to relieve skin irritation and pruritus.

col·loid car·ci·no·ma (kol´oyd kahr´si-nō´mă) SYN mucinous carcinoma.

col·loid cor·pus·cle (kol´oyd kōr´pŭs-ĕl) SYN corpus amylaceum.

col·loid cyst (kol´oyd sist) Lesion with gelatinous contents.

col·loid mil·i·um (kol´oyd mil´ē-ŭm) Yellow papules developing in sun-damaged skin of the head and backs of the hands, composed of colloid material in the dermis resembling amyloid but with a different ultrastructure. SYN colloid acne, colloid pseudomilium.

col·lum, gen. and pl. **col·la** (kol´ŭm, -ă) SYN neck.

col·lyr·i·um (kŏ-lir´ē-ŭm) Originally, any preparation for the eye; now, an eyewash.

colo- Combining form denoting the colon.

col·o·bo·ma (kol´ō-bō´mă) Any defect—congenital, pathologic, or artificial—especially of the eye due to incomplete closure of the optic fissure.

co·lo·cen·te·sis (kō´lō-sen-tē´sis) Surgical puncture of the colon with a trochar or scalpel to relieve distention. SYN colopuncture.

co·lo·cho·le·cys·tos·to·my (kō´lō-kō-lē-sis-tos´tŏ-mē) SYN cholecystocolostomy.

co·lo·co·los·to·my (kō´lō-kō-los´tŏ-mē) Surgical establishment of a communication between two noncontinuous segments of the colon.

co·lon (kō´lŏn) [TA] The division of the large intestine extending from the cecum to the rectum.

co·lon·ic (kō-lon´ik) Relating to the colon.

col·o·ni·za·tion (kol´ŏn-ī-zā´shŭn) SYN innidiation.

col·on·og·ra·phy, col·og·ra·phy (kō-lŏn-og´ra-fē, kō-log´ră-fē) Imaging study of the colon, most often using CT or MRI. SEE ALSO barium enema.

co·lon·os·co·py, co·los·co·py, co·lon·sco·py (kō´lŏn-os´kŏ-pē, kō-los´kŏ-pē, kō´lŏn-skop´ē) Visual examination of the inner surface of the colon by means of a colonoscope.

co·lon·scope (kō´lŏn-skōp) Instrument used to examine the colon. Also called colonoscope.

col·o·ny (kol´ō-nē) **1.** A group of cells growing on a solid nutrient surface, each arising from the multiplication of an individual cell; a clone. **2.** A group of people with similar interests, living in a particular location or area.

col·o·ny-stim·u·la·ting fac·tors (CSF) (kol´ŏ-nē-stim´yū-lāt-ing fak´tŏrz) A group of glycoprotein growth factors regulating differentiation in myeloid cell lines.

col·o·pex·y (kō´lō-pek-sē) Attachment of a portion of the colon to the abdominal wall.

co·lo·pli·ca·tion (kō´lō-pli-kā´shŭn) Reduction of the lumen of a dilated colon by making folds or tucks in its walls.

co·lo·proc·tos·to·my (kō´lō-prok-tos´tŏ-mē) Establishment surgically of a communication between the rectum and a discontinuous segment of the colon. SYN colorectostomy.

co·lop·to·sis, co·lop·to·si·a (kō´lop-tō´sis, -tō´sē-ă) Downward displacement, or prolapse, of the colon, especially of the transverse portion.

co·lo·punc·ture (kō´lō-pŭngk´shŭr) SYN colocentesis.

col·or (kŏl´ŏr) **1.** That aspect of the appearance of objects and light sources that may be specified as to hue, lightness (brightness), and saturation. **2.** That portion of the visible (370–760 nm) electromagnetic spectrum specified as to wavelength, luminosity, and purity. SYN colour.

col·or blind·ness (kŏl´ŏr blīnd´nĕs) Misleading term for anomalous or deficient color vision; complete color blindness is the absence of one of the primary cone pigments of the retina. SEE protanopia, deuteranopia, tritanopia. SYN colour blindness.

col·or chart (kŏl´ŏr chahrt) An assembly

of chromatic samples used in checking color vision. SYN chromatic chart.

co·lo·rec·tos·to·my (kō′lō-rek-tos′tŏ-mē) SYN coloproctostomy.

col·ored vi·sion (VC) (kŏl′ŏrd vizh′ŭn) SYN chromatopsia, coloured vision.

col·or hear·ing (kŏl′ŏr hēr′ing) Subjective perception of color produced by certain sounds. SYN chromatic audition.

col·or·im·e·ter (kŏl′ŏr-im′ĕ-tĕr) An optic device for determining the color and/or intensity of the color of a liquid. SYN colourimeter.

co·lor·rha·gi·a (kō′lŏr-rā′jē-ă) An abnormal discharge from the colon.

co·lor·rha·phy (kō-lōr′ă-fē) Suture of the colon.

col·or sco·to·ma (kŏl′ŏr skō-tō′mă) An area of depressed color vision in the visual field. SYN colour scotoma.

col·or sense (C) (kŏl′ŏr sens) Ability to perceive variations in hue, luminosity, and saturation of light.

co·los·co·py (kō-los′kŏ-pē) SYN colonoscopy.

co·lo·sig·moi·dos·to·my (kō′lō-sig-moy-dos′tŏ-mē) Establishment surgically of an anastomosis between any other part of the colon and the sigmoid colon.

co·los·to·my (kō-los′tŏ-mē) Establishment surgically of an artificial cutaneous opening into the colon.

co·los·to·my bag (kō-los′tŏ-mē bag) Container worn over a surgically produced connection between the colon and the skin to collect feces.

co·los·tric (kō-los′trik) Relating to the colostrum.

co·los·tror·rhe·a (kō-los′trōr-ē′ă) Abnormally profuse secretion of colostrum. SYN colostrorrhoea.

colostrorrhoea [Br.] SYN colostrorrhea.

co·los·trum (kŏ-los′trŭm) A thin white opalescent fluid, the first milk secreted at the termination of pregnancy. SYN foremilk.

co·lot·o·my (kō-lot′ŏ-mē) Incision into the colon.

colour [Br.] SYN color.

colour blindness [Br.] SYN color blindness.

coloured vision [Br.] SYN colored vision.

colour hearing [Br.] SYN color hearing.

colourimeter [Br.] SYN colorimeter.

Col·our In·dex (CI) (kŏl′ŏr in′deks) A publication concerned with the chemistry of dyes, with each listed dye identified by a five-digit Colour Index number, e.g., methylene blue is Colour Index 52015.

colour scotoma [Br.] SYN color scotoma.

co·lo·ves·i·cal fis·tu·la (kō′lō-ves′i-kăl fis′tyū-lă) Fistulous passage connecting the colon and urinary bladder. SYN vesicocolic fistula.

♻ **colp-** SEE colpo-.

col·pa·tre·si·a (kol′pă-trē′zē-ă) SYN vaginal atresia.

col·pec·ta·sis, col·pec·ta·si·a (kol-pek′tă-sis, -pek-tā′zē-ă) Distention of the vagina.

col·pec·to·my (kol-pek′tŏ-mē) SYN vaginectomy.

♻ **colpo-, colp-** Combining forms meaning the vagina. SEE ALSO vagino-.

col·po·cele (kol′pō-sēl) SYN colpoptosis.

col·po·clei·sis (kol′pō-klī′sis) Operation for obliterating the lumen of the vagina.

col·po·cys·to·cele (kol′pō-sis′tō-sēl) SYN cystocele.

col·po·cys·to·plas·ty (kol′pō-sis′tō-plas-tē) Plastic surgery to repair the vesicovaginal wall.

col·po·hys·ter·ec·to·my (kol′pō-his′-tĕr-ek′tŏ-mē) SYN vaginal hysterectomy.

col·po·mi·cro·scope (kol′pō-mī′krŏ-skōp) Special microscope for direct visual examination of the cervical tissue.

col·po·per·i·ne·or·rha·phy (kol′pō-per-i-nē-ōr′ă-fē) SYN vaginoperineorrhaphy.

col·po·pex·y (kol′pō-pek-sē) SYN vaginofixation.

col·po·pto·sis, col·po·pto·si·a (kol′pō-tō′sis, -sē-ă) Prolapse of the vaginal walls. SYN colpocele (2).

col·por·rha·gi·a (kol′pōr-ā′jē-ă) A vaginal hemorrhage.

col·por·rha·phy (kol-pōr′ă-fē) Repair of a rupture of the vagina by excision and suturing of the edges of the tear.

col·por·rhex·is (kol′pō-rek′sis) Tearing of the vaginal wall.

col·po·scope (kol′pō-skōp) Endoscopic instrument that magnifies cells of the vagina and cervix in vivo to allow direct observation and study of these tissues.

col·po·spasm (kol′pō-spazm) Spasmodic contraction of the vagina.

col·po·ste·no·sis (kol′pō-stĕ-nō′sis) Narrowing of the lumen of the vagina.

col·po·ste·not·o·my (kol′pō-stĕ-not′ŏ-mē) Surgical correction of a colpostenosis.

col·pot·o·my (kol-pot′ŏ-mē) A cutting operation in the vagina. SYN coleotomy, vaginotomy.

col·po·xe·ro·sis (kol′pō-zēr-ō′sis) Abnormal dryness of the vaginal mucous membrane.

col·u·mel·la, pl. **col·u·mel·lae** (kol′yū-mel′ă, -ē) 1. A small column. SYN columnella. 2. In fungi, a sterile invagination of a sporangium, as in Zygomycetes.

col·u·mel·la na·si (kol′yū-mel′ă nā′zī) The nasal skin investing the medial crura of the lower lateral cartilages and separating the nostrils.

col·umn (kol′ŭm) *Avoid the common mispronunciation koll′yum.* [TA] 1. An anatomic part or structure in the form of a pillar or cylindric funiculus. SYN columna [TA]. 2. A vertical object (usually cylindric), mass, or formation. SEE ALSO fascicle.

co·lum·na, gen. and pl. **co·lum·nae** (kō-lŭm′nă, -nē) [TA] SYN column (1).

co·lum·nar (kŏ-lŭm′năr) Pertaining to any form or body part that is higher than it is wide.

co·lum·nar ep·it·he·li·um (CE) (kŏ-lŭm′năr ep′i-thē′lē-ŭm) Epithelium formed of a single layer of prismatic cells taller than they are wide. SYN cylindric epithelium.

co·ma (kō′mă) 1. A state of profound unconsciousness from which one cannot be roused; may result from trauma, disease, or the action of an ingested toxic substance or of one formed in the body. 2. An aberration of spheric lenses; occurring in cases of oblique incidence (e.g., the image of a point becomes comet shaped).

co·ma scale (kō′mă skāl) A clinical measurement to assess impaired consciousness; may include motor responsiveness, verbal performance, and eye opening, as in the Glasgow (Scotland) Coma Scale, or the same three items and dysfunction of cranial nerves, as in the Maryland (U.S.) Coma Scale.

com·bi·na·tion che·mo·ther·a·py (kom-bi-nā′shŭn kē-mō-thār′ă-pē) Therapy using more than a single drug to exploit the varying levels of toxicity for the patient's benefit.

com·bined glau·co·ma (kŏm-bīnd′ glaw-kō′mă) Ocular disorder with angle-closure and open-angle mechanisms in the same eye.

com·bined preg·nan·cy (kŏm-bīnd′ preg′năn-sē) Coexisting uterine and ectopic pregnancy.

com·bined sys·tem dis·ease (CSD)

(kŏm-bīnd´ sis´tĕm di-zēz´) SYN sub-acute combined degeneration of the spinal cord.

com·bined ver·sion (kom-bīnd´ ver´ zhŭn) Bipolar obstetric version by means of one hand in the vagina, the other on the abdominal wall during childbirth.

com·bus·tion (kŏm-bŭs´chŭn) Burning.

Com·by sign (kom´bē sīn) Early symptom of measles, consisting of thin, whitish patches on the gums and buccal mucous membrane, formed of desquamating epithelial cells.

com·e·do, pl. **com·e·dos**, pl. **com·e·do·nes** (kom´ĕ-dō, -dōz, -dō´nēz) A dilated hair follicle infundibulum filled with keratin squamae, bacteria, particularly *Propionibacterium acnes*, and sebum; primary lesion of acne vulgaris.

com·e·do·gen·ic (kom´ĕ-dō-jen´ik) Tending to promote the formation of comedones.

co·mes, pl. **com·i·tes** (kō´mēz, -mi-tēz) A blood vessel accompanying another vessel or a nerve; the veins accompanying an artery, often two in number, are called venae comitantes or venae comites.

com·fort zone (kŭm´fŏrt zōn) Temperature range between 28–30°C at which the naked body is able to maintain the heat balance without either shivering or sweating; in the clothed body the range is from 13–21°C.

com·i·tant (kom´i-tănt) Having comitance. SYN concomitant.

com·i·tant stra·bis·mus (kom´i-tănt stră-biz´mŭs) A condition in which the degree of strabismus is the same in all directions of gaze.

com·man·do pro·ce·dure (kŏ-man´dō prŏ-sē´jŭr) Operation for malignant tumors of the floor of the oral cavity, involving resection of portions of the mandible in continuity with the oral lesion and radical neck dissection. SYN commando operation.

com·men·sal (kŏ-men´săl) 1. Pertaining to or characterized by commensalism. 2.

An organism participating in commensalism.

com·mi·nut·ed (com) (kom´i-nū´tĕd) Broken into several pieces; denoting especially a fractured bone.

com·mi·nut·ed frac·ture (kom´i-nū´tĕd frak´shŭr) A fracture in which the bone is broken into pieces.

com·mis·su·ra for·ni·cis (kom´i-sū´ră fōr´ni-sis) The triangular subcallosal plate of commissural fibers resulting from the converging of the right and left fornix bundles that exchange numerous fibers and that curve back in the contralateral fornix to end in the hippocampus of the opposite side.

com·mis·sur·al fi·bers (kom-i-shŭr´ăl fī´bĕrz) Nerve fibers crossing the midline and connecting two corresponding parts or regions of the nervous system.

com·mis·su·ra pos·te·ri·or (kom´i-sū´ ră pos-tēr´ē-ŏr) A thin band of white matter composed of fibers interconnecting the left and right pretectal region and related cell groups of the midbrain.

com·mis·su·ra su·pra·op·ti·ca dor·sa·lis (kom´i-sū´ră sū´pră-op´ti-kă dōr-sā´lis) The commissural fibers that lie above and behind the optic chiasm. SYN Gudden commissure.

com·mis·sur·ot·o·my (kom´i-shŭr-ot´ ŏ-mē) 1. Surgical division of any commissure, fibrous band, or ring via an incision or disruption, e.g., balloon inflation. 2. SYN midline myelotomy.

com·mit·ment (com) (kŏ-mit´mĕnt) Legal consignment, by certification, or voluntarily, of a patient to a mental hospital or institution.

com·mon ac·ne (kom´ŏn ak´nē) Dermatologic condition with eruptions of comedones, papules, pustules, and cysts of various types and sizes. SYN acne vulgaris.

com·mon a·cute lymph·o·blas·tic leu·ke·mia an·ti·gen (CALLA) (kom´ ŏn ă-kyūt´ lim-fō-blas´tik lū-kē´mē-ă an´ ti-jen) Agent that detects this disease and the related lymphoblastic lymphomas.

com·mon an·ti·gen (CA) (kom´ŏn an´ ti-jen) Cross-reacting antigen (epitope);

occurs in two or more different molecules or organisms.

com·mon atri·um (kom′ŏn ā′trē-ŭm) A single abnormal atrium in a three-chambered heart in which the interatrial septum is absent. SYN cor triloculare biventriculare.

com·mon bald·ness (kom′ŏn bawld′nĕs) SYN androgenic alopecia.

com·mon ba·sal vein (kom′ŏn bā′săl vān) [TA] The tributary to the inferior pulmonary vein (right and left) that receives blood from the superior and inferior basal veins.

com·mon ca·rot·id ner·vous plex·us (kom′ŏn kă-rot′id nĕr′vŭs plek′sŭs) [TA] An autonomic plexus accompanying the artery of the same name formed by fibers from the middle cervical ganglion. SYN plexus (nervosus) caroticus communis [TA].

com·mon coch·le·ar ar·te·ry (kom′ŏn kok′lē-ăr ahr′tĕr-ē) [TA] *Origin,* as a terminal branch, with the anterior vestibular artery, of the labyrinthine artery; *distribution,* runs in the cochlear axis of modiolus serving the spiral ganglia; sends the proper cochlear artery to the cochlear duct and supplies the apical two turns of the spiral modiolar artery. SYN arteria cochlearis communis [TA].

com·mon cold (kom′ŏn kōld) SYN cold.

com·mon fa·cial vein (kom′ŏn fā′shăl vān) A short vessel formed by the union of the facial vein and the retromandibular vein, emptying into the jugular vein.

com·mon he·pat·ic ar·te·ry (kom′ŏn he-pat′ik ahr′tĕr-ē) [TA] *Origin,* celiac; *branches,* right gastric, gastroduodenal, and proper hepatic. SYN arteria hepatica communis.

com·mon he·pat·ic duct (CHD) (kom′ŏn he-pat′ik dŭkt) [TA] Section of the biliary duct system formed by the confluence of right and left hepatic ducts. SYN ductus hepaticus communis [TA], hepatocystic duct.

com·mon il·i·ac vein (CIV) (kom′ŏn il′ē-ak vān) [TA] Formed by the union of the external and internal iliac veins at the brim of the pelvis, it passes upward

posterior to the internal iliac artery to the right side of the body of the fifth lumbar vertebra where it unites with its fellow of the opposite side to form the inferior vena cava. SYN vena iliaca communis [TA].

com·mon in·ter·os·se·ous ar·te·ry (kom′ŏn in′tĕr-os′ē-ŭs ahr′tĕr-ē) [TA] *Origin,* ulnar; *branches,* anterior and posterior interosseous. SYN arteria interossea communis.

com·mon pal·mar dig·i·tal ar·te·ry (kom′ŏn pahl′măr dij′i-tăl ahr′tĕr-ē) [TA] One of three arteries arising from the superficial palmar arch and running to the interdigital clefts where each divides into two proper palmar digital arteries. SYN arteria digitalis palmaris communis.

com·mon path·way of co·ag·u·la·tion (kom′ŏn path′wă kō-ag′yū-lā′shŭn) A part of the coagulation system where the intrinsic and extrinsic pathways converge to activate factor X.

com·mon plan·tar dig·i·tal nerves (kom′ŏn plan′tahr dij′i-tăl nĕrvz) [TA] Three nerves derived from the medial plantar nerve and the other the lateral plantar nerve that supply the skin overlying the metatarsals and terminate as proper plantar digital nerves to the side of each toe. SYN nervi digitales plantares communes.

com·mon var·i·a·ble im·mu·no·de·fi·cien·cy (CVI, CVID) (kom′ŏn var′ē-ă-bĕl im′yū-nō-dĕ-fish′ĕn-sē) Immunodeficiency of unknown cause, and usually unclassifiable; usual onset after age 15 years but may occur at any age in either sex. SYN acquired agammaglobulinemia, acquired hypogammaglobulinemia.

com·mo·tio re·ti·nae (kō-mō′shē-ō ret′in-ē) Disruption or disorganization of photoreceptors caused by edema resulting from blunt trauma.

com·mu·ni·ca·ble (comm, commun) (kŏ-myūn′i-kă-bĕl) Capable of being communicated or transmitted; said especially of disease.

com·mu·ni·ca·ble dis·ease (kŏ-myūn′i-kă-bĕl di-zēz′) Any disorder that is transmissible by infection or contagion directly or indirectly or through the agency of a vector.

com·mu·ni·cans, pl. **com·mu·ni·can·tes** (kŏ-myū'ni-kanz, -kan'tēz) Communicating; connecting or joining.

com·mu·ni·cat·ing branch (kŏ-myū'ni-kāt-ing branch) [TA] Bundle of nerve fibers passing from one named nerve to join another. SYN ramus communicans [TA].

com·mu·ni·cat·ing branch of fib·u·lar ar·te·ry (kŏ-myūn'i-kāt-ing branch fib'yū-lăr ahr'tĕr-ē) [TA] The communicating branch of the fibular (peroneal) artery.

com·mu·ni·ty (kŏ-myūn'i-tē) A given segment of a society or a population.

com·mu·ni·ty health nurse (kŏ-myū' ni-tē helth nŭrs) SYN public health nurse.

com·mu·ni·ty men·tal health cen·ter (CMHC) (kŏ-myū'ni-tē men'tăl helth sen'tĕr) A facility located in a neighborhood catchment area close to the homes of patients, introduced in the 1960s under new U.S. federal legislation designed to replace the large state hospitals, which usually were located in remote rural areas.

Com·mu·ni·ty Pe·ri·o·don·tal In·dex of Treat·ment Needs (CPITN) (kŏ-myūn'i-tē per'ē-ō-don'tăl in'deks trēt' mĕnt nēdz) An assessment of periodontal treatment needs that divides the mouth into sextants; is used for a standard procedure for examinations.

com·mu·ni·ty psy·ch·i·a·try (kŏ-myū' ni-tē sī-kī'ă-trē) Mental health care focusing on the detection, prevention, early treatment, and rehabilitation of patients with emotional disorders and social deviance as they develop in the community rather than as encountered one-on-one, in private practice, or at larger centralized psychiatric facilities.

com·mu·ni·ty psy·chol·o·gy (kŏ-myū' ni-tē sī-kol'ŏ-jē) The application of psychology to community programs, e.g., in the schools, correctional and welfare systems, and community mental health care centers.

co·mor·bid (kō-mōr'bid) Denotes additional intercurrent disease states that occur in relation to a primary disease state.

com·pact bone (kŏm-pakt' bōn) [TA] The noncancellous portion of bone that consists largely of concentric lamellar osteons and interstitial lamellae. SYN substantia compacta [TA], compact substance.

com·pan·i·on an·i·mal (kŏm-pan'yŭn an'i-măl) Pet kept for enjoyment and friendship.

com·par·a·tive a·nat·o·my (kŏm-par' ă-tiv ă-nat'ŏ-mē) The comparative study of animal structure with regard to homologous organs or parts.

com·par·a·tive pa·thol·o·gy (kŏm-par'ă-tiv pă-thol'ŏ-jē) Study of diseases of animals, especially in relation to human pathology.

com·par·a·tive phys·i·ol·o·gy (kŏm-par'ă-tiv fiz-ē-ol'ŏ-jē) Science concerned with the differences in the vital processes in different species of organisms, particularly with a view to the adaptation of the processes to the specific needs of the species, to illuminating the evolutionary relationships among different species, or to establishing other interspecific generalizations and relationships.

com·par·a·tive psy·chol·o·gy (kŏm-par'ă-tiv sī-kol'ŏ-jē) Mental health discipline concerned with the study and comparison of the behavior of organisms at different levels of phylogenic development to discover developmental trends.

com·part·ment syn·drome (kŏm-pahrt' mĕnt sin'drōm) Condition in which increased intramuscular pressure in a confined anatomic space brought on by overactivity or trauma impedes blood flow and function of tissues within that space. SYN compression syndrome (2).

com·pat·i·bil·i·ty (kŏm-pat'i-bil'i-tē) The condition or state of being compatible.

com·pat·i·ble (kŏm-pat'i-bĕl) **1.** Capable of being mixed without undergoing destructive chemical change or exhibiting mutual antagonism; said of the elements in a properly constructed pharmaceutical mixture. **2.** Denoting the ability of two biologic entities to exist together without nullification of, or deleterious effects on, the function of either; e.g., blood, tissues, or organs that cause no reaction when transfused or no rejection when transplanted. **3.** Denoting satisfactory relationships between two or more people as in work or in marriage or in other activities.

com·pen·sat·ed a·ci·do·sis (kom'pĕn-sāt-ĕd as'i-dō'sis) An acidosis in which the pH of body fluids is normal; compensation is achieved by respiratory or renal mechanisms.

com·pen·sat·ed al·ka·lo·sis (kom'pĕn-sāt-ĕd al'kă-lō'sis) Disorder in which there is a change in bicarbonate but the pH of body fluids remains normal; respiratory alkalosis may be compensated by increased production of metabolic acids or increased renal excretion of bicarbonate; metabolic alkalosis is rarely compensated by hypoventilation.

com·pen·sa·ted heart fail·ure (kom'pĕn-sāt-ĕd hahrt fāl'yŭr) Condition in which the damaged heart continues to produce sufficient cardiac output.

com·pen·sa·tion (kom'pĕn-sā'shŭn) An unconscious mechanism by which one tries to make up for fancied or real deficiencies.

com·pen·sa·to·ry (kŏm-pen'să-tōr-ē) Providing compensation; making up for a deficiency or loss.

com·pen·sa·to·ry cir·cu·la·tion (kŏm-pen'să-tōr-ē sĭr-kyū-lā'shŭn) Circulation established in dilated collateral vessels when the main vessel of the part is obstructed.

com·pen·sa·to·ry move·ment (kŏm-pen'să-tōr-ē mūv'mĕnt) Movement used habitually to achieve functional motor skills when a normal movement pattern has not been established or is unavailable.

com·pen·sa·to·ry pause (kŏm-pen'să-tōr-ē pawz) Delay following an extrasystole, when long enough to compensate for the prematurity of the extrasystole.

com·pen·sa·to·ry pol·y·cy·the·mi·a (kŏm-pen'să-tōr-ē pol'ē-sī-thē'mē-ă) A

secondary increase in red blood cell count resulting from anoxia.

com·pe·tence, com·pe·ten·cy (kom'pĕ-tĕns, -tĕn-sē) **1.** The quality of being competent or capable of performing an allotted function. **2.** In psychiatry, the mental ability to distinguish right from wrong and to manage one's own affairs, or to assist one's counsel in a legal proceeding.

com·pe·ti·tion (kom'pĕ-tish'ŭn) The process by which the activity or presence of one substance interferes with, or suppresses, the activity of another substance with similar affinities.

com·pet·i·tive in·hi·bi·tion (kŏm-pet'i-tiv in'hi-bish'ŭn) Blocking of the action of an enzyme by a compound that binds to the free enzyme, preventing the substrate from binding and thus preventing the enzyme from acting on that substrate. SYN selective inhibition.

com·plaint (kŏm-plānt') A disorder, disease, or symptom, or the description of it.

com·ple·ment (kom'plĕ-mĕnt) The thermolabile substance, normally present in serum, which is destructive to certain bacteria and other cells sensitized by a specific complement-fixing antibody.

com·ple·men·ta·ry and al·ter·na·tive med·i·cine (CAM) (kom'plĕ-men'tăr-ē awl-tĕr'nă-tiv med'i-sin) Collective term referring to a heterogeneous group of hygienic, diagnostic, and therapeutic philosophies and practices whose principles and techniques diverge from those of modern scientific medicine. SEE ALSO allopathy, alternative medicine. SYN holistic medicine (2).

com·ple·men·ta·ry colors (kom-plĕ-men'tăr-ē kŏl'ŏrz) Pairs of different colors of light that produce white light when combined.

com·ple·men·ta·ry DNA (cDNA) (kom'plĕ-men'tăr-ē) **1.** Single-stranded DNA that is complementary to messenger RNA. **2.** DNA that has been synthesized from mRNA by the action of reverse transcriptase.

com·ple·men·ta·tion (kom'plĕ-men-tā'shŭn) **1.** Interaction between two defective viruses permitting replication under conditions inhibitory to the single virus. **2.** Interaction between two genetic units, one or both of which are defective, permitting the organism containing these units to function normally, whereas it could not do so if either unit were absent.

com·plete a·bor·tion (kŏm-plēt′ ă-bōr′ shŭn) **1.** Total expulsion or extraction from its mother of a fetus or embryo. **2.** Total expulsion of any other product of gestation. (e.g., blighted oocyte).

com·plete AV block (kŏm-plēt′ blok) SEE atrioventricular block.

com·plete blood count (cbc, CBC) (kŏm-plēt′ blŭd kownt) Diagnostic combination of the following determinations: red blood cell count, white blood cell count, erythrocyte indices, hematocrit, differential blood count, and sometimes platelet count.

com·plete car·cin·o·gen (kŏm-plēt′ kahr-sin′ō-jen) Chemical carcinogen that is able to induce cancer without provocation by a tumor-promoting agent introduced during therapy.

com·plete den·ture (kom′plēt den′chŭr) Dental prosthesis that is a substitute for the lost natural dentition and associated structures of the maxillae or mandible.

com·plete frac·ture (kŏm-plēt′ frak′ shŭr) A break in a bone with total separation of the fragments.

com·plete he·mi·a·no·pi·a (kŏm-plēt′ hem′ē-ă-nō′pē-ă) SYN absolute hemianopia.

com·plete her·ni·a (kŏm-plēt′ hĕr′nē-ă) An indirect inguinal hernia in which the contents extend into the tunica vaginalis.

com·plete hy·ster·ec·to·my (kŏm-plēt′ his′tĕr-ek′tŏ-mē) Surgical excision of the uterus and cervix. SYN total hysterectomy.

com·plete·ly in the ca·nal (CIC) hear·ing aid (kŏm-plēt′lē kă-nal′ hēr′ing ād) A hearing aid that fits entirely in the external auditory canal and is not visible at the surface of the body.

com·plex (kom′pleks, kŏm-pleks′) **1.** PSYCHIATRY an organized constellation of feelings, thoughts, perceptions, and memories that may be in part unconscious but may strongly influence associations and attitudes. **2.** CHEMISTRY the relatively stable combination of two or more compounds into a larger molecule without covalent binding. **3.** A composite of chemical or immunologic structures. **4.** An anatomic structure made up of three or more interrelated parts. **5.** An informal term used to denote a group of individual structures known or believed to be anatomically, embryologically, or physiologically related. **6.** Atrial or ventricular systole as it appears on an electrocardiographic tracing.

com·plex frac·ture (kŏm-pleks′ frak′ shŭr) A fracture with significant soft tissue injury.

com·plex·ion (kŏm-plek′shŭn) The color, texture, and general appearance of the skin of the face.

com·plex joint (kŏm-pleks′ joynt) Articulation with three or more skeletal elements. SYN composite joint.

com·plex motor seiz·ure (kŏm-pleks′ mō′tŏr sē′zhŭr) Seizure characterized by muscles of each limb contracting asynchronously and sequentially to produce a movement that may resemble voluntary activity.

com·plex o·don·to·ma (kŏm-pleks′ ō-don-tō′mă) An odontoma in which the various odontogenic tissues are organized in a haphazard arrangement with no resemblance to teeth.

com·plex par·tial seiz·ure (CPS) (kŏm-pleks′ pahr′shăl sē′zhŭr) One with impairment of consciousness, occurring in a patient with focal epilepsy.

com·plex pleu·ral ef·fu·sion (kŏm-pleks′ plūr′ăl ĕ-fyū′zhŭn) One without actual infection but with signs of a high degree of inflammation (e.g., low pH, low glucose, high lactate dehydrogenase, many white blood cells).

com·plex pre·cip·i·tat·ed ep·i·lep·sy (kŏm-pleks′ prĕ-sip′i-tā-tĕd ep′i-lep′sē) Type of reflex epilepsy initiated by specialized sensory stimuli.

com·pli·ance (kŏm-plī′ăns) **1.** The consistency and accuracy with which a patient follows the regimen prescribed by a physician or other health care professional. Cf. adherence (2), maintenance. **2.** PHYSIOLOGY a measure of the ease with which a hollow viscus (e.g., lung, urinary bladder, gallbladder) may be distended, i.e., the volume change resulting from the application of a unit pressure differential between the inside and outside of the organ or sac; the reciprocal of elastance. **3.** Observance of rules or guidelines, such as those governing provision of medical services and billing for them; fulfillment of a requirement. **4.** A term considered prejudicial in distinguishing more or less aggressive patients. **5.** A measure of the distensibility of a chamber expressed as a change in volume per unit change in pressure.

com·pli·cat·ed (kom′pli-kā′ted) Made complex; denoting a disease on which a morbid process or event has been superimposed, thus altering symptoms and modifying its course for the worse.

com·pli·cat·ed cat·a·ract (kom′pli-kā′tĕd kat′ă-rakt) SYN secondary cataract (1).

com·pli·ca·ted frac·ture (kom′pli-kā′tĕd frak′shŭr) Breakage in an osseous structure such that the sharp edges of the bone have pierced an organ or bodily structure.

com·pli·ca·tion (kom′pli-kā′shŭn) A morbid process or event occurring during a disease that is not an essential part of the disease, although it may result from it or from independent causes.

com·po·nent (kŏm-pō′nĕnt) An element forming a part of the whole.

com·pos·ite (kŏm-poz′it) A colloquial term for resin materials used in restorative dentistry.

com·pos·ite flap, com·pound flap (kŏm-poz′it flap, kom′pownd) Flap containing two or more tissue elements, usually skin, muscle, bone, or cartilage.

com·pos·ite joint (kŏm-poz′it joynt) SYN complex joint.

com·pos·ite res·in (kŏm-poz′it rez′in) Synthetic form usually acrylic based, to which a glass or natural silica filter has been added. Used mainly in dental restorative procedures.

com·pos men·tis (kom′pos men′tis) Of sound mind; usually used in its negative form, non compos mentis.

com·pound an·eu·rysm (kom′pownd an′yūr-izm) An aneurysm in which some of the coats of the artery are ruptured, others intact.

com·pound gland (kom′pownd gland) A gland the larger excretory ducts of which branch repeatedly into smaller ducts, which ultimately drain secretory units.

com·pound hy·per·o·pic astig·ma·tism (kom′pownd hī′pĕr-ō′pik ă-stig′mă-tizm) Ocular disorder in which all meridians are hyperopic but to different degrees.

com·pound joint (kom′pownd joynt) Articulation made up of three or more skeletal elements, or in which two anatomically separate joints function as a unit.

com·pound mi·cro·scope (kom′pownd mī′krŏ-skōp) A microscope having two or more magnifying lenses.

com·pound my·o·pic astig·ma·tism (kom′pownd mī-op′ik ă-stig′mă-tizm) Ocular disorder in which all meridians are myopic but to different degrees.

com·pound ne·vus (kom′pownd nē′vŭs) Nevus with nests of melanocytes in the epidermal-dermal junction and in the dermis.

com·pound odon·to·ma (kom′pownd ō-don-tō′mă) An odontoma in which the odontogenic tissues are organized and resemble anomalous teeth.

com·pound pres·en·ta·tion (kom′pownd prez′ĕn-tā′shŭn) Prolapse of an extremity, usually a hand, along the presenting part, with both in the pelvis simultaneously.

com·pound pro·tein (kom′pownd prō′tēn) SYN conjugated protein.

com·pre·hen·sive med·i·cal care (kom′prē-hen′siv med′i-kăl kăr) Concept that includes not only the traditional care of the acutely or chronically ill patient, but also the prevention and early detection of disease and the rehabilitation of the disabled.

com·press (kom′pres) A pad of gauze or other material applied for local pressure.

com·pressed sponge (kŏm-prest′ spŭnj) One treated with a thin layer of acacia mucilage; used to dilate sinuses during surgery.

com·pres·sion (kŏm-presh′ŭn) Squeezing together; the exertion of pressure on a body to tend to increase its density; the decrease in a dimension of a body under the action of two external forces directed toward one another.

com·pres·sion cy·a·no·sis (kŏm-presh′ŭn sī-ă-nō′sis) Discolored skin accompanied by edema and petechial hemorrhages over the head, neck, and upper part of the chest, as a venous reflex resulting from severe compression of the thorax or abdomen; the conjunctiva and retinas are similarly affected.

com·pres·sion pa·ral·y·sis (kŏm-presh′ŭn păr-al′i-sis) Paralysis due to external pressure on a nerve.

com·pro·mised host (kom′prŏ-mīzd hōst) Patient with acquired or congenital immunologic deficiency at increased risk for infectious disease complications.

Comp·ton ef·fect, Comp·ton scat·ter·ing (komp′tŏn e-fekt′, skat′ĕr-ing) Change in wavelength of x-rays or gamma rays due to interaction of electron orbiting nucleus and incidental photon, resulting in scattered photons of lower energy and recoil electrons.

com·pul·sion (kŏm-pŭl′shŭn) Uncontrollable thoughts or impulses to perform an act, often repetitively, as an unconscious mechanism to avoid unacceptable ideas and desires that, by themselves, arouse anxiety; the anxiety becomes fully manifest if performance of the compulsive act is prevented. SEE ALSO fixed idea.

com·pul·sive per·son·al·i·ty dis·or·der (kŏm-pŭl′siv pĕr′sŏn-al′i-tē dis-ōr′dĕr) Anxiety-related condition characterized by rigid and oftentimes repetitive adherence to rituals in an attempt to eradicate intrusive thoughts. SYN obsessive compulsive disorder (OCD).

com·put·ed ra·di·og·ra·phy (CR) (kŏm-pyū′tĕd rā′dē-og′ră-fē) Converting transmitted x-rays into light, using a solid-state imaging device such as a photostimulable phosphor plate, and recovering and processing the image using a digital computer; the image may then be printed on film or displayed on a computer screen.

com·put·ed to·mog·ra·phy (CT) (kŏm-pyū′tĕd tŏ-mog′ră-fē) Imaging anatomic information from a cross-sectional plane of the body, each image generated by a computer synthesis of x-ray transmission data obtained in many different directions in a given plane.

com·pu·ter-based pa·tient re·cord (CPR) (kŏm-pyū′tĕr-bāst pā′shĕnt rek′ŏrd) Electronic health care record that integrates patient information into a database for accessibility; the CPR supports patient care, decision making, and research.

co·na·tion (kō-nā′shŭn) The conscious tendency to act, usually an aspect of mental process.

con·ca·nav·a·lin A (Con A) (kon-kă-nav′ă-lin) A phytomitogen, extracted from the jack bean (*Canavalia ensiformis*) that agglutinates the blood of mammals and reacts with glucosans; like other phytohemagglutinins, it stimulates T lymphocytes more vigorously than it does B lymphocytes.

Con·ca·to dis·ease (kon-kah′tō di-zēz′) SYN polyserositis.

con·cave (kon′kāv) Having a depressed or hollowed surface.

con·ca·vo·con·cave (kon-kā′vō-kon′kāv) SYN biconcave.

con·ca·vo·con·vex (kon-kā′vō-kon′veks) Concave on one surface and convex on the opposite surface.

con·ca·vo·con·vex lens (kon-kā′vō-kon′veks lenz) A converging meniscus lens that is concave on one surface and convex on the opposite surface.

con·ceal·ed con·duc·tion (kŏn-sēld′

kŏn-dŭk′shŭn) Transmission of an impulse through a part of the heart without direct evidence of its presence in the electrocardiogram.

con·ceal·ed pe·nis (kŏn-sēld′ pē′nis) Usually a complication of circumcision wherein the anastomotic line between shaft skin and preputial collar closes like an iris or cicatrix over the glans; equated by some to a buried penis.

con·ceive (kŏn-sēv′) To become pregnant, i.e., to achieve implantation of the blastocyst, ideally in the endometrium.

con·cen·tra·tion gra·di·ent (kon′sĕn-trā′shŭn grā′dē-ĕnt) SYN density gradient.

con·cen·tric (kŏn-sen′trik) Having a common center; said of two or more circles or spheres having a common center.

con·cen·tric fi·bro·ma (kŏn-sen′trik fī-brō′mă) Benign neoplasm, actually a leiomyoma, which occupies the entire circumference of the wall of the uterus.

con·cen·tric la·mel·la (kŏn-sen′trik lă-mel′ă) One of the concentric tubular layers of bone surrounding the central canal in an osteon. SYN haversian lamella.

con·cept (kon′sept) 1. An abstract idea or notion. 2. An explanatory variable or principle in a scientific system. SYN conception (1).

con·cep·tion (kŏn-sep′shŭn) 1. SYN concept. 2. Act of forming a general idea or notion. 3. Fertilization of oocyte by a sperm.

con·cep·tu·al frame·work (kŏn-sep′chū-ăl frām′wŏrk) Set of interrelated theories that form the basis for a research study. SYN theoretical framework.

con·cep·tus, pl. **con·cep·tus** (kŏn-sep′tŭs) The products of conception (i.e., fetus, placenta, embryo, and fetal membranes).

con·cha, pl. **con·chae** (kong′kă, -kē) [TA] ANATOMY a structure similar to a shell in shape, as the auricle or pinna of the ear or a turbinate bone in the nose.

con·cha bul·lo·sa (kong′kă bŭl-ō′să) Abnormal pneumatization of the middle turbinate that may interfere with normal ventilation of sinus ostia and can result in recurrent sinusitis.

con·cha of au·ri·cle (kong′kă awr′i-kĕl) [TA] Large hollow, or floor of the auricle, between the anterior portion of the helix and the antihelix; divided by the crus of the helix into cymba above and cavum below. Also called concha of ear.

con·com·i·tant (kŏn-kom′i-tănt) SYN comitant.

con·com·i·tant stra·bis·mus (kŏn-kom′i-tănt stră-biz′mŭs) SYN comitant strabismus.

con·cor·dance (kŏn-kōr′dăns) Agreement in the types of data that occur in natural pairs.

con·cor·dance rate (kŏn-kōr′dăns rāt) Proportion of a random sample of pairs that are concordant for a trait of interest.

con·cor·dant al·ter·na·tion (kŏn-kōr′dănt awl′tĕr-nā′shŭn) Alternation in either the mechanical or electrical activity of the heart, occurring in both systemic and pulmonary circulations.

con·cor·dant changes e·lec·tro·car·di·o·gram (kŏn-kōr′dănt chān′jĕz ĕ-lek′trō-kahr′dē-ō-gram) Presence of more than one waveform change, each in the same direction (polarity).

con·cres·cence (kŏn-kres′ĕns) 1. SYN coalescence. 2. DENTISTRY the union of the roots of two adjacent teeth by cementum.

con·cre·tio cor·dis (kon-krē′shē-ō kōr′dis) Extensive adhesion between parietal and visceral layers of the pericardium with partial or complete obliteration of the pericardial cavity. SYN internal adhesive pericarditis.

con·cre·tion (kŏn-krē′shŭn) Formation of solid material by the aggregation of discrete units or particles.

con·cus·sion (kŏn-kŭsh′ŭn) 1. A violent shaking or jarring. 2. An injury of a soft structure, as the brain, resulting from a blow or violent shaking. SYN commotio.

con·den·sa·tion (kon′dĕn-sā′shŭn) 1.

Making more solid or dense. **2.** The change of a gas to a liquid, or of a liquid to a solid. **3.** PSYCHOANALYSIS an unconscious mental process in which one symbol stands for a number of others. **4.** DENTISTRY the process of packing a filling material into a cavity, using such force and direction that no voids or gaps result.

con·dens·er (kŏn-den'sĕr) **1.** An apparatus for cooling a gas to a liquid or a liquid to a solid. **2.** DENTISTRY a manual or powered instrument used for packing a plastic or unset material into a prepared tooth cavity; variation in size and shape permit conformation of the mass to the cavity outline. **3.** Simple or compound lens on a microscope is used to supply sufficient illumination necessary to view the specimen under observation. **4.** SYN capacitor.

con·dens·ing os·te·i·tis (kŏn-dens'ing os-tē-ī'tis) SYN sclerosing osteitis.

con·di·tion (kŏn-dish'ŭn) **1.** To train; to undergo conditioning. **2.** BEHAVIORAL PSYCHOLOGY a certain response elicited by a specifiable stimulus or emitted in the presence of certain stimuli with reward of the response during prior occurrence. **3.** Referring to several classes of learning in the behavioristic branch of psychology.

con·di·tioned re·flex (Cr) (kŏn-dish'ŭnd rē'fleks) A reflex that is gradually developed by training and association through the frequent repetition of a definite stimulus. SEE conditioning.

con·di·tioned re·sponse (cond resp, CR) (kŏn-dish'ŭnd rĕ-spons') SEE conditioning. SYN conditioned reflex.

con·di·tioned stim·u·lus (kŏn-dish'ŭnd stim'yū-lŭs) **1.** A stimulus applied to one of the sense organs that are an essential and integral part of the neural mechanism underlying a conditioned reflex. **2.** A neutral stimulus, when paired with the unconditioned stimulus in simultaneous presentation to an organism, capable of eliciting a given response.

con·di·tion·ing (kŏn-dish'ŭn-ing) The process of acquiring, developing, educating, establishing, learning, or training new responses in a person; a change in the frequency or form of behavior as a result of the influence of the environment.

con·dom (kon'dŏm) Sheath or cover for the penis or vagina, for use in the prevention of conception or infection during coitus.

con·duc·tance (kŏn-dŭk'tăns) The ease with which a fluid or gas enters and flows through a conduit, air passage, or respiratory tract; the flow per unit pressure difference.

con·duct dis·or·der (kon'dŭkt dis-ōr'dĕr) A mental disorder of childhood or adolescence characterized by a persistent pattern of violating societal norms and the rights of others.

con·duct·ing air·way (kŏn-dŭkt'ing ăr'wā) Airway from the nasal cavity to a terminal bronchiole.

con·duc·tion (kŏn-dŭk'shŭn) **1.** The act of transmitting or conveying certain forms of energy, such as heat, sound, or electricity, from one point to another, without evident movement in the conducting body. **2.** The transmission of stimuli of various sorts by living protoplasm. **3.** The process by which a nerve impulse is transmitted.

con·duc·tion an·al·ge·sia (kŏn-dŭk'shŭn an'ăl-jē'zē-ă) SYN regional anesthesia.

con·duc·tion apha·sia (kŏn-dŭk'shŭn ă-fā'zē-ă) A form of aphasia in which the patient understands spoken and written words, is aware of her deficit, and can speak and write, but skips or repeats words, or substitutes one word for another (paraphasia); word repetition is severely impaired. The responsible lesion is in the associate tracts connecting the various language centers. SYN associative aphasia.

con·duc·tion block (kŏn-dŭk'shŭn blok) Failure of impulse transmission at some point along a nerve fiber, although conduction along the segments proximal and distal to it are unaffected; clinically, most often the result of an area of focal demyelination or, less often, transient ischemia; when caused by focal trauma involving the periperal nervous system, called neurapraxia.

con·duc·tive hear·ing im·pair·ment (kŏn-dŭk′tiv hēr′ing im-pār′mĕnt) A form of hearing impairment due to a lesion in the external auditory canal or middle ear.

con·duc·tive heat (kŏn-dŭk′tiv hēt) A rise in temperature conveyed from one structure or appliance to another in which the warmer affects the cooler by conduction.

con·duc·tiv·i·ty (kon′dŭk-tiv′i-tē) **1.** The power of transmission or conveyance of certain forms of energy, such as heat, sound, and electricity, without perceptible motion in the conducting body. **2.** The property, inherent in living protoplasm, of transmitting a state of excitation; e.g., in muscle or nerve.

con·duc·tor (kŏn-dŭk′tŏr) **1.** A probe or sound with a groove along which a knife is passed in slitting open a sinus or fistula; a grooved director. **2.** Any substance possessing conductivity.

con·du·it (kon′dū-it) A channel.

con·dy·lar ca·nal (kon′di-lăr kă-nal′) [TA] Inconstant opening through the occipital bone posterior to the condyle on each side that transmits the occipital emissary vein. SYN canalis condylaris [TA], condyloid canal, posterior condyloid foramen.

con·dy·lar fos·sa (kon′di-lăr fos′ă) [TA] A depression behind the condyle of the occipital bone in which the posterior margin of the superior facet of the atlas lies in extension.

con·dy·lar joint (kon′di-lăr joynt) [TA] SYN ellipsoid joint.

con·dy·lar·thro·sis (kon′dil-ahr-thrō′sis) A joint, like that of the knee, formed by condylar surfaces.

con·dyle (C) (kon′dīl) [TA] A rounded articular surface at the extremity of a bone. SYN condylus [TA].

con·dy·lec·to·my (kon′di-lek′tŏ-mē) Excision of a condyle.

con·dyl·i·on (cd) (kon-dil′ē-on) A point on the lateral outer or medial inner surface of the condyle of the mandible.

con·dy·loid (kon′di-loyd) Relating to or resembling a condyle.

con·dy·loid ca·nal (kon′di-loyd kă-nal′) SYN condylar canal.

con·dy·lo·ma (kon-di-lō′mă) A wartlike excrescence on the skin of the genitals, perineum, or anus, usually sexually transmitted.

con·dy·lo·ma a·cu·mi·na·tum (kon-di-lō′mă ă-kū-mi-nā′tŭm) A warty growth on the external genitals or at the anus.

con·dy·lo·ma la·tum (kon-di-lō′mă lā′tŭm) A secondary syphilitic eruption of flat-topped papules, found at the anus and wherever contiguous folds of skin produce heat and moisture. SYN flat condyloma (1).

con·dy·lot·o·my (kon′di-lot′ŏ-mē) Division, without removal, of a condyle.

con·dy·lus (kon′di-lŭs) [TA] SYN condyle.

-cone Suffix indicating the cusp of a tooth in the upper jaw.

cone (kōn) **1.** A surface joining a circle to a point above the plane containing the circle. **2.** Metallic cylinder or truncated cone, either circular or square in cross-section, used to confine a beam of x-rays. SYN conus (1).

cone bi·op·sy (kōn bī′op-sē) Surgical excision of a conic section of cervical tissue. SYN conization.

cone of light (kōn līt) SYN light reflex (3).

con·fab·u·la·tion (kŏn-fab′yū-lā′shŭn) The making of bizarre and incorrect responses, and a readiness to give a fluent but tangential answer, with no regard whatever to facts, to any question put.

con·fi·dence co·ef·fi·cient, con·fi·dence lev·el (kon′fi-dĕns kō′ĕ-fish′ĕnt, lev′ĕl) Degree of certainty with which one can state an estimated statistical range is correct.

con·fi·dence in·ter·val (CI) (kon′fi-dĕns in′tĕr-văl) Range of values for a variable of interest, constructed so that this range has a specified probability of including the true value of the variable.

con·fi·den·ti·al·i·ty (kon'fi-den-shē-al'i-tē) The statutorily protected right and duty of health care professionals not to disclose information acquired during consultation with a patient.

con·flict (kon'flikt) Tension or stress experienced by an organism when satisfaction of a need, drive, motive, or wish is thwarted by the presence of other attractive or unattractive needs, drives, or motives.

con·flu·ence (kon'flū-ĕns) [TA] A flowing together; a joining of two or more streams. SYN confluens [TA].

con·flu·ence of si·nus·es (kon'flū-ĕns sī'nŭs-ĕz) [TA] A meeting place, at the internal occipital protuberance, of the superior sagittal, straight, and occipital sinuses, drained by the two transverse sinuses of the dura mater. SYN confluens sinuum [TA].

con·fron·ta·tion (kon'frŏn-tā'shŭn) The act by the therapist, or another patient in a therapy group, of openly interpreting a patient's resistances, attitudes, feelings, or effects on either the therapist, the group, or its member(s).

con·fu·sion (kŏn-fyū'zhŭn) A mental state in which reactions to environmental stimuli are inappropriate because the person is bewildered, perplexed, or unable to orientate herself or himself.

con·fu·sion col·ors (kŏn-fyū'zhŭn cŏl'ŏrz) A set of colors (usually colored wools), cream, buff, pale blue, others; used to test color blindness.

con·ge·ner (kon'jĕ-nĕr) **1.** One of two or more things of the same kind, as of animal or plant with respect to classification. **2.** One of two or more muscles with the same function. **3.** Any member of a specified genus.

con·gen·ic (kŏn-jen'ik) Relating to an inbred strain of animals produced by repeated crossing of one gene line onto another inbred (isogenic) line.

con·gen·i·tal (kŏn-jen'i-tăl) Existing at birth, referring to mental or physical traits, anomalies, malformations, or diseases, which may be either hereditary or due to an influence occurring during gestation up to the moment of birth. USAGE NOTE often misused as a synonym of hereditary.

con·gen·i·tal adre·nal hy·per·pla·sia (CAH) (kŏn-jen'i-tăl ă-drē'năl hī'pĕr-plā'zē-ă) Group of autosomal recessively inherited disorders associated with a deficiency of one of the enzymes involved in cortisol biosynthesis, resulting in elevation of adrenocorticotropic hormone levels and overproduction and accumulation of cortisol precursors proximal to the block.

con·gen·i·tal a·nom·a·ly (kŏn-jen'i-tăl ă-nom'ă-lē) A structural abnormality present at birth. SEE ALSO birth defect.

con·gen·i·tal cat·a·ract (CC) (kŏn-jen'i-tăl kat'ăr-akt) Cataract, usually bilateral, present at birth; most are sporadic, some the result of prematurity, intrauterine infection, drug-related toxicity, injury, chromosomal, or metabolic disorders.

con·gen·i·tal di·a·phrag·mat·ic her·nia (kŏn-jen'i-tăl dī'ă-frag-mat'ik hĕr'nē-ă) Defective development of the pleuroperitoneal membrane (usually left) results in a posterolateral defect in the diaphragm and allows the abdominal viscera to protrude into the thorax. SYN Bochdalek hernia.

con·gen·i·tal glau·co·ma (kŏn-jen'i-tăl glaw-kō'mă) SYN buphthalmia.

con·gen·i·tal hip dys·pla·sia (kŏn-jen'i-tăl hip dis-plā'zē-ă) A developmental abnormality in which a neonate's hips easily become dislocated; etiology is complex, with mechanical, familial, hormonal, and obstetric factors all contributing; female predominance is 9:1. SYN developmental hip dysplasia.

con·gen·i·tal lo·bar em·phy·se·ma (CLE) (kŏn-jen'i-tăl lō'bahr em-fi-sē'mă) Common cause of neonatal respiratory distress which usually involves the left upper lobe.

con·gen·i·tal ne·vus (kŏn-jen'i-tăl nē'vŭs) A melanocytic nevus that is visible at birth, is often larger than an acquired nevus, and more frequently involves deeper structures.

con·gen·i·tal ny·stag·mus (CN) (kŏn-jen′i-tăl nis-tag′mŭs) **1.** Nystagmus present at birth or caused by lesions sustained in utero or at the time of birth; **2.** Inherited nystagmus, usually X-linked, without associated neurologic lesions and nonprogressive. **3.** Disorder associated with albinism, achromatopsia, and hypoplasia of the macula.

con·gen·i·tal par·a·my·o·to·ni·a (kŏn-jen′i-tăl par′ă-mī-ō-tō′nē-ă) Nonprogressive muscular disorder caused by exposure of muscles to cold. SYN Eulenberg disease.

con·gen·i·tal ru·bel·la syn·drome (CRS) (kŏn-jen′i-tăl rū-bel′ă sin′drŏm) Fetal infection with rubella virus during the first trimester of pregnancy resulting in a series of congenital abnormalities including heart disease, deafness, and blindness.

con·gen·i·tal spas·tic par·a·ple·gi·a (kŏn-jen′i-tăl spas′tik par′ă-plē′jē-ă) A type of cerebral palsy characterized by spastic paralysis of the lower extremities. Syn: Little disease.

con·gen·i·tal stri·dor (kŏn-jen′i-tăl strī′dŏr) Crowing inspiration occurring at birth or within the first few months of life; sometimes without apparent cause and sometimes due to abnormal flaccidity of epiglottis or arytenoids.

con·gen·i·tal syph·il·is (kŏn-jen′i-tăl sif′i-lis) Venereal disease acquired by the fetus in utero, thus present at birth.

con·gen·i·tal tox·o·plas·mo·sis (kŏn-jen′i-tăl tok′sō-plaz-mō′sis) Parasitic disease in an infected mother transmitted in utero to the fetus, observed as three syndromes: acute, subacute, and chronic, usually not recognized during the newborn period, but chorioretinitis and cerebral lesions may be detected weeks to years later.

con·ges·tion (kŏn-jes′chŭn) Presence of an abnormal amount of fluid in the vessels or passages of a part or organ; especially, of blood due either to increased influx or to an obstruction to the return flow. SEE ALSO hyperemia.

con·ges·tive car·di·o·my·op·a·thy (CCM) (kŏn-jes′tiv kahr′dē-ō-mī-op′ă-thē) SYN dilated cardiomyopathy.

con·ges·tive heart fail·ure (CHF) (kŏn-jes′tiv hahrt fāl′yŭr) SYN heart failure (1).

con·ges·tive splen·o·meg·a·ly (kŏn-jes′tiv splē-nō-meg′ă-lē) Enlargement of the spleen due to passive congestion.

con·glo·ba·tion (kon′glō-bā′shŭn) An aggregation of numerous particles into one rounded mass.

con·glu·ti·nant (kŏn-glŭ′ti-nănt) Adhesive, promoting the union of a wound.

con·glu·ti·na·tion (kŏn-glŭ′ti-nā′shŭn) **1.** SYN adhesion (1). **2.** Agglutination of antigen(erythrocyte)-antibody-complement complex by normal bovine serum (and certain other colloidal materials); the procedure provides a means of detecting the presence of nonagglutinating antibody.

con·go·phil·ic (kong′gō-fil′ik) Denoting any substance that takes a Congo red stain.

con·gru·ous hem·i·a·no·pia (kon′grŭ-ŭs hem′ē-ă-nō′pē-ă) Hemianopia in which the visual field defects in both eyes are completely symmetric in extent and intensity.

-conid Suffix meaning the cusp of a tooth in the lower jaw.

Co·nid·i·o·bo·lus (kō-nid′ē-ō-bō′lŭs) Fungal genus widely distributed in soil and among plants, insects, and amphibians; causes conidiobolomycosis, a chronic granulomatous disease of submucosal and subcutaneous tissues.

co·nid·i·um, pl. **co·nid·ia** (kō-nid′ē-ŭm, -ă) A fungal sexual spore borne externally in various ways.

co·ni·o·fi·bro·sis (kŏ′nē-ō-fī-brō′sis) Fibrosis produced by dust, especially in the lungs due to inhaled dust.

co·ni·o·sis (kŏ′nē-ō′sis) Any disease or morbid condition caused by inhalation of dust.

con·i·za·tion (kon′i-zā′shŭn) Excision of a cone of tissue, e.g., mucosa of the cervix uteri.

con·joined (kŏn-joynd′) Attached.

con·joined an·as·to·mo·sis (kŏn-joynd ă-nas'tŏ-mō'sis) The joining together of two small blood vessels by side-to-side elliptic connection to create a single larger stoma for subsequent end-to-end anastomosis.

con·joined twins (kŏn-joynd' twinz) Monozygotic twins with varying extent of union and different degrees of residual duplication.

con·ju·gant (kon'jŭ-gănt) A member of a mating pair of organisms or gametes undergoing conjugation.

con·ju·ga·ta (kon-jū-gā'tă) [TA] Any conjugate diameter of the pelvis. SEE conjugate.

con·ju·gate (kon'jŭ-găt) [TA] 1. Joined or paired. SYN conjugated. 2. A conjugate diameter of the pelvis. The distance between any two specified points on the periphery of the pelvic canal. SEE conjugata.

con·ju·gat·ed bil·i·ru·bin (bili-c, CBIL, CB) (kon'jŭ-gā-tĕd bil-i-rū'bin) SYN direct reacting bilirubin.

con·ju·gat·ed es·tro·gen (CE) (kon'jŭ-gā-tĕd es'trō-jĕn) Amorphous preparation of naturally occurring, water-soluble, conjugated forms of mixed estrogens obtained from the urine of pregnant horses.

con·ju·gate de·vi·a·tion of the eyes (kon'jŭ-găt dē-vē-a'shŭn īz) 1. Rotation of the eyes equally and simultaneously in the same direction, as occurs normally. 2. Condition in which both eyes are turned to the same side as a result of either paralysis or muscular spasm.

con·ju·gat·ed pro·te·in (kon'jŭ-gā-tĕd prō'tēn) Protein attached to some other molecule or molecules (not amino acid in nature) otherwise than as a salt. SEE ALSO prosthetic group, simple protein. SYN compound protein.

con·ju·gate for·a·men (kon'jŭ-găt fōr-ā'mĕn) Opening formed by the notches of two bones in apposition.

con·ju·gate gaze (kon'jŭ-găt gāz) Binocular movement with parallel ocular visual axes.

con·junc·ti·va, pl. **con·junc·ti·vae** (kŏn-jŭngk'tiv-ă, -vē) [TA] The mucous membrane investing the anterior surface of the eyeball and the posterior surface of the lids.

con·junc·ti·val re·flex (kŏn-jŭngk'ti-văl rē'fleks) Closure of the eyes in response to irritation of the conjunctiva.

con·junc·ti·val ring (kŏn-jŭngk'ti-văl ring) [TA] Anulus at the junction of the corneal periphery with the conjunctiva.

con·junc·ti·val sac (kŏn-jŭngk'ti-văl sak) [TA] Area bound by the conjunctival membrane between the palpebral and bulbar conjunctiva, into which the lacrimal fluid is secreted; closed space when eye closed; when eye is open, the sac is open anteriorly through the palpebral fissure. SYN saccus conjunctivalis [TA].

con·junc·ti·vi·tis (kŏn-jŭngk'ti-vī'tis) Disorder in which the conjunctivae are reddened. The eyes tear and produce exudate along the eyelid; may progress to drooping of the eyelid such that abnormal tissue may form.

con·junc·ti·vo·chal·a·sis (kŏn-jŭngk'ti-vō-kăl'ă-sis) Condition in which redundant bulbar conjunctiva billows over the eyelid margin or covers the lower punctum.

con·junc·ti·vo·ma (kŏn-jŭngk'ti-vō'mă) Tumor of the anterior surface of the eyeball or posterior surface of the eyelids.

con·junc·ti·vo·plas·ty, con·junc·ti·vi·plas·ty (kŏn-jŭngk'ti-vō-plas-tē, -vi-plas'tē) Plastic surgery on the conjunctiva.

con·nect·ing stalk (kŏ-nekt'ing stawk) Extraembryonic precursor of the umbilical cord by which the caudal end of the embryo is attached to the chorion. SYN body stalk.

con·nect·ing tu·bule (kŏ-nekt'ing tū'byūl) Narrow arching tubule of the kidney joining the distal convoluted tubule and the collecting tubule.

con·nec·tion (kŏ-nek'shŭn) A union of elements or things. SYN connexus.

con·nec·tive tis·sue (kŏ-nek'tiv tish'ū)

The supporting or framework tissue of the animal body, formed of fibrous and ground substance with more or less numerous cells of various kinds. SYN interstitial tissue.

con·nec·tive-tis·sue dis·ease (kŏ-nek'tiv-tish'ū di-zēz') Generalized disorders affecting connective tissue, especially those not inherited as mendelian characteristics. SEE ALSO collagen disease.

con·nec·tive tu·mor (kŏ-nek'tiv tū'mŏr) Any lesion of the connective tissue group, such as osteoma, fibroma, sarcoma.

con·nec·tor (kŏ-nek'tŏr) DENTISTRY a part of a partial denture that unites its components.

con·nex·in 26 (kon-eks'in) The gap junction protein that accounts for a major portion of recessive nonsyndromic hearing impairment.

con·nex·us (ko-nek'sŭs) SYN connection.

Conn syn·drome (kon sin'drōm) SYN primary aldosteronism.

co·noid (kō'noyd) 1. A conic structure. 2. Part of the apical complex characteristic of the protozoan subphylum, Apicomplexa.

co·noid lig·a·ment (kō'noyd lig'ă-mĕnt) [TA] Medial part of the coracoclavicular ligament that attaches to the conoid tubercle of the clavicle. SYN ligamentum conoideum [TA].

co·noid tu·ber·cle (kō'noyd tū'bĕr-kĕl) Prominence near the lateral end of the inferior surface of the clavicle that gives attachment to the conoid ligament.

con·san·guin·i·ty (kon-sang-gwin'i-tē) Kinship because of common ancestry. SYN blood relationship.

con·sci·en·tious·ness (kon'shē-en'shŭs-nĕs) Behavior based on one's conscience whereby one is meticulous and careful.

con·scious (cs, CS) (kon'shŭs) 1. Aware; having present knowledge or perception of oneself, one's acts, and surroundings. 2. Denoting something occur-

ring with the perceptive attention of the individual.

con·scious·ness (kon'shŭs-nĕs) The state of being aware, or perceiving physical facts or mental concepts.

con·scious se·da·tion (kon'shŭs sĕ-dā'shŭn) A medically controlled state of depressed consciousness that preserves airway patency, protective reflexes, and the ability to respond to stimulation.

con·sen·su·al val·i·da·tion (kon-sen'shū-ăl val-i-dā'shŭn) Confirmation of experience or judgment of one person by another.

con·ser·va·tion of en·er·gy (kon-sĕr-vā'shŭn en'ĕr-jē) Tenet that the total amount of energy in a closed system remains always the same, none being lost or created in any process or conversion of one kind of energy into another.

con·ser·va·tive (cons) (kŏn-sĕr'vă-tiv) Denoting treatment by gradual, limited, or well-established procedures, as opposed to radical.

con·ser·va·tive treat·ment (kŏn-sĕr'vă-tiv trēt'mĕnt) Course of therapeutic action designed to avoid harm, with less possibility of benefit than more risky actions.

con·sis·ten·cy prin·ci·ple (kŏn-sis'tĕn-sē prin'si-pĕl) In psychology, the desire of the human being to be consistent, especially in attitudes and beliefs.

con·sol·i·da·tion (kŏn-sol'i-dā'shŭn) Solidification into a firm dense mass.

con·spi·cu·i·ty (kon'spi-kyū'i-tē) The visibility of a structure of interest on a radiograph, a function of the inherent contrast of the structure and the complexity (noise) of the surrounding image.

con·stant (kon'stănt) A quantity that, under stated conditions, does not vary with changes in the environment.

con·sti·pa·tion (kon'sti-pā'shŭn) A condition in which bowel movements are infrequent or incomplete.

con·sti·tu·tion (kon'sti-tū'shŭn) The physical makeup of a body, including the mode of performance of its functions, the activity of its metabolic processes, the manner and degree of its reactions to stimuli, and its power of resistance to the attack of pathogenic organisms.

con·sti·tu·tion·al psy·chol·o·gy (kon-sti-tū´shŭn-ăl sī-kol´ŏ-jē) Someone's mental estimate of personal body habitus.

con·sti·tu·tion·al re·ac·tion (kon´sti-tū´shŭn-ăl rē-ak´shŭn) Generalized response in contrast to a focal or local reaction.

con·sti·tu·tive (kon´sti-tū-tiv) In genetics, denotes genes controlled by constantly active promoters.

con·sti·tu·tive en·zyme (kon´sti-tū-tiv en´zīm) One produced by cells, constantly regardless of the growth conditions. SEE ALSO induced enzyme.

con·stric·tion (kŏn-strik´shŭn) [TA] **1.** Any normally or pathologically narrowed portion of lumen. SYN constrictio [TA]. **2.** The process of binding or contracting, becoming narrowed. **3.** Subjective sensation of pressure or tightness. SEE ALSO stricture, stenosis.

con·struct va·lid·i·ty (kon´strŭkt vă-lid´i-tē) Extent to which a test or procedure appears to measure a higher order or inferred theoretical construct. SEE construct (2).

con·sul·ta·tion (kon´sŭl-tā´shŭn) Meeting of two or more physicians or surgeons to evaluate a case's nature and progress.

con·sult·ing staff (kŏn-sŭlt´ing staf) Specialists affiliated with a hospital who serve only in an advisory capacity to the attending staff.

con·sump·tion co·ag·u·lop·a·thy (kŏn-sŭmp´shŭn kō-ag´yū-lop´ă-thē) A disorder in which marked reductions develop in blood concentrations of platelets with exhaustion of the coagulation factors in the peripheral blood as a result of disseminated intravascular coagulation.

con·tact (kon´takt) **1.** The touching or apposition of two surfaces. **2.** Someone exposed to a contagious disease. **3.** DENTISTRY the area of two teeth in an arch where mesial and distal surfaces touch.

con·tac·tant (kŏn-tak´tănt) Any allergen that elicits manifestations of hypersensitivity by direct contact with skin or mucosa.

con·tact chei·li·tis (kon´takt kī-lī´tis) Lip inflammation resulting from contact with a primary irritant or specific allergen. SYN cheilitis venenata.

con·tact der·ma·ti·tis (kon´takt dĕr´mă-tī´tis) Inflammatory rash marked by itching and redness resulting from cutaneous contact with a specific allergen or irritant.

con·tact hy·per·sen·si·tiv·i·ty (CHS) (kon´takt hī´pĕr-sen-si-tiv´i-tē) **1.** SYN contact dermatitis. **2.** SYN delayed reaction.

con·tact in·hi·bi·tion (kon´takt in´hi-bish´ŭn) Cessation of replication of dividing cells that come into contact.

con·tact i·so·la·tion (kon´takt ī´sŏ-lā´shŭn) Isolation in which anyone entering the patient's room or in direct contact with the patient must don gloves and gown.

con·tact lens (kon´takt lenz) A lens that fits over the cornea and sclera or cornea only; used to correct refractive errors.

con·tact pre·cau·tions (kon´takt prĕ-kaw´shŭnz) Procedures that reduce the risk of spread of infections through direct or indirect contact. Transmission occurs with physical contact of the infected patient or handling of a contaminated object in the infected patient's room.

con·tact ul·cer (kon´takt ŭl´sĕr) Ulceration of the vocal folds due to abuse along their posterior borders, overlying vocal processes of arytenoid cartilages; produces hoarseness.

con·ta·gion (kŏn-tā´jŭn) Transmission of infection by direct contact, droplet spread, or contaminated fomites. SYN infectious (2).

con·ta·gious (kŏn-tā´jŭs) Relating to contagion. SYN infectious (2).

con·tam·i·nant (kŏn-tam´i-nănt) Any impurity or foreign matter associated with a chemical, pharmaceutical preparation, physiologic principle, or infectious agent.

con·tam·i·na·tion (kŏn-tam′i-nā′shŭn) **1.** The presence of an infectious agent on a body surface or on or in clothes, bedding, toys, surgical instruments or dressings, or other inanimate articles or substances including water, milk, and food, or that infectious agent itself. **2.** That portion of a chemical, biologic, or radiologic agent that remains on (external contamination) or in (internal contamination) a victim or inanimate object. **3.** EPIDEMIOLOGY States that exists when a population being studied for one condition or factor also possesses others that modify study results.

con·tent (kon′tent) **1.** That which is contained within something else. **2.** PSYCHOLOGY form of a dream as presented to consciousness. **3.** Ambiguous usage for concentration (3).

con·tent va·lid·i·ty (kon′tent vă-lid′i-tē) Extent to which the items of a test or procedure are in fact a representative sample of that which is to be measured.

con·ti·gu·i·ty, spa·tial con·ti·gu·ity (kon′ti-gyū′i-tē, spā′shăl) **1.** Contact without actual continuity (q.v.). **2.** Occurrence of two or more objects, events, or mental impressions together in space or time.

con·ti·nence (kon′ti-nĕns) **1.** Moderation, temperance, or self-restraint, especially sex. **2.** The ability to retain urine and/or feces until a proper time for their discharge.

con·tin·u·ing ed·u·ca·tion (kŏn-tin′yū-ing ed′yū-kā′shŭn) Opportunity to gain additional training and/or knowledge in a given field.

con·ti·nu·i·ty (kon′ti-nū′i-tē) Absence of interruption; a succession of parts intimately united. Cf. contiguity.

con·tin·u·ous in·ter·leaved sam·pling (kŏn-tin′yū-ŭs in′tĕr-lēvd sam′pling) A strategy in speech processing for cochlear implants in which brief pulses are presented to each electrode in a nonoverlapping sequence.

con·tin·u·ous man·da·to·ry ven·ti·la·tion (CMV) (kŏn-tin′yū-ŭs man′dă-tōr-ē ven′ti-lā′shŭn) SYN controlled mechanical ventilation.

con·tin·u·ous mur·mur (CM) (kŏn-tin′yū-ŭs mŭr′mŭr) Uninterrupted sound perceptible throughout systole and into diastole.

con·tin·u·ous pas·sive mo·tion (CPM) (kŏn-tin′yū-ŭs pas′iv mō′shŭn) A technique in which a joint, usually the knee, is moved constantly through a variable range of motion to prevent stiffness and to increase the range of motion; most often accomplished using a motorized device specifically designed also to relieve pain after surgery or injury to major joints of upper and lower extremities.

con·tin·u·ous phase (kŏn-tin′yū-ŭs fāz) SYN external phase.

con·tin·u·ous spon·ta·ne·ous ven·ti·la·tion (CSV) (kŏn-tin′yū-ŭs spon-tā′nē-ŭs ven′ti-lā′shŭn) A mode of mechanical ventilation in which every breath is spontaneous.

con·tin·u·ous su·ture (kŏn-tin′yū-ŭs sū′chŭr) An uninterrupted series of stitches using a single suture.

con·tin·u·ous trem·or (kŏn-tin′yū-ŭs trem′ŏr) SYN persistent tremor.

con·tin·u·ous ve·no·ven·ous he·mo·di·a·fil·tra·tion (CVVHD) (kŏn-tin′yū-us vē-no-vē′nŭs hē′mō-dī′ă-fil-trā′shŭn) Therapy that uses a diffusion solution clearance as a modality.

con·tin·u·ous ve·no·ve·nous he·mo·di·al·y·sis (CVVHD) (kŏn-tin′yū-ŭs vē-nō-vē′nŭs hē′mō-dī-al′i-sis) Process in which blood is pumped from a vein to the dialyzing unit and then returned to the venous circulation once treated.

con·tin·u·ous ve·no·ve·nous he·mo·fil·tra·tion (CVVH) (kŏn-tin′yū-ŭs vē-nō-vē′nŭs hē′mō-fil-trā′shŭn) Process in which blood is pumped from a vein to the filtration unit and then returned to the venous circulation.

con·tin·u·um, pl. **con·tin·ua** (kŏn-tin′yū-ŭm, -ă) Range across a spectrum.

con·tour (kon′tūr) **1.** Outline; surface configuration. **2.** DENTISTRY to restore the normal outlines of a broken or otherwise misshapen tooth.

contra- Prefix meaning opposed, against. SEE ALSO anti-.

con·tra·cep·tion (kon'tră-sep'shŭn) Prevention of conception or impregnation.

con·tra·cep·tive (kon'tră-sep'tiv) **1.** An agent to prevent conception. **2.** Relating to any measure or agent designed to prevent conception.

con·tra·cep·tive de·vice (kon'tră-sep'tiv dĕ-vīs') Something used to prevent pregnancy (e.g., occlusive diaphragm, condom).

con·tra·cep·tive meth·od (kon'tră-sep'tiv meth'ŏd) Means to prevent conception. SYN birth control.

con·tract (kŏn-trakt', kon'trakt) **1.** To shorten; to become reduced in size. **2.** To acquire by contagion or infection. **3.** An explicit bilateral commitment by psychotherapist and patient to a defined course of therapeutic action.

con·tract·ed pel·vis (kŏn-trakt'ĕd pel'vis) One with smaller than normal measurements in any diameter.

con·trac·tile (kon-trak'tīl) Having the property of contracting.

con·trac·til·i·ty (kon'trak-til'i-tē) The ability or property of a substance, of shortening or reducing in size.

con·trac·tion (C) (kŏn-trak'shŭn) **1.** A shortening or increase in tension; denoting the normal function of muscle. **2.** A shrinkage or reduction in size.

con·trac·tion band (kŏn-trak'shŭn band) A microscopic change in myocardial cells in which excessive contraction, associated with elevated intracellular calcium and serum norepinephrine, causes the formation of transverse amorphous bands in the fibers, which are then incapable of recontracting. SYN contraction band necrosis.

con·trac·tion band nec·ro·sis (kŏn-trak'shŭn band nĕ-krō'sis) SYN contraction band.

con·trac·tion stress test (kŏn-trak'

shŭn stres test) SYN oxytocin challenge test.

con·trac·ture (kŏn-trak'shŭr) Static muscle shortening due to tonic spasm or fibrosis, to loss of muscular balance, or to a loss of motion of an adjacent joint.

con·tra·fis·sura (kon'tră-fi-shŭr'ă) Fracture of a bone, as in the skull, at a point opposite that where the blow was received. SEE ALSO contrecoup injury of brain.

con·tra·in·di·cate (kon'tră-in'di-kāt) To avoid a protocol or treatment based on specific prevailing circumstances.

con·tra·in·di·ca·tion (kon'tră-in-di-kā'shŭn) Any special symptom or circumstance that renders the use of a remedy or the carrying out of a procedure inadvisable, due to risk.

con·tra·lat·er·al (kon'tră-lat'ĕr-ăl) Relating to the opposite side. SYN heterolateral.

con·tra·lat·er·al hem·i·ple·gi·a (kon'tră-lat'ĕr-ăl hem'ē-plē'jē-ă) Paralysis occurring opposite to the causal central lesion.

con·trast (kon'trast) A comparison in which differences are demonstrated or enhanced.

con·trast bath (kon'trast bath) One in which a body part is immersed in hot water for a period of a few minutes and then in cold, at intervals; used to increase the blood flow.

con·trast ech·o·car·di·og·ra·phy (kon'trast ek'ō-kahr'dē-og'ră-fē) Injection of contrast media of high echo reflectants (e.g., bubbles) to outline a chamber or delineate a shunt within the heart.

con·trast en·e·ma (CE) (kon'trast en'ĕ-mă) One using barium sulfate or a water-soluble contrast medium for radiographic purposes.

con·tre·coup frac·ture (kŏn'trĕ-kū' frak'shŭr) A fracture of the cranial vault occurring at a site approximately opposite the point of impact.

con·trol (kŏn-trōl') **1.** (v.) To regulate,

restrain, correct, restore to normal. **2.** (n.) Ongoing operations or programs aimed at reducing a disease. **3.** (n.) Members of a comparison group who differ in disease experience or allocation to a regimen from the subjects of a study.

con·trol an·i·mal (kŏn-trōl′ an′ĭ-măl) In research, an animal submitted to the same conditions as the others used for the experiment, but with the crucial factor (e.g., injection of antitoxin, the administration of a drug) omitted. SEE ALSO control, control experiment.

con·trol ex·per·i·ment (kŏn-trōl′ eks-per′i-mĕnt) One used to check another, to verify a result, or demonstrate what would have occurred had the factor under study been omitted. SEE ALSO control, control animal.

con·trol gene (kŏn-trōl′ jēn) SEE operator gene, regulator gene.

con·trolled me·chan·i·cal ven·ti·la·tion (kon-trōld′ mĕ-kan′ĭ-kăl ven′ti-lā′shŭn) A form of artificial respiration in which positive pressure is applied to the airway. SYN continuous mandatory ventilation.

con·trolled sub·stance (kŏn-trōld′ sŭb′stăns) One subject to the U.S. Controlled Substances Act (1970), which regulates the prescribing and dispensing, as well as the manufacturing, storage, sale, or distribution of substances assigned to five schedules according to their 1) potential for or evidence of abuse, 2) potential for psychic or physiologic dependence, 3) contribution to a public health risk, 4) harmful pharmacologic effect, or 5) role as a precursor of other controlled substances.

con·tuse (kŏn-tūz′) To injure a tissue without laceration. SYN bruise (2).

con·tu·sion (kŏn-tū′zhŭn) Any mechanical injury (usually caused by a blow) resulting in hemorrhage beneath unbroken skin. SEE ALSO bruise.

co·nus, pl. **co·ni** (kŏ′nŭs, -nī) **1.** SYN cone. **2.** Posterior staphyloma in myopic choroidopathy.

con·va·les·cence (kon′vă-les′ĕns) A period between the end of a disease and

the patient's restoration to complete health.

con·va·les·cent car·ri·er (kon-vă-les′ĕnt kar′ē-ĕr) Someone clinically recovered from an infectious disease but still capable of transmitting the infectious agent.

con·vec·tion (kŏn-vek′shŭn) Conveyance of heat in liquids or gases by movement of the heated particles, as when the layer of water at the bottom of a heated pot rises or the warm air of a room ascends to the ceiling.

con·vec·tive heat (kŏn-vek′tiv hēt) A rise in temperature conveyed from one structure or appliance to another in which the warmer affects the cooler by convection.

con·ver·gence (kŏn-vĕr′jĕns) **1.** The tending of two or more objects toward a common point. **2.** The direction of the visual lines to a near point.

con·ver·gence ex·cess (kŏn-vĕr′jĕns eks′es) Optic condition in which esophoria or esotropia is greater for near than far vision.

con·ver·gence in·suf·fi·cien·cy (kŏn-vĕr′jĕns in′sŭ-fish′ĕn-sē) Optic condition in which esophoria or esotropia is greater for far than near vision.

con·ver·gent ev·o·lu·tion (kŏn-vĕr′jĕnt ev′ŏ-lū′shŭn) Evolutionary development of similar structures in two or more species, often widely separated phylogenetically, in response to similarities of environment.

con·ver·gent stra·bis·mus (kŏn-vĕr′jĕnt stră-biz′mŭs) SYN esotropia.

con·ver·sion (kŏn-vĕr′zhŭn) **1.** SYN transmutation. **2.** Psychological defense mechanism in which unconscious conflict or repressed thought is expressed symbolically, or somatically. **3.** In virology, the acquisition by bacteria of a new property associated with the presence of a prophage.

con·ver·sive heat (kŏn-vĕr′siv hēt) That produced in a body by the absorption of waves that are not themselves hot.

con·ver·tase (kon′vĕr-tās) Proteases of complement that convert one component into another.

con·ver·tin (kon-věr'tin) Active form of factor VII designated VIIa.

con·vex (Cx) (kon'veks) Denotes surface that is evenly curved outward.

con·vex·o·con·cave lens (kon-vek'sō-kon'kāv lenz) A minus power lens having one surface convex and the opposite surface concave, with the latter having the greater curvature.

con·vex·o·con·vex (kon-vek'sō-kon'veks) SYN biconvex.

con·vo·lute (kon'vŏ-lūt') Rolled together with one part over the other; in the shape of a roll or scroll. SYN convoluted.

con·vo·lut·ed (kon'vŏlūt'ed)kon' SYN convolute.

con·vo·lu·tion (kon'vŏ-lū'shŭn) 1. A coiling or rolling of an organ. 2. Specifically, a gyrus of the cerebral or cerebellar cortex.

con·vul·sion (kŏn-vŭl'shŭn) 1. A violent spasm or series of jerkings of the face, trunk, or extremities. 2. SYN seizure (2).

con·vul·sive seiz·ure (kŏn-vŭl'siv sē'zhŭr) One with clonic or tonic-clonic motor activity.

con·vul·sive ther·a·py (kŏn-vŭl'siv thār'ă-pē) SYN electroshock therapy.

con·vul·sive tic (kŏn-vŭl'siv tik) SYN facial tic.

Coo·ley a·ne·mi·a (koo'lē ă-nē'mē-ă) SYN thalassemia major.

Coo·lidge tube (kū'lij tūb) X-ray tube, in which the cathode consists of a tungsten wire spiral surrounded by a focusing cup.

Coombs di·rect test (kūmz dīr-ekt' test) Laboratory test using erythrocytes to detect antibodies to them or to complement.

Coombs in·di·rect test (kūmz in'dīr-ekt' test) Laboratory test using serum that contains an antibody that may be used for erythrocyte typing.

Coop·er tes·tis (kū'pĕr tĕs'tis) Neuralgic testicular pain.

co·or·di·nate co·val·ent bond (kō-ōr'di-năt kō-vā'lĕnt bond) SYN semipolar bond.

co·or·di·na·tion (coord) (kō-ōr'di-nā'shun) The harmonious working together, especially of several muscles or muscle groups in the execution of complicated movements.

co·pay (kō'pā) A fixed or set amount paid for each health care or medical service; the remainder is paid by the health insurance plan. SEE ALSO coinsurance, cost sharing. SYN out-of-pocket costs, out-of-pocket expenses.

cope (kōp) 1. The upper half of a flask in the casting art; hence applicable to the upper or cavity side of a denture flask. 2. An act that enables one to adjust to setbacks.

cop·ing (kōp'ing) 1. A thin metal covering or cap. 2. An adaptive or otherwise successful method of dealing with individual or environmental situations that involve psychological or physiologic stress or threat.

co·pol·y·mer (kō'pol'i-měr) A polymer in which two or more monomers or base units are combined.

co·pol·y·mer-1 (kō'pol'i-měr) Acetate polypeptide salt; used to reduce relapse rate with relapsing-remitting multiple sclerosis.

cop·per (Cu) (kop'ĕr) A metallic element, atomic no. 29, atomic wt. 63.546; several of its salts are used in medicine.

cop·per·head (kop'ĕr-hed) A U.S. poisonous snake of the genus *Agkistrodon*.

cop·per sul·fate, cop·per sul·phate (kop'ĕr sŭl'fāt) SYN cupric sulfate.

cop·rem·e·sis (kop-rem'ĕ-sis) SYN fecal vomiting.

cop·ro·an·ti·bod·ies (kop'rō-an'ti-bod-ēz) Antibodies found in the intestine and in feces.

cop·ro·la·li·a (kop'rō-lā'lē-ă) Involuntary utterances of vulgar or obscene words; found in Tourette syndrome (q.v.). SYN coprophrasia.

cop·ro·lith (kop'rō-lith) A hard mass of inspissated feces. SYN fecalith, stercolith.

cop·rol·o·gy (kop-rol'ŏ-jē) Study of feces for physiologic and diagnostic purposes. SYN scatology.

cop·ro·ma (kop-rō'mă) An accumulation of inspissated feces in the colon or rectum mimicking an abdominal tumor. SYN fecaloma, stercoroma.

cop·ro·pha·gi·a, cop·ro·pha·gy (kop'rō-fā'jē-ă, -fā-jē) The eating of excrement. SYN scatophagy.

cop·ro·pho·bi·a (kop'rō-fō'bē-ă) Morbid fear of defecation and feces.

cop·ro·por·phyr·i·a (kop'rō-pōr-fir'ē-ă) Presence of coproporphyrins in the urine, as in variegate porphyria.

cop·ro·por·phy·rin (kop'rō-pōr'fir-in) One of two porphyrin compounds found normally in feces as a decomposition product of bilirubin (hence, from hemoglobin).

cop·ro·prax·ia (kop'rō-prak'sē-ă) Obscene gesturing.

cop·ro·zo·a (kop'rō-zō'ă) Protozoa that can be cultivated in fecal matter, although not necessarily living in feces within the intestine.

cop·u·la·tion (kop'yū-lā'shŭn) SYN coitus.

cop·u·line (kop'yū-lĭn) Any of several pheromones that occur in vaginal secretions; men who were exposed to copulines rated women as more attractive, especially those women considered less attractive by controls tested with water.

cor, gen. cor·dis (kōr, kōr'dis) [TA] SYN heart.

cor·a·cid·i·um (kor'ă-sid'ē-ŭm) The ciliated first-stage aquatic embryo of pseudophyllid and other cestodes with aquatic cycles.

cor·a·co·a·cro·mi·al lig·a·ment (kōr'ă-kō-ă-krō'mē-ăl lig'ă-mĕnt) [TA] Heavy arched fibrous band that passes between the coracoid process and the acromion above the shoulder joint. SYN ligamentum coracoacromiale [TA].

cor·a·co·bra·chi·a·lis mus·cle (kōr'ă-kō-brā-kē-ā'lis mŭs'ĕl) [TA] *Origin*, coracoid process of scapula; *insertion*, middle of medial border of humerus; *action*, adducts and flexes the arm; resists downward dislocation of shoulder joint; *nerve supply*, musculocutaneous. SYN musculus coracobrachialis [TA].

cor·a·co·cla·vic·u·lar (kōr'ă-kō-klă-vik'yū-lăr) Relating to the coracoid process and the clavicle. SYN scapuloclavicular (2).

cor·a·co·cla·vic·u·lar lig·a·ment (kōr'ă-kō-klă-vik'yū-lăr lig'ă-mĕnt) [TA] The strong ligament that unites the clavicle to the coracoid process. SYN ligamentum coracoclaviculare [TA].

cor·a·co·hu·mer·al (kōr'ă-kō-hyū'mĕr-ăl) Relating to the coracoid process and the humerus.

cor·a·coid (kōr'ă-koyd) Shaped like a crow's beak; denoting a process of the scapula.

cor·a·coid pro·cess (kōr'ă-koyd pros'es) [TA] A long curved projection from the neck of the scapula overhanging the glenoid cavity.

cor ad·i·po·sum (kōr ad-i-pō'sŭm) SYN fatty heart (2).

cord (kōrd) [TA] 1. ANATOMY any long, ropelike structure. SYN fasciculus (2) [TA], funiculus [TA], funicle. 2. SEE ALSO chorda.

cor·date (kōr'dāt) Heart-shaped.

cord blood (kōrd blŭd) Blood present in the umbilical vessels at the time of delivery.

cor·dec·to·my (kōr-dek'tŏ-mē) Excision of a part or whole of a cord.

cor·do·cen·te·sis (kōr'dō-sen-tē'sis) Transabdominal blood sampling of the fetal umbilical cord, performed under ultrasound guidance. SYN funipuncture.

cor·do·pexy (kōr'dō-pek-sē) 1. Operative fixation of any displaced anatomic cord. 2. Lateral fixation of one or both vocal cords to correct glottic stenosis.

cor·dot·o·my (kōr-dot'ŏ-mē) 1. Any operation on the spinal cord. **2.** Division of tracts of the spinal cord, which may be performed percutaneously (stereotactic cordotomy) or after laminectomy (open cordotomy) by various techniques such as incision or radio frequency coagulation. **3.** Incision through the membranous vocal fold to widen the posterior glottis in bilateral vocal paralysis. SYN chordotomy.

core-, coreo-, coro- Combining forms denoting the pupil (of the eye).

cor·ec·to·pi·a (kōr'ek-tō'pē-ă) Eccentric location of the pupil so that it is not in the center of the iris.

cor·e·o·plas·ty (kōr'ē-ō-plas-tē) Procedure to correct a misshapen or occluded pupil.

cor·e·pexy (kōr'ē-pek-sē) A suturing of the iris to modify the shape or size of the pupil.

cor·e·praxy (kōr'ē-prak'sē) A procedure designed to widen a small pupil.

co·re·pres·sor (kō-rĕ-pres'ŏr) A molecule, usually a product of a specific metabolic pathway, which combines with and activates a repressor produced by a regulator gene.

core tem·per·a·ture (kōr tem'pĕr-ă-chŭr) The temperature of the interior of the body.

co·ri·um, pl. **co·ri·a** (kō'rē-ŭm, -ă) SYN dermis.

corn (kōrn) **1.** The foodstuff, *Zea mays*. **2.** A hard or soft hyperkeratosis of the human foot secondary to friction and pressure. SYN clavus (1).

cor·nea (kōr'nē-ă) [TA] Transparent tissue constituting the anterior sixth of the outer wall of the eye, with a 7.7-mm radius of curvature as contrasted with the 13.5-mm of the sclera. It consists of stratified squamous epithelium continuous with that of the conjunctiva, a substantia propria, regularly arranged collagen imbedded in mucopolysaccharide, and an inner layer of endothelium.

cor·ne·al a·bra·sion (kōr-nē-ăl ă-brā'zhŭn) Scrape or scratch to the outer surface of the eyeball.

cor·ne·al a·stig·ma·tism (kōr'nē-ăl ă-stig'mă-tizm) Ocular disorder due to a defect in the curvature of the corneal surface.

cor·ne·al cor·pus·cles (kōr'nē-ăl kōr'pŭs-ĕlz) Connective tissue cells found between the laminae of fibrous tissue in the cornea.

cor·ne·al lim·bus (kōr'nē-ăl lim'bŭs) SYN corneoscleral junction.

cor·ne·al re·flex (kōr'nē-ăl rē'fleks) **1.** A contraction of the eyelids when the cornea is lightly touched. **2.** Reflection of light from the surface of the cornea.

cor·ne·al space (kōr'nē-ăl spās) One of the stellate spaces between the lamellae of the cornea, each of which contains a cell or corneal corpuscle.

cor·ne·al staph·y·lo·ma (kōr'nē-ăl staf'i-lō'mă) SYN anterior staphyloma.

cor·ne·al ul·cer (kōr'nē-ăl ŭl'sĕr) Lesion of the outer surface of the eyeball.

cor·ne·o·bleph·a·ron (kōr'nē-ō-blef'ă-ron) Adhesion of the eyelid margin to the cornea.

cor·ne·o·scle·ra (kōr'nē-ō-skler'ă) Combined cornea and sclera considered as forming the eyeball's external coat.

cor·ne·o·scle·ral junc·tion (kōr'nē-ō-skler'ăl jŭngk'shŭn) The margin of the cornea that is overlapped by the sclera. SYN corneal limbus.

cor·nic·u·late (kōr-nik'yū-lăt) **1.** Resembling a horn. **2.** Having horns or horn-shaped appendages.

cor·nic·u·lum (kōr-nik'yū-lŭm) A cornu of small size.

cor·ni·fi·ca·tion (kōr'ni-fi-kā'shŭn) SYN keratinization.

corn oil (kōrn oyl) The refined fixed oil expressed from the embryo of *Zea mays* (family Gramineae); a solvent. SYN maize oil.

cor·nu, gen. **cor·nus**, pl. **cor·nu·a** (kōr'nū, -nūs, -nū-ă) [TA] **1.** SYN horn. **2.** Any structure composed of horny substance. **3.** One of the coronal extensions of the dental pulp underlying a cusp or lobe. **4.** The major subdivisions of the lateral ventricle in the cerebral hemisphere (the frontal horn, occipital horn, and temporal horn). **5.** The major divisions of the gray columns of the spinal cord (anterior horn, lateral horn, posterior horn).

cor·nu·al (kōr′nū-ăl) Relating to a cornu.

cor·nu·al preg·nan·cy (kōr′nū-ăl preg′ năn-sē) The implantation and development of the impregnated oocyte in one of the cornua of the uterus.

cor·nu cu·ta·ne·um (kōr′nū kyū-tā′nē-ŭm) SYN cutaneous horn.

co·ro·na, gen. and pl. **co·ro·nae** (kŏ-rō′nă, -nē) [TA] SYN crown.

cor·o·nad (kōr′ŏ-nad) In a direction toward any corona.

co·ro·nal plane (kōr′ŏ-năl plān) A vertical plane at right angles to a sagittal plane, dividing the body into anterior and posterior portions, or any plane parallel to the central coronal plane. SYN Frontal plane.

cor·o·nal su·ture (kōr′ŏ-năl sū′chŭr) [TA] The line of junction of the frontal with the two parietal bones of the skull.

cor·o·nary (kōr′ŏ-nār-ē) **1.** Relating to or resembling a crown. **2.** Specifically, denoting the coronary blood vessels of the heart; colloquially, myocardial infarction or coronary thrombosis.

cor·o·nar·y an·gi·og·ra·phy (kōr′ŏ-nār-ē an′jē-og′ră-fē) Imaging myocardial circulation by injection of contrast medium.

cor·o·nar·y ar·te·ries (kōr′ŏ-nār-ē ahr′tĕr-ēz) A pair of arteries that branch from the aorta and supply blood to the myocardium.

cor·o·nar·y ar·ter·i·tis (kōr′ŏ-nā-rē ahr′tĕr-ī′tis) Inflammation of any or all of the layers of coronary artery walls.

cor·o·nar·y ar·te·ry by·pass graft (CABG) (kōr′ŏ-nār-ē ahr′tĕr-ē bī′pās graft) A surgical procedure in which damaged sections of the coronary arter-

ies are replaced with new articular or venous graftings to increase rate of cardiac blood flow; sometimes colloquially known as a 'cabbage procedure.'

cor·o·nar·y ar·te·ry dis·ease (CAD) (kōr′ŏ-nār-ē ahr′tĕr-ē di-zēz′) Narrowing of the lumen of one or more of the coronary arteries, usually due to atherosclerosis; myocardial ischemia.

cor·o·nar·y care unit (CCU) (kōr′ŏ-nār-ē kār yū′nit) A group of beds within a hospital set aside for the care of patients having or suspected of having acute cardiac episodes.

cor·o·nar·y cat·a·ract (kōr′ŏ-nār-ē kat′ăr-akt) Peripheral cortical developmental cataract occurring just after puberty.

cor·o·nar·y em·bo·lism (kōr′ŏ-nar-ē em′bŏ-lizm) Sudden occlusion of a coronary vessel caused by foreign matter (e.g., blood clot).

cor·o·nar·y heart dis·ease (kōr′ŏ-nar-ē hahrt di-zēz′) SYN coronary artery disease.

cor·o·nar·y in·suf·fi·cien·cy (kōr′ŏ-nār-ē in′sŭ-fish′ĕn-sē) Inadequate coronary circulation leading to anginal pain.

cor·o·nar·y oc·clu·sion (kōr′ŏ-nār-ē ŏ-klū′zhŭn) Blockage of a coronary vessel, usually by thrombosis or atheroma, often leading to myocardial infarction.

cor·o·nar·y throm·bo·sis (kōr′ŏ-nār-ē throm-bō′sis) Coronary occlusion by thrombus formation, usually the result of atheromatous changes in the arterial wall and usually leading to myocardial infarction.

co·ro·na ve·ne·ris (kŏ-rō′nă vē-ner′is) Papular syphilitic lesions (secondary eruption) along the anterior margin of the scalp or on the back of the neck.

Co·ro·na·vi·rus (kō-rō′nă-vī′rŭs) Viral genus associated with upper respiratory tract infections (i.e., the common cold) and possibly gastroenteritis in humans.

cor·o·ner (COR) (kōr′ŏ-nĕr) An official whose duty it is to investigate sudden, suspicious, or violent death to determine its cause; in some communities, office replaced by medical examiner.

cor·o·noid (kōr′ŏ-noyd) *Do not confuse this word with coronal or coronary.* Shaped like a crow's beak; denoting certain processes and other parts of bones.

cor·o·noi·dec·to·my (kōr′ŏ-noyd-ek′tŏ-mē) Surgical removal of the coronoid process of the mandible.

cor·o·noid pro·cess (kōr′ŏ-noyd pros′es) Coronoid process of the mandible, the triangular anterior process of the mandibular ramus, giving attachment to the temporal muscle; coronoid process of the ulna, a bracketlike projection from the anterior portion of the proximal extremity of the ulna.

cor·o·noid pro·cess of the ul·na (kōr′ŏ-noyd pros′es ŭl′nă) [TA] Bracketlike projection from the anterior portion of the proximal extremity of the ulna. SYN processus coronoideus ulnae [TA].

cor·ot·o·my (kŏr-ot′ŏ-mē) Incision of the iris to create a pseudopupil. SYN iridotomy.

cor·pora bi·gem·i·na (kōr-pōr′ă bī-jem′i-nă) SYN bigeminal bodies.

cor·pus, gen. **cor·po·ris** (kōr′pŭs, kōr-pō′ris) [TA] 1. SYN body. 2. The main part of an organ or other anatomic structure, as distinguished from the head or caudal region. SEE ALSO shaft, soma.

cor·pus ad·i·po·sum buc·cae (kōr′pŭs ad-i-pō′sŭm bŭk′ē) [TA] SYN buccal fat-pad.

cor·pus al·bi·cans (CA) (kōr′pŭs al′bikanz) [TA] Retrogressed corpus luteum characterized by increasing cicatrization and shrinkage of the cicatricial core with an amorphous, convoluted, completely hyalinized lutein zone surrounding the central plug of scar tissue. SYN albicans (2), atretic corpus luteum, corpus candicans.

cor·pus amyg·da·loi·de·um (kōr′pŭs ă-mig-di-loyd′ē-ŭm) [TA] SYN amygdaloid body.

cor·pus am·y·la·ce·um, pl. **cor·po·ra am·y·la·cea** (kōr′pŭs am-i-lā′shē-ŭm, kōr-pōr′ă am′i-lā′shē-ă) One of a number of small ovoid or rounded, sometimes granular, laminated, bodies found in nervous tissue, in the prostate, and in pulmonary alveoli. SYN amnionic corpuscle.

cor·pus cal·lo·sum (kōr′pŭs ka-lō′sŭm) [TA] The great commissural plate of nerve fibers interconnecting the cortical hemispheres (with the exception of most of the temporal lobes, which are interconnected by the anterior commissure).

cor·pus cav·er·no·sum pe·nis (kōr′pŭs kav′ĕr-nō′sŭm pē′nis) [TA] One of two parallel columns of erectile tissue forming the dorsal part of the body of the penis; they are separated posteriorly, forming the crura of the penis.

cor·pus·cle (kōr′pŭs-ĕl) 1. A small mass or body. 2. A blood cell. SYN corpusculum.

cor·pus·cu·lar lymph (kōr-pŭs′kyū-lăr limf) SYN aplastic lymph.

cor·pus·cu·lum, pl. **cor·pus·cu·la** (kōr-pŭs′kyū-lŭm, -lă) SYN corpuscle.

cor·pus fem·o·ris (kōr-pŭs fem′ō-ris) SYN shaft of femur.

cor·pus he·mor·rha·gi·cum (kōr′pŭs hem-ŏ-raj′i-kŭm) A hematoma within an ovarian follicle; gradual resorption of the blood elements leaves a cavity filled with a clear fluid.

cor·pus spon·gi·o·sum pe·nis (kōr′pŭs spŏn-jē-ō′sŭm pē′nis) [TA] The median column of erectile tissue located between and ventral to the two corpora cavernosa penis; posteriorly it expands into the bulbus penis and anteriorly it terminates as the enlarged glans penis. It is traversed by the urethra.

cor·pus stri·a·tum (kōr′pŭs strī-ā′tŭm) [TA] SYN striate body.

cor·pus u·ter·i (kōr-pŭs yū′tĕr-ī) [TA] SYN body of uterus.

cor·pus vit·re·um (kōr′pŭs vit′rē-ŭm) [TA] SEE ALSO vitreous. SYN vitreous body.

cor·rec·tion (cor) (kŏr-ek′shŭn) The act of reducing a fault; the elimination of an unfavorable quality.

cor·re·la·tion (CR) (kōr′ĕ-lā′shŭn) 1. The mutual or reciprocal relation of two or more items or parts. **2.** The act of bringing into such a relation. **3.** The degree to which variables change together.

cor·re·la·tion co·ef·fi·cient (r) (kōr´ĕ-lā´shŭn kō´ĕ-fish´ĕnt) Measure of association that indicates the degree to which two variables have a linear relationship.

cor·rel·a·tive dif·fer·en·ti·a·tion (kōr´ĕ-lā-tiv dif´ĕr-en-shē-ā´shŭn) That due to the interaction of different parts of an organism.

Cor·re·ra line (kōr-rār´ă līn) Outline of lung fields seen on plain film radiograph of thorax.

cor·re·spon·dence (kōr´ĕ-spon´dĕns) OPTICS the points on each retina that have the same visual direction.

Cor·ri·gan dis·ease (kōr´i-găn di-zēz´) SYN aortic regurgitation.

Cor·ri·gan pulse (kōr´i-găn pŭls) That marked by a sharp rise to full expansion then collapse; seen in aortic insufficiency.

Cor·ri·gan sign (kōr´i-găn sīn) **1.** A purple line at the junction of teeth and gingiva in chronic copper poisoning. **2.** Expanding pulsatile mass seen in abdominal aortic aneurysm.

cor·rin (kōr´in) The cyclic system of four pyrrole rings forming corrinoids, which are the central structure of the vitamins B12 and related compounds.

cor·ro·sion (COR) (kŏr-ō´zhŭn) **1.** Gradual deterioration or consummation of a substance by another, especially by biochemical or chemical reaction. Cf. erosion. **2.** The product of corroding, such as rust.

cor·ro·sive (kŏr-ō´siv) **1.** Causing corrosion. **2.** An agent that produces corrosion (e.g., a strong acid or alkali).

cor·ro·sive gas·tri·tis (kŏr-ō´siv gas-trī´tis) Inflammation of the inner lining of the stomach that may be caused by ingestion of strong acids or alkalies.

cor·tex, gen. **cor·ti·cis** (kōr´teks, -ti-sis) [TA] Outer portion of an organ, as distinguished from the inner, or medullary, portion.

cor·tex len·tis (kōr´teks len´tis) [TA] SYN cortex of lens.

cor·tex of lens (kōr´teks lenz) [TA] Softer, more superficial part of the lens of the eye that encloses the central part or nucleus; its refractive power is less than that of the nucleus. SYN cortex lentis [TA].

cor·tex of thy·mus (kōr´teks thī´mŭs) [TA] Outer part of a thymus lobule; surrounds the medulla and is composed of masses of closely packed lymphocytes. SYN cortex thymi [TA].

Cor·ti arch (kōr´tē ahrch) That formed by the junction of the heads of Corti inner and outer pillar cells, in the inner ear.

cor·ti·cal ar·te·ries (kōr´ti-kăl ahr´tĕr-ēz) Branches of the anterior, middle, and posterior cerebral arteries that supply the cerebral cortex.

cor·ti·cal au·di·om·e·try (kōr´ti-kăl aw´dē-om´ĕ-trē) Measurement of the potentials that arise in the auditory system above the level of the brainstem.

cor·ti·cal bone (kōr´ti-kăl bōn) [TA] The superficial thin layer of compact bone. SYN substantia corticalis [TA], cortical substance.

cor·ti·cal deaf·ness (kōr´ti-kăl def´nĕs) Hearing impairment resulting from bilateral lesions of the primary receptive area of the temporal lobe.

cor·ti·cal hor·mones (kōr´ti-kăl hōr´mōnz) Steroid hormones produced by the cortex of the suprarenal gland.

cor·ti·cal lab·y·rinth (kōr´ti-kăl lab´ĭr-inth) [TA] Region of renal cortex consisting of glomeruli and convoluted uriniferous tubules. SYN labyrinthus corticis [TA], convoluted part of renal cortex, pars convoluta corticis renalis.

cor·ti·cec·to·my (kōr´ti-sek´tŏ-mē) Removal of a specific portion of the cerebral cortex.

cor·ti·cif·u·gal, cor·ti·co·fu·gal (kōr-ti-sif´yū-găl, -kof´yū-găl) Passing in a direction away from the outer surface.

cor·ti·cip·e·tal (kōr-ti-sip´ĕ-tăl) Passing in a direction toward the outer surface;

denoting nerve fibers conveying impulses toward the cerebral cortex. SYN corticoafferent.

cor·ti·coid, cor·ti·co·ste·roid (kōr'ti-koyd, -kō-ster'oyd) **1.** Having an action similar to that of a hormone of the cortex of the suprarenal gland. **2.** Any substance exhibiting this action. **3.** SYN glucocorticoid (3).

cor·ti·cos·ter·one (kōr'ti-kos'tĕr-ōn) A corticosteroid that induces some deposition of glycogen in the liver, sodium conservation, and potassium excretion; the principal glucocortoid in the rat.

cor·ti·co·troph (kōr'ti-kō-trōf) A cell of the adenohypophysis that produces adrenocorticotropic hormone.

cor·ti·co·tro·pin·re·leas·ing hor·mone (CRH) (kōr'ti-kō-trō'pin-rĕ-lēs'ing hōr'mōn) Factor secreted by the hypothalamus that stimulates pituitary to release adrenocorticotropic hormone. SYN corticoliberin.

cor·ti·lymph (kōr'ti-limf) The fluid in the Corti tunnel.

cor·ti·sol (kōr'ti-sol) SYN hydrocortisone.

cor·ti·sone (kōr'ti-sōn) A glucocorticoid not normally secreted in significant quantities by the human cortex of the suprarenal gland.

cor tri·at·ri·a·tum (kōr trī-at-rī-ā'tŭm) A congenital anomaly characterized by a heart with three atrial chambers.

cor tri·lo·cu·la·re (kōr trī-lok-yū-lā'rē) Three-chambered heart due to absence of the interatrial or the interventricular septum.

cor tri·lo·cu·la·re bi·a·tri·a·tum (kōr trī-lok-yū-lā'rē bī-ā-trī-ā'tŭm) Absence of the interventricular septum.

cor tri·lo·cu·la·re bi·ven·tri·cu·la·re (kōr trī-lok-yū-lā'rē bi-ven-trik'yū-lā'rē) SYN common atrium.

Cor·vi·sart fa·cies (kōr'vē-sahr' fash'ē-ēz) Characteristic facies seen in cardiac insufficiency or aortic regurgitation.

co·rym·bi·form (kōr-im'bi-fōrm) Denot-

ing flowerlike clustering configuration of skin lesions in granulomatous diseases.

Cor·y·ne·bac·te·ri·um (kŏ-rī'nē-bak-tēr'ē-ŭm) A widely distributed genus of nonmotile (except for some plant pathogens), aerobic to facultatively anaerobic bacteria containing irregularly staining, gram-positive, straight to slightly curved, often club-shaped rods.

Cor·y·ne·bac·te·ri·um diph·the·ri·ae (kŏ-rī'nē-bak-tēr'ē-ŭm diph-thē'rē-ē) Bacterial cause of diphtheria. SYN Löffler bacillus.

co·ry·za (kō-rī'ză) SYN acute rhinitis.

cos·me·sis (koz-mē'sis) A concern in therapeutics for the appearance of the patient; i.e., an operation that improves appearance.

cos·met·ic (koz-met'ik) **1.** Referring to surgical procedures intended to improve appearance; specifically relates to correction of deformities that result from heredity or aging and *not* caused by congenital anomalies, disease, trauma, or tumors. **2.** Relating to the use of cosmetics.

cos·met·ic der·ma·ti·tis (koz-met'ik dĕr'mă-tī'tis) Cutaneous eruption that results from application of a cosmetic; due to allergic sensitization or primary irritation.

cos·ta, gen. and pl. **cos·tae** (kos'tă, -tē) [TA] **1.** SYN rib [I–XII]. **2.** A rodlike internal supporting organelle that runs along the base of the undulating membrane of certain flagellate parasites such as *Trichomonas.* SYN basal rod.

cos·tal an·gle (kos'tăl ang'gĕl) Abrupt change in curvature of the body of a rib posteriorly, such that the neck and head of the rib are directed upward.

cos·tal·gi·a (kos-tal'jē-ă) SYN pleurodynia.

cos·tive (kos'tiv) Pertaining to or causing constipation.

costo- Prefix meaning the ribs.

cos·to·ax·il·lary vein (kos'tō-aks'i-lar-ē vān) One of a number of anastomotic veins connecting the intercostal veins of the first to seventh intercostal spaces with the lateral thoracic or the thoracoepigastric vein.

cos·to·cer·vi·cal (kos'tō-sĕr'vi-kăl) Pertaining to the ribs and neck.

cos·to·cer·vi·cal (ar·te·ri·al) trunk (kos'tō-sĕr'vi-kăl ahr-tēr'ē-ăl trŭngk) A short artery that arises from the subclavian artery on each side and divides into deep cervical and superior intercostal branches, the latter dividing usually to form the first and second posterior intercostal arteries. SYN costocervical artery.

cos·to·cer·vi·cal ar·te·ry (kos'tō-sĕr' vi-kăl ahr'tĕr-ē) SYN costocervical (arterial) trunk.

cos·to·chon·dral (kos'tō-kon'drăl) Relating to the costal cartilages. SYN chondrocostal.

cos·to·chon·dri·tis (kos'tō-kŏn-drī'tis, kos'tō-kon-drī'tis) Inflammation of one or more costal cartilages, characterized by local tenderness and pain of the anterior chest wall that sometimes radiates. SYN Tietze syndrome.

cos·to·cla·vic·u·lar (kos'tō-klă-vik'yū-lăr) Relating to the ribs and the clavicle.

cos·to·cla·vic·u·lar lig·a·ment (kos' tō-klă-vik'yū-lăr lig'ă-mĕnt) [TA] The ligament that connects the first rib and the clavicle near its sternal end; limits elevation of shoulder (at sternoclavicular joint). SYN ligamentum costoclaviculare [TA], rhomboid ligament.

cos·to·gen·ic (kos'tō-jen'ik) Arising from a rib.

cos·to·phren·ic (CP) (kos'tō-fren'ik) Involving or denoting the ribs and diaphragm.

cos·to·ster·no·plas·ty (kos'tō-stĕr'nō-plas-tē) Surgery to correct a malformation of the anterior chest wall.

cos·tot·o·my (kos-tot'ŏ-mē) Division of a rib.

cos·to·trans·ver·sec·to·my (kos'tō-trans-vĕr-sek'tŏ-mē) Excision of a proximal portion of a rib and the articulating transverse process.

cos·to·ver·te·bral (kos'tō-vĕr'tĕ-brăl) Relating to the ribs and the bodies of the thoracic vertebrae with which they articulate. SYN vertebrocostal (1).

cos·to·ver·te·bral an·gle (kos'tō-vĕr' tĕ-brăl ang'gĕl) The acute angle formed between the twelfth rib and the vertebral column.

Co·tard syn·drome (kō-tahr' sin'drōm) Psychotic depression involving delusion of the existence of one's body, along with ideas of negation and suicidal impulses.

cot death (kot deth) SYN sudden infant death syndrome.

co·trans·port (kō'trans'pōrt) Movement of a substance across a membrane, coupled with the simultaneous transport of another substance across the same membrane in the same direction.

Cot·te op·e·ra·tion (kut'ē op-ĕr-ā'shŭn) SYN presacral neurectomy.

cot·ton (kot'ŏn) SYN gossypol.

cot·ton·seed oil (kot'ŏn-sēd oyl) The refined fixed oil obtained from the seed of cultivated plants of various varieties of *Gossypium hirsutum* or of other species of *Gossypium*; a solvent.

cot·ton-wool patch·es (kot'ŏn-wul pach'ĕz) White, fuzzy areas on retinal surface (accumulations of cellular organelles) caused by damage (usually infarction) to the retinal fiber layer.

cot·y·le·don (kot'i-lē'dŏn) 1. In plants, a seed leaf, the first leaf to grow from a seed. 2. Irregular convex area of the fetal part of the placenta composed of stem villi.

cot·y·loid (kot'i-loyd) 1. Cup-shaped; cuplike. 2. Relating to the cotyloid cavity or acetabulum.

cot·y·loid cav·i·ty (kot'i-loyd kav'i-tē) SYN acetabulum.

cot·y·loid lig·a·ment (kot'i-loyd lig'ă-mĕnt) SYN acetabular labrum.

cough (kawf) 1. A sudden expulsion of air through the glottis, occurring immediately on opening the previously closed glottis, and excited by mechanical or chemical irritation of the trachea or bronchi, or by pressure from adjacent structures. **2.** To force air through the glottis by a series of expiratory efforts.

cough frac·ture (CF) (kawf frak´shŭr) Breakage of a rib or cartilage, usually the fifth or seventh, from vigorous coughing.

cough re·flex (kawf rē´fleks) The reflex that mediates coughing in response to irritation of the larynx or tracheobronchial tree.

cough syn·co·pe (kawf sin´kŏ-pē) Fainting as a result of a coughing spell. SYN Charcot vertigo, laryngeal vertigo, tussive syncope.

cou·lomb (C, Q) (kū´lom) The SI unit of radiation and electrical charge. SEE ALSO roentgen.

cou·ma·rin (kū´mă-rin) Fragrant neutral principle obtained from the Tonka bean, *Dypterix odorata*, and also made synthetically from salicylic aldehyde; used to disguise unpleasant odors. SYN coumaric anhydride, cumarin.

Cou·mel tach·y·car·di·a (kū´mel tak´i-kahr´dē-ă) A persistent junctional reciprocating tachycardia that usually uses a slowly conducting posteroseptal pathway for the retrograde journey.

count (kownt) **1.** A reckoning, enumeration, or accounting. **2.** To enumerate or score. **3.** A tally of instruments and materials performed at the beginning of a surgical operation and again before the incision is closed, to ensure that no foreign object remains in the patient.

count·er·cur·rent (kownt´ĕr-kŭr´ĕnt) **1.** Flowing in an opposite direction. **2.** A current flowing in a direction opposite to another current.

count·er·cur·rent mech·a·nism (kownt´ĕr-kŭr´ĕnt mek´ă-nizm) A system in the renal medulla that facilitates concentration of the urine as it passes through the renal tubules.

count·er·ex·ten·sion (kown´tĕr-eks-ten´shŭn) SYN countertraction.

count·er·in·ci·sion (kown´tĕr-in-sizh´ ŭn) A second incision adjacent to a primary incision.

count·er·ir·ri·ta·tion (kown´tĕr-ir-i-tā´ shŭn) Irritation or mild inflammation (redness, vesication, or pustulation) of the skin excited for the purpose of relieving symptoms of an inflammation of the deeper structures.

count·er·pul·sa·tion (kown´tĕr-pŭl-sā´ shŭn) A means of assisting the failing heart by automatically removing arterial blood just before and during ventricular ejection and returning it to the circulation during diastole; a balloon catheter is inserted into the aorta and activated by an automatic mechanism triggered by the electrocardiographic device.

count·er·shock, count·er-shock (CS) (kown´tĕr-shok) Electric shock applied to heart to stop disturbances of its rhythm.

count·er·trac·tion (kown´tĕr-trak´shŭn) The resistance, or back-pull, made to traction or pulling on a limb. SYN counterextension.

count·er·trans·port (kown´tĕr-trans´ pōrt) Movement of one substance across a membrane, coupled with the simultaneous transport of another substance across the same membrane in the opposite direction.

count·ing cham·ber (kown´ting chām´ bĕr) A standardized ruled-glass slide (hemocytometer) used for counting cells (especially erythrocytes and leukocytes) and other particulate material in a measured volume of fluid.

coup de sa·bre (kū dĕ sahb´) Linear scleroderma of the scalp, face, or forehead with scarring alopecia.

coup in·ju·ry of brain (kū in´jŭr-ē brān) An injury occurring directly beneath the skull at the area of impact.

cou·ple (kŭp´ĕl) To copulate; to perform coitus.

cou·plet (kŭp´lĕt) A series of two consecutive premature ventricular contractions.

cou·pling (kŭp´ling) **1.** The repeated pairing of a normal sinus beat with a ventricular extrasystole. **2.** A condition in which one or more products of a reaction are the subsequent reactants (or substrates) of a second reaction.

cou·pling in·ter·val (kŭp'ling in'tĕr-văl) Duration expressed in milliseconds, between a normal sinus beat and the ensuing premature beat.

Cour·nand dip (kūr-nahn' dip) In constrictive pericarditis, rapid early diastolic fall and reascent of the ventricular pressure curve to an elevated plateau (square root configuration).

Cour·voi·si·er gall·blad·der (kūr-vwah'zē-ā' gawl'blad-ĕr) Enlarged, often palpable gallbladder in a patient with carcinoma of the head of the pancreas; associated with jaundice due to obstruction of the common bile duct. SEE Courvoisier law.

co·va·lence (kō-vā'lĕns) Number of pairs of electrons an atom can share with other atoms.

cov·er glass (kŭv'ĕr glas) A thin glass disc or plate covering an object examined under the microscope. SYN coverslip.

cov·er·slip (kŭv'ĕr-slip) SYN cover glass.

cov·ert sen·si·ti·za·tion (kō-vĕrt' sen'si-tī-zā'shŭn) Aversive conditioning or training to abolish an unwanted behavior, during which the patient is taught to imagine unpleasant and related aversive consequences while engaging in the unwanted habit.

Cow·dry type A in·clu·sion bo·dies (kow'drē tīp in-klū'zhŭn bod'ēz) Dropletlike masses of acidophilic material surrounded by clear halos within nuclei, with margination of chromatin on the nuclear membrane as seen in human-herpesvirus-infected cells.

Cow·per cyst (kow'pĕr sist) Lesion in the bulbourethral gland.

Cow·per gland (kow'pĕr gland) SYN bulbourethral gland.

cow·per·i·tis (kow'pĕr-ī'tis) Inflammation of a bulbourethral or Cowper gland.

cow·pox virus (CPV) (kow'poks vī'rŭs)

Virus of the genus *Orthopoxvirus* that causes cowpox.

coxa, gen. and pl. **coxae** (kok'să, -sē) SYN hip joint.

cox·al·gi·a (koks-al'jē-ă) SYN coxodynia.

cox·a mag·na (kok'să mag'nă) Enlargement and often deformation of the femoral head; usually refers to a sequela of Legg-Calvé-Perthes disease or osteoarthritis.

cox·a pla·na (kok'să plă'nă) SYN Legg-Calvé-Perthes disease.

Cox·i·el·la (kok-sē-el'ă) A genus of filterable bacteria containing small, pleomorphic, rod-shaped or coccoid, gram-negative cells that occur intracellularly in the cytoplasm of infected cells and possibly extracellularly in infected ticks.

cox·o·dyn·i·a (kok'sō-din'ē-ă) Pain in the hip joint. SYN coxalgia.

cox·o·fem·o·ral (kok'sō-fem'ŏr-ăl) Relating to the hip bone and the femur.

cox·o·tu·ber·cu·lo·sis (kok'sō-tū-bĕr-kyū-lō'sis) Tuberculous hip-joint disease.

Cox·sack·ie en·ceph·a·li·tis (kok-sak'ē en-sef'ă-lī'tis) A viral encephalitis, seen mainly in infants and involving principally the gray matter of the medulla and cord.

cox·sack·ie·vi·rus (kok-sak'ē-vī'rŭs) A group of picornaviruses causing myositis, paralysis, and death in young mice, and responsible for a variety of diseases in humans, although inapparent infections are common. May cause aseptic meningitis, myocarditis, pericarditis, and acute onset juvenile diabetes.

CPM ma·chine (mă-shēn') Abbreviation for continuous passive motion machine.

crack (krak) **1.** A fissure. **2.** SEE crack cocaine.

crack co·caine (krak kō-kān') A derivative of cocaine, usually smoked, producing brief, intense euphoria. Crack cocaine is relatively inexpensive and extremely addictive; dependency can develop in less than 2 weeks. Like snorted or injected cocaine, it has both acute and chronic adverse effects, including heart and nasopharyngeal damage, seizures, sudden death, and psychosis. SEE ALSO street drug.

crac·kle (krak′ĕl) Short, sharp, or rough breath sounds heard with a stethoscope over the chest caused by excessive fluid within the airways.

crack·ling rale (krak′ling rahl) Fine sounds produced by fluid in small airways in pneumonia or congestive heart failure.

cra·dle (krā′dĕl) A frame used to keep bedclothes from coming in contact with a patient.

cra·dle cap (krā′dĕl kap) Colloquialism for seborrheic dermatitis of the scalp of the newborn.

Craig test (krāg test) Technique to assess forward torsion of femur or femoral anteversion.

cramp (kramp) **1.** A painful muscle spasm caused by prolonged tetanic contraction. **2.** A localized muscle spasm related to occupational use, qualified according to the occupation of the sufferer (e.g., writer's cramp).

Cramp·ton test (kramp′tŏn test) Assessment of physical condition and resistance; a record is made of the pulse and the blood pressure in the recumbent and standing positions, and the difference is graded from the theoretic perfection of 100 (seldom attained) downward; high values indicate a good physical resistance but low ones indicate a nonconditioned state.

Cran·dall syn·drome (kran′dăl sin′drŏm) Disorder characterized by pili torti, sensorineural deafness, and hypogonadism. SEE ALSO Björnstad syndrome.

cra·ni·ad (krā′nē-ad) Situated nearer the head in relation to a specific reference point; opposite of caudad. SEE ALSO superior.

cra·ni·al (krā′nē-ăl) **1.** Relating to the cranium or head. SYN cephalic. **2.** SYN superior (2). SEE ALSO cephalad.

cra·ni·al ar·ter·i·tis (krā′nē-ăl ahr′tĕr-ī′tis) SYN temporal arteritis.

cra·ni·al cav·i·ty (krā′nē-ăl kav′i-tē) [TA] The space within the skull occupied by the brain, its coverings, and cerebrospinal fluid.

cra·ni·al fi·brous joints (krā′nē-ăl fī′brŭs joynts) [TA] Those of the cranium, including the cranial syndesmoses, cranial sutures, and dentoalveolar syndesmoses (gomphoses). SYN juncturae fibrosae cranii [TA].

cra·ni·al flex·ure (krā′nē-ăl flek′shŭr) SYN cephalic flexure.

cra·ni·al su·tures (krā′nē-ăl sū′chŭrz) [TA] The sutures between the bones of the skull.

cra·ni·al syn·chon·dro·ses (krā′nē-ăl syn′kon-drŏ′sēz) [TA] Cartilaginous joints of the skull. SYN synchondroses cranii [TA].

♻ **cranio-, crani-** Combining forms meaning the cranium. Cf. cerebro-.

cra·ni·o·car·po·tar·sal dys·tro·phy (krā′nē-ō-kahr′pō-tahr′săl dis′trŏ-fē) Syndrome characterized by specific facial features with sunken eyes, hypertelorism, long philtrum, small nose, and small mouth with pursing of lips as in whistling, and skeletal malformations with ulnar deviation of hands, camptodactyly, talipes equinovarus, and frontal bone defects; autosomal dominant inheritance.

cra·ni·o·cele (krā′nē-ō-sēl) SYN encephalocele.

cra·ni·o·cer·vical (krā′nē-ō-sĕr′vi-kăl) Pertaining to the skull and neck.

cra·ni·o·did·y·mus (krā′nē-ō-did′i-mŭs) Conjoined twins with fused bodies but with two heads.

cra·ni·o·fa·cial (krā′nē-ō-fā′shăl) Relating to both the face and the cranium.

cra·ni·o·fa·cial dys·junc·tion frac·ture (krā′nē-ō-fā′shăl dis-jŭngk′shŭn frak′shŭr) A complex fracture in which the facial bones are separated from the cranial bones. SYN Le Fort III fracture.

cra·ni·o·fe·nes·tria (krā′nē-ō-fĕ-nes′trē-ă) SYN craniolacunia.

cra·ni·o·la·cu·ni·a (krā′nē-ō-lă-kū′nē-ă) Incomplete formation of the bones of the vault of the fetal cranium so that there are nonossified areas in the calvaria. SYN craniofenestria.

cra·ni·ol·o·gy (krā′nē-ol′ō-jē) The science concerned with variations in size, shape, and proportion of the cranium, especially with the variations characterizing the different races of humans.

cra·ni·o·ma·la·ci·a (krā′nē-ō-mă-lā′shē-ă) Softening of the bones of the cranium.

cra·ni·om·e·try (krā′nē-om′ĕ-trē) Measurement of the dry skull after removal of the soft parts and study of its topography.

cra·ni·op·a·gus (krā-nē-op′ă-gus) A type of conjoined twin united on any portion of the cranial vault or calvarium not involving the foramen magnum, skull base, face, or vertebrae.

cra·ni·op·a·thy (krā′nē-op′ă-thē) Any pathologic condition of the cranial bones.

cra·ni·o·pha·ryn·gi·o·ma (krā′nē-ō-făr-in′jē-ō′mă) A suprasellar neoplasm that develops from the Rathke pouch. SYN Rathke pouch tumor.

cra·ni·or·a·chis·chis·is (krā′nē-ō-ră-kis′ki-sis) Congenital defect of the central nervous system and accessory structures (e.g., cranium) due to neural tube closure during the first trimester of pregnancy.

cra·ni·os·chi·sis (krā′nē-os′ki-sis) Congenital malformation with incomplete closure of the cranium; often accompanied by grossly defective development of the brain.

cra·ni·o·scle·ro·sis (krā′nē-ō-skler-ō′sis) Thickening of the skull.

cra·ni·o·ste·no·sis (krā′nē-ō-stĕ-nō′sis) Premature closure of cranial sutures resulting in malformation of the cranium.

cra·ni·os·to·sis (krā′nē-os-tō′sis) SYN craniosynostosis.

cra·ni·o·syn·os·to·sis (krā′nē-ō-sin′os-tō′sis) Premature ossification of the cranium and obliteration of the sutures. The particular sutures involved determine the resultant shape of the malformed head. SYN craniostosis.

cra·ni·o·ta·bes (krā′nē-ō-tā′bēz) A disease marked by areas of thinning and softening in the bones of the skull and widening of the sutures and fontanelles.

cra·ni·ot·o·my (krā′nē-ot′ŏ-mē) Opening into the skull, either by attached or detached craniotomy or by trephination.

cra·ni·o·tym·pan·ic (krā′nē-ō-tim-pan′ik) Relating to the skull and the middle ear.

cra·ni·um, pl. **cra·ni·a** (krā′nē-ŭm, -ă) [TA] The bones of the head collectively. SEE skull.

cra·ni·um bi·fi·dum, bi·fid cra·ni·um (krā′nē-ŭm bī′fi-dŭm, bī′fid krā′nē-ŭm) SYN encephalocele.

crash cart (krash kahrt) A movable collection of emergency equipment and supplies meant to be readily available for resuscitative effort. It includes medication as well as the equipment for defibrillation, intubation, intravenous medication, and passage of central lines.

cra·ter (krā′tĕr) The most depressed, usually central portion of an ulcer.

C-re·ac·tive protein (CRP) (rē-ak′tiv prō′tēn) A β-globulin found in the serum of various people with certain inflammatory, degenerative, and neoplastic diseases; although the protein is not a specific antibody, it precipitates in vitro the C polysaccharide present in all types of pneumococci.

cream, creme (krēm) **1.** Upper fatty layer that forms in milk on standing or is separated from it by centrifugation; contains about the same amount of sugar and protein as milk, but 12–40% more fat. **2.** Any whitish viscid fluid resembling cream. **3.** A semisolid emulsion of either the oil-in-water or the water-in-oil type, ordinarily intended for topical use.

crease (krēs) A line or linear depression as produced by a fold. SEE ALSO fold, groove, line.

cre·a·tine (krē′ă-tin) Agent that occurs in urine, sometimes as such, but generally as creatinine, and in muscle, generally as phosphocreatine; elevated in urine in muscular dystrophy; synthesized in liver and pancreas from amino acids; absorbed in bloodstream, it is deposited in tissue (e.g., muscles, brain).

cre·a·tine ki·nase (CK) (krē'ă-tin kī'nās) An enzyme catalyzing the reversible transfer of phosphate from phosphocreatine to adenosine diphosphate, forming creatine and adenosine triphosphate.

cre·a·tine phos·phate (CrP, CP) (krē'ă-tin fos'fāt) SYN phosphocreatine.

cre·a·tine phos·pho·ki·nase (CPK, CP) (krē'ă-tin fos'fō-kī'nās) SYN creatine kinase.

cre·at·i·nine (Cr) (krē-at'i-nin) A component of urine and the final product of creatine catabolism.

cre·at·i·nine clear·ance (krē-at'i-nin klēr'ăns) A mathematical calculation of the total amount of creatinine excreted in the urine over a denoted period of time.

cre·at·i·nu·ri·a (krē'ă-ti-nyūr'ē-ă) Urinary excretion of increased amounts of creatine.

creep (krēp) Any time-dependent strain developing in a material or an object in response to the application of a force or stress.

creep·ing erup·tion (krēp'ing ē-rŭp'shŭn) SYN cutaneous larva migrans.

crem·as·ter·ic (krem'as-ter'ik) Relating to the cremaster.

cre·na, pl. **cre·nae** (krē'nă, -nē) A V-shaped cut or the space created by such a cut.

cre·na·tion (krē-nā'shŭn) The process of forming a scalloped edge.

cre·no·cyte (krē'nō-sīt) A red blood cell with serrated edges.

cre·o·sol (krē'ō-sol) A slightly yellowish aromatic liquid distilled from guaiac or from beechwood tar; a constituent of creosote. Cf. cresol.

cre·o·sote (krē'ō-sōt) A mixture of phenols (chiefly methyl guaiacol, guaiacol, and creosol) obtained during the distillation of wood-tar, preferably that derived from beechwood; used as a disinfectant and wood preservative.

crep·i·tant (krep'i-tănt) **1.** Relating to or characterized by crepitation. **2.** Denoting a fine bubbling noise (rale) produced by air entering fluid in lung tissue; heard in pneumonia and in certain other conditions. **3.** The sensation imparted to the palpating finger by gas or air in the subcutaneous tissues.

crep·i·ta·tion (krep'i-tā'shŭn) **1.** Crackling; the quality of a fine bubbling sound (rale) that resembles noise heard on rubbing hair between the fingers. **2.** The sensation felt on placing the hand over the seat of a fracture when the broken ends of the bone are moved, or over tissue, in which gas gangrene is present. **3.** Noise or vibration produced by rubbing bone or irregular cartilage surfaces together as by movement of patella against femoral condyles in arthritis and other conditions. SYN crepitus (1).

cres·cent (kres'ĕnt) **1.** Any figure in the shape of the moon in its first quarter. The figure made by the gray columns or cornua on cross-section of the spinal cord.

cres·cent sign (kres'ĕnt sīn) **1.** RADIOGRAPHY in the lung, a crescent of gas near the top of a mass lesion, signifying cavitation with a space above the debris; seen in aspergilloma, hydatidoma. **2.** COMPUTED TOMOGRAPHY a high attenuating layer of new blood in an aneurysm; indicates a ruptured abdominal aortic aneurysm. **3.** DIAGNOSTIC ULTRASOUND a sonolucent crescentic layer in a tumor mass, typically necrosis in stromal tumors of the small bowel. **4.** OSTEORADIOLOGY a subcortical lucent crescent in the femoral head, signifying osteonecrosis. SYN meniscus sign.

cre·sol (krē'sol) A mixture of the three isomeric methyl phenols, *o-*, *m-*, and *p-*cresol, obtained from coal tar. Its properties are similar to those of phenol, but it is less poisonous; used as an antiseptic and disinfectant. SYN tricresol.

crest (krest) [TA] A ridge, especially a bony ridge. SYN crista [TA].

CREST syn·drome (krest sin′drōm) An acronymic designation for a variant of scleroderma characterized by *c*alcinosis, *R*aynaud phenomenon, *e*sophageal motility disorders, *s*clerodactyly, and *t*elangiectasia.

cres·yl blue, cres·yl blue bril·liant (kres′il blū, bril-yănt) A basic oxazin dye used for staining the reticulum in young erythrocytes (reticulocytes); also used in vital staining and as a selective stain for gastric surface epithelial mucin and other acid mucopolysaccharides.

Creutz·feldt-Ja·kob dis·ease (CJD) (kroyts′felt-yah′kōp di-zēz′) A progressive neurologic disorder, one of the subacute spongiform encephalopathies caused by prions. SEE ALSO bovine spongiform encephalopathy.

crev·ice (krev′is) A crack or small fissure, especially in a solid substance.

cre·vic·u·lar (krĕ-vik′yū-lăr) **1.** Relating to any crevice. **2.** DENTISTRY relating especially to the gingival crevice or sulcus.

crib death (krib deth) SYN sudden infant death syndrome.

cri·bra·tion (kri-brā′shŭn) **1.** Sifting; passing through a sieve. **2.** The condition of being cribrate or numerously pitted or punctured.

crib·ri·form (krib′ri-fōrm) [TA] Sievelike; containing many perforations. SYN cribrate, polyporous.

cri·coid (krī′koyd) Ring-shaped; denoting the cricoid cartilage.

cri·coid·ec·to·my (krī′koyd-ek′tŏ-mē) Excision of cricoid cartilage.

cri·co·thy·roid (krī′kō-thī′royd) Relating to the cricoid and thyroid cartilages.

cri·co·thy·rot·o·my, cri·co·thy·roid·ot·o·my (krī′kō-thī-rot′ŏ-mē, -thī′roydot′ŏ-mē) Incision through the skin and cricothyroid membrane for relief of respiratory obstruction; used before or in place of tracheotomy in certain emergency respiratory obstructions. SYN intercricothyrotomy.

cri·co·tra·che·ot·o·my (krī′kō-trā′kē-ot′ ŏ-mē) Surgical incision of the trachea through the cricoid cartilage.

cri-du-chat syn·drome, cat-cry syn·drome (krē-dū-shah′ sin′drōm, kat′krī) A disorder due to deletion of the short arm of chromosome 5, characterized by microcephaly, hypertelorism, antimongoloid palpebral fissures, epicanthal folds, micrognathia, strabismus, mental and physical retardation, and a characteristic high-pitched catlike whine.

Crig·ler-Naj·jar syn·drome (krig′lĕr nah′jahr sin′drōm) A rare defect in ability to form bilirubin glucuronide due to deficiency of bilirubin-glucuronide glucuronosyltransferase; characterized by familial nonhemolytic jaundice and, in its severe form, by irreversible brain damage in infancy that resembles kernicterus and may be fatal; autosomal recessive inheritance, caused by mutation in the uridine diphosphate glycosyltransferase 1 gene (*UGT1*) on chromosome 1q. There is an autosomal dominant form called Gilbert syndrome, also caused by mutation in the *UGT1* gene. SYN Crigler-Najjar disease.

Cri·me·an-Con·go hem·or·rhag·ic fe·ver (CCHF, C-CHFV) (krī-mē′ăn-kong′gō hem′ŏr-aj′ik fē′vĕr) Hemorrhagic fever distinct from Omsk hemorrhagic fever, occurring in central Russia, transmitted by species of the tick *Hyalomma*, and caused by Crimean-Congo hemorrhagic fever virus, a member of the Bunyaviridae family. SYN African tick fever.

crim·i·nal a·bor·tion (krim′i-năl ă-bōr′ shŭn) Termination of pregnancy without legal justification.

crim·i·nal psy·chol·o·gy (krim′i-năl sī-kol′ŏ-jē) The study of the mind and its workings in relation to crime.

crin·o·gen·ic (krin′ō-jen′ik) Causing secretion; stimulating a gland to increased function.

cri·sis, pl. **cri·ses** (krī′sis, -sēz) **1.** A sudden change, usually for the better, in the course of an acute disease, in contrast to gradual improvement by lysis. **2.** A paroxysmal pain in an organ or circumscribed region of the body occurring in the course of tabetic neurosyphilis. **3.** A convulsive attack.

cris·ta, pl. **cris·tae** (kris′tă, -tē) [TA] SYN crest.

cris·ta am·pul·la·ris (kris′tă am-pul-ā′ris) [TA] SYN ampullary crest.

cris·tae cu·tis (kris′tē kyū′tis) [TA] SYN dermal ridges.

cris·ta gal·li (kris′tă gal′ē) [TA] The triangular midline process of the ethmoid bone extending superiorly from the cribriform plate; it gives anterior attachment to the falx cerebri.

crit·i·cal (crit) (krit′ĭ-kăl) **1.** Denoting or of the nature of a crisis. **2.** Denoting a morbid condition in which death is possible. **3.** In sufficient quantity as to constitute a turning point.

crit·i·cal care unit (CCU) (krit′i-kăl kār yū′nit) SYN intensive care unit.

crit·i·cal con·trol point (krit′i-kăl kŏn-trōl′ poynt) A step or procedure in cooking at which controls can be applied and a food safety hazard can be prevented, eliminated, or reduced to acceptable levels.

crit·i·cal point (krit′i-kăl poynt) Stage at which two phases become identical; thus, at a given critical temperature and critical pressure, the liquid and gaseous states of a particular substance can no longer be differentiated.

crit·i·cal pres·sure (krit′i-kăl presh′ūr) Minimal pressure required to liquefy a gas at the critical temperature.

crit·i·cal tem·per·a·ture (krit′i-kăl tem′pĕr-ă-chŭr) The temperature of a gas above which it is no longer possible by use of any pressure, however great, to convert it into a liquid.

Crocq dis·ease (krok di-zēz′) SYN acrocyanosis.

Crohn dis·ease (krōn di-zēz′) SYN regional enteritis.

Cronk·hite-Can·a·da syn·drome (kron′kīt kan′ă-dă sin′drōm) Sporadic disorder of gastrointestinal polyps with diffuse alopecia and nail dystrophy.

Crooke gra·nules (kruk gran′yūlz) Lumpy masses of basophilic material in the basophil cells of the anterior lobe of the pituitary, associated with Cushing disease, or following the administration of adrenocorticotropic hormone.

cross (kraws) **1.** Any figure or structure characterized by the intersection of two lines. SYN crux. **2.** A method of hybridization or the hybrid so produced.

cross ag·glu·ti·na·tion (kraws ă-glū′ti-nā′shŭn) SYN group agglutination.

cross·bite (X) (kraws′bīt) An abnormal relationship of one or more teeth of one arch to the opposing tooth or teeth of the other arch due to labial, buccal, or lingual deviation of tooth position, or to abnormal jaw position.

cross-bite tooth (kraws′bīt tūth) A posterior tooth designed to permit the modified cusp of the upper tooth to be positioned in the fossae of the lower tooth.

cross·breed·ing (kraws′brēd-ing) SYN hybridization.

cross·ed an·es·the·sia (krawst an-es-thē′zē-ă) That affecting one side of the head and the other side of the body due to a brainstem lesion.

crossed dip·lo·pi·a (krawst di-plō′pē-ă) Diplopia in which the image seen by the right eye is to the left of the image seen by the left eye.

cross·ed em·bo·lism (krawst em′bŏlizm) SYN paradoxical embolism.

cross·ed eyes, cross-eye (krawst īz, kraws′ī) SYN strabismus.

cross·ed lat·er·al·i·ty (krawst lat′ĕr-al′ĭ-tē) Right dominance of some members' functions (e.g., use of upper limb or sighting with eye) and left dominance of others.

cross·ed re·flex (krawst rē′fleks) A reflexive movement on one side of the body in response to a stimulus on the other.

cross-flap (kraws′flap) A skin flap transferred from one part of the body to a corresponding part, as from one arm to the other.

cross-hybridisation [Br.] SYN crosshybridization.

cross·hy·brid·i·za·tion (kraws-hī′brid-ī-zā′shŭn) Annealing of a DNA probe to an imperfectly matching DNA molecule. SYN cross-hybridisation.

cross·in·fec·tion (kraws in-fek′shŭn) That spread from one source to another, (e.g., person to person, animal to person).

cross·ing-o·ver, cross-o·ver (kraws′ing-ō′vĕr, kraws′ō-vĕr) Reciprocal exchange of material between two paired chromosomes during meiosis, resulting in the transfer of a block of genes from each chromosome to its homologue.

cross-link (kraws′lingk) A covalent linkage between two polymers or between two different regions of the same polymer.

cross-match·ing (kraws′mach′ing) 1. A test for incompatibility between donor and recipient blood, carried out before a transfusion to avoid potentially lethal hemolytic reactions between the donor's red blood cells and antibodies in the recipient's plasma, or the reverse. 2. In allotransplantation of solid organs, a test for identification of antibody in the serum of potential allograft recipients that reacts directly with the lymphocytes or other cells of a potential allograft donor.

cross-re·ac·tion (kraws′rē-ak′shŭn) A specific reaction between an antiserum and an antigen complex other than the antigen complex that evoked the various specific antibodies of the antiserum.

cross-sec·tion (kraws sek′shŭn) 1. Planar or two-dimensional view, diagram, or image of the internal structure of the body, part of the body, or any anatomic structure afforded by slicing, actually or through imaging (e.g., radiographic, magnetic resonance, or microscopic) techniques, the body or structure along a particular plane. 2. Slice or section of a given thickness created by actual serial parallel cuts through a structure or by the application of imaging technique.

cross-sec·tion·al (kraws′sek′shŭn-ăl) 1. In histology, a sectioning of a tissue or organ perpendicular to its longitudinal axis. 2. Relating to planar sections of an anatomic or other structure. SEE synchronic.

cross-ta·per (kraws tā′pĕr) PHARMACOTHERAPY Practice of lowering the dosage of one medication while simultaneously increasing the dosage of another.

cross-tol·er·ance (kraws tol′ĕr-ăns) The resistance to one or more effects of a compound as a result of tolerance developed to a pharmacologically similar compound.

Crot·a·lus (krot′ă-lŭs) A genus of rattlesnakes native to North America, with large fangs and a venom that is both neurotoxic and hemolytic. The largest species are the diamondbacks of the southern and western states; the smallest the pigmy rattlers.

croup (krūp) 1. Laryngotracheobronchitis in infants and young children caused by parainfluenza viruses 1 and 2. 2. Any infection of the larynx in children, characterized by difficult and noisy respiration and a hoarse cough.

croup·ous mem·brane (krū′pŭs mem′brān) SYN false membrane.

crowd·ing (krowd′ing) A condition in which the teeth are pushed together, assuming altered positions (e.g., bunching, overlapping, displacement in various directions, torsiversion).

Crowe-Da·vis mouth gag (krō-dā′vis mowth gag) Instrument used for opening the mouth, depressing the tongue, maintaining the airway, and transmitting volatile anesthetics during tonsillectomy or other oropharyngeal surgery.

Crow-Fu·ka·se syn·drome (krō fū-kah′sē sin′drōm) SYN POEMS syndrome.

crow·ing in·spi·ra·tion (krō′ing in′spir-ā′shŭn) Noisy breathing associated with respiratory obstruction, usually at the larynx. SEE inspiratory stridor.

crown (CR) (krown) [TA] 1. Any structure, normal or pathologic, resembling or suggesting a crown or a wreath. 2. DENTISTRY that part of a tooth that is covered with enamel, or an artificial substitute for that part. SYN corona [TA].

crown-heel length (CHL) (krown-hēl length) Length of an outstretched 8-week embryo or fetus from the vertex of the cranium to the heel. SEE ALSO crown-rump length.

crown·ing (krown'ing) **1.** Preparation of the natural crown of a tooth and covering the prepared crown with a veneer of suitable dental material (gold or nonprecious metal casting, porcelain, plastic, or combinations). **2.** That stage of childbirth when the fetal head has negotiated the pelvic outlet and the largest diameter of the head is encircled by the vulvar ring.

crown-rump length (Cr, CRL) (krown-rŭmp length) A measurement from the vertex of the cranium to the midpoint between the apices of the buttocks of an embryo or fetus, which permits approximation of embryonic or fetal age. SEE ALSO crown-heel length.

cru·ci·ate (krū'shē-āt) Shaped like, or resembling, a cross.

cru·ci·ate a·nas·to·mo·sis, cru·cial a·nas·to·mo·sis (krū'shē-āt ă-nas'tŏ-mō'sis, krū'shăl ă-nas'tŏ-mō'sis) A four-way anastomosis between branches of the first perforating branch of the deep femoral, inferior gluteal, and medial and lateral circumflex femoral arteries, located posterior to the upper part of the femur.

cru·ci·ate lig·a·ment of the at·las (krū'shē-āt lig'ă-mĕnt at'lăs) [TA] Strong ligament that lies posterior to the dens of the axis holding it against the anterior arch of the atlas. SYN ligamentum cruciforme atlantis [TA], crucial ligament (3), cruciform ligament of atlas, ligamentum cruciatum atlantis.

cru·ci·ate lig·a·ments of knee (krū'shē-āt lig'ă-mĕnts nē) Those that pass from the intercondylar area of the tibia to the intercondylar fossa of the femur. SEE anterior cruciate ligament. SEE ALSO anterior cruciate ligament. SYN crucial ligament (2), ligamenta cruciata genus.

cru·ci·ate mus·cle (krū'shē-āt mŭs'ĕl) General type in which the muscles or bundles of muscle fibers cross in an X-shaped configuration. SYN musculus cruciatus.

cru·ci·ble (krū'si-bĕl) A vessel used as a container for reactions or experimental procedures at high temperatures.

cru·or (krū'ōr) Coagulated blood.

cru·ra ant·hel·i·cis (krū'ră ant-hel'i-sis) SYN crura of antihelix.

cru·ral sheath (krūr'ăl shēth) SYN femoral sheath.

cru·ra of an·ti·he·lix (krūs an'tē-hē'liks) Two ridges, inferior and superior, bounding the triangular fossa, by which the antihelix begins at the upper part of the auricle. SYN crura antihelicis [TA].

crus, gen. **cru·ris** (krūs, krū'ris) [TA] **1.** SYN leg. **2.** Any anatomic structure resembling a leg; usually (in the plural) a pair of diverging bands or elongated masses. SEE ALSO limb.

crus ce·re·bri (krūs sĕ-rē'brī) [TA] Specifically, the massive bundle of corticofugal nerve fibers passing longitudinally on the ventral surface of the midbrain on each side of the midline. SEE ALSO cerebral peduncle.

crus for·ni·cis (krūs fōr'ni-sis) [TA] That part of the fornix that rises in a forward curve behind the thalamus to continue forward as the body for fornix ventral to the corpus callosum. SYN crus of fornix

crush syn·drome (krŭsh sin'drōm) The shocklike state that follows release of a limb or limbs or the trunk and pelvis after a prolonged period of compression, as by a heavy weight; characterized by suppression of urine, probably the result of damage to the renal tubules by myoglobin from the damaged muscles. SYN compression syndrome (1).

crus of for·nix (krūs fōr'niks) [TA] SYN crus fornicis.

crust (krŭst) **1.** A hard outer layer or covering; cutaneous crusts are often formed by dried serum or pus on the surface of a ruptured blister or pustule. **2.** A scab. SYN crusta.

crus·ta, pl. **crus·tae** (krŭs'tă, -tē) SYN crust.

Crus·ta·ce·a (krŭs-tā'shē-ă) A large

class of aquatic animals (phylum Arthropoda) with a chitinous exoskeleton and jointed appendages; some are parasitic; others serve as intermediate hosts for parasitic worms that cause disease in humans and various other vertebrates.

crus·ta lac·te·a (krŭs'tă lak'shē-ă) Seborrhea of the scalp in an infant. SYN milk crust.

crutch (krŭch) A device used singly or in pairs to assist in walking when the act is impaired by a lower limb disability; transfers all or part of weight-bearing to the upper extremity.

crutch pal·sy (krŭch pawl'zē) SYN crutch paralysis.

Cru·veil·hier-Baum·gar·ten mur·mur (krū-vāl-yā' bahm'gahr-těn mŭr'mŭr) Venous murmur heard over collateral veins, connecting portal, and caval venous systems, on the abdominal wall.

Cru·veil·hier dis·ease (krū-vāl-yā' di-zēz') SYN amyotrophic lateral sclerosis.

Cru·veil·hier ul·cer (krū-vāl-yā' ŭl'sĕr) SYN gastric ulcer.

crux, pl. **cru·ces** (krŭks, krū'sēz) A junction or crossing. SYN cross (1).

crux of heart (krŭks hahrt) Zone of junction of the interatrial and interventricular septa, the atrioventricular valves, and of the four chambers of the heart, as observed using ultrasonography. SYN cross (2).

cryaesthesia [Br.] SYN cryesthesia.

cry·al·ge·si·a (krī'al-jē'zē-ă) Pain caused by cold. SYN crymodynia.

cryanaesthesia [Br.] SYN cryanesthesia.

cry·an·es·the·si·a (krī'an-es-thē'zē-ă) Inability to perceive cold. SYN cryanaesthesia.

cry·es·the·si·a (krī'es-thē'zē-ă) **1.** A subjective sensation of cold. **2.** Sensitiveness to cold. SYN cryaesthesia.

crymo- Prefix meaning cold.

cry·mo·dyn·i·a (krī'mō-din'ē-ă) SYN cryalgesia.

cry·mo·phil·ic (krī'mō-fil'ik) Preferring cold; denoting microorganisms that thrive best at low temperatures. SYN cryophilic.

cry·mo·phy·lac·tic (krī'mō-fi-lak'tik) Resistant to cold, said of certain microorganisms that are not destroyed even by freezing temperatures. SYN cryophylactic.

cryo-, cry- Combining forms meaning cold.

cry·o·an·es·the·si·a (krī'ō-an-es-thē'zē-ă) Localized application of cold as a means of producing regional anesthesia. SYN refrigeration anesthesia.

cry·o·bi·ol·o·gy (krī'ō-bī-ol'ŏ-jē) The study of the effects of low temperatures on living organisms.

cry·o·cau·ter·y (krī'ō-kaw'tĕr-ē) Any substance, such as liquid nitrogen or carbon dioxide snow, or a low temperature instrument, the application of which destroys tissue by freezing it. SYN cold cautery.

cry·o·ex·trac·tion (krī'ō-ek-strak'shŭn) Removal of cataracts by the adhesion of a freezing probe to the lens; now rarely done.

cry·o·ex·trac·tor (krī'ō-ek-strak'tŏr, -tōr) An instrument, artificially cooled, for extraction of the lens by freezing contact; not currently in use.

cry·o·fi·brin·o·gen (krī'ō-fī-brin'ō-jen) An abnormal type of fibrinogen very rarely found in human plasma; precipitated on cooling, but redissolves when warmed to room temperature.

cryofibrinogenaemia [Br.] SYN cryofibrinogenemia.

cry·o·fi·brin·o·gen·e·mi·a (krī'ō-fī-brin'ō-jĕ-nē'mē-ă) The presence in the blood of cryofibrinogens. SYN cryofibrinogenaemia.

cry·o·gen·ic (krī'ō-jen'ik) **1.** Denoting or characteristic of a cryogen. **2.** Relating to cryogenics.

cryoglobulinaemia [Br.] SYN cryoglobulinemia.

cry·o·glob·u·lin·e·mi·a (krī′ō-glob′yū-li-nē′mē-ă) The presence of abnormal quantities of cryoglobulin in blood plasma. SYN cryoglobulinaemia.

cry·o·glob·u·lins (krī′ō-glob′yū-linz) Abnormal plasma proteins characterized by precipitating, gelling, or crystallizing when serum or solutions containing them are cooled.

cry·o·hy·po·phys·ec·to·my (krī′ō-hī-pof′i-sek′tŏ-mē) Destruction of hypophysis by the application of extreme cold.

cry·o·ki·net·ics (krī′ō-ki-net′iks) The combination of cryotherapy with exercise. SEE ALSO cryotherapy.

cry·ol·y·sis (krī-ol′i-sis) Destruction by cold.

cry·op·a·thy (krī-op′ă-thē) A morbid condition in which exposure to cold is an important factor. SYN frigorism.

cry·o·pex·y (krī′ō-pek-sē) In retinal detachment surgery, sealing the sensory retina to the pigment epithelium and choroid by a freezing probe applied to the sclera.

cry·o·phil·ic (krī′ō-fil′ik) SYN cryomophilic.

cry·o·pre·cip·i·tate (krī′ō-prĕ-sip′i-tăt) Precipitate that forms when soluble material is cooled, especially with reference to the precipitate that forms in normal blood plasma subjected to cold precipitation.

cry·o·pres·er·va·tion (krī′ō-prez-ĕr-vā′shŭn) Maintenance of the viability of excised tissues or organs at extremely low temperatures.

cry·o·probe (krī′ō-prōb) An instrument used in cryosurgery to apply extreme cold to a selected area.

cry·o·pro·tein (krī′ō-prō′tēn) A protein that precipitates from solution when cooled and redissolves upon warming.

cry·os·co·py (krī-os′kŏ-pē) The determination of the freezing point of a fluid, usually blood or urine, compared with that of distilled water.

cry·o·stat (krī′ō-stat) A freezing chamber.

cry·o·sur·gery (cryo) (krī′ō-sŭr′jĕr-ē) An operation using freezing temperatures (achieved by liquid nitrogen or carbon dioxide) alone or in an instrument to destroy tissue.

cry·o·thal·a·mec·to·my (krī′ō-thal′ă-mek′tŏ-mē) Destruction of the thalamus by the application of extreme cold.

cry·o·ther·a·py (cryo) (krī′ō-thār′ă-pē) The use of cold in the treatment of disease.

crypt (kript) [TA] A pitlike depression or tubular recess.

cryp·ta, gen. and pl. **cryp·tae** (krip′tă, -tē) [TA] SYN crypt.

crypt ab·sces·ses (kript ab′ses-ĕz) Lesions in the intestines, a characteristic feature of ulcerative colitis.

cryp·tec·to·my (krip-tek′tŏ-mē) Excision of a tonsillar or other crypt.

cryp·tic (krip′tik) Hidden; occult; larvate.

cryp·ti·tis (krip-tī′tis) Inflammation of a follicle or glandular tubule, particularly in the rectum.

♻ **crypto-, crypt-** Combining forms meaning hidden, obscure; without apparent cause.

cryp·to·coc·co·sis (krip′tō-kok-ō′sis) Infection by *Cryptococcus neoformans*, causing a pulmonary, disseminated, or meningeal mycosis. SYN Busse-Buschke disease.

Cryp·to·coc·cus (krip′tō-kok′ŭs) A genus of yeastlike fungi that reproduce by budding.

cryp·to·gen·ic (krip′tō-jen′ik) Of obscure, indeterminate etiology or origin, in contrast to phanerogenic.

cryp·to·gen·ic sep·ti·ce·mi·a (krip′tō-jen′ik sep′ti-sē′mē-ă) A form of the disorder in which no primary focus of infection can be found.

cryp·to·lith (krip′tō-lith) A concretion in a gland follicle.

cryp·to·men·or·rhe·a (krip′tō-men-ŏr-ē'ă) Occurrence each month of the general symptoms of the menses without any flow of blood, as in cases of imperforate hymen.

cryptomenorrhoea [Br.] SYN cryptomenorrhea.

cryp·toph·thal·mos, cryp·toph·thal·mia (krip'tof-thal'mŏs, -thal'mē-ă) Congenital absence of eyelids, with the skin passing continuously from the forehead onto the cheek over a rudimentary eye.

cryp·to·po·di·a (krip'tō-pō'dē-ă) A swelling of the lower part of the leg and the foot.

cryp·tor·chi·dism, cryp·tor·chism (kript-ōr'ki-dizm, -ōr'kizm) Failure of one or both testes to descend.

cryp·tor·chi·do·pex·y (kript-ōr'ki-dō-pek-sē) SYN orchiopexy.

cryp·tor·chid tes·tis (kript-ōr'kid tes'tis) SYN undescended testis.

cryp·to·spo·rid·i·o·sis (krip'tō-spōr-id'ē-ō'sis) An enteric disease that is transferred by waterborne or fecal contamination routes; disease in immunocompetent people is usually manifest as a self-limiting diarrhea, whereas in immunocompromised people as a prolonged severe diarrhea that can be fatal.

Cryp·to·spo·rid·i·um (krip'tō-spō-rid'ē-ŭm) A genus of coccidian sporozoans that are common opportunistic parasites of humans that flourish under conditions of compromised immune function; can cause self-limiting diarrhea in immunocompetent people.

crys·tal (kris'tăl) A solid of regular shape and, for any given compound, characteristic angles, formed when an element or compound solidifies slowly enough, as a result either of freezing from the liquid form or of precipitating out of solution, to allow the individual molecules to take up regular positions with respect to one another.

crys·tal·line (kris'tă-lēn) 1. Clear; transparent. 2. Relating to a crystal or crystals.

crys·tal·line lens (kris'tă-lēn lenz) SYN lens (2).

crys·tal·lized tryp·sin (kris'tă-līzd trip'sin) Purified preparation of the pancreatic enzyme; used as an adjunct to surgery for débridement of necrotic wounds and ulcers.

crys·tal·lu·ri·a (kris-tăl-yūr'ē-ă) The excretion of crystalline materials in the urine.

crys·tal vi·o·let (CV) (kris'tăl vī'ŏ-lĕt) A compound that has been used in the external treatment of burns, wounds, and fungal infections of skin and mucous membranes, and internally for pinworm and certain fluke infections; used as a stain for chromatin, amyloid, platelets in blood, fibrin, and neuroglia; used also to differentiate bacteria. SYN methylrosaniline chloride.

Cs Abbreviation for cesium.

C-sec·tion (sek'shŭn) SEE cesarean section.

C-spine (spīn) First seven bones of the spinal column; neck bones. SYN cervical verbebrae, cervical spine.

Cte·no·ce·phal·i·des (tē-nō-se-fal'i-dēz) A genus of fleas. *Ctenocephalides canis* (dog flea) and *Ctenocephalides felis* (cat flea) are nearly universal ectoparasites of household pets; will attack humans when starving if pets are absent.

Cu Symbol for copper.

cu·bic cen·ti·me·ter (cc, c.c.) (kyū'bik sen'ti-mē-tĕr) One thousandth of a liter; 1 milliliter. SYN cubic centimetre.

cubic centimetre [Br.] SYN cubic centimeter.

cu·bi·tal tun·nel syn·drome (kyū'bi-tăl tŭn'ĕl sin'drōm) A group of symptoms that develop from compression of the ulnar nerve within the cubital tunnel at the elbow.

cu·bi·tus, ul·na, gen. and pl. **cu·bi·ti** (kyū'bi-tŭs, ŭl'nă, kyū'bi-tī), [TA] 1. SYN elbow (2). 2. SYN ulna.

cu·bi·tus val·gus (kyū'bi-tŭs val'gŭs) Deviation of the extended forearm to the outer (radial) side of the axis of the limb.

cu·bi·tus va·rus (kyū'bi-tŭs vā'rŭs) Deviation of the extended forearm to the inward (ulnar) side of the axis of the limb.

cu·boid, cu·boi·dal (kyū′boyd, kyū-boy′dăl) [TA] **1.** Resembling a cube in shape. **2.** Relating to the os cuboideum.

cu·boi·dal ep·i·the·li·um (kyū-boy′dăl ep′i-thē′lē-ŭm) Simple epithelium with cells appearing as squares in a vertical section but as polyhedra in surface view.

cuff (kŭf) Any structure with a gap that nearly encircles some extension or outgrowth, thus, anything shaped like a cuff.

cuff·ing (kŭf′ing) **1.** A perivascular accumulation of various leukocytes seen in infectious, inflammatory, or autoimmune diseases. **2.** To surround a structure with fluid or cells, as with a cuff; in chest radiography, thickening of bronchial walls on the image.

cui·rass (kwi-ras′) The anterior surface of the thorax in relation to symptoms or disease changes.

cui·rass ven·ti·la·tor (kwi-ras′ ven′ti-lă-tŏr) Rigid breast plate that fits over the anterior portion of the chest and by application and release of negative pressure moves the chest wall, thus ''breathing'' for the patient. SYN cuirass respirator.

cul-de-sac (CDS), pl. **culs-de-sac** (kul-dĕ-sahk′) *This word is correctly spelled with two hyphens.* **1.** A blind pouch or tubular cavity closed at one end. **2.** SYN rectouterine pouch.

cul·do·cen·te·sis (kŭl′dō-sen-tē′sis) Aspiration of fluid from the cul-de-sac by puncture of the vaginal vault near the midline between the uterosacral ligaments.

cul·dos·co·py (kŭl-dos′kŏ-pē) Introduction of an endoscope through the posterior vaginal wall for viewing the rectovaginal pouch and pelvic viscera.

cul·dot·o·my (kŭl-dot′ŏ-mē) **1.** Cutting through the posterior vaginal wall into the cul-de-sac of Douglas. **2.** SYN vaginal celiotomy.

Cu·lex (kū′leks) A genus of mosquitoes

including over 2000 species. Largely tropical but worldwide in distribution; vectors for many diseases of humans and of domestic and wild animals and birds.

Cu·lex ni·gri·pal·pus (kū′leks nī-gri-pal′pŭs) Mosquito species that is a vector of St. Louis encephalitis within the U.S.

cu·li·ci·dal (kū-li-sī′dăl) Destructive to mosquitoes.

cu·li·cide (kū′li-sīd) An agent that destroys mosquitoes.

cu·lic·i·fuge (kū-lis′i-fūj) **1.** Driving away gnats and mosquitoes. **2.** An agent that keeps mosquitoes from biting.

Cu·li·coi·des (kū′li-koy′dēz) A genus of biting blood-sucking midges that transmit numerous pathogens of humans and animals.

Cul·len sign (kŭl′lĕn sīn) Periumbilical darkening of the skin from blood, a sign of intraperitoneal hemorrhage, especially in ruptured ectopic pregnancy.

cul·men, pl. **cul·mi·na** (kŭl′men, kŭl-mī′nă) [TA] The anterior prominent portion of the monticulus of the vermis of the cerebellum. SYN lobulus culminis.

cul·ture (kŭl′chŭr) **1.** The propagation of microorganisms on or in various media. **2.** A mass of microorganisms on or in a medium. **3.** The propagation of mammalian cells, i.e., cell culture. SEE cell culture.

cul·ture me·di·um (kŭl′chŭr mē′dē-ŭm) A substance, either solid or liquid, used for the cultivation, isolation, identification, or storage of microorganisms. SYN medium (3).

cum (kum) With.

cu·mu·la·tive (kyūm′yŭ-lă-tiv) Tending to accumulate or pile up, as with certain drugs that may have a cumulative effect.

cu·mu·la·tive dose (CD) (kyūm′yŭ-lă-tiv dōs) Total dose resulting from repeated exposures to radiation or chemotherapy of the same part of the body or of the whole body.

Cu·mu·la·tive In·dex to Nur·sing and Al·lied Health Li·ter·a·ture (CI-

NAHL) (kyūm´yŭ-lă-tiv in´deks nŭrs´ing al´ĭd helth lit´ĕr-ă-chŭr) Database of major English language nursing journal publications from the American Nursing Association and the National League for Nursing as well as other professional journals including occupational and physical therapy citations.

cu·mu·la·tive trau·ma dis·or·der (CTD) (kyūm´yŭ-lă-tiv traw´mă dis-ōr´dĕr) Any of the chronic disorders involving tendon, muscle, joint, and nerve damage, often resulting from work-related physical activities. CTDs, including repetitive motion disorders and carpal tunnel syndrome, result when the body is subjected to direct pressure, vibration, or repetitive movements for prolonged periods. SYN repetitive strain disorder.

cu·mu·lus, pl. **cu·mu·li** (kyū´myū-lŭs, -lī) A collection of cells.

cu·ne·ate (kyū´nē-āt) Wedge-shaped.

cu·ne·ate nu·cle·us (kyū´nē-āt nū´klē-ŭs) [TA] The larger Burdach nucleus; one of the three nuclei of the posterior column of the spinal cord.

cu·ne·i·form (kyū´ne-i-fōrm) *Avoid the mispronunciation cune´iform.* Wedge-shaped.

cu·ne·o·cu·boid (kyū´nē-ō-kyū´boyd) Relating to the lateral cuneiform and the cuboid bones.

cu·ne·o·na·vic·u·lar (kyū´nē-ō-nă-vik´yū-lăr) Relating to the cuneiform and the navicular bones.

cu·ne·us, pl. **cu·ne·i** (kyū´nē-ŭs, -ī) [TA] That region of the medial aspect of the occipital lobe of each cerebral hemisphere bounded by the parietooccipital fissure and the calcarine fissure.

cu·nic·u·lus (kū-nik´yū-lŭs) The burrow of the scabies mite in the epidermis.

cun·ni·lin·gus (kŭn´i-ling´gŭs) Oral stimulation of the vulva or clitoris.

cup (kŭp) An excavated or cup-shaped structure, either anatomic or pathologic.

cup:disc ra·tio (kŭp disk rā´shē-ō) The ratio between the diameter of the cupped or depressed central zone of the optic disc and the diameter of the entire disc; normally lower than 1:3, it is increased in glaucoma.

Cu·pid's bow (kyu´pidz bō) Contour of the superior margin of the upper lip.

cu·pric (kyū´prik) Pertaining to copper, particularly to copper in the form of a doubly charged positive ion.

cu·pric sul·fate (kyū´prik sŭl´fāt) A blue salt highly poisonous to algae, it is a prompt and active emetic, and is used as an irritant, astringent, and fungicide. SYN copper sulfate, copper sulphate.

cu·prous (kū´prŭs) Pertaining to copper.

cu·pu·la, cu·po·la, pl **cu·pu·lae** (kū´pū-lă, -ŏ-lă, -pū-lē) [TA] A cup-shaped or domelike structure. SYN cupola.

cu·pu·lar (kyū´pyū-lăr) **1.** Relating to a cupula. **2.** Dome-shaped. SYN cupuliform.

cu·pu·li·form (kyū´pyū-li-fōrm) SYN cupular (2).

cu·pu·li·form cat·a·ract (kū´pū-li-fōrm kat´ă-rakt) Common form of senile cataract often confined to a region just within the posterior capsule. SYN saucer-shaped cataract.

cu·pu·lo·gram (kyū´pū-lō-gram) A graphic representation of vestibular function relative to normal performance.

cu·ra·re (kyū-rah´rē) An extract of various plants, which produces nondepolarizing paralysis of skeletal muscle after intravenous injection by blocking transmission at the myoneuronal junction. SYN arrow poison (1).

cu·ra·ri·za·tion (kyū-rah´ri-zā´shŭn) Induction of muscular relaxation or paralysis by the administration of curare or related compounds that have the ability to block nerve impulse transmission at the myoneural junction.

cu·ra·tive (kyūr´ă-tiv) **1.** That which heals or cures. **2.** Tending to heal or cure.

cu·ra·tive dose (CD) (kyūr´ă-tiv dōs) **1.** The quantity of any substance required to effect the cure of a disease or that will correct the manifestations of a deficiency of a particular factor in the diet. **2.** Effective dose used with therapeutically applied compounds.

cure (kyūr) **1.** To heal; to make well. **2.** A restoration to health. **3.** A special method or course of treatment. **4.** Hardening of certain materials with time or by the application of heat, light, or chemical agents, e.g., polymerization of acrylic denture-based material.

cu·ret·tage, cu·ret·te·ment (kyūr-e-tahzh´, kyūr-et´mĕnt) A scraping, usually of the interior of a cavity or tract, for the removal of new growths or other abnormal tissues, or to obtain material for tissue diagnosis.

cu·rette, cu·ret (kyūr-et´) Instrument in the form of a loop, ring, or scoop with sharpened edges attached to a rod-shaped handle, used for curettage.

cu·rie (C, c, Ci) (kyūr´ē) A unit of measurement of radioactivity; superseded by the S.I. unit, the becquerel.

cur·ing (kyūr´ing) **1.** The act of accomplishing a cure. **2.** A process by which something is prepared for use, as by heating, aging, etc.

cur·rant jel·ly clot (kŭr´ănt jel´ē klot) Jellylike mass of red blood cells and fibrin formed by in vitro or postmortem clotting of whole or sedimented blood.

cur·rent (kŭr´rĕnt) A stream or flow of fluid, air, or electricity.

cur·rent of in·ju·ry (kŭr´ĕnt in´jūr-ē) Current generated when an injured part of a nerve, muscle, or other excitable tissue is connected through a conductor with the uninjured region; the injured tissue is negative to the uninjured. SYN demarcation current.

Cur·rent Pro·ce·du·ral Ter·min·o·lo·gy (CPT) (kŭr´rĕnt prō-sē´jūr-ăl tĕr-mi-nol´ŏ-jē) A coding system for professional medical procedures and services, published by the American Medical Association and revised annually.

cur·va·ture, cur·va·tu·ra (kŭr´vă-chŭr, -tū´ră) A bending or flexure.

cur·va·ture my·o·pia (kŭr´vă-chŭr mī-ō´pē-ă) Nearsightedness due to refractive errors resulting from excessive corneal curvature.

curve (kŭrv) **1.** A nonangular continuous bend or line. **2.** A chart or graphic representation, by means of a continuous line connecting individual observations, of the course of a physiologic activity, of the number of cases of a disease in a given period, or of any entity that might be otherwise presented by a table of figures. SYN chart (2).

cur·vi·lin·e·ar (kŭr´vi-lin´ē-ăr) Pertaining to curved lines.

Cur·vu·la·ri·a (kŭr-vyū-lār´ē-ă) An opportunistic fungus widely spread in nature; in humans, has been associated with sinusitis, keratitis, pulmonary infections, and in the immunocompromised patient, occasionally, disseminated disease.

Cush·ing dis·ease (kush´ing di-zēz´) Adrenal hyperplasia (Cushing syndrome) caused by an adrenocorticotropic-hormone-secreting basophil adenoma of the pituitary. SYN Cushing pituitary basophilism.

Cush·ing neu·ro·ma (kush´ing nūr-ō´mă) An acoustic lesion with a 3:1 female predilection. Therapy is usually surgical removal.

Cush·ing syn·drome (kush´ing sin´drōm) A disorder resulting from increased adrenocortical secretion of cortisol (giving a clinical picture of Cushing disease), due to any one of several sources.

cush·ion (kush´ŭn) ANATOMY Any structure resembling a pad or cushion.

cusp (kŭsp) [TA] **1.** DENTISTRY a conic elevation arising on the surface of a tooth from an independent calcification center. **2.** A leaflet of a cardiac valve. SYN cuspis [TA].

cusp-and-groove pat·tern (kŭsp grūv pat´ĕrn) The arrangement of the cusps and grooves on molars; in the lower molars there are four principal ones, Y-5, Y-4, +5, and +4.

cusp height (kŭsp hīt) **1.** Shortest distance between the tip of a cusp and its base plane. **2.** Shortest distance between the deepest part of the central fossa of a posterior tooth and a line connecting the points of the cusps of the tooth.

cus·pid (kŭs'pid) **1.** Having but one cusp. **2.** SYN canine tooth.

cus·pid tooth, cus·pi·date tooth (kŭs'pid tūth, kŭs'pi-dāt) SYN canine tooth.

cus·pis, pl. **cus·pi·des** (kŭs'pis, -pi-dēz) [TA] SYN cusp.

cusp·less tooth (kŭsp'lĕs tūth) **1.** One devoid of cusp formation. **2.** Severe abrasion of an occlusal surface. **3.** Type of artificial denture tooth.

cusp ridge (kŭsp rij) An elevation extending both mesially and distally from the cusp tip of molars and premolars, thus forming the lingual and buccal boundaries of the occlusal surface.

cus·to·di·al care (kŭs-tō'dē-ăl kār) Nonskilled personal care to assist with activities of daily living.

cut (kŭt) **1.** MOLECULAR BIOLOGY a hydrolytic cleavage of two opposing phosphodiester bonds in a double-stranded nucleic acid. Cf. nick. **2.** To sever or divide. **3.** To separate into fractions. **4.** An informal term for a fraction.

cu·ta·ne·ous (kyū-tā'nē-ŭs) Relating to the skin.

cu·ta·ne·ous an·thrax (kyū-tā'nē-ŭs an' thraks) Dermatologic infection produces a characteristic lesion that begins as a papule and soon becomes a vesicle and breaks, discharging a bloody serum; the seat of this vesicle, in about 36 hours, becomes a bluish black necrotic mass; constitutional symptoms of septicemia are severe: high fever, vomiting, profuse sweating, and extreme prostration; the infection is often fatal. SYN malignant pustule.

cu·ta·ne·ous horn (kyū-tā'nē-ŭs hōrn) A protruding keratotic growth of the skin.

cu·ta·ne·ous lar·va mi·grans (kyū-tā'nē-ŭs lahr'vă mī'granz) An advancing creeping or netlike tunneling in the skin, with marked pruritus, caused by wandering hookworm larvae not adapted to intestinal maturation in humans.

cu·ta·ne·ous lu·pus er·y·the·ma·to·sus (kyū-tā'nē-ŭs lū'pŭs er'i-thē-mă-tō'sis) **1.** Skin disease seen in patients with a discoid form of lupus erythematosus. **2.** Various skin lesions seen in systemic lupus erythematosus.

cu·ta·ne·ous mus·cle (kyū-tā'nē-ŭs mŭs'ĕl) [TA] One lies in the subcutaneous tissue and attaches to the skin; it may or may not have a bony attachment. The muscles of expression are the chief examples in humans.

cu·ta·ne·ous nerve (kyū-tā'nē-ŭs nĕrv) [TA] A mixed nerve supplying a region of the skin, including its sensory endings, blood vessels, smooth muscle, and glands.

cu·ta·ne·ous T-cell lym·pho·ma (CTCL) (kyū-tā'nē-ŭs sel lim-fō'mă) SEE Sézary syndrome.

cu·ta·ne·ous tu·ber·cu·lo·sis (kyū-tā'nē-ŭs tū-bĕr'kyū-lō'sis) Pathologic lesions of the skin caused by *Mycobacterium tuberculosis*.

cu·ta·ne·ous vas·cu·li·tis (kyū-tā'nē-ŭs vas'kyū-lī'tis) An acute form that may affect the skin only, but also may involve other organs, with a polymorphonuclear infiltrate in the walls of and surrounding small (dermal) vessels. SEE ALSO leukocytoclastic vasculitis.

cut·down (kŭt'down) Dissection of a vein for insertion of a cannula or needle for the administration of intravenous fluids or medication. SYN venostomy.

cu·ti·cle (kyū'ti-kĕl) **1.** An outer thin layer, usually of a horny composition. SYN cuticula (1). **2.** The layer, chitinous in some invertebrates, which occurs on the surface of epithelial cells. **3.** SYN epidermis.

cu·tic·u·la, pl. **cu·tic·u·lae** (kyū-tik'yū-lă, -lē) **1.** SYN cuticle (1). **2.** SYN epidermis.

cu·ti·re·ac·tion (kyū'ti-rē-ak'shŭn) Inflammatory reaction to a skin test in a sensitive (allergic) subject.

cu·tis (kyū'tis) [TA] SYN skin.

cu·tis an·se·ri·na (kyū'tis an-sĕ-rī'nă) Contraction of the arrectores pilorum produced by cold or other stimulus, causing the follicular orifices to become prominent. SYN gooseflesh.

cu·tis lax·a (CL) (kyū′tis lak′să) [TA] SYN dermatochalasis.

cu·tis ver·ti·cis gy·ra·ta (CVG) (kyū′ tis věr′ti-sis jī-rā′tă) Congenital condition in which the skin of the scalp is hypertrophied and thrown into folds forming anterior to posterior furrows.

CW agent (ā′jěnt) Abbreviation for chemical-warfare agent.

CX NATO code for phosgene oxime.

cy·a·nide (sī′ăn-īd) 1. The radical -CN or ion (CN-). The ion is extremely poisonous, forming hydrocyanic acid in water; inhibits respiratory enzymes. 2. A salt of HCN. 3. A molecule containing a cyanide group. 4. A class of toxic chemical-warfare agents. SEE ALSO blood agent, hydrogen cyanide, cyanogen chloride.

♻ **cyano-** Combining form denoting blue.

Cy·a·no·bac·te·ria (sī′ă-nō-bak-tēr′ē-ă) A division of the kingdom Prokaryotae consisting of unicellular or filamentous bacteria that are either nonmotile or possess a gliding motility, reproduce by binary fission, and perform photosynthesis with the production of oxygen. SYN Cyanophyceae.

cy·a·no·co·bal·a·min (sī′ă-nō-kō-bal′ ă-min) A complex of cyanide and cobalamin, as in vitamin B12.

cy·an·o·phil, cy·an·o·phile (sī-an′ō-fil, -fīl) A cell or element that is colored blue by a staining procedure differentially.

Cy·a·no·phy·ce·ae (sī′ă-nō-fī′shē-ē) SYN Cyanobacteria.

cy·a·nop·si·a, cy·a·no·pia (sī′ă-nop′ sē-ă, -nō′pē-ă) A condition in which all objects appear blue; may temporarily follow cataract extraction.

cy·a·no·sis (C) (sī′ă-nō′sis) A dark bluish or purplish discoloration of the skin and mucous membrane due to deficient oxygenation of the blood, evident when reduced hemoglobin in the blood exceeds 5 g/100 mL.

cy·a·no·sis ret·i·nae (sī′ă-nō′sis ret′ inē) Venous congestion of the retina.

cy·a·not·ic (sī′ă-not′ik) Relating to or marked by cyanosis.

cy·cla·mate (sī′klă-māt) A salt or ester of cyclamic acid; the calcium and sodium are noncaloric artificial sweetening agents.

cyc·lar·thro·sis (sī′klahr-thrō′sis) A joint capable of rotation.

cy·clase (sī′klās) Descriptive name applied to an enzyme that forms a cyclic compound.

cy·cle (sī′kěl) 1. A recurrent series of events. 2. A recurring period of time. 3. One successive compression and rarefaction of a wave, as of a sound wave.

cy·clec·to·my (sī-klek′tŏ-mē) Excision of a portion of the ciliary body. SYN ciliectomy.

cy·cle length al·ter·nans (sī′kěl length awl-těr′nanz) A succession of alternately long and short diastolic intervals.

cy·clen·ceph·a·ly, cy·clen·ce·pha·lia (sī-klen-sef′ă-lē, -se-fā′lē-ă) Condition in a malformed fetus characterized by poor development and a varying degree of fusion of the two cerebral hemispheres. SYN cyclocephaly, cyclocephalia.

cy·cles per sec·ond (cps) (sī′kělz pěr sek′ŏnd) The number of successive compressions and rarefactions per second of a sound wave. The preferred designation for this unit of frequency is the hertz.

cy·clic, cy·cli·cal (sik′lik, sik′lī-kăl) 1. Pertaining to, or characteristic of, a cycle; occurring periodically, denoting the course of the symptoms in certain diseases or disorders. 2. CHEMISTRY pertaining to a molecule containing a ring of atoms; denoting a cyclic compound.

cy·clic AMP (sik′lik) SYN adenosine 3′, 5′-cyclic monophosphate.

cy·clic gua·no·sine 3′,5′-mon·o·phos·phate, cy·clic GMP (cGMP) (sik′lik gwah′nō-sēn mon′ō-fos′făt) Analogue of cyclic adenosine monophosphate; a second messenger for atrial natriuretic factor. SYN cyclic GMP.

cy·clic neu·tro·pe·ni·a (sik´lik nū-trō-pē´nē-ă) SYN periodic neutropenia.

cy·clin (sī´klin) A class of proteins involved in regulation of the cell cycle.

cy·clist's pal·sy (sī´klists pawl´zē) Paresthesia of the ulnar nerve in cyclists resulting from leaning on the handlebars for an extended period. SYN ulnar nerve compression syndrome.

cy·cli·tis (sik-lī´tis) Inflammation of the ciliary body.

cyclo-, cycl- 1. Combining forms meaning a circle or cycle; the ciliary body. 2. CHEMISTRY prefix meaning a molecule consisting of atoms in a ring.

cy·clo·cho·roid·i·tis (sī´klō-kōr´oyd-ī´tis) Inflammation of the ciliary body and the choroid.

cy·clo·cry·o·ther·a·py (sī´klō-krī´ō-thār´ă-pē) Transscleral freezing of the ciliary body in the treatment of glaucoma.

cy·clo·di·a·ther·my (sī´klō-dī´ă-thĕr-mē) Diathermy applied to the sclera adjacent to the ciliary body in the treatment of glaucoma.

cy·cloid (sī´kloyd) Suggesting cyclothymia; a term applied to personality traits associated with cyclothymia.

cy·clo·ox·y·gen·ase (COX, CLO) (sī´klō-oks´i-jĕn-ās) SYN prostaglandin endoperoxide synthase.

cy·clo·pho·ri·a (sī´klō-fōr´ē-ă) Abnormal tendency for each eye to rotate around its anteroposterior axis, the rotation being prevented by visual fusional impulses.

cy·clo·phos·pha·mide (sī´klō-fos´fă-mīd) An alkylating agent with antitumor activity and uses similar to those of its parent compound, nitrogen mustard (mechlorethamine hydrochloride); also a suppressor of B-cell activity and antibody formation.

cy·clo·pho·to·co·ag·u·la·tion (sī´klō-fō´tō-kō-ag´yŭ-lā´shŭn) Photocoagula-

tion of the ciliary processes to reduce the secretion of aqueous humor in glaucoma.

cy·clo·ple·gi·a (sī´klō-plē´jē-ă) Loss of power in the ciliary muscle of the eye; may be due to denervation or by pharmacologic action.

cy·clo·ple·gic (sī´klō-plē´jik) 1. Relating to cycloplegia. 2. A drug that paralyzes the ciliary muscle and thus the power of accommodation.

cy·clo·pro·pane (sī´klō-prō´pān) An explosive gas of characteristic odor; in the past, widely used to produce general anesthesia. SYN trimethylene.

cy·clops (sī´klops) A person with cyclopia. SYN monoculus (1), monops.

cy·clo·ser·ine (CS) (sī´klō-ser´ēn) An antibiotic produced by strains of *Streptomyces orchidaceus* or *S. garyphalus* with a wide spectrum of antibacterial activity. SYN orientomycin.

cy·clo·spor·i·a·sis (sī´klō-spōr-ī´ă-sis) Infection with *Cyclospora*.

cy·clo·spor·ine (sī´klō-spōr´in) A cyclic oligopeptide immunosuppressant produced by the fungus *Tolypocladium inflatum Gams;* used to inhibit organ transplant rejection.

cy·clo·thy·mi·a (sī´klō-thī´mē-ă) A mental disorder characterized by marked swings of mood from depression to hypomania but not to the degree that occurs in bipolar disorder.

cy·clo·thy·mic per·son·al·i·ty (sī´klō-thī´mik pĕr-sŏn-al´i-tē) A personality disorder in which a person experiences regularly alternating periods of elation and depression, usually not related to external circumstances.

cy·clot·o·my (sī-klot´ŏ-mē) Operation of cutting the ciliary muscle.

cyl·in·der (C) (sil´in-dĕr) 1. A cylindric or rodlike renal cast. 2. A cylindric metal container for gases stored under high pressure.

cy·lin·dric lens (C) (si-lin´drik lenz) A lens in which one of the surfaces is curved in one meridian and less curved in the opposite meridian; commonly used to correct the visual distortion resulting from astigmatism. SYN astigmatic lens.

cyl·in·droid (sil'in-droyd) SYN false cast.

cyl·in·dro·ma (sil'in-drŏ'mă) A histologic type of epithelial neoplasm, frequently malignant, characterized by islands of neoplastic cells embedded in a hyalinized stroma. SYN cylindroadenoma.

cyl·in·dru·ri·a (sil'in-drūr'ē-ă) The presence of renal cylinders or casts in the urine.

cym·bo·ceph·a·ly (sim'bō-sef'ă-lē) SYN scaphocephaly.

cy·no·ceph·a·ly (sī'nō-sef'ă-lē) Craniostenosis in which the skull slopes back from the orbits, producing a resemblance to the head of a dog.

cy·no·pho·bi·a (sī'nō-fō'bē-ă) Morbid fear of dogs.

CYP Abbreviation for cytochrome P450 enzymes; usually followed by an arabic numeral, a letter, and another arabic numeral (e.g., CYP 2D6); found in and on the smooth endoplasmic reticulum of liver and other cells and responsible for a large number of drug biotransformation reactions.

Cys Abbreviation for cysteine (half-cystine) or its mono- or diradical.

cyst (sist) 1. An abnormal sac containing gas, fluid, or a semisolid material, with a membranous lining. SEE ALSO pseudocyst. 2. Larval stage of some cestodes.

cyst·ad·e·no·car·ci·no·ma (sist-ad'ĕ-nō-kahr'si-nō'mă) A malignant neoplasm derived from glandular epithelium, in which cystic accumulations of retained secretions are formed.

cyst·ad·e·no·ma (sist'ad-ĕ-nō'mă) A histologically benign neoplasm derived from glandular epithelium, in which cystic accumulations of retained secretions are formed. SYN cystoadenoma.

cyst·al·gi·a (sist-al'jē-ă) Pain in a bladder, especially the urinary bladder.

cys·ta·thi·o·nine (sis'tă-thī'ō-nēn) An intermediate in the conversion of L-methionine to L-cysteine; cleaved by cystathionases.

cys·ta·thi·o·nine gam·ma (γ)-ly·ase (sis'tă-thī'ō-nēn gam'ă lī'ās) A liver enzyme that catalyzes the hydrolysis of L-cystathionine to L-cysteine and 2-ketobutyrate. A deficiency of this enzyme results in cystathioninuria. SYN cystathionase.

cys·ta·thi·o·ni·nu·ri·a (sis'tă-thī'ō-nin-yū'rē-ă) A disorder characterized by inability to metabolize cystathionine, normally due to deficiency of cystathionase, with high concentration of the amino acid in blood, tissue, and urine.

cys·te·a·mine (sis-tē'ă-mēn) 2-Aminoethanethiol; a sulfhydryl compound used experimentally to produce ulcers in rats and as a radioprotective agent; antidote to acetaminophen overdose.

cys·tec·ta·si·a, cys·tec·ta·sy (sis'tek-tā'zē-ă, sis-tek'tă-sē) Dilation of the bladder.

cys·tec·to·my (sis-tek'tŏ-mē) 1. Excision of the urinary bladder. 2. Excision of the gallbladder (cholecystectomy). 3. Removal of a cyst.

cys·te·ic ac·id (sis-tē'ik as'id) An oxidation product of cysteine, and a precursor of taurine and isethionic acid.

cys·te·ine (C, Cys) (sis-tē'in) An amino acid found in most proteins; especially abundant in keratin.

cys·tic (sis'tik) 1. Relating to the urinary bladder or gallbladder. 2. Relating to a cyst. 3. Containing cysts.

cys·tic ac·ne (sis'tik ak'nē) Severe form in which the predominant lesions are follicular cysts that rupture and scar.

cys·tic ar·te·ry (sis'tik ahr'tĕr-ē) [TA] *Origin*, right branch of hepatic; *distribution*, gall bladder and visceral surface of the liver. SYN arteria cystica [TA].

cys·tic bile (sis'tik bīl) Concentrated bile located in the gallbladder.

cys·tic car·ci·no·ma (sis'tik kahr'si-nō'mă) One in which true epithelium-lined cysts are formed, or degenerative changes may result in cystlike spaces.

cys·tic duct, cys·tic gall duct (sis´tik dŭkt, gawl) [TA] The ductus leading from the gallbladder; it joins the hepatic duct to form the common bile duct.

cys·ti·cer·co·sis (sis´ti-sĕr-kō´sis) Disease caused by encystment of cysticercus larvae (e.g., *Taenia solium* or *T. saginata*) in subcutaneous, muscle, or central nervous system tissues.

Cys·ti·cer·cus (sis´ti-sĕr´kŭs) The encysted larva of taenioid tapeworms.

cys·tic fi·bro·ma (sis´tik fī-brō´mă) A tumor composed mainly of fibrous or fully developed connective tissue.

cys·tic fi·bro·sis, cys·tic fi·bro·sis of the pan·cre·as (sis´tik fī-brō´sis, pan´krē-ăs) A congenital metabolic disorder, inherited as an autosomal trait, in which secretions of exocrine glands are abnormal; excessively viscid mucus causes obstruction of passageways (including pancreatic and bile ducts, intestines, and bronchi), and the sodium and chloride content of sweat are increased throughout the patient's life; symptoms usually appear in childhood and include meconium ileus, poor growth despite good appetite, malabsorption and foul bulky stools, chronic bronchitis with cough, recurrent pneumonia, bronchiectasis, emphysema, clubbing of the fingers, and salt depletion in hot weather.

cys·tic gall duct (sis´tik gawl dŭkt) SYN cystic duct.

cys·tic hy·gro·ma (sis´tik hī-grō´mă) Lymphangioma hygroma, poorly encapsulated tumor composed of lymph-filled endothelial-lined cysts, usually found around the neck, but may occur in the axilla, groin, or elsewhere. SYN lymphangioma hygroma.

cys·tic kid·ney (sis´tik kid´nē) General term used to indicate a kidney that contains one or more cysts, including polycystic disease, solitary cyst, multiple simple cysts, and retention cysts.

cys·tic mas·ti·tis (sis´tik mas-tī´tis) The presence of one or more cysts in a breast.

cys·tic tu·mor (sis´tik tū´mŏr) A lesion with cavities or sacs containing semisolid or liquid material.

cys·tic veins (sis´tik vānz) [TA] Veins, usually anterior and posterior, which drain the neck of the gallbladder and cystic duct.

cys·tine cal·cu·lus (sis´tēn kal´kyū-lŭs) A soft and faintly radiopaque urinary tract stone composed of cystine.

cys·ti·no·sis (sis´ti-nō´sis) A lysosomal storage disorder with various forms, all with autosomal recessive inheritance. SYN cystine storage disease.

cys·ti·nu·ria (sis´ti-nyūr´ē-ă) Excessive urinary excretion of cystine, along with lysine, arginine, and ornithine, arising from defective transport systems for these acids in the kidney and intestine; renal function is sometimes compromised by cystine crystalluria and nephrolithiasis.

cys·ti·tis (sis-tī´tis) Inflammation of the urinary bladder.

cys·ti·tis col·li (sis-tī´tis kol´ē) Inflammation of the neck of the bladder.

cys·ti·tis glan·du·la·ris (sis-tī´tis glan-dyū-lā´ris) Chronic cystitis with glandlike metaplasia of transitional epithelium.

cysto-, cysti-, cyst- Combining forms relating to the bladder; the cystic duct; a cyst. Cf. vesico-.

cys·to·cele (sis´tō-sēl) Hernia of the bladder usually into the vagina and introitus. SYN colpocystocele, vesicocele.

cys·to·du·o·de·nal lig·a·ment (sis´tō-dū-ō-dē´năl lig´ă-mĕnt) A peritoneal fold that sometimes passes from the gallbladder to the first part of the duodenum.

cys·to·fi·bro·ma (sis´tō-fī-brō´mă) A fibroma in which cysts or cystlike foci have formed.

cys·to·gas·tros·to·my (CGY) (sis´tō-gas-tros´tō-mē) Drainage of a pancreatic pseudocyst into the stomach.

cys·to·gram (sis´tō-gram) Radiographic demonstration of the bladder filled with contrast medium.

cys·tog·ra·phy (sis-tog′ră-fē) Radiography of the bladder following injection of a radiopaque substance.

cys·toid (sis′toyd) **1.** Bladderlike, resembling a cyst. SYN cystiform, cystomorphous. **2.** A tumor resembling a cyst, with fluid, granular, or pulpy contents, but without a capsule.

cys·toid mac·u·lar e·de·ma (CME) (sis′toyd mak′yū-lăr ĕ-dē′mă) Swelling of the posterior pole of the eye secondary to abnormal permeability of capillaries of the central sensory retina.

cys·toid mac·u·lop·a·thy (sis′toyd mak′yū-lop′ă-thē) Cystic degeneration of the central retina that may occur after cataract extraction, in senile macular degeneration, and in other retinal abnormalities.

cys·to·je·ju·nos·to·my (sis′tō-je-jū-nos′tŏ-mē) Drainage of a pancreatic pseudocyst into the jejunum.

cys·to·li·thi·a·sis (sis′tō-li-thī′ă-sis) The presence of a vesical calculus. SYN vesicolithiasis.

cy·sto·lith·o·la·pax·y (sis′tō-lith′ō-lā-paks-ē) Removal of bladder calculi by intravesical crushing and then irrigating to remove fragments.

cys·to·li·thot·o·my (sis′tō-li-thot′ŏ-mē) Removal of a stone from the bladder through an incision or endoscopic puncture in its wall. SYN vesical lithotomy.

cys·to·mor·phous (sis′tō-mōr′fŭs) SYN cystoid (1).

cys·to·pan·en·dos·co·py (sis′tō-pan-en-dos′kŏ-pē) Inspection of the interior of the bladder and urethra by means of specially designed endoscopes introduced in retrograde fashion through the urethra and into the bladder.

cys·to·pex·y (sis′tō-pek-sē) Surgical attachment of the gallbladder or of the urinary bladder to the abdominal wall or to other supporting structures.

cys·to·plas·ty (sis′tō-plas-tē) Any reconstructive operation on the urinary bladder. Cf. ileocystoplasty, colocystoplasty.

cys·to·ple·gi·a (sis′tō-plē′jē-ă) Paralysis of the bladder. SYN cystoparalysis.

cys·to·pros·ta·tec·to·my (sis′tō-pros′tă-tek′tŏ-mē) Surgical removal of bladder, prostate, and seminal vesicles simultaneously.

cys·top·to·sis, cys·to·pto·si·a (sis′tō-tō′sis, sis-tō-tō′sē-ă) Prolapse of the vesical mucous membrane into the urethra.

cys·to·py·e·li·tis (sis′tō-pī-ĕl-ī′tis) Inflammation of both the bladder and the pelvis of the kidney.

cys·to·py·e·lo·ne·phri·tis (sis′tō-pī′ĕl-ō-nef-rī′tis) Inflammation of the bladder, the pelvis of the kidney, and the kidney parenchyma.

cys·tor·rhe·a (sis′tōr-ē′ă) A mucous discharge from the bladder. SYN cystorrhoea.

cystorrhoea [Br.] SYN cystorrhea.

cys·to·sar·co·ma (sis′tō-sahr-kō′mă) A lesion in which cysts or cystlike foci have formed.

cys·tos·co·py (sis-tos′kŏ-pē) The inspection of the interior of the bladder by means of a cystoscope.

cys·tos·to·my (sis-tos′tŏ-mē) Creation of an opening into the urinary bladder.

cys·to·tome, cys·ti·tome (sis′tō-tōm, -ti-tōm) **1.** An instrument for incising the urinary bladder or gallbladder. **2.** A surgical instrument used for incising the capsule of a lens. SYN capsulotome.

cys·tot·o·my (sis-tot′ŏ-mē) Incision into urinary bladder or gallbladder.

cys·to·u·re·ter·i·tis (sis′tō-yūr′ē-tĕr-ī′tis) Inflammation of the bladder and of one or both ureters.

cys·to·u·re·ter·og·ra·phy (sis′tō-yūr′ĕ-tĕr-og′ră-fē) Radiography of the bladder and ureters.

cys·to·u·re·thri·tis (sis′tō-yūr′ē-thrī′tis) Inflammation of the bladder and of the urethra.

cys·to·u·re·thro·gram (sis′tō-yūr-ē′

thrō-gram) An x-ray image made during voiding and with the bladder and urethra filled with contrast medium to demonstrate the urethra. SYN voiding cystogram.

cys•to•u•re•throg•ra•phy (sis′tō-yūr′ĕ-throg′ră-fē) Radiography of the bladder and urethra during voiding, after the bladder has been filled with a radiopaque contrast medium either by intravenous injection or retrograde catheterization.

cys•to•u•re•thro•scope (sis′tō-yūr-ē′thrō-skōp) An instrument combining the uses of a cystoscope and a urethroscope, whereby both the bladder and urethra can be visually inspected.

cy•ta•pher•e•sis (sī′tă-fĕr-ē′sis) A procedure in which various cells can be separated from the withdrawn blood and retained, with the plasma and other formed elements retransfused into the donor.

-cyte Suffix meaning cell.

cyto-, cyt- Combining forms meaning a cell.

cy•to•ar•chi•tec•ture (sī′tō-ahr′ki-tek-shŭr) The arrangement of cells in a tissue. SYN architectonics.

cy•to•cen•trum (sī′tō-sen′trŭm) A zone of cytoplasm containing one or two centrioles but devoid of other organelles; usually located near the nucleus of a cell. SYN centrosome

cy•to•chem•is•try (sī′tō-kem′is-trē) The study of intracellular distribution of chemicals, reaction sites, and enzymes, often by means of staining reactions, radioactive isotope uptake, selective metal distribution in electron microscopy, or other methods. SYN histochemistry.

cy•to•chrome (sī′tō-krōm) A class of hemoprotein the principal biologic function of which is electron or hydrogen transport by virtue of a reversible valency change of the heme iron.

cy•to•chrome P-450 sys•tem (sī′tō-krōm sis′tĕm) A heterogeneous group of enzymes that catalyze various oxidative reactions in the human liver, intestine, kidney, lung, and central nervous system; these enzymes are involved in the metabolism of many endogenous and exogenous substrates, including drugs, toxins, hormones, and natural plant products.

cy•to•ci•dal (sī′tō-sī′dăl) Causing the death of cells.

cy•to•cide (sī′tō-sīd) An agent that destroys cells.

cy•toc•la•sis (sī-tok′lă-sis) Fragmentation of cells.

cy•to•cle•sis (sī′tō-klē′sis) The influence of one cell on another. SYN cytobiotaxis.

cy•to•di•er•e•sis (sī′tō-dī-ĕr′ē-sis) SYN cytokinesis.

cy•to•gene (sī′tō-jēn) SYN plasmagene.

cy•to•gen•e•sis (sī′tō-jen′ĕ-sis) The origin and development of cells.

cy•to•gen•et•ic map (sī′tō-jĕ-net′ik map) Schematic in which the classical bonding pattern of a chromosome is shown.

cy•to•ge•net•ics (sī′tō-jĕ-net′iks) The branch of genetics concerned with the structure and function of the cell, especially the chromosomes.

cy•to•gen•ic (sī′tō-jen′ik) Relating to cytogenesis.

cy•tog•e•nous (sī-toj′ĕ-nŭs) Denotes cell-forming.

cy•to•glu•co•pe•ni•a (sī′tō-glū-kō-pē′nē-ă) An intracellular deficiency of glucose.

cy•toid (sī′toyd) Resembling a cell.

cy•to•kine (sī′tō-kīn) Hormonelike proteins, secreted by many cell types, which regulate the intensity and duration of immune responses and are involved in cell-to-cell communication. SEE ALSO interferon, interleukin, lymphokine.

cy•to•kine net•work (sī′tō-kīn net′wŏrk) Group of cytokines that act together to modulate and regulate key cellular functions.

cy•to•ki•ne•sis (sī′tō-ki-nē′sis) Changes

occurring in the protoplasm of the cell outside the nucleus during cell division.

cy·tol·o·gy (sī-tol′ŏ-jē) The study of the anatomy, physiology, pathology, and chemistry of the cell. SYN cellular biology.

cy·tol·y·sin (sī-tol′i-sin) A substance, i.e., an antibody, which effects partial or complete destruction of an animal cell; may require complement.

cy·tol·y·sis (sī-tol′i-sis) The dissolution of a cell.

cy·to·ly·so·some (sī′tō-lī′sō-sōm) A variety of secondary lysosome that contains the remnants of mitochondria, ribosomes, or other organelles. SYN autophagic vacuole.

cy·to·me·ga·lic (sī′tō-mĕ-gā′lik) Denoting or characterized by markedly enlarged cells.

Cy·to·meg·a·lo·vi·rus (CMV) (sī′tō-meg′ă-lō-vī′rŭs) A group of viruses in the family Herpesviridae infecting humans and other animals; many have a special affinity for salivary glands; all forms are species specific and include salivary virus, inclusion body rhinitis virus of pigs, and others. SYN visceral disease virus.

cy·to·met·a·pla·si·a (sī′tō-met-ă-plā′zē-ă) Change of form or function of a cell, other than that related to neoplasia.

cy·tom·e·ter (sī-tom′ĕ-ter) A device used to count and measure cells, especially blood cells, either visually (with a microscope) or automatically (as in flow cytometry).

cy·tom·e·try (sī-tom′ĕ-trē) The counting of cells, especially blood cells, using a cytometer or hemocytometer.

cy·to·mor·phol·o·gy (sī′tō-mōr-fol′ŏ-jē) The study of the structure of cells.

cy·to·mor·pho·sis (sī′tō-mōr-fō′sis) Changes that the cell undergoes during the various stages of its existence. SEE ALSO prosoplasia.

cy·to·path·ic (sī′tō-path′ik) Pertaining to or exhibiting cytopathy.

cy·to·path·o·gen·e·sis (sī′tō-path′ŏ-jen′ĕ-sis) Process of production of pathologic changes in cells.

cy·to·path·o·gen·ic (sī′tō-path-ŏ-jen′ik) Pertaining to an agent or substance that causes a diseased condition in cells, in contrast to histologic changes.

cy·to·path·o·gen·ic virus (sī′tō-path-ŏ-jen′ik vī′rŭs) A virus the multiplication of which leads to degenerative changes in the host cell.

cy·to·path·o·log·ic, cy·to·path·o·log·i·cal (sī′tō-path-ŏ-loj′ik, -loj′i-kăl) **1.** Denoting cellular changes in disease. **2.** Relating to cytopathology.

cy·to·pa·thol·o·gist (sī′tō-pă-thol′ŏ-jist) A physician, usually skilled in anatomic pathology, who is specially trained and experienced in cytopathology.

cy·to·pa·thol·o·gy (sī′tō-pă-thol′ŏ-jē) **1.** The study of disease changes within individual cells or cell types. **2.** SYN exfoliative cytology.

cy·to·pe·ni·a (sī′tō-pĕ′nē-ă) A reduction, i.e., hypocytosis, or a lack of cellular elements in the circulating blood.

cy·toph·a·gy (sī-tof′ă-jē) Devouring of other cells by phagocytes.

cy·to·phil·ic (sī′tō-fil′ik) SYN cytotropic.

cy·to·phil·ic an·ti·body (sī′tō-fil′ik an′ti-bod-ē) SYN cytotropic antibody.

cy·to·phy·lax·is (sī′tō-fī-lak′sis) Protection of cells against lytic agents.

cy·to·pi·pette (sī′tō-pī-pet′) A slightly curved, blunt end tube usually made of glass and fitted with a rubber bulb to provide gentle negative pressure for the collection of vaginal secretions for cytologic examination.

cy·to·plasm (sī′tō-plazm) The substance of a cell, exclusive of the nucleus, that contains various organelles and inclusions within a colloidal protoplasm. SEE ALSO protoplasm, hyaloplasm, cytosol.

cy·to·pro·tec·tive (sī′tō-prō-tek′tiv) Descriptive of a drug or agent protecting cells from damage expected to occur.

cy·to·sine (Cyt) (sī'tō-sēn) A pyrimidine found in nucleic acids.

cy·to·skel·e·ton (sī'tō-skel'ĕ-tŏn) The tonofilaments, keratin, desmin, neurofilaments, or other intermediate filaments serving as supportive cytoplasmic elements to stiffen cells or to organize intracellular organelles.

cy·to·sol (sī'tō-sol) Cytoplasm exclusive of the mitochondria, endoplasmic reticulum, and other membranous components.

cy·to·some (sī'tō-sōm) **1.** The cell body exclusive of the nucleus. **2.** One of the osmiophilic bodies that are 1 mcm or less in diameter, have concentric lamellae, and occur in the great alveolar cells of the lung. SYN multilamellar body.

cy·tos·ta·sis (sī-tos'tă-sis) The slowing of movement and accumulation of blood cells, especially polymorphonuclear leukocytes, in the capillaries, as in a region of inflammation.

cy·to·stat·ic (sī'tō-stat'ik) Characterized by cytostasis.

cy·to·stome (sī'tō-stōm) The cell ''mouth'' of certain complex protozoa, usually with a short gullet or cytopharynx leading food into the organism.

cy·to·tax·is, cy·to·tax·i·a, pos·i·tive cy·to·tax·is, neg·a·tive cy·to·tax·is (sī'tō-tak'sis, -sē-ă, poz'i-tiv, neg'ă-tiv) The attraction (positive cytotaxis) or repulsion (negative cytotaxis) of cells for one another.

cy·toth·e·sis (sī-toth'ĕ-sis) The repair of injury in a cell; the restoration of cells.

cy·to·tox·ic drug (sī'tō-tok'sik drŭg) Pharmacotherapeutic agent that has a deleterious effect on cells.

cy·to·tox·ic·i·ty (sī'tō-tok-sis'i-tē) The quality or state of being cytotoxic.

cy·to·tox·ic re·ac·tion (sī'tō-tok'sik rē-ak'shŭn) An immunologic (allergic) reaction in which noncytotropic IgG or IgM antibody combines with a specific antigen on cell surfaces.

cy·to·tox·in (sī'tō-tok'sin) A specific substance, which may or may not be an antibody, which inhibits or prevents the functions of cells, causes destruction of cells, or both.

cy·to·tro·pho·blast (CTB) (sī'tō-trō'fō-blast) The inner cellular layer of the trophoblast of a blastocyst. SYN Langhans layer.

cy·to·tro·pho·blas·tic cells (sī'tō-trō'fō-blas'tik selz) Stem cells that fuse to form the overlying syncytiotrophoblast of placental villi. SYN Langhans cells (2).

cy·to·tro·pic (sī'tō-trō'pik) Having an affinity for cells. SYN cytophilic.

cy·to·tro·pic an·ti·bod·y (sī'tō-trō'pik an'ti-bod-ē) Antibody that has an affinity for certain kinds of cells, in addition to and unrelated to its specific affinity for the antigen that induced it, because of the properties of the Fc portion of the heavy chain.

cy·tot·ro·pism (sī-tot'rŏ-pizm) **1.** Affinity for cells. **2.** Affinity for specific cells, especially the ability of viruses to localize in and damage specific cells.

cy·to·zo·ic (sī'tō-zō'ik) Living in a cell; denoting certain parasitic protozoa.

cy·tu·ria (sī-tyūr'ē-ă) The passage of cells in unusual numbers in the urine.

Cza·pek so·lu·tion agar (shŏ'pek sŏ-lū'shŭn ā'gahr) Culture medium used for the cultivation of fungal species and identification of *Aspergillus* and *Penicillium* species. SYN Czapek-Dox medium.

D

D- Prefix indicating a chemical compound to be dextrorotatory; should be avoided when (+) or (−) could be used. Cf. L-, lambda.

dacryo-, dacry- Combining forms meaning tears; lacrimal sac or duct.

dac·ry·o·cys·tal·gi·a (dak′rē-ō-sis-tal′ jē-ă) Pain in the lacrimal sac.

dac·ry·o·cys·tec·to·my (dak′rē-ō-sis-tek′tŏ-mē) Surgical removal of the lacrimal sac.

dac·ry·o·cys·ti·tis (dak′rē-ō-sis-tī′tis) Inflammation of the lacrimal sac.

dac·ry·o·cys·to·cele (dak′rē-ō-sis′tō-sēl) Enlargement of the lacrimal sac with fluid.

dac·ry·o·cys·tot·o·my (dak′rē-ō-sis-tot′ŏ-mē) Incision of the lacrimal sac.

dac·ry·o·cyte (dak′rē-ō-sīt) An abnormally shaped red blood cell with a single point or elongation; also called a teardrop cell.

dacryohaemorrhoea [Br.] SYN dacryohemorrhea.

dac·ry·o·hem·or·rhe·a (dak′rē-ō-hem-ŏr-ē′ă) Bloody tears. SYN dacryohaemorrhoea.

dac·ry·o·lith (dak′rē-ō-lith) A concretion in the lacrimal apparatus. SYN tear stone.

dac·ry·ops (dak′rē-ops) **1.** Excess of tears in the eye. **2.** A cyst of a duct of the lacrimal gland.

dac·ry·o·py·or·rhe·a (dak′rē-ō-pī′ŏr-ē′ ă) The discharge of tears containing leukocytes. SYN dacryopyorrhoea.

dacryopyorrhoea [Br.] SYN dacryopyorrhea.

dac·ry·o·ste·no·sis (dak′rē-ō-stĕ-nō′sis) Stricture of a lacrimal or nasal duct.

dac·ti·no·my·cin (DACT) (dak′ti-nō-mī′sin) An antineoplastic antibiotic produced by several species of *Streptomyces* (e.g., *S. parvulus*). SYN actinomycin D.

dac·tyl (dak′til) SYN digit.

dactylo-, dactyl- Combining forms meaning the fingers, and (less often) toes.

dac·ty·lo·camp·sis (dak′ti-lō-kamp′sis) Permanent flexion of the fingers.

dac·ty·lo·gry·po·sis (dak′ti-lō-gri-pō′ sis) Permanent curvature or deformity of the fingers.

dac·ty·lol·y·sis (dak′ti-lol′i-sis) Spontaneous loss of digits, seen in leprosy, ainhum, and in utero when hair firmly wraps around the finger or toe, resulting in an amputation.

dac·ty·los·co·py (dak′ti-los′kŏ-pē) An examination of the markings in prints made from the fingertips; employed as a method of personal identification.

dac·ty·lus, pl. **dac·ty·li** (dak′ti-lŭs, -lī) SYN digit.

DAF (daf) Acronym for delayed auditory feedback.

Da·kin so·lu·tion (dā′kin sŏ-lū′shŭn) A bactericidal wound irrigant. SYN Dakin fluid.

dal·ton (Da, D) (dawl′tŏn) Term unofficially used to indicate a unit of mass equal to 1/12 the mass of a carbon-12 atom, 1.0000 in the atomic mass scale; numerically, but not dimensionally, equal to molecular or particle weight (atomic mass units).

dam (dam) **1.** Any barrier to the flow of fluid. **2.** In surgery and dentistry, a sheet of thin rubber arranged so as to shut off the operative site from the access of fluid.

da·na·zol (dā′nă-zol) A synthetic steroid used to treat endometriosis, fibrocystic breast disease, and angioedema. Indirectly reduces estrogen production by lowering levels of follicle-stimulating hormone and luteinizing hormone.

Dance sign (dans sīn) Slight retraction in the area of the right iliac fossa in some cases of intussusception.

dan·der (dan′dĕr) **1.** A fine scaling of the skin and scalp. SEE ALSO dandruff. **2.** A normal effluvium of animal hair or coat capable of causing allergic responses in atopic people.

dan·druff (dan′drŭf) The presence, in varying amounts, of white or gray scales in the hair of the scalp, due to exfoliation of the epidermis. SEE ALSO seborrheic dermatitis. SYN scurf, seborrhea sicca (2).

Dan·dy-Walk·er syn·drome (dan′dē waw′kĕr sin′drōm) Developmental anomaly of the fourth ventricle associated with atresia of the foramina of Luschka and Magendie that results in cerebellar hypoplasia, hydrocephalus, and posterior fossa cyst formation.

Dane par·ti·cles (dān pahr′ti-kĕlz) The larger spheric forms of hepatitis-associated antigens.

Dan·forth sign (dan′fōrth sīn) Shoulder pain on inspiration, due to irritation of the diaphragm by a hemoperitoneum in ruptured ectopic pregnancy.

D an·ti·gen (an′ti-jen) One of six antigens that comprise the Rh locus. Antibody induced by D antigen is the most frequent cause of hemolytic disease of the newborn.

dap·sone (dap′sōn) An antibiotic used to treat leprosy and other cutaneous diseases.

Da·ri·er sign (dah-rē-ā′ sīn) Urtication on stroking of cutaneous lesions of urticaria pigmentosa (mastocytosis).

dark-a·dapt·ed eye (dahrk-ă-dap′tĕd ī) One that has been in darkness or semidarkness and has undergone regeneration of rhodopsin (visual purple), which renders it more sensitive to reduced illumination. SYN scotopic eye.

dar·to·ic tis·sue (dahr-tō′ik tish′ū) That resembling tunica dartos.

dar·tos (dahr′tōs) SEE dartos fascia, dartos muscle.

dar·tos fa·sci·a (dahr′tōs fash′ē-ă) [TA] A superficial fascial layer incorporating smooth muscular tissue in the integument of the scrotum; it also forms the scrotal septum. SEE ALSO dartos muscle. SYN superficial fascia of scrotum, membrana carnosa, tunica carnea.

dar·tos mus·cle (dahr′tōs mŭs′ĕl) Smooth muscle fibers interspersed within the dartos fascia (superficial fascia of scrotum), causing contraction of the scrotum, as when experiencing a cool environmental temperature. SEE ALSO dartos fascia.

dar·win·i·an ref·lex (dahr-win′ē-ăn rē′ fleks) The tendency of young infants to grasp a bar and hang suspended. SEE ALSO grasping reflex.

dar·win·i·an the·o·ry (dahr-win′ē-ăn thē′ŏr-ē) Theory of the origin of species and of the development of higher organisms from lower forms through natural selection (survival of the fittest in the struggle for existence), and of the evolution of humans and apes from a common ancestor.

dar·win·i·an tu·ber·cle (dahr-win′ē-ăn tū′bĕr-kĕl) SYN auricular tubercle.

DASH di·et (dash dī′ĕt) The DASH (Dietary Approach to Stop Hypertension) diet is based on an eating plan that favors fruits, vegetables, and low- or nonfat dairy products.

da·ta (dā′tă) *This is a plural noun; datum is the singular form.* **1.** Facts (usually established by observation, measurement, or experiment) used as a basis for inference, testing, or models. **2.** Information collected about a patient, family, or community, often during intake of nursing history.

date boil, Del·hi boil, Jer·i·cho boil (dāt boyl, del′ē, jer′i-kō) The lesion occurring in cutaneous leishmaniasis.

date of ser·vice (DOS) (dāt sĕr′vis) In health care finance, the day when a therapy was initially provided; often of great importance in verifying charges covered with a third-party payer.

daugh·ter (daw′tĕr) In nuclear medicine, an isotope that is the disintegration product of a radionuclide.

daugh·ter cell (daw′tĕr sel) One of the two or more cells formed in the division of a parent cell.

dau·no·ru·bi·cin (daw′nō-rū′bi-sin) SYN rubidomycin.

dawn phe·nom·e·non (dawn fĕ-nom′ĕ-non) Abrupt increases in fasting levels of plasma glucose concentrations between 5–9 AM in the absence of antecedent hypoglycemia; occurs in diabetic patients receiving insulin therapy.

day blind·ness (dā blīnd′nĕs) SYN hemeralopia.

day health care ser·vices (dā helth kār sĕr′vis-ĕz) The provision of hospitals, nursing homes, or other facilities for health-related services to adult patients (e.g., physical therapy, counseling).

day hos·pi·tal (DH) (dā hos′pi-tăl) Special facility, or an arrangement within a hospital setting, which enables the patient to come to the hospital for treatment during the day and return home or to another facility at night. SEE ALSO night hospital.

DD Abbreviation meaning date dictated; developmental disability.

de- Prefix meaning away from, cessation, without; sometimes has an intensive force.

de·ac·ti·va·tion (dē′ak-ti-vā′shŭn) Process of rendering or of becoming inactive.

de·ac·yl·ase (dē-as′il-ās) A member of the subclass of hydrolases (EC class 3), especially of that subclass of esterases, lipases, lactonases, and hydrolases (EC subclass 3.1).

dead (d, D) (ded) **1.** Without life. SEE ALSO death. **2.** Numb.

dead fe·tus syn·drome (ded fē′tŭs sin′drōm) Disorder characterized by lengthy intrauterine retention of a dead fetus usually longer than 4 weeks with development of hypofibrinogenemia and occasionally disseminated intravascular coagulopathy.

dead·ly night·shade (ded′lē nīt′shād) SYN belladonna.

dead on ar·ri·val (DOA) (ded ă-rī′văl) Charting notation used in the emergency department stating the patient has not survived the trip to the hospital.

dead space (ded spās) A cavity, potential or real, remaining after the closure of a wound that is not obliterated by the operative technique. SEE physiologic dead space.

deaf (def) Unable to hear.

de·af·fer·en·ta·tion (dē-af′ĕr-ĕn-tā′shŭn) A loss of the sensory input from a portion of the body, usually caused by interruption of the peripheral sensory fibers.

deaf·ness (def′nĕs) General term for inability to hear.

de·am·i·nase (dē-am′i-nās) Any enzyme that removes an amino group from a compound.

Dean fluor·o·sis in·dex (dēn flūr-ō′sis in′deks) A measure of the degree of mottled enamel (fluorosis) in teeth; used most often in epidemiologic field studies.

death an·xi·e·ty (deth ang-zī′ĕ-tē) A state of restlessness and agitation caused by fears of the end of life.

death in·stinct (deth in′stingkt) The instinct of all living creatures toward self-destruction, death, or a return to the inorganic lifelessness from which they arose.

death rate (deth rāt) An estimate of the proportion of the population that dies during a specified period, usually a year. SYN mortality rate, mortality (2).

death trance (deth trans) State of suspended animation, marked by unconsciousness and barely perceptible respiration and heart action.

Dea·ver in·ci·sion (dē′vĕr in-si′zhŭn) An incision in the right lower abdominal quadrant, with medial displacement of the rectus muscle.

De·Bak·ey clas·si·fi·ca·tion of a·or·tic dis·sec·tion (dĕ-bā′kē klas′i-fi-kā′shŭn ā-ōr′tik di-sek′shŭn) Consists of three types: type I extends into the transverse arch and distal aorta and type II is confined to the ascending aorta; type III dissections begin in the descending aorta, with type IIIA extending toward the diaphragm and type IIIB extending below it.

De·Bak·ey for·ceps (dĕ-bā′kē fōr′seps) Nontraumatic tool used to pick up blood vessels; also known as "magics." SYN magic forceps.

de·bil·i·tat·ing (dĕ-bil'i-tāt-ing) Denoting or characteristic of a morbid process that causes weakness.

de·bil·i·ty (debil) (dĕ-bil'i-tē) Weakness.

de·bond (dē-bond') To separate a dental appliance such as an orthodontic band from the tooth to which it has been attached or bonded by a resin cement.

dé·bride·ment (dā-brēd-mawn[h]') Excision of devitalized tissue and foreign matter from a wound.

de·bulk·ing op·er·a·tion (dē-bŭlk'ing op-ĕr-ā'shŭn) Excision of a major part of a malignant tumor that cannot be completely removed, so as to enhance the effectiveness of subsequent radio- or chemotherapy.

deca- (da) Prefix used in the S.I. and metric system to signify 10. Also spelled deka-.

de·cal·ci·fi·ca·tion (dē-kal'si-fi-kā'shŭn) **1.** Removal of calcium salts from bones and teeth, either in vitro or as a result of a pathologic process. **2.** Precipitation of calcium from blood as by oxalate or fluoride, or the conversion of blood calcium to an un-ionized form as by citrate, thus preventing or delaying coagulation.

de·cal·ci·fy·ing (dē-kal'si-fī-ing) Denoting an agent, measure, or process that causes decalcification.

de·can·nul·a·tion (dē-kan'yū-lā'shŭn) Planned or accidental removal of a tracheostomy tube.

de·cant (dec, DEC) (dē-kant') To pour off gently the upper clear portion of a fluid, leaving the sediment in the vessel.

de·cap·i·ta·tion (dē-kap'i-tā'shŭn) Removal of a head.

de·cap·su·la·tion (dē-kap'sū-lā'shŭn) Incision and removal of a capsule or enveloping membrane.

de·car·box·yl·ase (dē'kahr-bok'sil-ās) Any enzyme (EC subclass 4.1.1) that removes a molecule of carbon dioxide from a carboxylic group.

de·cay (dē-kā') **1.** Destruction of an organic substance by slow combustion or gradual oxidation. **2.** SYN putrefaction. **3.** To deteriorate; to undergo slow combustion or putrefaction. **4.** DENTISTRY caries.

de·cayed, miss·ing, or filled tooth sur·faces (dmfs, DMFS) (dē-kād' mis'ing fild tūth sur'fā-sĕz) Denotes a survey by dentists of the state of a patient's teeth before beginning a course of therapy; part of a written health care record.

de·cel·er·a·tion (DECEL) (dē-sel'ĕr-ā' shŭn) **1.** The act of decelerating. **2.** The rate of decrease in velocity per unit of time.

de·cen·tered lens (dē-sen'tĕrd lenz) One so mounted that the visual axis does not pass through the axis of the lens.

de·cer·e·brate (dē-ser'ĕ-brāt) **1.** To cause decerebration. **2.** Denoting an animal so prepared, or a patient whose brain has suffered an injury that renders the patient, in neurologic behavior, comparable to a decerebrate animal.

de·cho·les·ter·ol·i·za·tion (dē'kŏ-les' tĕr-ol-ī-zā'shŭn) Therapeutic reduction of the cholesterol concentration of the blood.

deci- (d) Prefix used in the SI and metric system to signify one tenth (10^{-}).

dec·i·bel (dB, db) (des'i-bel) *Avoid mispronunciation des'i-b'l.* One tenth of a bel; unit for expressing the relative intensity of sound on a logarithmic scale.

de·cid·ua (dē-sij'ū-ă) The endometrium of the uterus in a pregnant woman.

de·cid·ua ba·sa·lis (dē-sij'ū-ă bā-sā'lis) [TA] The area of endometrium between the implanted chorionic sac and the myometrium, which develops into the maternal part of the placenta. SYN decidua serotina.

de·cid·ua cap·su·lar·is (dē-sij'ū-ă kap-sū-lā'ris) [TA] Layer of endometrium overlying the implanted chorionic vesicle. SYN membrana adventitia (2).

de·cid·u·al en·do·me·tri·tis (dē-sid' yū-ăl en'dō-mē-trī'tis) Inflammation of the decidual mucous membrane of the gravid uterus.

de·cid·ua pa·ri·e·tal·is (dē-sij´ū-ă pă-rī-ĕ-tā´lis) The altered endometrium lining the main cavity of the pregnant uterus other than at the site of attachment of the chorionic sac.

de·cid·ua po·ly·po·sa (dē-sij´ū-ă pol-i-pō´să) Decidua parietalis showing polypoid projections of the endometrial surface.

de·cid·ua spon·gi·o·sa (dē-sij´ū-ă spŏn-jē-ō´să) The portion of the decidua basalis attached to the myometrium.

de·cid·u·ate pla·cen·ta (dē-sid´yū-ăt plă-sen´tă) One in which the decidua is cast off with the fetal placenta.

de·cid·u·a·tion (dĕ-sij´ū-ā-ā´shŭn) Shedding of endometrial tissue during menstruation.

de·cid·u·ous (dĕ-sij´ū-ŭs) **1.** Not permanent; denoting that which eventually falls off. **2.** DENTISTRY referring to the first or primary dentition. SEE deciduous tooth.

de·cid·u·ous tooth, de·cid·u·ous den·ti·tion (dē-sij´ū-ŭs tūth, den-tī´shŭn) [TA] One of the first set of teeth, comprising 20 in all, which erupts between the mean ages of 6 and 28 months of life. SYN dens deciduus [TA], baby tooth, milk dentition, milk tooth, primary dentition, temporary tooth.

dec·i·gram (dg, dgm, d) (des´i-gram) One tenth of a gram.

dec·i·li·ter (dL) (des´i-lē´tĕr) One tenth of a liter.

de·clamp·ing phe·nom·e·non (dē-klamp´ing fē-nom´ĕ-non) Shock or hypotension following abrupt release of clamps from a large portion of the vascular bed, as from the aorta.

dec·li·na·tion (dek´li-nā´shŭn) A bending, sloping, or other deviation from a normal vertical position.

de·coc·tion (decoct) (dē-kok´shŭn) **1.** The process of boiling. **2.** The pharmacopeial name for preparations made by boiling crude vegetable drugs, and then straining, in the proportion of 50 g of the drug to 1000 mL of water. SYN apozem, apozema.

de·col·or·a·tion (dē-kŏ´lŏr-ā´shŭn) The natural loss or removal of color, such as caused by bleaching.

de·com·pen·sa·tion (dē-kom´pĕn-sā´shŭn) **1.** A failure of compensation in heart disease. **2.** The appearance or exacerbation of a mental disorder due to failure of defense mechanisms.

de·com·po·si·tion (dē-kŏm´pŏ-zish´ŭn) SYN putrefaction.

de·com·pres·sion (dē-kŏm-presh´ŭn) Removal of pressure.

de·com·pres·sion sick·ness (dē-kŏm-presh´ŭn sik´nĕs) A symptom complex caused by the escape from solution in the body fluids of nitrogen bubbles absorbed originally at high atmospheric pressure, as a result of abrupt reduction in atmospheric pressure (either rapid ascent to high altitude or return from a compressed-air environment); characterized by headache; pain in the arms, legs, joints, and epigastrium; itching of the skin; vertigo; dyspnea; coughing; choking; vomiting; weakness; sometimes paralysis; and severe peripheral circulatory collapse. SYN caisson disease.

de·con·ges·tant (dē-kŏn-jes´tănt) **1.** Having the property of reducing congestion. **2.** An agent that reduces congestion.

de·con·tam·i·na·tion (dē-kŏn-tam´i-nā´shŭn) Removal or neutralization of poisonous gas or other injurious agents from the environment, or from victims of such agents.

de·cor·ti·cate ri·gid·i·ty (dē-kōr´ti-kāt ri-jid´i-tē) A unilateral or bilateral postural change, in which the upper extremities are flexed and adducted and the lower extremities are held in rigid extension; due to structural lesions of the thalamus, internal capsule, or cerebral white matter.

de·cor·ti·ca·tion (dē-kōr´ti-kā´shŭn) **1.** Removal of the cortex, or external layer, beneath the capsule from any organ or structure. **2.** An operation to remove a clot and scar tissue that formed after a hemothorax or neglected empyema.

dec·re·ment (dek´rĕ-mĕnt) **1.** Decrease.

2. Decrease in conduction velocity at a particular point; a result of altered properties at that point. SEE ALSO decremental conduction.

dec·re·men·tal con·duc·tion (dek-rĕ-men′tăl kŏn-dŭk′shŭn) Impaired conduction in a portion of a fiber because of progressively lessening response of the unexcited portion of the fiber to the action potential coming toward it.

de·cru·des·cence (dē-krū-des′ĕns) Abatement of the symptoms of disease.

de·cu·bi·tus (dē-kyū′bi-tŭs) **1.** The position of the patient in bed; e.g., dorsal decubitus, lateral decubitus. SEE ALSO decubitus film. **2.** Sometimes used to mean a decubitus ulcer (q.v.).

de·cu·bi·tus film (dē-kyū′bi-tŭs film) A radiograph exposed with the subject in the decubitus position; named for the side that is dependent.

de·cu·bi·tus pa·ral·y·sis (dē-kyū′bi-tŭs păr-al′i-sis) The loss of the power of voluntary motion caused by damage to nerves that remained too long in the same position.

de·cu·bi·tus ul·cer (dē-kyū′bi-tŭs ŭl′sĕr) Focal ischemic necrosis of skin and underlying tissues at sites of constant pressure or recurring friction in patients confined to bed or immobilized by illness; malnutrition worsens the prognosis. SEE decubitus. SYN bedsore, pressure sore, pressure ulcer.

de·cus·sa·ti·o, pl. **de·cus·sa·ti·o·nes** (dē′kŭ-sā′shē-ō, -nēz) [TA] **1.** In general, any crossing over or intersection of parts. **2.** The intercrossing of two homonymous fiber bundles as each crosses over to the opposite side of the brain in the course of its ascent or descent through the brainstem or spinal cord. Also called decussation.

de·cus·sa·tion of me·di·al lem·nis·cus (dē-kŭs-ā′shŭn mē′dē-ăl lem-nis′kŭs) The intercrossing of the fibers of the left and right medial lemniscus ascending from the gracile and cuneate nuclei, immediately rostral to the level of the decussation of the pyramidal tracts in the medulla oblongata. SYN decussatio lemniscorum.

de·cus·sa·tion of pyr·a·mids (dē-kŭs-ā′shŭn pir′i-midz) [TA] Intercrossing of the bundles of corticospinal fibers at the lower border region of the medulla oblongata. SYN decussatio pyramidum [TA], decussatio motoria, motor decussation.

de·cus·sa·tion of su·pe·ri·or cer·e·bel·lar pe·dun·cles (dē-kŭs-ā′shŭn sū-pēr′ē-ŏr ser′ĕ-bel′ăr pĕ-dŭng′kĕlz) [TA] The decussation of the left and right superior cerebellar peduncles in the tegmentum of the caudal mesencephalon.

de·dif·fer·en·ti·a·tion (dē-dif′ĕr-en′shē-ā′shŭn) **1.** The return of parts to a more homogeneous state. **2.** SYN anaplasia.

deep (dēp) [TA] Situated at a lower level in relation to a specific reference point. Cf. superficialis.

deep au·ric·u·lar ar·ter·y (dēp awr-ik′yū-lăr ahr′tĕr-ē) [TA] *Origin*, first part of maxillary; *distribution*, articulation of jaw, parotid gland, and external acoustic meatus and external tympanic membrane; *anastomoses*, auricular branches of superficial temporal and posterior auricular. SYN arteria auricularis profunda.

deep brach·i·al ar·ter·y (dēp brā′kē-ăl ahr′tĕr-ē) SYN profunda brachii artery.

deep brain stim·u·la·tion (DBS) (dēp brān stim-yū-lā′shŭn) Functional neurosurgery in which stimulating electrodes are placed in the basal ganglia for management of movement disorders, including parkinsonism dystonia and tremor.

deep ce·re·bral veins (dēp ser′ĕ-brăl vānz) [TA] The numerous veins draining the deep structures of the cerebral hemispheres; they empty into the tributaries of the great cerebral vein. SYN venae profundae cerebri [TA].

deep cir·cum·flex il·i·ac ar·ter·y (dēp sir′kŭm-fleks il′ē-ak ahr′tĕr-ē) [TA] *Origin*, external iliac; *distribution*, muscles and skin of lower abdomen, sartorius, and tensor fasciae latae; *anastomoses*, lumbar, inferior epigastric, superior gluteal, iliolumbar, and superficial circumflex iliac. SYN arteria circumflexa iliaca profunda.

deep in·gui·nal ring (dēp ing′gwi-năl ring) [TA] The opening in the transversalis fascia through which the ductus deferens (or round ligament in the female) and gonadal vessels enter the inguinal canal.

deep la·mel·lar en·do·the·li·al ker·a·to·plas·ty (DLEK) (dēp lă-mel'ăr en'dō-thē'lē-ăl ker'ă-tō-plas-tē) A surgical procedure whereby only the inner retinal layers are subject to transplantation.

deep par·tial-thick·ness burn (dēp pahr'shăl-thik'nĕs bŭrn) A burn (q.v.) or thermal injury that destroys cells from the epidermis to the deep dermal layer.

deep pe·tro·sal nerve (dēp pĕ-trō'săl nĕrv) [TA] A branch of the internal carotid plexus, which joins the greater petrosal nerve at the entrance of the pterygoid canal forming the nerve of the pterygoid canal and thus provides postsynaptic fibers to the pterygopalatine ganglion. SYN nervus petrosus profundus [TA], sympathetic root of pterygopalatine ganglion.

deep re·flex (dēp rē'fleks) An involuntary muscular contraction following percussion of a tendon or bone. SYN jerk (2).

deep sen·si·bil·i·ty (dēp sens'ĭ-bil'ĭ-tē) SYN kinesthetic sense.

deep vein throm·bo·sis (DVT) (dēp vān throm-bō'sis) Formation of one or more thrombi in the deep veins, usually of the lower extremity or in the pelvis. Carries a high risk of pulmonary embolism. SEE ALSO thrombophlebitis.

defaecation [Br.] SYN defecation.

DEF car·ies in·dex (def kar'ēz in'deks) An index of past caries experience that includes *d*ecayed, *e*xtracted, and *f*illed deciduous teeth; sometimes the extracted portion (e) is not included.

def·e·ca·tion (def-ĕ-kā'shŭn) The discharge of feces from the rectum. SYN defaecation, movement (3).

def·e·cog·ra·phy (def'ĕ-kog'ră-fē) Radiographic examination of the act of defecation of a radiopaque stool.

de·fect (dē'fekt) An imperfection, anomaly, malformation, dysfunction, or absence; a qualitative departure from what

is expected. USAGE NOTE often confused with deficiency, which is a quantitative shortcoming.

de·fec·tive vi·rus (dĕ-fek'tiv vī'rŭs) Viral particle that contains insufficient nucleic acid to provide for production of all essential viral components.

defence [Br.] SYN defense.

de·fense (dĕ-fens') **1.** The psychological mechanisms used to control anxiety, e.g., rationalization, projection. **2.** Any protective posture, drug, or device. SYN defence.

de·fense re·flex (dĕ-fens' rē'fleks) SYN flexor reflex.

de·fen·sins (dĕ-fen'sinz) A class of basic antibiotic polypeptides, found in neutrophils, which kills bacteria by causing membrane damage. These cytotoxic peptides contain 29–38 amino acid residues.

def·er·ent (def'ĕr-ĕnt) Carrying away.

def·er·en·tial (def'ĕr-en'shăl) Relating to the ductus deferens.

def·er·en·ti·tis (def'ĕr-en-tī'tis) Inflammation of the ductus deferens.

def·er·ves·cence (def'ĕr-ves'ĕns) Lowering an elevated temperature; abatement of fever.

de·fib·ril·la·tion (dē-fib'ri-lā'shŭn) The arrest of fibrillation of the cardiac muscle (atrial or ventricular) with restoration of the normal rhythm.

de·fib·ril·la·tor (dē-fib'ri-lā-tŏr) **1.** Any agent or measure (e.g., electric shock) that arrests fibrillation of the atria or ventricles and restores the normal rhythm. **2.** The machine designed to administer a defibrillating electric shock.

de·fi·bri·na·tion (dē-fī'bri-nā'shŭn) Removal of fibrin from the blood, usually by means of constant agitation while the blood is collected in a container with glass beads or chips.

de·fi·cien·cy (dĕ-fish'ĕn-sē) An insufficient quantity of a substance (as in dietary deficiency, hemoglobin deficiency as in marrow aplasia), organization (as in mental deficiency), activity (as in enzyme deficiency or reduced oxygen-carrying capacity of the blood), or other process or component of which the amount present is of decreased quantity.

def·i·cit (def'i-sit) The result of consuming or losing something faster than it is replenished or replaced.

de·fin·i·tive (dĕ-fin'i-tiv) Fully differentiated or developed.

de·fin·i·tive host (dĕ-fin'i-tiv hōst) One in which a parasite reaches the adult or sexually mature stage.

de·fin·i·tive pros·the·sis (dĕ-fin'i-tiv pros-thē'sis) Dental prosthesis to be used over a prescribed period of time.

de·flec·tion (dĕ-flek'shŭn) *Do not confuse this word with deflexion.* **1.** A moving to one side. **2.** In the electrocardiogram, a deviation of the curve from the isoelectric base line; any wave or complex of the electrocardiogram.

de·flex·ion (dĕ-flek'shŭn) Term used to describe the position of the fetal head in relation to the maternal pelvis in which the head is descending in a nonflexed or extended attitude.

de·flu·vi·um (dĕ-flū'vē-ŭm) *Do not confuse this word with effluvium.* SYN defluxion.

de·flux·ion (dĕ-flŭk'shŭn) **1.** A falling down or out, as of the hair. SEE ALSO effluvium. **2.** A flowing down or discharge of fluid. SYN defluvium.

de·form·a·bil·i·ty (dĕ-fōrm'ă-bil'i-tē) The ability of cells to change shape as they pass through narrow spaces.

de·for·ma·tion (dĕ-fōr-mā'shŭn) **1.** Deviation of form from normal. **2.** In rheology, the change in the physical shape of a mass by applied stress.

de·for·mi·ty (dĕ-fōrm'i-tē) *Negative or pejorative connotations of this word may render it offensive in some contexts.* A permanent structural deviation from the normal shape or size, resulting in disfigurement; may be congenital or acquired. SYN deformation (2).

de·gen·er·ate (dĕ-jen'ĕr-āt) **1.** To pass to a lower level of mental, physical, or

moral state; to fall below the normal or acceptable type or state. **2.** Below the normal or acceptable; that which has passed to a lower level.

de·gen·er·a·tion (dĕ-jen'ĕr-ā'shŭn) **1.** Deterioration; passing from a higher to a lower level or type. **2.** A worsening of mental, physical, or moral qualities. **3.** A retrogressive pathologic change in cells or tissues, in consequence of which their functions are often impaired or destroyed; sometimes reversible.

de·gen·e·ra·tive disc dis·ease (dĕ-jen'ĕr-ă-tiv disk di-zēz') Protrusion, herniation, or fragmentation of an intervertebral disc beyond its borders with potential compression of a nerve root, the cauda equina in the lumbar region, or the spinal cord at higher levels.

de·gen·e·ra·tive dis·ease (dĕ-jen'ĕr-ă-tiv di-zēz') Any disorder (e.g., arteriosclerosis, diabetes mellitus, osteoarthritis) marked by progressively worsening changes in tissue.

de·gen·er·a·tive joint dis·ease (DJD) (dĕ-jen'ĕr-ă-tiv joynt di-zēz') SYN osteoarthritis.

de·glov·ing (dē-glŏv'ing) **1.** Intraoral surgical exposure of the anterior mandible used in various orthognathic surgical operations such as genioplasty or mandibular alveolar surgery. **2.** SEE degloving injury.

de·glov·ing in·ju·ry (dē-glŏv'ing in'jŭr-ē) Avulsion of the skin of the hand (or foot) in which the part is skeletonized by removal of most or all of the skin and subcutaneous tissue.

de·glu·ti·tion (dē-glū-tish'ŭn) The act of swallowing.

de·glu·ti·tion ap·nea (dē'glū-tish'ŭn ap'nē-ă) Inhibition of breathing during swallowing.

de·glu·ti·tion syn·co·pe (dē-glū-tish'ŭn sing'kŏ-pē) Faintness or unconsciousness on swallowing; nearly always due to excessive vagal effect on a heart with bradycardia or atrioventricular block.

deg·ra·da·tion (deg'ră-dā'shŭn) The change of a chemical compound into a less complex compound.

de·gran·u·la·tion (dē-gran′yū-lā′shŭn) Disappearance or loss of cytoplasmic granules from a cell or activation of granulocytic cells (e.g., neutrophils, mast cells, basophils, eosinophils).

de·gus·ta·tion (dē-gŭs-tā′shŭn) 1. The act of tasting. 2. The sense of taste.

De·hi·o test (dĕ-hē′ō test) If an injection of atropine relieves bradycardia, the condition is due to action of the vagus; if it does not, the condition may be due to an affliction of the heart itself.

de·his·cence (dē-his′ĕns) A bursting open, splitting, or gaping along natural or sutured lines.

de·hu·man·i·za·tion (dē-hyū′măn-ī-zā′shŭn) Loss of human characteristics; brutalization by either mental or physical means; stripping one of self-esteem.

de·hy·dra·tase (dē-hī′dră-tās) A subclass (EC 4.2.1) of lyases (hydrolyases) that remove hydrogen and the hydroxyl ion as water from a substrate, leaving a double bond, or add a group to a double bond by the elimination of water from two substances to form a third.

de·hy·drate (dē-hī′drāt) 1. To extract water from. 2. To lose water.

de·hy·drat·ed al·co·hol (dē-hī′drā-tĕd al′kŏ-hol) SYN absolute alcohol (2).

de·hy·dra·tion (dehyd) (dē-hī-drā′shŭn) *Avoid the jargonistic use of this word as a synonym of thirst.* 1. Deprivation of water. SYN anhydration. 2. Reduction of water content. 3. SYN exsiccation (2). 4. Used commonly in emergency departments to describe a state of water loss sufficient to cause intravascular volume deficits leading to orthostatic symptoms.

de·hy·dra·tion fe·ver (dē′hī-drā′shŭn fē′vĕr) SYN thirst fever.

11-de·hy·dro·cor·ti·co·ster·one (DHC) (dē-hī′drō-kōr-ti-kos′tĕr-ōn) A metabolite of corticosterone.

de·hy·dro·ep·i·an·dos·ter·one (DHEA, DHEA-S) (dē-hī′drō-ep′ē-an-dos′tĕr-ōn) A steroid secreted by the cortex of the suprarenal gland and the testis; a precursor of testosterone.

de·hy·dro·gen·ase (dē-hī′drō-jen-ās) Class name for those enzymes that oxidize substrates by catalyzing removal of hydrogen from metabolites (hydrogen donors) and transferring it to other substances (hydrogen acceptors).

de·hy·dro·gen·ate (dē′hī-droj′ĕ-nāt) To subject to dehydrogenation.

Dei·ters cells (dī′tĕrz selz) 1. SYN phalangeal cell. 2. SYN astrocyte.

de·jec·tion (dĕ-jek′shŭn) SYN depression (4).

De·je·rine-Klump·ke syn·drome (dĕ-zhĕ-rēn′ klump′kĕ sin′drōm) Injury or lesion of the inner cord of the brachial plexus; marked by numbness, hyperesthesia, pain on the ulnar side of the arm, and atrophy of hand muscles with eventual paralysis.

De·je·rine sign (dĕ-zhĕ-rēn′ sīn) Aggravation of symptoms of root irritation by the acts of coughing, sneezing, or straining to defecate.

De·je·rine-Sot·tas dis·ease (dĕ-zhĕ-rēn′ sō-tahz′ di-zēz′) Familial type of demyelinating sensorimotor polyneuropathy that begins in early childhood and is slowly progressive; clinically characterized by foot pain and paresthesias, followed by symmetric weakness and wasting of the distal limbs.

de·lam·i·na·tion (dē-lam′i-nā′shŭn) Division into separate layers.

de Lang·e syn·drome (dĕ lahng′ĕ sin′drōm) Multiple congenital anomaly syndrome characterized by mental retardation, distinctive facies with microcephaly, synophrys, low anterior hairline, depressed nasal bridge, anteverted nares, long philtrum, carp mouth, thin upper lip and low-set ears, prenatal and postnatal growth retardation, hirsutism, and frequently, limb anomalies. SYN Amsterdam syndrome, Cornelia de Lange syndrome.

de·layed al·ler·gy (dĕ-lād′ al′ĕr-jē) A type IV allergic reaction; so called because in a sensitized subject the reaction becomes evident hours after contact with the allergen (antigen), reaches its peak after 36–48 hours, then recedes slowly. SEE ALSO delayed reaction, immediate allergy.

de·layed au·di·tor·y feed·back (DAF) (dĕ-lād′ aw′di-tōr-ē fēd′bak) **1.** A time-lapsed auditory signal that is recorded and then played back with a delay of a set number of milliseconds. **2.** A system used for speech and stuttering treatment in which the subject's voice is recorded and played back, through an earpiece, with a time delay. The distraction caused by the altered feedback enhances fluency and slows speech rate for some users.

de·layed den·ti·tion (dĕ-lād′ den-tish′ŭn) Delayed eruption of the teeth.

de·layed flap (dĕ-lād′ flap) A flap raised in its donor area in two or more stages to increase its chances of survival after transfer.

de·layed graft (dĕ-lād′ graft) Application of a skin graft after waiting several days for healthy granulations to form.

de·layed hy·per·sen·si·ti·vi·ty (DHS, DH) (dĕ-lād′ hī′pĕr-sen′si-tiv′i-tē) **1.** SYN cell-mediated immunity. **2.** SYN delayed reaction.

de·layed re·ac·tion (dĕ-lād′ rē-ak′shŭn) A local or generalized immune response that begins 24–48 hours after exposure to an antigen. SYN delayed hypersensitivity. SEE cell-mediated reaction.

de·layed u·nion (dĕ-lād′ yū′nyŭn) Healing of a fracture that takes longer than expected.

de-lead (dē-led′) To cause the mobilization and excretion of lead deposited in the bones and other tissues, as by the administration of a chelating agent.

del·e·te·ri·ous (del′ĕ-tēr′ē-ŭs) Injurious; noxious; harmful.

de·le·tion (dĕ-lē′shŭn) GENETICS Any spontaneous elimination of part of the normal genetic complement, whether cytogenetically visible (chromosomal deletion) or inferred from phenotypic evidence (point deletion).

del·i·ques·cence (del′i-kwes′ĕns) Becoming damp or liquid by absorption of water from the atmosphere; a property of certain salts, such as calcium chloride.

de·lir·i·um, pl. **de·lir·i·a** (dĕ-lir′ē-ŭm) An altered state of consciousness, consisting of confusion, distractibility, disorientation, disordered thinking and memory, defective perception (illusions and hallucinations), prominent hyperactivity, agitation, and autonomic nervous system overactivity.

de·lir·i·um tre·mens (DTs) (dĕ-lir′ē-ŭm trē′mĕnz) A severe, sometimes fatal, form of delirium due to alcoholic withdrawal after a period of sustained intoxication.

de·liv·er·y (dĕ-liv′ĕr-ē) Passage of the fetus and the placenta from the genital canal into the external world.

del·le (del′ĕ) The central lighter-colored portion of the erythrocyte, as observed in a stained film of blood.

del·len (del′ĕn) Shallow, saucerlike, clearly defined excavations at the margin of the cornea, about 1.5 by 2 mm, due to localized dehydration; also called Fuchs dellen.

De·lorme op·er·a·tion (dĕ-lōrm′ op-ĕr-ā′shŭn) Surgical correction of rectal prolapse by plicaton of redundant mucosa rather than resection.

del·ta, δ (Δ, δ) (del′tă) **1.** Fourth letter of the Greek alphabet. **2.** ANATOMY a triangular surface.

delta (δ)-a·mi·no·lev·u·lin·ic ac·id (ALA) (del′tă ă-mē′nō-lev-yū-lin′ik as′id) An acid formed by δ-aminolevulinate synthase from glycine and succinyl-coenzyme A; a precursor of porphobilinogen, hence an important intermediate in the biosynthesis of hematin.

del·ta bi·li·ru·bin (del′tă bil′i-rū′bin) The fraction of bilirubin covalently bound to albumin.

del·ta hep·a·ti·tis (del′tă hep′ă-tī′tis) SYN viral hepatitis type D.

del·ta rhythm (del′tă ridh′ŭm) A wave pattern in the electroencephalogram in the frequency band of 1.5–4.0 Hz. SYN delta wave (2).

del·ta test (del′tă test) Comparison between the current results of a laboratory test and the previous test results for the same patient.

del·ta wave (del'tă wāv) **1.** A premature upstroke of the QRS complex due to an atrioventricular bypass tract as in Wolff-Parkinson-White syndrome. **2.** SYN delta rhythm.

del·toid (del'toyd) Resembling the Greek letter delta (Δ); triangular.

del·toid lig·a·ment (del'toyd lig'ă-měnt) Compound ligament consisting of four component ligaments that pass downward from the medial malleolus of the tibia to the tarsal bones. SYN ligamentum deltoideum.

del·toid tu·ber·os·i·ty (del'toyd tū'běr-os'i-tē) The prominence at the middle section of the lateral humerus that marks the point of attachment for the deltoid muscle.

de·lu·sion (del) (dĕ-lū'zhŭn) *Do not confuse this word with hallucination or illusion.* A false belief or wrong judgment, sometimes associated with hallucinations, held with conviction despite evidence to the contrary.

de·lu·sion·al dis·or·der (DD) (dĕ-lū'zhŭn-ăl dis-ŏr'děr) Severe mental illness characterized by the presence of delusions; may be related to paranoid, grandiose, somatic, or erotic themes.

de·lu·sion of con·trol, de·lu·sion of be·ing con·trolled (dĕ-lū'zhŭn kŏn-trōl', bē'ing kŏn-trōld') One in which one experiences one's feelings, impulses, thoughts, or actions as not one's own, but as being imposed on by some external force. SYN delusion of passivity.

de·lu·sion of ne·ga·tion (dĕ-lū'zhŭn nĕ-gā'shŭn) A delusion in which one imagines that the world and all that relates to it have ceased to exist.

de·lu·sion of ref·er·ence (dĕ-lū'zhŭn ref'ěr-ĕns) Erroneous notion that external events refer to the self.

de·mand ox·y·gen de·liv·er·y de·vice (dĕ-mand' ok'si-jĕn dĕ-liv'ěr-ē dĕ-vīs') Apparatus that conserves oxygen by sensing the initiation of an inspiratory effort and then delivering oxygen only during the inspiratory phase; usually attached to a nasal cannula.

de·mand pace·ma·ker (dĕ-mand' pās'mă-kěr) A form of artificial pacemaker usually implanted into cardiac tissue because its output of electrical stimuli can be inhibited by endogenous cardiac electrical activity; stimulates heart when that organ's impulses are not sufficient.

de·mar·ca·tion (dē'mahr-kā'shŭn) A setting of limits; a boundary.

de·mar·ca·tion cur·rent (dē'mahr-kā'shŭn kŭr'ĕnt) SYN current of injury.

de·ment·ed (dĕ-ment'ĕd) Suffering from dementia.

de·men·ti·a (dĕ-men'shē-ă) The loss, usually progressive, of cognitive and intellectual functions, without impairment of perception or consciousness; caused by a variety of disorders including severe infections and toxins, but most commonly associated with structural brain disease. Characterized by disorientation, impaired memory, judgment, and intellect, and a shallow labile affect. SYN amentia.

demi- Combining form meaning half, lesser. SEE ALSO hemi-, semi-.

dem·i·gaunt·let ban·dage (dem'ē-găwnt'lĕt ban'dăj) A gauntlet bandage that covers only the hand, leaving the fingers exposed.

de·min·er·al·i·za·tion (dē-min'ěr-ăl-ī-zā'shŭn) A loss or decrease of the mineral constituents of the body or individual tissues, especially of bone.

Dem·o·dex (dem'ō-deks) A genus of tiny mites that inhabit the skin and are usually found in the sebaceous glands and hair follicles.

de·mo·di·co·sis (dem'ō-di-kō'sis) Infestation by mites of the species *Demodex*, chiefly involving hair follicles and characterized by varying degrees of local inflammation and immune response.

de·mog·ra·phy (dĕ-mog'ră-fē) The study of populations, especially with reference to size, density, fertility, mortality, growth rate, age distribution, migration, and vital statistics.

De Mor·gan spot (dĕ mōr′găn spot) SYN senile hemangioma.

de·mul·cent (dĕ-mŭl′sĕnt) **1.** Soothing; relieving irritation. **2.** An agent, such as a mucilage or oil, which soothes and relieves irritation, especially of the mucous surfaces.

de·my·e·li·nat·ing dis·ease (dĕ-mī′ĕ-li-nāt-ing di-zēz′) Generic term for a group of diseases, of unknown cause, in which there is extensive loss of the myelin in the central nervous system, as in multiple sclerosis.

de·my·e·li·na·tion, de·my·e·lin·i·za·tion (dĕ-mī′e-lin-ā′shŭn, -ī-zā′shŭn) Loss of myelin with preservation of the axons or fiber tracts.

de·na·tur·a·tion (dĕ-nā′chŭr-ā′shŭn) The process of becoming denatured.

de·na·tured al·co·hol (dĕ-nā′chŭrd al′kŏ-hol) Ethyl alcohol rendered unfit for consumption as a beverage by the addition of one or several chemicals for commercial purposes (e.g., methanol, aldehol, sucrose octa-acetate). SYN industrial methylated spirit, methylated spirit.

de·na·tured pro·tein (dĕ-nā′chŭrd prō′tēn) One with characteristics or properties that have been altered in some way, as by heat, enzyme action, or chemicals, and in so doing has lost its biologic activity.

den·dri·form (den′dri-fōrm) Tree-shaped, or branching. SYN arborescent, dendritic (1), dendroid.

den·dri·form ker·a·ti·tis, den·drit·ic ker·a·ti·tis (den′dri-fōrm ker′ă-tī′tis, den-drit′ik) A form of herpetic keratitis.

den·drite (den′drīt) **1.** One of the two types of branching protoplasmic processes of the nerve cell (the other being the axon). SYN dendritic process, dendron, neurodendrite, neurodendron. **2.** A crystalline treelike structure formed during the freezing of an alloy.

den·drit·ic (den-drit′ik) **1.** SYN dendriform. **2.** Relating to the dendrites of nerve cells.

den·drit·ic cal·cu·lus (den-drit′ik kal′kyū-lŭs) SYN staghorn calculus.

den·drit·ic cor·ne·al ul·cer (den-drit′ik kōr′nē-ăl ŭl′sĕr) Keratitis caused by herpes simplex virus.

den·drit·ic spines (den-drit′ik spīnz) Variably long excrescences of nerve cell dendrites, varying in shape from small knobs to thornlike or filamentous processes. SYN gemmule (2).

den·dron (den′dron) SYN dendrite (1).

de·ner·va·tion (dĕ′nĕr-vā′shŭn) Loss of nerve supply.

den·gue, den·gue hem·or·rhag·ic fe·ver (den-gā′, hem′ŏr-aj′ik fē′vĕr) A disease of many tropic and subtropic regions that can occur epidemically; caused by dengue virus, a member of the family Flaviviridae. SYN Aden fever, bouquet fever, breakbone fever, dandy fever, date fever, exanthesis arthrosia, polka fever, scarlatina rheumatica, solar fever (1).

de·ni·al (dĕ-nī′ăl) An unconscious defense mechanism used to allay anxiety by denying the existence of important conflicts, troublesome impulses, events, actions, or illness. SYN negation.

Den·is Browne pouch (den′is brown powch) A pocket formed between scarpa and external oblique fascia adjacent to external inguinal ring; a common lodging site for an undescended testis (as in cryptorchism).

Den·is Browne splint (den′is brown splint) A light aluminum splint applied to the lateral aspect of the leg and foot; used for clubfoot.

de·ni·tro·gen·a·tion (dē-nī-troj′ĕ-nā′shŭn) Elimination of nitrogen from lungs and body tissues by breathing gases devoid of nitrogen.

Den·nie-Mor·gan fold, Den·nie line (den′ē mōr′găn fold, den′ē līn) Line below both lower eyelids caused by edema in atopic dermatitis.

De·non·vil·liers fa·sci·a (dĕ-nōn[h]-vē-ā′ fash′ē-ă) Extension of endopelvic fascia covering anterior extraperitoneal rectum and lying between prostate and rectum; important landmark in radical prostatectomy.

dens (denz) [TA] **1.** SYN tooth. **2.** A strong

toothlike process projecting upward from the body of the axis (second cervical vertebra), or epistropheus, around which the atlas rotates. SYN dens axis [TA], odontoid process of epistropheus, odontoid process.

dens in den•te (denz den′tē) A developmental disturbance in tooth formation resulting from invagination of the epithelium associated with crown development into the area destined to become pulp space.

den•si•tom•e•try (dens′i-tom′ĕ-trē) A procedure using a densitometer.

den•si•ty (dens′i-tē) **1.** The compactness of a substance. **2.** CLINICAL RADIOLOGY a less-exposed area on a film, corresponding to a region of greater x-ray attenuation (radiopacity) in the subject; the more light transmitted by the film, the greater the density of the subject.

den•si•ty gra•di•ent (den′si-tē grā′dē-ĕnt) Solution in which the concentration (density) of a solute increases in a continuous fashion from top to bottom, or end to end, of a container. SYN concentration gradient.

♻ **dent-, denti-, dento-** Combining forms meaning teeth; dental. SEE ALSO odonto-.

den•tal (den′tăl) Relating to the teeth.

den•tal ac•qui•red pel•li•cle (den′tăl ă-kwīrd′ pel′i-kĕl) A thin membranous layer, amorphous, acellular, and organic, which forms on exposed tooth surfaces, dental restorations, and dental calculus deposits.

den•tal an•ky•lo•sis (den′tăl ang′ki-lō′sis) Rigid fixation of a tooth to the surrounding alveolus as a result of ossification of the ligament; prevents eruption and orthodontic movement.

den•tal arch (den′tăl ahrch) The curved structure formed by the natural dentition and the residual ridge, which remains after the loss of some or all of the natural teeth.

den•tal bi•o•mech•a•nics (den′tăl bī′ō-mĕ-kan′iks) SYN dental biophysics.

den•tal bulb (den′tăl bŭlb) Papilla, derived from mesoderm, which forms part of the primordium of a tooth that is situated within the cup-shaped enamel organ.

den•tal cal•cu•lus (den′tăl kal′kyū-lŭs) **1.** Calcified deposits formed around the teeth; may appear as subgingival or supragingival calculus. **2.** SYN tartar (1).

den•tal car•ies (den′tăl kar′ēz) Localized, progressively destructive tooth disease that starts at the external surface (usually the enamel) with the apparent dissolution of the inorganic components by organic acids that are produced in immediate proximity to the tooth by the enzymatic action of masses of microorganisms (in the bacterial plaque) on carbohydrates. SYN saprodontia.

den•tal cast (den′tăl kast) Positive likeness of a part or parts of the oral cavity.

den•tal ce•ment (den′tăl sĕ-ment′) SEE cement (2).

den•tal cu•rette (den′tăl kyūr-et′) A curved dental instrument used for scaling, root planing, and gingival curettage.

den•tal en•gine (den′tăl en′jin) The motive power of a dental handpiece that causes it to rotate.

den•tal eth•ics (den′tăl eth′iks) Professional standards related to care of the teeth.

den•tal fis•tu•la (den′tăl fis′tyū-lă) SYN gingival fistula.

den•tal fol•li•cle (den′tăl fol′i-kĕl) The dental sac with its enclosed odontogenic organ and developing tooth.

den•tal for•ceps (den′tăl fŏr′seps) Device used to luxate teeth and to remove them from the alveolus. SYN extracting forceps.

den•tal for•mu•la (den′tăl fŏrm′yū-lă) A statement in tabular form of the number of each kind of teeth in the jaw.

den•tal ger•i•at•rics (den′tăl jer′ē-at′riks) Treatment of dental problems peculiar to advanced age. SYN gerodontics, gerodontology.

den•tal hy•gien•ist (den′tăl hī-jē′nist) A licensed, professional auxiliary in dentistry who is both an oral health educator and a clinician, and who uses preventive, therapeutic, and educational methods for the control of oral diseases.

den·tal iden·ti·fi·ca·tion (den′tăl ī-den′ti-fi-kā′shŭn) Using forensic evidence related to teeth to identify a cadaver.

den·tal im·pac·tion (den′tăl im-pak′shŭn) Confinement of a tooth in the alveolus and prevention of its eruption into normal position. SEE ALSO impacted tooth.

den·tal pa·pil·la, den·ti·nal pa·pil·la (den′tăl pă-pil′ă, den′ti-năl) [TA] Projection of the mesenchymal tissue of the developing jaw into the cup of the enamel organ; its outer layer becomes a layer of specialized columnar cells, the odontoblasts, which form the dentin of the tooth. SYN papilla dentis [TA], dentinal papilla.

den·tal path·ol·o·gy (den′tăl pă-thol′ŏ-jē) SYN oral pathology.

den·tal plaque (den′tăl plak) **1.** The noncalcified accumulation, mainly of oral microorganisms and their products, which adheres tenaciously to the teeth and is not readily dislodged. **2.** SYN bacterial plaque.

den·tal pros·the·sis (DP) (den′tăl prosthē′sis) Artificial replacement of one or more teeth and/or associated structures. SEE ALSO denture.

den·tal pulp, den·ti·nal pulp (den′tăl pŭlp, den′ti-năl) [TA] The soft tissue within the pulp cavity, consisting of connective tissue containing blood vessels, nerves, and lymphatics, and at the periphery a layer of odontoblasts capable of internal repair of the dentin. SYN pulp (2), tooth pulp.

den·tal ridge (den′tăl rij) The prominent border of a cusp or margin of a tooth.

den·tal sac (den′tăl sak) Outer investment of ectomesenchymal tissue surrounding a developing tooth; involved in formation of the periodontal ligament, alveolus, and cementum. SEE ALSO dental follicle.

den·tal seal·ant (den′tăl sēl′ănt) SYN fissure sealant.

den·tal sy·ringe (den′tăl sir-inj′) Breechloading metal cartridge syringe into which fits a hermetically sealed glass cartridge containing the anesthetic solution.

den·tal tu·bules (den′tăl tū′byūlz) SYN canaliculi dentales.

den·tal var·nish (den′tăl vahr′nish) Solutions of natural resins and gums in a suitable solvent; a thin coating is applied over the surfaces of the cavity preparations before placement of restorations; used to protect tooth against the constituents of restorative materials. SYN vernix.

den·tate (den′tāt) Notched; toothed; cogged.

den·tate gyrus (den′tāt jī′rŭs) [TA] One of the two interlocking gyri composing the hippocampus, the other one being the Ammon horn.

den·ti·a (den′shē-ă) The process of tooth development or eruption. Also serves to denote a relationship to the teeth.

den·ti·cle (den′ti-kĕl) **1.** SYN endolith. **2.** A toothlike projection from a hard surface.

den·tic·u·late, den·tic·u·lat·ed (den-tik′yū-lăt, -lāt-ed) **1.** Finely dentated, notched, or serrated. **2.** Having small teeth.

den·ti·frice (den′ti-fris) Any preparation used in the cleansing of the teeth, e.g., a tooth powder, toothpaste, or tooth wash.

den·tig·er·ous (den-tij′ĕr-ŭs) Arising from or associated with teeth.

den·tig·er·ous cyst (den-tij′ĕr-ŭs sist) An odontogenic cyst derived from the reduced enamel epithelium surrounding the crown of an impacted, unerupted, or embedded tooth. SYN follicular cyst (2).

den·ti·la·bi·al (den′ti-lā′bē-ăl) Relating to the teeth and lips.

den·ti·lin·gual (den′ti-ling′gwăl) Relating to the teeth and tongue.

den·tin (den′tin) The ivory forming the mass of the tooth. Calcified tissue that is not as hard as enamel but harder than cementum.

den·ti·nal·gi·a (den′ti-nal′jē-ă) Dentinal sensitivity or pain.

den·ti·nal la·mi·na cyst (den′ti-năl lam′i-nă sist) A small keratin-filled cyst, usually multiple, on the alveolar ridge of newborn infants; it is derived from remnants of the dental lamina.

den·ti·nal tu·bules (den′ti-năl tū′byūlz) SYN canaliculi dentales.

den·tin bridge (den′tin brij) A deposit of reparative dentin or other calcific substances that forms across and reseals exposed tooth pulp tissue.

den·tin dys·pla·si·a (den′tin dis-plā′zē-ă) A hereditary disorder of the teeth, involving both primary and permanent dentition, in which the clinical morphology and color of the teeth are normal, but the teeth radiographically exhibit short roots, obliteration of the pulp chambers and canals, mobility, and premature exfoliation.

den·tin·o·ce·ment·al (den′ti-nō-sĕ-men′tăl) Relating to the dentin and cementum of teeth.

den·tin·o·ce·ment·al junc·tion (den′ti-nō-sĕ-men′tăl jŭngk′shŭn) SYN cementodentinal junction.

den·tin·o·e·nam·el (den′ti-nō-ĕ-nam′ĕl) Relating to the dentin and enamel of teeth. SYN amelodentinal.

den·tin·o·gen·e·sis (den′ti-nō-jen′ĕ-sis) The process of dentin formation in the development of teeth.

den·tin·o·gen·e·sis im·per·fec·ta (den′ti-nō-jen′ĕ-sis im-pĕr-fek′tă) A hereditary disorder of the teeth characterized by translucent gray to yellow-brown teeth involving both primary and permanent dentition.

den·ti·no·ma (den′ti-nō′mă) A benign odontogenic tumor consisting microscopically of dysplastic dentin and strands of epithelium within a fibrous stroma. SYN dentinoid (2).

den·tist (den′tist) A legally qualified practitioner of dentistry.

den·tis·try (den′tis-trē) The healing science and art concerned with the structure and function of the orofacial complex, and with the prevention, diagnosis, and treatment of deformities, pathoses, and traumatic injuries thereof. SYN odontology, odontonosology.

den·ti·tion (den-tish′ŭn) The natural teeth, as considered collectively, in the dental arch; may be deciduous, permanent, or mixed.

den·to·al·ve·o·lar (den′tō-al-vē′ŏ-lăr) Usually, denoting that portion of the alveolar bone immediately about the teeth; used also to denote the functional unity of teeth and alveolar bone.

den·to·fa·cial (den′tō-fā′shăl) Of or relating to the dentition and face.

den·tu·lous (den′tyū-lŭs) Having natural teeth present in the mouth.

den·ture (den′chŭr) 1. An artificial substitute for missing natural teeth and adjacent tissues. SYN artificial dentition. 2. Sometimes used to denote the dentition of animals.

den·ture base (den′chŭr bās) 1. That part of a denture that rests on the oral mucosa and to which teeth are attached. 2. That part of a complete or partial denture that rests on the basal seat and to which teeth are attached.

den·ture bor·der (den′chŭr bōr′dĕr) 1. Limit or boundary or circumferential margin of a denture base. 2. Margin of the denture base at the junction of the polished surface with the impression (tissue) surface. 3. Extreme edges of a denture base at the buccolabial, lingual, and posterior limits. SYN periphery (2).

den·ture flask (den′chŭr flask) Sectional metal boxlike case in which a sectional mold is made of plaster of Paris or artificial stone for the purpose of compressing and curing dentures or other resinous restorations. SYN crown flask.

den·ture foun·da·tion (den′chŭr fowndā′shŭn) That portion of the oral structures that is available to support a denture.

den·ture pack·ing (den′chŭr pak′ing) Filling and compressing a denture base material into a mold in a flask.

den·ture sta·bil·i·ty (den′chŭr stă-bil′i-tē) Quality of a denture to be firm, steady, constant, and resistant to change of position when functional forces are applied.

den·u·da·tion (dē′nū-dā′shŭn) Depriving of a covering or protecting layer; the act of laying bare, as in the removal of the epithelium from an underlying surface.

Den·ver clas·si·fi·ca·tion (den′vĕr klas′i-fi-kā′shŭn) System of nomenclature for human mitotic chromosomes, based on length and position of the centromere.

de·o·dor·ant (dē-ō′dŏr-ănt) **1.** Eliminating or masking a smell, especially an unpleasant one. **2.** An agent having such an action, especially a cosmetic combined with an antiperspirant. SYN deodorizer.

de·or·sum·duc·tion (dē-ōr′sŭm-dŭk′shŭn) *Avoid the misspelling/mispronunciation dorsumduction.* Rotation of one eye downward. SYN infraduction.

de·os·si·fi·ca·tion (dē-os′i-fi-kā′shŭn) Removal of the mineral constituents of bone.

de·ox·i·di·zer (dē-ok′si-dī-zĕr) Any agent or process used to remove oxygen.

deoxy- Prefix to chemical names of substances that indicates replacement of an –OH by an H. The older desoxy- has been retained in some instances.

de·ox·y·cho·lic ac·id (dē-oks′ē-kō′lik as′id) A bile acid and choleretic; used in biochemical preparations as a detergent.

deoxyhaemoglobin [Br.] SYN deoxyhemoglobin.

de·ox·y·he·mo·glob·in (dē-oks′ē-hē′mō-glō-bin) The reduced form of hemoglobin, resulting when oxyhemoglobin loses its oxygen. SYN deoxyhaemoglobin.

de·ox·y·ri·bo·nu·cle·ase (DNase) (dē-oks′ē-rī′bō-nū′klē-ās) Any enzyme (phosphodiesterase) hydrolyzing phosphodiester bonds in DNA. SEE ALSO endonuclease, nuclease.

de·ox·y·ri·bo·nu·cle·ic ac·id (DNA) (dē-oks′ē-rī′bō-nū-klē′ik as′id) The type of nucleic acid containing deoxyribose as the sugar component found principally in the nuclei (chromatin, chromosomes) and mitochondria of animal and plant cells, usually loosely bound to protein (hence the term deoxyribonucleoprotein); considered to be the autoreproducing component of chromosomes and of many viruses, and the repository of hereditary characteristics.

de·ox·y·ri·bo·nu·cle·o·side (dē-oks′ē-rī′bō-nū′klē-ō-sīd) **1.** Nucleoside component of DNA. **2.** Condensation product of deoxy-D-ribose with purines or pyrimidines.

de·ox·y·ri·bo·nu·cle·o·tide (dē-oks′ē-rī′bō-nū′klē-ō-tīd) **1.** Nucleotide component of DNA. **2.** Phosphoric ester of deoxyribonucleoside; formed in nucleotide biosynthesis.

de·ox·y·ri·bose (dē-oks′ē-rī′bōs) A deoxypentose, 2-deoxy-D-ribose being the most common example, occurring in deoxyribonucleic acid and reason for its name.

de·ox·y·ri·bo·vi·rus (dē-ok′sē-rī′bō-vī′rŭs) SYN DNA virus.

de·ox·y·ur·i·dine (dē-oks′ē-yūr′i-dēn) A derivative of uridine in which one or more of the hydroxyl groups on the ribose moiety has been replaced by a hydrogen.

de·pen·dence, de·pen·den·cy (dē-pen′dĕns, -dĕn-sē) **1.** The quality or condition of relying on, being influenced by, or being subservient to a person, object, or substance, thus reflecting a particular need. **2.** In psychiatry, seen as an issue for a patient who has made a decision that others are responsible for that patient's personal well-being. SEE ALSO dependent personality disorder.

de·pen·dent (dē-pen′dĕnt) In health care finance, a patient, other than the insured, who is entitled to coverage under the insured's policy.

de·pen·dent drain·age (dē-pen′dĕnt drān′ăj) Drainage from the lowest part into a receptacle at a level even lower than the structure being drained.

de·pen·dent e·de·ma (dē-pen′dĕnt ĕ-dē′mă) A clinically detectable increase in extracellular fluid volume localized in a dependent area, as of a limb, characterized by swelling or pitting.

de·pen·dent per·son·al·i·ty dis·or·der (dĕ-pen'dĕnt pĕr'sŏn-al'ĭ-tē dis-ōr'dĕr) Enduring and pervasive pattern in adulthood characterized by submissive and clinging behavior and excessive reliance on others to meet one's emotional, social, or economic needs.

de·pen·dent var·i·a·ble (DV) (dĕ-pen'dĕnt var'ē-ă-bĕl) In experiments, a variable influenced by or dependent on changes in the independent variable.

depersonalisation [Br.] SYN depersonalization.

de·per·son·al·i·za·tion (dē-pĕr'sŏn-ăl-ĭ-zā'shŭn) A state in which someone loses the feeling of his own identity in relation to others in his family or peer group, or loses the feeling of his own reality. SYN depersonalisation.

de·per·son·al·i·za·tion dis·or·der (dē-pĕr'sŏn-ăl-ĭ-zā'shŭn dis-ōr'dĕr) Disorder characterized by persistent or recurrent experiences of detachment from one's mental processes or body, as if one is an automaton, an outside observer, or in a dream.

de Pez·zer cath·e·ter (dĕ-pĕ-zā' kath'ĕ-tĕr) A self-retaining catheter with a bulbous extremity.

de·phas·ing (dē-fāz'ing) MAGNETIC RESONANCE gradual loss of orientation of the magnetic atomic nuclei due to random molecular energy transfer or relaxation due to alignment by a radiofrequency pulse.

dep·i·late (dep'i-lāt) To remove hair by any means. Cf. epilate.

dep·i·la·tion (dep'i-lā'shŭn) SYN epilation.

de·ple·tion (dē-plē'shŭn) 1. The removal of accumulated fluids or solids. 2. A reduced state of strength from too many free discharges. 3. Excessive loss of a constituent, usually essential, of the body, e.g., salt, water.

de·ple·tion·al hy·po·na·tre·mi·a (dĕ-plē'shŭn-ăl hī'pō-nă-trē'mē-ă) Decreased serum sodium concentration associated with loss of sodium from the circulating blood through the gastrointestinal tract, kidney, skin, or into the "third space." Accompanied by hypovolemic and hypotonic state. SYN dilutional hyponatremia.

de·po·lar·i·za·tion (dē-pō'lăr-ĭ-zā'shŭn) The destruction, neutralization, or change in direction of polarity.

depolymerisation [Br.] SYN depolymerization.

de·po·lym·er·i·za·tion (dē-pol'i-mĕr-ĭ-zā'shŭn) The dismantling of a polymer into individual monomers. SYN depolymerisation.

de·pos·it (dep) (dĕ-poz'it) 1. A sediment or precipitate. 2. A pathologic accumulation of inorganic material in a tissue.

de·pres·sant (dĕ-pres'ănt) 1. Diminishing functional tone or activity. 2. An agent that reduces nervous or functional activity, such as a sedative or anesthetic.

de·pressed (depr) (dĕ-prest') 1. Flattened from above downward. 2. Below the normal level or the level of the surrounding parts. 3. Below the normal functional level. 4. Dejected; lowered in spirits. Cf. depression.

de·pressed frac·ture (dĕ-prest' frak'shŭr) SYN depressed skull fracture.

de·pressed skull frac·ture (dĕ-prest' skŭl frak'shŭr) Breakage with inward displacement of a part of the calvarium; may be associated with disruption of the underlying dura or cerebral cortex.

de·pres·sion (dĕ-presh'ŭn) [TA] 1. Reduction of the level of functioning. 2. A hollow or sunken area. 3. Displacement of a part downward or inward. 4. A mental state or chronic mental disorder characterized by feelings of sadness, loneliness, despair, low self-esteem, and self-reproach; accompanying signs include psychomotor retardation or less frequently agitation, withdrawal from social contact, and vegetative states such as loss of appetite and insomnia. SYN dejection.

de·pres·sion of op·tic disc (dĕ-presh'ŭn op'tik disk) The normal pit found in the center of the optic disc.

de·pres·sive re·ac·tion (dĕ-pres´iv rē-ak´shŭn) SYN depression (4).

de·pres·sor (dĕ-pres´ŏr) **1.** A muscle that flattens or lowers a part. **2.** Anything that depresses or retards functional activity. **3.** An instrument or device used to push bodily structures out of the way during an operation or examination. **4.** An agent that decreases blood pressure.

de·pres·sor fibers (dĕ-pres´ŏr fī´bĕrz) Sensory nerve fibers with pressure-sensitive nerve endings in arterial walls capable of activating blood-pressure-lowering brainstem mechanisms when stimulated by increased intraarterial pressure.

dep·ri·va·tion (dep´ri-vā´shŭn) Absence, loss, or withholding of something needed.

depth (depth) Distance from the surface downward.

depth dose (Ed) (depth dōs) Radiation dose at a distance beneath the surface, including secondary radiation or scatter, in proportion to the dose at the surface.

depth psy·chol·o·gy (depth sī-kol´ŏ-jē) Study of the unconscious, especially in contrast with older (19th-century) academic psychology dealing only with conscious mentation.

de Quer·vain dis·ease (dĕ kār´vahn[h]´ di-zēz´) Fibrosis of the sheath of a tendon of the thumb.

de Quervain frac·ture (dĕ kār´vahn[h]´ frak´shŭr) Break of the scaphoid bone of the wrist with volar subluxation of fragments and lunate.

de Quer·vain ten·o·syn·o·vi·tis (dĕ kār´vahn[h]´ ten´ō-sin-ō-vī´tis) Inflammation of the tendons of the first dorsal compartment of the wrist, which includes the abductor pollicis longus and extensor pollicis brevis; diagnosed by a specific provocative test (Finkelstein test).

de·rail·ment (dē-rāl´mĕnt) A symptom of a thought disorder in which one constantly gets "off the track" in one's thoughts and speech; similar to loosening of association.

der·by hat frac·ture (dĕr´bē hat frak´shŭr) Regular cranial concavity in infants; may or may not be associated with fracture.

Der·cum dis·ease (der´kŭm di-zēz´) SYN adiposis dolorosa.

de·re·al·i·za·tion (dē-rē´ă-lī-zā´shŭn) An alteration in one's perception of the environment such that things that are ordinarily familiar seem strange, unreal, or two-dimensional.

de·re·ism (dē-rē´izm) Mental activity in fantasy in contrast to reality.

de·re·is·tic (dē´rē-is´tik) Living in imagination or fantasy with thoughts that are incongruent with logic or experience.

der·en·ceph·a·ly (der´en-sef´ă-lē) Cervical rachischisis and meroanencephaly; a malformation involving an open cranial vault with a rudimentary brain usually crowded back toward bifid cervical vertebrae.

de·riv·a·tive (dē-riv´ă-tiv) **1.** Relating to or producing derivation. **2.** Something produced by modification of something preexisting. **3.** Specifically, a chemical compound produced from another compound in one or more steps.

de·rived protein (dĕ-rivd´ prō´tēn) A derivative of protein effected by chemical change, e.g., hydrolysis.

derm-, derma-, dermat-, dermato- Combining forms meaning the skin; corresponds to the L. *cut-*.

der·ma·bra·sion (dĕrm´ă-brā´zhŭn) Operative procedure used to remove acne scars or pits performed with sandpaper, rotating wire brushes, or other abrasive materials.

Der·ma·cen·tor (dĕr-mă-sen´tŏr) An ornate, characteristically marked genus of hard ticks with 11 festoons; consists of some 20 species with members that commonly attack dogs, humans, and other mammals.

Der·ma·cen·tor va·ri·a·bi·lis (dĕr-mă-sen´tŏr vā-rē-ă-bil´is) American dog tick; a vector of tularemia; principal vector of *Rickettsia rickettsii* that causes Rocky Mountain spotted fever in the central and eastern U.S.; may also cause tick paralysis.

der·mal (dĕr′măl) Relating to the skin. SYN dermatic, dermatoid (2), dermic.

der·mal duct tu·mor (dĕr′măl dŭkt tū′mŏr) Benign small lesion derived from the intradermal part of eccrine sweat gland ducts.

der·mal graft (dĕr′măl graft) A graft of dermis, made from skin by cutting away a thin split-thickness graft.

der·mal ridg·es (dĕr′măl rij′ĕz) [TA] Surface ridges of the epidermis of the palms and soles, where the sweat pores open. SYN cristae cutis [TA], papillary ridges, epidermal ridges, skin ridges.

der·mal si·nus (dĕr′măl sī′nŭs) Sinus lined with epidermis and skin appendages extending from the skin to some deeper-lying structure, most frequently the spinal cord.

der·ma·ti·tis, pl. **der·ma·tit·i·des** (dĕr′mă-tī′tis) Inflammation of the skin.

der·ma·ti·tis ar·te·fac·ta (dĕr′mă-tī′tis ahr-tĕ-fak′tă) Self-induced skin lesions resulting from habitual rubbing, scratching or hair-pulling, malingering, or mental disturbance.

der·ma·ti·tis ex·fo·li·a·ti·va in·fan·tum, der·ma·ti·tis ex·fo·li·a·ti·va ne·o·na·to·rum (dĕr′mă-tī′tis eks-fō-lē-a-tī′vă in-fan′tŭm, nē-ō-nā-tō′rŭm) Generalized pyoderma accompanied by exfoliative dermatitis, with constitutional symptoms, affecting young infants, which may due to Leiner disease, or staphylococcal scalded skin syndrome. SYN impetigo neonatorum (1).

der·ma·ti·tis gan·gre·no·sa in·fan·tum (dĕr′mă-tī′tis gang-grē-nō′să in-fan′tŭm) Bullous or pustular eruption, leading to necrotic ulcers or extensive gangrene in children younger than 2 years of age; untreated, death may result from hematogenous infection. SYN pemphigus gangrenosus (1).

der·ma·ti·tis her·pet·i·for·mis (DH) (dĕr′mă-tī′tis hĕr-pet-i-fŏr′mis) Chronic skin disease marked by a symmetric itching eruption of vesicles and papules that occur in groups; relapses common; associated with gluten-sensitive enteropathy and IgA together with neutrophils be-

neath the epidermis of lesional and perilesional skin. SYN Duhring disease.

der·ma·ti·tis re·pens (dĕr′mă-tī′tis rē′penz) SYN pustulosis palmaris et plantaris.

Der·ma·to·bi·a (dĕr′mă-tō′bē-ă) A genus of flies (family Oestridae) found in tropical areas of the Americas.

der·ma·to·cel·lu·li·tis (dĕr′mă-tō-sel′yū-lī′tis) Inflammation of the skin and subcutaneous connective tissue.

der·ma·to·cha·la·sis (dĕr′mă-tō-kal′ă-sis) An acquired condition characterized by undue looseness or pendulousness of the eyelid skin due to degeneration of elastic fibers. SYN cutis laxa [TA], pachydermatocele, blepharochalasis.

der·ma·to·cyst (dĕr′mă-tō-sist) A cyst of the skin.

der·mat·o·fi·bro·sar·co·ma pro·tu·ber·ans (DFSP) (dĕr′mă-tō-fī′brō-sahr-kō′mă prō-tū′bĕr-anz) Dermal neoplasm consisting of one or several firm nodules covered by dark red-blue skin, which tends to be fixed to the palpable masses; histologically, resembles a cellular dermatofibroma with a pronounced storiform pattern; metastases are unusual, but the incidence of recurrence is fairly high.

der·ma·to·glyph·ics (dĕr′mă-tō-glif′iks) **1.** The configurations of the characteristic ridge patterns of the volar surfaces of the skin; in the human hand, the distal segment of each digit has three types of configurations: whorl, loop, and arch. SEE ALSO fingerprint. **2.** The science or study of these configurations or patterns.

der·ma·tog·ra·phism (dĕr′mă-tog′ră-fizm) Urticaria in which wheals occur in the site and configuration of application of stroking (pressure, friction) of skin. SYN dermographia, dermographism.

der·ma·toid (dĕr′mă-toyd) **1.** Resembling skin. SYN dermoid (1). **2.** SYN dermal.

der·ma·tol·o·gy (dĕr′mă-tol′ŏ-jē) The branch of medicine concerned with the study of the skin, diseases of the skin, and the relationship of cutaneous lesions to systemic disease.

der·ma·tol·y·sis (dĕr′mă-tol′i-sis) Loosening or atrophy of the skin by disease; erroneously used as a synonym for cutis laxa.

der·ma·to·ma (dĕr′mă-tō′mă) A circumscribed thickening or hypertrophy of the skin.

der·ma·to·mere (dĕr′mă-tō-mēr) A metameric area of the embryonic integument.

der·ma·to·my·co·sis (dĕr′mă-tō-mī-kō′sis) Fungal skin infection caused by dermatophytes and yeasts. Cf. dermatophytosis.

der·ma·to·my·o·ma (dĕr′mă-tō-mī-ō′mă) SYN leiomyoma cutis.

der·ma·to·my·o·si·tis (dĕr′mă-tō-mī′ō-sī′tis) Progressive condition characterized by symmetric proximal muscular weakness with elevated muscle enzyme levels and a rash, typically a purplish-red or heliotrope erythema on the face, and edema of the eyelids and periorbital tissue.

der·ma·to·neu·ro·sis (dĕr′mă-tō-nūr-ō′sis) Any cutaneous eruption due to emotional stimuli.

der·ma·to·pa·thol·o·gy (dĕr′mă-tō-pă-thol′ŏ-jē) Histopathology of the skin and subcutis; study of the causes of skin disease.

der·ma·top·a·thy, der·ma·to·sis (dĕr′mă-top′ă-thē, -tō′sis) Any disease of the skin. SYN dermopathy.

der·ma·to·phy·lax·is (dĕr′mă-tō-fi-lak′sis) Protection of the skin against potentially harmful agents; e.g., infection, excessive sunlight, noxious agents.

der·ma·to·phyte (dĕr′mă-tō-fīt) A fungus that causes superficial infections of the skin, hair, and nails, i.e., keratinized tissues.

der·ma·to·phy·tid (dĕr′mă-tō-tof′i-tid) An allergic manifestation of dermatophytosis at a site distant from that of the primary fungal infection.

der·ma·to·phy·to·sis (dĕr′mă-tō-fī-tō′sis) Infection of the hair, skin, or nails caused by dermatophytes; lesions characterized by erythema, small papular vesicles, fissures, and scaling. Common sites of infection are the feet (tinea pedis), nails (onychomycosis), and scalp (tinea capitis). Cf. dermatomycosis.

der·mat·o·plas·ty (dĕr′mă-tō-plas-tē) Surgical repair of the skin, as by skin grafting. SYN dermoplasty.

der·ma·to·sis, gen. and pl. **der·ma·to·ses** (dĕr′mă-tō′sis, -sēz) Nonspecific term used to denote any cutaneous abnormality or eruption.

der·ma·to·sis pa·pu·lo·sa nig·ra (DPN) (dĕr′mă-tō′sis pap-yū-lō′să nī′gră) Dark brown papular lesions, observed in black people, on the face and upper trunk; histologically and clinically, they resemble seborrheic keratoses.

der·ma·to·tro·pic (dĕr′mă-tō-trō′pik) Having an affinity for the skin. SYN dermotropic.

der·ma·to·zo·on (dĕr′mă-tō-zō′on) An animal parasite of the skin.

der·mis, der·ma (dĕr′mis, -mă) [TA] Skin layer composed of a superficial thin layer that interdigitates with the epidermis, stratum papillare, and stratum reticulare; contains blood and lymphatic vessels, nerves and nerve endings, glands, and, except for glabrous skin, hair follicles. SYN corium, cutis vera.

Der·mo·bac·ter (dĕr′mō-bak′tĕr) A bacterial genus of nonmotile, non-spore-bearing gram-positive rods, recovered on human skin. *D. hominis* associated with positive blood cultures.

der·mo·blast (dĕr′mō-blast) One of the mesodermal cells from which the corium is developed.

der·moid (dĕr′moyd) 1. SYN dermatoid (1). 2. SYN dermoid cyst.

der·moid cyst (dĕr′moyd sist) A tumor consisting of displaced ectodermal structures along lines of embryonic fusion, the wall being formed of epithelium-lined connective tissue, including skin appendages and containing keratin, sebum, teeth, and hair. SYN dermoid tumor, dermoid (2).

der·mop·a·thy (dĕr-mop′ă-thē) SYN dermatopathy.

der·mo·vas·cu·lar (dĕr'mō-vas'kyū-lăr) Pertaining to the blood vessels of the skin.

des- CHEMISTRY a prefix indicating absence of some component of the principal part of the name; largely replaced by de- (e.g., deoxyribonucleic acid, dehydro-).

de·sat·u·ra·tion (dē-sach'ŭr-ā'shŭn) The act, or the result of the act, of making something less completely saturated; more specifically, the percentage of total binding sites remaining unfilled; e.g., when hemoglobin is 70% saturated with oxygen and nothing else, its desaturation is 30%. Cf. saturation (5).

De·sault ban·dage (dĕ-sō' ban'dăj) Dressing for fracture of the clavicle; elbow is bound to the side, with a pad placed under the arm.

des·ce·me·ti·tis (des'ĕ-mĕ-tī'tis) Inflammation of Descemet membrane.

des·ce·met·o·cele (des'ĕ-met'ō-sēl) Bulging forward of the Descemet membrane due to destruction of cornea substance.

de·scend·ing (desc) (dē-send'ing) Running downward or toward the periphery.

de·scend·ing a·or·ta (dē-send'ing ā-ōr'tă) [TA] Part of the aorta continuing distal (inferior) to the aortic arch, further divided into the thoracic aorta and the abdominal aorta. SYN pars descendens aortae [TA], aorta descendens, descending part of aorta.

de·scend·ing co·lon (dē-send'ing kō'lŏn) [TA] The part of the colon extending from the left colic flexure to the pelvic brim.

de·scend·ing de·gen·er·a·tion (dē-send'ing dē-jen'ĕr-ā'shŭn) **1.** Orthograde degeneration of an injured nerve fiber. **2.** Degeneration caudal to level of a spinal cord lesion.

de·scend·ing neu·ri·tis (dē-send'ing nūr-ī'tis) Inflammation progressing along a nerve trunk toward the periphery.

de·scen·sus (dē-sen'sŭs) *The plural of this word is descensus, not descensi.* A falling away from a higher position. SYN descent (1).

de·scen·sus tes·tis (dē-sen'sŭs tes'tis) [TA] Descent of the testis from the abdomen into the scrotum during the seventh and eighth months of intrauterine life. SEE ALSO ptosis, procidentia. SYN descensus, descent (1).

de·scrip·tive a·na·t·o·my (dē-skrip'tiv ă-nat'ŏ-mē) Description of, especially a treatise describing, physical structure (vs. merely identifying it), more particularly that of humans. SYN systematic anatomy.

desensitisation [Br.] SYN desensitization.

de·sen·si·tiz·a·tion (dē-sen'si-tī-zā'shŭn) **1.** The reduction or abolition of allergic sensitivity or reactions to the specific antigen (allergen). SYN antianaphylaxis. **2.** The act of removing an emotional complex. SYN desensitisation.

de·sert sore (dez'ĕrt sōr) Chronic nonspecific cutaneous ulcers, most commonly on the shins, knees, hands, and forearms, and probably a variant of ecthyma; seen in tropical and desert areas. SYN veldt sore.

des·flu·rane (des-flūr'ān) An inhalation anesthetic with physical characteristics that provide rapid induction of and recovery from anesthesia.

des·ic·cant (des'i-kănt) **1.** Drying; causing or promoting dryness. SYN desiccative. **2.** An agent that absorbs moisture; a drying agent. SYN exsiccant.

des·ig·na·ted do·nor (dez'ig-nāt-ĕd dō'nŏr) In health care, someone who has agreed to donate bone marrow, blood, or tissue to someone else who requires such therapy or has ordered donation of her organs at death.

des·lan·o·side (des-lan'ō-sīd) A rapidly acting steroid glycoside obtained from lanatoside C (*Digitalis lanata*) by alkaline hydrolysis; a cardiotonic.

Des·mar·res re·trac·tor (dā-mahr' rĕ-trak'tŏr) Instrument used to withdraw an eyelid.

des·mi·tis (des-mī'tis) Inflammation of a ligament.

desmo-, desm- Combining forms meaning fibrous connection; ligament.

des·mo·cra·ni·um (des′mō-krā′nē-ŭm) [TA] The mesenchymal primordium of the cranium.

des·mo·den·ti·um, des·mo·don·ti·um (des′mō-den′tē-ŭm, -don′tē-ŭm) [TA] The collagen fibers, running from the cementum to the alveolar bone, which suspend a tooth in its socket; include apical, oblique, horizontal, and alveolar crest fibers.

des·mog·e·nous (des-moj′ĕ-nŭs) Of connective tissue or ligamentous origin or causation; e.g., denoting a deformity due to contraction of ligaments, fascia, or a scar.

des·mog·ra·phy (des-mog′ră-fē) A description of, or treatise on, the ligaments.

des·moid (des′moyd) 1. Fibrous or ligamentous. 2. A nodule or mass of firm scarlike connective tissue resulting from active proliferation of fibroblasts, occurring most frequently in the abdominal muscles of women who have borne children. SYN desmoid tumor.

des·moid tu·mor (des′moyd tū′mŏr) SYN desmoid (2).

des·mop·a·thy (des-mop′ă-thē) Any disease of the ligaments.

des·mo·pla·si·a (des′mō-plā′zē-ă) Hyperplasia of fibroblasts and disproportionate formation of fibrous connective tissue, especially in the stroma of a carcinoma.

des·mo·plas·tic (des′mō-plas′tik) 1. Causing or forming adhesions. 2. Causing fibrosis in the vascular stroma of a neoplasm.

des·mo·plas·tic fi·bro·ma (des′mō-plas′tik fī-brō′mă) A benign fibrous tumor of bone affecting children and young adults; cortical destruction may result.

des·mo·plas·tic small cell tu·mor (des′mō-plas′tik smawl sel tū′mŏr) High-grade malignant lesion found most often in the abdomen of male adolescents; typically contain both desmin and keratin, i.e., show hybrid features like fetal mesothelial cells.

des·mo·pres·sin (DDAVP) (des′mō-pres′in) An analogue of vasopressin (antidiuretic hormone, ADH) with powerful antidiuretic activity.

des·mo·pres·sin ac·e·tate (DDAVP, dDAVP) (des′mō-pres′in as′ĕ-tāt) Synthetic analogue of vasopressin and an antidiuretic hormone.

des·mo·some (des′mō-sōm) A site of adhesion between two epithelial cells, consisting of a dense attachment plaque separated from a similar structure in the other cell by a thin layer of extracellular material. SYN macula adherens.

desoxy- SEE deoxy-.

des·qua·ma·tion (des′kwă-mā′shŭn) The shedding of the cuticle in scales or of the outer layer of any surface.

des·qua·ma·tive in·flam·ma·to·ry va·gi·ni·tis (des-kwah′mă-tiv in-flam′ă-tōr-ē vaj′i-nī′tis) Acute inflammation of the vagina of unknown cause, characterized by grayish pseudomembrane, pus discharge, and easy bleeding on trauma.

des·qua·ma·tive in·ter·sti·tial pneu·mo·ni·a (DIP) (des-kwah′mă-tiv in′tĕr-stish′ăl nū-mō′nē-ă) Diffuse proliferation of alveolar epithelial cells, which desquamate into the air sacs and become filled with macrophages, accompanied by interstitial cellular infiltration and fibrosis.

de·struc·tive dis·till·a·tion (dĕ-strŭk′tiv dis′ti-lā′shŭn) SYN dry distillation.

de·tach·ment (dĕ-tach′mĕnt) 1. A voluntary or involuntary feeling or emotion that accompanies a sense of separation from normal associations or environment. 2. Separation of a structure from its support.

de·tec·tor (dĕ-tek′tŏr) The component of a laboratory instrument that detects the chemical or physical signal indicating the presence or quantity of the substance of interest.

de·ter·gent (dĕ-tĕr′jĕnt) 1. Cleansing. 2. A cleansing or purging agent, usually salts of long-chain aliphatic bases or acids. SYN detersive.

de·ter·mi·nant (dĕ-tĕr′mi-nănt) The factor that contributes to the generation of a trait.

de·ter·mi·nate clea·vage (dĕ-tĕr′mi-n* klē′văj) That resulting in blastomeres each capable of developing only into a particular embryonic structure.

de·ter·mi·na·tion (dĕ-tĕr′mi-nā′shŭn) **1.** A change, which could be for the better or for the worse, in the course of a disease. **2.** A general move toward a given point. **3.** The measurement or estimation of any quantity or quality in any type of scientific or laboratory investigation. **4.** Discernment of a state or category (e.g., in diagnosis). **5.** A process, both necessary and sufficient, whereby an effect or result is caused. **6.** Judicial decision resolving controversy.

de·ter·mi·nism (dĕ-tĕr′mi-nizm) The proposition that all behavior is caused exclusively by genetic and environmental influences with no random component, and independent of free will.

de·tox·i·fi·ca·tion (dĕ-tok′si-fi-kā′shŭn) **1.** Recovery from drug effects. **2.** Removal of toxins from a poison. **3.** Metabolic conversion of pharmacologically active to pharmacologically less active principles. SYN detoxication.

de·tox·i·fi·ca·tion ther·a·py (dĕ-tok′si-fi-kā′shŭn thār′ă-pē) Helping patients get over substance dependency and likely adverse effects of withdrawal from such agents.

de·tri·tion (dĕ-trish′ŭn) A wearing away by use or friction.

de·tri·tus (dĕ-trī′tŭs) *Avoid the mispronunciation det′ritus.* Any broken-down material, carious or gangrenous matter, and gravel.

de·tru·sor (dĕ-trū′sŏr) A muscle that has the action of expelling a substance.

de·tru·sor a·re·flex·i·a (dĕ-trū′sŏr ā-rē-flek′sē-ă) Failure of the detrusor muscle to contract even though the bladder has reached or exceeded its capacity.

de·tru·sor hy·per·re·flex·i·a (dĕ-trū′sŏr hī′pĕr-rē-flek′sē-ă) SYN hyperreflexic bladder.

de·tru·sor in·sta·bili·ty (DI) (dĕ-trū′sŏr in′stă-bil′ĭ-tē) Uninhibitable bladder contractions that typically occur at bladder volumes below capacity.

de·tru·sor pres·sure (dĕ-trū′sŏr presh′ŭr) Component of intravesical pressure created by the tension (active and passive) exerted by the bladder wall.

de·tru·sor·rha·phy (dĕ-trū-sŏr′ă-fē) Surgery in which bladder muscle is reconstructed around ureterovesical junction to form a competent one-way valve. SYN extravesical reimplantation.

de·tu·mes·cence (dĕ′tū-mes′ĕns) Subsidence of a swelling.

deu·ter·a·nom·a·ly (dū′tĕr-ă-nom′ă-lē) Anomalous trichromatism due to a defect of the green-sensitive retinal cones.

deu·ter·an·o·pi·a, deu·ter·an·op·si·a (dū′tĕr-ă-nō′pē-ă, -op′sē-ă) Congenital retinal abnormality with two rather than three retinal cone pigments (dichromatism) and complete insensitivity to middle wavelengths (green).

deu·te·ri·um (dū-tēr′ē-ŭm) SYN hydrogen (2).

♻ **deutero-, deut-** Combining forms meaning second, secondary.

deu·ter·op·a·thy (dū′tĕr-op′ă-thē) A secondary disease or symptom.

de·vas·cu·lar·i·za·tion (dē-vas′kyū-lăr-ī-zā′shŭn) Occlusion of all or most of the blood vessels to any part or organ.

de·vel·op·ment (dē-vel′ŏp-mĕnt) **1.** The act or process of natural progression in physical and psychological maturation from a previous, lower, or embryonic stage to a later, more complex, or adult stage. **2.** The process of chromatography.

de·vel·op·men·tal a·nat·o·my (dĕ-vel′ŏp-men′tăl ă-nat′ŏ-mē) Anatomy of structural changes of a person from fertilization to adulthood.

de·vel·op·men·tal a·nom·a·ly (dĕ-vel′ŏp-men′tăl ă-nom′ă-lē) Defect established during intrauterine life.

de·vel·op·men·tal aprax·ia of speech (DAS) (dĕ-vel′ŏp-men′tăl ă-prak′sē-ă spēch) Severe articulatory disturbance in childhood characterized by inconsistent errors in production of voluntary sequences of phonemes, not due to weakness or spasticity of speech musculature. SYN childhood apraxia.

de·vel·op·men·tal dis·a·bil·i·ty (DD) (dĕ-vel′ŏp-men′tăl dis′ă-bil′i-tē) Loss of function brought on by prenatal and postnatal events in which the predominant disturbance is in the acquisition of cognitive, language, motor, or social skills.

de·vel·op·men·tal mile·stones (dĕ-vel′ŏp-men′tăl mīl′stōnz) The stages in the neuromuscular, mental, or social maturation of an infant or young child, generally marked by the attainment of a capacity or skill, such as rolling over, sitting with good head control, smiling spontaneously, laughing, and following moving objects with the eyes.

de·vel·op·men·tal psy·chol·o·gy (dĕ-vel′ŏp-men′tăl sī-kol′ŏ-jē) The study of the life-long psychological, physiologic, and behavioral changes in an organism.

de·vi·ant (dē′vē-ănt) **1.** Denoting or indicative of deviation. SYN aberrant (3), abnormal (2). **2.** A person exhibiting deviation, especially sexual.

de·vi·a·tion (dē′vē-ā′shŭn) **1.** A turning away or aside from the normal point or course. **2.** An abnormality. **3.** PSYCHIATRY, BEHAVIORAL SCIENCES a departure from an accepted norm, role, or rule. **4.** STATISTICS a measurement representing the difference between an individual value in a set of values and the mean value in that set.

de·vice (dĕ-vīs′) An appliance, usually mechanical, designed to perform a specific function (e.g., prosthesis or orthosis).

de·vi·om·e·ter (dē′vē-om′ĕ-tĕr) A form of strabismometer.

de·vi·tal·ize (dē-vī′tăl-īz) To deprive of vitality or of vital properties.

dex·a·meth·a·sone (dek′să-meth′ă-sōn)

A potent synthetic analogue of cortisol; used as an antiinflammatory agent.

dex·pan·the·nol (deks-pan′thĕ-nol) Pantothenic acid with –CH2OH replacing the terminal –COOH; a cholinergic agent and a dietary source of pantothenic acid. SYN pantothenyl alcohol.

dex·ter (deks′tĕr) Located on or relating to the right side.

dextro-, dextr- Combining forms meaning to the right, the right side.

dex·trad (deks′trad) Toward the right side.

dex·tral (deks′trăl) SYN right-handed.

dex·tral·i·ty (deks-tral′i-tē) Right-handedness; preference for the right hand in performing manual tasks.

dex·tran (DX) (deks′tran) Any of several water-soluble high molecular weight glucose polymers; used in isotonic sodium chloride solution for the treatment of shock, and in distilled water for the relief of the edema of nephrosis; lower molecular weight dextran.

dex·trin (deks′trin) A mixture of oligo (α-1,4-D-glucose) molecules formed during the enzymic or acid hydrolysis of starch, amylopectin, or glycogen.

dex·tri·no·sis (deks′trin-ō′sis) SYN glycogenosis.

dex·tri·nu·ri·a (deks′tri-nyūr′ē-ă) The passage of dextrin in the urine.

dex·tro·car·di·a, dex·i·o·car·di·a (deks′trō-kahr′dē-ă, deks′ē-ō-) Displacement of the heart to the right.

dex·tro·car·di·a with si·tus in·ver·sus (deks′trō-kahr′dē-ă sī′tis in-vĕr′sŭs) Displacement of the heart to the right side of the thorax with mirror transposition of the cardiac chambers together with transposition of the abdominal viscera.

dex·tro·car·di·o·gram (deks′trō-kahr′dē-ō-gram) That part of the electrocardiogram that is derived from the right ventricle.

dex·tro·gas·tri·a (deks′trō-gas′trē-ă)

Condition in which the stomach is displaced to the right; may represent either simple displacement or situs inversus.

dex·tro·gy·ra·tion (deks'trō-jī-rā'shŭn) A twisting to the right.

dex·tro·man·u·al (deks'trō-man'yū-ăl) SYN right-handed.

dex·tro·meth·or·phan hy·dro·bro·mide (deks'trō-mĕ-thōr'fan hī'drō-brō'mīd) A synthetic morphine derivative used as an antitussive agent.

dex·trop·e·dal (deks-trop'ĕ-dăl) Denoting one who uses the right leg in preference to the left. SYN right-footed.

dex·tro·po·si·tion (deks'trō-pŏ-zish'ŭn) Abnormal right-sided location or origin of a normally left-sided structure, e.g., origin of the aorta from the right ventricle.

dex·tro·ro·ta·to·ry (deks'trō-rō'tă-tōr-ē) Denoting dextrorotation, or certain crystals or solutions capable of such action; as a chemical prefix, usually abbreviated *d*- or D. Cf. levorotatory.

dex·trose (deks'trōs) SEE glucose.

dex·tro·si·nis·tral (deks'trō-sin'is-trăl) In a direction from right to left.

dex·tro·tor·sion (deks'trō-tōr'shŭn) A twisting to the right.

dex·tro·ver·sion (deks'trō-vĕr-zhŭn) **1.** Version toward the right. **2.** In ophthalmology, a conjugate rotation of both eyes to the right.

DHT Abbreviation for dihydrotestosterone.

♻ **di- 1.** Prefix meaning two, twice. **2.** CHEMISTRY often used in place of bis- when not likely to be confusing; e.g., dichloro compounds.

♻ **dia-** Prefix meaning through, throughout, completely.

di·a·be·tes (dī-ă-bē'tēz) Either diabetes insipidus or diabetes mellitus; a condition in which the pituitary gland increases urinary output (diabetes insipidus) or a disorder in which the pancreas produces defects in insulin production or

action, thus inducing hyperglycemia (diabetes mellitus). Both diseases have in common the symptom polyuria; when used without qualification, refers to diabetes mellitus.

di·a·be·tes in·sip·i·dus (DI) (dī-ă-bē' tēz in-sip'i-dŭs) Chronic excretion of very large amounts of pale urine of low specific gravity, causing dehydration and extreme thirst; ordinarily results from inadequate output of pituitary antidiuretic hormone. SEE ALSO nephrogenic diabetes insipidus.

di·a·be·tes in·ter·mit·tens (dī-ă-bē'tēz in-tĕr-mit'enz) Diabetes mellitus with periods of relatively normal carbohydrate metabolism followed by relapses to the previous diabetic state.

di·a·be·tes mel·li·tus (DM) (dī-ă-bē'tēz mel'i-tŭs) A metabolic disease in which carbohydrate use is reduced and that of lipid and protein enhanced; caused by an absolute or relative deficiency of insulin and is characterized, in more severe cases, by chronic hyperglycemia, glycosuria, water and electrolyte loss, ketoacidosis, and coma; long-term complications include neuropathy, retinopathy, nephropathy, generalized degenerative changes in large and small blood vessels, and increased susceptibility to infection. SEE ALSO Type 1 diabetes, Type 2 diabetes.

di·a·bet·ic (dī-ă-bet'ik) Relating to or having diabetes.

di·a·bet·ic a·ci·do·sis (dī-ă-bet'ik as-i-dō'sis) Decreased pH and bicarbonate concentration in the body fluids caused by accumulation of ketone bodies in diabetes mellitus. SEE ALSO diabetic ketoacidosis.

di·a·bet·ic am·y·o·tro·phy (dī-ă-bet'ik ă'mī-ot'rŏ-fē) Diabetic neuropathy that primarily affects elderly patients with diabetes mellitus; clinically characterized by unilateral or bilateral anterior thigh pain, weakness, and atrophy.

di·a·bet·ic co·ma (dī-ă-bet'ik kō'mă) State that develops in severe and inadequately treated diabetes mellitus and is commonly fatal, unless appropriate therapy is instituted promptly.

di·a·bet·ic di·et (dī-ă-bet'ik dī'ĕt) A dietary adjustment for patients with diabetes mellitus intended to decrease the need for insulin or oral diabetic agents and control weight by adjusting caloric and carbohydrate intake.

di·a·bet·ic gan·grene (dī′ă-bet′ik gang-grēn′) Necrosis due to arteriosclerosis associated with diabetes.

di·a·bet·ic glo·mer·u·lo·scler·o·sis (dī-ă-bet′ik glŏ-mer′yū-lō-skler-ō′sis) Rounded hyaline or laminated nodules in the periphery of the glomeruli with capillary basement membrane thickening and increased mesangial matrix occurring in long-standing diabetes, proteinuria, and ultimately renal failure. SYN intercapillary glomerulosclerosis.

di·a·bet·ic ke·to·a·ci·do·sis (DKA) (dī-ă-bet′ik kē′tō-as′i-dō′sis) Buildup of ketones in blood due to breakdown of stored fats for energy; a complication of diabetes mellitus. Untreated, can lead to coma and death.

di·a·bet·ic ne·phrop·a·thy (dī-ă-bet′ik nĕ-frop′ă-thē) A syndrome occurring in people with diabetes mellitus; associated with damage to blood vessels that supply the glomerula at the kidney; characterized by albuminuria, hypertension, and progressive renal insufficiency.

di·a·bet·ic neu·rop·a·thy (dī-ă-bet′ik nūr-op′ă-thē) A generic term for any diabetes mellitus–related disorder of the peripheral nervous system, autonomic nervous system, and some cranial nerves. This most commonly occurring of the chronic complications of diabetes takes two forms, peripheral (with dulling of the sensations of pain, temperature, and pressure, especially in the lower legs and feet), and autonomic (with alternating bouts of diarrhea and constipation, impotence, and reduced cardiac function).

di·a·bet·ic ret·i·nop·a·thy (dī-ă-bet′ik ret′i-nop′ă-thē) Optic changes occurring in chronic diabetes, marked by hemorrhages, microaneurysms, and waxy deposits.

di·a·be·to·gen·ic (dī-ă-bet′ō-jen′ik) Causing diabetes.

di·a·be·tog·en·ous (dī′ă-bē-toj′ĕn-ŭs) Caused by diabetes.

di·ac·e·tyl·mor·phine (DAM) (dī-as′ĕ-til-mōr′fēn) SYN heroin.

di·a·chron·ic study (dī-ă-kron′ik stŭd′ē) SYN longitudinal study.

di·ac·la·sis, di·a·cla·si·a (dī-ak′lă-sis, dī-ă-klă′zē-ă) SYN osteoclasis.

di·a·crit·ic, di·a·crit·i·cal (dī-ă-krit′ik, -i-kăl) Distinguishing; diagnostic; allowing of distinction.

di·ac·yl·glyc·er·ol (dī-as′il-glis′ĕr-ol) Intermediate in the synthesis of triacylglycerols and of lecithin; also serves as a second messenger in stimulating the activity of protein kinase C.

diaeretic [Br.] SYN dieretic.

di·ag·nose (dī-ăg-nōs′) To make a diagnosis.

di·ag·no·sis (dī-ăg-nō′sis) The determination of the nature of a disease, injury, or congenital defect. SEE ALSO nursing diagnosis. SYN diacrisis.

***Di·ag·nos·tic and Sta·tis·ti·cal Man·u·al of Men·tal Dis·or·ders* (DSM)** (dī-ăg-nos′tik stă-tis′ti-kăl man′yū-ăl men′tăl dis-ōr′dĕrz) An American Psychiatric Association publication that classifies mental illnesses; provides health care practitioners with a comprehensive system for diagnosing mental illnesses based on specific ideational and behavioral symptoms.

di·ag·nos·tic an·es·the·si·a (dī′ăg-nos′tik an-es-thē′zē-ă) That induced for evaluation of the mechanism responsible for a painful condition.

di·ag·nos·ti·cian (dī′ăg-nos-tish′ăn) One who is skilled in making diagnoses.

di·a·gram (diag) (dī′ă-gram) A simple, graphic depiction of an idea or object.

di·a·ki·ne·sis (dī′ă-ki-nē′sis) Final stage of prophase in meiosis I, in which the chromosomes continue to shorten and the nucleolus and nuclear membrane disappear.

di·al (dī′ăl) A clock face or instrument resembling a clock face.

di·al·y·sance (dī-al′i-săns) The number

of milliliters of blood completely cleared of any substance by an artificial kidney or by peritoneal dialysis in a unit of time.

di·al·y·sate (dī-al′i-sāt) That part of a mixture that passes through a dialyzing membrane. SYN diffusate.

di·al·y·sis (dī-al′i-sis) **1.** Filtration to separate crystalloid from colloid substances (or smaller molecules from larger ones) in a solution by interposing a semipermeable membrane between the solution and water. SYN diffusion (2). **2.** The separation of substances across a semipermeable membrane on the basis of particle size and/or concentration gradients. **3.** A method of providing artificial kidney function.

di·al·y·sis dis·e·qui·lib·ri·um syndrome (DDS) (dī-al′i-sis dis-ē′kwi-lib′rē-ŭm) Nausea, vomiting, and hypertension, occasionally with convulsions, developing within several hours after starting hemodialysis for renal failure.

di·al·y·sis en·ceph·a·lop·a·thy syndrome, di·al·y·sis de·men·ti·a (dī-al′i-sis en-sef′ă-lop′ă-thē sin′drōm, dĕ-men′shē-ă) A progressive, often fatal, diffuse encephalopathy occurring in long-term hemodialysis patients.

di·al·ysis ret·i·nae (dī-al′i-sis ret′i-nē) Congenital or traumatic separation of the peripheral sensory retina from the retinal pigment epithelium at the ora serrata, often causing a retinal detachment.

di·al·y·sis shunt (dī-al′i-sis shŭnt) Arteriovenous shunt connecting the arterial and venous cannulas in arm or leg.

di·a·lyz·er (dī′ă-lī-zĕr) The apparatus for performing dialysis; a membrane used in dialysis.

di·a·me·li·a (dī-ă-mē′lē-ă) Absence of two limbs.

di·am·e·ter (dī-am′ĕ-tĕr) **1.** A straight line connecting two opposite points on the surface of a more or less spheric or cylindric body, or at the boundary of an opening or foramen, passing through the center of such body or opening. **2.** The distance measured along such a line.

di·am·ni·ot·ic (dī′am-nē-ot′ik) Exhibiting two amniotic sacs.

di·a·pause (dī′ă-pawz) A period of biologic quiescence or dormancy with decreased metabolism; an interval in which development is arrested or greatly slowed.

di·a·pe·de·sis (dī′ă-pĕ-dē′sis) The passage of blood, or any of its formed elements, through the intact walls of blood vessels. SYN migration (2).

di·a·per der·ma·ti·tis (dī′ă-pĕr dĕr′mă-tī′tis) Colloquially referred to as diaper, ammonia, or napkin rash; dermal condition of thighs and buttocks resulting from exposure to urine and feces in infants′ diapers.

di·a·phan·og·ra·phy (dī-ă-fă-nog′ră-fē) Examination of a body part by transillumination, especially for the detection of breast cancer.

di·a·phe·met·ric (dī′ă-fĕ-met′rik) Relating to the determination of the degree of tactile sensibility.

di·a·pho·re·sis (dī′ă-fŏr-ē′sis) SYN perspiration (1).

di·a·pho·ret·ic (dī′ă-fŏr-et′ik) **1.** Relating to, or causing, perspiration. **2.** An agent that increases perspiration.

di·a·phragm (dī′ă-fram) [TA] **1.** Musculomembranous partition between the abdominal and thoracic cavities. SYN diaphragma (2) [TA], midriff. **2.** A thin disc pierced with an opening, used in a microscope, camera, or other optic instrument to shut out the marginal rays of light, thus giving a more direct illumination. **3.** Flexible ring covered with a dome-shaped sheet of elastic material placed in the vagina to prevent pregnancy. **4.** RADIOGRAPHY a grid (2).

di·a·phrag·ma, pl. **di·a·phrag·ma·ta** (dī-ă-frag′mă, -mă-tă) **1.** [TA] A thin partition separating adjacent regions. **2.** [TA] SYN diaphragm (1).

di·a·phrag·mat·ic (dī′ă-frag-mat′ik) Relating to a diaphragm. SYN phrenic (1).

di·a·phrag·mat·ic flut·ter (dī′ă-frag-mat′ik flŭt′ĕr) Rapid rhythmic contractions (average, 150 per minute) of the diaphragm, simulating atrial flutter clinically.

di·a·phrag·mat·ic her·ni·a (dī′ă-frag-mat′ik hĕr′nē-ă) Protrusion of abdominal contents into the chest through a weakness in the respiratory diaphragm; a common type is the hiatal hernia.

di·a·phrag·mat·ic per·i·to·ni·tis (dī′ă-frag-mat′ik per′ĭ-tŏ-nī′tis) Disorder affecting mainly the peritoneal surface of the diaphragm.

di·a·phy·sec·to·my (dī′ă-fi-sek′tŏ-mē) Partial or complete removal of the shaft of a long bone.

di·a·phys·i·al, di·a·phys·e·al (dī-ă-fiz′ē-ăl) Relating to a diaphysis.

di·aph·y·sis, pl. **di·aph·y·ses** (dī-af′i-sis, -sēz) [TA] SYN shaft.

di·aph·y·si·tis (dī′af-i-sī′tis) Inflammation of the shaft of a long bone.

di·a·pi·re·sis (dī′ă-pī-rē′sis) Passage of colloidal or other small particles of suspended matter through the unruptured walls of the blood vessels. SEE ALSO diapedesis.

di·ar·rhe·a (dī′ă-rē′ă) An abnormally frequent discharge of semisolid or fluid fecal matter from the bowel. SYN diarrhoea.

di·ar·rhe·a·gen·ic (dī′ă-rē-ă-jen′ik) Pertains to diarrhea-causing microorganisms (e.g., *Escherichia coli*).

di·ar·rhe·a pan·cre·at·i·ca (dī′ă-rē′ă pan-krē-at′i-kă) Diarrhea characterized by severe, watery, secretory diarrhea and hyperkalemia; most patients have hypercalcemia, many have hyperglycemia; results from excessive secretion of vasoactive intestinal peptide by an islet cell tumor of the pancreas. Sometimes called WDHA syndrome.

diarrhoea [Br.] SYN diarrhea.

di·ar·thric (dī-ahr′thrik) Relating to two joints. SYN biarticular, diarticular.

di·ar·thro·di·al joint (dī′ahr-thrō′dē-ăl joynt) SYN synovial joint.

di·ar·thro·sis, pl. **di·ar·thro·ses** (dī′ahr-thrō′sis, -sēz) SYN synovial joint.

di·ar·tic·u·lar (dī-ahr-tik′yū-lăr) SYN diarthric.

di·as·chi·sis (dī-as′ki-sis) A sudden inhibition of function produced by an acute focal disturbance in a portion of the brain at a distance from the original seat of injury, but anatomically connected with it through fiber tracts.

di·a·scope (dī′ă-skōp) A flat glass plate through which one can examine superficial skin lesions by means of pressure.

di·a·stal·sis (dī′ă-stal′sis) Peristalsis in which area of inhibition precedes contraction wave, as seen in the intestinal tract.

di·a·stase (dī′ă-stās) A mixture, obtained from malt that converts starch into dextrin and maltose.

di·as·ta·sis (dī-as′tă-sis) 1. Simple separation of normally joined parts. SYN divarication. 2. Midportion of diastole when blood enters the ventricle slowly or ceases to enter before atrial systole; duration is in inverse proportion to heart rate and absent at high heart rates.

di·as·tat·ic fer·men·ta·tion (dī′ă-stat′ik fĕr′men-tā′shŭn) Conversion of starch to glucose by action of ptyalin.

di·a·ste·ma, pl. **di·a·ste·ma·ta** (dī′ă-stē′mă, -mă-tă) [TA] 1. Fissure or abnormal opening in any part, especially if congenital. 2. Space between two adjacent teeth in the same dental arch. 3. A space between teeth not due to missing teeth. SYN space (2).

di·a·ste·ma·to·cra·ni·a (dī′ă-stē′mă-tō-krā′nē-ă) Congenital sagittal fissure of the cranium.

di·a·ste·ma·to·my·e·li·a (dī′ă-stē′mă-tō-mī-ē′lē-ă) Complete or incomplete sagittal division of the spinal cord by an osseous or fibrocartilaginous septum.

di·as·to·le (dī-as′tŏ-lē) Normal postsystolic dilation of the heart cavities, during which they fill with blood; diastole of the atria precedes that of the ventricles.

di·a·sto·lic blood pres·sure (dī′ă-stol′ik blŭd presh′ŭr) Intracardiac pressure during or due to diastolic relaxation in a cardiac chamber.

di·a·stol·ic pres·sure (dī′ă-stol′ik presh′

ŭr) Intracardiac pressure during or due to diastolic relaxation of a cardiac chamber.

di·a·stol·ic thrill (dī′ă-stol′ik thril) Vibration palpable over the precordium or over a blood vessel during ventricular diastole.

di·a·stroph·ic dys·pla·si·a (dī′ă-strō′fik dis-plā′zē-ă) A skeletal dysplasia characterized by scoliosis, hitchhiker's thumb due to shortening of the first metacarpal bone, cleft palate, malformed ear with calcification, chondritis, shortening of the Achilles tendon, clubbed foot, and characteristic radiologic findings.

di·a·tax·i·a (dī′ă-tak′sē-ă) Ataxia affecting both sides of the body.

di·a·ther·ma·nous (dī′ă-thĕr′mă-nŭs) Permeable by heat rays. SYN transcalent.

di·a·ther·mic (dī′ă-thĕr′mik) Relating to, characterized by, or affected by diathermy.

di·a·ther·my (dī′ă-thĕr-mē) Therapeutic use of short or ultrashort waves of electromagnetic energy to heat muscular tissue.

di·a·tom (dī′ă-tom) An individual of microscopic unicellular algae, the shells of which comprise a sedimentary infusorial earth.

di·a·to·ma·ceous (dī′ă-tō-mā′shŭs) Pertaining to diatoms or their fossil remains.

di·az·e·pam (DZ, DZP, DIAZ) (dī-az′ĕ-pam) A benzodiazepine skeletal muscle relaxant, sedative, and antianxiety agent; also used in parenteral treatment of status epilepticus.

♻ **diazo-** Prefix denoting a compound containing the ≡C–N≡N–X grouping, where X is not carbon (except for CN), or the grouping N_2 attached by one atom to carbon. Cf. azo-.

di·az·o·tize (dī-az′ō-tīz) To introduce the diazo group into a chemical compound, usually through the treatment of an amine with nitrous acid.

di·ba·sic (dī-bā′sik) Having two replaceable hydrogen atoms, denoting an acid with two ionizable hydrogen atoms.

di·ba·sic po·tas·si·um phos·phate (DKP) (dī-bā′sik pŏ-tas′ē-ŭm fos′fāt) SYN potassium phosphate.

di·ba·sic so·di·um phos·phate (DSP) (dī-bā′sik sō′dē-ŭm fos′fāt) SYN sodium phosphate.

di·bu·caine (dib′yū-kān) A potent local anesthetic with a long duration of action used by injection or topically on skin or mucous membranes.

di·cen·tric (dī-sen′trik) Having two centromeres, an abnormal state.

di·cho·ri·al, di·cho·ri·on·ic (dī-kōr′ē-ăl, -ē-on′ik) Showing evidence of two chorions.

di·chot·o·my, di·chot·o·mi·za·tion (dī-kot′ŏ-mē, -mī-zā′shŭn) Division into two parts.

di·chro·ism (dī′krō-izm) The property of seeming to be differently colored when viewed from emitted light and from transmitted light.

di·chro·mat·ic (dī′krō-mat′ik) **1.** Having or exhibiting two colors. **2.** Relating to dichromatism (2).

di·chro·ma·tism (dī-krō′mă-tizm) **1.** The state of being dichromatic (1). **2.** The abnormality of color vision in which only two of the three retinal cone pigments are present, as in protanopia, deuteranopia, and tritanopia. SYN dichromatopsia.

di·chro·mic (dī-krō′mik) Having, or relating to, two colors.

Dick test (dik test) An intracutaneous test of susceptibility to the erythrogenic toxin of *Streptococcus pyogenes* responsible for the rash and other manifestations of scarlet fever.

di·crot·ic notch (dī-krot′ik noch) The acute drop in arterial pressure pulse curves following the systolic peak, corresponding to the incisura of the displacement pulse curve.

di·crot·ic pulse (dī-krot′ik pŭls) One marked by a double beat, the second, due to a palpable dicrotic wave, being weaker than the first.

di·cro·tism (dī′krŏ-tizm) Form in which

a double beat can be appreciated at any arterial pulse for each beat of the heart; due to accentuation of the dicrotic wave.

dicta- Prefix meaning two hundred.

dic·ty·o·ma (dik′tē-ō′mă) A benign tumor of the ciliary epithelium with a netlike structure resembling embryonic retina. SYN embryonal medulloepithelioma.

dic·ty·o·tene (dik′tē-ō-tēn) The state of meiosis at which the oocyte is arrested during the several years between late fetal life and menarche.

di·cu·ma·rol (dī-kū′mă-rol) An anticoagulant that acts in the liver to block synthesis of vitamin K and vitamin K–dependent coagulation factors; discovered as the causative agent in spoiled hay, which causes bleeding in cattle (sweet clover disease).

di·cy·clo·mine hy·dro·chlor·ide (dī-sī′klō-mēn hī′drŏ-klōr′īd) An anticholinergic agent.

di·dac·ty·lism (dī-dak′ti-lizm) Congenital condition of having only two fingers on a hand or two toes on a foot.

di·del·phic (dī-del′fik) Having or relating to a double uterus.

did·y·mi·tis (did-i-mī′tis) Testicular inflammation.

-didymus Suffix meaning a conjoined twin, with the first element of the complete word designating fused parts.

di·e·cious (dī-ē′shŭs) Denoting animals or plants that are sexually distinct, the individuals being of one or the other sex.

di·el·drin (dī-el′drin) A chlorinated hydrocarbon used as an insecticide; may cause toxic effects.

di·en·ceph·a·lon, pl. **di·en·ceph·a·la** (dī′en-sef′ă-lon, -lă) [TA] That part of the prosencephalon composed of the epithalamus, dorsal thalamus, subthalamus, and hypothalamus.

die·ner (dē′nĕr) A laboratory worker who assists in cleaning; most commonly applied to laboratory workers who assist in the performance of autopsies and maintenance of morgues.

Di·ent·a·moe·ba frag·i·lis (dī′ent-ă-mē′bă fră-jil′ŭs) Small amebalike flagellates related to *Trichomonas,* parasitic in the large intestine of humans and certain monkeys; sometimes causes low-grade inflammation with mucous diarrhea.

di·er·e·sis (dī-er′ĕ-sis) SYN solution of continuity.

di·e·ret·ic (dī′ĕr-et′ik) **1.** Relating to dieresis. **2.** Dividing; ulcerating; corroding.

di·es·trus (dī-es′trŭs) A period of sexual quiescence intervening between two periods of estrus. SYN dioestrus.

di·et (dī′ĕt) **1.** Food and drink in general. **2.** A prescribed course of eating and drinking in which the amount and kind of food, as well as the times at which it is to be taken, are regulated for therapeutic purposes. **3.** Reduction of caloric intake so as to lose weight.

di·e·tar·y fi·ber (dī′ĕ-tār-ē fī′bĕr) The plant polysaccharides and lignin that are resistant to hydrolysis by human digestive enzymes.

di·e·tet·ic (dī′ĕ-tet′ik) **1.** Relating to the diet. **2.** Descriptive of food that, natural or processed, has a low caloric content.

di·e·tet·ics (dī′ĕ-tet′iks) The practical application of diet in the prophylaxis and treatment of disease.

di·eth·yl·ene·tri·a·mine pen·ta·a·ce·tic ac·id (DTPA) (dī-eth′il-ēn-trī′ă-mēn pen′tă-ă-sē′tik as′id) An important chelating agent used in therapy and in metal-containing diagnostic agents for magnetic resonance imaging and nuclear scanning.

di·eth·yl·stil·bes·trol (DES) (dī-eth′il-stil-bes′trol) A synthetic nonsteroidal estrogenic compound; sometimes previously used as a postcoital antipregnancy agent to prevent implantation of the fertilized oocyte.

di·e·ti·tian (dī′ĕ-tish′ŭn) An expert in dietetics.

dif- (L.) Prefix meaning separation, taking apart, in two, reversal, not, or un-.

dif·fer·ence (dif'ĕr-ĕns) Degree of variation found in the comparison of two similar items.

dif·fer·en·tial di·ag·no·sis (dif'ĕr-en' shăl dī-ăg-nō'sis) The determination of which of two or more diseases with similar symptoms is the one the patient has, by a systematic comparison and contrasting of the clinical findings. SYN differentiation (2).

dif·fer·en·tial growth (dif'ĕr-en'shăl grōth) Varying rates of growth in associated tissues or structures; used especially in embryology when the differences in growth rates result in changing the original proportions or relations.

dif·fer·en·tial thresh·old (dif'ĕr-en' shăl thresh'ōld) Lowest limit at which two stimuli can be differentiated. SYN threshold differential.

dif·fer·en·ti·ate (dif'ĕr-en'shē-āt) To make a distinction between two or more things in terms of characteristics inherent to each.

dif·fer·en·ti·a·tion (dif'ĕr-en-shē-ā'shŭn) **1.** The acquisition or possession of one or more characteristics or functions different from that of the original type. SYN specialization (2). **2.** SYN differential diagnosis. **3.** Partial removal of a stain from a histologic section to accentuate the staining differences of tissue components.

dif·frac·tion (di-frak'shŭn) Deflection of the rays of light from a straight line in passing by the edge of an opaque body or in passing an obstacle of about the size of the wavelength of the light.

dif·fu·sate (di-fyū'zāt) SYN dialysate.

dif·fuse (di-fyūz', di-fyūs') **1.** To disseminate; to spread about. **2.** Disseminated; spread about; not restricted.

dif·fuse ab·scess (di-fyūs' ab'ses) A collection of pus not circumscribed by a well-defined capsule.

dif·fuse glo·mer·u·lo·neph·ri·tis (DGN) (di-fyūs' glō-mer'yū-lō-nef-rī'tis) Glomerulonephritis affecting most of the renal glomeruli; it may lead to azotemia.

dif·fuse goi·ter (di-fyūs' goy'tĕr) One in which the morbid process involves the whole gland, as opposed to nodular goiter or thyroid adenoma.

dif·fuse hy·per·ker·a·to·sis of palms and soles (di-fyūs' hī'pĕr-ker'a-tō'sis pahlmz sōlz) Disorder with onset in early infancy; characterized by hyperkeratotic, scaling plaques and hyperhidrosis on the palms and soles. SYN Unna-Thost syndrome.

dif·fuse in·ju·ries (di-fyūs' in'jŭr-ēz) Extensive bodily damage due to encounters with low velocity–high mass forces.

dif·fuse la·mel·lar ker·a·ti·tis (DLK) (di-fyūs' lă-mel'ăr ker'ă-tī'tis) Inflammation in the interface of a surgically induced lamellar cut in the cornea in laser-assisted in situ keratomileusis surgery. SYN sands of Sahara.

dif·fuse Lewy body dis·ease (di-fyūs' lā've bod'ē di-zēz') A degenerative cerebral disorder of old people, characterized initially by progressive dementia or psychosis, and subsequently by parkinsonian findings. SYN Lewy body dementia.

dif·fuse per·i·to·ni·tis (di-fyūs' per'i-tō-nī'tis) SYN general peritonitis.

dif·fuse wax·y spleen (di-fyūs' waks'ē splēn) A condition of amyloid degeneration of the spleen, affecting chiefly the extrasinusoidal tissue spaces of the pulp.

dif·fus·i·ble (di-fyūz'i-bĕl) Capable of diffusing.

dif·fus·i·ble stim·u·lant (di-fyūz'i-bĕl stim'yū-lănt) A stimulant that produces a rapid but temporary effect.

dif·fu·sion (di-fyū'zhŭn) **1.** The random movement of molecules or ions or small particles in solution or suspension toward a uniform distribution throughout the available volume. **2.** SYN dialysis (1).

dif·fu·sion co·ef·fi·cient (dĕ-fyū'zhŭn kō'ĕ-fish'ĕnt) The mass of material diffusing across a unit area in time unit under a concentration gradient of unity.

dif·fu·sion con·stant (di-fyū'zhŭn kon' stănt) SYN diffusion coefficient.

dif·fu·sion res·pi·ration (di-fyū'zhŭn res'pir-ā'shŭn) Maintenance of oxygenation during apnea by intratracheal insufflation of oxygen at high flow rates.

di·gas·tric (dī-gas′trik) **1.** Having two bellies; denoting especially a muscle with two fleshy parts separated by an intervening tendinous part. **2.** Relating to the digastric muscle; denoting a fossa or groove with which it is in relation and a nerve supplying its posterior belly.

di·gas·tric fos·sa (dī-gas′trik fos′ă) [TA] A hollow on the posterior surface of the base of the mandible, on either side of the median plane, giving attachment to the anterior belly of the digastric muscle.

di·gas·tri·cus (dī-gas′tri-kŭs) **1.** SYN digastric. **2.** Denoting the digastric muscle.

di·ge·net·ic (dī′jĕ-net′ik) **1.** Pertaining to or characterized by digenesis. SYN heteroxenous. **2.** Pertaining to the digenetic fluke.

di·ges·tion (di-jes′chŭn) The mechanical, chemical, and enzymatic process whereby ingested food is converted into material suitable for assimilation for synthesis of tissues or liberation of energy.

di·ges·tive en·zyme (di-jes′tiv en′zīm) The enzymes that break down carbohydrates, protein, and fats from ingested foods.

di·ges·tive fe·ver (di-jes′tiv fē′vĕr) Slight rise of body temperature occurring during the period of digestion.

di·ges·tive sys·tem (di-jes′tiv sis′tĕm) The total digestive tract extending from the mouth to the anus with all its associated glands and organs (i.e., pharynx, esophagus, stomach, and intestine). SYN alimentary canal, alimentary tract.

dig·it (dij′it) [TA] A finger or toe. SYN digitus [TA], dactyl, dactylus.

dig·i·tal (dij′i-tăl) **1.** Relating to or resembling a digit or digits or an impression made by them. **2.** Based on numeric methodology.

dig·i·tal crease (dij′i-tăl krēs) One of the grooves on the palmar surface of a finger, at the level of an interphalangeal joint.

dig·i·tal fluor·os·co·py (DF) (dij′i-tăl flōr-os′kŏ-pē) Using a solid-state radia-

tion detector and electronic processing with a computer monitor for display.

dig·i·tal fur·row (dij′i-tăl fŭr′ō) SYN digital crease.

Dig·i·tal Imag·ing and Com·mu·ni·ca·tions in Med·i·cine (DICOM) (dij′i-tăl im′ăj-ing kŏ-myū′ni-kā′shŭnz med′i-sin) A joint standard of the American College of Radiology and National Equipment Manufacturers Association; specifies entities (or objects) and functions (or services) to allow communication between various image sources and other computer devices.

Di·gi·ta·lis (dij′i-tā′lis) A perennial flowering plant that is the main source for some cardioactive steroid glycosides useful in therapy for congestive heart failure and other cardiac disease.

dig·i·tal ra·di·og·ra·phy (DR) (dij′i-tăl rā′dē-og′ră-fē) Direct conversion of transmitted x-rays into a digital image using an array of solid-state detectors with computer processing and display of the image. SEE digital subtraction angiography.

dig·i·tate (dig) (dij′i-tāt) Marked by a number of fingerlike processes or impressions.

dig·i·tate wart (dij′i-tāt wōrt) SYN verruca digitata.

dig·i·ta·tion (dij′i-tā′shŭn) A process resembling a finger.

dig·i·tox·in (DT, DIG) (dij′i-tok′sin) A cardioactive glycoside obtained from the leaves of *Digitalis purpurea;* it is more completely absorbed from the gastrointestinal tract than is digitalis. SYN crystalline digitalin.

dig·i·tus, pl. **dig·i·ti** (dij′i-tŭs, -tī) [TA] SYN digit.

di·glos·si·a (dī-glos′ē-ă) A developmental defect that results in a longitudinal split in the tongue. SEE ALSO bifid tongue.

dig·na·thus (dig-nā′thŭs) A malformed fetus with a double mandible. SYN augnathus.

di·gox·in (DIG, DO, dig, dig.) (dī-gok′

sin) A cardioactive steroid glycoside obtained from *Digitalis lanata*.

di·hy·brid (dī-hī′brid) The offspring of parents differing in two characters.

di·hy·drate (dī-hī′drāt) A compound with two molecules of water of crystallization.

di·hy·dro·ta·chys·ter·ol (DHT, AT10) (dī-hī′drō-tă-kis′těr-ol) SEE tachysterol.

di·hy·drox·y·ac·e·tone (dī′hī-drok′sē-as′ĕ-tōn) The simplest ketose.

di·i·o·do·ty·ro·sine (DIT) (dī-ī′ŏ-dō-tī′rō-sēn) An intermediate in the biosynthesis of thyroid hormone.

di·lac·er·a·tion (dī-las′ĕr-a′shŭn) Displacement of some portion of a developing tooth, which is then further developed in its new relation, resulting in a tooth with sharply angulated root(s).

di·la·tan·cy (dī-lă′tăn-sē) An increasing viscosity with increasing rate of shear accompanied by volumetric expansion.

di·late (dī′lāt) To perform or undergo dilation.

di·lat·ed car·di·o·my·op·a·thy (dī′lāt-ĕd kahr′dē-ō-mī-op′ă-thē) Decreased function of the left ventricle associated with its dilation; most patients have global hypokinesia, although discrete regional wall movement abnormalities may occur; usually manifested by signs of overall cardiac failure, with congestive findings, as well as by fatigue indicative of a low output state. SYN congestive cardiomyopathy.

di·la·tion, dil·a·ta·tion (dī-lā′shŭn, dil′ă-tā′shŭn) **1.** Physiologic or artificial enlargement of a hollow structure or opening. **2.** The act of stretching or enlarging an opening or the lumen of a hollow structure.

di·la·tion and cu·ret·tage (D & C) (dī-lā′shŭn kyūr′ĕ-tahzh′) Dilation of the cervix and curettement of the endometrium.

di·la·tion and ex·trac·tion (dī-lā′shŭn ek-strak′shŭn) Abortion in which the cervix is dilated and the fetus extracted in pieces using surgical forceps; technique used to complete a second trimester

spontaneous abortion or as a form of induced abortion.

di·la·tor, dil·a·ta·tor (dī′lā-tŏr, dil′ă-tā-tŏr) **1.** An instrument designed to enlarge a hollow structure or opening. **2.** A muscle that opens an orifice. **3.** A substance that dilates or enlarges an opening or the lumen of a hollow structure. SEE ALSO bougie.

di·la·tor mus·cle (dī′lā-tŏr mŭs′ĕl) [TA] One that opens an orifice or dilates the lumen of an organ; the dilating or opening component of a pylorus (the other component is the sphincter muscle).

di·lep·tic sei·zure (dī-lep′tik sē′zhŭr) Attack characterized by impaired awareness of, interaction with, or memory of ongoing events.

dil·u·ent (dil′yū′ĕnt) *Avoid the incorrect forms diluent and dilutant.* Ingredient in a medicinal preparation that lacks pharmacologic activity but is pharmaceutically necessary or desirable. In tablet or capsule dosage forms, this may be lactose or starch; it is particularly useful in increasing the bulk of potent drug substances with a mass too small for dosage to allow manufacture or administration.

di·lute Rus·sell vi·per ven·om test (DRVVT) (dī-lūt′ rŭs′ĕl vī′pĕr ven′ŏm test) A test used to confirm the presence of a lupus anticoagulant.

di·lu·tion (di-lū′shŭn) **1.** The act of being diluted. **2.** A diluted solution or mixture. **3.** MICROBIOLOGY a method for counting the number of viable cells in a suspension.

di·lu·tion·al hy·po·na·tre·mi·a (di-lū′shŭn-ăl hī′pō-nā-trē′mē-ă) SYN depletional hyponatremia.

di·me·li·a (dī-mē′lē-ă) Congenital duplication of the whole or a part of a limb.

di·men·sion·al sta·bil·ity (di-men′shŭn-ăl stă-bil′i-tē) The property of a material to retain its size and form.

di·mer (dī′měr) A compound or unit produced by the combination of two like molecules.

di·mer·cap·rol (dī′měr-kap′rol) A chelating agent, developed as an antidote for lewisite and other arsenical poisons; also used as an antidote for antimony, bismuth, chromium, mercury, gold, and nickel. SYN antilewisite, British anti-Lewisite.

di·meth·i·cone (dī-meth′i-kōn) A silicone oil consisting of dimethylsiloxane polymers, usually incorporated into a petrolatum base or a nongreasy preparation and used for the protection of normal skin against various, chiefly industrial, skin irritants; may also be used to prevent diaper dermatitis.

di·meth·yl sul·fox·ide (DMSO) (dī-meth′il sŭl-foks′īd) **1.** A penetrating solvent, enhancing absorption of therapeutic agents from the skin. **2.** An industrial solvent that has been proposed as an effective analgesic and antiinflammatory agent in arthritis and bursitis.

dimethyl sulphoxide [Br.] SYN dimethyl sulfoxide.

di·mor·phic (dī-mōr′fik) MYCOLOGY growth and reproduction in two forms: mold and yeast.

di·mor·phism (dī-mōr′fizm) Existence in two shapes or forms; denoting a difference of crystalline form exhibited by the same substance, or a difference in form or outward appearance between individuals of the same species.

dim·ple (dim′pĕl) **1.** A natural indentation, usually small and circular, in the chin, cheek, or sacral region. **2.** A depression of similar appearance to a dimple, resulting from trauma or the contraction of scar tissue.

din·ner pad (din′ĕr pad) Moderately thick dressing placed over the pit of the stomach before the application of a plaster jacket; after the plaster has set, the pad is removed, leaving space for varying degrees of abdominal distention.

Di·no·fla·gell·i·da (dī′nō-flă-jel′i-dă) An order in the phylum Sarcomastigophora characterized by the presence of two flagella so placed as to cause the organism to have a whirling motility.

di·no·prost (dī′nō-prost) An oxytocic agent. SYN prostaglandin $F_{2\alpha}$.

di·nu·cle·o·tide (dī-nū′klē-ō-tīd) A compound containing two nucleotides.

Di·oc·to·phy·ma (dī-ok′tō-fī′mă) A genus of very large nematode worms infecting the kidney.

dioestrus [Br.] SYN diestrus.

di·op·ter, di·op·tre (D, Δ, δ) (dī-op′tĕr) The unit of refracting power of lenses, denoting the reciprocal of the focal length expressed in meters.

di·op·trics (dī-op′triks) The branch of optics concerned with the refraction of light.

di·ot·ic (dī-ot′ik) Simultaneous presentation of the same sound to each ear.

di·ov·u·lar (dī-ov′yū-lăr) Relating to two oocytes. SYN biovular.

di·ov·u·la·to·ry (dī-ōv′yŭ-lă-tōr-ē) Releasing two oocytes in one ovarian cycle.

di·ox·ide (dī-ok′sīd) A molecule containing two atoms of oxygen; e.g., carbon dioxide.

di·pep·ti·dase (dī-pep′ti-dās) A hydrolase catalyzing the hydrolysis of a dipeptide to its constituent amino acids.

Di·pet·a·lo·ne·ma (dī-pet′ă-lō-nē′mă) A genus of nematode filariae in humans and many other mammals; as with other filarial worms, produces microfilariae in blood or tissue fluids, with adults found in deep connective tissue, membranes, or visceral surfaces.

di·pha·sic (dī-fā′zik) Occurring in or characterized by two phases or stages.

di·phen·yl (dī-fen′il) Colorless liquid used as a heat transfer agent, frequently as a polychlorinated biphenyl (PCB); used as fungistat for oranges and in organic syntheses. Produces convulsions and central nervous system depression. SYN biphenyl, phenylbenzene.

diph·the·ri·a (dif-thēr′ē-ă) A specific infectious disease due to *Corynebacterium diphtheriae* and its highly potent toxin; marked by severe inflammation with formation of a thick membranous coating of the pharynx, the nose, and sometimes the tracheobronchial tree; the toxin produces degeneration in peripheral nerves, heart muscle, and other tissues.

diph·the·ri·a an·ti·tox·in (DIPant, DAT) (dif-thēr′ē-ă an′tē-tok′sin) Antitoxin specific for the toxin of *Corynebacterium diphtheriae*.

diph·the·ri·al, diph·the·rit·ic (dif-thēr′ē-ăl, dif′thĕ-rit′ik) Relating to diphtheria, or the membranous exudate characteristic of this disease.

diph·the·ri·a toxin (DT) (dif-thēr′ē-ă tok′sin) SEE *Corynebacterium diphtheriae*.

diph·the·ri·a tox·oid, tet·a·nus tox·oid, and per·tus·sis vac·cine (dif-thēr′ē-ă toks′oyd tet′ă-nŭs toks′oyd pĕr-tŭs′is vak-sēn′) A vaccine available in three forms: 1) diphtheria and tetanus toxoids plus pertussis vaccine (DTP); 2) tetanus and diphtheria toxoids, adult type (Td); and 3) tetanus toxoid (T).

diph·ther·oid (dif′thĕ-royd) **1.** One of a group of local infections suggesting diphtheria, but caused by microorganisms other than *Corynebacterium diphtheriae*. **2.** Any microorganism resembling *Corynebacterium diphtheriae*.

di·phyl·lo·both·ri·a·sis (dī-fil′ō-both-rī′ă-sis) Infection with the cestode *Diphyllobothrium latum;* human infection is caused by ingestion of raw or inadequately cooked fish infected with the plerocercoid larva.

Di·phyl·lo·both·ri·um (dī-fil′lō-both′rē-ŭm) A large genus of tapeworms (order Pseudophyllidea) characterized by a spatulate scolex with dorsal and ventral sucking grooves, or bothria. Several species are found in humans.

di·phy·o·dont (dī-fī′ō-dont) Developing two successive sets of teeth, as occurs in humans and most other mammals.

dip·la·cu·sis (dip′lă-kyū′sis) Abnormal perception of sound, either in time or in pitch, so that one sound is heard as two.

di·ple·gi·a (dī-plē′jē-ă) Paralysis of corresponding parts on both sides of the body.

♻ **diplo-** Double, twofold. SEE haplo-.

dip·lo·ba·cil·lus (dip′lō-bă-sil′ŭs) Two rod-shaped bacterial cells linked end to end.

dip·lo·bac·te·ri·a (dip′lō-bak-tēr′ē-ă) Bacterial cells linked together in pairs.

dip·lo·co·ri·a (dip′lō-kōr′ē-ă) The occurrence of two pupils in the eye. SYN dicoria.

dip·lo·ë (dip′lŏ-wē) [TA] The central layer of spongy bone between the two layers of compact bone, outer and inner plates, or tables, of the flat cranial bones.

dip·lo·gen·e·sis (dip′lō-jen′ĕ-sis) Production of a double fetus or of one with some parts doubled.

di·plo·ic vein (dip-lō′ik vān) One of the veins in the diploë of the cranial bones, connected with the cerebral sinuses by emissary veins; the main diploic veins are the frontal, anterior temporal, posterior temporal, and occipital.

dip·loid (dip′loyd) Denoting the state of a cell containing two haploid sets derived from the father and from the mother respectively; the normal chromosome complement of somatic cells (in humans, 46 chromosomes).

dip·loid nu·cle·us (dip′loyd nū′klē-ŭs) A nucleus containing the diploid or normal double complement of chromosomes for one somatic cell.

dip·lo·my·e·li·a (dip′lō-mī-ē′lē-ă) Complete or incomplete doubling of the spinal cord; may be accompanied by a bony septum of the vertebral canal.

dip·lop·a·gus (dip-lop′ă-gŭs) General term for conjoined twins, each with fairly complete bodies, although one or more internal organs may be shared in common. SEE conjoined twins.

di·plo·pho·ni·a (dip′lō-fō′nē-ă) Vibration of both the ventricular folds and the vocal folds, producing two simultaneous voice tones.

di·plo·pi·a (dip-lō′pē-ă) The condition in which a single object is perceived as two objects. SYN double vision.

dip·lo·some (dip′lō-sōm) Paired allosomes; the pair of centrioles of mammalian cells.

dip·lo·so·mi·a (dip′lō-sō′mē-ă) Condition in which twins who seem functionally independent are joined at one or more points. SEE conjoined twins.

di·po·di·a (dī-pō′dē-ă) A developmental anomaly involving complete or incomplete duplication of a foot.

di·po·lar ions (dī-pō′lăr ī′onz) Ions possessing both a negative charge and a positive charge, each localized at a different point in the molecule, which thus has both positive and negative "poles." SYN zwitterions.

di·pole (dī′pōl) A pair of separated electrical charges, one or more positive and one or more negative; or a pair of separated partial charges. SYN doublet (2).

dip·se·sis, dip·so·sis (dip-sē′sis, -sō′sis) An abnormal or excessive thirst, or a craving for unusual forms of drink.

-dipsia, -dipsy Combining forms indicating thirst.

dip·so·ther·a·py (dip′sō-thār′ă-pē) Treatment of certain diseases by abstention, as far as possible, from liquids.

dip·stick (dip′stik) A strip of plastic or paper bearing one or more dots or squares of reagent, used to perform qualitative or semiquantitative tests on urine. Results of tests are seen in color changes.

Dip·ter·a (dip′tĕr-ă) Important insect order (two-winged flies and gnats); includes many significant disease vectors (e.g., mosquito, tsetse fly, sandfly, biting midge).

dip·ter·ous (dip′tĕr-ŭs) **1.** Having two wings. **2.** Relating to or characteristic of the order Diptera.

di·rect Coombs test (DCT) (dĭr-ekt′ kūmz test) SEE Coombs direct test.

di·rect cur·rent (DC) (dĭr-ekt′ kŭr′ĕnt) Current that flows in only one direction, e.g., that is derived from a battery; sometimes referred to as galvanic current. SEE ALSO galvanism.

di·rect flap (dĭr-ekt′ flap) A flap raised completely and transferred at the same stage.

di·rect frac·ture (dĭr-ekt′ frak′shŭr) A

fracture, especially of the skull, occurring at the point of injury.

di·rec·tion·al ath·er·ec·to·my (DCA) (dĭr-ek′shŭn-ăl ath′thĕr-ek′tŏ-mē) Excision of an atheroma with a motor-driven shaver mounted on an arterial catheter.

di·rect lead (dĭr-ekt′ lēd) In electrocardiography, a unipolar lead recorded with the exploring electrode placed directly on the surface of the exposed heart.

di·rect oph·thal·mo·scope (dĭr-ekt′ of-thal′mŏ-skōp) An instrument designed to visualize the interior of the eye, with the instrument placed relatively close to the subject's eye and the observer viewing an upright magnified image.

di·rec·tor (DIR) (dĭr-ek′tŏr) **1.** A smoothly grooved instrument used with a knife to limit the incision of tissues. **2.** The head of a service or specialty division.

di·rect re·act·ing bil·i·ru·bin (dĭr-ekt′ rē-akt′ing bil′i-rū′bin) The fraction of serum bilirubin that has been conjugated with glucuronic acid in the liver cell to form bilirubin diglucuronide.

di·rect trans·fu·sion (dĭr-ekt′ trans-fyū′zhŭn) Transfusion of blood from the donor to the recipient, either through a tube connecting their blood or by suturing the vessels together. SYN immediate transfusion.

di·rect vi·sion (dĭr-ekt′ vizh′ŭn) SYN central vision.

di·rect wet mount ex·am·i·na·tion (dĭr-ekt′ wet mownt eg-zam′i-nā′shŭn) Microscopic review at low (100×) and high dry (400×) total magnifications of a saline and fresh fecal specimen to detect parasites, including motile protozoan trophozoites.

Di·ro·fi·la·ri·a (dī′rō-fi-lā′rē-ă) A genus of filaria usually found in mammals other than humans, but rare examples of human infection are known, as by *D. immitis*.

dis·a·bil·i·ty (dis′ă-bil′i-tē) **1.** Diminished capacity to perform within a prescribed range. **2.** An impairment or defect of one or more organs or members.

dis·a·bil·i·ty-ad·just·ed life years

(DALYs) (dis´ă-bil´i-tē ă-jŭs´tĕd līf yērz) A measure of the burden of disease on a defined population, based on adjustment of life expectancy to allow for long-term disability as estimated from official statistics.

di·sac·char·i·dase (dī-sak´ăr-īd-ās) An enzyme that catalyzes disaccharides to monosaccharides.

di·sac·cha·ride (dī-sak´ă-rīd) A condensation product of two monosaccharides by elimination of water.

dis·ag·gre·ga·tion (dis-ag´rĕ-gā´shŭn) 1. A breaking up into component parts. 2. An inability to coordinate various sensations and failure to comprehend their mutual relations.

dis·ap·pear·ing bone dis·ease (dis-ă-pēr´ing bōn di-zēz´) Extensive decalcification of a single bone; of unknown cause, sometimes associated with angioma. SYN Gorham disease, Gorham syndrome.

dis·ar·tic·u·la·tion (dis´ahr-tik´yū-lā´shŭn) Amputation of a limb through a joint, without cutting of bone.

disc, disk (disk) 1. A round, flat plate; any approximately flat circular structure. 2. DENTISTRY a circular piece of thin paper or other material, coated with an abrasive substance, used for cutting and polishing teeth and fillings. 3. MICROBIOLOGY a plate coated with an antibiotic to measure susceptibility and resistance. 4. The optic nerve head as viewed during ophthalmoscopy.

disc·ec·to·my, disk·ec·to·my (disk-ek´tŏ-mē) Excision, in part or whole, of an intervertebral disc. SYN discotomy.

dis·charge (DC) (dis´chahrj) 1. That which is emitted or evacuated, as an excretion or a secretion. 2. The activation or firing of a neuron.

disc her·ni·a·tion (disk hĕr´nē-ā´shŭn) Extension of disc material beyond the posterior anulus fibrosus and posterior longitudinal ligament and into the spinal canal.

dis·ci·form, dis·ki·form (dis´ki-fōrm) Disc-shaped.

dis·ci·form de·gen·er·a·tion (dis´ki-

fōrm dĕ-jen´ĕr-ā´shŭn) Subretinal neovascularization with retinal separation and hemorrhage leading finally to a circular mass of fibrous tissue with marked loss of visual acuity. Also called disciform macular degeneration.

dis·cis·sion (di-sizh´ŭn) 1. Incision or cutting through a part. 2. In ophthalmology, opening of the capsule and breaking up of the cortex of the lens with a needle knife or laser.

dis·clos·ing a·gent (dis-klōz´ing ā´jĕnt) A selective dye in solution or tablet form used to visualize and identify soft debris, pellicle, and bacterial plaque on the surfaces of the teeth. Also called disclosing solution.

♻ **disco-** Combining form meaning disc.

dis·co·blas·tu·la (dis´kō-blas´tyū-lă) A blastula of the type produced by the meroblastic discoidal cleavage of a large-yolked oocyte.

dis·co·gen·ic, dis·ko·gen·ic (dis´kō-jen´ik) Denoting a disorder originating in or from an intervertebral disc.

dis·coid (dis´koyd) 1. Resembling a disc. 2. In dentistry, an excavating or carving instrument having a circular blade with a cutting edge around the periphery.

dis·coid lu·pus er·y·the·ma·to·sus (dis´koyd lū´pŭs er´ă-thē-mă-tō´sŭs) A form of lupus erythematosus in which cutaneous lesions appear on the face and elsewhere.

dis·con·nec·tion syn·drome (dis-kŏ-nek´shŭn sin´drōm) General term for various neurologic disorders (e.g., transcortical dysphasia) due to interruption of various association pathways located in either one cerebral hemisphere or linking both.

dis·cop·a·thy (dis-kop´ă-thē) Disease of a disc, particularly an invertebral disc.

dis·co·pla·cen·ta (dis´kō-plă-sen´tă) A placenta of discoid shape.

dis·cor·dance (dis-kōr´dăns) Dissociation of two characteristics in the members of a sample from a population; used as a measure of dependence.

dis·cor·dant al·ter·na·tion (dis-kōr´

dănt awl'tĕr-nā'shŭn) Alternation in cardiac activities of either the systemic or the pulmonary circulation, but not of both, or in both but oppositely directed in each.

dis·crete (dis-krēt') Separate; distinct; not joined to or incorporated with another; denoting especially certain lesions of the skin.

dis·crim·i·na·tion (dis-krim'i-nā'shŭn) **1.** The act of distinguishing between different things; ability to perceive different things as different, or to respond to them differently. **2.** PSYCHOLOGY responding differently, as when the subject responds in one way to a reinforced stimulus and in another to an unreinforced stimulus. **3.** Acting differently toward some people on the basis of the social class or category to which they belong rather than their individual qualities.

dis·crim·i·na·tion score (dis-krim'i-nā'shŭn skōr) The percentage of words that a subject can repeat correctly from a list of phonetically balanced words presented at 25–40 dB above the speech reception threshold.

dis·cus, pl. **dis·ci** (dis'kŭs, dis'sī) [TA] SYN lamella (2).

dis·cus ar·ti·cu·la·ris (dis'kŭs ahr-tik-yū-lā'ris) [TA] SYN articular disc.

dis·cu·ti·ent (dis-kyū'shĕnt) An agent that helps to break down necrotic tissue.

dis·ease (di-zēz') **1.** An interruption, cessation, or disorder of body functions, systems, or organs. SYN illness, morbus, sickness. **2.** A morbid entity characterized usually by at least two of these criteria: recognized etiologic agent(s), identifiable group of signs and symptoms, or consistent anatomic alterations. SEE ALSO syndrome.

dis·ease de·ter·mi·nants (di-zēz' dĕ-tĕr'mi-nănts) Variables that influence frequency of occurrence and/or distribution of any disease; include specific disease agents, host characteristics, and environmental factors.

dis·ease-mod·i·fy·ing an·ti·rheu·ma·tic drugs (DMARD) (di-zēz' mod'i-fī-ing an'tē-rū-mat'ik drŭgz) Agents that apparently alter the course and progression

of rheumatoid arthritis, as opposed to more rapidly acting substances that suppress inflammation and decrease pain, but do not prevent cartilage or bone erosion or progressive disability.

dis·en·gage·ment (dis-ĕn-gāj'mĕnt) **1.** Setting free or extricating; in childbirth, the emergence of the head from the vulva. **2.** Ascent of the presenting part from the pelvis after the inlet has been negotiated.

dis·e·qui·lib·ri·um, dys·e·quil·i·bri·um (dis-ē-kwi-lib'rē-ŭm) A disturbance or absence of balance.

dis·flu·en·cy (dis-flū'ĕn-sē) Inability to produce a smooth flow of speech sounds in connected discourse; the flow of speech is characterized by frequent interruptions and repetitions. SEE stuttering.

dis·ger·mi·no·ma (dis-jĕr'mi-nō'mă) SYN dysgerminoma.

dis·im·pac·tion (dis-im-pak'shŭn) **1.** Separation of impaction in a fractured bone. **2.** Removal of impacted feces, usually manually.

dis·in·fec·tant (dis-in-fek'tănt) **1.** Capable of destroying pathogenic microorganisms or inhibiting their growth. **2.** An agent that possesses the capacity to disinfect.

dis·in·hi·bi·tion (dis'in-hi-bish'ŭn) **1.** Removal of an inhibition, such as by a toxic or organic process. **2.** Removal of an inhibitory effect by a stimulus, as when a conditioned reflex has undergone extinction but is restored by some extraneous stimulus.

dis·in·te·gra·tion (dis-in'tĕ-grā'shŭn) **1.** Loss or separation of the component parts of a substance, as in catabolism or decay. **2.** Disorganization of psychic and behavioral processes. SYN decay (7).

dis·lo·ca·tion frac·ture (dis-lō-kā'shŭn frak'shŭr) A fracture of a bone near a joint with concomitant dislocation from that joint.

dis·lo·ca·tions (dis-lō-kā'shŭnz) Displacements of an organ or any part; specifically disturbance or disarrangement of the normal relation of the bones entering into the formation of a joint. SYN luxation (1).

dis·or·der (dis-ōr′dĕr) A disturbance of function or structure, resulting from a genetic or embryologic failure in development or from exogenous factors such as poison, trauma, or disease.

dis·order of sleep (dis-ōr′dĕr slēp) Any of a range of problems that interfere with sleep (e.g., insomnia, sleep apnea).

dis·or·ga·ni·za·tion (dis-ōr′găn-i-zā′shŭn) Destruction of an organ or tissue with consequent loss of function.

dis·o·ri·en·ta·tion (dis-ōr′ē-ĕn-tā′shŭn) Loss of the sense of familiarity with one's surroundings (time, place, and person); loss of one's bearings.

dis·pen·sa·ry (dis-pen′săr-ē) 1. A physician's office, especially the office of one who dispenses medicines. 2. The office of a hospital pharmacist, where medicines are distributed on physicians' orders. 3. An outpatient department of a hospital.

dis·pense (disp) (dis-pens′) To give out medicine and other necessities to the sick; to fill a medical prescription.

di·sper·my, di·sperm·i·a (dī′spĕr-mē, -mē-ă) Entrance of two sperms into one oocyte.

dis·perse (dis-pĕrs′) To dissipate, to cause disappearance of, to scatter, to dilute.

dis·per·sion (dis-pĕr′zhŭn) 1. The act of dispersing or of being dispersed. 2. Incorporation of the particles of one substance into the mass of another, including solutions, suspensions, and colloidal dispersions (solutions). 3. Specifically, what is usually called a colloidal solution. 4. The extent or degree to which values of a statistical frequency distribution are scattered about a mean or median value.

dis·per·sion col·loid (dis-pĕr′zhŭn kol′oyd) SYN dispersoid.

dis·per·soid (dis-pĕr′soyd) A colloidal solution in which the dispersed phase can be concentrated by centrifugation. SYN dispersion colloid.

dis·place·ment (dis-plās′mĕnt) 1. Removal from the normal location or position. 2. The adding to a fluid (particularly a gas) in an open vessel one of greater density whereby the first is expelled. 3. CHEMISTRY a change in which one element, radical, or molecule is replaced by another, or in which one element exchanges electric charges with another by reduction or oxidation. 4. PSYCHIATRY the transfer of impulses from one expression to another, as from fighting to talking.

dis·pro·por·tion (dis′prŏ-pōr′shŭn) Lack of proportion or symmetry.

dis·sect (di-sekt′) 1. To cut apart or separate the tissues of the body for study. 2. SURGERY to separate structures along natural lines or planes of cleavage.

dis·sec·tion (di-sek′shŭn) The act of dissecting. SYN anatomy (3), necrotomy (1).

dis·sem·i·nat·ed (di-sem′i-nā-tĕd) Widely scattered throughout an organ, tissue, or the body.

dis·sem·i·nat·ed in·tra·vas·cu·lar co·ag·u·la·tion (DIC) (di-sem′i-nā′tĕd in′tră-vas′kyū-lăr kō-ag′yū-lā′shŭn) A hemorrhagic syndrome that occurs following the uncontrolled activation of clotting factors and fibrinolytic enzymes throughout small blood vessels; fibrin is deposited, platelets and clotting factors are consumed, and fibrin degradation products inhibit fibrin polymerization, resulting in tissue necrosis and bleeding. SEE ALSO consumption coagulopathy.

dis·sem·i·nat·ed scler·o·sis (DS) (di-sem′i-nā-tĕd skler-ō′sis) SYN multiple sclerosis.

dis·sem·i·nat·ed tu·ber·cu·lo·sis (di-sem′i-nā-tĕd tū-bĕr′kyū-lō′sis) SYN acute tuberculosis.

dis·sim·u·la·tion (di-sim′yū-lā′shŭn) Concealment of the truth about a situation, especially about a state of health or during a mental status examination, as by a malingerer or someone with a factitious disorder.

dis·so·ci·at·ed an·es·the·si·a (dis-sō′sē-ā-tĕd an′es-thē′zē-ă) Loss of some types of sensation with persistence of others; most often used in context of nerve blocks, wherein a loss of sensation for pain and temperature occurs without loss of tactile sense.

dis·so·ci·at·ed ver·ti·cal de·vi·a·tion (di-sō′sē-āt-ĕd vĕr′ti-kăl dē-vē-ā′shŭn) A tendency, often associated with congenital esotropia, in which an eye elevates, abducts, and extorts when covered, in violation of Hering law.

dis·so·ci·a·tion, dis·as·so·ci·a·tion (di-sō′sē-ā′shŭn, dis′ă-) **1.** Separation, or a dissolution of relations. **2.** The change of a complex chemical compound into a simpler one by any lytic reaction, by ionization, by heterolysis, or by homolysis. **3.** An unconscious separation of a group of mental processes from the rest. **4.** A state used as an essential part of a technique for healing in psychology and psychotherapy, for instance in hypnotherapy or the neurolinguistic programming technique of time-line therapy. SEE ALSO Time-Line therapy. **5.** The translocation between a large chromosome and a small supernumerary one. **6.** Separation of the nuclear components of a heterokaryotic dikaryon.

dis·so·ci·a·tion move·ment (di-sō′sē-ā′shŭn mūv′mĕnt) **1.** Physical movement that evidences the ability to differentiate among movements of different parts of the body. **2.** Stabilization of one part of the body or movement of one part in the opposite direction of another (e.g., pelvic trunk as used in ambulation).

dis·so·ci·a·tive dis·or·ders (di-sō′sē-ă-tiv dis-ōr′dĕrz) Group of mental states characterized by disturbances in the functions of identity, memory, consciousness, or perception of the environment.

dis·so·ci·a·tive i·den·ti·ty dis·or·der (di-sō′sē-ă-tiv ī-den′ti-tē dis-ōr′dĕr) Condition in which two or more distinct conscious personalities alternately prevail in someone, sometimes without one personality being aware of the other(s).

dis·so·ci·a·tive re·ac·tion (di-sō′sē-ă-tiv rē-ak′shŭn) Reaction characterized by such dissociative behavior as amnesia, fugues, sleepwalking, and dream states.

dis·so·lut·ion (dis′ō-lū′shŭn) The act of breaking down into component parts.

dis·solve (di-zolv′) To change or cause to change from a solid to a dispersed form by immersion in a fluid of suitable properties.

dis·tal (dis′tăl) [TA] **1.** Situated away from the center of the body, or from the point of origin; specifically applied to the extremity or distant part of a limb or organ. **2.** DENTISTRY away from the median sagittal plane of the face, following the curvature of the dental arch. SYN distalis.

dis·tal ac·i·nar em·phy·se·ma (dis′tăl as′i-năr em-fi-sē′mă) SYN paraseptal emphysema.

dis·tal an·gle (dis′tăl ang′gĕl) That formed by the meeting of the distal with the labial, buccal, or lingual surface of a tooth.

dis·tal end (dis′tăl end) The posterior extremity of a dental appliance. SYN heel(2).

dis·tal il·e·i·tis, ter·mi·nal il·e·i·tis (dis′tăl il′ē-ī′tis, tĕr′mi-năl il′ē-ī′tis) SYN regional enteritis.

dis·tal in·ter·pha·lan·ge·al joints (DIP) (dis′tăl in′tĕr-fă-lan′jē-ăl joynts) The synovial joints between the middle and distal phalanges of the fingers and of the toes.

dis·ta·lis (dis-tā′lis) [TA] SYN distal.

dis·tal my·op·a·thy (dis′tăl mī-op′ă-thē) Neurologic disorder affecting predominantly the distal portions of the limbs; onset is usually after age 40 years, with weakness and wasting of small muscles of the hands.

dis·tal part of pros·ta·tic u·re·thra (dis′tăl pahrt pros-tat′ik yū-rē′thră) [TA] Portion of prostatic urethra inferior to the merging of the urinary and genital tracts at the openings of the ejaculatory ducts. SYN pars distalis urethrae prostaticae [TA].

dis·tant flap (dis′tănt flap) A flap in which the donor site is distant from the recipient area.

dis·ten·tion, dis·ten·sion (dis-ten′shŭn) The act or state of being distended or stretched. SEE ALSO dilation.

dis•ti•chi•a•sis (dis'ti-kī'ă-sis) A congenital, abnormal, accessory row of eyelashes.

dis•til•la•tion (dis'ti-lā'shŭn) Volatilization of a liquid by heat and subsequent condensation of the vapor; in a liquid mixture, a means of separating the volatile from the nonvolatile, or the more volatile from the less volatile part.

dis•tilled wa•ter (DW, aq. dist) (distild´ waw´tĕr) Water purified by distillation.

dis•to•buc•co•oc•clu•sal (dis'tō-bŭk'ŏ-ŏ-klū'zăl) Relating to the distal, buccal, and occlusal surfaces of a premolar or molar tooth; denoting especially the angle formed by the junction of these surfaces.

dis•to•buc•co•pul•pal (dis'tō-bŭk'ŏ-pŭl'păl) Relating to the point (trihedral) angle formed by the junction of a distal, buccal, and pulpal walls of a cavity.

dis•to•cer•vi•cal (dis'tō-sĕr'vi-kăl) Relating to the line angle formed by the junction of the distal and cervical (gingival) walls of a class V cavity.

dis•to•clu•sion, dis•to•oc•clu•sion (dis'tō-klū'zhŭn, dis'tō-ŏ-klū'zhŭn) A malocclusion in which the mandibular arch articulates with the maxillary arch in a position distal to normal.

dis•to•lin•gual (dis'tō-ling'gwăl) Relating to the distal and lingual surfaces of a tooth; denoting the angle formed by their junction.

dis•to•lin•guo•oc•clu•sal (dis'tō-ling' gwŏ-ŏ-klū'zăl) Relating to the distal, lingual, and occlusal surfaces of a bicuspid or molar tooth.

dis•to•mi•a•sis, dis•to•ma•to•sis (dis'tō-mī'ă-sis, -mă-tō'sis) Presence in any of the organs or tissues of digenetic flukes formerly classified as *Distoma* or *Distomum;* in general, infection by any parasitic trematode or fluke.

dis•to•mo•lar (dis'tō-mō'lăr) A supernumerary tooth located in the region posterior to the third molar tooth.

dis•tor•tion (dis-tōr'shŭn) **1.** PSYCHIATRY a defense mechanism that helps to repress or disguise unacceptable thoughts.

2. DENTISTRY permanent deformation of the impression material after the registration of an imprint. **3.** A twisting out of normal shape or form. **4.** OPHTHALMOLOGY unequal magnification over a field of view.

dis•trac•tion (dis-trak'shŭn) **1.** Difficulty or impossibility of concentration or fixation of the mind. **2.** Manipulation or traction of a limb to separate bony fragments or joint surfaces.

dis•trac•tion os•te•o•gen•e•sis (dis-trak'shŭn os'tē-ō-jen'ĕ-sis) A technique of inducing new bone formation by dividing a bone and applying tension through an external fixation device to lengthen the bone.

dis•trib•ut•ing ar•te•ry (dis-trib´yūt-ing ahr´tĕr-ē) SYN muscular artery.

dis•tri•bu•tion (dis'tri-byū'shŭn) **1.** The passage of the branches of arteries or nerves to the tissues and organs. **2.** The area in which the branches of an artery or a nerve terminate, or the area supplied by such an artery or nerve. **3.** Passage of an agent through blood or lymph to body sites remote from the site(s) of contact and absorption; thus called systemic distribution. **4.** The relative numbers of people in each of various categories or populations, such as in different age, sex, or occupational samples. **5.** The pattern of occurrence of a substance within or between cells, tissues, organisms, or taxa.

dis•trix (dis'triks) Splitting of the hairs at their ends.

di•sul•fide bridge (dī-sul'fīd brij) **1.** Linkage between two cysteinyl residues in a polypeptide or oligopeptide or in a protein. **2.** Any disulfide linkage between any thiol-containing moieties of a larger molecule. SYN cystine bridge.

di•sul•fi•ram (DSF) (dī-sŭl'fi-ram) An antioxidant that interferes with the normal metabolic degradation of alcohol in the body, resulting in increased acetaldehyde concentrations in blood and tissues. Used in the treatment of chronic alcoholism; when taken regularly in chronic alcoholism, it can lower the risk of relapse by inducing severe malaise and nausea if alcohol is consumed. Also used as a chelator in copper and nickel poisoning. SYN tetraethylthiuram disulfide.

Ditt·rich plug (dit′rik plŭg) A minute, dirty-grayish, foul-smelling mass of bacteria and fatty acid crystals in the sputum in pulmonary gangrene and fetid bronchitis.

di·u·re·sis (dī-yūr-ē′sis) Excretion of urine; commonly denotes production of unusually large volumes.

di·u·ret·ic (dī-yūr-et′ik) **1.** Promoting excretion of urine. **2.** An agent that increases the amount of urine excreted.

di·ur·nal (dī-ūr′năl) **1.** Pertaining to the daylight hours; opposite of nocturnal. **2.** Repeating once each 24 hours (e.g., a diurnal variation or a diurnal rhythm). Cf. circadian.

di·ur·nal en·ur·e·sis (dī-ūr′năl en-yūr-ē′sis) Urinary accidents during wakefulness.

di·va·lent (dī-vā′lĕnt) SYN bivalent (1).

di·var·i·ca·tion (dī′var-i-kā′shŭn) SYN diastasis (1).

di·ver·gence (di-věr′jĕns) **1.** A moving or spreading apart or in different directions. **2.** The spreading of branches of the neuron to form synapses with several other neurons.

di·ver·gence in·suf·fi·cien·cy (di-věr′jĕns in′sŭ-fish′ĕn-sē) That condition in which an exophoria or exotropia is more marked for near vision than for far vision.

di·ver·gence pa·re·sis (di-věr′jĕns pă-rē′sis) An esodeviation of the eyes that is greater in the distance than near, which may be a sign of central nervous system disease or a mild bilateral sixth cranial nerve palsy.

di·ver·gent stra·bis·mus (di-věr′jĕnt stră-biz′mŭs) SYN exotropia.

di·ver·sion (di-věr′zhŭn) The process of rerouting an ambulance to another facility other than the closest appropriate facility.

di·ver·tic·u·lar (dī′věr-tik′yū-lăr) Relating to a diverticulum.

di·ver·tic·u·lar dis·ease (dī-věr-tik′yū-lăr di-zēz′) Symptomatic congenital or acquired diverticula of any portion of the gastrointestinal tract.

di·ver·tic·u·lec·to·my (dī′věr-tik′yū-lek′tŏ-mē) Excision of a diverticulum.

di·ver·tic·u·li·tis (dī′věr-tik′yū-lī′tis) Inflammation of a diverticulum, especially of the small pockets in the colon wall that fill with stagnant fecal material and become inflamed.

di·ver·tic·u·lum, pl. **di·ver·tic·u·la** (dī′věr-tik′yū-lŭm, -lă) [TA] A pouch or sac opening from a tubular or saccular organ, such as the gut or bladder.

di·vid·ed dose (di-vīd′ĕd dōs) A definite fraction of a full dose; given at shorter intervals than a full dose.

div·ing goi·ter (dīv′ing goy′tĕr) A freely movable goiter that is sometimes above and sometimes below the sternal notch.

di·vi·sion (div) (di-vizh′ŭn) A separating into two or more parts. SEE ALSO ramus.

di·vi·sion·al block (di-vizh′ŭn-ăl blok) Arrested impulse in one of the assumed two main divisions of the left branch of the atrioventricular bundle. SYN hemiblock.

di·vulse (di-vŭls′) To tear away or apart.

di·vul·sion (di-vŭl′shŭn) **1.** Removal of a part by tearing. **2.** Forcible dilation of the walls of a cavity or canal.

di·vul·sor (di-vŭl′sŏr) An instrument for forcible dilation of the urethra or other canal or cavity.

Dix-Hall·pike ma·neu·ver (diks-hawl′pīk mă-nū′věr) Test for eliciting paroxysmal vertigo and nystagmus in which the patient is brought from the sitting to the supine position with the head hanging over the examining table and turned to the right or left.

di·zy·got·ic, di·zy·gous (DZ, diz) (dī-zī-got′ik, dī-zī′gŭs) Relating to twins derived from two separate zygotes, i.e., bearing the same genetic relationship as full sibs but sharing a common intrauterine environment.

di·zy·got·ic twins (dī-zī-got′ik twinz)

Twins derived from two zygotes. SYN fraternal twins.

diz·zi·ness (dĭz′ĕ-nĕs) Imprecise term commonly used by patients in an attempt to describe various symptoms such as faintness, vertigo (q.v.), or disequilibrium.

♻ DL- Prefix (in small capital letters) denoting a substance consisting of equal quantities of the two enantiomorphs, D and L; replaces the older *dl-* (in lower case italics) as a more exact definition of structure.

DNA li·gase (lī′gās) Enzyme that leads to formation of a phosphodiester bond at a break of one strand in duplex DNA.

DNA mar·kers (mahr′kĕrz) Segments of chromosomal DNA known to be linked with heritable traits or diseases.

DNA pol·ym·er·ase (pŏ-lim′ĕr-ās) SEE nucleotidyltransferases. SEE ALSO polymerase.

DNA vi·rus (vī′rŭs) A major group of animal viruses in which the core consists of deoxyribonucleic acid (DNA); includes parvoviruses, papovaviruses, adenoviruses, herpesviruses, poxviruses, and other unclassified DNA viruses. SYN deoxyribovirus.

DNR Abbreviation for do not resuscitate. SEE do not attempt resuscitation.

DO Abbreviation for Doctor of Osteopathy. SEE osteopathy.

doc·tor (dok′tŏr) 1. A title conferred by a university on one who has followed a prescribed course of study, or given as a title of distinction; as doctor of medicine, laws, philosophy, and other disciplines. 2. A physician, especially one on whom has been conferred the degree of M.D. or D.O. degree. More generally, an independent practitioner in any health care profession (e.g., dentistry, optometry, podiatry).

Doc·tor of Phys·i·cal Ther·a·py (D.P.T.) (dok′tŏr fiz′i-kăl thār′ă-pē) Highest degree conferred on students in the profession of physical therapy.

dol (dōl) A unit measure of pain.

♻ **dolicho-** Prefix meaning long.

doll's eye sign (dolz ī sīn) Reflex movement of the eyes in the opposite direction to that in which the head is moved, e.g., the eyes being lowered as the head is raised, and the reverse (Cantelli sign); an indication of functional integrity of the brainstem tegmental pathways and cranial nerves involved in eye movement.

do·lor (dō′lŏr) Pain, as one of the four signs of inflammation (d., calor, rubor, tumor) enunciated by Celsus.

do·lor·if·ic (dō-lŏr-if′ik) Pain-producing.

do·lor·im·e·try (dō-lŏr-im′ĕ-trē) The measurement of pain.

do·main (dō-mān′) 1. Homologous unit of 110–120 amino acids, groups of which make up the light and heavy chains of the immunoglobulin molecule; each serves a specific function. 2. A region of a protein having some distinctive physical feature or role. 3. An independently folded, globular structure composed of one section of a polypeptide chain.

dom·i·nance (dom′i-năns) The state of being dominant.

dom·i·nant (dom′i-nănt) 1. Ruling or controlling. 2. GENETICS denoting an allele possessed by one of the parents of a hybrid that is expressed in the latter to the exclusion of a contrasting allele (the recessive) from the other parent.

dom·i·nant al·lele (dom′i-nănt ă-lēl′) Variant gene form that remains capable of expression although carried by only one of a genetic pair.

dom·i·nant hem·i·sphere (dom′i-nănt hem′is-fēr) That cerebral hemisphere containing the representation of speech and controlling the arm and leg used preferentially in skilled movements; usually the left hemisphere.

dom·i·nant i·de·a (dom′i-nănt ī-dē′ă) An idea that governs all one's actions and thoughts.

Don·ders law (don′dĕrz law) The rotation of the eyeball is determined by the distance of the object from the median plane and the line of the horizon.

Done no·mo·gram (dōn nō′mō-gram) One in common use that describes toxicity resulting from salicylate overdose based on blood levels sampled at a fixed timepoint postingestion (usually 6 hours). Regarded by some clinicians as unreliable.

do·nor (dō′nŏr) **1.** A person from whom blood, tissue, or an organ is taken for transplantation. **2.** A compound that will transfer an atom or a radical to an acceptor. **3.** An atom that readily yields electrons to an acceptor.

do·nor in·sem·i·na·tion (DI) (dō′nŏr in-sem′i-nā′shŭn) SYN heterologous insemination.

do not at·tempt re·sus·ci·ta·tion (DNAR) (dū not ă-tempt′ rē-sus′i-tā′ shŭn) Directive to health care workers from a patient who has expressed in writing a wish not to be resuscitated in the event of cardiac or respiratory arrest.

do·pa (dō′pă) An intermediate in the catabolism of L-phenylalanine and L-tyrosine, and in the biosynthesis of norepinephrine, epinephrine, and melanin; the L form, levodopa, is biologically active.

do·pa·mine (DM) (dō′pă-mēn) An intermediate in tyrosine metabolism and precursor of norepinephrine and epinephrine.

do·pa·mine hy·dro·chlor·ide (dō′pă-mēn hī′drŏ-klōr′īd) Biogenic amine and neural transmitter substance, used as a vasopressor agent for treatment of shock.

do·pa·min·er·gic (dō′pă-min-ĕr′jik) Pertaining to the action of dopamine or to neural or metabolic pathways in which it functions as a transmitter.

dope (dōp) **1.** Any drug, either stimulating or depressing, administered for its temporary effect, or taken habitually or addictively. **2.** To administer or take such a drug.

Dopp·ler ech·o·car·di·og·ra·phy (dop′ lĕr ek′ō-kahr-dē-og′ră-fē) Use of Doppler ultrasonography techniques to augment two-dimensional echocardiography by allowing velocities to be registered in the echocardiographic image. SEE ALSO duplex ultrasonography, Doppler ultrasonography.

Dopp·ler ef·fect (dop′lĕr e-fekt′) Change

in frequency observed when the sound source and observer are in relative motion away from or toward each other. SEE ALSO Doppler shift.

Dopp·ler op·er·a·tion (dop′lĕr op′ĕr-ā′shŭn) Destruction of periarterial sympathetic nerves by local injection of phenol. SYN chemical sympathectomy.

Dopp·ler shift (dop′lĕr shift) The magnitude of the frequency change in hertz when sound and observer are in relative motion away from or toward each other. SEE ALSO Doppler effect.

Dopp·ler ul·tra·son·og·ra·phy (dop′ lĕr ŭl′tră-sŏ-nog′ră-fē) Application of the Doppler effect in ultrasound to detect movement of scatterers (usually red blood cells) by the analysis of the change in frequency of the returning echoes.

Dor fun·dop·li·ca·tion (dōr fŭn′dō-pli-kā′shŭn) A partial (180 degree) and anterior fundoplication, popular in Europe and South America; often used with myotomy to treat achalasia.

dor·sad (dōr′sad) Toward or in the direction of the back.

dor·sal (dōr′săl) **1.** Pertaining to the back or any dorsum. **2.** SYN posterior (2).

dor·sal de·cu·bi·tus (dōr′săl dĕ-kyū′bi-tŭs) Lying on one's back; supine.

dor·sal flex·ure (dōr′săl flek′shŭr) A flexure in the middorsal region in the embryo.

dor·sal plate (dōr′săl plāt) SEE roof plate.

dor·sal re·cum·bent po·si·tion (dōr′ săl rē-kŭm′bĕnt pŏ-zish′ŭn) SYN supine.

dor·si·flex·ion (dōr′si-flek′shŭn) Turning upward of the foot or toes or of the hand or fingers.

dor·si·spi·nal (dōr′si-spī′năl) Relating to the vertebral column, especially to its dorsal aspect.

dor·so·ceph·a·lad (dōr′sō-sef′ă-lad) Toward the occiput, or back of the head.

dor·so·lat·er·al (dōr′sō-lat′ĕr-ăl) Relating to the back and the side.

dor·sum (dōr´sŭm) [TA] **1.** The back of the body. **2.** The upper or posterior surface, or the back, of any part.

dor·sum sel·lae (dōr´sŭm sel´ē) [TA] Square portion of bone on the body of the sphenoid posterior to the sella turcica or hypophysial fossa. SYN dorsum ephippii.

dos·age (dō´săj) **1.** The giving of medicine or other therapeutic agent in prescribed amounts. **2.** The size, frequency, and number of doses of medicine to be given. USAGE NOTE sometimes incorrectly used for dose. Cf. dose.

dose (dōs) **1.** The quantity of a drug or other remedy to be taken or applied all at one time or in fractional amounts within a given period. USAGE NOTE Sometimes incorrectly used for dosage (q.v.). **2.** NUCLEAR MEDICINE amount of energy absorbed per unit mass of irradiated material (absorbed dose). **3.** RADIATION THERAPY the energy absorbed per unit mass of irradiated material.

dose cal·i·bra·tions (dōs kal´i-brā´shŭnz) Adjustments in dosage of a pharmacotherapeutic agent as required by circumstances.

dose e·quiv·a·lent (dōs ē-kwiv´ă-lĕnt) In radiation therapy, product of absorbed dose and the quality factor; the SI unit of dose equivalent is sievert (Sv).

dose rate (dōs rāt) In radiation therapy, rate at which radiation is delivered.

dose-re·sponse re·la·tion·ship (dōs rē-spons´ rē-lā´shŭn-ship) Direct association between a stimulus and a desired outcome (e.g., quantity of physical activity and good health).

do·sim·e·try (dō-sim´ĕ-trē) Measurement of radiation exposure, especially x-rays or gamma rays; calculation of radiation dose from internally administered radionuclides.

dot (dot) A small spot.

dou·ble a·or·tic arch (DAA) (dŭb´ĕl ā-ōr´tik ahrch) Congenital malformation of the aorta that splits and has a right and a left arch instead of a single arch.

dou·ble blind ex·per·i·ment (dŭb´ĕl blīnd eks-per´i-mĕnt) An investigation conducted with neither experimenter nor subjects knowing which experiment is the control; prevents bias in recording results.

dou·ble-chan·nel cath·e·ter (dŭb´ĕl-chan´ĕl kath´ĕ-tĕr) A catheter with two lumens, allowing irrigation and aspiration.

dou·ble el·e·va·tor pal·sy (dŭb´ĕl el´ĕ-vā-tŏr pawl´zē) Limited elevation of an eye in abduction and adduction, implying paresis of the superior rectus and inferior oblique muscles, although many cases are due to restriction of the inferior rectus muscle.

dou·ble he·lix (dŭb´ĕl hē´liks) SYN Watson-Crick helix.

dou·ble pneu·mo·ni·a (dŭb´ĕl nū-mō´nē-ă) Lobar pneumonia involving both lungs.

dou·ble re·frac·tion (dŭb´ĕl rē-frak´shŭn) The property of having more than one refractive index according to the direction of the transmitted light. SYN birefringence.

dou·ble ring sign (dŭb´ĕl ring sīn) Two concentric rings around the optic nerve characteristic of optic nerve hypoplasia.

dou·ble vi·sion (dŭb´ĕl vizh´ŭn) SYN diplopia.

dou·ble void (dŭb´ĕl voyd) A urinalysis procedure in which the first sample is discarded; a second, obtained 30 to 45 minutes later, is tested.

dou·bly armed su·ture (dŭb´lē ahrmd sū´chŭr) A suture with a needle attached at both ends. SYN cobbler's suture.

douche (dūsh) **1.** A current of water, gas, or vapor directed against a surface or projected into a cavity. **2.** An instrument for giving a douche. **3.** To apply a douche.

Doug·las bag (dŭg´lăs bag) A large sack in which expired gas is collected for several minutes to determine oxygen consumption in humans under conditions of actual work.

Doug·las pouch, Doug·las space

(dug′lăs powch, spās) Rectouterine pouch lined with parietal peritoneum; mass in this area is palpable during rectal examination.

dow·a·ger hump (dow′ă-jěr hŭmp) Postmenopausal cervical kyphosis of older women due to osteoporosis and compression fractures of vertebra.

dow·el (dow′ěl) **1.** A cast gold or preformed metal pin placed into a root canal for the purpose of providing retention for a crown. **2.** A preformed metal pin placed in a copper-plated die to provide a die stem. **3.** A pin or rod that aligns or joins two structures by fitting into holes in both of them; dowels of various materials are used in orthopaedic surgery and dentistry.

down reg·u·la·tion (down′ reg′yū-lā′shŭn) Development of a refractory or tolerant state consequent on repeated administration of a pharmacologically or physiologically active substance; often accompanied by an initial decrease in affinity of receptors for the agent and a subsequent diminution in the number of receptors.

Down syn·drome (down sin′drōm) A chromosomal dysgenesis syndrome consisting of a variable constellation of abnormalities caused by triplication or translocation of chromosome 21. The abnormalities include mental retardation, retarded growth, flat hypoplastic face with short nose, prominent epicanthic skin folds, small, low-set ears with prominent antihelix, fissured and thickened tongue, laxness of joint ligaments, pelvic dysplasia, broad hands and feet, stubby fingers, and transverse palmar crease. Lenticular opacities and heart disease are common. SYN trisomy 21 syndrome.

dox·o·ru·bi·cin (DOX) (doks′ō-rū′bi-sin) An antineoplastic antibiotic isolated from *Streptomyces peucetius;* also used in cytogenetics to produce Q-type chromosome bands.

dox·y·cy·cline (DO, doxy) (doks′ē-sī′klēn) A broad-spectrum antibiotic.

DP Abbreviation for Doctor of Pharmacy; Doctor of Podiatry.

DPH Abbreviation for Doctor of Public Health; Doctor of Public Hygiene; Diploma of Public Health.

dra·cun·cu·li·a·sis, dra·cun·cu·lo·sis (dră-kŭng′kyū-lī′ă-sis, -kyū-lō′sis) Infection with *Dracunculus medinensis*.

Dra·cun·cu·lus (dră-kŭng′kyū-lŭs) A genus of nematodes with some resemblance to true filarial worms; adults are larger and the intermediate host is a freshwater crustacean rather than an insect.

drain (drān) **1.** To remove fluid from a cavity (e.g., to drain an abscess). **2.** A device, usually in the shape of a tube or wick, for draining fluid as it collects in a cavity, especially a wound cavity.

drain·age (drān′ăj) Continuous flow or withdrawal of fluids from a wound or other cavity.

drain·age tube (drān′ăj tūb) A tube introduced into a wound or cavity to facilitate removal of a fluid.

dream (drēm) Mental activity during sleep in which events, thoughts, emotions, and images are experienced as real.

dress·ing (dres′ing) The material applied, or the application itself of material, to a wound for protection, absorbance, and drainage.

dress·ing for·ceps (dres′ing fōr′seps) A forceps for general use in dressing wounds, removing fragments of necrotic tissue, small foreign bodies, and other functions.

Dress·ler beat (dres′lěr bēt) Fusion beat interrupting a ventricular tachycardia and producing a normally narrow QRS complex as a result of the fusion of two impulses, one impulse from the ventricular tachycardia and the other from a supraventricular focus; presence strongly supports diagnosis of ventricular tachycardia by interruption of it.

dried yeast (drīd yēst) Cells of a suitable strain of *Saccharomyces cerevisiae;* brewers' dried yeast, debittered brewers' dried yeast, or primary dried yeast are the sources of dried yeast; it contains not less than 45% of protein, and in 1 g not less than 0.3 mg of nicotinic acid, 0.04 mg riboflavin, and 0.12 mg thiamin hydrochloride; used as a dietary supplement.

drift (drift) **1.** A gradual movement, as from an original position. **2.** A gradual change in the value of a random variable over time as a result of various factors, some random and some systematic effects of trend or manipulation.

Drin·ker res·pi·ra·tor (dringk'ĕr res'pir-ā'tŏr) Mechanical respirator in which the body (except the head) is encased within a metal tank, which is sealed at the neck with an airtight gasket; artificial respiration is induced by making the air pressure inside negative. SYN iron lung, tank respirator.

drip (drip) **1.** To flow a drop at a time. **2.** A flowing in drops; often associated with intravenous infusion.

Dripps clas·si·fi·ca·tion (drips klas'i-fi-kā'shŭn) System used by anesthesiologists to describe physical status of patient. SYN ASA classification.

driv·ing (drīv'ing) The induction of a frequency in the electroencephalogram by sensory stimulation at this frequency.

drom·e·da·ry hump (drom'ĕ-dār-ē hŭmp) Supernumerary mass of nonpathologic tissue found on the lateral portion of the left kidney.

drom·o·graph (drom'ō-graf) An instrument for recording the rapidity of the blood circulation.

drom·o·ma·ni·a (drom'ō-mā'nē-ă) An uncontrollable impulse to wander or travel.

dro·mo·tro·pic (drom'ō-trō'pik) Influencing the velocity of conduction of excitation, as in nerve or cardiac muscle fibers.

dro·nab·i·nol (drō-nab'i-nol) A major psychoactive substance present in *Cannabis sativa*, used therapeutically as an antinauseant to control the nausea and vomiting associated with cancer chemotherapy.

droop·ing lil·y sign (drūp'ing lil'ē sīn) In urography, a sign of a double renal collecting system, with an obstruction of the upper system depressing the opacified calyces of the lower system, so they appear to droop.

drop (drop) **1.** To fall, or to be dispensed or poured in globules. **2.** A liquid globule. **3.** A volume of liquid regarded as a unit of dosage, equivalent in the case of water to about 1 minim (20 drops are equal to 1 mL).

drop at·tack (drop ă-tak') An episode of sudden falling that occurs during standing or walking, without warning and without loss of consciousness, vertigo, or postictal behavior. The patients are usually elderly and have normal findings on electroencephalograms; of unknown cause.

drop·foot, drop foot (drop'fut, drop fut) SEE footdrop.

drop hand (drop hand) SYN wrist-drop.

drop·let in·fec·tion (drop'lĕt in-fek'shŭn) Infection acquired through the inhalation of droplets or aerosols of saliva or sputum containing virus or other microorganisms expelled by another person during sneezing, coughing, laughing, or talking.

drop·let pre·cau·tions (drop'lĕt prĕ-kaw'shŭnz) Procedures that reduce the risk of droplet-borne infections. Transmission through droplets occurs when the droplets contact the conjunctivae or the nasal or oral mucous membranes of a susceptible patient. Masks as well as standard precautions must be used when in the infected patient's room. SEE standard precautions, Universal Precautions.

drop·per (drop'ĕr) SYN instillator.

drop·sy (drop'sē) Older term for generalized edema, most often associated with cardiac failure.

drown·ing (drow'ning) Death from suffocation induced by immersion in water or other fluid, with filling of pulmonary air spaces and passages with fluid to the detriment of gas exchange.

drug (drŭg) **1.** A therapeutic agent; any substance, other than food, used in the prevention, diagnosis, alleviation, treatment, or cure of disease. SEE ALSO agent, medication. **2.** To administer or take a drug, usually implying that an excessive quantity or a narcotic is involved. **3.** General term for any substance, stimulating or depressing, which can be habituating or addictive, especially a narcotic.

drug a·buse (drŭg ă-byūs´) Habitual use of drugs not needed for therapeutic purposes (e.g., such as solely to alter one's mood, affect, or state of consciousness) or to affect a body function unnecessarily (e.g., laxative abuse); nonmedical use of drugs.

drug ad·dic·tion (drŭg ă-dik´shŭn) Disorder marked by a consuming urge to continue consuming a drug or substance regardless of consequence.

drug al·ler·gy (drŭg al´ĕr-jē) Sensitivity (hypersensitivity) to a drug or other chemical.

drug e·rup·tion (drŭg ē-rŭp´shŭn) One caused by ingestion, injection, or inhalation of a drug, most often due to allergic sensitization; reactions to drugs applied to the cutaneous surface are not generally designated as drug eruption, but as contact-type dermatitis. SYN dermatitis medicamentosa, dermatosis medicamentosa, drug rash, medicinal eruption.

drug-fast (drŭg-fast) Pertaining to microorganisms that resist or become tolerant to an antibacterial agent.

drug fe·ver (drŭg fē´vĕr) One resulting from an allergic reaction to a drug that clears rapidly on discontinuation of the drug.

drug·gist (drŭg´ist) Older but still common term for pharmacist.

drug-in·duced lu·pus (DIL) (drŭg-in-dūst´ lū´pŭs) Syndrome of systemic lupus erythematosus induced by exposure to drugs, especially procainamide or hydralazine, and characterized by antihistone antibodies. More benign than the usual disease, with less renal involvement. The syndrome clears after stopping the offending drug. SYN hydralazine syndrome.

drug-in·duced ter·at·o·gen·e·sis (drŭg-in-dūst´ ter´ă-tō-jen´ĕ-sis) Congenital anomalies that produce toxic effects on the developing fetus.

drug me·tab·o·lism (drŭg mĕ-tab´ŏ-lizm) The series of chemical changes that take place in an organism, by means of which food is manufactured and utilized and waste materials are eliminated.

drug re·sis·tance (drŭg rĕ-zis´tăns) Capacity of disease-causing pathogens to withstand drugs previously toxic to them; achieved by spontaneous mutation or through selective pressure after exposure to the drug in question.

drug use re·view (drŭg yūs rĕ-vyū´) An authorized, structured, ongoing program that collects, analyzes, and interprets drug use patterns to improve the quality of drug use and patient outcomes. SYN clinical drug trial.

Drum·mond sign (drŭm´ŏnd sīn) In certain cases of aortic aneurysm, a puffing sound, synchronous with cardiac systole, heard from the nostrils, when the mouth is closed.

drunk·en·ness (drungk´ĕn-nĕs) Intoxication, usually alcoholic.

dru·sen (drū´sĕn) Small bright structures seen in the retina and in the optic disc.

dry ab·scess (drī ab´ses) The remains of an abscess after the pus has been absorbed.

dry cough (drī kawf) A cough not accompanied by expectoration; a nonproductive cough.

dry dis·til·la·tion (drī dis-ti-lā´shŭn) Submission of an organic substance to heat in a closed vessel so that oxygen is absent and combustion prevented with the objective of effecting its decomposition with release of volatile constituents and the formation of new substances. SYN destructive distillation.

dry dress·ing (DD) (drī dres´ing) Dry gauze or other material applied to a wound.

dry eye syn·drome (drī ī sin´drōm) SYN keratoconjunctivitis sicca.

dry gan·grene (drī gang-grēn´) A form of gangrene in which the involved part is dessicated and shriveled. SYN mummification (1).

dry ice (drī īs) SYN carbon dioxide snow.

dry joint (drī joynt) Articulation affected with atrophic desiccating changes.

dry pleu·ri·sy (drī plūr'i-sē) Pleurisy with a fibrinous exudation, without an effusion of serum, resulting in adhesion between the opposing surfaces of the pleura. SYN adhesive pleurisy, fibrinous pleurisy, plastic pleurisy.

dry rale (drī rahl) A harsh or musical breath sound produced by a constriction in a bronchial tube or the presence of a viscid secretion narrowing the lumen.

dry socket (drī sok'ĕt) SYN alveoalgia.

dry sy·no·vit·is (drī sin'ō-vī'tis) Synovial inflammation with little serous or purulent effusion.

dry vom·it·ing (drī vom'it-ing) SYN retching.

DTaP Abbreviation for diphtheria, tetanus, and acellular pertussis vaccine.

du·al per·son·al·i·ty (dū'ăl pĕr'sŏ-nal'i-tē) Mental disturbance in which a person assumes alternately two different identities without either personality being consciously aware of the other.

du·al x-ray ab·sorp·ti·om·e·try (DXA) (dū'ăl eks'rā ăb-sorp'shē-om'ĕ-trē) Use of low-dose x-radiation of two different energies to measure bone mineral content at different anatomic sites.

Duane syn·drome (dwān sin'drōm) SYN retraction syndrome.

Du·bo·witz score (dū'bŏ-wits skōr) A method of clinical assessment of gestational age in the newborn that includes neurologic criteria for the infant's maturity and other physical criteria to determine the gestational age of the infant; useful from birth to 5 days of life.

Du·chenne-A·ran dis·ease (dū-shen' ah-rahn' di-zēz') SYN amyotrophic lateral sclerosis.

Du·chenne dys·tro·phy, Du·chenne dis·ease, Du·chenne mus·cu·lar dys·tro·phy (dū-shen' dis'trŏ-fē, diz-ēz', mŭs-kyū'lăr) The most common childhood muscular dystrophy, with onset usually before age 6 years.

Du·chenne sign (dū-shen' sīn) Falling in of the epigastrium during inspiration in paralysis of the diaphragm.

duck wad·dle (dŭk wah'dĕl) A peculiar pattern of walking associated with congenital hip dysplasia.

Duck·worth phe·nom·e·non (dŭk' wŏrth fē-nom'ĕ-non) Respiratory arrest before cardiac arrest as a result of intracranial disease.

duct (dŭkt) [TA] A tubular structure giving exit to the secretion of a gland, or conducting any fluid. SEE ALSO canal. SYN ductus [TA].

duc·tal an·eu·rysm (dŭk'tăl an'yūr-izm) Aneurysm of the patent ductus arteriosus; occurs either in infants or adults. SYN ductus diverticulum.

duct car·ci·no·ma, duc·tal car·ci·no·ma (dŭkt kahr'si-nō'mă, dŭk'tăl) Lesion derived from epithelium of ducts, e.g., in the breast or pancreas.

duct·less glands (dŭkt'lĕs glandz) SYN endocrine glands.

duct of ep·i·did·y·mis (dŭkt ep-i-did'i-mis) [TA] Convoluted tube into which the efferent ductules open; terminates in the ductus deferens.

duct of sweat glands (dŭkt swet glandz) Superficial portion of the sweat gland that passes through the corium and epidermis, opening on the surface by the porus sudoriferus or sweat pore. SYN sudoriferous duct.

duct of Va·ter (dŭkt fah'tĕr) SYN His canal.

duc·tule (dŭk'tyūl) A minute duct. SYN ductulus [TA].

duc·tu·lus, gen. and pl. **duc·tu·li** (dŭk' tyū-lŭs, -lī) [TA] SYN ductule.

duc·tus, gen. and pl. **duc·tus** (dŭk'tŭs) [TA] SYN duct.

duc·tus de·fer·ens (dŭk'tŭs def'ĕr-enz) The secretory duct of the testicle.

due dil·i·gence (dū dil′i-jĕns) In health care, making certain that rules and procedures are followed to avoid harm to patients and staff.

Du·gas test (dū-gah′ test) In the case of an injured shoulder, if the elbow cannot be made to touch the chest while the hand rests on the opposite shoulder, the injury is a dislocation and not a fracture of the humerus.

Du·hot line (dū-ō′ līn) Hypothetic demarcation running from the sacral apex to the superior iliac spine.

Duh·ring dis·ease (dū′ring di-zēz′) SYN dermatitis herpetiformis.

Dukes clas·s·i·fi·ca·tion (dūks klas′i-fi-kā′shŭn) A classification of the extent of invasion of a resected adenocarcinoma of the colon or rectum.

Duke test (dūk test) Procedure to measure bleeding time.

dull (dŭl) Not sharp or acute, in any sense; qualifying a surgical instrument, the action of the mind, pain, a sound (especially the percussion note), or other qualities.

dull·ness (dŭl′nĕs) The character of the sound obtained by percussing over a solid part incapable of resonating; usually applied to an area containing less air than those that can resonate.

dump·ing syn·drome (dŭmp′ing sin′drōm) A syndrome that occurs after eating, most often seen in patients with shunts of the upper alimentary canal; characterized by flushing, sweating, dizziness, weakness, and vasomotor collapse, occasionally with pain and headache; results from rapid passage of large amounts of food into the small intestine, with an osmotic effect removing fluid from plasma and causing hypovolemia. SYN early dumping syndrome, postgastrectomy syndrome.

du·o·de·nal (dū′ō-dē′năl, dū-od′ĕ-năl) Relating to the duodenum.

du·o·de·nal bulb (DB) (dū′ō-dē′năl bŭlb) SYN duodenal cap.

du·o·de·nal cap (dū′ō-dē′năl kap) The first portion of the duodenum, as seen in a roentgenogram or by fluoroscopy.

du·o·de·nal di·ges·tion (dū′ō-dē′năl di-jes′chŭn) Phase of digestion carried on in the duodenum.

du·o·de·nal glands (dū′ō-dē′năl glandz) [TA] Small, branched, coiled tubular glands that occur mostly in the submucosa of the first third of the duodenum; they secrete an alkaline mucoid substance that serves to neutralize gastric juice.

du·o·de·nal ul·cer (DU) (dū′ō-dē′năl ŭl′sĕr) Lesion of the duodenum; 90% associated with *Helicobacter pylori* infection. SEE ALSO peptic ulcer.

du·o·de·nec·to·my (dū′ō-dĕ-nek′tŏ-mē) Excision of the duodenum.

du·od·e·ni·tis (dū-od′ĕ-nī′tis) Inflammation of the duodenum.

duodeno- Combining form relating to the duodenum.

du·o·de·no·cho·lan·gi·tis (dū′ō-dē′nō-kō-lan-jī′tis) Inflammation of the duodenum and common bile duct.

du·o·de·no·cho·led·o·chot·o·my (dū′ō-dē′nō-kō′led-ō-kot′ō-mē) Incision into the common bile duct and the adjacent portion of the duodenum.

du·o·de·no·en·ter·os·to·my (dū′ō-dē′nō-en-tĕr-os′tŏ-mē) Establishment of communication between the duodenum and another part of the intestinal tract.

du·o·de·no·je·ju·nal (dū-od′ē-nō-jē-jū′năl) Pertaining to the duodenum and the jejunum.

du·o·de·no·je·ju·nal flex·ure (dū′ō-dē′nō-jĕ-jū′năl flek′shŭr) [TA] An abrupt bend in the small intestine at the junction of the duodenum and jejunum. SYN flexura duodenojejunalis [TA].

du·o·de·no·je·ju·nos·to·my (dū′ō-dē′nō-jĕ-jū-nos′tŏ-mē) Operative formation of an artificial communication between the duodenum and the jejunum.

du·o·de·nol·y·sis (dū′ō-dĕ-nol′i-sis) Incision of adhesions to the duodenum.

du·o·de·nos·to·my (dū′ō-dĕ-nos′tŏ-mē)

Establishment of a fistula into the duodenum.

du•o•de•not•o•my (dū´ō-dĕ-not´ŏ-mē) Incision of the duodenum.

du•o•de•num, gen. **du•o•de•ni,** pl. **du•o•de•na** (dū´ō-dē´nŭm, -nī, -nă) [TA] The first division of the small intestine, about 25 cm in length, extending from the pylorus to the junction with the jejunum at the level of the first or second lumbar vertebra on the left side.

du•plex trans•mis•sion (dū´pleks transmish´ŭn) Passage of impulses in both directions through a nerve trunk.

du•plex u•ter•us (dū´pleks yū´tĕr-ŭs) Any uterus with two lumina (uterus didelphys, uterus bicornis bicollis, or septate uterus).

du•pli•ca•tion (dū´pli-kā´shŭn) **1.** A doubling. SEE ALSO reduplication. **2.** GENETICS Inclusion of two copies of the same genetic material in a genome.

du•pli•ca•tion cyst (dū´pli-kā´shŭn sist) Congenital cystic malformation attached to or originating from any part of the alimentary canal, from the base of the tongue to the anus, which reproduces the structure of the adjacent alimentary tract.

Du•puy•tren am•pu•ta•tion (dū-pwē´ trahn[h] amp´yū-tā´shŭn) Surgical removal of the arm at the shoulder joint.

Du•puy•tren ca•nal (dū-pwē´trahn[h] kă-nal´) SYN diploic vein.

Du•puy•tren con•trac•ture (dū-pwē´ trahn[h] kŏn-trak´shŭr) A disease of the palmar fascia resulting in thickening and shortening of fibrous bands on the palmar surface of the hand and fingers resulting in a characteristic flexion deformity of the fourth and fifth digits.

Du•puy•tren frac•ture (dū-pwē´trahn[h] frak´shŭr) A break in the lower part of fibula, with ankle dislocation.

Du•puy•tren sign (dū-pwē´trahn[h] sīn) **1.** In congenital dislocation, free up-and-down movement of the head of the femur occurs on intermittent traction. **2.** A crackling sensation on pressure over the bone in certain cases of sarcoma.

dur•a•ble pow•er of at•tor•ney (dūr´ă-bĕl pow´ĕr ă-tŏr´nē) SYN living will.

du•ral (dūr´ăl) Relating to the dura mater.

du•ral ca•ver•nous si•nus fis•tu•la (dūr´ăl kav´ĕr-nŭs sī´nŭs fis´tyū´lă) A vascular shunt between the meningeal branches of the internal or external carotid arteries and the cavernous sinus.

du•ral sac (dūr´ăl sak) Continuation of the dura mater below the termination of the spinal cord (L2 vertebral level), surrounding the lumbar cistern, cauda equina, and filum terminale.

du•ral sheath (dūr´ăl shēth) An extension of the dura mater that ensheathes the roots of spinal nerves or, more particularly, the vagina externa nervi optici.

Dur•ham rule (dūr´ăm rūl) A U.S. test of criminal responsibility (1954): ''an accused is not criminally responsible if his unlawful act was the product of mental disease or mental defect.''

Dur•ham tube (dūr´ăm tūb) Jointed tracheostomy tube.

Du•ro•zi•ez dis•ease (dū-rō´zē-ā´ di-zēz´) Congenital stenosis of the mitral valve.

Du•ro•zi•ez mur•mur (dū-rō´zē-ā´ mŭr´ mŭr) A two-phase murmur over peripheral arteries, especially the femoral artery, due to rapid ebb and flow of blood during aortic insufficiency; audible when pressure is applied to the area just distal to the stethoscope.

dust cell (dŭst sel) SYN alveolar macrophage.

Dut•ton dis•ease (dŭt´ŏn di-zēz´) African tick-borne relapsing fever caused by *Borrelia duttonii* and spread by a soft tick, *Ornithodoros moubata.*

Dut•ton re•lap•sing fe•ver (dŭt´ŏn rē-lap´sing fē´vĕr) SYN Dutton disease.

Du•ver•ney frac•ture (dū-ver-nā´ frak´ shŭr) Break in the ilium below the anterior superior spine.

DVM Abbreviation for Doctor of Veterinary Medicine. SEE veterinarian; veterinary medicine.

dwarf (D) (dwōrf) *Negative or pejorative connotations of this word may render it offensive in some contexts.* An abnormally undersized person with disproportion among the body parts. SEE dwarfism.

Dwy•er os•te•o•to•my (dwī′er os′tē-ot′ ŏ-mē) A surgical procedure to correct clubfoot.

Dy Abbreviation for dysprosium.

dy•ad (dī′ad) **1.** A pair. SYN diad (2). **2.** In chemistry, a bivalent element, molecule, or ion. **3.** Two people in an interactional situation, e.g., patient and therapist, husband and wife. **4.** The double chromosome resulting from division in meiosis. **5.** Two units treated as one. **6.** A pair of cells resulting from the first meiotic division. **7.** The transverse tubule and a terminal cisterna in cardiac muscle cells.

dye (dī) A stain or coloring matter; a compound consisting of chromophore and auxochrome groups attached to one or more benzene rings, its color being due to the chromophore and its dyeing affinities to the auxochrome.

dy•nam•ic con•stant ex•ter•nal re•sis•tance train•ing (dī-nam′ik kon′ stănt eks-tĕr′năl rē-zis′tăns trān′ing) Physical training in which external resistance does not change; joint flexion and extension occur with each repetition. Formerly (but incorrectly) referred to as isotonic exercise.

dy•nam•ic e•qui•lib•ri•um (dī-nam′ik ē′kwi-lib′rē-ŭm) SYN equilibrium (2).

dy•nam•ic gait in•dex (DGI) (dī-nam′ik gāt in′deks) Assessment tool to measure a patient's ability to change gait with varying demands.

dy•nam•ic il•e•us (dī-nam′ik il′ē-ŭs) Intestinal obstruction due to spastic contraction of a segment of the bowel.

dy•nam•ic psy•chi•a•try (dī-nam′ik sī-kī′ă-trē) SYN psychoanalytic psychiatry.

dy•nam•ic psy•chol•o•gy (dī-nam′ik sī-kol′ŏ-jē) Therapy that concerns itself with the causes of behavior.

dy•nam•ics (dyn) (dī-nam′iks) **1.** The science of motion in response to forces. **2.** In psychiatry, used as a contraction of psychodynamics. **3.** In the behavioral sciences, any of the numerous intrapersonal and interpersonal influences or phenomena associated with personality development and interpersonal processes.

dy•nam•ic splint (dī-nam′ik splint) A splint using springs or elastic bands that aids in movements initiated by the patient by controlling the plane and range of motion. SYN active splint, functional splint (1).

dynamo- Combining form denoting force, energy.

dy•na•mo•gen•e•sis (dī′nă-mō-jen′ĕ-sis) The production of force, especially of muscular or nervous energy.

dy•nam•o•graph (dī-nam′ŏ-graf) An instrument for recording the degree of muscular power.

dy•na•mom•e•ter (dī′nă-mom′ĕ-tĕr) An instrument for measuring the degree of muscular power. SYN ergometer (1).

dyn•ein (dīn′ēn) A protein associated with motile structures, exhibiting adenosine triphosphatase activity; it forms "arms" on the outer tubules of cilia and flagella. SEE ALSO tubulin.

-dynia Suffix denoting pain.

dys- Prefix meaning bad, difficult, un-, mis-; opposite of eu-. Cf. dis-.

dys•a•cu•sis, dys•a•cu•si•a, dys•a•cou•si•a (dis-ă-kyū′sis, -zē-ă, -kū′zē-ă) **1.** Any impairment of hearing involving difficulty in processing details of sound as opposed to any loss of sensitivity to sound. **2.** Pain or discomfort in the ear from exposure to sound.

dysaesthesia [Br.] SYN dysesthesia.

dys•a•phi•a (dis-ā′fē-ă) Impairment of the sense of touch.

dys•ar•thri•a (dis-ahr′thrē-ă) A disturbance of speech due to paralysis, incoordination, or spasticity of the muscles used for speaking. SYN dysarthrosis (1).

dys•ar•thro•sis (dis′ahr-thrō′sis) **1.** SYN

dysarthria. **2.** Malformation of a joint. **3.** A false joint.

dys·au·to·no·mi·a (dis'aw-tō-nō'mē-ă) Abnormal functioning of the autonomic nervous system.

dys·bar·ism (dis'băr-izm) General term for the symptom complex resulting from exposure to decreased or changing barometric pressure.

dys·ba·si·a, dys·ba·sis (dis-bā'sē-ă, -sis) **1.** Difficulty in walking. **2.** The difficult or distorted walking that occurs in people with certain mental disorders.

dys·ce·pha·li·a, dys·ceph·a·ly (dis'sĕ-fā'lē-ă, -sef'ă-lē) Malformation of the head and face.

dys·chei·ri·a, dys·chi·ri·a (dis-kī'rē-ă) A disorder of sensory processing in which the patient is unable to tell which side of the body has been touched (acheiria) or refers the stimulus to the wrong side (allocheiria) or to both sides (syncheiria).

dys·che·zi·a (dis-kē'zē-ă) Difficulty in defecation.

dys·chon·dro·gen·e·sis (dis'kon-drō-jen'ĕ-sis) Abnormal development of cartilage.

dys·chon·dros·te·o·sis (dis'kon-dros'tē-ō'sis) Skeletal genetic dysplasia involving the radius, ulna, elbows, wrist and other findings.

dys·chro·ma·top·si·a (dis'krō-mă-top'sē-ă) A condition in which the ability to perceive colors is not fully normal. Cf. dichromatism, monochromatism, chromatopsia.

dys·chro·mi·a (dis-krō'mē-ă) Any abnormality in skin color.

dys·con·trol (dis'kŏn-trōl') SYN intermittent explosive disorder.

dys·co·ri·a (dis-kōr'ē-ă) Abnormality in the shape of the pupil.

dys·cra·si·a (dis-krā'zē-ă) A morbid general state resulting from the presence of abnormal material in the blood, usually applied to diseases affecting blood cells or platelets.

dys·cra·sic, dys·crat·ic (dis-krā'sik, -krat'ik) Pertaining to or affected with dyscrasia.

dys·en·ter·ic (dis'en-ter'ik) Relating to or suffering from dysentery.

dys·en·ter·y (dis'ĕn-ter'ē) A disease marked by frequent watery stools, often with blood and mucus; characterized clinically by pain, tenesmus, fever, and dehydration.

dys·er·e·thism (dis-er'ĕ-thizm) A condition of slow response to stimuli.

dys·er·gi·a (dis-ĕr'jē-ă) Lack of harmonious action between the muscles concerned in executing any definite voluntary movement.

dys·es·the·si·a (dis'es-thē'zē-ă) **1.** Impairment of sensation short of anesthesia. **2.** A condition in which a disagreeable sensation is produced by ordinary stimuli; caused by lesions of the sensory pathways, peripheral or central. **3.** Abnormal sensations experienced in the absence of stimulation.

dysfibrinogenaemia [Br.] SYN dysfibrinogenemia.

dys·fi·brin·o·ge·ne·mi·a (dis'fī-brin'ō-jĕ-nē'mē-ă) An autosomal dominant disorder of qualitatively abnormal fibrinogens of various types, resulting in abnormalities of coagulation tests; symptoms vary from none to abnormal bleeding and excessive clotting. SYN dysfibrinogenaemia.

dys·flu·en·cy, dis·flu·en·cy (dis-flū'ĕn-sē) Speech interrupted in its forward flow by hesitations, repetitions, or prolongations of sounds; common manifestation of a stuttering disorder; present in normal speech, particularly during speech development in young children. SEE stuttering.

dys·func·tion (dis-fŭngk'shŭn) Abnormal or difficult function.

dys·func·tion·al (dis-fungk'shŭn-ăl) Unable to behave or act normally.

dysgammaglobulinaemia [Br.] SYN dysgammaglobulinemia.

dys·gam·ma·glob·u·lin·e·mi·a (dis-

gam′ă-glob′yū-li-nē′mē-ă) An immunoglobulin abnormality, especially a disturbance of the percentage distribution
of γ-globulins. SYN dysgammaglobulinaemia.

dys·gen·e·sis, dys·ge·ne·si·a (dis-
jen′ĕ-sis, -jĕ-nē′zē-ă) Defective development.

dys·ger·mi·no·ma (dis′jĕr-mi-nō′mă) A
malignant neoplasm of the ovary composed of undifferentiated gonadal germinal cells and occurring more frequently
in patients younger than 20 years of age.

dys·geu·si·a (dis-gū′sē-ă) Impairment or
perversion of the gustatory sense.

dys·gnath·i·a (dis-gnā′thē-ă) Any abnormality that extends beyond the teeth and
includes the maxilla or mandible, or
both.

dys·gno·si·a (dis-gnō′zē-ă) Any cognitive disorder, i.e., any mental illness.

dys·graph·i·a (dis-graf′ē-ă) 1. Difficulty
in writing. 2. SYN writer's cramp.

dyshaematopoiesis [Br.] SYN dys-
hematopoiesis.

**dys·hem·a·to·poi·e·sis, dys·he·mo·
poi·e·sis** (dis-hē′mă-tō-poy-ē′sis, -mō-
poy-ē′sis) Defective formation of the
blood.

**dys·hi·dro·sis, dys·i·dro·sis, dys·
hy·dro·sis, dys·hi·drot·ic ec·ze·
ma** (dis′hi-drō′sis, dis′i-, dis′hī-, dis′hi-
drot′ik ek′sĕ-mă) A vesicular or vesicopustular eruption, which is of unknown
cause, chiefly involving the volar surfaces of the hands and feet; self-limited
but may be recurrent. SYN cheiropom-
pholyx, chiropompholyx, dyshidria, pom-
pholyx.

dys·kar·y·o·sis (dis-kar′ē-ō′sis) Abnormal maturation seen in exfoliated cells
that have normal cytoplasm but hyper-
chromatic nuclei, or irregular chromatin
distribution; may be followed by the development of a malignant neoplasm.

dys·ker·a·to·ma (dis-ker′ă-tō′mă) A
skin tumor exhibiting dyskeratosis.

dys·ker·a·to·sis (dis-ker′ă-tō′sis) 1. Premature keratinization in individual epithelial cells that have not reached the
keratinizing surface layer; dyskeratotic
cells generally become rounded and they
may break away from adjacent cells and
fall off. 2. Epidermalization of the conjunctival and corneal epithelium. 3. A
disorder of keratinization.

**dys·ki·ne·si·a, dys·ki·ne·sis, dys·
ci·ne·si·a** (dis′ki-nē′sē-ă, -nē′sis) Difficulty in performing voluntary movements.

dys·ki·ne·si·a in·ter·mit·tens (dis′ki-
nē′sē-ă in-tĕr-mit′enz) Intermittent disability of the limbs due to impairment of
circulation.

dys·ki·ne·si·a syn·drome (dis′ki-nē′
sē-ă sin′drōm) SYN primary ciliary dyskinesia.

dys·lex·i·a (dis-lek′sē-ă) Impaired reading ability with a competence level
below that expected on the basis of the
person's level of intelligence, and in the
presence of normal vision, letter recognition, and normal recognition of the meaning of pictures and objects.

dys·lex·ic (dis-lek′sik) Relating to, or
characterized by, dyslexia.

dys·lip·i·de·mi·a (dis-lip′i-dē′mē-ă) Any
biochemical disorder characterized by
one or more abnormal levels of blood
lipids.

dys·lo·gi·a (dis-lō′jē-ă) Impairment of
speech and reasoning as the result of a
mental disorder.

dys·ma·tu·ri·ty (dis′mă-chŭr′i-tē) Syndrome of an infant born with relative absence of subcutaneous fat, wrinkling of
the skin, prominent finger and toe nails,
and meconium staining of skin and placental membranes; often associated with
postmaturity or placental insufficiency.

dys·ma·tu·ri·ty syn·drome (dis′mă-
chŭr′i-tē sin′drōm) SYN Ballantyne disease.

dys·me·li·a (dis-mē′lē-ă) Congenital abnormality characterized by missing or
foreshortened limbs, sometimes with associated vertebral column abnormalities;
caused by metabolic disturbance at the
time of primordial limb development.
SEE amelia, phocomelia.

dys·men·or·rhe·a (dis-men′ŏr-ē′ă) Difficult and painful menstruation. SYN menorrhalgia.

dysmenorrhoea [Br.] SYN dysmenorrhea.

dys·met·ri·a (dis-mē′trē-ă) An aspect of ataxia, in which the ability to control the distance, power, and speed of an act is impaired. SEE ALSO hypermetria, hypometria.

dys·mne·sic syn·drome (dis-nē′sik sin′drōm) SYN Korsakoff syndrome.

dys·mor·phism, dys·mor·phi·a (dis-mŏr′fizm, -fē-ă) Abnormality of shape.

dys·mor·phol·o·gy (dis′mŏr-fol′ŏ-jē) The study of developmental structural defects. A branch of clinical genetics.

dys·my·e·li·na·tion (dis′mī-ĕ-li-nā′shŭn) Improper breakdown of a myelin sheath of a nerve fiber; caused by abnormal myelin metabolism.

dys·my·o·to·ni·a (dis′mī-ō-tō′nē-ă) Abnormal muscular tonicity (either hyper- or hypo-). SEE dystonia.

dys·nys·tax·is (dis′nis-tak′sis) A condition of half sleep. SYN light sleep.

dys·o·don·ti·a·sis (dis′ō-don-tī′ă-sis) **1.** Difficulty or irregularity in the eruption of the teeth. **2.** An imperfect dentition.

dys·on·to·gen·e·sis (dis′on-tō-jen′ĕ-sis) Defective embryonic development.

dys·o·rex·i·a (dis′ŏr-ek′sē-ă) Diminished or perverted appetite, associated with emotional or psychological disorders.

dys·os·mi·a (dis-oz′mē-ă) Altered sense of smell.

dys·os·te·o·gen·e·sis, dys·os·to·sis (dis-os′tē-ō-jen′ĕ-sis, -os-tō′sis) Defective bone formation. SYN dysostosis.

dys·os·to·sis mul·ti·plex (dis-os-tō′sis mul′tē-pleks) Specific pattern of radiographic changes observed in many lysosomal storage disorders.

dys·pa·reu·ni·a (dis′păr-ū′nē-ă) Pain experienced during sexual intercourse.

dys·pep·si·a (dis-pep′sē-ă) Impaired gastric function or "upset stomach" due to some stomach disorder; characterized by epigastric pain, burning, nausea, and belching. SYN gastric indigestion.

dys·pha·gi·a, dys·pha·gy (dis-fā′jē-ă, dis′fă-jē) Difficulty in swallowing.

dys·pha·si·a (dis-fā′zē-ă) Impairment in the production of speech and failure to arrange words clearly; caused by brain lesion. SYN dysphrasia.

dys·phe·mi·a (dis-fē′mē-ă) Disordered phonation, articulation, or hearing due to emotional or mental deficits.

dys·pho·ni·a (dis-fō′nē-ă) Any disorder of phonation affecting voice quality or ability to produce voice. SEE aphonia.

dys·pho·ri·a (dis-fōr′ē-ă) A mood of general dissatisfaction, restlessness, depression, and anxiety; a feeling of unpleasantness or discomfort.

dys·phy·lax·i·a (dis′fi-lak′sē-ă) Inability to remain asleep.

dys·pig·men·ta·tion (dis-pig′měn-tā′shŭn) Any abnormality in the formation or distribution of pigment, especially in the skin; usually applied to an abnormal reduction in pigmentation (depigmentation).

dys·pla·si·a (dis-plā′zē-ă) Abnormal tissue development. SEE ALSO heteroplasia.

dys·plas·tic mel·a·not·ic ne·vi (dis-plas′tik mel-ă-not′ik nē′vī) Cutaneous pigmented lesions with notched, irregular borders; considered premalignant and marker for increased risk of melanoma.

dys·plas·tic ne·vus syn·drome, dys·plas·tic ne·vus (dis-plas′tik nē′vŭs sin′drōm, dis-plas′tik nē′vŭs) Clinically atypical skin malformation with variable pigmentation and ill-defined borders, with an increased risk for development of cutaneous malignant melanoma.

dysp·ne·a (disp-nē′ă) Shortness of breath, a subjective difficulty or distress in breathing, usually associated with disease of the heart or lungs.

dysp·ne·ic (disp-nē′ik) Out of breath; relating to or suffering from dyspnea.

dyspnoea [Br.] SYN dyspnea.

dys·prax·i·a (dis-prak′sē-ă) Difficulty in performing motor tasks.

dys·pro·sod·y, dys·pro·sod·i·a (dis-pros′ŏ-dē, dis′prō-sŏ′dē-ă) Impairment in ability to apply normal speech intonation patterns. SEE ALSO aprosody.

dysproteinaemia [Br.] SYN dysproteinemia.

dys·pro·tein·e·mi·a (dis-prō′tēn-ē′mē-ă) An abnormality in plasma proteins, usually in immunoglobulins. SYN dysproteinaemia.

dys·ra·phism, dys·raph·i·a (dis′rǎ-fizm, -raf′ē-ă) Defective fusion, especially of the neural folds, resulting in status dysraphicus or neural tube defect.

dys·rhyth·mi·a (dis-ridh′mē-ă) Defective rhythm. SEE ALSO arrhythmia.

dys·som·ni·a (dis-som′nē-ă) Disturbance of normal sleep or rhythm pattern.

dys·sta·si·a (dis-stā′sē-ă) Difficulty in standing.

dys·stat·ic (dis-tat′ik) Marked by difficulty in standing.

dys·syn·er·gi·a, dys·syn·er·gy (dis′sin-ěr′jē-ă, -syn′ěr′jē) An aspect of ataxia, in which an act is not performed smoothly or accurately because of lack of harmonious association of its various components; usually used to describe abnormalities of movement caused by cerebellar disorders.

dys·syn·er·gia cer·e·bel·lar·is my·o·clo·ni·ca (DCM) (dis′sin-ěr′jē-ă ser′ě-bel-ā′ris mī-ŏ′klŏ′ni-kă) Familial disorder beginning in late childhood, characterized by progressive cerebellar ataxia, action myoclonus and preserved intellect. Probably due to multiple causes, of which mitochondrial abnormalities are one. SYN dentatorubral cerebellar atrophy with polymyoclonus.

dys·thy·mi·a (dis-thī′mē-ă) Chronic mood disorder manifested as depression for most of the day, more days than not, accompanied by some of the following symptoms: poor appetite or overeating, insomnia or hypersomnia, low energy or fatigue, low self-esteem, poor concentration, difficulty making decisions, and feelings of hopelessness. SEE endogenous depression, exogenous depression.

dys·thy·mic (dis-thī′mik) Relating to dysthymia.

dys·thy·mic dis·or·der (dis-thī′mik dis-ōr′děr) A chronic disturbance of mood characterized by mild depression or loss of interest in usual activities. SEE depression.

dys·to·ci·a (dis-tō′sē-ă) Difficult childbirth.

dys·to·ni·a (dis-tō′nē-ă) A state of abnormal (either hypo- or hyper-) tonicity in any tissue, particularly skeletal muscle. SYN dysmyotonia, torsion spasm.

dys·ton·ic re·ac·tion (dis-ton′ik rē-ak′shŭn) Abnormal tension or muscle tone, similar to dystonia, produced as an adverse effect of certain antipsychotic medication; a severe form, in which the eyes appear to roll up into the head, is called oculogyric crisis.

dys·to·pi·a (dis-tō′pē-ă) Faulty or abnormal position of a part or organ. SYN malposition.

dys·tro·phi·a (dis-trō′fē-ă) SYN dystrophy.

dys·tro·phic cal·ci·fi·ca·tion (dis-trō′fik kal′si-fi-kā′shŭn) Hardening of degenerated or necrotic tissue, as in hyalinized scars, degenerated foci in leiomyomas, and caseous nodules.

dys·tro·phin (dis-trō′fin) A protein found in the sarcolemma of normal muscle. SYN distropin, dystropin.

dys·tro·phy, dys·tro·phi·a (dis′trŏ-fē, dis-trō′fē-ă) Abnormal development or growth of a tissue or organ, usually resulting from nutritional deficiency. SYN dystrophia.

dys·tro·pin (dis-trō′pin) SYN dystrophin.

dys·u·ri·a, dys·ur·y (dis-yūr′ē-ă, dis′yūr-ē) Difficulty or pain in urination. SYN dysury.

dys·ver·sion (dis-věr′zhŭn) A turning in any direction, less marked than inversion.

E

E1 Symbol for estrone.

E2 Symbol for estradiol.

ear (ēr) [TA] The organ of hearing: composed of the external ear, which includes the auricle and the external acoustic, or auditory, meatus; the middle ear, or the tympanic cavity with its ossicles; and the internal ear or inner ear, or labyrinth, which includes the semicircular canals, vestibule, and cochlea. SEE ALSO auricle. SYN auris [TA].

ear lobe crease (ēr lōb krēs) A diagonal crease found on one or both earlobes with a possible connection to coronary heart disease in males.

ear·ly de·cel·er·a·tion (ĕr′lē dē-sel-ĕr-ā′shŭn) Slowed fetal heart rate early in the uterine contraction phase, denoting compression of the fetal head.

ear·ly re·cep·tor po·ten·tial (ERP) (ĕr′lē rĕ-sep′tŏr pō-ten′shăl) Voltage arising across the eye from a charge displacement within photoreceptor pigment, in response to an intense flash of light.

ear wax, ear·wax (ēr waks, ēr′waks) SYN cerumen.

East·ern e·quine en·ceph·a·lo·my·e·li·tis (EEE) (ēs′tĕrn ē′kwīn en-sef′ă-lō-mī-ĕ-lī′tis) Form of mosquito-borne equine encephalomyelitis seen in the eastern U.S. caused by the eastern equine encephalomyelitis virus, a species of alphavirus.

eat·ing dis·or·ders (ēt′ing dis-ōr′dĕrz) A class of mental disorders including anorexia nervosa, bulimia nervosa, and pica.

eat·ing ep·i·lep·sy (ēt′ing ep′i-lep′sē) Epileptic seizures provoked by eating; a type of reflex epilepsy.

Ea·ton-Lam·bert syn·drome (ē′tŏn lam′bĕrt sin′drōm) SYN Lambert-Eaton myasthenic syndrome.

E·berth lines (ā′bĕrt līnz) Lines appearing between the cells of the myocardium when stained with silver nitrate.

E·bo·la vi·rus (ē-bō′lă vī′rŭs) A virus morphologically similar to but antigenically distinct from Marburg virus, which causes viral hemorrhagic fever.

Eb·stein a·nom·a·ly, Eb·stein dis·ease (eb′shtīn ă-nom′ă-lē, di-zēz′) Congenital downward displacement of the tricuspid valve into the right ventricle; causes fatigue, palpitations, and dyspnea.

Eb·stein sign (eb′shtīn sīn) In pericardial effusion, obtuseness of the cardiohepatic angle on percussion.

eb·ur·na·tion (ē-bŭr-nā′shŭn) A change in exposed subchondral bone in degenerative joint disease in which it is converted into a dense substance with a smooth surface like ivory.

e·bur·ni·tis (ē-bŭr-nī′tis) Increased density and hardness of the dentin, which may occur after the dentin is exposed.

ec- Prefix meaning out of, away from.

e·cau·date (ē-kaw′dāt) Tailless.

ec·cen·tric (ek-sen′trik) 1. Abnormal or peculiar in ideas or behavior. 2. Situated away from a center or proceeding from a center. Cf. centrifugal (2). 3. SYN peripheral.

ec·cen·tric hy·per·tro·phy (EH) (ek-sen′trik hī-pĕr′trō-fē) Thickening of the wall of the heart or other cavity, with dilation.

ec·cen·tric oc·clu·sion (ek-sen′trik ŏ-klū′zhŭn) Occlusion other than centric that results in premature tooth contact.

ec·chon·dro·ma, ec·chon·dro·sis (ek-kon-drō′mă, -drō′sis) 1. A neoplasm arising from cartilage as a mass protruding from the articular surface of a bone. 2. An enchondroma that has burst through the shaft of a bone and become pedunculated.

ec·chy·mo·ma (ek-i-mō′mă) A slight hematoma following a bruise.

ec·chy·mo·sis (ek-i-mō′sis) A purplish patch caused by extravasation of blood into the skin, differing from petechiae only in size (larger than 3 mm diameter).

ec·crine (ek′rin) 1. SYN exocrine (1). 2. Denoting the flow of sweat.

ec·crine gland (ek'rin gland) A type of coiled tubular sweat gland (other than apocrine glands) that occurs in the skin on almost all parts of the body.

ec·cri·sis (ek'ri-sis) 1. The removal of waste products. 2. Any waste product; excrement.

ec·crit·ic (e-krit'ik) 1. Promoting the expulsion of waste matter. 2. An agent that promotes excretion.

ec·cy·e·sis (ek-sī-ē'sis) SYN ectopic pregnancy.

ec·dem·ic (ek-dem'ik) Denoting a disease brought into a region from another region.

ec·go·nine (ek'gō-nēn, -nin) A product of the hydrolysis of cocaine; a topical anesthetic; basis of many coca alkaloids.

echin- SEE echino-.

e·chin·a·ce·a (ek'i-nā'shē-ă) (*Echinacea angustifolia, E. pallida, E. purpurea*) A widely used herbal supplement claimed to act against infectious diseases; some clinical studies suggest value in preventing and treating the common cold; severe adverse reactions include anaphylaxis and angiooedema. SYN comb flower, cornflower, snakeroot.

echino-, echin- Combining forms meaning prickly, spiny.

e·chi·no·coc·co·sis, e·chi·no·coc·ci·a·sis (ĕ-kī'nō-kok-kō'sis, -kok-sē-ā'sis) Infection with *Echinococcus;* larval infection is called hydatid disease. SYN echinococciasis, echinococcus disease.

e·chi·no·coc·cus cyst (ĕ-kī'nō-kok'ŭs sist) SYN hydatid cyst.

e·chi·no·cyte (echino) (ĕ-kī'-nō-sīt) A crenated red blood cell.

ech·o (ek'ō) 1. A reverberating sound sometimes heard during auscultation of the chest. 2. In ultrasonography, the acoustic signal received from scattering or reflecting structures or the corresponding pattern of light on a cathode ray tube or ultrasonogram. 3. In magnetic resonance imaging, the signal detected following an inverting pulse.

ech·o·a·cou·si·a (ek'ō-ă-kyū'zē-ă) A subjective disturbance of hearing in which a sound seems to be repeated.

ech·o·a·or·tog·ra·phy (ek'ō-ă-ōr-tog'ră-fē) Application of ultrasound techniques to the diagnosis and study of the aorta.

ech·o beat (ek'ō bēt) Extrasystole produced by the return of an impulse in the heart retrograde to a focus near its origin, which then returns antegradely to produce a second depolarization.

ech·o·car·di·o·gram (ek'ō-kahr'dē-ō-gram) The ultrasonic record obtained by echocardiography. SEE ultrasonography.

ech·o·car·di·og·ra·phy (ek'ō-kahr-dē-og'ră-fē) The use of ultrasound in the investigation of the structure and motion of the heart and great vessels and diagnosis of cardiovascular lesions. SYN ultrasound cardiography.

ech·o·graph·i·a (ek'ō-graf'ē-ă) A form of agraphia in which one cannot write spontaneously but can write from dictation or copy.

ech·og·ra·phy (e-kog'ră-fē) SYN ultrasonography.

ech·o·kin·e·sis, ech·o·kin·e·si·a (ek'ō-ki-nē'sis, -sē-ă) Copying someone else's motions; a form of mental disorder.

ech·o·la·li·a (ek'ō-lā'lē-ă) Involuntary parrotlike repetition of a word or sentence just spoken by someone else; usually seen with schizophrenia. SYN echophrasia.

e·chop·a·thy (e-kop'ă-thē) A form of psychopathology, usually associated with schizophrenia, in which the words (echolalia) or actions (echopraxia) of another are imitated and repeated. SYN echomimia.

ech·o·prax·i·a, ech·o·prax·is (ek'ō-prak'sē-ă, -prak'sis) Involuntary imitation of movements made by another. SEE echopathy. SYN echomotism.

ECHO vi·rus, ech·o·vi·rus (ek'ō vī'rŭs) An enterovirus isolated from humans; although there are many inapparent infections, certain of the several serotypes are associated with fever and aseptic meningitis, and some appear to cause mild respiratory disease.

ec·lamp·si·a (ĕ-klamp′sē-ă) Occurrence of one or more convulsions, not attributable to other cerebral conditions such as epilepsy or cerebral hemorrhage, in a patient with preeclampsia.

ec·lamp·to·gen·ic, ec·lamp·tog·e·nous (ĕ-klamp′tō-jen′ik, -toj′ĕ-nŭs) Causing eclampsia.

ec·lec·tic (eclec) (ek-lek′tik) Picking out from different sources what appears to be the best or most desirable.

e·clipse pe·ri·od (ē-klips′ pēr′ē-ŏd) The time between infection by (or induction of) a bacteriophage, or other virus, and the appearance of mature virus within the cell; an interval of time during which infective viral material cannot be recovered.

ECM Abbreviation for erythema chronicum migrans.

♻ **eco-** Prefix meaning related to the environment.

e·con·o·my (ē-kon′ŏ-mē) System; the body regarded as an aggregate of functioning organs.

e·co·tax·is (ēk′ō-tak′sis) Migration of lymphocytes "homing" from the thymus and bone marrow into tissues possessing an appropriate microenvironment.

ec·o·tro·pic vi·rus (ek′ō-trō′pik vī′rŭs) An oncornavirus that does not produce disease in its natural host but does replicate in tissue culture cells derived from the host species.

ec·phy·ma (ek-fī′mă) A warty growth or protuberance.

ec·sta·sy (ek′stă-sē) A drug of abuse used especially at clubs and raves; increases energy, heightens sexual urges, and induces euphoria. Even small recreational dosage *can* lead to hazardous reactions.

ec·tad (ek′tad) Outward.

♻ **-ectasia, -ectasis** Combining forms meaning dilation, expansion.

ec·ta·si·a, ec·ta·sis (ek-tā′zē-ă, ek′tă-sis) Dilation of a tubular structure.

ec·tat·ic em·phy·se·ma (ek-tat′ik em′fi-sē′mă) Obstructive airway disease with areas of dilatation of alveoli acini. SEE panlobular emphysema.

ect·eth·moid (ekt-eth′moyd) SYN ethmoidal labyrinth.

ec·thy·ma (ek-thī′mă) A pyogenic infection of the skin initiated by β-hemolytic streptococci characterized by adherent crusts beneath which ulceration occurs; the ulcers heal with scar formation.

♻ **ecto-, ect-** Combining forms meaning outer, on the outside. SEE ALSO exo-.

ec·to·an·ti·gen (ek′tō-an′ti-jen) Any toxin or other excitor of antibody formation, separate or separable from its source. SYN exoantigen.

ec·to·car·di·a (ek′tō-kahr′dē-ă) Congenital displacement of the heart. SYN exocardia.

ec·to·derm (ek′tō-dĕrm) The outer layer of cells in the embryo, after establishment of the three primary germ layers (e.g., ectoderm, mesoderm, endoderm).

ec·to·der·mal clo·a·ca (ek-tō-dĕr′măl klō-ā′kă) Proctodeum of the embryo.

ec·to·der·mal dys·pla·si·a (ED) (ek-tō-dĕr′măl dis-plā′zē-ă) Congenital defect of ectodermal tissues, including the skin and its appendages; associated with dental dysplasia and hyperthermia. SEE anhidrotic ectodermal dysplasia, hidrotic ectodermal dysplasia.

ec·to·der·mo·sis (ek′tō-dĕr-mō′sis) A disorder of any organ or tissue developed from the ectoderm. SYN ectodermatosis.

ec·to·en·tad (ek′tō-en′tad) From without inward; in an inward direction.

ec·to·en·zyme (ek′tō-en′zīm) One excreted externally that acts outside the organism.

ec·tog·e·nous (ek-toj′ĕ-nŭs) SYN exogenous.

ec·to·mere (ek'tō-mēr) A blastomere involved in ectoderm formation.

-ectomy Suffix meaning removal of an anatomic structure. SEE ALSO -tomy.

ec·top·a·gus (ek-top'ă-gŭs) Conjoined twins whose bodies are joined laterally. SEE conjoined twins.

ec·to·pi·a, ec·to·py (ek-tō'pē-ă, ek'tō-pē) Congenital displacement or malposition of any organ or part of the body. SYN heterotopia (1).

ec·to·pi·a len·tis (ek-tō'pē-ă len'tis) Displacement of the lens of the eye. SYN dislocation of lens.

ec·to·pi·a pu·pil·lae con·gen·i·ta (ek-tō'pē-ă pyū-pil'ē kon-jen'i-tă) Displacement of the pupil present at birth.

ec·top·ic (ect) (ek-top'ik) **1.** Out of place; said of an organ not in its proper position, or of a pregnancy occurring elsewhere than in the cavity of the uterus. SYN heterotopic (1). **2.** In cardiography, denoting a heartbeat that has its origin in some abnormal focus; developing from a focus other than the sinuatrial node.

ec·top·ic bone (ek-top'ik bōn) Proliferation of bone in an abnormal place.

ec·top·ic fo·cus (ek-top'ik fō'kŭs) An irritable zone of myocardium capable of initiating ectopic beats or assuming the function of a pacemaker.

ec·top·ic hor·mone (ek-top'ik hōr'mōn) One formed by tissue outside the normal endocrine site of production. SYN inappropriate hormone.

ec·top·ic im·pulse (ek-top'ik im'pŭls) One from an area of the heart other than the sinus node.

ec·top·ic preg·nan·cy (EP) (ek-top'ik preg'năn-sē) Implantation and development of a blastocyst outside the uterine cavity. SYN eccyesis, extrauterine pregnancy, heterotopic pregnancy, paracyesis.

ec·top·ic rhythm (ek-top'ik ridh'ŭm) Any cardiac rhythm arising from a center other than the normal pacemaker, the sinus node.

ec·top·ic ur·e·ter·o·cele (ek-top'ik yūr-ē'tĕr-ō-sēl) A ureterocele extending distal to the bladder neck.

ec·to·plasm (ek'tō-plazm) The peripheral, more viscous cytoplasm of a cell; it contains microfilaments but is lacking in other organelles. SYN exoplasm.

ec·tos·te·al (ek-tos'tē-ăl) Relating to the external surface of a bone.

ec·tos·to·sis (ek'tos-tō'sis) Ossification in cartilage beneath the perichondrium, or formation of bone beneath the periosteum.

ec·to·thrix (ek'tō-thriks) A sheath of spores (conidia) on the outside of a hair.

ectro- Prefix meaning congenital absence of a part.

ec·tro·dac·ty·ly, ec·tro·dac·tyl·i·a, ec·tro·dac·tyl·ism (ECD) (ek'trō-dak'ti-lē, -dak-til'ē-ă, -dak'ti-lizm) Congenital absence of all or part of one or more fingers or toes.

ec·trog·e·ny (ek-troj'ĕ-nē) Congenital absence or defect of any body part.

ec·tro·me·li·a (ek'trō-mē'lē-ă) Congenital hypoplasia or aplasia of one or more limbs.

ec·tro·pi·on, ec·tro·pi·um (ek-trō'pē-on, -trō'pē-ŭm) A rolling outward of the margin of a part, e.g., of an eyelid.

ec·tro·pi·on u·ve·ae (ek-trō'pē-on ū've-ē) Eversion of the pigmented posterior epithelium of the iris at the pupillary margin.

ec·trop·o·dy (ek-trop'ŏ-dē) Total or partial absence of a foot.

ec·tro·syn·dac·ty·ly (ek'trō-sin-dak'ti-lē) Congenital anomaly marked by the absence of one or more fingers or toes and the fusion of others.

ec·ze·ma (ek'sĕ-mă) Generic term for inflammatory conditions of the skin, particularly with vesiculation in the acute stage, typically erythematous, edematous, papular, and crusting; followed often by lichenification and scaling and occasionally by duskiness of the erythema and, infrequently, hyperpigmentation.

ec•ze•ma her•pe•t•i•cum (ek'sĕ-mă her-pet'i-kŭm) Febrile condition caused by cutaneous dissemination of herpes virus type 1, occurring most commonly in children, consisting of a widespread eruption of vesicles that rapidly become umbilicated pustules; clinically indistinguishable from a generalized vaccinia.

ec•ze•ma•toid (ek-sem'ă-toyd) Resembling eczema in appearance.

EDC Abbreviation for expected date of confinement.

e•de•ma (ĕ-dē'mă) An accumulation of an excessive amount of watery fluid in cells, tissues, or serous cavities. SYN oedema.

e•de•ma•to•gen•ic (e-dem'ă-tō-jen'ik) Causing swelling of a body part.

e•den•tu•lous (ē-den'tyū-lŭs) Toothless, having lost natural teeth. SYN edentate.

Ed•er-Pus•tow bou•gie (ed'ĕr pus'tof bū-zhē') A metal olive-shaped bougie with a flexible metal dilating system (for esophageal stricture).

ed•e•tate (ed'ĕ-tāt) Contraction for ethylenediaminetetraacetate approved by the U.S. Adopted Names Council.

e•det•ic ac•id (ĕ-det'ik as'id) SYN ethylenediaminetetraacetic acid.

edge (ej) A line at which a surface terminates. SEE ALSO border, margin.

edge-to-edge bite (ej ej bīt) SYN edge-to-edge occlusion.

edge-to-edge oc•clu•sion (ej ej ŏ-klū'zhŭn) One in which the anterior teeth of both jaws meet along their incisal edges when the teeth are in centric occlusion. SYN end-to-end bite.

edge•wise ap•pli•ance (ej'wīz ă-plī'ăns) Fixed, multibanded orthodontic appliance using an attachment bracket the slot of which receives a rectangular archwire horizontally, which gives precise control of tooth movement in all three planes of space.

e•dis•y•late (e-dis'i-lāt) USAN-approved

contraction for 1,2-ethanedisulfonate, $^{-}O_3S(CH_2)_2SO_3^{-}$.

ed•ro•pho•ni•um chlor•ide (ed'rō-fō'nē-ŭm klōr'īd) A rapid-acting, short-duration cholinesterase inhibitor used as an antidote for curariform drugs, as a diagnostic agent in myasthenia gravis, and in myasthenic crisis.

Ed•ward•si•el•la (ed'wărd-sē-el'lă) A genus of gram-negative, facultatively anaerobic bacteria containing motile, peritrichous, nonencapsulated rods; etiologic agent of gastroenteritis in humans.

ef•face•ment (e-fās'mĕnt) The thinning out of the cervix just before or during labor.

ef•fec•tive con•ju•gate (e-fek'tive kon'jŭ-găt) The internal conjugate measured from the nearest lumbar vertebra to the symphysis, in spondylolisthesis. SYN false conjugate (2).

ef•fec•tive dose (ED) (e-fek'tiv dōs) Dose that produces a specific effect; when followed by a subscript (generally "ED_{50}"), it denotes the dose having such an effect on a certain percentage (e.g., 50%) of the test animals; ED_{50} is the median effective dose.

ef•fec•tive half-life (e-fek'tiv haf'līf) Time required for the body burden of an administered quantity of radioactivity to decrease by half through a combination of radioactive decay and biologic elimination.

ef•fec•tive re•nal blood flow (ERBF) (e-fek'tiv rē'năl blŭd flō) The amount of blood flowing to the parts of the kidney involved with production of constituents of urine.

ef•fec•tive re•nal plas•ma flow (ERPF) (e-fek'tiv rē'năl plaz'mă flō) Amount of plasma flowing to kidney parts that function in production of constituents of urine.

ef•fec•tor (e-fek'tŏr) **1.** A peripheral tissue that receives nerve impulses and reacts by contraction (muscle), secretion (gland), or a discharge of electricity (electric organ of certain bony fishes). **2.** A small metabolic molecule that, by combining with a repressor gene, depresses the activity of an operon. **3.** A small molecule that binds to a protein and, in so doing, alters the activity of that protein. **4.** A substance, technique, procedure, or individual that causes an effect.

ef•fec•tor cell (e-fek′tŏr sel) Terminally differentiated leukocyte that performs one or more specific functions. SEE ALSO effector.

ef•fer•ent (ef′ĕr-ĕnt) Conducting outward from an organ or part; e.g., the efferent connections of a group of nerve cells, efferent blood vessels, or the excretory duct of an organ.

ef•fer•ent fi•bers (ef′ĕr-ĕnt fī′bĕrz) Those conveying impulses peripheral to effector tissues (smooth, cardiac, or striated muscle, or glands).

ef•fer•ent nerve (ef′ĕr-ĕnt nĕrv) One conveying impulses from the central nervous system to the periphery. SYN centrifugal nerve, exodic nerve.

ef•fer•vesce (ef-ĕr-ves′) To boil up or cause bubbles to rise to the surface of a fluid in large numbers.

ef•fer•ves•cent (ef′ĕr-ves′ĕnt) Boiling; bubbling.

ef•fi•ca•cy (ef′i-kă-sē) The limit or extent to which a specific intervention, procedure, regimen, pharmacotherapy, or service produces a beneficial result under ideal conditions.

ef•fleu•rage (ef-lūr-ahzh′) A form of massage consisting of superficial or deep long, unbroken strokes in which the hand conforms to the surface and follows the fiber direction of underlying structures. SEE ALSO pétrissage.

ef•flor•es•cent (ef-flōr-es′ĕnt) Denoting a crystalline body that gradually changes to a powder by losing its water of crystallization on exposure to a dry atmosphere.

ef•flu•vi•um, pl. **ef•flu•vi•a** (ĕ-flū′vē-ŭm, -ē-ă) Shedding of hair. SEE ALSO defluxion (1).

ef•fort throm•bo•sis (ef′ŏrt throm-bō′sis) Stress-induced blood clot that occurs in the subclavian or axillary vein.

ef•fu•sion (eff) (e-fyū′zhŭn) **1.** The escape of fluid from the blood vessels or lymphatics into the tissues or a cavity. **2.** A collection of the fluid effused.

e•ges•ta (ē-jes′tă) Unabsorbed food residues that are discharged from the digestive tract.

egg (eg) The female sexual cell or gamete. (This term is *not* used in relation to humans.) SEE ALSO oocyte.

egg mem•brane, sec•on•dar•y egg mem•brane, ter•ti•ar•y egg mem•brane (eg mem′brān, sek′ŏn-dar-ē, tĕr′shē-ăr-ē) A primary egg membrane is produced from ovarian cytoplasm (e.g., a vitelline membrane); a secondary egg membrane is the product of the ovarian follicle (e.g., the zona pellucida); a tertiary egg membrane is secreted by the lining of the oviduct (e.g., a shell).

egg•shell cal•ci•fi•ca•tion (eg′shel kal′si-fi-kā′shŭn) A thin layer around an intrathoracic lymph node, usually in silicosis, seen on a chest radiograph.

e•glan•du•lous (ē-glan′dyū-lŭs) Without glands.

e•go (ē′gō) In freudian psychoanalysis, ego, along with id and superego, are the three components of the psychic apparatus. It perceives from moment to moment external reality, needs of the self (both physical and psychological), integrates the perceptions and uses of logical, abstract, secondary process thinking, and the mechanisms of defense available to it to formulate a response.

e•go•bron•choph•o•ny (ē′gō-brong-kof′ŏ-nē) Egophony with bronchophony.

e•go•cen•tric (ē′gō-sen′trik) Marked by extreme concentration of attention on oneself. SYN egotropic.

e•go•dys•ton•ic (ē′gō-dis-ton′ik) Repugnant to or at variance with the aims of the ego and related psychologic needs of the individual (e.g., an obsessive thought or compulsive behavior); the opposite of ego-syntonic.

e•go i•de•al (ē′gō ī-dēl′) The part of the personality that comprises the goals, aspirations, and aims of the self, usually growing out of the emulation of a significant person with whom one has identified.

e·go·ma·ni·a (ē'gō-mā'nē-ă) Extreme self-centeredness, self-appreciation, or self-content.

e·goph·o·ny (ē-gof'ŏ-nē) A peculiar broken quality in voice sounds, like the bleating of a goat, heard about the upper level of the fluid in association with cases of pleurisy with effusion.

E·gyp·tian oph·thal·mi·a (ē-jip'shŭn of-thal'mē-ă) SYN trachoma.

Ehl·ers-Dan·los syn·drome (ā'lerz dahn'lōs sin'drōm) An inherited disorder of connective tissue characterized by fragile hyperelastic skin and hypermobility of the joints. At least 14 variant forms have been identified and named.

Ehr·lich·i·a (er-lik'ē-ă) A genus of small, often pleomorphic, coccoid to ellipsoidal, nonmotile, gram-negative bacteria that occur either singly or in compact inclusions in circulating mammalian leukocytes; species are the etiologic agents of ehrlichiosis and are transmitted by ticks. The type species is *Ehrlichia canis*.

Ehr·lich·i·e·ae (er-lik'ē-ē) Members of the Rickettsiaceae family; obligate intracellular parasites of peripheral blood leukocytes.

Ehr·lich in·ner bod·y (er-lik in'ĕr bod'ē) A round oxyphil body found in the red blood cell in hemolysis due to a specific blood poison. SYN Heinz-Ehrlich body.

ehr·lich·i·o·sis (er-lik'ē-ō'sis) A tick-borne infection of humans, dogs, and many other mammals caused by bacteria from the *Neorickettsia*, *Anaplasma*, and *Ehrlichia* groups; produces manifestations similar to those of Rocky Mountain spotted fever.

Eich·horst cor·pus·cles (īk'hōrst kōr'pŭs-ĕlz) The globular forms sometimes occurring in the poikilocytosis of pernicious anemia.

ei·det·ic (ī-det'ik) **1.** Relating to the power of visualization of and memory for objects previously seen that peaks in children aged 8–10. **2.** A person possessing this power to a high degree.

ei·det·ic im·age (ī-det'ik im'ăj) Vivid mental picture in the form of a dream, fantasy, or an unusual power of memory and visualization of objects previously seen or imagined.

Ei·ken·el·la cor·ro·dens (ī-kĕ-nel'ă kō-rō'denz) A species of nonmotile, rod-shaped, gram-negative, facultatively anaerobic bacteria that is part of the normal flora of the adult human oral cavity but may be an opportunistic pathogen, especially in immunocompromised hosts.

Ei·sen·men·ger com·plex (ī'zĕn-meng'ĕr kom'pleks) The combination of ventricular septal defect with pulmonary hypertension and consequent right-to-left shunt through the defect, with or without an associated overriding aorta.

Ei·sen·men·ger syn·drome (ī'zĕn-meng'ĕr sin'drōm) Cardiac failure with significant right-to-left shunt producing cyanosis due to higher pressure on the right side of the shunt.

e·jac·u·la·tion, e·jac·u·la·ti·o (ē-jak'yū-lā'shŭn, -shē-ō) The process that results in propulsion of semen from the genital ducts and urethra to the exterior; caused by the rhythmic contractions of the muscles surrounding the internal genital organs and the ischiocavernous and bulbocavernous muscles, resulting in an increase in pressure on the semen in the internal genital glands and the internal urethra.

e·jac·u·la·tor·y duct (ē-jak'yū-lă-tōr-ē dŭkt) [TA] The duct formed by the union of the deferent duct and the excretory duct of the seminal vesicle, which opens into the prostatic urethra.

e·jec·tion (ē-jek'shŭn) **1.** The act of driving or throwing out by physical force from within. **2.** That which is ejected. SYN ejecta.

e·jec·tion click (EC) (ē-jek'shŭn klik) Clicking ejection sound. SEE sound.

e·jec·tion frac·tion (EF) (ē-jek'shŭn frak'shŭn) The fraction of blood contained in the ventricle at the end of diastole that is expelled during its contraction.

e·jec·tion mur·mur (ē-jek´shŭn mŭr´ mŭr) A diamond-shaped systolic murmur produced by the ejection of blood into the aorta or pulmonary artery and ending by the time of the second heart sound component produced, respectively, by closing of the aortic or pulmonic valve.

e·jec·tion pe·ri·od (ē-jek´shŭn pēr´ē-ŏd) SYN sphygmic interval.

e·jec·tion sounds (ē-jek´shŭn sowndz) Clicks audible during ejection from a hypertensive aorta or pulmonary artery or associated with stenosis (particularly congenital) of the aortic or pulmonic valve.

el·a·pid (el´ă-pid) Any member of the snake family Elapidae.

E·lap·i·dae (ē-lap´i-dē) A family of highly venomous snakes characterized by a pair of comparatively short, permanently erect deeply grooved fangs at the front of the mouth. There are over 150 species, including cobras, kraits, mambas, and coral snakes.

e·las·tance (E) (ē-las´tăns) A measure of the tendency of a structure to return to its original form after removal of a deforming force. In medicine and physiology, usually a measure of the tendency of a hollow viscus (e.g., lung, urinary bladder) to recoil toward its original dimensions on removal of a distending or compressing force, the recoil pressure resulting from a unit distention or compression of the viscus.

e·las·tic (ē-las´tik) 1. Having the property of returning to the original shape after being stretched, compressed, bent, or otherwise distorted. 2. A rubber or plastic band used in orthodontics as either a primary or adjunctive source of force to move teeth.

e·las·tic bou·gie (ē-las´tik bū-zhē´) Investigative instrument made of rubber, latex, or other similarly flexible material.

e·las·tic fi·bers (ē-las´tik fī´bĕrz) Fibers that are 0.2–2 mcm in diameter but may be larger in some ligaments; they branch and anastomose to form networks and fuse to form fenestrated membranes. SYN yellow fibers.

e·las·tic lam·i·nae of ar·te·ries (ē-las´ tik lam´i-nē ahr´tĕr-ēz) External: the layer of elastic connective tissue lying immediately outside the smooth muscle of the tunica media. Internal: a fenestrated layer of elastic tissue of the tunica intima. SYN elastic layers of arteries.

e·las·tic mem·brane (ē-las´tik mem´ brān) One formed of elastic connective tissue, present as fenestrated lamellae in the coats of the arteries and elsewhere.

e·las·tic tis·sue (ē-las´tik tish´ū) A form of connective tissue in which elastic fibers predominate.

e·las·tin (ē-las´tin) A yellow elastic fibrous mucoprotein that is the major connective tissue protein of elastic structures (large blood vessels, tendons, and ligaments). SYN elasticin.

e·las·to·fi·bro·ma (ē-las´tō-fī-brō´mă) A nonencapsulated slow-growing mass of poorly cellular, collagenous, fibrous, and elastic tissue.

e·las·toid de·gen·er·a·tion (ē-las´toyd dē-jen´ĕr-ā´shŭn) 1. SYN elastosis (2). 2. Hyaline degeneration of the elastic tissue of the arterial wall, seen during involution of the uterus.

e·las·tol·y·sis (ē-las-tol´i-sis) Dissolution of elastic fibers.

e·las·to·ma (ē-las-tō´mă) A tumorlike deposit of elastic tissue.

e·las·tor·rhex·is (ē-las´tō-rek´sis) Fragmentation of elastic tissue in which the normal wavy strands appear shredded and clumped and take a basophilic stain.

e·las·to·sis (ē-las-tō´sis) 1. Degenerative change in elastic tissue. 2. Degeneration of collagen fibers, with altered staining properties resembling elastic tissue, or formation by fibroblast-activated ultraviolet or mast cell mediators of abnormal fibers. SYN elastoid degeneration (1), elastotic degeneration.

e·las·tot·ic (ē´las-tot´ik) Pertaining to elastosis.

e·la·tion (ē-lā´shŭn) The feeling or expression of excitement or gaiety; if prolonged and inappropriate, a characteristic of mania.

el·bow (el′bō) [TA] **1.** The region of the upper limb between arm and forearm surrounding the elbow joint, especially posteriorly. **2.** The joint between the arm and the forearm. SYN cubitus (1) [TA]. **3.** An angular body resembling a flexed elbow.

el·bow jerk (EJ) (el′bō jĕrk) SYN triceps reflex.

el·bow joint (el′bō joynt) [TA] Compound hinge synovial articulation between the humerus and the bones of the forearm; consists of the articulatio humeroradialis and the articulatio humeroulnaris. SYN articulatio cubiti [TA], elbow (2) [TA], cubital joint.

el·bow re·flex (el′bō rē′fleks) SYN triceps reflex.

el·der, el·der flow·ers (el′dĕr, flow′ĕrz) SYN sambucus.

el·der a·buse (el′dĕr ă-byūs′) Physical or emotional abuse, including financial exploitation, of an elderly person, by one or more of the person's children, caregivers, or others.

E·lec·tra com·plex (ĕ-lek′tră kom′pleks) Unresolved conflicts during childhood toward the father that subsequently influence a woman's relationships with men.

e·lec·tret (el-ek′tret) A type of insulator that carries a permanent charge similar to that found in a magnet.

e·lec·tri·cal al·ter·nans (ĕ-lek′tri-kăl awl-tĕr′nanz) Alternation in the amplitude of P waves, QRS complexes, or T waves as observed by electrocardiography.

e·lec·tri·cal al·ter·na·tion of heart (ĕ-lek′tri-kăl awl-tĕr-nā′shŭn hahrt) A disorder in which the ventricular or atrial complexes or both are regular in time but of alternating pattern.

e·lec·tri·cal di·as·to·le (ĕ-lek′tri-kăl dī-as′tŏ-lē) Period from end of T wave to beginning of next Q wave.

e·lec·tri·cal sys·to·le (ĕ-lek′tri-kăl sis′tŏ-lē) The duration of the QRS-T complex (i.e., from the earliest Q wave to the end of the latest T wave on the electrocardiogram).

e·lec·tric an·es·the·si·a (ĕ-lek′trik anes-thē′zē-ă) Anesthesia, usually general, produced by application of an electrical current.

e·lec·tric cat·a·ract (ĕ-lek′trik kat′ă-rakt) One caused by contact with a high-power electric current or a lightning bolt. SYN cataracta electrica.

electro- Combining form meaning electric, electricity.

e·lec·tro·a·cu·punc·ture (ĕ-lek′trō-ak′yū-pŭngk-shŭr) Acupuncture in which needles are attached to a source of electric current.

e·lec·tro·an·al·ge·si·a (ĕ-lek′trō-an-ăl-jē′zē-ă) Analgesia induced by the passage of an electric current.

e·lec·tro·car·di·o·gram (ECG) (ĕ-lek′trō-kahr′dē-ō-gram) Graphic record of cardiac action currents obtained with the electrocardiograph.

e·lec·tro·car·di·og·ra·phy (ECG) (ĕ-lek′trō-kahr-dē-og′ră-fē) **1.** A method of recording the electrical activity of the heart: impulse formation, conduction, depolarization, and repolarization of atria and ventricles. **2.** The study and interpretation of electrocardiograms.

e·lec·tro·ca·tal·y·sis (ĕ-lek′trō-că-tal′i-sis) Breaking down tissues chemically by introducing an electric current into the tissues.

e·lec·tro·cau·ter·i·za·tion (ĕ-lek′trō-kaw′tĕr-ī-zā′shŭn) Cauterization by passage of high frequency current through tissue or by metal that has been electrically heated.

e·lec·tro·cau·ter·y (EC), electric cautery (ĕ-lek′trō-kaw′tĕr-ē, ĕ-lek′trik kaw′tĕr-ē) An instrument for directing a high frequency current through a local area of tissue.

e·lec·tro·ce·re·bral si·lence (ECS) (ĕ-lek′trō-ser′ĕ-brăl sī′lĕns) Flat or isoelectric encephalogram; an electroencephalogram with absence of cerebral activity from symmetrically placed electrode pairs.

e·lec·tro·chem·i·cal (ĕ-lek′trō-kem′i-kăl)

Denoting chemical reactions involving electricity, and the mechanisms involved.

e·lec·tro·chem·i·cal gra·di·ent (ĕ-lek´trō-kem´i-kăl grā´dē-ĕnt) Measure of ionic tendency to move passively from one point to another, taking into consideration the differences in its concentration and in the electrical potentials between the two points.

e·lec·tro·che·mo·ther·a·py (ECT) (ĕ-lek´trō-kē´mō-thār´ă-pē) Anticancer therapy used to treat dermal basal cell carcinoma; this alternative therapy to surgical excision has demonstrated 98% effectiveness.

e·lec·tro·co·ag·u·la·tion (ĕ-lek´trō-kō-ag´yū-lā´shŭn) That produced by an electrocautery.

e·lec·tro·co·chle·og·ra·phy (ĕ-lek´trō-kok-lē-og´ră-fē) A measurement of the electrical potentials generated in the inner ear as a result of sound stimulation.

e·lec·tro·con·trac·til·i·ty (ĕ-lek´trō-kŏn-trak-til´i-tē) The power of contraction of muscular tissue in response to an electrical stimulus.

e·lec·tro·con·vul·sive (ĕ-lek´trō-kŏn-vŭl´siv) Denoting a convulsive response to an electrical stimulus. SEE electroshock therapy.

e·lec·tro·con·vul·sive ther·a·py (ECT, ECVT) (ĕ-lek´trō-kŏn-vŭl´siv thār´ă-pē) SYN electroshock therapy.

e·lec·tro·cor·ti·co·gram (ĕ-lek´trō-kōr´ti-kō-gram) Direct record of electrical activity from the cerebral cortex.

e·lec·tro·cor·ti·cog·ra·phy (ĕ-lek´trō-kor-ti-kog´ră-fē) The technique of recording the electrical activity of the cerebral cortex by means of electrodes placed directly on it.

e·lec·trode (ĕ-lek´trōd) Device to record one of two extremities of an electric circuit; one of two poles of an electric battery or of the end of the connected conductors.

e·lec·trode cath·e·ter ab·la·tion (ĕ-lek´trōd kath´ĕ-tĕr ăb-lā´shŭn) A method of removing the site of origin of arrhythmias whereby high energy electric shocks are delivered by intravascular catheters.

e·lec·tro·der·mal (ĕ-lek´trō-dĕr´măl) Pertaining to electric properties of the skin, usually referring to altered resistance.

e·lec·tro·der·mal au·di·om·e·try (ĕ-lek´trō-dĕr´măl aw´dē-om´ĕ-trē) A form of electrophysiologic audiometry used to determine hearing thresholds by measuring changes in skin resistance as a conditioned response to noise stimuli.

e·lec·tro·des·ic·ca·tion (ĕ-lek´trō-des-i-kā´shŭn) Destruction of lesions or sealing blood vessels (usually of the skin, but also of available surfaces of mucous membrane) by monopolar high-frequency electric current.

e·lec·tro·dy·nam·ics (ĕ-lek´trō-dī-nam´iks) The study of the movement of electrostatic charges.

e·lec·tro·en·ceph·a·lo·gram (EEG) (ĕ-lek´trō-en-sef´ă-lō-gram) The record obtained by means of the electroencephalograph.

e·lec·tro·en·ceph·a·lo·graph (EEG) (ĕ-lek´trō-en-sef´ă-lō-graf) A system for recording the electric potentials of the brain via scalp electrodes.

e·lec·tro·en·ceph·a·log·ra·phy (EEG) (ĕ-lek´trō-en-sef´ă-log´ră-fē) Registration of the electrical potentials recorded by an electroencephalograph.

e·lec·tro·gas·trog·ra·phy (ĕ-lek´trō-gas-trog´ră-fē) The recording of the electrical phenomena associated with gastric secretion and motility.

e·lec·tro·gram (ĕ-lek´trō-gram) **1.** Any record on paper or film made by an electrical event. **2.** ELECTROPHYSIOLOGY surface recording taken directly with unipolar or bipolar leads.

electrohaemostasis [Br.] SYN electrohemostasis.

e·lec·tro·he·mo·sta·sis (ĕ-lek´trō-hē-mos´tă-sis) Arrest of hemorrhage by means of an electrocautery. SYN electrohaemostasis.

e·lec·tro·hy·draul·ic shock wave lith·o·trip·sy (ESWL) (ĕ-lek´trō-hīdrawl'ik shok wāv lith'ō-trip-sē) De-struction of calculi (urinary tract or other) by fragmentation using shock waves sent transcutaneously via ultra-sound transducers.

e·lec·tro·im·mu·no·dif·fu·sion (EID) (ĕ-lek'trō-im'yū-nō-di-fyū'zhŭn) An im-munochemical method that combines electrophoretic separation with immuno-diffusion by incorporating antibody into the support medium.

e·lec·trol·y·sis (ĕ-lek-trol'i-sis) **1.** De-composition of a salt or other chemical compound by means of an electric cur-rent. **2.** Destruction of certain hair folli-cles by means of galvanic electricity.

e·lec·tro·lyte (ĕ-lek'trō-līt) Any com-pound that, in solution, conducts electric-ity and is decomposed by it; an ionizable substance in solution.

e·lec·tro·lyte im·bal·ance (ĕ-lek'trō-līt im-bal'ăns) Physiologic disorder in which there are fewer or more than normal levels of serum electrolytes.

e·lec·tro·mag·net (ĕ-lek'trō-mag'nĕt) A bar of soft iron rendered magnetic by an electric current encircling it.

e·lec·tro·mag·net·ic in·duc·tion (ĕ-lek'trō-mag-net'ik in-dŭk'shŭn) Genera-tion of an electrical current in a conduc-tor when it is moved across a magnetic field.

e·lec·tro·me·chan·i·cal sys·to·le (ĕ-lek'trō-mĕ-kan'i-kăl sis'tō-lē) The period from the beginning of the QRS complex to the first (aortic) vibration of the second heart sound. SYN QS₂ interval.

e·lec·tro·mo·til·i·ty (ĕ-lek'trō-mō-til'i-tē) Movement of the cochlear outer hair cells in response to electrical stimula-tion.

e·lec·tro·mo·tive force (EMF) (ĕ-lek'trō-mō'tiv fōrs) The force (measured in volts) that causes the flow of electricity from one point to another.

e·lec·tro·my·o·gram (EMG) (ĕ-lek'trō-mī'ō-gram) Graphic representation of electric currents associated with muscu-lar action.

e·lec·tro·my·o·graph·ic (EMG) syn·

drome (ĕ-lek'trō-mī'ō-graf'ik sin'drōm) SYN Beckwith-Wiedemann syndrome.

e·lec·tro·my·og·ra·phy (EMG) (ĕ-lek'trō-mī-og'ră-fē) **1.** The recording of elec-trical activity generated in muscle for di-agnostic purposes. **2.** Umbrella term for the entire electrodiagnostic study per-formed in the EMG laboratory, including not only needle electrode examination, but also nerve conduction studies.

e·lec·tron (ĕ-lek'tron) One of the nega-tively charged subatomic particles dis-tributed in the positive nucleus and with it constitute the atom.

e·lec·tro·nar·co·sis (ĕ-lek'trō-nahr-kō'sis) Production of insensibility to pain by the use of electrical current.

e·lec·tron beam to·mog·ra·phy (EBT) (ĕ-lek'tron bēm tŏ-mog'ră-fē) Computed tomography in which the circular motion of the x-ray tube is replaced by rapid elec-tronic positioning of the cathode ray a-round a circular anode.

e·lec·tro·neg·a·tive (ĕ-lek'trō-neg'ă-tiv) Relating to or charged with negative elec-tricity.

e·lec·tro·neu·ro·my·og·ra·phy (ĕ-lek'trō-nūr'ō-mī-og'ră-fē) A method of mea-suring changes in a peripheral nerve by combining electromyography of a muscle with electrical stimulation of the nerve trunk carrying fibers to and from it.

e·lec·tron·ic fe·tal mon·i·tor (ĕ-lek-tron'ik fē'tăl mon'i-tŏr) Instrument for continuous monitoring of the fetal heart before or during labor.

e·lec·tron mi·cro·scope (ĕ-lek'tron mī'krŏ-skōp) A visual and photographic mi-croscope in which electron beams with wavelengths shorter than visible light are used instead of light, thereby allowing much greater resolution and magnifica-tion.

e·lec·tron ra·di·og·ra·phy (ĕ-lek'tron rā'dē-og'ră-fē) Radiographic imaging in which x-radiation is converted to a latent image and subsequently printed out.

e·lec·tro·nys·tag·mog·ra·phy (ENG) (ĕ-lek'trō-nis-tag-mog'ră-fē) Nystag-mography based on electrooculography; skin electrodes are placed at outer canthi to register horizontal nystagmus, or above and below each eye for vertical nystagmus.

e·lec·tro·oc·u·log·ra·phy (EOG) (ĕ-lek'trō-ok'yū-log'ră-fē) Oculography in which electrodes placed on the skin adjacent to the eyes measure changes in standing potential between the front and back of the eyeball as the eyes move.

e·lec·tro·ol·fac·to·gram (EOG) (ĕ-lek'trō-ōl-fak'tŏ-gram) An electronegative wave of potential occurring on the surface of the olfactory epithelium in response to stimulation by an odor.

e·lec·tro·pher·o·gram, e·lec·tro·pho·ret·o·gram (ĕ-lek'trō-fer'ŏ-gram, -fŏret'ŏ-gram) The densitometric or colorimetric pattern obtained from filter paper or similar porous strips on which substances have been separated by electrophoresis; may also refer to the strips themselves. SYN electrophoretogram.

e·lec·tro·pho·re·sis (ĕ-lek'trō-fŏr-ē'sis) The movement of particles in an electric field toward anode or cathode. SEE ALSO electropherogram. SYN ionophoresis, phoresis (1).

e·lec·tro·phren·ic (ĕ-lek'trō-fren'ik) Denoting electrical stimulation of the phrenic nerve usually at its motor point in the neck. SEE ALSO electrophrenic respiration.

e·lec·tro·phren·ic res·pi·ra·tion (ĕ-lek'trō-fren'ik res'pir-ā'shŭn) The rhythmic electrical stimulation of the phrenic nerve by an electrode applied to the skin at the motor points of the phrenic nerve; it is used in paralysis of the respiratory center resulting from acute bulbar poliomyelitis.

e·lec·tro·phys·i·ol·o·gy (EP) (ĕ-lek'trō-fiz'ē-ol'ŏ-jē) Science concerned with electrical phenomena that are associated with physiologic processes.

e·lec·tro·por·a·tion (ĕ-lek'trō-pōr-ā'shŭn) A technique in which a brief electric shock is applied to cells; momentary holes open briefly in the plasma membrane, allowing the entry of macromolecules (e.g., a way of introducing new DNA into a cell).

e·lec·tro·po·ra·tion ther·a·py (EPT) (ĕ-lek'trō-pōr-ā'shŭn thār'ă-pē) Investigational therapy involving use of electric fields to open pores in human cells; provides for easier and more efficient entry of genes or pharmaceutical products.

e·lec·tro·pos·i·tive (ĕ-lek'trō-pos'i-tiv) 1. Relating to or charged with positive electricity. 2. Referring to an element whose atoms tend to lose electrons.

e·lec·tro·ret·i·no·gram (ERG) (ĕ-lek'trō-ret'i-nō-gram) Record of the retinal action currents produced in the retina by light stimulus.

e·lec·tro·scis·sion (ĕ-lek'trō-sizh'ŭn) Division of tissues by means of an electrocautery knife.

e·lec·tro·shock ther·a·py (EST) (ĕ-lek'trō-shok' thār'ă-pē) A form of treatment of mental disorders in which convulsions are elicited by the passage of an electric current through the brain. SYN electroconvulsive therapy.

e·lec·tro·sur·ger·y (ĕ-lek'trō-sŭr'jĕr-ē) Division of tissues by high frequency current applied locally with a metal instrument or needle. SEE ALSO electrocautery.

e·lec·tro·tax·is (ĕ-lek'trō-tak'sis) Reaction of plant or animal protoplasm to either an anode or a cathode. SEE ALSO tropism. SYN electrotropism.

e·lec·tro·ton·ic (ĕ-lek'trō-ton'ik) Relating to electrotonus.

e·lec·tro·ton·ic cur·rent (ĕ-lek'trō-ton'ik kŭr'ent) SEE electrotonus.

e·lec·tro·val·ence (ĕ-lek'trō-vā'lĕns) Ability of an element to blend with another through sharing of electrons.

el·ec·tro·vi·bra·to·ry mas·sage (ĕ-lek'trō-vī'bră-tōr-ē mă-sazh') Use of an electronic vibrating device in massage.

el·e·ment (el'ĕ-mĕnt) A substance composed of atoms of only one kind, i.e., of identical atomic (proton) number, which therefore cannot be decomposed into two or more elements.

eleo- Prefix meaning oil. SEE ALSO oleo-.

el·e·o·ma (el'ē-ō'mă) SYN lipogranuloma.

el·e·phan·ti·a·sis (el'ĕ-fan-tī'ă-sis) Hypertrophy and fibrosis of the skin and subcutaneous tissue, especially of the lower extremities and genitalia, caused by long-standing obstruction of lymphatic vessels, most commonly after years of infection by the filarial worms *Wuchereria bancrofti* or *Brugia malayi*, coupled with secondary bacterial infection alone or combined with a fungal infection.

el·e·phan·toid fe·ver (el'ĕ-fan'toyd fē' vĕr) Lymphangitis and an elevation of temperature marking the beginning of endemic elephantiasis (filariasis).

el·e·va·tor (el'ĕ-vā-tŏr) 1. An instrument for prying up a sunken part. 2. A surgical instrument used to luxate and remove teeth and roots that cannot be engaged by the beaks of a forceps, or to loosen teeth and roots prior to forceps application.

e·lev·enth cra·ni·al nerve [CN XI] (ĕ-lev'ĕnth krā'nē-ăl nĕrv) SYN accessory nerve [CN XI].

e·lim·i·na·tion di·et (ĕ-lim'i-nā'shŭn dī' ĕt) One designed to detect what ingredient of the food causes allergic manifestations in the patient; items to which the patient may be sensitive are withdrawn separately and successively from the diet until the allergenic item is discovered.

e·lix·ir (elix.) (ĕ-lik'sĭr) A clear, sweetened, hydroalcoholic liquid intended for oral use.

el·lip·sis (ĕ-lip'sis) Omission of words or ideas, leaving the whole to be completed by the reader or listener.

el·lip·soi·d joint, el·lip·soi·dal joint (ĕ-lip'soyd joynt, ĕ-lip-soy'dăl) SYN condylar joint.

el·lip·tic am·pu·ta·tion (ĕ-lip'tik amp' yū-tā'shŭn) Circular amputation in which the sweep of the knife is not exactly vertical to the axis of the limb.

El Tor vib·ri·o (el tōr vib'rē-ō) Bacterium regarded as a biovar of *Vibrio cholerae*. It was originally isolated from six pilgrims who died of dysentery or gangrene of the colon at the Tor quarantine station on the Sinai Peninsula.

el·u·ate (el'yū-āt) The solution emerging from a column or paper in chromatography. SEE ALSO elution.

el·u·ent (el'yū-ĕnt) The mobile phase in chromatography. SEE ALSO elution. SYN developer (2).

e·lu·tion, e·lu·tri·a·tion (ē-lū'shŭn, -trē-ā'shŭn) 1. The separation, by washing, of one solid from another. 2. The removal, by means of a suitable solvent, of one material from another that is insoluble in that solvent, as in column chromatography. 3. The removal of antibodies absorbed onto the erythrocyte surface.

E·ly sign (ē'lī sīn) Indicator of femoral nerve irritation, lateral thigh contracture, or tightness of the rectus femoris muscle if when the prone patient flexes the calf onto the thigh, the gluteus muscles retract and the hip abducts.

elytro- Prefix meaning the vagina. SEE ALSO colpo-.

e·ma·ci·a·tion (ē-mā'shē-ā'shŭn) Becoming abnormally thin from extreme loss of flesh. SYN wasting (1).

e·mas·cu·la·tion (ē-mas'kyū-lā'shŭn) Castration of the male by removal of the testes and/or penis.

Emb·den-Mey·er·hof path·way (em' dĕn mī'ĕr-hof path'wā) The anaerobic glycolytic pathway by which D-glucose (most notably in muscle) is converted to lactic acid. Cf. glycolysis.

em·bo·le (em'bŏ-lē) Formulation of the gastrula by invagination.

em·bo·lec·to·my (em'bō-lek'tŏ-mē) Removal of an embolus.

em·bol·ic (em-bol'ik) Relating to an embolus or to embolism.

em·bol·ic gan·grene (em-bol'ik gang' grēn) Gangrene resulting from obstruction of an artery by an embolus.

em·bol·i·form (em-bol'i-fŏrm) Shaped like an embolus.

em·bol·i·form nu·cle·us (em-bol'i-fōrm nū′klē-ŭs) A small wedge-shaped nucleus in the central white substance of the cerebellum just internal to the hilus of the dentate nucleus. SYN embolus (2).

embolisation [Br.] SYN embolization.

em·bo·lism (em′bŏ-lizm) Obstruction or occlusion of a vessel by an embolus.

em·bo·li·za·tion (em′bŏl-ī-zā′shŭn) **1.** The formation and release of an embolus into the circulation. **2.** Therapeutic introduction of various substances into the circulation to occlude vessels, either to arrest or prevent hemorrhaging, to devitalize a structure, tumor, or organ by occluding its blood supply, or to reduce blood flow to an arteriovenous malformation.

em·bo·lus, gen. and pl. **em·bo·li** (em′bŏ-lŭs, -lī) **1.** A plug, composed of a detached thrombus or vegetation, mass of bacteria, quantity of air or gas, or foreign body, which occludes a vessel. **2.** SYN emboliform nucleus.

em·bo·ly (em′bŏ-lē) SYN embole (2).

em·bra·sure (em-brā′shŭr) In dentistry, an opening that widens outwardly or inwardly; specifically, that space adjacent to the interproximal contact area that spreads toward the facial, gingival, lingual, occlusal, or incisal aspect.

em·bry·o (em′brē-ō) **1.** An organism in the early stages of development. **2.** In humans, the developing organism from conception until the end of the eighth week; developmental stages from this time to birth are commonly designated as fetal. **3.** A primordial plant within a seed.

embryo- Prefix denoting related to the embryo.

em·bry·o·blast (em′brē-ō-blast) The mass of cells at the embryonic pole of the blastocyst that forms the embryo and some extraembryonic or adnexal tissues. SYN inner cell mass.

em·bry·o·car·di·a (em′brē-ō-kahr′dē-ă) A condition in which the cadence of the heart sounds resembles that of the fetus, the first and second sounds becoming alike and evenly spaced; a sign of serious myocardial disease.

em·bry·o·gen·e·sis (em′brē-ō-jen′ĕ-sis) That phase of prenatal development involved in establishment of the characteristic configuration of the embryonic body; in humans, embryogenesis is usually regarded as extending from the end of the second week, when the embryonic disc is formed, to the end of the eighth week, after which the conceptus is usually spoken of as a fetus.

em·bry·o·gen·ic, em·bry·o·ge·net·ic (em′brē-ō-jen′ik, -jĕ-net′ik) Producing an embryo; relating to the formation of an embryo.

em·bry·oid (em′brē-oyd) SYN embryonoid.

em·bry·ol·o·gy (em′brē-ol′ŏ-jē) Science of the origin and development of the organism from fertilization of the oocyte to the end of the eighth week and, by extension, all subsequent stages up to birth.

em·bry·o·nal (em′brē-ōn′ăl) Relating to an embryo.

em·bry·o·nate (em′brē-ō-nāt) **1.** SYN embryonal. **2.** Containing an embryo. **3.** Impregnated.

em·bry·on·i·form (em′brē-on′i-fōrm) SYN embryonoid.

em·bry·on·i·za·tion (em′brē-ŏn-ī-zā′shŭn) Reversion of a cell or tissue to an embryonic form.

em·bry·o·noid (em′brē-ŏ-noyd) Resembling an embryo or a fetus. SYN embryoid, embryoni form.

em·bry·o·path·ic cat·a·ract (em′brē-ō-path′ik kat′ăr-akt) Congenital cataract as a result of intrauterine infection.

em·bry·op·a·thy (em′brē-op′ă-thē) A morbid condition in the embryo or fetus. SYN fetopathy.

em·bry·o·plas·tic (em′brē-ō-plas′tik) **1.** Producing an embryo. **2.** Relating to the formation of an embryo.

em·bry·ot·o·my (em′brē-ot′ŏ-mē) Any mutilating operation on the fetus to make possible its removal when delivery is impossible by natural means.

em·bry·o·tox·ic·i·ty (em'brē-ō-tok-sis'i-tē) Injury to the embryo, which may result in death or abnormal development of a part, owing to substances that enter the placental circulation.

em·bry·o·tox·on (em'brē-ō-tok'son) Congenital opacity of the corneal periphery.

em·bry·o trans·fer (ET) (em'brē-ō trans'fĕr) After in vitro artificial insemination, the embryo is transferred at the morula or blastocyst stage to the recipient's uterus or uterine tube.

em·bry·o·tro·phic (em'brē-ō-trō'fik) Relating to any process or agency involved in the nourishment of the embryo.

e·med·ul·late (ē-med'yū-lāt) To extract any marrow.

e·mer·gen·cy (emer, EMG, emerg) (ē-mĕr'jĕn-sē) A patient's condition requiring immediate treatment.

e·mer·gen·cy con·tra·cep·tive (ē-mĕr'jĕn-sē kon'tră-sep'tiv) SYN morning after pill.

e·mer·gen·cy de·part·ment (ē-mĕr'jĕn'sē dĕ-pahrt'mĕnt) That section of a hospital or other health care facility that is designed, staffed, and equippped to treat injured people and those afflicted with sudden, severe illness.

e·mer·gen·cy doc·trine (ē-mĕr'jĕn-sē dok'trin) In medical jurisprudence, an assumption that a disabled or nonresponsive patient will agree to life-saving measures.

emer·gen·cy med·i·cal tech·ni·cian– ba·sic (EMT-B) (ē-mĕr'jĕn-sē med'i-kăl tek-nish'ăn-bā'sik) A certified prehospital provider who can perform basic life support (BLS); uses assessment-based approach to patient management. Minimum level of certification required to staff a BLS ambulance.

emer·gen·cy med·i·cal tech·ni·cian– par·a·med·ic (EMT-P) (ē-mĕr'jĕn-sē med'i-kăl tek-nish'ăn-par'ă-med'ik) A licensed prehospital provider who can perform all aspects of advanced life support; usually works according to standing orders or protocols and uses a diagnostic approach to patient management.

emer·gen·cy med·i·cine (ē-mĕr'jĕn-sē med'i-sin) That branch of health care involved with remediation or therapy of patients who are acutely ill or traumatized.

e·mer·gent (ē-mĕr'jĕnt) 1. Arising suddenly and unexpectedly, calling for quick judgment and prompt action. 2. Coming out; leaving a cavity or other part.

e·mer·gent ev·o·lu·tion (ē-mĕr'jĕnt ev-ō-lū'shŭn) Appearance of a property in a complex system e.g., organism that could have been predicted only with difficulty, or perhaps not at all, from a knowledge and understanding of the individual genotype changes taken separately.

em·er·y (em'ĕr-ē) An abrasive containing aluminum oxide and iron.

-emesis Suffix denoting vomiting, vomitus.

em·e·sis (em'ĕ-sis) 1. SYN vomiting. 2. Combining form, used as a suffix, for vomiting.

em·e·sis ba·sin, kid·ney ba·sin (em'ĕ-sis bā'sin, kid'nē) A kidney-shaped container, usually plastic, intended to catch vomitus at the bedside.

em·e·sis grav·i·da·rum (em'ĕ-sis grav'i-dā'rŭm) Vomiting due to pregnancy.

e·met·ic (ē-met'ik) 1. Relating to or causing vomiting. 2. An agent that causes vomiting.

em·e·tine (em'ĕ-tēn) The principal alkaloid of ipecacuanha (q.v.), used as an emetic; its salts are used in amebiasis; available as the hydrochloride.

em·e·to·ca·thar·tic (em'ĕ-tō-kă-thahr'tik) 1. Both emetic and cathartic. 2. An agent that causes both vomiting and purging.

-emia Suffix meaning blood.

em·i·gra·tion (em-i-grā'shŭn) The passage of white blood cells through the endothelium and wall of small blood vessels.

em·i·nence (em'i-nĕns) [TA] A circumscribed area raised above the general level of the surrounding surface, particularly on a bone surface. SYN eminentia [TA].

em·i·nen·ti·a, pl. **em·i·nen·ti·ae** (em-i-nen'shē-ă, -ē) [TA] SYN eminence.

em·i·o·cy·to·sis, **em·ei·o·cy·to·sis** (ē'mē-ō-sī-tō'sis) SYN exocytosis (2).

em·is·sa·ry (em'i-sar-ē) **1.** Relating to, or providing, an outlet or drain. **2.** SYN emissary vein.

em·is·sa·ry vein (em'i-sar-ē vān) [TA] A channel of communication between the venous sinuses of the dura mater and the veins of the diploë and the scalp. SYN vena emissaria [TA], emissarium, emissary (2).

e·mis·sion (ē-mish'ŭn) A discharge; usually referring to a discharge of the male internal genital organs into the internal urethra. Cf. ejaculation.

em·me·tro·pi·a (em'ĕ-trō'pē-ă) The state of refraction of the eye in which parallel rays, when the eye is at rest, are focused exactly on the retina.

Em·mon·si·a (e-mon'sē-ă) A filamentous soil fungus, one species of which (*E. parva*) occasionally causes pneumonitis in rodents and humans; infection worse in immunocompromised hosts.

e·mol·li·ent (ē-mol'ē-ĕnt) **1.** Soothing to the skin or mucous membrane. **2.** An agent that softens the skin or soothes irritation in the skin or mucous membrane.

e·mo·tion (emot) (ē-mō'shŭn) A strong feeling, aroused mental state, or intense state of drive or unrest, which may be directed toward a definite object and is evidenced in both behavior and in psychological changes, with accompanying autonomic nervous system manifestations.

e·mo·tion·al age (ē-mō'shŭn-ăl āj) Measure of emotional maturity by comparison with average emotional development.

emo·tion·al a·men·or·rhe·a (ē-mō'shŭn-ăl ă-men-ōr-ē'ă) Menstrual hiatus caused by a strong emotional disturbance, e.g., fright, grief.

emo·tion·al dep·ri·va·tion (ē-mō'shŭn-ăl dep'ri-vā'shŭn) Lack of adequate and appropriate interpersonal or environmental experiences, or both, usually in the early developmental years.

emo·tion·al glu·co·su·ri·a (ē-mō'shŭn-ăl glū'kō-syūr'ē-ă) A fluctuating increase in urinary sugar levels caused by anxiety.

em·pa·thy (em'pă-thē) The ability to sense the emotions, feelings, and reactions intellectually and emotionally that another person is experiencing and to communicate that understanding to the person effectively. SEE ALSO sympathy (3).

em·phy·se·ma (em'fi-sē'mă) **1.** Presence of air in the interstices of the connective tissue of a part. **2.** A condition of the lung characterized by increase beyond the normal in the size of air spaces distal to the terminal bronchiole (those parts containing alveoli), with destructive changes in their walls and reduction in their number.

em·pir·i·cism (em-pir'i-sizm) A looking to experience as a guide to practice or to the therapeutic use of any remedy.

em·pir·ic for·mu·la (em-pir'ik fōr'myū-lă) CHEMISTRY a formula indicating the kind and number of atoms in the molecules of a substance, or its composition, but not the relation of the atoms to each other or the intimate structure of the molecule. SYN molecular formula.

em·pir·ic treat·ment (em-pir'ik trēt'mĕnt) Therapy based on experience, usually without adequate data to support its use.

em·pros·thot·o·nos, **em·pros·thot·o·nus** (em'pros-thot'ŏ-nos, -nŭs) A tetanic contraction of the flexor muscles, curving the back with concavity forward.

em·py·e·ma, pl. **em·py·e·ma·ta** (em'pī-ē'mă, -tă) Pus in a body cavity; when used without qualification, refers specifically to pyothorax.

em·py·e·mic (em'pī-ē'mik) Relating to empyema.

EMT Abbreviation for Emergency Medical Technician.

e·mul·gent (ē-mŭl′jĕnt) Denoting a straining, extracting, or purifying process.

e·mul·si·fi·ca·tion (ē-mŭl′si-fi-kā′shŭn) Partial dissolution of lipidinous matter.

emul·si·fi·er (ē-mŭl′si-fī-ĕr) An agent (e.g., gum arabic or egg yolk), used to make an emulsion of a fixed oil. Soaps, detergents, steroids, and proteins can act as emulsifiers.

e·mul·sion (ē-mŭl′shŭn) A system containing two immiscible liquids in which one is dispersed, in the form of very small globules (internal phase), throughout the other (external phase).

e·nam·el (ĕ-nam′ĕl) [TA] The hard, acellular, inert substance covering the tooth. Also called enamelum.

e·nam·el cap (ĕ-nam′ĕl kap) The hard substance covering the crown of a tooth.

e·nam·el cell (ĕ-nam′ĕl sel) SYN ameloblast.

e·nam·el crypt (ĕ-nam′ĕl kript) The narrow, mesenchyme-filled space between the dental ledge and an enamel organ. Also called enamel niche.

e·nam·el fis·sure (ĕ-nam′ĕl fish′ŭr) Deep cleft between adjoining cusps affording retention to caries-producing agents.

e·nam·el germ (ĕ-nam′ĕl jĕrm) The enamel organ of a developing tooth.

e·nam·el hy·po·pla·si·a (ĕ-nam′ĕl hī′pō-plā′zē-ă) Developmental disturbance of teeth characterized by deficient or defective enamel matrix formation.

e·nam·el·ins (ĕ-nam′ĕl-inz) Proteins that form the organic matrix of mature tooth enamel.

e·nam·el lay·er (ĕ-nam′ĕl lā′ĕr) SYN ameloblastic layer.

e·nam·el mem·brane (ĕ-nam′ĕl mem′brăn) Internal layer of the enamel organ formed by the ameloblasts.

e·nam·el·o·ma, e·nam·el pearl (ĕ-nam′ĕl-ō′mă, ĕ-nam′ĕl pĕrl) A developmental anomaly in which there is a small nodule of enamel below the cementoenamel junction, usually at the bifurcation of molar teeth. SYN enamel drop, enamel nodule.

e·nam·el or·gan (ĕ-nam′ĕl ōr′găn) A circumscribed mass of ectodermal cells budded off from the dental lamina; it develops the ameloblast layer of cells, which produces the enamel cap of a developing tooth. SYN dental organ.

en·an·ti·o·mer (en-an′tē-ō-mĕr) One of a pair of molecules that are nonsuperimposable mirror images of each other; neither molecule has an internal plane of symmetry.

en·an·ti·o·morph (en-an′tē-ō-mōrf′) A crystal enantiomer.

en·ar·thro·di·al joint (en′ahr-thrō′dē-ăl joynt) SYN ball-and-socket joint.

en·ar·thro·sis (en′ahr-thrō′sis) SYN ball-and-socket joint.

en bloc (on[h] blok) In a lump; as a whole; referring to a surgical or autopsy procedure in which organs or tissues are removed from the body in continuity, without prior dissection.

en·cap·su·lat·ed (en-kap′sŭ-lā-tĕd) Enclosed in a capsule or sheath. SYN encapsuled.

♲ **encephal-** SEE encephalo-.

en·ceph·a·lal·gi·a (en-sef′ă-lal′jē-ă) SYN headache.

en·ceph·a·lat·ro·phy (en-sef′ă-lat′rŏ-fē) Atrophy of the brain.

en·ce·phal·ic (en′se-fal′ik) Relating to the brain, or to the structures within the cranium.

en·ceph·a·li·tis, pl. **en·ceph·a·lit·i·des** (en-sef′ă-lī′tis, -lit′i-dēz) Inflammation of the brain parenchyma. Cf. meningoencephalitis. SYN cephalitis.

en·ceph·a·li·to·gen·ic (en-sef′ă-li-tō-jen′ik) Producing encephalitis; typically by hypersensitivity mechanisms.

En·ceph·a·li·to·zo·on hel·lem (en-sef′ă-lit-ō-zō′on hel′ĕm) A species of *En-*

cephalitozoon described in human ophthalmic infections; causes punctate keratopathy and corneal ulceration in AIDS patients.

En·ceph·a·li·to·zo·on in·tes·ti·na·le (en-sef′ă-lit-ō-zō′on in-tes-ti-nā′lē) A diarrheogenic microsporidian described in HIV-infected patients; disease may be localized to the gastrointestinal tract or may disseminate intravascularly.

encephalo-, encephal- Combining forms denoting the brain. Cf. cerebro-.

en·ceph·a·lo·cele (en-sef′ă-lō-sēl) A congenital gap in the cranium with herniation of brain substance. SYN craniocele, cranium bifidum, bifid cranium.

en·ceph·a·lo·cys·to·cele (en-sef′ă-lō-sis′tō-sēl) SYN hydrencephalocele.

en·ceph·a·lo·dys·pla·si·a (en-sef′ă-lō-dis-plā′zē-ă) Any congenital abnormality of the brain.

en·ceph·a·loid (en-sef′ă-loyd) Resembling brain substance; denoting a carcinoma of soft, brainlike consistency.

en·ceph·a·lo·lith (en-sef′ă-lō-lith) A concretion in the brain or one of its ventricles.

en·ceph·a·lo·ma (en-sef′ă-lō′mă) Herniation of brain substance. SYN cerebroma.

en·ceph·a·lo·ma·la·ci·a (en-sef′ă-lō-mă-lā′shē-ă) Abnormal softness of the cerebral parenchyma often due to ischemia or infarction. SYN cerebromalacia.

en·ceph·a·lo·men·in·gi·tis (en-sef′ă-lō-men-in-jī′tis) SYN meningoencephalitis.

en·ceph·a·lo·me·nin·go·cele (en-sef′ă-lō-me-ning′gō-sēl) SYN meningoencephalocele.

en·ceph·a·lo·mere (en-sef′ă-lō-mēr) SYN neuromere.

en·ceph·a·lom·e·ter (en-sef′ă-lom′ĕ-tĕr) An apparatus to indicate cranial cortical centers.

en·ceph·a·lo·my·e·li·tis (en-sef′ă-lō-

mī′ĕ-lī′tis) Inflammation of the brain and spinal cord.

en·ceph·a·lo·my·el·o·cele (en-sef′ă-lō- mī′ĕ-lō-sēl) Congenital cranial defect usually in the occipital region and cervical vertebrae, with herniation of the meninges and neural tissue.

en·ceph·a·lo·my·e·lo·neu·rop·a·thy (en-sef′ă-lō-mī′ĕ-lō-nūr-op′ă-thē) A disease involving the brain, spinal cord, and peripheral nerves.

en·ceph·a·lo·my·e·lo·ra·dic·u·li·tis (en-sef′ă-lō-mī′ĕ-lō-ră-dik′yū-lī′tis) SYN encephalomyeloradiculopathy.

en·ceph·a·lo·my·e·lo·ra·dic·u·lop·a·thy (en-sef′ă-lō-mī′ĕ-lō-ră-dik′yū-lop′ă-thē) Disorder involving the brain, spinal cord, and spinal roots. SYN encephalomyeloradiculitis.

en·ceph·a·lo·my·o·car·di·tis (en-sef′ă-lō-mī′ō-kahr-dī′tis) Associated encephalitis and myocarditis; often caused by a viral infection such as in poliomyelitis.

en·ceph·a·lo·my·o·car·di·tis vi·rus (en-sef′ă-lō-mī′ō-kahr-dī′tis vī′rŭs) A picornavirus, probably of rodents; occasionally causes febrile illness with central nervous system involvement in humans.

en·ceph·a·lon, pl. **en·ceph·a·la** (en-sef′ă-lon, -lă) [TA] That portion of the cerebrospinal axis contained within the cranium, composed of the prosencephalon, mesencephalon, and rhombencephalon.

en·ceph·a·lop·a·thy, en·ceph·a·lo·pa·thi·a (en-sef′ă-lop′ă-thē, -lō-path′ē-ă) 1. Any brain disorder. 2. A disorder of the brain parenchyma. SYN cephalopathy, cerebropathy, encephalosis.

en·ceph·a·lo·py·o·sis (en-sef′ă-lō-pī-ō′sis) Term for purulent inflammation of the brain.

en·ceph·a·lo·scle·ro·sis (en-sef′ă-lō-skler-ō′sis) A sclerosis, or hardening, of the brain. SEE ALSO cerebrosclerosis.

en·ceph·a·lo·sis (en-sef′ă-lō′sis) SYN encephalopathy.

en·ceph·a·lot·o·my (en-sef′ă-lot′ŏ-mē) Dissection or incision of the brain.

en·ceph·a·lo·tri·gem·i·nal an·gi·o·ma·to·sis (en-sef'ă-lō-trī-jem'i-năl an'jē-ō-mă-tō'sis) SYN Sturge-Weber syndrome.

en·chon·dro·ma, pl. **en·chon·dro·ma·ta** (en'kon-drō'mă, -tă) A benign cartilaginous growth starting within the medullary cavity of a bone originally formed from cartilage; may distend the cortex, especially of small bones and be solitary or multiple (endochondromatosis).

en·clave (en'klāv, on') Detached mass of tissue enclosed in tissue of another kind; seen especially as isolated masses of gland tissue detached from the main gland.

en·cop·re·sis (en'kōp-rē'sis) The repeated, generally involuntary passage of feces into inappropriate places (e.g., clothing).

end (end) [TA] An extremity, or the most remote point of an extremity.

end·an·gi·i·tis, end·an·ge·i·tis (end-an'jē-ī'tis) Inflammation of the intima of a blood vessel. SYN endovasculitis.

end·a·or·ti·tis, end·o·a·or·ti·tis (end'ā-ōr-tī'tis, en'dō-) Inflammation of the intima of the aorta.

end·ar·ter·ec·to·my (end'ahr-tĕr-ek'tŏ-mē) Excision of atheromatous deposits, along with the diseased endothelium and media or most of the media of an artery, so as to leave a smooth lining, mostly consisting of adventitia.

end·ar·te·ri·tis, end·o·ar·ter·it·is (end'ahr-tĕr-ī'tis, en'dō-) Inflammation of the intima of an artery.

end·ar·ter·it·is ob·li·te·rans, ob·lit·er·at·ing end·ar·ter·it·is (end'ahr-tĕr-ī'tis ob-lit'ĕr-anz, ob-lit-ĕr-ā'ting) An extreme degree of endarteritis proliferans closing the lumen of the artery. SYN arteritis obliterans.

end ar·te·ry (end ahr'tĕr-ē) An artery with insufficient anastomoses to maintain viability of the tissue supplied if occlusion of the artery occurs. SYN terminal artery.

end·au·ral (end-awr'ăl) Within the ear.

end bud (end bŭd) SYN caudal eminence.

en·dem·ic (en-dem'ik) Present in a community or among a group of people; said of a disease prevailing continually in a region. Cf. epidemic, sporadic.

en·dem·ic goi·ter (en-dem'ik goy'tĕr) One of usual simple type, prevalent in certain regions where dietary intake of iodine is suboptimal.

en·dem·ic he·ma·tu·ri·a (en-dem'ik hē'mă-tyūr'ē-ă) SYN schistosomiasis haematobium.

en·dem·ic sy·phil·is (en-dem'ik sif'i-lis) SYN nonvenereal syphilis.

en·dem·ic ty·phus (en-dem'ik tī'fŭs) SYN murine typhus.

en·dem·o·ep·i·dem·ic (en-dem'ō-ep-i-dem'ik) Denoting a temporary large increase in the number of cases of an endemic disease.

end·er·gon·ic (en'dĕr-gon'ik) Referring to a chemical reaction that takes place with absorption of energy from its surroundings (i.e., a positive change in Gibbs free energy).

♻ **endo-, end-** Combining forms indicating within, inner, absorbing, or containing. SEE ALSO ento-.

en·do·an·eu·rys·mor·rha·phy (en'dō-an-yūr-iz-mōr'ă-fē) SYN aneurysmoplasty.

en·do·ap·pen·di·ci·tis (en'dō-ă-pen'di-sī'tis) Simple catarrhal inflammation, limited more or less strictly to the mucosal surface of the vermiform appendix.

en·do·blast (en'dō-blast) Entoderm.

en·do·bron·chi·al (en'dō-brong'kē-ăl) SYN intrabronchial.

en·do·bron·chi·al tube (en'dō-brong'kē-ăl tūb) A single- or double-lumen tube with an inflatable cuff at the distal end that, after being passed through the larynx and trachea, is positioned so that ventilation is restricted to one lung.

en·do·car·di·ac, en·do·car·di·al (en'

dō-kahr′dē-ak, -dē-ăl) **1.** SYN intracardiac. **2.** Relating to the endocardium.

en·do·car·di·al cush·ions (en′dō- kahr′dē-ăl kush′ŭnz) SYN atrioventricular canal cushions.

en·do·car·di·al mur·mur (en′dō-kahr′ dē-ăl mŭr′mŭr) Cardiac murmur arising, from any cause.

en·do·car·di·tis (en′dō-kahr-dī′tis) Inflammation of the endocardium.

en·do·car·di·um, pl. **en·do·car·di·a** (en′dō-kahr′dē-ŭm, -ă) [TA] The innermost tunic of the heart, which includes endothelium and subendothelial connective tissue; in the atrial wall, smooth muscle and numerous elastic fibers also occur.

en·do·cer·vi·ci·tis (en′dō-sĕr-vi-sī′tis) Inflammation of the columnar epithelium cervix uteri.

en·do·cer·vix (en′dō-sĕr′viks) The mucous membrane of the cervical canal.

en·do·chon·dral (en′dō-kon′drăl) SYN intracartilaginous.

en·do·chon·dral bone (en′dō-kon′drăl bōn) A bone that develops in a cartilage environment after the latter is partially or entirely destroyed by calcification and subsequent resorption. SYN cartilage bone.

en·do·chon·dral os·si·fi·ca·tion (en′ dō-kon′drăl os′i-fi-kā′shŭn) Formation of osseous tissue by the replacement of calcified cartilage; long bones grow in length by endochondral ossification at the epiphysial cartilage plate where osteoblasts form bone trabeculae on a framework of calcified cartilage.

en·do·co·li·tis (en′dō-kō-lī′tis) Simple catarrhal inflammation of the colon.

en·do·cra·ni·al (en′dō-krā′nē-ăl) **1.** Within the cranium. **2.** Relating to the endocranium.

en·do·cra·ni·um (en′dō-krā′nē-ŭm) The lining membrane of the cranium, or dura mater of the brain.

en·do·crine (en′dō-krin) **1.** Secreting internally, most commonly into the sys-

temic circulation; of or pertaining to such secretion. Cf. paracrine. **2.** The internal or hormonal secretion of a ductless gland. **3.** Denoting a gland that furnishes an internal secretion.

en·do·crine glands (en′dō-krin glandz) [TA] Glands that have no ducts, their secretions being absorbed directly into the blood. SYN ductless glands.

en·do·crine sys·tem (en′dō-krin sis′ tĕm) Collective designation for those tissues capable of secreting hormones.

en·do·cri·nol·o·gy (endocr, ENDO, END) (en′dō-kri-nol′ŏ-jē) The science and medical specialty concerned with the internal or hormonal secretions and their physiologic and pathologic relations.

en·do·cri·nop·a·thy (en′dō-kri-nop′ă- thē) A disorder in the function of an endocrine gland and the consequences thereof.

en·do·cy·to·sis (en′dō-sī-tō′sis) Internalization of substances from the extracellular environment through the formation of vesicles formed from the plasma membrane. SEE ALSO phagocytosis. Cf. exocytosis (2).

en·do·derm (en′dō-dĕrm) The innermost of the three primary germ layers of the embryo (ectoderm, mesoderm, endoderm). SYN entoderm, hypoblast.

en·do·der·mal, en·do·der·mic (en′dō- dĕr′măl, -mik) Denotes association with the three inner embryonic layers.

en·do·der·mal clo·a·ca (en′dō-dĕr′măl klō-ā′kă) Terminal portion of the hindgut internal to the cloacal membrane of the embryo.

en·do·don·ti·a (en′dō-don′shē-ă) SYN endodontics.

en·do·don·tics, en·do·don·ti·a, en· do·don·tol·o·gy (ENDO) (en′dō-don′ tiks, -shē-ă, -don-tol′ŏ-jē) A field of dentistry concerned with the diseases and injuries of the dental pulp and periapical tissues, and with the prevention, diagnosis, and treatment of diseases and injuries in these tissues.

en·do·don·tol·o·gy (en′dō-don-tol′ŏ-jē) SYN endodontics.

en·dog·a·my (en-dog′ă-mē) Reproduction by conjugation between sister cells, the descendants of one original cell.

en·dog·e·nous, en·do·gen·ic (E) (en-doj′ĕ-nŭs, en′dō-jen′ik) Originating or produced within the organism or one of its parts. SYN endogenic.

en·dog·e·nous de·pres·sion (en-doj′ĕ-nŭs dĕ-presh′ŭn) A descriptive syndrome for a cluster of symptoms and features occurring in the absence of external precipitants and believed to have a biologic origin.

en·do·la·ryn·ge·al (en′dō-lă-rin′jē-ăl) Within the larynx.

en·do·lith (en′dō-lith) Calcified body found in the pulp chamber of a tooth. SYN denticle (1), pulp stone.

en·do·lymph (en′dō-limf) [TA] The fluid contained within the membranous labyrinth of the inner ear.

en·do·lym·phat·ic duct (en′dō-lim-fat′ik dŭkt) [TA] Small membranous tube, connecting with both saccule and utricle of the membranous labyrinth, passing through the aqueduct of vestibule, and terminating in a dilated blind extremity, the endolymphatic sac, located on the posterior surface of the petrous portion of the temporal bone beneath the dura mater. SYN ductus endolymphaticus [TA].

en·do·me·tri·al (en′dō-mē′trē-ăl) Relating to or composed of endometrium.

en·do·me·tri·al ab·la·tion (en′dō-mē′trē-ăl ăb-lā′shŭn) Therapeutic selective endometrial destruction.

en·do·me·tri·al cyst (en′dō-mē′trē-ăl sist) Lesion resulting from endometrial implantation outside the uterus, as in endometriosis.

en·do·me·tri·oid (en′dō-mē′trē-oyd) Microscopically resembling endometrial tissue.

en·do·me·tri·oid car·ci·no·ma (en′dō-mē′trē-oyd kahr′si-nō′mă) Adenocarcinoma of the ovary or prostate resembling endometrial adenocarcinoma, possibly arising from ovarian foci of endometriosis.

en·do·me·tri·o·ma (en′dō-mē-trē-ō′mă) Circumscribed mass of ectopic endometrial tissue in endometriosis.

en·do·me·tri·o·sis (EMS) (en′dō-mē-trē-ō′sis) Ectopic occurrence of endometrial tissue. SYN endometrial implants.

en·do·me·tri·tis (en′dō-mē-trī′tis) Inflammation of the endometrium.

en·do·me·tri·um, pl. **en·do·me·tri·a** (en′dō-mē′trē-ŭm, -ă) [TA] The mucous membrane forming the inner layer of the uterine wall; it consists of a simple columnar epithelium and a lamina propria that contains simple tubular uterine glands. The structure, thickness, and state of the endometrium undergo marked change with the menstrual cycle.

en·do·mi·to·sis (en′dō-mī-tō′sis) SYN endopolyploidy.

en·do·morph (en′dō-mōrf) A constitutional body type or build (biotype or somatotype) in which tissues that originated in the endoderm prevail; from a morphologic standpoint, the trunk predominates over the limbs.

en·do·my·o·car·di·al (en′dō-mī-ō-kahr′dē-ăl) Relating to the endocardium and the myocardium.

en·do·my·o·car·di·al fi·bro·sis (EMF) (en′dō-mī-ō-kahr′dē-ăl fī-brō′sis) Thickening of the ventricular endocardium by fibrosis, involving the subendocardial myocardium, and sometimes the atrioventricular valves, with mural thrombosis, leading to progressive right and left ventricular failure with mitral and tricuspid insufficiency. SYN Davies disease, endomyocardial fibroelastosis.

en·do·my·o·car·di·tis (en′dō-mī′ō-kahr-dī′tis) Inflammation of both endocardium and myocardium.

en·do·mys·i·um (en′dō-mis′ē-ŭm) [TA] The fine connective tissue sheath surrounding a muscle fiber.

en·do·neu·ri·um (en′dō-nūr′ē-ŭm) [TA] The innermost connective tissue supportive structure of nerve trunks, surrounding individual myelinated and unmyelinated nerve fibers. SYN Henle sheath, sheath of Key and Retzius.

en·do·nu·cle·ase (en′dō-nū′klē-ās) A nuclease (phosphodiesterase) that cleaves polynucleotides (nucleic acids) at interior bonds, thus producing polynucleotide or oligonucleotide fragments of varying size. Cf. exonuclease.

en·do·pep·ti·dase (en′dō-pep′ti-dās) Enzyme that catalyzes hydrolysis of a peptide chain at points well within the chain, but not near either terminus; (e.g., pepsin, trypsin).

en·do·per·i·car·di·tis (en′dō-per′i-kahr-dī′tis) Simultaneous inflammation of the endocardium and pericardium.

en·do·per·i·my·o·car·di·tis (en′dō-per′i-mī′ō-kahr-dī′tis) Simultaneous inflammation of the heart muscle and of the endocardium and pericardium. SYN pancarditis.

en·do·per·i·to·ni·tis (en′dō-per′i-tŏ-nī′tis) Superficial inflammation of the peritoneum.

en·doph·thal·mi·tis, en·doph·thal·mi·a (en′dof-thal-mī′tis, -thal′mē-ă) Inflammation of the tissues within the eyeball.

en·do·phyte (en′dō-fīt) A plant parasite living within another organism.

en·do·phyt·ic (en′dō-fit′ik) 1. Pertaining to an endophyte. 2. Referring to an infiltrative, invasive tumor.

en·do·plasm (E) (en′dō-plazm) The inner or medullary part of the cytoplasm, as opposed to the ectoplasm, containing the cell organelles. SYN entoplasm.

en·do·plas·mic re·tic·u·lum (ER) (en′dō-plas′mik rĕ-tik′yū-lŭm) Network of cytoplasmic tubules or flattened sacs (cisternae) with (rough ER) or without (smooth ER) ribosomes on the surface of their membranes in eukaryotes. SYN endomembrane system.

en·do·pol·y·ploid (en′dō-pol′ē-ployd) Relating to endopolyploidy.

en·do·pol·y·ploi·dy (en′dō-pol′ē-ploy′dē) The process or state of duplication of the chromosomes without accompanying spindle formation or cytokinesis, resulting in a polyploid nucleus. SYN endomitosis.

en·do·pros·the·sis, pl. **en·do·pros·the·ses** (en-dō-pros-thē′sis, -sēz) A synthetic insert, such as a stent, to maintain patency of a hollow structure.

en·do·re·du·pli·ca·tion (en′dō-rē-dū-pli-kā′shŭn) A form of polyploidy or polysomy by redoubling of chromosomes, giving rise to four-stranded chromosomes at prophase and metaphase.

en·dor·phin (ĕn-dōr′fĭn) A natural substance produced in the brain that binds to opioid receptors, thus dulling the perception of pain; postulated to trigger ''exercise high,'' a state of euphoria and exhilaration during intense exercise.

en·do·sal·pin·gi·tis (en′dō-sal-pin-jī′tis) Inflammation of the lining membrane of the pharyngotympanic or the uterine tube.

en·do·sal·pinx (en′dō-sal′pingks) The mucosa of the uterine tube.

en·do·scope (en′dŏ-skōp) An instrument for the examination of the interior of a tubular or hollow organ.

en·do·scop·ic bi·op·sy (en′dŏ-skop′ik bī′op-sē) Biopsy obtained by instruments passed through an endoscope or obtained by a needle introduced under endoscopic guidance.

en·do·scop·ic ret·ro·grade chol·an·gi·o·pan·cre·a·tog·ra·phy (ERCP) (en′dŏ-skop′ik ret′rō-grād kō-lan′jē-ō-pan′krē-ă-tog′ră-fē) A method of cholangiopancreatography using an endoscope to inspect and cannulate the hepatopancreatic ampulla, with injection of contrast medium for radiographic examination of the pancreatic, hepatic, and common bile ducts.

en·dos·co·py (en-dos′kŏ-pē) Examination of the interior of a canal or hollow viscus by means of a special instrument, such as an endoscope. SEE endoscope.

en·do·skel·e·ton (en′dō-skel′ĕ-tŏn) The internal bony framework of the body; the skeleton in its usual context as distinguished from the exoskeleton.

en·do·some (en′dō-sōm) A more or less central body in the vesicular nucleus of certain Feulgen-negative protozoa (e.g., trypanosomes, parasitic amebae, and phytoflagellates), with the chromatin lying between the nuclear membrane and the endosome. Cf. nucleolus.

en·do·so·nos·co·py (en′dŏ-sŏ-nos′kŏ-pē) A sonographic study carried out by transducers inserted into the body as miniature probes in the esophagus, urethra, bladder, vagina, or rectum.

en·dos·se·ous im·plant (en-dos′sē-ŭs im′plant) One that is inserted into the alveolar and/or basal bone and protrudes through the mucoperiosteum. SYN endosteal implant.

en·dos·te·al, en·dos·se·ous (en-dos′tē-ăl, -dos′ē-ŭs) Relating to the endosteum.

en·dos·te·al im·plant (en-dos′tē-ăl im′plant) SYN endosseous implant.

en·dos·te·i·tis (end-os′tē-ī′tis) Inflammation of the endosteum or of the medullary cavity of a bone. SYN central osteitis.

en·dos·te·o·ma (en-dos′tē-ō′mă) A benign neoplasm of bone tissue in the medullary cavity of a bone. SYN endostoma.

en·dos·te·um, pl. **en·dos·tea** (en-dos′tē-ŭm, -ă) [TA] A layer of cells lining the inner surface of bone in the central medullary cavity. SYN medullary membrane.

en·dos·to·ma (en′dos-tō′mă) SYN endosteoma.

en·do·ten·din·e·um (en′dō-ten-din′ē-ŭm) The fine connective tissue surrounding secondary fascicles of a tendon.

en·do·the·li·al (en′dō-thē′lē-ăl) Relating to the endothelium.

en·do·the·li·al cell (en′dō-thē′lē-ăl sel) One of the simple squamous cells forming the lining of blood and lymph vessels and the inner layer of the endocardium.

en·do·the·lin (ET) (en′dō-thē′lin) A 21-amino acid peptide originally derived from endothelial cells; extremely potent vasoconstrictor.

en·do·the·li·o·ma (en′dō-thē-lē-ō′mă) Generic term for a group of neoplasms, benign or malignant, derived from the endothelial tissue of blood vessels or lymphatic channels.

en·do·the·li·o·sis, pl. **en·do·the·li·o·ses** (en′dō-thē-lē-ō′sis, -sēz) Proliferation of endothelium.

en·do·the·li·um (en′dō-thē′lē-ŭm) [TA] A layer of flat cells lining, especially blood and lymphatic vessels and the heart.

en·do·ther·mic (en′dō-thĕr′mik) Denoting a chemical reaction during which heat (enthalpy) is absorbed. Cf. exothermic (1).

en·do·tho·rac·ic fa·scia (en′dō-thōr-as′ik fash′ē-ă) [TA] Extrapleural fascia that lines the walls of the thorax.

en·do·thrix (en′dō-thriks) Fungal spores invading the interior of a hair shaft.

endotoxaemia [Br.] SYN endotoxemia.

en·do·tox·e·mi·a (en′dō-tok-sē′mē-ă) Presence in the blood of endotoxins, rod-shaped bacteria, may cause a generalized Shwartzman phenomenon with shock. SYN endotoxaemia.

en·do·tox·in (en′dō-tok′sin) A bacterial toxin not freely liberated into the surrounding medium, in contrast to exotoxin.

en·do·tox·in shock (en′dō-tok′sin shok) That induced by release of endotoxin from gram-negative bacteria, especially *Escherichia coli.*

en·do·tra·che·al (en′dō-trā′kē-ăl) Within the trachea.

en·do·tra·che·al in·tu·ba·tion (en′dō-trā′kē-ăl in-tū-bā′shŭn) Passage of a tube through the nose or mouth into the trachea for maintenance of the airway during anesthesia or for maintenance of an imperiled airway.

en·do·tra·che·al tube (ET) (en′dō-trā′kē-ăl tūb) SYN tracheal tube.

en·do·u·rol·o·gy (en′dō-yūr-ol′ŏ-jē) Genitourinary operative procedures (diagnostic and therapeutic) performed through instruments; may be cystoscopic, pelviscopic, celioscopic, laparoscopic, percutaneous, or ureteroscopic.

en·do·vas·cu·li·tis (en′dō-vas′kyū-lī′tis) SYN endangiitis.

end·plate, end-plate (end′plāt) The ending of a motor nerve fiber in relation to a skeletal muscle fiber.

end prod·uct (end prod′ŭkt) Final point in a metabolic pathway.

end-stage dis·ease (end′stāj di-zēź) Generalized term for any disorder that is likely to lead to death in a short time.

end-stage re·nal dis·ease (ESRD) (end′stāj rē′năl di-zēz′) SYN renal failure.

end-sys·tol·ic vol·ume (ESV) (end-sis-tol′ik vol′yūm) Capacity or amount of blood in the ventricle at the end of the ventricular ejection period and immediately preceding the beginning of ventricular relaxation.

end-ti·dal (end-tī′dăl) At the end of a normal expiration.

end-to-end an·as·to·mo·sis (EEA) (end end ă-nas′tŏ-mō′sis) Surgical union performed after cutting each structure to be joined in a plane perpendicular to the ultimate structural flow.

end-to-end bite (end end bīt) SYN edge-to-edge occlusion.

en·e·ma (en′ĕ-mă) A rectal injection to cleanse the bowel or to administer drugs or food.

en·er·gy (E) (en′ĕr-jē) The exertion of power; the capacity to do work, taking the forms of kinetic energy, potential energy, chemical energy, electrical energy, and other types.

en·er·va·tion (en′ĕr-vā′shŭn) Failure of nervous force.

en·large·ment (en-lahrj′mĕnt) An increase in size; an anatomic swelling, enlargement, or prominence. SYN intumescentia.

en·oph·thal·mos, en·oph·thal·mi·a (en′of-thal′mos, -thal′mē-ă) Recession of the eyeball within the orbit.

en·os·to·sis (en′os-tō′sis) A mass of proliferating bone tissue within a bone.

en·ox·ap·a·rin (ē-noks′ă-par′in) A low-molecular-weight heparin.

en·si·form (en′si-fōrm) SYN xiphoid.

ENT Abbreviation for ears, nose, and throat. SEE otorhinolaryngology.

en·tad (en′tad) Toward the interior.

en·ta·me·bi·a·sis (ent′ă-mē-bī′ă-sis) Infection with *Entamoeba histolytica*. SEE amebiasis, amebic dysentery.

Ent·a·moe·ba (ent′ă-mē′bă) A genus of ameba parasitic in the oral cavity, cecum, and large bowel of humans and other primates and in many domestic and wild mammals and birds.

Ent·a·moe·ba his·to·ly·t·i·ca (ent′ă-mē′bă his′tō-lit′i-kă) Species of ameba that is the only distinct pathogen in the species; causes amebic dysentery.

entamoebiasis [Br.] SYN entamebiasis.

en·ter·al, en·ter·ic (en′tĕr-ăl, en-ter′ik) Within, or by way of, the intestine or gastrointestinal tract, especially as distinguished from parenteral.

en·ter·al·gi·a (en′tĕr-al′jē-ă) Severe abdominal pain accompanying spasm of the bowel.

en·ter·al nu·tri·tion (en′tĕr-ăl nū-trish′ŭn) Alimentation provided by means of a tube into the intestine or gastrointestinal tract.

en·ter·ic ba·cil·lus (en-ter′ik bă-sil′ŭs) A bacterium, resident in the intestines, which is potentially pathogenic.

en·ter·ic-coat·ed tab·let (en-ter′ik kō′tĕd tab′lĕt) A tablet covered with a substance that delays release of the medication until the tablet has passed through the stomach and into the intestine.

en·ter·ic fe·ver (en-ter′ik fē′vĕr) 1. SYN typhoid fever. 2. The group of typhoid and paratyphoid fevers.

en·ter·ic tu·ber·cu·lo·sis (en-ter′ik tū-bĕr′kyū-lō′sis) Complication of cavitary pulmonary tuberculosis usually resulting from expectoration and swallowing of bacilli that then infect areas of the diges-

E

tive tract where there is relative stasis or abundant lymphoid tissue. SEE ALSO tuberculous enteritis.

en·ter·i·tis (en'tĕr-ī'tis) Inflammation of the intestine, especially of the small intestine.

entero-, enter- Combining forms indicating the intestines.

En·ter·o·bac·ter (en'tĕr-ō-bak'tĕr) A genus of aerobic, facultatively anaerobic, non-spore-forming, motile bacteria containing gram-negative rods; somewhat resistant to antibiotics.

En·ter·o·bac·ter clo·a·cae (en'tĕr-ō-bak'tĕr klō-ā'sē) Bacterial species found in the feces of humans and other animals and in sewage, soil, and water; serious cause of nosocomial infection.

En·ter·o·bac·te·ri·a·ce·ae (en'tĕr-ō-bak-ter'ē-ā'sē-ē) A family of aerobic, facultatively anaerobic, non-spore-forming bacteria containing gram-negative rods. These organisms grow well on artificial media; type genus is *Escherichia*.

en·ter·o·bi·a·sis (en'tĕr-ō-bī'ă-sis) Infection with *Enterobius vermicularis*, the human pinworm.

en·ter·o·cele (en'tĕr-o-sēl) 1. A hernial protrusion through a defect in the rectovaginal or vesicovaginal pouch. 2. SYN abdominal cavity. 3. An intestinal hernia.

en·ter·o·cen·te·sis (en'tĕr-ō-sen-tē'sis) Puncture of the intestine with a hollow needle (trocar and cannula) to withdraw substances.

en·ter·o·chro·maf·fin cells (en'tĕr-ō-krō'maf-in selz) SYN enteroendocrine cells.

en·ter·o·ci·dal (en'tĕr-ō-sī'dal) An agent that kills parasites residing in the gastrointestinal tract.

en·ter·o·clei·sis (en'tĕr-ō-klī'sis) Occlusion of the lumen of the alimentary canal.

en·ter·o·coc·cem·i·a (en'tĕr-ō-kok-sē'mē-ă) A blood-borne disease, occasionally leading to septicemia, due to mem-

bers of the group D streptococci, *Enterococcus faecalis* or *E. faecium*.

En·ter·o·coc·cus (E) (en'tĕr-ō-kok'ŭs) Genus of facultatively anaerobic, generally nonmotile, non-spore-forming, gram-positive bacteria; found in the intestinal tract of humans and animals; cause of intraabdominal, wound, and urinary tract infections.

en·ter·o·coc·cus (E), gen. and pl. **en·ter·o·coc·ci** (en'tĕr-ō-kok'ŭs, -sī) An intestinal streptococcus.

En·ter·o·coc·cus fae·ca·lis (en'tĕr-ō-kok'ŭs fē-kā'lis) Bacterium found in human feces; occasionally found in urinary infections and in blood and heart lesions in subacute endocarditis; a major cause of nosocomial infection.

En·ter·o·coc·cus fae·ci·um (en'tĕr-ō-kok'ŭs fē'shē-ŭm) Bacterial species recovered in human infection; has low-level resistance to ampicillin, and in the U.S. and other countries where vancomycin is used frequently, resistant strains have been rapidly appearing as nosocomial infections.

en·ter·o·co·li·tis (en'tĕr-ō-kŏ-lī'tis) Inflammation of the mucous membrane of a greater or lesser extent of both small and large intestines. SYN coloenteritis.

en·ter·o·co·los·to·my (en'tĕr-ō-kŏ-los'tŏ-mē) Establishment of a new communication between the small intestine and the colon.

en·ter·o·cu·ta·ne·ous fis·tu·la (en'tĕr-ō-kyū-tā'nē-ŭs fis'tyū-lă) Fistulous passage connecting the intestine and skin of the abdomen.

en·ter·o·cyst, en·ter·o·cys·to·ma (en'tĕr-ō-sist, -sis-tō'mă) A cyst of the wall of the intestine.

en·ter·o·cys·to·cele (en'tĕr-ō-sis'tō-sēl) A hernia of both intestine and bladder wall.

en·ter·o·cys·to·plas·ty (en'tĕr-ō-sis'tō-plas'tē) Surgical procedure to the urinary bladder using tissue from the intestine.

en·ter·o·en·do·crine cells (en'tĕr-ō-end'ŏ-krin selz) A family of cells with argyrophilic granules occurring throughout the digestive tract and believed to produce at least 20 gastrointestinal hormones and neurotransmitters.

en·ter·o·gas·tric re·flex (en′tĕr-ō-gas′ trik rē′fleks) Peristaltic contraction of the small intestine induced by the entrance of food into the stomach. SEE ALSO gastrocolic reflex.

en·ter·og·e·nous (en′tĕr-oj′ĕ-nŭs) Of intestinal origin.

en·ter·og·e·nous cy·a·no·sis (en′tĕr-oj′ĕ-nŭs sī′ă-nō′sis) Apparent cyanosis caused by the absorption of nitrites or other toxic materials from the intestine with the formation of methemoglobin or sulfhemoglobin.

en·ter·og·ra·phy (en′tĕr-og′ră-fē) The making of a graphic record delineating the intestinal muscular activity.

en·ter·o·he·pat·ic (en′tĕr-ō-he-pat′ik) Denotes association with both the liver and the intestine.

en·ter·o·hep·a·ti·tis (en′tĕr-ō-hep-ă-tī′ tis) Inflammation of both the intestine and the liver.

en·ter·o·in·va·sive *Esch·e·rich·i·a co·li* (EIEC) (en′tĕr-ō-in-vā′siv esh-ĕ-rik′ē-ă kō′lī) Strain of *E. coli* that penetrates gut mucosa and multiplies in colon epithelial cells, resulting in shigellosislike changes of the mucosa; produces a severe diarrheal illness.

en·ter·o·ki·nase (EK) (en′tĕr-ō-kī′nās) SYN enteropeptidase.

en·ter·o·ki·ne·sis (en′tĕr-ō-ki-nē′sis) Muscular contraction of the alimentary canal. SEE ALSO peristalsis.

en·ter·o·lith (en′tĕr-ō-lith) An intestinal calculus formed of layers of soaps and earthy phosphates surrounding a nucleus of some hard body, such as a swallowed fruit stone or other indigestible substance.

en·ter·ol·o·gy (en′tĕr-ol′ŏ-jē) The branch of medical science concerned especially with the intestinal tract.

en·ter·ol·y·sis (en′tĕr-ol′i-sis) Division of intestinal adhesions.

en·ter·o·my·co·sis (en′tĕr-ō-mī-kō′sis) An intestinal disease of fungal origin.

en·ter·o·path·ic ar·thri·tis (en′tĕr-ō-path′ik ahr-thrī′tis) Inflammatory disease sometimes resembling rheumatoid arthritis that may complicate the course of ulcerative colitis, Crohn disease, or other intestinal disease, including bacterial enteritis.

en·ter·o·path·o·gen·ic (en′tĕr-ō-path′ŏ-jen′ik) Capable of producing disease in the intestinal tract.

en·ter·o·path·o·gen·ic *Esch·e·rich·i·a co·li* (EPEC, EEC) (en′tĕr-ō-path′ŏ-jen′ik esh-ĕ-rik′ē-ă kō′lī) Strain of *E. coli* in which organisms adhere to small-bowel mucosa and produce characteristic changes in the microvilli; produces symptomatic, sometimes serious, gastrointestinal illnesses, especially severe in neonates and young children.

en·ter·op·a·thy (en′tĕr-op′ă-thē) An intestinal disease.

en·ter·o·pep·ti·dase (en′tĕr-ō-pep′ti-dās) An intestinal proteolytic glycoenzyme from the duodenal mucosa that converts trypsinogen into trypsin. SYN enterokinase.

en·ter·o·pex·y (en′tĕr-ō-pek-sē) Fixation of a segment of the intestine to the abdominal wall.

en·ter·op·to·sis, en·ter·op·to·si·a (en′ tĕr-op-tō′sis, -tō′sē-ă) Abnormal descent of the intestines in the abdominal cavity.

en·ter·or·rha·gi·a (en′tĕr-ōr-ā′jē-ă) Bleeding within the intestinal tract.

en·ter·o·scope (en′tĕr-ō-skōp′) A speculum for inspecting the inside of the intestine in surgically.

en·ter·o·sep·sis (en′tĕr-ō-sep′sis) Sepsis occurring in or derived from the alimentary canal.

en·ter·o·spasm (en′tĕr-ō-spazm) Increased, irregular, and painful peristalsis.

en·ter·o·sta·sis (en′tĕr-ō-stā′sis) Intestinal stasis; a retardation or arrest of the passage of the intestinal contents.

E

en·ter·o·ste·no·sis (en'tĕr-ō-stĕn-ō'sis) Narrowing of the lumen of the intestine.

en·ter·os·to·my (en'tĕr-os'tŏ-mē) An artificial anus or fistula into the intestine through the abdominal wall.

enterotoxaemia [Br.] SYN enterotoxemia.

en·ter·o·tox·e·mi·a (en'tĕr-ō-tok-sē'mē-ă) The presence of an enterotoxin in the blood. SYN enterotoxaemia.

en·ter·o·tox·in (en'tĕr-ō-tok'sin) A cytotoxin specific for the cells of the intestinal mucosa.

en·ter·o·tro·pic (en'tĕr-ō-trō'pik) Attracted by or affecting the intestine.

en·ter·o·ves·i·cal fis·tu·la (en'tĕr-ō-ves'i-kăl fis'tyū-lă) Fistulous passage connecting the intestine and the bladder.

En·te·ro·vi·rus **(EV)** (en'tĕr-ō-vī'rŭs) A large and diverse group of viruses that includes poliovirus types 1 to 3, Coxsackie viruses A and B, echoviruses, and the enteroviruses identified since 1969 and assigned type numbers.

en·ter·o·zo·on (en'tĕr-ō-zō'on) An animal parasite in the intestine.

♻ **ento-, ent-** Combining forms meaning inner, or within. SEE ALSO endo-.

en·to·blast (en'tō-blast) **1.** Pertaining to entoderm. **2.** Cell nucleolus.

en·to·cho·roi·de·a (en'tō-kōr-oyd'ē-ă) SYN choriocapillary layer.

en·to·co·nid (en'tō-kō'nid) The distolingual cusp of human lower molars.

en·to·derm (en'tō-dĕrm) SYN endoderm.

en·to·mi·on (en-tō'mē-on) The tip of the mastoid angle of the parietal bone.

en·to·mol·o·gy (en'tŏ-mol'ŏ-jē) The science concerned with the study of insects.

En·to·moph·thor·al·es (en-tō-mof'thō-rā'lēz) An order of the fungal class Zygomycetes. The genera include *Conidiobolus,* which causes a chronic granulomatous inflammation of a nasal and paranasal sinus mucosa and *Basidiobolus,* which causes a chronic subcutaneous granuloma.

en·top·ic (en-top'ik) Placed within; occurring or situated in the normal place; opposed to ectopic.

en·top·tic (en-top'tik) Within the eyeball.

en·to·ret·i·na (en'tō-ret'i-nă) The layers of the retina from the outer plexiform to the nerve fiber layer inclusive. SYN Henle nervous layer.

en·to·zo·on, pl. **en·to·zo·a** (en'tō-zō'on, -ă) An animal parasite with a habitat in any of the internal organs or tissues.

en·trap·ment neu·rop·a·thy (en-trap'mĕnt nūr-op'ă-thē) A focal nerve lesion produced by constriction or mechanical distortion of the nerve, within a fibrous or fibroosseous tunnel.

en·tro·pi·on, en·tro·pi·um (en-trō'pē-on, -ŭm) **1.** Inversion or turning inward of a part. **2.** The infolding of the margin of an eyelid.

en·tro·py (S) (en'trŏ-pē) That fraction of heat (energy) content not available for the performance of work, usually because (in a chemical reaction) it has been used to increase the random motion of the atoms or molecules in the system.

e·nu·cle·a·tion (e-nū'klē-ā'shŭn) **1.** Removal of an entire structure without rupture, as one shells the kernel of a nut. **2.** Removal or destruction of the nucleus of a cell.

en·u·re·sis (en-yūr-ē'sis) Involuntary discharge or leakage of urine.

en·ve·lope (en'vĕ-lōp) ANATOMY any structure that encloses or covers.

en·vi·ron·men·tal med·i·cine (en-vī'rŏn-men'tăl med'i-sin) That branch of health care involved with therapy of patients who are afflicted by causes related to the environment (e.g., duststorms, heat, overcrowding); also studies effect of diet and environmental allergens on health and illness.

en·zy·got·ic (en'zī-got'ik) Derived from

a single fertilized oocyte; denoting twins so derived.

en·zyme (en′zīm) A protein that acts as a catalyst to induce chemical changes in other substances, while remaining apparently unchanged itself by the process.

enzyme im·mu·no·as·say (EIA, EI) (en′zīm im′yū-nō-as′ā) Any of several immunoassay methods that use an enzyme covalently linked to an antigen or antibody as a label; the most common types are enzyme-linked immunosorbent assay (ELISA) (q.v.) and enzyme-multiplied immunoassay technique (EMIT) (q.v.).

en·zyme ki·net·iks (en′zīm ki-net′iks) Study of enzyme-catalyzed reactions.

en·zyme-linked im·mu·no·sor·bent as·say (ELISA) (en′zīm-lingkt im′yū-nō-sōr′bĕnt as′ā) A sensitive method for serodiagnosis of specific infectious diseases; an in vitro competitive binding assay in which an enzyme and its substrate rather than a radioactive substance serve as the indicator system.

en·zyme-mul·ti·plied im·mu·no·as·say tech·nique (EMIT) (en′zīm-mŭl′ti-plīd im′yū-nō-as′ā tek-nēk′) A type of test in which the ligand is labeled with an enzyme.

en·zyme re·pres·sion (en′zīm rĕ-presh′ŭn) Inhibition of enzyme synthesis by a metabolite.

en·zy·mop·a·thy (en′zi-mop′ă-thē) Any disturbance of enzyme function, including genetic deficiency or defect in specific enzymes.

e·o·sin (ē′ō-sin) A derivative of fluorescein used as a fluorescent acid dye for cytoplasmic stains and counterstains in histology and in Romanowsky-type blood stains.

e·o·sin·o·pe·ni·a (ē′ō-sin-ō-pē′nē-ă) An abnormally small number of eosinophils in the peripheral bloodstream.

e·o·sin·o·phil, e·o·sin·o·phile (ē′ō-sin′ō-fil, -fīl) SYN eosinophilic leukocyte.

e·o·sin·o·phil cat·i·on·ic pro·tein (ECP) (ē′ō-sin′ō-fil kat′ī-on′ik prō′tēn) A protein the level of which in serum of clotted blood reflects the rate of activation of circulating eosinophils.

e·o·sin·o·phil gran·ule (ē-ō-sin′ō-fil gran′yūl) One that stains with eosin.

e·o·sin·o·phil·i·a (ē′ō-sin-ō-fil′ē-ă) SYN eosinophilic leukocytosis.

e·o·sin·o·phil·ic (ē′ō-sin-ō-fil′ik) Staining readily with eosin dyes; denoting such cell or tissue elements.

e·o·sin·o·phil·ic gas·tri·tis (ē′ō-sin′ō-fil′ik gas-trī′tis) SYN eosinophilic gastroenteritis.

e·o·sin·o·phil·ic gas·tro·en·ter·i·tis (EGE, EG, EOG) (ē′ō-sin-ō-fil′ik gas′trō-en-tĕr-ī′tis) Disorder comprising abdominal pain, malabsorption, often obstructive symptoms, associated with peripheral eosinophilia and areas of eosinophilic infiltration of the stomach, small intestine, and colon. SYN eosinophilic gastritis.

e·o·sin·o·phil·ic gran·u·lo·ma (ē′ō-sin-ō-fil′ik gran′yū-lō′mă) A lesion observed more frequently in children and adolescents, occasionally in young adults, which occurs chiefly as a solitary focus in one bone, although multiple involvement is sometimes observed and similar foci may develop in the lung.

e·o·sin·o·phil·ic leu·ke·mi·a, eo·sin·o·phil·o·cyt·ic leu·ke·mi·a (ē′ō-sin-ō-fil′ik lū-kē′mē-ă, ē′ō-sin′ō-fil-ō-sit′ik) A form of granulocytic leukemia in which there are conspicuous numbers of eosinophilic granulocytes in the tissues and circulating blood, or in which such cells are predominant.

e·o·sin·o·phil·ic leu·ko·cyte (ē′ō-sin-ō-fil′ik lū′kŏ-sīt) A polymorphonuclear white blood cell characterized by prominent cytoplasmic granules that are bright yellow-red or orange when treated with Wright stain. SYN eosinophil, eosinophile, oxyphil (2), oxyphile, oxyphilic leukocyte.

e·o·sin·o·phil·ic leu·ko·cy·to·sis (ē′ō-sin-ō-fil′ik lū′kō-sī-tō′sis) A form of relative leukocytosis in which the greatest proportionate increase is in the eosinophils. SYN eosinophilia.

e·o·sin·o·phil·ic leu·ko·pe·ni·a (ē'ō-sin-ō-fil'ĭk lū'kō-pē'nē-ă) A decrease in the number of eosinophilic granulocytes normally present in the circulating blood.

e·o·sin·o·phil·ic men·in·gi·tis (ē'ō-sin-ō-fil'ĭk men-in-jī'tis) Form of the disorder meningitis in which meningeal signs predominate.

e·o·sin·o·phil·ic pus·tu·lar fol·lic·u·li·tis (ē'ō-sin-ō-fil'ĭk pŭs'chū-lăr fŏ-lik'yū-lī'tis) A dermatosis characterized by sterile pruritic papules and pustules that coalesce to form plaques with papulovesicular borders; has been reported in AIDS, and a possibly separate form of eosinophilic pustular folliculitis occurs in infants. SYN Ofuji disease.

e·o·sin·o·phi·lu·ri·a (ē'ō-sin'ō-fil-yūr'ē-ă) Presence of eosinophils in the urine.

e·pac·tal (ē-pak'tăl) SYN supernumerary.

ep·ax·i·al (ep-ak'sē-ăl) Above or behind any axis, such as the spinal axis or the axis of a limb.

e·pen·dy·ma (ĕ-pen'di-mă) [TA] The cellular membrane lining the central canal of the spinal cord and the brain ventricles. SYN endyma.

e·pen·dy·mo·blast (ĕ-pen'di-mō-blast) An embryonic ependymal cell.

e·pen·dy·mo·cyte (ĕ-pen'di-mō-sīt) An ependymal cell.

e·pen·dy·mo·ma (ĕ-pen'di-mō'mă) A glioma derived from relatively undifferentiated ependymal cells; may originate from the lining of any of the ventricles or the spinal cord central canal.

e·phed·rine (ĕ-fed'rin, ef'ĕ-drin) An alkaloid from the leaves of *Ephedra equisetina, E. sinica,* and other species (family Gnetaceae), or produced synthetically; an adrenergic (sympathomimetic) agent with actions similar to those of epinephrine.

e·phe·lis, pl. **e·phe·li·des** (ĕ-fē'lis, -li-dēz) SYN freckles.

♻ **epi-** Prefix meaning on, following, or subsequent to.

ep·i·an·dros·ter·one (ep'i-an-dros'tĕr-ōn) Inactive isomer of androsterone; found in urine and in testicular and ovarian tissue.

ep·i·bleph·a·ron (ep'i-blef'ă-ron) A congenital horizontal skin fold near the margin of the eyelid, caused by abnormal insertion of muscle fibers.

ep·i·bul·bar (ep'i-bŭl'bahr) On a bulb of any kind; specifically, on the eyeball.

ep·i·con·dy·lal·gi·a (ep'i-kon-di-lal'jē-ă) Pain in an epicondyle of the humerus or in the tendons or muscles originating therefrom.

ep·i·con·dyle (ep'i-kon'dīl) [TA] A projection from a long bone near the articular extremity above or on the condyle. SYN epicondylus [TA].

ep·i·con·dy·lus, pl. **ep·i·con·dy·li** (ep'i-kon'di-lŭs, -lī) [TA] SYN epicondyle.

ep·i·cra·ni·um (ep'i-krā'nē-ŭm) The muscle, aponeurosis, and skin covering the cranium.

ep·i·cri·sis (ep'i-krī-sis) A secondary crisis; a crisis terminating a recrudescence of morbid symptoms following a primary crisis.

ep·i·crit·ic, ep·i·crit·ic sen·si·bil·i·ty (ep'i-krit'ik, sens'i-bil'i-tē) The aspect of somatic sensation that permits the discrimination and the topographic localization of the finer degrees of touch and temperature stimuli. Cf. protopathic.

ep·i·cys·ti·tis (ep'i-sis-tī'tis) Inflammation of the cellular tissue around the bladder.

ep·i·cyte (ep'i-sīt) A cell membrane, especially of protozoa; the external layer of cytoplasm in gregarine parasites.

ep·i·dem·ic (ep'i-dem'ik) The occurrence in a community or region of cases of an illness, specific health-related behavior, or other health-related events clearly in excess of normal expectancy. Cf. endemic, sporadic.

ep·i·dem·ic cer·e·bro·spi·nal men·in·gi·tis (ep'i-dem'ik ser'ĕ-brō-spī'năl men-in-jī'tis) SYN meningococcal meningitis.

ep·i·dem·ic ros·e·o·la (ep'i-dem'ik rō' zē-ō'lă) SYN rubella.

ep·i·dem·ic ty·phus (ep'i-dem'ik tī'fŭs) Form caused by *Rickettsia prowazekii* and spread by body lice; marked by high fever, mental and physical depression, and a macular and papular eruption. SYN European typhus, hospital fever, louse-borne typhus, prison fever typhus.

ep·i·dem·ic vom·it·ing (ep'i-dem'ik vom'it-ing) Symptom caused by Norwalk virus; strikes suddenly and without prodromal illness or malaise, is intense while it lasts, but ceases abruptly after 24–48 hours; symptoms are headache, abdominal pain, giddiness, and diarrhea in most cases, but extreme prostration in about 75%. SYN epidemic nausea.

ep·i·de·mi·ol·o·gist (ep'i-dē'mē-ol'ŏ-jist) An investigator who studies the occurrence of disease or other health-related conditions, states, or events in specified populations; the control of disease usually is considered a task of the epidemiologist.

ep·i·de·mi·ol·o·gy (ep'i-dē'mē-ol'ŏ-jē) The study of the distribution and determinants of health-related states or events in specified populations, and the application of this study to control of health problems.

ep·i·der·mal cyst (ep'i-dĕr'măl sist) Lesion formed of a mass of epidermal cells that, as a result of trauma, has been pushed beneath the epidermis. SYN implantation cyst, inclusion cyst (1), inclusion dermoid.

ep·i·der·mal growth fac·tor (ep'i-dĕr'mal grōth fak'tŏr) **(EGF)** Heat-stable antigenic protein isolated from the submaxillary glands of male mice; when injected into newborn animals, it accelerates eyelid opening and tooth eruption, stimulates epidermal growth and keratinization, and, in larger doses, inhibits body growth and hair development and produces fatty livers.

ep·i·der·mal growth fac·tor re·cep·tor (EGFR) (ep'i-dĕr'măl grōth fak'tŏr rĕ-sep'tŏr) Receptor often upregulated in epithelial tumors.

ep·i·der·mi·dal·i·za·tion (ep'i-dĕr'mid-ăl-ī-zā'shŭn) SYN squamous metaplasia.

ep·i·der·mis, pl. **ep·i·derm·i·des** (ep'i-dĕrm'is, -i-dēz) [TA] **1.** Superficial epithelial portion of the skin (cutis). **2.** In botany, the outermost layer of cells in leaves and the young parts of plants. SYN cuticle (3), cuticula (2), epiderm, epiderma.

ep·i·der·mi·tis (ep'i-der-mī'tis) Inflammation of the epidermis or superficial layers of the skin.

ep·i·der·mo·dys·pla·si·a (ep'i-dĕr'mō-dis-plā'zē-ă) Faulty growth or development of the epidermis.

ep·i·der·moid (ep'i-dĕr'moyd) **1.** Resembling epidermis. **2.** A cholesteatoma or other cystic tumor arising from aberrant epidermal cells.

ep·i·der·moid car·ci·no·ma (ep'i-dĕr'moyd kahr'si-nō'mă) Squamous cell carcinoma of the skin.

ep·i·der·moid cyst (ep'i-dĕr'moyd sist) A spheric, unilocular dermal lesion, composed of encysted keratin and sebum.

ep·i·der·mol·y·sis (ep'i-dĕr-mol'i-sis) A condition in which the epidermis is loosely attached to the corium, readily exfoliating or forming blisters.

ep·i·der·mol·y·sis bul·lo·sa, der·mal type, ep·i·der·mal type, junc·tion·al type (ep'i-dĕr-mol'i-sis bul-ō'să, dĕr'măl tīp, ep'i-dĕr'măl, jŭngk'shŭn'ăl) A group of inherited chronic noninflammatory skin diseases in which large bullae and erosions result from slight mechanical trauma; a form limited to the hands and feet is also called Weber-Cockayne syndrome.

Ep·i·der·mo·phy·ton (ep'i-dĕr-mof'i-ton, -dĕr-mō-fī'ton) A genus of fungi wih macroconidia that are clavate and smooth-walled; common cause of tinea pedis and tinea cruris.

ep·i·did·y·mec·to·my (ep'i-did-i-mek'tŏ-mē) Operative removal of the epididymis.

ep·i·did·y·mis, pl. **ep·i·did·y·mi·des** (ep'i-did'i-mis, -i-dēz) [TA] An elongated structure connected to the posterior surface of the testis, consisting of the head, body, and tail, which turns sharply on itself to become the ductus deferens;

transports, stores, and matures sperms between testis and ductus deferens (vas deferens). SYN parorchis.

ep·i·did·y·mi·tis (ep'i-did'i-mī'tis) Inflammation of the epididymis.

ep·i·did·y·mo·or·chi·tis (ep'i-did'i-mō-ōr-kī'tis) Simultaneous inflammation of both epididymis and testis.

ep·i·did·y·mo·plas·ty (ep'i-did'i-mō-plas-tē) Surgical repair of the epididymis.

ep·i·du·ral (ep'i-dūr'ăl) On (or outside) the dura mater.

ep·i·dural ab·scess (ep-i-dūr'ăl ab'ses) Lesion found between the cranium and dura mater; often due to infection in mastoid and frontal sinuses, to trauma, and, in the context of emergency medicine, to illicit injecting drug use.

ep·i·du·ral an·es·the·sia (ep'i-dūr'ăl an'es-thē'zē-ă) Regional anesthesia produced by injection of local anesthetic solution into the peridural space. SYN peridural anesthesia.

ep·i·du·ral block (ep'i-dūr'ăl blok) An obstruction in the epidural space; used *inaccurately* to mean epidural anesthesia.

ep·i·du·ral cav·i·ty (ep'i-dūr'ăl kav'i-tē) The space between the walls of the vertebral canal and the dura mater of the spinal cord.

ep·i·du·ral he·ma·to·ma (ep'i-dū'răl hē-mă-tō'mă) SEE extradural hemorrhage.

ep·i·du·ral in·jec·tion (ep'i-dūr'ăl in-jek'shŭn) Subcutaneous or intramuscular injection of a pharmacotherapeutic or anesthetic agent into the epidural space.

ep·i·du·ral space (ep'i-dūr'ăl spās) Area between the walls of the vertebral canal and the dura mater of the spinal cord. SYN extradural space [TA], spatium extradurale, cavum epidurale, epidural cavity.

ep·i·fas·ci·al (ep'i-fash'ē-ăl) On the surface of a fascia; denoting a method of injecting drugs in which the solution is put on the fascia lata instead of injected into the substance of the muscle.

ep·i·gas·tral·gi·a (ep'i-gas-tral'jē-ă) Pain in the epigastric region.

ep·i·gas·tric fossa (ep'i-gas'trik fos'ă) [TA] Slight midline depression just inferior to the sternae xiphoid process.

ep·i·gas·tric her·nia (ep'i-gas'trik hěr'nē-ă) Hernia through the linea alba above the navel.

ep·i·gas·tric re·flex (ep-i-gas'trik rē'fleks) Contraction of the upper portion of the rectus abdominis muscle when the skin of the epigastrium above is scratched. SYN supraumbilical reflex (1).

ep·i·gen·e·sis (ep'i-jen'ě-sis) **1.** Development of offspring from a zygote. Cf. preformation theory. **2.** Regulation of the expression of gene activity without alteration of genetic structure.

ep·i·ge·net·ic (ep'i-jě-net'ik) Relating to epigenesis.

ep·i·glot·tic val·le·cu·la (ep'i-glot'ik vă-lek'yū-lă) [TA] Depression immediately posterior to the root of the tongue between the median and lateral glosso-epiglottic folds on either side.

ep·i·glot·ti·dec·to·my (ep'i-glot-i-dek'tŏ-mē) Excision of the epiglottis.

ep·i·glot·tis (ep'i-glot'is) [TA] A leaf-shaped plate of elastic cartilage, covered with mucous membrane, at the root of the tongue, which serves as a diverter valve over the superior aperture of the larynx during the act of swallowing.

ep·i·la·tion (ep'i-lā'shŭn) The act or result of removing hair. SYN depilation.

e·pil·a·to·ry (e-pil'ă-tōr-ē) Pertaining to hair removal that removes the entire hair shaft, as in the application of heated wax products that harden, allowing the patient to remove an entire mass of hair.

ep·i·lem·ma (ep'i-lem'ă) The connective tissue sheath of nerve fibers near their termination.

ep·i·lep·sy, ep·i·lep·sia, grand mal (ep'i-lep'sē, -lep'sē-ă, grawn[h] mahl) A chronic disorder characterized by paroxysmal brain dysfunction due to excessive neuronal discharge; usually associated with some alteration of consciousness; clinical manifestations of the attack may vary from complex abnormalities of behavior including generalization or focal convulsions to momentary spells of impaired consciousness. SYN fit (3), seizure disorder.

ep·i·lep·tic (ep'i-lep'tik) Relating to, characterized by, or suffering from epilepsy.

ep·i·lep·tic de·men·tia (ep'i-lep'tik dĕ-men'shē-ă) Mental disorder in someone afflicted with epilepsy, thought due to prolonged seizures, the epileptogenic brain lesion, or antiepileptic drugs.

ep·i·lep·tic spasm (ep'i-lep'tik spazm) Muscle contraction characterized by a sudden flexion-extension, or mixed extension-flexion, predominantly proximal (including truncal muscles), which is usually more sustained than a myoclonic movement but not as sustained as a tonic seizure.

ep·i·lep·ti·form (ep'i-lep'ti-fōrm) SYN epileptoid.

ep·i·lep·to·gen·ic, ep·i·lep·tog·e·nous (ep'i-lep-tō-jen'ik, ep'i-lep-toj'ĕ-nŭs) Causing epilepsy.

ep·i·lep·to·gen·ic zone (ep'i-lep-tō-jen'ik zōn) A cortical region that on stimulation reproduces the patient's spontaneous epileptic seizure or aura.

ep·i·lep·toid (ep'i-lep'toyd) Resembling epilepsy; denoting certain convulsions, especially of functional nature. SYN epileptiform.

ep·i·man·dib·u·lar (ep'i-man-dib'yū-lăr) On the lower jaw.

ep·i·men·or·rhe·a (ep'i-men-ōr-ē'ă) Too frequent menstruation, occurring at any time, but particularly at the beginning and end of menstrual life.

ep·i·mer (ep'i-mĕr) One of two molecules (having more than one chiral center) differing only in the spatial arrangement about a single chiral atom. SEE sugars. Cf. anomer.

ep·i·mor·pho·sis (ep'i-mōr-fō'sis) Regeneration of a part of an organism by growth at the cut surface.

ep·i·mys·i·ot·o·my (ep'i-mis-ē-ot'ŏ-mē) Incision of the sheath of a muscle.

ep·i·mys·i·um (ep'i-mis'ē-ŭm) [TA] The fibrous connective tissue envelope surrounding a skeletal muscle.

ep·i·neph·rine (ep'i-nef'rin) A catecholamine that is the chief neurohormone of the medulla of the suprarenal gland; affects heart rate and force of contraction, vasoconstriction or vasodilation, and other metabolic effects. SYN adrenaline.

ep·i·neph·ros (ep'i-nef'ros) SYN suprarenal gland.

ep·i·neu·ral (ep'i-nūr'ăl) On a neural arch of a vertebra.

ep·i·neu·ri·um (ep'i-nūr'ē-ŭm) [TA] The outermost supporting structure of peripheral nerve trunks, consisting of a condensation of areolar connective tissue.

ep·i·ot·ic (ep'ē-ot'ik) A component of the otic capsule of some vertebrates.

ep·i·ot·ic cen·ter (ep'ē-ot'ik sen'tĕr) The center of ossification of the petrous part of the temporal bone that appears posterior to the posterior semicircular canal.

ep·i·pas·tic (ep'i-pas'tik) 1. Usable as a dusting powder. 2. A dusting powder.

ep·i·phe·nom·e·non (ep'i-fĕ-nom'ĕ-non) A symptom appearing during the course of a disease, not of usual occurrence, and not necessarily associated with the disease.

e·piph·o·ra (ē-pif'ōr-ă) An overflow of tears on the cheek, due to imperfect drainage by the tear-conducting passages or excess lacrimal production.

ep·i·phys·i·al, ep·i·phys·e·al (ep'i-fiz'ē-ăl) *Avoid the mispronunciation epiphyse'al*. Relating to an epiphysis.

ep·i·phys·i·al car·ti·lage (ep'i-fiz'ē-ăl kahr'ti-lăj) [TA] Particular type of new cartilage produced by the epiphysis of a growing long bone. SEE ALSO epiphysial plate.

ep·i·phys·i·al frac·ture, e·phys·e·al frac·ture (ep'i-fiz'ē-ăl frak'shŭr) Separation of the epiphysis of a long bone, caused by trauma.

ep·i·phys·i·al line (ep'i-fiz'ē-ăl līn) [TA] The line of junction of the epiphysis and diaphysis of a long bone where growth in length occurs. SYN linea epiphysialis [TA].

ep·i·phys·i·al plate (ep'i-fiz'ē-ăl plāt) [TA] The disc of cartilage between the metaphysis and the epiphysis of an immature long bone permitting growth in length. SYN cartilago epiphysialis [TA], growth plate.

e·piph·y·sis, pl. **e·piph·y·ses** (e-pif'i-sis, -sēz) [TA] A part of a long bone developed from a center of ossification distinct from that of the shaft and separated at first from the latter by a layer of cartilage.

ep·i·phy·sis ce·re·bri (e-pif'i-sis ser'ē-brī) SYN pineal body.

e·piph·y·si·tis (e-pif'i-sī'tis) Inflammation of an epiphysis.

♻ **epiplo-** Combining form meaning omentum.

e·pip·lo·on (e-pip'lō-on) SYN greater omentum.

ep·i·scle·ra (ep'i-skler'ă) The connective tissue between the sclera and the conjunctiva.

ep·i·scle·ral (ep'i-skler'ăl) **1.** On the sclera. **2.** Relating to the episclera.

ep·i·scle·ral veins (ep'i-skler'ăl vānz) [TA] A series of small venules in the sclera close to the corneal margin that empty into the anterior ciliary veins.

ep·i·scle·ri·tis, ep·i·scler·o·ti·tis (ep'i-skler-ī'tis, -ō-tī'tis) Inflammation of the episcleral connective tissue. SEE ALSO scleritis.

♻ **episio-** Prefix meaning the vulva. SEE ALSO vulvo-.

ep·i·si·o·per·i·ne·or·rha·phy (e-piz'ē-ō-per'i-nē-ōr'ă-fē) Repair of an incised or a ruptured perineum and lacerated vulva or repair of a surgical incision of the vulva and perineum.

ep·i·si·o·plas·ty (e-piz'ē-ō-plas-tē) Surgical repair of the vulva.

ep·i·si·or·rha·phy (e-piz'ē-ōr'ă-fē) Repair of a lacerated vulva or an episiotomy.

ep·i·si·o·ste·no·sis (e-piz'ē-ō-stē-nō'sis) Narrowing of the vulvar orifice.

ep·i·si·ot·o·my (EPIS) (e-piz'ē-ot'ŏ-mē) Surgical incision of the vulva to prevent laceration at the time of delivery or to facilitate vaginal surgery.

ep·i·sode (ep'i-sōd) An important event or series of events taking place in the course of continuous events (e.g., an episode of depression).

ep·i·so·dic hy·per·ten·sion (ep'i-sod'ik hī'pĕr-ten'shŭn) Hypertension manifested intermittently, triggered by anxiety or emotional factors. SYN paroxysmal hypertension.

ep·i·some (ep'i-sōm) An extrachromosomal element (plasmid) that may either integrate into the bacterial chromosome of the host or replicate and function stably when physically separated from the chromosome.

ep·i·spa·di·as (ep'i-spā'dē-ăs) A malformation in which the urethra opens on the penile dorsum.

ep·i·sple·ni·tis (ep'i-splē-nī'tis) Inflammation of the capsule of the spleen.

ep·i·stax·is (ep'i-stak'sis) Profuse bleeding from the nose. SYN nosebleed.

ep·i·sten·o·car·di·ac per·i·car·di·tis (ep'i-sten-ō-kahr'dē-ak per'i-kahr-dī'tis) Pericardial inflammation with transmural myocardial infarction limited to the area over the infarct.

ep·i·stro·phe·us (ep'i-strō'fē-ŭs) SYN axis (5).

ep·i·ten·din·e·um (ep'i-ten-din'ē-ŭm) The white fibrous sheath surrounding a tendon.

ep·i·thal·a·mus (ep'i-thal'ă-mŭs) [TA] A small dorsomedial area of the thalamus corresponding to the habenula and its associated structures, the medullary stria, pineal body, and habenular commissure.

ep·i·the·li·al (ep'i-thē'lē-ăl) Relating to or consisting of epithelium.

ep·i·the·li·al can·cer (ep-i-thē′lē-ăl kan′sĕr) Any malignant neoplasm originating from epithelium, i.e., a carcinoma.

ep·i·the·li·al dys·tro·phy (ep′i-thē′lē-ăl dis′trŏ-fē) Corneal dystrophy affecting primarily the epithelium and its basement membrane.

ep·i·the·li·al·i·za·tion, ep·i·the·li·za·tion (ep′i-thē′lē-ăl-ī-zā′shŭn, -thē′li-zā′shŭn) Formation of epithelium over a denuded surface.

ep·i·the·li·al lam·i·na (ep′i-thē′lē-ăl lam′i-nă) The layer of modified ependymal cells that forms the inner layer of the tela choroidea, facing the ventricle.

ep·i·the·li·al plug (ep′i-thē′lē-ăl plŭg) A mass of epithelial cells temporarily occluding an embryonic opening; most commonly used with reference to the external nares.

ep·i·the·li·al tis·sue (ep-i-thē′lē-ăl tish′ū) SEE epithelium.

ep·i·the·li·oid (ep′i-thē′lē-oyd) Resembling or having some of the characteristics of epithelium.

ep·i·the·li·o·lyt·ic (ep′i-thē′lē-ō-lit′ik) Destructive to epithelium.

ep·i·the·li·op·a·thy (ep′i-thē′lē-op′ă-thē) Disease involving epithelium.

ep·i·the·li·um, pl. **ep·i·the·li·a** (ep′i-thē′lē-ŭm, -ă) [TA] The purely cellular avascular layer covering all the free surfaces, cutaneous, mucous, and serous, including the glands and other structures derived therefrom.

ep·i·tope (ep′i-tōp) The simplest form of an antigenic determinant, on a complex antigenic molecule, that can combine with antibody or T-cell receptor.

ep·i·trich·i·um (ep′i-trik′ē-ŭm) SYN periderm.

ep·i·tym·pan·ic (ep′i-tim-pan′ik) Above, or in the upper part of, the tympanic cavity or membrane.

ep·i·tym·pa·num, ep·i·tym·pan·ic re·cess (ep′i-tim′pă-nŭm, ep′i-tim-pan′ik rē′ses) The upper portion of the tympanic cavity or middle ear above the tympanic

membrane; contains the head of the malleus and the body of the incus. SYN recessus epitympanicus [TA], attic, epitympanic space, Hyrtl epitympanic recess, tympanic attic.

ep·i·zo·ic (ep′i-zō′ik) Living as a parasite on the skin surface.

ep·o·nych·i·a (ep′ŏ-nik′ē-ă) Infection involving the proximal nail fold.

ep·o·nym (ep′ŏ-nim) The name of a disease, structure, operation, or procedure, usually derived from the name of the person who first discovered or described it. SYN eponymic (2).

ep·o·prost·en·ol, ep·o·prost·en·ol so·di·um (ep′ō-prost′en-ol, sō′dē-ŭm) SYN prostacyclin.

e·pox·y (ē-pok′sē) Chemical term describing an oxygen atom bound to two linked carbon atoms. Generally, any cyclic ether, but commonly applied to a three-membered ring; important chemical intermediates, and the basis of epoxy resins (polymers) formed from epoxy monomers.

Ep·stein-Barr vi·rus (EBV, EB virus) (ep′stīn bahr vī′rŭs) A herpesvirus that causes infectious mononucleosis and is also found in cell cultures of Burkitt lymphoma; associated with nasopharyngeal carcinoma. SYN human herpesvirus 4.

Ep·stein sign (ep′stīn sīn) Lid retraction in an infant giving it a frightened expression and a "wild glance."

ep·u·lis (ep-yū′lis) A nonspecific exophytic gingival mass.

e·qua·tion (ē-kwā′zhŭn) A statement expressing the equality of two things, usually by means of mathematical or chemical symbols.

e·qua·tor (ē-kwā′tŏr) [TA] A line encircling a globular body, equidistant at all points from the two poles; the periphery of a plane cutting a sphere at the midpoint of, and at right angles to, its axis.

e·qua·to·ri·al (ēk′wă-tō′rē-ăl) Situated, like the earth's equator, equidistant from either end.

e·qua·to·ri·al staph·y·lo·ma (ek′wă-tōr′ē-ăl staf′i-lō′mă) A staphyloma occurring in the area of exit of the vortex veins.

e·qui·ax·i·al (ē′kwē-ak′sē-ăl) Having axes of equal length.

e·quil·i·bra·tion (ē-kwil′i-brā′shŭn) **1.** The act of maintaining an equilibrium or balance. **2.** The act of exposing a liquid (e.g., blood or plasma) to a gas at a certain partial pressure until the partial pressures of the gas within and without the liquid are equal. **3.** DENTISTRY modification of occlusal forms of the teeth by grinding, with the intent of equalizing occlusal stress, producing simultaneous occlusal contacts, or harmonizing cuspal relations. **4.** CHROMATOGRAPHY the saturation of the stationary phase with the vapor of the elution solvent to be used.

e·qui·lib·ri·um (ē′kwi-lib′rē-ŭm) **1.** The condition of being evenly balanced; a state of repose between two or more antagonistic forces that exactly counteract each other. **2.** CHEMISTRY a state of apparent repose created by two reactions proceeding in opposite directions at equal speed; in chemical equations, sometimes indicated by two opposing arrows (↔). SYN dynamic equilibrium.

e·qui·lib·ri·um di·a·ly·sis (ē′kwi-lib′ rē-ŭm dī-al′i-sis) IMMUNOLOGY Method to determine association constants for hapten-antibody reactions in a system in which the hapten (dialyzable) and antibody (nondialyzable) solutions are separated by semipermeable membranes.

e·quine in·fec·tious a·ne·mi·a (ē′ kwīn in-fek′shŭs ă-nē′mē-ă) A worldwide disease of horses and other equids, caused by equine infectious anemia virus and a member of the family Retroviridae, marked by general debility, remittent fever, staggering gait, progressive anemia, and loss of flesh. SYN swamp fever (1).

e·qui·no·val·gus (ē-kwī′nō-val′gŭs) SYN talipes equinovalgus.

e·quiv·a·lence, e·quiv·a·len·cy (ē-kwiv′ă-lĕns, -lĕn-sē) The property of an element or radical of combining with or displacing, in definite and fixed proportion, another element or radical in a compound.

e·quiv·a·lent (ē-kwiv′ă-lĕnt) **1.** Equal in any respect. **2.** Having the capability to counterbalance or neutralize each other. **3.** Having equal valences. **4.** SYN gram equivalent.

e·quiv·a·lent weight (ē-kwiv′ă-lĕnt wāt) SYN gram equivalent.

e·quiv·o·cal symp·tom (ē-kwiv′ō-kăl simp′tŏm) One that points definitely to no particular disease, being associated with any one of a number of morbid states, or one with a presence that remains uncertain.

Er Symbol for erbium.

e·rad·i·ca·tion (ĕ-rad′i-kā′shŭn) Referring to disease, the termination of all transmission of infection by extermination of the infectious agent through surveillance and containment; global eradication has been achieved for smallpox, regional eradication for malaria, and perhaps in some places for measles.

Erb dis·ease (erb di-zēz′) SYN progressive bulbar palsy.

Erb pal·sy, Erb pa·ral·y·sis (erb pawl′ zē, păr-al′i-sis) Brachial palsy in which there is paralysis of the muscles of the upper arm and shoulder girdle (deltoid, biceps, brachialis, and brachioradialis muscles) due to a lesion of the upper trunk of the brachial plexus or of the roots of the fifth and sixth cervical roots. SYN Duchenne-Erb paralysis.

e·rec·tile (ĕ-rek′tīl) Capable of erection.

e·rec·tile dys·func·tion (ED) (ĕ-rek′tīl dis-fŭngk′shŭn) Inability to achieve or maintain penile tumescence sufficient for sexual intromission or for achieving orgasm.

e·rec·tile tis·sue (ĕ-rek′tīl tish′ū) A tissue with numerous vascular spaces that may become engorged with blood.

e·rec·tion (ĕ-rek′shŭn) The condition of erectile tissue when filled with blood, which then becomes hard and unyielding; denoting especially this state of the penis.

e·rec·tor (ĕ-rek′tŏr) **1.** One who or that which raises or makes erect. **2.** Denoting specifically certain muscles having such action. SYN arrector.

er·e·this·mic, er·e·this·tic, er·e·thit·ic (er'ĕ-thiz'mik, -this'tik, -thit'ik) Excited; marked by or causing erethism; irritable.

erg (ĕrg) The unit of work in the CGS system; the amount of work done by 1 dyne acting through 1 cm, 1 g cm² s⁻²; in the SI, 1 erg equals 10^{-7} joule.

er·gas·to·plasm (ĕr-gas'tō-plazm) SYN granular endoplasmic reticulum.

ergo- Combining form indicating work.

er·go·cal·cif·er·ol (ĕr'gō-kal-sif'ĕr-ol) Activated ergosterol, the vitamin D of plant origin; it arises from ultraviolet irradiation of ergosterol; used in prophylaxis and treatment of vitamin D deficiency. SYN calciferol, vitamin D2.

er·go·gen·ic aid (ĕr'gō-jen'ik ād) Ergogenic aids have been classified as nutritional, pharmacologic, physiologic, or psychological; methods to enhance athletic performance range from use of accepted techniques such as carbohydrate loading to illegal and unsafe approaches such as use of anabolic-androgenic steroids.

erg·o·lyt·ic (ĕr'gō-lit'ik) Pertaining to any substance that impairs exercise performance.

er·go·nom·ics (ĕr'gŏ-nom'iks) The science of workplace, tools, and equipment designed to reduce worker discomfort, strain, and fatigue and to prevent work-related injuries.

er·go·no·vine (er'gō-nō'vēn) An alkaloid from ergot; on hydrolysis it yields D-lysergic acid and L-2-aminopropanol; stimulates uterine contractions. SYN ergobasine, ergometrine, ergostetrine.

er·go·no·vine ma·le·ate (EM) (ĕr'gō-nō'vēn mal'ē-āt) Powerful oxytocic agent; this action is more prominent, and other actions of ergot (e.g., vasoconstriction, central nervous system stimulation, adrenergic blockade) are less prominent than for other ergot alkaloids; effective orally and parenterally. SYN ergometrine maleate.

er·got (ĕr'got) The resistant, overwintering stage of the parasitic ascomycetous fungus *Claviceps purpurea*, a pathogen of cereal rye that transforms the seed of rye into a compact spurlike mass of fungal pseudotissue (the sclerotium) containing five or more optically isomeric pairs of alkaloids. The levoratory isomers induce uterine contractions, control bleeding, and alleviate certain localized vascular disorders (migraine headaches). SEE ALSO ergotism. SYN rye smut.

er·got al·ka·loids (ĕr'got al'kă-loydz) Any of a large number of alkaloids obtained from the ergot fungus *Claviceps purpurea* or semisynthetically derived; examples include ergotamine, ergonovine, dihydroergotamine, lysergic acid diethylamide (LSD), methysergide.

er·got·a·mine (er-got'ă-mēn) An alkaloid from ergot, used to relieve migraine; it is a potent stimulant of smooth muscle, particularly of the blood vessels and the uterus, and produces adrenergic blockade (chiefly of the alpha receptors); hydrogenated ergotamine, dihydroergotamine, is less toxic and has fewer side effects. Also available as ergotamine tartrate.

er·got·ism (ĕr'got-izm) Poisoning by a toxic substance contained in the sclerotia of the fungus *Claviceps purpura*, growing on cereal rye; characterized by necrosis of the extremities (gangrene) due to contraction of the peripheral vascular bed. SYN ergot poisoning, Saint Anthony fire (1).

er·go·tro·pic (ĕr'gō-trō'pik) Mechanisms and the functional status of the nervous system that favor the organism's capacity to expend energy.

Er·len·mey·er flask (er'len-mī-er flask) A glass container with a flat base and a funnel-shaped body, the top of which forms the pour spout, usually with a wide opening.

e·rog·e·nous (ĕ-roj'ĕ-nŭs) *Do not confuse this word with aerogenous*. Capable of producing sexual excitement when stimulated.

e·rog·e·nous zone, er·o·to·gen·ic zone (ĕ-roj'ĕ-nŭs zōn, er'ō-tō-jen'ik zōn) Areas of the body, such as genitals and nipples, which elicit sexual arousal when stimulated.

e·ro·sion (ē-rō'zhŭn) **1.** A shallow ulcer;

in the stomach and intestine, an ulcer limited to the mucosa. **2.** The wearing away of a tooth by nonbacterial chemical action; when the cause is unknown, called idiopathic erosion. SYN odontolysis.

e·rot·ic (ĕ-rot'ik) Lustful; relating to sexual passion; having the quality to produce sexual arousal.

er·o·tism, er·ot·i·cism (er'ō-tizm, ĕ-rot'i-sizm) A condition of sexual excitement.

er·o·to·gen·ic (ĕ-rot'ō-jen'ik) Capable of causing sexual excitement or arousal.

er·o·to·ma·ni·a (ĕ-rot'ō-mā'nē-ă) **1.** Excessive or morbid inclination to erotic thoughts and behavior. **2.** The delusional belief that one is involved in a relationship with another, generally of higher socioeconomic status.

er·o·top·a·thy (er'ō-top'ă-thē) Any abnormality of the sexual impulse.

er·o·to·pho·bi·a (ĕ-rot'ŏ-fō'bē-ă) Morbid aversion to the thought of sexual love and to its physical expression.

er·rat·ic (ĕ-rat'ik) **1.** SYN eccentric (1). **2.** Denoting symptoms that vary in intensity, frequency, or location.

er·ror (er'ŏr) **1.** A defect in structure or function. **2.** BIOSTATISTICS a mistaken decision, as in hypothesis testing or classification by a discriminant function; or the difference between the true value and the observed value of a variate, ascribed to randomness or misreading by an observer. **3.** A false or mistaken belief; in biomedical and other sciences, there are many varieties of error, for example due to bias, inaccurate measurements, or faulty instruments.

er·ror of the first kind (er'ŏr fĭrst kīnd) In a Neyman-Pearson test of a statistical hypothesis the probability of rejecting the null hypothesis when it is true. SYN alpha error.

er·ror of the sec·ond kind (er'ŏr sek'ŏnd kīnd) In a Neyman-Pearson test of a statistical hypothesis, the probability of accepting the null hypothesis when it is false; the complement of the power of the test.

e·ruc·ta·tion (ē-rŭk-tā'shŭn) The voiding of gas or of a small quantity of acidic fluid from the stomach through the mouth. SYN belching, ructus.

e·rup·tion (ĕr-up'shŭn) **1.** A breaking out, especially the appearance of lesions on the skin. **2.** The passage of a tooth through the alveolar process and perforation of the gums. SEE ALSO emergence.

e·rup·tive fe·ver (ĕ-rŭp'tiv fē'vĕr) SYN Mediterranean spotted fever.

e·rup·tive xan·tho·ma (ĕr-ŭp'tiv zan-thō'mă) Sudden appearance of groups of 1–4 mm waxy yellow or yellowish-brown papules with an erythematous halo, especially over extensors of the elbows and knees, and on the back and buttocks of patients with severe hyperlipemia, often familial or, more rarely, in cases of severe diabetes.

er·y·sip·e·las (er'i-sip'ĕ-lăs) A specific, acute, cutaneous inflammatory disease caused by β-hemolytic streptococci and characterized by hot, red, edematous, brawny, and sharply defined eruptions.

er·y·sip·e·loid (er'i-sip'ĕ-loyd) An erythematous specific, usually self-limiting, cellulitis of the hand caused by *Erysipelothrix rhusiopathiae*. SYN blubber finger, crab hand, pseudoerysipelas, seal fingers, whale fingers.

Er·y·sip·e·lo·thrix (er'i-sip'ĕ-lō-thriks) A genus of bacteria containing nonmotile, gram-positive, rod-shaped organisms that have a tendency to form long filaments.

er·y·the·ma (er'i-thē'mă) Redness of the skin due to capillary dilatation.

er·y·the·ma an·u·la·re (er'i-thē'mă an-yū-lā'rē) Rounded or ringed lesions.

er·y·the·ma an·u·lare cen·tri·fu·gum (EAC) (er'i-thē'mă an-yū-lā'rē sen-trif' fyū-gŭm) A chronic, recurring erythematous eruption consisting of small and large anular lesions, with a scant marginal scale, usually of unknown cause. SYN erythema figuratum perstans.

er·y·the·ma chro·ni·cum mi·grans (er'i-thē'mă kron'i-kŭm mī'granz) A raised erythematous ring with advancing indurated borders and central clearing, radiating from the site of a tick bite such as that by *Ixodes scapularis;* the characteristic skin lesion of Lyme disease, due to the spirochete *Borrelia burgdorferi.*

er•y•the•ma dose (er'i-thē'mă dōs) The minimum dose of x-rays or other forms of radiation sufficient to produce erythema.

er•y•the•ma in•du•ra•tum (er'i-thē'mă in-dū-rā'tŭm) Recurrent hard subcutaneous nodules that frequently break down and form necrotic ulcers, usually on the calves and less frequently on the thighs or arms of middle-aged women. SYN Bazin disease.

er•y•the•ma in•fec•ti•o•sum (er'i-thē'mă in-fek-shē-ō'sŭm) A mild infectious exanthema of childhood characterized by an erythematous maculopapular eruption, resulting in a lacelike facial rash or "slapped cheek" appearance. SYN fifth disease.

er•y•the•ma mul•ti•for•me (er'i-thē'mă mŭl-ti-fōr'mē) An acute eruption of macules, papules, or subdermal vesicles presenting a multiform appearance, the characteristic lesion being the target or iris form of lesion over the dorsal aspect of the hands and forearms; its origin may be allergic, seasonal, or from drug sensitivity, and the eruption, although usually self limited, may be recurrent or may run a severe course, sometimes even death (Stevens-Johnson syndrome). SYN herpes iris (2).

er•y•the•ma ne•o•na•to•rum (er'i-thē'mă nē-ō-nā-tō'rŭm) SYN erythema toxicum.

er•y•the•ma no•do•sum (er'i-thē'mă nō-dō'sŭm) A panniculitis marked by the sudden formation of painful nodes on the extensor surfaces of the lower extremities, with lesions that are self limiting but tend to recur; associated with arthralgia and fever.

er•y•the•ma per•stans (er'i-thē'mă pĕr' stanz) Probably a chronic form of erythema multiforme in which the relapses recur so persistently that the eruption is almost permanent.

er•y•the•ma•to•ve•sic•u•lar (er'i-thē'mă-tō-vĕ-sik'yū-lăr) Denoting a condition characterized by erythema and ve-

siculation, as in allergic contact dermatitis.

er•y•the•ma tox•i•cum (er'i-thē'mă tok' si-kŭm) Flushing of the skin due to allergic reaction to some toxic substance. SYN erythema neonatorum.

er•y•the•ma tox•i•cum ne•o•na•to• rum (er'i-thē'mă tok'si-kŭm nē-o-nā-tō'rŭm) A common transient idiopathic eruption of erythema, small papules, and occasionally pustules filled with eosinophilic leukocytes overlying hair follicles of the newborn.

erythr- SEE erythro-.

erythraemia [Br.] SYN erythremia.

er•y•thras•ma (er'i-thraz'mă) An eruption of well-circumscribed reddish brown patches, in the axillae and groin especially, due to the presence of *Corynebacterium minutissimum* in the stratum corneum.

er•y•thre•mi•a (er'i-thrē'mē-ă) SYN polycythemia vera, erythraemia.

er•y•thrism (er'i-thrizm) Redness of the hair with a ruddy, freckled complexion.

erythro-, erythr- 1. Combining forms denoting red or red blood cell; corresponds to L. *rub-*. 2. Indicates the structure of erythrose in a larger sugar; used as such, it is italicized (e.g., 2-deoxy-D-*erythro*-pentose).

e•ryth•ro•blast (ĕ-rith'rō-blast) The first generation of cells in the red blood cell series that can be distinguished from precursor endothelial cells. In normal maturation, four stages of development can be recognized: pronormoblast, basophilic normoblast, polychromatic normoblast, and orthochromatic normoblast.

erythroblastaemia [Br.] SYN erythroblastemia.

eryth•ro•blas•te•mi•a (ĕ-rith'rō-blas-tē'mē-ă) The presence of nucleated red blood cells in peripheral blood. SYN erythroblastaemia.

e•ryth•ro•blas•to•pe•ni•a (EBP) (ĕ-rith'rō-blas-tō-pē'nē-ă) A primary deficiency of erythroblasts in bone marrow.

e•ryth•ro•blas•to•sis (ĕ-rith'rō-blas-tō'

e·ryth·ro·chro·mi·a (ĕ-rith′rō-krō′mē-ă) A red coloration or staining.

er·y·throc·la·sis (er′i-throk′lă-sis) Fragmentation of the red blood cells.

e·ryth·ro·clas·tic (ĕ-rith′rō-klas′tik) Pertaining to erythroclasis; destructive to red blood cells.

e·ryth·ro·cy·a·no·sis (ĕ-rith′rō-sī-ă-nō′sis) A condition seen in girls and young women in which exposure of the limbs to cold causes them to become swollen and dusky red; it results from direct exposure to cold, but not freezing, temperatures.

e·ryth·ro·cyte (ĕ-rith′rō-sīt) A mature red blood cell. SYN hemacyte, red blood cell, red cell, red corpuscle.

e·ryth·ro·cyte in·di·ces (ĕ-rith′rō-sīt in′di-sēz) Calculations for determining the average size, hemoglobin content, and concentration of hemoglobin in red blood cells, specifically mean cell volume, mean cell hemoglobin, and mean cell hemoglobin concentration.

e·ryth·ro·cyte sed·i·men·ta·tion rate (ESR, sed rate) (ĕ-rith′rō-sīt sed′i-mĕn-tā′shŭn rāt) The rate of settling of red blood cells in anticoagulated blood; increased rates are often associated with anemia or inflammatory states.

erythrocythaemia [Br.] SYN erythrocythemia.

e·ryth·ro·cy·the·mi·a (ĕ-rith′rō-sī-thē′mē-ă) SYN polycythemia, erythrocythaemia.

e·ryth·ro·cyt·ic (ĕ-rith′rō-sit′ik) Pertaining to an erythrocyte.

e·ryth·ro·cyt·ic cy·cle (ĕ-rith′rō-sit′ik sī′kĕl) That pathogenic portion of the vertebrate phase of the life cycle of malarial organisms that takes place in the red blood cells.

e·ryth·ro·cyt·ic se·ries (ĕ-rith′rō-sit′ik sēr′ēz) The cells in the various stages of development in the red bone marrow leading to the formation of the erythrocyte, e.g., erythroblasts, normoblasts, erythrocytes.

e·ryth·ro·cy·tol·y·sis (ĕ-rith′rō-sī-tol′i-sis) SYN hemolysis.

e·ryth·ro·cy·to·pe·ni·a (ĕ-rith′rō-sī′tō-pē′nē-ă) SYN erythropenia.

e·ryth·ro·cy·tos·chi·sis (ĕ-rith′rō-sī-tos′ki-sis) A breaking up of the red blood cells into small particles that morphologically resemble platelets.

e·ryth·ro·cy·to·sis (ĕ-rith′rō-sī-tō′sis) Polycythemia, especially that which occurs in response to some known stimulus.

e·ryth·ro·der·ma des·qua·ma·ti·vum (ĕ-rith′rō-dĕr′mă des-kwah′mă-tī′vŭm) Severe, extensive seborrheic dermatitis with exfoliative dermatitis, generalized lymphadenopathy, and diarrhea in the newborn; frequently occurs in undernourished, cachectic children. SYN Leiner disease.

e·ryth·ro·der·ma pso·ri·at·i·cum (ĕ-rith′rō-dĕr′mă sōr-ē-at′i-kŭm) Extensive exfoliative dermatitis simulating psoriasis.

e·ryth·ro·don·ti·a (ĕ-rith′rō-don′shē-ă) Reddish discoloration of the teeth, as may occur in porphyria.

e·ryth·ro·gen·ic (ĕ-rith′rō-jen′ik) **1.** Producing redness, as causing an eruption or a red color sensation. **2.** Pertaining to the formation of red blood cells.

er·y·throid (ĕ-rith′royd) Of a reddish color.

e·ryth·ro·ker·a·to·der·mi·a (ĕ-rith′rō-ker-ă-tō-dĕr′mē-ă) A neurocutaneous syndrome characterized by papulosquamous erythematous plaques with onset shortly after birth.

e·ryth·ro·ker·a·to·der·mia va·ri·a·bi·lis (ĕ-rith′rō-ker-ă-tō-dĕr′mē-ă vă-rē-ă-bil′is) A dermatosis characterized by hyperkeratotic plaques of bizarre, geographic configuration, associated with erythrodermic areas that may vary remarkably in size, shape, and position from day to day; hair, nails, and teeth are not affected.

e·ryth·ro·ki·net·ics (ĕ-rith′rō-ki-net′iks) The kinetics of erythrocytes from their generation to destruction.

erythroleukaemia [Br.] SYN erythroleukemia.

e·ryth·ro·leu·ke·mi·a (FAB M6, EL) (ĕ-rith′rō-lū-kē′mē-ă) Simultaneous neoplastic proliferation of erythroblastic and leukoblastic tissues.

e·ryth·ro·mel·al·gi·a (ĕ-rith′rō-mel-al′jē-ă) Paroxysmal throbbing and burning pain in the skin often precipitated by exertion or heat, affecting the hands and feet, accompanied by a dusky mottled redness of the parts with increased skin temperature; may be associated with myeloproliferative disorders. SYN red neuralgia.

e·ryth·ro·my·cin (E, EM, ETM, ERYTH) (ĕ-rith′rō-mī′sin) *Avoid the mispronunciation ĕ-rith-rō-mī″ă-sin.* A macrolide antibiotic agent obtained from cultures of a strain of *Streptomyces erythraeus* found in soil; active against *Corynebacterium diphtheriae* and several other species of *Corynebacterium*, Group A hemolytic streptococci, *Streptococcus pneumoniae*, *Legionella*, *Mycoplasma pneumoniae*, and *Bordetella pertussis*; used as a substitute antibiotic in penicillin-allergic patients.

e·ryth·ro·ne·o·cy·to·sis (ĕ-rith′rō-nē-ō-sī-tō′sis) The presence in the peripheral circulation of regenerative forms of red blood cells.

e·ryth·ro·pe·ni·a (ĕ-rith′rō-pē′nē-ă) Deficiency in the number of red blood cells. SYN erythrocytopenia.

e·ryth·ro·pha·gi·a (ĕ-rith′rō-fā′jē-ă) Phagocytic destruction of red blood cells.

e·ryth·ro·phag·o·cy·to·sis (ĕ-rith′rō-fag′ō-sī-tō′sis) Phagocytosis of erythrocytes.

e·ryth·ro·phil (ĕ-rith′rō-fil) **1.** Staining readily with red dyes. SYN erythrophilic. **2.** A cell or tissue element that stains red.

e·ryth·ro·pla·ki·a (ĕ-rith′rō-plā′kē-ă) A red, velvety, plaquelike lesion of mucous membrane that often represents malignant change.

e·ryth·ro·pla·si·a (ĕ-rith′rō-plā′zē-ă) Erythema and dysplasia of the epithelium.

e·ryth·ro·poi·e·sis (ĕ-rith′rō-poy-ē′sis) The formation of red blood cells.

e·ryth·ro·poi·et·ic por·phy·ria (ĕ-rith′rō-poy-et′ik pōr-fir′ē-ă) A classification of porphyria that includes congenital erythropoietic porphyria and erythropoietic protoporphyria.

e·ryth·ro·poi·e·tin (ĕ-rith′rō-poy′ĕ-tin) A protein that enhances erythropoiesis by stimulating formation of proerythroblasts and release of reticulocytes from bone marrow; secreted by the kidney and possibly by other tissues.

e·ryth·ro·pros·o·pal·gi·a (ĕ-rith′rō-pros-ō-pal′jē-ă) A disorder similar to erythromelalgia, but with facial pain and redness.

er·y·throp·si·a, e·ryth·ro·pi·a (er′ith-rop′sē-ă er′i-thrō′pē-ă) An abnormality of vision in which all objects appear to be tinged with red.

ESADDI Abbreviation for estimated safe and adequate daily dietary intake.

es·cape (es-kāp′) Term used to describe the situation when a pacemaker defaults or atrioventricular conduction fails and another, usually lower pacemaker, assumes the function of pacemaking for one or more beats.

es·cape beat, es·caped beat (es-kāp′ bēt, es-kāpt′) An automatic beat, usually arising from the atrioventricular junction or ventricle, occurring after the next expected normal beat has defaulted; it is therefore always a late beat, terminating a longer cycle than the normal.

es·cape in·ter·val (es-kāp′ in′tĕr-văl) Duration between the last beat of the patient's basic rhythm (ectopic or sinus beat) and a beat from a spontaneous escape focus or the initial electronic pacemaker impulse (a preset interval in the circuitry).

es·cape rhythm (es-kāp′ ridh′ŭm) Three or more consecutive impulses at a rate not exceeding the upper limit of the inherent pacemaker.

es·char (es′kahr) A thick, coagulated crust or slough that develops following a thermal burn or chemical or physical cauterization of the skin.

es·cha·rot·ic (es′kă-rot′ik) Caustic or corrosive.

Esch·e·rich·i·a (esh-ĕ-rik′ē-ă) A genus of aerobic, facultatively anaerobic bacteria containing short, motile or nonmotile, gram-negative rods; found in feces; some are pathogenic to humans.

Esch·e·rich·i·a co·li (esh-ĕ-rik′ē-ă kō′lī) A bacterial species that occurs normally in the intestines of humans and other vertebrates, is widely distributed in nature, and is a frequent cause of infections of the urogenital tract and of diarrhea in infants.

es·cutch·eon (es-kŭch′ŏn) Pattern of distribution of pubic hair.

-esis (ē′sis) Combining form denoting condition, action, or process.

Es·march ban·dage (es′mark ban′dăj) Rubber tourniquet that is wrapped around an extremity from distal to proximal before starting a surgical procedure to exsanguinate the limb before the inflation of a proximally placed pneumatic tourniquet.

e·soph·a·ge·al (ĕ-sof′ă-jē′ăl) Relating to the esophagus.

e·soph·a·ge·al a·cha·la·si·a (ĕ-sof′ă-jē′ăl ak′ă-lā′zē-ă) An obstruction to the passage of food that develops in the terminal esophagus; caused by an autonomic nervous system abnormality. SYN achalasia of the cardia, cardiospasm, oesophageal achalasia.

e·soph·a·ge·al dys·func·tion (ĕ-sof′ă-jē′ăl dis-fŭngk′shŭn) Any disorder that adversely affects esophageal function.

e·soph·a·ge·al hi·a·tus (ĕ-sof′ă-jē′ăl hī-ā′tŭs) [TA] The opening in the right crus of the diaphragm, between the central tendon and the hiatus aorticus, through which pass the esophagus and the two vagus nerves. SYN oesophageal hiatus.

e·soph·a·ge·al ner·vous plex·us (ĕ-sof′ă-jē′ăl nĕrv′ŭs pleks′ŭs) One of two nervous plexuses, posterior and anterior, on the walls of the esophagus. SYN plexus gulae, plexus nervosus esophageus.

e·soph·a·ge·al spasm (ĕ-sof′ă-jē′ăl spazm) Disorder of the motility of the esophagus characterized by pain or forceful belches after swallowing food. Esophageal muscle contractions are of excessive force and duration. Chest pain can be confused with symptoms of cardiac or other origin. SYN oesophageal spasm.

e·soph·a·ge·al speech (ĕ-sof′ă-jē′ăl spēch) A technique for speaking after total laryngectomy; phonation results from introducing air into the upper esophagus to allow vibration of the pharyngoesophageal (PE) segment. SYN oesophageal speech.

e·soph·a·ge·al veins (ĕ-sof′ă-jē′ăl vānz) [TA] Series of veins draining the submucous venous plexus of the esophagus. SYN oesophageal veins.

e·soph·a·ge·al web (ē-sof′ă-jē′ăl web) Congenital or acquired transverse fold of the mucous membrane and sometimes the deeper layers of the esophagus, often causing dysphagia. SYN oesophageal web.

e·soph·a·gec·ta·sis, e·soph·a·gec·ta·si·a (ĕ-sof′ă-jek′tă-sis, -jek-tā′zē-ă) Dilation of the esophagus. SYN oesophagectasis.

e·soph·a·gi·tis (ĕ-sof′ă-jī′tis) Inflammation of the esophagus. SYN oesophagitis.

e·soph·a·go·car·di·o·plas·ty (ĕ-sof′ă-gō-kahr′dē-ō-plas-tē) Surgical repair of the esophagus and cardiac end of the stomach. SYN oesophagocardioplasty.

e·soph·a·go·cele (ĕ-sof′ă-gō-sēl) Protrusion of the mucous membrane of the esophagus through a tear in the muscular coat. SYN oesophagocele.

e·soph·a·go·du·o·den·os·to·my (ĕ-sof′ă-gō-dū′ō-dĕ-nos′tŏ-mē) Surgical formation of a direct communication between the esophagus and the duodenum, with or without removal of the stomach. SYN oesophagoduodenostomy.

e·soph·a·go·dyn·i·a (ĕ-sof'ă-gō-din'ē-ă) SYN esophagalgia.

e·soph·a·go·en·ter·os·to·my (ĕ-sof'ă-gō-en-tĕr-os'tŏ-mē) Surgical formation of a direct communication between the esophagus and intestine.

e·soph·a·go·gas·trec·to·my (ĕ-sof'ă-gō-gas-trek'tŏ-mē) Removal of a portion of the lower esophagus and proximal stomach for treatment of neoplasms or strictures of those organs. SYN oesophagogastrectomy.

e·soph·a·go·gas·tric junc·tion (ĕ-sof'ă-gō-gas'trik jŭngk'shŭn) Terminal end of esophagus and beginning of stomach at the cardiac orifice; site of the physiologic inferior esophageal sphincter. SYN oesophagogastric junction.

e·soph·a·go·gas·tro·du·o·de·nos·co·py (EGD) (ĕ-sof'ă-gō-gas'trō-dū'ŏ-dĕ-nos'kŏ-pē) Endoscopic examination of the esophagus, stomach, and duodenum. SYN oesophagogastroduodenoscopy.

e·soph·a·go·gas·tro·plas·ty (ĕ-sof'ă-gō-gas'trō-plas-tē) SYN cardioplasty, oesophagogastroplasty.

e·soph·a·go·gas·tros·to·my (ĕ-sof'ă-gō-gas-tros'tŏ-mē) Anastomosis of esophagus to stomach, usually following esophagogastrectomy. SYN esophagogastroanastomosis, gastroesophagostomy, oesophagogastrostomy.

e·soph·a·go·gram (ĕ-sof'ă-gō-gram) A radiograph of the esophagus. SYN oesophagogram.

e·soph·a·go·ma·la·ci·a (ĕ-sof'ă-gō-mă-lā'shē-ă) Softening of the walls of the esophagus. SYN oesophagomalacia.

e·soph·a·go·my·ot·o·my (ĕ-sof'ă-gō-mī-ot'ŏ-mē) Treatment of esophageal achalasia by longitudinal division of the lowest part of the esophageal muscle down to the submucosal layer. SYN oesophagomyotomy.

e·soph·a·go·plas·ty (ĕ-sof'ă-gō-plas-tē) Surgical repair of the wall of the esophagus. SYN oesophagoplasty.

e·soph·a·go·pli·ca·tion (ĕ-sof'ă-gō-pli-kā'shŭn) Reduction in size of a dilated esophagus or of a pouch within it by making longitudinal folds or tucks in its wall.

e·soph·a·go·pto·sis, e·soph·a·gop·to·si·a (ĕ-sof'ă-gō-tō'sis, -gop-tō'zē-ă) Relaxation and downward displacement of the walls of the esophagus. SYN oesophagoptosis.

e·soph·a·go·scope (ĕ-sof'ă-gō-skōp) An endoscope for inspecting the interior of the esophagus.

e·soph·a·gos·co·py (ĕ-sof'ă-gos'kŏ-pē) Inspection of the interior of the esophagus by means of an endoscope. SYN oesophagoscopy.

e·soph·a·go·ste·no·sis (ĕ-sof'ă-gō-stĕ-nō'sis) Stricture or a general narrowing of the esophagus. SYN oesophagostenosis.

e·soph·a·got·o·my (ĕ-sof'ă-gō-got'ŏ-mē) An incision through the wall of the esophagus.

e·soph·a·gus, gen. and pl. **e·soph·a·gi** (ĕ-sof'ă-gŭs, -jī) [TA] The 25-cm portion of the digestive canal between the pharynx and stomach. SYN oesophagus.

es·o·pho·ri·a (es'ō-fōr'ē-ă) A tendency for the eyes to turn inward, prevented by binocular vision.

es·o·tro·pi·a (es'ō-trō'pē-ă) The form of strabismus in which the visual axes converge; may be paralytic or concomitant, monocular or alternating, accommodative or nonaccommodative. SYN convergent strabismus.

es·sence (ess) (es'ĕns) **1.** The true characteristic or substance of a body. **2.** An element. **3.** A fluidextract. **4.** An alcoholic solution, or spirit, of the volatile oil of a plant. **5.** Any volatile substance responsible for odor or taste of the organism (usually a plant) producing it; by extension, synthetic perfumes or flavors.

es·sen·tial (ĕ-sen'shăl) **1.** Necessary, indispensable (e.g., essential amino acids, essential fatty acids). **2.** Characteristic of. **3.** Determining. **4.** Of unknown etiology. **5.** Relating to an essence (e.g., essential oil). **6.** SYN intrinsic.

es·sen·tial a·mi·no acids (ĕ-sen'shăl ă-mē′nō as′idz) The α-amino acids nutritionally required by an organism that must be supplied in its diet (i.e., cannot be synthesized by the organism), either as free amino acid or in proteins.

es·sen·tial fat·ty acid (EFA) (ĕ-sen′ shăl fat′ē as′id) The 18-carbon fatty acids that are nutritionally required by humans and must be consumed through dietary sources.

es·sen·tial fruc·to·su·ri·a (ĕ-sen′shăl fruk′tŏ-syūr′ē-ă) Benign, asymptomatic inborn error of metabolism due to deficiency of fructokinase, the first enzyme in the specific fructose pathway. SYN benign fructosuria, fructokinasedeficiency.

es·sen·tial oil (ĕ-sen′shăl oyl) A plant product, usually somewhat volatile, giving the odors and tastes characteristic of the particular plant. SEE ALSO volatile oil.

es·sen·tial throm·bo·cy·to·pe·ni·a (ĕ-sen′shăl throm′bō-sī-tō-pē′nē-ă) A primary form of this disorder (in contrast to secondary forms that are associated with metastatic neoplasms, tuberculosis, and leukemia involving the bone marrow, or with direct suppression of bone marrow by the use of chemical agents, or with other conditions).

es·sen·tial trem·or (ET) (ĕ-sen′shăl trem′ŏr) Action tremor of 4–8 Hz frequency that usually begins in early adult life and is limited to the upper limbs and head; called familial when it appears in several family members.

EST Abbreviation for electroshock therapy.

es·ter·ase (ES, EST) (es′tĕr-ās) A generic term for enzymes (EC class 3.1, hydrolases) that catalyze the hydrolysis of esters.

es·ter·i·fied es·tro·gens (es-ter′i-fīd es′trŏ-jenz) A mixture of the sodium salts of sulfate esters of estrogenic substances.

esthesio- Prefix meaning sensation, perception. SYN aesthesio-.

es·the·si·od·ic (es-thē′zē-od′ik) Conveying sensory impressions.

es·the·si·ol·o·gy (es-thē′zē-ol′ŏ-jē) The science concerned with sensory phenomena.

es·the·si·om·e·ter (es-thē′zē-om′ĕ-tĕr) An instrument for determining the state of tactile and other forms of sensibility.

es·thet·ics (es-thet′iks) The branch of philosophy concerned with art and beauty, especially with the components thereof. SYN aesthetics.

es·ti·mate (es′ti-măt) 1. A measurement or a statement about the value of some quantity that is known, believed, or suspected to incorporate some degree of error. 2. The result of applying any estimator to a random sample of data. It is not a random variable but a realization of one, a fixed quantity, and it has no variance although commonly it also furnishes an estimate of what the variance of the estimator is.

es·ti·ma·tor (es′ti-mā′tŏr) A prescription for obtaining an estimate from a random sample of data.

es·tra·di·ol (es′tră-dī′ol) The most potent naturally occurring estrogen, formed by the ovary, placenta, testes, and possibly the cortex of the suprarenal gland. SYN oestradiol.

es·trange·ment (es-trānj′mĕnt) Failure to bond between mother and infant due to illness in either patient or a congenital disorder in the infant that mandates separation.

es·tro·gen (es′trŏ-jen) Generic term for any substance, natural or synthetic, which exerts biologic effects characteristic of estrogenic hormones; formed by the ovary, placenta, testes, and possibly the cortex of the suprarenal gland, as well as by certain plants. SYN oestrogen.

es·tro·gen·ic (es′trŏ-jen′ik) 1. Causing estrus in animals. 2. Having an action similar to that of an estrogen. SYN oestrogenic.

es·tro·gen re·cep·tor (es′trŏ-jen rĕ-sep′tŏr) Receptor for estrogens; its presence conveys a better prognosis for breast cancers. SYN oestrogen receptor.

es·tro·gen re·place·ment ther·a·py (ERT) (es′trŏ-jen rĕ-plās′mĕnt thār′ă-pē) Administration of sex hormones to women after menopause or oophorectomy. SYN hormone replacement therapy, oestrogen replacement therapy.

es·trone (es′trōn) A metabolite of 17β-estradiol, commonly found in urine, ovaries, and placenta, with considerably less biologic activity than the parent hormone. SYN oestrone.

es·trous (es′trŭs) Pertaining to estrus. SYN estrual.

es·trus, es·tru·a·tion (es′trŭs, es′trū-ā′shŭn) That portion or phase of the sexual cycle of female animals characterized by willingness to permit coitus; readily detectable behavioral and other signs are exhibited by animals during this period. SYN estruation, heat (2), oestrus.

é·tat cri·blé (ā-tah′ krē′blā) In neuropathology, a term describing perivascular atrophy of cerebral tissue, producing lacunae.

eth·a·cryn·ic ac·id (EA, ECA) (eth′ă-krin′ik as′id) An unsaturated ketone derivative of aryloxyacetic acid; a potent loop diuretic and a weak antihypertensive.

eth·a·nol (eth′ăn-ol) SYN alcohol (2).

e·ther (ē′thĕr) 1. Any organic compound in which two carbon atoms are independently linked to a common oxygen atom, thus containing the group –C–O–C–. SEE ALSO epoxy. 2. Loosely used to refer to diethyl ether.

e·the·re·al (ĕ-thēr′ē-ăl) Relating to or containing ether.

eth·i·nyl es·tra·di·ol (EE) (eth′ĭ-nil es-trā-dī′ol) SYN ethynyl estradiol.

eth·i·o·dized oil (eth-ī′ō-dīzd oyl) A radiopaque medium used for lympangiography and hysterosalpingography.

ethmo- Combining form denoting: 1. Ethmoid. 2. The ethmoid bone.

eth·mo·car·di·tis (eth′mō-kahr-dī′tis) Long-term inflammation of cardiac interstitial tissue.

eth·mo·fron·tal (eth′mō-frŏn′tăl) Relating to the ethmoid and the frontal bones.

eth·moid (ETH) (eth′moyd) [TA] SEE ethmoid bone. SYN os ethmoidale [TA].

eth·moid air cells (eth′moyd ār selz) SYN ethmoid cells.

eth·moi·dal cells (eth-moy′dăl selz) [TA] SYN ethmoid cells.

eth·moi·dal in·fun·dib·u·lum (eth-moy′dăl in′fŭn-dib′yū-lŭm) [TA] Passage from the middle meatus of the nose communicating with the anterior ethmoidal cells and frontal sinus. SYN infundibulum ethmoidale [TA], ethmoid infundibulum.

eth·moi·dal lab·y·rinth (eth-moy′dăl lab′i-rinth) [TA] Mass of air cells with thin bony walls forming part of the lateral wall of the nasal cavity. SYN labyrinthus ethmoidalis [TA], ectoethmoid, lateral mass of ethmoid bone.

eth·moi·dal si·nus·es (eth-moy′dăl sī′nŭs-ēz) SYN ethmoid cells.

eth·moid cells (eth′moyd selz) Ethmoidal air cells; evaginations of the mucous membrane of the middle and superior meatus of the nasal cavity into the ethmoidal labyrinth forming multiple small paranasal sinuses; they are subdivided into anterior, middle and posterior ethmoidal sinuses. SYN ethmoidal sinuses.

eth·moid crest (eth′moyd krest) Bony ridge that articulates with, or provides attachment for, any part of the ethmoid bone, especially the middle nasal concha.

eth·moi·dec·to·my (eth′moy-dek′tŏ-mē) Removal of all or part of the mucosal lining and bony partitions between the ethmoid sinuses.

eth·moid fo·ra·men (eth′moyd fōr-ā′mĕn) Either of two foramina formed by grooves on either edge of the ethmoidal notch of the frontal bone and completed by similar grooves on the ethmoid bone.

eth·moid in·fun·dib·u·lum (eth′moyd in′fŭn-dib′yū-lŭm) A passage from the middle meatus of the nose communicating with the anterior ethmoid cells and frontal sinus.

eth·moid lab·y·rinth (eth′moyd lab′i-rinth) A mass of air cells with thin bony walls forming part of the lateral wall of the nasal cavity; the cells are arranged in three groups, anterior, middle, and posterior, and are closed laterally by the orbital plate, which forms part of the wall of the orbit.

eth·mo·max·il·lar·y (eth′mō-mak′si-lar-ē) Relating to the ethmoid and the maxillary bones.

eth·mo·tur·bi·nals (eth′mō-tŭr′bi-nălz) The conchae of the ethmoid bone.

eth·no·bot·a·ny (eth′nō-bot′ă-nē) A study of the role of plants in the life of early humankind.

eth·nol·o·gy (eth-nol′ŏ-jē) The science that compares human culture and/or races; cultural anthropology.

eth·no·phar·ma·col·o·gy (eth′nō-fahrm′ă-kol′ŏ-jē) The study of differences in response to drugs based on varied ethnicity; pharmacogenetics.

eth·yl (Et) (eth′il) The hydrocarbon radical CH_3CH_2-.

eth·yl al·co·hol (eth′il al′kŏ-hol) SYN alcohol (2).

eth·yl·cel·lu·lose (eth′il-sel′yū-lōs) An ethyl ether of cellulose used as a tablet binder.

eth·yl chlo·ride (eth′il klōr′ĭd) Volatile explosive liquid (under increased pressure); when sprayed on the skin, produces local anesthesia by superficial freezing, but also is a potent inhalation anesthetic. SYN chloroethane.

eth·yl·ene (eth′il-ēn) An explosive constituent of ordinary illuminating gas; hastens ripening of fruit.

eth·yl·ene·di·a·mine (ED) (eth′il-ēn-dī′ă-mēn) A volatile colorless liquid of ammoniac odor and caustic taste; the dihydrochloride is used as a urinary acidifier.

eth·yl·ene·di·a·mine·tet·ra·a·ce·tic ac·id (EDTA) (eth′i-lēn-dī′ă-mēn-tet′ră-ă-sē′tik as′id) A chelating agent and anticoagulant; added to blood specimens for hematologic and other tests.

eth·yl·ene gly·col (eth′il-ēn glī′kol) SEE glycol (2).

eth·yl·ene ox·ide (EtO, EO, ETOX, ETO) (eth′i-lēn ok′sīd) Fumigant, used for cold sterilization of surgical instruments. SYN oxirane.

eth·yl·i·dene (eth′il-i-dēn) The radical $CH_3CH=$. SYN ethidene.

eth·yl ox·ide (eth′il ok′sīd) SYN diethyl ether.

eth·y·nyl es·tra·di·ol (eth′i-nil es-trā′dē-ol) Semisynthetic derivative of 17β-estradiol; active by mouth, with a long half-life, it is among the most potent of known estrogenic compounds; used in oral contraceptive preparations. SYN ethinyl estradiol.

e·ti·o·la·tion (ē′tē-ō-lā′shŭn) 1. Pallor resulting from absence of light. 2. The process of blanching, bleaching, or making pale by withholding light.

e·ti·ol·o·gy (ē′tē-ol′ŏ-jē) 1. The science and study of the causes of disease and their mode of operation. Cf. pathogenesis. 2. The science of causes, causality; in common usage, cause. SYN aetiology.

Eu Symbol for europium.

eu- Good, well; opposite of dys-, caco-.

eu·bi·ot·ics (yū′bī-ot′iks) The science of hygienic living.

eu·ca·lyp·tol (yū′kă-lip′tol) SYN cineole.

eu·cap·ni·a (yū-kap′nē-ă) A state in which the arterial carbon dioxide pressure is optimal. SEE ALSO normocapnia.

eu·car·y·ot·ic (yū′kar-ē-ot′ik) SYN eukaryotic.

eu·cho·li·a (yū-kō′lē-ă) A normal state of the bile as regards quantity and quality.

eu·chro·ma·tin (yū-krō′mă-tin) The parts of chromosomes that during interphase are uncoiled dispersed threads and not stained by ordinary dyes.

eu·ge·nol (yū′jĕ-nol) Analgesic obtained

from oil of cloves; used in dentistry with zinc oxide as a base for impression materials; also used in perfume manufacture as a substitute for oil of cloves. SYN eugenic acid.

eu·glob·u·lin (yū-glob′yū-lin) That fraction of the serum globulin less soluble in ammonium sulphate solution than the pseudoglobulin fraction.

euglycaemia [Br.] SYN euglycemia.

eu·gly·ce·mi·a (yū′glī-sē′mē-ă) A normal blood glucose concentration. SYN euglycaemia, normoglycemia.

eu·gly·ce·mic (yū′glī-sē′mik) Denoting, characteristic of, or promoting euglycemia.

eu·gon·ic (yū-gon′ik) A term used to indicate that the growth of a bacterial culture is rapid and relatively luxuriant.

eu·kar·y·on (yū-kar′ē-on) Complicated cellular nucleus enrobed by a nuclear membrane.

eu·kar·y·ote, eu·car·y·ote (yū-kar′ē-ōt) 1. A cell containing a membrane-bound nucleus with chromosomes of DNA, RNA, and proteins, with cell division involving a form of mitosis in which mitotic spindles (or some microtubule arrangement) are involved; mitochondria are present, and, in photosynthetic species, plastids are found. 2. Common name for members of the Eukaryotae.

eu·kar·y·ot·ic, eu·car·y·ot·ic (yū′kar-ē-ot′ik) Pertaining to or characteristic of a eukaryote.

Eu·len·burg dis·ease (oy′lĕn-bĕrg di-zēz′) SYN congenital paramyotonia.

eu·me·tri·a (yū-mē′trē-ă) Graduation of the strength of nerve impulses to match the need.

eu·nuch (yū′nŭk) A male whose testes have been removed or have never developed.

eu·nuch·ism (yū′nŭk-izm) 1. The state of being a eunuch; absence of the testes or failure of the gonads to develop or function with consequent lack of reproductive and sexual function and of devel-

opment of secondary sex characteristics. 2. SYN eunuchoidism.

eu·nuch·oid gi·gan·tism (yū′nŭ-koyd jī-gant′izm) Gigantism with deficient development of sexual organs.

eu·nuch·oid·ism (yū′nŭ-koyd-izm) A state in which testes are present but fail to function normally. SYN eunuchism (2).

eu·pep·si·a, eu·pep·sy (yū-pep′sē-ă, -pep′sē) Good digestion.

eu·pep·tic (yū-pep′tik) Digesting well; having a good digestion.

eu·pho·ri·a (yū-fōr′ē-ă) A feeling of well-being, commonly exaggerated and not necessarily well founded.

eu·phor·i·ant (yū-fōr′ē-ănt) 1. Having the capability to produce a sense of well-being. 2. An agent with such a capability.

eu·plas·tic lymph (yū-plas′tik limf) Lymph that contains relatively few leukocytes but a comparatively high concentration of fibrinogen.

eu·ploid (yū′ployd) Relating to euploidy.

eup·ne·a (yūp-nē′ă) Easy, free respiration; the type observed in a normal individual under resting conditions.

eu·prax·i·a (yū-prak′sē-ă) Normal ability to perform coordinated movements.

eu·rhyth·mi·a (yū-ridh′mē-ă) Harmonious body relationships of the separate organs.

eury- Prefix meaning broad, wide; opposite of steno-.

eu·ry·bleph·a·ron (yūr′ē-blef′ă-ron) A congenital anomaly characterized by sagging of the lateral aspect of the lower eyelid away from the eye.

eu·ry·ce·phal·ic, eu·ry·ceph·a·lous (yūr′ē-sē-fal′ik, -sef′ă-lŭs) Having an abnormally broad head.

eu·ryg·nath·ic (yūr′ig-nath′ik) Having a wide jaw.

eu·ry·on (yūr′ē-on) The extremity, on

eu·tha·na·si·a (yū´thă-nā´zē-ă) **1.** A quiet, painless death. **2.** The intentional putting to death of a person with an incurable or painful disease intended as an act of mercy.

eu·ther·mic (yū-thĕr´mik) At an optimal temperature.

eu·thy·mi·a (yū-thī´mē-ă) **1.** Joyfulness; mental peace and tranquility. **2.** Moderation of mood, not manic or depressed.

eu·thy·mic (yū-thī´mik) Relating to, or characterized by, euthymia.

eu·to·ci·a (yū-tō´sē-ă) Normal childbirth, characterized by uterine contractions that result in progressive cervical dilatation and fetal descent.

eu·to·pic (yū-top´ik) Located in the proper place.

eu·tro·phi·a (yū-trō´fē-ă) A state of normal nourishment and growth.

e·vac·u·ant (ē-vak´yū-ănt) Promoting an excretion, especially of the bowels.

e·vac·u·ate (EVAC) (ē-vak´yū-āt) To accomplish evacuation.

e·vag·i·na·tion (ē-vaj´i-nā´shŭn) Protrusion of some part or organ from its normal position.

e·val·u·a·tion (ē-val´yū-ā´shŭn) **1.** NURSING determining whether expected outcomes were met; measuring effectiveness of nursing care, medical care, and forms of health care by other providers. **2.** Synthesis of examination findings into a defined cluster of diagnostic classifications.

Eval·u·a·tion and Man·age·ment codes (E&M codes) (ē-val´yū-ā´shŭn man´ăj-mĕnt kōdz) Current procedure terminology (CPT) codes that describe patient encounters with health care professionals; used to evaluate and manage health.

ev·a·nes·cent (ev´ă-nes´ĕnt) Of short duration.

Ev·ans syn·drome (ev´ănz sin´drōm) Acquired hemolytic anemia and thrombocytopenia.

e·ven ech·o re·phas·ing (ē´vĕn ek´ō rē-fāz´ing) Use of evenly spaced echoes to reduce artifact in magnetic resonance imaging.

e·ven·ing prim·rose oil (ēv´ning prim´rōz oyl) An herbal supplement used to treat female disorders, skin disorders, and heart disease; serious adverse effects reported; contraindicated in preganant patients.

e·ven·tra·tion (ē´ven-trā´shŭn) **1.** Protrusion of omentum and/or intestine through an opening in the abdominal wall. SYN evisceration (2). **2.** Removal of the contents of the abdominal cavity.

ev·er·green con·tract (ev´ĕr-grēn kon´trakt) An agreement for health care contract that is renewed anually unless efforts are made to request changes in coverage.

e·ver·sion (ē-vĕr´zhŭn) A turning outward, as of the eyelid or foot.

e·vis·cer·a·tion (ē-vis´ĕr-ā´shŭn) **1.** Removal of the contents of the eyeball, leaving the sclera and sometimes the cornea. **2.** SYN eventration (1).

e·vo·ca·tion (ev´ō-kā´shŭn) Induction of a particular tissue produced by the action of an evocator during embryogenesis.

e·vo·ca·tor (ev´ō-kā-tŏr) A factor in the control of morphogenesis in the early embryo.

e·voked po·ten·tial (EP) (ē-vōkt´ pŏ-ten´shăl) Event-related potential, elicited by, and time-locked to, a stimulus.

ev·o·lu·tion (ev´ō-lū´shŭn) **1.** A continuing process of change from one state, condition, or form to another. **2.** A progressive distancing between the genotype and the phenotype in a line of descent.

e·vul·sion (ē-vŭl´shŭn) A forcible pulling out or extraction. Cf. avulsion.

Ew·art sign (yu´ărt sīn) In large pericardial effusions, an area of dullness with bronchial breathing and bronchophony below the angle of the left scapula. SYN Pins sign.

Ew·ing sign (yū′ing sīn) Tenderness at the upper inner angle of the orbit at the point of attachment of the pulley of the superior oblique muscle, denoting closure of the outlet of the frontal sinus.

Ew·ing tu·mor (yū′ing tū′mŏr) A malignant neoplasm that occurs usually before the age of 20 years, about twice as frequently in males, and in about 75% of patients involves bones of the extremities, including the shoulder girdle, with a predilection for the metaphysis. SYN endothelial myeloma, Ewing sarcoma.

ex- Prefix meaning out of, from, away from.

exa- (E) Prefix used in the SI and metric system to signify a multiple of one quintillion (10^{18}).

exaemia [Br.] SYN exemia.

ex·am·i·na·tion, ex·am (eg-zam′i-nā′shŭn, eg-zam′) Any investigation or inspection made for the purpose of diagnosis; usually qualified by the method used.

ex·an·the·ma, ex·an·them (ek-san′thĕ-mă, ek-san′thĕm) Skin eruption as a symptom of an acute viral or coccal disease. SYN exanthem.

ex·an·the·ma su·bi·tum (ek′san-thē′mă sū′bī-tŭm) A disease due to human herpesvirus-6 of infants and young children. SYN Dukes disease, roseola infantilis, roseola infantum, sixth disease.

ex·an·them·a·tous (ek′san-them′ă-tŭs) Relating to an exanthema.

ex·ar·tic·u·la·tion (eks′ahr-tik-yū-lā′shŭn) SYN disarticulation.

ex·cal·a·tion (eks′kă-lā′shŭn) Absence, suppression, or failure of development of one of a series of structures, as of a digit or vertebra.

ex·ca·va·ti·o (eks-kă-vā′shē-ō) [TA] SYN excavation (1).

ex·ca·va·tion (eks′kă-vā′shŭn) **1.** A natural cavity, pouch, or recess; a sunken or depressed area. SYN depression (2)

[TA], excavatio. **2.** A cavity formed artificially or as the result of a pathologic process.

ex·ce·men·to·sis (ek′sē-men-tō′sis) A nodular outgrowth of cementum on the root surface of a tooth.

ex·cess (XS) (ek′ses) That which is more than the usual or specified amount.

ex·change (exch) (eks-chānj′) To substitute one thing for another, or the act of such substitution.

ex·change list for meal plan·ning (eks-chānj′ list mēl plan′ing) Nutritional plan, often used in treatment of diabetes, in which food is sorted by groups and portion sizes.

ex·change trans·fu·sion (ET, EXT) (eks-chānj′ trans-fyū′zhŭn) Removal of most of a patient's blood followed by introduction of an equal amount from donors. SYN exsanguination transfusion, total transfusion.

ex·ci·mer la·ser (ek′si-mĕr lā′zĕr) Laser used particularly for refractive optical procedures.

ex·cip·i·ent (ek-sip′ē-ĕnt) Mostly inert substance added in a prescription as a diluent or vehicle or to give form or consistency when the remedy is given in pill form.

ex·cise (ek′sīz) To cut out. SEE ALSO resect.

ex·ci·sion (ek-sizh′ŭn) **1.** The act of cutting out; the surgical removal of part or all of a structure or organ. SYN resection (3). **2.** MOLECULAR BIOLOGY a recombination event in which a genetic element is removed. SEE ALSO resection.

ex·cit·a·ble (ek-sī′tă-bĕl) **1.** Capable of quick response to a stimulus; having potentiality for emotional arousal. Cf. irritable. **2.** NEUROPHYSIOLOGY referring to a tissue, cell, or membrane capable of undergoing excitation in response to an adequate stimulus.

ex·cit·ant (ek-sī′tănt) SYN stimulant.

ex·ci·ta·tion (ek′sī-tā′shŭn) **1.** The act of increasing the rapidity or intensity of the physical or mental processes. **2.** In neurophysiology, the complete all-or-none response of a nerve or muscle to an adequate stimulus, ordinarily including propagation of excitation along the membranes of the cell or cells involved. SEE ALSO stimulation.

ex•ci•ta•to•ry a•mi•no ac•ids (ek-sī'tă-tōr-ē ă-mē'nō as'idz) Group of organic acids that affect the central nervous system.

ex•cit•ing eye (ek-sī'ting ī) The injured eye in sympathetic ophthalmia.

ex•ci•tor (ek-sī'tŏr, -tōr) SYN stimulant (2).

ex•ci•to•re•flex nerve (ek-sī'tō-rē'fleks nĕrv) A visceral nerve the special function of which is to cause reflex action.

ex•ci•tor nerve (ek-sī'tŏr nĕrv) A nerve conducting impulses that stimulate to increase function.

ex•clave (eks-klāv') An outlying, detached portion of a gland or other part, such as the thyroid or pancreas; an accessory gland.

ex•clu•sion (eks-klū'zhŭn) A shutting out; disconnection from the main portion.

ex•clu•sive pro•vid•er or•gan•i•za•tion (EPO) (eks-klū'siv prŏ-vī'dĕr ōr'găn-ī-zā'shŭn) U.S. managed care plan in which enrollees must receive their care from affiliated providers; treatment provided outside the approved network must be paid for by policyholders. SEE ALSO managed care.

ex•co•ri•ate (eks-kōr'ē-āt) To scratch or otherwise strip off the skin by physical means.

ex•co•ri•a•tion (eks-kōr'ē-ā'shŭn) A scratch mark; a linear break in the skin surface, usually covered with blood or serous crusts.

ex•cre•ment (eks'krĕ-mĕnt) Waste matter or any excretion cast out of the body.

ex•cres•cence (eks-kres'ĕns) Any outgrowth from a surface.

ex•cre•ta (eks-krē'tă) SYN excretion (2).

ex•crete (eks-krēt') 1. To separate from the blood and cast out. 2. To perform excretion.

ex•cre•tion (eks-krē'shŭn) 1. The process whereby the undigested residue of food and the waste products of metabolism are eliminated, material is removed to regulate the composition of body fluids and tissues, or substances are expelled to perform functions on an exterior surface. 2. The product of a tissue or organ that is material to be passed out of the body. SYN excreta. SEE excrement. Cf. secretion.

ex•cre•to•ry duct (eks'krĕ-tōr-ē dŭkt) A duct carrying the secretion from a gland or a fluid from any reservoir.

ex•cur•sion (eks-kŭr'zhŭn) Any movement from one point to another, usually with the implied idea of returning again to the original position.

ex•cy•clo•pho•ri•a (eks-sī'klō-fōr'ē-ă) A cyclophoria in which the upper poles of each cornea tend to rotate laterally.

ex•cy•clo•tro•pi•a (ek'sī-klō-trō'pē-ă) A cyclotropia in which the upper poles of the corneas are rotated outward (laterally) relative to each other.

ex•cys•ta•tion (eks'sis-tā'shŭn) The action of an encysted organism in escaping from its envelope.

ex•e•mi•a (ek-sē'mē-ă) A condition, as in shock, in which a considerable portion of the blood is removed from the main circulation but remains within blood vessels in certain areas where it is stagnant. SYN exaemia.

ex•en•ceph•a•ly, ex•en•ceph•a•li•a (eks'en-sef'ă-lē, -se-fā'lē-ă) Condition in which the neurocranium is defective with the brain exposed or extruding.

ex•en•ter•a•tion (eks-en'tĕr-ā'shŭn) Removal of internal organs and tissues, usually radical removal of the contents of a body cavity.

ex•en•ter•i•tis (eks-en'tĕr-ī'tis) Inflammation of the peritoneal covering of the intestine.

ex•er•cise (ek'sĕr-sīz) 1. *Active:* Planned repetitive physical activity structured to improve and maintain physical fitness. **2.** *Passive:* motion of limbs without effort by the patient.

ex·er·cise-in·duced a·men·or·rhe·a (ek´sĕr-sīz-in-dūst´ ă-men´ōr-rē´ă) Temporary cessation of menstrual discharge due to overly rigorous exercise regimens.

ex·er·cise-in·duced as·thma (EIA), ex·er·cise-in·duced bron·cho·spasm (eks´ĕr-sīz-in-dūst´ az´mă, brong´kō-spazm) Bronchial spasm, edema, and mucus secretion brought about by exercise, particularly in cool, dry environment. Recovery usually occurs spontaneously within 90 minutes. SEE ALSO asthma.

ex·er·tio·nal head·ache (eg-zĕr´shŭn-ăl hed´ăk) The form of headache brought on by physical exercise.

ex·fo·li·a·tion (eks-fō´lē-ā´shŭn) **1.** Detachment and shedding of superficial cells from any tissue surface. **2.** Scaling or desquamation of the horny layer of epidermis. **3.** Loss of deciduous teeth following physiologic loss of root structure.

ex·fo·li·a·tive cy·tol·o·gy (eks-fō´lē-ă-tiv sī-tol´ŏ-jē) The examination, for diagnostic purposes, of cells denuded from a neoplasm or an epithelial surface, recovered from exudate, secretions, or washings from tissue. SYN cytopathology (2).

ex·fo·li·a·tive der·ma·ti·tis (eks-fō´lē-ă-tiv dĕr´mă-tī´tis) Generalized exfoliation with dermal scaling and usually with erythema (erythroderma); may be a drug reaction or associated with various benign dermatoses, lupus erythematosus, lymphomas, or of undetermined cause. SYN pityriasis rubra, Wilson disease (2).

ex·fo·li·a·tive gas·tri·tis (eks-fō´lē-ă-tiv gas-trī´tis) Gastritis with excessive shedding of mucosal epithelial cells.

ex·fo·li·a·tive psor·i·a·sis (eks-fō´lē-ă-tiv sōr-ī´ă-sis) Shedding dermatitis developing from chronic psoriasis, sometimes resulting from overtreatment of psoriasis.

ex·ha·la·tion (eks´hă-lā´shŭn) **1.** Breathing out. SYN expiration (1). **2.** The giving forth of gas or vapor. **3.** Any exhaled or emitted gas or vapor.

ex·hale (eks-hāl´) **1.** To breathe out. SYN expire (1). **2.** To emit a gas, vapor, or odor.

ex·haus·tion (eg-zaws´chŭn) **1.** Extreme fatigue; inability to respond to stimuli. **2.** Removal of contents; depletion of a supply of anything. **3.** Extraction of the active constituents of a drug by treating with water, alcohol, or other solvent.

ex·haus·tion psy·cho·sis (eg-zaws´ chŭn sī-kō´sis) Delirium and other mental findings related to overt physical exhaustion.

ex·hi·bi·tion·ism (ek´si-bish´ŭn-izm) A morbid compulsion to expose a part of the body, especially the genitals, with the intent of provoking sexual interest in the viewer.

ex·hi·bi·tion·ist (ek´si-bish´ŭn-ist) One who engages in exhibitionism.

ex·it block (eg´zit blok) Inability of an impulse to leave its point of origin, the mechanism for which is conceived as an encircling zone of refractory tissue denying passage to the emerging impulse.

ex·it dose (ED) (eg´zit dōs) Exposure dose of radiation leaving a body opposite the portal of entry.

Ex·ner plex·us (eks´nĕr plek´sŭs) Network formed by tangential nerve fibers in the superficial plexiform or molecular layer of the cerebral cortex.

exo- *Do not confuse this prefix with eco-.* Exterior, external, or outward. SEE ALSO ecto-.

ex·o·crine (ek´sō-krin) **1.** Denoting glandular secretion delivered onto the body surface. SYN eccrine (1). **2.** Denoting a gland that secretes outwardly through excretory ducts.

ex·o·cy·to·sis (ek´sō-sī-tō´sis) **1.** The appearance of migrating inflammatory cells in the epidermis. **2.** The process whereby secretory granules or droplets are released from a cell. SYN endocytosis, emeiocytosis, emiocytosis.

ex·o·de·vi·a·tion (ek'sō-dē-vē-ā'shŭn) **1.** SYN exophoria. **2.** SYN exotropia.

ex·o·en·zyme (ek'sō-en-zīm) SYN extracellular enzyme.

ex·og·a·my (eks-og'ă-mē) Sexual reproduction with conjugation of two gametes of different ancestry.

ex·o·gas·tru·la (eks'ō-gas'trū-lă) An abnormal embryo in which the primordial gut is everted.

ex·og·e·nous (eks-oj'ĕ-nŭs) Originating or produced outside of the organism. SYN ectogenous, exogenetic.

ex·og·e·nous de·pres·sion (eks-oj'ĕ-nŭs dĕ-presh'ŭn) Disorder with signs and symptoms similar to those of endogenous depression but its precipitating factors are social or environmental and outside the person.

ex·og·e·nous fi·bers (eks-oj'ĕ-nŭs fī'bĕrz) Nerve fibers by which a given region of the central nervous system is connected with other regions.

ex·og·e·nous he·mo·chro·ma·to·sis (eks-oj'ĕ-nŭs hē'mō-krō-mă-tō'sis) Hemosiderosis due to repeated blood transfusions.

ex·og·e·nous hy·per·lip·e·mi·a (eks-oj'ĕ-nŭs hī'pĕr-li-pē'mē-ă) Supraphysiolgic hematologic fat levels, usually related to dietary excess.

ex·om·pha·los, mac·ro·glos·si·a, and gi·gan·tism syn·drome (EMG) (eks-om'fă-lŏs, mak'rō-glaws'ē-ă, ji-gan'tizm sin'drōm) **1.** Protrusion of the umbilicus. SYN exumbilication (1). **2.** SYN umbilical hernia. **3.** SYN omphalocele.

ex·on (ek'son) A portion of a DNA that codes for a section of the mature messenger RNA from that DNA, and is therefore expressed ("translated" into protein) at the ribosome.

ex·o·nu·cle·ase (eks'ō-nū'klē-ās) A nuclease that releases one nucleotide at a time, serially, beginning at one end of a polynucleotide (nucleic acid). Cf. endonuclease.

ex·o·pep·ti·dase (eks'ō-pep'ti-dās) An enzyme that catalyzes the hydrolysis of the terminal amino acid of a peptide chain (e.g., carboxypeptidase). SEE ALSO endopeptidase.

Ex·o·phi·a·la (eks-ō-fī-ā'lă) A fungal species that causes tinea nigra.

ex·o·pho·ri·a (EXO, X, XP) (eks'ō-fōr'ē-ă) *Do not confuse this word with esophoria.* Tendency of the eyes to deviate outward when fusion is suspended. SYN exodeviation (1).

ex·oph·thal·mic goi·ter (eks'of-thal'mik goy'tĕr) Any of the various forms of hyperthyroidism in which the thyroid gland is enlarged and exophthalmos is present.

ex·oph·thal·mic oph·thal·mo·ple·gi·a (eks'of-thal'mik of-thal'mō-plē'jē-ă) Condition causing protrusion of the eyeballs due to increased water content of orbital tissues incidental to thyroid disorders, usually hyperthyroidism.

ex·oph·thal·mos, ex·oph·thal·mus (eks'of-thal'mos, -thal'mŭs) Protrusion of one or both eyeballs.

ex·o·phyt·ic (eks'ō-fit'ik) **1.** Pertaining to an exophyte. **2.** Denoting a neoplasm or lesion that grows outward from an epithelial surface.

ex·o·se·ro·sis (eks'ō-sĕ-rō'sis) Serous exudation from the skin surface, as in eczema or abrasions.

ex·o·skel·e·ton (eks'ō-skel'ĕ-tŏn) All hard parts (e.g., hair, teeth, nails, feathers, dermal plates, scales), developed from the ectoderm or somatic mesoderm in vertebrates.

ex·os·to·sis, ex·os·to·ses, pl. **ex·os·to·ses** (eks'os-tō'sis, -sēz) A cartilage-capped bony projection arising from any bone that develops from cartilage. SEE ALSO osteochondroma. SYN hyperostosis (2), poroma (2).

ex·os·to·sis car·ti·la·gi·ne·a (eks-os-tō'sis kahr-ti-la-ji-nē'ă) Ossified chondroma arising from the epiphysis or joint surface of a bone.

ex·o·ther·mic (eks'ō-thĕr'mik) **1.** Denoting a chemical reaction during which heat (i.e., enthalpy) is emitted. Cf. endothermic. **2.** Relating to the external warmth of the body.

ex·o·tox·in (eks'ō-tok'sin) A specific, soluble, antigenic, usually heat labile, injurious substance elaborated by certain bacteria; it is formed within the cell but is released into the environment where it is rapidly active in extremely small amounts. SYN extracellular toxin.

ex·o·tro·pi·a (ek'sō-trō'pē-ă) Form of strabismus in which the visual axes diverge. SYN divergent strabismus.

ex·pand·ed dis·a·bil·i·ty sta·tus scale (EDSS) (eks-pand'ĕd dis'ă-bil'i-tē stat'ŭs skāl) A commonly used rating system for evaluating the degree of neurologic impairment in multiple sclerosis, based on neurologic findings, and not symptoms. SYN Kurtzke multiple sclerosis disability scale.

ex·pan·sion (eks-pan'shŭn) **1.** An increase in size as of chest or lungs. **2.** The spreading out of any structure, as a tendon. **3.** An expanse; a wide area.

ex·pec·to·rant (eks-pek'tŏr-ănt) **1.** Promoting secretion from the mucous membrane of the air passages or facilitating its expulsion. **2.** An agent (e.g., guaifenesin) that thins respiratory tract mucus and promotes its removal from the tracheobronchial passages.

ex·pec·to·ra·tion (eks-pek'tŏr-ā'shŭn) **1.** The act of coughing and spitting out mucus from the lower respiratory tract. **2.** Mucus or other material so expelled.

ex·pe·ri·en·tial au·ra (eks-pēr'ē-en' shăl awr'ă) Epileptic aura characterized by altered perception of one's internal or external environment; may involve auditory, visual, olfactory, gustatory, somatosensory, or emotional altered perceptions. SEE ALSO aura (1).

ex·per·i·ment (eks-per'i-mĕnt) **1.** A study in which the investigator intentionally alters one or more factors under controlled conditions to study the effects of doing so. **2.** MAGNETIC RESONANCE pulse sequence.

ex·per·i·men·tal em·bry·ol·o·gy (ek-sper'i-men'tăl em'brē-ol'ŏ-jē) Clinical examination of embryonic development.

ex·per·i·men·tal med·i·cine (eks-per' i-men'tăl med'i-sin) The scientific investigation of medical problems by experimentation on animals or by clinical research.

ex·per·i·men·tal psy·chol·o·gy (eks-per'i-men'tăl sī-kol'ŏ-jē) A subdiscipline concerned with the study of conditioning, learning, perception, motivation, emotion, language, and thinking.

ex·per·i·ment·er ef·fects (eks-per'i-men'tĕr e-fekts') Influence of the experimenter's behavior, personality traits, or expectancies on the results of that person's own research. SEE double-blind study.

ex·pi·ra·tion (eks'pir-ā'shŭn) **1.** SYN exhalation (1). **2.** Death.

ex·pi·ra·to·ry cen·ter (ek-spīr'ă-tōr-ē sen'tĕr) Region of the medulla oblongata that is electrically active during expiration and where electrical stimulation produces sustained expiration.

ex·pi·ra·to·ry re·serve vol·ume (ERV) (eks-pīr'ă-tōr-ē rĕ-zĕrv' vol'yūm) The maximal volume of air (about 1000 mL) that can be expelled from the lungs after a normal expiration. SYN reserve air, supplemental air.

ex·pi·ra·to·ry stri·dor (eks-pīr'ă-tōr-ē strī'dŏr) A singing sound due to the semi-approximated vocal folds offering resistance to the escape of air.

ex·pire (eks-pīr') **1.** SYN exhale (1). **2.** To die.

ex·plant (eks-plant') Living tissue transferred from an organism to an artificial medium for culture.

ex·plo·ra·tion (eks'plŏr-ā'shŭn) An active examination, usually involving endoscopy or a surgical procedure, to ascertain conditions present as an aid in diagnosis.

ex·plor·a·to·ry sur·gery (eks-plōr'ă-tōr-ē sŭr'jĕr-ē) Surgical investigation to diagnose cause of a disorder or condition.

ex·plor·er (eks-plōr'ĕr) A sharp pointed probe used to investigate natural or restored tooth surfaces to detect caries or other defects.

ex·plo·sion (eks-plō′zhŭn) A sudden and violent increase in volume accompanied by noise and release of energy, as from a chemical change, nuclear reaction, or escape of gases or vapors under pressure.

ex·plo·sive speech (ek-splō′siv spēch) Loud, sudden way of speaking related to injury of the nervous system. SYN logospasm.

ex·po·sure (eks-pō′zhŭr) Contact of a compound with an epithelial barrier such as the skin, eyes, respiratory tract, or gastrointestinal tract before absorption occurs.

ex·po·sure dose (eks-pō′zhŭr dōs) The radiation dose, expressed in roentgens, delivered at a point in free air.

ex·po·sure ker·a·ti·tis (eks-pō′zhŭr ker′ă-tī′tis) Inflammation of the cornea resulting from irritation caused by inability to close the eyelids.

ex·pressed skull frac·ture (eks-prest′ skŭl frak′shŭr) A fracture with outward displacement of a part of the cranium.

ex·pres·sion (eks-presh′ŭn) **1.** Squeezing out; expelling by pressure. **2.** Mobility of the features giving a particular emotional significance to the face. SYN facies (3) [TA]. **3.** Something that manifests something else.

ex·pres·sion vec·tor (eks-presh′ŭn vek′tŏr) An agent (plasmid, yeast, or animal virus genome) used experimentally to introduce foreign genetic material into a propagatable host cell to replicate and amplify the foreign DNA sequences as a recombinant molecule (recombinant DNA cloning of sequences).

ex·pres·sive a·pha·si·a (eks-pres′iv ă-fā′zē-ă) A type of aphasia in which the greatest deficit is in speech production or language output. SYN Broca aphasia (2), motor aphasia, nonfluent aphasia.

ex·pres·sive lan·guage dis·or·der (eks-pres′iv lang′gwăj dis-ōr′dĕr) Any problem related to oral communication; may have physical or emotional causes.

ex·pres·siv·i·ty (eks′pres-siv′i-tē) In clinical genetics, the degree of severity in which a gene is manifested.

Ex·ser·o·hi·lum (eks′ĕr-ō-hī′lŭm) A genus of fungi; a cause of human phaeohyphomycosis; found in the environment, on grasses, and on other plants.

ex·sic·ca·tion (ek′si-kā′shŭn) The removal of water of crystallization. SYN dehydration (3).

ex·sorp·tion (ek-sōrp′shŭn) Movement of substances from the blood into the lumen of the gut.

ex·stro·phy (eks′trŏ-fē) Congenital eversion of a hollow organ.

ex·tend·ed-care fa·cil·i·ty (eks-ten′ dĕd-kār fă-sil′i-tē) Health care supplier of skilled care after hospitalization or severe illness or injury. SYN nursing home.

ex·tend·ed me·di·as·ti·nos·co·py (eks-ten′dĕd mē′dē-ă-sti-nos′kŏ-pē) Cervical mediastinoscopy in which, in addition to the standard pre- and paratracheal exploration, the mediastinoscope is passed anterior to the innominate artery and aortic arch to provide access to the subaortic (aortopulmonary window) and anterior mediastinal lymph nodes.

ex·ten·der (eks-tend′ĕr) A person who or thing that spreads, stretches, or increases.

ex·ten·sion bridge (ek-sten′shŭn brij) SYN cantilever bridge.

ex·ten·sor (eks-ten′sŏr) [TA] A muscle the contraction of which causes movement at a joint with the consequence that the limb or body assumes a straighter line, or so that the distance between the parts proximal and distal to the joint is increased or extended; the antagonist of a flexor. SEE muscle.

ex·ten·sor ap·o·neu·ro·sis (ek-sten′ sŏr ap-ō-nūr-ō′sis) SYN extensor digital expansion.

ex·ten·sor dig·i·tal ex·pan·sion (eks-ten′sŏr dij′i-tăl eks-pan′shŭn) Triangular tendinous aponeurosis including the tendon of the extensor digitorum centrally, interosseus tendons on each side, and a lumbrical tendon laterally. It covers the dorsal aspect of the metacarpophalangeal joint and the proximal phalanx. SYN extensor aponeurosis.

ex·ten·sor ex·pan·sion (ek-sten´sŏr ek-span´shŭn) SYN extensor digital expansion.

ex·ten·sor thrust (eks-ten´sŏr thrŭst) SEE tonic spasm.

ex·te·ri·or dig·i·tal ex·pan·sion (eks-ten´sŏr dij´i-tăl eks-pan´shŭn) Triangular tendinous aponeurosis in the region of the extensor digitorum. SYN extensor expansion.

ex·tern (eks´tĕrn) An advanced student or recent graduate who assists in the medical or surgical care of hospital patients; formerly, one who lived outside of the institution.

ex·ter·nal (eks-tĕr´năl) [TA] On the outside or farther from the center; often incorrectly used to mean lateral. SYN externus.

ex·ter·nal ab·sorp·tion (eks-tĕr´năl ăb-sŏrp´shŭn) Absorption of substances through skin, mucocutaneous surfaces, or mucous membranes.

ex·ter·nal cap·sule (eks-tĕr´năl kap´sŭl) [TA] A thin lamina of white substance separating the claustrum from the putamen. It joins the internal capsule at either extremity of the putamen, forming a capsule of white matter external to the lenticular nucleus. SYN capsula externa [TA].

ex·ter·nal ca·rot·id ner·ves (eks-tĕr´năl kă-rot´id nĕrvz) [TA] A number of sympathetic nerve fibers conveyed through the cephalic arterial ramus of the sympathetic trunk that extends from the superior cervical ganglion to the external carotid artery, forming the external carotid plexus. SYN nervi carotici externi [TA].

ex·ter·nal ear (eks-tĕr´năl ēr) SEE ear. SEE ALSO auricle, pinna.

ex·ter·nal fix·a·tion (eks-tĕr´năl fik-sā´shŭn) Care of fractured bones with splints, plastic dressings, or transfixion pins.

ex·ter·nal gen·i·tal·i·a (eks-tĕr´năl jen´i-tā´lē-ă) The vulva and clitoris in the female, and the penis and scrotum in the male.

ex·ter·nal il·i·ac ar·te·ry (EIA) (eks-tĕr´năl il´ē-ak ahr´tĕr-ē) [TA] *Origin*, as terminal branch (with internal iliac artery of common iliac; *branches*, inferior epigastric, deep circumflex iliac; becomes the femoral at the inguinal ligament. SYN arteria iliaca externa [TA].

ex·ter·nal il·i·ac vein (EIV) (eks-tĕr´năl il´ē-ak vān) [TA] Direct continuation of the femoral vein superior to the inguinal ligament, uniting with the internal iliac vein to form the common iliac vein. SYN vena iliaca externa [TA].

ex·ter·nal jug·u·lar vein (EJV) (eks-tĕr´năl jŭg´yū-lăr vān) [TA] Superficial vein formed inferior to the parotid gland by the junction of the posterior auricular vein and the retromandibular vein, and passing down the side of the neck crossing to the sternocleidomastoid muscle vertically to empty into the subclavian vein. SYN vena jugularis externa [TA].

ex·ter·nal nose (eks-tĕr´năl nōz) The visible portion of the nose that forms a prominent feature of the face; it consists of a root, dorsum, and apex from above downward and is perforated inferiorly by two nostrils separated by a septum. SYN nasus (1).

ex·ter·nal oc·cip·i·tal crest (eks-tĕr´năl ok-sip´i-tăl krest) [TA] A ridge extending from the external occipital protuberance to the border of the foramen magnum.

ex·ter·nal oph·thal·mop·a·thy (eks-tĕr´năl of´thăl-mop´ă-thē) Any disease of ocular conjunctiva, cornea, or adnexa.

ex·ter·nal oph·thal·mo·ple·gi·a (eks-tĕr´năl of´thăl-mō-plē´jē-ă) SYN ophthalmoplegia externa.

ex·ter·nal pace·ma·ker (eks-tĕr´năl păs´mă-kĕr) Artificial cardiac pacemaker of which the electrodes for delivering rhythmic electric stimuli to the heart are placed on the chest wall.

ex·ter·nal phase (eks-tĕr´năl fāz) The medium or fluid in which a dispersant is suspended. SYN dispersion medium.

ex·ter·nal pin fix·a·tion, bi·phase (eks-tĕr′năl pin fik-sā′shŭn, bī′fāz) In oral surgery, stabilization of fractures of the mandible, maxilla, or zygoma by pins or screws drilled into the bony part through the overlying skin and connected by a metal bar.

ex·ter·nal res·pi·ra·tion (eks-tĕr′năl res′pir-ā′shŭn) The exchange of respiratory gases in the lungs as distinguished from internal or tissue respiration.

ex·ter·nal ta·ble of cal·var·i·a (eks-tĕr′năl tā′bĕl kal-var′ē-ă) Outer compact layer of the cranial bones.

ex·ter·nal u·re·thral or·i·fice (eks-tĕr′năl yūr-ē′thrăl ŏr′i-fis) [TA] **1.** Slitlike opening of the urethra in the glans penis. **2.** External orifice of the urethra (in the female) in the vestibule, usually upon a slight elevation, the papilla urethrae. SYN ostium urethrae externum [TA], external urinary meatus, external opening of urethra, meatus urinarius, orificium urethrae externum.

ex·ter·nus (eks-ter′nŭs) [TA] SYN external.

ex·ter·o·cep·tive (eks′tĕr-ō-sep′tiv) Relating to the exteroceptors; denoting the surface of the body containing the end organs adapted to receive impressions or stimuli from without.

ex·ter·o·cep·tor (eks′tĕr-ō-sep′tŏr) One of the peripheral end organs of the afferent nerves in the skin or mucous membrane that respond to stimulation by external agents.

ex·ter·o·fec·tive (eks′tĕr-ō-fek′tiv) Pertaining to the response of the nervous system to external stimuli.

ex·tinc·tion (eks-tingk′shŭn) In behavior modification, progressive decrease in the frequency of a response is not positively reinforced; the withdrawal of reinforcers known to maintain an undesirable behavior. SEE conditioning.

ex·tor·sion (eks-tōr′shŭn) **1.** Outward rotation of a limb or of an organ. **2.** Conjugate rotation of the upper poles of each cornea outward.

♻ **extra-** Prefix meaning without, outside of.

ex·tra·ar·tic·u·lar (eks′tră-ahr-tik′yū-lăr) Outside of a joint.

ex·tra·ax·i·al (eks′tră-aks′ē-ăl) Off the axis; applied to intracranial lesions that do not arise from the brain itself.

ex·tra·cap·su·lar (EC) (eks′tră-kap′sŭlăr) Outside a joint capsule.

ex·tra·cap·su·lar an·ky·lo·sis (eks′tră-kap′sŭ-lăr ang′ki-lō′sis) Joint stiffness due to induration or heterotopic ossification of the surrounding tissues; surgical technique in which a joint is fused by bridging tissues surrounding it. SYN spurious ankylosis.

ex·tra·cap·su·lar frac·ture (ek′stră-kap′sŭ-lăr frak′shŭr) Breakage near a joint, but outside the line of attachment of the joint capsule.

ex·tra·cel·lu·lar (eks′tră-sel′yŭ-lăr) Outside the cells.

ex·tra·cel·lu·lar en·zyme (eks′tră-sel′yŭ-lăr en′zīm) An enzyme performing its functions outside a cell (e.g., the various digestive enzymes). SYN exoenzyme.

ex·tra·cel·lu·lar ma·trix (ECM) (ek′stră-sel′yŭ-lăr mā′triks) Aggregate of cellular proteins.

ex·tra·cel·lu·lar tox·in (eks′tră-sel′yŭ-lăr tok′sin) SYN exotoxin.

ex·tra·chro·mo·som·al (eks′tră-krō′mŏ-sōm′ăl) Outside or separated from, a chromosome; especially DNA separated from a chromosome.

ex·tra·cor·o·nal re·tain·er (ek′stră-kōr′ŏ-năl rē-tā′nĕr) Dental appliance that depends on contact with the outer circumference of the crown of a tooth for its retentive qualities.

ex·tra·cor·po·re·al (eks′tră-kōr-pōr′ē-ăl) Outside, or unrelated to, the body or any anatomic corpus.

ex·tra·cor·po·re·al cir·cu·la·tion (eks′tră-kōr-pōr′ē-ăl sĭr′kyū-lā′shŭn) The circulation of blood outside of the body through a machine that temporarily assumes an organ's functions (e.g., through a heart-lung machine or artificial kidney).

ex·tra·cor·po·re·al shock wave lith·o·trip·sy (ESWL) (eks′tră-kōr-pōr′ē-ăl shok wāv lith′ō-trip′sē) Breaking up of renal or ureteral calculi by focused ultrasound energy.

ex·tra·cra·ni·al (EC) (eks′tră-krā′nē-ăl) Outside of the cranial cavity.

ex·tract (eks′trakt, ek-strakt′) **1.** A concentrated preparation of a drug obtained by removing the active constituents with suitable solvents, evaporating all or nearly all of the solvent, and adjusting the residual mass or powder to the prescribed standard. **2.** To perform extraction.

ex·trac·tion (ek-strak′shŭn) **1.** Luxation and removal of a tooth from its alveolus. **2.** Partitioning of material (solute) into a solvent. **3.** The active portion of a drug; the making of an extract. **4.** Surgical removal by pulling out. **5.** Removal of the fetus from the uterus or vagina at or near the end of pregnancy, either manually or with instruments. **6.** Removal by suction of the products of conception before a menstrual period has been missed.

ex·trac·tor (ek-strak′tŏr) Instrument for use in drawing or pulling out any natural part, as a tooth, or a foreign body.

ex·tra·du·ral (eks′tră-dū′răl) **1.** On the outer side of the dura mater. **2.** Unconnected with the dura mater. SEE ALSO epidural.

ex·tra·du·ral an·es·the·si·a (ek′stră-dūr′ăl an-es-thē′zē-ă) Anesthetization, by local anesthetics, of nerves near the spinal canal external to the dura mater; often refers to epidural anesthesia, but may include paravertebral anesthesia.

extradural haemorrhage [Br.] SYN extradural hemorrhage.

ex·tra·du·ral hem·or·rhage (eks′tră-dūr′ăl hem′ŏr-ăj) An accumulation of blood between the skull and the dura mater. SYN extradural haemorrhage.

ex·tra·em·bry·on·ic (eks′tră-em′brē-on′ik) Outside the embryonic body.

ex·tra·me·dul·la·ry (eks′tră-med′ŭ-lar-ē) Outside of, or unrelated to, any medulla, especially the medulla oblongata.

ex·tra·med·ul·la·ry my·e·lo·ma (eks′tră-med′ŭ-lar-ē mī′ĕ-lō′mă) A plasma cell tumor that arises from the bone marrow.

ex·tra·mu·ral (eks′tră-myū′răl) Outside, not in the substance of, the wall of a part.

ex·tra·ne·ous (eks-trā′nē-ŭs) Outside the organism and not belonging to it.

ex·tra·nu·cle·ar (eks′tră-nū′klē-ăr) Located outside, or not involving, a cell nucleus.

ex·tra·oc·u·lar (EO) (eks′tră-ok′yū-lăr) Adjacent to but outside the eyeball.

ex·tra·oc·u·lar mus·cles (eks′tră-ok′yū-lăr mŭs′ĕlz) [TA] The muscles within the orbit including the four rectus muscles (superior, inferior, medial, and lateral), two oblique muscles (superior and inferior), and the levator of the superior eyelid (levator palpebrae superioris).

ex·tra·per·i·to·ne·al (eks′tră-per′i-tŏ-nē′ăl) Outside of the peritoneal cavity.

ex·tra·per·i·to·ne·al fas·ci·a (eks′tră-per′i-tŏ-nē′ăl fash′ē-ă) [TA] The thin layer of fascia and adipose tissue between the peritoneum and fascia transversalis. SYN fascia subperitonealis [TA].

ex·tra·pla·cen·tal (eks′tră-plă-sen′tăl) Unrelated to the placenta.

ex·tra·pleu·ral pneu·mo·thor·ax (ek′stră-plūr′ăl nū′mō-thōr′aks) Presence of a gas between the endothoracic fascia–pleural layer and the adjacent chest wall.

ex·tra·pul·mo·na·ry (eks′tră-pul′mŏ-nar-ē) Outside or having no relation to, the lungs.

ex·tra·py·ram·i·dal (eks′tră-pir-am′i-dăl) Other than the pyramidal tract. SEE extrapyramidal motor system.

ex·tra·py·ram·i·dal dis·ease (eks′tră-pir-am′i-dăl di-zēz′) General term for disorders caused by abnormalities of the basal ganglia or certain brainstem or thalamic nuclei. SYN extrapyramidal motor system disease.

ex·tra·py·ram·i·dal dys·ki·ne·si·a

(eks'tră-pir-am'i-dăl dis'ki-nē'zē-ă) Abnormal involuntary movement attributed to pathologic states of one or more parts of the striate body and characterized by insuppressible, stereotyped, automatic movements that cease only during sleep (e.g., Parkinson disease; chorea; athetosis; hemiballism).

ex·tra·py·ram·i·dal mo·tor sys·tem (eks'tră-pir-am'i-dăl mō'tŏr sis'tĕm) Literally, all brain structures that affect bodily (somatic) movement, excluding the motor neurons, the motor cortex, and the pyramidal (corticobulbar and corticospinal) tract; more often used to denote in particular the striate body (basal ganglia), its associated structures (substantia nigra, subthalamic nucleus), and its descending connections with the midbrain.

ex·tra·py·ram·i·dal syn·drome (EPS) (ek'stră-pir-am'i-dăl sin'drōm) Abnormalities of movement related to injury of motor pathways other than the pyramidal tract.

ex·tra·sac·cu·lar her·ni·a (eks'tră-sak'yŭ-lăr hĕr'nē-ă) SYN sliding hernia.

ex·tra·sys·to·le, ex·tra·sys·to·le (ES) (eks'tră-sis'tŏ-lē) A nonspecific word for an ectopic beat from any source in the heart.

ex·tra·thor·a·cic air·way ob·struc·tion (eks'tră-thōr-as'ik ār'wā ŏb-strŭk'shŭn) Form of airway obstruction in which the site of airway narrowing is above the thoracic inlet.

ex·tra·thy·roi·dal hy·per·me·tab·o·lism (ek'stră-thī-roy'dăl hī'pĕr-mĕ-tab'ŏ-lizm) Increased metabolic rate with normal levels of thyroid hormone production.

ex·tra·u·ter·ine (eks'tră-yū'tĕr-in) Outside the uterus.

ex·tra·u·ter·ine preg·nan·cy (EUP) (ek'stră-yū'tĕr-in preg'năn-sē) SYN ectopic pregnancy.

ex·trav·a·sate (eks-trav'ă-sāt) **1.** To exude or pass out of a vessel into the tissues, said of blood, lymph, or urine. **2.** The substance thus exuded. SYN suffusion (4).

ex·trav·a·sa·tion (eks-trav'ă-sā'shŭn) The act of extravasating.

ex·tra·vert (eks'tră-vĕrt) *Avoid the misspelling/mispronunciation* extrovert. A gregarious person whose chief interests lie outside the self, and who is socially self-confident and involved in the affairs of others. Cf. introvert.

ex·tra·ves·i·cal re·im·plan·ta·tion (eks'tră-ves'i-kăl rē'im-plan-tā'shŭn) SYN detrusorrhaphy.

ex·tre·mal quo·tient (eks-trē'măl kwō'shĕnt) The ratio of the rate in the jurisdiction with the highest rate of interventions, such as surgical procedures, to the rate in the jurisdiction with the lowest rate.

ex·trem·i·ty, ex·trem·i·tas (eks-trem'i-tē, -tăs) [TA] One of the ends of an elongated or pointed structure. Incorrectly but widely used to mean limb. [TA].

ex·trin·sic (eks-trin'sik) Originating outside of the part where found or on which it acts; denoting especially a muscle, such as extrinsic muscles of hand.

ex·trin·sic al·ler·gic al·ve·o·li·tis (eks-trin'sik ă-lĕr'jik al've-ŏ-lī'tis) Pneumoconiosis resulting from hypersensitivity to organic dust, usually specified according to occupational exposure.

ex·trin·sic co·a·gu·la·tion path·way (eks-trin'sik kō-ag'yŭ-lā'shŭn path'wā) A part of the coagulation pathway, activated by contact of factor VII in the blood with tissue factor (TF).

ex·trin·sic fac·tor (EF) (eks-trin'sik fak'tŏr) Dietary vitamin B12.

ex·tro·ver·sion, ex·tra·ver·sion (eks'trō-vĕr'zhŭn, eks'tră-) **1.** A turning outward. **2.** A personality patterned on the presence of others. Cf. introversion. SYN extraversion.

ex·trude (eks-trūd') To thrust, force, or press out.

ex·tu·ba·tion (eks'tū-bā'shŭn) Removal of a tube from an organ, structure, or orifice. Often associated with removal of the endotracheal tube after ventilation or surgical procedure.

ex·u·ber·ant (eg-zū'bĕr-ănt) Denoting excessive proliferation or growth.

ex·u·date (eks′yū-dāt) Any fluid that has drained out of a tissue or its capillaries because of injury or inflammation. Cf. transudate.

ex·u·da·tion cyst (eks′yū-dā′shŭn sist) Lesion due to distention of a closed cavity by an excessive secretion of its normal fluid contents.

ex·u·da·tive in·flam·ma·tion (eks-yū′dă-tiv in′flă-mā′shŭn) Inflammation in which the conspicuous or distinguishing feature is an exudate, which may be chiefly serous, serofibrinous, fibrinous, or mucous (e.g., relatively few cells are present), or may be characterized by relatively large numbers of neutrophils, eosinophils, lymphocytes, monocytes, or plasma cells, frequently with one or two types being predominant.

ex·um·bil·i·ca·tion (eks′ŭm-bil′i-kā′shŭn) **1.** SYN exomphalos (1). **2.** SYN umbilical hernia. **3.** SYN omphalocele.

ex vi·vo (eks vē′vō) Referring to the use or positioning of a tissue or cell after removal from an organism while the tissue or cells remain viable.

eye (ī) [TA] **1.** The organ of vision that consists of the eyeball and the optic nerve. SYN oculus [TA]. **2.** The area of the eye, including lids and other accessory organs of the eye; the contents of the orbit (common).

eye·ball (ī′bawl) [TA] The eye proper without appendages. SYN bulbus oculi [TA], bulb of eye, globe of eye.

eye·brow (ī′brow) [TA] The crescentic line of hairs at the superior edge of the orbit. SYN supercilium (1) [TA].

eye-clo·sure pu·pil re·ac·tion (ī-klō′zhŭr pyū′pil rē-ak′shŭn) A constriction of both pupils when an effort is made to close eyelids forcibly held apart. A variant of the pupil response to near vision. SYN Galassi pupillary phenomenon, Gifford reflex, Westphal pupillary reflex.

eye·glass·es (ī′glas-ĕz) SYN spectacles.

eye·lash (ī′lash) One of the stiff hairs projecting from the margin of the eyelid. SYN cilium (1).

eye·lid (ī′lid) [TA] One of two movable folds that cover the front of the eyeball when closed; formed of a fibrous core (tarsal plate) and the palpebral portions of the orbicularis oculi muscle covered with skin on the superficial, anterior surface and lined with conjunctiva on the deep, posterior surface; rapid contraction of the contained muscle fibers produces blinking. SYN palpebra [TA], blepharon, lid.

eye·piece (ī′pēs) The compound lens at the end of the microscope tube nearest the eye; magnifies objective lens image.

eye soc·ket (ī sok′ĕt) Commonly the orbit, although the true "socket" for the eyeball, into which a prosthetic eye would be inserted, is formed by the fascial sheath of the eyeball. SYN orbit.

E

F

Fab SEE Fab fragment.

fa·bel·la (fă-bel´lă) A sesamoid bone in the tendon of the lateral head of the gastrocnemius muscle.

Fa·ber syn·drome (fah´bĕr sin´drōm) SYN achlorhydric anemia.

Fab fragment (fab frag´mĕnt) The antigen-binding fragment of an immunoglobulin molecule, consisting of both a light chain and part of a heavy chain.

fab·ri·ca·tion (fab´ri-kā´shŭn) Telling false tales as true; e.g., the malingering of symptoms or illness or feigning an incorrect response during a mental status examination.

Fa·bry dis·ease (fah´brē di-zēz´) Deficiency of α-galactosidase characterized by abnormal accumulations of neutral glycolipids (e.g., globotriaosylceramide) in endothelial cells in blood vessel walls. Clinical findings, include angiokeratomas on the thighs, buttocks, and genitalia; hypohidrosis; paresthesia in the extremities, cornea verticillata, and spoke-like posterior subcapsular cataracts.

F.A.C.C.P. Abbreviation for Fellow of the American College of Chest Physicians.

F.A.C.D. Abbreviation for Fellow of the American College of Dentists.

face (fās) [TA] **1.** The front portion of the head; the visage including the eyes, nose, mouth, forehead, cheeks, and chin, but not the ears. SYN facies (1) [TA]. **2.** SYN surface.

face-bow (fās´bō) A caliperlike device used to record the relationship of the jaws to the temporomandibular joints.

fac·et, fa·cette (fas´ĕt, fă-set´) [TA] **1.** A small, smooth area on a bone or other firm structure. **2.** A worn spot on a tooth, produced by chewing or grinding.

fac·e·tec·to·my (fas´ĕ-tek´tŏ-mē) Surgical intervention involving excision of a facet.

fa·cial (fā´shăl) Relating to the face.

fa·cial ca·nal (fā´shăl kă-nal´) [TA] Bony passage in the temporal bone through which the facial nerve passes.

fa·cial cleft (fā´shăl kleft) That resulting from incomplete fusion of embryonic facial processes normally uniting in facial formation, e.g., cleft lip palate. SYN prosopoanoschisis.

fa·cial di·ple·gi·a (fā´shăl dī-plē´jē-ă) Paralysis of both sides of the face, with unaffected limb muscle.

fa·cial hem·i·ple·gi·a (fā´shăl hem´ē-plē´jē-ă) Paralysis of one side of the face, with unaffected limb muscle.

fa·cial mus·cles (fā´shăl mŭs´ĕlz) [TA] The numerous muscles supplied by the facial nerve that are attached to and move the skin of the face. SYN musculi faciei [TA], mimetic muscles, muscles of facial expression.

fa·cial nerve [CNVII] (fā´shăl nĕrv) [TA] Nerve with its origin in the tegmentum of the lower portion of the pons. SYN nervus facialis [CN VII] [TA], motor nerve of face, seventh cranial nerve [CN VII].

fa·cial neu·ral·gi·a (fā´shăl nūr-al´jē-ă) SYN trigeminal neuralgia.

fa·cial pal·sy (fā´shăl pawl´zē) SYN facial paralysis.

fa·cial pa·ral·y·sis (fā´shăl păr-al´i-sis) Paresis of the facial muscles, usually unilateral, due to either a lesion involving the nucleus or the facial nerve or a supranuclear lesion in the cerebrum or upper brainstem. SYN facial palsy, facioplegia, prosopoplegia.

fa·cial re·cess ap·proach (fā´shăl rē ses ă-prōch´) Surgical entry to the middle ear from the mastoid through a recess lateral to facial nerve canal.

fa·cial tic (fā´shăl tik) Involuntary twitching of the facial muscles, sometimes unilateral. SYN palmus (1), prosopospasm.

fa·cial tri·an·gle (fā´shăl trī´ang-gĕl) Area formed by lines connecting the basion, prosthion, and nasion.

-facient Generally, a combining form meaning causing; one who or that which brings something about.

fa·ci·es, pl. **fa·ci·es** (fash´ē-ēz) [TA] **1.**

SYN face (1). **2.** SYN surface. **3.** SYN expression (2).

fa·cil·i·ta·tion (fă-sil′i-tā′shŭn) Enhancement or reinforcement of a reflex or other nervous activity by the arrival at the reflex center of other excitatory impulses.

fa·cil·i·ta·tive (fă-sil′i-tā-tiv) Accentuation or diminution one or more factors to improve overall function.

facio- Combining form meaning the face. SEE ALSO prosopo-.

fa·ci·o·lin·gual (fā′shē-ō-ling′gwăl) Relating to the face and the tongue, often denoting a paralysis affecting these parts.

fa·ci·o·plas·ty (fā′shē-ō-plas-tē) Surgical repair involving the face.

fa·ci·o·ple·gi·a (fā′shē-ō-plē′jē-ă) SYN facial paralysis.

F.A.C.O.G. Abbreviation for Fellow of the American College of Obstetricians and Gynecologists.

F.A.C.P. Abbreviation for Fellow of the American College of Prosthodontists.

F.A.C.P. Abbreviation for Fellow of the American College of Physicians.

F.A.C.S. Abbreviation for Fellow of the American College of Surgeons.

F.A.C.S.M. Abbreviation for Fellow of the American College of Sports Medicine.

fac·ti·tious (fak-tish′ŭs) *Do not confuse this word with factitial.* Artificial; self-induced; not naturally occurring.

fac·ti·tious dis·or·der (fak-tish′ŭs dis-ŏr′dĕr) A mental condition in which the patient intentionally induces symptoms of illness for psychological reasons.

fac·tor (fak′tŏr) **1.** A contributing cause in any action. **2.** One of the components that, by multiplication, make up a number or expression. **3.** SYN gene. **4.** A vitamin or other essential element. **5.** An event, characteristic, or other definable entity that brings about a change in a health condition. **6.** A categoric independent variable used to identify, by means of numeric codes, membership in a qualitatively identifiable group.

fac·tor H (fak′tŏr) **1.** Vitamin B12 analogue or precursor. **2.** Glycoprotein that regulates the activity of complement factor C3b.

fac·tor P (fak′tŏr) Chemical, formed in ischemic skeletal or cardiac muscle, thought responsible for the pain of intermittent claudication and angina pectoris. SYN P substance of Lewis.

fac·tor I (fak′tŏr) In the clotting of blood, a factor that is converted to fibrin through thrombin's action. SEE ALSO fibrinogen.

fac·tor II (fak′tŏr) A glycoprotein converted in the clotting of blood to thrombin by factor Xa, platelets, calcium ions, and factor V. SEE ALSO prothrombin.

fac·tor III (fak′tŏr) In the clotting of blood, tissue factor, or thromboplastin, initiates the extrinsic pathway by reacting with factor VII and calcium to form factor VIIa. SEE ALSO thromboplastin.

fac·tor IV (fak′tŏr) In the clotting of blood, calcium ions.

fac·tor V (fak′tŏr) In the clotting of blood, also known as: proaccelerin, labile or plasma labile factor, plasma accelerator globulin, thrombogene, prothrombokinase, plasmin prothrombins conversion factor, component A of prothrombin, prothrombin accelerator, cofactor of thromboplastin, and accelerator factor. SYN accelerator factor, labile factor, plasma accelerator globulin, plasma labile factor, plasmin prothrombin conversion factor, proaccelerin, prothrombokinase, thrombogene.

fac·tor VII (fak′tŏr) A plasma factor in blood coagulation, forms a complex with tissue thromboplastin and calcium to activate factor X; accelerates the conversion of prothrombin to thrombin, in the presence of tissue thromboplastin, calcium, and factor V. SYN cothromboplastin, proconvertin, serum accelerator, serum prothrombin conversion accelerator.

fac·tor VIII (fak′tŏr) A plasma factor in blood coagulation; participates in the clotting of the blood by forming a com-

F

plex with factor IXa, platelets, and calcium and enzymatically catalyzing the activation of factor X; deficiency is associated with classic hemophilia A. SYN antihemophilic factor A, antihemophilic globulin A, proserum prothrombin conversion accelerator.

fac·tor IX (fak'tŏr) In the clotting of blood, required for the formation of intrinsic blood thromboplastin; deficiency causes hemophilia B. SYN antihemophilic globulin B, Christmas factor, plasma thromboplastin component.

fac·tor X (fak'tŏr) A plasma coagulation factor that assists in the conversion of prothrombin to thrombin. Deficiency impairs blood coagulation. SYN Stuart-Prower factor.

fac·tor XI (fak'tŏr) A plasma coagulation factor; a component of the contact system that is absorbed from plasma and serum by glass and similar surfaces. Deficiency of factor XI results in a hemorrhagic tendency.

fac·tor XII (fak'tŏr) A plasma coagulation factor. Deficiency greatly prolongs clotting time of venous blood, but only rarely in a hemorrhagic tendency. SYN Hageman factor.

fac·tor XIII (fak'tŏr) A plasma coagulation factor catalyzed by thrombin into its active form, factor XIIIa, which cross-links subunits of the fibrin clot to form insoluble fibrin. SYN Laki-Lorand factor.

fac·tor IX com·plex (fak'tŏr kom'pleks) A hemostatic containing factors II, VII, IX, and X.

fac·ul·ta·tive (fak'ŭl-tā'tiv) Able to live under more than one specific set of environmental conditions.

faecal [Br.] SYN fecal.

faecal examination [Br.] SYN fecal examination.

faecal fistula [Br.] SYN fecal fistula.

faecalith [Br.] SYN fecalith.

faecaloid [Br.] SYN fecaloid.

faecaluria [Br.] SYN fecaluria.

faecal vomiting [Br.] SYN fecal vomiting.

faeces [Br.] SYN feces.

Fahr·en·heit scale (far'ĕn-hīt skăl) Thermometer in which the freezing point of water is 32°F and the boiling point of water 212°F; 0°F indicates the lowest temperature G.D, Fahrenheit could obtain by a mixture of ice and salt in 1724; °C = (5/9)(°F − 32).

fail·ure to thrive (fāl'yŭr thrīv) A condition in which an infant's weight gain and growth are far below usual levels for age.

faint (fānt) **1.** Extremely weak; threatened with syncope. **2.** An episode of syncope. SEE ALSO syncope.

fal·cial (fal'shăl) Relating to a falx. SYN falcine.

fal·ci·form (fal'si-fōrm) Having a crescentic or sickle shape.

fal·ci·form lig·a·ment (fal'si-fōrm lig'ă-mĕnt) SYN falciform process.

fal·ci·form lig·a·ment of liv·er (fal'si-fōrm lig'ă-mĕnt liv'ĕr) [TA] A crescentic fold of peritoneum extending to the surface of the liver from the diaphragm and anterior abdominal wall. SYN ligamentum falciforme hepatis [TA].

fal·ci·form pro·cess (fal'si-fōrm pros'es) A continuation of the inner border of the sacrotuberous ligament upward and forward on the inner aspect of the ramus of the ischium. SYN processus falciformis [TA], falciform ligament.

fal·cip·a·rum ma·la·ri·a (fal-sip'ă-rŭm mă-lar'ē-ă) Disease caused by *Plasmodium falciparum* characterized by paroxysms that typically occur every 48 hours with acute cerebral, renal, or gastrointestinal manifestations in severe cases, chiefly caused by the large number of red blood cells affected and the tendency for such infected red blood cells to become sticky and block capillaries. SYN aestivoautumnal fever, falciparum fever, malignant tertian fever, malignant tertian malaria, pernicious malaria.

fal·cu·lar (fal'kyū-lăr) **1.** Resembling a

sickle or falx. **2.** Relating to the falx cerebelli or cerebri.

fal·lo·pi·an ca·nal (fă-lō′pē-ăn kă-nal′) SYN facial canal.

Fal·lot tet·rad (fă-lō′ tet′rad) SYN tetralogy of Fallot.

false an·eu·rysm (fawls an′yŭr-izm) **1.** Pulsating, encapsulated hematoma in communication with the lumen of a ruptured vessel. **2.** Ventricular pseudoaneurysm, a cardiac rupture contained and loculated by pericardium, which forms its external wall. **3.** One with walls that consist of adventitia, periarterial fibrous tissue, and hematoma.

false an·ky·lo·sis (fawls ang′ki-lō′sis) SYN fibrous ankylosis.

false cast (fawls kast) An elongated, ribbonlike mucous thread with poorly defined edges and pointed or split ends, often confused with a true urinary cast. SYN cylindroid.

false he·ma·tu·ri·a (fawls hē′mă-tyūr′ē-ă) SYN pseudohematuria.

false herm·aph·ro·di·tism (fawls hĕr-maf′rō-dīt-izm) SYN pseudohermaphroditism.

false im·age (fawls im′ăj) The image in the deviating eye in strabismus.

false joint (fawls joynt) SYN pseudarthrosis.

false la·bor (fawls lā′bŏr) Braxton Hicks contraction that causes the patient physical discomfort. SEE ALSO Braxton Hicks contraction. Cf. false pains.

false mem·brane (fawls mem′brān) Thick, tough fibrinous exudate on the surface of a mucous membrane or the skin. SYN croupous membrane, neomembrane, plica (2), pseudomembrane.

false neg·a·tive (fawls neg′ă-tiv) A test result that erroneously excludes a person from a specific diagnostic or reference group.

false neu·ro·ma (fawls nūr-ō′mă) SYN traumatic neuroma.

false pains (fawls pānz) Ineffective uterine contractions, preceding and sometimes resembling true labor, but distinguishable from it by the lack of progressive effacement and dilation of the cervix. Cf. false labor.

false pel·vis (fawls pel′vis) SYN greater pelvis.

false pos·i·tive (FP) (fawls poz′i-tiv) A test result that erroneously assigns a patient to a specific diagnostic or reference group, due particularly to insufficiently exact methods of testing.

false preg·nan·cy (fawls preg′năn-sē) A condition in which some signs and symptoms suggest pregnancy, although the woman is not pregnant. SYN pseudopregnancy (1).

false ribs (fawls ribz) [TA] Five lower ribs on either side that do not articulate with the sternum directly. SYN costae spuriae [TA].

false su·ture (fawls sū′chŭr) One with opposing margins that are smooth or present only a few ill-defined projections. SYN sutura notha.

false ver·te·brae (fawls vĕr′tĕ-brē) Fused vertebral segments of the sacrum and coccyx. SYN vertebrae spuriae.

false wa·ters (fawls waw′tĕrs) Fluid leak before or at beginning labor, before rupture of the amnion.

fal·si·fi·ca·tion (fawl′si-fi-kā′shŭn) Deliberate misrepresentation so as to deceive.

falx (fawlks) [TA] A sickle-shaped structure.

falx ce·re·bel·li (fawlks ser-ĕ-bel′ī) [TA] A short process of dura mater projecting forward from the internal occipital crest below the tentorium. SYN falcula.

falx ce·re·bri (fawlks ser′ĕ-brī) [TA] Scythe-shaped fold of dura mater in the longitudinal fissure between the two cerebral hemispheres. SYN cerebral falx.

fa·mil·i·al, fa·mil·i·ar (fă-mil′ē-ăl, -ăr) Affecting more members of the same family than can be accounted for by chance, usually within a single sibship;

commonly but *incorrectly* used to mean genetic.

fa·mil·i·al ad·e·no·ma·tous pol·y·po·sis (FAP) (fă-mil´ē-ăl ad´ĕ-nō´mă-tŭs pol´i-pō´sis) Appearance of colonic polyps that usually begins in childhood; polyps increase in number, causing symptoms of chronic colitis; pigmented retinal lesions are frequently found; carcinoma of the colon almost invariably develops in untreated cases. SYN familial polyposis coli.

fa·mil·i·al ag·gre·ga·tion (fă-mil´ē-ăl ag´rĕ-gā´shŭn) Occurrence of a trait in more members of a family than can be readily accounted for by chance; presumptive but not cogent evidence of the operation of genetic factors.

fa·mil·i·al am·y·loid neu·rop·a·thy (fă-mil´ē-ăl am´i-loyd nūr-op´ă-thē) A disorder in which various peripheral nerves are infiltrated with amyloid and their functions disturbed, an abnormal prealbumin is also formed and is present in the blood; characteristically, it begins during mid-life and is found largely in people of Portuguese descent.

fa·mil·i·al e·ryth·ro·pha·go·cy·tic lymph·o·his·ti·o·cy·to·sis (FEL) (fă-mil´ē-ăl ă-rith´rō-făg´ō-sit´ik lim´fō-his´tē-ō-sī-tō´sis) SYN familial hemophagocytic lymphohistiocytosis.

fa·mil·i·al fat-in·duced hy·per·li·pe·mi·a (fă-mil´ē-ăl fat´in-dūst´ hī´pĕr-li-pē´mē-ă) SYN type I familial hyperlipoproteinemia.

fa·mil·i·al he·mo·pha·go·cy·tic lymph·o·his·ti·o·cy·to·sis (FMLH) (fă-mil´ē-ăl hē´mō-făg´ō-sit´ik lim´fō-his´tē-ō-sī-tō´sis) An extremely rare, usually fatal disease of childhood characterized by multiorgan infiltration with activated macrophages and lymphocytes. SYN familial erythrophagocytic lymphohistiocytosis.

fa·mil·i·al high-den·si·ty lip·o·pro·tein de·fi·cien·cy (fă-mil´ē-ăl hī-den´si-tē lip´ō-prō´tēn dĕ-fish´ĕn-sē) SYN analphalipoproteinemia.

fa·mil·i·al hy·po·phos·pha·tem·ic ric·kets (FHR) (fă-mil´ē-ăl hī´pō-fos-fă-tē´mik rik´ĕts) SYN vitamin D–resistant rickets.

fa·mil·i·al Med·i·ter·ra·ne·an fe·ver (FMF) (fă-mil´ē-ăl med´i-tĕr-ā´nē-ăn fē´vĕr) SYN familial paroxysmal polyserositis.

fa·mil·i·al non·he·mo·lyt·ic jaun·dice (fă-mil´ē-ăl non´hē-mō-lit´ik jawn´dis) Mild form of the hepatic disorder due to increased amounts of unconjugated bilirubin in the plasma without evidence of liver damage, biliary obstruction, or hemolysis. SYN Gilbert disease.

fa·mil·i·al par·ox·ys·mal pol·y·ser·o·si·tis (fă-mil´ē-ăl păr-ok-siz´măl pol´ē-sēr´ō-sī´tis) Transient recurring attacks of abdominal pain, fever, pleurisy, arthritis, and rash; the condition is asymptomatic between attacks. SYN familial Mediterranean fever.

fa·mil·i·al par·tial lip·o·dys·tro·phy (fă-mil´ē-ăl pahr´shăl lip´ō-dis´trŏ-fē) Characterized by symmetric lipoatrophy of the trunk and limbs but not face; with full rounded face, xanthomata, acanthosis nigricans, and insulin-resistant hyperglycemia; fat collects at neck, shoulders, and genitalia. SYN Kobberling-Dunnigan syndrome.

fa·mil·i·al per·i·od·ic pa·ral·y·sis (fă-mil´ē-ăl pēr´ē-od´ik păr-al´i-sis) Inherited muscle disorder manifested as recurrent episodes of marked generalized weakness. SEE hyperkalemic periodic paralysis, hypokalemic periodic paralysis, normokalemic periodic paralysis.

fa·mil·i·al pseu·do·in·flam·ma·to·ry mac·u·lar de·gen·er·a·tion (fă-mil´ē-ăl sū´dō-in-flam´ă-tōr-ē mak´yŭ-lăr dē-jen´ĕr-ā´shŭn) Ocular disease that occurs during the fifth decade of life, with sudden development of a central scotoma in one eye soon followed by a similar lesion in the other. SYN Sorsby macular degeneration.

fam·i·ly (fam´i-lē) **1.** A group of two or more people linked by blood, adoptive, or marital ties, or the common-law equivalent. **2.** In biologic classification, a taxonomic grouping at the level intermediate between the order and the tribe or genus.

fam·i·ly dy·nam·ics (fam´i-lē dī-nam´iks) Intrafamily conditions that must be considered in diagnosis of disorders.

fam·i·ly his·to·ry (fam´i-lē his´tŏr-ē) A

written documentation made after questioning the patient about the presence or absence of diseases or conditions that might have an effect on the health of the patient, generally involves a form filled out by a new patient (or surrogate) during intake.

fam·i·ly med·i·cine (fam′i-lē med′i-sin) The medical specialty concerned with providing continuous comprehensive care to all age groups, from first patient contact to terminal care, with special emphasis on care of the family as a unit.

fam·i·ly of or·i·gin (fam′i-lē ōr′i-jin) Birth family.

fam·i·ly phy·si·cian (FP, fam phys) (fam′i-lē fi-zish′ăn) Doctor who specializes in family practice.

fam·i·ly prac·tice (FP) (fam′i-lē prak′tis) Medical specialty in which the physician takes responsibility for the health and medical care of all members of a family group, regardless of age or gender, but usually also does limited amounts of obstetrics and surgery.

fam·i·ly ther·a·py (fam′i-lē thār′ă-pē) Group psychotherapy in which a family in conflict meets as a group with the therapist to explore its relationships and processes; focus is on the resolution of current issues between members rather than on individual members' issues.

Fan·co·ni a·ne·mi·a (FA) (fahn-kō′nē ă-nē′mē-ă) A type of idiopathic refractory anemia characterized by pancytopenia, hypoplasia of the bone marrow, and congenital anomalies, occurring in members of the same family (an autosomal recessive trait in at least five nonallelic types); the anemia is normocytic or slightly macrocytic, macrocytes and target cells may be found in the circulating blood, and the leukopenia usually is due to neutropenia. Congenital anomalies include short stature; microcephaly; hypogenitalism; strabismus; anomalies of the thumbs, radii, kidneys, and urinary tract; mental retardation; and microphthalmia. SYN Fanconi syndrome (1).

Fan·co·ni syn·drome (fahn-kō′nē sin′drŏm) **1.** SYN Fanconi anemia. **2.** A group of conditions with characteristic disorders of renal tubular function, which may be classified as: cystinosis, an autosomal recessive disease of early childhood.

fang (fang) **1.** A long tooth or tusk, usually a canine. **2.** The hollow tooth of a snake through which the venom is ejected.

fan·ta·sy, phan·ta·sy (fan′tă-sē) Imagery that is more or less coherent, as in dreams and daydreams, yet unrestricted by reality. SYN phantasia.

Far·a·beuf am·pu·ta·tion (fahr′ă-buf amp′yū-tā′shŭn) **1.** Surgical removal of the leg, the flap being large and on the outer side. **2.** Surgical removal of the foot.

far·ad (F) (fahr′ăd) A practical unit of electrical capacity, the capacity of a condenser having a charge of 1 coulomb under an electromotive force of 1 volt.

far·a·day, Fa·ra·day (F, F) (far′ă-dā) Amount of electricity required to reduce one equivalent of a monovalent ion.

Far·ber dis·ease, Far·ber syn·drome (fahr′bĕr di-zēz′, sin′drŏm) SYN disseminated lipogranulomatosis.

far·del (fahr′del) The total measurable risk incurred due to occurrence of a genetic disease in one individual; one of two major quantitative considerations in the prognostic aspects of genetic counseling, the other is occurrence.

farm·er's lung (fahr′mĕrz lŭng) A hypersensitivity pneumonitis characterized by fever and dyspnea, caused by inhalation of organic dust from moldy hay containing spores of actinomycetes and certain true fungi.

far point (fahr poynt) That point in conjugate focus of the retina when the eye is not accommodating.

Farr test (fahr test) Measures capacity of radiolabeled antigen to bind with antibody (which is precipitated using ammonium sulfate); can be used for all classes of immunoglobulin.

far sight (fahr sīt) SYN hyperopia.

far·sight·ed·ness (fahr′sīt′ĕd-nĕs) SYN hyperopia.

fas·ci·a, pl. **fas·ci·ae** (fash′ē-ă, -ē) [TA]

A sheet of fibrous tissue that envelops the body beneath the skin.

fas·ci·a ad·he·rens (fash'ē-ă ad-hē' renz) A broad intercellular junction in the intercalated disc of cardiac muscle that anchors actin filaments.

fas·ci·a graft (fash'ē-ă graft) A graft of fibrous tissue, usually the fascia lata.

fas·ci·cle, fas·ci·cu·lum, pl. **fas·ci·cu·la** (fas'i-kĕl, fă-sik'yū-lŭm, -lă) A band or bundle of fibers, usually of muscle or nerve fibers; a nerve fiber tract. SYN fasciculus (1) [TA].

fas·cic·u·lar (fă-sik'yū-lăr) Relating to a fasciculus; arranged in the form of a bundle or collection of rods. SYN fasciculate, fasciculated.

fas·cic·u·lar de·gen·er·a·tion (fă-sik' yū-lăr dĕ-jen'ĕr-ā'shŭn) Breakdown restricted to certain fascicles of nerves or muscles.

fas·cic·u·lar graft (fă-sik'yū-lăr graft) One in which each bundle of fibers is approximated and sutured separately.

fas·cic·u·la·tion (fasc) (fă-sik'yū-lā' shŭn) 1. An arrangement in the form of fasciculi. 2. Involuntary contractions, or twitchings, of groups (fasciculi) of muscle fibers.

fas·cic·u·lus, gen. and pl. **fas·cic·u·li** (fă-sik'kyū-lŭs, -lī) [TA] 1. SYN fascicle. 2. SYN cord (1). 3. [TA] SYN bundle.

fas·ci·ec·to·my (fash'ē-ek'tŏ-mē) Excision of strips of fascia.

fas·ci·i·tis, fas·ci·tis (fash-ē-ī'tis, fash-ī'tis) Fascial inflammation.

♻ **fascio-** Prefix indicating a fascia.

fas·ci·od·e·sis (fash'ē-od'ĕ-sis) Surgical attachment of a fascia to another fascia or a tendon.

Fas·ci·o·la (fa-shē'lă) Genus of large, leaf-shaped, digenetic mammalian liver flukes.

fas·ci·o·la, pl. **fas·ci·o·lae** (fash'ē-ō'lă, -lē) A small band or group of fibers.

fas·ci·o·li·a·sis (fash'ē-ō-lī'ă-sis) Infection with a species of *Fasciola*.

fas·ci·o·lop·si·a·sis (fash'ē-ō-lop-sī'ă-sis) Parasitization by any of the flukes of the genus *Fasciolopsis*.

Fas·ci·o·lop·sis (fash'ē-ō-lop'sis) A genus of large intestinal fasciolid flukes.

Fas·ci·o·lop·sis bus·ki (fash'ē-ō-lop' sis bŭs'kī) Large intestinal fluke, a species found in the intestine of humans in eastern and southern Asia.

fas·ci·o·plas·ty (fash'ē-ō-plas-tē) Plastic surgery of a fascia.

fas·ci·or·rha·phy (fash'ē-ōr'ă-fē) Suture of a fascia or aponeurosis. SYN aponeurorrhaphy.

fas·ci·o·scap·u·lo·hu·mer·al mus·cu·lar dys·tro·phy (fash'ē-ō-skap'yū-lō-hyū'mĕr-ăl mŭs'kyū-lăr dis'trŏ-fē) Hereditary diorder with youthful onset; characterized by muscular wasting and weakness.

fas·ci·ot·o·my (fash'ē-ot'ŏ-mē) Incision through a fascia.

fas·ci·tis (fa-shī'tis) SYN fasciitis.

fast (fast) 1. Durable; resistant to change; applied to stained microorganisms that cannot be decolorized. SEE ALSO acid-fast. 2. Abstinence from ingesting food.

fast com·po·nent of ny·stag·mus (fast kŏm-pō'nĕnt nis-tag'mŭs) Compensatory movement of the eyes in the vestibuloocular reflex.

fast-neu·tron ra·di·a·tion ther·a·py (fast-nū'tron rā'dē-ā'shŭn thār'ă-pē) Treatment using high-energy neutrons from cyclotrons or proton accelerators.

fast-twitch fi·bers (fast-twich fī'bĕrz) Histologically distinct skeletal muscle fibers that generate energy rapidly and are active in quick, powerful actions. SYN fast glycolytic (FG) fibers, fast-oxidative-glycolytic (FOG) fibers, Type II fibers.

fat (fat) 1. Common term for obese. 2. A greasy, soft-solid material, found in animal tissues and many plants, composed of a mixture of glycerol esters; together with oils, fats comprise the homolipids.

fa·tal (fā′tăl) Pertaining to or causing death; denoting especially inevitability or inescapability of death.

fa·tal fa·mil·i·al in·som·ni·a (FFI) (fā′tăl fă-mil′ē-ăl in-som′nē-ă) A progressive neuropathy with worsening insomnia and thalamic lesions.

fa·tal·i·ty (fă-tal′i-tē) **1.** A condition, disease, or disaster ending in death. **2.** An individual instance of death.

fa·tal·i·ty rate (fă-tal′i-tē rāt) Number of deaths seen in a designated series of people affected by a simultaneous event such as a disaster.

fat cell (fat sel) A connective tissue cell distended with one or more fat globules, the cytoplasm usually being compressed into a thin envelope. SYN adipocyte, adipose cell.

fate map (fāt map) Determination in very young embryos of the cellular origin of specific organs or structures. SYN germinal localization.

fat em·bo·lism (fat em′bŏ-lizm) Occurrence of fat globules in the circulation following fractures of a long bone, in burns, in parturition, and in association with fatty degeneration of the liver.

fat-free bod·y mass (FFM) (fat′frē bod′ē mas) That devoid of storage fat; theoretic entity that contains the small percentage of non-sex-specific essential fat equivalent to approximately 3% of body mass (located in the central nervous system, bone marrow, and internal organs). SYN lean body mass.

fa·ther com·plex (fah′dhĕr kom′pleks) SYN Electra complex.

fat her·ni·a (fat hĕr′nē-ă) One in which the tissue protruding out of its normal location is composed only of fat.

fat·i·ga·bil·i·ty (fat′i-gă-bil′i-tē) A condition in which tiredness is easily induced.

fa·tigue (fă-tēg′) **1.** That state, following a period of mental or bodily activity, characterized by a lessened capacity for work and reduced efficiency of accomplishment, usually accompanied by a feeling of weariness, sleepiness, or irritability; may also supervene when, from any cause, energy expenditure outstrips restorative processes and may be confined to a single organ. **2.** Sensation of lassitude due to absence of stimulation, monotony, or lack of interest.

fat in·di·ges·tion (fat in′di-jes′chŭn) SYN steatorrhea.

fat me·tab·o·lism (fat mĕ-tab′ŏ-lizm) Oxidation, decomposition, and synthesis of fats in the tissues.

fat ne·cro·sis (fat nĕ-krō′sis) Death of adipose tissue, characterized by the formation of small (1–4 mm), dull, chalky, gray or white foci that are calcium soaps formed in the affected tissue when fat breaks down into glycerol and fatty acids. SYN steatonecrosis.

fat over·load syn·drome (fat ō′vĕr-lōd sin′drōm) Constellation of symptoms related to overingestion of fats, frequently related to total parenteral nutrition.

fat-sol·u·ble vi·ta·mins (fat-sol′yū-bĕl vī′tă-minz) Those vitamins, soluble in fat solvents (nonpolar solvents) and relatively insoluble in water, marked in chemical structure by the presence of large hydrocarbon moieties in the molecule.

fat-stor·ing cell (fat′stōr′ing sel) A multilocular fat-filled cell present in the perisinusoidal space in the liver. SYN lipocyte.

fat tide (fat tīd) Increase in the fat content of blood and lymph after eating a meal.

fat·ty (fat′ē) Oily or greasy; relating in any sense to fat.

fat·ty ac·id (FA) (fat′ē as′id) Any acid derived from fats by hydrolysis or any long-chain monobasic organic acid.

ω-3 fat·ty ac·ids (fat′ē as′idz) Those with a double bond of three carbons from the methyl moiety; reportedly, they play a role in lowering cholesterol. SYN omega-3 fatty acids.

fat·ty al·co·hol (fat′ē al′kŏ-hol) Long-chain alcohol, analogous to the fatty acids, of which the fatty alcohol may be viewed as a reduction product.

fat·ty cir·rho·sis (fat′ē sir-ō′sis) Early nutritional cirrhosis, especially in people with alcoholism, in which the liver is enlarged by fatty change, with mild fibrosis.

fat·ty di·ar·rhe·a (fat′ē dī-ă-rē′ă) Intestinal disorder seen in malabsorption syndromes including chronic pancreatic disease, characterized by foul-smelling stools with increased fat content that usually float in water. SYN pimelorrhea.

fat·ty heart (fat′ē hahrt) Myocardial degeneration. SYN cor adiposum.

fat·ty in·fil·tra·tion (fat′ē in′fil-trā′shŭn) Abnormal accumulation of fat droplets in cell cytoplasm, particularly extracellular fat. SEE ALSO fatty degeneration.

fat·ty kid·ney (fat′ē kid′nē) One with fatty metamorphosis of the parenchymal cells, especially fatty degeneration.

fat·ty li·ver (fat′ē liv′ĕr) Yellow discoloration of the liver due to fatty degeneration of liver parenchymal cells.

fat·ty met·a·mor·pho·sis (fat′ē met′ă-mōr′fŏ-sis) Appearance of microscopically visible droplets of fat in cell cytoplasm. SEE ALSO fatty degeneration.

fat·ty oil (fat′ē oyl) An oil derived from both animals and plants, which is permanent and not capable of distillation.

fat·ty stool (fat′ē stūl) Feces containing excessive amounts of fat.

fau·ces, pl. **fau·ces** (faw′sēz) [TA] The space between oral cavity and pharynx, bounded by the soft palate and lingual base.

fa·ve·o·late (fă-vē′ō-lāt) Pitted.

fa·ve·o·lus (fă′vē-ō′lŭs) A small pit or depression.

fa·vid (fā′vid) An allergic reaction in the skin observed in patients who have favus, which is a type of tinea capitis.

fa·vism (fā′vizm) An acute condition seen following the ingestion of certain species of beans, e.g., *Vicia faba*, or inhalation of the pollen of its flower, in patients with genetic erythrocytic deficiency of glucose 6-phosphate dehydrogenase; characterized by fever, headache, abdominal pain, severe anemia, prostration, and coma.

Fav·re-Ra·cou·chot dis·ease (fahv′rĕ-rah-kū-shō′ di-zēz′) Comedones developing on sun-damaged skin due to obstruction of pilosebaceous follicles by solar elastosis. SYN solar comedo.

Fc fragment, Fc (frag′mĕnt) The crystallizable fragment of an immunoglobulin molecule composed of part of the heavy chains and responsible for binding to antibody receptors on cells and the Clq component of complement.

F.D.I. den·tal no·men·cla·ture (den-tăl nō′mĕn-klā-chŭr) A system of identifying teeth; used worldwide, which identifies each dental quadrant (1–4 for the permanent teeth and 5–8 for the deciduous teeth) and each tooth with a number indicating its location from the midline. SEE ALSO Palmer dental nomenclature.

Fe Symbol for iron.

fear (fēr) Apprehension; dread; alarm; by having an identifiable stimulus, fear is differentiated from anxiety, which has no easily identifiable stimulus.

feath·er edge (fedh′ĕr ej) The thinnest area of a blood smear, where the differential count is performed.

feb·ri·fa·cient (feb′ri-fā′shĕnt) **1.** Causing or favoring the development of fever. SYN febriferous, febrific. **2.** Anything that produces fever. SEE ALSO pyrogenic. SYN febricant.

fe·brif·u·gal (fĕ-brif′yŭ-găl) SYN antipyretic (1).

feb·rile (feb′ril) Denoting or relating to fever. SYN feverish (1), pyretic.

feb·rile con·vul·sion (feb′ril kŏn-vŭl′shŭn) A brief seizure, lasting less than 15 minutes, seen in a neurologically normal infant or young child, associated with fever. SYN febrile seizure.

feb·rile u·rine (feb′ril yūr′in) Dark concentrated urine of strong odor, passed by one suffering from fever. SYN feverish urine.

fe·cal (fē′kăl) Relating to feces. SYN faecal.

fe·cal ex·am·i·na·tion (fē′kăl eg-zam′i-nā′shŭn) Microscopic review of direct wet mounts, concentration methods, and permanent stained smears to recover and identify parasites from stool specimens.

fe·cal fis·tu·la (fē′kăl fis′tyū-lă) SYN intestinal fistula, faecal fistula.

fe·cal im·pac·tion (fē′kăl im-pak′shŭn) Immovable collection of compressed or hardened feces in the colon or rectum.

fe·ca·lith (fē′kă-lith) SYN coprolith, faecalith.

fe·cal·oid (fē′kă-loyd) Resembling feces. SYN faecaloid.

fe·ca·lu·ri·a (fē′kăl-yūr′ē-ă) Mixing feces with urine in people with a fistula connecting the intestinal tract and bladder. SYN faecaluria.

fe·cal vom·it·ing (fē′kăl vom′it-ing) Vomitus with appearance or odor of feces suggestive of long-standing distal small-bowel or colonic obstruction. SYN copremesis, faecal vomiting, stercoraceous vomiting.

fe·ces (fē′sēz) The matter discharged from the bowel during defecation, consisting of the undigested residue of food, epithelium, intestinal mucus, bacteria, and waste material from the food. SYN faeces, stercus.

fec·u·lent (fek′yū-lĕnt) Foul.

fe·cun·da·tion (fek′ŭn-dā′shŭn) The act of rendering fertile. SEE ALSO fertilization, impregnation.

fe·cun·di·ty (fē-kŭn′di-tē) Ability to produce live offspring.

feed·back (fēd′bak) **1.** In a given system, the return, as input, of some of the output, as a regulatory mechanism. **2.** An explanation for the learning of motor skills. **3.** The feeling evoked by another person's reaction to oneself. SEE biofeedback.

feed·ing cen·ter (fēd′ing sen′tĕr) Region of the lateral zone of the hypothalamus, electrical stimulation of which in the rat elicits uninterrupted eating; its chronic destruction causes anorexia.

feed·ing tube (fēd′ing tūb) Tube passed through the pharynx into the esophagus and stomach, through which liquid food is fed.

feel·ing (fēl′ing) **1.** Any kind of conscious experience of sensation. **2.** The mental perception of a sensory stimulus. **3.** A quality of any mental state or mood, whereby it is recognized as pleasurable or the reverse. **4.** A bodily sensation that is correlated with a given emotion.

Feer dis·ease (fār di-zēz′) SYN acrodynia (2).

Feh·ling so·lu·tion (fā′ling sŏ-lū′shŭn) An alkaline copper tartrate solution formerly used for detection of reducing sugars. SYN Fehling reagent.

Feiss line (fīs līn) Line running from the medial malleolus to the plantar aspect of the first metatarsophalangeal joint.

fel·la·ti·o (fĕ-lā′shē-ō) Oral stimulation of the penis; a type of oral-genital sexual activity; contrasted with cunnilingus, which is the oral stimulation of the vulva or clitoris. SYN irrumation.

fel·low (fel′ō) A board-qualified specialist pursuing subspecialty training.

Fel·low of the Roy·al Col·lege of Phy·si·cians (FRCP) (fel′ō roy′ăl kol′ĕj fi-zish′ănz) A doctor who is a member of the British medical professional group.

fel·on (fel′ŏn) In medicine, purulent infection or abscess involving the bulbous distal end of a finger. SYN whitlow.

felt·work (felt′wŏrk) **1.** A fibrous network. **2.** A close plexus of nerve fibrils.

fe·male (fē′māl) ZOOLOGY denoting the gender that produces oocytes (or ova) and thus bears the young.

fe·male cath·e·ter (fē′māl kath′ĕ-tĕr) A

short, nearly straight catheter for passage into the female bladder.

fe·male cir·cum·ci·sion (fē′măl sǐr′kŭm-si′zhŭn) A broad term referring to many forms of female genital cutting, ranging from removal of the clitoral prepuce to the removal of the clitoris, labia minora, and parts of the labia majora, and of infibulation; done for cultural, not medical, reasons.

fe·male con·dom (fē′măl kon′dŏm) An intravaginal bag, usually latex, which lines the vulva and vagina and is intended to prevent contraception during coitus.

fe·male pat·tern al·o·pe·ci·a (fē′măl pat′ĕrn al′ŏ-pē′shē-ă) Diffuse partial hair loss in the centroparietal area of the scalp, with preservation of the frontal and temporal hair lines; the most frequent type of androgenic alopecia in women.

fe·male ster·i·li·ty (fē′măl stĕr-il′ĭ-tē) Inability of female to conceive, due to inadequacy in structure or function of the genital organs. SYN infecundity.

fe·male u·re·thra (fē′măl yūr-ē′thră) [TA] 4-cm canal passing from the bladder, close to the anterior vaginal wall and with a long axis that parallels that of the vagina, opening in the vaginal vestibule posterior to the clitoris and anterior to the vaginal orifice. SYN urethra feminina [TA], urethra muliebris.

fem·i·nin·i·ty com·plex (fem′i-nin′i-tē kom′pleks) In psychoanalysis, the unconscious fear, in boys and men, of castration at the hands of the mother with resultant identification with the aggressor and envious desire for breasts and vagina.

fem·i·ni·za·tion (fem′i-nī-zā′shŭn) Development of what are superficially external female characteristics by a male.

fem·o·ral (fem′ŏr-ăl) Relating to the femur or thigh.

fem·o·ral ca·nal (fem′ŏr-ăl kă-nal′) [TA] The medial compartment of the femoral sheath. SYN canalis femoralis [TA].

fem·o·ral e·piph·y·sis (fem′ŏr-ăl e-pif′

i-sis) Secondary osseous structure of the femur.

fem·o·ral her·ni·a (fem′ŏr-ăl hĕr′nē-ă) Hernia through the femoral ring. SYN femorocele.

fem·o·ral re·flex (fem′ŏr-ăl rē′fleks) Scratching the skin of the upper part of the front of the thigh causes extension of the knee and flexion of the foot.

fem·o·ral ring (fem′ŏr-ăl ring) [TA] Superior opening of the femoral canal, bounded anteriorly by the inguinal ligament, posteriorly by the pectineus muscle, medially by the lacunar ligament, and laterally by the femoral vein. Passageway by which many lymphatics from lower limb pass to abdomen. SYN anulus femoralis [TA], crural ring.

fem·o·ral sept·um (fem′ŏr-ăl sep′tŭm) [TA] Mass of connective tissue that occupies the femoral canal, effectively closing the canal but permitting the passage of lymphatics draining the lower limb. SYN septum femorale [TA], Cloquet septum, crural septum.

fem·o·ral sheath (fem′ŏr-ăl shēth) The fascia enclosing the femoral vessels. SYN crural sheath.

fem·o·ral tri·an·gle (fem′ŏr-ăl trī′anggĕl) [TA] A triangular space at the upper part of the thigh, bounded by the sartorius and adductor longus muscles and the inguinal ligament, with a floor formed laterally by the iliopsoas muscle and medially by the pectineus muscle. SYN trigonum femorale [TA], Scarpa triangle.

fem·o·ro·ab·dom·i·nal re·flex (fem′ŏ-rō-ăb-dom′ĭ-năl rē′fleks) Contraction of the abdominal muscles upon stroking the inner aspect of the thigh; in association with the cremasteric reflex. SYN hypogastric reflex.

fem·o·ro·cele (fem′ŏr-ō-sēl) SYN femoral hernia.

femto- (f) Prefix indicating unit of measure in the SI and metric system signifying one quadrillionth (10^{-15}).

fe·mur, gen. **fe·mo·ris**, pl. **fem·o·ra** (fē′mŭr, fem′ŏr-is, -ă) [TA] **1.** The thigh. **2.** The long bone of the thigh, articulating with the hip bone proximally and the tibia and patella distally. SYN thigh bone.

fe·nes·tra, pl. **fe·nes·trae** (fĕ-nes′tră, -trē) [TA] **1.** An anatomic aperture, often closed by a membrane. **2.** An opening left in a cast or other form of fixed dressing to permit access to a wound or inspection of the part. **3.** The opening in one of the blades of an obstetric forceps. **4.** A lateral opening in the sheath of an endoscopic instrument that allows lateral viewing or operative maneuvering through the sheath. **5.** Openings in the wall of a tube, catheter, or trocar designed to promote better flow of air or fluids. SYN window.

fe·nes·tra co·chle·ae (fĕ-nes′tră kōk′lē-ē) [TA] An opening on the medial wall of the middle ear leading into the cochlea, closed in life by the secondary tympanic membrane.

fen·es·trat·ed (fen′ĕs-trāt-ĕd) Having fenestrae or windowlike openings.

fen·es·trat·ed mem·brane (fen′ĕs-trāt-ĕd mem′brān) An elastic membrane, as in elastic laminae of arteries.

fen·es·tra·tion (fen′ĕs-trā′shŭn) **1.** The presence of openings in a body part. **2.** Making openings in a dressing to allow inspection of the parts. **3.** In dentistry, a surgical perforation of the mucoperiosteum and alveolar process to expose the root tip of a tooth to permit drainage of tissue exudate. **4.** An operation to create an opening in the horizontal semicircular canal to improve hearing in otosclerosis.

fe·nes·tra ves·tib·u·li (fĕ-nes′tră vestib′yū-lī) [TA] An oval opening on the medial wall of the tympanic cavity leading into the vestibule, closed by the foot of the stapes.

feng shui (fŭng shwā) Chinese esthetic belief system used to configure one's living or work environment to promote health, happiness, and prosperity, by enhancement of energy flow (chi).

fen·nel (fen′ĕl) Fennel seed, the dried ripe fruit of cultivated varieties of *Foeniculum vulgare*, a diaphoretic and carminative.

fen·u·greek (fen′yū-grēk) (*Trigonella foenum-graecum*) Purported therapeutic use in gastrointestinal disorders; also used topically; may cause bleeding disorders and hypoglycemia. SYN Greek hay.

Fer·gus·son in·ci·sion (fĕr′gŭ-sŏn in-sizh′ŭn) An incision used in maxillectomy, along the junction of the nose and cheek, and bisecting the upper lip.

fer·men·ta·tion (fĕr′mĕn-tā′shŭn) **1.** A chemical change induced in a complex organic compound by the action of an enzyme, whereby the substance is split into simpler compounds. **2.** BACTERIOLOGY the anaerobic dissimilation of substrates with the production of energy and reduced compounds; the mechanism of fermentation does not involve a respiratory chain or cytochrome, hence oxygen is not the final electron acceptor as it is in oxidation.

fer·ment·a·tive dys·pep·si·a (fĕr-men′tă-tiv dis-pep′sē-ă) Stomach upset accompanied by fermentation, usually occurring in gastric dilation.

fer·mi·um (Fm) (fĕr′mē-ŭm) Radioactive element, artificially prepared in 1955; atomic no. 100, atomic wt. 257.095; ^{257}Fm has the longest known half-life (100.5 days).

fern·ing (fĕrn′ing) **1.** A term used to describe the pattern of arborization produced by cervical mucus, secreted at midcycle, on crystallization, when it somewhat resembles a fern or a palm leaf. **2.** SYN filigree burn.

fern test (fĕrn test) **1.** Assessment for estrogenic activity; cervical mucus smears form a fern pattern when estrogen secretion is elevated, as at the time of ovulation. **2.** Means to detect ruptured amniotic membranes.

fer·re·dox·ins (Fd) (fer′ĕ-dok′sinz) Proteins containing iron and (labile) sulfur in equal amounts, displaying electron-carrier activity but no classical enzyme function.

Fer·rein va·sa a·ber·ran·ti·a (fer-ān[h]′ vă′să ă-ber-an′shē-ă) Biliary canaliculi that are not connected with hepatic lobules.

ferri- Prefix designating the presence of a ferric ion in a compound.

fer·ric (fer'ik) **1.** Relating to iron in its valence state of 3 + (Fe^{3+}). **2.** A compound in which iron exists in its valence state of Fe^{3+}.

fer·ri·tin (fer'i-tin) An iron protein complex, containing up to 23% iron formed by the union of ferric iron with apoferritin; found in the intestinal mucosa, spleen, bone marrow, reticulocytes, and liver.

fer·ro·ki·net·ics (fer'ō-ki-net'iks) The study of iron metabolism using radioactive iron.

fer·rous (fer'ŭs) Relating to iron in its valence state, Fe^{2+}.

fer·ru·gi·na·tion (fĕ-rū'ji-nā'shŭn) Deposition of mineral deposits including iron in the walls of small blood vessels and at the site of a dead neuron.

fer·ru·gi·nous (fĕ-rū'ji-nŭs) **1.** Iron bearing; associated with or containing iron. **2.** Of the color of iron rust.

fer·ru·gi·nous bod·ies (fĕ-rū'ji-nŭs bod'ēz) In the lungs, foreign inorganic or organic fibers coated by complexes of hemosiderin and glycoproteins; believed to be formed by macrophages that have phagocytized the fibers. SEE ALSO asbestos bodies.

Fer·ry line (fer'ē līn) An iron line occurring in the corneal epithelium anterior to a filtering bleb.

fer·til·i·ty (fert) (fer-til'i-tē) The actual production of live offspring.

fer·til·i·za·tion (fer'til-ī-zā'shŭn) The process beginning with penetration of the secondary oocyte by the sperm and completed by fusion of the male and female pronuclei.

fer·til·i·za·tion age (fer'til-ī-zā'shŭn āj) [TE] Age of embryo or fetus defined by the time elapsed since fertilization of the oocyte. SYN conceptual age.

fer·til·i·za·tion mem·brane (fer'ti-lī-zā'shŭn mem'brān) Viscous membrane formed on the inner surface of the vitelline membrane from the cytoplasm of the egg cell after entry of the sperm to prevent entry of additional sperms.

fer·ves·cence (fer-ves'ĕns) An increase of fever.

fes·ter (fes'tĕr) **1.** To form pus or putrefy. **2.** To make inflamed.

fes·ti·nat·ing gait, fes·ti·na·tion (fes'ti-nā'ting gāt, fes'ti-nā'shŭn) Way of walking in which the trunk is flexed, legs are flexed at the knees and hips, but stiff; the steps are short and progressively more rapid; characteristic of parkinsonism (1) and other neurologic diseases.

fes·toon (fes-tūn') **1.** A carving in the base material of a denture that simulates the contours of the natural tissue replaced by the denture. **2.** A distinguishing characteristic of certain hard tick species, consisting of small rectangular areas separated by grooves along the posterior margin of the dorsum.

fe·tal (fē'tăl) **1.** Relating to a fetus. **2.** Development in utero after the eighth week. SYN foetal.

fe·tal al·co·hol syn·drome (FAS) (fē'tăl al'kŏ-hol sin'drōm) Malformation or alteration present in varying degrees that includes growth deficiency, hyperactivity, craniofacial anomalies, and limb defects, found among offspring of mothers with long-term alcoholism during pregnancy.

fe·tal as·pi·ra·tion syn·drome (fē'tăl as'pir-ā'shŭn sin'drōm) Sign resulting from fetal aspiration of amnionic fluid and meconium, caused by hypoxia that often leads to aspiration pneumonia. SYN meconium aspiration syndrome.

fe·tal at·ti·tude (fē'tăl at'i-tūd) SYN lie.

fe·tal bra·dy·car·di·a (fē'tăl brad'ē-kahr'dē-ă) Fetal heart rate below 120 beats/min.

fe·tal cir·cu·la·tion (fē'tăl sĭr'kyū-lā'shŭn) Circulation of the fetus in utero, with the placental circuit responsible for supplying oxygen and nutritive material and for eliminating carbon dioxide and nitrogenous wastes.

fe·tal dis·tress (FD) (fē'tăl dis-tres') SYN nonreassuring fetal status.

fe·tal growth re·stric·tion (fē'tăl grōth

rĕ-strik'shŭn) Fetal weight in the fifth percentile or lower for gestational age.

fe·tal growth re·tar·da·tion (fē'tăl grōth rē'tahr-dā'shŭn) Fetal weight that is much below the norm.

fe·tal hy·dan·to·in syn·drome (FHS) (fē'tăl hī-dan'tō-in sin'drōm) Disorder due to maternal ingestion of hydantoin analogue (e.g., phenytoin), characterized by growth and mental deficiency, dysmorphic facies, cleft palate and/or lip, cardiac defects, and abnormal genitalia.

fe·tal hy·drops, hy·drops fe·ta·lis (fē'tăl hī'drops, fē-tā'lis) Abnormal accumulation of serous fluid in fetal tissues.

fe·tal med·i·cine (fē'tăl med'i-sin) Study of the growth, development, care, and treatment of the fetus, and of environmental factors harmful to the fetus. SYN fetology.

fe·tal pla·cen·ta, pla·cen·ta fe·ta·lis (fē'tăl plă-sen'tă, fē-tā'lis) Chorionic portion of the placenta, containing the fetal blood vessels, from which the umbilical cord develops. SYN pars fetalis placentae.

fe·tal scalp stim·u·la·tion (fē'tăl skalp stim'yŭ-lā'shŭn) Intrapartum test for fetal well-being; acceleration of fetal heart rate in response to digital or forceps stimulation of scalp is associated with a normal scalp blood pH.

fe·tal souf·fle (fē'tăl sū'fĕl) A blowing murmur, synchronous with the fetal heart beat, sometimes only systolic and sometimes continuous, heard on auscultation over the pregnant uterus.

fe·tal tach·y·car·di·a (fē'tăl tak'i-kahr'dē-ă) Fetal heart rate above 160 beats/min.

fe·ta·tion (fē-tā'shŭn) SYN pregnancy.

fe·ti·cide (fē'ti-sīd) Destruction of the embryo or fetus in the uterus.

fet·id (fet'id) Foul-smelling.

fet·ish (fet'ish) An inanimate object or nonsexual body part that is regarded as endowed with magic or erotic qualities.

fet·ish·ism (fet'ish-izm) The act of wor-

shipping or using for sexual arousal and gratification that which is regarded as a fetish.

fe·tol·o·gy (fē-tol'ŏ-jē) SYN fetal medicine.

fe·tom·e·try (fē-tom'ĕ-trē) Estimation of fetal size, especially cranial, before delivery.

fe·top·a·thy (fē-top'ă-thē) SYN embryopathy.

fe·to·pro·tein, al·pha (α)-fe·to·pro·tein (AFP), gam·ma (γ)-fe·to·pro·tein, be·ta (β)-fe·to·pro·tein (fē'tō-prō'tēn, al'fă, gam'ă, bā'tă) Fetal proteins found in small amounts in adults in the following forms: 1) AFP increases in maternal blood during pregnancy; when detected by amniocentesis, is an important indicator of neural tube defects, used as a tumor marker in adults with hepatocellular carcinoma; 2) beta (β)-fetoprotein, although a fetal liver protein, has been detected in adult patients with liver disease; and 3) gamma (γ)-fetoprotein occurs in association with various neoplasms. SEE ALSO fetoglobulins.

fe·tor (fē'tŏr) A very offensive odor.

fe·tor he·pat·i·cus (fē'tŏr hē-pat'i-kŭs) A peculiar breath odor to people with severe liver disease.

fe·to·scope (fē'tō-skōp) 1. A fiberoptic endoscope used in fetology. 2. A stethoscope designed for listening to fetal heart sounds.

fe·tu·in (fē-tū'in) A low molecular-weight globulin that constitutes nearly the total globulin in fetal blood.

fe·tus, pl. **fe·tus·es** (fē'tŭs, -ĕz) 1. The unborn young of a viviparous animal after it has taken form in the uterus. 2. In humans, the product of conception from the end of the eighth week to the moment of birth. SYN foetus.

fe·tus in fe·tu (FIF) (fē'tŭs fē'tū) Disorder in which a small, imperfectly formed fetus is contained within another fetus.

fe·tus pap·y·ra·ce·us (fē'tŭs pap-i-rā'shē-ŭs) One of twin fetuses that has died and been pressed flat against the uterine wall by the growth of the living fetus.

fe·ver (fē′vĕr) A complex physiologic response to disease mediated by pyrogenic cytokines and characterized by a rise in core temperature, generation of acute phase reactants, and activation of immunologic systems. SYN pyrexia.

fe·ver blis·ter (fē′vĕr blis′tĕr) Colloquialism for herpes simplex of the lips.

fe·ver·few (fē′vĕr-fyū) Herbal agent used in migraine headache and fever. Associated with ulceration of oral cavity, labial edema, and hypersensitivity reactions. SYN bachelor's button, Santa Maria.

fe·ver·ish (fē′vĕr-ish) 1. SYN febrile. 2. Having a fever.

fe·ver of un·known origin (FUO) (fē′vĕr ŭn′nōn ōr′i-jin) A sustained elevation of temperature, lasting 2 weeks or longer, for which no explanation can be found despite vigorous diagnostic evaluation. SYN pyrexia of unknown origin.

F fac·tor (fak′tŏr) SYN F plasmid.

fi·ber, fi·bra (fī′bĕr, fī′bră) [TA] 1. A strand or filament. 2. The nerve cell axon with its glial envelope. 3. Elongated, hence threadlike, cells such as muscle cells and the epithelial cells composing the major part of the eye lens. 4. Dietary nutrients not digested by gastrointestinal enzymes. SYN fibre.

fi·ber·op·tics (fī′bĕr-op′tiks) An optic system in which flexible glass or plastic fibers are used to transmit light around curves and corners; of particular use in endoscopy. SYN fibre-optics.

fib·ric ac·id (fīb′rik as′id) Drug used to treat hypercholesterolemia.

fibre [Br.] SYN fiber.

fibre-optics [Br.] SYN fiberoptics.

fi·bril, fi·bril·la (fī′bril, fī-bril′ă) A minute fiber or component of a fiber. SYN fibrilla.

fi·bril·lar·y as·tro·cyte, fi·brous as·tro·cyte (fī′bri-lar-ē as′trō-sīt, fī′brŭs) A stellate astrocytic cell with long processes found mainly in the white matter of the brain and spinal cord; origin of most astrocytomas.

fi·bril·lar·y con·trac·tions (fī′bri-lar-ē kŏn-trak′shŭnz) Those occurring spontaneously in individual muscle fibers; they are seen commonly a few days after damage to the motor nerves supplying the muscle; distinguished from fasciculation, which is related to activation of motor units.

fi·bril·lar·y waves (fī′bri-lar-ē wāvz) SYN f wave.

fi·bril·late (fī′bri-lāt) 1. To make or to become fibrillar. 2. SYN fibrillated. 3. To be in a state of fibrillation (3).

fi·bril·lat·ed (fī′bri-lā-tĕd) Composed of fibrils. SYN fibrillate (2).

fi·bril·la·tion (fī′bri-lā′shŭn) 1. The condition of being fibrillated. 2. The formation of fibrils. 3. Exceedingly rapid contractions or twitching of muscular fibrils, but not of the muscle as a whole.

fi·bril·lin (fī′bril-in) A microfibrillar protein in connective tissue with a wide distribution in the body.

fi·brin (FIB) (fī′brin) An elastic filamentous protein derived from fibrinogen by the action of thrombin, which releases fibrinopeptides A and B from fibrinogen in the coagulation of blood.

fi·brin cal·cu·lus (fī′brin kal′kyū-lŭs) A urinary stone formed largely from fibrinogen in blood.

fibrino- Combining form meaning fibrin.

fi·brin·o·gen (fī-brin′ō-jen) Blood plasma globulin converted into fibrin by the action of thrombin in the presence of ionized calcium to produce coagulation of the blood; the only coagulable protein in the blood plasma of vertebrates.

fi·bri·no·gen·ic, fi·bri·nog·e·nous (fī′brin-ō-jen′ik, fī′brin-noj′ĕ-nŭs) 1. Pertaining to fibrinogen. 2. Producing fibrin.

fi·brin·o·gen·ol·y·sis (fī-brin′ō-jĕ-nol′i-sis) The inactivation or dissolution of fibrinogen in the blood.

fi·brin·oid (fī′bri-noyd) 1. Resembling fibrin. 2. A deeply or brilliantly acidophilic, homogeneous, proteinaceous material that is frequently formed in blood vessel walls and connective tissue of patients with such diseases as disseminated lupus erythematosus, polyarteritis nodosa, scleroderma, dermatomyositis, and rheumatic fever.

fi·brin·oid de·gen·er·a·tion, fi·brin·ous de·gen·er·a·tion (fī′bri-noyd dē-jen′ĕr-ā′shŭn, fī′brin-ŭs) A process resulting in acidophilic refractile deposits with staining reactions that resemble fibrin, occurring in connective tissue, blood vessel walls, and other sites.

fi·bri·no·ki·nase (fī′brin-ō-kī′nās) SYN plasminogen activator, fibrinolysokinase.

fi·bri·nol·y·sin (fī′brin-ol′i-sin) SYN plasmin.

fi·bri·nol·y·sis (fī′bri-nol′i-sis) Hydrolysis of fibrin.

fi·bri·no·ly·so·ki·nase (fī′brin-ō-lī′sō-kī′nās) SEE plasminogen activator.

fi·bri·no·lyt·ic pur·pu·ra (fī′brin-ō-lit′ik pŭr′pyŭr-ă) A disorder in which bleeding is associated with rapid fibrinolysis of the clot.

fi·brin·o·pep·tide (fī′brin-ō-pep′tīd) One of two pairs of peptides (A and B) released from the amino-terminal ends of 2α- and 2β-chains of fibrinogen by the action of thrombin to form fibrin; has a vasoconstrictive effect.

fi·bri·no·pu·ru·lent (fī′brin-ō-pyūr′yū-lĕnt) Pertaining to pus or suppurative exudate that contains a relatively large amount of fibrin.

fi·brin·ous, fi·brous (fī′brin-ŭs, fī′brŭs) Pertaining to or composed of fibrin.

fi·brin·ous in·flam·ma·tion (fī′brin-ŭs in′flă-mā′shŭn) An exudative inflammation in which there is a disproportionately large amount of fibrin.

fi·brin·ous lymph (fī′bri-nŭs limf) A euplastic or croupous lymph.

fi·brin·ous per·i·car·di·tis (fī′brin-ŭs per′i-kahr-dī′tis) Acute pericarditis with fibrinous exudate.

fi·brin·ous pleu·ri·sy (fī′brin-ŭs plūr′i-sē) SYN dry pleurisy.

fi·brin·sta·bi·liz·ing fac·tor (fī′brin-stā′bi-līz-ing fak′tŏr) SYN factor XIII.

fi·bri·nu·ri·a (fī′bri-nyūr′ē-ă) The passage of urine that contains fibrin.

fibro-, fibr- Combining forms meaning fiber.

fi·bro·ad·e·no·ma (fī′brō-ad-ĕ-nō′mă) A benign neoplasm derived from glandular epithelium, in which there is a conspicuous stroma of proliferating fibroblasts and connective tissue elements; commonly occurs in breast tissue. SYN fibroid adenoma, adenoma fibrosum.

fi·bro·ad·i·pose (fī′brō-ad′i-pōs) Relating to or containing both fibrous and fatty structures. SYN fibrofatty.

fi·bro·a·re·o·lar (fī′brō-ă-rē′ō-lăr) Denoting connective tissue that is both fibrous and areolar in character.

fi·bro·blast (fī′brō-blast) A stellate or spindle-shaped cell with cytoplasmic processes present in connective tissue, capable of forming collagen fibers.

fi·bro·bron·chi·tis (fī′brō-brong-kī′tis) SEE fibrinous bronchitis.

fi·bro·cal·ci·fic (fī′brō-kal-sif′ik) Pertaining to sharply defined linear and nodular opacities containing calcifications, seen on a chest radiographic image, usually due to earlier granulomatous disease.

fi·bro·car·ci·no·ma (fī′brō-kahr-si-nō′mă) SYN scirrhous carcinoma.

fi·bro·car·ti·lage (fī′brō-kahr′ti-lăj) Cartilage that contains visible type I collagen fibers; appears as a transition between tendons or ligaments or bones. SYN fibrocartilago.

fi·bro·car·ti·lag·i·nous joint (fī′brō-kahr-ti-laj′i-nŭs joynt) SYN symphysis.

fi·bro·chon·dri·tis (fī′brō-kon-drī′tis) Inflammation of a fibrocartilage.

fi·bro·cys·tic (FC) (fī′brō-sis′tik) Pertaining to or characterized by the presence of fibrocysts.

fi·bro·cys·tic breast dis·ease (fī′brō-sis′tik brest di-zēz′) Common benign female breast disorder of unknown etiology. It can be manifest by multiple dense breast masses and multiple tiny lumps. Masses enlarge and shrink with menstrual cycle.

fi·bro·cys·tic dis·ease of pan·cre·as (fī′brō-sis′tik di-zēz′ pan′krē-ŭs) SYN cystic fibrosis.

fi·bro·cys·to·ma (fī′brō-sis-tō′mă) A benign neoplasm, usually derived from glandular epithelium, characterized by cysts within a conspicuous fibrous stroma.

fi·bro·dys·pla·si·a (fī′brō-dis-plā′zē-ă) Abnormal development of fibrous connective tissue.

fi·bro·e·las·tic (fī′brō-ĕ-las′tik) Composed of collagen and elastic fibers.

fi·bro·e·las·to·sis (fī′brō-ĕ′las-tō′sis) Excessive proliferation of collagenous and elastic fibrous tissue.

fi·bro·ep·i·the·li·o·ma (FE) (fī′brō-ep′i-thē-lē-ō′mă) A skin tumor composed of fibrous tissue intersected by thin anastomosing bands of basal cells of the epidermis, enclosing keratin cysts. SYN Pinkus tumor.

fi·bro·fol·lic·u·lo·ma (FF) (fī′brō-fŏ-lik′yū-lō′mă) Small papular hamartomas of the fibrous sheath of the hair follicle, with solid extensions of the epithelium of the follicular infundibulum; multiple fibrofolliculomas may be familial.

fi·bro·gli·o·sis (fī′brō-glī-ō′sis) A cellular reaction within the brain, usually in response to a penetrating injury.

fi·broid (fī′broyd) Resembling or composed of fibers or fibrous tissue. SYN fibroleiomyoma.

fi·broid cat·a·ract, fi·brin·ous cat·a·ract (fī′broyd kat′ăr-akt, fī′brin-ŭs) Sclerotic hardening of the capsule of the lens due to exudative iridocyclitis.

fi·broid·ec·to·my (fī′broyd-ek′tŏ-mē) Removal of a fibroid tumor.

fi·bro·la·mel·lar liv·er cell car·ci·no·ma (fī′brō-lam′ĕ-lăr liv′ĕr sel kahr′si-nō′mă) Primary hepatic carcinoma in

which malignant hepatocytes are intersected by fibrous lamellated bands. SYN oncocytic hepatocellular tumor.

fi·bro·lei·o·my·o·ma (fī′brō-lī′ō-mī-ō′mă) A leiomyoma containing nonneoplastic collagenous fibrous tissue, which may make the tumor hard; usually arises in the myometrium; proportion of fibrous tissue increases with age. SYN fibroid (3), leiomyofibroma.

fi·bro·li·po·ma (fī′brō-li-pō′mă) A lipoma with an abundant stroma of fibrous tissue.

fi·bro·ma (fī-brō′mă) A benign neoplasm derived from fibrous connective tissue.

fi·bro·ma·toid (fī-brō′mă-toyd) A focus, nodule, or mass (of proliferating fibroblasts) that resembles a fibroma but is not regarded as neoplastic.

fi·bro·ma·to·sis (fī-brō′mă-tō′sis) **1.** A condition characterized by the occurrence of many fibromas, with a relatively large distribution. **2.** Abnormal hyperplasia of fibrous tissue.

fi·bro·mus·cu·lar (fī′brō-mŭs′kyū-lăr) Both fibrous and muscular; relating to both fibrous and muscular tissues.

fi·bro·mus·cu·lar dys·pla·si·a (FMD) (fī′brō-mŭs′kyū-lăr dis-plā′zē-ă) Idiopathic nonatherosclerotic disease leading to stenosis of arteries, usually renal, and hypertension.

fi·bro·my·al·gi·a, fi·bro·my·al·gi·a syn·drome (fī′brō-mī-al′jē-ă, sin′drōm) A condition involving lack of stage IV sleep and chronic diffuse widespread aching and stiffness of muscles and soft tissues; diagnosis requires 11 of 18 specific tender points.

fi·bro·my·ec·to·my (fī′brō-mī-ek′tŏ-mē) Excision of a fibromyoma.

fi·bro·my·i·tis (fī′brō-mī-ī′tis) Muscular inflammation with concurrent fibrous degeneration.

fi·bro·my·o·ma (fī′brō-mī-ō′mă) A leiomyoma that contains a relatively abundant amount of fibrous tissue.

fi·bro·myx·o·ma (fī′brō-mik-sō′mă) A myxoma that contains a relatively abundant amount of mature fibroblasts and connective tissue.

fi·bro·nec·tin (fī'brō-nek'tin) Any of various glycoproteins found on cell membranes and in blood and other body fluids; thought to function as adhesive ligandlike molecules.

fi·bro·pap·il·lo·ma (fī'brō-pap-i-lō'mă) Lesion characterized by a conspicuous amount of fibrous connective tissue at the base and forming cores on which the neoplastic epithelial cells are massed.

fi·bro·pla·si·a (fī'brō-plā'zē-ă) Production of fibrous tissue.

fi·bro·re·tic·u·late (fī'brō-re-tik'yū-lăt) Relating to or consisting of a network of fibrous tissue.

fi·bro·sar·co·ma (fī'brō-sahr-kō'mă) A malignant neoplasm derived from deep fibrous tissue, characterized by bundles of immature proliferating fibroblasts arranged in a distinctive herringbone pattern with variable collagen formation.

fi·brose (fī'brōs) To form fibrous tissue.

fi·bros·ing al·ve·o·li·tis (FA) (fī-brōs'ing al'vē-ō-lī'tis) SYN idiopathic pulmonary fibrosis.

fi·bros·ing co·lon·op·a·thy (fī-brōs'ing kō'lŏn-op'ă-thē) Colonic fibrosis seen in cystic fibrosis patients.

fi·bros·ing me·di·a·stin·i·tis (fī-brōs'ing me'dē-as-ti-nī'tis) SYN mediastinal fibrosis.

fi·bro·sis (fī-brō'sis) Formation of fibrous tissue as a reparative or reactive process.

fi·bro·sit·ic head·ache (fī'brō-sit'ik hed'āk) Headache centered in the occipital region due to fibrositis of the occipital muscles.

fi·bro·tho·rax (fī'brō-thōr'aks) Fibrosis of the pleural space.

fi·brous (fī'brŭs) Denotes a body structure composed of or containing fibroblasts, and also the fibrils and fibers of connective tissue formed by such cells.

fi·brous an·ky·lo·sis (fī'brŭs ang'ki-lō'sis) Stiffening of a joint due to the presence of fibrous bands between and about the bones forming the joint. SYN false ankylosis, pseudankylosis.

fi·brous ar·tic·u·lar cap·sule (fī'brŭs ahr-tik'yū-lăr kap'sŭl) The outer fibrous part of the capsule of a synovial joint, which may in places be thickened to form capsular ligaments.

fi·brous cap·sule of kid·ney (fī'brŭs kap'sŭl kid'nē) [TA] A fibrous membrane ensheathing the kidney.

fi·brous cap·sule of liv·er (fī'brŭs kap'sŭl liv'ĕr) [TA] A layer of connective tissue ensheathing the hepatic artery, portal vein, and bile ducts as these ramify within the liver. SYN capsula fibrosa perivascularis hepatis [TA], Glisson capsule.

fi·brous cor·ti·cal de·fect (fī'brŭs kōr'ti-kăl dē'fekt) A common 1–3 cm defect in the cortex of a bone, most commonly the lower femoral shaft of a child, filled with fibrous tissue. SYN nonosteogenic fibroma.

fi·brous de·gen·er·a·tion (fī'brŭs dē-jen'ĕr-ā'shŭn) Not a decline in itself, but rather a reparative process; cells and foci of tissue previously affected with degenerative processes and necrosis are replaced by cellular fibrous tissue.

fi·brous dys·pla·si·a of bone (fī'brŭs dis-plā'zē-ă bōn) A disturbance in which bone undergoing physiologic destruction is replaced by abnormal fibrous tissue, resulting in asymmetric distortion and expansion of bone.

fi·brous goi·ter (fī'brŭs goy'tĕr) A firm hyperplasia of the thyroid and its capsule.

fi·brous ha·mar·to·ma of in·fan·cy (fī'brŭs ham'ahr-tō'mă in'făn-sē) Tumor appearing in the upper arm or shoulder in the first 2 years of life; consists of cellular fibrous tissue infiltrating the subcutis.

fi·brous joint (fī'brŭs joynt) [TA] A union of two bones by fibrous tissue such that there is no joint cavity and almost no motion possible; types include sutures, syndesmoses, and gomphoses. SYN immovable joint, synarthrodial joint (1).

fi·brous per·i·car·di·tis (fī′brŭs per′ĭ-kahr-dī′tis) Scarring, usually with adhesions, of all or most of the pericardium.

fi·brous tis·sue (fī′brŭs tish′ū) A tissue composed of bundles of collagenous white fibers between which are rows of connective tissue cells; the tendons, ligaments, aponeuroses, and some membranes, such as the dura mater.

fi·brous tu·ber·cle (fī′brŭs tū′bĕr-kĕl) Nodule in which fibroblasts proliferate about the periphery, eventually resulting in a rim or wall of cellular fibrous tissue or collagenous material around it.

fi·brous un·ion (fī′brŭs yūn′yŭn) Union of fracture by fibrous tissue. SEE nonunion, vicious union. SYN faulty union.

fi·bro·xan·tho·ma, fi·brous xan·tho·ma (fī′brō-zan-thō′mă, fī′brŭs) A fibrohistiocytic neoplasm.

fib·u·la (fib′yū-lă) [TA] The lateral and smaller of the two bones of the leg; it does not bear weight and articulates with the tibia above and the tibia and talus below. SYN calf bone.

fib·u·lar (fib′yū-lăr) [TA] 1. Relating to the fibula. SYN fibularis [TA], peroneal, peronealis. 2. Lateral in position within the leg.

fib·u·lo·cal·ca·ne·al (fib′yū-lō-kal-kā′nē-ăl) Relating to the fibula and the calcaneus.

fi·cin, fi·cain (fī′sin, fī′kān) 1. A cysteine endopeptidase isolated from figs; used in industry as a protein digestant; has a wide specificity for protein substrates; an anthelmintic. 2. The crude dried latex from *Ficus* spp.

Fi·coll-Hy·paque tech·nique (fī′kol-hī′pāk tek-nēk′) A density-gradient centrifugation technique for separating lymphocytes from other formed elements in the blood.

Fied·ler my·o·car·di·tis (fēd′ler mī′ō-kahr-dī′tis) SYN acute isolated myocarditis.

field (fēld) A definite area of plane surface, considered in relation to some specific object.

field block (fēld blok) Regional anesthesia produced by infiltration of local anesthetic solution into tissues surrounding an operative field.

field fe·ver (fēld fē′vĕr) A leptospirosis caused by *Leptospira*.

field of view (FOV) (fēld vyū) Area of anatomy included in an image.

field test (fēld test) An evaluation of physical fitness performed outside the laboratory environment that can be easily administered to large numbers of subjects with little or no equipment (e.g., 6-minute walk test, 1.5 mile run test, step test).

fifth dis·ease (fifth di-zēz′) SYN erythema infectiosum.

fig·ure (fig.) (fig′yŭr) 1. A form or shape. 2. A person representing the essential aspects of a particular role (e.g., relating to one's male boss as a father figure or to one's female teacher as a mother figure). 3. A form, shape, outline, or representation of an object or person.

fil·a·ment, fil·a·men·tum, pl. **fil·a·men·ta** (fil′ă-mĕnt, fil-ă-men′tŭm, -tă) A fine threadlike form, unsegmented or segmented without constrictions; any fibrous structure.

fil·a·men·tous (fil′ă-men′tŭs) 1. Threadlike in structure. SYN filiform (1). 2. Composed of filaments or threadlike structures. SYN filaceous, filar (2).

fi·la·ri·a (fi-lar′ē-ă) Common name for nematodes that live as adults in the blood, tissue fluids, tissues, or body cavities of many vertebrates.

fi·lar·i·cide (fi-lar′i-sīd) An agent that kills filariae.

Fil·a·tov-Dukes dis·ease (fē′lah-tof-dūks′ di-zēz′) An exanthem-producing infectious childhood disease of unknown etiology. SYN fourth disease.

file (fīl) A tool for smoothing, grinding, or cutting.

fil·gras·tim (fil-gras′tim) Human granulocyte-stimulating factor produced by recombinant DNA technology.

fil·i·al (fil′ē-ăl) Denoting the relationship

of offspring to parents. SEE filial generation.

fi·li·form (fil'i-fōrm) **1.** SYN filamentous (1). **2.** BACTERIOLOGY denoting an even growth along the line of inoculation, either stroke or stab.

fi·li·form bou·gie (fil'i-fōrm bū-zhē') A very slender probe used for gentle exploration of strictures or sinus tracts of small diameter where false passages can be encountered or created.

fi·li·form pa·pil·lae (fil'i-fōrm pă-pil'ē) [TA] Numerous elongated conic keratinized projections on the dorsum of the tongue. SYN papillae filiformes [TA].

fil·let (fil'et) **1.** SYN lemniscus. **2.** A skein, loop of cord, or tape used for making traction on a part of the fetus.

fill·ing (fil'ing) Colloquial term for a dental restoration.

film (film) **1.** A thin sheet of flexible material coated with a light-sensitive or x-ray-sensitive substance used in taking photographs or radiographs. **2.** A thin layer or coating. **3.** A radiograph (colloq.).

film badge (film baj) Small packet of x-ray film and filters worn by radiation workers to monitor exposure to radiation on a monthly basis. SEE ALSO pocket dosimeter, thermoluminescent dosimeter.

fi·lo·pres·sure (fī'lō-presh'ŭr) Temporary pressure on a blood vessel by a ligature, which is removed when the flow of blood has ceased.

Fi·lo·vi·ri·dae (fī'lō-vir'i-dē) A family of filamentous, single-stranded, negative sense RNA viruses with an enveloped nucleocapsid; associated with hemorrhagic fever; natural reservoir is unknown. SEE Ebola virus.

fil·ter (fil'tĕr) **1.** A porous substance through which a liquid or gas is passed to separate it from contained particulate matter or impurities. SYN filtrum. **2.** To use or to subject to the action of a filter. **3.** RADIOLOGY a device, used in both diagnostic and therapeutic radiology, which permits passage of useful x-rays and absorbs those with a lower and less desirable energy. **4.** A device used in spectrophotometric analysis to isolate a segment of the spectrum. **5.** A mathematic algorithm applied to image data for the purpose of enhancing image quality, usually by suppression of high spatial frequency noise. **6.** A passive electronic circuit or device that selectively permits passage of electrical signals. **7.** A device placed in the inferior vena cava to prevent pulmonary embolism from low extremity clot. **8.** RADIATION PHYSICS material placed in an x-ray beam used to improve the beam's quality by removing low-energy beams.

fil·ter·ing bleb (fil'tĕr-ing bleb) A blister of conjunctiva resulting from glaucoma surgery by which a flap of sclera is created in the eye wall, allowing aqueous humor to percolate out of the eye and underneath the conjunctiva, thus lowering intraocular pressure.

fil·ter·ing op·er·a·tion (fil'tĕr-ing op-ĕr-ā'shŭn) Surgical procedure to create a fistula between the anterior chamber of the eye and the subconjunctival space to treat glaucoma.

fil·trate (fil'trāt) That which has passed through a filter.

fil·tra·tion (fil-trā'shŭn) **1.** The process of passing a liquid or gas through a filter. **2.** RADIOLOGY the process of attenuating and hardening a beam of x-rays or gamma rays by interposing a filter (3) between the radiation source and the object being irradiated. SYN percolation (1).

fil·tra·tion frac·tion (FF) (fil-trā'shŭn frak'shŭn) The portion of the plasma entering the kidney that filters into the lumen of the renal tubules, determined by dividing the glomerular filtration rate by the renal plasma flow; normally, it is around 0.17.

fi·lum, fi·la, pl. **fi·la** (fī'lum, fī'lă) [TA] A structure of filamentous or threadlike appearance.

fi·lum of spi·nal du·ra mat·er (fī'lŭm spī'năl dūr'ă ma'tĕr) The threadlike termination of the spinal dura mater, surrounding and fused to the filum terminale of the cord, and attached to the deep dorsal sacrococcygeal ligament.

fi·lum ter·mi·na·le (fī'lum ter-mē-nā'lē) [TA] The slender threadlike termination of the spinal cord.

fim·bri·a, pl. **fim·bri·ae** (fim′brē-ă, -ē) **1.** Any fringelike structure. **2.** SYN pilus (2).

fim·bri·ec·to·my (fim′brē-ek′tŏ-mē) Excision of fimbriae.

fim·bri·o·cele (fim′brē-ō-sēl) Hernia of the corpus fimbriatum of the oviduct.

fim·bri·o·plas·ty (fim′brē-ō-plas′tē) Corrective operation on the tubal fimbriae.

fi·nal host (fī′năl hōst) SYN definitive host.

find·ing (fīnd′ing) A clinically significant observation, usually used in relation to one found on physical examination or laboratory test.

fine mo·tor co·or·di·na·tion (FMC) (fīn mō′tŏr kō-ōr′di-nā′shŭn) Ability to perform delicate manipulations with the hand requiring steadiness, muscle control, and simultaneous discrete finger movements. SYN fine coordination, fine motor control.

fine nee·dle bi·op·sy (fīn nē′dĕl bī′op-sē) Removal of tissue or suspensions of cells through a small needle.

fine trem·or (fīn trem′ŏr) Shaking in which the amplitude is small and the frequency is usually greater than 12 Hz.

fin·ger-nose test (fing′gĕr-nōz test) A test of voluntary eye-motor coordination of the upper limb(s); the subject is asked to slowly touch the tip of the nose with the extended index finger; assesses cerebellar function.

fin·ger·print (fing′gĕr-print) **1.** An impression of the inked bulb of the distal phalanx of a finger, showing the configuration of the surface ridges, used as a means of identification. **2.** In genetics, the analysis of DNA fragments to determine the identity of a person or the paternity of a child.

fin·ger-to-fin·ger test (fing′gĕr fing′gĕr test) Test for coordination and position sense of the upper limbs; the subject is asked to approximate the ends of the index fingers; assesses cerebellar function.

Fin·kel·stein test (fing′kĕl-shtīn test) Assay to detect de Quervain tenosynovitis in which the thumb is flexed into the palm and is covered by the remaining four digits; the wrist is then bent toward the ulna; positive result of test produces pain and crepitus along the path of the involved tendon.

first aid (fĭrst ād) Immediate assistance administered in the case of injury or sudden illness by a bystander or other lay person, before the arrival of trained medical personnel.

first and sec·ond pos·te·ri·or in·ter·cos·tal ar·te·ries (fĭrst sek′ŏnd postēr′ē-ŏr in′tĕr-kos′tăl ahr′tĕr-ēz) [TA] Terminal branches of the superior intercostal artery (from costocervical trunk) supplying upper two intercostal spaces. SYN arteriae intercostales posteriores I et II, posterior intercostal arteries 1–2.

first-de·gree AV block (fĭrst-dĕ-grē′ blok) SEE atrioventricular block.

first-de·gree burn (fĭrst-dĕ-grē′ bŭrn) SYN superficial burn.

first-de·gree pro·lapse (fĭrst dĕ-grē′ prō′laps) Form of cervical prolapse where the cervix of the prolapsed uterus is well within the vaginal orifice.

first heart sound (S1) (fĭrst hahrt sownd) Occurs with ventricular systole and is mainly produced by closure of the atrioventricular valves.

first-pass me·tab·o·lism, first-pass ef·fect (FPM) (fĭrst-pas mĕ-tab′ŏ-lizm, e-fekt′) Intestinal and hepatic degradation or alteration of a drug or substance taken by mouth, after absorption, removing some of the active substance from the blood before it enters the general circulation.

first re·spon·der (fĭrst rĕ-spon′dĕr) **1.** The first trained person to arrive at the emergency scene (medical incident or trauma) to assist the patient or render immediate life-sustaining aid. **2.** The basic level of training and certification for prehospital medical responders (i.e., fire fighters and law enforcement personnel).

fis·sion (fish′ŭn) **1.** The act of splitting. **2.** Splitting of the nucleus of an atom.

fis·sip·a·rous (fi-sip′ă-rŭs) Reproducing or propagating by fission.

fis·su·la (fis-sū′lă) Diminutive form of fissure; a small fissure or cleft.

fis·su·la an·te fe·nes·tram (fis-sū′lă an′tē fen-es′tram) Minute, slitlike passage in the labyrinthine wall of the tympanic cavity, extending obliquely from the region of the cochleiform process to the vestibule of the bony labyrinth, anterior to the oval window.

fis·su·ra, pl. **fis·su·rae** (fis-sū′ră, -rē) [TA] **1.** [TA] SYN fissure. **2.** NEUROANATOMY a particularly deep sulcus of the surface of the brain or spinal cord. SYN fissure (1).

fis·sur·al an·gi·o·ma (fish′ŭr-ăl an′jē-ō′mă) Lesion made up of enlarged blood vessels on the facial areas in an embryonal fissure.

fis·sure (fish′ŭr) [TA] **1.** A deep furrow, cleft, or slit. SYN fissura (2). **2.** DENTISTRY a developmental break or fault in the tooth enamel. SEE ALSO sulcus. SYN fissura (1).

fis·sured tongue (fish′ŭrd tŭng) Painless condition characterized by numerous dorsal grooves or furrows.

fis·sure seal·ant (fish′ŭr sēl′ănt) Dental material usually made from interaction between bisphenol A and glycidyl methacrylate; such sealants are used to seal nonfused, noncarious pits and fissures on surfaces of teeth. SYN dental sealant.

fis·tu·la, pl. **fis·tu·lae**, pl. **fis·tu·las** (fis′tyū-lă, -lē, -lăz) An abnormal passage from one epithelialized surface to another, either congenital, caused by disease or injury, or created surgically.

fis·tu·la·tion, fis·tu·li·za·tion (fis′tyū-lā′shŭn, -lī-ză′shŭn) Formation of a fistula in a part; becoming fistulous.

fis·tu·la·tome (fis′tyū-lă-tōm) A long, thin-bladed, probe-pointed knife for slitting open a fistula. SYN fistula knife, syringotome.

fit (fit) **1.** An attack of an acute disease or the sudden appearance of some symptom, such as coughing. **2.** A convulsion. **3.** SYN epilepsy. **4.** DENTISTRY the adaptation of any dental restoration, e.g., of an inlay to the cavity preparation in a tooth, or of a denture to its basal seat.

fix·a·tion (fik-sā′shŭn) **1.** The condition of being firmly attached or set. **2.** HISTOLOGY the rapid killing of tissue elements and their preservation and hardening to retain as nearly as possible the same relations they had in the living body. SYN fixing. **3.** CHEMISTRY the conversion of a gas into solid or liquid form by chemical reactions, with or without the help of living tissue. **4.** PSYCHOANALYSIS the quality of being firmly attached to a particular person or object or period in one's development. **5.** PHYSIOLOGIC OPTICS the coordinated positioning and accommodation of both eyes that results in bringing or maintaining a sharp image of a stationary or moving object on the fovea of each eye.

fix·a·tion ny·stag·mus (fik-sā′shŭn nis-tag′mŭs) Rolling of eyes aggravated or induced by ocular fixation, arising as optokinetic nystagmus, or resulting from midbrain lesions.

fix·a·tive (fik′să-tiv) **1.** Serving to fix, bind, or make firm or stable. **2.** A substance used to preserve gross and histologic specimens of tissue or individual cells. SEE ALSO fluid, solution.

fixed coup·ling (fikst kŭp′ĕl-ing) where several premature beats are seen, the interval between each of them and the preceding normal beat is constant. SYN constant coupling.

fixed dress·ing (fikst dres′ing) Bandage stiffened with a substance that when dry produces immobilization.

fixed end (fikst end) [TA] In motion, the end of a bone that is held stationary (as a consequence of attachment or muscular fixation) while the other end of the bone (the mobile end) moves in response to muscle activity or gravity. SYN punctum fixum.

fixed i·de·a (fikst ī-dē′ă) **1.** An exaggerated notion, belief, or delusion that persists, despite evidence to the contrary, and controls the mind. **2.** The obstinate conviction of a psychotic person regarding the correctness of a delusion.

fixed oil (fikst oyl) SYN fatty oil.

fixed pu·pil (fikst pyū′pil) A stationary pupil unresponsive to all stimuli.

fixed-rate pace·ma·ker (fikst-rāt pās′ mā-kĕr) An artificial pacemaker that emits electrical stimuli at a constant frequency.

fixed tor·ti·col·lis (fikst tŏr′ti-kol′is) Persistent contracture of cervical muscles on one side.

fixed vi·rus (fikst vī′rŭs) Rabies virus the virulence of which for rabbits has been stabilized by numerous passages through this experimental host. SEE ALSO street virus.

flac·cid (flak′sid) Relaxed, flabby, or without tone.

flac·cid blad·der (flak′sid blad′ĕr) Absence of sense of urinary filling that can lead to failure of urinary retention.

flac·cid dys·arth·ri·a (flak′sid dis-ahr′ thrē-ă) Dysarthria associated with peripheral muscle weakness usually due to lower motor neuron disorders, causing hypernasality, imprecise consonants, breathy voice, and monotony of pitch. SEE hypernasality.

flac·cid·i·ty (flak-sid′i-tē) The condition or state of being flaccid.

flac·cid pa·ral·y·sis (flak′sid pă-ral′i-sis) Paralysis with a loss of muscle tone. Cf. spastic diplegia.

flac·cid part of tym·pan·ic mem·brane (flak′sid pahrt tim-pan′ik mem′ brăn) Loose triangular part of tympanic membrane located within the maleolar folds.

fla·gel·lar (flă-jel′ăr) Relating to a flagellum or to the extremity of a protozoan.

fla·gel·lar an·ti·gen (flă-jel′ăr an′ti-jen) The heat-labile antigens associated with bacterial flagella, in contrast to somatic antigen. SEE ALSO H antigen.

flag·el·late (flaj′ĕ-lāt) 1. Possessing one or more flagella. 2. A member of the class Mastigophora.

flag·el·la·tion (flaj′ĕ-lā′shŭn) 1. Whipping either oneself or another as a means of arousing or heightening sexual feel-

ing. 2. The pattern of formation of flagella.

flag·el·lin (flaj′ĕ-lin) Any member of a class of proteins that constitute subunits of the flagella and that contain the amino acid ε-N-methyllysine.

flag·el·lo·sis (flaj′ĕ-lō′sis) Infection with flagellated protozoa in the intestinal or genital tract, e.g., trichomoniasis.

fla·gel·lum, pl. **fla·gel·la** (flă-jel′ŭm, -lă) A whiplike locomotory organelle of constant structural arrangement consisting of nine double peripheral microtubules and two single central microtubules; it arises from a deeply staining basal granule.

flail chest (flāl chest) Flapping chest wall; condition in which three or more consecutive ribs on the same side of the chest have been fractured in at least two places, with resulting instability of the chest wall, paradoxic respiratory movements of the injured segment, and loss of respiratory efficiency.

flail mi·tral valve (flāl mī′trăl valv) SEE mitral valve prolapse.

flange (flanj) That part of the denture base that extends from the cervical ends of the teeth to the border of the denture.

flank (flangk) [TA] SYN latus.

flank po·si·tion (flangk pŏ-zish′ŏn) Lateral recumbent position, but with the lower leg flexed, the upper leg extended, and convex extension of the upper side of the body; used for nephrectomy.

flap (flap) 1. Mass of partially detached tissue. SEE ALSO pedicle flap, distant flap. 2. An uncontrolled movement, as of the hands. SEE asterixis.

flam·ma·ble (flam′ă-bĕl) *This word is preferred to inflammable; the prefix in- is sometimes mistaken for a sign of negation.* The property of burning readily and quickly. SYN inflammable.

flap am·pu·ta·tion (flap amp′yū-tā′ shŭn) An amputation in which flaps of the muscular and cutaneous tissues are shaped to cover the end of the bone. SYN flap operation (1).

flap·less am·pu·ta·tion (flap′lĕs amp′ yū-tā′shŭn) An amputation without any tissue to cover the stump.

flap op·er·a·tion (flap op-ĕr-ā′shŭn) SYN flap amputation. SEE ALSO flap.

flap·ping trem·or (flap′ing trem′ŏr) SYN asterixis.

flare (flār) **1.** A gradual tapering or spreading outward. **2.** A diffuse redness of the skin extending beyond the local reaction to the application of an irritant; due to dilation of the arterioles and capillaries. SEE ALSO triple response.

flash blind·ness (flash blīnd′nĕs) A temporary loss of vision produced when retinal light-sensitive pigments are bleached by light more intense than that to which the retina is physiologically adapted at that moment.

flash burn (flash bŭrn) One due to very brief exposure to intense radiant heat; the typical burn produced by atomic explosion.

flask (flask) A small receptacle, usually glass, used for holding liquids, powder, or gases.

flask clo·sure (flask klō′zhŭr) In dentistry, the procedure of bringing the two halves or parts of a flask together.

flask·ing (flask′ing) The process of investing the cast and a wax denture in a flask preparatory to molding the denture-base material into the form of the denture.

flat af·fect (flat a′fekt) Absence of or diminution in the amount of emotional tone or outward emotional reaction (e.g., facial expression, posture) typically shown by oneself or others under similar circumstances; may include lack of vocal expression; often a symptom of mental disorders; a milder form is termed blunted affect.

Fla·tau law (flah′tow law) Rule concerning the position of the long tracts of the spinal cord: the further the nerve fibers run lengthwise in the cord, the more they are situated toward the periphery.

flat bone (flat bōn) [TA] A type of bone characterized by its thin, flattened shape,

such as the scapula or certain of the cranial bones.

flat chest (flat chest) A thorax in which the anteroposterior diameter is shorter than the average.

flat con·dy·lo·ma (flat kon′di-lō′mă) **1.** SYN condyloma latum. **2.** Warty lesion of the uterine cervix or other site caused by human papillomavirus infection.

flat·foot (flat′fut) SYN talipes planus.

flat pel·vis (flat pel′vis) One in which the anteroposterior diameter is uniformly abnormally shortened, the sacrum being dislocated forward between the iliac bones. SYN pelvis plana.

flat·u·lence (flat′yū-lĕns) Presence of an excessive amount of gas in the stomach and intestines.

fla·tus (flā′tŭs) Gas or air in the gastrointestinal tract that may be expelled through the anus.

flat wart (flat wŏrt) SYN verruca plana.

flat·worm (flat′wŏrm) A member of the phylum Platyhelminthes, including the parasitic tapeworms and flukes.

Fla·vi·vi·ri·dae (flā′vi-vir′i-dē) A family of enveloped single-stranded positive sense RNA viruses 40–60 mm in diameter formerly classified as the "group B" arboviruses, including yellow fever and dengue viruses; maintained in nature by transmission from arthropod vectors to vertebrate hosts.

Fla·vi·vi·rus (flā′vi-vī′rŭs) A genus in the family Flaviviridae that includes yellow fever, dengue, and St. Louis encephalitis viruses.

Fla·vo·bac·te·ri·um (flā′vō-bak-tēr′ē-ŭm) A genus of aerobic to facultatively anaerobic, non-spore-forming, motile and nonmotile bacteria containing gramnegative rods; characteristically produce yellow, orange, red, or yellow-brown pigments; found in soil and fresh and salt water. Some species are pathogenic.

fla·vo·en·zyme (flā′vō-en′zīm) Any enzyme that possesses a flavin nucleotide as coenzyme.

fla·vone (flā′vōn) **1.** A plant pigment that is the basis of the flavonoids; it is a potent inhibitor of prostaglandin biosynthesis. **2.** One of a class of compounds based on flavone (1).

fla·vo·noid (flā′vŏ-noyd) Metabolite from plant matter; ingestion may have benefits as antioxidant.

flea (flē) An insect marked by lateral compression, sucking mouthparts, extraordinary jumping powers, and ectoparasitic adult life in the hair and feathers of warm-blooded animals.

Flech·sig tract (flek′sig trakt) SYN posterior spinocerebellar tract.

Fleisch·mann bur·sa (flīsh′mahn bŭr′ să) SYN sublingual bursa.

flesh (flesh) **1.** Living tissue, especially soft tissues as contrasted with bone. **2.** SYN muscular tissue. **3.** The meat of animals used for food.

Flet·cher fac·tor (flech′ĕr fak′tŏr) SYN prekallikrein.

flex·i·bil·i·tas ce·re·a (flek-si-bil′i-tahs sē′rē-ă) The rigidity of catalepsy that may be overcome by slight external force, but that returns at once, holding the limb firmly in the new position.

flex·i·bil·i·ty (fleks′i-bil′i-tē) Range of motion about a joint dependent on the condition of surrounding structures. SEE range of motion.

flex·i·ble col·lo·di·on (fleks′i-bĕl kŏ-loyd′ē-ŏn) Mixture of camphor, castor oil, and collodion, or a mixture of castor oil, Canada turpentine, and collodion, used for the same purposes as collodion, but its film possesses the advantage, for certain conditions, of not contracting.

flex·i·ble en·do·scope (fleks′i-bĕl en′dŏ-skōp) An optic instrument that transmits light and carries images back to the observer through a flexible bundle of small (about 10 mcm) transparent fibers; used to inspect interior portions of the body. SEE ALSO fiberoptics.

flex·i·ble hys·ter·o·scope (fleks′i-bĕl his′tĕr-ŏ-skōp) Steerable flexible small diameter instrument for operative or diagnostic procedures that does not require an outer sheath, has fiberoptics for visualization, and must be used with a distending gas.

flex·ion (flek′shŭn) [TA] **1.** The act of flexing or bending. **2.** The condition of being flexed or bent. SYN open-packed position (2).

flex·ion crease (flek′shŭn krēs) Permanent skin fold on the flexor aspect of a movable joint.

flex·ion-ex·ten·sion in·ju·ry (flek′ shŭn-eks-ten′shŭn in′jŭr-ē) Forceful application of a forward and backward movement of the unsupported head that may produce an injury to the cervical spine or the brain.

flex·or (fleks′ŏr) [TA] A muscle the action of which is to flex a joint.

flex·or re·flex (fleks′ŏr rē′fleks) Flexion of ankle, knee, and hip when the foot is painfully stimulated.

flex·or re·ti·nac·u·lum of low·er limb (flek′sŏr ret′i-nak′yū-lŭm lō′ĕr lim) [TA] A wide band passing from the medial malleolus to the medial and upper border of the calcaneus and to the plantar surface as far as the navicular bone.

flex·u·ral psor·i·a·sis (flek′shŭr-ăl sōr-ī′ă-sis) Skin disease involving intertriginous folds (e.g., axillary and inguinal skin); may resemble seborrheic dermatitis.

flex·ure, flex·u·ra (flek′shŭr, flek-shŭr′ă) [TA] A bend, as in an organ or structure.

flicks (fliks) Rapid, involuntary fixation movements of the eye of 5–10 minutes of arc. SYN flick movements.

Fli·e·ring·a ring (flēr-ing′gă ring) A stainless steel ring sutured to the sclera to prevent collapse of the globe in difficult intraocular operations.

flight blind·ness (flīt blīnd′nĕs) Visual blackout in aviators. SEE ALSO amaurosis fugax.

flight of i·de·as (FOI) (flīt ī-dē′ăz) Uncontrollable symptom of the manic phase of a bipolar depressive disorder in which streams of unrelated words and ideas occur to the patient at a rate that is difficult to vocalize despite a marked increase in the person's overall output of words. SEE ALSO mania, manic episode.

Flint ar·cade (flint ahr-kād´) A series of vascular arches at the bases of the pyramids of the kidney.

flint dis·ease (flint di-zēz´) SYN chalicosis.

Flint mur·mur (flint mŭr´mŭr) A diastolic murmur, similar to that of mitral stenosis, heard best at the cardiac apex. SYN bicuspid murmur.

float·er (flōt´ĕr) **1.** Colloquial term for a cadaver removed from a body of water. **2.** An object in the field of vision that originates in the vitreous body.

float·ing kid·ney (flōt´ing kid´nē) The abnormally mobile kidney in nephroptosis. SYN wandering kidney.

float·ing spleen (flōt´ing splēn) One palpable because of excessive mobility from a relaxed or lengthened pedicle rather than enlargement. SYN lien mobilis, movable spleen.

floc·cil·la·tion (flok´si-lā´shŭn) An aimless plucking at the bedclothes, as if one were picking off threads or tufts of cotton.

floc·cose (flok´ōs) BACTERIOLOGY describes a growth of short, curving filaments or chains closely but irregularly disposed.

floc·cu·lar (flok´yū-lăr) Relating to a flocculus of any sort, and specifically to the flocculus of the cerebellum.

floc·cu·lent (flok´yū-lĕnt) Resembling tufts of cotton or wool; denoting a fluid, such as urine, containing numerous shreds or fluffy particles of gray-white or white mucus or other material.

floc·cu·lus, pl. **floc·cu·li** (flok´yū-lŭs, -lī) [TA] **1.** A tuft or shred of cotton or wool or anything resembling it. **2.** [TA] A small lobe of the cerebellum at the posterior border of the middle cerebellar peduncle anterior to the biventer lobule; associated with the nodulus of the vermis; together, these two structures compose the vestibular part of the cerebellum.

flood·ing (flŭd´ing) **1.** Profuse bleeding from the uterus, especially after childbirth or in severe cases of menorrhagia. **2.** A type of behavior therapy; a therapeutic strategy at the beginning of therapy in which the patients imagine the most anxiety-producing scene and fully immerse (flood) themselves in it.

floor (flōr) [TA] The lower inner surface of an open space or hollow organ.

floor plate (flōr plāt) Ventral midline thinning of the developing neural tube, a continuity between the basal plates of either side; opposite of roof plate.

flop·py in·fant (flop´ē in´fănt) A young child afflicted with neuromuscular or muscular disorders such that the limbs cannot move independently.

flo·ra (flō´ră) **1.** Plant life, usually of a certain locality or district. **2.** The population of microorganisms inhabiting the internal and external surfaces of healthy conventional animals.

flor·id (flōr´id) **1.** Of a bright red color; denoting certain cutaneous lesions. **2.** Fully developed.

flor·id os·se·ous dys·pla·si·a, ce·ment·al dys·pla·si·a (flōr´id os´ē-ŭs dis-plā´zē-ă, sĕ-men´tăl) SYN sclerotic cemental mass.

flow (flō) **1.** To bleed from the uterus less profusely than in flooding. **2.** The menstrual discharge. **3.** Movement of a liquid or gas; specifically, the volume of liquid or gas passing a given point per unit of time. **4.** RHEOLOGY A permanent deformation of a body that proceeds with time.

flow-con·trol·led ven·ti·la·tor (flō´ kŏn-trōld´ ven´ti-lā-tŏr) A device designed to deliver mandatory breaths with a preset flow waveform.

flow cy·to·me·try (flō sī-tom´ĕ-trē) A method of measuring fluorescence from stained cells that are in suspension and flowing through a narrow orifice, usually with one or two lasers to activate the dyes; used to measure cell size, number, viability, and nucleic acid content.

flow·me·ter, flow me·ter (FM) (flō´

mē′tĕr) A device for measuring velocity or volume of flow of liquids or gases.

flow-vol·ume curve (flō-vol′yūm kŭrv) Graphic produced by plotting the instantaneous flow of respiratory gas against the simultaneous lung volume, usually during maximal forced expiration.

flu (flū) SYN influenza.

fluc·tu·ate (flŭk′shū-āt) 1. To move in waves. 2. To vary, to change from time to time.

fluc·tu·a·tion (flŭk′shū-ā′shŭn) 1. The act of fluctuating. 2. A wavelike motion felt on palpating a cavity with nonrigid walls, especially one containing fluid. SYN fluctuancy.

flu·ent (flū′ĕnt) Relating to fluency.

flu·ent a·pha·si·a (flū′ĕnt ă-fā′zē-ă) SYN receptive aphasia.

flu·id (flū′id) 1. A nonsolid substance, such as a liquid or gas, which tends to flow or conform to the shape of the container. 2. Consisting of particles or distinct entities that can readily change their relative positions; tending to move or capable of flowing.

flu·id bal·ance chart (flū′id bal′ăns chahrt) Record used to monitor input and output of fluids. Input includes oral fluids and infused intravenous fluids and blood products. Output includes fluid loss as urine, emesis, and wound drainage. SYN input and output record.

flu·id·ex·tract (flū′id-eks′trakt) *Avoid the incorrect form fluid extract.* Pharmacopeial liquid preparation of vegetable drugs, made by percolation, containing alcohol as a solvent or as a preservative, or both, and so made that each 1 mL contains the therapeutic constituents of 1 g of the standard drug that it represents. SYN liquid extract.

flu·id o·ver·load (flū′id ō′vĕr-lōd) Fluid that remains in the body due to either impaired clearance or overconsumption.

flu·ma·ze·nil (FMZ) (flū′mă-zē′nil) Benzodiazepine with antagonist properties at the benzodiazepine recognition site of the benzodiazepine gamma-aminobutyric acid–chloride channel complex. Used to treat overdose with benzodiazepine-type central nervous system depressants or controlled reversal of anesthesia induced by such agents.

flu·men, pl **flu·mi·na** (flū′mĕn, -mi-nă) A flowing, or stream.

flu·mi·na pi·lo·rum (flū′mi-nă pī-lō′rŭm) SYN hair streams.

fluor-, fluoro- Combining forms meaning fluorine.

fluor·ap·a·tite (flōr-ap′ă-tīt) Hydroxyapatite (q.v) in which fluoride ions have replaced some of the hydroxyl ions; as a component of teeth, it resists acids from plaque-forming bacteria and high carbohydrate intake. SEE ALSO apatite.

fluor·es·ce·in (flōr-es′ē-in) [C.I. 45350] An orange-red crystalline powder that yields a bright green fluorescence in solution, and is reduced to fluorescin; a nontoxic, water-soluble indicator used diagnostically to trace water flow and to visualize corneal abrasions or ulcers.

fluor·es·ce·in in·stil·la·tion test (flōr-es′sē-in in′sti-lā′shŭn test) A test for patency of the lacrimal system; fluorescein instilled in the conjunctival sac can be recovered from the inferior nasal meatus. SYN dye disappearance test, Jones test.

fluor·es·ce·in i·so·thi·o·cy·a·nate (FITC) (flōr-es′sē-in ī′sō-thī-ō-sī′ă-nāt) Fluorochrome dye frequently coupled to antibodies that are used to locate and identify specific antigens.

fluor·es·cence (flōr-es′ĕns) Emission of a longer wavelength radiation by a substance as a consequence of absorption of energy from a shorter wavelength radiation, continuing only as long as the stimulus is present.

fluor·es·cence mi·cros·co·py (flōr-es′ĕns mī-kros′kŏ-pē) A procedure based on the fact that fluorescent materials emit visible light when they are irradiated with ultraviolet or violet-blue visible rays.

fluor·es·cent an·ti·bod·y tech·nique (flōr-es′ĕnt an′ti-bod-ē tek-nēk′) A procedure to test for antigen with a fluorescent antibody.

fluor·es·cent trep·o·ne·mal an·ti·bod·y-ab·sorp·tion test (flōr-es'ĕnt trep'ŏ-nē'măl an'ti-bod-ē-ăb-sōrp'shŭn test) A sensitive and specific serologic assay for syphilis using a suspension of the Nichols strain of *Treponema pallidum* as antigen.

fluor·i·da·tion (flōr'i-dā'shŭn) Addition of fluorides to a community water supply, usually 1 ppm or less, to reduce incidence of dental decay.

fluor·ine (F) (flōr-ēn') A gaseous chemical element, atomic no. 9, atomic wt. 18.9984032; ^{18}F (half-life of 1.83 h) is used as a diagnostic aid in various tissue scans.

fluor·o·chrome (flōr'ō-krōm) Any fluorescent dye used to label or stain.

fluor·om·e·ter (flōr-om'ĕ-tĕr) A device employing an ultraviolet source, monochromators for selection of wavelength, and a detector of visible light; used in fluorometry.

fluor·om·e·try (flōr-om'ĕ-trē) An analytic method for detecting fluorescent compounds, using a beam of ultraviolet light that excites the compounds and causes them to emit visible light.

fluor·o·pho·tom·e·try (flōr'ō-fō-tom'ĕ-trē) Photomultiplier tube measurement of fluorescence emitted from the interior of the eye after intravenous administration of fluorescein; used to measure the rate of formation of aqueous humor or integrity of the retinal vasculature.

fluor·o·quin·o·lone (flōr'ō-kwin'ŏ-lōn) A class of antibiotics with a broad spectrum of antimicrobial activity, well absorbed orally, with good tissue penetration and long duration of action.

fluor·os·co·py (flōr-os'kŏ-pē) Examination of the tissues and deep structures of the body by x-ray, using a fluoroscope.

fluor·o·sis (flōr-ō'sis) A condition caused by an excessive intake of fluorides, characterized mainly by mottling, staining, or hypoplasia of the enamel of the teeth.

fluor·o·u·ra·cil (FU, FUra) (flōr'ō-yū'ră-sil) An antineoplastic effective in the treatment of some carcinomas.

flush (flŭsh) **1.** To wash out with a full stream of fluid. **2.** A transient erythema due to heat, exertion, stress, or disease. **3.** Flat, or even with another surface, as a flush stoma.

flux (J) (flŭks) **1.** The discharge of a fluid material in large amounts from a cavity or surface of the body. SEE ALSO diarrhea. **2.** Material discharged from the bowels. **3.** A material used to remove oxides from the surface of molten metal and to protect it during casting; serves a similar purpose in soldering operations. **4.** The moles of a substance crossing through a unit area of a boundary layer or membrane per unit of time. **5.** Bidirectional movement of a substance at a membrane or surface. **6.** DIAGNOSTIC RADIOLOGY photon fluence per unit of time.

fly (flī) A two-winged insect in the order Diptera.

Fm Symbol for fermium.

foam (fōm) **1.** Masses of small bubbles on the surface of a liquid. **2.** To produce such bubbles. **3.** Masses of air cells in a solid or semisolid, as in foam rubber.

foam cells (fōm selz) Cells with abundant, pale-staining, finely vacuolated cytoplasm, usually histiocytes that have ingested or accumulated material that dissolves during tissue preparation, especially lipids. SEE ALSO lipophage.

fo·cal der·mal hy·po·pla·si·a (FDH) (fō'kăl dĕr'măl hī'pō-plā'zē-ă) Pathologic condition of the skin and, in some cases, the mucosa inherited as an X-linked dominant with in utero lethality in males; characterized by linear areas of dermal atrophy or hypoplasia, herniation of fat through the dermal defects, and papillomas of the mucous membranes or skin. SYN Goltz syndrome.

fo·cal dis·tance (fō'kăl dis'tăns) The distance from the center of a lens to its focus.

fo·cal ep·i·lep·sy (fō'kăl ep'i-lep'sē) Neural disorder characterized by focal seizures or secondarily generalized tonic-clonic seizures. SYN cortical epilepsy, local epilepsy, localization-related epilepsy (2), partial epilepsy.

fo·cal-film dis·tance (FFD) (fō'kăl-film

dis′tăns) The distance from the source of
radiation (the focal spot of the x-ray tube)
to the film or other image-receptor. SYN
source-to-image distance.

fo•cal in•fec•tion (fō′kăl in-fek′shŭn)
Local infection that can serve as a source
of disseminated or metastatic infection.

fo•cal in•ju•ry (fō′kăl in′jŭr-ē) Trauma
to a small, concentrated area, usually
caused by high velocity–low mass
forces.

fo•cal ne•cro•sis (fō′kăl nĕ-krō′sis) Occurrence of numerous, relatively small or
tiny, fairly well-circumscribed, usually
spheroid portions of tissue that manifest
coagulative, caseous, or gummatous necrosis and are characteristically associated with agents that are hematogenously
disseminated.

fo•cal re•ac•tion (fō′kăl rē-ak′shŭn) One
that occurs at the point of entrance of an
infecting organism or of an injection.

**fo•cal seg•men•tal glo•mer•u•lo•
scler•o•sis** (fō′kăl seg-men′tăl glŏm-
er′yū-lō-skler-ō′sis) Segmental collapse of glomerular capillaries with
thickened basement membranes and increased mesangial matrix.

fo•cus (F), pl. **fo•ci** (fō′kŭs, -sī) **1.** The
point at which the light rays meet after
passing through a convex lens. **2.** The
center, or the starting point, of a disease
process.

fo•cused grid (fō′kŭst grid) SEE grid
(2).

foetal [Br.] SYN fetal.

foetus [Br.] SYN fetus.

fog (fawg) **1.** Droplets dispersed in the
atmosphere or a respiratory device.
2. Areas of an x-ray clouded by stray
light during processing.

**Fo•gar•ty cath•e•ter, Fo•gar•ty em•
bo•lec•to•my cath•e•ter** (fō′găr-tē
kath′ĕ-tĕr, em′bŏ-lek′tŏ′mē) A catheter
with an inflatable balloon at its tip; commonly used to remove arterial emboli
and thrombi from major veins or to remove stones from the biliary ducts.

fog•ging (fawg′ing) A method of refrac-

tion in which accommodation is relaxed
by overcorrection with a convex spherical lens.

foil (F) (foyl) An extremely thin pliable
sheet of metal.

fo•late (fō′lāt) A salt or ester of folic acid.

fold (fōld) **1.** A ridge or margin apparently
formed by the doubling back of a lamina.
SEE ALSO plica. **2.** In the embryo, a
transient elevation or reduplication of tissue in the form of a lamina.

fold•able in•tra•oc•u•lar lens (fōld′ă-
bĕl in′tră-ok′yū-lăr lenz) A lens usually
made of silicone or an acrylic polymer
that may be doubled over for implantation into the eye following cataract removal.

Fo•ley cath•e•ter (fō′lē kath′ĕ-tĕr) A urethral catheter with a retaining balloon;
used to drain the bladder.

fo•li•a•ceous (fō′lē-ā′shŭs) SYN foliate.

fo•li•ate (fō′lē-ăt) Pertaining to or resembling a leaf or leaflet. SYN foliaceous,
foliar, foliose.

fo•lic ac•id (fō′lik as′id) Pteroylmonoglu-
tamic acid, a member of the vitamin B
complex necessary for the production of
red blood cells; present in liver, green
vegetables, and yeast; used to treat folate
deficiency and megaloblastic anemia.

fo•lic ac•id an•tag•o•nist (fō′lik as′id
an-tag′ŏ-nist) Modified pterins that interfere with the action of folic acid and thus
produce the symptoms of folic acid deficiency; used in cancer chemotherapy.

fo•lic ac•id de•fi•cien•cy a•ne•mi•a
(fō′lik as′id dĕ-fish′ĕn-sē ă-nē′mē-ă)
Form of megaloblastic anemia due to dietary folic acid deficiencies.

fo•lie à deux (fō-lē ah du) Mental disorder in which a delusion develops in a
person in a relationship with another person with an established delusion.

fo•lie gé•mel•laire (fō-lē zhā-mel-ār′)
Psychotic disorder appearing simultaneously, or nearly so, in twins, who are not
necessarily living together or intimately
associated at the time.

fo·lin·ic ac·id (fō-lin'ik as'id) The active form of folic acid, which acts as a formyl group carrier in transformylation reactions.

fo·li·um, pl. **fo·li·a** (fō'lē-ŭm, -ă) [TA] A broad, thin, leaflike structure.

folk med·i·cine (fōk med'i-sin) Treatment of ailments with remedies and simple measures based on experience and knowledge handed on from generation to generation.

fol·lib·er·in (fo-lib'ĕr-in) A decapeptide of hypothalamic origin capable of accelerating pituitary secretion of follitropin.

fol·li·cle (fol'i-kĕl) [TA] 1. A more or less spheric mass of cells usually containing a cavity. 2. A crypt or minute cul-de-sac. SYN folliculus [TA].

fol·lic·u·lar ad·e·no·ma (fŏ-lik'yū-lăr ad-ĕ-nō'mă) Thyroid lesion with a simple glandular pattern.

fol·lic·u·lar an·trum (fŏ-lik'yū-lăr an'trŭm) Cavity of an ovarian follicle filled with liquor folliculi.

fol·lic·u·lar cyst (fŏ-lik'yū-lăr sist) 1. An odontogenic lesion that arises from the epithelium of a tooth bud and dental lamina. 2. SYN dentigerous cyst.

fol·lic·u·lar cys·ti·tis (fŏ-lik'yū-lăr sis-tī'tis) Chronic cystitis characterized by small nodules due to lymphocytic infiltration.

fol·lic·u·lar goi·ter (fŏ-lik'yū-lăr goy'tĕr) SYN parenchymatous goiter.

fol·lic·u·lar lym·pho·ma (fŏ-lik'yū-lăr lim-fō'mă) SYN nodular lymphoma.

fol·lic·u·lar stig·ma (fŏ-lik'yū-lăr stig'mă) Blanched spot where the vesicular ovarian follicle is about to rupture on the surface of the ovary. SYN stigma (2).

fol·lic·u·lar vul·vi·tis (fŏ-lik'yū-lăr vŭl-vī'tis) Inflammation of the vulvar hair follicles.

fol·li·cu·li lym·phat·i·ci rec·ti (fŏ-lik'yū-lī lim-fat'i-sī rek'tī) Scattered collections of lymphoid tissue in the wall of the rectum. SYN lymphatic follicles of rectum.

fol·lic·u·li·tis (fŏ-lik'yū-lī'tis) An inflammatory reaction in hair follicles; the lesions may be papules or pustules.

fol·li·cu·li·tis de·cal·vans (fŏ-lik'yū-lī'tis dē-kal'vanz) A papular or pustular inflammation of the hair follicles of the scalp seen mostly in men, resulting in scarring and loss of hair in the affected area.

fol·lic·u·lose (fŏ-lik'yū-lōs) Denotes anything composed of follicles.

fol·lic·u·lo·sis (fŏ-lik'yū-lō'sis) Presence of lymph follicles in abnormally great numbers.

fol·lic·u·lus, pl. **fol·lic·u·li** (fŏ-lik'yū-lŭs, -lī) [TA] SYN follicle.

Fol·ling dis·ease (fol'ing di-zēz') SYN phenylketonuria.

fol·li·stat·in (fol'i-stat'in) A peptide synthesized by granulosa cells in response to follitropin, which suppresses follitropin's activity, probably by binding activins.

fol·li·tro·pin-re·leas·ing hor·mone (FRH) (fol'i-trō'pin rĕ-lēs'ing hōr'mōn) A hypothalamic hormone that stimulates release of follitropin and luteotropin by the adenohypophysis.

fol·low-up, fol·low·up (fol'ō-ŭp) Noun or adjective meaning the act of providing continuing or further attention to something.

fo·men·ta·tion (Fo) (fō'men-tā'shŭn) 1. A warm application. SEE ALSO poultice, stupe. 2. Application of warmth and moisture in the treatment of disease.

fo·mes, pl. **fom·i·tes** (fō'mēz, -mi-tēz) Objects, such as clothing, towels, and utensils that possibly harbor a disease agent and are capable of transmitting it; usually used in the plural. SYN fomite.

Fon·se·cae·a (fon-sē'sē-ă) A genus of fungi of which at least two species, *Fonsecaea pedrosoi* and *Fonsecaea compacta*; causes chromoblastomycosis.

Fon·se·cae·a pe·dro·so·i (fon-sē'sē-ă ped-rō'sō-ī) A slow-growing dematiaceous fungal species that produces skin and subcutaneous tissue infections usually during trauma.

fon·ta·nelle, fon·ta·nel (fon'tă-nel') [TA] One of several membranous intervals at the margins of the cranial bones in the infant. SYN fonticulus [TA].

fon·tic·u·lus, pl. **fon·tic·u·li** (fon-tik'yū-lŭs, -lī) [TA] SYN fontanelle.

food ad·di·tives (fūd ad'i-tivz) Natural and chemical agents added to prepared foods to enhance some aspect of the food (e.g., shelf life, appearance, nutrition levels).

food chain (fūd chān) Description of the feeding relationships among the organisms present in an ecosystem.

Food Guide Py·ra·mid (fūd gīd pir'ă-mid) U.S. Department of Agriculture guidelines for sound nutrition that emphasize grains, vegetables, and fruits and downplay food sources high in animal protein, lipids, and dairy products. SYN MyPyramid.

food poi·son·ing (fūd poy'zŏn-ing) Illness related to the ingestion of a foodstuff tainted by pathogens of any type.

food ser·vice ad·min·is·tra·tor (fūd sĕr'vis ăd-min'i-strā'tŏr) A nutrition specialist with a professional certificate or an associate degree who is trained to manage alimentation in an institutional operation.

food ser·vice de·part·ment (fūd sĕr'vis dĕ-pahrt'mĕnt) Office concerned with preparation and delivery of meals to the patients in a facility.

foot, pl. **feet** (fut, fēt) [TA] **1.** The distal part of the leg. SYN pes (1) [TA]. **2.** A unit to measure length, containing 12 inches, equal to 30.48 cm.

foot-and-mouth dis·ease (FMD) (fut mowth di-zēz') Highly infectious disease of worldwide distribution and great economic importance, occurring in cattle, swine, sheep, goats, and all wild and domestic cloven-hoofed animals caused by a picornavirus and characterized by vesicular eruptions in the mouth, tongue, hoofs, and udder; humans are rarely affected. SYN aftosa.

foot·board (fut'bōrd) A flat or vertical structure placed at the end of the patient's bed to maintain the feet in a functional position.

foot can·dle (fut kan'dĕl) Illumination or brightness equivalent to 1 lumen/square foot.

foot·drop (fut'drop) Partial or total inability to dorsiflex the foot, as a consequence of which the toes drag on the ground during walking unless a steppage gait is used; most often ultimately due to weakness of the dorsiflexor muscles of the foot (especially the tibialis anterior), but has many causes, including central nervous system disorders.

foot·ling breech (fut'ling brēch) An abnormal fetal position that causes the presenting part to be the foot of the fetus.

foot·plate, foot-plate, foot plate (fut'plāt) SYN base of stapes.

foot·print·ing (fut'print-ing) A method for determining the area of DNA covered by protein binding.

fo·ra·men, pl. **fo·ram·i·na** (fōr-ā'mĕn, fōr-am'i-nă) [TA] An aperture or perforation through a bone or a membranous structure.

Forbes-Al·bright syn·drome (fōrbz-awl'brīt sin'drōm) Pituitary tumor in a patient without acromegaly, which secretes excessive amounts of prolactin (PRL) and produces persistent lactation.

force (F) (fōrs) **1.** That which tends to produce motion in a body. **2.** Application of energy to initiate motion.

forced beat (fōrst bēt) **1.** An extrasystole supposedly precipitated in some way by the preceding normal beat to which it is coupled. **2.** An extrasystole caused by artificial stimulation of the heart.

forced ex·pi·ra·to·ry flow (FEF) (fōrst ek-spīr'ă-tōr-ē flō) Expiratory flow during measurement of forced vital capacity; subscripts specify the exact parameter measured.

forced ex·pi·ra·to·ry vi·tal ca·pa·ci·ty (fōrst ek-spīr'ă-tōr-ē vī'tăl kă-pas'i-tē) SYN forced expiratory volume.

forced ex·pi·ra·to·ry vol·ume (FEV) (fōrst ek-spīr'ă-tōr-ē vol'yūm) The maximal volume that can be expired in a specific time interval when starting from maximal inspiration. SYN forced expiratory vital capacity.

forced feed·ing, forc·i·ble feed·ing (fōrst fēd'ing, fōr'si-bĕl) **1.** Giving liquid food through a nasal tube that passes into the stomach. **2.** Forcing a person to eat more food than desired.

forced vi·tal ca·pa·ci·ty (FVC) (fōrst vī'tăl kă-pas'i-tē) Vital capacity measured with the subject exhaling as rapidly as possible.

for·ceps (fōr'seps) [TA] **1.** An instrument for seizing a structure and making compression or traction. Cf. clamp. **2.** [TA] Bands of white fibers in the brain, major forceps and minor forceps.

for·ceps de·li·ver·y (fōr'seps dĕ-liv'ĕr-ē) Assisted birth of the child by an instrument designed to grasp the fetal head.

for·ceps ma·jor (fōr'seps mā'jŏr) [TA] SYN major forceps.

for·ceps mi·nor (fōr'seps mī'nŏr) [TA] SYN minor forceps.

for·ci·ble in·spi·ra·tion (fōr'si-bĕl in'spir-ā'shŭn) Continuing inhalation beyond the amount of air moved in normal inspiration to achieve maximum lung capacity. SYN inspiratory reserve volume.

for·ci·pate (fōr'si-pāt) Shaped like a forceps.

For·dyce spots, For·dyce gran·ules, For·dyce dis·ease (fōr'dīs spots, gran'yūlz, di-zēz') Condition marked by the presence of numerous small, yellowish-white bodies or granules on the inner surface and vermilion border of the lips.

fore·arm (fōr'ahrm) [TA] The segment of the upper limb between the elbow and the wrist. SYN antebrachium [TA].

fore·brain (fōr'brān) SYN prosencephalon.

fore·con·scious (fōr'kon-shŭs) Denoting memories, not at present in the consciousness, which can be evoked from time to time, or an unconscious mental process that becomes conscious only on the fulfillment of certain conditions. Cf. preconscious.

fore·fin·ger (fōr'fing-gĕr) SYN index finger.

fore·foot (fōr'fut) The part of the foot containing the metatarsal bones and phalanges; the front part of the foot.

fore·gut (fōr'gŭt) The cephalic portion of the primordial digestive tube in the embryo. From its endoderm arise the epithelial lining of the pharynx, trachea, lungs, esophagus, and stomach, the first part and cranial half of the second part of the duodenum, and the parenchyma of the liver, gallbladder, and pancreas. SYN headgut.

fore·head (fōr'hed) [TA] The part of the face between the eyebrows and the hairy scalp. SYN brow (2), frons.

for·eign bod·y ob·struc·tion (fōr'ĕn bod'ē ŏb-strŭk'shŭn) Blockage of a passageway by something external; for example, food blocking the trachea, which prevents passage of air.

for·eign bod·y re·ac·tion (fōr'ĕn bod'ē rē-ak'shŭn) Protective response by the immune system to a foreign body; includes chronic inflammation and granulomatous formations around the intrusive object.

for·eign se·rum (fōr'ĕn sēr'ŭm) One derived from an animal and injected into an animal of another species or into humans.

fo·ren·sic (fōr-en'sik) Pertaining or applicable to personal injury, murder, and other legal proceedings.

fo·ren·sic med·i·cine (FM) (fōr-en'sik med'i-sin) **1.** Relation and application of medical facts to legal matters. **2.** The law in its bearing on the practice of medicine. SYN legal medicine, medical jurisprudence.

fo·ren·sic psy·chi·a·try, le·gal psy·chi·a·try (fōr-en'sik sī-kī'ă-trē, lē'găl) The application of psychiatry in courts of law, e.g., in determinations for involuntary commitment, competency, fitness to stand trial, responsibility for crime.

fore·play (fōr'plā) Stimulative sexual activity preceding sexual intercourse.

fore·quar·ter am·pu·ta·tion (fōr′kwôr-tĕr amp′yū-tā′shŭn) Amputation of the arm with removal of the scapula and a portion of the clavicle.

fore·skin (fōr′skin) SYN prepuce.

fore·wa·ters (fōr′waw′tĕrz) Colloquialism for the bulging fluid-filled amnionic membrane presenting in front of the fetal head.

for·give·ness fa·cil·i·ta·tion (fŏr-giv′nĕs fă-sil′i-tā′shŭn) Nursing term: helping a patient give up a negative response to someone and replace it with a positive response.

fork (fôrk) A pronged instrument used for holding or lifting.

For·mad kid·ney (fōr′mad kid′nē) An enlarged and deformed kidney sometimes seen in chronic alcoholism.

for·mal·de·hyde (HCHO) (fōr-mal′dĕ-hīd) A pungent gas, HCHO, used as an antiseptic, disinfectant, and histologic fixative, usually in an aqueous solution. SYN formic aldehyde, methyl aldehyde.

for·mal·de·hyde so·lu·tion (fōr-mal′dĕ-hīd sŏ-lū′shŭn) The liquid form of the simplest aldehyde, often used as a fixative for preservation of tissue samples; a pollutant in tobacco smoke, automobile exhaust, and smog.

for·ma·lin (fōr′mă-lin) A 37% aqueous solution of formaldehyde.

for·ma·lin-e·ther sed·i·men·ta·tion con·cen·tra·tion (fōr′mă-lin-ē′thĕr sed′i-mĕn-tā′shŭn kon′sĕn-trā′shŭn) A sedimentation method to separate parasitic elements from fecal debris through centrifugation and the use of ether to trap debris in a separate layer from the parasites.

for·mal op·er·a·tions (fōr′măl op′ĕr-ā′shŭnz) Stage of development in thinking, occurring approximately between 11–15 years of age, when a child becomes capable of reasoning about abstract situations.

for·mant (fōr′mănt) Tones and their overtones resulting from the production of vowel phonemes.

for·mate (fōr′māt) A salt or ester of formic acid; i.e., the monovalent radical HCOO– or the anion HCOO⁻.

for·ma·ti·o, pl. **for·ma·ti·o·nes** (fōr-mā′shē-ō, -ō′nēz) [TA] A structure of definite shape or cellular arrangement.

form·a·tive (fōr′mă-tiv) Capable of producing new cells or tissues; capable of causing growth or development to follow a certain pattern.

form·board (fōrm′bōrd) Neuropsychological test with a board containing cutouts in various shapes, into which blocks of corresponding shape are to be fitted.

forme fruste, pl. **formes frustes** (fōrm frŭst) A partial, arrested, or inapparent form of disease.

for·mic ac·id (fōr′mik as′id) The smallest carboxylic acid; a strong caustic, used as an astringent and counterirritant.

for·mi·ca·tion (fōr′mi-kā′shŭn) A form of paresthesia or tactile hallucination; a sensation as if ants were creeping under the skin.

for·mim·i·no·glu·tam·ic ac·id (FIGLU) (fōr-mim′i-nō-glū-tam′ik as′id) An intermediate metabolite in ʟ-histidine catabolism in the conversion of ʟ-histidine to ʟ-glutamiate; it may appear in the urine of patients with folic acid or vitamin B12 deficiency, or liver disease.

for·mu·la (fōrm′yū-lă) **1.** A recipe or prescription containing directions for the compounding of a medicinal preparation. **2.** CHEMISTRY a symbol or collection of symbols expressing the number of atoms of the element or elements forming one molecule of a substance, together with, on occasion, information such as the arrangement of the atoms within the molecule, their electronic structure, their charge, and the nature of the bonds within the molecule. **3.** An expression by symbols and numbers of the normal order or arrangement of parts or structures.

for·mu·lar·y (F) (fōrm′yŭ-lār-ē) A collection of formulas for the compounding of medicinal preparations. SEE National Formulary.

for·mu·late (fōrm′yŭ-lāt) To develop an

for·mu·la·tion (fōrm´yū-lā´shŭn) Process of developing a concept or formula.

idea; to express in systematic terms; to produce a substance chemically.

for·myl (f) (fōr´mil) The radical, HCO–.

for·ni·cate gy·rus (fōr´ni-kāt jī´rŭs) The horseshoe-shaped cortical convolution bordering the hilus of the cerebral hemisphere. SYN gyrus fornicatus (1).

for·ni·ca·tion (fōr´ni-kā´shŭn) Sexual intercourse between partners when unmarried to each other.

for·nix, gen. **for·ni·cis**, pl. **for·ni·ces** (fōr´niks, -ni-sis, -ni-sēz) [TA] **1.** [TA] In general, an arch-shaped structure; often the arch-shaped roof (or roof portion) of an anatomic space. **2.** The compact, white fiber bundle by which the hippocampus of each cerebral hemisphere projects to the contralateral hippocampus and to the septum, anterior nucleus of the thalamus, and mammillary body.

for·nix of sto·mach (fōr´niks stŏm´ăk) [TA] The domed or pocketlike portion of the stomach that lies superior to and to the left of the cardial orifice, in which, in the upright position, gas is often contained.

Forsch·heim·er spots (for´shī-mer spots) Petechiae on the soft palate.

Forss·man an·ti·bod·y (fōrs´măn an´ti-bod´ē) Molecule found in the blood of patients with infectious mononucleosis. SYN heterophil antibody, heterophile antibody.

Forss·man an·ti·gen (fōrs´măn an´ti-jen) Heterogenetic antigen found in dogs, horses, sheep, cats, turtles, eggs of some fish, in certain bacteria (e.g., some strains of enteric organisms and pneumococci), and varieties of corn; usually found in the tissues and organs (not in blood), but is present in sheep erythrocytes, though not in this animal's tissues; antibody that develops in infectious mononucleosis of humans reacts specifically with it.

För·ster u·ve·i·tis (fĕr´ster yū´vē-ī´tis) Syphilitic inflammation, with diffuse nodules involving the choroid and retinal vasculitis.

for·ti·fied milk (fōr´ti-fīd milk) Milk to which some essential nutrient, usually vitamin D, has been added.

for·ward-bend·ing ma·neu·ver (fōr´wărd-bend´ing mă-nū´vĕr) **1.** Examination method for neoplastic changes in the breast; patient bends forward from the waist with head held up and arms extended toward the examiner; if retraction is present, an asymmetry will be evident. **2.** Assessment position useful in diagnosis of scoliosis.

for·ward chain·ing (fōr´wărd chān´ing) System of reasoning used in artificial intelligence; starts with available data and uses inference rules to extract more data until the solution is reached.

for·ward heart fail·ure (fōr´wărd hahrt fāl´yŭr) A concept that maintains that the phenomena of congestive heart failure result from the inadequate cardiac output, and especially from the consequent inadequacy of renal blood flow with resulting retention of sodium and water. Cf. backward heart failure.

fos·sa, gen. and pl. **fos·sae** (fos´ă, -ē) [TA] A depression usually more or less longitudinal below the level of the surface of a part.

fos·su·la, pl. **fos·su·lae** (fos´yū-lă, -lē) [TA] **1.** A small fossa. **2.** A minor fissure or slight depression on the surface of the cerebrum.

Fos·ter frame (faws´tĕr frăm) A reversible bed similar to a Stryker frame.

Fou·chet stain (fū-shā´ stān) Reagent employed to demonstrate bile pigments.

fou·lage (fū-lahz[h]´) Kneading and pressure of the muscles, constituting a form of massage.

foun·da·tion (fown-dā´shŭn) A base; a supporting structure.

four-hand·ed den·tis·try (fōr´hand´ĕd den´tis-trē) A technique of dental procedure in which the dentist and dental assistant work closely together, reducing the stress and fatigue felt by a dentist practicing alone.

Fou·ri·er a·nal·y·sis, Fou·ri·er trans·form (fūr-ē-ā´ ă-nal´i-sis, trans´fōrm) A mathematical approximation of a function as the sum of periodic functions (sine waves) of different frequencies; used in reconstruction of magnetic resonance images and computed tomographs and analysis of any kind of signal for its frequency content.

Four·ni·er gan·grene (fūr-nē-ā´ gang´ grēn) SYN Fournier disease.

four-post·er or·tho·sis (for´pō´stĕr ōr-thō´sis) A rigid cervical brace that consists of a chest harness, two front posts, two back posts, and a headpiece to told the cervical spine in fixed position.

four-tailed band·age (fōr´tāld ban´dăj) Strip of cloth split in two except for a central portion placed under the chin, with four tails tied over the head; used to limit motion of the mandible.

fourth cra·ni·al nerve [CN IV] (fōrth krā´nē-ăl nĕrv) SYN trochlear nerve [CN IV].

fourth dis·ease (fōrth di-zēz´) SYN Filatov-Dukes disease.

fourth heart sound (S4) (fōrth hahrt sownd) The sound produced in late diastole in association with ventricular filling due to atrial systole and related to reduced ventricular compliance.

fourth lum·bar nerve [L4] (fōrth lŭm´ bahr nĕrv) The ventral branch of the nerve is forked to enter into the formation of both lumbar and sacral plexuses.

fourth stage of la·bor (fōrth stäj lā´bŏr) The period after the delivery of the fetus and the placenta when the mother's pulse, blood pressure, and body temperature stabilize and the uterus clamps down to control blood loss.

fo·ve·a, pl. **fo·ve·ae** (fō´vē-ă, -ē) [TA] Any natural depression on the surface of the body, such as the axilla, or on the surface of a bone. Cf. dimple.

fo·ve·a ca·pi·tis (fō´vē-ă kap´i-tis) The point of attachment of the ligamentum teres femoris on the head of the femur.

fo·ve·ate, fo·ve·at·ed (fō´vē-āt, -ā-ted) Pitted; having foveae or depressions on the surface.

fo·ve·a·tion (fō-vē-ā´shŭn) Pitted scar formation, as in chickenpox.

fo·ve·o·la, pl **fo·ve·o·lae** (fō-vē´ō-lă, -ē) [TA] *Avoid the mispronunciation foveo´la.* A minute fovea or pit.

Fo·ville syn·drome (fō-vēl´ sin´drōm) Ipsilateral facial and abducens nerve paralysis, and contralateral hemiplegia, due to a lesion (usually infarction) within the tegmentum of the pons.

Fow·ler po·si·tion (fowl´ĕr pŏ-zish´ŭn) SYN semirecumbent.

Fow·ler test (fowl´ĕr test) Measurement of anterior shoulder instability; the supine patient's shoulder is abducted and externally rotated while posterior force is applied to the humerus. If movement is detected, the test is positive and instability is presumed to be present.

Fox-For·dyce dis·ease (foks fōr´dīs, di-zēz´) Chronic pruritic eruption of dry papules and distended ruptured apocrine glands, seen mostly in women, with follicular hyperkeratosis of the nipples, axillae, and pubic and sternal regions. SYN apocrine miliaria.

F plas·mid (plaz´mid) The prototype conjugative plasmid associated with conjugation in the K-12 strain of *Escherichia coli.* SYN F factor.

frac·tion (frak´shŭn) **1.** The quotient of two quantities. **2.** An aliquot portion or any portion.

frac·tion·al dis·til·la·tion (frak´shŭn-ăl dis´ti-lā´shŭn) That of a compound liquid at varying degrees of heat whereby the components of different boiling points are collected separately.

frac·tion·a·ted dose (frak´shŭn-āt-ĕd dōs) The portion of the total daily dosage of a medication or radiation to be given at specified intervals.

frac·tion·a·tion (frak´shŭn-ā´shŭn) **1.** To separate components of a mixture. **2.** The administration of a course of therapeutic radiation of a neoplasm in a planned series of fractions of the total dose, most often once a day for several weeks, in order to minimize radiation damage of contiguous normal tissues.

frac·ture (Fx, frac, fract, frx, fx, FXR, Fr, FX) (frak′shŭr) **1.** To break. **2.** A break, especially the breaking of a bone or cartilage.

frac·ture blis·ter (frak′shŭr blis′tĕr) Superficial epidermolysis that occurs in association, most commonly, with fractures of the leg and ankle and forearm and wrist.

frac·ture by con·tre·coup (frak′shŭr kŏn′trĕ-kū′) Skull fracture at a point distant from the site of impact.

frac·ture-dis·lo·ca·tion (frak′shŭr-dis′ lō-kā′shŭn) A severe injury in which breaking of a bone and movement out of alignment occur simultaneously.

frag·ile X chro·mo·some (fraj′il krō′ mŏ-sōm) An X chromosome with a weak (i.e., fragile) site near the end of the long arm, resulting in the appearance of an almost detached fragment.

fra·gi·li·tas cri·ni·um (fră-jil′i-tahs krī′ nē-ŭm) Brittleness of the hair; in which the hair of the head or face tends to split or break off.

fra·gil·i·tas os·si·um (fră-jil′i-tahs os′ē-ŭm) Brittle bone disease, which results from a genetic defect.

fra·gil·i·tas un·gui·um (fră-jil′i-tahs ŭng′ gwē-ŭm) A disorder that produces brittle nails.

fra·gil·i·ty (frag) (fră-jil′i-tē) Liability to break, burst, or disintegrate. SYN fragilitas.

fra·gi·li·ty of blood (fră-jil′i-tē blŭd) SYN osmotic fragility.

Fra·ley syn·drome (frā′lē sin′drōm) Dilation of the upper pole renal calyces due to stenosis of the upper infundibulum, usually caused by compression from vessels supplying the upper and middle segments of the kidney.

fram·be·si·a (fram-bē′zē-ă) SYN framboesia.

fram·be·si·o·ma (fram-bē′zē-ō′mă) SYN mother yaw.

framboesia [Br.] SYN frambesia.

frame (frām) A structure made of parts fitted together.

frame of ref·er·ence (frām ref′ĕr-ĕns) In psychology, a set of standards or beliefs governing perceptual evaluation of social behavior.

Fran·ces·chet·ti syn·drome (frahn-ses-ket′ē sin′drōm) Mandibulofacial dysostosis, when complete or nearly complete.

Fran·ci·sel·la (fran-si-sel′lă) A genus of nonmotile, non-spore-forming, aerobic bacteria that contain small, gram-negative cocci and rods. These organisms are highly pleomorphic; they do not grow on plain agar or in liquid media without special enrichment; they are pathogenic and cause tularemia in humans.

Fran·ci·sel·la tu·la·ren·sis (fran-si-sel′lă tū-lă-ren′sis) A bacterial species that causes tularemia in humans, transmitted from wild animals by bloodsucking insects or by contact with infected animals such as rabbits and ticks; can penetrate unbroken skin to cause infection.

fran·ci·um (Fr) (fran′sē-ŭm) Radioactive element of the alkali metal series; atomic no. 87; half-life of most stable known isotope, ^{223}Fr, is 21.8 minutes.

Franc·ke nee·dle (frahng′kĕ nē′dĕl) Small, lancet-shaped, spring-activated needle, used to evacuate a small effusion of blood.

Fränt·zel mur·mur (frent′sel mŭr′mŭr) Murmur of mitral stenosis when louder at its beginning and end than in its midportion.

fra·ter·nal twins (fră-tĕr′năl twinz) SYN dizygotic twins.

Fraun·hof·er lines (frown′hō-fer līnz) SYN absorption lines.

Fra·zier nee·dle (frā′zhĕr nē′dĕl) One used to drain lateral ventricles of brain.

F.R.C.S. Abbreviation for Fellow of the Royal College of Surgeons.

freck·le (frek′ĕl) Yellowish or brownish macules developing on the exposed parts of the skin, especially in people with light complexions. SEE ALSO lentigo. SYN ephelis.

Fred·rick·son clas·si·fi·ca·tion (fred′ rik-sŏn klas′i-fi-kā′shŭn) Five-point scale for hyperlipoproteinemia that uses plasma appearance, triglyceride values, and total cholesterol values. SEE ALSO hyperlipoproteinemia.

free as·so·ci·a·tion (frē ă-sō′sē-ā′shŭn) An investigative psychoanalytic technique in which the patient verbalizes, without reservation or censorship, the passing contents of his or her mind; the conflicts verbalized are the basis of the psychoanalyst's interpretations.

free-bas·ing (frē′bās-ing) Smoking drugs, especially cocaine or heroin, in a purified or concentrated form.

free en·er·gy (F, F) (frē en′ĕr-jē) A thermodynamic function symbolized as F, or G (Gibbs free energy), $= H - TS$, where H is the enthalpy of a system, T the absolute temperature, and S the entropy.

free fat·ty ac·id (frē fat′ē as′id) A blood product that occurs due to the digestion of triglycerides.

free flap (frē flap) One in which donor vessels are divided, the tissue is transported to another area, and the flap is revascularized by anastomosis of vessels in the recipient bed to the artery and vein(s) of the flap.

free-float·ing an·xi·e·ty (frē′flōt-ing ang-zī′ĕ-tē) In psychoanalysis, a pervasive unrealistic expectation unattached to a clearly formulated concept or object of fear; observed particularly in anxiety neurosis and may be seen in some cases of latent schizophrenia.

free gin·gi·va (frē jin′ji-vă) That portion of the gingiva that surrounds the tooth but is not directly attached to the tooth surface.

free gin·gi·val groove (frē jinj′i-văl grūv) A shallow linear depression between attached and marginal gingiva.

free in·duc·tion de·cay (FID) (frē in-dŭk′shŭn dĕ-kā′) MAGNETIC RESONANCE IMAGING the decay curve that is detected by the radiofrequency coil after the application of an excitation pulse, without additional pulses (free).

free nerve end·ings (frē nĕrv end′ingz) A form of peripheral ending of sensory nerve fibers in which the terminal filaments end freely in the tissue.

free rad·i·cal (frē rad′i-kăl) A radical in its (usually transient) uncombined state; an atom or atom group carrying an unpaired electron and no charge. SYN radical (4).

free-rad·i·cal the·o·ry of ag·ing (frē′ rad′i-kăl thē′ŏr-ē āj′ing) The proposition that organisms age because they accumulate free radicals, which are the products of oxidation reactions, over the course of time.

free thy·rox·ine in·dex (FTI, FT₄I) (frē thī-rok′sēn in′deks) Arbitrary value obtained by multiplying the triiodothyronine uptake by the serum thyroxine concentration.

free wa·ter (frē waw′tĕr) Water in the body that can be removed by ultrafiltration and in which substances can be dissolved.

freeze-dry·ing (frēz′drī′ing) SYN lyophilization.

freeze frac·ture (frēz frak′shŭr) A procedure for preparing cells or other biologic samples for electron microscopy during which the sample is frozen quickly and then broken with a sharp blow. SYN cryofracture.

freez·ing point (fp, FP) (frēz′ing poynt) Temperature at which a liquid solidifies.

Frei·berg dis·ease (frī′bĕrg di-zēz′) Osteonecrosis of second metatarsal head.

frem·i·tus (frem′i-tŭs) A vibration imparted to the hand resting on the chest or other part of the body. SEE ALSO thrill.

frem·i·tus pec·to·ral·is (frem′i-tŭs pek-tō-rā′lis) Vibration on the chest wall produced by phonation.

French-A·mer·i·can-Bri·tish clas·si·fi·ca·tion sys·tem (FAB) (french′ ă-mer′i-kăn-brit′ish klas′i-fi-kāshŭn sis′ tĕm) A classification and nomenclature system for acute leukemias based on morphologic characteristics and cytochemical stain reactions. SEE ALSO myelodysplastic syndrome.

French scale (Fr) (french skāl) Assessment tool for grading sizes of sounds, tubules, and catheters as based on a measurement of 1/3 mm and equaling 1 Fr on the scale (e.g., 3 Fr = 1 mm).

Fren·kel ex·er·cis·es (frengk′ĕl ek′sĕr-sīz-ĕz) A system of therapeutic actions intended to palliate the effects of ataxic cerebral palsy.

fren·u·lo·plasty, fre·no·plas·ty (fren′yū-lō-plas-tē, fren′ō-plast-tē) Correction of an abnormally attached frenum by surgically repositioning it.

fren·u·lum, fre·num (fren′yū-lŭm, frē′nŭm) [TA] A small frenum or bridle. SYN habenula (1) [TA], frenum (3).

fre·num, pl. **fre·nums** (frē′nŭm, -nŭmz)
1. A narrow reflection or fold of mucous membrane passing from a more fixed to a movable part, serving to check undue movement of the part. **2.** An anatomic structure resembling such a fold. **3.** SYN frenulum.

fre·quen·cy (ν) (frē′kwĕn-sē) **1.** The number of regular recurrences in a given time, e.g., heartbeats, sound vibrations. **2.** ACOUSTICS the number of cycles of compression and rarefaction of a sound wave that occur in 1 second, expressed in hertz (Hz). **3.** The rate of vocal fold vibration (i.e., the number of times the glottis opens and closes in 1 second) during phonation.

fresh fro·zen plas·ma (FFP) (fresh frō′zĕn plaz′mă) Separated plasma, frozen within 6 hours of collection, used in hypovolemia and coagulation factor deficiency.

freud·i·an (froyd′ē-ăn) Relating to or described by the Viennese psychiatrist Sigmund Freud (1856–1939).

freud·i·an psy·cho·a·nal·y·sis (froyd′ē-ăn sī′kō-ă-nal′i-sis) The theory and practice of psychoanalysis and psychotherapy as developed by Sigmund Freud, based on: 1) his theory of personality, which postulates that psychic life is made up of instinctual and socially acquired forces, or the id, the ego, and a superego;

2) his discovery that the free-associated technique of verbalizing for the analyst all thoughts reveals the areas in conflict within a patient's personality; 3) that the vehicle for gaining this insight and readjusting one's personality is the learning a patient does, first developing a stormy emotional bond with the analyst (transference relationship) and next successfully learning to break this bond.

freu·di·an slip (froyd′ē-ăn slip) A mistake in speech or deed that presumably suggests some underlying motive, often sexual or aggressive.

Freund ad·ju·vant (froynd ad′jū-vănt) SEE adjuvant.

Freund a·nom·a·ly (froynd ă-nom′ă′lē) A narrowing of the upper aperture of the thorax by shortening the first rib and its cartilage.

Freund oper·a·tion (froynd op-ĕr-ā′shŭn) **1.** Total abdominal hysterectomy for uterine cancer. **2.** Chondrotomy to relieve Freund anomaly.

fri·a·ble (frī′ă-bĕl) **1.** Said of tissue that readily tears, fragments, or bleeds when gently palpated or manipulated. **2.** Easily reduced to powder. **3.** BACTERIOLOGY denoting a dry and brittle culture falling into powder when touched or shaken.

fric·tion (frik′shŭn) **1.** The act of rubbing the surface of an object against that of another; especially rubbing the limbs of the body to aid circulation. **2.** Force required for relative motion of two bodies in contact. **3.** Movements in massage intended to move superficial layers over deeper structures, to reach deeper tissues, or to create heat. Includes static, cross-fiber, and circular frictions.

fric·tion burn (frik′shŭn bŭrn) An injury caused by rubbing against a rough surface, which removes layers of the skin.

fric·tion force (frik′shŭn fōrs) Pressure resisting the relative motion of two surfaces in contact or a surface in contact with a fluid.

fric·tion frem·i·tus (frik′shŭn frem′i-tŭs) A palpable vibration felt by the physician's hand, which is placed on the patient's chest during the patient's coughing.

F

fric·tion sound (frik′shŭn sownd) Noise heard on auscultation made by the rubbing of two opposed serous surfaces roughened by an inflammatory exudate, or, if chronic, by nonadhesive fibrosis.

Fried·län·der pneu·mo·ni·a (frēd′lān-der nū-mō′nē-ă) A form of pneumonia caused by infection with *Klebsiella pneumoniae*, characteristically severe and lobar in distribution.

Fried·man test (frēd′măn test) A nonparametric measurement that compares three or more paired groups.

Fried·reich a·tax·i·a (frēd′rīk ă-tak′sē-ă) A neurologic disorder characterized by ataxia, dysarthria, scoliosis, high-arched foot or pes cavus, and paralysis of the muscles, especially of the lower extremities; onset usually in childhood or youth with sclerosis of the posterior and lateral columns of the spinal cord.

Fried·reich sign (frēd′rīk sīn) In adherent pericardium, sudden collapse of the previously distended veins of the neck at each diastole of the heart.

Fried rule (frēd rūl) A method to calculate the pediatric dose of a medication: multiply the child's age in months by the adult dose of the medication and divide the result by 150.

frig·id (frij′id) **1.** SYN cold. **2.** Temperamentally, especially sexually, unresponsive.

fri·gid·i·ty (fri-jid′i-tē) **1.** Inability in the female to achieve orgasm or any other satisfactory level of sexual response. **2.** The state of being frigid (2).

frit (frit) **1.** The material from which the glaze for artificial teeth is made. **2.** A powdered pigment material used in coloring the porcelain of artificial teeth.

Fröh·lich dwarf·ism (froy′lik dwŏrf′izm) Dwarfism with Fröhlich syndrome.

frôle·ment (frol-mawn[h]′) **1.** Light friction or massage with the palm of the hand. **2.** A rustling sound heard in auscultation.

frons, gen. **fron·tis** (fronz, fron′tis) [TA] SYN forehead.

front·ad (frŏn′tad) Toward the front.

fron·tal, fron·ta·lis (frŏn′tăl, frŏn-tā′lis) [TA] In front, relating to the anterior part of the body.

fron·tal cortex (frŏn′tăl kōr′teks) Cortex of the frontal lobe of the cerebral hemisphere. SYN frontal area.

fron·tal crest (frŏn′tăl krest) [TA] Ridge ascending from the foramen cecum to the origin of the sagittal sulcus on the cerebral surface of the frontal bone. SYN crista frontalis [TA].

fron·tal lobe de·men·ti·a (frŏn′tăl lōb dĕ-men′shē-ă) Progressive mental disorder with atrophy of the frontal and temporal lobes of the brain, affecting mainly behavior and language and characterized by gradual personality changes, speech impairment, and eventual dementia. SYN Pick disease, frontal-temporal dementia.

fron·tal lobe ep·i·lep·sy (frŏn′tăl lōb ep′i-lep-sē) A disorder with seizures originating in the frontal lobe of the brain.

fron·tal lobe of cer·e·brum (frŏn′tăl lōb ser′ĕ-brŭm) [TA] The portion of each cerebral hemisphere anterior to the central sulcus. Sometimes called frontal lobe.

fron·tal lobe syn·drome (frŏn′tăl lōb sin′drōm) Constellation of symptoms associated with damage to the frontal lobe of the brain that includes impairment of planning function, lack of inhibition, hypomania, depression, apathy, and neglect of personal appearance.

fron·tal lo·bot·o·my (frŏn′tăl lō-bot′ŏ-mē) A surgical treatment for severe psychiatric disorders that reduces distress but often blunts emotion and personality.

fron·tal nerve (frŏn′tăl nĕrv) [TA] A branch of the ophthalmic nerve that divides within the orbit into the supratrochlear and the supraorbital nerves. SYN nervus frontalis [TA].

fron·tal pole (frŏn′tăl pōl) [TA] SYN frontal pole [TA] of cerebrum.

fron·tal pole of cer·e·brum (frŏn′tăl

pōl ser'ĕ-brŭm) The most anterior promontory of each cerebral hemisphere.

fron·tal pro·cess of max·il·la (frŏn'tăl pros'es mak-sil'ă) Upward extension from the maxillary body, which articulates with the frontal bone.

fron·tal si·nus (frŏn'tăl sī'nŭs) [TA] A hollow paranasal sinus formed on either side in the lower part of the squama of the frontal bone; it communicates by the ethmoidal infundibulum with the middle meatus of the nasal cavity of the same side.

fron·tal tri·an·gle (frŏn'tăl trī'ang-gĕl) Area bounded above by the maximum frontal diameter and laterally by lines joining the extremities of this diameter with the glabella.

fron·to·an·te·ri·or po·si·tion (frŏn'tō-an-tēr'ē-ŏr pŏ-zish'ŏn) A cephalic presentation of the fetus with its forehead directed toward the right (right frontoanterior, RFA) or to the left (left frontoanterior, LFA) of the acetabulum of the mother.

fron·to·max·il·lar·y (frŏn'tō-mak'si-lar-ē) Relating to the frontal and the maxillary bones.

fron·to·na·sal dys·pla·si·a (frŏn'tō-nā'zăl dis-plā'zē-ă) An uncommon disorder characterized by abnormalities affecting the head and facial region including widely spaced eyes, broad flat nose, and a vertical groove down the middle of the face. SYN median cleft face syndrome.

fron·to·na·sal prom·i·nence, fron·to·na·sal pro·cess (frŏn'tō-nā'zăl prom'i-nĕns, pro'ses) Unpaired embryonic prominence formed by the tissues surrounding the forebrain vesicle. SYN forebrain eminence, forebrain prominence.

fron·to·oc·cip·i·tal (frŏn'tō-ok-sip'i-tăl) Relating to the frontal and the occipital bones, or to the forehead and the occiput.

fron·to·pa·ri·e·tal (FP) (frŏn'tō-păr-ī'ĕ-tăl) Relating to the frontal and the parietal bones.

fron·to·pos·te·ri·or po·si·tion (frŏn'tō-pos-tēr'ē-ŏr pŏ-zish'ŏn) Fetal cephalic presentation with its forehead directed toward the right (right frontoposterior, RFP) or to the left (left frontoposterior, LFP) sacroiliac articulation of the mother.

fron·to·tem·po·ral (frŏn'tō-tem'pŏr-ăl) Relating to the frontal and the temporal bones.

fron·to·trans·verse po·si·tion (frŏn'tō-tranz-vĕrs' pŏ-zish'ŏn) A cephalic presentation of the fetus with its forehead directed toward the right (right frontotransverse, RFT) or to the left (left frontotransverse, LFT) iliac fossa of the mother.

front-tap re·flex (frŏnt'tap rē'fleks) Contraction of the gastrocnemius muscle when the shin is struck. SYN front-tap contraction, Gowers contraction.

frost (frawst) A deposit resembling that of frozen vapor or dew.

frost·bite (frawst'bīt) Local tissue destruction resulting from exposure to extreme cold; in mild cases, produces superficial, reversible freezing followed by erythema and slight pain (frostnip); in severe cases, can be painless or paresthetic and result in blistering, edema, and gangrene; currently treated by rapid rewarming.

frost·ed branch an·gi·i·tis (frawst'ĕd branch an'jē-ī'tis) Inflammation of blood vessels with sheathing giving the appearance of branches on a tree.

frost·ed liv·er (frawst'ĕd liv'ĕr) Hyaloserositis of the liver.

Frost su·ture (frawst sū'chŭr) Intermarginal suture between the eyelids to protect the cornea.

frot·tage (fraw-tahzh') 1. The rubbing movement in massage. 2. SYN frotteurism.

frot·teur (fraw-tur') One sexually excited by frottage.

frot·teur·ism (fraw'tur-izm) Sexual gratification derived from rubbing a bodily area against another person, often a stranger, in an inappropriate way. SYN frottage (1).

fro·zen pel·vis (frō′zĕn pel′vis) Disorder in which the true pelvis is indurated throughout, especially by carcinoma. SYN hardened pelvis.

fro·zen sec·tion (FS, FZ, FX, F/S) (frō′zĕn sek′shŭn) Thin slice of tissue cut from a frozen specimen, used for rapid microscopic diagnosis.

F.R.S.C. Abbreviation for Fellow of the Royal Society (Canada).

fructo- Chemical prefix denoting the fructose configuration.

fruc·to·fu·ra·nose (fruk′tō-fūr′ă-nōs) Fructose in furanose form.

fruc·to·ki·nase (fruk′tō-kī′nās) A liver enzyme that catalyzes the reaction of adenosine triphosphate and D-fructose to form fructose-6-phosphate and adenosine diphosphate; deficient in patients with essential fructosuria (hepatic fructokinase deficiency).

fructosaemia [Br.] SYN fructosemia.

fruc·to·sa·mine test (fruk-tō′să-mēn test) Assessment to help control the blood sugar levels of a diabetic patient during rapid changes in treatment, pregnancy, and erythrocyte loss. SYN glycated serum protein, glycated albumin.

fruc·tose (fruk′tōs) A ketohexose; the D-isomer (also called fruit sugar, levulose, and D-*arabino*-2-hexulose) found in fruits and honey and is a product of sucrose hydrolysis. It can be metabolized or converted to glucose.

fruc·tose in·tol·er·ance (fruk′tōs in-tol′ĕr-ăns) A digestive disorder of the small intestine in which the fructose carrier in enterocytes is deficient. SYN fructose malabsorption, dietary fructose intolerance.

fruc·tose in·tol·er·ance breath test (fruk′tōs in-tol′ĕr-ăns breth test) An assessment used to determine inability to digest fructose.

fruc·to·se·mi·a (fruk′tō-sē′mē-ă) Presence of fructose in the circulating blood.

fruc·to·side (fruk′tō-sīd) Fructose in –C–O– linkage where the –C–O–

group is the original 2 group of the fructose.

fruc·to·su·ri·a (fruk′tō-syūr′ē-ă) Excretion of fructose in the urine.

FTA-ABS test (test) SEE fluorescent treponemal antibody-absorption test.

Fuchs ad·e·no·ma (fūks ad′ĕ-nō′mă) A benign epithelial tumor of the nonpigmented epithelium of the ciliary body, rarely exceeding 1 mm in diameter.

fuch·sin (fūk′sin) A nonspecific term referring to any of several red rosanilin dyes used as stains in histology and bacteriology.

fuch·sin·o·phil granule (fūk-sin′ō-fil gran′yūl) A granule that has an affinity for fuchsin.

Fuchs syn·drome (fūks sin′drŏm) Condition characterized by corneal degeneration, heterochromia of the iris, iridocyclitis, keratic precipitates, and cataract. SYN Fuchs heterochromic cyclitis.

Fuchs u·ve·i·tis (fūks yū′vē-ī′tis) SYN heterochromic uveitis.

fu·cose (Fuc) (fū′kōs) 6-Deoxygalactose; a methylpentose, the L-configuration of which occurs in the mucopolysaccharides of the blood group substances, in human milk (as a polysaccharide), and elsewhere in nature. SYN rhodeose.

fu·co·si·do·sis (fū′kō-si-dō′sis) A metabolic storage disease characterized by accumulation of fucose-containing glycolipids and deficiency of the enzyme α-fucosidase; progressive neurologic deterioration begins after the first year of life, accompanied by spasticity, tremor, and mild skeletal changes.

fu·gac·i·ty (f) (fyū-gas′i-tē) Tendency of fluid molecules, as a result of all forces acting on them, to exit a given site in the body; the escaping tendency of a fluid, as in diffusion, evaporation, and the like.

-fugal Suffix meaning movement away from the part indicated by the main portion of the word.

-fuge Suffix meaning flight, denoting the place from which flight takes place or that which is put to flight.

fugue (fyūg) Psychological disorder in which a person suddenly abandons a present activity or lifestyle and starts a new and different one, often in a different city; afterward, alleges amnesia for events occurring during the fugue state, although earlier events are remembered and habits and skills are usually unaffected.

Fu·ku·ya·ma type mus·cu·lar dys·tro·phy (fū-kū-yah´mah tīp mŭs´kyū-lăr dis´trŏ-fē) A rare inherited muscle-wasting disease found primarily in Japan and characterized by mental retardation and muscle weakness that begins in infancy.

ful·gu·ra·tion, di·rect ful·gu·ra·tion, in·di·rect ful·gu·ra·tion (fulg) (ful´gŭr-ā´shŭn, dĭr-ekt, in-dĭr-ekt´) Destruction of tissue by means of a high-frequency electric current.

full liq·uid diet (ful lik´wid dī´ĕt) Nutritional regimen involving clear liquids and soft foods, including juices, broth, ice cream, yogurt, honey, jelly, milk, liquid meal replacements, milk shakes, pudding, and similar foods.

full-risk HMO (ful-risk) A health care company fully capitated to include a wide range of benefits across preventive, primary, and acute care services.

full-thick·ness burn (ful-thik´nĕs bŭrn) One involving destruction of the entire skin; deep full-thickness burns extend into subcutaneous tissue, muscle, or bone and often cause much scarring. SYN third-degree burn.

full-thick·ness graft (ful-thik´nĕs graft) A graft of the full thickness of mucosa and submucosa or of skin and subcutaneous tissue.

full-weight-bear·ing (ful wāt bār´ing) Denotes a patient's ability to place entire body weight on the feet.

ful·mi·nant hep·a·ti·tis (ful´mi-nănt hep-ă-tī´tis) Severe, rapidly progressive loss of hepatic function due to viral infection or other cause of inflammatory destruction of liver tissue with associated coagulopathy and encephalopathy.

ful·mi·nate (ful´mi-nāt) Denotes violently explosive, (e.g., a chemical compound containing the fumanate ion or friction-sensitive explosives.

ful·mi·na·ting ap·pen·di·ci·tis (ful´mi-nāt-ing ă-pen´di-sī´tis) A form of the disorder that develops suddenly and severely.

fu·ma·rate hy·dra·tase, fu·ma·rase (fū´măr-āt hī´drā-tās, fū´mă-rās) An enzyme catalyzing the reversible interconversion of fumaric acid and water to malic acid; deficiency leads to mental retardation.

fu·mar·ic ac·id (fyū-mar´ik as´id) A trans-butanedioic acid; an unsaturated dicarboxylic acid occurring as an intermediate in the tricarboxylic acid cycle.

fu·mi·ga·tion (fyū´mi-gā´shŭn) Fumigating; use of a fumigant.

fum·ing (fyūm´ing) Giving forth a visible vapor, a property of concentrated nitric, sulfuric, and hydrochloric acids, and of certain other substances.

func·ti·o lae·sa (fŭnk´shē-ō lē´să) Impaired function; a fifth sign of inflammation added by Galen to those enunciated by Celsus (rubor, tumor, calor, and dolor).

func·tion (fŭngk´shŭn) **1.** The special action or physiologic property of an organ or other part of the body. **2.** To perform its special work or office, said of an organ or other part of the body. **3.** The general properties of any substance, depending on its chemical character and relation to other substances, according to which it may be grouped among acids, bases, alcohols, esters, or other groups. **4.** A particular reactive grouping in a molecule; e.g., a functional group, such as the –OH group of an alcohol. **5.** A quality, trait, or fact that is so related to another as to be dependent on and to vary with this other.

func·tion·al (fŭngk´shŭn-ăl) **1.** Relating to a function. **2.** Not organic in origin; denoting a disorder with no known or detectable organic basis to explain the symptoms. SEE neurosis.

func·tion·al ac·ti·vi·ty (fŭngk´shŭn-ăl ak-tiv´i-tē) **1.** A task or act that allows one to meet the demands of the environment and daily life. **2.** Activity essential to support the physical, social, and psychological well-being of a person.

func·tion·al age (fŭngk´shŭn-ăl āj) A patient who manifests the development and behaviors of a particular age group, which are not necessarily typical of the chronologic age of the person.

func·tion·al blind·ness (fŭngk´shŭn-ăl blīnd´nĕs) Apparent loss of vision without discernible physical cause.

func·tion·al cas·tra·tion (fŭngk´shŭn-ăl kast-rā´shŭn) Gonadal atrophy produced by prolonged treatment with sex hormones or gonadotropin-releasing hormone superagonists or antagonists. SYN medical castration.

func·tion·al con·ges·tion (fŭngk´shŭn-ăl kŏn-jes´chŭn) Hyperemia occurring during functional activity of an organ.

func·tion·al dis·or·der, func·tion·al dis·ease (fŭngk´shŭn-ăl dis-ōr´dĕr, di-zēz´) A physical disorder with no known or detectable organic basis to explain the symptoms. SEE behavior disorder, neurosis. SYN functional illness.

func·tion·al dys·pep·si·a (fŭngk´shŭn-ăl dis-pep´sē-ă) 1. SYN atonic dyspepsia. 2. SYN nervous dyspepsia.

func·tion·al e·lec·tric stim·u·la·tion (FES) (fŭngk´shŭn-ăl ĕ-lek´trik stim´yū-lā´shŭn) A multiple-channel electrotherapeutic modality that uses pulsatile waveforms to activate a muscle or group of muscles in an activity (e.g., walking, reaching up).

func·tion·al ge·nom·ics (fŭngk´shŭn-ăl jē-nō´miks) The study of expressed genes in organisms, including the identity of the genes and the factors that control differential expression.

func·tion·al hear·ing loss (fŭngk´shŭn-ăl hēr´ing laws) Acoustic disorder involving a psychological or emotional problem, rather than physical damage to the hearing pathway; the person does not seem to hear or understand but in reality has normal hearing.

func·tion·al im·ag·ing (fŭngk´shŭn-ăl im´āj-ing) Modality for measurement of changes in metabolism, blood flow, regional chemical composition, and absorption in an organ or tissue. SYN functional medical imaging.

func·tion·al mag·net·ic re·so·nance im·ag·ing (fMRI, f-MRI) (fŭngk´shŭn-ăl mag-net´ik rez´ŏ-năns im´āj-ing) Brain activity revealed by manipulating the MR signal to show regional oxygen uptake.

func·tion·al neu·ro·sur·gery (fŭngk´shŭn-ăl nūr´ō-sŭr´jĕr-ē) Destruction or chronic excitation of a part of the brain to treat disordered behavior or function.

func·tion·al oc·clu·sal har·mo·ny (fŭngk´shŭn-ăl ŏ-klū´zăl hahr´mŏ-nē) Relationship of opposing teeth in all functional ranges and movements so as to provide the greatest masticatory efficiency without causing undue strain or trauma on the supporting tissues, teeth, and muscles.

func·tion·al oc·clu·sion (fŭngk´shŭn-ăl ŏ-klū´zhŭn) 1. Any tooth contacts made within the functional range of the opposing teeth surfaces. 2. Occlusion that occurs during function.

func·tion·al path·ol·o·gy (fŭngk´shŭn-ăl pă-thol´ŏ-jē) Pathology pertaining to abnormalities in function of a tissue, organ, or part, with or without associated changes in structure.

func·tion·al pro·gres·sion (fŭngk´shŭn-ăl prŏ-gresh´ŏn) 1. A program of exercises designed to develop balanced mobility, active stability, and integrated strength in rehabilitation of a muscle group. 2. In mental health, the measurement of increase or decrease of intellectual function.

func·tion·al re·sid·u·al ca·pa·ci·ty (FRC) (fŭngk´shŭn-ăl rĕ-zid´yū-ăl kă-pas´i-tē) Volume of gas remaining in the lungs at the end of a normal expiration; sum of expiratory reserve volume and residual volume. SYN functional residual air.

func·tion·al splint (fŭngk´shŭn-ăl splint) 1. SYN dynamic splint. 2. The joining of two or more teeth into a rigid unit by means of fixed restorations that cover all or part of the abutment teeth.

fun·dal pla·cen·ta (fŭn´dăl plă-sen´tă)

Placenta implanted at the base (fundus) of the uterus.

fun·da·men·tal fre·quen·cy (F0) (fŭn′dă-men′tăl frē′kwĕn-sē) **1.** ACOUSTICS basic frequency of a vibrating object or sound as opposed to its harmonics, or the principal component of a complex sound wave. **2.** Frequency of vocal fold vibration at the glottis, unaffected by resonance. SEE ALSO optimal pitch.

fun·dec·to·my (fŭn-dek′tŏ-mē) SYN fundusectomy.

fun·di·form (fŭn′di-fōrm) Looped; sling-shaped.

fun·do·pli·ca·tion (fŭn′dō-pli-kā′shŭn) Suture of the fundus of the stomach completely or partially around the gastroesophageal junction to treat gastroesophageal reflux disease.

fun·dus, pl. **fun·di** (fŭn′dŭs, -dī) [TA] The bottom or lowest part of a sac or hollow organ; that part farthest removed from the opening or exit; occasionally a broad cul-de-sac.

fun·du·scope (fŭn′dŭ-skōp) SYN ophthalmoscope.

fun·du·sec·to·my (fŭn′dŭ-sek′tŏ-mē) Excision of the fundus of an organ. SYN fundectomy.

fungaemia [Br.] SYN fungemia.

fun·gal, fun·gous (fŭng′găl, -gŭs) Relating to a fungus. SYN fungous.

fun·gal in·fec·tion of nails (fŭng′găl in-fek′shŭn nālz) Thickened discolored toenails and fingernails caused by othogenic fungi on the nail bed, matrix, or plate. SYN onychomycosis.

fun·gate (fŭng′gāt) To grow exuberantly like a fungus or spongy growth.

fun·ge·mi·a (fŭn-jē′mē-ă) Fungal infection disseminated by way of the bloodstream. SYN fungaemia.

Fun·gi (fŭn′jī) A kingdom of eukaryotic organisms that grow in irregular masses, without roots, stems, or leaves, and are devoid of chlorophyll or other pigments capable of photosynthesis; reproduce sexually or asexually (spore formation), and may obtain nutrition from other living organisms as parasites or from dead organic matter as saprobes (saprophytes). SEE ALSO kingdom.

fun·gi·ci·dal (fŭn-ji-sī′dăl) Having a killing action on fungi.

fun·gi·cide (fŭn′ji-sīd) Any substance that has a killing action on fungi.

fun·gi·form (fŭn′ji-fōrm) Shaped like a fungus or mushroom; applied to any structure with a broad, often branched, free portion and a narrower base.

fun·gi·form pa·pil·lae (fŭn′ji-fōrm pă-pil′ē) [TA] Numerous minute elevations on the dorsum of the tongue with tips being broader than bases; epithelium of many such papillae has taste buds.

fun·gi·sta·sis (fŭn′ji-stā′sis) Inhibition of the growth of fungi.

fun·gi·stat (fŭn′ji-stat) An agent having fungistatic action.

fun·gi·stat·ic (fŭn′ji-stat′ik) Having an inhibiting action on the growth of fungi. SYN mycostatic.

fun·gi·tox·ic (fŭn′ji-tok′sik) Poisonous or in any way deleterious to the growth of fungi.

fun·goid (fŭng′goyd) Resembling a fungus; denoting an exuberant morbid growth on the surface of the body.

fun·gus, pl. **fun·gi** (fŭng′gŭs, fŭn′jī) A general term used to encompass the diverse morphologic forms of yeasts and molds. Originally classified as primitive plants without chlorophyll, the fungi are placed in the kingdom Fungi and some in the kingdom Protista, along with algae, protozoa, and slime molds.

fun·gus ball (fŭng′gŭs bawl) Compact mass of fungal mycelium and cellular debris, 1–5 cm in diameter, residing within a lung cavity, paranasal sinus, or urinary tract.

fu·nic (fyū′nik) Relating to the funis, or umbilical cord. SYN funicular (2).

fu·ni·cle (fyū′ni-kĕl) SYN cord.

fu·nic pre·sen·ta·tion (fyū′nik prez′ĕn-tā′shŭn) A birth presentation in which the umbilical cord is between the presenting part of the fetus and the internal os of the uterine cervix, potentially cutting off circulation in the umbilical cord; also called cord presentation. SYN umbilical cord prolapse.

fu·nic souf·fle, fu·nic·u·lar souf·fle (fyū′nik sū′fĕl, fŭ-nik′yū-lăr) SYN fetal souffle.

fu·nic·u·lar graft (fŭn-ik′yū-lăr graft) Nerve graft in which each funiculus (composed of two or more fasciculi) is approximated separately.

fu·ni·cu·lar her·ni·a (fŭn-ik′yū-lăr hĕr′nē-ă) An indirect inguinal hernia that includes part of the umbilical or spermatic cord.

fu·nic·u·lar part of duc·tus def·e·rens (fŭn-ik′yū-lăr pahrt dŭk′tŭs def′ĕr-enz) [TA] Portion of the ductus deferens contained within the spermatic cord. SYN pars funicularis ductus deferentis [TA].

fu·nic·u·lar pro·cess (fŭn-ik′yū-lăr pros′es) Tunica vaginalis surrounding the spermatic cord.

fu·nic·u·li·tis (fŭn-ik′yū-lī′tis) 1. Inflammation of a funiculus, especially of the spermatic cord. 2. Inflammation of the umbilical cord usually associated with chorioamnionitis.

fu·nic·u·lo·ep·i·di·dy·mi·tis (fŭn-ik′yū-lō-ep′i-did-i-mī′tis) Inflammation of the spermatic cord and the epididymis.

fu·nic·u·lus, pl. **fu·nic·u·li** (fŭn-ik′yū-lŭs, -lī) [TA] SYN cord (1).

fu·nic·u·lus sper·mat·i·cus (fŭn-ik′yū-lŭs spĕr-mat′i-kŭs) [TA] SYN spermatic cord.

fu·ni·form (fyū′ni-fōrm) Ropelike.

fu·nis (fyū′nis) 1. SYN umbilical cord. 2. A cordlike structure.

fu·ni·si·tis (fyū′ni-sī′tis) Inflammation of the umbilical cord.

fun·nel breast, fun·nel chest (fŭn′ĕl brest, chest) SYN pectus excavatum.

fun·ny bone (fŭn′ē bōn) Colloquial name for tip of olecranon.

fu·ra·nose (fyūr′ă-nōs) A saccharide unit or molecule containing the furan grouping.

fur·cal (fŭr′kăl) Forked.

fur·cal nerve (fŭr′kăl nĕrv) SYN fourth lumbar nerve [L4].

fur·ca·tion (fŭr-kā′shŭn) 1. A forking, or a forklike part or branch. 2. In dental anatomy, the region of a multirooted tooth at which the roots divide.

fur·fu·ra·ceous (fŭr′fŭr-ā′shŭs) Branny, or composed of small scales; denoting a form of desquamation. SYN pityroid.

fu·ror ep·i·lep·ti·cus (fyūr′ŏr ep′i-lep′ti-kŭs) Bursts of anger to which people with epilepsy are occasionally subject, occurring without apparent provocation or disturbance of consciousness.

fu·ro·se·mide (fyū-rō′sĕ-mīd) Loop diuretic that inhibits reabsorption of sodium and chloride in the ascending loop of Henle. SYN frusemide.

fur·row (fŭr′ō) A groove or sulcus.

fur·rowed tongue (fŭr′ōd tŭng) A painless condition marked by numerous longitudinal grooves on the lingual surface. SYN scrotal tongue.

fu·run·cle, fu·run·cu·lus (fŭr-ŭng′kĕl, -kyū-lŭs) A localized pyogenic infection, most frequently by *Staphylococcus aureus*, originating deep in a hair follicle. SYN boil, furunculus.

fu·run·cu·lar (fū-rŭng′kyū-lăr) Relating to a furuncle. SYN furunculous.

fu·run·cu·lo·sis (fŭr-ŭng′kyū-lō′sis) A condition marked by the presence of furuncles, often chronic and recurrent.

fu·run·cu·lous (fŭr-ŭng′kyū-lŭs) SYN furuncular.

Fu·sar·i·um (fyū-sā′rē-ŭm) A genus of rapidly growing fungi producing characteristic sickle-shaped, multiseptate macroconidia that can be mistaken for those produced by some dermatophytes; some species produce corneal ulcers; some are common colonizers of burned skin.

fused kid·ney (fyūzd kid′nē) A single,

anomalous organ resulting from fusion of the two primordia of the kidneys.

fused vul·va (fyūzd vŭl´vă) Condition in which a girl's labia are stuck together, leaving either a small opening or none; normally resolves without treatment. SYN fused labia.

fu·si·form (fyū´si-fŏrm) Spindle-shaped; tapering at both ends.

fu·si·form mus·cle (fyū´si-fŏrm mŭs´ĕl) [TA] One with a fleshy belly, tapering at either extremity. SYN musculus fusiformis [TA], spindle-shaped muscle.

fu·si·mo·tor (fyū´si-mō´tŏr) Pertaining to the efferent innervation of intrafusal muscle fibers by gamma motor neurons. SEE ALSO neuromuscular spindle.

fu·sion (fyū´zhŭn) **1.** Liquefaction, as by melting by heat. **2.** Union, as by joining together. **3.** The blending of slightly different images from each eye into a single perception. **4.** The joining of two or more adjacent teeth during their development by a dentinal union. SEE ALSO concrescence. **5.** Joining of two genes, often neighboring genes. **6.** The joining of two bones into a single unit, thereby obliterating motion between the two.

fu·sion pro·tein (fyū´zhŭn prō´tēn) Biotechnologic product targeting malignant cells and some normal lymphocytes containing interleukin-2 receptors; used to treat patients with advanced and recurrent cutaneous T-cell lymphoma.

Fu·so·bac·te·ri·um **(FB)** (fū´zō-bak-tēr´ē-ŭm) A genus of bacteria containing gram-negative, non-spore-forming, obligately anaerobic rods that produce butyric acid as a major metabolic product; found in cavities of humans and other animals; some species are pathogenic.

Fu·so·bac·te·ri·um   nu·cle·a·tum (fū´zō-bak-tēr´ē-ŭm nū-klē-ā´tŭm) A species that is found indigenously in gingival crevices; involved in infections of the upper respiratory tract and pleural cavity. SYN Vincent bacillus.

fu·so·cel·lu·lar (fyū´zō-sel´yū-lăr) Spindle-celled.

fu·so·spi·ro·chet·al dis·ease (fyū´zō-spī´rō-kē´tăl di-zēz´) Infection of the mouth and/or pharynx associated with fusiform bacilli and spirochetes, commonly part of the normal flora of the mouth. SEE ALSO necrotizing ulcerative gingivitis.

fu·so·spi·ro·chet·al gin·gi·vi·tis (fyū´zō-spī-rō-kē´tăl jin´ji-vī´tis) SYN necrotizing ulcerative gingivitis.

Fut·cher line (fuch´ĕr līn) A dorsoventral line of pigmentation occurring symmetrically and bilaterally for about 10 cm along the lateral edge of the biceps muscle.

fu tzu (fū tsū) SYN aconite.

F waves (wāvz) The waves of atrial flutter usually best seen in electrocardiographic leads 2, 3, and AVF. (A lowercase f indicates atrial fibrillation).

G

γ 1. Third letter in the Greek alphabet, gamma. **2.** In chemistry, denotes the third in a series, the fourth carbon in an aliphatic acid, or position 2 removed from the α position in the benzene ring. **3.** Symbol for 10^{-4} gauss; surface tension; activity coefficient; microgram.

G1 Symbol for gap_1 period.

G2 Symbol for gap_2 period.

Ga Symbol for gallium.

gad·o·lin·i·um (Gd) (gad′ō-lin′ē-ŭm) An element of the lanthanide group; magnetic properties of this element are used in contrast media for magnetic resonance imaging.

gag (gag) **1.** To retch; to cause to retch or heave. **2.** To prevent from talking. **3.** An instrument adjusted between the teeth to keep the mouth from closing during operations in the mouth or throat.

gag re·flex (gag rē′fleks) Contact of a foreign body with the mucous membrane of the fauces causing retching or gagging.

gain (gān) **1.** Profit; advantage. **2.** The ratio of output to input of an amplifying system, generally expressed in decibels.

gait (gāt) Manner of walking, characterized by rhythm, cadence, step length, stride length, and velocity.

Gait As·sess·ment Rat·ing Scale (gāt ă-ses′mĕnt rāt′ing skāl) A measure used to assess ambulation and associated risk of falling.

ga·lac·ta·gogue (gă-lak′tă-gog) An agent that promotes the secretion and flow of milk.

ga·lac·tan (gă-lak′tan) A polymer of galactose occurring naturally, along with galacturonans and arabans, in pectins, e.g., agar. SYN galactosans.

♻ **galacto-, galact-** Prefix denoting milk.

ga·lac·to·cele (gă-lak′tō-sēl) Retention cyst caused by occlusion of a lactiferous duct. SYN lactocele.

ga·lac·tog·ra·phy (gal′ak-tog′ră-fē) Mammographic imaging of lactiferous ducts using retrograde introduction of contrast material. SYN ductography.

ga·lac·to·ki·nase (gă-lak′tō-kī′nās) An enzyme (phosphotransferase) that, in the presence of adenosine triphosphate, catalyzes the phosphorylation of D-galactose to D-galactose-1-phosphate.

ga·lac·to·ki·nase de·fi·cien·cy (gă-lak′tō-kī′nās dĕ-fish′ĕn-sē) Inborn error of metabolism due to congenital deficiency of galactokinase (GALK), resulting in increased blood galactose concentration (galactosemia), cataracts, hepatomegaly, and mental deficiency.

ga·lac·to·phore (gă-lak′tō-fōr) SYN lactiferous ducts.

ga·lac·to·pho·ri·tis (gă-lak′tō-fōr-ī′tis) Inflammation of the milk ducts.

gal·ac·toph·o·rous (gal′ak-tof′ŏr-ŭs) Conveying milk.

ga·lac·to·poi·e·sis (gă-lak′tō-poy-ē′sis) Milk production.

ga·lac·to·poi·et·ic (gă-lak′tō-poy-et′ik) Pertaining to galactopoiesis.

ga·lac·tor·rhe·a (gă-lak′tŏr-ē′ă) **1.** Any persistent white discharge from the nipple that looks like milk. **2.** Continued discharge of milk from the breasts between intervals of nursing or after the child has been weaned. SYN incontinence of milk, lactorrhea.

galactorrhoea [Br.] SYN galactorrhea.

galactosaemia [Br.] SYN galactosemia.

ga·lac·tose (Gal) (gă-lak′tōs) An aldohexose found (in D form) as a constituent of lactose, cerebrosides, gangliosides, mucoproteins, in galactoside or galactosyl combination.

ga·lac·tose breath test (gă-lak′tōs breth test) An accurate and noninvasive assessment of liver function.

ga·lac·tose cat·a·ract (gă-lak′tōs kat′ăr-akt) A neonatal cataract associated with intralenticular accumulation of galactose alcohol. SEE galactosemia.

ga·lac·to·se·mi·a (gă-lak′tō-sē′mē-ă)

An inborn error of galactose metabolism. SYN galactosaemia.

ga·lac·tose tol·er·ance test (GALTT) (gă-lak′tōs tol′ĕr-ăns test) Liver function test, based on the ability of the liver to convert galactose to glycogen, measured by the rate of excretion of galactose following ingestion or intravenous injection of a known amount.

ga·lac·to·side (gă-lak′tō-sīd) A compound in which the H of the OH group on carbon-1 of galactose is replaced by an organic radical.

gal·ac·to·sis (gă-lak-tō′sis) Formation of milk by the lacteal glands.

ga·lac·to·ther·a·py (gă-lak′tō-thār′ă-pē) Treatment of disease by means of an exclusive or nearly exclusive milk diet.

ga·le·a (gā′lē-ă) **1.** A body structure shaped like a helmet. **2.** A form of bandage covering the head. **3.** SYN caul (1).

Gal·e·a·ti glands (gahl-ā-ah′tē glandz) SYN intestinal glands.

ga·len·i·cals (gă-len′i-kălz) **1.** Herbs and other vegetable drugs, as distinguished from the mineral or chemical remedies. **2.** Crude drugs and the tinctures, decoctions, and other preparations made from them, as distinguished from the alkaloids and other active principles. **3.** Remedies prepared according to an official formula.

gall (gawl) **1.** SYN bile. **2.** An excoriation or erosion.

gal·la·mine tri·eth·i·o·dide (gal′ă-mēn trī′eth-ī′ō-dīd) A triple quaternary ammonium compound with action comparable with that of curarine.

gall·blad·der (gawl′blad-ĕr) [TA] A pear-shaped receptacle located on the inferior surface of the liver, in a hollow between the right lobe and the quadrate lobe; it serves as a storage reservoir for bile in the organ. SYN cholecystis.

Gal·lie trans·plant (gal′ē trans′plant) Narrow strips of the femoral fascia lata used for suture material.

gal·li·um (Ga) (gal′ē-ŭm) A rare metal, atomic no. 31, atomic wt. 69.723.

gal·li·um scan (gal′ē-ŭm skan) A nuclear medicine test that uses a special camera to take pictures of specific tissues in the body after a radioactive tracer has been administered to make them more visible.

gal·lon (gal, gal., GAL) (gal′ŏn) A measure of U.S. liquid capacity containing 4 quarts, 231 in^3, or 8.3293 pounds of distilled water at 20°C; it is the equivalent of 3.785412 L. The British imperial gallon contains 277.4194 cu. in.

gal·lop, gal·lop rhythm (G) (gal′ŏp, ridh′ŭm) Triple cadence to heart sounds; due to an abnormal third or fourth heart sound being heard in addition to the first and second sounds; usually indicates of serious disease. SYN bruit de galop, cantering rhythm, Traube bruit.

gall·stone (gawl′stōn) A concretion in the gallbladder or a bile duct, composed chiefly of a mixture of cholesterol, calcium bilirubinate, and calcium carbonate. SYN cholelith.

gall·stone colic (gawl′stōn kol′ik) SYN biliary colic.

gal·oche chin (ga-lōsh′ chin) A chin that is exceptionally narrow and protuberant.

gal·van·ic (Galv, galv) (gal-van′ik) Pertaining to galvanism. SYN voltaic.

gal·van·ic cur·rent (gal-van′ik kŭr′rĕnt) Low-voltage direct current.

gal·van·ic skin re·sponse (GSR) (gal-van′ik skin rĕ-spons′) A measure of changes in emotional arousal recorded by attaching electrodes to any part of the skin and recording changes in moment-to-moment perspiration and related autonomic nervous system activity.

gal·va·nism (Galv) (gal′vă-nizm) **1.** Direct current electricity produced by chemical action, as by a battery. **2.** Oral manifestations of direct current electricity occurring when dental restorations with dissimilar electric potentials (e.g., silver and gold) are placed in the mouth. SYN voltaism.

gal·va·no·con·trac·til·i·ty (gal′vă-nō-kon′trak-til′i-tē) The capability of a muscle of contracting under the stimulus of a galvanic (direct) current.

gal·va·nom·e·ter (gal'vă-nom'ĕ-ter) An instrument for measuring the strength of an electric current.

Gal·ves·ton Or·i·en·ta·tion and Am·ne·si·a Test (gal'vĕs-tŏn ōr'ē-ĕn-tā' shŭn am-nē'zĕ-ă test) An assessment developed to evaluate cognition serially during the subacute phase of recovery from closed head injury; measures orientation to person, place, time, and memory for events before and after the injury.

gam·ete (gam'ēt) **1.** One of two haploid cells that can undergo karyogamy. **2.** Any germ cell, whether oocyte or sperm.

gam·ete in·tra·fal·lo·pi·an trans·fer (GIFT) (gam'ēt in'trā-fă-lō'pē-ăn trans' fĕr) Placement of the oocyte and sperm into the ampulla of the uterine tube; a form of assisted reproduction.

ga·me·tic phase (gă-met'ik fāz) In a diploid individual, the original allelic combinations that an individual received from its parents; a particular association of alleles at different loci on the same chromosome.

♻ **gameto-** Combining form meaning a gamete.

ga·me·to·cide (gă-mē'tō-sīd) An agent destructive of gametes, specifically the malarial gametocytes.

ga·me·to·cyte (gă-mē'tō-sīt) A cell capable of dividing to produce gametes, e.g., a spermatocyte or oocyte.

gam·e·to·gen·e·sis (gam'ĕ-tō-jen'ĕ-sis) The process of formation and development of gametes.

gam·e·to·phyte (gă-mē'tō-fīt) In plants and algae that undergo alternation of generations, the multicellular structure or phase that is haploid, containing a single set of chromosomes.

gam·ma (γ)-a·mi·no·bu·tyr·ic ac·id (GABA) (gam'ă ă-mē'nō-byū-tir'ik as' id) 4-aminobutyric acid; The principal inhibitory neurotransmitter, used in the treatment of epilepsy.

gam·ma (γ) ben·zene hex·a·chlor·ide (GBH) (gam'ă ben'zēn heks'ă-klōr'īd) One of the purified isomers of hexachlorobenzene that is used as a scab-icide and pediculicide applied topically to the skin in various lotions, creams, and shampoos; GBH can be absorbed through the skin. Resembles DDT in its actions but is less persistent. SYN hexachlorocyclohexane.

gam·ma cam·er·a (gam'ă kam'ĕr-ă) A scintigraphic camera that simultaneously records counts from the entire field of view.

gam·ma fi·bers (gam'ă fī'bĕrz) Nerve fibers that have a conduction rate of 15–40 m/sec.

gam·ma glob·u·lins (gam'ă glob'yū-linz) A class of proteins the most significant of which are immunoglobulins; a serum is made from these immunoglobulins that may be administered to boost a patient's immunity to disease.

Gam·ma·her·pes·vir·i·nae (gam'ă-her'pĕz-vir'i-nē) A subfamily of *Herpesviridae* containing Epstein-Barr virus and others that cause lymphoproliferation.

gam·ma (γ)-hy·drox·y·bu·ty·rate (GHB) (gam'ă hī-drok'sē-byū'tir-āt) A naturally occurring short-chain fatty acid, a metabolite of γ-aminobutyric acid (GABA) found in all body tissues, with the highest concentration in the brain; it affects levels of GABA, dopamine, 5-hydroxytryptamine, and acetylcholine, and may itself be a neurotransmitter. SYN 4-hydroxybutyrate.

gam·ma knife (gam'ă nīf) A minimally invasive radiosurgical system used to treat benign and malignant intracranial neoplasms and arteriovenous malformations.

gam·ma ra·di·a·tion (gam'ă ră'dē-ā' shŭn) Ionizing electromagnetic radiation resulting from nuclear processes, such as radioactive decay or fission.

gam·ma rays (gam'ă rāz) Electromagnetic radiation emitted from radioactive substances; they are high-energy x-rays but originate from the nucleus rather than the orbital shell and are not deflected by a magnet.

gam·mop·a·thy (gă-mop'ă-thē) A primary disturbance in immunoglobulin synthesis.

Gam·na dis·ease (gahm′nă di-zēz′) A form of chronic splenomegaly characterized by conspicuous thickening of the capsule and the presence of multiple, small, rustlike, brown foci (Gamna-Gandy bodies), which contain iron.

gam·o·gen·e·sis (gam′ō-jen′ĕ-sis) SYN sexual reproduction.

Gan·dy-Gam·ma nod·ules (gan′dē-gam′ă nod′yūlz) Nodules of hemosiderin-laden macrophages with calcium deposits and fibrosis that are usually seen in conjunction with hepatic sclerosis.

gan·gli·at·ed nerve (gang′glē-ā-tĕd nĕrv) A sympathetic nerve.

gan·gli·form (gang′gli-fōrm) Having the form or appearance of a ganglion. SYN ganglioform.

gan·gli·o·blast (gang′glē-ō-blast) An embryonic cell from which develop ganglion cells.

gan·gli·o·cy·to·ma (gang′glē-ō-sī-tō′mă) A rare lesion that contains neuronal (ganglion) cells in a sparse glial stoma. SYN central ganglioneuroma.

gan·gli·o·form (gang′glē-ŏ-fōrm) SYN gangliform.

gan·gli·o·gli·o·ma (gang′glē-ō-glī-ō′mă) A rare tumor consisting of a glioma component and an atypical neuronal (ganglion) cell component; in younger patients often associated with seizures.

gan·gli·o·gli·o·neur·o·ma (gang′glē-ō-glī′ō-nūr-ō′mă) A benign neoplasm composed of nerve fibers and mature ganglion cells. SYN ganglioma.

gan·gli·ol·y·sis (gang′glē-ol′i-sis) The dissolution or breaking up of a ganglion.

gan·gli·o·ma (gang′glē-ō′mă) SYN ganglioneuroma.

gan·gli·on, pl. **gan·gli·a, gan·gli·ons** (gang′glē-ŏn, -ă, -ŏnz) [TA] **1.** [TA] Aggregation of nerve cell bodies located in the peripheral nervous system. SYN neuroganglion. **2.** A cyst with mucopolysaccharide-rich fluid in a fibrous capsule; usually attached to a tendon sheath in the hand, wrist, or foot, or connected with the underlying joint. SYN myxoid cyst, synovial cyst.

gan·gli·on·at·ed (gang′glē-ŏ-nā-tĕd) SYN gangliate.

gan·gli·on cell (gang′glē-ŏn sel) A neuron the cell body of which is located outside the limits of the brain and spinal cord, hence forming part of the peripheral nervous system. SYN gangliocyte.

gan·gli·on·ec·to·my (gang′glē-ō-nek′tŏ-mē) Excision of a ganglion. SYN gangliectomy.

gan·gli·o·neur·o·blas·to·ma (gang′lē-ō-nūr′ō-blas-tō′mă) A tumor of mixed cellular type, with elements of neuroblastoma and ganglioneuroma.

gan·glio·neu·ro·ma (GN) (gang′glē-ō-nūr-ō′mă) Benign neoplasm composed of mature ganglionic neurons, in varying numbers, scattered singly or clumped within a relatively abundant and dense stroma of neurofibrils and collagenous fibers. SYN ganglioma.

gan·gli·on·ic (gang) (gang′glē-on′ik) Relating to a ganglion. SYN ganglial.

gan·gli·on im·par (gang′glē-ŏn im′pahr) [TA] A cluster of nerve cells in front of the sacrum and coccyx joint; overactivity causes chronic coccyx pain.

gan·gli·on·i·tis (gang′glē-ŏn-ī′tis) **1.** Inflammation of a lymphatic ganglion. **2.** Inflammation of a nerve ganglion. SYN gangliitis.

gan·gli·o·nos·to·my (gang′glē-ŏn-os′tŏ-mē) Making an opening into a ganglion (2).

gan·gli·o·ple·gic (gang′glē-ō-plē′jik) A pharmacologic compound that paralyzes an autonomic ganglion, usually for a relatively short time.

gan·gli·o·side (gang′glē-ō-sīd) A glycosphingolipid chemically similar to cerebrosides but containing one or more sialic (*N*-acetylneuraminic or *N*-glycolylneuraminic) acid residues; found principally in nerve tissue, spleen, and thymus. SYN sialoglycosphingolipid.

gan·gli·o·si·do·sis (gang′glē-ō-si-dō′sis) Any disease characterized, in part, by the abnormal accumulation within the nervous system of specific gangliosides (e.g., G_{M2} gangliosidosis, Tay-Sachs disease).

gang rape (gang răp) Forcible sexual congress involving intrusive contact perpetrated by a group (nearly always male) on a nonconsenting victim.

gan·grene (gang′grēn) *Avoid the mispronunciation gang-grēn′.* **1.** Necrosis due to obstruction, loss, or diminution of blood supply; may be localized to a small area or involve an entire extremity or organ, may be wet or dry. SYN mortification. **2.** Extensive necrosis from any cause.

gan·o·blast (gan′ō-blast) SYN ameloblast.

Gan·ser syn·drome (gahn′ser sin′drōm) Psychoticlike condition, without the symptoms and signs of a traditional psychosis, occurring typically in prisoners who feign insanity. SEE malingering, factitious disorder. SYN nonsense syndrome, syndrome of approximate relevant answers, syndrome of deviously relevant answers.

Gant clamp (gant klamp) A right-angled clamp used in hemorrhoidectomy.

gan·try (gan′trē) A frame housing the x-ray tube, collimators, and detectors in a computed tomography machine, with a large opening into which the patient is inserted; a mechanical support for mounting a device to be moved in a circular path.

gap (G) (gap) **1.** A hiatus or opening in a structure. **2.** An interval or discontinuity in any series or sequence. **3.** A period in the cell cycle.

gap junc·tion (GJ) (gap jŭngk′shŭn) Intercellular junction formerly considered to be a tight, membrane-to-membrane junction (macula occludens) but now shown to have a 2-nm gap between apposed cell membranes; the gap is not void but contains subunits in the form of polygonal lattices, which are the intercellular aspects of the two connexons that fit together, forming a channel between the cytoplasms of the two cells.

Gard·ner·el·la vag·i·na·lis vag·i·

ni·tis (gahrd′něr-el′ă vaj′i-nā′lis vaj′i-nī′tis) SEE bacterial vaginosis.

gar·gle (gahr′gěl) **1.** To rinse the fauces with fluid through which expired breath is forced to produce a bubbling effect while the head is held far back. **2.** A medicated fluid used for gargling; a throat wash.

gar·goyl·ism (gahr′goyl-izm) A grossly offensive term describing appearance of patients suffering the constellation of symptoms and findings associated with Hurler syndrome (q.v.).

Gar·land tri·an·gle (gahr′lănd trī′anggěl) A triangular area of relative resonance in the lower back near the spine, found on the same side as a pleural effusion.

gar·lic (gahr′lik) A herbal product promoted for treatment of vascular disease, dyslipidemias, and hypertension.

Gar·ré dis·ease (gah-rā′ di-zēz′) SYN sclerosing osteitis.

Garré os·te·o·my·e·li·tis (gah-rā′ os′tē-ō-mī′ě-lī′tis) **1.** Chronic osteomyelitis with proliferative periostitis. **2.** Inflammation of bone marrow.

GARS (gahrz) Acronym for Gilliam Autism Rating Scale.

Gart·ner cyst (gahrt′něr sist) A lesion of the principal duct in the vestigial structures of the paroophoron in the cervix or anterolateral vaginal wall, corresponding to the sexual portion of mesonephros in the male. SYN Gartner duct cyst.

Gärt·ner meth·od (gärt′něr meth′ŏd) Means to measure venous pressure, based on the Gärtner vein phenomenon; considered highly inaccurate, especially in elderly patients.

Gärt·ner to·nom·e·ter (gärt′ner tō-nom′ě-těr) An apparatus for estimating the blood pressure by noting the force, expressed by the height of a column of mercury, needed to arrest pulsation in a finger encircled by a compressing ring.

gas (gas) **1.** Fluid, like air, capable of indefinite expansion but convertible by compression and cold into a liquid and, eventually, a solid. **2.** In clinical practice, a substance entirely in its vapor phase at 1 atmosphere of pressure because ambient temperature is above its boiling point.

gas ab·scess (gas ab′ses) Lesion containing gas; frequently caused by gas-forming organisms such as *Enterobacter aerogenes* or *Escherichia coli*.

gas chro·ma·togra·phy (GC) (gas krō′mă-tog′ră-fē) A chromatographic procedure in which the mobile phase is a mixture of gases or vapors, which are separated in the process by their differential adsorption on a stationary phase.

gas gan·grene (gas gang′grēn) Necrosis occurring in a wound infected with various anaerobic spore-forming bacteria, especially *Clostridium perfringens* and *C. novyi*, which cause rapidly advancing crepitation of the surrounding tissues, due to gas liberated by bacterial fermentation, and constitutional toxic and septic symptoms including cytotoxic damage to kidney, liver, and other organs. SYN clostridial myonecrosis, emphysematous gangrene, gangrenous emphysema, progressive emphysematous necrosis.

gas-liq·uid chro·ma·tog·ra·phy (GLC) (gas-lik′wid krō′mă-tog′ră-fē) A chromatographic technique in which the mobile phase is an inert gas and the stationary phase is liquid rather than solid.

gas mask (gas mask) A device worn over the nose and mouth as protection against airborne toxic gases.

gas·o·met·ric (gas′ō-met′rik) Relating to gasometry.

gas ret·i·no·pex·y (gas ret′i-nō-pek′sē) A retinal detachment repair in which the retina is held in place by an expandable gas.

gas·ser·i·an gan·gli·on (gă-sēr′ē-ăn gang′glē-on) SYN trigeminal ganglion.

gas ster·i·li·za·tion (gas ster′i-lĭ-zā′shŭn) A technique for killing all microorganisms using ethylene oxide gas under pressure; used only for material and supplies that cannot withstand steam sterilizing.

gas·ter (gas′tĕr) [TA] SYN stomach.

gas ther·mom·e·ter (gas thĕr-mom′ĕ-tĕr) A thermometer filled with dry air or a gas, the expansion or increased pressure of which indicates the degree of heat; used to measure high temperatures.

gas·trad·e·ni·tis, gas·tro·ad·e·ni·tis (gas′trad-ĕ-nī′tis, gas′trō-) Inflammation of the glands of the stomach.

gas·trec·ta·sis, gas·trec·ta·si·a (gas-trek′tă-sis, gas-trek-tā′zē-ă) Dilation of the stomach.

gas·trec·to·my (gas-trek′tŏ-mē) Excision of a part or all of the stomach.

gas·tric (G) (gas′trik) Relating to the stomach. SYN gastricus.

gas·tric band·ing (gas′trik band′ing) SYN bariatric surgery.

gas·tric by·pass (gas′trik bī′pas) High division of the stomach, anastomosis of the small upper pouch of the stomach to the jejunum, and closure of the distal part of the stomach that is retained; used for treatment of morbid obesity.

gas·tric di·ges·tion (gas′trik di-jes′chŭn) That part of digestion, chiefly of the proteins, carried on in the stomach by the enzymes of the gastric juice.

gas·tric fis·tu·la (gas′trik fis′tyū-lă) A fistulous tract from the stomach to the abdominal wall.

gas·tric folds (gas′trik fōldz) [TA] Characteristic folds of the gastric mucosa, especially evident when the stomach is contracted. SYN plicae gastricae [TA], gastric rugae, ruga gastrica, rugae of stomach.

gas·tric in·di·ges·tion (gas′trik in′di-jes′chŭn) SYN dyspepsia.

gas·tric in·hib·i·tor·y pol·y·pep·tide, gas·tric in·hib·i·to·ry pep·tide (GIP) (gas′trik in-hib′i-tōr-ē pol′ē-pep′tīd, pep′tīd) Hormone secreted by the stomach; GIP inhibits secretion of acids and of pepsin and stimulates insulin release as part of the digestion. SYN gastric inhibitory peptide.

gas·tric juice (GJ) (gas′trik jūs) Digestive fluid secreted by stomach glands.

G

gas·tric mo·til·i·ty (gas′trik stā′pĕl-ing) Contractions of the smooth muscle of the stomach that help to liquefy food into chyme and force it through the pyloric canal into the small intestine (i.e., gastric emptying).

gas·tric mu·cin (gas′trik myū′sin) Agent used to treat peptic ulcer due to its protective and lubricating action.

gas·tric re·sec·tion (gas′trik rē-sek′shŭn) A surgical procedure to remove a portion of the stomach; most often undertaken because of disease-related damage.

gas·tric stap·ling (gas′trik stāp′ling) Partitioning of the stomach by rows of staples; used to treat morbid obesity.

gas·tric tet·a·ny (gas′trik tet′ă-nē) Tetany associated with a gastric disorder, especially with loss of hydrochloric acid by vomiting.

gas·tric ul·cer (gas′trik ŭl′sĕr) An ulcer of the stomach. SYN Cruveilhier ulcer.

gas·tric ver·ti·go (gas′trik vĕr′ti-gō) Sensation of imbalance symptomatic of disease of the stomach.

gas·trin·o·ma (gas′tri-nō′mă) A gastrin-secreting tumor associated with the Zollinger-Ellison syndrome.

gas·trins (gas′trinz) Hormones secreted in the pyloric-antral mucosa of the mammalian stomach that stimulate secretion of hydrochloric acid by the parietal cells of the gastric glands.

gas·trin test (gas′trin test) Assessment of the level of gastrin in the blood.

gas·tri·tis (gas-trī′tis) Inflammation, especially mucosal, of the stomach.

♻ **gastro-, gastr-** Combining forms denoting the stomach or abdomen.

gas·tro·a·nas·to·mo·sis (gas′trō-an-as-tŏ-mō′sis) Anastomosis of the cardiac and antral segments of the stomach, for relief from marked hour-glass contraction of the stomach. SYN gastrogastrostomy.

gas·tro·cam·e·ra (gas′trō-kam′ĕr-ă) A camera on an endoscope used to examine and photograph the inside of the stomach.

gas·tro·cele (gas′trō-sēl) Hernia of part of the stomach.

gas·tro·coel (gas′trō-sēl) SYN primordial gut.

gas·tro·co·lic (gas′trō-kol′ik) Relating to the stomach and the colon.

gas·tro·co·lic o·men·tum (gas′trō-kol′ik ō-men′tŭm) SYN greater omentum.

gas·tro·co·lic re·flex (gas′trō-kol′ik rē′fleks) Mass movement of the contents of the colon, frequently preceded by a similar movement in the small intestine, which sometimes occurs immediately after the entrance of food into the stomach.

gas·tro·co·li·tis (gas′trō-kŏ-lī′tis) Inflammation of both stomach and colon.

gas·tro·co·los·to·my (gas′trō-kŏ-los′tŏ-mē) Establishment of a communication between stomach and colon.

gas·tro·cys·to·plas·ty (gas′trō-sis′tō-plas′tē) Augmentation of the bladder by a piece of vascularized stomach.

gas·tro·du·o·de·nal (GD) (gas′trō-dū-ō-dē′năl) Relating to the stomach and duodenum.

gas·tro·du·od·e·ni·tis (gas′trō-dū′ō-dĕ-nī′tis) Inflammation of both stomach and duodenum.

gas·tro·du·o·de·nos·co·py (gas′trō-dū′ō-dĕ-nos′kŏ-pē) Visualization of the interior of the stomach and duodenum by a gastroscope.

gas·tro·du·o·de·nos·to·my (gas′trō-dū′ō-dĕ-nos′tŏ-mē) Establishment of a communication between the stomach and the duodenum.

gas·tro·en·ter·al·gi·a (gas′trō-en′tĕr-al′jē-ă) Pain in the stomach and intestines.

gas·tro·en·ter·i·tis (GE) (gas′trō-en′tĕr-ī′tis) Inflammation of the mucous membrane of both stomach and intestine. SYN enterogastritis.

gas·tro·en·ter·o·a·nas·to·mo·sis

(gas′trō-en′těr-ō-an-as′tŏ-mō′sis) Surgical attachment of the stomach to a section of the small intestine.

gas·tro·en·ter·o·co·li·tis (gas′trō-en′těr-ō-kŏ-lī′tis) Inflammatory disease involving the stomach and intestines.

gas·tro·en·ter·op·a·thy (gas′trō-en-těr-op′ă-thē) Any disorder of the alimentary canal.

gas·tro·en·ter·o·plas·ty (gas′trō-en′těr-ō-plas-tē) Operative repair of defects in the stomach and intestine.

gas·tro·en·ter·op·to·sis (gas′trō-en-těr-op-tō′sis) Downward displacement of the stomach and a portion of the intestine.

gas·tro·en·ter·ot·o·my (gas′trō-en-těr-ot′ŏ-mē) Surgical incision into both stomach and intestine.

gas·tro·ep·i·plo·ic (gas′trō-ep-i-plō′ik) Relating to the stomach and greater omentum (epiploon).

gas·tro·e·soph·a·ge·al (gas′trō-ĕ-sof′ă-jē′ăl) Relating to both stomach and esophagus. SYN gastro-oesophageal.

gas·tro·e·soph·a·ge·al her·ni·a (gas′trō-ĕ-sof′ă-jē′ăl hěr′nē-ă) A hiatal hernia into the thorax. SYN gastro-oesophageal hernia.

gas·tro·e·soph·a·ge·al re·flux dis·ease (GERD) (gas′trō-ĕ-sof′ă-jē′ăl rē′flŭks di-zēz′) A syndrome of chronic or recurrent epigastric or retrosternal pain, accompanied by varying degrees of belching, nausea, cough, or hoarseness, due to reflux of acid gastric juice into the lower esophagus; results from malfunction of the lower esophageal sphincter and disordered gastric motility. SYN gastro-oesophageal reflux disease.

gas·tro·e·soph·a·gi·tis (gas′trō-ĕ-sof′ă-jī′tis) Inflammation of the stomach and esophagus. SYN gastro-oesophagitis.

gas·tro·gas·tros·to·my (gas′trō-gas-tros′tŏ-mē) Anastomosis between two parts of the stomach usually to bypass an area of narrowing. SYN gastroanastomosis.

gas·tro·ga·vage (gas′trō-gă-vahzh′) SYN gavage (1).

gas·tro·gen·ic (gas′trō-jen′ik) Deriving from or caused by the stomach.

gas·tro·he·pat·ic (gas′trō-he-pat′ik) Relating to the stomach and the liver.

gas·tro·il·e·ac re·flex (gas′trō-il′ē-ak rē′fleks) Opening of the ileocolic valve induced by entrance of food into the stomach.

gas·tro·il·e·i·tis (gas′trō-il-ē-ī′tis) Inflammation of the alimentary canal in which the stomach and ileum are primarily involved.

gas·tro·il·e·os·to·my (gas′trō-il-ē-os′tŏ-mē) A surgical joining of stomach to ileum; most commonly used in the treatment of severe obesity.

gas·tro·in·tes·ti·nal (GI) (gas′trō-in-tes′ti-năl) Relating to the digestive tract from mouth to anus. SYN gastroenteric.

gas·tro·in·tes·ti·nal au·to·no·mic nerve tu·mor (GANT) (gas′trō-in-tes′ti-năl aw′tŏ-nom′ik něrv tū′mŏr) Benign or malignant lesion of stomach and small intestine histogenetically related to myenteric plexus; may be familial and related to gastrointestinal neuronal dysplasia.

gas·tro·in·tes·ti·nal (GI) tract (gas′trō-in-tes′ti-năl trakt) Stomach, small intestine, and large intestine; often used to mean digestive tract.

gas·tro·in·tes·ti·nal stro·mal tu·mor (gas′trō-in-tes′ti-năl strō′măl tū′mŏr) Benign or malignant tumor composed of unclassifiable spindle cells.

gas·tro·je·ju·no·co·lic (gas′trō-jĕ-jū′nŏ-kol′ik) Referring to the stomach, jejunum, and colon.

gas·tro·je·ju·nos·to·my (gas′trō-jĕ-jū-nos′tŏ-mē) Establishment of a direct communication between the stomach and the jejunum.

gas·tro·li·e·nal (gas′trō-lī′en-ăl) SYN gastrosplenic.

gas·trol·y·sis (gas-trol′i-sis) Division of perigastric adhesions.

gas·tro·ma·la·ci·a (gas′trō-mă-lā′shē-ă) Softening of the walls of the stomach.

gas·tro·meg·a·ly (gas'trō-meg'ă-lē) **1.** Enlargement of the stomach. **2.** Enlargement of the abdomen.

gas·tro·myx·or·rhe·a (gas'trō-mik-sō-rē'ă) Excessive secretion of mucus in the stomach. SYN gastromyxorrhea.

gastromyxorrhoea [Br.] SYN gastromyxorrhea.

gastro-oesophageal [Br.] SYN gastroesophageal.

gastro-oesophageal hernia [Br.] SYN gastroesophageal hernia.

gastro-oesophageal reflux disease [Br.] SYN gastroesophageal reflux disease.

gastro-oesophagitis [Br.] SYN gastroesophagitis.

gas·tro·pa·ral·y·sis (gas'trō-păr-al'i-sis) Paralysis of the muscular coat of the stomach.

gas·tro·pa·re·sis (gas'trō-păr-ē'sis) A slight degree of gastroparalysis.

gas·trop·a·thy (gas-trop'ă-thē) Any disease of the stomach.

gas·tro·pex·y (gas'trō-pek-sē) Attachment of the stomach to the abdominal wall or diaphragm.

gas·tro·phren·ic (gas'trō-fren'ik) Relating to the stomach and the diaphragm.

gas·trop·to·sis, gas·trop·to·si·a (gas'trō-tō'sis, -tō'zē-ă) *In the diphthong pt, the p is silent only at the beginning of a word.* Downward displacement of the stomach. SYN bathygastry, descensus ventriculi, ventroptosis, ventroptosia.

gas·tro·py·lor·ec·to·my (gas'trō-pī-lōr-ek'tō-mē) SYN pylorectomy.

gas·tro·py·lor·ic (gas'trō-pī-lōr'ik) Relating to the stomach and to the pylorus.

gas·tror·rha·gi·a (gas'trō-rā'jē-ă) Hemorrhage from the stomach.

gas·tror·rha·phy (gas-trōr'ă-fē) Suture of a perforation of the stomach.

gas·tror·rhe·a (gas'trōr-ē'ă) Excessive secretion of gastric juice or of mucus (gastromyxorrhea) by the stomach. SYN gastrorrhoea.

gastrorrhoea [Br.] SYN gastrorrhea.

gas·tros·chi·sis (gas-tros'ki-sis) A defect in the anterior abdominal wall; usually accompanied by protrusion of viscera.

gas·tros·co·py (gas-tros'kŏ-pē) Inspection of the inner surface of the stomach through an endoscope.

gas·tro·spasm (gas'trō-spazm) Spasmodic contraction of the walls of the stomach.

gas·tro·splen·ic (gas'trō-splen'ik) Relating to the stomach and spleen. SYN gastrolienal.

gas·tro·ste·no·sis (gas'trō-stě-nō'sis) Diminution in size of the cavity of the stomach.

gas·tros·to·ga·vage (gas-tros'tō-gă-vahzh') SYN gavage (1).

gas·tros·to·la·vage (gas-tros'tō-lă-vahzh') Lavage of the stomach through a gastric fistula.

gas·tros·to·my (GT, G) (gas-tros'tŏ-mē) Establishment of a new opening into the stomach.

gas·tros·to·my feed·ing (gas-tros'tŏ-mē fēd'ing) Providing liquid nourishment through a tube permanently inserted through the abdominal wall into the stomach. SYN G-tube feeding, PEG tube feeding.

gas·tros·to·my tube (gas-tros'tŏ-mē tūb) SYN percutaneous endoscopic gastrostomy tube.

gas·tro·tro·pic (gas'trō-trō'pik) Affecting the stomach.

Gatch bed (gach bed) One with divided sections for independent elevation of a patient's head and knees.

gate (gāt) **1.** To close an ion channel by electrical or chemical action. **2.** Action of a special nerve fiber to block the transmission of impulses through a synapse.

3. A device that can be switched electronically to control the passage of a signal.

gate·con·trol the·o·ry (gāt′kŏn-trōl′ thē′ŏr-ē) Concept to explain the mechanism of pain; small-fiber afferent stimuli, particularly painful, entering the substantia gelatinosa can be modulated by large-fiber afferent stimuli and descending spinal pathways so that their transmission to ascending spinal pathways is blocked (gated).

gat·ed ra·di·o·nu·clide an·gi·o·car·di·og·ra·phy (gāt′ĕd rā′dē-ō-nū′klĭd an′jē-ō-kahr-dē-og′ră-fē) Radionuclide imaging using cardiac gating to combine images from several cardiac cycles to improve the quality of the images of separate phases (e.g., systole and diastole).

gate·way drugs (gāt′wā drŭgz) The concept that the use of less addictive drugs such as marijuana can lead to the use of harder drugs such as cocaine and heroin.

gat·ing (gāt′ing) 1. In a biologic membrane, the opening and closing of a channel, believed to be associated with changes in integral membrane proteins. 2. A process in which electrical signals are selected by a gate, which passes such signals only when the gate pulse is present to act as a control signal, or passes only the signals that have certain characteristics. SEE gate.

Gauch·er cells (gō-shā′ selz) Large, finely and uniformly vacuolated cells derived from the reticuloendothelial system; found especially in the spleen, lymph nodes, liver, and bone marrow of patients with Gaucher disease.

Gauch·er dis·ease (gō-shā′ di-zēz′) A lysosomal storage disease resulting from glycocerebroside accumulation due to a genetic deficiency of glucocerebrosidase; may occur in adults but occurs most severely in infants.

gaunt·let band·age (gawnt′lĕt ban′dăj) A figure-of-8 bandage covering the hand and fingers.

gauss (G) (gows) A unit of magnetic field intensity, equal to 10^{-4} T.

gauss·i·an dis·tri·bu·tion (gaw′sē-ăn dis′tri-bū′shŭn) The statistical distribution of members of a population around the population mean. In a gaussian distribution, 68.2% of values fall within $\pm$ 1 standard deviation (SD); 95.4% fall within $\pm$ 2 SD of the mean; and 99.7% fall within $\pm$ 3 SD of the mean.

Gauss sign (gows sīn) Marked mobility of the uterus in the early weeks of pregnancy.

gauze (gawz) A bleached cotton cloth used for dressings, bandages, and absorbent sponges.

ga·vage (gă-vahzh′) 1. Forced feeding by stomach tube. SYN gastrogavage. 2. Therapeutic use of a high-potency diet administered by stomach tube.

Gay Nurs·es' Al·li·ance (gā nŭr′sĕz ă-lī′ăns) A professional organization for gay nurses that is recognized by the American Nurse's Association.

Gay/Straight Al·li·ance (GSA) (gā-strāt′ ă-lī′ăns) U.S. organization that is involved in issues related to sexuality.

gaze nys·tag·mus (gāz nis-tag′mŭs) An involuntary bouncing or jerking of the eye that occurs when the eyes are fixed on an object or image; usually caused by neural disruption.

gaze pa·ret·ic nys·tag·mus (gāz pă-ret′ik nis-tag′mŭs) Ocular jerking occurring in partial gaze paralysis when an attempt is made to look in the direction of the gaze paresis.

GB vi·rus·es (GBV) (vī′rŭs-ĕz) Members of the family Flaviviridae; GBV-A and GBV-B have been isolated from tamarins (small South American monkeys) infected with human viral agents; GBV-C is a human pathogen related to hepatitis G virus.

G cells (selz) Enteroendocrine cells that secrete gastrin, found primarily in the mucosa of the pyloric antrum of the stomach.

Gd Symbol for gadolinium.

GDNF Neurotrophic factors that promote survival of dopaminergic neurons; studied as potential treatment for parkinsonism.

Ge Symbol for germanium.

Gei·ger-Muel·ler coun·ter (gī'ger-mil'er kown'tĕr) An instrument used to detect and monitor radiation. (Mueller is a variant spelling for Müller.)

gel (jel) **1.** A jelly, or the solid or semisolid phase of a colloidal solution. **2.** To form a gel or jelly; to convert a solution into a gel.

Gel and Coombs clas·si·fi·ca·tion (jel kūmz klas'i-fi-kā'shŭn) A system that differentiates anaphylactic reactions, cytotoxic reactions, immune complex reactions, and cell-mediated/delayed hypersensitivity reactions.

gel·a·tin (jel'ă-tin) A derived protein formed from the collagen of tissues by boiling in water; it swells up when put in cold water, but dissolves only in hot water; used as a hemostat, plasma substitute, and protein food adjunct to treat malnutrition.

ge·lat·i·nous sub·stance (jĕ-lat'i-nŭs sub'stăns) [TA] The apical part of the posterior horn of the spinal cord's gray matter, composed mostly of small nerve cells; appearance is due to its very low content of myelinated nerve fibers.

ge·lat·i·nous tis·sue (jĕ-lat'i-nŭs tish'ū) SYN mucous connective tissue.

ge·la·tion (jĕ-lā'shŭn) COLLOIDAL CHEMISTRY the transformation of a solution into a gel.

gel dif·fu·sion (jel di-fyū'zhŭn) Diffusion in a gel, as in the case of gel diffusion precipitin tests in which the immune reactants diffuse in agar. SEE ALSO immunodiffusion.

gel fil·tra·tion (jel fil-trā'shŭn) Separation of molecular sizes by passage of a mixture through columns of beads of cross-linked dextrans or similar relatively inert material of a well-defined pore size range.

Gé·ly su·ture (zhā-lē' sū'chŭr) Cobbler's stitch used in closing intestinal wounds.

Ge·mel·la (jĕ-mel'ă) A genus of motile, aerobic, facultatively anaerobic, coccoid bacteria that occur singly or in pairs, with flattened adjacent sides. They are gram indeterminate but have a cell wall like that of gram-positive bacteria, and are parasitic on mammals.

ge·mel·lol·o·gy (jem'el-ol'ŏ-jē) The study of twins and the phenomenology of twinning.

gem·i·nate (jem'i-năt) Occurring in pairs. SYN geminous.

gem·ma (jem'ă) Any budlike or bulblike body, especially a taste bud or end bulb.

gem·ma·tion (jem-ā'shŭn) A form of fission in which the parent cell does not divide but puts out a small budlike process (daughter cell) with its proportionate amount of chromatin; the daughter cell then separates to begin independent existence.

gem·mule (jem'yūl) **1.** A small bud that projects from the parent cell, and finally becomes detached, forming a cell of a new generation. **2.** SYN dendritic spines.

-gen Suffix meaning ''precursor of.'' SEE ALSO pro- (2).

ge·nal (jē'năl) Relating to the gena, or cheek.

gen·der (jen'dĕr) Category to which a person is assigned by self or others, on the basis of sex. Cf. sex, gender role.

gen·der i·den·ti·ty (jen'dĕr i-den'ti-tē) The sex role adopted by a person; the degree to which a person acts out a stereotypical masculine or feminine role in everyday behavior. Cf. gender role, sex role.

gen·der i·den·ti·ty dis·or·der (jen'dĕr ī-den'ti-tē dis-or'dĕr) Persistent feeling of identification with the opposite gender and discomfort with one's own sex.

gen·der role (jen'dĕr rōl) The sex of a child assigned by a parent; when opposite to the child's anatomic sex (e.g., due to genital ambiguity at birth or to the parents' strong wish for a child of the opposite sex), the basis is set for postpubertal dysfunctions. SEE sex role.

gene (jēn) A functional unit of heredity that occupies a specific place (locus) on a chromosome, is capable of reproducing itself exactly at each cell division, and directs the formation of an enzyme or other protein. In organisms reproducing sexually, genes normally occur in pairs in all cells except gametes, as a consequence of the fact that all chromosomes are paired except the sex chromosomes (X and Y) of the male. SYN factor (3).

gene ex·pres·sion (jēn eks-presh'ŭn) **1.** The detectable effect of a gene. **2.** Appearance of an inherited trait; for many reasons, a gene may not be expressed at all.

gene li·brar·y (jēn lī'brăr-ē) A haphazard assembly of cloned DNA fragments inside of a vector, which may contain genetic information about a species.

gene pool (jēn pūl) Set of the genes available for inheritance in a particular mating population.

gen·er·al an·es·the·si·a (jen'ĕr-ăl an'es-thē'zē-ă) Loss of ability to perceive pain associated with loss of consciousness produced by intravenous or inhalation anesthetic agents.

generalised [Br.] SYN generalized.

gen·er·al·ized (jen'ĕr-ă-līzd) Not highly differentiated or adapted to a particular environment; widespread; nonspecific.

gen·er·al·ized anx·i·e·ty dis·or·der (jen'ĕr-ă-līzd ang-zī'ĕ-tē dis-ŏr'dĕr) Chronic, repeated episodes of anxiety or dread accompanied by autonomic changes. SEE ALSO anxiety.

gen·er·al·ized ep·i·lep·sy (GE) (jen'ĕr-ă-līzd ep'i-lep-sē) Major category of epilepsy syndromes characterized by one or more types of generalized seizures.

gen·er·al·ized ton·ic-clo·nic sei·zure, gen·er·al·ized ton·ic-clo·nic ep·i·lep·sy (jen'ĕr-ăl-īzd ton'ik-klon'ik sē'zhŭr, ep'i-lep'sē) Seizure characterized by the sudden onset of tonic contraction of the muscles often associated with a cry or moan, and frequently resulting in a fall. The tonic phase gradually gives way to clonic convulsive movements occurring bilaterally and synchronously before slowing and eventually stopping, followed by a variable period of unconsciousness and gradual recovery. SYN grand mal.

gen·er·al pa·re·sis (GP) (jen'ĕr-ăl pă-rē'sis) SYN paretic neurosyphilis.

gen·er·al per·i·to·ni·tis (jen'ĕr-ăl per'i-tŏ-nī'tis) Peritonitis throughout the peritoneal cavity. SYN diffuse peritonitis.

gen·er·al prac·tice (jen'ĕr-ăl prak'tis) SEE family practice.

gen·er·al stim·u·lant (jen'ĕr-ăl stim'yū-lănt) A stimulant that affects the entire body.

gen·er·a·tion (GEN) (jen'ĕr-ā'shŭn) **1.** SYN reproduction (1). **2.** A discrete stage in succession of descent; e.g., father, son, and grandson are three generations.

gen·er·a·tor (jen'ĕr-ā-tŏr) An apparatus for conversion of chemical, mechanical, atomic, or other forms of energy into electricity.

gene re·pres·sion (jēn rĕ-presh'ŭn) The normal silencing of a gene such that its effect is not shown by the cell containing it; at any given time, about 90% of the genes contained within a cell are silent; this is necessary for the health of the organism.

ge·ner·ic name (jĕ-ner'ik nām) **1.** CHEMISTRY a noun that indicates the class or type of a single compound (e.g., salt, saccharide (sugar), hexose, alcohol, aldehyde, lactone, acid, amine, alkane, steroid, vitamin). "Class" is more appropriate and more often used than is "generic." **2.** In the pharmaceutical and commercial fields, a common misnomer for nonproprietary name. **3.** BIOLOGIC SCIENCES the first part of the scientific name (Latin binary combination or binomial) of an organism; written with an initial capital letter and in italics. **4.** BACTERIOLOGY the species name consists of two parts (comprising one name): the generic name and the specific epithet; in other biologic disciplines, the species name is regarded as being composed of two names: the generic name and the specific name.

gen·e·sis (jen'ĕ-sis) An origin or beginning process; also used as combining form in suffix position.

gene ther·a·py (jēn thār'ă-pē) The process of inserting a gene into an organism to replace or repair gene function to treat a disease or genetic defect.

ge·net·ic (jĕ-net´ik) Pertaining to genetics.

ge·net·ic ad·ap·ta·tion (jĕ-net´ik ad´ap-tā´shŭn) Change in a biologic organism in response to change in the environment, making survival of the organism possible.

ge·net·ic af·fin·i·ty (jĕ-net´ik ă-fin´i-tē) A genetic or hereditary relationship between populations. SYN genetic genealogy.

ge·net·ic am·pli·fi·ca·tion (jĕ-net´ik amp´li-fi-kā´shŭn) A process for producing an increase in pertinent genetic material, particularly for increasing the proportion of plasmid DNA to that of bacterial DNA.

ge·net·ic car·ri·er (jĕ-net´ik kar´ē-ĕr) Someone heterozygous for a mutant allele that, in homozygous form, causes a recessive condition.

ge·net·ic code (jĕ-net´ik kōd) The genetic information carried by the specific deoxyribonucleic acid (DNA) molecules of the chromosomes; specifically, the system whereby particular combinations of three consecutive nucleotides in a DNA molecule control the insertion of a given amino acid in equivalent places in a protein molecule.

ge·net·ic col·on·i·za·tion (jĕ-net´ik kol´ŏ-nī-zā´shŭn) Propagation of a gene by a host into which the gene has been introduced, naturally or artificially.

ge·net·ic death (jĕ-net´ik deth) Demise of the bearer of a gene at any age before generating living offspring. May be compatible with good health and long life.

ge·net·ic de·fect (jĕ-net´ik dē´fekt) Any disease or disorder that is inherited. SYN genetic abnormality, inherited genetic disease, genetic disorder, hereditary condition, hereditary disease, inherited disease, inherited disorder.

ge·net·ic de·ter·mi·nant (jĕ-net´ik dĕ-tĕr´mi-nănt) Any antigenic determinant or identifying characteristic, particularly those of allotypes.

ge·net·ic drift (jĕ-net´ik drift) Change in the frequencies of genetic traits or allele frequencies over generations.

ge·net·ic en·gi·neer·ing (jĕ-net´ik en-ji-nēr´ing) Internal manipulation of basic genetic material of an organism to modify biologic heredity or to produce peptides of high purity.

ge·net·ic ep·i·de·mi·ol·o·gy (jĕ-net´ik ep´i-dē-mē-ol´ŏ-jē) The branch of epidemiology that studies the role of genetic factors and their interactions with environmental factors in the occurrence of disease in various populations.

ge·net·ic e·quil·ib·ri·um (jĕ-net´ik ē´kwi-lib´rē-ŭm) State of a dynamic genetic system in which the several rates of change between all possible pairs of parts are such that the composition is invariant.

ge·net·ic fin·ger·print (jĕ-net´ik fing´gĕr-print) SYN fingerprint (3).

ge·net·ic ho·me·o·sta·sis (jĕ-net´ik hō´mē-ō-stā´sis) SYN Lerner homeostasis.

ge·net·ic i·so·late (jĕ-net´ik ī´sō-lăt) SYN isolate (6).

ge·net·ic map (jĕ-net´ik map) An abstract representation of the ordered array of genetic loci such that the interval between entries has algebraic signs and magnitude proportional to the expected number of crossings over between them and distances are algebraically additive.

ge·net·ic pol·y·mor·phism (jĕ-net´ik pol´ē-mōr´fizm) Occurrence in the same population of multiple discrete alletic states of which at least two have high frequency (conventionally of 1% or more).

ge·net·ics (jĕ-net´iks) **1.** Science concerned with the means and consequences of transmission and generation of the components of biologic inheritance. **2.** Genetic features and constitution of any one or more organisms.

Ge·net·ics So·ci·e·ty of Am·er·i·ca (GSA) (jĕ-net´iks sŏ-sī´e-tē ă-měr´i-kă) Professional organization composed of members of various disciplines related to inheritance; also publishes books and learned journals.

ge·net·o·tro·phic (jĕ-net′ō-trō′fik) Relating to inherited individual distinctions in nutritional requirements.

gene trans·fer (jēn trans′fĕr) Any process in which an organism (usually a bacterium) transfers genetic material to another cell that is not its offspring. SYN lateral gene transfer, horizontal gene transfer.

ge·ni·al, ge·ni·an (jĕ-nī′ăl, -ăn) SYN mental (2).

-genic Suffix meaning producing, forming; produced, formed by.

ge·nic·u·lar (jĕ-nik′yū-lăr) Pertaining to the knee or to a structure that is bent like a knee.

ge·nic·u·lar ar·te·ries (jĕ-nik′yū-lăr ahr′tĕr-ēz) Blood vessels contributing to the articular vascular plexus of the knee.

ge·nic·u·late (jĕ-nik′yū-lăt) 1. Bent like a knee. 2. Referring to the geniculum of the facial nerve, denoting the ganglion there present. 3. Denoting the lateral or medial geniculate body.

ge·nic·u·late gan·gli·on (jĕ-nik′yū-lăt gang′glē-on) [TA] A ganglion of the nervus intermedius fibers conveyed by the facial nerve, located within the facial canal at the genu of the canal and containing the sensory neurons innervating the taste buds on the anterior two thirds of the tongue and a small area on the external ear.

ge·nic·u·late neu·ral·gi·a (jĕ-nik′yū-lăt nūr-al′jē-ă) Severe paroxysmal lancinating pain deep in the ear, on the anterior wall of the external meatus, and on a small area just in front of the pinna. SYN geniculate otalgia, Hunt neuralgia, neuralgia facialis vera.

ge·nic·u·lum, pl. **ge·nic·u·la** (jĕ-nik′ yū-lŭm, -lă) [TA] 1. A small genu or angular kneelike structure. 2. A knotlike structure.

ge·ni·o·plas·ty (jē′nē-ō-plas-tē) Surgical correction of the bony contour of the chin.

gen·i·tal (jen′i-tăl) 1. Relating to reproduction or generation. 2. Relating to the primary female or male sex organs or genitals. 3. Relating to or characterized by genitality.

gen·i·tal am·bi·gu·i·ty (jen′i-tăl am′bi-gyū′i-tē) Incomplete development of fetal genitalia as a result of excessive androgen action on a female fetus or inadequate amounts of androgen in a male fetus.

gen·i·tal cor·pus·cles (jen′i-tăl kōr′ pŭs-ĕlz) Special encapsulated nerve endings found in the skin of the genitalia and nipples. SYN corpuscula genitalia [TA].

gen·i·tal cri·sis of new·born (jen′i-tăl krī′sis nū′bōrn) Birth of an infant with ambiguous genitalia in whom sex cannot be accurately determined. SYN ambiguous genitalia of the newborn.

gen·i·tal fur·row (jen′i-tăl fŭr′ō) SYN urethral groove.

gen·i·tal her·pes (jen′i-tăl hĕr′pēz) Herpetic lesions on the penis of the male or on the cervix, perineum, vagina, or vulva of the female, caused by herpes simplex virus type 2. SYN herpes genitalis.

gen·i·ta·li·a (jen′i-tă′lē-ă) [TA] The organs of reproduction or generation, external and internal. SYN genitals.

gen·i·tal stage (jen′i-tăl stāj) Psychic organization derived from, and which is characteristic of, the genital period of the infant's psychosocial organization in Freud's original conception. SEE ALSO orality.

gen·i·tal sys·tem (jen′i-tăl sis′tĕm) The complex system consisting of the male or female gonads, associated ducts, and external genitalia dedicated to the function of reproducing the species. SYN reproductive system.

gen·i·tal tract, gen·i·tal duct (jen′i-tăl trakt, dŭkt) The genital passages of the urogenital apparatus. SYN genital tract.

gen·i·tal wart (jen′i-tăl wōrt) SYN condyloma acuminatum.

gen·i·to·fem·o·ral (jen′i-tō-fem′ŏr-ăl) Relating to the genitalia and the thigh; denoting the genitofemoral nerve.

G

gen·i·to·u·ri·nar·y fis·tu·la (jen´i-tō-yūr´i-nar-ē fis´tyū-lă) Fistulous opening into the urogenital tract. SYN urogenital fistula.

gen·i·to·u·ri·nar·y sys·tem (GUS) (jen´i-tō-yūr´i-nar-ē sis´těm) SYN urogenital system.

gen·o·cide (jen´ŏ-sīd) Aggressive acts committed with intent to destroy a national, ethnic, racial, or religious group.

ge·no·der·ma·to·sis (jen´ō-děr-mă-tō´sis) A skin condition of genetic origin.

ge·no·gram (jē´nō-gram) A diagram resembling a family tree with expanded relationships among individual family members and information related to their medical histories.

ge·nome (jē´nōm) **1.** A complete set of chromosomes derived from one parent, the haploid number of a gamete. **2.** The total gene complement of a set of chromosomes found in higher life forms (the haploid set in a eukaryotic cell), or the functionally similar but simpler linear arrangements found in bacteria and viruses.

ge·nome se·quenc·ing cen·ter (GSC) (jē´nōm sěk´wěn-sing sen´těr) Laboratory and clinical offices that study the genomes of one or more species.

ge·nom·ics (jē-nō´miks) Study of the structure of the genome of particular organisms, including mapping and sequencing.

ge·no·spe·cies (jē´nō-spē-shēz) A group of organisms in which interbreeding is possible, as evidenced by genetic transfer and recombination.

ge·no·tox·ic (jē´nō-toks´ik) Denoting a substance that by damaging DNA may cause mutation or cancer.

gen·o·type (jē´nō-tīp) **1.** The genetic constitution of an individual. **2.** Gene combination at one specific locus or any specified combination of loci.

♻ **-genous** Suffix meaning the condition of causing or the condition of starting.

gen·ta·mi·cin (jen´tă-mī´sin) *Avoid the misspelling gentamycin.* A broad spectrum antibiotic of the aminoglycoside class, which inhibits growth of both gram-positive and gram-negative bacteria; sulfate salt is also used medicinally.

gen·tian, gen·tian root (jen´shŭn, rūt) The dried rhizome and roots of *Gentiana lutea* (family Gentianaceae), an herb of southern and central Europe; a simple bitter.

gen·tian vi·o·let (jen´shŭn vī´ŏ-lět) An unstandardized dye mixture of violet rosanilins.

ge·nu, pl. **gen·u·a** (jē´nyū, -ă) [TA] **1.** The joint between the thigh and the leg. SYN knee (1) [TA]. **2.** Any structure of angular shape resembling a flexed knee. SEE ALSO knee joint, geniculum.

gen·u·al (jen´yū-ăl) Relating to the knee.

ge·nu re·cur·va·tum (jē´nyū rē-kŭr-vā´tŭm) Hyperextension of the knee, the lower limb having a forward curvature. SYN back-knee.

ge·nus, pl. **gen·er·a** (jē´nŭs, jen´ěr-ă) In natural history classification, the taxonomic level of division between the family, or tribe, and the species; a group of species alike in the broad features of their organization but different in detail, and incapable of fertile mating.

ge·nu val·gum (jē´nyū val´gŭm) A deformity marked by lateral angulation of the leg in relation to the thigh. SYN knock-knee, tibia valga.

ge·nu va·rum (jē´nyū vā´rŭm) A deformity marked by medial angulation of the leg in relation to the thigh; an outward bowing of the lower limbs. SYN bowleg, bow-leg, tibia vara.

♻ **geo-** Prefix indicating the earth, soil.

ge·ode (jē´ōd) A cystlike space (or spaces) with or without an epithelial lining, observed radiologically in subarticular bone, usually in arthritic disorders.

ge·o·grap·hic ret·i·nal at·ro·phy (jē´ŏ-graf´ik ret´i-năl at´rŏ-fē) A pattern of well-demarcated retinal pigment epithelial atrophy associated with choriocapillary layer and photoreceptor atrophy leading to vision loss.

ge·o·graph·ic tongue (jē'ŏ-graf'ik tŭng) Idiopathic, asymptomatic erythematous circinate macules, often bounded peripherally by a white band, due to atrophy of the filiform papillae. SYN glossitis areata exfoliativa, lingua geographica, pityriasis linguae.

ge·o·tax·is (jē'ŏ-tak'sis) A form of positive barotaxis in which there is a tendency to growth or movement toward or into the earth. SYN geotropism.

ge·o·tri·cho·sis (jē'ŏ-tri-kō'sis) An opportunistic systemic hyalohyphomycosis caused by *Geotrichum candidum;* ascribed symptoms are diverse and suggestive of secondary or mixed infections.

Ge·ot·ri·chum (jē-ot'ri-kŭm) A genus of yeastlike fungi that produce arthroconidia but rarely blastoconidia. *Geotrichum candidum* was once thought to cause infection in humans.

ge·ot·ro·pism (jē-ot'rŏ-pizm) SYN geotaxis.

ge·phy·rin (je-fir'in) A protein in the ataxia telangiectasia mutation-related family, essential for glycine receptor clustering on neuronal membranes.

ger·i·at·ric (jer'ē-at'rik) Relating to old age.

ger·i·at·rics (jer'ē-at'riks) The branch of medicine concerned with the medical problems and care of old people.

germ (jĕrm) 1. A microbe; a microorganism. 2. A primordium; the earliest trace of a structure within an embryo.

ger·ma·ni·um (Ge) (jĕr-mā'nē-ŭm) A metallic element, atomic no. 32, atomic wt. 72.61.

Ger·man mea·sles (jĕr'măn mē'zĕlz) SYN rubella.

ger·mi·nal ar·e·a, ar·e·a ger·mi·na·ti·va (jĕr'mi-năl ār'ē-ă, jĕr'mi-nā-tī'vă) The place in the blastoderm where the embryo begins to be formed.

ger·mi·nal cen·ter (GC) (jĕr'mi-năl sen'tĕr) Area in a lymph node or other tissue such as the liver (in infection with hepatitis C virus) and synovium (in patients with rheumatoid arthritis) in which there is a rapid clonal expansion of antigen-specific B cells.

ger·mi·nal disc, germ disc (jĕr'mi-năl disk, jĕrm) The point in a telolecithal oocyte where the embryo begins to form.

ger·mi·nal lo·cal·i·za·tion (jĕr'mi-năl lō'kăl-ī-zā'shŭn) SYN fate map.

ger·mi·nal stage (jĕr'mi-năl stāj) A period of development beginning at conception and lasting through the first 8 weeks, characterized by rapid cell division; implantation occurs; the placenta and body systems form.

ger·mi·na·tion (jĕr'mi-nā'shŭn) Sprouting; formation of a new plant from a seed.

ger·mi·no·ma (jĕr'mi-nō'mă) A neoplasm of the germinal tissue of gonads, mediastinum, or pineal region, such as seminoma.

germ the·o·ry (jĕrm thē'ŏr-ē) Doctrine that infectious diseases are due to the presence and functional activity of microorganisms within the body.

gero-, geront-, geronto- Combining forms meaning old age or old people. SEE ALSO presby-.

ger·o·der·ma (jer'ō-dĕr'mă) 1. The atrophic skin of the aged. 2. Any condition in which the skin is thinned and wrinkled, resembling the integument of old age.

ger·o·don·tics, ger·o·don·tol·o·gy (jer'ō-don'tiks, -don-tol'ŏ-jē) SYN dental geriatrics.

ger·o·ma·ras·mus (jer'ō-mă-raz'mŭs) SYN senile atrophy.

geronto- SEE gero-.

ger·on·to·gen (jer-on'tō-jen) Agent that causes aging, especially premature aging (e.g., tobacco smoke).

Ger·on·to·log·ic·al So·ci·e·ty of Am·er·i·ca (jer'ŏn-tŏ-loj'i-kăl sŏ-sī'ĕ-tē ă-mer'i-kă) A multidisciplinary organization for professionals in the field of care of aging patients.

ger·on·tol·o·gist (Geront) (jer'ŏn-tol'

ŏ-jist) One who specializes in gerontology.

ger·on·tol·o·gy (Geront, geront) (jer'ŏn-tol'ŏ-jē) The scientific study of the clinical, sociologic, biologic and psychological phenomena related to aging. SYN geratology.

ger·on·to·ther·a·peu·tics (jer-on'tō-thār'ă-pyū'tiks) The science concerned with treatment of the aged.

Ge·ro·ta meth·od (gă-rō'tah meth'ŏd) Injection of the lymphatics with a dye that is soluble in chloroform or ether but not in water.

Gerst·mann-Sträuss·ler-Schein·ker syn·drome (gerst'mahn-stris'lĕr-shīn'kĕr sin'drōm) Chronic cerebellar form of spongiform encephalopathy.

Ges·sell De·vel·op·men·tal Ob·ser·va·tion (GDO) (ges'ĕl dĕ-vel'ŏp-men'tăl ob'sĕr-vā'shŭn) A standard procedure for direct observation of a child's growth and development in which the examiner makes discriminating observations and compares them with normative patterns for each developmental age.

ges·ta·gen (jes'tă-jen) Any of several gestagenic substances, which are usually steroid hormones.

ge·stalt, ge·stalt phe·nom·e·non (ge-stahlt', fĕ-nom'ĕ-non) A perceived entity so integrated as to constitute a functional unit with properties not derivable from its parts. SEE gestaltism.

ges·ta·tion (jes-tā'shŭn) SYN pregnancy.

ges·ta·tion·al age (jes-tā'shŭn-ăl āj) The age of a fetus expressed in elapsed time since the first day of the last normal menstrual period.

ges·ta·tion·al di·a·be·tes (jes-tā'shŭn-ăl dī'ă-bē'tēz) High blood sugar in a pregnant female never known to have diabetes; affects about 4% of all pregnant women; cause unknown, but may be related to the placental hormones blocking insulin action.

ges·ta·tion·al e·de·ma (jes-tā'shŭn-ăl ĕ-dē'mă) Generalized and excessive accumulation of fluid in the tissues of greater than 1+ pitting after 12 hours'

bed rest, or of a weight gain of 5 pounds or more in 1 week due to the influence of pregnancy.

ges·ta·tion·al hy·per·ten·sion (jes-tā'shŭn-ăl hī'pĕr-ten'shŭn) Hypertension during pregnancy in a previously normotensive woman or aggravation of hypertension during pregnancy in a hypertensive woman.

ges·ta·tion·al pro·tein·u·ri·a (jes-tā'shŭn-ăl prō'tē-nyūr'ē-ă) The presence of protein in urine during or under the influence of pregnancy in the absence of hypertension, edema, renal infection, or known intrinsic renovascular disease.

ges·ta·tion·al ring (jes-tā'shŭn-ăl rīng) White anulus identified by pulse echosonography that signals an early stage of pregnancy.

ges·ta·tion·al sac (GS) (jes-tā'shŭn-ăl sak) Cystic structure of early pregnancy that represents the amnionic sac, fluid, and placenta.

ges·ta·tion·al tro·pho·blas·tic dis·ease (GTD) (jes-tā'shŭn-ăl trof'ō-blas'tik di-zēz') SYN hydatidiform mole.

ges·to·sis, pl. **ges·to·ses** (jes-tō'sis, -sēz) Any disorder of pregnancy.

Ghon tu·ber·cle, Ghon com·plex, Ghon fo·cus (gon tū'bĕr-kĕl, kom'pleks, fō'kŭs) Calcification seen in pulmonary parenchyma (usually midlung) resulting from earlier, usually childhood, infection with tuberculosis.

ghost (gōst) A hemoglobin-depleted erythrocyte that has also lost most, if not all, of its internal proteins.

ghost cell (gōst sel) A dead cell in which the outline remains visible, but without other cytoplasmic structures or stainable nucleus.

ghrel·in (grel'in) A peptide hormone secreted by endocrine cells in the gastrointestinal tract; acts as a growth hormone secretagogue and as an orexigenic agent.

Gian·ot·ti-Cros·ti syn·drome (jyah-nawt'tē-krōs'tē sin'drōm) A cutaneous manifestation of hepatitis B infection occurring in young children. SYN papular acrodermatitis of childhood.

gi·ant cell (GC) (jī′ănt sel) Large cell, often with many nuclei.

gi·ant cell ar·ter·i·tis (jī′ănt sel ahr′tĕr-ī′tis) SYN temporal arteritis.

gi·ant cell ep·u·lis (jī′ănt sel ep-yū′lis) SYN giant cell granuloma.

gi·ant cell fi·bro·ma (jī′ănt sel fī-brō′mă) A tumor of the oral mucosa composed of fibrous connective tissue with large stellate and multinucleate fibroblasts. Cf. giant cell granuloma.

gi·ant cell gli·o·blas·to·ma mul·ti·for·me (jī′ănt sel glī′ō-blas-tō′mă mŭl-ti-fōr′mē) A histologic form of glioblastoma with large, often multinucleated, bizarre tumor cells.

gi·ant cell gran·u·lo·ma (jī′ănt sel gran′yū-lō′mă) A nonneoplastic lesion characterized by a proliferation of granulation tissue containing numerous multinucleated giant cells; it occurs on the gingiva and alveolar mucosa (occasionally on other soft tissues) where it presents as a soft red-blue hemorrhagic nodular swelling; it also occurs within the mandible or maxilla as a unilocular or multilocular radiolucency. SEE ALSO giant cell tumor of bone. Cf. giant cell fibroma.

gi·ant cell my·e·lo·ma (jī′ănt sel mī′ĕ-lō′mă) SYN giant cell tumor of bone.

gi·ant cell my·o·car·di·tis (GCM) (jī′ănt sel mī′ō-kahr-dī′tis) Acute isolated myocarditis characterized by infiltration by granulomas with giant cells.

gi·ant cell pneu·mo·ni·a (jī′ănt sel nū-mō′nē-ă) A rare complication of measles, with a postmortem finding of multinucleated giant cells lining alveoli. SYN interstitial pneumonia.

gi·ant cell sar·co·ma (jī′ănt sel sahr-kō′mă) Malignant giant cell tumor of bone.

gi·ant cell tu·mor of bone (GCTB) (jī′ănt sel tū′mŏr bōn) Soft, reddish-brown, sometimes malignant, osteolytic tumor composed of multinucleated giant cells and ovoid or spindle-shaped cells, occurring most frequently at the end of a long tubular bone of young adults. SYN giant cell myeloma, osteoclastoma.

gi·ant chro·mo·some (jī′ănt krō′mŏ-sōm) SYN lampbrush chromosome.

gi·ant con·dy·lo·ma (jī′ănt kon′di-lō′mă) Large condyloma acuminatum found in the anus, vulva, or preputial sac of the penis of middle-aged, uncircumcised men.

gi·ant hair·y ne·vus (jī′ănt hār′ē nē′vŭs) SEE congenital nevus.

gi·ant pig·men·ted ne·vus (jī′ănt pig′men-tĕd nē′vŭs) SYN bathing trunks nevus.

gi·ant ur·ti·car·i·a (jī′ănt ŭr′ti-kar′ē-ă) SYN angioedema.

Gi·ar·di·a (jē-ahr′dē-ă) A genus of flagellates that parasitize the small intestine of human beings, domestic and wild mammals, and birds.

gi·ar·di·a·sis (jē′ahr-dī′ă-sis) Infection with the protozoan parasite *Giardia; G. lamblia* may cause diarrhea, dyspepsia, and occasionally malabsorption in humans. SYN lambliasis.

gib·bos·i·ty (gi-bos′i-tē) Something that bulges out from a flatter bodily formation or structure.

gib·bous (gib′ŭs) Humped; humpbacked; denoting a sharp angle in the flexion of the spine.

Gibbs free en·er·gy (gibz frē en′ĕr-jē) SEE free energy.

Gib·ney boot (gib′nē būt) Adhesive tape treatment of a sprained ankle or similar condition, applied in a basket-weave fashion under the sole of the foot and around the back of the lower leg; also called Gibney fixation bandage.

Gib·son ban·dage (gib′sŏn ban′dăj) A bandage, resembling a Barton bandage, for stabilizing fracture of the mandible.

Gib·son mur·mur (gib′sŏn mŭr′mŭr) SYN machinery murmur.

Gib·son walk·ing splint (gib′sŏn wawk′ing splint) A modification of the Thomas splint used to treat malformations of the lower limbs.

Giem·sa stain (gēm′să stān) Compound

of methylene blue–eosin and methylene blue used for demonstrating Negri bodies, *Tunga* species, spirochetes and protozoans, and differential staining of blood smears; also used for chromosomes.

giga- (G) Prefix used in the SI and metric system to signify one billion (10^9).

gi·ga·hertz (GHz) (gig′ă-hĕrts) Equal to one billion (10^9) hertz; used in ultrasound.

gi·gan·ti·form ce·men·to·ma (jī-gan′ti-fōrm sem-en-tō′mă) Familial occurrence of cemental masses in the jaws.

gi·gan·tism, gi·ant·ism (jī-gant′izm, jī′ăn-tizm) A condition of abnormal size or overgrowth of the entire body or of any of its parts. SYN giantism.

giganto- Prefix meaning huge, gigantic.

gi·gan·to·mas·ti·a (jī-gan′tō-mas′tē-ă) Massive hypertrophy of the breast.

Gig·li saw (jē′lyē saw) A hand-held wire saw for use in craniotomy.

Gil·bert dis·ease, Gil·bert syn·drome (zhēl′bār di-zēz, sin′drōm) SYN familial nonhemolytic jaundice.

Gil·christ dis·ease (gil′krist di-zēz′) SYN blastomycosis.

Gilles de la Tou·rette dis·ease (zhēl dĕ lah tū-ret′ di-zēz′) SYN Tourette syndrome.

Gil·les·pie syn·drome (gi-les′pē sin′drōm) Congenital absence of the iris, mental retardation, and cerebellar ataxia.

Gil Ver·net tech·nique (hēl fer′net tek-nēk′) A surgical reimplantation technique used to treat unilateral vesicoureteric reflux.

gin·ger (zz.) (jin′jĕr) The dried rhizome of *Zingiber officinale*, known in commerce as Jamaica ginger, African ginger, and Cochin ginger. The outer cortical layers often are either partially or completely removed; used as a carminative and flavoring agent. SYN zingiber.

gin·gi·va, gen. and pl. **gin·gi·vae** (jin′ji-vă, -vē) [TA] The dense fibrous tissue, covered by mucous membrane, which envelops the alveolar processes of the upper and lower jaws and surrounds the necks of the teeth. SYN gum (2).

gin·gi·val crev·ice (GC) (jin′ji-văl krev′is) SYN gingival sulcus.

gin·gi·val fes·toon (jin′ji-văl fes-tūn′) Arcuate enlargement of marginal gingiva.

gin·gi·val fis·tu·la (jin′ji-văl fis′tyū-lă) A sinus tract originating in a peripheral abscess and opening into the oral cavity on the gingiva. SYN dental fistula.

gin·gi·val hy·per·pla·si·a (GH) (jin′ji-văl hī′pĕr-plā′zē-ă) Enlargement of gums due to proliferation of fibrous connective tissue. SYN gingival proliferation.

gin·gi·val line (jin′ji-văl līn) The position of the margin of the gingiva in relation to the teeth in the dental arch. SYN gum line.

gin·gi·val mar·gin (GM) (jin′ji-văl mahr′jin) **1.** Most coronal portion of the gingiva surrounding the tooth. **2.** Edge of the free gingiva. SYN cervical margin (1), gingival crest.

Gin·gi·val-Per·i·o·don·tal In·dex (GPI) (jin′ji-văl per′ē-ō-don′tăl in′deks) An index of gingivitis, gingival irritation, and advanced periodontal disease.

gin·gi·val sul·cus (jin′ji-văl sŭl′kŭs) [TA] SYN sulcus (4).

gin·gi·vec·to·my (GVTY, GING, GV) (jin′ji-vek′tō-mē) Surgical resection of unsupported gingival tissue. SYN gum resection.

gin·gi·vi·tis (jin′ji-vī′tis) Inflammation of the gingiva as a response to bacterial plaque on adjacent teeth; characterized by erythema, edema, and fibrous enlargement of the gingiva without resorption of the underlying alveolar bone.

gingivo- Combining form denoting human gums.

gin·gi·vo·glos·si·tis (jin′ji-vō-glos-ī′tis) Inflammation of both the tongue and gingival tissues. SEE ALSO stomatitis.

gin·gi·vo·os·se·ous (jin′ji-vō-os′ē-ŭs) Referring to the gingiva and its underlying bone.

gin·gi·vo·sis (jin′ji-vō′sis) SYN chronic desquamative gingivitis.

gin·gi·vo·sto·ma·ti·tis (jin′ji-vō-stō′mă-tī′tis) Inflammation of the gingiva and other oral mucous membranes.

gin·glym·o·ar·thro·di·al (jing′gli-mō-ahr-thrō′dē-ăl) Denoting a joint having the form of both ginglymus and arthrodia, or hinge joint and sliding joint.

gin·gly·moid (jing′gli-moyd) Relating to or resembling a hinge joint. SYN ginglyform.

gin·gly·moid joint (jing′gli-moyd joynt) SYN hinge joint.

gin·gly·mus (jing′gli-mŭs) [TA] SYN hinge joint.

Gink·go bi·lo·ba (ging′kō bi-lō′bă) Extremely widely used herbal native to China; claimed to improve vascular insufficiency and palliate symptoms of Alzheimer disease; adverse effects include subdural hematoma and bleeding disorders.

gin·seng (jin′seng) (*Panax quinquefolius*) Herbal with dozens of purported therapeutic properties (e.g., antidepressant, aphrodisiac, sleep aid, systemic panacea); used worldwide.

gir·dle (gĭr′dĕl) [TA] A belt; a zone. A structure that has the form of a belt or girdle. SYN cingulum (1) [TA].

gir·dle an·es·the·si·a (gĭr′dĕl an′es-thē′zē-ă) Anesthesia distributed as a band encircling the trunk.

gir·dle sen·sa·tion (gĭr′dĕl sen-sā′shŭn) SYN zonesthesia.

gla·bel·la (glă-bel′ă) [TA] **1.** A smooth prominence, more marked in the male, on the frontal bone above the root of the nose. **2.** The most forward projecting point of the forehead in the midline at the level of the supraorbital ridges. SYN intercilium, mesophryon. SEE ALSO antinion.

gla·brous, gla·brate (glā′brŭs, -brāt)

Smooth or hairless; denoting areas of the body where hair does not normally grow, i.e., palms or soles.

gla·brous skin (glā′brŭs skin) That normally devoid of hair.

gla·cial a·ce·tic ac·id (GAA) (glā′shăl ă-sē′tik as′id) A caustic for removal of corns and warts.

gla·di·o·lus (glă-dī-ō′lŭs) *Although the correct pronunciation is gladi′olus, the word is often pronounced gladio′lus in the U.S.* SYN body of sternum.

gland (gland) [TA] An organized aggregation of cells functioning as a secretory or excretory organ. SYN glandula (1).

glan·ders (glan′dĕrz) A chronic debilitating disease of horses and other equids, as well as some members of the cat family, caused by *Pseudomonas mallei* and transmissible to humans.

glan·di·lem·ma (glan′di-lem′ă) The capsule of a gland.

glan·du·la, gen. and pl. **glan·du·lae** (glan′dyū-lă, -lē) [TA] **1.** SYN gland. **2.** SYN glandule.

glan·du·lar ep·i·the·li·um (glan′dyū-lăr ep′i-thē′lē-ŭm) Epithelium composed of secretory cells.

glan·dule (glan′dyūl) A small gland. SYN glandula (2).

glans, gen. **glan·dis,** pl. **glan·des** (glanz, glan′dis, -dēz) [TA] A conic acorn-shaped structure.

glans of clit·o·ris (glanz klit′ŏr-is) [TA] Small mass of highly sensitized erectile tissue capping the body of the clitoris.

glans pe·nis (glanz pē′nis) [TA] The conic expansion of the corpus spongiosum that forms the head of the penis.

glan·u·lar (glan′yū-lăr) Pertaining to the glans penis.

Glanz·mann throm·bas·the·ni·a (glahnts′ mahn throm′bas-thē′nē-ă) A hemorrhagic diathesis characterized by normal or prolonged bleeding time, normal coagulation time, defective clot retraction, and normal platelet count but morphologic or functional abnormality of platelets.

Glas·gow Co·ma Scale (glas′gō kō′mǎ skāl) A measure used to assess level of consciousness and reaction to stimuli in a neurologically impaired patient based on performance in three categories: eye opening, verbal response-performance, and motor responsiveness.

Glas·gow sign (glas′gō sīn) Systolic murmur heard over the brachial artery in aneurysm of the aorta.

glass (vitr) (glas) A transparent substance composed of silica and oxides of various bases.

glass·es (glas′ĕz) SYN spectacles.

Glau·ber salt (glow′bĕr sawlt) SYN sodium sulfate.

glau·co·ma (glaw-kō′mǎ) Ocular disease associated with increased intraocular pressure and excavation and atrophy of the optic nerve; produces defects in the visual field and may result in blindness; may be primary or secondary, acute or chronic, open or closed.

glau·co·ma·to·cy·clit·ic cri·sis (glaw-kō′mǎ-tō-si-klit′ik krī′sis) Type of monocular secondary open-angle glaucoma due to recurrent mild cyclitis.

glau·co·ma·tous cat·a·ract (glaw-kō′mǎ-tŭs kat′ăr-akt) A nuclear opacity usually seen in absolute glaucoma.

glau·co·ma·tous cup (glaw-kō′mǎ-tŭs kŭp) A deep depression of the optic disc combined with optic atrophy; caused by glaucoma. SYN glaucomatous excavation.

glau·co·ma·tous ha·lo (glaw-kō′mǎ-tŭs hā′lō) 1. A yellowish white ring surrounding the optic disc, indicating atrophy of the choroid in glaucoma. 2. A halo surrounding lights, caused by corneal edema in closed-angle granule closure glaucoma.

Glea·son tu·mor grade (glē′sŏn tū′mŏr grād) A five-step classification of adenocarcinoma of the prostate by evaluation of the pattern of glandular differentiation; the tumor grade, known as Gleason score, is the sum of the dominant and secondary patterns.

Glenn op·er·a·tion (glen op-ĕr-ā′shŭn) Anastomosis between the superior vena cava and the right main pulmonary artery to increase pulmonary blood flow as a palliative correction for tricuspid atresia.

gle·no·hu·mer·al (GH) (glē′nō-hyū′mĕr-ăl) Relating to the glenoid cavity and the humerus.

gle·no·hu·mer·al lig·a·ments (glē′nō-hyū′mĕr-ăl lig′ă-mĕnts) [TA] Three fibrous bands that reinforce the anterior part of the articular capsule of the shoulder joint. SYN ligamenta glenohumeralia [TA].

gle·noid (glē′noyd) Resembling a socket.

gle·noid fos·sa (glē′noyd fos′ă) SYN glenoid cavity of scapula.

gle·noid la·brum (glē′noyd lā′brŭm) Soft tissue lip around the periphery of the glenoid fossa that widens and deepens the shoulder joint to aid in the achievement of stability.

glen·oid la·brum of scap·u·la (glē′noyd lā′brŭm skap′yŭ-lă) A ring of fibrocartilage attached to the margin of the glenoid cavity of the scapula to increase its depth. SYN glenoid ligament.

gle·noid lig·a·ment (glē′noyd lig′ă-mĕnt) SYN glenoid labrum of scapula.

gli·a (glī′ă) SYN neuroglia.

gli·a·cyte (glī′ă-sīt) A neuroglia cell. SEE neuroglia.

gli·a·din (glī′ă-din) A class of protein, separable from wheat and rye glutens, which contains up to 40% L-glutamine.

gli·al (glī′ăl) Pertaining to glia or neuroglia.

gli·al-cell-de·rived neu·ro·tro·phic fac·tor (GDNF) (glī′ăl sel dĕ-rīvd′ nūr′ō-trō′fik fak′tŏr) A small protein that assists survival of many types of neurons.

gli·al fib·ril·la·ry a·cid·ic pro·tein (glī′ăl fī′bri-lar-ē ă-sid′ik prō′tēn) A 51-kD cytoskeletal protein found in fibrous astrocytes.

glid·ing joint (glīd′ing joynt) SYN plane joint.

glio- Prefix meaning glue, gluelike (relating specifically to the neuroglia).

gli·o·blas·to·ma mul·ti·for·me (glī′ō-blas-tō′mă mŭl′ti-fōr′mē) A glioma consisting chiefly of undifferentiated anaplastic cells of glial origin that show marked nuclear pleomorphism, necrosis, and vascular endothelial proliferation.

gli·o·ma (glī-ō′mă) Any neoplasm derived from one of the various types of cells that form the interstitial tissue of the brain, spinal cord, pineal gland, posterior pituitary gland, and retina.

gli·o·ma·to·sis (glī′ō-mă-tō′sis) Neoplastic growth of neuroglial cells in the brain or spinal cord; especially a relatively large neoplasm. SYN neurogliomatosis.

gli·o·sis (glī-ō′sis) Overgrowth of the astrocytes in an area of damage in the brain or spinal cord.

Glis·son cap·sule (glis′ĕn kap′sŭl) SYN fibrous capsule of liver.

Glis·son cir·rho·sis (glis′ĕn sir-ō′sis) Chronic perihepatitis with thickening and subsequent contraction, resulting in atrophy and deformity of the liver.

glis·so·ni·tis (glis′ŏ-nī′tis) Inflammation of Glisson capsule, or the connective tissue surrounding the portal vein and the hepatic artery and bile ducts.

glit·ter cells (glit′ĕr selz) Polymorphonuclear leukocytes observed in urine sediment; characteristic of pyelonephritis.

glo·bal a·pha·si·a (glō′băl ă-fā′zē-ă) Disorder in which all aspects of speech and communication are severely impaired. At best, patients can understand or speak only a few words or phrases; they can neither read nor write. SYN mixed aphasia, total aphasia.

glo·bi (glō′bī) Brown bodies sometimes found in the granulomatous lesions of leprosy.

glo·bin (glō′bin) The protein of hemoglobin; α-globin and β-globin represent the two types of chains found in adult hemoglobin. SYN hematohiston.

glo·boid cell (glō′boyd sel) Large cell of mesodermal origin found clustered in intracranial tissues in globoid cell leukodystrophy.

glo·bo·side (glō′bō-sīd) A glycosphingolipid isolated from kidney and erythrocytes.

glob·u·lar pro·tein (glob′yū-lăr prō′tēn) Any protein soluble in water, usually with added acid, alkali, salt, or ethanol, and roughly so classified (albumins, globulins, histones, and protamines).

glob·ule (glob′yūl) **1.** A small spheric body of any kind. **2.** A fat droplet in milk.

glob·u·lin (glob′yū-lin) A family of proteins precipitated from plasma by ammonium sulfate; may be further fractionated by solubility, electrophoresis, ultracentrifugation, and other separation methods.

glob·u·li·nu·ri·a (glob′yū-li-nyūr′ē-ă) The excretion of globulin in the urine.

glob·u·lo·max·il·lar·y cyst (GMC) (glō′byū-lō-maks′il-lar-ē sist) Odontogenic lesion found between the roots of the maxillary lateral incisor and canine teeth.

glo·bus, pl. **glo·bi** (glō′bŭs, -bī) A round body; ball.

glo·bus hys·ter·i·cus (glō′bŭs his-ter′i-kŭs) Difficulty in swallowing; a sensation as if a ball was in the throat or as if the throat compressed; a symptom of conversion disorder.

glo·bus pal·li·dus (glō′bŭs pal′i-dŭs) [TA] The inner and lighter gray portion of the lentiform nucleus. SEE ALSO paleostriatum. SYN pallidum.

glo·man·gi·o·ma (glō-man′jē-ō′mă) A variant of glomus tumor, characterized often by multiple tumors resembling cavernous hemangioma. SEE ALSO glomus.

glo·man·gi·o·sis (glō-man′jē-ō′sis) The occurrence of multiple complexes of small vascular channels, each resembling a glomus.

glo·mec·to·my (glō-mek'tŏ-mē) Excision of a glomus tumor.

glom·er·a a·or·ti·ca (glom'ĕr-ă ā-ōr'ti-kă) SYN paraaortic bodies.

glo·mer·u·lar, glo·mer·u·lose (glō-mer'yū-lăr, -yū-lōs) Relating to or affecting a glomerulus or the glomeruli.

glo·mer·u·lar cap·sule (glō-mer'yū-lăr kap'sŭl) [TA] Expanded beginning of a nephron with inner and outer layers.

glo·mer·u·lar cyst (glō-mer'yū-lăr sist) Lesion formed by dilation of Bowman capsule, found in rare cases of congenital polycystic kidneys.

glo·mer·u·lar neph·ri·tis (glō-mer'yū-lăr nĕ-frī'tis) SYN glomerulonephritis.

glo·mer·u·lo·scler·o·sis (glō-mer'yū-lō-skler-ō'sis) Hyaline deposits in the renal glomeruli.

glo·mer·u·li·tis (glō-mer'yū-lī'tis) Inflammation of a glomerulus, specifically of the renal glomeruli.

glo·mer·u·lo·ne·phri·tis, pl. **glo·mer·u·lo·ne·phrit·i·des** (glō-mer'yū-lō-nĕ-frī'tis, -frit'i-dēz) Renal disease characterized by inflammatory changes in glomeruli not due to infection of the kidneys. SYN glomerular nephritis.

glo·mer·u·lop·a·thy (glō-mer'yū-lop'ă-thē) Glomerular disease of any type.

glo·mer·u·lo·scle·ro·sis (glō-mer'yū-lō-skler-ō'sis) Hyaline deposits or scarring within the renal glomeruli.

glo·mer·u·lus, gen. and pl. **glo·mer·u·li** (glō-mer'yū-lŭs, -lī) **1.** A plexus of capillaries. **2.** A tuft formed of capillary loops at the beginning of each nephric tubule in the kidney. **3.** The twisted secretory portion of a sweat gland. **4.** A cluster of dendritic ramifications and axon terminals forming a complex synaptic relationship and surrounded by a glial sheath. SYN glomerule.

glo·mus, pl. **glo·mer·a** (glō'mŭs, glom'ĕr-ă) [TA] **1.** A small globular body. **2.** A highly organized arteriolovenular anastomosis forming a tiny nodular focus in the nailbed, pads of the fingers and

toes, ears, hands, and feet and many other organs of the body.

glo·mus ca·ro·ti·cum (glō'mŭs kă-rot'i-kŭm) [TA] SYN carotid body.

glo·mus cell (glō'mŭs sel) A peripheral chemoreceptor located in the carotid artery or aorta that is involved with regulation of breathing.

glo·mus cho·roi·de·um (glō'mŭs kō-roy'dē-ŭm) [TA] SYN choroid enlargement.

glo·mus tu·mor (glō'mŭs tū'mŏr) An painful, unusual vascular neoplasm composed of specialized pericytes, usually in nodular masses, which occurs almost exclusively in the skin. SEE ALSO glomangioma.

glo·mus tym·pan·i·cum tu·mor (glō'mŭs tim-pan'i-kŭm tū'mŏr) A glomus tumor of the medial wall of the middle ear.

glos·sal (glos'ăl) SYN lingual (1).

glos·sec·to·my,   glos·so·ster·e·sis (glos-ek'tŏ-mē, glos'ō-ster-ē'sis) Resection or amputation of the tongue. SYN lingulectomy (1).

Glos·si·na (glos-ī'nă) African genus of bloodsucking Diptera (tsetse flies).

glos·si·tis (glos-ī'tis) Inflammation of the tongue.

glos·si·tis ar·e·a·ta ex·fo·li·a·ti·va (glos-ī'tis ar-ē-ā'tă eks-fō-lē-ă-tī'vă) SYN geographic tongue.

🔹 **glosso-, gloss-** Combining forms indicating language; corresponds to L. *linguo-*. Cf. linguo-.

glos·so·cele (glos'ō-sēl) Swelling and protrusion of the tongue from the mouth. SEE ALSO macroglossia.

glos·so·dyn·i·a (glos'ō-din'ē-ă) A condition characterized by burning or painful tongue. SYN burning tongue, glossalgia.

glos·so·ep·i·glot·tic,   glos·so·ep·i·glot·tid·e·an (glos'ō-ep-i-glot'ik, glos' ō-ep-i-glŏ-tid´ē-ăn) Relating to the tongue and the epiglottis.

glos·so·graph (glos´ō-graf) An instrument to record movements of the tongue in speaking.

glos·sol·o·gy (glos-ol´ō-jē) Medical science concerned with the tongue and its diseases. SYN glottology.

glos·son·cus (glos-ong´kŭs) Any swelling involving the tongue, including neoplasms.

glos·so·pha·ryn·ge·al (glos´ō-făr-in´ jē-ăl) Relating to the tongue and the pharynx.

glos·so·pha·ryn·ge·al breath·ing (GPB) (glos´ō-făr-in´jē-ăl brēdh´ing) Respiration unaided by the usual primary muscles of respiration; the air is forced into the lungs by use of the tongue and muscles of the pharynx.

glos·so·pha·ryn·ge·al nerve [CN IX] (glos´ō-făr-in´jē-ăl něrv) [TA] Ninth cranial nerve, which emerges from the rostral end of the medulla, through the retro-olivary groove, and passes through the jugular foramen to supply sensation (including taste) to the pharynx and posterior third of the tongue. SYN nervus glossopharyngeus [CN IX] [TA], ninth cranial nerve [CN IX].

glos·so·pha·ryn·ge·al neu·ral·gi·a (GPN) (glos´ō-fă-rin´jē-ăl nūr-al´jē-ă) Paroxysmal sharp pain in throat or palate. SYN glossopharyngeal tic.

glos·so·plas·ty (glos´ō-plas-tē) Surgical repair of the tongue.

glos·sop·to·sis, glos·sop·to·si·a (glos´ op-tō´sis, -op-tō´sē-ă) Displacement of the tongue toward the pharynx.

glos·so·py·ro·sis (glos´ō-pī-rō´sis) SYN burning tongue.

glos·sor·rha·phy (glos-ōr´ă-fē) Suture of a wound of the tongue.

glot·tal at·tack (glot´ăl ă-tak´) Excessive glottal closure before phonation resulting in loud and sudden voice onset.

glot·tal fry (glot´ăl frī) Vocal fold vibra-

tion in the lowest part of the pitch range, characterized by a creaky, pulsed type of phonation. SYN gravel voice.

glot·tal stop (glot´ăl stop) A stop and then a release of sound at the point of the glottis (e.g., Clint-N).

glot·tis, pl. **glot·ti·des** (glot´is, glot´i-dēz) [TA] The vocal apparatus of the larynx, consisting of the vocal folds of mucous membrane investing the vocal ligament and vocal muscle on each side, the free edges of which are the vocal cords, and of a median fissure, the rima glottidis.

glove an·es·the·si·a (glŏv an´es-thē´zē-ă) Loss of sensation in the distal upper limb, i.e., the hand and fingers.

glu·ca·gon (glū´kă-gon) A hormone produced by pancreatic alpha cells.

glu·ca·gon·like in·su·li·no·tro·pic pep·tide (GLIP) (glū´kă-gon-līk in´sŭ-lin-ō-trō´pik pep´tīd) An insulinotropic substance originating in the gastrointestinal tract and released into the circulation following ingestion of a meal containing glucose.

glu·ca·gon·like pep·tide (GLP-1) (glū´kă-gon-līk pep´tīd) A gut hormone that slows gastric emptying and stimulates insulin secretion.

glu·ca·gon·o·ma (glū´kă-gon-ō´mă) A glucagon-secreting tumor, usually derived from pancreatic islet cells.

glu·ca·gon·o·ma syn·drome (glū´kă-gon-ō´mă sin´drōm) Necrolytic migratory erythema or intertriginous and periorofacial dermatitis, stomatitis, anemia, weight loss, and hyperglycemia resulting from glucagon-secreting pancreatic islet cell tumors.

glu·can (glū´kan) A polyglucose; e.g., callose, cellulose, starch amylose, glycogen amylose.

glu·cep·tate (glū-sep´tāt) *USAN*-approved contraction for glucoheptonate.

gluco- Combining form meaning glucose. SEE ALSO glyco-.

glu·co·am·y·lase (GA) (glū´kō-am´i-lās) SYN exo-1, 4-α-d-glucosidase.

glu·co·cer·e·bro·side (glū'kō-ser'ĕ-brō-sīd) SYN glucosylceramide.

glu·co·cor·ti·coid (glū'kō-kōr'ti-koyd) **1.** Any steroidlike compound capable of significantly influencing intermediary metabolism such as promotion of hepatic glycogen deposition. Cortisol (hydrocortisone) is the most potent of the naturally occurring glucocorticoids. **2.** SYN corticoid.

glu·co·fu·ra·nose (glū'kō-fyūr'ă-nōs) Glucose in furanose form.

glu·co·gen·e·sis (glū'kō-jen'ĕ-sis) Formation of glucose.

glu·co·ki·nase (GK) (glū'kō-kī'nās) Phosphotransferase that catalyzes the conversion of D-glucose and adenosine triphosphate to D-glucose 6-phosphate and adenosine diphosphate.

glu·co·ki·net·ic (glū'kō-ki-net'ik) Tending to mobilize glucose; usually evidenced by reduced glycogen stores in tissues to increase the concentration of blood glucose.

glu·com·e·ter (glū-kom'ĕ-tĕr) A device used to measure sugar levels in blood.

glu·co·ne·o·gen·e·sis (glū'kō-nē'ō-jen'ĕ-sis) The formation of glucose from noncarbohydrates, such as protein or fat. Cf. glyconeogenesis.

glu·con·ic ac·id (glū-kon'ik as'id) The hexonic (aldonic) acid derived from glucose by oxidation of the –CHO group to –COOH.

glu·co·pyr·a·nose (glū'kō-pir'ă-nōs) Glucose in its pyranose form.

glu·co·sa·mine (GlcN, GS) (glū-kō'să-mēn) An amino sugar found in chitin, cell membranes, and mucopolysaccharides generally.

glu·co·san (glū'kō-san) A polysaccharide yielding glucose on hydrolysis (e.g., callose, cellulose, glycogen, starch, dextrins).

glu·cose (glū'kōs) A dextrorotatory monosaccharide found in a free form in fruits and other parts of plants, and in combination in glucosides, glycogen, disaccharides, and polysaccharides (starch cellulose); the chief source of energy in human metabolism, the final product of carbohydrate digestion, and the principal sugar of the blood. SYN d-glucose.

gluc·ose-de·pen·dent in·su·lin·o·tro·pic pol·y·pep·tide (glū'kōs-dĕ-pen'dĕnt in'sŭ-lin-ō-trō'pik pol'ē-pep'tīd) Insulinotropic substance originating in the gastrointestinal tract and released into the circulation following ingestion of a meal containing glucose.

glu·cose in·tol·er·ance (glū'kōs in-tol'ĕr-ăns) Sometimes called "prediabetes," usually diagnosed by measuring fasting blood sugar levels.

glu·cose tol·er·ance test (GTT) (glū'kōs tol'ĕr-ăns test) A test for diabetes, or for hypoglycemic states, after ingestion of 75 g of glucose while the patient is fasting, the blood sugar promptly rises and then falls to normal within 2 hours; in diabetic patients, the increase is greater and the return to normal unusually prolonged; in hypoglycemic patients, depressed glucose levels may be observed in 3-, 4-, or 5-hour measurements.

glu·cose trans·port max·i·mum (glū'kōs trans'pōrt mak'si-mŭm) The maximal rate of reabsorption of glucose from the glomerular filtrate; approximately 320 mg/minute in humans.

glu·co·si·dase in·hib·i·tors (glū-kō'si-dās in-hib'i-tŏrz) Agents that reduce gastrointestinal absorption of carbohydrates. This group of drugs, known popularly as "starch blockers," lowers plasma glucose levels and tend to cause weight loss. Flatulence is a limiting adverse effect.

glu·co·side, gly·co·side (glū'kō-sīd) A compound of glucose with an alcohol or other R–OH compound involving loss of the H atom of the 1-OH (hemiacetal) group of the glucose, yielding a –C–O–R link from the C-1 of the glucose.

glu·co·su·ri·a, gly·co·su·ri·a (glū'kō-syūr'ē-ă, glī'-) The urinary excretion of glucose, usually in enhanced quantities. SYN glycuresis (1).

glu·co·syl (glū'kō-sil) The radical of glucose that has lost its hemiacetal (C-1) OH.

glu·co·syl·cer·a·mide (glū′kō-sil-ser′ ă-mīd) A neutral glycolipid containing equimolar amounts of fatty acid, glucose, and sphingosine. SYN glucocerebroside.

glu·cu·ro·nide, glu·cu·ro·no·side (glucur) (glū-kyūr′ō-nīd, glū′kyūr-on′ō-sīd) A glycoside of glucuronic acid; many foreign chemicals, as well as catabolic products of normal body constituents (e.g., steroid hormones), are commonly excreted in the urine as D-glucuronides. This conjugation is known to take place in the liver. SYN glucuronoside.

glue ear (glū ēr) Middle ear inflammation with thick mucoid effusion caused by long-standing pharyngotympanic (auditory) tube obstruction.

glue-sniff·ing (glū′snif-ing) Inhalation of fumes from plastic cements; solvents, which include toluene, xylene, and benzene, induce central nervous system stimulation followed by depression.

glu·ta·mate (glū′tă-māt) A salt or ester of glutamic acid.

glu·tam·ic ac·id (E, Glu) (glū-tam′ik as′id) Amino acid that occurs in proteins. Cf. glutamate.

glu·ta·min·ase (glū-tam′in-ās) An enzyme in kidney and other tissues that catalyzes the hydrolysis of L-glutamine to ammonia and L-glutamic acid.

glu·ta·mine (Gln, Q) (glū′tă-mēn) The δ-amide of glutamic acid, derived by oxidation from proline in the liver or by the combination of glutamic acid with ammonia.

glu·tar·ic ac·id (glū-tar′ik as′id) An intermediate in tryptophan catabolism; accumulates in glutaric acidemia.

glu·ta·thi·one (GSH) (glū′tă-thī′ōn) The principal low molecular weight thiol compound of living plant cells; used in the course of intermediary metabolism as a donor of thiol (SH) groups; essential for detoxification of acetaminophen overdose or abuse.

glu·te·al (glū′tē-ăl) Relating to the buttocks.

glu·te·al cleft (glū′tē-ăl kleft) SYN intergluteal cleft.

glu·te·al fold, glu·te·al fur·row (glū′tē-ăl fōld, fŭr′ō) [TA] Prominent fold that marks the upper limit of the thigh from the lower limit of the buttocks. SYN sulcus gluteus [TA].

glu·te·al line (glū′tē-ăl līn) One of three curved lines on the outer surface of the ala of the ilium, which provide attachments for the gluteus minimus and gluteus medius muscles.

glu·te·al re·flex (glū′tē-ăl rē′fleks) Contraction of the gluteal muscles following irritation of the skin of the buttocks.

glu·te·al re·gion (glū′tē-ăl rē′jŏn) [TA] The region of the buttocks. SYN regio glutealis [TA].

glu·ten (glū′tĕn) The insoluble protein (prolamines) constituent of wheat and other grains; a mixture of gliadin, glutenin, and other proteins; involved in celiac disease.

glu·ten a·tax·i·a (glū′tĕn ă-tak′sē-ă) Neural disorder due to immunologic damage to the cerebellum, posterior spinal columns, and peripheral nerves in people sensitive to gluten.

glu·ten en·ter·o·pa·thy (glū′tĕn en′tĕr-op′ă-thē) SYN celiac disease.

glu·ti·nous (glū′tin-ŭs) Sticky.

glu·ti·tis (glū-tī′tis) Inflammation of the muscles of the buttock.

glycaemia [Br.] SYN glycemia.

gly·can (glī′kan) SYN polysaccharide.

gly·cate (glī′kāt) The product of the nonenzymic reaction between a sugar and the free amino group(s) of proteins in which it is not known whether the sugar is attached by a glycosyl or a glycoside linkage, or whether it has instead formed a Schiff base.

gly·ca·ted he·mo·glo·bin (glī′kāt-ĕd hē′mŏ-glō-bin) Any one of four hemoglobin A fractions to which glucose and related monosaccharides bind; concentrations are increased in the erythrocytes of patients with diabetes mellitus. SYN glycohemoglobin.

gly·ce·mi·a (glī-sē'mē-ă) The presence of glucose in the blood. SYN glycaemia.

glyc·er·al·de·hyde (glis'ĕr-al'dĕ-hīd) A triose and the simplest optically active aldose; the dextrorotatory isomer is taken as the structural reference point for all D compounds, the levorotatory isomer for all L compounds.

gly·cer·ic ac·id (glī-ser'ik as'id) The fatty acid analogue of glycerol; occurs particularly as phosphorylated derivatives as an intermediate in glycolysis. SYN 2, 3-dihydroxypropranoic acid.

glyc·er·ol, glyc·er·in (glis'ĕr-ol, -in) Sweet oily fluid obtained by saponification of fats and fixed oils; used as a solvent, skin emollient, in suppository form for constipation, orally to reduce ocular tension, and as sweetening agent.

gly·cer·ol de·hy·dra·tion test (glis'ĕr-ol dē'hī-drā'shŭn test) Transient hearing improvement in some patients with Ménière disease after an oral glycerol dose resulting in an osmotic diuresis.

gly·cer·ol ki·nase (GK) (glis'ĕr-ol kī'nās) Enzyme that catalyzes a reaction between adenosine triphosphate and glycerol to yield sn-glycerol 3-phosphate and adenosine diphosphate. SYN glycerokinase.

glyc·er·yl (glis'ĕr-il) The trivalent radical, $C_3H_5^{3-}$, of glycerol; often used in error for glycero- or glycerol.

glyc·er·yl mon·o·ste·a·rate (GMS) (glis'ĕr-il mon'ō-stē'ăr-āt) Agent used in the manufacture of cosmetic creams and dermatologic preparations.

glyc·er·yl tri·ni·trate (GTN) (glis'ĕr-il trī-nīt'rāt) SYN nitroglycerin.

gly·cine (G, Gly) (glī'sēn) The simplest amino acid; a major component of gelatin and silk fibroin.

♻ **glyco-** Combining form denoting relationship to sugars or to glycine. SEE ALSO gluco-.

gly·co·ca·lyx (glī'kō-kā'liks) A filamentous coating on the apical surface of certain epithelial cells, composed of carbohydrate moieties of proteins that protrude from the free surface of the plasma membrane.

gly·co·cho·late (glī'kō-kō'lāt) A salt or ester of glycocholic acid.

gly·co·cho·lic ac·id (glī'kō-kō'lik as'id) N-cholylglycine; this is one of the major bile acid conjugates, formed by condensation of the —COOH group of cholic acid and also by the amino group of glycine.

gly·co·gen (glī'kō-jen) A glucosan of high molecular weight, resembling amylopectin in structure [with α(1,4) linkages] but with even more highly branched [α(1,6) linkages, as well as a small number of α(1,3) linkages], found in most of the tissues of the body, especially those of the liver and muscles. SYN animal starch.

gly·co·gen·e·sis (glī'kō-jen'ĕ-sis) Formation of glycogen from D-glucose by means of glycogen synthase and dextrin dextranase.

gly·co·gen·ol·y·sis (glī'kō-jĕ-nol'i-sis) The hydrolysis of glycogen to glucose.

gly·co·ge·no·sis (glī'kō-jĕ-nō'sis) Any glycogen deposition disease (six forms exist) characterized by accumulation of glycogen of normal or abnormal chemical structure in tissue; there may be enlargement of the liver, heart, or striated muscle, including the tongue, with progressive muscular weakness. SYN dextrinosis.

gly·co·gen phos·phor·y·lase (glī'kō-jen fos-fōr'i-lās) SYN phosphorylase.

gly·co·geu·si·a (glī'kō-gū'sē-ă) A subjective sweet taste.

gly·col (glī'kol) 1. A compound containing two alcohol groups. 2. Ethylene glycol.

gly·col·ic ac·id (glī-kol'ik as'id) An intermediate in the interconversion of glycine and ethanolamine.

gly·col·ic ac·i·du·ri·a (glī-kol'ik as'i-dyūr'ē-ă) Excessive excretion of glycolic acid in the urine.

gly·co·lip·id (glī′kō-lip′id) A lipid with one or more covalently attached sugars.

gly·col·y·sis (glī-kol′i-sis) The energy-yielding conversion of D-glucose to lactic acid (instead of pyruvate oxidation products) in various tissues, notably muscle, when sufficient oxygen is not available (as in an emergency). SYN glucolysis.

gly·co·ne·o·gen·e·sis (glī′kō-nē′ō-jen′ĕ-sis) Formation of glycogen from noncarbohydrates, such as protein or fat, by conversion of the latter to D-glucose. SEE ALSO glycogenesis. Cf. gluconeogenesis.

gly·co·pe·ni·a (glī′kō-pē′nē-ă) A deficiency of any or all sugars in an organ or tissue.

gly·co·pep·tide (GP) (glī′kō-pep′tīd) A compound containing sugar(s) linked to amino acids (or peptides), with the latter preponderant, as in bacterial cell walls. Cf. peptidoglycan.

gly·co·phil·i·a (glī′kō-fil′ē-ă) State with a distinct tendency to develop hyperglycemia, even after ingestion of a relatively small quantity of glucose.

gly·co·pho·rin (glī′kō-fōr′in) A membrane-spanning protein of red blood cells that transports sugar molecules.

gly·co·pro·tein (glī′kō-prō′tēn) One of a group of protein-carbohydrate compounds (conjugated proteins), among which the most important are the mucins, mucoid, and amyloid. SEE ALSO mucoprotein.

gly·cor·rhe·a (glī′kōr-ē′ă) A discharge of sugar from the body, especially in large quantities.

glycorrhoea [Br.] SYN glycorrhea.

gly·cos·am·i·no·gly·can (GAG) (glī′kōs-am′i-nō-glī′kan) SEE mucopolysaccharide.

gly·co·se·cre·to·ry (glī′kō-sĕ-krē′tŏr-ē) Causing or involved in the secretion of glycogen.

gly·co·se·mi·a (glī′kō-sē′mē-ă) Denotes presence of glucose in the blood; it does not imply abnormally high or low levels of blood glucose. SYN glycemia.

gly·co·si·a·li·a (glī′kō-sī-ā′lē-ă) Presence of sugar in the saliva. SYN glycoptyalism.

gly·co·si·a·lor·rhe·a (glī′kō-sī′-ă-lōr-ē′ă) An excessive secretion of saliva that contains sugar. SYN glycosialorrhoea.

glycosialorrhoea [Br.] SYN glycosialorrhea.

gly·co·side (glī′kō-sīd) Condensation product of a sugar with any other radical involving the loss of the OH of the hemiacetal or hemiketal of the sugar, leaving the anomeric carbon as the link.

gly·co·sphin·go·lip·id (glī′kō-sfing′gō-lip′id) Ceramide linked to one or more sugars through the terminal OH group; included are cerebrosides, gangliosides, and ceramide oligosaccharides (oligoglycosylceramides). The prefix glycmay be replaced by gluc-, galact-, and lact-.

gly·co·stat·ic (glī′kō-stat′ik) Indicating property of certain extracts of the anterior hypophysis that permits the body to maintain glycogen stores in muscle and other tissues.

gly·co·su·ria (glī′kō-syūr′ē-ă) **1.** SYN glucosuria. **2.** Urinary excretion of carbohydrates. SYN glycuresis (2).

gly·co·syl (glī′kō-sil) The radical resulting from detachment of the OH of the hemiacetal or hemiketal of a saccharide. Cf. glycoside.

gly·co·sy·la·tion (glī′kō-si-lā′shŭn) Formation of linkages with glycosyl groups. SEE ALSO glycosylated hemoglobin.

gly·co·tro·pic, gly·co·tro·phic (glī′kō-trō′pik, -trō′fik) Pertaining to a principle in extracts of the anterior lobe of the pituitary that antagonizes the action of insulin and causes hyperglycemia.

gly·co·tro·pic fac·tor (glī′kō-trō′pik fak′tŏr) A principle in extracts of the anterior lobe of the hypophysis that raises the blood sugar and antagonizes the action of insulin. SYN insulin-antagonizing factor.

glyc·yr·rhi·za (glis'i-rī'ză) The dried rhizome and root of *Glycyrrhiza glabra* and allied species; a demulcent, mild laxative, and expectorant; also used to disguise the taste of other remedies. SYN licorice, liquorice.

gly·ox·yl·ic ac·id (glī'oks-il'ik as'id) Produced by the action of glycine dehydrogenases on glycine or sarcosine, or from allantoic acid by the action of allantoicase, or through alanine:glyoxylate aminotransferase. SYN oxoacetic acid.

G_{M1} gan·gli·o·si·do·sis (gang'glē-ō-si-dō'sis) Three forms exist: infantile, generalized; juvenile; and adult. SYN generalized gangliosidosis.

G_{M2} gan·gli·o·si·do·sis (gang'glē-ō-si-dō'sis) A hereditary metabolic disorder; several forms exist, including Tay-Sachs disease, Sandhoff disease, AB variant, and adult onset; characterized by accumulation of a specific metabolite, G_{M2} ganglioside, due to deficiency of hexosaminidase A or B, or G_{M2} activator factor.

gnat (nat) A midge; general term applied to several species of minute insects, including species of *Simulium* (buffalo gnat) and *Hippelates* (eye gnat).

gnath·i·on (nath'ē-on) The most inferior point of the mandible in the midline.

gnath·i·tis (nath-ī'tis) Inflammation of the jaw.

gnatho-, gnath- Combining forms denoting the jaw.

gnath·o·dy·nam·ics (nath'ō-dī-nam'iks) The study of the relationship of the magnitude and direction of the forces developed by and on the components of the masticatory system during function.

gnath·o·dy·na·mom·e·ter (nath'ō-dī'nă-mom'ĕ-tĕr) A device for measuring biting pressure.

gnath·o·plas·ty (nath'ō-plas-tē) Plastic and reconstructive surgery of the jaw.

gnath·os·chi·sis (nath-os'ki-sis) SYN cleft jaw.

gnath·o·stat·ic cast (nath'ō-stat'ik kast) An impression of the teeth trimmed so that the occlusal plane is in its normal position in the mouth when the cast is set on a plane surface.

Gnath·os·to·ma (nath-os'tō-mă) A genus of nematode worms characterized by several rows of cuticular spines about the head and by multiple-host aquatic life cycles.

-gnosia Combining form denoting perception of something.

gno·si·a (nō'sē-ă) The faculty of perceiving and recognizing.

gno·to·bi·ol·o·gy (nō'tō-bī-ol'ŏ-jē) The study of "germ-free" animals.

gno·to·bi·o·ta (nō'tō-bī-ō'tă) Living colonies or species assembled from pure isolates.

gno·to·bi·ote (GN) (nō'tō-bī'ōt) An individual organism from a group assembled from pure isolates.

goal (gōl) In psychology, any object or objective that an organism seeks to attain or achieve.

gob·let cell (GC) (gob'lĕt sel) Epithelial cell that distends with a large accumulation of mucinogen-containing secretory granules at its apex, making it look like a goblet. SYN beaker cell, caliciform cell, chalice cell.

goi·ter (goy'tĕr) A chronic enlargement of the thyroid gland, not due to a neoplasm, occurring endemically in certain localities, especially regions where glaciation occurred and the soil is low in iodine, and sporadically elsewhere. SYN goitre, struma.

goitre [Br.] SYN goiter.

gold (Au) (gōld) A yellow metallic element, atomic no. 79, atomic wt. 196.96654; ^{198}Au (half-life of 2.694 days) is used in the treatment of certain tumors and in imaging. SYN aurum.

gold 198 (gōld) An isotope of gold used in medical treatment of tumors by direct injection into the tumor.

Gold·blatt hy·per·ten·sion (gōld'blat hī'pĕr-ten'shŭn) Increased blood pressure after obstruction of blood flow to one kidney.

gol·den·seal (gōld′ĕn sēl) (*Hydrastis canadensis*) Herbal remedy that claims unsubstantiated benefit in treatment of anorexia nervosa, cancer, and other conditions. Widely reported adverse effects (e.g., seizures, cardiac problems, respiratory depression). Death has been reported after overdose. SYN eye balm, yellow paint, yellow puccoon.

gold foil (gōld foyl) Pure gold rolled into extremely thin sheets; used in the restoration of carious or fractured teeth.

gold in·lay (G) (gōld in′lā) Restoration fabricated by casting in a mold made from a wax pattern; the restoration is sealed in the prepared cavity with dental cement.

Gold·man e·qua·tion (gōld′man ē-qwā′zhŭn) Means to predict membrane potentials using membranous permeability and concentrations. SYN constant field equation.

Gold·mann ap·pla·na·tion to·no·me·ter (gōld′mahn ap′lă-nā′shŭn tō-nom′ĕ-tĕr) An applanation tonometer that flattens only 3 sq. mm of cornea, used with a slitlamp; used to measure intraocular pressure.

Gold·mann-Fav·re syn·drome (gōld′mahn fahv′rĕ sin′drōm) An autosomal recessive, progressive vitreotapetoretinal degeneration.

Gold·schei·der test (gōlt′shī-der test) Determination of the temperature sense by touching the skin with a sharp-pointed metallic rod heated to varying degrees.

Gold·stein toe sign (gōld′stīn tō sīn) Increased space between the great toe and its neighbor, seen in Down syndrome, occasionally in cretinism, and as a normal variant.

Gol·gi ap·pa·ra·tus, bod·y, com·plex (gol′jē ap′ă-rat′ŭs, bod′ē, kom′pleks) A membranous system of cisternae and vesicles located between the nucleus and the secretory pole or surface of a cell.

Gol·gi neu·rons (gol′jē nūr′onz) **1.** Pyramidal cells with long axons that exit gray matter of the central nervous system and terminate in the periphery. **2.** Stellate neurons with short axons in the cerebral and cerebellar cortices and in the retina.

Gol·gi stain (gol′jē stān) Any of several methods for staining nerve cells, nerve fibers, and neuroglia using fixation and hardening in formalin-osmic-dichromate combinations for various times, followed by impregnation in silver nitrate.

Gol·gi ten·don or·gan (GTO) (gol′jē ten′dŏn ōr′găn) Proprioceptive sensory nerve ending embedded among the fibers of a tendon, often near the musculotendinous junction. SYN neurotendinous organ, neurotendinous spindle.

Gol·gi ten·don or·gan re·flex (gol′jē ten′dŏn ōr′găn rē′fleks) The relaxation or inhibitory response in muscles to protect them from excessive force or speed: elicited by Golgi tendon organs. Cf. myotactic reflex.

go·mit·o·li (gō-mit′ō-lī) Intricately coiled and looped capillary vessels present in the upper infundibular stem of the pituitary gland stalk; comprise part of pituitary portal circulation.

gom·pho·sis (gom-fō′sis) [TA] Fibrous joint in which a peglike process fits into a hole.

go·nad (gō′nad) An organ that produces sex cells; a testis or an ovary.

go·nad·al a·gen·e·sis (gō-nad′ăl ā-jen′ĕ-sis) Absence of one or both gonads.

go·nad·al a·pla·si·a (gō-nad′ăl ă-plā′zē-ă) Congenital absence of essentially all gonadal tissue.

go·nad·al dose (gō-nad′ăl dōs) SYN gonad dose.

go·nad·al dys·gen·e·sis (gō-nad′ăl dis-jen′ĕ-sis) Defective gonadal development; types include gonadal aplasia or agenesis, rudimentary gonads, congenitally defective gonads, and true hermaphroditism.

go·nad dose (gō′nad dōs) The exposure dose to the male or female gonad, usually from incidental secondary radiation in diagnostic or therapeutic irradiation, or from whole-body irradiation. SYN gonadal dose.

go·nad·ec·to·my (gon'ă-dek'tŏ-mē) Excision of ovary or testis.

♻ **gonado-, gonad-** Combining forms indicating the gonads.

go·nad·o·troph (gō-nad'ō-trōf) An endocrine cell of the adenohypophysis that affects certain cells of the ovary or testis.

go·nad·o·tro·pin, go·nad·o·tro·phin, go·nad·o·tro·pic hor·mone (gō-nad'ō-trō'pin, -fin, gō-nad'ō-trō'pik hōr'mōn) **1.** Hormone that promotes gonadal growth and function; such effects, as exerted by a single hormone, usually are limited to discrete functions or histologic gonadal components. **2.** Any hormone that increases or stimulates gonadal function. **3.** Any substance that has the combined effects of both the follicle-stimulating hormone and luteinizing hormone.

go·nad·o·tro·pin-re·leas·ing hor·mone (GnRH) (gō-nad'ō-trō'pin-rē-lēs'ing hōr'mōn) SYN gonadoliberin (1).

gon·an·gi·ec·to·my (gon'an-jē-ek'tŏ-mē) SYN vasectomy.

gon·ar·thri·tis (gon'ahr-thrī'tis) Inflammation of the knee joint.

gon·ar·throt·o·my (gon'ahr-throt'ŏ-mē) Incision into the knee joint.

♻ **gonio-** Combining form denoting an angle.

go·ni·om·e·ter (gō'nē-om'ĕ-tĕr) **1.** An instrument for measuring joint angles. **2.** An appliance used in the static test of labyrinthine disease. **3.** A calibrated device used to measure the arc or range of motion of a joint. SYN arthrometer, flexometer.

go·ni·om·e·try (gō'nē-om'ĕ-trē) Measurement of the angles created by the bones of the body at the joints.

go·ni·on (Go), pl. **go·ni·a** (gō'nē-on, -ă) [TA] The lowest posterior and most outward point of the angle of the mandible.

go·ni·o·punc·ture (gō'nē-ō-pŭngk-shŭr) An operation for congenital glaucoma in which a puncture is made in the filtration angle of the anterior chamber.

go·ni·o·scope (gō'nē-ŏ-skōp) A lens designed to study the angle of the anterior chamber of the eye.

go·ni·os·co·py (gō'nē-os'kŏ-pē) Examination of the angle of the anterior chamber of the eye with a gonioscope or with a contact prism lens.

go·ni·o·sy·nech·i·a (gō'nē-ō-si-nek'ē-ă) Adhesion of the iris to the posterior corneal surface in the anterior chamber angle.

go·ni·ot·o·my (gō'nē-ot'ŏ-mē) Surgical opening of the trabecular meshwork in congenital glaucoma.

gon·o·cele (gon'ō-sēl) Lesion of the epididymis or rete testis due to obstruction.

gonococcaemia [Br.] SYN gonococcemia.

gon·o·coc·cal con·junc·ti·vi·tis (gon'ō-kok'ăl kŏn-jŭngk'ti-vī'tis) A type of hyperacute, purulent conjunctivitis.

gon·o·coc·ce·mi·a (gon'ō-kok-sē'mē-ă) The presence of gonococci in the circulating blood.

gon·o·coc·cus (GC, GN), pl. **gon·o·coc·ci** (gon'ō-kok'ŭs, -sī) SYN *Neisseria gonorrhoeae.*

gon·o·cyte (gon'ō-sīt) SYN primordial germ cell.

gon·o·phore, gon·oph·o·rus (gon'ō-fōr, gō-nof'ŏr-ŭs) Any structure that stores or conducts sex cells; oviduct, spermatic duct, uterus, or seminal vesicle.

gon·or·rhe·a (gon'ŏr-ē'ă) A contagious catarrhal inflammation of the genital mucous membrane, acquired through sexual contact and due to *Neisseria gonorrhoeae;* may involve the lower or upper genital tract, especially the urethra, endocervix, and uterine tubes, or may spread to the peritoneum and rarely to the heart, joints, or other structures by way of the bloodstream. SYN gonorrhoea.

gon·or·rhe·al oph·thal·mi·a (gon'ŏr-ē'ăl of-thal'mē-ă) Acute purulent conjunctivitis due to *Neisseria gonorrhoeae.* SYN gonorrhoeal ophthalmia.

gon·or·rhe·al proc·ti·tis (gon'ŏr-ē'ăl

prok-tī′tis) Rectal infection by *Neisseria gonorrhoeae* due to anal intercourse.

gonorrhoea [Br.] SYN gonorrhea.

gonorrhoeal conjunctivitis [Br.] SYN gonorrheal ophthalmia.

gonorrhoeal ophthalmia [Br.] SYN gonorrheal ophthalmia.

Gon·y·au·lax cat·a·nel·la (gon′ē-aw′ laks kat′ă-nel′ă) Marine protozoan that produces a toxin in mussels that may poison humans when the shellfish are eaten.

gon·y·o·cele (gon′ē-ō-sēl) Inflammation of the synovial membrane of the femorotibial joint.

gon·y·on·cus (gon′ē-ongk′ŭs) Tumor of the femorotibial joint.

Good·ell sign (gud′el sīn) Softening of the cervix and vagina as being usually indicative of pregnancy.

Good·e·nough-Har·ris draw·ing test (gud′ē-nō-har′is draw′ing test) Refinement of Goodenough draw-a-person test that evaluates inclusion of body details and clothing.

Good·man syn·drome (gud′măn sin′ drōm) An autosomal recessive genetic syndrome characterized by birth defects of the head and fingers, including extra fingers, fusion of the fingers, and ulnar deviation.

Good·pas·ture syn·drome (gud′paschŭr sin′drōm) Glomerulonephritis of the anti-basement membrane type associated with or preceded by hemoptysis.

goose flesh (gūs flesh) SYN cutis anserina.

Gop·a·lan syn·drome (gō′pah-lahn sin′ drōm) Severe discomfort of the feet associated with elevated skin temperature and excessive sweating.

Gor·don re·flex (gōr′dŏn rē′fleks) Dorsal flexion of the great toe produced by firm lateral pressure on the calf muscles. SYN paradoxic flexor reflex.

gor·get (gōr′jet) A director or guide with wide groove for use in lithotomy.

Gor·ham dis·ease (gōr′ăm di-zēz′) SYN disappearing bone disease, Gorham-Stout disease.

Gor·lin sign (gōr′lin sīn) Unusual ease in touching the tip of the nose with the tongue; seen in Ehlers-Danlos syndrome.

gos·er·e·lin (gō′sĕr-el′in) A synthetic decapeptide agonist analogue of luteinizing hormone–releasing hormone that inhibits pituitary gonadotropin secretion and is used to treat prostate cancer, breast cancer, and endometriosis.

Gos·se·lin frac·ture (gō-slen[h]′ frak′ shŭr) V-shaped fracture of distal end of tibia.

gos·sy·pol (gos′i-pol) (*Gossypium hirsutum*) This plant's parts are thought to be of value as a male contraceptive (clinical studies done); other uses are as an antineoplastic and vaginal spermicide. Adverse effects reported include heart failure, hepatotoxicity, nephrotoxicity, and, with oral ingestion of seeds, death by poisoning. SYN cotton.

Gou·ley cath·e·ter (gū′lē kath′ĕ-tĕr) A solid curved steel instrument grooved on its inferior surface so that it can be passed over a guide through a urethral stricture.

gout (gowt) A disorder of purine metabolism, occurring especially in men, characterized by a raised but variable blood uric acid level and severe recurrent acute arthritis of sudden onset resulting from deposition of crystals of sodium urate in connective tissues and articular cartilage.

gou·ty ar·thri·tis (gow′tē ahr-thrī′tis) Inflammation of the joints in gout.

gou·ty neph·rop·a·thy (gowt′ē nūrop′ă-thē) A chronic kidney disease associated with the abnormal production and excretion of uric acid.

gou·ty to·phus (gow′tē tō′fŭs) A deposit of uric acid and urates in periarticular fibrous tissue, cartilage of the external ear, or kidney, in gout.

Gow·ers syn·drome (gow′ĕrz sin′drōm) Palpitation, chest pain, respiratory difficulties, and disturbances with gastric motility; considered psychogenic (anxiety neurosis).

Gow·ers tract (gow′ĕrz trakt) SYN anterior cerebellar tract.

Goy·rand in·ju·ry (gwah-rōn[h] in′jŭr-ē) Eponymic usage for pulled elbow.

G6PD de·fi·cien·cy (dĕ-fish′ĕn-sē) Disorder involving lack of the enzyme glucose-6-phosphate, which helps erythrocytes function normally; can cause hemolytic anemia.

gra·cile nu·cle·us (gras′il nū′klē-ŭs) The medial one of the three nuclei of the dorsal column, the other two being the cuneate nucleus and the accessory cuneate nucleus, which corresponds to the clava. It receives dorsal-root fibers conveying sensory innervation of the leg and lower trunk and projects, by way of the medial lemniscus, to the ventral nucleus posterior nucleus of the thalamus.

gra·cile tu·ber·cle (gras′il tū′bĕr-kĕl) Expanded upper end of the gracile fasciculus, corresponding to the position of the gracile nucleus. SYN clava, tuberculum gracile.

grac·i·lis (gras′i-lis) Slender; denoting a thin or slender structure.

gra·ded ex·er·cise test (GXT) (grād′ĕd eks′ĕr-sīz test) Multistage exercise testing (usually on treadmill or bicycle ergometer) in which exercise intensity is progressively increased (graded) through levels that bring the test subject to a self-imposed fatigue level. SEE stress test.

Gra·de·ni·go syn·drome (grah-dā-nē′gō sin′drōm) Disorder consisting of otorrhea, headache, diplopia, and retroorbital pain in petrositis due to an epidural abscess at the apex of the anterior surface of the petrous pyramid causing compression of the abducens nerve in the Dorello canal and irritation of the trigeminal ganglion.

gra·di·ent (grā′dē-ĕnt) Rate of change of temperature, pressure, or other variable, as a function of factors of distance or time.

gra·di·ent ech·o pulse se·quence (grā′dē-ĕnt ek′ō pŭls sē′kwĕns) MAG-NETIC RESONANCE IMAGING modality that uses a gradient to regenerate an echo.

gra·di·ent-re·called ac·qui·si·tion in the stea·dy state (GRASS) (grā′dē-ĕnt-rē-kawld′ ak′wi-zish′ŏn sted′ē stāt) A type of gradient echo sequence with free induction decay sampling in magnetic resonance imaging.

grad·u·at·ed (graj′ū-āt′ĕd) **1.** Marked by lines or in other ways to denote capacity, degrees, percentages, or other discrete instruments. **2.** Divided or arranged in levels, grades, or successive steps.

grad·u·at·ed ten·ot·o·my (graj′ū-āt′ĕd te-not′ŏ-mē) Partial incisions of the tendon of an eye muscle for correction of strabismus.

grad·u·ate nurse (GN) (graj′ū-ăt nŭrs) One granted a degree by a state-certified nursing program but who has not yet passed a licensing examination.

Grae·fe knife (grā′fĕ nīf) Narrow-bladed knife used in making a section of the cornea.

Grae·fe op·er·a·tion (grā′fĕ op-ĕr-ā′shŭn) **1.** Removal of cataract by a limbal incision with capsulotomy and iridectomy. **2.** Iridectomy for glaucoma.

Grae·fe sign (grā′fĕ sīn) In Graves disease, lag of the upper eyelid as it follows the rotation of the eyeball downward. SYN von Graefe sign.

graft (gr) (graft) **1.** Any tissue or organ used for transplantation. **2.** To transplant such structures. SEE ALSO flap, implant, transplant.

graft-ver·sus-host dis·ease (GVHD) (graft vĕr′sŭs hōst di-zēz′) An incompatibility reaction (which may be fatal) in a subject (host) of low immunologic competence (deficient lymphoid tissue) who has been the recipient of immunologically competent lymphoid tissue from a donor who lacks at least one antigen possessed by the recipient host.

graft-ver·sus-host re·ac·tion (GVHR) (graft vĕr′sŭs hōst rē-ak′shŭn) Clinical and histologic changes of graft-versus-host disease occurring in a specific organ.

Gra·ham Steell mur·mur (grā′ăm stēl

mŭr′mŭr) An early diastolic sound of pulmonic insufficiency due to pulmonary hypertension. SYN Steell murmur.

grain itch (grān ich) Wheallike cutaneous eruption occasionally noted in farmers and grain handlers due to *Pyemotes ventricosus*.

-gram Suffix meaning a recording, usually by an instrument. Cf. -graph.

gram (g) (gram) A unit of weight in the metric or centesimal system, the equivalent of 15.432358 grains or 0.03527 avoirdupois ounce.

gram e·qui·va·lent (gram ĕ-kwiv′ă-lĕnt) 1. The weight in grams of an element that combines with or replaces 1 gram of hydrogen. 2. The weight of a substance contained in 1 liter of normal solution; a variant of (1). SYN equivalent (5).

gram·i·ci·din (gram′i-sī′din) Polypeptide antibiotic that is bacteriostatic in action against gram-positive cocci and bacilli.

gram-neg·a·tive (gram-neg′ă-tiv) Refers to the inability of a bacterium to resist decolorization with alcohol after being treated with Gram crystal violet. SEE Gram stain.

gram-pos·i·tive (gram-poz′i-tiv) Refers to the ability of a bacterium to resist decolorization with alcohol after being treated with Gram crystal violet stain. SEE Gram stain.

Gram stain (gram stān) A method for differential staining of bacteria; useful in bacterial taxonomy and identification and to show fundamental differences in cell wall structure.

gra·na (grā′nă) Bodies within the chloroplasts of plant cells that contain layers composed of chlorophyll and phospholipids.

grand·daugh·ter cyst (grand′daw-tĕr sist) Tertiary lesion sometimes developed within a daughter cyst.

gran·di·ose (gran′dē-ōs) Pertaining to feelings of great importance, expansiveness, or delusions of grandeur.

grand mal (GM) (grŏn[h] mal) SYN generalized tonic-clonic seizure.

grand mal seiz·ure (grŏn[h] mahl sē′zhŭr) SYN generalized tonic-clonic seizure.

Gran·ger line (grān′jĕr līn) On lateral skull radiographs, line produced by the groove of the optic chiasm or sulcus prechiasmaticus.

gran·u·lar (gran′yū-lăr) 1. Composed of or resembling granules or granulations. 2. Particles with strong affinity for nuclear stains, seen in bacterial species.

gran·u·lar cast (GC) (gran′yū-lăr kast) Dark, dense urinary cast of particulate cellular debris and other proteinaceous material, frequently seen in chronic renal disease. SEE ALSO waxy cast.

gran·u·lar cell tu·mor (gran′yū-lăr sel tū′mŏr) A microscopically specific, generally benign lesion, often involving peripheral nerves in skin, mucosa, or connective tissue, derived from Schwann cells.

gran·u·lar cor·ne·al dys·tro·phy (gran′yū-lăr kōr′nē-ăl dis′trŏ-fē) An autosomal dominant disorder characterized by hyaline deposits in the corneal stroma.

gran·u·lar en·do·plas·mic ret·ic·u·lum (gran′yū-lăr en′dō-plaz′mik rĕ-tik′yū-lŭm) Endoplasmic reticulum in which ribosomal granules are applied to the cytoplasmic surface of the cisternae; involved in the synthesis and secretion of protein through membrane-bound vesicles to the extracellular space. SYN ergastoplasm.

gran·u·lar fo·ve·o·lae (gran′yū-lăr fō′vē-ō′lē) Pits on the inner surface of the skull, along the course of the superior sagittal sinus, in which the arachnoidal granulations are lodged.

gran·u·lar leu·ko·cyte (gran′yū-lăr lū′kō-sīt) A polymorphonuclear leukocytes, especially a neutrophilic one. SEE ALSO granulocyte, basophilic leukocyte, eosinophilic leukocyte.

gran·u·lar pits (gran′yū-lăr pits) Indentations on cranial inner surface, along the course of the superior sagittal sinus.

gra·nu·la·ti·o, pl. **gran·u·la·ti·o·nes**

(gran'yū-lā'shē-ō, -ō'nēz) SYN granulation.

gran·u·la·tion (gran'yū-lā'shŭn) **1.** Formation into grains or granules. **2.** A granular mass in or on the surface of any organ or membrane. **3.** The formation of minute, rounded, fleshy connective tissue projections on the surface of a wound, ulcer, or inflamed tissue surface in the process of healing. **4.** In pharmacy, the formation of crystals by constant agitation of a supersaturated solution of a salt. SYN granulatio.

gran·u·la·tion tis·sue (gran'yū-lā'shŭn tish'ū) Vascular connective tissue forming granular projections on the surface of a healing wound, ulcer, or inflamed surface. SEE ALSO granulation.

gran·ule (gran'yūl) **1.** A grainlike particle. **2.** A very small pill, usually gelatin- or sugar-coated, containing a drug to be given in a small dose. **3.** A colony of the bacterium or fungus causing a disease or colonizing the tissues of the patient.

gran·ule cells (gran'yūl selz) **1.** Small nerve cell bodies in the external and internal granular layers of the cerebral cortex. **2.** Small nerve cell bodies in the granular layer of the cerebellar cortex.

♻ **granulo-** Combining form denoting granular, granules.

gran·u·lo·cyte (GR) (gran'yū-lō-sīt) A mature granular leukocyte; includes neutrophilic, acidophilic, and basophilic types of polymorphonuclear leukocytes; respectively, neutrophils, eosinophils, and basophils.

gran·u·lo·cyte col·o·ny-stim·u·lat·ing fac·tor (G-CSF, GCSF) (gran'yū-lō-sīt kol'ŏ-nē stim'yū-lā-ting fak'tŏr) Glycoproteins synthesized by a variety of cells that stimulate production of neutrophils from hematopoietic stem cells. SEE ALSO colony-stimulating factors.

gran·u·lo·cyte-mac·ro·phage col·o·ny-stim·u·lat·ing fac·tor (GM-CSF) (gran'yū-lō-sīt-mak'rō-fāzh kol'ŏ-nē-stim'yū-lā-ting fak'tŏr) Glycoprotein secreted by macrophages or bone stromal cells that functions as a growth factor for myeloid progenitor cells.

gran·u·lo·cyt·ic leu·ke·mi·a (gran'yū-lō-sit'ik lū-kē'mē-ă) A form of the hematologic disorder characterized by an uncontrolled proliferation of myelopoietic cells in bone marrow and extramedullary sites, and the presence of large numbers of immature and mature granulocytic forms in various tissues (and organs) and in the circulating blood. SYN myelocytic leukemia, myelogenic leukemia, myelogenous leukemia, myeloid leukemia.

gran·u·lo·cyt·ic sar·co·ma (gran'yū-lō-sit'ik sahr-kō'mă) A malignant tumor of immature myeloid cells. SYN myeloid sarcoma.

gran·u·lo·cyt·ic se·ries (gran'yū-lō-sit'ik sēr'ēz) Cells in the several stages of development in the bone marrow leading to the mature granulocyte of the circulation (e.g., myeloblasts, granulocytes).

gran·u·lo·cy·to·pe·ni·a (gran'yū-lō-sī'tō-pē'nē-ă) Fewer granular leukocytes in the blood than normal. SYN granulopenia.

gran·u·lo·cy·to·poi·e·sis (gran'yū-lō-sī'tō-poy-ē'sis) SYN granulopoiesis.

gran·u·lo·cy·to·sis (gran'yū-lō-sī-tō'sis) A condition characterized by more granulocytes in the circulating blood or in the tissues than normal.

gran·u·lo·ma, pl. **gran·u·lo·ma·ta** (gran'yū-lō'mă, -mă-tă) A nodule consisting of epithelioid macrophages and other inflammatory and immune cells and matrix formed when the immune system fends off and isolates an antigen.

gran·u·lo·ma an·u·la·re (GA) (gran'yū-lō'mă an-yū-lā'rē) Chronic or recurrent, usually self-limited papular eruption that tends to develop on the distal portions of the limbs and over prominences, although the condition may be generalized.

gran·u·lo·ma in·gui·na·le (gran'yū-lō'mă ing-gwī-nā'lē) A specific granuloma, classified as a sexually transmitted disease and caused by *Calymmatobacterium granulomatis*. SYN donovanosis, granuloma venereum, ulcerating granuloma of pudenda.

gran·u·lo·ma·to·sis (gran'yū-lō'mă-tō'

sis) Any condition characterized by the presence of granulomas.

gran·u·lo·ma·to·sis si·de·ro·ti·ca (gran′yū-lō′mă-tō′sis sid-ĕr-ot′i-kă) Disorder in which firm, brown foci that contain iron pigment are present in an enlarged spleen.

gran·u·lom·a·tous (gran′yū-lom′ă-tŭs) Having the characteristics of a granuloma.

gran·u·lom·a·tous co·li·tis (GC) (gran′yū-lom′ă-tŭs kŏ-lī′tis) Colonic changes, identical to those of regional enteritis.

gran·u·lom·a·tous en·ceph·a·lo·my·e·li·tis (gran′yū-lom′ă-tŭs en-sef′a-lō-mī′ĕ-lī′tis) Inflammation of brain and spinal cord accompanied by granulomas.

gran·u·lom·a·tous in·flam·ma·tion (gran′yū-lom′ă-tŭs in′flă-mā′shŭn) A form of proliferative inflammation. SEE ALSO granuloma.

gran·u·lo·mere (gran′yū-lō-mēr) The central part of a blood platelet. SYN chromomere (2).

gran·u·lo·pe·ni·a (gran′yū-lō-pē′nē-ă) SYN granulocytopenia.

gran·u·lo·plas·tic (gran′yū-lō-plas′tik) Forming granules.

gran·u·lo·poi·e·sis (gran′yū-lō-poy-ē′sis) Production of granulocytes. In adults, granulocytes are produced chiefly in the red bone marrow of flat bones. SYN granulocytopoiesis.

gran·u·lo·sa cell tu·mor (GCT) (gran′yū-lō′să sel tū′mŏr) A pale benign or malignant ovarian lesion arising from the membrana granulosa of the vesicular ovarian follicle and frequently secreting estrogen. SYN folliculoma (1).

-graph **1.** Suffix indicating something written, as in monograph, radiograph. **2.** Suffix indicating the instrument for making a recording, as in kymograph.

graph (graf) **1.** A line or tracing denoting varying values of commodities, temperatures, or urinary output. **2.** Visual display of the relationship between two variables, in which the values of one are plot-

ted on the horizontal axis, the values of the other on the vertical axis.

graph·es·the·si·a, graph·an·es·the·si·a (graf′es-thē′zē-ă, graf′an-es-thē′zē-ă) Tactual ability to recognize writing on the skin.

-graphia Suffix denoting relationship to writing.

graph·ite (graf′īt) A crystallizable soft black form of carbon. SYN black lead, plumbago.

-graphy Suffix indicating a writing, a description.

grasp·ing for·ceps (grasp′ing fōr′seps) A twin-bladed medical instrument used to seize and hold objects firmly in surgical, obstetric, and dental procedures.

grasp·ing re·flex, grasp re·flex (grasp′ing rē′fleks, grasp) Involuntary flexion of the fingers to tactile or tendon stimulation on the palm of the hand, producing an uncontrollable grasp.

grasp pat·tern (grasp pat′ĕrn) Coordinated movements used to pick up and hold an object in the hand; during the first year of life, it develops steadily in complexity and in the degree of motor control required.

Gras·set phe·nom·e·non (grah-sā′ fĕ-nom′ĕ-non) In organic paralysis of the lower limb, the supine patient can raise either limb separately, but not both together. SYN Grasset-Gaussel phenomenon.

Gras·set sign (grah-sā′ sīn) Normal contraction of the sternocleidomastoid muscle on the paralyzed side in cases of hemiplegia.

grat·tage (gră-tazh′) Scraping or brushing an ulcer or surface with sluggish granulations to stimulate the healing process.

grav·el (grav′ĕl) Small concretions, usually of uric acid, calcium oxalate, or phosphates, formed in the kidney and passed through the ureter, bladder, and urethra.

Graves dis·ease (grāvz di-zēz′) **1.** Toxic goiter characterized by diffuse hyperplasia of the thyroid gland, a form of hyper-

G

thyroidism; exophthalmos is a common, but not invariable, concomitant. **2.** Thyroid dysfunction and all or any of its clinical associations. **3.** An organ-specific autoimmune disease of the thyroid gland.

Graves oph·thal·mo·pa·thy (GO) (grāvz of′thal-mop′ă-thē) Exophthalmos caused by increased water content of retroocular orbital tissues; associated with thyroid disease, usually hyperthyroidism.

Graves op·tic neu·ro·pa·thy (grāvz op′tik nūr-op′ă-thē) Visual dysfunction due to optic nerve compression in Graves ophthalmopathy.

grav·id (gr, GR, G) (grav′id) SYN pregnant.

grav·i·da (G, grav) (grav′i-dă) A pregnant woman. With a prefix indicating number for the total number of times a woman has been pregnant, including live births, still births, and abortions (e.g., primigravida, one pregnancy).

gra·vid·i·ty (gră-vid′i-tē) The number of pregnancies (complete or incomplete) experienced by a woman.

gra·vid·o·car·di·ac (grav′i-dō-kahr′dē-ak) Pertaining to heart disease during pregnancy.

grav·id u·ter·us (grav′id yū′tĕr-ŭs) The condition of the uterus in pregnancy.

grav·i·met·ric (grav′i-met′rik) Relating to or determined by weight.

grav·i·ta·tion·al in·se·cu·ri·ty (grav′i-tă′shŭn-ăl in′sĕ-kyūr′i-tē) Excessive reaction to or fear of ordinary movement or change in head position; avoidance or pronounced emotional response to situations normally requiring adjustment of sense of balance. SYN postural insecurity.

grav·i·ta·tion·al ul·cer (grav′i-tă′shŭn-ăl ŭl′sĕr) A chronic lesion of the leg with impaired healing because of the incompetence of the valves of varicose veins. SEE ALSO varicose ulcer.

gray (Gy) (grā) The SI unit of absorbed dose of ionizing radiation, equivalent to 1 J/kg of tissue; 1 Gy = 100 rad.

gray cat·a·ract (grā kat′ăr-akt) A cataract of gray color, usually seen in senile, mature, or cortical cataract.

gray col·umns (grā kol′ŭmz) The three somewhat ridge-shaped masses of gray matter that extend longitudinally through the center of each lateral half of the spinal cord. SYN columnae griseae [TA].

gray de·gen·er·a·tion (grā dĕ-jen′ĕr-ā′shŭn) Breakdown of the white substance of the spinal cord, the fibers of which lose their myelin sheaths and become darker in color.

gray fi·bers (grā fī′bĕrz) SYN unmyelinated fibers.

gray he·pa·ti·za·tion (grā hep′ă-tī-zā′shŭn) The second stage of hepatization in pneumonia, when exudate degenerates before breaking down.

gray in·dur·a·tion (grā in′dūr-ā′shŭn) Pulmonary condition during and after pneumonic processes in which there is failure of resolution.

gray mat·ter, gray sub·stance (grā mat′ĕr, sŭb′stăns) [TA] Colloquial usage for nonmyelinated neural tissue of the central nervous system.

gray scale (grā skāl) SEE gray-scale ultrasonography. SYN latitude.

gray·scale dis·play (grā′skāl dis-plā′) A high-resolution view screen used in radiology, mammography, and medical imaging.

gray syn·drome, gray ba·by syn·drome (grā sin′drōm, bā′bē sin′drōm) Dingy appearance of an infant at birth and during the neonatal period that can be caused by transplacental toxic effects of the drug chloramphenicol taken by the mother during late pregnancy.

great·er a·lar car·ti·lage (grā′tĕr ā′lăr kahr′ti-lăj) One of a pair of cartilages that form the tip of the nose.

great·er cur·va·ture of stom·ach (grā′tĕr kŭr′vă-chŭr stŏm′ăk) [TA] Border of the stomach to which the greater omentum is attached. SYN curvatura ventriculi major [TA].

great·er o·men·tum (grā'tĕr ō-men'tŭm) [TA] A peritoneal fold passing from the greater curvature of the stomach to the transverse colon, hanging like an apron in front of the intestines. SYN caul (2), cowl, velum (3).

great·er pal·a·tine ca·nal (grā'tĕr pal'ă-tīn kă-nal') [TA] Passage formed between the maxilla and palatine bones.

great·er pal·a·tine for·a·men (grā'tĕr pal'ă-tīn fōr-ā'mĕn) [TA] An opening in the posterolateral corner of the hard palate opposite the last molar tooth.

great·er pel·vis (grā'tĕr pel'vis) [TA] The expanded portion of the pelvis above the brim. SYN false pelvis.

great·er su·pra·cla·vic·u·lar fos·sa (grā'tĕr sū'pră-klă-vik'yū-lăr fos'ă) [TA] A depressed area above the middle of the clavicle, lateral to the sternocleidomastoid muscle, overlying the omoclavicular triangle.

great toe (grāt tō) The first digit of the foot.

great ves·sels (grāt ves'ĕlz) Collective term for the venae cavae, pulmonary artery, pulmonary veins, and aorta.

Greek hay (grēk hā) SYN fenugreek.

green blind·ness (grēn blīnd'nĕs) Impaired perception of shades of green.

Green·field dis·ease (grēn'fēld di-zēz') The late infantile form of metachromatic leukodystrophy.

green fluor·es·cent pro·tein (GFP) (grēn flōr-es'ĕnt prō'tēn) A fluorescent marker used in biology and neuroscience.

green·house ef·fect (grēn'hows ef-ekt') The process in which the emission of infrared radiation warms the atmosphere of a planet's surface.

green soap (grēn sōp) SYN medicinal soft soap.

green soap tinc·ture (grēn sōp tingk'shŭr) Liquid preparation containing potassium soaps and alcohol; frequently advocated in skin cleansing, particularly after exposure to plant toxins such as poison ivy.

green·stick frac·ture (grēn'stik frak'shŭr) One in which the bone is partially broken and partially bent; a type of incomplete fracture that occurs primarily in children.

green tea (grēn tē) Chinese and Japanese tea purported to have health benefits, including reduction of risk of certain cancers and improvement in rheumatoid arthritis, elevated cholesterol, cardiovascular disease, infections, and immune function.

green to·bac·co sick·ness (grēn tŏ-bak'ō sik'nĕs) Illness in tobacco harvest workers characterized by headache, dizziness, and vomiting.

grenz rays (grenz rāz) A type of ultrasoft radiation used to treat skin conditions (e.g., dermatitis, warts, psoriasis, eczema).

Greu·lich-Pyle meth·od (groy'lish-pīl meth'ŏd) Assessment to determine the bone age of a child.

grid (grid) **1.** A chart with horizontal and perpendicular lines for plotting curves. **2.** X-RAY IMAGING a device formed of lead strips for preventing scattered radiation from reaching the x-ray film.

grid ra·ti·o (grid rā'shē-ō) In a radiographic scatter-absorbing grid, the relationship of the height to the width of the gaps between lead strips.

grief (grēf) A normal emotional response to an external loss; distinguished from a depressive disorder because it usually subsides after a reasonable time.

grief work fa·cil·i·ta·tion (grēf wŏrk fă-sil'i-tā'shŭn) Process of assisting patients to work through the process of grief and loss with the assistance of counselors or support personnel; a nursing intervention.

Grie·sing·er dis·ease (grē'zing-ger di-zēz') Severe form of louse-borne relapsing fever caused by *Borrelia recurrentis*.

Grie·sing·er sign (grē'zing-ger sīn) Erythema and edema over the posterior part of the mastoid process due to septic thrombosis of the mastoid emissary vein and indicating thrombophlebitis of the sigmoid sinus.

grind·er's dis·ease (grīnd´ĕrz di-zēz´) SYN silicosis.

grip, grippe (grip) SYN influenza.

gris·e·o·ful·vin (gris´ē-ō-ful´vin) A fungistatic agent used to treat superficial fungal infections caused by dermatophytes, which inhibits microtubule assembly.

Gris·wold brace (griz´wawld brās) An adjustable orthopedic device for the back with two sections that telescope together and can be locked in varying positions of longitudinal and rotational adjustment.

Grit·ti-Stokes am·pu·ta·tion (grēt´tē stōks amp´yū-tā´shŭn) Supracondylar amputation of the femur, the patella being preserved and applied to the end of the bone, its articular cartilage being removed so as to obtain union. SYN Gritti operation.

Groc·co sign (grok´kō sīn) 1. Acute dilation of the heart following a muscular effort; also occurring in various forms of myocardiopathy. 2. Extension of liver dullness several centimeters to the left of the midspinal line in cases of enlargement of that organ.

Groe·nouw cor·ne·al dys·tro·phy (grer´nō kor´nē-ăl dis´trŏ-fē) 1. A granular type of corneal dystrophy. 2. A progressive macular type of corneal dystrophy, characterized by punctate opacities and episodes of photophobia, corneal erosion, and foreign body sensation.

groin (groyn) [TA] 1. Topographic area of the inferior abdomen related to the inguinal canal, lateral to the pubic region. SYN inguen [TA], regio inguinalis, iliac region. 2. Sometimes used to indicate only the crease in the junction of the thigh with the trunk.

groove (grūv) [TA] A narrow elongated depression or furrow on any surface. SEE ALSO sulcus.

gross (grōs) Coarse or large; large enough to be visible to the naked eye.

gross an·at·o·my (grōs ă-nat´ŏ-mē) General study of the body, so far as it can be done without the use of the microscope; commonly used to denote the study of anatomy by dissection of a cadaver. SYN macroscopic anatomy.

gross mo·tor skills (grōs mō´tŏr skilz) Those abilities and actions related to activity controlled by the large muscle groups.

ground-glass pat·tern (grownd-glas pat´ĕrn) Radiographic or computed tomographic appearance of hazy opacity that does not obscure underlying anatomic detail.

ground itch (grownd ich) SYN cutaneous larva migrans.

ground la·mel·la (grownd lă-mel´ă) SYN interstitial lamella.

ground sub·stance (grownd sub´stăns) Amorphous material in which structural elements occur. SYN substantia fundamentalis.

group (grūp) 1. A number of similar or related objects. 2. CHEMISTRY a radical.

group ag·glu·ti·na·tion (grūp ă-glū´ti-nā´shŭn) Clumping by antibodies specific for minor (group) antigens common to several microorganisms, each of which possesses its own major specific antigen.

group ag·glu·ti·nin (grūp ă-glū´ti-nin) An immune agglutinin specific for a group antigen. SYN cross-reacting agglutinin.

group A strep·to·coc·cal (GAS) nec·ro·tiz·ing fas·ci·i·tis (grūp strep´tŏ-kok´ăl gas nek´rō-tīz-ing fash´ē-ī´tis) A complication of infection with GAS in which the bacteria attack and destroy muscle tissue.

group dy·nam·ics (grūp dī-nam´iks) The study of underlying features of group behavior, e.g., motives, attitudes; concerned with group change rather than with static characteristics.

group med·i·cine (grūp med´i-sin) Therapy in which health care is provided by individual physicians who have allied themselves as a collective, usually with practitioners of various disciplines located within a building or complex.

group mod·el HMO (grūp mod'ĕl) An HMO that contracts with a single medical practice to be the sole source of care for its subscribers; two types of practice exist under this model: the ''captive'' group, which is formed by an HMO to serve its subscribers, and the ''independent'' group, a previously independent practice that contracts with the HMO.

group prac·tice (grūp prak'tis) The cooperative practice of medicine by a group of physicians, each of whom as a rule specializes in some particular field; such a group often shares a common suite of consulting rooms, laboratories, staff, equipment, and like facilities.

group ther·a·py (grūp thār'ă-pē) A meeting in which several patients with the same condition meet with a single counselor to discuss a condition or problem shared by all patients; generally thought helpful because patients may share perceptions and understandings.

grow·ing frac·ture (grō'ing frak'shŭr) Linear skull crack in a young child that grows due to an associated dural tear and arachnoid cyst formation within the fracture line.

grow·ing pains (grō'ing pānz) Aching pains, frequently felt at night, in the limbs of growing children; attributed variously to growth, rheumatic state, faulty posture, fatigue, or ill-defined psychic causes.

growth (grōth) The increase in size of a living being or any of its parts occurring in the process of development; as measured in increments of weight, volume, or linear dimensions.

growth and de·vel·op·ment, de·lay·ed (grōth dĕ-vel'ŏp-mĕnt, dĕ-lād') Poor or abnormally slow gains in weight or height in a child younger than 5 years old.

growth ar·rest lines (grōth ă-rest' līnz) Dense lines parallel to the growth plates of long bones on radiographs, representing temporary slowing or cessation of longitudinal growth. SYN Harris lines.

growth chart (grōth chahrt) A diagram used by pediatricians and other health care providers to follow a child's growth

over time and compare it with normal ranges by age group.

growth curve (grōth kŭrv) Graphic representation of the change in size of an individual or a population over a period of time.

growth fac·tor (grōth fak'tŏr) A naturally occurring protein capable of stimulating cellular proliferation and cellular differentiation.

growth fac·tor re·cep·tor (grōth fak'tŏr rĕ-sep'tŏr) A cell surface site capable of accepting attachment of growth factor.

growth hor·mone (GH) (grōth hōr'mōn) SYN somatotropin.

growth hor·mone–in·hib·it·ing hor·mone (GIH) (grōth-hōr'mōn-in-hib'i-ting hōr'mōn) SYN somatostatin.

growth hor·mone–re·leas·ing fac·tor (GHRF, GH-RF) (grōth hōr'mōn-rĕ-lēs'ing fak'tŏr) SYN somatoliberin.

growth hor·mone–re·leas·ing hor·mone (GHRH, GH-RH) (grōth hōr'mōn-rĕ-lēs'ing hōr'mōn) SYN somatoliberin.

growth plate (grōth plāt) SYN epiphysial plate.

growth rate (grōth rāt) Absolute or relative growth increase, expressed per unit of time.

growth re·tar·da·tion (grōth rē'tahr-dā'shŭn) A slower than normal pattern of growth caused by a variety of factors including heredity, growth hormone deficiency, thyroid disorders, chronic illness, poor nutrition, and emotional stress.

gru·mous (grū'mŭs) Thick and lumpy, as clotting blood.

Gru·nert spur (grū'nĕrt spŭr) Epithelial outgrowth of the dilator muscle of the pupil at the junction of the iris and the ciliary body; part of the origin of the iris dilator muscle.

gry·po·sis (grip-ō'sis) An abnormal curvature.

guai·ac (G) (gwī'ak) Nauseant, diaphoretic, stimulant, and reagent used in testing for occult blood. SYN guaiac gum.

guai·fen·e·sin (gwī-fen'ĕ-sin) An expectorant that allegedly reduces the viscosity of sputum, thus facilitating its elimination. SYN glyceryl guaiacolate, guaiacol glyceryl ether.

guan·i·dine (G) (gwahn'i-dēn) A strongly basic compound, usually found (in some plants and lower animals) as the hydrochloride; a constituent of creatine and arginine.

guan·ine (G) (gwah'nēn) One of the two major purines (the other being adenine) occurring in all nucleic acids.

guan·o·sine (G, Guo) (gwah'nō-sēn) A major constituent of RNA and of guanine nucleotides.

guan·o·sine 5'-tri·phos·phate (GTP) (gwah'nō-sēn trī-fos'fāt) An immediate precursor of guanine nucleotides in RNA; similar to ATP; has a crucial role in microtubule formation.

gua·nyl·ic ac·id (GMP) (gwă-nil'ik as'id) A major component of ribonucleic acids. SYN guanine ribonucleotide.

guar gum (GG) (gwahr gŭm) Legume used in pharmaceutical jelly formulations.

Guar·ni·er·i bod·ies (gwahr-nē-er'ē bod'ēz) Intracytoplasmic acidophilic inclusion bodies observed in epithelial cells in variola (smallpox) and vaccinia infections.

Gub·bay Test of Mo·tor Pro·fi·cien·cy (gŭ-bā' test mō'tŏr prŏ-fish'ĕn-sē) An assessment tool for evaluating coordination and muscle skills in children.

gu·ber·nac·u·lar cord (gū'bĕr-nak'yū-lăr kōrd) Contents of the gubernacular canal, usually composed of remnants of dental lamina and connective tissue.

gu·ber·nac·u·lum (gū'bĕr-nak'yū-lŭm) **1.** A fibrous cord connecting two structures. **2.** A mesenchymal column of tissue that connects the fetal testis to the developing scrotum. SYN gubernaculum testis [TA].

gu·ber·nac·u·lum den·tis (gū'bĕr-nak' yū-lŭm den'tis) A connective tissue band uniting the tooth sac with the gum.

gu·ber·nac·u·lum tes·tis (gū'bĕr-nak' yū-lŭm tes'tis) [TA] SYN gubernaculum (2).

Gud·den com·mis·sure (gūd'en kom'ĭ-shŭr) SYN commissura supraoptica dorsalis.

Gue·del signs (gū-del' sīnz) A system for determining the stages of anesthesia; originally developed for use with ether.

gug·gul (gŭg'gĕl) A plant used in herbal medicine to treat a wide variety of conditions including rheumatism and obesity; contraindicated for use in pregnant patients.

guide (gīd) **1.** To lead in a set course. **2.** Any device or instrument by which another is led into its proper course, e.g., a grooved director, a catheter guide.

guid·ed im·a·gery (gī'dĕd im'ăj-rē) Theoretic therapy that posits the power of the mind to affect physiology directly; used in a variety of medical settings to reduce stress, calm the mind, decrease pain, stimulate the immune system, and slow the heart rate.

guide dog (gīd dawg) Personal-assistance dog trained to lead blind or visually impaired people.

guid·ed tis·sue re·gen·er·a·tion (gīd' ĕd tish'ū rē-jen'ĕr-ā'shŭn) Regeneration of tissue directed by the physical presence or chemical activities of a biomaterial; often involves placement of barriers to exclude one or more cell types during healing or regeneration of tissue.

guide plane (gīd plān) A fixed or removable device used to displace a single tooth, an arch segment, or an entire arch toward an improved relationship.

guide·wire, guide wire (gw, GW) (gīd'wīr) A wire or spring used as a guide for placement of a larger device or prosthesis, such as a catheter or intramedullary pin.

Guil·lain-Bar·ré syn·drome (gē-yan [h]' bă-rā' sin'drōm) An acute, immune-mediated disorder of peripheral nerves, spinal roots, and cranial nerves, commonly presenting as a rapidly progressive, areflexive, relatively symmetric ascending weakness of the limb, truncal, respiratory, pharyngeal, and facial musculature, with variable sensory and autonomic dysfunction; typically reaches its nadir within 2–3 weeks, followed initially by a plateau period of similar duration, and then subsequently by gradual but complete recovery in most cases. SYN acute idiopathic polyneuritis, acute inflammatory polyneuropathy, infectious polyneuritis, Landry paralysis, Landry syndrome, Landry-Guillain-Barré syndrome, postinfectious polyneuritis.

guil·lo·tine (gē'ŏ-tēn) An instrument in the shape of a metal ring through which runs a sliding knifeblade, used in excising a tonsil.

guil·lo·tine am·pu·ta·tion (gē'ŏ-tēn ampyū-tā'shŭn) SYN circular amputation.

guilt work fa·cil·i·ta·tion (gilt wŏrk făsil'i-tā'shŭn) A nursing intervention to assist families in dealing with stress and feelings of responsibility during prolonged illness of a family member.

Gui·nea worm (gin'ē wŏrm) A waterborne parasite that causes infection, primarily in Africa. SYN dracunculiasis.

Gull dis·ease (gŭl di-zēz') A form of hypothyroidism characterized by decrease in sweating, cold hypersensitivity, dry cold skin, weight gain, fatigue, decreased activity, constipation, mental dullness, prolonged reflex time, carotinuria, and prolonged menses. SYN adult cretinism.

gul·let (gŭl'ĕt) SYN throat (1).

gum (gŭm) **1.** The dried exuded sap from a number of trees and shrubs, forming an amorphous brittle mass; often used as a suspending agent in liquid preparations of insoluble drugs. **2.** SYN gingiva. **3.** Water-soluble glycans, often containing uronic acids, found in many plants.

gum line (gŭm līn) SYN gingival line.

gum·ma, pl. **gum·ma·ta,** pl. **gum·mas** (gŭm'ă, -ă-tă, -ăz) An infectious granuloma that is characteristic of tertiary syphilis, but does not always develop, and that may be solitary (as large as 8–10 cm in diameter) or multiple and diffusely scattered (1 mm or less in diameter). As they age, an irregular scar or rounded fibrous nodule persists.

Gunn sign (gŭn sīn) **1.** Compression of the underlying vein at arteriovenous crossings seen ophthalmoscopically in arteriolar sclerosis. Also called Gunn crossing sign. **2.** On alternate stimulation with light, the pupil of an eye with optic nerve transmission defect constricts poorly or even dilates when stimulated (a relative afferent pupillary defect).

Gun·son meth·od (gŭn'sŏn meth'ŏd) Procedure that involves having an x-ray of the throat taken when the patient is swallowing.

gun·stock de·form·i·ty (gŭn'stok dĕförm'i-tē) Cubitus varus resulting from condylar fracture at the elbow in which the axis of the extended forearm is not continuous with that of the arm but is displaced toward midline.

gur·gling rale (gŭr'gling rahl) Coarse sound heard over large cavities or over a trachea nearly filled with secretions.

gur·ney (gŭr'nē) A stretcher or cot with wheels used to transport hospital patients.

gus·ta·tion (gŭs-tā'shŭn) **1.** The act of tasting. **2.** The sense of taste.

gus·ta·to·ry ag·no·si·a (gŭs'tă-tōr-ē ag-nō'zē-ă) Inability to classify or identify a tastant, even though the ability to distinguish between or recognize tastants may be normal; may be general, partial, or specific.

gus·ta·to·ry au·ra (gŭs'tă-tōr-ē awr'ă) Epileptic aura characterized by illusions or hallucinations of physical taste. SEE ALSO aura (1).

gus·ta·to·ry cells (gŭs'tă-tōr-ē selz) SYN taste cells.

gus·ta·to·ry hyp·er·es·the·si·a (gŭs'tă-tōr-ē hī'pĕr-es-thē'zē-ă) SYN hypergeusia.

gus·ta·to·ry hy·per·hi·dro·sis (gŭs'tă-tōr-ē hī'pĕr-hī-drō'sis) Excessive sweating of the lips, nose, and forehead after eating certain foods.

gus·ta·to·ry pa·pil·lae (gus'tă-tōr-ē pă-pil′ē) Raised structures tongue that contain the taste buds.

gut·as·so·ci·at·ed lym·phoid tis·sue (GALT) (gŭt′ă-sō′sē-ā-tĕd lim′foyd tish′ū) Lymphoid tissue of the gastrointestinal mucosa that contains both B and T cells. This tissue is responsible for localized immunity to pathogens such as bacteria, viruses, and parasites.

Guth·rie bac·te·ri·al in·hib·i·tion as·say (gŭth′rē bak-tēr′ē-ăl in′hi-bish′ŭn as′ā) Bacterial inhibition assay for direct measurement of serum phenylalanine; widely used to detect phenylketonuria. SYN Guthrie test.

Guth·rie test (gŭth′rē test) Assessment done in infants soon after birth to detect the presence of a metabolic disorder called phenylketonuria (q.v.). SYN Guthrie bacterial inhibition assay.

gut·ta (gt), pl. **gut·tae** (gŭt′ă, -ē) **1.** A drop. (abbrev. gt, [sing.], gtt. [pl.]. **2.** A rubberlike polyterpene found in gutta-percha. Cf. gutta-percha.

gut·ta-per·cha (gut′ă-pĕr′chă) Dental filling material, especially in root canals in endodontics, and in the manufacture of splints and electrical insulators.

gut·tate psor·i·a·sis (gŭt′āt sōr-ī′ă-sis) A skin condition with a finding of small salmon-pink droplike lesions.

gut·ter frac·ture (gŭt′ĕr frak′shŭr) A long, narrow, depressed fracture of the skull.

gut·ter wound (gŭt′ĕr wūnd) A tangential wound that makes a furrow without perforating the skin.

Gutt·man scale (gūt′mahn skāl) A measurement scale that ranks categories of responses to a question, with each unit representing an increasingly strong expression of an attribute such as pain or disability.

gut·tur·al (gŭt′ŭr-ăl) Relating to the throat.

Gu·yon sign (gē-yōn[h]′ sīn) **1.** Ballottement of the kidney in cases of nephroptosis, especially when there is also a renal tumor. **2.** The hypoglossal nerve lies directly on the external carotid artery, whereby this vessel may be distinguished from the internal carotid when ligation is necessary.

Gu·yon tun·nel syn·drome (gē-yōn[h]′ tūn′el sin′drōm) Entrapment or compression of the ulnar nerve within the Guyon canal as the ulnar nerve passes into the wrist.

gym·nas·tics (jim-nas′tiks) Muscular exercise, performed indoors, as distinguished from athletics, and usually by means of special apparatus.

Gym·no·din·i·um (jim-nŏ-din′ē-ŭm) Genus of marine dinoflagellates that includes the unicellular organism that causes red tide.

gyn-, gyne-, gyneco-, gyno-, gy·ne·co- Combining forms meaning female.

gynae- [Br.] SYN gyne-.

gynaecic [Br.] SYN gynecic.

gynaecoid [Br.] SYN gynecoid.

gynaecoid pelvis [Br.] SYN gynecoid pelvis.

gynaecologic [Br.] SYN gynecologic.

gynaecologist [Br.] SYN gynecologist.

gynaecology [Br.] SYN gynecology.

gynaecomastia [Br.] SYN gynecomastia.

gynaephobia [Br.] SYN gynephobia.

gy·nan·drism (gī-nan′drizm) A developmental abnormality characterized by hypertrophy of the clitoris and union of the labia majora, simulating in appearance the penis and scrotum. SEE hermaphroditism, female pseudohermaphroditism.

gy·nan·dro·blas·to·ma (gī-nan′drō-blas-tō′mă) SYN Sertoli-Leydig cell tumor.

gy·nan·droid (gī-nan′droyd) A person exhibiting gynandrism.

gy·nan·dro·mor·phism (gī-nan′drō-mōr′fizm) An abnormal combination of male and female characteristics.

gy·nan·dro·mor·phous (gī-nan′drōmôr′fŭs) Having both male and female characteristics.

gy·ne·cic (gī-nē′sik) Pertaining to or associated with women. SYN gynaecic.

gy·ne·coid (gī′nĕ-koyd) **1.** Resembling a woman in form and structure. **2.** OBSTETRICS referring to the shape of the normal female pelvis. SYN gynaecoid.

gy·ne·coid pel·vis (gī′nĕ-koyd pel′vis) Normal female pelvis.

gy·ne·co·log·ic, gy·ne·co·log·i·cal (gī′nĕ-kŏ-loj′ik, -loj′i-kăl) Relating to gynecology. SYN gynaecologic.

gy·ne·col·o·gist (gī′nĕ-kol′ŏ-jist) A physician specializing in gynecology. SYN gynaecologist.

gy·ne·col·o·gy (GYN) (gī′nĕ-kol′ŏ-jē) The medical specialty concerned with diseases of the female genital tract, as well as endocrinology and reproductive physiology of the female. SYN gynaecology.

gy·ne·co·mas·ti·a, gy·ne·co·mas·ty (gī′nĕ-kō-mas′tē-ă, -mas′tē) Excessive development of the male mammary glands, due to ductal proliferation with periductal edema; mild gynecomastia may occur in normal adolescents. SYN gynaecomastia.

gy·ne·pho·bi·a (gī′nĕ-fō′bē-ă) Morbid fear of women or of the female sex. SYN gynaephobia.

gy·no·gen·e·sis (gī′nō-jen′ĕ-sis) Oocyte development activated by a sperm, in which the male gamete contributes no genetic material.

gy·no·plas·ty (gī′nō-plas-tē) Reparative or plastic surgery of the female genital organs.

gyp·sum (jip′sŭm) The natural hydrated form of calcium sulfate used in dentistry.

gy·rase (jī′rās) The prokaryotic topoisomerase II that uses ATP to generate negative supercoils of DNA.

gy·rate (jī′rāt) **1.** Of a convoluted or ring shape. **2.** To revolve.

gy·ra·tion (jī-rā′shŭn) **1.** A circular motion or revolution. **2.** Arrangement of convolutions or gyri in the cerebral cortex.

gy·rec·to·my (jī-rek′tŏ-mē) Excision of a cerebral gyrus.

Gy·ro·mi·tra es·cu·len·ta (jī-rō-mī′tră es-kyū-len′tă) A mushroom that may produce a monomethylhydrazine toxin that causes nausea, diarrhea, and sometimes death.

gy·rose (jī′rōs) Marked by irregular curved lines like the surface of a cerebral hemisphere.

gy·ro·spasm (jī′rō-spazm) Spasmodic rotary movements of the head.

gy·rus, pl. **gy·ri** (jī′rŭs, -rī) [TA] One of the prominent rounded elevations or convolutions that form the cerebral hemispheres, each consisting of an exposed superficial portion and a portion hidden from view in the wall and floor of the sulcus.

gy·rus lon·gus in·su·lae (jī′rŭs long′gŭs in′sū-lē) [TA] SYN long gyrus of insula.

H

H⁺ Abbreviation for hydrogen ion, the proton.

Haa·se rule (hah′sĕ rūl) Fetal length in centimeters, divided by 5, is the duration of pregnancy in months, i.e., fetal age.

ha·be·na, pl. **ha·be·nae** (hă-bē′nă, -nē)
1. A frenum or restricting fibrous band. **2.** A restraining bandage. **3.** SYN habenula (2).

ha·ben·u·la, pl. **ha·ben·u·lae** (hă-ben′yū-lă, -lē) [TA] **1.** SYN frenulum. **2.** Pineal gland, [TA] circumscript cell mass in the caudal and dorsal aspect of the dorsal thalamus, embedded in the posterior end of the medullary stria from which it receives most of its afferent fibers. SYN habena (3).

ha·bil·i·ta·tion (hă-bil′i-tā′shŭn) Educating people with functional limitations so that they can live in society more easily.

hab·it (hab′it) An act, behavioral response, practice, or custom established in one's repertoire by frequent repetition of the same activity.

hab·i·tat (hab′i-tat) **1.** An ecologic area that is inhabited by a particular species. **2.** Physical environment that surrounds a population of a given species.

hab·it cough (hab′it kawf) Persistent cough due to a tic or to psychological causes.

hab·it spasm (hab′it spazm) SYN tic.

hab·it tic (hab′it tik) Habitual repetition of a grimace, shrug of the shoulder, twisting or jerking of the head, or the like.

ha·bit·u·al (hă-bich′ū-ăl) Done automatically, mechanically.

ha·bit·u·a·tion (hă-bich′ū-ā′shŭn) **1.** The process of forming a habit, referring generally to psychological dependence on the continued use of a drug to maintain a sense of well-being, which can result in drug addiction. **2.** The method by which the nervous system reduces or inhibits responsiveness during repeated stimulation.

hab·i·tus (hab′i-tŭs) The physical characteristics of a person.

HACEK group (has′ek grūp) A group of gram-negative bacteria that includes *Haemophilus aphrophilus*, *Actinobacillus actinomycetemcomitans*, *Cardiobacterium hominis*, *Eikenella corrodens*, and *Kingella kingae*. Bacteria in this group have in common a culture requirement of an enhanced carbon dioxide atmosphere and ability to infect human heart valves.

Ha·der·up den·tal no·men·cla·ture (hah′der-ŭp den′tăl nō′měn-klă-chŭr) **1.** European system of identifying teeth by use of a number for each permanent tooth and a + or − sign to indicate the position of each tooth, e.g., 6 + is the upper right first permanent molar. **2.** A system for deciduous teeth analogous to that for the permanent teeth in which a 0 is added before the tooth number, e.g., 03 + is the upper right deciduous canine.

haem [Br.] SYN heme.

haem- SEE hem-.

haem- [Br.] SYN hem-.

haema- [Br.] SYN hem-.

haemachrome [Br.] SYN hemachrome.

haemacyte [Br.] SYN hemacyte.

haemacytometer [Br.] SYN hemacytometer.

Hae·ma·dip·sa cey·lon·i·ca (hē′mă-dip′să sā-lon′i-kă) A land leech that attaches itself to the skin of animals or humans; bite is painful and may cause anemia.

haemagglutination [Br.] SYN hemagglutination.

haemagglutinin [Br.] SYN hemagglutinin.

haemal [Br.] SYN hemal.

haemanalysis [Br.] SYN hemanalysis.

haemangiectasis [Br.] SYN hemangiectasis.

haemangio- [Br.] SYN hemangio-.

haemangioblastoma [Br.] SYN hemangioblastoma.

haemangioendothelioblastoma [Br.] SYN hemangioendothelioblastoma.

haemangioendothelioma [Br.] SYN hemangioendothelioma.

haemangiofibroma [Br.] SYN hemangiofibroma.

haemangioma [Br.] SYN hemangioma.

haemangiomatosis [Br.] SYN hemangiomatosis.

haemangiopericytoma [Br.] SYN hemangiopericytoma.

haemangiosarcoma [Br.] SYN hemangiosarcoma.

haemarthrosis [Br.] SYN hemarthrosis.

haemastatic [Br.] SYN hemostatic.

haemat- [Br.] SYN hemat-.

haematein [Br.] SYN hematein.

haematemesis [Br.] SYN hematemesis.

haematic [Br.] SYN hematic.

haematidrosis [Br.] SYN hematidrosis.

haematin [Br.] SYN hematin.

haematinic [Br.] SYN hematinic.

haemato- [Br.] SYN hemato-.

haematocele [Br.] SYN hematocele.

haematocephaly [Br.] SYN hematocephaly.

haematochezia [Br.] SYN hematochezia.

haematochyluria [Br.] SYN hematochyluria.

haematocolpometra [Br.] SYN hematocolpometra.

haematocolpos [Br.] SYN hematocolpos.

haematocystis [Br.] SYN hematocystis.

haematogenic [Br.] SYN hematogenic.

haematoidin [Br.] SYN hematoidin.

haematology [Br.] SYN hematology.

haematolymphangioma [Br.] SYN hematolymphangioma.

haematolysis [Br.] SYN hematolysis.

haematolytic [Br.] SYN hematolytic.

haematoma [Br.] SYN hematoma.

haematometra [Br.] SYN hematometra.

haematomphalocele [Br.] SYN hematomphalocele.

haematomyelia [Br.] SYN hematomyelia.

haematomyelopore [Br.] SYN hematomyelopore.

haematopathology [Br.] SYN hematopathology.

haematoplast [Br.] SYN hematoplast.

haematoplastic [Br.] SYN hematoplastic.

haematopoiesis [Br.] SYN hematopoiesis.

haematopoietic gland [Br.] SYN hematopoietic gland.

haematopsia [Br.] SYN hematopsia.

haematorrhachis [Br.] SYN hematorrhachis.

haematosalpinx [Br.] SYN hematosalpinx.

haematosin [Br.] SYN hematosin.

haematosis [Br.] SYN hematosis.

haematospermatocele [Br.] SYN hematospermatocele.

haematostatic [Br.] SYN hematostatic.

haematostaxis [Br.] SYN hematostaxis.

haematosteon [Br.] SYN hematosteon.

haematotherma [Br.] SYN hematotherma.

H

haematothorax [Br.] SYN hemothorax.

haematotropic [Br.] SYN hematotropic.

haematoxylin [Br.] SYN hematoxylin.

haematuria [Br.] SYN hematuria.

haemerythrin [Br.] SYN hemerythrin.

haemic [Br.] SYN hemic.

haemic murmur [Br.] SYN hemic murmur.

haemin [Br.] SYN hemin.

haemo- [Br.] SYN hemo-.

haemobilia [Br.] SYN hemobilia.

haemoblast [Br.] SYN hemoblast.

haemoblastosis [Br.] SYN hemoblastosis.

haemocatheresis [Br.] SYN hemocatheresis.

Haemoccult test [Br.] SYN Hemoccult test.

haemochorial placenta [Br.] SYN hemochorial placenta.

haemochromatosis [Br.] SYN hemochromatosis.

haemochrome [Br.] SYN hemochrome.

haemochromogen [Br.] SYN hemochromogen.

haemochromometer [Br.] SYN hemochromometer.

haemoconcentration [Br.] SYN hemoconcentration.

haemocyanin [Br.] SYN hemocyanin.

haemocyte [Br.] SYN hemocyte.

haemocytocatheresis [Br.] SYN hemocytocatheresis.

haemocytolysis [Br.] SYN hemocytolysis.

haemocytoma [Br.] SYN hemocytoma.

haemocytometry [Br.] SYN hemocytometry.

haemocytotrypsis [Br.] SYN hemocytotripsis.

haemodiafiltration [Br.] SYN hemodiafiltration.

haemodiagnosis [Br.] SYN hemodiagnosis.

haemodialyser [Br.] SYN hemodialyzer.

haemodialysis [Br.] SYN hemodialysis.

haemodilution [Br.] SYN hemodilution.

haemodynamics [Br.] SYN hemodynamics.

haemoendothelial placenta [Br.] SYN hemoendothelial placenta.

haemofiltration [Br.] SYN hemofiltration.

haemoflagellate [Br.] SYN hemoflagellate.

haemofuscin [Br.] SYN hemofuscin.

haemogenesis [Br.] SYN hemogenesis.

haemoglobin [Br.] SYN hemoglobin.

haemoglobinolysis [Br.] SYN hemoglobinolysis.

haemoglobinopathy [Br.] SYN hemoglobinopathy.

haemoglobinophilic [Br.] SYN hemoglobinophilic.

haemoglobin S [Br.] SYN hemoglobin S.

haemoglobins [Br.] SYN hemoglobin.

haemoglobinuria [Br.] SYN hemoglobinuria.

haemoglobinuric nephrosis [Br.] SYN hemoglobinuric nephrosis.

haemohistioblast [Br.] SYN hemohistioblast.

haemolith [Br.] SYN hemolith.

haemolutein [Br.] SYN hemolutein.

haemolymph [Br.] SYN hemolymph.

haemolysate [Br.] SYN hemolysate.

haemolysin [Br.] SYN hemolysin.

haemolysinogen [Br.] SYN hemolysinogen.

haemolysis [Br.] SYN hemolysis.

haemolytic anaemia [Br.] SYN hemolytic anemia.

haemolytic disease of newborn [Br.] SYN hemolytic disease of newborn.

haemolytic jaundice [Br.] SYN hemolytic jaundice.

haemolytic uremic syndrome [Br.] SYN hemolytic uremic syndrome.

haemometra [Br.] SYN hemometra.

haemonchiasis [Br.] SYN hemonchiasis.

haemopathology [Br.] SYN hemopathology.

haemopathy [Br.] SYN hemopathy.

haemoperfusion [Br.] SYN hemoperfusion.

haemopericardium [Br.] SYN hemopericardium.

haemopexin [Br.] SYN hemopexin.

haemophagocyte [Br.] SYN hemophagocyte.

haemophil [Br.] SYN hemophil.

haemophilia [Br.] SYN hemophilia.

haemophilia A [Br.] SYN hemophilia A.

haemophilia B [Br.] SYN hemophilia B.

haemophiliac [Br.] SYN hemophiliac.

haemophilic [Br.] SYN hemophilic.

Hae·moph·i·lus **(H)** (hē-mof'i-lŭs) *Avoid the misspelling Hemophilus.* A genus of aerobic to facultatively anaerobic, nonmotile bacteria containing minute, gram-negative, rod-shaped cells that sometimes form threads and are pleomorphic; occur in various lesions and secretions, as well as in normal respiratory tracts, of vertebrates.

Hae·moph·i·lus in·flu·en·zae (hē-mof'i-lŭs in-flū-en'zē) A bacterial species found in the respiratory tract that causes acute respiratory infections including pneumonia, acute conjunctivitis, bacterial meningitis, and purulent meningitis in children, rarely in adults. SYN Pfeiffer bacillus, Weeks bacillus.

Hae·moph·i·lus in·flu·en·zae **type B** (hē-mof'i-lŭs in-flū-en'zē) The most virulent serotype (there are six, A–F, based on antigenic typing of the polysaccharide capsule); bacterial species responsible for meningitis and respiratory infections in young children.

haemophoresis [Br.] SYN hemophoresis.

haemophthalmia [Br.] SYN hemophthalmia.

haemoplastic [Br.] SYN hemoplastic.

haemopoiesis [Br.] SYN hemopoiesis.

haemopoietic [Br.] SYN hemopoietic.

haemoporphyrin [Br.] SYN hemoporphyrin.

haemoprecipitin [Br.] SYN hemoprecipitin.

haemoprotein [Br.] SYN hemoprotein.

haemoptysis [Br.] SYN hemoptysis.

hae·mor·rha·chis [Br.] SYN hemorrachis.

haemorrhage [Br.] SYN hemorrhage.

haemorrhagic cystitis [Br.] SYN hemorrhagic cystitis.

haemorrhagic disease of the newborn [Br.] SYN hemorrhagic disease of the newborn.

H

haemorrhagic infarct [Br.] SYN hemorrhagic infarct.

haemorrhagic measles [Br.] SYN hemorrhagic measles.

haemorrhagins [Br.] SYN hemorrhagins.

haemorrhoid [Br.] SYN hemorrhoid.

haemorrhoidectomy [Br.] SYN hemorrhoidectomy.

haemosiderin [Br.] SYN hemosiderin.

haemosiderosis [Br.] SYN hemosiderosis.

haemospermia [Br.] SYN hemospermia.

haemostasis [Br.] SYN hemostasis.

haemostat [Br.] SYN hemostat.

haemostatic [Br.] SYN hemostatic.

haemotherapy [Br.] SYN hemotherapy.

haemothorax [Br.] SYN hemothorax.

haemotoxic [Br.] SYN hemotoxic.

haemotoxin [Br.] SYN hemotoxin.

haemotroph [Br.] SYN hemotroph.

haemotropic [Br.] SYN hemotropic.

haemotympanum [Br.] SYN hemotympanum.

haemoximeter [Br.] SYN hemoximeter.

haem protein [Br.] SYN heme protein.

haemprotein [Br.] SYN heme protein.

haf·ni·um (Hf) (haf′nē-ŭm) A rare chemical element, atomic no. 72, atomic wt. 178.49.

Hage·man fac·tor (hāg′măn fak′tŏr) SYN factor XII.

H ag·glu·ti·nin (ă-glŭ′ti-nin) Agglutinin formed as the result of stimulation by, and which reacts with, the thermolabile antigen(s) in the flagella of motile strains of microorganisms. SYN flagellar agglutinin.

Hag·lund dis·ease, Hag·lund de·form·i·ty (hahg′lŭnd di-zēz′, dĕ-fōrm′i-tē) An abnormal prominence of the posterior superior lateral aspect of the os calcis.

hair (hār) [TA] **1.** One of the fine, keratinized filamentous epidermal growths arising from the skin of the body of mammals except the palms, soles, and flexor surfaces of the joints. **2.** One of the fine, hairlike processes of the auditory cells of the labyrinth and of other sensory cells.

hair anal·y·sis (hār ă-nal′i-sis) Testing for retrospective purposes when blood and urine can no longer be expected to contain a particular contaminant; most widely used in forensic toxicology and environmental toxicology; used controversially in alternative medicine.

hair cells (hār selz) Sensory epithelial cells present in the spiral organ, maculae, and cristae of the membranous labyrinth of the ear. SEE Corti cells.

hair cy·cle (hār sī′kĕl) Phases of growth (anagen), regression (catagen), and quiescence (telogen) in the life of a hair.

hair fol·li·cle (hār fol′i-kĕl) [TA] Tubelike invagination of the epidermis from which the hair shaft develops and into which the sebaceous glands open. SYN folliculus pili [TA].

hair pa·pil·la (hār pă-pil′ă) SYN papilla pili.

hair streams (hār strēmz) The curved lines along which the hairs are arranged on the head and various parts of the body, especially noticeable in the fetus. SYN flumina pilorum.

hair trans·plan·ta·tion (hār tranz′plantā′shŭn) Relocating baldness-resistant hair follicles from the back and sides of the head to bald or thinning areas elsewhere on the head.

hair whorls (hār wōrlz) [TA] A spiral arrangement of the hairs, as at the crown of the head.

hair·y cell (hār′ē sel) Medium-sized leukocytes that have features of reticuloendothelial cells and multiple cytoplasmic projections (hairs) on the cell surface, but may be a variety of B lymphocyte; found in hairy cell leukemia.

hair·y cell leu·ke·mi·a (hār'ē sel lū-kē'mē-ă) A rare, usually chronic disorder characterized by proliferation of hairy cells in reticuloendothelial organs and blood.

hair·y tongue (hār'ē tŭng) One with abnormal elongation of the filiform papillae, resulting in a thickened furry appearance. SYN trichoglossia.

ha·la·tion (hă-lā'shŭn) Blurring of the visual image by glare.

Hal·dane ef·fect (hawl'dān e-fekt') The promotion of carbon dioxide dissociation by oxygenation of hemoglobin.

half-life (haf'līf) **1.** The period in which the radioactivity or number of atoms of a radioactive substance decreases by half; similarly applied to any substance whose quantity decreases exponentially with time. Cf. half-time. **2.** Time required for the serum concentration of a drug to decline by 50%.

half-nor·mal sa·line (haf-nōr'măl sā-lēn') An intravenous solution containing sodium chloride at about half the concentration found in blood.

half-way house (haf'wā hows) A facility for patients who no longer require the complete facilities of a hospital or institution but are not yet prepared to return to independent living.

ha·lis·te·re·sis (hă-lis'těr-ē'sis) Osseous deficiency of lime salts. SYN halosteresis.

hal·i·to·sis (hal'i-tō'sis) Foul mouth odor. SYN fetor oris, ozostomia, stomatodysodia.

hal·i·tus (hal'i-tŭs) Any exhalation, as of a breath or vapor.

Hal·ler·vor·den-Spatz syn·drome, Hal·ler·vor·den-Spatz dis·ease (hahf'lĕr-fōr'den-shpahts sin'drōm, di-zēz') A disorder characterized by dystonia with other extrapyramidal dysfunctions appearing in the first two decades of life.

Hal·lo·peau dis·ease (ah-lō-pō' di-zēz') SYN pemphigus vegetans (2).

Hall·pike ma·neu·ver (hawl'pīk mă-nū'věr) Test for vertigo.

hal·lu·ci·na·to·ry neu·ral·gi·a (hă-lū'si-nă-tōr-ē nūr-al'jē-ă) Sense of local pain persisting after an attack of neuralgia has ceased.

hal·lu·ci·no·gen (hă-lū'si-nō-jen) A mind-altering chemical, drug, or agent.

hal·lu·ci·no·gen·ic (hă-lū'si-nō-jen'ik) SYN psychedelic.

hal·lu·ci·no·sis (hă-lū'si-nō'sis) A syndrome, usually of organic origin (e.g., alcoholic hallucinosis characterized by more or less persistent hallucinations), in which the patient perceives as real things that do not, in fact, exist.

hal·lux, pl. **hal·lu·ces** (hal'ŭks, -ū-sēz) [TA] The great toe; the first digit of the foot.

hal·lux do·lo·ro·sus (hal'ŭks dō-lō-rō'sŭs) A condition, usually associated with flatfoot, in which walking causes severe pain in the metatarsophalangeal joint of the great toe.

hal·lux flex·us (hal'ŭks flek'sŭs) Hammer toe involving the great toe.

hal·lux ri·g·i·dus (hal'ŭks rij'i-dŭs) A condition in which stiffness in the first metatarsophalangeal joint.

hal·lux val·gus (hal'ŭks val'gŭs) A deviation of the tip of the great toe, or main axis of the toe, toward the outer or lateral side of the foot.

hal·lux va·rus (hal'ŭks vā'rŭs) Deviation of the distal portion of the great toe at the metatarsophalangeal joint to the inner side of the foot away from the second toe.

ha·lo (hā'lō) **1.** A reddish yellow ring surrounding the optic disc, due to a widening of the scleral ring making the deeper structures visible. **2.** An angular flare of light surrounding a luminous body or a depigmented ring around a mole. SEE halo nevus. **3.** SYN areola (4). **4.** A circular metal band used in a halo cast or halo brace, attached to the skull with pins.

H

hal·o·gen (Hal) (hal'ŏ-jen) One of the chlorine group (fluorine, chlorine, bromine, iodine, astatine) of elements.

hal·o·gen ac·ne (hal'ŏ-jen ak'nē) Acneform eruption due to bromides or iodides.

ha·lom·e·ter (hal-om'ĕ-tĕr) An instrument used to measure the diffraction halo of a red blood cell.

ha·lo ne·vus (hā'lō nē'vŭs) A benign, sometimes multiple, melanocytic nevus in which involution occurs with a central brown mole surrounded by a uniformly depigmented zone or halo. SYN Sutton nevus.

ha·lo sign (hā'lō sīn) Elevation of the subcutaneous fat layer over the fetal skull in a dead or dying fetus.

Hal·stead for·ceps (hawl'sted fōr'seps) A small surgical grasping instrument used for clamping small vessels or narrow-gauge tubing.

Hal·sted su·ture (hawl'sted sū'chŭr) Stitch placed through the subcuticular fascia; used for exact skin approximation.

ha·mar·ti·a (ham-ahr'shē-ă) A localized developmental disturbance characterized by abnormal arrangement and/or combinations of the tissues normally present in the area.

ham·ar·to·ma (ham'ahr-tō'mă) A focal malformation that resembles a neoplasm, grossly and even microscopically, but due to faulty development, with a disproportion or abnormal mixture of tissue elements normally present at the site.

Ham·il·ton-Stew·art meth·od (ham'ĭl-tŏn-stū'ărt meth'ŏd) Formula to calculate cardiac output after intravenous indicator dye injection. SYN indicator dilution method.

Ham·man-Rich syn·drome (ham'ăn-rich' sin'drōm) SYN idiopathic pulmonary fibrosis.

ham·mer fin·ger (ham'ĕr fing'gĕr) SYN mallet finger.

ham·mer toe, ham·mer·toe (ham'ĕr tō)

Permanent flexion at the midphalangeal joint of one or more of the toes.

Ham·mond dis·ease (ham'ŏnd di-zēz') SYN athetosis.

ham·ster (Ha) (ham'stĕr) Any of four genera of small rodents widely used in research and as pets. *Cricetus*, *Cricetulus*, *Mesocricetus*, and *Phodopus*.

Ham test (ham test) SYN acidified serum test.

ham·u·lus, gen. and pl. **ham·u·li** (ham'yū-lŭs, -lī) [TA] Any hooklike structure. SYN hook (2).

Han·cock am·pu·ta·tion (han'kok amp'yū-tā'shŭn) Surgical removal of the foot through the astragalus (talus).

hand (hand) [TA] The portion of the upper limb distal to the radiocarpal joint, comprising the wrist, palm, and fingers. SYN manus [TA].

hand-foot-and-mouth dis·ease (hand-fut-mowth di-zēz') An exanthematous eruption of small, pearl-gray vesicles of the fingers, toes, palms, and soles, accompanied by painful vesicles and ulceration of the buccal mucous membrane and the tongue and by slight fever; the disease lasts 4–7 days, and is usually caused by Coxsackie virus type A-16.

hand·i·cap (hand'ē-kap) 1. A physical, mental, or emotional condition that interferes with normal functioning. 2. Reduction in the capacity to fulfill a social role as a consequence of an impairment, inadequate training for the role, or other circumstances. SEE ALSO disability.

han·dle of mal·le·us (han'dĕl mal'lē-ŭs) Major elongated process extending inferiorly and slightly posteriorly, and medially from the neck of the malleus.

hand·piece (HDPC) (hand'pēs) A powered dental instrument held in the hand, used to hold rotary cutting, grinding, or polishing implements while they revolve.

Hand-Schül·ler-Chris·tian dis·ease (hahnt shēl'er kris'chăn di-zēz') The chronic disseminated form of Langerhans cell histiocytosis. SYN Christian disease (1), Christian syndrome, Schüller syndrome.

hang·man's frac·ture (hang′mănz frak′ shŭr) A break in the cervical spine through the pedicles of C-2.

Han·hart syn·drome (han′hahrt sin′ drōm) SYN peromellia.

Han·sen ba·cil·lus (hahn′sen bă-sil′ŭs) SYN *Mycobacterium leprae.*

Han·sen dis·ease (hahn′sen di-zēz′) SYN leprosy.

Han·ta·vi·rus (hahn′tă-vī′rŭs) A genus of Bunyaviridae responsible for pneumonia and hemorrhagic fevers. Four members of the genus are recognized thus far: Hantaan, Puumala, Seoul, and Prospect Hill; the first three are known human pathogens, and Hantaan virus causes Korean hemorrhagic fever.

H an·ti·gen (HA) (an′ti-jen) Antigen in the flagella of motile bacteria.

haph·al·ge·si·a (haf′al-jē′zē-ă) Pain caused by the merest touch. SYN Pitres sign (1).

haplo- Combining form meaning simple, single.

hap·loid (hap′loyd) Denoting the number of chromosomes in sperm or oocytes, which is half the number in somatic (diploid) cells. SYN monoploid.

hap·lo·scope (hap′lō-skōp) An instrument for presenting separate views to each eye so that they may be seen as one.

hap·lo·type (hap′lō-tīp) Genetic constitution of an individual with respect to one member of a pair of allelic genes; individuals are of the same haplotype (but of different genotypes) if alike with respect to one allele of a pair but different with respect to the other allele of a pair.

hap·py pup·pet syn·drome (hap′ē pŭp′ĕt sin′drŏm) Disorder characterized by mental retardation, ataxia, hypotonia, epileptic seizures, easily provoked and prolonged spasms of laughter, prognathism, and an open-mouthed expression.

hap·ten (hap′tĕn) A molecule that is incapable, alone, of causing the production of antibodies but can, however, combine with a larger antigenic molecule called a carrier. SYN incomplete antigen, partial antigen.

hap·tic (hap′tik) 1. Of or pertaining to the sensation of touch or tactile sense. 2. The flexible, looping extension attached to an artificial intraocular lens that stabilizes and centers it within the eye.

hap·tic hal·lu·ci·na·tion (hap′tik hă-lū′si-nā′shŭn) The sensation of touch in the absence of stimuli; may be seen in alcoholic delirium tremens.

hap·tics (hap′tiks) The science concerned with the tactile sense.

hap·to·glo·bin (HP, HAPTO, Hp, Hpt) (hap′tō-glō′bin) A group of $α_2$-globulins in human serum, so called because of their ability to combine with hemoglobin, preventing loss in urine.

Ha·ra·da syn·drome, Ha·ra·da dis·ease (hah-rah′dah sin′drōm, di-zēz′) Bilateral retinal edema, uveitis, choroiditis, and retinal detachment, with temporary or permanent deafness, graying of the hair (poliosis), and alopecia.

hard chan·cre (hahrd shang′kĕr) SYN chancre.

hard corn (HD) (hahrd kŏrn) Usual form of corn over a toe joint. SYN heloma durum.

har·den·ing of the ar·te·ries (hahr′ dĕn-ing ahr′tĕr-ēz) SYN arteriosclerosis.

hard pal·ate (hahrd pal′ăt) [TA] The anterior part of the palate, consisting of the bony palate covered above by the mucous membrane of the floor of the nasal cavity and below by the mucoperiosteum of the roof of the mouth that contains the palatine vessels, nerves, and mucous glands.

hard par·aff·in (hahrd par′ă-fin) Purified mixture of solid hydrocarbons derived from petroleum. SYN paraffin (2).

hard pulse (hahrd pŭls) One that strikes forcibly against the tip of the finger and is with difficulty compressed, suggesting hypertension.

hard soap (hahrd sōp) One made with

olive oil, or some other suitable oil or fat, and sodium hydroxide.

hard wa·ter (hahrd waw′tĕr) That containing ions, such as Mg^{2+} and Ca^{2+}, that form insoluble salts with fatty acids so that ordinary soap will not lather in it.

hare·lip (HL) (hār′lip) SYN cleft lip.

har·le·quin fe·tus (hahr′lĕ-kwin fē′tŭs) Severe and fatal form of deforming collodion in a newborn, usually premature.

Har·ring·ton rods (har′ing-tŏn rodz) Metal stabilizing rods used in surgery to lessen scoliosis.

Har·ris-Ben·e·dict e·qua·tion (har′is-ben′ĕ-dikt ē-kwā′zhŭn) An equation based on a person's height, age, and weight that is used for estimating caloric needs.

Har·ris lines (har′is līnz) SYN growth arrest lines.

Har·ri·son groove (har′i-sŏn grūv) Rib deformity due to the pull of the diaphragm on ribs weakened by rickets.

Har·ris tube (har′is tūb) A single-lumen tube about 6 feet long that ends in with a mercury balloon; used to treat bowel obstruction.

Hart·mann op·er·a·tion (hahrt′măn op-ĕr-ā′shŭn) Resection of the sigmoid colon beginning at or just above the peritoneal reflexion and extending proximally, with closure of the rectal stump and end-colostomy.

Hart·nup dis·ease, Hart·nup syn·drome (hahrt′nŭp di-zēz′, sin′drōm) A congenital metabolic disorder consisting of aminoaciduria due to a defect in renal tubular absorption of neutral α-amino acids and urinary excretion of tryptophan derivatives, which occurs because defective intestinal absorption leads to bacterial degradation of unabsorbed tryptophan in the gut.

har·vest (hahr′vĕst) To obtain cells, tissues, or organs for grafting or transplantation, from either a donor or the patient.

Ha·shi·mo·to thy·roid·i·tis, Ha·shi·mo·to stru·ma (HT) (hah-shē-mō′tō thī-royd-ī′tis, strū′mă) Diffuse infiltra-

tion of the thyroid gland with lymphocytes, resulting in diffuse goiter, progressive destruction of the parenchyma and hypothyroidism. Also called Hashimoto disease. SYN autoimmune thyroiditis, chronic lymphadenoid thyroiditis, chronic lymphocytic thyroiditis, lymphocytic thyroiditis, struma lymphomatosa.

hash·ish (hah-shēsh′) A form of cannabis that consists largely of resin from the flowering tops and sprouts of cultivated female hemp plants of the species *Cannabis sativa*.

Has·sall bod·ies, Has·sall con·cen·tric cor·pus·cle (has′ăl bod′ēz, kŏn-sen′trik kōr′pŭs-ĕl) SYN thymic corpuscle.

haus·tra of co·lon, haus·tra co·li (haws′tră kō′lŏn, kō′lī) [TA] Sacculations of the colon, caused by the teniae, or longitudinal bands, which are slightly shorter than the gut so that the latter is thrown into tucks or pouches. SYN sacculation of colon.

haus·tra·tion (haws-trā′shŭn) **1.** The process of formation of a haustrum. **2.** An increase in prominence of the haustra.

haus·trum, haus·tra (haws′trŭm, -ă) [TA] One of a series of saccules or pouches, so called because of a fancied resemblance to the buckets on a water wheel.

haus·tus (h) (haw′stŭs) A potion; medicinal beverage.

Ha·ver·hill fe·ver (hav′ĕr-hil fē′ver) An infection by *Streptobacillus moniliformis*, usually due to a rat bite, marked by initial chills and high fever (gradually subsiding), by arthritis usually in the larger joints and spine, and by a rash occurring chiefly over the joints and on the extensor surfaces of the extremities. SYN erythema arthriticum epidemicum.

ha·ver·si·an ca·n·al·ic·u·lus (ha-vĕr′shăn kan′ă-lik′yū-lŭs) One of many tiny passages leading from the pits of bone tissue to larger haversian canals.

ha·ver·si·an ca·nals (ha-vĕr′shăn kă-nalz′) Vascular canals that run longitudinally in the center of haversian systems of compact osseous tissue.

ha·ver·si·an gland (ha-věr´shăn gland) SYN synovial villi.

ha·ver·si·an la·mel·la (ha-věr´shăn lă-mel´ă) SYN concentric lamella.

ha·ver·si·an sys·tem (ha-věr´shăn sis´těm) SYN osteon.

Haw·ley re·tain·er (haw´lē rē-tān´ĕr) Removable wire and acrylic palatal appliance used to retain or stabilize the teeth in their new position following orthodontic tooth movement. SYN Hawley appliance.

Ha·yem so·lu·tion (āh´yem sŏ-lū´shŭn) A blood diluent used before red blood cells are counted.

hay fe·ver (hā fē´vĕr) Form of seasonal, allergic atopy characterized by an acute irritative inflammation of the mucous membranes of the eyes and upper respiratory passages accompanied by itching and profuse watery secretion, followed occasionally by bronchitis and asthma.

Hay·flick lim·it (hā´flik lim´it) The limit of human cell division in subcultures; such cells typically divide only about 50 times before dying out.

Hay·garth nodes (hā´gahrth nōdz) Exostoses from the margins of the articular surfaces and from the periosteum and bone in the neighborhood of the joints of the fingers, leading to ankylosis and associated with lateral deflection of the fingers toward the ulnar side, which occur in rheumatoid arthritis.

Haz·ard A·nal·y·sis Crit·i·cal Con·trol Point (HACCP) (haz´ărd ă-nal´ă-sis krit´i-kăl kon´trōl poynt) A food safety system that identifies points in food production where risk of bacterial contamination is high.

H band (band) Paler area in the center of the A band of a striated muscle fiber; the central portion of thick filaments overlapped by thin filaments. SYN H disc, Hensen disc, Hensen line.

hCG Abbreviation for human chorionic gonadotropin.

hCG ra·di·o·re·cep·tor as·say (rā´dē-ō-rĕ-sep´tŏr as´ā) A rapid test done in cases of suspected ectopic pregnancy;

has the highest true-positive rate for this condition.

H chain (chān) SYN heavy chain.

He Symbol for helium.

head (hed) [TA] **1.** The upper or anterior extremity of the animal body, containing the brain and the organs of sight, hearing, taste, and smell. **2.** The upper, anterior, or larger extremity, expanded or rounded, of any body, organ, or other anatomic structure. **3.** The rounded extremity of a bone. **4.** That end of a muscle that is attached to the less movable part of the skeleton.

head·ache (HA) (hed´āk) Pain in various parts of the head, not confined to the area of distribution of any nerve. SEE ALSO cephalodynia. SYN encephalalgia.

head bang·ing (hed bang´ing) Behavior that appears in up to 20% of normal children in the latter half of the first year of life and ends spontaneously by about 4 years of age; more common in boys.

head cap (hed kap) A device fitted closely to the skull; used for fixed anchorage in external traction.

head fold (hed fōld) Ventral folding of the cephalic end of the embryonic disc, so that the brain lies rostrad to the mouth and pericardium.

head·gear (hed´gēr) A removable extraoral appliance used as a source of traction to apply force to the teeth and jaws.

head mir·ror (hed mir´ŏr) Circular concave mirror with a hole in its center to look through attached to a head band, used to project a beam of light into a cavity, for examination and to permit binocular vision.

head pro·cess (hed pros´es) Primordium of the notochord.

heads-up tilt ta·ble test (HUT) (hedz-ŭp´ tilt tā´bĕl test) Assessment to determine the cause of syncope (fainting or loss of consciousness). SYN tilt table test.

head-tilt/chin-lift ma·neu·ver (hĕd´tilt-chin´lift mă-nū´vĕr) Basic procedure used in cardiopulmonary resuscitation to open the patient's airway. Rescuer's one hand tilts head back while other hand is placed under the chin to lift the mandible and displace the tongue. SYN manual airway maneuver, rescue breathing.

heal (hēl) **1.** To restore to health, especially to cause a wound to cicatrize or unite. **2.** To become well, to be cured.

heal·ing (hēl'ing) **1.** Restoring to health; promoting the closure of wounds and ulcers. **2.** The process of a return to health. **3.** Closing of a wound. SEE ALSO union.

heal·ing by first in·ten·tion (hēl'ing fĭrst in-ten'shŭn) Healing by fibrous adhesion, without suppuration or granulation tissue formation. SYN primary adhesion, primary union.

heal·ing by sec·ond in·ten·tion (hēl' ing sek'ŏnd in-ten'shŭn) Delayed closure of two granulating surfaces. SYN secondary union.

heal·ing by third in·ten·tion (hēl'ing thĭrd in-ten'shŭn) The slow filling of a wound cavity or ulcer by granulations, with subsequent cicatrization.

health (helth) **1.** The state of an organism when it functions optimally without evidence of disease or abnormality. **2.** A state characterized by anatomic, physiologic, and psychological integrity. **3.** Complete physical, mental, and social well-being, not just the absence of disease, as defined by the World Health Organization.

health be·ha·vior (helth bē-hāv'yŏr) Combination of knowledge and practices that together contribute to motivate actions taken regarding health.

health be·lief mod·el (HBM) (helth bĕ-lēf' mod'ĕl) A psychological precept that attempts to explain and predict health behaviors by focusing on the attitudes and beliefs of individual patients.

health care con·su·mer (helth kār kŏn-sū'mĕr) One who participates in health care services as a patient, client, or family member.

Health·care In·fec·tion Con·trol Prac·ti·ces Ad·vi·so·ry Com·mit·tee (HICPAC) (helth'kār in-fek'shŭn kŏn-trōl' prak'tis-ĕz ad-vī'zŏr-ē kŏ-mit'ē) A U.S. federal government appointed panel of experts in infection control who provide advice and guidance to the Centers for Disease Control and the Secretary of the Department of Health.

health cen·ter (helth sen'tĕr) An institution or group of institutions providing all types of medical care and preventive services to a population.

health cer·ti·fi·cate (helth sĕr-tif'i-kăt) An official statement issued by a physician giving the state of health of a patient.

health haz·ard (helth haz'ărd) Any substance that causes measurable changes in the body; employees so exposed must be informed of the possible change in body function and its symptoms.

health in·for·ma·tics (helth in'fŏr-mat' iks) The practice and technology of collecting, storing, and analyzing health care data electronically and transferring data between computer systems.

health in·for·ma·tion ad·min·i·stra·tor (helth in'fŏr-mā'shŭn ad-min'i-strā-tŏr) A trained professional responsible for maintenance of patient records in a hospital or other health care facility.

Health Lev·el 7 (HL-7) (helth lev'ĕl) A medical informatics standard that facilitates communication among different digital systems.

health main·te·nance or·gan·i·za·tion (HMO) (helth mān'tĕn-ăns ŏr'găn-ī-zā'shŭn) A comprehensive prepaid system of managed health care with emphasis on the prevention and early detection of disease and continuity of care. HMOs may be nonprofit or profit-making ventures; along with preferred provider organizations (PPOs) and other managed care plans, they dominate the health care market. HMOs generally offer a package of services; however, the choice of physician is frequently limited to those participating in the HMO. SEE ALSO managed care, preferred provider organization.

health rec·ord (helth rek'ŏrd) A comprehensive compilation of information traditionally placed in the medical record but also covering aspects of the patient's physical, mental, and social health that do not necessarily relate directly to the condition under treatment.

health screen•ing (helth skrēn'ing) Tests or examinations done to diagnose a condition before symptoms begin, including physical examinations, Papanicolaou smears, mammograms, colonoscopies, diabetes screening, blood pressure checks, cholesterol screening, osteoporosis screening, prostate cancer screening, among countless other modalities.

hear•ing (hēr'ing) The ability to perceive sound; the sensation of sound as opposed to vibration. SYN -acousis (2), -acusis, audition.

hear•ing aid (hēr'ing ād) An electronic amplifying device designed to bring sound more effectively into the ear; it consists of a microphone, amplifier, and receiver. SYN hearing instrument.

hear•ing con•ser•va•tion pro•gram (hēr'ing kon'sĕr-vā'shŭn prō'gram) Measures taken to protect workers who are exposed to high noise levels in the workplace.

Hear•ing Han•di•cap In•ven•tory for the El•der•ly (HHIE-S) (hēr'ing hand'ē-kap in'vĕn-tōr-ē el'dĕr-lē) Screening test that uses a communication scale to determine whether older adults have difficulty hearing and understanding speech.

hear•ing im•pair•ment, hear•ing loss (hēr'ing im-pār'mĕnt, laws) A reduction in the ability to perceive sound; may range from slight inability to complete deafness. SEE ALSO deafness.

heart (hahrt) [TA] A hollow chambered muscular organ that receives the blood from the veins and propels it into the arteries. SYN cor [TA], coeur.

heart beat (hahrt bēt) Complete cardiac cycle, including spread of the electrical impulse and the consequent mechanical contraction. SYN ictus cordis.

heart block (hb, HB) (hahrt blok) SYN atrioventricular block.

heart•burn (hahrt'bŭrn) SYN pyrosis.

heart dis•ease risk fac•tors (hahrt di-zēz' risk fak'tŏrz) Conditions that increase the risk of developing heart disease, including increasing age, being male, heredity and race, tobacco smoke, high blood cholesterol, high blood pressure, physical inactivity, obesity and overweight, and diabetes mellitus.

heart fail•ure (hahrt fāl'yŭr) **1.** Inadequacy of the heart so that as a pump it fails to maintain the circulation of blood, with the result that congestion and edema develop in the tissues. SYN cardiac insufficiency, congestive heart failure, myocardial insufficiency. **2.** Resulting clinical syndromes including shortness of breath, pitting edema, enlarged tender liver, engorged neck veins, and pulmonary rales in various combinations. SEE ALSO forward heart failure, backward heart failure, right ventricular failure, left ventricular failure.

heart fail•ure cell (hahrt fāl'yŭr sel) Macrophage in the lung during left heart failure that often carries large amounts of hemosiderin. SEE ALSO siderophore.

heart-lung ma•chine (hahrt-lŭng mă-shēn') A device incorporating a blood pump (artificial heart) and a blood oxygenator (artificial lung) to provide extracorporeal circulation and oxygenation of the blood during cardiac surgery.

heart mas•sage (hahrt mă-sahzh') Rhythmic stroking of the heart either in an open chest or through the chest wall to renew failed circulation during cardiac resuscitation. SYN cardiac massage.

heart mur•mur (hahrt mŭr'mŭr) A colloquialism for cardiac murmur (q.v.).

heart rate (hahrt rāt) Velocity of the heart's beat, recorded as the number of beats per minute.

heart scan (hahrt skan) A specialized computed tomography scan that measures calcium in the coronary arteries to identify areas of plaque build up; this technique is controversial.

heart sounds (HS) (hahrt sowndz) Noise made by muscle contraction and the closure of the heart valves during the cardiac cycle. SEE first heart sound, second heart sound, third heart sound, fourth heart sound. SYN cardiac sound, heart tones.

heart trans•plan•ta•tion (HT, HTx, HTX) (hahrt trans-plan-tā'shŭn) Replacement of a severely damaged heart with a normal heart from a brain-dead donor.

heart valves (hahrt valvz) Flaps between the atria and the ventricles and at the entrances to aorta and pulmonary artery that maintain the direction of blood flow.

heart·worm (hart′wŏrm) SYN *Dirofilaria immitis.*

heat (hēt) **1.** A high temperature. **2.** SYN estrus.

heat ca·pa·ci·ty (hēt kǎ-pas′i-tē) The quantity of heat required to raise the temperature of a system 1°C.

heat cramps (hēt kramps) Painful muscle spasms resulting from excessive water and electrolyte loss. SEE hyperthermia. SEE ALSO dehydration.

heat ex·haus·tion (hēt eg-zaws′chŭn) Reaction to heat marked by prostration, weakness, and collapse, due to severe dehydration. SYN heat prostration.

heat hy·per·py·rex·i·a (hēt hī′pĕr-pī-rek′sē-ă) SYN heatstroke.

heat pros·tra·tion (hēt pros-trā′shŭn) SEE heat exhaustion.

heat rash (hēt rash) SYN miliaria rubra.

heat stress in·dex (hēt stres in′deks) Measure of environment's potential to cause heat injury.

heat·stroke (hēt′strōk) A severe and often fatal illness produced by exposure to excessively high temperatures, especially when accompanied by marked exertion. SYN malignant hyperpyrexia.

heav·y chain (hev′ē chān) A polypeptide chain of high molecular weight determining the class and subclass of an immunoglobulin.

heav·y met·al (hev′ē met′ăl) One with a high specific gravity, typically larger than 5, e.g., Fe, Co, Cu, Mn, Mo, Zn, V.

Heb·er·den nodes (hē′bĕr-dĕn nōdz) Exostoses no larger than a pea found on the terminal phalanges of the fingers in osteoarthritis. SYN tuberculum arthriticum (1).

he·bet·ic (hē-bet′ik) Pertaining to youth.

heb·e·tude (heb′ĕ-tūd) SYN moria (1).

hec·a·ter·o·mer·ic (hek′ă-ter′ō-mer′ik) Denoting a spinal neuron the axon of which divides and gives off processes to both sides of the cord. SYN hecatomeral, hecatomeric.

hecto- (h) Prefix used in the SI and metric system to signify one hundred (10^2).

hec·to·me·ter (hm) (hek′tō-mē-tĕr) 100 meters.

hectometre [Br.] SYN hectometer.

he·don·ism (hē′dŏn-izm) Philosophy that pleasure is of utmost importance.

hed·ro·cele (hed′rō-sēl) Anal prolapse of the intestine.

heel (hēl) **1.** Proximal portion of the plantar surface of the foot. **2.** SYN calx (2). **3.** SYN distal end.

heel bone (hēl bōn) SYN calcaneus (1).

heel cup (hēl kŭp) A silicone gel device for cushioning the heel to reduce shock in patients with plantar fasciitis and other conditions that affect the feet.

heel-knee test (hēl-nē′ test) A neurologic evaluation of coordination in which a patient is asked to lie on his or her back, to put one heel on the knee of the other leg, and then to move the heel downward toward the foot. SYN heel-shin test.

heel lift (hēl lift) An orthotic device put into a shoe to even out unequal leg length.

heel punc·ture (hēl pŭngk′shŭr) Phlebotomy technique for collecting blood specimens from a newborn.

heel spur (hēl spŭr) An abnormal bony growth on the calcaneus. SYN calcaneal spur.

HEENT Abbreviation for head, eyes, ears, nose, and throat; the medical specialty dealing with those body systems.

Heer·fordt dis·ease (hār′fŏrt di-zēz′) SYN uveoparotid fever.

He·gar sign (hā′gahr sīn) Softening and compressibility of the lower segment of the uterus in early pregnancy (about the seventh week) that, on bimanual examination, is felt by the finger in the vagina as though the neck and body of the uterus were separated, or connected by only a thin band of tissue.

Heg·glin a·nom·a·ly (heg′lin ă-nom′ă-lē) A disorder in which neutrophils and eosinophils contain basophilic structures known as Döhle or Amato bodies and in which there is faulty maturation of platelets, with thrombocytopenia. SYN May-Hegglin anomaly.

Hei·den·hain i·ron he·ma·tox·y·lin stain (hī′den-hīn ī′ŏrn hē′mă-toks′i-lin stān) Stain used in turning muscle striations and mitotic structures blue-black.

height (h) (hīt) The distance from the lowest point to the highest point on an object or part.

height of con·tour (hīt kon′tūr) Greatest elevation on the crown of a tooth on the buccal and lingual surfaces (i.e., bulge).

height ver·ti·go (hīt vĕr′ti-gō) Dizziness experienced when looking down from a great height or in looking up at a high building or cliff. SYN vertical vertigo (1).

Heim·lich ma·neu·ver (hīm′lik mă-nū′vĕr) Action designed to expel an obstructing bolus of food from the throat by placing a fist on the abdomen between the navel and the costal margin, grasping the fist from behind with the other hand, and forcefully thrusting it inward and upward to force the diaphragm upward, forcing air up the trachea to dislodge the obstruction.

Heinz bod·ies (hīnz bod′ēz) Intracellular inclusions usually attached to the red blood cell membrane, composed of denatured hemoglobin; they occur in various diseases.

Heinz-Ehr·lich bod·y (hīnts-er′lik bod′ē) SYN Ehrlich inner body.

He·La cells (hē′lă selz) The first continuously cultured human malignant cells, derived from a cervical carcinoma of a patient, Henrietta Lacks; used in the cultivation of viruses.

hel·i·cal (hel′i-kăl) **1.** Relating to a helix. SYN helicine (2). **2.** SYN helicoid.

hel·i·cal com·put·ed to·mog·ra·phy (HCT) (hel′i-kăl kŏm-pyū′tĕd tŏ-mog′-ră-fē) SYN spiral computed tomography.

hel·i·cine (hel′i-sēn) **1.** Coiled. **2.** SYN helical (1).

Hel·i·co·bac·ter (hel′i-kō-bak′tĕr) A genus of gram-negative helical, curved, or straight microaerophilic bacteria with rounded ends and numerous sheathed flagella with terminal bulbs. Found in gastric mucosa. Some species are associated with gastric and peptic ulcers and predispose to gastric carcinoma. The type species is *H. pylori.*

***Hel·i·co·bac·ter py·lor·i* (H. pylori, HP, Hp)** (hel′i-kō-bak′ter pī-lō′rī) Bacterial species that produces urease and causes gastritis and nearly all peptic ulcer disease of the stomach and duodenum.

hel·i·coid (hel′i-koyd) Resembling a helix. SYN helical (2).

hel·i·co·pod gait (hel′i-kō-pod gāt) A gait, seen in some conversion reactions or hysteric disorders, in which the feet move in half circles. SYN helicopodia.

hel·i·co·tre·ma (hel′i-kō-trē′mă) [TA] A semilunar opening at the apex of the cochlea through which the scala vestibuli and the scala tympani of the cochlea communicate with one another.

he·li·en·ceph·a·li·tis (hē′lē-en-sef′ă-lī′tis) Inflammation of the brain following sunstroke.

he·li·um (He) (hē′lē-ŭm) A gaseous element present in minute amounts in the atmosphere; used as a diluent of medicinal gases, particularly oxygen.

he·lix, pl. **hel·ix·es,** pl. **hel·i·ces** (hē′liks, -ĕz, hel′i-sēz) **1.** [TA] *Often mistakenly applied to a spiral.* The margin of the auricle; a folded rim of cartilage forming the upper part of the anterior, the superior, and the greater part of the posterior edges of the auricle. **2.** A line in the shape of a coil, each point being equidistant from a straight line that is the axis of the cylinder in which each point of the helix lies.

H

Hel·ler plex·us (hel'ĕr plek'sŭs) Nidus of small arteries in the wall of the intestine.

Hel·lin law (hel'in law) Twins occur once in 89 births, triplets once in 89^2, and quadruplets once in 89^3.

hel·met cell (hel'mĕt sel) SEE keratocyte.

hel·minth (hel'minth) Any intestinal vermiform parasite, primarily nematodes, cestodes, trematodes, and acanthocephalans.

hel·min·tha·gogue (hel-minth'ă-gog) SYN anthelmintic (1).

hel·min·them·e·sis (hel'min-them'ĕ-sis) The vomiting or expelling of intestinal worms through the mouth.

hel·min·thi·a·sis, hel·minth·ism (hel'min-thī'ă-sis, -min-thizm) The condition of having intestinal vermiform parasites. SYN invermination.

hel·min·thic (hel-min'thik) 1. Helmintic. 2. SYN anthelmintic (1).

hel·min·thol·o·gy (hel'min-thol'ŏ-jē) The branch of science concerned with worms. SYN scolecology.

he·lo·ma (hē-lō'mă) SYN clavus.

he·lo·ma du·rum (hē-lō'mă dū'rŭm) SYN hard corn.

he·lo·ma mol·le (hē-lō'mă mol'ē) SYN soft corn.

he·lot·o·my (hē-lot'ŏ-mē) Surgical treatment of corns.

help·er cells (hel'pĕr selz) SYN T-helper cells.

help·er virus (hel'pĕr vī'rŭs) One with replication that renders it possible for a defective virus or a virusoid to develop into a fully infectious agent.

HELPP syn·drome (help sin'drōm) Condition of pregnancy characterized by raised liver enzymes, hemolysis, and low platelet count with preeclampsia.

Hel·weg-Lars·sen syn·drome (hel'weg lahr'sen sin'drōm) Disorder characterized by anhidrotic ectodermal dysplasia and hearing loss.

🕭 **hem-, hema-** Combining forms meaning blood. SEE ALSO hemat-, hemato-, hemo-. SYN haem-.

he·ma·chrome (hē'mă-krōm) The coloring matter of the blood, hemoglobin, or hematin. SYN haemachrome.

he·ma·cyte (hē'mă-sīt) SYN erythrocyte, haemacyte.

he·ma·cy·tom·e·ter (hē'mă-sī-tom'ĕ-tĕr) SYN haemacytometer.

he·mag·glu·ti·na·tion (hē'mă-glū-ti-nā'shŭn) The agglutination of red blood cells. SYN haemagglutination.

he·mag·glu·ti·na·tion in·hi·bi·tion (HAI, HI) (hē'mă-glū-ti-nā'shŭn in'hi-bish'ŭn) Repression of nonimmune hemagglutination by an antibody specific for it.

he·mag·glu·ti·nin (hē'mă-glū'ti-nin) Substance that causes hemagglutination. SYN haemagglutinin.

he·mal (hē'măl) 1. Relating to the blood or blood vessels. 2. Referring to the ventral side of the vertebral bodies or their precursors, where the heart and great vessels are located, as opposed to neural (2).

he·ma·nal·y·sis (hē'mă-nal'i-sis) Analysis of blood, especially with chemical methods.

🕭 **hemangi-, hemangio-** Combining forms meaning blood vessel.

he·man·gi·ec·ta·sis, he·man·gi·ec·ta·si·a (hē-man'jē-ek'tă-sis, hē-man'jē-ek-tā'zē-ă) Dilation of blood vessels. SYN haemangiectasis.

he·man·gi·o·blas·to·ma (hē-man'jē-ō-blas-tō'mă) Slow-growing benign cerebellar neoplasm composed of capillary vessel-forming endothelial cells and stromal cells. SYN angioblastoma, haemangioblastoma, Lindau tumor.

he·man·gi·o·en·do·the·li·o·blas·to·ma (hē-man'jē-ō-en'dō-thē'lē-ō-blas-tō'mă) One in which endothelial cells seem to be especially immature. SYN haemangioendothelioblastoma.

he·man·gi·o·en·do·the·li·o·ma (hē-man′jē-ō-en′dō-thē′lē-ō′mă) A neoplasm derived from blood vessels, characterized by numerous prominent endothelial cells that occur singly, in aggregates, and as the lining of congeries of vascular tubes or channels. SYN haemangioendothelioma.

he·man·gi·o·fi·bro·ma (hē-man′jē-ō-fī-brō′mă) A hemangioma with an abundant fibrous tissue framework. SYN haemangiofibroma.

he·man·gi·o·ma (hē-man′jē-ō′mă) A congenital anomaly, in which proliferation of blood vessels leads to a mass that resembles a neoplasm. SEE ALSO nevus. SYN haemangioma.

he·man·gi·o·ma throm·bo·cy·to·pe·ni·a syn·drome (hē-man′jē-ō′mă throm′bō-sī-tō-pē′nē-ă sindrōm) SYN Kasabach-Merritt syndrome.

he·man·gi·o·ma·to·sis (hē-man′jē-ō-mă-tō′sis) A condition with numerous hemangiomas. SYN haemangiomatosis.

he·man·gi·o·per·i·cy·to·ma (hē-man′jē-ō-per′i-sī-tō′mă) A vascular, usually benign, neoplasm composed of round and spindle cells derived from pericytes and surrounding endothelium-lined vessels. SYN haemangiopericytoma.

he·man·gi·o·sar·co·ma (hē-man′jē-ō-sahr-kō′mă) A malignant neoplasm characterized by rapidly proliferating, extensively infiltrating, anaplastic cells derived from blood vessels and lining irregular blood-filled or lumpy spaces. SYN haemangiosarcoma.

he·ma·pher·e·sis (hē′mă-fĕr-ē′sis) Laboratory procedure of separating blood into its component parts and removing cells from the blood to treat hematologic, oncologic, and neurologic disorders.

he·mar·thro·sis (hēm′ahr-thrō′sis) Blood in a joint. SYN haemarthrosis.

hemat- Combining form meaning blood. SEE ALSO hem-, hemato-, hemo-. SYN haemat-.

he·ma·te·in (hē′mă-tē′in) An oxidation product of hematoxylin. SYN haematein.

he·ma·tem·e·sis (hematem) (hē′mă-tem′ĕ-sis) Vomiting of blood. SYN vomitus cruentes.

he·mat·ic (hē-mat′ik) **1.** Relating to blood. SYN hemic. **2.** SYN hematinic (2). SYN haematic.

he·ma·ti·dro·sis (hē′mă-tid-rō′sis) Excretion of blood or blood pigment in the sweat. SYN haematidrosis, hemidrosis (1).

he·ma·tin (hē′mă-tin) Heme in which the iron is Fe(III) (Fe^{3+}); the prosthetic group of methemoglobin. SYN ferriheme, haematin, hematosin, oxyheme, oxyhemochromogen.

he·ma·tin·ic (hē′mă-tin′ik) Improving the condition of the blood. SYN hematic (2). SYN haematinic.

hemato- Combining form denoting blood. SEE ALSO hem-, hemat-, hemo-.

he·ma·to·cele (hē′mă-tō-sēl) **1.** SYN hemorrhagic cyst. **2.** Effusion of blood into a canal or a cavity of the body. **3.** Swelling due to effusion of blood into the tunica vaginalis testis. SYN haematocele.

he·ma·to·ceph·a·ly (hē′mă-tō-sef′ă-lē) Intracranial effusion of blood, commonly in a fetus. SYN haematocephaly.

he·ma·to·che·zi·a (hē′mă-tō-kē′zē-ă) Passage of bloody stools, in contradistinction to melena, or tarry stools.

he·ma·to·chy·lu·ri·a (hē′mă-tō-kī-lyūr′ē-ă) Presence of blood and chyle in the urine. SYN haematochyluria.

he·ma·to·col·po·me·tra (hē′mă-tō-kol′pō-mē′tră) Accumulation of blood in the uterus and vagina due to an imperforate hymen or other lower vaginal obstruction. SYN haematocolpometra.

he·ma·to·col·pos (hē′mă-tō-kol′pŏs) Vaginal accumulation of menstrual blood due to imperforate hymen or other obstruction. SYN haematocolpos, retained menstruation.

he·ma·to·cys·tis (hē′mă-tō-sis′tis) An effusion of blood into the bladder. SYN haematocystis.

he·ma·to·cyte (hē′mă-tō-sīt) SYN hemocyte.

he·ma·to·gen·ic, he·ma·tog·e·nous (hē′mă-tō-jen′ik, -toj′ĕ-nŭs) **1.** SYN hemopoietic. **2.** Pertaining to anything produced from, derived from, or transported by the blood. SYN haematogenic.

he·ma·tog·e·nous pig·ment (hem-ă-toj′ĕ-nŭs pig′mĕnt) Color derived from the hemoglobin of the red blood cells.

he·ma·tog·e·nous tu·ber·cu·lo·sis (hem′ă-toj′ĕ-nŭs tū-bĕr′kyū-lō′sis) Tuberculosis of the synovial joints.

he·ma·toi·din (hē-mă-toy′din) A pigment derived from hemoglobin that contains no iron but is closely related to or identical to bilirubin. SYN blood crystals, hematoidin crystals.

he·ma·tol·o·gy (hē′mă-tol′ŏ-jē) Medical specialty involving the anatomy, physiology, pathology, symptomatology, and therapeutics related to blood and blood-forming tissues. SYN haematology.

he·ma·to·lymph·an·gi·o·ma (hē′mă-tō-limf′an-jē-ō′mă) Congenital anomaly consisting of numerous, closely packed, variably sized lymphatic vessels and larger channels, in association with a moderate number of blood vessels of a similar type. SYN haematolymphangioma.

he·ma·tol·y·sis (hē′mă-tol′i-sis) SYN hemolysis, haematolysis.

he·ma·to·lyt·ic (hē′mă-tō-lit′ik) SYN hemolytic, haematolytic.

he·ma·to·ma (hē′mă-tō′mă) A localized mass of extravasated blood that is relatively or completely confined within an organ or tissue, a space, or a potential space.

he·ma·to·me·di·a·sti·num (hē′mă-tō-mē′dē-ă-stī′nŭm) Blood in the mediastinum.

he·ma·to·me·tra, he·mo·me·tra (hē′mă-tō-mē′tră, hē-mō-mē′tră) A collection or retention of blood in the uterine cavity. SYN haematometra.

he·ma·tom·e·try (hē′mă-tom′ĕ-trē) Examination of the blood to determine any

or all of the following: 1) the total number, types, and relative proportions of various blood cells; 2) the number or proportion of other formed elements; 3) the percentage of hemoglobin. SYN hemometry.

he·mat·om·pha·lo·cele (hē′mat-om-fal′ō-sēl) Umbilical hernia into which an effusion of blood has taken place. SYN haematomphalocele.

he·ma·to·my·e·li·a (hē′mă-tō-mī-ē′lē-ă) Hemorrhage into the substance of the spinal cord. SYN haematomyelia, hematorrhachis interna, myelapoplexy, myelorrhagia.

he·ma·to·my·e·li·tis (hē′mă-tō-mī′ĕ-lī′tis) Inflammation of the spinal cord with effusion of blood.

he·ma·to·my·e·lo·pore (hē′mă-tō-mī′ĕ-lō-pōr) Formation of porosities in the spinal cord due to hemorrhages. SYN haematomyelopore.

he·ma·to·pa·thol·o·gy (hē′mă-tō-pă-thol′ŏ-jē) The division of pathology concerned with diseases of the blood and of hemopoietic and lymphoid tissues. SYN haematopathology, hemopathology.

he·ma·to·pha·gi·a (hē′mă-tō-fā′jē-ă) Living on the blood of another animal, as does the vampire bat or a leech. SYN hemophagia.

he·ma·toph·a·gous (hē′mă-tof′ă-gŭs) Subsisting on blood.

he·ma·to·plast (hē′mă-tō-plast) SYN hemocytoblast, haematoplast.

he·ma·to·plas·tic (hē′mă-tō-plas′tik) SYN hemopoietic, haematoplastic.

he·ma·to·poi·e·sis (hē′mă-tō-poy-ē′sis) SYN hemopoiesis.

he·ma·to·poi·et·ic (hē′mă-tō-poy-et′ik) SYN hemopoietic, haematopoietic.

he·ma·to·poi·et·ic gland (hē′mă-tō-poy-et′ik gland) Blood-forming organ. SYN haematopoietic gland.

he·ma·to·por·phy·ri·nu·ri·a (hē′mă-tō-pōr′fī-ri-nyū′rē-ă) Used to designate enhanced urinary excretion of porphyrins.

he·ma·top·si·a (hē'mă-top'sē-ă) SYN hemophthalmia, haematopsia.

he·ma·tor·rha·chis, he·mor·rha·chis (hē'mă-tōr'ă-kis, hē-mōr'ă-kis) A spinal hemorrhage.

he·ma·to·sal·pinx, he·mo·sal·pinx (hē'mă-tō-sal'pingks, hē'mō-sal'pingks) Collection of blood in a body tube. SYN haematosalpinx.

he·ma·to·sin (hē'mă-tō'sin) SYN hematin, haematosin.

he·ma·to·sis (hē'mă-tō'sis) Oxygenation of venous blood in the lungs. Cf. hemopoiesis. SYN haematosis.

he·ma·to·sper·mat·o·cele (hē'mă-tō-spĕr-mat'ō-sēl) A spermatocele that contains blood.

he·ma·to·sper·mi·a (hē'mă-tō-spĕr'mē-ă) The presence of blood in seminal ejaculate.

he·ma·to·stat·ic (hē'mă-tō-stat'ik) **1.** Variant of hemostatic. **2.** Due to stagnation or arrest of blood flow. SYN haematostatic.

he·ma·to·stax·is (hē'mă-tō-stak'sis) Spontaneous bleeding due to a disease of the blood. SYN haematostaxis.

he·ma·tos·te·on (hē'mă-tos'tē-on) Bleeding in the medullary cavity of a bone.

hem·a·to·ther·ma (hē'mă-tō-thĕr'mă) The warm-blooded vertebrates (birds and mammals). SYN haematotherma.

he·ma·to·tro·pic (hē'mă-tō-trō'pik) SYN hemotropic.

he·ma·tox·y·lin (hē'mă-toks'i-lin) [C.I. 75290] A crystalline compound, containing the coloring matter of *Haematoxylon campechianum*; used as a dye in histology.

he·ma·tu·ri·a (HEM) (hē'mă-tyūr'ē-ă) Presence of blood or red blood cells in the urine.

heme (hēm) **1.** The porphyrin chelate of iron in which the iron is Fe(II) (Fe^{2+}); the oxygen-carrying, color-furnishing, prosthetic group of hemoglobin. **2.** Iron complexed with nonporphyrins but related tetrapyrrole structures (e.g., biliverdin heme). SYN haem, reduced hematin.

heme pro·tein (hēm prō'tēn) Any protein containing an iron-porphyrin (heme) prosthetic group resembling that of hemoglobin. SYN haem protein, haemprotein.

hem·er·a·lo·pi·a, hem·er·a·no·pi·a (hem'ĕr-ă-lō'pē-ă, -nō'pē-ă) Inability to see as distinctly in a bright light as in reduced illumination; seen in patients with impaired cone function. SYN day blindness.

hem·e·ryth·rin (hēm'ĕ-rith'rin) An iron-containing, oxygen-binding circulatory protein in certain invertebrates. SYN haemerythrin.

hemi- Combining form meaning one half. Cf. semi-.

hem·i·a·chro·ma·top·si·a (hem'ē-ă-krō'mă-top'sē-ă) Monocular color blindness caused by brain damage.

hem·i·a·geu·si·a, hem·i·a·geu·sti·a, hem·i·geu·si·a (hem'ē-ă-gū'sē-ă, -gūs'tē-ă, hem'ē-gū'sē-ă) Loss of sense of taste from one side of the tongue.

hemianaesthesia [Br.] SYN hemianesthesia.

hem·i·an·al·ge·si·a (hem'ē-an-ăl-jē'zē-ă) Analgesia affecting one side of the body.

hem·i·an·es·the·si·a (hem'ē-an-es-thē'zē-ă) Anesthesia on one side of the body. SYN hemianaesthesia, unilateral anesthesia.

hem·i·an·es·the·si·a cru·ci·ate (hem'ē-an'es-thē'zē-ă krū'she-āt) SYN crossed hemianesthesia.

hem·i·a·no·pi·a, hem·i·an·op·si·a (hem'ē-ă-nō'pē-ă, -nop'sē-ă) Loss of vision for one half of the visual field of one or both eyes.

hem·i·a·nop·ic sco·toma (hem'ē-ă-nop'ik skō-tō'mă) Blind spot involving half of the central field.

hem·i·an·os·mi·a (hem′ē-an-oz′mē-ă) Loss of the sense of smell on one side.

hem·i·a·prax·i·a (hem′ē-ă-prak′sē-ă) Apraxia affecting one side of the body.

hem·i·ar·thro·plas·ty (hem′ē-ahr′thrō-plas′tē) Arthroplasty in which one joint surface is replaced with artificial material, usually metal.

hem·i·a·tax·i·a (hem′ē-ă-tak′sē-ă) Ataxia affecting one side of the body.

hem·i·ath·e·to·sis (hem′ē-ath-ĕ-tō′sis) Athetosis affecting one hand, or one hand and foot, only.

hem·i·at·ro·phy (hem′ē-at′rŏ-fē) Atrophy of one lateral half of a part or of an organ, as the face or tongue.

hem·i·az·y·gos vein (hem′ē-az′i-gŏs vān) [TA] A vein that supplies the thoracic area.

hem·i·bal·lis·mus, hem·i·bal·lism (hem′ē-bal-iz′mŭs, -bal′izm) Jerking movement involving one side of the body.

hem·i·block (hem′ē-blok) Arrest of the impulse in one of the two main divisions of the left branch of the bundle of His.

he·mic (hē′mik) SYN hematic (1), haemic.

hem·i·cen·trum (hem′ē-sen′trŭm) One of the two lateral halves of the centrum of a vertebra.

hem·i·ceph·al·al·gi·a (hem′ē-sef-ă-lal′jē-ă) The unilateral headache characteristic of migraine. SYN hemicrania (2).

hem·i·ce·pha·li·a (hem′ē-sĕ-fā′lē-ă) Congenital failure of the cerebrum to develop normally. SYN partial anencephaly.

hem·i·cer·e·brum (hem′ē-ser′ĕ-brŭm) One side of the cerebrum.

he·mic mur·mur (hē′mik mŭr′mŭr) SYN haemic murmur.

hem·i·cra·ni·a (hem′ē-krā′nē-ă) **1.** SYN migraine. **2.** SYN hemicephalalgia.

hem·i·cra·ni·o·sis (hem′ē-krā-nē-ō′sis) Enlargement of one side of the cranium.

hem·i·des·mo·somes (hem′ē-des′mō-sōmz) Adhering junctions that occur on the basal surface of the stratum basale of stratified squamous epithelium.

hem·i·di·a·pho·re·sis (hem′ē-dī-ă-fŏr-ē′sis) Diaphoresis, or sweating, on one side of the body. SYN hemidrosis (2), hemihidrosis.

hem·i·di·a·phragm (hem′ē-dī′ă-fram) Half of the diaphragm.

hem·i·dro·sis (hem′ē-drō′sis) SYN hemidiaphoresis.

hemidysaesthesia [Br.] SYN hemidysesthesia.

hem·i·dys·es·the·si·a (hem′ē-dis-es-thē′zē-ă) Dysesthesia affecting one side of the body. SYN hemidysaesthesia.

hem·i·fa·cial (hem′ē-fā′shăl) Pertaining to one side of the face.

hem·i·gas·trec·to·my (hem′ē-gas-trek′tŏ-mē) Excision of the distal half of the stomach.

hem·i·geu·si·a (hem′ē-gū′sē-ă) SYN hemiageusia.

he·mi·glo·bin (hem′ē-glō-bin) SYN methemoglobin.

hem·i·glos·sal (hem′ē-glos′ăl) SYN hemilingual.

hem·i·glos·sec·to·my (hem′ē-glos-ek′tŏ-mē) Surgical removal of half of the tongue.

hem·i·hi·dro·sis (hem′ē-hī-drō′sis) SYN hemidiaphoresis.

hemihypaesthesia [Br.] SYN hemihypesthesia.

hem·i·hy·pal·ge·si·a (hem′ē-hīp′al-jē′zē-ă) Hypalgesia affecting one side of the body.

hem·i·hy·per·hi·dro·sis (hem′ē-hī′pĕr-hī-drō′sis) Excessive sweating confined to one side of the body.

hem·i·hy·per·tro·phy (hem′ē-hī-pĕr′trŏ-fē) Muscular or osseous hypertrophy of one side of the face or body.

hem·i·hy·pes·the·si·a, hem·i·hy·po·es·the·sia (hem'ē-hīp'es-thē'zē-ă, -hī pō-es-thē'zē-ă) Diminished sensibility in one side of the body. SYN hemihypaesthesia.

hem·i·hy·po·pla·si·a (hem'ē-hī'pō-plā' zē-ă) Lack of development of one side of the body or bodily structure.

hem·i·hy·po·to·ni·a (hem'ē-hī-pō-tō' nē-ă) Partial loss of muscular tonicity on one side of the body.

hem·i·kar·y·on (hem'i-kar'ē-on) A cell nucleus containing a haploid set of chromosomes.

hem·i·ke·tal (hem'ē-kē'tăl) Product of the addition of an alcohol to a ketone.

hem·i·lam·i·nec·to·my (hem'ē-lam-i-nek'tŏ-mē) Removal of a portion of a vertebral lamina.

hem·i·lat·er·al (hem'ē-lat'ĕr-ăl) Relating to one lateral half.

he·min (hēm'in) **1.** Chloride of heme in which Fe^{2+} has become Fe^{3+}. **2.** Any coordination complex of chloro(porphyrinato)iron(III). SYN chlorohemin, factor X for Haemophilus, ferriheme chloride, ferriporphyrin chloride, ferriprotoporphyrin, hematin chloride.

hem·i·ple·gi·a (hem'ē-plē'jē-ă) Paralysis of one side of the body.

He·mip·ter·a (hem-ip'tĕr-ă) An arthropod order of the class Insecta that includes many plant lice and other true bugs (e.g., bedbugs).

hem·i·spasm (hem'ē-spazm) A spasm affecting one or more muscles of one side of the face or body.

hem·i·sphere (H, hemi) (hem'is-fēr') [TA] Half a spheric structure. SYN hemispherium [TA].

hem·i·sphe·ri·um (hem'is-fēr'ē-ŭm) [TA] **1.** SYN cerebral hemisphere. **2.** SYN hemisphere of cerebellum H II–H X.

hem·i·ver·te·bra (hem'ē-věr'tĕ-bră) A congenital defect of a vertebra in which one side of a vertebra fails to develop completely.

hem·i·zo·na as·say (HZA) (hem'ē-zō' nă as'ā) Diagnostic test evaluating the binding capacity of a sperm to the zona pellucida.

hem·i·zy·gos·i·ty (hem'ē-zī-gos'i-tē) The state of being hemizygous.

hem·i·zy·gote (hem'ē-zī'gōt) An individual hemizygous with respect to one or more specified loci.

hem·i·zy·gous (hem'ē-zī'gŭs) In human beings, refers to genes on the X chromosome in males, which are expressed whether dominant or recessive. SYN hemizygotic.

hemo- Combining form denoting blood. SEE ALSO hem-, hemat-, hemato-. SYN haemo-.

he·mo·bil·i·a, he·ma·to·bi·li·a (hē' mō-bil'ē-ă, -mă-tō-bil'ē-ă) The presence of blood in the bile. SYN haemobilia.

he·mo·blast (hē'mō-blast) SYN hemocytoblast.

he·mo·blas·to·sis (hē'mō-blas-tō'sis) A proliferative condition of the hematopoietic tissues in general. SYN haemoblastosis.

he·mo·cath·e·re·sis (hē'mō-kă-ther'ĕ-sis) Destruction of the blood cells, especially of erythrocytes. SYN haemocatheresis.

Hem·oc·cult test (hēm'ō-kŭlt' test) A qualitative assay for occult blood in stool based on detecting the peroxidase activity of hemoglobin. SYN Haemoccult test.

he·mo·cho·ri·al pla·cen·ta (hē'mō-kōr'ē-ăl plă-sen'tă) One, as in humans and some rodents, in which maternal blood is in direct contact with the chorion.

he·mo·chro·ma·to·sis (hē'mō-krō-mă-tō'sis) A disorder of iron metabolism characterized by excessive absorption of ingested iron, saturation of iron-binding protein, and deposition of hemosiderin in tissue, particularly in the liver, pancreas, and skin. SYN haemochromatosis.

he·mo·chrome (hē'mō-krōm) SYN hemochromogen.

he·mo·chro·mo·gen (hē′mō-krō′mō-jen) Any compound in which 1 mol of ferro- or ferriporphyrin is combined with 2 mol of a nitrogenous base or protein. SYN haemochromogen, hemochrome.

he·mo·chro·mo·me·ter (hē′mō-krō-mom′ĕ-tĕr) SYN haemochromometer.

he·mo·con·cen·tra·tion (hē′mō-kon′sĕn-trā′shŭn) Decrease in the volume of plasma in relation to the number of red blood cells.

he·mo·cy·a·nin (hē′mō-sī′ă-nin) An oxygen-carrying pigment in some mollusks, crustacea, and arthropods; used as an experimental antigen. SYN haemocyanin.

he·mo·cyte (hē′mō-sīt) Any cell or formed element of the blood. SYN haemocyte.

he·mo·cy·to·ca·ther·e·sis (hē′mō-sī′tō-kă-ther′ĕ-sis) Hemolysis or other type of destruction of red blood cells.

he·mo·cy·tol·o·gy (hē′mō-sī-tol′ŏ-jē) The study of blood cells.

he·mo·cy·tol·y·sis (hē′mō-sī-tol′i-sis) The dissolution of blood cells, including hemolysis. SYN haemocytolysis.

he·mo·cy·to·ma (hē′mō-sī-tō′mă) A tumor made up of undifferentiated blood cells. SYN haemocytoma.

he·mo·cy·tom·e·try (hē′mō-sī-tom′ĕ-trē) The counting of red blood cells. SYN haemocytometry.

he·mo·cy·to·trip·sis (hē′mō-sī′tō-trip′sis) Fragmentation or disintegration of blood cells by means of mechanical trauma, e.g., compression between hard surfaces. SYN haemocytotrypsis.

he·mo·di·a·fil·tra·tion (HDF) (hē′mō-dī′ă-fil-trā′shŭn) The combination of hemodialysis and hemofiltration, performed either simultaneously or sequentially.

he·mo·di·ag·no·sis (hē′mō-dī′ăg-nō′sis) Diagnosis by means of examination of the blood.

he·mo·di·al·y·sis (hē′mō-dī-al′i-sis) Dialysis of soluble substances and water from the blood by diffusion through a semipermeable membrane. SYN haemodialysis.

he·mo·di·a·lyz·er (hē′mō-dī′ă-līz-ĕr) A machine for hemodialysis in acute or chronic renal failure. SYN artificial kidney, haemodialyser.

he·mo·di·lu·tion (hē′mō-di-lū′shŭn) Increase in the volume of plasma in relation to red blood cells; reduced concentration of red blood cells in the circulation. SYN haemodilution.

he·mo·dy·nam·ics (hē′mō-dī-nam′iks) The study of the dynamics of blood circulation. SYN haemodynamics.

he·mo·en·do·the·li·al pla·cen·ta (hē′mō-en′dō-thē′lē-ăl plă-sen′tă) The type of placenta, in which the trophoblast becomes so attenuated that, by light microscopy, maternal blood appears to be separated from fetal blood only by the endothelium of the chorionic capillaries. SYN haemoendothelial placenta.

he·mo·fil·tra·tion (hē′mō-fil-trā′shŭn) A process, similar to hemodialysis, by which blood is dialyzed using ultrafiltration and simultaneous reinfusion of physiologic saline solution. SYN haemofiltration.

he·mo·flag·el·late (hē′mō-flaj′ĕ-lāt) Protozoan flagellates that are parasitic in the blood; they include the genera *Leishmania* and *Trypanosoma*, several species of which are important pathogens. SYN haemoflagellate.

he·mo·fus·cin (hē′mō-fŭs′in) A brown pigment derived from hemoglobin that occurs in urine occasionally along with hemosiderin, usually indicative of increased red blood cell destruction. SYN haemofuscin.

he·mo·gen·e·sis (hē′mō-jen′ĕ-sis) SYN hemopoiesis, haemogenesis.

he·mo·gen·ic (hē′mō-jen′ik) Pertaining to or related to the formation of blood cells. SYN hematopoietic.

he·mo·glo·bin (Hgb, Hb) (hē′mō-glō′bin) The red respiratory protein of erythrocytes. SYN haemoglobin, haemoglobins.

he·mo·glo·bi·nol·y·sis (hē′mō-glō′bi-nol′i-sis) Destruction or chemical splitting of hemoglobin. SYN haemoglobinolysis.

he·mo·glo·bi·nom·e·ter (hē′mō-glō′bi-nom′ĕ-tĕr) A laboratory device for measuring the level of hemoglobin in the blood.

he·mo·glo·bi·nop·a·thy (hē′mō-glō′bi-nop′ă-thē) A disorder or disease caused by or associated with the presence of abnormal hemoglobins in the blood, e.g., sickle cell disease, hemoglobin C, D, E, H, or I disorders.

he·mo·glo·bi·no·phil·ic (hē′mō-glō′bi-nō-fil′ik) Denoting certain microorganisms that cannot be cultured except in the presence of hemoglobin. SYN haemoglobinophilic.

he·mo·glo·bin Port·land (hē′mō-glō′bin pōrt′lănd) Form of embryonic hemoglobin containing the ζ chains of hemoglobin Gower-1 and the γ chains of Hb F, thus having the formula $\zeta_2\gamma_2$.

he·mo·glo·bin S (Hb S) (hē′mō-glō′bin) An abnormal form that renders erythrocytes subject to sickling and hemolysis at reduced oxygen tension; makes up 70–100% of hemoglobin in people with sickle cell anemia. SYN haemoglobin S, sickle cell hemoglobin.

he·mo·glo·bi·nu·ria (hē′mō-glō′bi-nyūr′ē-ă) The presence of hemoglobin in the urine. SYN haemoglobinuria.

he·mo·glo·bi·nu·ric ne·phro·sis (hē′mō-glō′bi-nyūr′ik nĕ-frō′sis) Acute oliguric renal failure associated with hemoglobinuria, due to massive intravascular hemolysis. SYN haemoglobinuric nephrosis.

he·mo·his·ti·o·blast (hē′mō-his′tē-ō-blast) A primordial type of mesenchymal cell believed to be capable of developing into all types of blood cells. SYN Ferrata cell, haemohistioblast.

he·mo·lith (hē′mō-lith) A concretion in the wall of a blood vessel. SYN haemolith.

he·mo·lu·te·in (hē′mō-lū′tē-in) A pigment derived from hemoglobin that contains no iron but is closely related to or similar to bilirubin. SYN hemolutein.

he·mo·lymph (hē′mō-limf) **1.** The blood and lymph, in the sense of a "circulating tissue." **2.** The nutrient fluid of certain invertebrates.

he·mol·y·sate (hē-mol′i-sāt) Preparation resulting from the lysis of erythrocytes. SYN haemolysate.

he·mol·y·sin (hē-mol′i-sin) **1.** Any substance elaborated by a living agent and capable of causing lysis of red blood cells and liberation of their hemoglobin. SYN erythrocytolysin, erythrolysin. **2.** A sensitizing (complement-fixing) antibody that combines with red blood cells of the antigenic type that stimulated formation of the hemolysin, a fixing complement with the antibody-cell union resulting in lysis of the cells.

he·mol·y·sin·o·gen (hē′mō-lī-sin′ŏ-jen) The antigenic material in red blood cells that stimulates the formation of hemolysin. SYN haemolysinogen.

he·mol·y·sin u·nit, he·mo·lyt·ic u·nit (hē-mol′i-sin yū′nit, hē′mō-lit′ik) The smallest quantity (highest dilution) of inactivated immune serum (hemolysin) that will sensitize the standard suspension of erythrocytes so that the standard complement will cause complete hemolysis. SYN haemolysin unit.

he·mol·y·sis (hē-mol′i-sis) Alteration, dissolution, or destruction of red blood cells in such a manner that hemoglobin is liberated into the medium in which the cells are suspended. SYN erythrocytolysis, erythrolysis, haemolysis, hematolysis.

he·mo·lyt·ic a·ne·mi·a (hē′mō-lit′ik ă-nē′mē-ă) Any anemia resulting from an increased rate of erythrocyte destruction. SYN haemolytic anaemia.

he·mo·lyt·ic cri·sis (hē-mō-lit′ik krī′sis) Massive hemolysis with severe anemia associated with hemolytic disease, such as sickle cell disease.

he·mo·lyt·ic jaun·dice (hē′mō-lit′ik jawn′dis) Hepatic disorder that results from increased production of bilirubin

H

from hemoglobin as a result of any process (e.g., toxic, genetic, or immune) causing increased destruction of erythrocytes. SYN haemolytic jaundice, hematogenous jaundice.

he·mo·lyt·ic u·re·mic syn·drome (hē′mō-lit′ik yūr-ē′mik sin′drōm) Combination of hemolytic anemia and thrombocytopenia that occurs with acute renal failure. SYN haemolytic uremic syndrome.

he·mo·lyze (hē′mō-līz) To produce hemolysis or liberation of the hemoglobin from red blood cells.

he·mo·me·tra (hē′mō-mē′tră) SYN hematometra, haemometra.

he·mon·chi·a·sis (hē′mong-kī′a-sĭs) Infestation with nematodes of the genus *Haemonchus*. SYN haemonchiasis.

he·mo·pa·thol·o·gy (hē′mō-pă-thol′ŏ-jē) SYN hematopathology.

he·mop·a·thy (hē-mop′ă-thē) Any abnormal condition or disease of the blood or hemopoietic tissues. SYN haemopathy.

he·mo·per·fu·sion (hē′mō-pĕr-fyū′zhŭn) Passage of blood through columns of adsorptive material, such as activated charcoal, to remove toxic substances. SYN haemoperfusion.

he·mo·per·i·car·di·um (hē′mō-per′i-kahr′dē-ŭm) Blood in the pericardial sac. SYN haemopericardium.

he·mo·pex·in (hē′mō-peks′in) A serum protein related to β-globulins, important in binding heme and porphyrins, preventing excretion, and perhaps regulating heme in drug metabolism. SYN haemopexin.

he·mo·phag·o·cyte (hē′mō-fag′ŏ-sīt) A cell that engulfs and destroys blood cells, especially erythrocytes. SYN haemophagocyte.

he·mo·phil, he·mo·phile (hē′mō-fil, -fīl) A microorganism growing preferably in media containing blood. SYN haemophil.

he·mo·phil·i·a (hemo, HEM) (hē′mō-fil′ē-ă) An inherited disorder of blood coagulation characterized by a permanent tendency to hemorrhages, spontaneous or traumatic.

he·mo·phil·i·a A (hē′mō-fil′ē-ă) The inherited blood disorder resulting from a deficiency of factor VIII. SYN classic hemophilia, haemophilia A.

he·mo·phil·i·a B (HEMB) (hē′mō-fil′ē-ă) Clotting disorder resembling hemophilia A, caused by hereditary deficiency of factor IX. SYN Christmas disease.

he·mo·phil·i·a C (hē′mō-fil′ē-ă) Hemophilia due to deficiency of factor XI.

he·mo·phil·i·ac (hē′mō-fil′ē-ak) A person suffering from hemophilia. SYN haemophiliac.

he·mo·phil·ic (hē′mō-fil′ik) Relating to hemophilia. SYN haemophilic.

he·mo·pho·re·sis (hē′mō-fŏr-ē′sis) Blood convection or irrigation of tissues. SYN haemophoresis.

he·moph·thal·mi·a, he·moph·thal·mus (hē′mof-thal′mē-ă, -mof-thal′mŭs) A blood-filled eye. SYN haemophthalmia, hematopsia.

he·mo·plas·tic (hē′mō-plas′tik) SYN hemopoietic, haemoplastic.

he·mo·poi·e·sis (hē′mō-poy-ē′sis) The process of formation and development of the various types of blood cells and other formed elements. SYN hematosis (1), hematopoiesis, hematosis (1), hemogenesis, sanguification.

he·mo·poi·et·ic (hē′mō-poy-et′ik) Pertaining to or related to the formation of blood cells. SYN hematopoietic.

he·mo·por·phy·rin (hē′mō-pōr′fir-in) SYN haemoporphyrin.

he·mo·pre·cip·i·tin (hē′mō-prē-sip′i-tin) An antibody that combines with and precipitates soluble antigenic material from erythrocytes.

he·mo·pro·tein (hē′mō-prō′tēn) Protein linked to a metal-porphyrin compound. SYN haemoprotein.

he·mop·so·nin (hē-mop'sŏ-nin) An antibody that makes red blood cells more liable to phagocytosis.

he·mop·ty·sis (hē-mop'ti-sis) Spitting blood derived from the lungs due to pulmonary or bronchial hemorrhage. SYN haemoptysis.

he·mor·rha·chis (hē-mōr'ă-kis) SYN hematorrhachis, haemorrhachis.

hem·or·rhage (hem'ŏr-ăj) 1. An escape of blood through ruptured or unruptured vessel walls. 2. To bleed. SYN haemorrhage.

hem·or·rhag·ic cyst (hem'ŏ-raj'ik sist) A cyst containing blood or resulting from the encapsulation of a hematoma. SYN hematocele.

hem·or·rhag·ic cys·ti·tis (hem'ŏr-aj'ik sis-tī'tis) Bladder inflammation with macroscopic hematuria. SYN haemorrhagic cystitis.

hem·or·rhag·ic dis·ease of the new·born (hem'ŏr-aj'ik di-zēz' nū'bōrn) A syndrome characterized by spontaneous internal or external bleeding accompanied by hypoprothrombinemia, slightly decreased platelet counts, and markedly elevated bleeding and clotting times, usually occurring between the third and sixth days of life and effectively treated with vitamin K. SYN haemorrhagic disease of the newborn.

hem·or·rhag·ic in·farct (hem'ŏr-aj'ik in'fahrkt) Red infarct from infiltration of blood from collateral vessels into the necrotic area. SYN hemorrhagic gangrene (1), red infarct.

hem·or·rhag·ic meas·les (hem'ŏr-aj'ik mē'zělz) Severe form in which the eruption is dark due to effusion of blood into affected areas of the skin. SYN black measles (1).

hem·or·rhag·ic pe·ri·car·di·tis (hem-ŏr-aj'ik per'i-kahr-dī'tis) Pericarditis with bloodstained effusion.

hem·or·rhag·ins (hem'ŏr-aj'inz) Cytolysins found in certain venoms and poisonous material from some plants, e.g., rattlesnake venom and ricin.

hem·or·rhoid (HEM) (hem'ŏr-oyd) *Avoid the misspelling hemroid and its many variants.* Denoting one of the tumors or varices constituting hemorrhoids.

hem·or·rhoi·dal tag (hem'ŏr-oyd'ăl tag) A skin polyp protruding from the anus after a hemorrhoid has healed.

hem·or·rhoid·al zone (hem'ŏ-roy'dăl zōn) Anal canal area that contains the rectal venous plexus. SYN zona hemorrhoidalis.

hem·or·rhoid·ec·to·my (hem'ŏr-oy-dek'tŏ-mē) Surgical removal of hemorrhoids.

hem·or·rhoids (ROIDS) (hem'ŏr-oydz) Varicosity of external hemorrhoidal veins causing painful anal swellings. SYN piles.

he·mo·sid·er·in (hē'mō-sid'ĕr-in) A yellow or brown protein produced by phagocytic digestion of hematin; found in most tissues, but especially in the liver. SYN haemosiderin.

he·mo·sid·er·o·sis (hē'mō-sid-ĕr-ō'sis) Accumulation of hemosiderin in tissue, particularly in liver and spleen. SEE hemochromatosis. SYN haemosiderosis.

he·mo·sta·sis, he·mo·sta·si·a (hē'mō-stā'sis, -stā'zē-ă) 1. The arrest of bleeding. 2. The arrest of circulation in a part. 3. Stagnation of blood. SYN haemostasis.

he·mo·stat (hē'mō-stat) 1. Any agent or instrument that arrests, chemically or mechanically the flow of blood from an open vessel. 2. SYN haemostat.

he·mo·stat·ic (hē'mō-stat'ik) 1. Arresting the flow of blood within the vessels. 2. SYN antihemorrhagic. SYN haemastatic, haemostatic.

he·mo·ther·a·py, he·mo·ther·a·peu·tics (hē'mō-thār'ă-pē, -thār-ă-pyū'tiks) Treatment of disease with blood or blood derivatives. SYN haemotherapy.

he·mo·tho·rax, pl. **he·mo·tho·ra·ces** (hē'mō-thōr'aks, -ă-sēz) Blood in the pleural cavity. SYN haematothorax, haemothorax.

he·mo·tox·ic, he·ma·to·tox·ic, he·ma·tox·ic (hē'mō-tok'sik, hē'mă-tō-toks'ik, hē'mă-toks'ik) 1. Causing blood poisoning. 2. SYN hemolytic. SYN haemotoxic.

he·mo·tox·in (hē'mō-tok'sin) Any substance that causes destruction of red blood cells, including various hemolysins. SYN hematotoxin, hematoxin.

he·mo·troph, he·mot·ro·phe (hē'mō-trŏf) The nutritive materials supplied to the embryos of placental mammals through the maternal bloodstream. Cf. embryotroph, histotroph.

he·mo·trop·ic (hē'mō-trō'pik) Pertaining to the mechanism by which a substance in or on blood cells, especially the erythrocytes, attracts phagocytic cells. SYN haemotropic, hematotropic.

he·mo·tym·pa·num, he·ma·to·tym·pa·num (hē'mō-tim'pă-nŭm, hē'mă-tō-) The presence of blood in the middle ear. SYN haemotympanum.

hem·ox·im·e·ter (hēm'oks-im'ĕ-ter) SYN oximeter, haemoximeter.

Hen·der·son-Has·sel·balch e·qua·tion (hen'dĕr-sŏn hahs'ĕl-bawlk ĕ-kwā'zhŭn) A formula relating the pH value of a solution to the pK_a value of the acid in the solution and the ratio of the acid and the conjugate base concentrations.

Hen·le fis·sure (hen'lē fish'ŭr) Tissue connecting the cardiac muscular fibers.

Hen·le lay·er (hen'lē lā'ĕr) Cells of the inner root sheath of the hair follicle.

Hen·le loop (hen'lē lūp) SYN nephron loop.

Hen·le re·ac·tion (hen'lē rē-ak'shŭn) Dark brown staining of the medullary cells of the suprenal gland when treated with the salts of chromium, the cortical cells remaining unstained.

Hen·le sheath (hen'lē shēth) SYN endoneurium.

Hen·ne·bert sign (en'ĕ-bār sīn) Nystagmus produced by pressure applied to a sealed external auditory canal.

He·noch-Schön·lein pur·pu·ra, He·noch pur·pu·ra (hen'awk shĕrn'līn pŭr'pyŭr-ă) An eruption of nonthrombocytopenic purpuric lesions due to dermal leukocytoclastic vasculitis associated with joint pain and swelling, and other findings. SYN Schönlein purpura.

hen·ry (H) (hen'rē) Unit of electrical inductance, when 1 V is induced by a change in current of 1 ampere/sec.

Hen·ry law (hen'rē law) At equilibrium, at a given temperature, the amount of gas dissolved in a given volume of liquid is directly proportional to the partial pressure of that gas in the gas phase.

Hen·sen cell (hen'sĕn sel) A supporting cell in the organ of Corti.

he·par, gen. **hep·a·tis** (hē'pahr, hĕ-pat'is) [TA] SYN liver.

hep·a·ran sul·fate (hep'ă-ran sŭl'fāt) A heteropolysaccharide that has the same repeating disaccharide as heparin but with fewer sulfates and more acetyl groups; accumulates in people with certain types of mucopolysaccharidosis. SYN heparitin sulfate.

hep·a·rin (H, HEP, HP) (hep'ăr-in) An anticoagulant. SYN heparinic acid.

hep·a·rin lock (hep'ăr-in lok) A small catheter positioned in a vein in the upper limb for easy access for administration of intravenous medication; capped when not in use so that it can be flushed with heparin to keep it open and the intravenous line can be disconnected.

hepat-, hepato-, hepatico- Combining forms meaning the liver.

hep·a·ta·tro·phi·a, hep·a·tat·ro·phy (hĕ-pat'ă-trō'fē-ă, hep'ă-tat'rŏ-fē) Atrophy of the liver.

he·pa·tic (hĕ-pat'ik) Relating to the liver.

he·pa·tic a·me·bi·a·sis (hĕ-pat''ik ă-mē-bī'ă-sis) Liver infection with *Entamoeba histolytica;* may occur with or without antecedent amebic dysentery.

he·pa·tic col·ic (hĕ-pat'ik kol'ik) SYN biliary colic.

he·pa·tic co·ma (hĕ-pat'ik kō'mă) State that occurs with advanced hepatic insufficiency and portal-systemic shunts, caused by elevated blood ammonia levels.

he·pa·tic duct (hĕ-pat'ik dŭkt) SEE common hepatic duct.

he·pa·tic en·ceph·a·lo·pa·thy (hĕ-pat′ik en-sef′ă-lop′ă-thē) **1.** SYN portal-systemic encephalopathy. **2.** SYN Reye syndrome.

he·pa·tic fis·tu·la (hĕ-pat′ik fis′tyū-lă) Fistulous passage leading to the liver.

he·pa·tic in·suf·fi·cien·cy (HI) (hĕ-pat′ik in′sŭ-fish′ĕn-sē) Defective functional activity of the liver cells.

he·pa·tic lobes (hĕ-pat′ik lōbz) The five lobes of the liver.

he·pat·i·co·do·chot·o·my (hĕ-pat′i-kō-dō-kot′ŏ-mē) Combined hepaticotomy and choledochotomy.

he·pat·i·co·li·thot·o·my (hĕ-pat′i-kō-li-thot′ŏ-mē) Removal of a stone from a hepatic duct.

he·pat·i·co·lith·o·trip·sy (hĕ-pat′i-kō-lith′ŏ-trip-sē) The crushing or fragmentation of a biliary calculus in the hepatic duct.

he·pat·i·cos·to·my (hĕ-pat′i-kos′tŏ-mē) Establishment of an opening into the hepatic duct.

he·pat·i·cot·o·my (hĕ-pat′i-kot′ŏ-mē) Incision into the hepatic duct.

he·pa·tic por·phy·ri·a (hĕ-pat′ik pōr-fir′ē-ă) A category of porphyria (q.v.) that includes porphyria cutanea tarda, variegate porphyria, and coproporphyria.

he·pa·tic sphinc·ter (hĕ-pat′ik sfingk′tĕr) The thickened area of the muscular coat of the hepatic veins about the entrance to the inferior vena cava.

hep·a·tit·ic (hep′ă-tit′ik) Relating to hepatitis.

hep·a·ti·tis (hep′ă-tī′tis) Inflammation of the liver.

hep·a·ti·tis A (hep′ă-tī′tis) SYN viral hepatitis type A.

hep·a·ti·tis A vi·rus (HAV) (hep′ă-tī′tis vī′rŭs) A ribonucleic acid virus, cause of viral hepatitis type A. SYN infectious hepatitis virus.

hep·a·ti·tis B (hep′ă-tī′tis) SYN viral hepatitis type B.

hep·a·ti·tis B con·ju·gate vac·cine (HbCV) (hep′ă-tī′tis kon′jŭ-gāt vak-sēn′) A type of vaccine used against the virus that combines proteins from a bacterium with elements of the virus.

hep·a·ti·tis B core an·ti·gen (hep′ă-tī′tis kōr an′ti-jen) That found in the core of the Dane particle and also in hepatocyte nuclei in hepatitis B infections.

hep·a·ti·tis B e an·ti·gen (hep′ă-tī′tis an′ti-jen) An antigen, or group of antigens, associated with hepatitis B infection and distinct from the surface antigen (HB_sAg) and the core antigen (HB_cAg).

hep·a·ti·tis B im·mune glob·u·lin (HBIG) (hep′ă-tī′tis i-myūn′ glob′yū-lin) A high-titer passive immune globulin directed against type B hepatitis virus.

hep·a·ti·tis B sur·face an·ti·gen (HB_sAg) (hep′ă-tī′tis sŭr′făs an′ti-jen) Antigen of the small (20 nm) spheric and filamentous forms of hepatitis B antigen, and a surface antigen of the larger (42 nm) Dane particle (complete infectious hepatitis B virus). SEE ALSO hepatitis B e antigen.

hep·a·ti·tis B vi·rus (HBV) (hep′ă-tī′tis vī′rŭs) A DNA virus, the causative agent of viral hepatitis type B. SYN serum hepatitis virus.

hep·a·ti·tis C vi·rus (HCV, HVC, HBC) (hep′ă-tī′tis vī′rŭs) A non-A, non-B ribonucleic acid virus causing posttransfusion hepatitis.

hep·a·ti·tis D (HD, HEP D) (hep′ă-tī′tis) SYN viral hepatitis type D.

hep·a·ti·tis D vi·rus, hep·a·ti·tis del·ta vi·rus (HDV) (hep′ă-tī′tis vī′rŭs, del′tă) A small "defective" ribonucleic acid virus that requires the presence of hepatitis B virus for replication. SYN delta agent.

hep·a·ti·tis E (hep′ă-tī′tis) Primarily tropical form transmitted by the fecal-oral route; has a higher mortality than hepatitis A, particularly in pregnancy.

hep·a·ti·tis G vi·rus (HGV) (hep′ă-tī′tis vī′rŭs) A ribonucleic acid virus related to the hepatitis C virus, which may cause coinfection with that agent.

hep·a·ti·za·tion (hep′ă-tī-zā′shŭn) Conversion of a loose tissue into a firm mass.

hep·a·to·bil·i·ary hep·a·ti·tis (hĕ-pat'ŏ-bil'ē-ar-ē hep'ă-tī'tis) Interruption of the normal bile flow with resulting inflammation of liver tissue; caused by cholelithasis or cholestasis.

hep·a·to·blas·to·ma (hep'ă-tō-blas-tō'mă) A malignant neoplasm occurring in young children, primarily in the liver.

hep·a·to·car·cin·o·gen (hep'ă-tō-kahr-sin'ŏ-jen) An agent capable of causing liver cancer.

hep·a·to·car·ci·no·ma (hep'ă-tō-kahr-si-nō'mă) SYN malignant hepatoma.

he·pa·to·cele (hĕ-pat'ŏ-sēl) Protrusion of part of the liver through the abdominal wall or the diaphragm.

hep·a·to·cel·lu·lar car·ci·no·ma (hep'ă-tō-sel'yū-lăr kahr'si-nō'mă) SYN malignant hepatoma.

he·pa·to·cel·lu·lar jaun·dice (hep'ă-tō-sel'yū-lăr jawn'dis) Liver disorder resulting from diffuse injury or inflammation or failure of function of the hepatic cells, usually due to viral or toxic hepatitis.

hep·a·to·cho·lan·gi·o·car·ci·no·ma (hep'ă-tō-kō-lan'jē-ō-kahr'si-nō'mă) A mixed neoplasm with hepatocellular and biliary epithelial differentiations.

hep·a·to·cho·lan·gi·o·je·ju·nos·to·my (hep'ă-tō-kō-lan'jē-ō-jĕ'jū-nos'tŏ-mē) Union of the hepatic duct to the jejunum.

hep·a·to·cys·tic (hep'ă-tō-sis'tik) Relating to the gallbladder, or to both liver and gallbladder.

hep·a·to·cyte (hep'ă-tō-sīt) A parenchymal liver cell.

hep·a·to·en·ter·ic (hep'ă-tō-en-ter'ik) Relating to the liver and the intestine.

he·pa·to·eryth·ro·poi·et·ic por·phy·ri·a (HEP) (hep'ă-tō-ĕ-rith'rō-poy-et'ik pōr-fir'ē-ă) Disorder with a deficiency or absence of uroporphyrinogen decarboxylase.

hep·a·to·gas·tric (hep'ă-tō-gas'trik) Relating to the liver and the stomach.

hep·a·to·gen·ic, he·pa·tog·e·nous (hep'ă-tō-jen'ik, -toj'ĕn-ŭs) Of hepatic origin; formed in the liver.

hep·a·to·gen·ic jaun·dice (hep'ă-tō-jen'ik jawn'dis) A yellowish discoloration of the skin, whites of the eyes, nail beds, and mucous membranes due to any hepatic disease or disorder.

hep·a·tog·ram (hep'ă-tō-gram) A radiograph of the liver.

hep·a·toid (hep'ă-toyd) Resembling or like the liver.

he·pa·to·jug·u·lar re·flux, he·pa·to·jug·u·lar re·flex (hep'ă-tō-jŭg'yū-lăr rē'flŭks, rē'fleks) An elevation of venous pressure visible in the jugular veins and measurable in the veins of the arm.

he·pa·to·len·tic·u·lar de·gen·er·a·tion (hep'ă-tō-len-tik'yū-lăr dĕ-jen'ĕr-ā'shŭn) **1.** A familial disorder characterized by copper deposition in the liver, causing chronic hepatitis and eventually cirrhosis. **2.** SYN Wilson disease (1).

hep·a·to·lith (hep'ă-tō-lith) A concretion in the liver.

hep·a·to·lith·ec·to·my (hep'ă-tō-li-thek'tŏ-mē) Removal of a calculus from the liver.

hep·a·to·li·thi·a·sis (hep'ă-tō-li-thī'ă-sis) Presence of calculi in the liver.

hep·a·tol·o·gist (hep'ă-tol'ŏ-jist) A medical specialist in hepatology.

hep·a·tol·o·gy (hep'ă-tol'ŏ-jē) Discipline concerned with diseases of the liver.

hep·a·tol·y·sin (hep'ă-tol'i-sin) A cytolysin that destroys parenchymal cells of the liver.

hep·a·tol·y·sis (hep'ă-tol'i-sis) Destruction of liver cells.

hep·a·to·ma (HEP) (hep'ă-tō'mă) SEE malignant hepatoma. SYN hepatocellular carcinoma.

hep·a·to·meg·a·ly, he·pa·to·me·ga·li·a (hep'ă-tō-meg'ă-lē, -mĕ-gā'lē-ă) Enlargement of the liver.

hep·a·to·mel·a·no·sis (hep'ă-tō-mel'ă-nō'sis) Heavy pigmentation of the liver.

hep·a·tom·pha·lo·cele, he·pa·tom·pha·los (hep'ă-tom'fă-lō-sēl, -fă-lōs) Umbilical hernia with involvement of the liver.

hep·a·to·ne·cro·sis (hep'ă-tō-nĕ-krō'sis)
Death of liver cells.

hep·a·to·path·ic (hep'ă-tō-path'ik) Damaging the liver.

hep·a·to·pex·y (hep'ă-tō-pek'sē) Anchoring the liver to the abdominal
wall.

**hep·a·to·pneu·mon·ic, hep·a·ti·co·
pul·mo·nar·y, hep·a·to·pul·mo·nar·
y** (hĕp'ă-tō-nū-mon'ik, he-pat'i-kō-pul'
mŏ-nār-ē, hep'ă-tō-) Relating to the liver
and lungs.

hep·a·to·por·tal (hep'ă-tō-pōr'tăl) Relating to the portal system of the liver.

**hep·a·to·pul·mo·nar·y syn·drome
(HPS)** (hep'ă-tō-pul'mŏ-nar-ē sin'drōm)
Constellation consisting of liver disease
(usually cirrhosis), hypoxemia, and the
presence of intrapulmonary vascular di-
latations.

hep·a·to·re·nal, hep·a·to·neph·ric
(hep'ă-tō-rē'năl, -nef-rik) Relating to the
liver and the kidney.

**hep·a·to·re·nal syn·drome, hep·a·
to·neph·ric syn·drome, hep·a·to·
ne·pho·ric syn·drome** (hep'ă-tō-rē'năl
sin'drōm, hep'ă-tō-nef'rik, -nĕ-fōr'ik) A-
cute renal failure in patients with disease of
liver or biliary tract.

hep·a·tor·rhex·is (hep'ă-tōr-ek'sis) Rupture of the liver.

hep·a·tos·co·py (hep'ă-tos'kŏ-pē) Examination of the liver.

hep·a·to·sis (hep'ă-tō'sis) Any disorder
of the liver.

hep·a·to·sple·ni·tis (hep'ă-tō-splē-nī'
tis) Inflammation of the liver and spleen.

hep·a·to·splen·o·meg·a·ly (hep'ă-tō-
splē-nō-meg'ă-lē) Enlargement of the
liver and spleen.

he·pa·to·sple·nop·a·thy (hep'ă-tō-splē-
nop'ă-thē) Disease of the liver and
spleen.

hep·a·tot·o·my (hep'ă-tot'ŏ-mē) Incision into the liver.

hepatotoxaemia [Br.] SYN hepatotox-
emia.

hep·a·to·tox·e·mi·a (hep'ă-tō-tok-sē'
mē-ă) Autointoxication assumed to be
due to improper functioning of the liver.
SYN hepatotoxaemia.

hep·a·to·tox·ic·i·ty (hep'ă-tō-tok-sis'i-
tē) The capacity of a drug, chemical, or
other exposure to produce injury to the
liver.

hepta-, hept- Combining forms denoting
seven. Cf. septi-, sept-.

hep·ta·chrom·ic (hep'tă-krō'mik) Being
able to see all seven colors of the spectrum; having seven colors in the following order: red, orange, yellow, green,
blue, indigo, and violet.

hep·tose (hep'tōs) A sugar with seven
carbon atoms in its molecule; e.g., sedo-
heptulose.

herbal (ĕr'băl) An imprecise but common
usage for any agent in any form intended
to improve or affect health; sold over the
counter, without prescription and without F.D.A. oversight about potency, ap-
propriateness, or purity. SEE ALSO naturopathic medicine.

herb bath (ĕrb bath) Immersion in a tub
of water that is used as an infusion to
cure dermatologic or other complaints.

herb·i·cide (ĕr-bi'sīd) Any chemical
compound designed to kill plants.

her·biv·o·rous (hĕr-biv'ŏr-ŭs) Feeding
exclusively on vegetable foods.

herd im·mu·ni·ty (hĕrd i-myū'ni-tē) Resistance to invasion and spread of an infectious agent in a group or community,
based on the resistance to infection of a
high proportion of individual members
of the group. SYN group immunity.

herd in·stinct (hĕrd in'stingkt) Tendency
or inclination to band together with and
share the customs of others of a group,
and to conform to the opinions and adopt
the views of the group.

her·ed·i·ta·bil·i·ty (hĕr-ed'i-tă-bil'i-tē)
1. Condition of being able to be passed
to future generations genetically. **2.** A
system for predicting the likelihood of
the occurrence of a trait in future generations.

he·red·i·tar·y (hered) (hĕr-ed'i-tar-ē)

Transmissible from parent to offspring by information encoded in the parental germ cell.

he·red·i·tar·y an·gi·o·e·de·ma (HAE) (hĕr-ed´i-tar-ē an´jē-ō-ĕ-dē´mă) Inherited disease characterized by episodic appearance of brawny nonpitting edema, most often affecting the limbs, but capable of involving other parts of the body.

he·red·i·tar·y cho·re·a (hĕr-ed´i-tar-ē kōr-ē´ă) SYN Huntington chorea.

he·red·i·ta·ry lymph·e·de·ma (hĕ-red´ i-tar-ē limf´ă-dē´mă) Permanent pitting edema usually confined to the legs.

he·red·i·ty (hĕr-ed´i-tē) **1.** The transmission of characteristics from parent to offspring by information encoded in the parental germ cells. **2.** Genealogy.

heredo- Prefix meaning heredity.

he·re·do·fa·mil·i·al (her´ĕ-dō-fă-mil´ē-ăl) Health issues occurring in families under circumstances that could suggest a genetic cause.

He·ring-Breu·er re·flex (her´ing broy´er rē´fleks) The effects of afferent impulses from the pulmonary vagi in the control of respiration.

He·ring test (her´ing test) A test of binocular vision.

her·i·ta·bil·i·ty (her´i-tă-bil´i-tē) **1.** PSYCHOMETRICS a statistical term used to denote the extent of variance of a subject's total score or response that is attributable to a presumed genetic component, in contrast to an acquired component. **2.** GENETICS a statistical term used to denote the proportion of phenotypic variance due to variance in genotypes that is genetically determined, denoted by the traditional symbol h^2.

Her·man·sky-Pud·lak syn·drome (hār-mahn´skē pūd´lahk sin´drōm) Oculocutaneous albinism with accumulation of ceroid in lysosomes with restrictive lung disease, granulomatous colitis, kidney failure, cardiomyopathy, and storage pool-deficient platelets. SEE ALSO oculocutaneous albinism.

her·maph·ro·dit·ism, her·maph·ro·dism (hĕr-maf´rō-dīt-izm, -frō-dizm) The presence in one person or animal of both ovarian and testicular tissue and ambiguous external genitalia; i.e., true hermaphroditism. SYN hermaphrodism.

her·met·ic (hĕr-met´ik) Airtight; denoting a vessel closed or sealed in such a way that air can neither enter it nor issue from it.

her·ni·a, pl. **her·ni·as,** pl. **her·ni·ae** (hĕr´nē-ă, -ăz, -ē) Protrusion of a part or structure through the tissues normally containing it. SYN rupture (1).

her·ni·al, her·ni·a·ted (hĕr´nē-ăl, -āt-ed) Relating to hernia.

her·ni·al sac (hĕr´nē-ăl sak) The peritoneal envelope of a hernia.

her·ni·at·ed (hĕr´nē-ā-tĕd) Denoting any structure protruded through a hernial opening.

her·ni·at·ed disc (hĕr´nē-ā-tĕd disk) Protrusion of a degenerated or fragmented intervertebral disc into the intervertebral foramen. SYN protruded disc, ruptured disc.

her·ni·a·tion (hĕr´nē-ā´shŭn) Protrusion of an anatomic structure from its normal anatomic position.

her·ni·a u·te·ri in·gui·na·lis (hĕr´nē-ă yū´tĕr-ī ing´gwi-nā´lis) Common persistent mullerian duct syndrome in males; produces cryptorchidism on one side with a contralateral inguinal hernia containing a testis, uterus, and uterine tube.

hernio- Prefix meaning a hernia.

her·ni·og·ra·phy (hĕr´nē-og´ră-fē) Radiographic examination of a hernia following injection of a contrast medium into the hernial sac.

her·ni·oid (hĕr´nē-oyd) Resembling hernia.

her·ni·o·plas·ty (hĕr´nē-ō-plas-tē) SYN herniorrhaphy.

her·ni·or·rha·phy (hĕr´nē-ōr´ă-fē) Surgical repair of a hernia. SYN hernioplasty.

her·ni·o·tome (her´nē-ō-tōm) SYN hernia knife.

her·ni·ot·o·my (hĕr-nē-ot′ŏ-mē) Surgical division of the constriction or strangulation of a hernia, often followed by herniorrhaphy.

her·o·in (her′ō-in) An alkaloid prepared from morphine by acetylation; formerly used for the relief of cough. Except for research, its use in the United States is prohibited by federal law because of its potential for abuse.

her·pan·gi·na (HA) (hĕr-pan′ji-nă) A disease caused by types of Coxsackievirus and marked by vesiculopapular lesions about 1–2 mm in diameter that are present around the fauces and soon break down to form grayish yellow ulcers.

her·pes (her′pēz) A papular, vesicular, or ulcerative eruption of skin or mucous membranes caused by local infection with herpesvirus 1 or 2 (herpes simplex) or reactivation of varicella-zoster virus. SYN serpigo (2).

her·pes en·ceph·a·li·tis (hĕr′pēz en-sef′ă-lī′tis) SYN herpes simplex encephalitis.

her·pes fe·bri·lis (hĕr′pēz fē-brī′lis) SYN herpes simplex.

her·pes gen·i·ta·l·is, gen·i·tal her·pes (HG) (hĕr′pēz jen-i-tā′lis, jen′i-tăl) Herpes simplex infection on the genitals, most commonly herpes simplex-2 virus.

her·pes la·bi·a·lis (hĕr′pēz lă-bē-ā′lis) SYN herpes simplex.

her·pes pro·gen·i·ta·lis (hĕr′pēz prō-jen-i-tā′lis) Genital herpes infection caused by herpes simplex virus.

her·pes sim·plex (HSV) (her′pēz sim′pleks) Recurring infections caused by herpesvirus types 1 and 2; type 1 infections are marked most commonly by the eruption of one or more groups of vesicles on the vermilion border of the lips or at the external nares, type 2 by such lesions on the genitalia. SYN herpes facialis, herpes febrilis, herpes labialis, Simplexvirus.

her·pes sim·plex en·ceph·a·li·tis vi·rus (HSE) (hĕr′pēz sim′pleks en-sef′ă-lī′tis) Most common type caused by herpes simplex virus 1; affects people of any age; preferentially involves the inferomedial portions of the temporal lobe and the orbital portions of the frontal lobes. SYN acute inclusion body encephalitis, herpes encephalitis.

her·pes sim·plex vi·rus en·ceph·a·li·tis (HSV) (hĕr′pēz sim′pleks en-sef′ă-lī′tis) The most common acute encephalitis, caused by HSV-1; affects people of any age; preferentially involves the inferomedial portions of the temporal lobe and the orbital portions of the frontal lobes; pathologically, severe hemorrhagic necrosis is present along with, in the acute stages, intranuclear eosinophilic inclusion bodies in the neurons and glial cells. SYN herpes encephalitis.

her·pes·vi·rus, her·pes vi·rus (HV) (hĕr′pēz-vī′rŭs) Any virus belonging to the family Herpesviridae.

her·pes zos·ter (HZ) (hĕr′pēz zos′tĕr) Self-limited infection by herpesvirus, characterized by an eruption of groups of vesicles on one side of the body following the course of a nerve due to inflammation of ganglia and dorsal nerve roots resulting from activation of the virus, which in many instances has remained latent for years following a primary chickenpox infection. SEE ALSO varicella. SYN zona (2) [TA], shingles, zoster.

her·pes zos·ter oph·thal·mi·cus (hĕr′pēz zos′tĕr of-thal′mi-kŭs) A herpetic involvement of the ophthalmic branch of the trigeminal nerve, which may lead to corneal ulceration.

her·pes zos·ter vi·rus (HZV) (hĕr′pēz zos′tĕr vī′rŭs) SYN varicella-zoster virus.

her·pet·ic (hĕr-pet′ik) **1.** Relating to or characterized by herpes. **2.** Relating to or caused by a herpetovirus or herpesvirus.

her·pet·ic whit·low (hĕr-pet′ik wit′lō) Painful herpes simplex virus infection of a finger from direct inoculation of the unprotected perionychial fold, often accompanied by lymphangitis and regional adenopathy, lasting up to several weeks.

Herr·mann syn·drome (hĕr′măn sin′drōm) A multisystem disorder beginning in late childhood or early adolescence, with photomyoclonus and hearing loss followed by diabetes mellitus, progressive dementia, pyelonephritis, and glomerulonephritis.

her·sage (ār-sahzh´) Separating the individual fibers of a nerve trunk.

Hert·wig sheath (hert´vig shēth) The merged outer and inner epithelial layers of the enamel organ that extends beyond the region of the anatomic crown and initiates formation of dentin in the root of a developing tooth.

hertz (Hz) (hĕrts) A unit of sound or alternating current frequency, 1 Hz is equivalent to 1 cycle per second.

Herx·hei·mer re·ac·tion (herks´hīm-er rē-ak´shŭn) Systemic inflammatory manifestation affecting skin, mucous membranes, nervous system, or viscera after antimicrobial treatment of treponemal disease. SYN Jarisch-Herxheimer reaction.

Hes·sel·bach her·ni·a (hes´ĕl-bahk hĕr´nē-ă) Hernia with diverticula through the cribriform fascia, presenting a lobular outline.

het·a·starch (het´ă-stahrch) A carbohydrate starch derivative used as a cryoprotective agent for erythrocytes; also used as an extender of blood plasma volume.

heteraesthesia [Br.] SYN heteresthesia.

het·er·e·ci·ous (het´ĕr-ē´shŭs) Having more than one host; said of a parasite passing different stages of its life cycle in different animals.

het·er·es·the·si·a (het´ĕr-es-thē´zē-ă) A change occurring in the degree (either plus or minus) of the sensory response to a cutaneous stimulus as the latter crosses a certain line on the surface. SYN heteraesthesia.

♻ **hetero-, heter-** Combining forms meaning the other, different; opposite of homo-.

het·er·o·ag·glu·ti·na·tion (het´ĕr-ō-ă-glū´ti-nā´shŭn) Clumping of particulate antigens of one kind by antibodies derived from a second antigen.

het·er·o·ag·glu·ti·nin (het´ĕr-ō-ă-glū´ti-nin) A form of hemagglutinin that agglutinates the red blood cells of species other than that in which the heteroagglutinin occurs.

het·er·o·al·lele (het´ĕr-ō-ă-lēl´) One of several forms of a gene that vary at nonidentical mutation sites.

het·er·o·an·ti·bod·y (het´ĕr-ō-an´ti-bod-ē) One heterologous with respect to antigen, in contradistinction to isoantibody.

het·er·o·an·ti·gen (het´ĕr-ō-an´ti-jen) An antigen that derives from a species other than that of the producer of the antibody.

het·er·o·an·ti·se·rum (het´ĕr-ō-an´tē-sēr´ŭm) One developed in one animal species against antigens of another.

het·er·o·blas·tic (het´ĕr-ō-blas´tik) Developing from more than a single type of tissue.

het·er·o·cel·lu·lar (het´ĕr-ō-sel´yū-lăr) Formed of cells of different kinds.

het·er·o·ceph·a·lus (het´ĕr-ō-sef´ă-lŭs) Conjoined twins with heads of unequal size.

het·er·o·chro·ma·tin (het´ĕr-ō-krō´mă-tin) Area of chromonema that remains tightly coiled and condensed during interphase and thus stains readily.

het·er·o·chro·mi·a (het´ĕr-ō-krō´mē-ă) A difference in coloration in two structures that are normally alike in color.

het·er·o·chro·mi·a ir·i·dis, het·er·o·chro·mi·a of i·ris (het´ĕr-ō-krō´mē-ă ī-rid´is, ī´ris) A difference in coloration of the irides.

het·er·o·chro·mic u·ve·i·tis (het´ĕr-ō-krō´mik yū´vē-ī´tis) Anterior uveitis and depigmentation of the iris. SYN Fuchs uveitis.

het·er·o·chro·mous (het´ĕr-ō-krō´mŭs) Having an abnormal difference in coloration.

het·er·o·chron·ic (het´er-ō-kron´ik) SYN heterochronous.

het·er·o·clad·ic (het´ĕr-ō-klad´ik) Denoting an anastomosis between branches of different arterial trunks, as distinguished from homocladic.

het·er·o·crine (het′ĕr-ō-krin) Denoting the secretion of two or more kinds of material.

het·er·o·cy·clic com·pounds (het′ĕr-ō-sik′lik kom′powndz) Organic compounds that contain a ring structure containing atoms as well as carbon as part of the ring.

het·er·o·cy·to·trop·ic (het′ĕr-ō-sī′tō-trō′pik) Having an affinity for cells of a different species.

het·er·o·dont (het′ĕr-ō-dont) Having teeth that are morphologically different, as in humans.

het·er·od·ro·mous (het′ĕr-od′rŏ-mŭs) Moving in the opposite direction.

het·er·o·du·plex (het′ĕr-ō-dū′pleks) **1.** A DNA molecule, the two constitutive strands of which derive from distinct sources and hence are likely to be somewhat mismatched. **2.** A DNA-RNA hybrid.

het·er·o·e·cious par·a·site (het′ĕr-ē′shŭs păr′ă-sīt) Pathogen that needs two or more hosts, one for the mature form and one or more others for the immature.

het·er·o·e·rot·i·cism, het·er·o·er·ot·ism (het′ĕr-ō-ĕ-rot′i-sism, -er′ō-tism) A condition of sexual excitement brought about by congress with a person of the opposite sex.

het·er·o·ga·met·ic (het′ĕr-ō-gă-met′ik) Having sex gametes of contrasting types; human males are heterogametic.

het·er·og·a·my (het′ĕr-og′ă-mē) **1.** Conjugation of unlike gametes. **2.** Bearing different types of flowers. **3.** Reproduction by indirect methods of pollination.

het·er·o·ge·ne·i·ty, het·er·o·ge·nic·i·ty (het′ĕr-ō-jĕ-nē′i-tē, -jĕ-nis′i-tē) Heterogeneous state or quality.

het·er·o·ge·ne·ous (het′ĕr-ō-jĕ′nē-ŭs) Comprising elements with various and dissimilar properties.

het·er·o·gen·e·sis (het′ĕr-ō-jen′ĕ-sis) **1.** Alternation of generations. **2.** SYN asexual generation. **3.** SYN spontaneous generation.

het·er·o·ge·net·ic (het′ĕr-ō-jĕ-net′ik) Relating to heterogenesis.

het·er·o·ge·net·ic an·ti·gen (het′ĕr-ō-jĕ-net′ik an′ti-jen) One possessed by a variety of phylogenetically unrelated species.

het·er·o·gen·ic, het·er·o·ge·ne·ic (het′ĕr-ō-jen′ik, -jĕ-nē′ik) Having different gene constitutions.

het·er·o·gon·ic life cy·cle (het′ĕr-ō-gon′ik līf sī′kĕl) Free-living stage of the life cycle of an organism (e.g., *Strongyloides stercoralis*) that also has a parasitic stage.

het·er·o·graft (het′ĕr-ō-graft) SYN xenograft.

het·er·o·ker·a·to·plas·ty (het′ĕr-ō-ker′ă-tō-plas′tē) Surgery in which the cornea from one species of animal is grafted to the eye of another species.

het·er·o·ki·ne·sis, het·er·o·ki·ne·si·a (het′ĕr-ō-ki-nē′sis, -ki-nē′zē-ă) Differential distribution of X and Y chromosomes during meiotic cell division.

het·er·ol·o·gous (het′ĕr-ol′ŏ-gŭs) **1.** Pertaining to cytologic or histologic elements occurring where they are not normally found. SEE ALSO xenogeneic. **2.** Derived from an animal of a different species.

het·er·ol·o·gous graft (het′ĕr-ol′ŏ-gŭs graft) SYN xenograft.

het·er·ol·o·gous in·sem·i·na·tion (het′ĕr-ol′ŏ-gŭs in-sem′i-nā′shŭn) Artificial insemination with semen from a donor who is not the woman's husband. SYN donor insemination.

het·er·ol·o·gous stim·u·lus (het′ĕr-ol′ŏ-gŭs stim′yū-lŭs) One that acts on any of the sensory apparatus or nerve tract.

het·er·ol·o·gous tu·mor (het′ĕr-ol′ŏ-gŭs tū′mŏr) Lesion composed of a tissue unlike that from which it springs.

het·er·ol·o·gous twins (het′ĕr-ol′ŏ-gŭs twinz) SYN dizygotic twins.

het·er·ol·y·sis (het′ĕr-ol′i-sis) Dissolution or digestion of cells or protein components from one species by a lytic agent from a different species.

H

het·er·o·lyt·ic (het′ĕr-ō-lit′ik) Pertaining to heterolysis or to the effect of a heterolysin.

het·er·o·mer·ic (het′ĕr-ō-mer′ik) **1.** Having a different chemical composition. **2.** Denoting spinal neurons that have processes passing over to the opposite side of the cord.

het·er·o·met·a·pla·si·a (het′ĕr-ō-met′ă-plā′zē-ă) Tissue transformation resulting in production of a tissue foreign to the part where produced.

het·er·o·met·ric (het′ĕr-ō-met′rik) Involving or depending on a change in size.

het·er·o·me·tro·pi·a (het′ĕr-ō-mĕ-trō′pē-ă) A condition in which the refraction is different in each eye. SYN anisometropia.

het·er·o·mor·pho·sis (het′ĕr-ō-mōr-fō′sis) **1.** Development of one tissue from tissue of another kind or type. **2.** Embryonic development of tissue or an organ inappropriate to its site.

het·er·o·mor·phous (het′ĕr-ō-mōr′fŭs) Differing from the normal form.

het·er·on·o·mous (het′ĕr-on′ŏ-mŭs) **1.** Different from the type; abnormal. **2.** Subject to the direction or control of another; not self-governing.

het·er·on·y·mous (het′ĕr-on′i-mŭs) Having different names.

het·er·on·y·mous dip·lo·pi·a (het′ĕr-on′i-mŭs di-plō′pē-ă) SYN crossed diplopia.

het·er·o·os·te·o·plas·ty (het′ĕr-ō-os′tē-ō-plas-tē) Surgical repair of a bone with osseous structures taken from an individual of a different species.

het·er·oph·a·gy (het′ĕr-of′ă-jē) Digestion within a cell of a substance phagocytized from without.

het·er·o·phil, het·er·o·phile (het′ĕr-ō-fil, -fīl) **1.** The neutrophilic leukocyte. **2.** Pertaining to heterogenetic antigens occurring in different species or to antibodies directed against such antigens.

het·er·o·pho·ri·a (het′ĕr-ō-fōr′ē-ă) A tendency for deviation of the eyes from parallelism, prevented by binocular vision.

het·er·o·pla·si·a (het′ĕr-ō-plā′zē-ă) **1.** Development of cytologic and histologic elements that are not normal for the organ or part in question (e.g., the growth of bone in a site where there is normally fibrous connective tissue). **2.** Malposition of otherwise normal tissue.

het·er·o·plas·tic graft (het′ĕr-ō-plas′tik graft) SYN xenograft.

het·er·o·pyk·no·sis (het′ĕr-ō-pik-nō′sis) Any state of variable density or condensation, usually in different chromosomes or between different regions of the same chromosome; a region may be attenuated or accentuated.

het·er·o·sis (het′ĕr-ō′sis) Beneficial effect on the phenotype of crossing (hybridization) on growth, vigor, and physical or mental qualities in a strain of plants or in animal stock; also referred to as hybrid vigor.

het·er·o·to·pi·a, het·er·o·to·py (het′ĕr-ō-tō′pē-ă, -ot′ō-pē) **1.** SYN ectopia. **2.** NEUROPATHOLOGY displacement of gray matter, typically into the deep cerebral white matter.

het·er·o·to·pic os·si·fi·ca·tion (het′ĕr-ō-top′ik os′i-fi-kā′shŭn) Growth of calcium deposits within soft tissue, usually at the site of a hematoma due to blunt trauma or in tissue atrophied due to central nervous system injury. SYN myositis ossificans.

het·er·o·top·ic preg·nan·cy (het′ĕr-ō-top′ik preg′năn-sē) SYN ectopic pregnancy.

het·er·o·trans·plan·ta·tion (het′ĕr-ō-trans-plan-tā′shŭn) Transfer of a heterograft (xenograft).

het·er·o·troph·ic (het′ĕr-ō-trō′fik) **1.** Relating to or exhibiting the properties of heterotrophy. **2.** Relating to a heterotroph.

het·er·o·tro·pi·a, het·er·ot·ro·py (het′ĕr-ō-trō′pē-ă, -ot′rŏ-pē) SYN strabismus.

het·er·o·typ·ic (het′ĕr-ō-tip′ik) Of a different or unusual type or form.

het·er·ox·e·nous (het′ĕr-oks′ĕ-nŭs) SYN digenetic (1).

het·er·o·zy·gos·i·ty, het·er·o·zy·go·sis (het′ĕr-ō-zī-gos′i-tē, -zī-gō′sis) The state of being heterozygous.

het·er·o·zy·gote (het′ĕr-ō-zī′gōt) A heterozygous individual.

het·er·o·zy·gous (het′ĕr-ō-zī′gŭs) Having different allelic genes at one locus or (by extension) many loci; heterotic.

heu·ris·tic (hyūr-is′tik) Denotes a trial-and-error method.

hexa-, hex- Combining forms meaning six.

hex·a·chlo·ro·phene (hek′să-klō′rŏ-fēn) A topical antibacterial formerly widely used in wound care and as a surgical scrub. Use is currently restricted to disinfection of intact adult skin. Products containing more than 0.1% hexachlorophene are available only by prescription.

hex·ad (heks′ad) A sexivalent element or radical.

hex·a·dac·ty·ly, hex·a·dac·tyl·ism (hek′să-dak′ti-lē, -lizm) The presence of six fingers or six toes on one or both hands or feet.

Hex·ad·no·vi·rus (heks-ad′nō-vī′rŭs) A genus in the family Hepadnaviridae, which is the cause of hepatitis B.

hex·o·ki·nase (HK) (heks′ō-kī′nās) A phosphotransferase present in yeast, muscle, brain, and other tissues that catalyzes the adenosine-triphosphate-dependent phosphorylation of D-glucose and other hexoses to form D-glucose 6-phosphate (or other hexose 6-phosphates).

hex·os·a·mine (heks-ōs′ă-mēn) The amine derivative (NH_2 replacing OH) of a hexose (e.g., glucosamine).

hex·os·a·min·i·dase (HEX) (heks-ōs′ă-min′i-dās) General term for enzymes hydrolyzing N-acetylhexose (e.g., N-acetylglucosamine) residues from gangliosidelike oligosaccharides.

hex·ose (heks′ōs) A monosaccharide containing six carbon atoms in the molecule (e.g., $C_6H_{12}O_6$); D-glucose is the principal hexose in nature.

hex·ur·on·ic ac·id (heks′yūr-on′ik as′id) The uronic acid of a hexose.

hex·yl·re·sor·ci·nol (hek′sil-rē-zōr′si-nol) A broad spectrum anthelmintic and antiseptic.

Hey am·pu·ta·tion (hā amp′yū-tā′shŭn) Amputation of the foot in front of the tarsometatarsal joint.

Heyde syn·drome (hād sin′drōm) Gastrointestinal disorder involving hemorrhage and anemia to aortic valve secondary stenosis.

Hey·er-Pu·denz valve (hī′ĕr-pū′denz valv) Type used in the shunting procedure for hydrocephaly.

Hg Symbol for mercury (hydrargyrum).

H gene SYN histocompatibility gene.

hi·a·tal her·ni·a, hi·a·tus her·ni·a (hī-ā′tăl hĕr′nē-ă, hī-ā′tŭs) Protrusion of a stomach part through the esophageal hiatus of the diaphragm.

hi·a·tus, pl. **hi·a·tus** (hī-ā′tŭs) [TA] An aperture, opening, or foramen.

hi·a·tus a·or·ti·cus (hī-ā′tŭs ā-ōr′ti-kŭs) [TA] SYN aortic hiatus.

Hick·man cath·e·ter (HC) (hik′măn kath′ĕ-tĕr) Long-term, central venous indwelling catheter with external port(s).

hi·drad·e·ni·tis (hī′drad-ĕ-nī′tis) Inflammation of the sweat glands.

hi·drad·e·ni·tis sup·pu·ra·ti·va (HS) (hī′drad-ĕ-nī′tis sŭp-yūr-ă-tī′vă) Chronic suppurative folliculitis of apocrine sweat gland–bearing skin of the perianal, axillary, and genital areas or under the breasts, developing after puberty and producing abscesses or sinuses with scarring.

hi·drad·e·no·ma, hy·drad·e·no·ma (hī′drad′ĕ-nō′mă) A benign neoplasm derived from epithelial cells of sweat glands.

hidro-, hidr- Combining forms meaning sweat, sweat glands. Cf. sudor-.

hi·dro·cys·to·ma (hī′drō-sis-tō′mă) A cystic form of hidradenoma, usually apocrine.

hi·dro·poi·e·sis (hī′drō-poy-ē′sis) The formation of sweat.

hi·dros·che·sis (hī-dros′kĕ-sis) Suppression of sweating.

hi·drot·ic ec·to·der·mal dys·pla·si·a (HED) (hī′drot′ik ek′tō-dĕr′măl dis-plā′zē-ă) Congenital dystrophy of the nails and hair with thickened nails and sparse or absent scalp hair.

high-den·si·ty lip·o·pro·tein (HDL) (hī-den′si-tē lip′ō-prō′tēn) Complex containing lipids and protein that carries cholesterol to the liver so that it may be excreted in bile.

high den·si·ty lip·o·pro·tein cho·les·ter·ol (HDL-C) (hī-den′si-tē lip′ō-prō′tēn-kŏ-les′tĕr-ol) So-called "good" cholesterol, which, because of its high protein:lipid ratio, is thought to be cardioprotective.

high-ef·fi·cien·cy par·tic·u·late air fil·ters (HEPA) (hī-ĕ-fish′ĕn-sē pahr-ti-k′yū-lăt ăr fil′tĕrz) A type used in health care settings that removes all but the very smallest potential irritants from recirculating air.

high-fi·ber di·et (HFD) (hī-fī′bĕr dī′ĕt) Regimen including much of the nondigestible part of plants, i.e., fiber, found in fruits, vegetables, whole grains, and legumes.

high- Fow·ler po·si·tion (hī-fowl′ĕr pŏ-zish′ŏn) Patient position in which the head of the bed is raised to a 90-degree angle.

high-frequency os·cil·la·tion (HFO) (hī-frē′kwĕn-sē os′i-lā′shŭn) A type of mechanical ventilation.

high-fre·quen·cy pos·i·tive pres·sure ven·ti·la·tion (HFPPV) (hī-frē′kwĕn-sē poz′i-tiv presh′ŭr ven′ti-lā′shŭn) Mechanical ventilatory support system that imposes a respiratory rate exceeding 60 cycles per minute.

high-fre·quen·cy ven·ti·la·tion (HFV) (hī-frē′kwĕn-sē ven′ti-lā′shŭn) Mechanical ventilation using "jet" administra-

tion of breaths at frequencies anywhere from 300–3,000 breaths per minute to avoid some complications of more conventional ventilation.

high-grade squa·mous in·tra·ep·i·the·li·al le·sion (HSIL, HGSIL) (hī′grād skwă′mŭs in′tră-ep-i-thē′lē-ăl lē′zhŭn) Term used in the Bethesda system for reporting cervical-vaginal cytologic diagnosis to describe a spectrum of findings.

high lith·ot·o·my (hī li-thot′ō-mē) SYN suprapubic lithotomy.

high·ly ac·tive an·ti·ret·ro·vi·ral ther·a·py (HAART) (hī′lē ak′tiv an′tē-ret′rō-vī′răl thār′ă-pē) A combination of anti-AIDS medications usually consisting of two nucleoside reverse transcription inhibitors (NRTIs) with one or two protease inhibitors, or two NRTIs with a nonnucleoside reverse transcription inhibitor (NNRTI).

high-per·for·mance liq·uid chro·ma·tog·ra·phy, high-pres·sure liq·uid chro·ma·tog·ra·phy (HPLC) (hī-pĕr-fōr′măns lik′wid krō′mă-tog′ră-fē, hī-presh′ŭr) A chromatographic technology used to separate and quantitate mixtures of substances in solution.

high-res·o·lu·tion com·put·ed to·mog·ra·phy (HRCT) (hī-rez′ō-lū′shŭn kŏm-pyū′tĕd tŏ-mog′ră-fē) Technique with narrow collimation to reduce volume-averaging and an edge-enhancing reconstruction algorithm to sharpen the image, sometimes with a restricted field of view to minimize the size of pixels in the region imaged; used particularly for lung imaging.

high-risk in·fant (hī′risk in′fănt) A newborn considered to be in greater danger of health problems than the norm in the first month of life. Premature infants are more likely to be so categorized than infants carried to term.

hil·lock (hil′lok) ANATOMY any small elevation or prominence.

Hill-Sachs le·sion (hil saks lē′zhŭn) An articular cartilage defect on the posterior aspect of the humeral head, often caused by injury to the humeral head by the rim of the glenoid fossa after anterior glenohumeral dislocation.

hi•lum (hī′lŭm) [TA] **1.** Organ part where nerves and vessels enter and leave. **2.** Depression resembling the hilum in cerebral olivary nucleus.

hind•brain (hīnd′brān) [TA] SYN rhombencephalon.

hind•foot (hīnd′fut) Calcaneus and talus of the foot.

hind•gut (hīnd′gŭt) **1.** The caudal or terminal part of the embryonic gut. **2.** Descending and sigmoid colon, rectum and superior two thirds of the anal canal. SYN endgut.

hinge ax•is (hinj ak′sis) SYN transverse horizontal axis.

hinge joint (hinj joynt) [TA] Uniaxial joint in which a broad, transversely cylindric convexity on one bone fits into a corresponding concavity on the other. SYN ginglymoid joint, ginglymus.

Hin•man syn•drome (hin′măn sin′drŏm) SYN nonneurogenic neurogenic bladder.

hip (hip) **1.** The lateral prominence of the pelvis from the waist to the thigh. **2.** The joint between femur and pelvis. **3.** Colloquially, the head, neck, and greater trochanter of femur, as found in the phrases ''hip fracture'' and ''hip replacement.''

hip bath (hip bath) SYN sitz bath.

hip joint (hip joynt) [TA] The ball-and-socket synovial joint between the head of the femur and the acetabulum. SYN coxa (2).

Hip•pel dis•ease (hip′el di-zēz′) SYN von Hippel-Lindau syndrome.

hip•po•cam•pus (HC, H), pl. **hip•po•cam•pi** (hip′ŏ-kam′pŭs, -pī) [TA] The complex, internally convoluted structure that forms the medial margin (''hem'') of the cortical mantle of the cerebral hemisphere, bordering the choroid fissure of the lateral ventricle, and composed of two gyri (Ammon horn and the dentate gyrus), together with their white matter, the alveus and fimbria hippocampi. SYN hippocampus major, major hippocampus.

Hip•poc•ra•tes (hi-pok′ră-tēz) An an-

cient Greek physician considered to be the father of modern medicine.

hip•po•crat•ic fa•ci•es, fa•ci•es hip•po•cra•ti•ca (hip′ŏ-krat′ik fash′ē-ēz, hip′ŏ-krat′ĭ-kă) Pinched facial expression with sunken eyes, concavity of cheeks and temples, relaxed lips, and leaden complexion.

Hip•po•crat•ic Oath (hip′ŏ-krat′ik ōth) An oath taken by physicians usually on receiving the doctoral degree, whereby they promise to observe ethical principles in the practice of medicine.

hip•po•crat•ic suc•cus•sion sound (hip′ŏ-krat′ik sŭ-kŭsh′ŭn sownd) A splashing sound elicited by shaking a patient with hydro- or pyopneumothorax, the physician's ear is applied to the chest.

hip point•er (hip poynt′ĕr) Traumatic subperiosteal hematoma of the pelvic girdle.

hip•pu•ric ac•id (HA) (hi-pyūr′ik as′id) A detoxification and excretory product of benzoate found in the urine of humans and many herbivorous animals. An organic acid in the urine of horses and other herbivores; a derivative, paraaminohippuric acid, is used in renal testing.

hip•pus (hip′ŭs) Intermittent pupillary dilation and constriction, independent of illumination, convergence, or psychic stimuli.

hip re•place•ment (hip rē-plās′mĕnt) Orthopedic surgery involving femoral head prosthetic replacement.

hir•ci (hĕr′sī) Plural of hircus.

Hirsch•berg test, meth•od (hĕrsh′berg test, meth′od) A test of binocular motor alignment by which a penlight is shone at the eyes and the position of the light reflex on the cornea observed, allowing an estimate of the amount of deviation, if present.

hir•sute (hir-sūt′) Relating to or characterized by hirsutism.

hir•sut•ism, hir•su•ti•es (hir′sū-tizm, hir-sū′tē-ēz) Presence of excessive bodily and facial terminal hair, in a male pattern, especially in women; may be pres-

H

ent in normal adults as an expression of an ethnic characteristic or develop in children or adults as the result of androgen excess due to tumors or nonandrogenetic drugs.

hir·u·din (hir-ū′din) An antithrombin substance from the leech that prevents blood coagulation.

Hir·u·din·e·a (hir′ū-din′ē-ă) The leeches, a class of worms (phylum Annelida) with flat, segmented bodies, a sucker at the posterior end, and often a smaller sucker at the anterior end; they are predatory on invertebrate tissues, or feed on blood and tissue exudates of vertebrates.

Hi·ru·do (hi-rū′dō) A genus of leeches; used in traditional medicine for bloodletting or as an antithrombin.

hir·u·log (hir′yū-log) A synthetic thrombin inhibitor. SYN bivalirudin.

✿ **–His** Combining form for histidino.

His bun·dle elec·tro·gram (HBE) (hiz bŭn′dĕl ĕ-lek′trō-gram) Image recorded from the His bundle, either in experimental animals or humans during electrophysiologic cardiac catheterization.

His ca·nal (hiz kă-nal′) Structural opening in a fetus between the posterior tongue and the developing thyroid. Distal part may form a thyroidal pyramidal lobe and the proximal part is usually obliterated. SYN Bochdalek duct, duct of His, duct of Vater, thyroglossal duct.

His-Pur·kin·je sys·tem (hiz-pŭr-kin′jē sis′tem) SEE atrioventricular bundle.

His·ta·log test (his′tă-lawg test) Measurement of maximal production of gastric acidity or anacidity; similar to the histamine test, but uses betazole hydrochloride, an analogue of histamine.

histaminaemia [Br.] SYN histaminemia.

his·ta·mine (his′tă-mēn) A depressor amine derived from histidine and present in ergot and in animal tissues. It is a powerful stimulant of gastric secretion, a constrictor of bronchial smooth muscle and a vasodilator (capillaries and arterioles) that causes a fall in blood pressure. Histamine is liberated in the skin as a result of injury;

when injected intradermally in high dilution, it causes the triple response.

his·ta·mine-block·ing a·gent (his′tă-mēn blok′ing ā′jĕnt) A substance that can slow or stop the action of histamine.

his·ta·mine head·ache (his′ta-mēn hed′āk) Intense episodic headaches usually related to changes in blood pressure.

his·ta·mi·ne·mi·a (his′tă-min-ē′mē-ă) The presence of histamine in the circulating blood.

his·ta·mine-re·leas·ing fac·tor (his′tă-mēn-rē-lēs′ing fak′tŏr) A lymphokine produced from antigen-stimulated lymphocytes that induces the release of histamine from basophils.

his·ta·mi·nu·ri·a (his′tă-mi-nyūr′ē-ă) The excretion of histamine in the urine.

his·ti·dine (His, H) (his′ti-dēn) The L-isomer is a basic amino acid found in most proteins.

his·ti·di·ne·mi·a (hist) (his′ti-di-nē′mē-ă) A metabolic disorder characterized by speech defects, growth deficiency, and mild mental retardation.

his·ti·di·nu·ri·a (his′ti-di-nyūr′ē-ă) Excretion of considerable amounts of histidine in the urine.

✿ **histio-** Combining form indicating tissue, especially connective tissue.

his·ti·o·cyte, his·to·cyte (his′tē-ō-sīt, his′tō-sīt) A tissue macrophage (e.g., hepatic Kupffer cells, alveolar macrophages, others). SYN histocyte.

his·ti·o·cyt·ic leu·ke·mi·a (his′te-ō-sit′ik lū-kē′mē-ă) Hematologic disease with monocytes and monoblasts in blood.

his·ti·o·cy·to·ma (his′tē-ō-sī-tō′mă) A tumor composed of histiocytes.

his·ti·o·cy·to·sis (his′tē-ō-sī-tō′sis) A generalized multiplication of histiocytes. SYN histocytosis.

his·ti·o·gen·ic (his′tē-ō-jen′ik) SYN histogenous.

✿ **histo-** Combining form meaning tissue.

his·to·chem·is·try (his′tō-kem′is-trē) SYN cytochemistry.

his·to·com·pat·i·bil·i·ty (his′tō-kŏm-pat′i-bil′i-tē) A state of immunologic similarity (or identity) that permits successful homograft transplantation.

his·to·com·pat·i·bil·i·ty gene (his′tō-kŏm-pat′ă-bil′i-tē jēn) In laboratory animals, a gene that can elicit an immune response and thereby cause rejection of a homograft when tissue is transplanted from one individual to another. SYN H gene.

his·to·com·pat·i·bil·i·ty test·ing (his′tō-kŏm-pat′i-bil′i-tē test′ing) A testing system for human leukocyte antigens of major importance in tissue transplantation.

his·to·dif·fer·en·ti·a·tion (his′tō-dif′ĕr-en-shē-ā′shŭn) The morphologic appearance of tissue characteristics during development.

his·to·gen·e·sis (his′tō-jen′ĕ-sis) The origin of a tissue. SYN histogeny.

his·to·ge·net·ic (his′tō-jĕ-net′ik) Relating to histogenesis.

his·tog·e·nous (his-toj′ĕ-nŭs) Formed by the tissues. SYN histiogenic.

his·to·gram (his′tō-gram) A bar chart representing a frequency distribution.

his·tog·ra·phy (his-tog′ră-fē) The written description of a tissue.

his·toid (his′toyd) Resembling in structure one of the tissues of the body.

his·to·in·com·pat·i·bil·i·ty (his′tō-in′kŏm-pat′i-bil′i-tē) A state of immunologic dissimilarity of tissues sufficient to cause rejection of a homograft when tissue is transplanted from one person to another.

his·to·log·ic, his·to·log·i·cal (his′tō-loj′ik, -i-kăl) Pertaining to histology.

his·tol·o·gy (his-tol′ŏ-jē) The science concerned with the minute structure of cells, tissues, and organs in relation to their function. SEE ALSO microscopic anatomy. SYN microanatomy.

his·tol·y·sis (his-tol′i-sis) Disintegration of tissue.

his·to·ma, his·ti·o·ma (his-tō′mă, -ē-ō′mă) A benign neoplasm in which the cytologic and histologic elements are closely similar to those of normal tissue from which the neoplastic cells are derived.

his·to·met·a·plas·tic (his′tō-met-ă-plas′tik) Exciting tissue metaplasia.

his·to·mo·ni·a·sis (his′tō-mŏ-nī′ă-sis) A turkey disease caused by *Histomonas meleagridis* characterized by liver lesions, acute onset, and a high mortality rate. SYN blackhead (2).

his·tone (his′tōn) One of a number of simple proteins (often found in the cell nucleus) that contains a high proportion of basic amino acids, are soluble in water, dilute acids, and alkalies, and are not coagulable by heat.

his·to·phys·i·ol·o·gy (his′tō-fiz′ē-ol′ŏ-jē) The microscopic study of tissues in relation to their functions.

his·to·plas·min (his′tō-plaz′min) An antigenic extract of *Histoplasma capsulatum*, used in immunologic tests to diagnose histoplasmosis.

his·to·plas·mo·ma (his′tō-plaz-mō′mă) An infectious granuloma caused by *Histoplasma capsulatum*.

his·to·plas·mo·sis (his′tō-plaz-mō′sis) A widely distributed infectious epidemic disease caused by *Histoplasma capsulatum* that has pulmonary and optic effects.

his·to·ry (his′tŏr-ē) In health care, record of a patient's symptoms, illness, and treatment thereof, and other health details.

his·to·tech·nol·o·gist (his′tō-tek-nol′ŏ-jist) Laboratory worker who prepares tissue for examination by pathologists, performs complex procedures for processing tissues, and evaluates the quality of the results.

his·to·throm·bin (his′tō-throm′bin) A clotting agent derived from connective tissue.

his·tot·o·my (his-tot′ŏ-mē) SYN microtomy.

his·to·tox·ic (his′tō-tok′sik) Relating to poisoning of the respiratory enzyme system of the tissues.

his·to·tox·ic a·nox·i·a (his′tō-tok′sik ă-nok′sē-ă) Poisoning the respiratory enzyme systems of the tissues.

his·to·troph·ic (his′tō-trō′fik) Providing nourishment for or favoring the formation of tissue.

his·tri·on·ic per·son·al·i·ty dis·or·der (his′trē-on′ik pĕr′sŏ-nal′i-tē dis-ōr′dĕr) In adults, a pattern of excessive emotional expression and attention-seeking behavior coupled with an extreme need for approval and inappropriate seductive behavior.

HIV-as·so·ci·a·ted en·ceph·a·lop·a·thy (ă-sō′sē-ă-tĕd en-sef′ă-lop′ă-thē)

HIV-as·so·ci·a·ted neph·rop·a·thy (HIVAN) (ă-sō′sē-ă-tĕd ne-frop′ă-thē) A serious renal complication of HIV and AIDS that causes chronic and eventually end-stage renal failure.

hives (hīvz) **1.** SYN urticaria. **2.** SYN wheal.

HLA com·plex (kom′pleks) The major histocompatibility complex in humans.

HMG-CoA re·duc·tase (rĕ-dŭk′tās) The enzyme that is thought to produce cholesterol.

HMG CoA-re·duc·tase in·hib·i·tors (rĕ-dŭk′tās in-hib′i-tŏrz) Drugs that interfere with the biosynthesis of cholesterol; used to treat hyperlipidemia.

H₂O Symbol for water.

Ho Symbol for holmium.

Hodg·kin dis·ease, Hodg·kin lym·pho·ma (hoj′kin di-zēz′, lim-fō′mă) A disease marked by chronic enlargement of the lymph nodes, often local at the onset and later generalized, together with enlargement of the spleen and often of the liver; considered to be a malignant neoplasm of lymphoid cells of uncertain origin.

Hodg·kin sar·co·ma (hoj′kin sahr-kō′mă) Lymphocyte depletion form of Hodgkin disease.

Hodg·son dis·ease (hoj′sŏn di-zēz′) An aneurysmal dilation of aortic arch associated with aortic valve insufficiency.

hol·an·dric gene (hol-an′drik jēn) SYN Y-linked gene.

hol·an·dric in·her·i·tance (hol-an′drik in-her′ĭ-tăns) SYN Y-linked inheritance.

Hol·i·day-Se·gar for·mu·la (hol′i-dā-sē′găr for′myū-lă) A system for calculating patients' daily fluid requirements.

ho·lism (hō′lizm) Principle that an organism, or one of its actions, is not equal to merely the sum of its parts but must be perceived or studied as an entity.

ho·lis·tic care (hō-lis′tik kār) Therapy that incorporates the whole of a person, that is, physical, psychological, emotional, and spiritual dimensions. SEE ALSO complementary and alternative medicine.

hol·low bone (hol′ō bōn) SYN pneumatic bone.

hol·low-cath·ode lamp (hol′ō-kath′ōd lamp) One consisting of a metal cathode and an inert gas that can emit a line spectrum of specific wavelength.

Holm·gren wool test (hōlm′gren wul test) A test for color blindness, in which the subject matches variously colored skeins of wool.

holo- Prefix meaning whole, entire, complete.

hol·o·blas·tic (hol′ō-blas′tik) Denoting involvement of the entire oocyte act of in cleavage.

ho·lo·blast·ic cleav·age (hol′ō-blas′tik klē′văj) Cleavage in which the blastomeres are completely separated; the entire egg participates in cell division. SYN total cleavage.

hol·o·ce·phal·ic (hol′ō-sē-fal′ik) Denoting a fetus with a complete head but also deficiencies in other body parts.

hol·o·crine gland (hol′ō-krin gland) A gland with a secretion that consists of disintegrated cells of the gland itself.

hol·o·di·a·stol·ic (hol'ō-dī-ă-stol'ik) Relating to or occupying the entire diastolic period.

hol·o·en·dem·ic (hol'ō-en-dem'ik) Endemic in the entire population.

hol·o·en·zyme (hol'ō-en'zīm) A complete enzyme, i.e., apoenzyme plus coenzyme, cofactor, metal ion, and/or prosthetic group.

hol·o·gram (hōl'ō-gram) A three-dimensional image produced by wavefront reconstruction and recorded on a photographic plate.

hol·og·ra·phy (hol-og'ră-fē) The process of creating a hologram.

hol·o·gyn·ic in·her·i·tance (hol'ō-jin'ik in-her'i-tăns) Transmission of a trait from mother to daughters but not to sons.

hol·o·pros·en·ceph·a·ly (hol'ō-pros-en-sef'ă-lē) Failure of the forebrain or prosencephalon to divide into hemispheres or lobes; cyclopia occurs in the severest form.

hol·o·ra·chis·chi·sis (hol'ō-ră-kis'ki-sis) Spina bifida of the entire spinal column.

Hol·ter mon·i·tor (HM) (hōl'tĕr mon'i-tŏr) Technique for long-term, continuous recording of electrocardiographic signals on magnetic tape for scanning and selection of significant but transient changes that might otherwise escape notice.

Holt·house her·ni·a (hōlt'hows hĕr'nē-ă) Inguinal hernia with extension of intestinal loop at the inguinal ligament.

Holt-Or·am syn·drome (HOS) (hōlt-ōr'ăm sin'drōm) Atrial septal defect in association with fingerlike or absent thumb and other deformities of the forearm.

Holtz·man Ink·blot test (HIT) (hōlts'măn ingk'blot test) A multivariable personality assessment designed to overcome the Rorschach test's limitations.

Ho·mans sign (hō'mănz sīn) Pain in the calf when the ankle is slowly and gently dorsiflexed (with the knee bent).

ho·mat·ro·pine (hō-mat'rō-pēn) An anticholinergic, mydriatic, and cycloplegic agent. SYN mandelytropine, tropine mandelate.

ho·max·i·al (hōm-ak'sē-ăl) Having all the axes alike, as in a sphere.

home as·sess·ment (hōm ă-ses'mĕnt) A tool for evaluating the need to modify a patient's residence to resolve problems related to decreased mobility.

home health care (hōm helth kār) Care of patients delivered within their residence rather than a clinical setting; usually provided by nurses, home health aides, and other professionals on a regularly scheduled visit.

home health care clas·si·fi·ca·tion (hōm helth kār klas'i-fi-kā'shŭn) A standardized nursing terminology that provides a framework for describing home care services.

home health nurse (hōm helth nŭrs) One responsible for a group of clients in the home setting; visits clients on a routine basis to assist client and family with care as needed and to teach family the care needed so that the client may remain at home.

homeo- Combining form meaning the same, alike. SEE ALSO homo- (1).

ho·me·o·met·ric (hō'mē-ō-met'rik) Without change in size.

ho·me·o·met·ric au·to·reg·u·la·tion (hō'mē-ō-met'rik aw'tō-reg-yŭ-lā'shŭn) Intrinsic regulation of strength of cardiac contraction in response to influences that do not depend on change in fiber length.

ho·me·o·path·ic (hō'mē-ō-path'ik) 1. Relating to homeopathy. SYN homeotherapeutic (1). 2. Denoting an extremely small dose of a pharmacologic agent, such as might be used in homeopathy; more generally, a dose believed to be too small to produce the effect usually expected from that agent. Cf. pharmacologic (2), physiologic (4).

Ho·me·o·path·ic Phar·ma·co·poeia of the United States (HPCUS) (hō'mē-ō-path'ik fahr'mă-kō-pē'ă yū-nī'tĕd stāts) Listing of substances used in homeopathic medicine that are recognized by the U.S. Food and Drug Administration.

ho·me·op·a·thy (Homeo) (hō′mē-op′ă-thē) A system of therapy developed by Samuel Hahnemann based on the "law of similia," from the aphorism, *similia similibus curantur* (likes are cured by likes), which holds that a medicinal substance that can evoke certain symptoms in healthy people may be effective in the treatment of illnesses having similar symptoms, if given in *very* small doses.

ho·me·o·pla·si·a, ho·moi·o·pla·si·a (hō′mē-ō-plā′zē-ă, hō′moy-ō-plā′zē-ă) The formation of new tissue of the same character as that already existing in the part.

ho·me·o·sta·sis (hō′mē-ō-stā′sis) **1.** The state of equilibrium (balance between opposing pressures) in the body with respect to various functions and to the chemical compositions of the fluids and tissues. **2.** The processes through which such bodily equilibrium is maintained.

ho·me·o·stat·ic (hō′mē-ō-stat′ik) Relating to homeostasis.

ho·me·o·ther·a·peu·tic (hō′mē-ō-thār′ă-pyū′tik) **1.** SYN homeopathic (1). **2.** Relating to homeotherapy.

ho·me·o·ther·a·py, ho·me·o·ther·a·peu·tics (hō′mē-ō-thār′ă-pē, -thār′ă-pyū′tiks) Treatment or prevention of a disease using the principles of homeopathy.

ho·me·o·ther·mic (hō′mē-ō-thĕr′mik) Denotes having a stable internal temperature.

ho·me·o·typ·i·cal (hō′mē-ō-tip′i-kăl) Of or resembling the usual type.

hom·i·cide (hom′i-sīd) The killing of one human being by another.

hom·i·nal phy·si·ol·o·gy (hom′i-năl fiz-ē-ol′ŏ-jē) That science as applied to the elucidation of the normal bodily functions of human beings.

hom·i·nid (hom′i-nid) A member of the family Hominidae, including extinct species of humans, as well as present-day chimpanzees, gorillas, bonobos, and orangutans.

Ho·mo (hō′mō) The genus of primates that includes humans.

homo- **1.** Prefix meaning the same, alike; opposite of hetero-. SEE ALSO homeo-. **2.** CHEMISTRY prefix used to indicate insertion of one more carbon atom in a chain (i.e., insertion of a methylene moiety).

ho·mo·car·no·sin·o·sis (hō′mō-kahr′nō-si-nō′sis) An inborn error in metabolism in which homocarnosine levels are elevated, particularly in the cerebrospinal fluid.

ho·mo·cit·rul·li·nu·ri·a (hō′mō-sit′rū-li-nyūr′ē-ă) An inherited disorder associated with elevated urinary levels of homocitrulline.

ho·mo·clad·ic (hō′mō-klad′ik) Denoting an anastomosis between branches of the same arterial trunk, as distinguished from heterocladic.

ho·mo·cys·te·ine test (hō′mō-sis′tē-ēn test) A controversial screening modality for patients at high risk for heart attack or stroke.

ho·mo·cys·ti·nu·ri·a (HCU, HC) (hō′mō-sis′ti-nyūr′ē-ă) A metabolic disorder characterized by sparse blond hair, long limbs, pectus excavatum, dislocation of lens, failure to thrive, mental retardation, psychiatric disturbances, and thromboembolic episodes.

ho·mo·cy·to·tro·pic (hō′mō-sī′tō-trō′pik) Having an affinity for cells of the same or a closely related species.

ho·mo·cy·to·tro·pic an·ti·bod·y (hō′mō-sī′tō-trō′pik an′ti-bod-ē) Antibody of the IgE class that has an affinity for tissues of the same or a closely related species.

ho·mod·ro·mous (hō-mod′rŏ-mŭs) Moving in the same direction.

ho·mo·ga·met·ic (hō′mō-gă-met′ik) Producing only one type of gamete with respect to sex chromosomes; in humans and most animals, the female is homogametic. SYN monogametic.

ho·mog·a·my (hŏ-mog′ă-mē) Similarity of husband and wife in a specific trait.

ho·mog·e·nate (hŏ-moj′ĕ-nāt) Tissue ground into a creamy consistency in which the cell structure is disintegrated (so-called cell-free).

ho·mo·ge·ne·ous (hŏ′mō-jĕ′nē-ŭs) Of uniform structure or composition throughout.

ho·mo·ge·ne·ous ra·di·a·tion (hŏ′mō-jĕ′nē-ŭs rā′dē-ā′shŭn) Radiation consisting of a narrow band of frequencies, the same energy, or a single type of particle.

ho·mo·ge·ne·ous sys·tem (hŏ′mō-jĕ′nē-ŭs sis′tĕm) CHEMISTRY one with parts that cannot be mechanically separated and is therefore uniform throughout.

ho·mo·gen·e·sis (hŏ′mō-jen′ĕ-sis) Production of offspring similar to the parents, in contrast to heterogenesis. SYN homogeny.

ho·mo·gen·et·ic (hŏ′mō-jĕ-net′ĭk) Denotes organisms that exhibit similarity of structure; this is taken as evidence of common ancestry.

ho·mog·e·nize (hŏ-moj′ĕ-nīz) **1.** To blend into a uniform mixture. **2.** To break down a substance into smaller particles and disperse them evenly throughout a liquid.

ho·mo·gen·tis·ic ac·id (hŏ′mō-jen-tis′ik as′id) An intermediate in L-phenylalanine and L-tyrosine catabolism; elevated levels are observed in patients with alcaptonuria. SYN alcapton, alkapton.

ho·mog·e·ny (hŏ-moj′ĕ-nē) SYN homogenesis.

ho·mo·graft (hŏ′mō-graft) SYN allograft.

ho·moi·o·pla·si·a (hŏ′moy-ō-plā′zē-ă) SYN homeoplasia.

ho·mo·lat·er·al limb syn·kin·e·sis (hŏ′mō-lat′ĕr-ăl lim sin′ki-nē′sis) Mutual dependency between upper and lower affected limbs; for example, when the arm flexes, the leg also flexes.

ho·mol·o·gous (hŏ-mol′ŏ-gŭs) **1.** In biology or zoology, denoting organs or parts corresponding in evolutionary origin and similar to some extent in structure, but not necessarily similar in function. **2.** In chemistry, denoting a single

chemical series, differing by fixed increments. **3.** In genetics, denoting chromosomes or chromosome parts identical with respect to their construction and genetic content. **4.** In immunology, denoting serum or tissue derived from members of a single species, or an antibody with respect to the antigen that produced it. **5.** Proteins having identical or similar functions (particularly with respect to proteins from different species).

ho·mol·o·gous an·ti·gen (hŏ-mol′ŏ-gŭs an′ti-jen) That which generates the formation of an antibody that in turn can react with that antigen.

ho·mol·o·gous chro·mo·somes (hŏ-mol′ŏ-gŭs krō′mō-sōmz) members of a single pair of chromosomes.

ho·mol·o·gous graft (hŏ-mol′ŏ-gŭs graft) SYN allograft.

ho·mol·o·gous in·sem·i·na·tion (hŏ-mol′ŏ-gŭs in-sem′i-nā′shŭn) Artificial insemination with the husband's semen.

ho·mol·o·gous re·com·bi·na·tion (hŏ-mol′ŏ-gŭs rē-kom′bi-nā′shŭn) Exchange of corresponding stretches of DNA between two sister chromosomes.

ho·mol·o·gous re·stric·tion fac·tor (hŏ-mol′ŏ-gŭs rē-strik′shŭn fak′tŏr) A regulatory protein that binds to the membrane attack complex in autologous cells and inhibits the final stages of complement activation.

ho·mol·o·gous stim·u·lus (hŏ-mol′ŏ-gŭs stim′yū-lŭs) A stimulus that acts only on the nerve terminations in a special sense organ.

ho·mol·o·gous tu·mor (hŏ-mol′ŏ-gŭs tū′mŏr) A tumor composed of tissue of the same sort as that from which it springs.

hom·o·logue, ho·mo·log (hom′ŏ-log) One of a homologous pair or series.

ho·mol·y·sin (hŏ-mol′i-sin) A sensitizing hemolytic antibody (hemolysin) formed as the result of stimulation by an antigen derived from an animal of the same species.

ho·mol·y·sis (hŏ-mol′i-sis) Lysis of red

blood cells by a homolysin and complement.

ho·mo·mor·phic (hŏ′mō-môr′fik) Denoting two or more structures of similar size and shape.

ho·mon·o·mous (hŏ-mon′ŏ-mŭs) Denoting parts with similar form and structure, arranged in a series.

ho·mon·y·mous (hŏ-mon′i-mŭs) Having the same name or expressed in the same terms.

ho·mon·y·mous dip·lo·pi·a (hŏ-mon′ŏ-mŭs di-plō′pē-ă) Visual defect in which the image observed by the right eye appears shifted to the right of the image observed by the left eye.

ho·mon·y·mous hem·i·a·no·pi·a, ho·mon·y·mous hem·i·a·nop·si·a (hŏ-mon′ŏ-mŭs hem′ē-ă-nō′pē-ă, -nop′sē-ă) Visual deficit affecting the same side (right or left) of each visual field. SYN homonymous hemianopsia.

ho·mo·phil·ic (hŏ′mō-fil′ik) Someone fascinated with gays and lesbians.

ho·mo·plas·tic (hŏ′mō-plas′tik) Similar in form and structure, but not in origin.

ho·mo·plas·tic graft (hŏ′mō-plas′tik graft) SYN allograft.

hom·or·gan·ic (hom′ôr-gan′ik) Produced by the same organs, or by homologous organs.

ho·mo·sex·u·al (H) (hŏ′mō-sek′shū-ăl) **1.** Relating to or characteristic of homosexuality. **2.** One whose interests and behavior are characteristic of homosexuality. SEE gay, lesbian.

ho·mo·sex·u·al·i·ty (hŏ′mō-sek′shū-al′i-tē) Erotic attraction, predisposition, or activity, including sexual congress, between people of the same sex, especially past puberty.

ho·mo·sex·u·al pan·ic (hŏ′mō-sek′shū-ăl pan′ik) Acute anxiety attack based on subconscious conflicts regarding homosexuality.

ho·mo·top·ic (hŏ′mō-top′ik) Pertaining to or occurring at the same place or part of the body.

ho·mo·type (hŏ′mō-tīp) Any part or organ of the same structure or function as another, especially as one on the opposite side of the body.

ho·mo·va·nil·lic ac·id (HVA) (hŏ′mō-vă-nil′ik as′id) A phenol found in human urine.

hon·ey·comb lung (hŏn′ē-kōm lŭng) The radiologic and gross appearance of the lungs resulting from interstitial fibrosis and cystic dilation of bronchioles and distal air spaces.

hood·ed fore·skin (hud′ĕd for′skin) A condition involving an unfused dorsal foreskin usually seen with hypospadias (q.v.).

hook (huk) **1.** An instrument curved or bent near its tip, used for fixation of a part or traction. **2.** SYN hamulus.

hook·worm (huk′wŏrm) Common name for bloodsucking nematodes, chiefly members of the genera *Ancylostoma* (Old World hookworm), *Necator*, and *Uncinaria*.

hook·worm a·ne·mi·a (huk′wŏrm ă-nē′mē-ă) Blood disease of heavy infestation by *Ancylostoma duodenale* or *Necator americanus*.

Hop·mann pa·pil·lo·ma (hop′mahn pap′i-lō′mă) Overgrowth of the nasal mucous membrane.

hops (hops) SYN humulus.

hor·de·o·lum (hōr-dē′ō-lŭm) A suppurative inflammation of a gland or hair follicle of the eyelid. SYN stye.

hor·de·o·lum ex·ter·num (hōr-dē′ō-lŭm ek-stĕr′nŭm) Inflammation of the sebaceous gland of an eyelash.

hor·i·zon·tal fis·sure of cer·e·bel·lum (hōr′i-zon′tăl fish′ŭr ser′ĕ-bel′ŭm) Line that bisects the ansiform lobule.

hor·i·zon·tal heart (hōr′i-zon′tăl hahrt) Description of the heart's electrical position.

hor·i·zon·tal lam·i·nar flow hood (hōr′i-zon′tăl lam′i-năr flō hud) One in which the air is pushed through a filter horizontally toward the user to maintain a sterile environment.

hor·i·zon·tal la·ryn·gec·to·my (hōr'i-zon'tăl lar'in-jek'tŏ-mē) SYN partial laryngectomy.

hor·i·zon·tal max·il·lary frac·ture (hōr'i-zon'tăl mak'si-lar-ē frak'shŭr) A horizontal fracture at the base of the maxillae above the apices of the teeth.

hor·i·zon·tal over·lap (hōr'i-zon'tăl ō' vĕr-lap) The projection of the upper anterior or posterior teeth beyond their antagonists in a horizontal direction.

hor·i·zon·tal re·sorp·tion (hōr'i-zon' tăl rĕ-sōrp'shŭn) SYN horizontal atrophy.

hor·i·zon·tal ver·ti·go (hōr'i-zon'tăl vĕr'ti-gō) Dizziness experienced when lying down.

hor·mic psy·chol·o·gy (hōr'mik sī-kol'ŏ-jē) The theory that goal-seeking is the primary motivation for human behavior.

hor·mi·on (hōr'mē-on) A craniometric point at the junction of the posterior border of the vomer with the sphenoid bone.

hor·mo·nal gin·gi·vi·tis (hōr-mōn'ăl jin'ji-vī'tis) Gingivitis in which the host response to bacterial plaque is presumably exacerbated by hormonal alterations occurring during puberty, pregnancy, oral contraceptive use, or menopause.

hor·mone (hōr'mōn) A chemical substance formed in a tissue or organ and carried in the blood; stimulates or inhibits the growth or function of one or more other tissues or organs.

hor·mone re·place·ment ther·a·py (HRT) (hōr'mōn rĕ-plās'mĕnt thār'ă-pē) SYN estrogen replacement therapy.

hor·mone-sen·si·tive lip·ase (hōr'mōn sen'si-tiv lip'ās) A protein found in cytosol and on lipid droplets of adipocytes; hydrolyzes triglycerides, thus freeing fatty acids and glycerols.

hor·mo·no·gen·e·sis, hor·mo·no·poi·e·sis (hōr-mō'nō-jen'ĕ-sis, -poy-ē'sis) The formation of hormones.

horn (hōrn) [TA] Any structure resembling a horn in shape. SYN cornu (1).

Hor·ner syn·drome (hōr'nĕr sin'drōm) Ptosis, miosis, and anhidrosis on the side of a sympathetic palsy. Enophthalmos is more apparent than real. The affected pupil is visibly slow to dilate in dim light; due to a lesion of the cervical sympathetic chain or its central pathways. Also called Bernard-Horner syndrome and ptosis sympathetica.

horn·y lay·er (hōr'nē lā'ĕr) SYN stratum corneum epidermidis.

ho·rop·ter (hŏ-rop'tĕr) The sum of the points in space, the images of which for a given fixation point fall on corresponding retinal points.

hor·ror (hōr'ŏr) Dread; fear.

hor·ror au·to·tox·i·cus (hōr'ŏr aw-tō-tok'si-kŭs) Tenet that immunity is directed against foreign materials but not against the constituents of one's own body; exceptions to this concept are the autoallergic reactions and diseases.

horse se·rum (hōrs sēr'ŭm) A serum made of equine blood that contains growth factors not found in other animal sera.

horse·shoe kid·ney (hōrs'shū kid'nē) Poles of the two kidneys, usually the inferior ones.

hos·pice (hos'pis) An institution that provides a centralized program of palliative and supportive services to dying patients and their families, in the form of physical, psychological, social, and spiritual care.

hos·pi·tal (hos'pi-tăl) A health care facility or institution equipped for medical diagnosis, treatment, and care for both inpatients and outpatients and for clinical training of physicians, nurses, and allied care personnel.

hos·pi·tal-ac·quired in·fec·tion (hos' pi-tăl-ă-kwīrd' in-fek'shŭn) SEE nosocomial (2).

hospitalisation [Br.] SYN hospitalization.

hos·pi·tal·ism (hos'pi-tăl-izm) The environmental factors that negatively affect the physical or mental health of hospital patients.

hos·pi·tal·i·za·tion (H, hosp, HX) (hos′-pi-tăl-ī-zā′shŭn) Confinement in a hospital as a patient for diagnostic study and treatment.

host (hōst) The organism in or on which a parasite lives, thus deriving its body substance or energy.

host de·fense mech·a·nisms (hōst dĕ-fens′ mek′ă-niz-ŭmz) Natural protections against infection including skin, mucous membranes, and specific and nonspecific immune responses.

hot com·press (hot kom′pres) A pad of flannel or gauze dipped in hot water or physiologic saline and firmly applied to a body surface to promote local pain relief, muscular relaxation, or pointing of an abscess.

hot flash, hot flush (hot flash, flŭsh) Colloquialism for one of the vasomotor symptoms of the climacteric that may involve the whole body as a flash of heat.

hot gan·grene (hŏt gang′grēn) The dermatogic disorder due to inflammation of a body part.

hot line (hot līn) In health care, a direct telephone link for emergency services.

Houns·field u·nit (Hu, HU, H) (hownz′fēld yū′nit) Normalized index of x-ray attenuation based on a scale of −1000 (air) to +1000 (bone), with water being 0; used in CT imaging.

hour·glass con·trac·tion (owr′glas kŏn-trak′shŭn) Constriction of the middle portion of a hollow organ, such as the stomach or the gravid uterus.

hour·glass stom·ach (owr′glas stŏm′ăk) Condition with a constriction of the stomach wall dividing it into two cavities, cardiac and pyloric. SYN bilocular stomach, ectasia ventriculi paradoxa.

house·maid's knee (hows′mādz nē) An adventitious occupational bursitis occurring over the tibial tuberosity, the area of contact when kneeling; not to be confused with infrapatellar bursitis.

house staff (hows staf) Physicians and surgeons in specialty training at a hospital who care for the patients under the direction and supervision of the attending staff.

Hous·ton-Har·ris syn·drome (hyū′stŏn-har′is sin′drŏm) SYN achondrogenesis type IA.

Hous·ton valves (how′stŏn valvz) Semilunar transverse folds in the rectal wall that protrude into the anal canal and support fecal matter.

Howe sil·ver pre·cip·i·ta·tion meth·od (how sil′vĕr prē-sip′i-tă′shŭn meth′ŏd) A dental technique of depositing silver in enamel and dentin by application of an ammoniacal silver nitrate solution and reduction with formalin or eugenol.

How·ship la·cu·nae (how′ship lă-kū′nē) Tiny depressions, pits, or irregular grooves in bone that is being resorbed by osteoclasts. SYN resorption lacunae.

H₁ re·cep·tor an·tag·o·nist; H₂ re·cep·tor an·tag·o·nists (rĕ-sep′tŏr an-tag′ŏ-nist, -nists) Agents that serve to inhibit the release of histamine.

H₁ re·cep·tors; H₂ re·cep·tors (rĕ-sep′tŏrz) Histamine-releasing sites found throughout the body on smooth muscle, on vascular endothelial cells, in the heart, and in the central nervous system.

Hru·by lens (rū′bē lenz) A non-contact lens mounted on a slitlamp used for evaluating the retina.

H sub·stance (sŭb′stăns) Diffusible substance in skin, indistinguishable in action from histamine, liberated by injury; causes the triple response. SYN released substance.

huang chi (hwahng chē) SYN *Astragalus*.

Hu an·ti·gen (hū an′ti-jen) A neuronal protein identified in the serum of patients with small-cell lung cancer and paraneoplastic encephalomyelitis.

Hub·bard tank (HT) (hŭb′ărd tangk) Large container, filled with warm water, used for therapeutic exercises in a program of physiotherapy.

huff·ing (hŭf′ing) **1.** Colloquial but general term for the inhalation abuse of volatile solvents (e.g., gasoline) to achieve intoxication or alter consciousness. **2.** SYN glue-sniffing.

Hughes-Sto·vin syn·drome (hyūhz stō′vin sin′drōm) Disorder characterized by aneurysms of the large and small pulmonary arteries and thrombosis of peripheral veins and dural sinuses.

Huh·ner test (HT) (hū′nĕr test) SYN postcoital test.

hum (hŭm) A low continuous murmur.

hu·man ac·ti·va·ted pro·tein C (HAPC) (hyū′măn ak′ti-vā-tĕd prō′tēn) A substance that inhibits coagulation by inactivating cofactors Va and VIIIa.

hu·man an·ti·he·mo·phil·ic fac·tor (hyū′măn an′tē-hē′mō-fil′ik fak′tŏr) Lyophilized concentrate of factor VIII, obtained from fresh normal human plasma; used as a hemostatic agent in hemophilia. SYN antihemophilic globulin (2).

hu·man ca·lor·im·e·ter (hyū′măn kal′ŏr- im′ĕ-tĕr) A device to measure the heat output of the human body during various levels of physical exertion.

hu·man cho·ri·on·ic so·ma·to·mam·mo·tro·pic hor·mone (HCS) (hyū′măn kōr′ē-on′ik sō′mă-tō-mam′ō-trō′pik hōr′mōn) SYN human placental lactogen.

hu·man dip·loid cell ra·bies vac·cine (HDCV) (hyū′măn dip′loyd sel rā′bēz vak-sēn′) SYN human diploid cell vaccine.

hu·man dip·loid cell vac·cine (hyū′măn dip′loyd sel vak-sēn′) An iodinated virus vaccine used for protection against rabies.

hu·man en·dog·e·nous ret·ro·vi·rus·es (HERVs) (hyū′măn en-doj′ĕ-nŭs ret′rō-vīr′ŭs-ĕz) Remnants of ancient viruses inherent in the human genome; associated with many diseases including cancers.

hu·man e·o·si·no·phil·ic en·ter·i·tis (hyū′măn ē′ō-sin-ō-fil′ik en′tĕr-ī′tis) Segmental eosinophilic inflammation of the gastrointestinal tract in humans; suspected etiologic agent is *Ancylostoma caninum*.

hu·man gam·ma glob·u·lin (hyū′măn gam′ă glob′yū-lin) A preparation of the proteins of liquid human plasma, containing the antibodies of normal adults; it is obtained from pooled liquid human plasma from a number of donors.

hu·man ge·net·ics (hyū′măn jĕ-net′iks) The study of the genetic aspects of humans as a species. Cf. medical genetics.

hu·man gran·u·lo·cyt·ic ehr·lich·i·o·sis (HGE) (hū′măn gran′yū-lō-sit′ik er-lik′ē-ō′sis) A febrile disease causing headache and myalgia and sometimes involving the respiratory, digestive, and central nervous systems.

hu·man growth fac·tor (HGF) (hyū′măn grōth fak′tŏr) Physiologic matter produced to regulate cell creation and activity.

hu·man her·pes·vi·rus 1 (hyū′măn hĕr′pēz-vī′rŭs) Herpes simplex virus, type 1. SEE herpes simplex.

hu·man her·pes·vi·rus 2 (hyū′măn hĕr′pēz-vī′rŭs) Herpes simplex virus, type 2. SEE herpes simplex.

hu·man her·pes·vi·rus 3 (hyū′măn hĕr′pēz-vī′rŭs) SYN varicella-zoster virus.

hu·man her·pes·vi·rus 4 (hyū′măn hĕr′pēz-vī′rŭs) SYN Epstein-Barr virus.

hu·man her·pes·vi·rus 5 (hyū′măn hĕr′pēz-vī′rŭs) SYN cytomegalovirus.

hu·man her·pes·vi·rus 6 (HHV6, HHV-6) (hyū′măn hĕr′pēz-vī-rŭs) Form found in certain lymphoproliferative disorders, replicates in a number of different types of leukocytes, and is associated with the childhood disease roseola (exanthema subitum).

hu·man her·pes·vi·rus 7 (hyū′măn hĕr′pēz-vī′rŭs) Virus found in association with human T lymphocytes; shed in saliva of most adults; however, a causal relationship to any known disease has not been determined.

hu·man her·pes·vi·rus 8 (hyū′măn hĕr′pēz-vī′rŭs) A linear double-stranded DNA virus that induces Kaposi sarcoma (KS) in immunodeficient people.

hu·man im·mu·no·de·fi·cien·cy vi·

H

rus (HIV) (hyū′măn im′yū-nō-dĕ-fish′ĕn-sē vī′rŭs) Human T-cell lymphotropic virus type III; a cytopathic retrovirus that is the etiologic agent of acquired immunodeficiency syndrome (AIDS) (q.v.).

hu·man·is·tic and ex·is·ten·tial ther·a·pies (hyū′mă-nis′tik eg′zis-ten′shăl thār′ă-pēz) Psychoanalytic theory that emphasizes understanding the totality of human experience and focuses on patients not symptoms.

hu·man·is·tic nurs·ing mod·el (hyū′mă-nis′tik nŭr′sing mod′ĕl) A philosophy of nursing practice that focuses on using real-world knowledge to develop nursing skills.

hu·man·is·tic psy·chol·o·gy (hyū′mă-nis′tik sī′kol-ŏ-gē) Existential approach to psychology that emphasizes human uniqueness, subjectivity, and capacity for psychological growth.

hu·man leu·ko·cyte an·ti·gen (HLA) (hyū′măn lū′kō-sīt an′ti-jen) Any of several members of a system consisting of the gene products of at least four linked loci (A, B, C, and D) and a number of subloci on the sixth human chromosome that have been shown to have a strong influence on human allotransplantation, transfusions in refractory patients, and certain disease associations.

hu·man men·o·pau·sal go·nad·o·tro·pin (HMG, hMG) (hyū′măn men′ŏ-paw′zăl gō-nad′ō-trō′pin) Pituitary hormone originally obtained from the urine of postmenopausal women but now produced synthetically; used to induce ovulation. SEE ALSO menotropins.

hu·man me·ta·pneu·mo·vi·rus (hyū′măn met′ă-nū′mō-vī′rus) A negative single-stranded RNA virus that may be the primary cause of lower respiratory tract infection in children.

hu·man mo·no·cy·tic ehr·lich·i·o·sis (HME) (hyū′măn mon′ō-sit′ik er-lik′ē-ō′sis) A febrile disease caused by *Ehrlichia chaffeensis* transmitted by the Lone Star tick (*Amblyomma americanum*); similar to human granulocytic ehrlichiosis.

hu·man pa·pil·lo·ma·vi·rus (HPV) (hyū′măn pap′i-lō′mă-vī′rŭs) DNA virus of the genus *Papillomavirus*; certain types cause cutaneous and genital warts in humans, including verruca vulgaris and condyloma acuminatum; other types are associated with severe cervical intraepithelial neoplasia and anogenital and laryngeal carcinomas. SYN infectious papillomavirus.

hu·man par·vo·vi·rus B19 (hyū′măn pahr′vō-vīr′ŭs) A virus linked to several autoimmune diseases including vasculitis and connective tissue disorders.

hu·man pla·cen·tal lac·to·gen (hyū′măn plă-sen′tăl lak′tŏ-jen) Any agent to stimulate human milk production that has been isolated from human placentas. SYN chorionic growth hormone-prolactin, human chorionic somatomammotropic hormone, placental growth hormone.

hu·man plas·ma pro·tein frac·tion (hyū′măn plaz′mă prō′tēn frak′shŭn) A solution of selected proteins used as a blood volume supporter.

hu·man T-cell lym·pho·ma leu·ke·mi·a vi·rus (HTLV) (hyū′măn sel lim-fō′mă lū-kē′mē-ă vī′rŭs) Lymphotropic viruses with selective affinity for helper/inducer cells; associated with adult T-cell leukemia and lymphoma.

hu·mec·tant (hyū-mek′tănt) An agent that promotes retention of moisture.

hu·mer·us, gen. and pl. hu·mer·i (hyū′mĕr-ŭs, -rī) [TA] Arm bone articulating with the scapula above and the radius and ulna below.

hu·mid·i·fi·ca·tion (hyū-mid′i-fi-kā′shŭn) Mechanical regulation of the content of water vapor in the air, either in room air or in oxygen and breathing devices.

hu·mid·i·fi·er lung (hyū-mid′i-fī-ĕr lŭng) Respiratory infection caused by inhaling contaminated droplets produced by a humidifier or air conditioner.

hu·mor (hyū′mŏr) [TA] 1. Any clear fluid or semifluid hyaline anatomic substance. 2. One of the elemental body fluids that were the basis of the physiologic and pathologic teachings of the hippocratic school: blood, yellow bile, black bile, and phlegm. SYN humour.

hu·mor·al im·mu·ni·ty (HI) (hyū′mŏr-ăl i-myū′ni-tē) That associated with circulating antibodies, in contradistinction to cellular immunity.

humour [Br.] SYN humor.

hump (hŭmp) A rounded protuberance or bulge.

hump·back (hŭmp′bak) Nonmedical term for kyphosis or gibbus.

hun·ger (hŭng′gĕr) **1.** A desire or need for food. **2.** Any appetite, strong desire, or craving.

Hun·ner ul·cer (hŭn′ĕr ŭl′sĕr) A focal and often multiple lesion involving all layers of the bladder wall in chronic interstitial cystitis.

hun·te·ri·an chan·cre (hŭn-ter′ē-ăn shang′kĕr) SYN chancre.

Hun·ting·ton cho·re·a, Hun·ting·ton dis·ease (hŭn′ting-tŏn kŏ-rē′ă, di-zēz′) A neurodegenerative disorder, with onset usually in the third or fourth decade, characterized by spasms and dementia. SYN hereditary chorea.

Hunt neu·ral·gi·a (hŭnt nūr-al′jē-ă) SYN geniculate neuralgia.

Hunt syn·drome (hŭnt sin′drŏm) An intention tremor beginning in one extremity, gradually increasing in intensity, and subsequently involving other parts of the body.

Hur·ler syn·drome (hĕr′lĕr sin′drŏm) Mucopolysaccharidosis with a deficiency of α-L-iduronidase, accumulation of an abnormal intracellular material, and urinary excretion of dermatan sulfate and heparan sulfate.

Hürth·le cell (hĕrt′lĕ sel) Large, granular eosinophilic cell derived from thyroid follicular epithelium by accumulation of mitochondria, e.g., in Hashimoto disease. SYN Askanazy cell.

Hürth·le cell car·ci·no·ma (hĕrt′lĕ sel kahr′si-nō′mă) A salivary or thyroid carcinoma composed of cells that have eosinophilic cytoplasm. SYN oncocytic carcinoma.

Hürthle cell tu·mor (hĕrt′lĕ sel tū′mŏr)

A neoplasm of the thyroid gland composed of polyhedral acidophilic cells, thought by some to be oncocytes; it may be benign or malignant, the behavior of the latter depending on the general microscopic pattern, whether follicular, papillary, or undifferentiated. Also called Hürthle cell carcinoma.

Husch·ke ca·nal (hūsh′kĕ kă-nal′) A passage formed by the tympanic ring tubercles.

Hutch blad·der di·ver·tic·u·lum (hŭch blad′ĕr dī′vĕr-tik′yū-lŭm) A defect in the urinary bladder near the ureterovesical junction, which weakens the detrusor muscle.

Hutch·in·son frac·ture (hŭch′in-sŏn frak′shŭr) Radial styloid fracture. SYN chauffeur's fracture.

Hutch·in·son-Gil·ford dis·ease (hŭch′in-sŏn gil′fŏrd di-zēz′) SYN progeria.

Hutch·in·son pu·pil (hŭch′in-sŏn pyū′pil) Dilation of the pupil on the side of the lesion as part of a third nerve palsy.

Hutch·in·son teeth (hŭch′in-sŏn tēth) Dental sign of congenital syphilis in which the incisal edge is notched and narrower than the cervical area. SYN notched teeth, screwdriver teeth, syphilitic teeth.

Hutch·in·son tri·ad (hŭch′in-sŏn trī′ad) Parenchymatous keratitis, labyrinthine disease, and Hutchinson teeth, signs of congenital syphilis.

Hutch·in·son-type neu·ro·blas·to·ma (hŭch′in-sŏn tīp nūr′ō-blas-tō′mă) Cancer that affects the suprarenal gland.

hy·a·lin (hī′ă-lin) A clear, eosinophilic, homogeneous substance occurring in degeneration (e.g., in arteriolar walls in arteriolar sclerosis and in glomerular tufts in diabetic glomerulosclerosis).

hy·a·line (hī′ă-lēn) Transparent or colorless. SYN hyaloid.

hy·a·line cast (HC) (hī′ă-lēn kast) Relatively transparent renal cast seen in urine of patients with renal disease or transiently with exercise, fever, congestive heart failure, and diuretic therapy.

H

hy·a·line de·gen·er·a·tion (hī'ă-lēn dĕ-jen'ĕr-ā'shŭn) A group of degenerative processes that affect various cells and tissues, resulting in rounded masses (''droplets'') or broad bands of substances that are homogeneous, translucent, refractile, and acidophilic.

hy·a·line mem·brane (hī'ă-lēn mem'brăn) **1.** The thin, clear basement membrane beneath certain epithelia. **2.** SYN glassy membrane (2).

hy·a·line mem·brane dis·ease (HMD) (hī'ă-lēn mem'brăn di-zēz') SYN respiratory distress syndrome of the newborn.

hy·a·line throm·bus (hī'ă-lēn throm'bŭs) Translucent colorless plug, partly or wholly filling a capillary or small artery or vein, formed by agglutination of red blood corpuscles. SYN agglutinative thrombus.

hy·a·lin·i·za·tion (hī'ă-lin-ī-zā'shŭn) The formation of hyalin.

hy·a·li·no·sis (hī'ă-li-nō'sis) Hyaline degeneration, especially that of relatively extensive degree.

hy·a·li·tis (hī'ă-lī'tis) SYN vitreitis.

hyalo-, hyal- Combining forms meaning glassy, hyalin; vitreous. Cf. vitreo-.

hy·al·o·gens (hī-al'ō-jenz) Substances similar to mucoids that are found in many animal structures (e.g., cartilage, vitreous humor, hydatid cysts) and yield sugars on hydrolysis.

hy·a·lo·hy·pho·my·co·sis (hī'ă-lō-hī'fō-mī-kō'sis) An infection caused by a fungus with hyaline (colorless) mycelia in tissue, usually with a decrease in body resistance due to surgery, indwelling catheters, steroid therapy, or immunosuppressive drugs or cytotoxins.

hy·a·loid (hī'ă-loyd) SYN hyaline.

hy·a·loid bod·y (hī'ă-loyd bod'ē) SYN vitreous body.

hy·a·lo·mere (hī'ă-lō-mēr) The clear periphery of a blood platelet.

Hy·a·lom·ma (hī'ă-lom'ă) An Old World genus (about 21 species) of large ixodid ticks with submarginal eyes, coalesced festoons, an ornate scutum, and a long rostrum. Adults parasitize all domestic animals and a wide variety of wild animals. Species harbor a great variety of pathogens of humans and animals and also cause considerable mechanical injury.

hy·a·lo·mu·coid (hī'ă-lō-myū'koyd) A mucoprotein found in the space behind the lens of the eye.

hy·a·lo·nyx·is (hī'ă-lō-nik'sis) Puncturing the space behind the ocular lens.

hy·a·lo·pha·gi·a, hy·a·loph·a·gy (hī'ă-lō-fā'jē-ă, -lof'ă-jē) The eating or chewing of glass.

hy·a·lo·plasm, hy·a·lo·plas·ma (hī'ă-lō-plazm, -plaz'mă) The protoplasmic fluid substance of a cell.

hy·a·lo·se·ro·si·tis (hī'ă-lō-sēr'ō-sī'tis) Inflammation of a serous membrane with a fibrinous exudate that eventually becomes hyalinized, resulting in a relatively thick, dense, opaque, glistening, white or gray-white coating; when the process involves the visceral serous membranes of various organs, the grossly apparent condition is sometimes colloquially termed icing liver, sugar-coated spleen, frosted heart, and so on, depending on the site.

hy·a·lo·sis (hī'ă-lō'sis) Degenerative changes in the vitreous body.

hy·al·o·some (hī-al'ō-sōm) An oval or round structure within a cell nucleus that stains faintly but otherwise resembles a nucleolus.

hy·a·lu·ro·nate (hī'ă-lūr'ō-nāt) A salt or ester of hyaluronic acid.

hy·a·lu·ron·ic ac·id (hī'ă-lūr-on'ik as'id) A mucopolysaccharide forming a gelatinous material in the tissue spaces and acting as a lubricant and shock absorbant; hydrolyzed by hyaluronidase.

hy·a·lu·ron·i·dase (hī'ă-lū-ron'i-dās) Term applied loosely to hyaluronate lyase, hyaluronoglucosaminidase, and hyaluronoglucuronidase, one or more of which are present in sperm, the testes, and other organs, bee and snake venoms, type II pneumonococci, and certain hemolytic streptococci.

H-Y an·ti·gen (an′ti-jen) An antigen factor, dependent on the Y chromosome, responsible for the differentiation of the human embryo into the male phenotype by inducing the initially bipotential embryonic gonad to develop into a testis.

hy·brid (hī′brid) An individual (plant or animal) with parents that are different varieties of the same species or belong to different but closely allied species. SYN crossbreed (1).

hybridisation [Br.] SYN hybridization.

hy·brid·i·za·tion (hī′brid-ī-zā′shŭn) **1.** The process of breeding a hybrid. **2.** Crossing over between related but nonallelic genes. **3.** The specific reassociation of complementary strands of polynucleic acids. **4.** The process or act of forming a macromolecular hybrid in which the subunits are obtained from different sources. SYN cross-breeding.

hy·brid·o·ma (hī′brid-ō′mă) A tumor of hybrid cells used in the production in vitro of specific monoclonal antibodies.

hy·da·tid (hī′dă-tid) A vesicular structure resembling an *Echinococcus* cyst.

hy·da·tid cyst (hī′dă-tid sist) Lesion of liver, brain, and many other body sites due to the larval metacestode stage of *Echinococcus*, chiefly in herbivores and humans. SYN echinococcus cyst.

hy·da·tid·i·form (hī′dă-tid′i-fōrm) Having the form or appearance of a hydatid.

hy·da·tid·i·form mole, hy·da·tid mole (hī′dă-tid′i-fōrm mōl, hī′dă-tid) A vesicular or polycystic mass due to proliferation of the trophoblast, with hydropic degeneration and avascularity of the chorionic villi.

hy·da·tid·o·sis (hī′dă-tid-ō′sis) The morbid state caused by the presence of hydatid cysts.

hy·da·ti·dos·to·my (hī′dă-ti-dos′tŏ-mē) Surgical evacuation of a hydatid cyst.

hy·dat·id thrill (hī′dă-tid thril) The peculiar trembling or vibratory sensation felt on palpation of a hydatid cyst. SYN Blatin syndrome.

hy·drad·e·ni·tis (hī′drad-ĕ-nī′tis) SYN hidradenitis.

hydraemia [Br.] SYN hydremia.

hy·dra·gogue (hī′dră-gog) Producing a discharge of watery fluid.

hy·dram·ni·os, hy·dram·ni·on (hī-dram′nē-os, -on) Presence of an excessive amount of amniotic fluid, usually over 2,000 mL.

hy·dran·en·ceph·a·ly (hī′dran-en-sef′ă-lē) Complete or nearly complete absence of cerebral hemispheres, which have been replaced by fluid-filled sacs lined by leptomeninges.

hy·drar·thro·sis (hī′drahr-thrō′sis) Effusion of a serous fluid into a joint cavity.

hy·drate (hī′drāt) An aqueous solvate (in older terminology, a hydroxide); a compound crystallizing with one or more molecules of water.

hy·dra·tion (hī-drā′shŭn) **1.** Chemically, the addition of water; differentiated from hydrolysis, where the union with water is accompanied by a splitting of the original molecule and the water molecule. **2.** Clinically, the taking in of water; used commonly in the sense of reduced hydration or dehydration.

hy·dra·zine (hī′dră-zēn) Oily liquid from which phenylhydrazine and similar products are derived. It is very toxic and possibly a carcinogen.

hy·dre·mi·a (hī-drē′mē-ă) A condition in which the blood volume is increased as a result of an increase in the water content of plasma. SYN hydraemia.

hy·dren·ceph·a·lo·cele, hy·dro·ceph·a·lo·cele, hy·dro·en·ceph·a·lo·cele (hī′dren-sef′ă-lō-sēl, hī′drō-sef′ă-lō-sēl, -en-sef′ă-lō-sēl) Protrusion, through a cleft in brain substance expanded into a sac that contains fluid. SYN encephalocystocele.

hy·dren·ceph·a·lo·me·nin·go·cele (hī′dren-sef′ă-lō-mĕ-ning′gō-sēl) Protrusion, through a defect in the cranium, of a sac containing meninges, brain substance, and cerebrospinal fluid.

hydro-, hydr- Combining forms meaning **1.** Water, watery. **2.** Containing or combined with hydrogen. **3.** A hydatid.

hy·dro·a (hī-drō'ă) Any bullous eruption.

hy·dro·bil·i·ru·bin (hī'drō-bil'i-rū'bin) A dark brown-red pigment that may be formed when bilirubin is reduced.

hy·dro·bro·mic ac·id (HBr) (hī'drō-brō'mik as'id) An aqueous solution of hydrogen bromide (HBr); its salts are bromides.

hy·dro·bro·mide (hī'drō-brō'mīd) A compound of hydrobromic acid and a base.

hy·dro·cal·y·co·sis (hī'drō-kal-i-kō'sis) A usually symptomless anomaly of the renal calyx dilated from obstruction of the infundibulum; usually discovered incidentally.

hy·dro·car·bon (hī'drō-kahr'bŏn) A compound containing only hydrogen and carbon.

hy·dro·cele (hī'drō-sēl) *Avoid the misspelling hydroseal.* Collection of serous fluid in a sacculated cavity.

hy·dro·ce·lec·to·my (hī'drō-sē-lek'tŏ-mē) Excision of a hydrocele.

hy·dro·ceph·a·lus, hy·dro·ceph·a·ly (hī'drō-sef'ă-lŭs, -sef'ă-lē) A condition marked by an excessive accumulation of cerebrospinal fluid resulting in dilation of the cerebral ventricles and raised intracranial pressure. SYN hydrocephaly.

hy·dro·chlor·ic ac·id (HCl) (hī'drō-klōr'ik as'id) The acid of gastric juice.

hy·dro·chlor·ide (hī'drō-klōr'īd) A compound formed by the addition of a hydrochloric acid molecule to an amine or related substance.

hy·dro·chlo·ro·thi·a·zide (HCTZ, HCT) (hī'drō-klōr'ō-thī'ă-zīd) A potent orally effective diuretic and antihypertensive agent related to chlorothiazide.

hy·dro·cho·le·re·sis (hī'drō-kō-lĕr-ē'sis) Increased output of a watery bile of low specific gravity, viscosity, and solid content.

hy·dro·co·done (HC) (hī'drō-kō'dōn) A potent analgesic derivative of codeine used as an antitussive and analgesic. Often used combined with aspirin or acetaminophen.

hy·dro·col·loid (hī'drō-kol'oyd) A gelatinous colloid in unstable equilibrium with its contained water, useful in dentistry for impressions because of its dimensional stability under controlled conditions.

hy·dro·cor·ti·sone (hī'drō-kōr'ti-sōn) A steroid hormone secreted by the cortex of suprarenal gland and the most potent of the naturally occurring glucocorticoids in humans. SYN cortisol.

hy·dro·cyst (hī'drō-sist) Lesion with clear, watery contents.

hy·dro·gen (H) (hī'drō-jen) **1.** A gaseous element, atomic no. 1, atomic wt. 1.00794. **2.** The molecular form (H_2) of the element. SYN dihydrogen.

hy·dro·gen 1 (hī'drō-jen) The common hydrogen-1 isotope, making up 99.985% of the hydrogen-1 atoms occurring in nature.

hy·dro·gen bond (hī'drō-jen bond) That arising from the sharing of a hydrogen atom, covalently bound to a strongly electronegative element (e.g., nitrogen, oxygen, or a halogen), with another strongly electronegative element (e.g., nitrogen, oxygen, or a halogen).

hy·dro·gen cy·a·nide (HCN) (hī'drō-jen sī'ăn-īd) A highly toxic cellular asphyxiant, HCN, used as a fumigant and also as a chemical-warfare agent. Its NATO code is AC.

hy·dro·gen ion (H+) (hī'drō-jen ī'on) A hydrogen atom minus its electron and therefore carrying a unit positive charge (i.e., a proton); in water, it combines with a water molecule to form hydronium ion, H_3O^+.

hy·dro·gen pe·rox·ide (HP, H_2O_2) (hī'drō-jen pĕr-ok'sīd) Unstable compound readily broken down to water and oxygen, a reaction catalyzed by various powdered metals and by the enzyme, catalase. SYN hydroperoxide.

hy·dro·gen sul·fide (hī'drō-jen sŭl'fīd) A fetid poisonous gas that smells like rotten eggs. SYN sulfureted hydrogen.

hy·dro·ki·net·ic (hī'drō-ki-net'ik) Pertaining to the motion of fluids and the forces giving rise to such motion.

hy·dro·ki·net·ics (hī′drō-ki-net′iks) That branch of kinetics concerned with fluids in motion.

hy·dro·las·es (hī′drō-lās-ĕz) Enzymes (EC class 3) cleaving substrates with addition of water at the point of cleavage.

hy·drol·y·sate (hī-drol′i-sāt) A solution containing the products of hydrolysis.

hy·drol·y·sis (hī-drol′i-sis) A chemical process whereby a compound is cleaved into two or more simpler compounds with the uptake of the H and OH parts of a water molecule on either side of the chemical bond cleaved. Cf. hydration.

hy·dro·lyze (hī′drō-līz) To subject to hydrolysis.

hy·dro·ma (hī-drō′mă) SYN hygroma.

hy·dro·me·nin·go·cele (hī′drō-mĕ-ning′gō-sēl) Protrusion of the meninges of brain or spinal cord through a defect in the cranium or vertebral column, the sac so formed containing cerebrospinal fluid.

hy·drom·e·ter (hī-drom′ĕ-tĕr) An instrument for determining the specific gravity or density of a liquid. SYN areometer, gravimeter.

hy·dro·me·tro·col·pos (hī′drō-me′trō-kol′pos) Distention of uterus and vagina by fluid other than blood or pus.

hy·dro·mor·phone hy·dro·chlor·ide (hī′drō-mōr′fōn hī′drō-klōr′īd) A synthetic derivative of morphine, with analgesic potency about 10 times that of morphine.

hy·dro·my·e·li·a (hī′drō-mī-ē′lē-ă) An increase of fluid in the dilated central canal of the spinal cord, or in congenital cavities elsewhere in the cord substance.

hy·dro·my·e·lo·cele (hī′drō-mī′ĕ-lō-sēl) Protrusion of a portion of the spinal cord, thinned out into a sac distended with cerebrospinal fluid, through a vertebral column.

hy·dro·my·e·lo·me·nin·go·cele (hī′drō-mī′ĕ-lō-mĕ-ning′gō-sēl) Spinal defect marked by protrusion of spinal cord membranes and tissue. Cf. spina bifida.

hy·dro·my·o·ma (hī′drō-mī-ō′mă) A leiomyoma that contains cystlike foci of proteinaceous fluid.

hy·dro·ne·phro·sis (hī′drō-nĕ-frō′sis) Dilation of the pelvis and calyces of one or both kidneys due to obstruction to the flow of urine. SYN pelvocaliectasis, uronephrosis.

hy·dro·ne·phrot·ic (hī′drō-nĕ-frot′ik) Relating to hydronephrosis.

hy·dro·pe·ni·a (hī′drō-pē′nē-ă) Reduction or deprivation of water.

hy·dro·per·i·to·ne·um, hy·dro·per·i·to·ni·a (hī′drō-per′i-tō-nē′ŭm, -tō′nē-ă) SYN ascites.

hy·dro·phil·i·a (hī′drō-fil′ē-ă) **1.** Associating freely with water. **2.** A tendency of the blood and tissues to absorb fluid.

hy·dro·phil·ic (hī′drō-fil′ik) Denoting the property of attracting or associating with water molecules, possessed by polar radicals or ions, as opposed to hydrophobic (2).

hy·dro·pho·bi·a (hī′drō-fō′bē-ă) SYN rabies.

hy·dro·pho·bic (hī′drō-fō′bik) **1.** Relating to or suffering from hydrophobia. **2.** Lacking an affinity for water molecules, as opposed to hydrophilic. SYN apolar (2). **3.** Tending not to dissolve in water. **4.** Nonpolar.

hy·drop·ic (hī-drop′ik) Containing water or a watery fluid.

hy·dro·pneu·ma·to·sis (hī′drō-nū′mă-tō′sis) Combined emphysema and edema; the presence of liquid and gas in tissues.

hy·dro·pneu·mo·go·ny (hī′drō-nū-mō′gŏ-nē) Injection of air into a joint to determine the amount of effusion.

hy·dro·pneu·mo·per·i·car·di·um (hī′drō-nū′mō-per′i-kahr′dē-ŭm) The presence of a serous effusion and of gas in the pericardial sac. SYN pneumohydropericardium.

hy·dro·pneu·mo·per·i·to·ne·um (hī′drō-nū′mō-per′i-tō-nē′ŭm) The presence of gas and serous fluid in the peritoneal cavity. SYN pneumohydroperitoneum.

hy·dro·pneu·mo·tho·rax, pneu·mo·hy·dro·thor·ax (hī′drō-nū′mō-thōr′aks, nū′mō-hī′drō-thōr′aks) The presence of both gas and fluids in the pleural cavity. SYN pneumoserothorax.

hy·drops, hy·drop·sy (hī′drops, -ē) An excessive accumulation of clear, watery fluid in any of the tissues or cavities of the body; synonymous, according to its character and location, with ascites, anasarca, or edema.

hy·dro·py·o·ne·phro·sis (hī′drō-pī′ō-nĕ-frō′sis) Presence of purulent urine in the pelvis and calyces of the kidney following obstruction of the ureter.

hy·dror·rhe·a (hī′drō-rē′ă) Profuse discharge of watery fluid from any body part. SYN hydrorrhea.

hy·dror·rhe·a grav·i·dae, hy·dror·rhe·a grav·i·da·rum (hī′drō-rē′ă grav′i-dē, -dā′rŭm) Discharge of a watery fluid from the vagina during pregnancy.

hydrorrhoea [Br.] SYN hydrorrhea.

hy·dro·sal·pinx (hī′drō-sal′pingks) Accumulation of serous fluid in the uterine tube, often an end result of pyosalpinx.

hy·dro·sol (hī′drō-sol) A colloid in aqueous solution, the particles being in the dispersed or internal phase and the water in the external or dispersion phase.

hy·dro·stat·ic pres·sure (HP) (hī′drō-stat′ik presh′ŭr) That exerted by a liquid as a result of its potential energy, ignoring its kinetic energy.

hy·dro·sta·tic weigh·ing (hī′drō-stat′ik wā′ing) SYN underwater weighing.

hy·dro·tax·is (hī′drō-tak′sis) The movement of cells or organisms in relation to water.

hy·dro·ther·a·py (hī′drō-thār′ă-pē) The external application of water as a liquid, solid, or vapor for therapeutic purposes.

hydrothionaemia [Br.] SYN hydrothionemia.

hy·dro·thi·o·ne·mi·a (hī′drō-thī′ō-nē′mē-ă) The presence of hydrogen sulfide in the circulating blood. SYN hydrothionaemia.

hy·dro·tho·rax (hī′drō-thōr′aks) Presence of fluid in one or both pleural cavities, usually resulting from cardiac failure.

hy·dro·tro·pism, pos·i·tive hy·dro·tro·pism, neg·a·tive hy·dro·tro·pism (hī′drō-trō′pizm, poz′i-tiv, neg′ă-tiv) The property in growing organisms of turning toward or away from a moist surface.

hy·dro·tu·ba·tion (hī′drō-tū-bā′shŭn) Injection of a liquid medication or saline solution through the cervix into the uterine cavity and uterine tubes for dilation and treatment.

hy·drous (hī′drŭs) SYN hydrated.

hy·drox·ide (hī-drok′sīd) A compound containing a potentially ionizable hydroxyl group; particularly a compound that liberates OH^- on dissolving in water.

hydroxy- Prefix indicating addition or substitution of the −OH group to or in the compound named after it. SEE ALSO oxo-, oxy-.

hy·drox·y ac·id (hī-drok′sē as′id) An organic acid containing both OH and COOH groups, e.g., lactic acid.

hy·drox·y·ap·a·tite, hy·drox·yl·ap·a·tite (hī-drok′sē-ap′ă-tīt, -il-ap′ă-tīt) A natural mineral structure resembling the crystal lattice of bones and teeth. SEE ALSO apatite.

hy·drox·y·co·bal·a·min (hī-drok′sē-kō-bal′ă-min) A chemical compound, also called vitamin B12a, which is the immediate precursor to cyanocobalamin (vitamin B12) in the body and that has also been investigated as an antidote in cyanide poisoning, although it is not currently approved for such use in the U.S. SEE ALSO sodium nitrite, sodium thiosulfate.

hy·drox·y·u·re·a (OHU, HU, HUR, HYD) (hī-drok′sē-yū-rē′ă) An oral antineoplastic agent that inhibits DNA synthesis; used to treat malignancies including melanoma, chronic myelocytic leukemia, and ovarian carcinoma.

hy·drox·y·zine (hī-drok′si-zēn) A mild sedative and minor tranquilizer used to treat neuroses; also used to prevent nausea and to enhance the effects of narcotics.

hy·giene (hī′jēn) **1.** The science of health and its maintenance. **2.** Cleanliness that promotes health and well-being, especially of a personal nature.

hygro-, hygr- Combining forms meaning moisture, humidity; opposite of xero-.

hy·gro·ma, hy·dro·ma (hī-grō′mă, -drō′mă) Cystic swelling containing a serous fluid.

hy·grom·e·ter (hī-grom′ĕ-tĕr) Any device for measuring the water vapor in the atmosphere, usually indicating relative humidity directly.

hy·grom·e·try (hī-grom′ĕ-trē) SYN psychrometry.

hy·gro·scop·ic (hī′grō-skop′ik) Denoting a substance capable of readily absorbing and retaining moisture.

hy·men (hī′mĕn) [TA] A thin membranous fold, highly variable in appearance, which partly occludes the ostium of the vagina before its rupture, which may occur for a variety of reasons. It is frequently absent, even in virgins, although remnants are commonly present as hymenal tags (ca... carunculae).

hy·me·nec·to·my (hī′mĕ-nek′tŏ-mē) Excision of the hymen.

hy·me·ni·tis (hī′mĕ-nī′tis) Inflammation of the hymen.

hy·me·no·le·pi·a·sis (hī′mĕ-nō-lĕ-pī′ă-sis) Illness produced by infection with tapeworms of the genus *Hymenolepis*.

Hy·me·nol·e·pis (hī′mĕ-nol′ĕ-pis) The largest genus of tapeworms; especially common parasites of rodents, shrews, and aquatic birds.

hy·me·nol·o·gy (hī′mĕ-nol′ŏ-jē) The branch of anatomy and physiology concerned with the membranes of the body.

Hy·me·nop·ter·a (hī′mĕ-nop′tĕr-ă) An order of insects, including bees, wasps, and ants, characterized by locked pairs of membranous wings and high development of social or colonial behavior.

hy·o·ep·i·glot·tic (hī′ō-ep′i-glot′ik) Relating to the hyoid bone and the epiglottis. SYN hyoepiglottia.

hy·o·ep·i·glot·tid·e·an (hī′ō-ep′i-glo-tid′ē-ăn) SYN hyoepiglottic.

hy·o·glos·sal (hī′ō-glos′ăl) *Do not confuse this word with hypoglossal.* Relating to the hyoid bone and the tongue. SYN glossohyal.

hy·oid (hī′oyd) U-shaped or V-shaped.

hy·o·scine (hī′ō-sēn) SYN scopolamine.

hy·o·scy·a·mine (hī′ō-sī′ă-mēn) An alkaloid used as an antispasmodic, analgesic, and sedative.

hyp- Variation of the prefix hypo-, often used before a vowel. Cf. sub-.

hy·pa·cu·sis, hy·po·a·cu·sis (hī′pă-kyū′sis, hī′pō-ă-kyū′sis) Hearing impairment of a conductive or neurosensory nature.

hypaesthesia [Br.] SYN hypesthesia.

hy·pal·ge·si·a, hy·po·al·ge·si·a, hyp·al·gi·a (hīp′al-jē′zē-ă, hī′pō-al-jē′zē-ă, hī-pal′jē-ă) Decreased sensibility to pain.

hy·par·te·ri·al (hī′pahr-tēr′ē-ăl) Below or beneath an artery.

hy·pax·i·al (hī-pak′sē-ăl, hip-ak′) Below any axis, such as the spinal axis or the axis of a limb. SEE hypomere.

hy·pax·ial mus·cles (hī-paks′ē-ăl mŭs′ĕlz) Those placed in a ventral position to the transverse vertebral processes.

hyper- Prefix meaning excessive, above normal; opposite of hypo-.

hy·per·a·cu·i·ty (hī′pĕr-ă-kyū′i-tē) Having better than normal perception or skill.

hy·per·a·cu·sis, hy·per·a·cu·si·a (hī′pĕr-ă-kyū′sis, -kyū′sē-ă) *The term is not synonymous with recruitment or hypersensitivity.* Heightened auditory acuity, sometimes accompanied by painful sensitivity to ordinary environmental sounds.

hy·per·ad·e·no·sis (hī′pĕr-ad′ē-nō′sis) Glandular enlargement, especially of the lymphatic glands.

hy·per·ad·i·po·sis, hy·per·ad·i·pos·i·ty (hī′pĕr-ad′i-pō′sis, -pos′i-tē) An extreme degree of adiposis or fatness.

hyperaesthesia [Br.] SYN hyperesthesia.

hy·per·al·do·ste·ron·ism (hī′pĕr-al-dos′tĕr-ōn-izm) SYN aldosteronism.

hy·per·al·i·men·ta·tion (hī′pĕr-al′i-men-tā′shŭn) Administration or consumption of nutrients beyond minimum normal requirements to replace nutritional deficiencies.

hy·per·al·pha·lip·o·pro·tein·e·mi·a (HALP) (hī′pĕr-al′fă-lip′ō-prō′tēn-ē′mē-ă) An inherited defect that results in elevated levels of high-density lipoproteins in the serum.

hy·per·am·mo·ne·mi·a, hy·per·am·mo·ni·e·mia (hī′pĕr-am′ō-nē′mē-ă, hī′pĕr-am′ō-nē-ē′mē-ă) Denotes having excessive hematologic levels of ammonia.

hy·per·an·a·ki·ne·si·a, hy·per·an·a·ki·ne·sis, hy·per·an·a·ci·ne·si·a, hy·per·an·a·ci·ne·sis (hī′pĕr-an′ă-ki-nē′zē-ă, -ki-nē′sis, -si-nē′zē-ă, -si-nē′sis) Excessive to-and-fro movement, e.g., of the stomach or intestine.

hy·per·a·phi·a (hī′pĕr-ā′fē-ă) Extreme sensitivity to touch.

hy·per·aph·ic (hī′pĕr-af′ik) Marked by hyperaphia.

hy·per·a·zo·te·mi·a (hī′pĕr-az′ō-tē′mē-ă) Presence in blood of abnormal amounts of urea.

hy·per·bar·ic (hī′pĕr-bar′ik) **1.** Pertaining to pressure of ambient gases exceeding 1 atmosphere. **2.** Concerning solutions, more dense than the diluent or medium.

hy·per·bar·ism (hī′pĕr-bar′izm) Disturbances in the body due to the pressure of ambient gases at greater than 1 atmosphere.

hy·per·be·ta·lip·o·pro·tein·e·mi·a (HBLP) (hī′pĕr-bā′tă-lip′ō-prō′tēn-ē′mē-ă) Enhanced concentration of β-lipoproteins in the blood.

hyperbilirubinaemia [Br.] SYN hyperbilirubinemia.

hy·per·bil·i·ru·bi·ne·mi·a (hī′pĕr-bil′i-rū-bi-nē′mē-ă) An abnormally large amount of bilirubin in the circulating blood. SYN hyperbilirubinaemia.

hypercalcaemia [Br.] SYN hypercalcemia.

hy·per·cal·ce·mi·a (hī′pĕr-kal-sē′mē-ă) An abnormally high concentration of calcium compounds in the circulating blood. SYN calcemia, hypercalcaemia.

hy·per·cal·ci·uri·a, hy·per·cal·ci·nu·ri·a, hy·per·cal·cu·ri·a (hī′pĕr-kal′sē-yūr′ē-ă, -si-nyūr′ē-ă, -kal-kyūr′ē-ă) Excretion of abnormally large amounts of calcium in the urine. SYN calcinuric diabetes.

hy·per·cap·ni·a, hy·per·car·bi·a (hī′pĕr-kap′nē-ă, hī′pĕr-kahr′bē-ă) Abnormally increased arterial carbon dioxide tension. SYN hypercarbia.

hy·per·cap·nic ac·id·o·sis (hī′pĕr-kap′nik as′i-dō′sis) SYN respiratory acidosis.

hy·per·ca·ro·te·ne·mi·a (hī′pĕr-kar′ō-tē-nē′mē-ă) Disorder marked by orange skin discoloration caused by excess carotenoids in the blood, usually from overconsumption of vegetables that contain Vitamin A (e.g., carrots). SYN carotenoderma.

hy·per·ca·tab·o·lism (hī′pĕr-kă-tab′ō-lizm) An increase in basal metabolic rate and in breakdown of muscle and adipose tissue as a result of injury, metabolic stress, or sepsis. SEE ALSO catabolism.

hy·per·ca·thar·sis (hī′pĕr-kă-thahr′sis) Excessive and frequent defecation.

hy·per·cel·lu·la·ri·ty (hī′pĕr-sel′yū-lar′i-tē) Condition of having an excessively large number of cells.

hyperchloraemia [Br.] SYN hyperchloremia.

hy·per·chlor·e·mi·a (hī′pĕr-klōr-ē′mē-ă) An abnormally large amount of chloride ions in the circulating blood. SYN chloremia (2).

hy·per·chlor·em·ic ac·id·o·sis (hī′

pĕr-klōr-ē´mik as´i-dō´sis) SYN renal tubular acidosis.

hy·per·chlor·hy·dri·a, hy·per·hy·dro·chlor·ia (hī´pĕr-klōr-hī´drē-ă, -hī-drŏ-klōr´ē-ă) Presence of an excessive amount of hydrochloric acid in the stomach. SYN chlorhydria.

hypercholesterolaemia [Br.] SYN hypercholesterolemia.

hy·per·cho·les·ter·ol·e·mi·a, hy·per·cho·les·ter·e·mi·a, hy·per·cho·les·ter·in·e·mi·a (hī´pĕr-kŏ-les´tĕr-ol-ē´mē-ă, -ē-mē-ă, -i-nē-mē-ă) The presence of an abnormally large amount of cholesterol in the blood.

hy·per·cho·li·a (hī´pĕr-kō´lē-ă) An abnormally large amount of bile in the liver.

hy·per·chro·mat·ic (hī´pĕr-krō-mat´ik) 1. Abnormally highly colored, excessively stained, or overpigmented. 2. Showing increased chromatin.

hy·per·chro·ma·tism, hy·per·chro·ma·si·a (hī´pĕr-krō´mă-tizm, hī´pĕr-krō-mā´zē-ă) 1. Excessive pigmentation. 2. Increased staining capacity. 3. An increase in chromatin in cell nuclei. SYN hyperchromia.

hyperchylomicronaemia [Br.] SYN hyperchylomicronemia.

hy·per·chy·lo·mi·cro·ne·mi·a (HCM) (hī´pĕr-kī´lō-mī´krō-nē´mē-ă) Increased plasma concentrations of chylomicrons.

hypercryaesthesia [Br.] SYN hypercryesthesia.

hy·per·cry·al·ge·si·a (hī´pĕr-krī´al-jē´zē-ă) SYN hypercryesthesia.

hy·per·cry·es·the·si·a (hī´pĕr-krī´es-thē´zē-ă) Extreme sensibility to cold. SYN hypercryaesthesia, hypercryalgesia.

hypercupraemia [Br.] SYN hypercupremia.

hy·per·cu·pre·mi·a (hī´pĕr-kyū-prē´mē-ă) An abnormally high level of plasma copper. SYN hypercupraemia.

hy·per·cy·a·not·ic (hī´pĕr-sī´ă-not´ik) Marked by extreme cyanosis.

hypercythaemia [Br.] SYN hypercythemia.

hy·per·cy·the·mi·a (hī´pĕr-sī-thē´mē-ă) The presence of an abnormally high number of red blood cells in circulating blood. SYN hypercythaemia, hypererythrocythemia.

hy·per·dy·na·mi·a (hī´pĕr-dī-nām´ē-ă) Denotes having excessive amounts of energy.

hy·per·e·cho·ic (hī´pĕr-ĕ-kō´ik) Denoting a region in an ultrasound image in which the echoes are stronger than normal or than surrounding structures.

hy·per·ek·plex·i·a (hī´pĕr-ek-pleks´ē-ă) A hereditary disorder with pathologic startle responses, i.e., protective reactions to unanticipated, potentially threatening, stimuli of any type, particularly auditory; the stimuli induce often widespread and violent sudden contractions of the head, neck, spinal, and sometimes, limb musculature, resulting in involuntary shouting, jerking, jumping, and falling. SYN kok disease, startle disease.

hy·per·em·e·sis (hī´pĕr-em´ĕ-sis) Excessive vomiting.

hy·per·em·e·sis grav·i·da·rum (hī´pĕr´em´ĕ-sis grā-vē´dā-rŭm) Nausea and vomiting during pregnancy severe enough to result in dehydration, acidosis, and weight loss. May require hospitalization; if untreated, can be fatal.

hy·per·e·mi·a (hī´pĕr-ē´mē-ă) The presence of an increased amount of blood in a part or organ. SEE ALSO congestion.

hy·per·en·dem·ic dis·ease (hī´pĕr-en-dem´ik di-zēz´) One that is constantly present at a high incidence and/or prevalence rate and affects all age groups equally.

hy·per·e·o·sin·o·phil·i·a (hī´pĕr-ē´ō-sin-ō-fil´ē-ă) A greater degree of increase in the number of eosinophilic granulocytes in the circulating blood or the tissues than would be expected in the disease or condition causing the increase.

hy·per·e·qui·lib·ri·um (hī´pĕr-ē´kwi-lib´rē-ŭm) Excessive capacity for feeling dizzy.

H

hypererythrocythaemia [Br.] SYN hypererythrocythemia.

hy·per·e·ryth·ro·cy·the·mi·a (hī′pĕr-ĕ-rith′rō-sī-thē′mē-ă) SYN hypercythemia, hypererythrocythaemia.

hy·per·es·the·si·a (hī′pĕr-es-thē′zē-ă) Abnormal acuteness of sensitivity to touch, pain, or other sensory stimuli. SYN hyperaesthesia, oxyesthesia.

hy·per·es·tro·gen·ism (hī′pĕr-es′trō-jĕn-izm) Having excess amounts of estrogen in the body.

hyperferraemia [Br.] SYN hyperferremia.

hy·per·fer·re·mi·a (hī′pĕr-fĕr-ē′mē-ă) High serum iron level; found in hemochromatosis. SYN hyperferraemia.

hyperfibrinogenaemia [Br.] SYN hyperfibrinogenemia.

hy·per·fi·brin·o·ge·ne·mi·a (hī′pĕr-fī-brin′ō-jĕ-nē′mē-ă) An increased level of fibrinogen in the blood. SYN fibrinogenemia, hyperfibrinogenaemia.

hy·per·flex·ion (hī′pĕr-flek′shŭn) Flexion of a limb or part beyond the normal limit.

hy·per·frac·tion·a·tion (hī′pĕr-frak-shŭn-ā′shŭn) Radiation therapy that occurs more than once daily.

hy·per·ga·lac·ti·a (hī′pĕr-gă-lak′shē-ă) Excessive milk production.

hypergammaglobulinaemia [Br.] SYN hypergammaglobulinemia.

hy·per·gam·ma·glob·u·lin·e·mi·a (hī′pĕr-gam′ă-glob′yū-lin-ē′mē-ă) An increased amount of the γ-globulins plasma, as observed in chronic infectious diseases.

hy·per·gen·e·sis (hī′pĕr-jen′ĕ-sis) Excessive development or redundant production of parts or organs of the body.

hy·per·ge·net·ic (hī′pĕr-jĕ-net′ik) Relating to hypergenesis.

hy·per·geu·si·a (hī′pĕr-gū′sē-ă, -jū′sē-ă) Abnormal acuteness of the sense of taste. SYN gustatory hyperesthesia

hyperglycaemia [Br.] SYN hyperglycemia.

hy·per·gly·ce·mi·a (hī′pĕr-glī-sē′mē-ă) An abnormally high concentration of glucose in the blood, a feature of diabetes mellitus. SYN hyperglycaemia.

hyperglyceridaemia [Br.] SYN hyperglyceridemia.

hy·per·glyc·er·i·de·mi·a (hī′pĕr-glis′ĕr-i-dē′mē-ă) Elevated plasma concentration of glycerides. SYN hyperglyceridaemia.

hy·per·gly·ci·nu·ri·a (hī′pĕr-glī′si-nyūr′ē-ă) Enhanced urinary excretion of glycine.

hy·per·gly·co·ge·nol·y·sis (hī′pĕr-glī′kō-jĕ-nol′i-sis) Excessive glycogenolysis.

hy·per·gly·cor·rha·chi·a (hī′pĕr-glī′kō-rā′kē-ă) Excessive sugar in the cerebrospinal fluid.

hy·per·go·nad·ism (hī′pĕr-gō′nad-izm) A clinical state resulting from enhanced secretion of gonadal hormones.

hy·per·go·nad·o·tro·pic, hy·per·go·nad·o·tro·phic (hī′pĕr-gō-nad′ō-trō′pik, -trō′fik) Indicating an increased production or excretion of gonadotropic hormones.

hy·per·go·nad·o·tro·pic eu·nuch·oid·ism (hī′pĕr-gō-nad′ō-trō′pik yū′nŭ-koyd-izm) Eunuchoidism of gonadal origin, commonly accompanied by enhanced levels of pituitary gonadotropins in the blood and urine.

hy·per·go·nad·o·tro·pic hy·po·go·nad·ism (hī′pĕr-gō-nad′ō-trō′pik hī′pō-gō′nad-izm) Defective gonadal development or function of the gonads, resulting in elevated levels of gonadotropins.

hy·per·hi·dro·sis, hy·per·i·dro·sis (hī′pĕr-hi-drō′sis, -id-rō′sis) Excessive or profuse sweating. SYN polyidrosis.

hy·per·hy·dra·tion (hī′pĕr-hī-drā′shŭn) Excess water content of the body.

hy·per·im·mune (hī′pĕr-im-yūn′) Having large quantities of specific antibodies in the serum from repeated immunizations or infections.

hyperinsulinaemia [Br.] SYN hyperinsulinemia.

hy·per·in·su·li·ne·mia, hy·per·in·su·lin·ism (hī′pĕr-in′sŭ-lin-ē′mē-ă) Increased levels of insulin in the plasma due to increased secretion of insulin by the beta cells of the pancreatic islets. SYN hyperinsulinaemia, hyperinsulinism.

hy·per·ir·rit·a·bil·i·ty (hī′pĕr-ir′i-tă-bil′i-tē) State of being agitated by stimuli to an extreme degree.

hy·per·i·so·ton·ic (hī′pĕr-ī′sō-ton′ik) SYN hypertonic.

hyperkalaemia [Br.] SYN hyperkalemia.

hy·per·ka·le·mi·a, hy·per·ka·li·e·mi·a (hyper K) (hī′pĕr-kă-lē′mē-ă, -kal′ē-ē′mē-ă) A greater than normal concentration of potassium ions in the circulating blood. SYN hyperkaliemia, hyperpotassemia.

hy·per·ker·a·to·sis, hy·per·ker·a·tin·i·za·tion (hī′pĕr-ker′ă-tō′sis, -ti-nī′ză′shŭn) Thickening of the horny layer of the epidermis or mucous membrane. SEE ALSO keratoderma, keratosis.

hyperketonaemia [Br.] SYN hyperketonemia.

hy·per·ke·to·ne·mi·a (hī′pĕr-kē′tō-nē′mē-ă) Elevated concentrations of ketone bodies in the blood.

hyperkinaemia [Br.] SYN hyperkinemia.

hy·per·ki·ne·mi·a (hī′pĕr-ki-nē′mē-ă) Increased circulation rate; increased volume flow through the circulation; supernormal cardiac output.

hy·per·ki·ne·sis, hy·per·ki·ne·si·a, hy·per·ci·ne·sis, hy·per·ci·ne·si·a (hī′pĕr-ki-nē′sis, -nē′zē-ă, -si-nē′sis, -si-nē′zē-ă) 1. Excessive motility. 2. Excessive muscular activity.

hy·per·ki·net·ic syn·drome (hī′pĕr-ki-net′ik sin′drōm) Condition marked by pathologically excessive energy seen sometimes in young children with brain injury, mental illness, and attention deficit disorder, and in epileptics.

hy·per·lac·ta·tion (hī′pĕr-lak-tā′shŭn) SYN superlactation.

hy·per·leu·ko·cy·to·sis (hī′pĕr-lū′kō-sī-tō′sis) An unusually great increase in the number and proportion of leukocytes in the circulating blood or the tissues.

hyperlipaemia [Br.] SYN hyperlipemia.

hy·per·li·pe·mi·a (hī′pĕr-li-pē′mē-ă) An elevated level of lipids in the blood. SEE ALSO lipemia. SYN hyperlipaemia.

hyperlipidaemia [Br.] SYN hyperlipidemia.

hy·per·lip·id·e·mi·a (hī′pĕr-lip′i-dē′mē-ă) Elevated levels of lipids in the blood plasma.

hyperlipoproteinaemia [Br.] SYN hyperlipoproteinemia.

hy·per·lip·o·pro·tein·e·mi·a (hī′pĕr-lip′ō-prō-tēn-ē′mē-ă) An increase in the lipoprotein concentration of the blood. SYN hyperlipoproteinaemia.

hy·per·li·thu·ri·a (hī′pĕr-li-thyūr′ē-ă) An excessive excretion of uric (lithic) acid in the urine.

hy·per·lor·do·sis (hī′pĕr-lōr-dō′sis) An abnormal anteriorly convex curvature of the spine, usually lumbar.

hy·per·lor·dot·ic (hī′pĕr-lōr-dot′ik) Having a pathologically exaggerated lordotic curve of the lumbar spine; colloquial term is ''swayback.''

hy·per·lu·cent lung (hī′pĕr-lū′sĕnt lŭng) The radiographic finding that a lung or portion thereof is less dense than normal, e.g., from air trapping by a bronchial foreign body, asymmetric emphysema, or decreasing blood flow.

hy·per·ly·si·nu·ri·a (hī′pĕr-lī-si-nyūr′ē-ă) The presence of abnormally high concentrations of lysine in the urine.

hy·per·mag·ne·se·mi·a (hī′pĕr-mag′nĕ-sē′mē-ă) Excessive magnesium in blood.

hy·per·mas·ti·a (hī′pĕr-mas′tē-ă) Excessively large breasts.

hy·per·ma·ture cat·a·ract (hī′pĕr-mă-chŭr′ kat′ăr-akt) A cataract in which the

H

lens cortex becomes liquid, with the nucleus gravitating within the capsule (Morgagni cataract).

hy·per·men·or·rhe·a (hī′pĕr-men-ŏr-ē′ă) *Do not confuse this word with polymenorrhea.* Excessively prolonged or profuse menses. SYN menorrhagia.

hypermenorrhoea [Br.] SYN hypermenorrhea.

hy·per·me·tab·o·lism (hī′pĕr-mĕ-tab′ŏ-lizm) Heat production by the body above normal, as in thyrotoxicosis.

hy·per·me·tro·pi·a (h, H, Hy) (hī′pĕr-mĕ-trō′pē-ă) SYN hyperopia.

hy·perm·ne·si·a (hī′pĕrm-nē′zē-ă) Extreme power of memory.

hy·per·mo·bil·i·ty (hī′pĕr-mō-bil′i-tē) Increased range of movement of joints, and joint laxity, occurring normally in children and adolescents or as a result of disease.

hy·per·morph (hī′pĕr-mōrf) Person whose sitting height is low in proportion to standing height, owing to excessive length of limb.

hy·per·mo·til·i·ty (hī′pĕr-mō-til′ĭ-tē) Excessive activity of the gastrointestinal tract. Cf. dumping syndrome.

hy·per·mo·tor sei·zure (hī′pĕr-mō′tŏr sē′zhŭr) Attack characterized by automatisms involving predominantly proximal limb muscles and producing marked limb displacement.

hy·per·my·ot·ro·phy (hī′pĕr-mī-ot′rŏ-fē) Muscular hypertrophy.

hy·per·na·sal·i·ty (hī′pĕr-nā-zal′i-tē) Speech produced with excessive resonance in the nasal cavity, often due to dysfunction of the soft palate. SYN hyperrhinophonia.

hypernatraemia [Br.] SYN hypernatremia.

hypernatraemic encephalopathy [Br.] SYN hypernatremic encephalopathy.

hy·per·na·tre·mi·a (hī′pĕr-nā-trē′mē-ă) Excessive plasma concentration of sodium ions. SYN hypernatraemia.

hy·per·na·tre·mic en·ceph·a·lop·a·thy (hī′pĕr-nă-trē′mik en-sef′a-lop′a-thē) Subarachnoid and subdural effusions in infants with hypernatremic dehydration. SYN hypernatraemic encephalopathy.

hy·per·ne·o·cy·to·sis (hī′pĕr-nē′ō-sī-tō′sis) Hyperleukocytosis with considerable numbers of immature and young cells.

hy·per·ne·phro·ma (hī′pĕr-ne-frō′mă) Cancerous growth in the kidney tubules.

hypernoea [Br.] SYN hypernoia.

hy·per·noi·a (hī′pĕr-noy′ă) Great rapidity of thought; excessive mental activity, as seen in the manic phase of bipolar disorder. SYN hypernoea.

hy·per·nu·tri·tion (hī′pĕr-nū-trish′ŭn) SYN supernutrition.

hy·per·on·cot·ic (hī′pĕr-on-kot′ik) Indicating an oncotic pressure higher than normal, e.g., of blood plasma.

hy·per·o·nych·i·a (hī′pĕr-ō-nik′ē-ă) Hypertrophy of the nails.

hy·per·o·pi·a (hī′pĕr-ō′pē-ă) An ocular condition in which only convergent rays can be brought to focus on the retina. SYN farsightedness, hypermetropia.

hy·per·or·chi·dism (hī′pĕr-ōr′ki-dizm) Increased size or functioning of the testes.

hy·per·or·ni·thi·ne·mi·a (hī′pĕr-ōr′ni-thi-nē′mē-ă) Elevated levels of ornithine in the serum; sometimes associated with hyperammonemia and homocitrullinuria.

hy·per·or·ni·thi·ne·mi·a-hy·per·am·mo·ne·mi·a-ho·mo·ci·trul·lin·u·ri·a syn·drome (HHH syndrome) (hī′pĕr-ōr′ni-thi-nē′mē-a-hī′pĕr-am′ō-nē′mē-ă-hō′mō-sit′rū-li-nyūr′e-ă sin′drōm) An uncommon genetic metabolic disorder in which ammonia builds up in the body; severity varies considerably.

hy·per·or·tho·cy·to·sis (hī′pĕr-ōr′thō-sī-tō′sis) Hyperleukocytosis in which the relative percentages of the various types of white blood cells are within the normal range.

hy·per·os·mo·lal·i·ty (hī′pĕr-oz′mō-lal′ i-tē) Increased concentration of a solution expressed as osmoles of solute per kilogram of serum solution.

hy·per·os·mo·lar (hy·per·gly·cem·ic) non·ke·tot·ic co·ma (hī′pĕr-oz-mō′ lăr hī′per-glī-sē′mik non′kē-tot′ik kō′mă) A complication seen in diabetes mellitus in which marked hyperglycemia occurs (e.g., levels exceeding 800 mg/dL), causing osmotic shifts in water in brain cells and resulting in coma; can be fatal or lead to permanent neurologic damage; ketoacidosis does not occur.

hy·per·os·mo·lar·i·ty (hī′pĕr-oz′mō-lar′ i-tē) An increase in the osmotic concentration of a solution expressed as osmoles of solute per liter of solution.

hy·per·os·mot·ic (hī′pĕr-oz-mot′ik) **1.** Having an osmolality greater than that of another fluid, ordinarily assumed to be plasma or extracellular fluid. **2.** Relating to increased osmosis.

hy·per·os·to·sis (hī′pĕr-os-tō′sis) **1.** Hypertrophy of bone. **2.** SYN exostosis.

hy·per·ox·i·a (hī′pĕr-ok′sē-ă) **1.** An increased amount of oxygen in tissues and organs. **2.** A greater oxygen tension than normal.

hy·per·par·a·site (hī′pĕr-par′ă-sīt) A secondary parasite capable of development within another parasite.

hy·per·par·a·thy·roid·ism (hī′pĕr-par′ ă-thī′royd-izm) Condition due to increased parathyroid secretion.

hy·per·phen·yl·al·a·nine·mi·a (MHP) (hī′pĕr-fen′il-al′ă-ni-nē′mē-ă) The presence of abnormally high blood levels of phenylalanine.

hy·per·pho·ne·sis (hī′pĕr-fō-nē′sis) An increase in the percussion sound or of the voice sound in auscultation.

hy·per·pho·ri·a (hī′pĕr-fōr′ē-ă) A tendency of the visual axis of one eye to deviate upward, prevented by binocular vision.

hy·per·phos·pha·ta·se·mi·a (hī′pĕr-fos′fă-tă-sē′mē-ă) Abnormally high content of alkaline phosphatase in the circulating blood.

hy·per·phos·pha·ta·si·a (hī′pĕr-fos′fă-tā′zē-ă) Skeletal dysplasia characterized by dwarfism, macrocranium and other findings.

hy·per·phos·pha·te·mi·a (hī′pĕr-fos′fă-tē′mē-ă) Elevation of phosphorus concentration in blood.

hy·per·phos·pha·tu·ri·a (hī′pĕr-fos′fă-tyūr′ē-ă) An increased excretion of phosphates in the urine.

hy·per·pig·men·ta·tion (hī′pĕr-pig-men-tā′shŭn) An excess of color in a tissue or part.

hy·per·pi·tu·i·ta·rism (hī′pĕr-pi-tū′i-tă-rizm) Excessive production of anterior pituitary hormones.

hy·per·pla·si·a (hī′pĕr-plā′zē-ă) An increase in the number of cells in a tissue or organ, excluding tumor formation, whereby the bulk of the part or organ may be increased.

hy·per·plas·tic in·flam·ma·tion (hī′ pĕr-plas′tik in′flă-mā′shŭn) SYN proliferative inflammation.

hy·per·ploid·y (hī′pĕr-ploy-dē) Presence of extra chromosomes in incomplete sets.

hy·per·pnea (hī′pĕrp-nē′ă) Breathing that is deeper and more rapid than is normal at rest. SYN hyperpnoea.

hyperpnoea [Br.] SYN hyperpnea.

hy·per·po·lar·i·za·tion (hī′pĕr-pō′lăr-ī-ză′shŭn) An increase in polarization of membranes of nerves or muscle cells; the reverse change from that associated with excitatory action.

hy·per·po·ne·sis (hī′pĕr-pō-nē′sis) Exaggerated activity within the motor portion of the nervous system.

hyperpotassaemia [Br.] SYN hyperpotassemia.

hy·per·po·tas·se·mi·a (hī′pĕr-pŏ-tas-ē′ mē-ă) SYN hyperkalemia, hyperpotassaemia.

hy·per·prax·i·a (hī′pĕr-prak′sē-ă) Overactivity; restlessness; agitation.

hyperprebetalipoproteinaemia [Br.] SYN hyperprebetalipoproteinemia.

H

hy·per·pre·be·ta·lip·o·pro·tein·e·mi·a (hī′pĕr-prē′bā′tă-lip′ō-prō′tēn-ē′mē-ă) Increased concentrations of pre-β-lipoproteins in blood. SYN hyperprebetalipoproteinaemia.

hyperproinsulinaemia [Br.] SYN hyperproinsulinemia.

hy·per·pro·in·su·li·ne·mi·a (hī′pĕr-prō-in′sŭl-i-nē′mē-ă) Elevated plasma levels of proinsulin or proinsulinlike material.

hy·per·pro·lac·ti·ne·mi·a (hī′pĕr-prō-lak′ti-nē′mē-ă) Elevated levels of prolactin in the blood; a normal physiologic reaction during lactation, but pathologic otherwise.

hy·per·pro·li·ne·mi·a (hī′pĕr-prō′li-nē′mē-ă) Metabolic disorder characterized by enhanced plasma proline concentrations and urinary excretion of proline, hydroxyproline, and glycine.

hy·per·pro·te·o·sis (hī′pĕr-prō′tē-ō′sis) A condition resulting from an excessive amount of protein in the diet.

hy·per·py·rex·i·a (hī′pĕr-pī-rek′sē-ă) Extremely high fever.

hy·per·re·ac·tiv·i·ty (hī′pĕr-rē-ak-tiv′i-tē) A reaction that seems excessive when considering the size of the irritant.

hy·per·re·flex·i·a (hī′pĕr-rĕ-flek′sē-ă) A condition in which the deep tendon reflexes are exaggerated.

hy·per·re·flex·ic blad·der (hī′pĕr-rĕ-flek′sik blad′ĕr) A bladder exhibiting uninhibitable contraction. SYN detrusor hyperreflexia.

hy·per·res·o·nance (hī′pĕr-rez′ŏ-năns) An extreme degree of resonance.

hy·per·rhi·no·pho·ni·a (hī′pĕr-rī′nō-fō′nē-ă) SYN hypernasality.

hy·per·sar·co·si·ne·mi·a (hī′pĕr-sahr′kō-si-nē′mē-ă) SYN sarcosinemia.

hy·per·sen·si·bil·i·ty (hī′pĕr-sen′-si-bil′i-tē) Pathologic response to stimuli.

hy·per·sen·si·tiv·i·ty (hī′per-sen′si-tiv′i-tē) Abnormal sensitivity with an exaggerated response by the body to the stimulus of a foreign agent. SEE allergy.

hy·per·som·ni·a (hī′pĕr-som′nē-ă) A condition in which sleep periods are excessively long, but the person responds normally in the intervals; distinguished from somnolence.

hy·per·splen·ism (hī′pĕr-splēn′izm) Any of a group of conditions in which the cellular components of the blood or platelets are removed at an abnormally high rate by the spleen, resulting in low circulating levels.

hy·per·sthe·ni·a (hī′pĕr-sthē′nē-ă) Excessive tension or strength.

hy·per·sthe·nu·ri·a (hī′pĕr-sthē-nyū′rē-ă) Excretion of urine with an unusually high specific gravity and concentration of solutes, usually resulting from loss or deprivation of water.

hy·per·sys·to·le (hī′pĕr-sis′tŏ-lē) Abnormal force or duration of the cardiac systole.

hy·per·tel·or·ism (hī′pĕr-tel′ŏr-izm) Abnormal distance between two paired organs.

hy·per·ten·sion (HTN) (hī′pĕr-ten′shŭn) Persisting high arterial blood pressure; generally established guidelines are values exceeding 140 mmHg systolic or exceeding 90 mmHg diastolic blood pressure. Despite many discrete and inherited but rare forms that have been identified, the evidence is that for the most part blood pressure is a multifactorial, perhaps galtonian, trait. Hypertension is considered a risk factor for heart disease, stroke, and kidney disease.

hy·per·ten·sive (HT) (hī′pĕr-ten′siv) 1. Marked by an increased blood pressure. 2. Denoting a person suffering from high blood pressure.

hy·per·ten·sive ar·ter·i·op·a·thy (hī′pĕr-ten′siv ahr-tēr′ē-op′ă-thē) Arterial degeneration resulting from hypertension.

hy·per·ten·sive cri·sis (hī′pĕr-ten′siv krī′sis) Condition in which blood pressure is sufficiently high that it may damage organs.

hy·per·ten·sive en·ceph·a·lop·a·thy (HE, HTE) (hī′pĕr-ten′siv en-sef′ă-lop′ă-thē) Metabolic encephalopathy caused by diffuse cerebral edema; follows abrupt elevation of blood pressure in a long-term hypertensive patient.

hy·per·ten·sive ret·i·nop·a·thy (HR) (hī′pĕr-ten′siv ret′i-nop′ă-thē) Retinal condition occurring in accelerated vascular hypertension.

hy·per·the·co·sis (hī′pĕr-thē-kō′sis) Diffuse hyperplasia of the theca cells of the graafian follicles.

hy·per·the·li·a (hī′pĕr-thē′lē-ă) SYN polythelia.

hy·per·ther·mal·ge·si·a (hī′pĕr-thĕrm′al-jē′zē-ă) Extreme sensitivity to heat.

hy·per·ther·mi·a (HT) (hī′pĕr-thĕr′mē-ă) Therapeutically or iatrogenically induced hyperpyrexia.

hy·per·thy·mi·a (hī′pĕr-thī′mē-ă) State of overactivity.

hy·per·thy·mism (hī′pĕr-thī′mizm) Excessive activity of the thymus gland. SYN hyperthymization.

hy·per·thy·roid·ism (hī′pĕr-thī′royd-izm) An abnormality of the thyroid gland in which secretion of thyroid hormone is usually increased and no longer under regulatory control of hypothalamic-pituitary centers; characterized by a hypermetabolic state, usually with weight loss, tremulousness, elevated plasma levels of thyroxin and/or triiodothyronine.

hy·per·ton·ic (hī′pĕr-ton′ik) Having a greater degree of tension. SYN spastic (1). SYN hyperisotonic.

hy·per·ton·ic blad·der (hī′pĕr-ton′ik blad′ĕr) One with poor compliance.

hy·per·to·nic·i·ty (hī′pĕr-tŏ-nis′i-tē) Abnormally increased muscle tone or strength. The condition is sometimes associated with genetic or central nervous system disorders and may be manifest in arm or leg deformities. SEE ALSO spasticity. SYN high muscle tone.

hy·per·ton·ic la·bor (hī′pĕr-ton′ik lā′bŏr) Labor in which the uterus does not relax between contractions and general myometrial spasm prevents expulsion of the fetus.

hy·per·tri·cho·sis (hī′pĕr-tri-kō′sis)

Growth of hair in excess of the normal. SEE ALSO hirsutism.

hypertriglyceridaemia [Br.] SYN hypertriglyceridemia.

hy·per·tri·glyc·er·i·de·mi·a (HTG) (hī′pĕr-trī-glis′ĕr-i-dē′mē-ă) Elevated triglyceride concentration in the blood.

hy·per·tro·phic ar·thri·tis (hī′pĕr-trō′fik ahr-thrī′tis) Variant of osteoarthritis characterized by periarticular osteophyte formation.

hy·per·tro·phic gas·tri·tis (hī′pĕr-trō′fik gas-trī′tis) SYN Ménétrier disease.

hy·per·tro·phic py·lor·ic ste·no·sis (hī′pĕr-trō′fik pī-lōr′ik stĕ-nō′sis) Muscular hypertrophy of the pyloric sphincter, associated with projectile vomiting beginning in the second or third week of life, usually in males. SYN congenital pyloric stenosis.

hy·per·tro·phic rhi·ni·tis (hī′pĕr-trō′fik rī-nī′tis) Chronic rhinitis with permanent thickening of the mucous membrane.

hy·per·tro·phy, hy·per·tro·phi·a (hī-pĕr′trō-fē, -ă) General increase in bulk of a part or organ, due to increase in size, but not in number, of the individual tissue elements. SEE ALSO hyperplasia.

hy·per·tro·pi·a (hī′pĕr-trō′pē-ă) An ocular deviation with one eye higher than the other.

hy·per·ty·ro·si·ne·mi·a (hī′pĕr-tī′rō-si-nē′mē-ă) SYN tyrosinemia.

hyperuricaemia [Br.] SYN hyperuricemia.

hy·per·u·ri·ce·mi·a (hī′pĕr-yūr′i-sē′mē-ă) Enhanced blood concentrations of uric acid.

hy·per·u·ric·u·ri·a (hī′pĕr-yūr′i-kyū′rē-ă, hī′pĕr-yūri-kyūrē′-ă) Increased uric acid secretion.

hypervalinaemia [Br.] SYN hypervalinemia.

hy·per·val·i·ne·mi·a (hī′pĕr-val′i-nē′mē-ă) Abnormally high plasma concentrations of valine, a common finding in maple syrup urine disease. SYN hypervalinaemia.

hy·per·ven·ti·la·tion (hī′pĕr-ven′ti-lā′ shŭn) Increased alveolar ventilation relative to metabolic carbon dioxide production, so that alveolar carbon dioxide pressure decreases to below normal.

hy·per·ven·ti·la·tion syn·drome (HVS) (hī′pĕr-ven-ti-lā′shŭn sin′drōm) SEE chronic hyperventilation syndrome.

hy·per·ven·ti·la·tion tet·a·ny (hī′pĕr-ven′ti-lā′shŭn tet′ă-nē) A neurologic disorder caused by forced overbreathing, due to reduced levels of carbon dioxide in the blood.

hy·per·vis·cos·i·ty syn·drome (HVS) (hī′pĕr-vis-kos′i-tē sin′drōm) Disorder due to increased viscosity of the blood; an increase in serum proteins may be associated with bleeding from mucous membranes, retinopathy, and neurologic symptoms, and is sometimes seen in Waldenström macroglobulinemia and in multiple myeloma.

hy·per·vi·ta·min·o·sis (hī′pĕr-vī′tă-mi-nō′sis) A condition resulting from the ingestion of an excessive amount of a vitamin preparation.

hy·per·vo·le·mi·a (hī′pĕr-vol-ē′mē-ă) Abnormally increased volume of blood. SYN plethora (1), repletion (1).

hyp·es·the·si·a, hy·po·es·the·si·a (hīp′es-thē′zē-ă, hī′pō-) Diminished sensitivity to stimulation.

hy·pha, pl. **hy·phae** (hī′fă, -fē) A branching tubular cell characteristic of the filamentous fungi (molds). Intercommunicating hyphae constitute a mycelium, the visible colony on natural substrates or artificial laboratory media.

hyphaema [Br.] SYN hyphema.

hyphaemia [Br.] SYN hyphemia.

hyp·he·do·ni·a (hīp′hē-dō′nē-ă) A habitually lessened or attenuated degree of pleasure from something that should normally give great pleasure.

hy·phe·ma (hī-fē′mă) *Do not confuse this word with hyphemia.* Blood in the anterior chamber of the eye.

hy·phe·mi·a (hī-fē′mē-ă) SYN hypovolemia, hyphaemia.

hyp·na·gog·ic (hip′nă-goj′ik) Denoting a transitional state, related to the hypnoidal, preceding sleep; applied also to various hallucinations that may manifest themselves at that time.

hyp·na·gogue (hip′nă-gog) An agent that induces sleep.

♻ **hypno-, hypn-** Combining forms meaning sleep, hypnosis.

hyp·no·a·nal·y·sis (hip′nō-ă-nal′i-sis) Psychoanalysis or other psychotherapy that employs hypnosis as an adjunctive technique.

hyp·no·don·tics (hip′nō-don′tiks) Use of hypnotism in dentistry.

hyp·no·gen·ic, hyp·nog·e·nous (hip′nō-jen′ik, -noj′ĕ-nŭs) **1.** Relating to hypnogenesis. **2.** An agent capable of inducing a hypnotic state. SEE hypnosis.

hyp·noid (hip′noyd) Resembling hypnosis; denoting the subwaking state, a mental condition intermediate between sleeping and waking. SEE hypnagogic. SYN hypnoidal.

hyp·no·pom·pic (hip′nō-pom′pik) Denoting the occurrence of visions or dreams during the drowsy state following sleep.

hyp·no·sis (hip-nō′sis) An artificially induced trancelike state, resembling somnambulism, in which the subject is highly susceptible to suggestion and responds readily to the commands of the hypnotist.

hyp·no·ther·a·py (HT) (hip′nō-thār′ă-pē) **1.** Psychotherapeutic treatment by means of hypnotism. **2.** Treatment of disease by inducing a trancelike sleep.

hyp·not·ic (hip-not′ik) **1.** Causing sleep. **2.** An agent that promotes sleep. **3.** Relating to hypnotism.

hyp·not·ic sug·ges·tion (hip-not′ik sŭg-jes′chŭn) Direction given to a hypnotized subject for an activity that occurs during the trance or after; subject is not aware of such order and is purported to follow it regardless. SYN posthypnotic suggestion.

hyp·not·ic trance (hip-not′ik trans) That

state of somnolence or dissociation experienced by someone subjected to hypnosis.

hyp·no·tism (hip′nŏ-tizm) **1.** The process or act of inducing hypnosis. **2.** The practice or study of hypnosis.

hyp·no·tize (hip′nŏ-tīz) To induct someone into hypnosis.

hypo- 1. Prefix meaning deficient, below normal. SEE ALSO hyp-. **2.** CHEMISTRY denoting the lowest, or least rich in oxygen, of a series of chemical compounds. Cf. sub-.

hy·po·a·cid·i·ty (hī′pō-ă-sid′i-tē) A subnormal degree of acidity as in gastric juice.

hy·po·ac·ti·vi·ty (hī′pō-ak-tiv′i-tē) A state in which there is less movement than expected.

hy·po·a·cu·sis (hī′pō-ă-kyū′sis) SYN hypacusis.

hy·po·a·dre·nal·ism (hī′pō-ă-drē′năl-izm) Reduced function of cortices and medullae of the suprarenal gland.

hy·po·al·i·men·ta·tion (hī′pō-al′i-mĕn-tā′shŭn) SYN subalimentation.

hy·po·az·o·tu·ri·a (hī′pō-az′ō-tyūr′ē-ă) Excretion of abnormally small quantities of nonprotein nitrogenous material (especially urea) in the urine.

hy·po·bar·ic (hī′pō-bar′ik) **1.** Pertaining to pressure of ambient gases less than 1 atmosphere. **2.** With respect to solutions, less dense than the diluent or medium.

hy·po·bar·ism (hī′pō-bar′izm) Dysbarism due to decreasing bodily barometric pressure without hypoxia.

hy·po·blast (hī′pō-blast) SYN endoderm.

hypocalcaemia [Br.] SYN hypocalcemia.

hy·po·cal·ce·mi·a (hī′pō-kal-sē′mē-ă) Abnormally low levels of calcium in the circulating blood. SYN hypocalcaemia.

hy·po·cap·ni·a, hy·po·car·bi·a (hī′pō-kap′nē-ă, -kahr′bē-ă) Abnormally decreased arterial carbon dioxide tension. SYN hypocarbia.

hypochloraemia [Br.] SYN hypochloremia.

hy·po·chlor·e·mi·a (hī′pō-klōr-ē′mē-ă) An abnormally low level of chloride ions in the circulating blood. SYN hypochloraemia.

hy·po·chlor·hy·dri·a (hī′pō-klōr-hī′drē-ă, -hid′rī-ă) Abnormally small amount of digestive hydrochloric acid.

hy·po·chlor·ite (hī′pō-klōr′īt) A salt of hypochlorous acid.

hy·po·chlor·ous ac·id (HOCl, HClO) (hī′pō-klōr′ŭs as′id) An acid having oxidizing and bleaching properties.

hy·po·cho·les·ter·e·mi·a (hī′pō-kŏ-les′tĕr-ē′mē-ă) SYN hypocholesterolemia.

hy·po·cho·les·ter·in·e·mi·a (hī′pō-kŏ-les′tĕr-in-ē-mē-ă) SYN hypocholesterolemia.

hy·po·cho·les·ter·ol·e·mi·a, hy·po·cho·les·ter·i·ne·mi·a (hī′pō-kŏ-les′tĕr-ol-ē′mē-ă, -tĕr-i-nē′mē-ă) The presence of abnormally small amounts of cholesterol in the circulating blood.

hy·po·chon·dri·ac (hī′pō-kon′drē-ak) **1.** A person with a somatic overconcern, including morbid attention to the details of bodily functioning and exaggeration of any symptoms no matter how insignificant. **2.** Beneath the ribs.

hy·po·chon·dri·a·cal mel·an·chol·i·a (hī′pō-kŏn-drī′ă-kăl mel′ăn-kō′lē-ă) Melancholia with many associated physical complaints, often with no identifiable physical cause.

hy·po·chon·dri·ac re·gion (hī′pō-kon′drē-ak rē′jŭn) The region on each side of the abdomen covered by the costal cartilages; it is lateral to the epigastric region. SYN hypochondrium.

hy·po·chon·dri·a·sis (hī′pō-kŏn-drī′ă-sis) A morbid concern about one's own health and exaggerated attention to any unusual bodily or mental sensations.

hy·po·chon·dri·um (hī′pō-kon′drē-ŭm) [TA] SYN hypochondriac region.

hy·po·chro·ma·si·a (hī′pō-krō-mā′zē-ă) SYN hypochromia.

H

hy·po·chro·mat·ic (hī′pō-krō-mat′ik) Containing a small amount of pigment, or less than the normal amount for the such tissue.

hy·po·chro·ma·tism (hī′pō-krō′mă-tizm) **1.** The condition of being hypochromatic. **2.** SYN hypochromia.

hy·po·chro·mi·a (hī′pō-krō′mē-ă) An anemic condition in which the percentage of hemoglobin in the red blood cells is less than the normal range. SYN hypochromasia, hypochromatism (2).

hy·po·cit·ra·tu·ria (hī′pō-si′tră-tyū′rē-ă) Abnormally low concentration of citrate in the urine.

hypocythaemia [Br.] SYN hypocythemia.

hy·po·cy·the·mi·a (hī′pō-sī-thē′mē-ă) Hypocytosis of the circulating blood, as observed in aplastic anemia. SYN hypocythaemia.

hy·po·der·mic (hī′pō-děr′mik) SYN subcutaneous.

hy·po·der·mic in·jec·tion (hī′pō-děr′mik in-jek′shŭn) The administration of a remedy in liquid form by injection into the subcutaneous tissues.

hy·po·der·mic nee·dle (hī′pō-děr′mik nē′děl) Hollow type, similar to but smaller than an aspirating needle, attached to a syringe.

hy·po·der·mic sy·ringe (hī′pō-děr′mik sir-inj′) A small syringe with a barrel (which may be calibrated), perfectly matched plunger, and tip; used with a hollow needle for subcutaneous injections and for aspiration.

hy·po·der·moc·ly·sis (HDC, clysis) (hī′pō-děr-mok′li-sis) Subcutaneous injection of a saline or other solution.

hy·po·dip·si·a (hī′pō-dip′sē-ă) A reduced sense of thirst.

hy·po·don·ti·a (hī′pō-don′shē-ă) A congenital or acquired condition of having fewer than the normal complement of teeth. SYN oligodontia.

hy·po·dy·nam·ic (hī′pō-dī-nam′ik) Possessing or exhibiting subnormal power or force.

hy·po·ec·cri·sis (hī′pō-ek′ri-sis) Reduced excretion of waste matter.

hy·po·ech·o·ic (hī′pō-ĕ-kō′ik) Pertaining to a region in an ultrasound image in which the echoes are weaker or fewer than normal or in the surrounding regions.

hy·po·es·o·pho·ri·a (hī′pō-es′ŏ-fŏr′ē-ă) A tendency of the visual axis of one eye to deviate downward and inward, prevented by binocular vision.

hy·po·ex·o·pho·ri·a (hī′pō-eks′ŏ-fŏr′ē-ă) A tendency of the visual axis of one eye to deviate downward and outward, prevented by binocular vision.

hypoferraemia [Br.] SYN hypoferremia.

hy·po·fer·re·mi·a (hī′pō-fěr-ē′mē-ă) A deficiency of iron in the circulating blood. SYN hypoferraemia.

hypofibrinogenaemia [Br.] SYN hypofibrinogenemia.

hy·po·fi·brin·o·ge·ne·mi·a (hī′pō-fī-brin′ŏ-jĕ-nē′mē-ă) Abnormally low concentration of fibrinogen in the circulating blood plasma.

hy·po·ga·lac·ti·a (hī′pō-gă-lak′shē-ă) Less than normal milk secretion.

hy·po·gam·ma·glo·bi·ne·mi·a (hī′pō-gam′ă-glō′bi-nē′mē-ă) SYN hypogammaglobulinemia.

hypogammaglobulinaemia [Br.] SYN hypogammaglobulinemia.

hy·po·gam·ma·glob·u·lin·e·mi·a (hī′pō-gam′ă-glob′yū-li-nē′mē-ă) Decreased gamma fraction of serum globulin; associated with increased susceptibility to pyogenic infections. SYN hypogammaglobulinaemia.

hy·po·gan·gli·on·o·sis (hī′pō-gang′glē-ŏ-nō′sis) A reduction in the number of ganglionic nerve cells.

hy·po·gas·tric (hī′pō-gas′trik) Relating to the hypogastrium.

hy·po·gas·tric re·flex (hī′pō-gas′trik rē′fleks) SYN femoroabdominal reflex.

hy·po·gas·tri·um (hī′pō-gas′trē-ŭm) [TA] SYN pubic region.

hy·po·gas·tros·chi·sis (hī′pō-gas-tros′ ki-sis) Congenital fissure of the anterior abdominal wall in the hypogastric region.

hy·po·gen·e·sis (hī′pō-jen′ĕ-sis) Congenital defect of growth with underdevelopment of parts or organs of the body.

hy·po·gen·i·tal·ism (hī′pō-jen′i-tăl-izm) Partial or complete failure of maturation of the genitalia.

hy·po·geu·si·a (hī′pō-gū′sē-ă) Blunting of the sense of taste.

hy·po·glos·sal, hy·po·glos·sus (hī′ pō-glos′ăl, -sŭs) **1.** Below the tongue. **2.** Relating to the twelfth cranial nerve, nervus hypoglossus.

hy·po·glos·sal ca·nal (hī′pō-glos′ăl kă-nal′) [TA] The canal through which the hypoglossal nerve emerges from the skull. SYN canalis hypoglossalis [TA], anterior condyloid foramen.

hy·po·glot·tis, hy·po·glos·sis (hī′pō-glot′is, -glos′is) The undersurface of the tongue.

hypoglycaemia [Br.] SYN hypoglycemia.

hypoglycaemic [Br.] SYN hypoglycemic.

hy·po·gly·ce·mi·a (HG) (hī′pō-glī-sē′ mē-ă) Symptoms resulting from low blood glucose (normal glucose range 60–100 mg/dL [3.3–5.6 mmol/L]), which are either autonomic or neuroglycopenic. Autonomic symptoms include sweating, trembling, feelings of warmth, anxiety, and nausea. SYN glucopenia.

hy·po·gly·ce·mic (hī′pō-glī-sē′mik) Pertaining to or characterized by hypoglycemia. SYN hypoglycaemic.

hy·po·gly·co·gen·ol·y·sis (hī′pō-glī′ kō-jĕ-nol′i-sis) Diminished ability of the liver to convert glycogen to glucose.

hy·po·gly·cor·rha·chi·a (hī′pō-glī-kōrā′kē-ă) Depressed concentration of glucose in the cerebrospinal fluid; a characteristic of bacterial, fungal, and tuberculous meningitis.

hy·po·gnath·ous (hī-pog′nă-thŭs) Having an abnormally small mandible.

hy·po·go·nad·ism (hī′pō-gō′nad-izm) Inadequate gonadal function, as manifested by deficiencies in gametogenesis or the secretion of gonadal hormones; results in atrophy or deficient development of secondary sexual characteristics and, when occurring in prepubertal males, in altered body habitus, characterized by a short trunk and long limbs.

hy·po·go·nad·ism with a·nos·mi·a (hī′pō-gō′nad-izm an-oz′mē-ă) Failure of sexual development secondary to inadequate secretion of pituitary gonadotrophins, associated with anosmia due to agenesis of the olfactory lobes of the brain. SYN Kallmann syndrome.

hy·po·gon·a·do·trop·ic, hy·po·gon·a·do·troph·ic (hī′pō-gon′ă-dō-trō′pik, -trō′fik) Indicating inadequate secretion of gonadotropins and its consequences.

hy·po·gon·a·do·trop·ic hy·po·go·nad·ism (HH, HHG) (hī′pō-gon′ă-dō-trōp′ik hī′pō-gō′nad-izm) Defective gonadal development or function, or both, due to inadequate secretion of pituitary gonadotropins. SYN secondary hypogonadism.

hy·po·hi·dro·sis, hy·phi·dro·sis (hī′ pō-hi-drō′sis, hī′fi-) Diminished perspiration.

hy·po·hy·dra·tion (hī′pō-hī-drā′shŭn) Decrease in body water content.

hy·po·in·su·lin·ism (hī′pō-in′sŭ-lin-izm) Diminished ability of the pancreas to secrete insulin.

hypokalaemia [Br.] SYN hypokalemia.

hy·po·ka·le·mi·a, hy·po·po·tas·se·mi·a (hī′pō-kă-lē′mē-ă, -pō-ta-sē′mē-ă) The presence of an abnormally small concentration of potassium ions in the circulating blood; occurs in familial periodic paralysis and in potassium depletion due to excessive loss from the gastrointestinal tract or kidneys. SYN hypokalaemia.

hy·po·ka·le·mic neph·rop·a·thy (hī′ pō-ka-lē′mik ne-frop′ă-thē) Vacuolation of the epithelial cytoplasm of renal convoluted tubules in people seriously depleted of potassium. SYN vacuolar nephrosis.

H

hy·po·ka·le·mic per·i·od·ic pa·ral·y·sis (HOKPP) (hī′pō-kă-lē′mik pēr′ē-od′ik păr-al′i-sis) Form of periodic paralysis in which the serum potassium level is low during attacks; onset usually occurs between the ages of 7–21 years; attacks may be precipitated by exposure to environmental cold, high carbohydrate meal, or alcohol, may last hours to days, and may cause respiratory paralysis.

hy·po·ki·net·ic dys·ar·thri·a (hī′pō-ki-net′ik dis-ahr′thrē-ă) Dysarthria associated with disorders of the extrapyramidal motor system resulting in reduction and rigidity of movement, causing monotony of pitch and loudness, reduced stress, and imprecise enunciation of consonants. SEE ALSO extrapyramidal motor system, parkinsonian dysarthria.

hy·po·lac·ta·si·a (hī′pō-lak-tā′zē-ă) Reduced intestinal production of lactase.

hypolakaemic periodic paralysis [Br.] SYN hypokalemic periodic paralysis.

hy·po·ley·dig·ism (hī′pō-lī′dig-izm) Subnormal secretion of androgens by the interstitial (Leydig) cells of the testes.

hy·po·lip·i·de·mi·a (hī′pō-lip′i-dē′mē-ă) Diminished hematologic levels of fat.

hypomagnesaemia [Br.] SYN hypomagnesemia.

hy·po·mag·ne·se·mi·a (hī′pō-mag′nē-sē′mē-ă) Deficiency of magnesium in blood; may be caused by chronic alcoholism, dehydration, diabetic acidosis, and chronic diarrhea, malabsorption syndrome, postoperative complication of bowel surgery, prolonged nasogastric suction, prolonged diuretic therapy, or starvation. SYN hypomagnesaemia.

hy·po·ma·ni·a (hī′pō-mā′nē-ă) A mild degree of mania.

hy·po·man·ic ep·i·sode (hī′pō-man′ik ep′i-sōd) **1.** Several days of elevated or irritable mood involving a lesser degree of some or all of the features of a manic episode. **2.** SEE ALSO bipolar disorder, cyclothymia.

hy·po·mas·ti·a, hy·po·ma·zi·a (hī′pō-mas′tē-ă, -mā′zē-ă) Atrophy or congenital smallness of the breasts.

hy·po·me·li·a (hī′pō-mē′lē-ă) General term for hypoplasia of some or all parts of one or more limbs.

hy·po·men·or·rhe·a (hī′pō-men-ōr-ē′ă) *Do not confuse this word with oligomenorrhea.* Reduced flow or a shortening of the duration of menstruation.

hy·po·met·ri·a (hī′pō-mē′trē-ă) Ataxia characterized by underreaching an object or goal; seen with cerebellar disease.

hy·pom·ne·si·a (hī′pom-nē′zē-ă) Impaired memory.

hy·po·mo·bile pa·tel·la (hī′pō-mō′bil pă-tel′ă) A range of patellar movement equal to one quadrant or less.

hy·po·mo·bil·i·ty (hī′pō-mō-bil′i-tē) Reduction in ability to move, whether by disease state or age.

hy·po·morph (hī′pō-mōrf) A person whose standing height is short in proportion to sitting height, owing to shortness of the lower limbs.

hy·po·mo·tor sei·zure (hī′pō-mō′tŏr sē′zhŭr) One characterized by complete or partial arrest of ongoing motor activity in a patient whose level of consciousness cannot be determined accurately.

hy·po·my·e·li·na·tion, hy·po·my·e·lin·o·gen·e·sis (hī′pō-mī′e-lin-ā′shun, -ō-jen′ē-sis) Defective formation of myelin in the spinal cord and brain; basis for several demyelinating diseases.

hy·po·my·o·to·ni·a (hī′pō-mī′ō-tō′nē-ă) Diminished muscular tonus.

hy·po·myx·i·a (hī′pō-mik′sē-ă) A condition in which the secretion of mucus is diminished.

hy·po·na·sal·i·ty (hī′pō-nā-zal′i-tē) Insufficient nasal resonance during speech, usually due to obstruction of the nasal tract. SYN hyporhinophonia.

hy·po·na·tre·mi·a (hī′pō-nă-trē′mē-ă) Abnormally low concentrations of sodium ions in the circulating blood.

hy·po·ne·o·cy·to·sis (hī′pō-nē′ō-sī-tō′sis) Leukopenia associated with the presence of immature and young leukocytes.

hy·po·noi·a (hī′pō-noy′ă) Deficient or sluggish mental activity or imagination.

hy·po·nych·i·al (hī′pō-nik′ē-ăl) **1.** SYN subungual. **2.** Relating to the hyponychium.

hy·po·nych·i·um (hī′pō-nik′ē-ŭm) [TA] The epithelium of the nail bed, particularly its proximal part near the nailroot and lunula, forming the nail matrix.

hy·pon·y·chon (hī-pon′i-kon) An ecchymosis beneath a fingernail or toenail.

hy·po·or·tho·cy·to·sis (hī′pō-ōr′thō-sī′-tō′sis) Leukopenia in which the relative numbers of the various types of white blood cells are within normal ranges.

hy·po·pan·cre·a·tism (hī′pō-pan′krē-ă-tizm) Diminished activity of pacreatic digestive enzyme secretion.

hy·po·par·a·thy·roid·ism (hī′pō-par′ă-thī′royd-izm) A condition due to diminution or absence of the secretion of the parathyroid hormones, with low serum calcium, tetany, and sometimes increased bone density.

hy·po·pha·lan·gism (hī′pō-fă-lan′jizm) Congenital absence of one or more of the phalanges of a finger or toe.

hy·po·pha·ryn·ge·al (hī′pō-fă-rin′jē-ăl) Located beneath the pharyngeal apparatus. SYN hypobranchial.

hy·po·phar·ynx (hī′pō-far′ingks) SYN laryngopharynx.

hy·po·pho·ne·sis (hī′pō-fō-nē′sis) In percussion or auscultation, a sound that is diminished or fainter than usual.

hy·po·pho·ni·a (hī′pō-fō′nē-ă) An abnormally weak voice due to incoordination of the muscles concerned in vocalization. SYN leptophonia, microphonia, microphony.

hy·po·pho·ri·a (hī′pō-fōr′ē-ă) A tendency of the visual axis of one eye to deviate downward, prevented by binocular vision.

hy·po·phos·pha·ta·si·a (hī′pō-fos′fă-tā′zē-ă) An abnormally low content of alkaline phosphatase in the circulating blood.

hy·po·phos·pha·te·mi·a (hī′pō-fos-fă-tē′mē-ă) Deficiency of phosphorus in blood; may be due to chronic diarrhea, deficiency of vitamin D, hyperparathyroidism with hypercalcemia, hypomagnesemia, malnutrition, chronic alcoholism, or malabsorption syndrome.

hy·po·phos·pha·tu·ri·a (hī′pō-fos′fă-tyūr′ē-ă) Reduced urinary excretion of phosphates.

hy·po·phos·pho·rous ac·id (hī′pō-fos′fŏr-ŭs as′id) An aqueous solution used as a stabilizing reducing agent in pharmaceutical preparations.

hy·poph·y·sec·to·my (hī-pof′i-sek′tŏ-mē) Surgical removal of the hypophysis or pituitary gland.

hy·po·phys·e·o·trop·ic (hī′pō-fiz′ē-ō-trō′pik) SYN hypophysiotropic.

hy·po·phy·si·al, hy·po·phy·se·al (hī′pō-fiz′ē-ăl) Relating to a hypophysis.

hy·po·phy·si·al ca·chex·i·a (hī′pō-fiz′ē-ăl kă-kek′sē-ă) SYN Simmonds disease, panhypopituitarism.

hy·po·phy·si·al fos·sa (hī′pō-fiz′ē-ăl fos′ă) [TA] Fossa of the sphenoid bone housing the pituitary gland. SEE ALSO sella turcica.

hy·po·phy·si·al in·fan·til·ism (hī′pō-fiz′ē-ăl in′făn-til-izm) Growth hormone deficiency due to failure of hypothalamic growth hormone–releasing hormone (also known as somatocrinin.)

hy·po·phys·i·o·por·tal sys·tem (hī′pō-fiz′ē-ō-pōr′tăl sis′těm) SYN portal hypophysial circulation.

hy·po·phys·i·o·priv·ic, hy·po·phy·se·o·priv·ic (hī′pō-fiz′ē-ō-priv′ik) Pertaining to absence or depressed function of the pituitary gland. SYN hypophyseoprivic.

hy·po·phys·i·o·sphe·noi·dal syn·drome (hī′pō-fiz′ē-ō-sfē-noy′dăl sin′drōm) Neoplastic invasion of cranial base near the sphenoidal sinus.

hy·po·phys·i·o·trop·ic, hy·po·phy·se·o·trop·ic (hī′pō-fiz′ē-ō-trō′pik) Denoting a stimulatory hormone that acts on the pituitary gland (hypophysis). SYN hypophyseotropic.

hy·poph·y·sis (hī-pof´i-sis) [TA] An unpaired compound gland suspended from the base of the hypothalamus by a short extension of the infundibulum, the infundibular or pituitary stalk. SYN pituitary gland.

hy·poph·y·sis ce·re·bri (hī-pof´i-sis ser´ĕ-brī) SYN pituitary gland.

hy·po·pi·tu·i·ta·rism (hī´pō-pi-tū´i-tăr-izm) A condition due to diminished activity of anterior hypophysial lobe of the hypophysis, with inadequate secretion of one or more anterior pituitary hormones.

hy·po·pla·si·a (hī´pō-plā´zē-ă) Underdevelopment or atrophy of a tissue or organ, usually due to a decrease in the number of cells.

hy·po·plas·tic a·ne·mi·a (hī´pō-plas´tik ă-nē´mē-ă) Progressive nonregenerative anemia resulting from greatly depressed, inadequately functioning bone marrow.

hy·po·ploid·y (hī´pō-ploy-dē) Loss of one or more chromosomes.

hy·pop·ne·a (hī-pop´nē-ă) Breathing that is shallower, or slower, than normal. SYN oligopnea.

hy·po·po·ro·sis (hī´pō-pōr-ō´sis) Lack of adequate formation of callus after osseous trauma.

hy·po·po·tas·se·mi·a (hī´pō-pō-ta-sē´mē-ă) SYN hypokalemia, hypopotassaemia.

hy·pop·ty·a·lism (hī´pop-tī´ă-lizm) SYN hyposalivation.

hy·po·py·on (hī-pō´pē-on) Presence of visibly layered leukocytes in the anterior chamber of the eye.

hyporeninaemia [Br.] SYN hyporeninemia.

hy·po·ren·i·ne·mi·a (hī´pō-rē´ni-nē´mē-ă) Low levels of renin in the circulating blood. SYN hyporeninaemia.

hy·po·sal·i·va·tion (hī´pō-sal´i-vā´shŭn) Reduced salivation. SYN hypoptyalism.

hy·po·scle·ral (hī´pō-skler´ăl) Beneath the sclerotic coat of the eyeball.

hy·po·se·cre·tion (hī´pō-sĕ-krē´shŭn) Lower than normal glandular output.

hy·po·sen·si·tive (hī´pō-sen´si-tiv) Reduced ability to respond to stimuli.

hy·po·sen·si·tiv·i·ty (hī´pō-sen´si-tiv´i-tē) A condition of subnormal sensitivity, in which the response to a stimulus is unusually delayed or lessened in degree.

hy·pos·mi·a (hī-poz´mē-ă) Diminished sense of smell.

hy·po·so·ma·to·tro·pism (hī´pō-sō-mat´ō-trō´pizm) Deficient secretion of pituitary growth hormone (somatotropin).

hy·po·som·ni·a (hī´pō-som´nē-ă) State of sleeping very little; insomnia.

hy·po·spa·di·ac (hī´pō-spā´dē-ak) Relating to hypospadias.

hy·po·spa·di·as (hī´pō-spā´dē-ăs) A developmental anomaly characterized by a defect on the ventral surface of the penis so that the urethral opening is more proximal than normal; may be associated with chordee. SYN urogenital sinus anomaly.

hy·po·sphyg·mi·a (hī´pō-sfig´mē-ă) Abnormally low blood pressure with sluggishness of the circulation.

hy·po·splen·ism (hī´pō-splēn´izm) Absent or reduced splenic function.

hy·pos·ta·sis (hī-pos´tă-sis) **1.** Formation of a sediment at the bottom of a liquid. **2.** SYN hypostatic congestion.

hy·po·stat·ic (hī´pō-stat´ik) **1.** Sedimentary; resulting from a dependent position. **2.** Relating to hypostasis.

hy·po·stat·ic con·ges·tion (hī´pō-stat´ik kŏn-jes´chŭn) That due to pooling of venous blood in a dependent part. SYN hypostasis (2).

hy·po·stat·ic ec·ta·si·a (hī´pō-stat´ik ek-tā´zē-ă) Dilation of a blood vessel, usually a vein, in a dependent body part.

hy·po·stat·ic pneu·mo·ni·a (hī´pō-stat´ik nū-mō´nē-ă) That due to infection developing in the dependent portions of the lungs due to decreased ventilation of those areas, with resulting failure to drain bronchial secretions.

hy·po·sthe·ni·a (hī′pos-thē′nē-ă) Weakness. SEE asthenia.

hy·pos·the·nu·ri·a (hī′pos-thĕ-nyūr′ē-ă) Excretion of urine of low specific gravity, due to inability of the tubules of the kidneys to produce a concentrated urine or in diabetes insipidus.

hy·po·sy·ner·gi·a (hī′pō-sin-ĕrjē-ă) Poor coordination. SYN dyssynergia.

hy·po·tel·or·ism (hī′pō-tel′ŏr-izm) Abnormal closeness of eyes.

hy·po·ten·sion (hī′pō-ten′shŭn) 1. Subnormal arterial blood pressure. SYN hypopiesis. 2. Reduced pressure or tension of any kind.

hy·po·ten·sive (hī′pō-ten′siv) Having lower than normal blood pressure.

hy·po·tha·lam·ic in·fun·dib·u·lum (hī′pō-thă-lam′ik in′fŭn-dib′yū-lŭm) The apical portion of the tuber cinereum extending into the stalk of the hypophysis.

hy·po·tha·lam·ic o·be·si·ty (hī′pō-thă-lam′ik ō-bē′si-tē) Obesity caused by disease of the hypothalamus.

hy·po·thal·a·mus (hī′pō-thal′ă-mŭs) [TA] The ventral and medial region of the diencephalon forming the walls of the ventral half of the third ventricle; delineated from the thalamus by the hypothalamic sulcus, lying medial to the internal capsule and subthalamus, continuous with the precommissural septum anteriorly and with the mesencephalic tegmentum and central gray substance posteriorly. SEE ALSO hypophysis.

hy·po·the·nar (hī′pō-thē′năr) [TA] Denoting any structure in relation with the hypothenar eminence or its underlying collective components.

hy·po·ther·mi·a (hī′pō-thĕr′mē-ă) A core body temperature significantly lower than 98.6°F (37°C).

hy·po·ther·mi·a blan·ket (hī′pō-thĕr′mē-ă blangk′ĕt) A cover or wrap used to cool the patient's body.

hy·po·ther·mi·a ther·a·py (hī′pō-thĕr′mē-ă thăr′ă-pē) Cooling the patient's body below normal body temperature to prevent cerebral damage after cardiac arrest or trauma.

hy·poth·e·sis (hī-poth′ĕ-sis) A conjecture cast in a form that is amenable to confirmation or refutation by experiment and the assembly of data. SEE ALSO postulate, theory.

hy·po·thy·mi·a (hī′pō-thī′mē-ă) Depression of spirits; the "blues."

hy·po·thy·mic (hī′pō-thī′mik) Denoting or characteristic of hypothymia.

hy·po·thy·roid·ism (hī′pō-thī′royd-izm) Diminished production of thyroid hormone, leading to clinical manifestations of thyroid insufficiency, including somnolence, slow mentation, hair loss, subnormal temperature, hoarseness, muscle weakness, delayed relaxation of tendon reflexes, and myxedema.

hy·po·to·ni·a, hy·pot·o·nus, hy·pot·o·ny (hī′pō-tō′nē-ă, hī-tot′ŏ-nŭs, -pot′ŏ-nē) 1. Reduced tension in any part, as in the eyeball. 2. Relaxation of the arteries. 3. A condition in which there is a diminution or loss of muscular tonicity.

hy·po·ton·ic (hī′pō-ton′ik) 1. Having a lesser degree of tension. 2. Having a lesser osmotic pressure than a reference solution, ordinarily plasma or interstitial fluid.

hy·po·tri·cho·sis (hī′pō-tri-kō′sis) A less than normal amount of hair on the head and/or body. SYN hypotrichiasis (1), oligotrichia, oligotrichosis.

hy·pot·ro·phy (hī′pot′rō-fē) Degeneration of an organ or limb due to lack of cells or inactivity.

hy·po·tro·pi·a (hī′pō-trō′pē-ă) An ocular deviation with one eye lower than the other.

hy·po·tym·pa·not·o·my (hī′pō-tim-pă-not′ŏ-mē) Operative procedure for the excision, without sacrifice of hearing, of small tumors confined to the bottom of the tympanic cavity.

hy·po·tym·pa·num (hī′pō-tim′pă-nŭm) Lower part of the tympanic cavity; separated by a bony wall from the jugular bulb.

H

hypouricaemia [Br.] SYN hypouricemia.

hy·po·u·ri·ce·mi·a (hī′pō-yūr′i-sē′mē-ă) Reduced blood concentration of uric acid. SYN hypouricaemia.

hy·po·ven·ti·la·tion (hī′pō-ven-ti-lā′shŭn) Reduced alveolar ventilation relative to metabolic carbon dioxide production, so that alveolar carbon dioxide pressure increases above normal. SYN underventilation.

hypovolaemia [Br.] SYN hypovolemia.

hypovolaemic shock [Br.] SYN hypovolemic shock.

hy·po·vo·le·mi·a (hī′pō-vŏ-lē′mē-ă) Decreased bodily blood volume. SYN hyphemia, hypovolaemia.

hy·po·vo·le·mic shock (hī′pō-vŏ-lē′mik shok) Shock caused by a reduction in volume of blood, as from hemorrhage or dehydration. SYN hypovolaemic shock.

hy·po·vo·li·a (hī′pō-vō′lē-ă) Diminished water content or volume of a given compartment; e.g., extracellular hypovolia.

hypoxaemia [Br.] SYN hypoxemia.

hy·po·xan·thine (hī′pō-zan′thēn) A purine present in the muscles and other tissues, formed during purine catabolism by deamination of adenine.

hy·pox·e·mi·a (hī′pok-sē′mē-ă) Subnormal oxygenation of arterial blood, short of anoxia. SYN hypoxaemia.

hy·pox·i·a (hī-pok′sē-ă) Lower than normal levels of oxygen in inspired gases, arterial blood, or tissue, short of anoxia.

hy·pox·ic hy·pox·i·a (hī-pok′sik hī-pok′sē-ă) Condition resulting from defective oxygenation in the lungs.

hy·pox·ic neph·ro·sis (hī-pok′sik nĕ-frō′sis) Acute oliguric renal failure following hemorrhage, burns, shock, or other causes of hypovolemia and reduced renal blood flow.

hyp·sa·rhyth·mi·a (hip′să-ridh′mē-ă) The abnormal and characteristically chaotic electroencephalogram in patients with infantile spasms.

hyp·si·brach·y·ce·phal·ic (hip′sē-brak′ē-sē-fal′ik) Denotes a human or animal with a high broad head.

hyp·so·dont (hip′sŏ-dont) Having long teeth.

hyp·so·kin·e·sis (hip′sō-ki-nē′sis) Falling backward when standing upright; seen in certain types of paralysis.

hys·ter·al·gi·a (his′tĕr-al′jē-ă) Pain in the uterus. SYN hysterodynia, metrodynia.

hys·ter·a·tre·si·a (his′tĕr-ă-trē′zē-ă) Atresia of the uterine cavity, usually due to inflammatory endocervical adhesions.

hys·ter·ec·to·my (his′tĕr-ek′tŏ-mē) Removal of the uterus; unless otherwise specified, usually denotes complete removal of the uterus.

hys·ter·e·sis (his′tĕr-ē′sis) Failure of either one of two related phenomena to keep pace with the other; or any situation in which the value of one depends on whether the other has been increasing or decreasing.

hys·ter·eu·ry·sis (his′tĕr-yūr-ē′sis) Dilation of the lower segment and cervical canal of the uterus.

hys·te·ri·a (his-ter′ē-ă) A somatoform disorder with altered or lost physical functioning that suggests a physical disorder, but is instead apparently an expression of a psychological conflict or need. SEE conversion disorder.

hys·ter·ic, hys·ter·i·cal (his-ter′ik, -i-kăl) Relating to or characterized by hysteria.

hys·ter·ic pa·ral·y·sis (his-ter′ik pă-ral′i-sis) Older term for paralysis based on conversion disorder (q.v.).

hys·ter·ic psy·cho·sis (his-ter′ik sī-kō′sis) **1.** A psychotic disturbance with predominantly hysteric symptoms. **2.** A mental disorder resembling conversion hysteria but of psychotic severity. **3.** A brief reactive psychosis, often culture bound.

hys·ter·ic syn·co·pe (his-ter′ik sin′kŏ-pē) Psychogenic form of fainting based on conversion.

hystero-, hyster- Combining forms, meaning, **1.** the uterus. SEE ALSO metr-, utero-. **2.** Hysteria. **3.** Later, following.

hys·ter·o·cat·a·lep·sy (his'tĕr-ō-kat'ă-lep-sē) Hysteria with cataleptic manifestations, including rigid body posture and a generalized trancelike state.

hys·ter·o·cele (his'tĕr-ō-sēl) **1.** An abdominal or perineal hernia containing part or all of the uterus. **2.** Protrusion of uterine contents into a weakened, bulging area of uterine wall.

hys·ter·o·clei·sis (his'tĕr-ō-klī'sis) Operative occlusion of the uterus.

hys·ter·o·dyn·i·a (his'tĕr-ō-din'ē-ă) SYN hysteralgia.

hys·ter·o·ep·i·lep·sy (his'tĕr-ō-ep'i-lep-sē) Hysteric convulsions.

hys·ter·o·gen·ic, hys·ter·og·en·ous (his'tĕr-ō-jen'ik, -oj'ē-nŭs) Causing hysteric symptoms or reactions.

hys·ter·og·ra·phy (his'tĕr-og'ră-fē) **1.** Radiographic examination of the uterine cavity filled with a contrast medium. **2.** Graphic procedure used to record uterine contractions.

hys·ter·o·lap·a·rot·o·my (his'tĕr-ō-lap'ă-rot'ŏ-mē) Surgical incision through the abdominal wall into the uterus.

hys·ter·o·lith (his'tĕr-ō-lith) A uterine calculus or stone.

hys·ter·ol·y·sis (his'tĕr-ol'i-sis) Breaking up of adhesions between the uterus and neighboring parts.

hys·ter·om·e·ter (his'tĕr-om'ē-tĕr) A graduated sound for measuring the depth of the uterine cavity.

hys·ter·o·my·o·ma (his'tĕr-ō-mī-ō'mă) A myoma of the uterus.

hys·ter·o·my·o·mec·to·my (his'tĕr-ō-mī'ō-mek'tŏ-mē) Operative removal of a uterine myoma.

hys·ter·o·my·ot·o·my (his'tĕr-ō-mī-ot'ŏ-mē) Incision into the muscles of the uterus.

hys·ter·o·o·oph·o·rec·to·my (his'tĕr-ō-ō-of'ŏr-ek'tŏ-mē) Surgical removal of the uterus and ovaries.

hys·ter·o·pex·y (his'tĕr-ō-pek-sē) Fixation of a displaced or abnormally movable uterus. SYN uterofixation, uteropexy.

hys·ter·o·plas·ty (his'tĕr-ō-plas-tē) SYN uteroplasty.

hys·ter·or·rha·phy (his'tĕr-ōr'ă-fē) Sutural repair of a lacerated uterus.

hys·ter·or·rhex·is (his'tĕr-ō-rek'sis) Rupture of the uterus.

hys·ter·o·sal·pin·gec·to·my (his'tĕr-ō-sal-pin-jek'tŏ-mē) Operation for the removal of the uterus and one or both uterine tubes.

hys·ter·o·sal·pin·gog·ra·phy (his'tĕr-ō-sal-ping-gog'ră-fē) Radiography of the uterus and uterine tubes after the injection of radiopaque material. SYN hysterotubography, metrosalpingography, uterosalpingography, uterotubography.

hys·ter·o·sal·pin·gos·to·my (his'tĕr-ō-sal-ping-gos'tŏ-mē) Operation to restore patency of a uterine tube.

hys·ter·o·scope (his'tĕr-ō-skōp) An endoscope used in direct visual examination of the uterine cavity. SYN metroscope, uteroscope.

hys·ter·o·spasm (his'tĕr-ō-spazm) Spasm of the uterus.

hys·ter·ot·o·my (his'tĕr-ot'ŏ-mē) Incision of the uterus.

H

♻ **-ia** A suffix used to form terms for states or conditions, often abnormal. Cf. -ism.

♻ **-iasis** Combining form meaning a condition or state, especially an unhealthy one.

i·at·ric (ī-at'rik) Pertaining to medicine or to a physician or healer.

♻ **-iatrist, -iatrician** Combining forms denoting a specialist in a given field of medicine.

♻ **iatro-** Combining form meaning physicians, medicine, treatment. Cf. medico-.

i·at·ro·gen·ic (ī-at'rō-jen'ik) Denoting response to medical or surgical treatment, usually unfavorable.

i·at·ro·gen·ic trans·mis·sion (ī-at'rō-jen'ik trans-mish'ŭn) Transmission of infectious agents due to medical interference (e.g., transmission by contaminated needles).

I band (band) A light band on each side of the Z line of striated muscle fibers, comprising a region of the sarcomere where thin filaments are not overlapped by thick filaments.

i·bu·pro·fen (IBU, IB) (ī'byū-prō'fĕn) A nonsteroidal analgesic and antiinflammatory agent derived from propionic acid.

♻ **-ic 1.** Suffix denoting of, pertaining to. **2.** Chemical suffix denoting an element in a compound in one of its highest valencies. Cf. -ous (1). **3.** Suffix indicating an acid.

I cell (sel) Cultured skin fibroblast containing membrane-bound inclusions. SYN inclusion cell.

ice pack (IP) (īs pak) A cold local application to limit or reduce swelling in recently traumatized tissues, usually in the form of a waterproof container for ice. Improvised means for containing ice (e.g., plastic bags, towels) are often employed.

i·chor·ous (ī'kōr-ŭs) Relating to or resembling ichor.

i·chor·rhe·a (ī'kō-rē'ă) A profuse ichorous discharge.

i·chor·rhe·mi·a, i·cho·re·mi·a (ī'kō-rē'mē-ă) Sepsis resulting from infection accompanied by an ichorous discharge.

ich·thy·ism (ik'thē-izm) Poisoning caused by eating stale or otherwise unfit fish.

♻ **ichthyo-** Combining form denoting fish.

ich·thy·oid (ik'thē-oyd) Fish-shaped.

ich·thy·o·sis (ik'thē-ō'sis) Congenital disorders of keratinization characterized by noninflammatory dryness and scaling of the skin, often associated with other defects and with abnormalities of lipid metabolism.

ich·thy·o·sis vul·ga·ris (IV) (ik'thē-ō'sis vŭl-gā'ris) One of the most common inherited dermatologic disorders that causes dry scaly skin. SYN common ichthyosis, fish-scale disease, hyperkeratosis congenita, ichthyosis simplex.

ich·thy·o·tox·ism (ik'thē-ō-tok'sizm) Poisoning caused by fish.

♻ **-ics** Suffix meaning organized knowledge, practice, treatment.

ic·tal (ik'tăl) Relating to or caused by a stroke or seizure.

♻ **ictero-** Combining form related to jaundice.

ic·ter·o·gen·ic (ik'tĕr-ō-jen'ik) Causing jaundice.

icterohaemorrhagic fever [Br.] SYN icterohemorrhagic fever.

ic·ter·o·hem·or·rhag·ic fe·ver (ik'tĕr-ō-hem'ŏr-aj'ik fē'vĕr) Infection with *Leptospira interrogans* serotype *icterohemorrhagiae*, characterized by fever, jaundice, hemorrhagic lesions, azotemia, and central nervous system manifestations. SYN leptospirosis icterohemorrhagica.

ic·ter·o·hep·a·ti·tis (ik'tĕr-ō-hep'ă-tī'tis) Inflammation of the liver with jaundice as a prominent symptom.

ic·ter·oid (ik'tĕr-oyd) Yellow or seemingly jaundiced.

ic·ter·us (ik'tĕr-ŭs) SYN jaundice.

ic·ter·us ne·o·na·to·rum (IN) (ik′tĕr-ŭs nē-ō-nā-tō′rŭm) Jaundice in the newborn. SYN jaundice of the newborn, physiologicicterus, physiologic jaundice.

ic·tus (ik′tŭs) **1.** A stroke or attack. **2.** A beat.

ic·tus cor·dis (ik′tŭs kōr′dis) SYN heart beat.

ICU psy·cho·sis (sī-kō′sis) Psychotic episode(s) occurring within 24 hours after entering the intensive care unit (ICU) in people with no previous history of psychosis; related to sleep deprivation, overstimulation, and time spent on life support systems.

-id Suffix denoting a state of sensitivity of the skin in which a part remote from the primary lesion reacts (''-id reaction'') to the pathogen, giving rise to a secondary inflammatory lesion.

id (id) PSYCHOANALYSIS one of three components of the psychic apparatus in the freudian structural framework, the other two being the ego and superego. It is completely in the unconscious realm, is unorganized, is the reservoir of psychic energy or libido.

ID₅₀ Median infective dose.

-ide 1. Combining form denoting the more electronegative element in a binary chemical compound. **2.** Combining form (in a sugar name) indicating substitution for the H of the hemiacetal OH; e.g., glycoside.

i·de·al·ized im·age (ī-dē′ă-līzd im′ăj) An overblown view of one's own virtues and abilities. SEE ALSO narcissism.

i·de·a of ref·er·ence (ī-dē′ă ref′rĕns) The misinterpretation that other people's statements or acts or neutral objects in the environment are directed toward one's self.

i·de·a·tion·al a·prax·i·a (ī-dē′ă′shŭn-ăl ă-prak′sē-ă) Dysfunctional voluntary movement in which objects are misused because the afflicted person has difficulty identifying the object's proper function.

i·dée fixe (ē-dā′ fēks) French for fixed idea (q.v.).

i·den·ti·cal twins (i-dent′ti-k′ăl twinz) SYN monozygotic twins.

i·den·ti·ty cri·sis (ī-dent′ti-tē krī′sis) A disorientation concerning one's sense of self, values, and role in society, often of acute onset and related to a particular and significant event in one's life.

ideo- Prefix meaning ideas; ideation Cf. idio-.

id·eo·ge·net·ic (id′ē-ō-jĕ-net′ĭk) Denotes thoughts formed from sensory impressions rather than words.

i·de·o·ki·net·ic a·prax·i·a, i·de·o·mo·tor a·prax·i·a (id′ē-ō-ki-net′ik ă-prak′sē-ă, id′ē-ō-mō′tŏr) A motor disorder in which simple acts are incapable of being performed, presumably because the connections between the cortical centers that control volition and the motor cortex are interrupted.

i·de·o·mo·tion (ī′dē-ō-mō′shŭn) Muscular movement executed under the influence of a dominant idea, being practically automatic and not volitional.

i·de·o·mo·tor (ī′dē-ō-mō′tŏr) Relating to ideomotion. SYN ideokinetic.

idio- Prefix meaning private, distinctive, peculiar to. Cf. ideo-.

id·i·o·cy (id′ē-ō-sē) An grossly offensive term denoting extreme mental retardation; no medical meaning; use to be avoided.

id·i·o·glos·si·a (id′ē-ō-glos′ē-ă) An extreme form of lalling or vowel or consonant substitution, by which the speech of a child may be made unintelligible and appear to be another language to one who does not have the key to the literal changes.

id·i·o·gram (id′ē-ō-gram) SYN karyotype.

id·i·o·het·er·o·ag·glu·ti·nin (id′ē-ō-het′ĕr-ō-ă-glū′ti-nin) An idioagglutinin occurring in the blood of one animal, but capable of combining with the antigenic material from another species.

id·i·o·het·er·o·ly·sin (id′ē-ō-het-ĕr-ol′i-sin) An idiolysin occurring in the blood of an animal of one species, but capable of combining with the red blood cells of another species, thereby causing hemolysis when complement is present.

id·i·o·mus·cu·lar con·trac·tion (id′ē-ō-mŭs′kyū-lăr kŏn-trak′shŭn) SYN myoedema.

id·i·o·no·dal rhythm (id′ē-ō-nōd′ăl ridh′ŭm) An independent cardiac rhythm.

id·i·o·path·ic (id′ē-ō-path′ik) Denoting a disease of unknown cause. SYN agnogenic.

id·i·o·path·ic dis·ease (id′ē-ō-path′ik di-zēz′)A disease of unknown cause or mechanism.

id·i·o·path·ic hy·per·tro·phic sub·a·or·tic ste·no·sis (id′ē-ō-path′ik hī′pĕr-trō′fik sŭb′ā-ōr′tik stĕ-nō′sis) Left ventricular outflow obstruction due to hypertrophy, usually congenital, of the ventricular septum.

id·i·o·path·ic meg·a·co·lon (id′ē-ō-path′ik meg′ă-kō-lŏn) Acquired megacolon, found in children and adults, without distal obstruction or absence of ganglion cells; the muscle of the dilated colon is thin.

id·i·o·path·ic pul·mo·nar·y fi·bro·sis (IPF) (id′ē-ō-path′ik pul′mŏ-nar-ē fĭ-brō′sis) Subacute form also called Hamman-Rich syndrome; an acute to chronic inflammatory process of the lungs, the healing stage of diffuse alveolar damage or acute interstitial pneumonia, either idiopathic or associated with collagen-vascular diseases. SYN cryptogenic fibrosing alveolitis, Hamman-Rich syndrome.

id·io·path·ic sub·glot·tic ste·no·sis (id′ē-ō-path′ik sŭb-glot′ik stĕ-nō′sis) Narrowing of the infraglottic lumen, of unknown cause; apparently occurring only in women.

id·i·o·path·ic throm·bo·cy·to·pe·nic pur·pu·ra (ITP) (id′ē-ō-path′ik throm′bō-sī-tō-pē′nik pŭr′pyŭr-ă) A systemic illness characterized by extensive ecchymoses and hemorrhages from mucous membranes and very low platelet counts; due to destruction in the spleen of platelets to which an autoimmune globulin is bound. SYN thrombopenic purpura.

id·i·o·phren·ic (id′ē-ō-fren′ik) Relating to, or originating in, the mind or brain alone, not reflex or secondary.

id·i·o·syn·cra·sy (id′ē-ō-singk′ră-sē) A characteristic, reaction, or physical finding peculiar to an individual.

id·i·o·syn·crat·ic drug ef·fect (id′ē-ō-sin-krat′ik drŭg e-fekt′) Drug reactions that occur only rarely and unpredictably.

id·i·o·tope (id′ē-ō-tōp) Single antigenic determinant of an idiotype. SYN idiotypic antigenic determinant.

id·i·o·troph·ic (id′ē-ō-trō′fik) Capable of choosing its own food.

id·i·ot-sa·vant (ē′dē-ō′sah-vawn[h]′) Someone of low general intelligence who possesses an unusual facility in performing some mental tasks that most normal people cannot do.

id·i·o·type (ID) (id′ē-ō-tīp) Collection of idiotopes within the variable region that confers on an immunoglobulin molecule an antigenic specificity and is frequently a unique attribute of a given antibody in a given animal. SEE idiotope.

id·i·o·typ·ic an·ti·bod·y (id′ē-ō-tip′ik an′ti-bod-ē) An antibody that binds to an idiotope of another antibody.

id·i·o·typ·ic an·ti·gen·ic de·ter·mi·nant (id′ē-ō-tip′ik an′ti-jen′ik dĕ-tĕr′mi-nănt) Single antigenic determinant of an idiotype. SYN idiotope.

id·i·o·ven·tric·u·lar rhythm (id′ē-ō-ven-trik′yū-lăr ridh′ŭm) A slow independent ventricular rhythm under control of an ectopic ventricular center; occurs in heart block and sinus arrest.

i·dox·ur·i·dine (ī′doks-yūr′i-dēn) A pyrimidine analogue that produces both antiviral and anticancer effects by interference with DNA synthesis; a topical agent.

i·fos·fa·mide (ī-fos′fă-mīd) A prodrug antineoplastic alkylating agent.

IgA de·fi·cien·cy (dē-fish′ĕn-sē) Lack of immunogloulin A, which protects against infections of the mucous membranes of the respiratory and digestive tracts. SYN selective immunoglobulin A (IgA) deficiency.

ig·bo-or·a vi·rus (ig´bō-ōr´ă vīr´ŭs) An alphavirus associated with a disease similar to dengue fever.

ig·ni-punc·ture (ig´ni-pŭngk-shŭr) The original procedure of closing a retinal separation by transfixation with cautery.

IHSS Abbreviation for idiopathic hypertrophic subaortic stenosis.

il·e·al, il·e·ac (il´ē-ăl, -ak) **1.** Relating to ileus. **2.** Relating to the ileum.

il·e·al a·tre·si·a (il´ē-ăl ă-trē´zē-ă) Failure of the ileum (last section of the small intestine) to form during fetal stage.

il·e·al con·duit (il´ē-ăl kon´dū-it) Isolated segment of ileum serving as a substitution for the urinary bladder, into which ureters can be implanted, the lumen of which is connected to the skin; used following total cystectomy or other loss of normal bladder function requiring supravesical diversion.

il·e·al di·ver·tic·u·lum (il´ē-ăl dī´vĕr-tik´yū-lŭm) SYN Meckel diverticulum.

il·e·al in·tus·sus·cep·tion (il´ē-ăl in´tŭs-sŭs-sep´shŭn) Process in which one portion of the ileum is ensheathed in another portion of the same bowel division.

il·e·al pouch-a·nal an·as·to·mo·sis (IPAA) (il´ē-ăl powch-ā´năl an-as´tŏ-mō´sis) Surgery that involves attaching the ileum to the anus after the entire colon and rectum have been removed, allowing the patient to pass stool normally and avoid colostomy.

il·e·i·tis (il´ē-ī´tis) Inflammation of the ileum.

ileo- Combining form denoting the ileum; bottom of the small intestine.

il·e·o·a·nal (il´ē-ō-ā´năl) Denoting a relationship to the ileum and the anus.

il·e·o·a·nal an·as·to·mo·sis (il´ē-ō-ā´năl ă-nas´tŏ-mō´sis) Surgical procedure that bypasses the large intestine and attaches the distal end of the small intestine directly to the anus.

il·e·o·a·nal pouch (il´ē-ō-ā´năl powch) One constructed from the ileum and anastomosed to the proximal anus for restoration of continence after proctocolectomy.

ile·o·a·nal pull-through (il´ē-ō-ā´năl pul´thrū) Surgcal removal of colon and inner lining of rectum, leaving rectal outer muscle intact, and pulling the ileum through it to join the anus; allows normal passage of stool.

il·e·o·a·nal res·er·voir (il´ē-ō-ā´năl rez´ĕr-vwahr) Two-stage restorative surgery that removes a section of the colon and uses the ileum to form a new reservoir for waste, which can be expelled through the anus.

ileocaecostomy [Br.] SYN ileocecostomy.

il·e·o·ce·cal (IC) (il´ē-ō-sē´kăl) Relating to both ileum and cecum.

il·e·o·ce·cal in·tus·sus·cep·tion (il´ē-ō-sē´kăl in´tŭ-sŭ-sep´shŭn) Act of taking up or reception in which the lower segment of the ileum passes through the valve of the colon into the cecum.

il·e·o·ce·cal junc·tion (ICJ) (il´ē-ō-sē´kăl jŭngk´shŭn) Point along the course of the gastrointestinal tract where the small intestine ends as it opens into the cecal portion of the large intestine; occurs within the iliac fossa, demarcated internally as the ileocecal orifice.

il·e·o·ce·co·cys·to·plas·ty (il´ē-ō-sē´kō-sis´tō-plas´tē) Bladder reconstruction and augmentation with an isolated vascularized segment of ileocecum.

il·e·o·ce·cos·to·my (il´ē-ō-sē-kos´tŏ-mē) Anastomosis of the ileum to the cecum. SYN cecoileostomy, ileocaecostomy.

il·e·o·co·lic, il·e·o·co·lon·ic (il´ē-ō-kol´ik, -kŏ-lon´ik) Relating to the ileum and the colon.

il·e·o·co·li·tis (il´ē-ō-kŏ-lī´tis) Inflammation of both ileum and colon.

il·e·o·co·los·to·my (il´ē-ō-kŏ-los´tŏ-mē) Establishment of a new communication between the ileum and the colon.

il·e·o·cys·to·plas·ty (il´ē-ō-sis´tō-plas-tē) Surgical reconstruction of the bladder involving the use of an isolated intestinal segment to augment bladder capacity.

il·e·o·cys·tos·to·my (il'ē-ō-sis-tos'tŏ-mē) Surgically adapting a segment of the ileum to create a passage for urine through an opening in the abdominal wall.

il·e·o·il·e·os·to·my (il'ē-ō-il-ē-os'tŏ-mē) **1.** Establishment of a communication between two segments of the ileum. **2.** The opening so established.

il·e·o·pex·y (il'ē-ō-pek-sē) Surgical fixation of the ileum.

il·e·or·rha·phy (il'ē-ōr'ă-fē) Suturing the ileum.

il·e·o·sig·moid·os·to·my (il'ē-ō-sig'moyd-os'tŏ-mē) Establishment of a communication between the ileum and the sigmoid colon.

il·e·os·to·my (il'ē-os'tŏ-mē) **1.** Establishment of a fistula through which the ileum discharges the bowel's contents directly to the outside of the body. **2.** A type of fecal diversion.

il·e·os·to·my bag (il'ē-os'tŏ-mē bag) Plastic or latex pouch attached to the body to collect urine or fecal material after surgical procedures.

il·e·ot·o·my (il'ē-ot'ŏ-mē) Incision into the ileum.

il·e·o·trans·verse co·los·to·my (il'ē-ō-tranz-vĕrs' kŏ-los'tŏ-mē) Anastomosis between the ileum and transverse colon.

il·e·o·ves·i·cos·to·my (il'ē-ō-ves'i-kos'tŏ-mē) Surgically adapting an ileal section to create a channel for passage of urine through an opening on the abdominal surface.

il·e·um, pl. **il·e·a** (il'ē-ŭm, -ă) [TA] The third portion of the small intestine, about 3.6 m (12 ft) in length, extending from the jejunum to the ileocecal opening.

il·i·ac (il'ē-ak) Relating to the ilium.

il·i·ac co·lon (il'ē-ak kŏ'lŏn) Portion of the descending colon that occupies the left iliac fossa between the crest of the left ilium and the pelvic brim.

il·i·ac crest (il'ē-ak krest) [TA] The long, curved upper border of the wing of the ilium.

ilio- Combining form meaning the ilium; top of hip bone.

il·i·o·coc·cyg·e·al (IC) (il'ē-ō-kok-sij'ē-ăl) Relating to the ilium and coccyx.

il·i·o·cos·tal (il'ē-ō-kos'tăl) Relating to the ilium and ribs; denoting muscles passing between the two parts.

il·i·o·fem·o·ral (il'ē-ō-fem'ŏr-ăl) Relating to the ilium and the femur.

il·i·o·in·gui·nal (il'ē-ō-ing'gwi-năl) Relating to the iliac region and the groin.

il·i·o·lum·bar (il'ē-ō-lŭm'bahr) Relating to the iliac and the lumbar regions.

il·i·o·lum·bar lig·a·ment (il'ē-ō-lŭm'bahr lig'ă-mĕnt) [TA] Strong ligament that connects the fourth and fifth lumbar vertebrae with the ilium, spanning the "notch" between the vertebral column and the wing of the ilium. SYN ligamentum iliolumbale [TA].

il·i·o·lum·bar vein (il'ē-ō-lŭm'bahr vān) [TA] Accompanying the artery of the same name, anastomosing with the lumbar and deep circumflex iliac veins, and emptying into the internal iliac vein. SYN vena iliolumbalis [TA].

il·i·o·pec·tin·e·al (il'ē-ō-pek-tin'ē-ăl) Relating to the ilium and the pubis.

il·i·o·tib·i·al (IT) (il'ē-ō-tib'ē-ăl) Relating to the ilium and tibia.

il·i·o·tib·i·al band fric·tion syn·drome (il'ē-ō-tib'ē-ăl band frik'shŭn sin'drōm) A painful condition affecting the hip, thigh, or knee; produced by irritation of the iliotibial tract as it glides over the greater trochanter, and other structures.

il·i·o·tro·chan·ter·ic (il'ē-ō-trō'kan-ter'ik) Relating to the ilium and the great trochanter of the femur.

il·i·um (il'ē-ŭm) [TA] The broad, flaring portion of the hip bone, distinct at birth but later becoming fused with the ischium and pubis. SYN iliac bone.

il·li·cit (il-is′it) Not permitted; unlawful, as in illicit drugs.

il·lit·er·ate (il-it′ĕr-ăt) Unable to read and write.

ill·ness (il′nĕs) SYN disease (1).

ill·ness ex·pe·ri·ence (il′nĕs eks-pēr′ē-ĕns) A patient's report of her/his illness, not just the clinical signs and symptoms; a concept in patient-centered interviewing.

il·lu·mi·na·tion (i-lū′mi-nā′shŭn) 1. Throwing light on the body or a part or into a cavity for diagnostic purposes. 2. Lighting an object under a microscope.

im·age (im′ăj) 1. Representation of an object made by the rays of light emanating or reflected from it. 2. Representation produced by x-rays, ultrasound, tomography, thermography, radioisotopes, or other modalities. 3. To produce such a representation.

im·age am·pli·fi·er (im′ăj am′pli-fī′ĕr) A device for converting a low light level fluoroscopic image to one that can be seen by the eye in a lighted environment; usually consists of an electronic light amplifier chained to a television tube.

im·age in·ten·si·fi·er (II) (im′ăj in-ten′si-fī′ĕr) SYN image amplifier.

im·ag·er·y (im′ăj-rē) A technique in behavior therapy in which patient is conditioned to substitute pleasant fantasies to counter anxiety.

im·ag·ing (im′ăj-ing) Production of a clinical image using x-rays, ultrasound, computed tomography, magnetic resonance, radionuclide scanning, or thermography; especially, cross-sectional imaging (e.g., ultrasonography, CT, MRI). SEE image.

i·ma·go, pl. **i·mag·i·nes** (i-mā′gō, i-mā′ji-nēz) The last stage of an insect after it has completed all its metamorphoses through the egg, larva, and pupa; the adult insect form.

im·a·tin·ib (im-ă-tin′ib) An oral agent important in the treatment of chronic myeloid leukemia and gastrointestinal stromal tumors.

im·bal·ance (im-bal′ăns) 1. Lack of equality between opposing forces. 2. Lack of equality in some aspect of binocular vision.

im·bi·bi·tion (im′bi-bish′ŭn) 1. Absorption of fluid by a solid body without resultant chemical change in either. 2. Taking up of water by a gel, thereby increasing its size.

im·bri·cate, im·bri·cat·ed (im′bri-kāt, -kāt′ĕd) Overlapping, like roof shingles.

ImD$_{50}$ Abbreviation meaning 50% of the dose required to cause immunity to a pathogen.

im·id·a·zole (i-mid′i-zōl) A five-membered heterocyclic compound occurring in L-histidine and other biologically important compounds.

im·ide (im′īd) The radical or group, =NH, attached to two –CO– groups.

imido- Prefix denoting the radical of an imide, formed by the loss of the H of the =NH group.

-imine Suffix denoting the group =NH.

im·ine (i-mēn′) A common substrate in a variety of chemical reactions.

imino- Prefix denoting the group =NH.

im·i·no ac·ids (im′i-nō as′idz) Compounds with molecules containing both an acid group and an imino group.

im·i·no·gly·ci·nu·ri·a (im′i-nō-glī′si-nyūr′ē-ă) A benign inborn error of amino acid transport in renal tubule and intestine.

im·i·pen·em (im′i-pen′em) A beta-lactam antibiotic derived from thienamycin with broad spectrum activity used, in combination with cilastin, to treat various infections.

im·i·qui·mod (im′i-kwi′mod) An immune response modifier used dermally to treat external genital and perianal warts.

Im·lach fat-pad (im′lăk fat′pad) Fat surrounding the round ligament of the uterus in the inguinal canal.

im·ma·ture (im′ă-chūr′) Not fully developed; in process.

im·ma·ture cat·a·ract (i′mă-chŭr′ kat′ ăr-akt) A stage of partial lens opacification.

im·me·di·ate al·ler·gy (i-mē′dē-ăt al′ĕr-jē) A type I allergic reaction; so called because in a sensitized subject the reaction becomes evident usually within minutes after contact with the allergen (antigen), reaches its peak within an hour or so, then rapidly recedes.

im·me·di·ate aus·cul·ta·tion, di·rect aus·cul·ta·tion (i-mē′dē-ăt aws′kŭl-tā′shŭn, dĭr-ekt′) Listening to body sounds by application of the ear or a stethoscope to the surface of the body.

im·me·di·ate flap (i-mē′dē-ăt flap) SYN direct flap.

im·me·di·ate hy·per·sen·si·tiv·i·ty (IH) (i-mē′dē-ăt hī′pĕr-sen-si-tiv′i-tē) Exaggerated immune response mediated by mast cell-bound immunoglobulin E antibodies occurring within minutes after exposing a sensitized individual to the approximate antigen; also called Type I hypersensitivity. SEE allergy. SYN immediate allergy, immediate hypersensitivity reaction.

im·me·di·ate per·cus·sion (i-mē′dē-ăt pĕr-kŭsh′ŭn) The striking of the part under examination directly with the finger or a plessor, without using another finger or plessimeter.

im·me·di·ate post·trau·mat·ic au·tom·a·tism (i-mē′dē-ăt pōst-traw-mat′ik aw-tom′ă-tizm) Posttraumatic state in which the patient performs automatically without immediate or later memory of that behavior.

im·me·di·ate trans·fu·sion (i-mē′dē-ăt trans-fyū′zhŭn) SYN direct transfusion.

im·mer·sion foot (i-mĕr′zhŭn fut) A condition resulting from prolonged exposure to damp and cold; the extremity is initially cold and anesthetic, but on rewarming becomes hyperemic, paresthetic, and hyperhidrotic; recovery is often slow. SYN immersion injury (2), trenchfoot.

im·mer·sion in·ju·ry (i-mĕr′zhŭn in′jŭr-ē) **1.** Trauma related to near drowning. **2.** SYN immersion foot.

im·mis·ci·ble (i-mis′i-bĕl) Incapable of mutual solution, e.g., oil and water.

immobilisation [Br.] SYN immobilization.

im·mo·bi·li·za·tion (i-mō′bi-lī-zā′shŭn) The act or process of fixing or rendering immobile. SYN immobilisation.

im·mo·bi·lize (i-mō′bi-līz) To render fixed or incapable of moving.

im·mor·tal·i·za·tion (i-mōr′tăl-ī-zā′shŭn) Conferring on normal cells cultured in vitro the property of an infinite lifespan, as from spontaneous mutation, by exposure to chemical carcinogens, or by viral infection.

im·mo·tile cil·i·a syn·drome (ICS) (i-mō′til sil′ē-ă sin′drōm) Inherited disorder characterized by recurrent sinopulmonary infections, reduced fertility in women, and sterility in men due to the inability of ciliated structures to beat effectively because of the absence of one or both dynein arms.

im·mov·a·ble joint (i-mū′vă-bĕl joynt) SYN fibrous joint.

im·mune (i-myūn′) **1.** Free from the possibility of acquiring a given infectious disease; resistant to an infectious disease. **2.** Pertaining to cell-mediated or humoral immunity, whereby an organism is so altered by previous contact with an antigen that it responds quickly and on specifically subsequent contact.

im·mune ad·her·ence (i-myūn′ ad-hēr′ ĕns) The binding of antigen-antibody complexes or cells coated with antibodies or complement to cells bearing the appropriate complement or Fc receptors.

im·mune ad·sorp·tion (i-myūn′ ad-sōrp′shŭn) **1.** Removal of antibody from antiserum by use of specific antigen. **2.** Removal of antigen by specific antiserum.

im·mune ag·glu·ti·nin (i-myūn′ ă-glū′ti-nin) SYN agglutinin (1).

im·mune com·plex (i-myūn′ kom′pleks) Antigen combined with specific antibody, to which complement may also be fixed and may precipitate or remain in solution. Frequently associated with autoimmune disease.

im·mune com·plex dis·ease (i-myūn′ kom′pleks di-zēz′) Immunologic category of diseases evoked by the deposition of antigen-antibody or antigen-antibody-complement complexes on cell surfaces, with subsequent development of vasculitis. SEE ALSO autoimmune disease.

im·mune de·vi·a·tion (i-myūn′ dē-vē-ā′shŭn) SYN split tolerance.

im·mune he·mol·y·sis (i-myūn′ hē-mol′i-sis) That caused by complement when erythrocytes have been sensitized by specific complement-fixing antibody. SYN conditioned hemolysis.

im·mune op·so·nin (i-myūn′ op′sŏ-nin) SYN specific opsonin.

im·mune pa·ral·y·sis (i-myūn′ păr-al′i-sis) The induction of tolerance due to injection of large amounts of antigen. The antigen is poorly metabolized and the paralysis remains only during the persistence of the above antigen.

im·mune pro·tein (i-myūn′ prō′tēn) SYN antibody.

im·mune re·ac·tion (i-myūn′ rē-ak′shŭn) Process mediated by humoral or cell-mediated immune mechanisms.

im·mune re·sponse (i-myūn′ rĕ-spons′) Any response of the immune system to an antigen including antibody production or cell-mediated immunity.

im·mune re·sponse genes (i-myūn′ rĕ-spons′ jĕnz) Those in the human leukocyte antigen-D region of the histocompatibility complex of human chromosome 6 that control the immune response to specific antigens.

im·mune se·rum (i-myūn′ sēr′ŭm) SYN antiserum.

im·mune se·rum glob·u·lin (ISG) (i-myūn′ sēr′ŭm glob′yū-lin) Sterile solution of globulins that contains many antibodies normally present in adult human blood.

im·mune sta·tus (i-myūn′ stat′ŭs) The ability of the body to demonstrate an im-

mune response or to defend itself against disease or foreign substances.

im·mune sur·veil·lance (i-myūn′ sŭr-vā′lăns) A theory that the immune system destroys tumor cells, which are constantly arising during the life of the individual.

im·mune sys·tem (i-myūn′ sis′tĕm) An intricate complex of interrelated cellular, molecular, and genetic components, which provides a defense against foreign organisms and aberrant native cells.

im·mu·ni·ty (i-myū′ni-tē) The status or quality of being immune (1). SYN insusceptibility.

im·mu·ni·za·tion (immun, IMM) (im′myū-nī-zā′shŭn) Protection of susceptible patients from communicable diseases by administration of a living modified agent, a suspension of killed organisms, a protein expressed in a heterologous organism, or an inactivated toxin. SEE ALSO vaccination.

im·mu·nize (im′yū-nīz) To render immune.

immuno- Combining form meaning immune, immunity.

im·mu·no·ab·la·tion (im′yū-nō-ă-blā′shŭn) The systematic weakening or destruction of a patient's immunoresponse, which is undertaken to prepare the patient for imminent organ transplantation.

im·mu·no·ab·sorp·tion (im′yū-nō-ăb-sōrp′shŭn) A technique for removing antibodies from a patient.

im·mu·no·ad·ju·vant (im′yū-nō-ad′jū-vănt) SEE adjuvant (2).

im·mu·no·as·say (im′yū-nō-as′ā) Detection and assay of substances by serologic (immunologic) methods.

im·mun·o·bi·ol·o·gy (im′yū-nō-bī-ōl′ŏ-jē) The study of the immune factors that affect the growth, development, and health of biologic organisms.

im·mu·no·blast (im′yū-nō-blast) An antigenically stimulated lymphocyte; a large cell with well-defined basophilic cytoplasm, a large nucleus with prominent nuclear membrane, distinct nucleoli, and clumped chromatin.

im·mu·no·blot, im·mu·no·blot·ting (im′yū-nō-blot′, -blot′ing) Process by which antigens can be separated by electrophoresis and blotted to nitrocellulose sheets, where they bind and are subsequently identified by staining with labeled antibodies.

im·mu·no·chem·is·try (im′yū-nō-kem′is-trē) The field of chemistry concerned with chemical aspects of immunologic phenomena.

im·mu·no·che·mo·ther·a·py (im′yū-nō-kē′mō-thār′ă-pē) Intercurrent use of immunotherapy and chemotherapy to treat or control diseases.

im·mu·no·com·pe·tence (im′yū-nō-kom′pĕ-tĕns) The ability to produce a normal immune response.

im·mu·no·com·plex (im′yū-nō-kom′pleks) SEE immune complex.

im·mu·no·com·pro·mised (IC) (im′yū-nō-kom′prŏ-mīzd) Denoting a person with an immunologic mechanism deficient either because of an immunodeficiency disorder or because it has been so rendered by immunosuppressive agents.

im·mu·no·con·glu·ti·nin (im′yū-nō-kŏn-glū′ti-nin) An autoantibodylike immunoglobulin (IgM) formed by an organism against its own complement, following injection of complement-containing complexes or sensitized bacteria.

im·mu·no·cyte (im′yū-nō-sīt) An immunologically competent leukocyte capable of producing antibodies or reacting in cell-mediated immunity reactions. SEE ALSO I cell.

im·mu·no·cy·to·ad·her·ence (im′yū-nō-sī′tŏ-ad-hēr′ĕns) A method for determining cell surface properties, in which immunoglobulin or receptors on the surface of one cell population cause cells with corresponding molecular configurations on their surface to adhere in rosettes.

im·mu·no·cy·to·chem·is·try (im′yū-nō-sī′tŏ-kem′is-trē) The study of cell constituents by immunologic methods.

im·mu·no·de·fi·cien·cy (im′yū-nō-dĕ-fish′ĕn-sē) A condition resulting from a defective immune mechanism; may be primary (due to a defect in the immune mechanism itself) or secondary (dependent on another disease process).

im·mu·no·de·fi·cien·cy dis·ease (im′yū-nō-dĕ-fish′ĕn-sē di-zēz′) A disorder or condition related to a defective or suppressed immune response.

im·mu·no·de·fi·cient (im′yū-nō-dĕ-fish′ĕnt) Lacking in some essential function of the immune system.

im·mu·no·di·ag·no·sis (im′yū-nō-dī′ag-nō′sis) The process of determining specified immunologic characteristics of individuals or of cells, sera, or other biologic specimens.

im·mu·no·dif·fu·sion (im′yū-nō-di-fyū′zhŭn) A technique of studying antigen-antibody reactions by observing precipitates formed by combination of specific antigen and antibodies that have diffused in a gel in which they have been separately placed.

im·mu·no·e·lec·tron mi·cros·co·py (im′yū-nō-ē-lek′tron mī-kros′kŏ-pē) Clinical technique employing antibodies to detect intracellular locations of structures or proteins at high-resolution electron microscopy.

im·mu·no·e·lec·tro·pho·re·sis (im′yū-nō-ĕ-lek′trō-fōr-ē′sis) A kind of precipitin test in which the components of one group of immunologic reactants are first separated on the basis of electrophoretic mobility, the separated components then being identified on the basis of precipitates formed by reaction with components of the other group of reactants.

im·mu·no·fer·ri·tin (im′yū-nō-fer′i-tin) Antibody-ferritin conjugate used to identify an antigen by electron microscopy.

im·mu·no·fluor·es·cence (im′yū-nō-flōr-es′ĕns) An immunohistochemical technique using labeling of antibodies by fluorescent dyes to identify bacterial, viral, or other antigenic material specific for the labeled antibody. SEE ALSO fluorescent antibody technique.

im·mu·no·gen (i-myū′nō-jen) SYN antigen.

im·mu·no·ge·net·ics (im'yū-nō-jĕ-net' iks) The study of the genetics of transplantation and tissue rejection, histochemical loci, immunologic response, immunoglobulin structure, and immunosuppression.

im·mu·no·ge·nic·i·ty (im'yū-nō-jĕ-nis' i-tē) SYN antigenicity.

im·mu·no·glob·u·lin (Ig, IG) (im'yū-nō-glob'yū-lin) One of a class of structurally related proteins, each consisting of two pairs of polypeptide chains, one pair of light (L) low molecular weight chains (κ or λ), and one pair of heavy (H) chains (γ, α, μ, δ, and ε), usually all four linked by disulfide bonds.

im·mu·no·glob·u·lin A (IgA) (im'yū-nō-glob'yū-lin) An antibody that provides mucosal immunity; the major antibody found in mucous secretions, and other excreted bodily solutions.

im·mu·no·glob·u·lin D (IgD) (im'yū-nō-glob'yū-lin) An antibody isotope present in small amounts in the body; it acts as part of the immune response.

im·mu·no·glob·u·lin E (IgE) (im'yū-nō-glob'yū-lin) An antibody that is vital in allergic and immune responses.

im·mu·no·glob·u·lin G (IgG) (im'yū-nō-glob'yū-lin) Most abundant immunoglobulin; active against various pathogenic agents including bacteria and fungi.

im·mu·no·glob·u·lin M (IgM) (im'yū-nō-glob'yū-lin) An antibody present in bodily fluids; largest antibody; activated first in presence of an allergic threat.

im·mu·no·he·ma·tol·o·gy (im'yū-nō-hē'mă-tol'ŏ-jē) Division of hematology concerned with immune, or antigen-antibody reactions, and with related changes in blood.

im·mu·no·log·ic, im·mu·no·log·ic·al (im'yū-nō-loj'ik, -loj'i-kăl) Pertaining to the study of bodily immunity.

im·mu·no·log·ic com·pe·tence (im'yū-nō-loj'ik kom'pĕ-tĕns) Capability of mounting an immunologic response.

im·mu·nol·o·gy (im'yū-nol'ŏ-jē) 1. The science concerned with the various phenomena of immunity, induced sensitivity, and allergy. 2. Study of the structure and function of the immune system.

im·mu·no·mod·u·la·to·ry (im'yū-nō-mod'yū-lă-tōr-ē) 1. Capable of modifying or regulating one or more immune functions. 2. An immunologic adjustment, regulation, or potentiation.

im·mu·no·pa·thol·o·gy (im'yū-nō-pă-thol'ŏ-jē) Study of diseases or conditions due to immune reactions.

im·mu·no·po·ten·ti·a·tion (im'yū-nō-pŏ-ten'shē-ā'shŭn) Enhancement of the immune response by increasing its rate or prolonging its duration.

im·mu·no·pre·cip·i·ta·tion (IPT) (im' yū-nō-prĕ-sip'i-tā'shŭn) The phenomenon of aggregation of sensitized antigen on addition of specific antibody (precipitin) to antigen in solution. SYN immune precipitation.

im·mu·no·pro·lif·er·a·tive dis·or·ders (im'myū-nō-prō-lif'ĕr-ă-tiv dis-ōr'dĕrz) Those with a continuing proliferation of cells of the immunocyte complex associated with autoallergic disturbances and immunoglobulin abnormalities.

im·mu·no·re·ac·tion (im'yū-nō-rē-ak'shŭn) Any immunologic activity, but especially those that occur in vitro between antigen and antibody.

im·mu·no·se·lec·tion (im'yū-nō-sĕ-lek'shŭn) 1. Selective death or survival of fetuses of different genotypes depending on immunologic incompatibility with the mother. 2. The survival of certain cells depending on their surface antigenicity.

im·mu·no·sor·bent (im'yū-nō-sōr'bĕnt) An antibody (or antigen) used to remove specific antigens (or antibodies) from solution or suspension.

im·mu·no·sup·pres·sant (im'yū-nō-sŭ-pres'ănt) An agent that induces immunosuppression. SYN immunosuppressive (2).

im·mu·no·sup·pres·sion (im'yū-nō-sŭ-presh'ŭn) Prevention or interference with the development of immunologic response; may reflect natural immunologic unresponsiveness (tolerance), may be artificially induced by chemical, biologic, or physical agents, or may be caused by disease.

im·mu·no·sup·pres·sive (im′yū-nō-sŭ-pres′iv) **1.** Denoting or inducing immunosuppression. **2.** SYN immunosuppressant.

im·mu·no·sup·pres·sive ther·a·py (im′yū-nō-sŭ-pres′iv thār′ă-pē) Medication given to patients to curb response by their immune systems.

im·mu·no·ther·a·py (im′yū-nō-thār′ă-pē) Originally, therapeutic administration of serum or immune globulin containing preformed antibodies produced by another person; currently, immunotherapy includes nonspecific systemic stimulation, adjuvants, active specific immunotherapy, and adoptive immunotherapy. New forms of immunotherapy include the use of monoclonal antibodies. SYN biologic immunotherapy.

im·mu·no·tox·in (im′yū-nō-tokśin) A molecule that combines an antibody or antigen and a toxin to kill specific cell types.

im·mu·no·trans·fu·sion (im′yū-nō-transfyŭ′zhŭn) An indirect transfusion in which the donor is first immunized by injections of antigen from microorganisms isolated from the recipient; later, the donor's blood is collected, defibrinated, and then administered to the patient; the latter is thus passively immunized by antibody formed in the donor.

im·pact·ed (im-pak′tĕd) Wedged or pressed closely so as to be immovable.

im·pact·ed fe·tus (im-pak′tĕd fē′tŭs) One that, because of its large size or narrowing of the pelvic canal, has become wedged and incapable of spontaneous advance or recession.

im·pact·ed frac·ture (im-pak′tĕd frak′shŭr) Breakage in which one of the fragments is driven into the cancellous bone of the other fragment.

im·pact·ed tooth (im-pak′tĕd tūth) **1.** A tooth the normal eruption of which is prevented by adjacent teeth or bone. **2.** A tooth that has been driven into the alveolar process or surrounding tissue as a result of trauma.

im·pac·tion (impx) (im-pak′shŭn) The process or condition of being impacted.

im·paired gas ex·change (im-pārd′ gas eks-chānj′) A nursing diagnosis for a patient suffering current or future problems with oxygen/carbon dioxide balance.

im·paired glu·cose tol·er·ance (IGT) (im-pārd′ glū′kōs tol′ĕr-ăns) A disordered state in which a patient does not process glucose properly but such activity does not confirm a diagnosis of diabetes mellitus. SEE ALSO Type 1 diabetes, Type 2 diabetes.

im·paired phys·ic·al mo·bil·ity (im-pārd′ fiz′i-kăl mō-bil′i-tē) A nursing diagnosis for a patient who is suffering from an inability to control physical movement.

im·paired skin in·teg·ri·ty (im-pārd′ skin in-teg′ri-tē) A nursing diagnosis indicating adverse dermal reactions, present or possible.

im·paired spon·ta·ne·ous ven·til·a·tion (im-pārd′ spon-tā′nē-ŭs ven′ti-lā′shŭn) A nursing diagnosis referring to a patient who is unable to maintain adequate vital respiration.

im·paired tis·sue in·teg·ri·ty (im-pārd′ tish′ū in-teg′ri-tē) A nursing diagnosis referring to current or possible skin damage, in hospitalized patients.

im·paired trans·fer a·bil·i·ty (im-pārd′ trans′fĕr ă-bil′i-tē) A nursing diagnosis referring to a patient's inability to move from one flat surface to another or to change position from standing up to sitting down.

im·paired ver·bal com·mu·ni·ca·tion (im-pārd′ vĕr′băl kŏ-myū′ni-kā′shŭn) A nursing diagnosis referring to current or possible speech difficulties.

im·paired wheel·chair mo·bil·ity (im-pārd′ wēl′chār mō-bil′i-tē) A nursing diagnosis referring to current or possible inability by a patient to use a wheelchair without difficulty.

im·pair·ment (im-pār′mĕnt) A physical or mental defect at the level of a body system or organ.

im·pal·pa·ble (im-pal′pă-bĕl) Denotes something that cannot be touched.

im·ped·ance (im-pē′dăns) **1.** Opposition to flow of gases, liquids, or electrical current. **2.** Resistance of an acoustic system to being set in motion.

im·ped·ance pleth·ys·mog·ra·phy (im-pē′dăns pleth′iz-mog′ră-fē) Recording changes in electrical impedance between electrodes placed on opposite sides of a part of the body, as a measure of volume changes in the path of the current. SYN dielectrography.

im·per·fect fun·gus (im-pĕr′fĕkt fŭng′gŭs) One in which the means of sexual reproduction is not yet recognized; these fungi generally reproduce by means of conidia.

im·per·fo·rate (im-pĕr′fŏr-ăt) SYN atretic.

im·per·fo·rate a·nus (im-pĕr′fŏr-ăt ā′nŭs) **1.** SYN anal atresia. **2.** SYN ectopic (1).

im·per·fo·rate hy·men (im-pĕr′fŏr-ăt hī′mĕn) Condition in which the membrane has no opening and completely occludes the vagina.

im·per·fo·ra·tion (im′pĕr-fŏr-ā′shŭn) Condition of being atretic, occluded, or closed.

im·per·me·a·ble (im-pĕr′mē-ă-bĕl) SEE atresia.

im·pe·ti·go (im-pĕ-tī′gō) Contagious superficial pyoderma, caused by *Staphylococcus aureus* and/or group A streptococci, which begins with a superficial flaccid vesicle that ruptures and forms a yellowish crust; most common in children. SYN impetigo contagiosa, impetigo vulgaris.

im·pe·ti·go her·pet·i·for·mis (im-pĕ-tī′gō hĕr-pet-i-fōr′mis) A pyoderma, most common in the third trimester of pregnancy as an eruption of small closely aggregated pustules accompanied by severe constitutional symptoms and fetal death.

im·pe·ti·go ne·o·na·to·rum (IN) (im-pĕ-tī′gō nē′ō-nă-tō′rŭm) **1.** SYN dermatitis exfoliativa infantum. **2.** SYN bullous impetigo of newborn.

im·pinge·ment syn·drome (im-pinj′mĕnt sin′drōm) Chronic shoulder pain and disability due to trauma to the rotator cuff (particularly the supraspinatus tendon) by surrounding bony processes and ligaments.

im·plant (im-plant′, im′plant) **1.** To graft or insert. **2.** (im′plant) Material inserted or grafted. SEE ALSO graft, transplant. **3.** ORTHOPAEDICS a device employed in joint reconstruction.

im·plant·a·ble car·di·o·ver·ter-de·fib·ril·la·tor (im-plant′ă-bĕl kahr′dē-ō-vĕr-tĕr-dē-fib′yū-lā-tŏr) A device surgically inserted into the thoracic area that monitors cardiac activity and is capable of adjusting current flow to deal with arrythmias.

im·plant·a·ble hear·ing de·vice (IHD) (im-plant′ă-bĕl hēr′ing dĕ-vīs′) Electronic instrument that is placed within the ear surgically to improve audition.

im·plan·ta·tion (im′plan-tā′shŭn) **1.** The process of placing a device or substance within the body. **2.** Insertion of a natural tooth into an artificially constructed alveolus. **3.** Tissue grafting.

im·plant den·ture (im′plant den′chŭr) A denture that receives its stability and retention from a substructure that is partially or wholly implanted under the soft tissues of the denture basal seat.

im·plo·sion (im-plō′zhŭn) **1.** A sudden collapse, as of an evacuated vessel, in which there is a bursting inward rather than outward as in an explosion. **2.** A type of behavior therapy, similar to flooding, during which the patient is given massive exposure to extreme anxiety-arousing stimuli by being asked to describe, and thus relive in imagination, those life events or situations typically producing these overwhelming emotional reactions. As the patient does so, the therapist attempts to extinguish the future influence of such unconscious material over the patient's behavior and feelings, and previous avoidance responses to the stimuli are replaced by more appropriate responses.

im·po·tence, im·po·ten·cy (im′pŏ-tĕns, -tĕn-sē) **1.** Weakness; lack of power. **2.** Inability of the male to achieve and/or maintain penile erection and thus engage in copulation; a manifestation of neurologic, vascular, or psychological dysfunction.

im·preg·na·tion (im′preg-nā′shŭn) **1.** The act of making pregnant. **2.** The process of diffusing or permeating with another substance. SEE ALSO saturation.

im·pres·sion, im·pres·si·o (im-presh′ŭn, -pres′ē-ō) [TA] **1.** A mark seemingly made by the pressure of one structure or organ on another, seen especially in cadaveric dissections. **2.** An effect produced on the mind by some external object acting through the organs of sense. **3.** An imprint or negative likeness; especially, the negative form of the teeth and/or other tissues of the oral cavity, made in a plastic material that becomes relatively hard while in contact with these tissues, made to reproduce a positive form or cast of the recorded tissues.

im·pres·sion ma·te·ri·al (im-presh′ŭn mă-tēr′ē-ăl) Substance or combination of substances used to make a negative reproduction.

im·pres·sion tray (im-presh′ŭn trā) A U-shaped receptacle that holds the material used for making a dental impression; can be metal or plastic, and prefabricated or custom made in the dental laboratory.

im·print·ed gene (im-print′ĕd jēn) A gene the expression of which varies according to which parent passed along its characteristics.

im·print·ing (im′print-ing) A particular kind of learning characterized by its occurrence in the first few hours of life, which determines species-recognition behavior.

im·pulse (im′pŭls) **1.** A sudden pushing or driving force. **2.** A sudden, often unreasoning, determination to perform some act. **3.** The action potential of a nerve fiber.

im·pulse con·trol dis·or·der (im′pŭls kŏn-trōl′ dis-ōr′dĕr) A class of mental disorders characterized by failure to resist an impulse to perform some act harmful to oneself or to others; includes pathologic gambling, pedophilia, kleptomania, pyromania, trichotillomania, and intermittent or isolated explosive disorders.

In 1. Symbol for indium. **2.** Abbreviation for inulin.

♻ **in-** Prefix meaning (1) Not, thus akin to G. *a-*, *an-* or Eng. *un-*; (2) In, within, inside; (3) Very; appears as *im-* before b, p, or m.

in·ac·ti·va·ted vac·cine (in-ak′ti-vāt-ĕd vak-sēn′) One prepared from a deactivated pathogen.

in·ac·ti·va·tion (in-ak′ti-vā′shŭn) The process of destroying or removing the activity or the effects of an agent or substance.

in·ac·tive re·pres·sor (in-ak′tiv rĕ-pres′ŏr) One that cannot combine with an operator gene until it has combined with a corepressor (usually a product of a protein pathway); after activation, it arrests production of the proteins controlled by the operator gene. SYN aporepressor.

in·an·i·mate (in-an′i-măt) Not alive.

in·a·ni·tion (in′ă-nish′ŭn) Severe weakness and wasting as results from lack of food, defect in assimilation, or neoplastic disease.

in·ap·pe·tence (in-ap′ĕ-tĕns) Lack of desire or of craving.

in·ar·tic·u·late (in′ahr-tik′yū-lăt) **1.** Not fluent in the form of intelligible speech. **2.** Unable to satisfactorily express oneself in words.

in ar·ti·cu·lo mor·tis (in ahr-tik′yū-lō mōr′tis) Latin expression meaning at the point or moment of death.

in·born (in′bōrn) Implanted during development in utero. SEE inborn errors of metabolism. SYN innate.

in·born er·rors of me·tab·o·lism (īn′bōrn er′ŏrz mĕ-tab′ŏ-lizm) A group of disorders, each of which involves a disorder of a single unique enzyme, genetic in origin and operating from birth; effects are ascribable to accumulation of the substrate on which the enzyme normally acts, to deficiency of the product of the enzyme, or to forced metabolism through an auxiliary pathway.

in·breed·ing (in′brēd-ing) **1.** Mating between organisms that are genetically more closely related than organisms selected at random from the population. **2.** A practice of mating animals that are closely related.

in·ca·pac·i·ta·ting Ct$_{50}$ (in′kă-pas′i-tā-ting) The concentration time (Ct) product required to produce incapacitation (temporary decrement in performance) in 50% of an exposed group.

in·ca·pac·i·ta·ting dose (in′kă-pas′i-tā-ting dōs) The dose of a chemical or biologic preparation likely to cause incapacitation.

in·car·cer·at·ed (in-kahr′sĕr-ā-tĕd) Confined; imprisoned; trapped.

in·cep·tion (in-sep′shŭn) Beginning; commencement.

in·cest (in′sest) **1.** Sexual relations between people closely related by blood, especially between parents and their children, and between sibs. **2.** The crime of sexual relations between people related by blood, where such cohabitation is prohibited by law.

in·ci·dence (in′si-dĕns) **1.** The number of specified new events, e.g., people falling ill with a specified disease, during a specified period in a specified population. **2.** optics intersection of a ray of light with a surface.

in·ci·dence rate (in′si-dĕns rāt) Velocity at which new events occur in a population. The numerator is the number of new events occurring in a defined period; the denominator is the population at risk of experiencing the event during this period.

in·ci·dent (in′si-dĕnt) **1.** Going toward; impinging on. **2.** An occurrence or event, generally an untoward, or unwelcome occurrence.

in·ci·dent·a·lo·ma (in′si-den′tă-lō′mă) Mass lesion, usually of the suprarenal gland, serendipitously noted during computed tomographic examinations performed for other reasons.

in·ci·den·tal par·a·site (in′si-den′tăl par′ă-sīt) A parasite that normally lives on a host other than its present host. SYN accidental parasite.

in·ci·pi·ent (in-sip′ē-ĕnt) Not fully formed; vestigial; beginning to appear.

in·ci·sal (in-sī′zăl) Cutting; relating to the cutting edges of the incisor and canine teeth.

in·ci·sal guide (in-sī′zăl gīd) In dentistry, that part of an articulator on which the anterior guide pin rests to maintain the vertical dimension of occlusion and the incisal guide angle as established by the incisal guidance. SYN anterior guide.

in·cise (in-sīz′) To cut with a knife.

in·cised wound (in-sīzd′ wūnd) A clean cut, as by a sharp instrument.

in·ci·sion (in-sizh′ŭn) A cut; a surgical wound; a division of the soft parts made with a knife.

in·ci·sion bi·op·sy (in-sizh′ŭn bī′op-sē) Removal of only a part of a lesion by incising into it.

in·ci·sive (in-sī′siv) **1.** Cutting; having the power to cut. **2.** Relating to the incisor teeth.

in·ci·sor tooth, in·ci·sor (in-sī′zŏr tūth) [TA] Tooth with a chisel-shaped crown and a single conic tapering root; there are four of these teeth in the anterior part of each jaw, in both the deciduous and the permanent dentitions. SYN dens incisivus [TA].

in·ci·su·ra, pl. **in·ci·su·rae** (in′si-sū′ră, -sū′rē) [TA] SYN notch.

in·ci·sure (in-sī′zhŭr) SYN notch.

in·cli·na·ti·o, pl. **in·cli·na·ti·o·nes** (in′kli-nā′shē-ō, -ō′nēz) [TA] SYN inclination.

in·cli·na·tion (in′kli-nā′shŭn) [TA] **1.** A leaning or sloping. **2.** DENTISTRY deviation of the long axis of a tooth from the perpendicular. SYN version (3).

in·clu·sion (in-klū′zhŭn) **1.** Any foreign or heterogeneous substance contained in a cell or in any tissue or organ, not due to trauma. **2.** The process by which a foreign or heterogeneous structure is misplaced in another tissue.

in·clu·sion bod·ies (in-klū′zhŭn bod′ēz) Distinctive structures frequently formed in the nucleus or cytoplasm (occasionally in both locations) in cells infected with certain filtrable viruses.

in·clu·sion cell (in-klū′zhŭn sel) SYN I cell.

in·clu·sion com·plex (in-klū′zhŭn kom′pleks) Unbonded amalgam in which one molecular substance is subsumed into those of a second substance.

in·clu·sion con·junc·ti·vi·tis (in-klū′zhŭn kŏn-jŭngk′ti-vī′tis) A follicular eye disorder caused by *Chlamydia trachomatis*.

in·co·her·ent (in′kō-hēr′ĕnt) Disjointed; confused; denoting a lack of connectedness in verbal expression.

in·com·pat·i·bil·i·ty (in′kŏm-pat′i-bil′i-tē) 1. The quality of being incompatible. 2. A means of classifying bacterial plasmids; two plasmids are incompatible if they cannot coexist in one host cell.

in·com·pat·i·ble (in′kŏm-pat′i-bĕl) 1. Not of suitable composition to be combined or mixed with another agent or substance, without resulting in an undesirable reaction. 2. Denoting those who are unable to associate with one another without resulting anxiety and conflict. 3. Having genotypes that put progeny at high risk of severe recessive disorders or that promote harmful maternal-fetal reaction. 4. Having antigenic nonidentity between a donor and a recipient.

in·com·pe·tence, in·com·pe·ten·cy (in-kom′pĕ-tĕns, -tĕn-sē) 1. The quality of being incompetent or incapable of performing the allotted function. SYN insufficiency (2). 2. FORENSIC PSYCHIATRY inability to distinguish right from wrong or to manage one's affairs. 3. Inability of the cervix to remain closed and thereby continue pregnancy to term.

in·com·pe·tent cer·vi·cal os (in-kom′pĕ-tĕnt sĕr′vi-kăl os) A defect in the strength of the internal os allowing premature dilation of the cervix.

in·com·plete ag·glu·ti·nin (in′kŏm-plēt′ ă-glū′ti-nin) Antibody that binds to antigen but does not induce agglutination.

in·com·plete an·ti·gen (in′kŏm-plēt′ an′ti-jen) SYN hapten.

in·com·plete dom·i·nance (in′kŏm-plēt′ dom′i-năns) A form of genetic inheritance in which neither allele produces true dominance.

in·com·plete frac·ture (in′kŏm-plēt′ frak′shŭr) Breakage in which the bone is not completely divided.

in·com·plete hem·i·a·no·pi·a (in′kŏm-plēt′ hem′ē-ă-nō′pē-ă) Ocular disorder involving less than half the visual field of each eye.

in·com·plete pro·tein (in′kŏm-plēt′ prō′tēn) A proteinaceous food that lacks all essential amino acids.

in·con·gru·ent com·mu·ni·ca·tion (in′kon-grū′ĕnt kŏ-myū′ni-kā′shŭn) Failing to be in agreement; out of synchronism.

in·con·ti·nence, in·con·ti·nen·ti·a (in-kon′ti-nĕns, -nen′shē-ă) 1. Inability to prevent the discharge of urine or feces. 2. Lack of restraint of the appetites, especially sexual.

in·con·ti·nence of fe·ces (in-kon′ti-nĕns fē′sēz) The involuntary voiding of feces into clothing or bedclothes, usually due to pathology affecting sphincter control or loss of cognitive functions.

in·cre·ment (in′krĕ-mĕnt) A change in the value of a variable; usually an increase, with ''decrement'' applied to a decrease, although ''increment'' can also correctly be applied to both.

in·cre·tin (in-krē′tin) Generic term for all insulinotropic substances originating in the gastrointestinal tract that are released into the circulation by meals containing glucose.

in·crus·ta·tion (in′krŭs-tā′shŭn) 1. Formation of a crust or a scab. 2. A coating of some adventitious material or an exudate; a scab.

in·cu·bate (in′kyū-bāt) To maintain an optimal physical environment for growth in some fashion.

in·cu·ba·tion (in′kyū-bā′shŭn) 1. Act of maintaining controlled environmental conditions to favor growth or development of microbial or tissue cultures or to maintain optimal conditions for a chemical or immunologic reaction. **2.** Maintenance of an artificial environment for an infant, usually a premature or hypoxic one, by providing proper temperature, humidity, and, usually, oxygen.

in·cu·ba·tion pe·ri·od (ICP, IP) (in'kyū-bā'shŭn pēr'ē-ŏd) **1.** Interval between invasion of the body by an infecting organism and the appearance of the first sign or symptom it causes; SYN incubative stage, latent period (2), latent stage, stage of invasion. **2.** In a disease vector, the period between entry of the disease organism and the time at which the vector is capable of transmitting the disease to another human host.

in·cu·ba·tor (in'kyū-bā-tŏr) **1.** A container in which controlled environmental conditions can be maintained. **2.** Apparatus to maintain an infant (usually premature) in an environment of proper oxygenation, humidity, and temperature.

in·cu·dal (in'kyū-dăl) Relating to the incus.

in·cu·do·mal·le·al (in-kyū'dō-mal'lē-ăl) Relating to the incus and the malleus; denoting the articulation between the incus and the malleus in the middle ear. SYN ambomalleal.

in·cu·do·sta·pe·di·al (in-kyū'dō-stā-pē'dē-ăl) Relating to the incus and the stapes; denoting the articulation between the incus and the stapes in the middle ear.

in·cur·a·ble (incur) (in-kyūr'ă-bĕl) Denoting a morbid process unresponsive to medical or surgical treatment.

in·cus, pl. **in·cu·des** (ing'kŭs, in-kyū'dēz) [TA] *Avoid the incorrect plural inci.* The middle of the three ossicles in the middle ear. SYN anvil.

in·cy·clo·pho·ri·a (in-sī'klō-fōr'ē-ă) A cyclophoria in which the 12-o'clock position in the iris tends to twist medially.

in·cy·clo·tro·pi·a (in-sī'klō-trō'pē-ă) A cyclotropia in which the upper poles of the corneas are rotated inward (medially) to each other.

in·den·ta·tion (in'den-tā'shŭn) **1.** The act of notching or pitting. **2.** A notch. **3.** A state of being notched.

in·de·pen·dent as·sort·ment (in'dĕ-pen'dĕnt ă-sōrt'mĕnt) Pattern of transmission of unlinked loci.

in·de·pen·dent liv·ing (in'dĕ-pen'dĕnt liv'ing) A philosophy for self-determination and equal opportunity for people with disabilities that includes the right to live with the same opportunities and choices as someone who does not have a disablility.

in·de·pen·dent med·i·cal e·val·u·a·tion (IME) (in'dĕ-pen'dĕnt med'i-kăl ĕ-val'yū-ā'shŭn) Used by insurers to determine a patient's diagnosis, need for continued treatment, degree and permanency of disability, or ability to return to work.

in·de·pen·dent prac·tice as·so·ci·a·tion (in'dĕ-pen'dĕnt prak'tis ă-sō'sē-ā'shŭn) Consortium of independent physicians or small groups of physicians formed to contract with one or more managed health care organizations. Member physicians provide medical services for patients enrolled in those organizations in their own offices and are allowed to maintain private practices.

in·de·pen·dent var·i·a·ble (in'dĕ-pen'dĕnt var'ē-ă-bĕl) STATISTICS a variable that is manipulated by the researcher and measured by the effect it has on the dependent variable or variables.

in·dex, gen. **in·di·cis,** pl. **in·di·ces,** pl. **in·dex·es** (in'deks, -di-sis, -di-sēz, -deks'ez) [TA] **1.** A guide, standard, indicator, symbol, or number denoting the relation in respect to size, capacity, or function, of one part or thing to another. **2.** A core or mold used to record or maintain the relative position of a tooth or teeth to one another or to a cast. **3.** A guide, usually made of plaster, used to reposition teeth, casts, or parts. **4.** EPIDEMIOLOGY a rating scale.

in·dex case (in'deks kās) The first patient in the investigation of the outbreak of a potentially epidemic disease.

in·dex fing·er (in'deks fing'gĕr) [TA] The second finger (the thumb being counted as the first).

in·dex my·o·pi·a (in′deks mī-ō′pē-ă) Shortsightedness related to the refractive index in the ocular media.

In·di·an Health Ser·vic·es (HIS) (in′ dē-ăn helth sēr′vis-ĕz) Branch of the U.S. Department of Health and Human Services that supplies medical and public health services to Native Americans and other indigenous peoples.

in·di·can·i·dro·sis (in′di-kan′i-drō′sis) Excretion of indican in the sweat.

in·di·ca·nu·ri·a (in′di-kan-yūr′ē-ă) An increased urinary excretion of indican, a derivative of indol formed chiefly in the intestine when protein is putrefied; indol is also formed during the putrefaction of protein in other sites.

in·di·ca·tor (in′di-kā-tŏr) **1.** CHEMICAL ANALYSIS a substance that changes color within a certain definite range of pH or oxidation potential, or in any way renders visible the completion of a chemical reaction (e.g., litmus, phenolsulfonphthalein). **2.** An isotope that is used as a tracer.

in·di·ca·tor di·lu·tion meth·od (in′di-kā-tŏr di-lū′shŭn meth′ŏd) SYN Hamilton-Stewart method.

in·dif·fer·ent el·ec·trode (in-dif′ĕr-ĕnt ĕ-lek′trōd) In unipolar electrocardiography, a remote electrode placed either on a single limb or connected with the central terminal and paired with an exploring electrode, the indifferent electrode is supposed to contribute little or nothing to the resulting record. SYN dispersing electrode, silent electrode.

in·dif·fer·ent tis·sue (in-dif′ĕr-ĕnt tish′ ū) Undifferentiated, nonspecialized, embryonic tissue.

in·dig·e·nous (in-dij′ĕ-nŭs) Native; natural to the country or region where found.

in·di·gent (in′di-jĕnt) Having insufficient income to pay for medical care or other living necessities.

in·di·ges·ti·ble (in′di-jes′ti-bĕl) Alimentation that is intractable to digestive-system enzymes.

in·di·ges·tion (in′di-jes′chŭn) Nonspe-

cific term for various symptoms resulting from a failure of proper digestion and absorption of food in the alimentary tract.

in·di·go (ind) (in′di-gō) [C.I. 73000] A blue dyestuff obtained from *Indigofera tinctoria*, and other species of *Indigofera* (family Leguminosae); also made synthetically. SYN indigo blue, indigotin.

in·di·go car·mine (in′di-gō kahr′mīn) [C.I. 73015] A blue dye used to measure kidney function and as a special stain for Negri bodies. SYN sodium indigotin disulfonate.

in·dig·o·tin (in-dig′ō-tin, in-di-gō′tin) SYN indigo.

in·di·rect bil·i·ru·bin (in′di-rekt′ bil′i-rū′bin) That fraction of bilirubin that does not conjugate with glucuronic acid in hepatic cells.

in·di·rect con·tact (in′di-rekt′ kon′takt) Exposure to potential pathogens by touching possibly infected domestic surfaces.

in·di·rect frac·ture (in′di-rekt′ frak′ shŭr) Breakage, especially of the skull, which occurs at a point other than the site of impact.

in·di·rect he·mag·glu·ti·na·tion test (in′di-rekt hē′mă-glū′ti-nā′shŭn test) SYN passive hemagglutination.

in·di·rect im·mu·no·flu·o·res·cence (in′di-rekt′ im′yū-nō-flōr-es′ĕns) Fluorescence microscopy of normal tissue after application of the patient's serum, to detect antibodies to normal tissue components (autoantibodies).

in·di·rect nurs·ing care (in′di-rekt′ nŭrs′ing kār) Management of nursing care that does not directly involve one-on-one patient care.

in·di·rect oph·thal·mo·scope (in′di-rekt′ of-thal′mŏ-skōp) An instrument designed to visualize the interior of the eye, with the instrument at arm's length from the subject's eye and the observer viewing an inverted image through a convex lens located between the instrument and the subject's eye.

in·di·rect re·act·ing bil·i·ru·bin (in′di-

rekt´ rē-ak´ting bil´i-rū´bin) The fraction of serum bilirubin that has not been conjugated with glucuronic acid in the liver cell.

in·di·rect res·to·ra·tions (in´di-rekt´ res´stŏr-ā´shŭnz) Dental replacement structures prepared outside the patient's mouth and then cemented into position.

in·di·rect re·tain·er (in´di-rekt´ rē-tā´něr) Part of a removable partial denture that assists the direct retainers in preventing occlusal displacement of the distal extension bases by functioning through lever action on the opposite side of the fulcrum line.

in·di·rect trans·fu·sion (in´di-rekt´ trans-fyū´zhŭn) Transfusion into a patient of blood previously obtained from a donor and stored in a suitable container.

in·di·rect vi·sion (in´di-rekt´ vizh´ŭn) SYN peripheral vision.

in·di·um (In) (in´dē-ŭm) A metallic element, atomic no. 49, atomic wt. 114.82.

In·di·um 111 (^{111}In, In-111) (in´dē-um) A cyclotron-produced radionuclide with a half-life of 2.8049 days and with gamma ray emissions of 171.2 and 245.3 kiloelectron volts.

in·di·vid·u·al ha·bil·i·ta·tion plan (I.H.P.) (in´di-vij´yū-ăl hab-il´i-tā´shŭn plan) A document that outlines the provision of services provided to people with disabilities who reside in a group living arrangement to promote engagement in activities of daily living and functional independence.

In·di·vid·u·al·ized Ed·u·ca·tion Pro·gram (IEP) (in´di-vij´yū-ăl-īzd ed´yū-kā´shŭn prŏ´gram) In the U.S., a program tailored to a particular student with a disability, the provision of which is mandated by law. Mandated by IDEA, an IEP has two parts; the plan itself and the written document supporting it.

in·di·vid·u·a·lized fam·i·ly ser·vice plan (IFSP) (in´di-vij´yū-ăl-īzd fam´i-lē sěr´vis plan) The written contract that identifies the early intervention services designed for individual children and their families who are eligible for these services under the IDEA.

in·di·vid·u·al prac·tice as·so·ci·a·tion (IPA) (in´di-vij´yū-ăl prak´tis ă-sō´sē-ā´shŭn) Form of HMO in which the patient does not need a referral or permission to see any physician in the plan.

in·di·vid·u·al prac·tice as·so·ci·a·tion mod·el (IPA) (in´di-vij´yū-ăl prak´tis ă-sō´sē-ā´shŭn mod´ĕl) A type of HMO in which the HMO contracts with an association of physicians to treat the patients of the HMO while continuing to see their own private patients.

in·do·cy·a·nine green (in´dō-sī´ă-nēn grēn) A tricarbocyanine dye that binds to serum albumin and is used in blood volume determinations and in liver function tests.

in·dol·a·mine (in-dol´ă-mēn) An indole or indole derivative containing a primary, secondary, or tertiary amine group.

in·dole (in´dōl) **1.** Basis of many biologically active substances (e.g., serotonin, tryptophan); formed in degradation of tryptophan. SYN ketole. **2.** Any of many alkaloids containing the indole (1) structure.

in·do·lent (in´dō-lĕnt) Inactive; sluggish; painless or nearly so.

in·dol·ic ac·ids (in-dō´lik as´idz) Metabolites of L-tryptophan formed within the body or by intestinal microorganisms.

in·do·meth·a·cin (in´dō-meth´ă-sin) A potent analgesic, antipyretic, and nonsteroidal antiinflammatory agent used to treat acute exacerbations of various joint diseases.

in·dox·yl (in-dok´sil) Product of intestinal bacterial degradation of indoleacetic acid; increased amounts are excreted in the urine in phenylketonuria.

in·duced en·zyme, in·duc·i·ble en·zyme (in´dŭst en´zīm, in-dū´si-bĕl) **1.** One that can be detected in a growing culture of a microorganism, after the addition of a particular substance (inducer) to the culture medium, but was not detectable prior to the addition and can act on the inducer. Cf. constitutive enzyme. **2.** One that has its rate of biosynthesis increased due to the presence of the substrate or other molecular entity. SYN adaptive enzyme.

in·duced fe·ver (in-dŭst´ fē´vĕr) SYN pyretotherapy.

in·duced la·bor (in-dŭst´ lā´bŏr) An obstetric procedure intended to hasten delivery through some form of medical intervention.

in·duced pha·go·cy·to·sis (in-dŭst´ fag´ŏ-sī-tō´sis) Process in which bacteria are subjected to the action of opsonins in blood and then brought in contact with leukocytes.

in·duced psy·chot·ic dis·or·der (in-dŭst´ sī-kot´ik dis-ōr´dĕr) Severe mental disorder brought about by a toxic agent.

in·duced ra·di·o·ac·ti·vi·ty (in-dŭst´ rā´dē-ō-ak-tiv´ĭ-tē) SYN artificial radioactivity.

in·duced trance (in-dŭst´ trans) Artificially induced state of hypnosis or of somnambulistic trance.

in·duced vom·it·ing (in-dŭst´ vom´it-ing) Emesis brought on by medication or physical intervention.

in·duc·er (in-dūs´ĕr) A molecule, usually a substrate of a specific enzyme pathway, which combines with and deactivates an active repressor; this allows an operator gene previously repressed to activate the structural genes controlled by it to resume enzyme production.

in·duc·tion (in-dŭk´shŭn) 1. Production or causation. 2. Production of an electric current or magnetic state in a body by electricity or magnetism in another body close to the first. 3. Period from the start of anesthesia to establishment of a depth of anesthesia adequate for a surgical procedure. 4. Causal analysis; method of reasoning in which an inference is made from one or more specific observations to a more general statement.

in·duc·tion che·mo·ther·a·py (ICT) (in-dŭk´shŭn kē´mō-thār´ă-pē) Use of chemotherapy as initial treatment before surgery or radiotherapy on a malignancy.

in·duc·tion pe·ri·od (in-dŭk´shŭn pēr´ē-ŏd) The interval between an initial injection of antigen and the appearance of demonstrable antibodies in the blood.

in·duc·tor (in-dŭk´tŏr) 1. That which

brings about induction. 2. EMBRYOLOGY an evocator or an organizer.

in·du·ra·tion (in´dŭr-ā´shŭn) 1. The process of extreme hardening or having such physical features. 2. A focus or region of indurated tissue. SYN sclerosis (1).

in·du·ra·tive my·o·car·di·tis (in-dŭr´ă-tiv mī´ō-kahr-dī´tis) Chronic form leading to hardening of the muscular wall of the heart.

in·dwell·ing cath·e·ter (IDC) (in´dwel-ing kath´ĕ-tĕr) One left in place in the bladder, usually a balloon catheter.

in·e·bri·a·tion (in-ē´brē-ā´shŭn) Intoxication, especially by alcohol. SEE inebriant.

in·ef·fec·tive air·way clear·ance (in-e-fek´tiv âr´wā klēr´ăns) A nursing diagnosis referring to inability to clear secretions of obstructions from the respiratory tract to maintain patency.

in·ef·fec·tive breath·ing pat·tern (in-e-fek´tiv brēdh´ing pat´ĕrn) A nursing diagnosis for a patient who cannot breathe spontaneously without assistance.

in·ef·fec·tive cop·ing (in-e-fek´tiv kōp´ing) Nursing diagnosis denoting a patient who fails in trying to cope with environmental or mental challenges.

in·ef·fec·tive health main·te·nance (in-e-fek´tiv helth mān´tĕn-ăns) Nursing diagnosis referring to inability to follow needed health measures.

in·ef·fec·tive in·fant feed·ing pat·tern (in-e-fek´tiv in´fănt fēd´ing pat´ĕrn) A nursing diagnosis referring to the state when an infant shows impaired ability to suck or swallow properly.

in·ef·fec·tive pro·tec·tion (in-e-fek´tiv prō-tek´shŭn) A nursing diagnosis for when a patient fails to guard against threats such as illness or injury.

in·ef·fec·tive role per·for·mance (in-e-fek´tiv rōl pĕr-fōr´măns) A nursing diagnosis referring to the inability of a patient to successfully fulfill an expected role in the family or larger social group.

in·ef·fec·tive sex·u·al·i·ty pat·terns (in-e-fek´tiv sek´shū-al´i-tē pat´ĕrnz) A nursing diagnosis referring to when a patient undergoes or is at risk for undergoing an alteration in sexual behavior or sexual health.

in·ef·fec·tive ther·mo·reg·u·la·tion (in-e-fek´tiv thĕr´mō-reg´yū-lā´shŭn) A nursing diagnosis for when a patient undergoes or is in danger of undergoing development of an inability to maintain a stable core normal body temperature when faced with adverse external factors.

in·ert (in-ĕrt´) **1.** Slow in action; sluggish; inactive. **2.** Devoid of active chemical properties, as the inert gases. **3.** Denoting a drug or agent having no pharmacologic or therapeutic action.

in·ert gas·es (in-ĕrt´ gas´ĕz) SYN noble gases.

in·er·ti·a (in-ĕr´shē-ă) **1.** The tendency of a physical body to oppose any force tending to move it from a position of rest or to change its uniform motion. **2.** Denoting inactivity or lack of force, lack of mental or physical vigor, or sluggishness of thought or action.

in·er·ti·a time (in-ĕr´shē-ă tīm) Interval elapsing between reception of the stimulus from a nerve and muscular contraction.

in ex·tre·mis (in eks-trē´mis) At the point of death.

in·fan·cy (inf) (in´făn-sē) Babyhood; the earliest period of extrauterine life; roughly, the first year of life.

in·fant (in´fănt) A child younger than 1 year of age; more specifically, a newborn baby.

in·fant death (ID) (in´fănt deth) Demise of a liveborn infant within the first year.

in·fant grasp re·flex (in´fănt grasp rē´fleks) SYN palmar reflex.

in·fan·tile ac·ro·pus·tu·lo·sis (in´făn-tīl ak´rō-pŭs´tyū-lo´sis) A recurrent papulopustular and crusting pruritic eruption, usually in black children.

in·fan·tile au·tism (IA) (in´făn-tīl aw´tizm) Severe emotional disturbance of childhood characterized by qualitative impairment in reciprocal social interaction and in communication, language, and social development.

in·fan·tile hem·i·ple·gi·a (in´făn-tīl hem´ē-plē´jē-ă) Acute hemiparesis that occurs in infancy; usually caused by a vascular accident; frequently associated with seizures.

in·fan·tile os·te·o·ma·la·ci·a, ju·ve·nile os·te·o·ma·la·ci·a (in´făn-tīl os´tē-ō-mă-lā´shē-ă, jū´vĕ-nil) SYN rickets.

in·fan·tile sex·u·al·i·ty (in´făn-tīl sek´shū-al´i-tē) PSYCHOANALYSIS body of theories concerning psychosexual development in infants and children; encompasses overlapping oral, anal, and phallic phases during the first 5 years of life.

in·fan·tile spasm (in´fan-tīl spazm) Brief (1–3 second) muscular spasms in infants with West syndrome, which often appear as nodding or salaam spasms.

in·fan·tile spi·nal mus·cu·lar at·ro·phy (in´făn-tīl spī´năl mŭs´kyū-lăr at´rŏ-fē) Progressive dysfunction of the anterior horn cells in the spinal cord and brainstem cranial nerves with profound weakness and bulbar dysfunction occurring in the first 2 years of life.

in·fan·ti·lism (in-fan´ti-lizm) **1.** A state marked by slow development of mind and body. SYN infantile dwarfism. **2.** Childishness, as characterized by a temper tantrum of an adolescent or adult. **3.** Underdevelopment of the sexual organs.

in·fant mor·tal·i·ty rate (in´fănt mōr-tal´i-tē rāt) Measure of the rate of deaths of liveborn infants before their first birthday; the numerator is the number of infants less than 1 year of age born alive in a defined region during a calendar year who die before they are 1 year old; the denominator is the total number of live births.

in·farct (inf) (in´fahrkt) An area of necrosis resulting from a sudden insufficiency of arterial or venous blood supply.

in·farc·tion (in-fahrk´shŭn) **1.** Sudden insufficiency of arterial or venous blood supply due to emboli, thrombi, vascular torsion, or pressure that produces a macroscopic area of necrosis. **2.** SYN infarct.

in·fect (in-fekt') **1.** To enter, invade, or inhabit another organism, causing infection or contamination. **2.** To dwell internally, endoparasitically.

in·fec·tion (in-fek'shŭn) Invasion of the body by organisms that have the potential to cause disease.

in·fec·tion con·trol (in-fek'shŭn kŏn-trōl') Measures taken to avoid spread of infection within a health care facility or larger area (e.g., neighborhood).

in·fec·tion con·trol nurse (in-fek'shŭn kŏn-trōl' nŭrs) SYN nurse epidemiologist.

in·fec·tion trans·mis·sion pa·ram·e·ter (in-fek'shŭn trans-mish'ŭn păr-am'ĕ-tĕr) Proportion of total possible contacts between infectious cases and susceptible people in a specific population that actually leads to new cases.

in·fec·tious (in-fek'shŭs) **1.** Capable of being transmitted by infection, with or without actual contact. **2.** Caused by infection of the body by pathogenic organisms. SYN contagion, contagious, infective.

In·fec·tious Dis·eas·es So·ci·e·ty of A·mer·i·ca (IDSA) (in-fek'shŭs di-zēz'ĕz sŏ-sī'ĕ-tē ă-mer'i-kă) Professional organization that offers informaion services and two learned journals to clinical specialists in various fields.

in·fec·tious gran·u·lo·ma (in-fek'shŭs gran-yū-lō'mă) Any such lesion known to be caused by a living agent; e.g., bacteria, fungi, helminths.

in·fec·tious mon·o·nu·cle·o·sis (in-fek'shŭs mon'ō-nū-klē-ō'sis) An acute febrile illness caused by the Epstein-Barr virus; frequently spread by saliva transfer; characterized by fever, sore throat, and enlargement of lymph nodes and spleen.

in·fec·tious nu·cle·ic ac·id (INA) (in-fek'shŭs nū-klē'ik as'id) Viral nucleic acid that can infect cells and bring about the production of viruses.

in·fec·tiv·i·ty (in'fek-tiv'i-tē) **1.** The characteristic of a disease agent that embodies its capability to enter, survive in, and multiply in a susceptible host. **2.** The proportion of exposures in defined circumstances that result in infection.

in·fer·i·or (in-fēr'ē-ŏr) **1.** Situated below or directed downward. **2.** ANATOMY situated nearer the soles of the feet in relation to a specific reference point; opposite of superior. **3.** Less useful or of poorer quality.

in·fer·i·or·i·ty com·plex (in-fēr'ē-ōr'i-tē kom'pleks) Sense of inadequacy expressed in extreme shyness, diffidence, or timidity, or in compensatory exhibitionism or aggressiveness.

in·fe·ri·or la·ryn·got·o·my (in-fēr'ē-ŏr lar-in-got'ŏ-mē) SYN cricothyrotomy.

in·fe·ro·lat·er·al (in'fĕr-ō-lat'ĕr-ăl) Below and to the side.

in·fer·o·me·di·al (in'fĕr-ō-mē'dē-ăl) Below and in or toward the middle.

in·fer·tile (in-fer'til) Denotes a woman unable to get pregnant after at least 1 year of effort.

in·fer·til·i·ty (in'fĕr-til'i-tē) Diminished or absent ability to produce offspring; in either the male or the female, not as irreversible as sterility.

in·fest (in-fest') To dwell on or in a host as a parasite.

in·fes·ta·tion (in'fes-tā'shŭn) Parasitization of a host; usually refers to multicellular parasites (worms, arthropods).

in·fib·u·la·tion (in-fib'yū-lā'shŭn) Closure of the vaginal vestibule by fusing the labia majora; typically done after excision of the labia minora and clitoris and incision of the labia majora to create raw surfaces that can be surgically joined by pinning so that they will eventually grow together; done for cultural, not medical, reasons. SEE ALSO female circumcision. Cf. mutilation.

in·fil·trate (in'fil-trāt) **1.** To perform or undergo infiltration. **2.** Infiltration in the lung as inferred from appearance of a localized, ill-defined opacity on a chest radiograph.

in·fil·tra·tion (in'fil-trā'shŭn) **1.** The act of permeating or penetrating into a substance, cell, or tissue; said of gases, fluids, or matter held in solution. **2.** The gas, fluid, or dissolved matter that has entered any substance, cell, or tissue. **3.** Extravasation of solutions intended for intravascular injection.

in•fil•tra•tion an•es•the•si•a (in′fil-trā′shŭn an′es-thē′zē-ă) Anesthesia produced by injection of local anesthetic solution directly into an area that is painful or about to be operated on.

in•firm (in-fĭrm′) Weak or feeble because of old age or disease.

in•fir•ma•ry (in-fĭr′măr-ē) A clinic or small hospital, especially in a school or college.

in•flam•ma•tion (in′flă-mā′shŭn) A fundamental, stereotyped complex of cytologic and chemical reactions that occur in affected blood vessels and adjacent tissues in response to an injury or abnormal stimulation caused by a physical, chemical, or biologic agent.

in•flam•ma•to•ry bow•el dis•ease (IBD) (in-flam′ă-tōr-ē bow′ĕl di-zēz′) General term for Crohn disease and ulcerative colitis, chronic disorders of the small and large intestine.

in•flam•ma•to•ry lymph (in-flam′ă-tōr-ē limf) A faintly yellow coagulable fluid that collects on the surface of an acutely inflamed membrane or cutaneous wound.

in•flam•ma•to•ry pap•il•lar•y hy•per•pla•si•a (in-flam′ă-tōr-ē pap′i-lar-ē hī′pĕr-plā′zē-ă) Closely arranged papules of the palatal mucosa underlying an ill-fitting denture.

in•flam•ma•to•ry pseu•do•tu•mor (in-flam′ă-tōr-ē sū′dō-tū′mŏr) A tumorlike mass composed of fibrous or granulation tissue infiltrated by inflammatory cells.

in•flam•mat•o•ry re•sponse (in-flam′ă-tōr-ē rĕ-spons′) Body's reaction to a threat in release of physiologic agents that induce swelling, fever, and other measures.

in•flam•ma•to•ry rheu•ma•tism (in-flam′ă-tōr-ē rū′mă-tizm) Rheumatoid arthritis or other cause of joint inflammation.

in•fla•tion (in-flā′shŭn) Distention by a fluid or gas.

in•flix•i•mab (in-fliks′i-mab) A chimeric antitumor necrosis factor (TNF)-α monoclonal antibody containing a murine TNF-α binding region and a human immunoglobulin G1 backbone.

in•flu•en•za, flu (in′flū-en′ză, flū) An acute infectious respiratory disease, caused by influenza viruses; attacks the respiratory epithelial cells and produces a catarrhal inflammation; characterized by sudden onset, chills, fever of short duration, severe prostration, headache, muscle aches, and a cough that usually is dry until secondary infection occurs. SYN grip, grippe.

in•flu•en•zal pneu•mo•ni•a (in′flū-en′zăl nū-mō′nē-ă) **1.** A pulmonary disorder complicating influenza. **2.** Any such disorder due to *Haemophilus influenzae.*

in•flu•en•za vac•cine (in′flū-en′ză vak-sēn′) An annual vaccine to guard against the specific influenza virus determined to be most prolific in a given 12-month period.

in•fold•ing (in′fold-ing) Act on enclosure within a fold, whether by surgical intervention or in the process of maturation of an embryo.

in•for•mal ad•mis•sion (in-fōr′măl ad-mish′ŭn) Entry of a patient into a psychiatric care facility voluntarily; such patients are free to leave without staff permission.

in•for•mat•ics (in′fŏr-mat′iks) **1.** The study of information and ways to process and handle it, especially by means of information technology, i.e., computers and other electronic devices for rapid transfer, processing, and analysis of large amounts of data. **2.** The science of arranging and organizing the results of genomic and functional genomic studies.

in•for•ma•tion pro•cess•ing (in-fŏr-mā′shŭn pros′es-ing) In cognitive psychology, theory that short-term memory is limited to five to nine 'chunks' or meaningful units of information.

in•formed con•sent (in-fōrmd′ kŏn-sent′) Voluntary agreement given by a person or a responsible proxy (e.g., a parent) for participation in a study, immunization program, or treatment regimen, after being informed of the purpose, methods, procedures, benefits, and risks. The essential criteria of informed consent are that the subject has both knowledge and comprehension, that consent is freely given without duress or undue influence, and that the right of withdrawal at any time is clearly communicated to the subject.

♻ **infra-** Prefix denoting a position below the part denoted by the word to which it is joined.

in·fra·cla·vic·u·lar (in′fră-klă-vik′yū-lăr) SYN subclavian (1).

in·fra·clu·sion, in·fra·oc·clu·sion (in′fră-klū′zhŭn, -ŏ-klū′zhŭn) The state wherein a tooth has failed to erupt to the maxillomandibular plane of interdigitation. SYN infraocclusion, infraversion (3).

in·fra·den·ta·le (Id) (in′fră-den-tā′lē) Apex of the septum between the mandibular central incisors. SYN lower alveolar point.

in·fra·di·an (in-frā′dē-ăn) Relating to biologic variations or rhythms occurring in cycles less frequent than every 24 hours. Cf. circadian, ultradian.

in·fra·duc·tion (in′fră-dŭk′shŭn) SYN deorsumduction.

in·fra·glen·oid (in′fră-glē′noyd) Inferior to the glenoid cavity of the scapula.

in·fra·glot·tic (in′fră-glot′ik) Inferior to the glottis.

in·fra·he·pat·ic (in′fră-he-pat′ik) Below the liver.

in·fra·hy·oid (in′fră-hī′oyd) Inferior to the hyoid bone.

in·fra·mam·mary (in′fră-mam′ă-rē) Below a mammary gland. SYN submammary (2).

in·fra·mam·ma·ry re·gion (in′fră-mam′ăr-ē rē′jŏn) [TA] Pectoral area inferior to the mammary gland. SYN regio inframammaria [TA].

in·fra·max·il·lar·y (in′fră-mak′si-lar-ē) SYN mandibular.

in·fra·nod·al ex·tra·sys·to·le (in′fră-nō′dăl eks′tră-sis′tŏ-lē) SYN ventricular extrasystole.

in·fra·or·bit·al (in′fră-ōr′bi-tăl) Below or beneath the orbit.

in·fra·pa·tel·lar (IP) (in′fră-pă-tel′ăr) Inferior to the patella; denoting especially a bursa, a pad of fat, or a synovial fold. SYN subpatellar (2).

in·fra·red (in′fră-red) That portion of the electromagnetic spectrum with wavelengths between 770–1000 nm.

in·fra·red mi·cro·scope (in′fră-red mī′krŏ-skōp) Device equipped with infrared transmitting optics that measures the infrared absorption of minute samples with the aid of photoelectric cells.

in·fra·red ther·a·py (in′fră-red thār′ă-pē) Controversial experimental treatment to relieve pain and promote healing through the use of infrared light.

in·fra·red ther·mog·ra·phy (IRT) (in′fră-red ther-mog′ră-fē) Measurement of the regional skin temperature with an infrared sensing device.

in·fra·red tym·pan·ic ther·mom·e·ter (in′fră-red tim-pan′ik thĕr-mom′ĕ-tĕr) One that uses infrared technology to measure the patient's temperature through use of light on the tympanic membrane within the external ear.

in·fra·son·ic (in′fră-son′ik) Denoting those frequencies that lie below the range of human hearing.

in·fra·spi·nous (in′fră-spī′nŭs) Below a spine or spinous process (e.g., fossa infraspinata). SYN subspinous (1).

in·fra·ster·nal (in′fră-stĕr′năl) Inferior to the sternum. SYN substernal (2).

in·fra·tem·po·ral (in′fră-tem′pŏ-răl) Below the temporal fossa.

in·fra·ver·sion (in′fră-vĕr′zhŭn) **1.** A turning (version) downward. **2.** PHYSIOLOGIC OPTICS rotation of both eyes downward. **3.** SYN infraclusion.

in·fun·dib·u·lar (in′fŭn-dib′yū-lăr) Relating to an infundibulum.

in·fun·dib·u·lar stem (in′fŭn-dib′yū-lăr stem) The neural component of the pituitary stalk that contains nerve tracts passing from the hypothalamus to the pars nervosa.

in·fun·dib·u·lec·to·my (in′fŭn-dib′yū-lek′tŏ-mē) Excision of the infundibulum, especially of hypertrophied ventricular septal myocardium encroaching on the ventricular outflow tract in the tetralogy of Fallot.

in·fun·dib·u·li·form (in′fŭn-dib′yū-li-fōrm′) SYN choanoid.

in·fun·dib·u·lo·ma (in′fŭn-dib′yū-lō′mă) A pilocytic astrocytoma arising in the neurohypophysis of the pituitary.

in·fun·dib·u·lum, pl. **in·fun·dib·u·la** (in′fŭn-dib′yū-lŭm, -lă) **1.** [TA] Any funnel or funnel-shaped structure or passage. **2.** Expanding portion of a calyx as it opens into the pelvis of the kidney. **3.** Termination of a bronchiole in the alveolus. **4.** Termination of the cochlear canal beneath the cupola. **5.** Funicular, unpaired prominence of the base of the hypothalamus behind the optic chiasm, enclosing the infundibular recess of the third ventricle and continuous below with the stalk of the hypophysis.

in·fu·sate (in-fyū′zāt) A fluid given intravenously over a period of time for therapeutic purposes.

in·fu·sion (in-fyū′zhŭn) **1.** The process of steeping a substance in water, either cold or hot (below the boiling point), to extract its soluble principles. **2.** A medicinal preparation obtained by steeping the crude drug in water. **3.** The introduction of fluid other than blood, e.g., saline solution, into a vein.

in·fu·sion pump (in-fyū′zhŭn pŭmp) A device that instills intravenous fluids into a patient's circulatory system at a set rate. SYN intravenous infusion pump.

in·ges·tant, in·ges·ta (in-jest′ănt, -tă) Anything taken into the gastrointestinal system.

in·ges·tion (in-jes′chŭn) **1.** Introduction of food and drink into the stomach. **2.** Incorporation of particles into the cytoplasm of a phagocytic cell by invagination of a portion of the cell membrane as a vacuole.

in·ges·tive (in-jes′tiv) Relating to ingestion.

in·gra·ves·cent (in′gră-ves′ĕnt) Increasing in severity.

in·grown hair (in′grōn hār) Hair that grows at more acute angles than is normal, and in all directions; it incompletely clears the follicle, turns back in, and causes pseudofolliculitis.

in·grown nail (in′grōn nāl) A toenail, one edge of which is overgrown by the nailfold, producing a pyogenic granuloma; due to faulty trimming of the toenails or pressure from a tight shoe.

in·guen (ing′gwen) [TA] SYN groin (1).

in·gui·nal (ing, ING) (ing′gwi-năl) Relating to the groin.

in·gui·nal her·ni·a (ing′gwi-năl hĕr′nē-ă) A hernia in the groin area.

in·gui·no·cru·ral her·ni·a, in·gui·no·fem·o·ral her·ni·a (in′gwin-nō-krūr′ăl hĕr′nē-ă, in′gwin-nō-fem′ŏr-ăl) Bilocular or double hernia, both inguinal and femoral.

in·gui·no·la·bi·al (ing′gwi-nō-lā′bē-ăl) Relating to the groin and the labium.

in·gui·no·per·i·to·ne·al (ing′gwi-nō-per′i-tō-nē′ăl) Relating to the groin and the peritoneum.

in·gui·no·scro·tal (ing′gwi-nō-skrŏ′tăl) Relating to the groin and the scrotum.

in·hal·ant (in-hā′lănt) **1.** That which is inhaled; a remedy given by inhalation. **2.** A drug (or combination of drugs) with high vapor pressure, carried by an air current into the nasal passage, where it produces its effect. **3.** Group of products consisting of finely powdered or liquid drugs that are carried to the respiratory passages by the use of special devices such as low-pressure aerosol containers. SYN insufflation (2).

in·ha·la·tion (in′hă-lā′shŭn) **1.** The act of drawing in the breath. SYN inspiration. **2.** Drawing a medicated vapor in with the breath. **3.** A solution of a drug or combination of drugs for administration as a nebulized mist intended to reach the respiratory tree.

in·ha·la·tion·al an·thrax (in'hă-lā'shŭn-ăl an'thraks) Disease acquired by breathing in spores of *Bacillus anthracis* in airborne particles less than 5 mcg. Early diagnosis of inhalational anthrax is difficult because initial symptoms are nonspecific chills, fever, muscle aches, cough. After 1–3 days, dyspnea, hypotension, high fever, and stridor become the primary symptoms; mortality nears 100%, even with treatment.

in·ha·la·tion an·es·the·si·a (in'hă-lā' shŭn an'es-thē'zē-ă) General anesthesia due to breathing of anesthetic gases.

in·ha·la·tion chal·lenge test (in'hă-lā' shŭn chal'ĕnj test) Assessment of velocity of inhaling and exhaling before and after taking a therapeutic investigative agent; a test for asthma.

in·ha·la·tion in·ju·ry (in'hă-lā'shŭn in' jŭr-ē) Trauma to the throat, lungs, and associated areas caused by fire, exposure to toxins, or lethal gases.

in·ha·la·tion ther·a·py (in'hă-lā'shŭn thār'ă-pē) Treatment with a substance introduced into patient's respiratory tract through breathing in.

in·hal·er (in-hāl'ĕr) An apparatus for administering medicines by inhalation. SYN metered-dose inhaler.

in·her·ent (in-her'ĕnt) Occurring as a natural part or consequence; intrinsic.

in·her·ent im·mu·ni·ty (in-her'ĕnt i-myū'ni-tē) Bodily defense against a pathogen that occurs from genetic bases rather than through exposure. SYN innate immunity, native immunity, nonspecific immunity, species immunity.

in·her·i·tance (in-her'i-tăns) 1. Characters or qualities that are transmitted from parent to offspring by coded cytologic data. 2. Cultural or legal endowment. 3. The act of inheriting.

in·her·it·ed char·ac·ter (in-her'it-ĕd kar'ăk-tĕr) A single attribute of an animal or plant that is transmitted at one locus from generation to generation in accordance with mendelian laws. SEE gene.

in·her·i·ted dis·or·der (in-her'i-tĕd dis-ōr'dĕr) An illness or disease that is derived from genetic aberration.

in·her·i·ted trait (in-her'i-tĕd trāt) Any characteristic that is passed from one generation to the next.

in·hib·in (in-hib'in) One of several proteins that participate in differentiation and growth.

in·hib·it (in-hib'it) To curb or restrain.

in·hi·bi·tion (in'hi-bish'ŭn) 1. Depression or arrest of a function. SEE ALSO inhibitor. 2. PSYCHOANALYSIS the restraining of instinctual or unconscious drives or tendencies, especially if they conflict with one's conscience or with societal demands. 3. PSYCHOLOGY the gradual attenuation, masking, and extinction of a previously conditioned response.

in·hib·i·tion the·o·ry (in'hi-bish'ŏn thē'ŏr-ē) Notion that during the performance of a mental task, a person alternates between states of distraction and attention.

in·hib·i·tor (in-hib'i-tŏr) 1. An agent that restrains or retards physiologic, chemical, or enzymatic action. 2. A nerve, stimulation of which represses activity. SEE ALSO inhibition.

in·hib·i·tor·y (in-hib'i-tōr-ē) Restraining; tending to inhibit.

in·hib·i·tor·y fi·bers (in-hib'i-tōr-ē fī'bĕrz) Nerve fibers that inhibit the activity of the nerve cells with which they have synaptic connections, or of the effector tissue (smooth muscle, heart muscle, glands) in which they terminate.

in·hib·i·tor·y nerve (in-hib'i-tōr-ē nĕrv) A nerve conveying impulses that diminish functional activity in a part.

in·hib·i·tor·y ob·ses·sion (in-hib'i-tōr-ē ŏb-sesh'ŭn) An obsession involving an impediment to action, usually representing a phobia.

in·hib·i·tor·y post·syn·ap·tic po·ten·tial (in-hib'i-tōr-ē pōst'si-nap'tik pŏ-ten'shăl) The change in potential produced in the membrane of the next neuron when an impulse that has an inhibitory influence arrives at the synapse.

in·i·on (In) (in′ē-on) [TA] A point located on the external occipital protuberance at the intersection of the midline with a line drawn tangent to the uppermost convexity of the right and left superior nuchal lines.

in·i·ti·a·tion (i-nish′ē-ā′shŭn) **1.** The first stage of tumor induction by a carcinogen; subtle alteration of cells by exposure to a carcinogenic agent so that they are likely to form a tumor on subsequent exposure to a promoting agent (promotion). **2.** Starting point of replication or translation in macromolecule biosynthesis. **3.** Start of chemical or enzymatic reaction.

in·i·ti·a·tion fac·tor (IF) (i-nish′ē-ā′shŭn fak′tŏr) One of several soluble proteins involved in the initiation of protein or RNA synthesis.

in·i·ti·a·tor (i-nish′ē-ā-tŏr) That which causes, elicits, or starts another thing or process.

in·i·tis (in-ī′tis) **1.** Inflammation of fibrous tissue. **2.** SYN myositis.

in·jec·tion (in-jek′shŭn) **1.** Introduction of a medicinal substance or nutrient material into the subcutaneous tissue, the muscular tissue, a vein, an artery, the rectum, or the vagina, the urethra, or other canals or cavities of the body. **2.** An injectable pharmaceutical preparation. **3.** Congestion or hyperemia.

in·jec·tion drug us·er (IDU) (in-jek′shŭn drŭg yū′zĕr) A person who uses a hypodermic to administer drugs, usually illegally; often leads to dermatologic and hematologic disorders due to unclean site or equipment; widely associated with transmission of HIV. SYN intravenous drug user.

in·ju·ry (in′jŭr-ē) Damage, harm, or loss, to a person particularly as the result of external force.

in·ju·ry se·ver·i·ty score (ISS) (in′jŭr-ē sĕ-ver′i-tē skōr) Therapeutic and diagnostic six-point assessment of amount of bodily damage due to trauma. (6 indicates injury that exceeds therapeutic means to deal with it); has largely replaced all others clinically.

ink·blot test (ingk′blot test) SYN Rorschach test.

in·lay (inl) (in′lā) **1.** In dentistry, a prefabricated restoration sealed in the cavity with cement. **2.** A graft of bone into a bone cavity. **3.** A graft of skin into a wound cavity for epithelialization. **4.** In orthopedics, an orthomechanical device inserted into a shoe; commonly called an arch support.

in·lay graft (in′lā graft) A skin graft wrapped (raw side out) around a bolus of dental compound and inserted into a prepared surgical pocket. SYN Esser graft.

in·let (in′lĕt) [TA] A passage leading into a cavity. SYN aditus [TA].

in lo·co pa·ren·tis (in lō′kō pă-ren′tis) Latin expression meaning in place of the parents; legal obligation of a nonparental authority to provide a level of care equal to that of parents.

INN Abbreviation for international nonproprietary names.

in·nate (i-nāt′) SYN inborn.

in·nate im·mu·ni·ty (i-nāt′ i-myū′ni-tē) Resistance manifested by an organism that has not been sensitized by previous infection or vaccination; innate immunity is nonspecific and is not stimulated by specific antigens. SEE ALSO self (3). SYN nonspecific immunity.

in·ner cell mass (in′ĕr sel mas) SYN embryoblast.

in·ner·va·tion (in′ĕr-vā′shŭn) The supply of motor and sensory nerve fibers functionally connected with an organ or region.

in·nid·i·a·tion (i-nid′ē-ā′shŭn) The growth and multiplication of abnormal cells in a location to which they have been transported by means of lymph or the blood stream, or both. SEE ALSO metastasis.

in·no·cent (in′ŏ-sĕnt) **1.** Not apparently harmful. **2.** Free from moral wrong.

ino-, in- Fiber, fibrous. SEE ALSO fibro-.

in·oc·u·la·bil·i·ty (i-nok′yū-lă-bil′i-tē) The quality of being inoculable.

in·oc·u·la·ble (i-nok′yū-lă-bĕl) **1.** Trans-

in·oc·u·late (i-nok′yū-lāt) **1.** To introduce the agent of a disease or other antigenic material into the subcutaneous tissue or a blood vessel, or through an abraded or absorbing surface for preventive, curative, or experimental purposes. **2.** To implant microorganisms or infectious material into or on culture media. **3.** To communicate a disease by transferring its virus.

in·oc·u·la·tion (INOC) (i-nok′yū-lā′shŭn) *Avoid the misspelling innoculation.* Introduction into the body of the causative organism of a disease. Also sometimes used, incorrectly, to mean immunization with any type of vaccine.

in·oc·u·lum, pl. **in·oc·u·la** (i-nok′yū-lŭm, -lă) The microorganism or other material introduced by inoculation.

in·op·er·a·ble (in-op′ĕr-ă-bĕl) Denoting that which cannot be operated on, or cannot be corrected or removed by an operation.

in·or·gan·ic (in′ōr-gan′ik) Not containing carbon nor formed by living organisms. SEE inorganic compound.

in·or·gan·ic ac·id (in′ōr-gan′ik as′id) One made up of molecules not containing organic radicals.

in·or·gan·ic che·mis·try (in′ōr-gan′ik kem′is-trē) The science concerned with compounds not involving carbon-containing molecules.

in·or·gan·ic com·pound (in′ōr-gan′ik kom′pownd) A compound in which the atoms or radicals consist of elements other than carbon and are typically held together by electrostatic forces rather than by covalent bonds.

inosaemia [Br.] SYN inosemia.

in·os·co·py (in-os′kŏ-pē) Microscopic examination of biologic materials after dissection or chemical digestion of the fibrillary elements and strands of fibrin.

in·o·se·mi·a (in′ō-sē′mē-ă) The presence of inositol in the circulating blood. SYN inosaemia.

in·o·sine (I, Ino) (in′ō-sēn) A nucleoside formed by the deamination of adenosine.

in·o·si·tol (in-ō′si-tol) A member of the vitamin B complex.

in·o·tro·pic (in′ō-trō′pik) Influencing the contractility of muscular tissue.

in·pa·tient (in′pā-shĕnt) Patient who is admitted to and is assigned a bed in a health care facility while undergoing diagnosis and receiving treatment and care.

in·pa·tient care u·nit (in′pā′shĕnt kār yū′nit) A nursing unit providing 24-hour patient care.

in·quest (in′kwest) A legal inquiry into the cause of sudden, violent, or mysterious death.

in·sa·lu·bri·ous (in′să-lū′brē-ŭs) Unwholesome; unhealthful; usually describes climate.

in·san·i·ty (in-san′i-tē) **1.** A nonmedical term referring to severe mental illness or psychosis. **2.** LAW that degree of mental illness that negates the person's legal responsibility or capacity.

in·sa·tia·ble (in-sā′shă-bĕl) Being unable to be satisfied in some need.

in·scrip·tion, in·scrip·ti·o (in-skrip′shŭn, -shē-ō) **1.** The main part of a prescription; that which indicates the drugs and the quantity of each to be used in the mixture. **2.** A mark, band, or line.

in·scrip·ti·o ten·din·e·a (in-skrip′shē-ō ten-din′ē-ă) SYN tendinous intersection.

In·sec·ta (in-sek′tă) The insects, the largest class of the phylum Arthropoda and the largest major grouping of living things, chiefly characterized by flight, great adaptability, vast speciation in terrestrial and freshwater environments, and possession of three pairs of jointed legs and, usually, two pairs of wings. Some are parasitic, others serve as intermediate hosts for parasites, including those that cause many human diseases. SYN Hexapoda.

in·sem·i·na·tion (in-sem′i-nā′shŭn) Deposit of seminal fluid within the vagina, normally during coitus.

in·sen·si·ble (in-sen′si-bĕl) **1.** SYN unconscious. **2.** Not appreciable by the senses.

in·ser·tion (in-sĕr′shŭn) **1.** A putting in. **2.** The attachment of a muscle to the more movable part of the skeleton, as distinguished from origin. **3.** DENTISTRY the intraoral placing of a dental prosthesis. **4.** Intrusion of fragments of any size from molecular to cytogenetic into the normal genome.

in·ser·vice ed·u·ca·tion (in′sĕr′vis ed′ yū-kā′shŭn) Training provided on premises by any type of health care facility to its staff.

in·sheathed (in-shēdhd′) Enclosed in a sheath or capsule.

in·sid·i·ous (in-sid′ē-ŭs) Treacherous; stealthy; denoting a disease that progresses gradually with inapparent symptoms.

in·sight (in′sīt) Self-understanding as to the motives and reasons behind one's own actions or those of another's.

in si·tu (in sit′ū) In position; not extending beyond the focus or level of origin.

in si·tu hy·brid·i·za·tion (in sit′ū hī′ brid-ī-zā′shŭn) A technique for annealing nucleic acid probes to cellular DNA for detection by autoradiography; key step in DNA fingerprinting.

in·sol·u·ble (in-sol′yū-bĕl) Incapable of dissolving in solution.

in·sol·u·ble fi·ber (in-sol′yū-bĕl fī′bĕr) That portion of a foodstuff (e.g., bran) that cannot be digested and is passed through the alimentary system without change.

in·som·ni·a (in-som′nē-ă) Inability to sleep, in the absence of external impediments during the period when sleep should normally occur; may vary in degree from restlessness or disturbed slumber to a curtailment of the normal length of sleep or to absolute wakefulness. SYN sleeplessness.

in·sorp·tion (in-sōrp′shŭn) Movement of substances from the lumen of the gut into the blood.

in·sper·sion (in-spĕr′zhŭn) Sprinkling with a fluid or a powder.

in·spi·ra·tion (in′spir-ā′shŭn) SYN inhalation (1).

in·spi·ra·to·ry (in′spīr-ă-tōr-ē) Relating to or timed during inhalation.

in·spi·ra·to·ry ca·pa·ci·ty (in′spīr-ă-tōr-ē kă-pas′i-tē) The volume of air that can be inspired after a normal expiration. SYN complementary air.

in·spi·ra·to·ry dys·pn·ea (in′spīr-ă-tōr-ē disp-nē′ă) Problems with inhalation phase of breathing; shortness of breath. SYN air hunger.

in·spi·ra·to·ry hold (in′spīr-ă-tōr-ē hōld) Therapeutic technique that requires a patient to hold air in the lungs for a given time before it is exhaled.

in·spi·ra·to·ry re·serve vol·ume (IRV) (in′spīr-ă-tōr-ē rĕ-zĕrv′ vol′yūm) The maximal volume of air that can be inspired after a normal inspiration. SYN complemental air.

in·spi·ra·to·ry stri·dor (in′spīr-ă-tōr-ē strī′dŏr) A crowing sound during the inspiratory phase of respiration due to pathology involving the epiglottis or larynx.

in·spired gas (I) (in-spīrd′ gas) **1.** Any gas that is being inhaled; **2.** Specifically, that gas after it has been humidified at body temperature.

in·spi·rom·e·ter (in′spi-rom′ĕ-tĕr) An instrument for measuring the force, frequency, or volume of inspirations.

in·spis·sa·tion (in′spi-sā′shŭn) **1.** The act of thickening or condensing, as by evaporation or absorption of fluid. **2.** An increased thickening or diminished fluidity.

in·sta·bil·i·ty (in′stă-bil′i-tē) **1.** The state of being unstable, or lacking stability. **2.** The abnormal tendency of a joint to subluxate or dislocate with normal activities and stresses. SEE ALSO laxity.

in·step (in′step) The arch, or highest part of the dorsum of the foot. SEE ALSO tarsus.

in·stil·la·tion (in'sti-lā'shŭn) Dropping liquid on or into a part.

in·stil·la·tor (in'sti-lā'tŏr) A device for performing instillation. SYN dropper.

in·stinct (in'stingkt) **1.** An enduring disposition or tendency to act in an organized and biologically adaptive manner. **2.** The unreasoning impulse to perform some purposive action without an immediate consciousness of the end to which that action may lead. **3.** PSYCHOANALYTIC THEORY the forces assumed to exist behind the tension caused by the needs of the id.

In·sti·tute of Med·i·cine (IOM) (in'sti-tūt med'i-sin) The IOM was chartered in 1970 as a component of the U.S. National Academy of Sciences; provides a vital service by working outside the framework of government to ensure scientifically informed analysis and independent guidance.

in·sti·tu·tion·al·ism (in'sti-tū′shŭn-ăl-izm) Maladaptation pattern seen in the mentally ill and others confined to group homes that renders it problematic for them to function outside such a setting.

in·sti·tu·tion·al·i·za·tion (in'sti-tū′shŭn-ăl-ĭ-zā′shŭn) Patient care within an institution for medium- or long-term durations.

in·sti·tu·tion·al li·cen·sure (in'sti-tū′shŭn-ăl lī′sĕn-shŭr) Credentials granted to a unitary institution, rather than to its individual practitioners, which allows such institution the right to provide health care services as specified and permitted by the operative authority.

In·sti·tu·tion·al Re·view Board (IRB) (in'sti-tū′shŭn-ăl rĕ-vyū′ bōrd) The standing committee in a hospital or other facility that is charged with responsibility for ensuring the safety and well-being of human subjects involved in research.

in·stru·ment (in'strŭ-mĕnt) A tool or implement.

in·stru·men·tal ac·tiv·i·ties of dai·ly liv·ing (IADL) (in'strŭ-men′tăl ak-tiv′i-tēz dā′lē liv′ing) Activities oriented to interactions with the environment, more complex than activities of daily living (ADL); usually optional or can be delegated.

in·stru·men·ta·tion (in'strŭ-mĕn-tā′shŭn) **1.** In dentistry, application of an armamentarium in a restorative procedure. **2.** The use of dental instruments.

in·su·date (in'sŭ-dāt) Fluid swelling within an arterial wall (ordinarily serous), differing from an exudate in that it does not come to lie extramurally.

in·suf·fi·cien·cy (in'sŭ-fish′ĕn-sē) **1.** Lack of completeness of function or power. **2.** SYN incompetence (1).

in·suf·fla·tion (in'sŭ-flā′shŭn) **1.** The act or process of insufflating. **2.** SYN inhalant (3).

in·suf·fla·tion an·es·the·si·a (in'sŭ-flā′shŭn an′es-thē′zē-ă) Maintenance of inhalation anesthesia by delivery of anesthetic gases or vapors directly to the airway of a spontaneously breathing patient.

in·su·la, gen. and pl. **in·su·lae** (in'sŭ-lă, -lē) [TA] **1.** An oval region of the cerebral cortex overlying the extreme capsule, lateral to the lenticular nucleus, buried in the depth of the fissura lateralis cerebri (sylvian fissure). SYN island of Reil. **2.** SYN island. **3.** Any circumscribed body or patch on the skin.

in·su·la·tion (in'sŭ-lā′shŭn) **1.** The act or state of insulating. **2.** The nonconducting substance so used.

in·su·lin (I, In, IN, INS) (in'sŭ-lin) A polypeptide hormone, secreted by β cells in the islets of Langerhans, which promotes glucose use, protein synthesis, and the formation and storage of neutral lipids; available in various preparations including genetically engineered human insulin, which is currently favored. Insulin is used parenterally in the treatment of diabetes mellitus.

insulinaemia [Br.] SYN insulinemia.

in·su·lin-an·tag·o·niz·ing fac·tor (in'sŭ-lin-an-tag′ŏ-nīz-ing fak′tŏr) SYN glycotropic factor.

in·su·lin an·ti·bod·y test (in'sŭ-lin an′ti-bod′ē test) Clinical assessment of allergic reaction to insulin.

in·su·li·nase (in'sŭ-lin-ās) Hepatic enzyme that deactivates insulin.

in·su·lin as·say test (in'sŭ-lin as'ā test) Clinical measurement of insulin resistance.

in·su·li·ne·mi·a (in'sŭ-li-nē′mē-ă) Literally, insulin in the circulating blood; usually connotes an abnormally large concentration of insulin. SYN insulinaemia.

in·su·lin·like ac·ti·vi·ty (ILA) (in'sŭ-lin-līk ak-tiv′i-tē) A measure of substances, usually in plasma, that exert biologic effects similar to those of insulin in various bioassays.

in·su·lin·like growth fac·tors (IGF) (in'sŭ-lin-līk grōth fak′tŏrz) Peptides with formation stimulated by growth hormone; can bring about peripheral tissue effects of that hormone and have high (about 70%) homology to human insulin.

in·su·lin lip·o·dys·tro·phy (in'sŭ-lin lip′ō-dis′trŏ-fē) Atrophy of subcutaneous tissues in diabetic patients at the site of frequent injections of insulin. SYN insulin lipoatrophy.

in·su·lin·o·gen·e·sis (in'sŭ-lin-ō-jen′ĕ-sis) Production of insulin.

in·su·lin·o·gen·ic, in·su·lo·gen·ic (in'sŭ-lin-ō-jen′ik, -lō-jen′ik) Relating to insulinogenesis.

in·su·li·no·ma (in'sŭ-li-nō′mă) An islet cell adenoma that secretes insulin.

in·su·lin pump (in'sŭ-lin pŭmp) Device used to deliver insulin subcutaneously by continuous basal infusion and intermittent bolus injections.

in·su·lin re·ac·tion (in'sŭ-lin re-ak′shŭn) Very low levels of blood sugar, which result from misdosage of insulin.

in·su·lin re·bound (in'sŭ-lin rē′bownd) The diabetic body's response to consuming too much sugar, which elevates blood glucose levels before they decline to a level lower than before the sugar was ingested.

in·su·lin re·sis·tance (in'sŭ-lin rĕ-zis′tăns) Diminished effectiveness of insulin in lowering blood sugar levels associated with obesity, ketoacidosis, infection, and certain rare conditions.

in·su·lin-re·sis·tance syn·drome (in'sŭ-lin rĕ-zis′tĕns sin′drŏm) SYN metabolic syndrome.

in·su·lin shock (in'sŭ-lin shok) Severe hypoglycemia produced by administration of insulin, manifested by sweating, tremor, anxiety, vertigo, and diplopia, followed by delirium, convulsions, and collapse. SYN wet shock.

in·su·lin zinc sus·pen·sion (IZS) (in'sŭ-lin zingk sŭ-spen′shŭn) Sterile buffered suspension with zinc chloride, usually containing 100 units per mL; the solid phase of the suspension consists of a mixture of seven parts of crystalline insulin and three parts of amorphous insulin. SYN lente insulin.

in·su·li·tis (in'sŭ-lī′tis) Inflammation of the islands of Langerhans, with lymphocytic infiltration that may result from viral infection and be the initial lesion of Type 1 diabetes mellitus.

in·sur·ance au·thor·i·za·tion (in-shur′ăns aw′thŏr-ī-zā′shŭn) SEE gatekeeper.

in·sus·cep·ti·bil·i·ty (in'sŭ-sep′ti-bil′i-tē) SYN immunity.

in·take (in′tāk) **1.** The act of consuming or absorbing anything. **2.** That which is taken in. Cf. output.

in·take and out·put (I and O; I&O) (in′tāk owt′put) Notations on a patient's hospital chart showing how much liquid was consumed and how much was eliminated in the form of urine.

in·te·gral dose (in′tĕ-grăl dōs) Total energy absorbed by the body, the product of the mass of tissue irradiated and the absorbed dose.

in·te·grat·ed de·liv·e·ry sys·tem (in'tĕ-grā-tĕd dĕ-liv′ĕr-ē sis′tĕm) Health care practice with individuals in different fields of specialization who work together to provide therapy and control costs. SYN integrated multispecialty group.

in·te·gra·tion (in'tĕ-grā′shŭn) **1.** The state of being combined, or the process of combining, into a complete and harmonious whole. **2.** In physiology, the process of building up. **3.** In mathematics, the process of ascertaining a function from its differential. **4.** In molecular biology, a recombination event in which a genetic element is inserted.

in·te·gra·tion of self (in'tĕ-grā'shŭn self) Psychological theory that one's integrity requires aggregating all facets of the self into harmony.

in·te·gra·tive med·i·cine (in'tĕ-grā-tiv med'i-sin) Combines mainstream medical therapies with complementary and alternative medical therapies for which there is some reliable scientific evidence of safety and effectiveness.

in·te·grin (in-teg'rin) Cell surface receptor that interacts with extracellular matrix in promulgation of the cell cycle.

in·teg·u·ment (in-teg'yū-mĕnt) [TA] **1.** The enveloping membrane of the body; includes, in addition to the epidermis and dermis, all of the derivatives of the epidermis, e.g., hairs, nails, sudoriferous and sebaceous glands, and mammary glands. **2.** The rind, capsule, or covering of any body or part. SYN integumentum commune [TA], tegument.

in·teg·u·men·ta·ry (in-teg'yū-mĕn'tăr-ē) Relating to the integument. SEE ALSO cutaneous, dermal.

in·tel·lect (in'tĕ-lekt) An ability to learn, reason, and think abstractly

in·tel·li·gence quo·tient (IQ) (in-tel'i-jĕns kwō'shĕnt) The psychologist's index of intelligence as one part of a two-part determination, the other part being an index of adaptive behavior.

in·tel·li·gence test (in-tel'i-jĕns test) Assessement using well-researched items and involving a systematic method of administration and scoring a person's general aptitude or level of potential competence.

in·tem·per·ance (in-tem'pĕr-ăns) Lack of proper self-control, usually in reference to the use of alcoholic beverages. Cf. incontinence (2).

in·ten·sive care u·nit (ICU) (in-ten'siv kār yū'nit) A hospital facility for provision of intensive nursing and medical care of critically ill patients, characterized by high quality and quantity of continuous nursing and medical supervision and by use of sophisticated monitoring and resuscitative equipment. SYN critical care unit.

in·ten·tion (in-ten'shŭn) **1.** An objective. **2.** In surgery, a process or operation.

in·ten·tion spasm (in-ten'shŭn spazm) A spasmodic contraction of the muscles occurring when a voluntary movement is attempted.

in·ten·tion trem·or (in-ten'shŭn trem'ŏr) One that occurs during performance of precise voluntary movements. SYN volitional tremor (2).

inter- *Do not confuse this word with intra-* or *intro-.* Combining form meaning among, between.

in·ter·ac·tion (in'tĕr-ak'shŭn) **1.** The reciprocal action between two entities in a common environment. **2.** The effects when two entities concur that would not be observed with either in isolation. **3.** STATISTICS, PHARMACOLOGY, QUANTITATIVE GENETICS the phenomenon that the combined effects of two causes differ from the sum of the effects separately (as in synergism and antagonism). **4.** STATISTICS the necessity for a product term in a linear model.

in·ter·ac·tive guid·ed im·ag·ery (in'tĕr-ak'tiv gīd'ĕd im'ăj-rē) A technique for facilitating the enhanced awareness of the unconscious imagery within the patient to bring about psychological and physiosociologic improvement.

in·ter·al·ve·o·lar (in'tĕr-al-vē'ŏ-lăr) Between any alveoli, especially the alveoli of the lungs.

in·ter·arch dis·tance (in'tĕr-ahrch dis'tăns) The vertical distance between the maxillary and mandibular arches under conditions of vertical dimensions that must be specified.

in·ter·ar·tic·u·lar (in'tĕr-ahr-tik'yū-lăr) **1.** Between two joints. Cf. intraarticular. **2.** Between two joint surfaces.

in·ter·ar·tic·u·lar fi·bro·car·ti·lage (in'tĕr-ahr-tik'yū-lăr fī'brō-kahr'ti-lăj) SYN articular disc.

in·ter·a·tri·al (in′tĕr-ā′trē-ăl) Between the atria of the heart. SYN interauricular (1).

in·ter·a·tri·al con·duc·tion time (in′tĕr-ā′trē-ăl kŏn-dŭk′shŭn tīm) SYN intraatrial conduction time (2).

in·ter·au·ral (in′tĕr-awr′ăl) Referring to differences between ears, particularly temporal events occurring in or emanating from the ears.

in·ter·ca·dent (in′tĕr-kā′dĕnt) Irregular in rhythm.

in·ter·ca·la·ted (in-tĕr′kă-lā-tĕd) Interposed between two others.

in·ter·ca·la·ted disc (in-tĕr′kă-lā-tĕd disk) A histologic feature of cardiac muscle, occurring at the junction of two myocardial cells; site of intercellular passage of ions and electrical impulses.

in·ter·ca·la·ted ducts (in-tĕr′kă-lā-tĕd dŭkts) The minute ducts of glands that lead from the acini.

in·ter·cap·il·lar·y (in′tĕr-kap′i-lar′ē) Between or among capillary vessels.

in·ter·cap·il·lar·y glo·mer·u·lo·scle·ro·sis (in′tĕr-kap′i-lar-ē glo-mer′yū-lō-skler-ō′sis) SYN diabetic glomerulosclerosis.

in·ter·ca·rot·id bod·y (in′tĕr-kă-rot′id bod′ē) SYN carotid body.

in·ter·car·pal (IC) (in′tĕr-kahr′păl) Between the carpal bones.

in·ter·car·pal joints (in′tĕr-kahr′păl joynts) SYN carpal joints.

in·ter·car·ti·lag·i·nous (in′tĕr-kahr′ti-laj′i-nŭs) Between or connecting cartilages. SYN interchondral.

in·ter·cav·er·nous (in′tĕr-kav′ĕr-nŭs) Between two cavities.

in·ter·cel·lu·lar (in′tĕr-sel′yū-lăr) Between or among cells.

in·ter·cel·lu·lar bridges (in′tĕr-sel′yū-lăr brij′ĕz) Slender cytoplasmic strands connecting adjacent cells. SYN cell bridges, cytoplasmic bridges.

in·ter·cel·lu·lar ca·na·lic·u·lus (in′tĕr-sel′yū-lăr kan′ă-lik′yū-lŭs) One of the fine channels between adjoining secretory cells, such as those between serous cells in salivary glands.

in·ter·cel·lu·lar junc·tions (in′tĕr-sel′yū-lăr jŭngk′shŭnz) Specializations of the cellular margins that contribute to the adhesion or allow for communication between cells.

in·ter·cep·tive or·tho·don·tics (in′tĕr-sep′tiv ŏr′thŏ-dont′iks) Dental practice of assessing children's occlusion early, even though normal, to avoid later need of prosthodontics.

in·ter·ce·re·bral (in′tĕr-ser′ĕ-brăl) Between the cerebral hemispheres.

in·ter·cos·tal (in′tĕr-kos′tăl) Between the ribs.

in·ter·cos·tal mem·branes (in′tĕr-kos′tăl mem′brănz) [TA] The membranous layers between ribs.

in·ter·cos·tal mus·cles (in′tĕr-kos′tăl mŭs′ĕlz) The internal and external muscles about the ribs.

in·ter·cos·tal neu·ral·gi·a (ICN) (in′tĕr-kos′tăl nūr-al′jē-ă) Pain in the chest wall due to neuralgia of one or more of the intercostal nerves. SYN abdominal cutaneous nerve entrapment syndrome.

in·ter·cos·tal space (in′tĕr-kos′tăl spās) [TA] An interval between the ribs, occupied by intercostal muscles, veins, arteries, and nerves.

in·ter·course (in′tĕr-kōrs) Communication or dealings between or among people. SEE ALSO coitus.

in·ter·cri·co·thy·rot·o·my (in′tĕr-krī′kō-thī-rot′ŏ-mē) SYN cricothyrotomy.

in·ter·cris·tal (in′tĕr-kris′tăl) Between two crests, as between the crests of the ilia, applied to one of the pelvic measurements.

in·ter·cur·rent (in′tĕr-kŭr′ĕnt) Intervening; said of a disease attacking a person already ill of another malady. SEE ALSO intercurrent disease.

in·ter·cur·rent dis·ease (in′tĕr-kŭr′ĕnt

di-zēz′) New disease occurring during the course of another disease, not related to the primary disease process. SEE ALSO intercurrent.

in·ter·cus·pa·tion (in′tĕr-kŭs-pā′shŭn) **1.** The cusp-to-fossa relation of the maxillary and mandibular posterior teeth to each other. **2.** The interlocking or fitting together of the cusps of opposing teeth. SYN interdigitation (4).

in·ter·cusp·ing (in′tĕr-kŭsp′ing) SYN intercuspation.

in·ter·den·tal (in′tĕr-den′tăl) Between the teeth.

in·ter·den·tal ca·nals (in′tĕr-den′tăl kă-nalz′) Those that extend vertically through interdental alveolar bone between roots of mandibular and maxillary incisors and maxillary bicuspid teeth. SYN Hirschfeld canals.

in·ter·den·tal sep·tum (in′tĕr-den′tăl sep′tŭm) The bony interval separating two adjacent teeth in a dental arch.

in·ter·den·ti·um (in′tĕr-den′shē-ŭm) The interval between any two contiguous teeth.

in·ter·dig·i·ta·tion (in′tĕr-dij′i-tā′shŭn) **1.** The mutual interlocking of toothed or fingerlike processes. **2.** The processes thus interlocked. **3.** Infoldings or plicae of adjacent cell or plasma membranes. **4.** SYN intercuspation (2).

in·ter·dis·charge in·ter·val (in′tĕr-dis′ chahrj in′tĕr-văl) Time elapsed between consecutive discharges of muscle fibers.

in·ter·dis·ci·pli·nar·y (in′tĕr-dis′i-pli-nar-ē) Denoting the overlapping interests of different fields of medicine and science.

in·ter·face (in′tĕr-fās) **1.** A surface that forms a common boundary of two bodies. **2.** The boundary between regions of different radiopacity, acoustic, or magnetic resonance properties.

in·ter·fas·cic·u·lar (in′tĕr-fă-sik′yū-lăr) Between fasciculi.

in·ter·fem·o·ral (in′tĕr-fem′ŏ-răl) Between the thighs.

in·ter·fe·ren·tial cur·rent (IFC) (in′tĕr-fĕr-en′shăl kŭr′rĕnt) An electrotherapeutic modality that employs the interference of two polyphasic sine waves to decrease the perception of pain.

in·ter·fer·on (IFN) (in′tĕr-fēr′on) A class of small protein and glycoprotein cytokines (15–28 kD) produced by T cells, fibroblasts, and other cells in response to viral infection and other biologic and synthetic stimuli. Interferons are divided into five major classes (alpha, beta, gamma, tau, and omega) and several subclasses (indicated by Arabic numerals and letters) on the basis of various properties.

in·ter·fer·on-al·pha (α) (in′tĕr-fēr′on-al′fă) The major interferon made by virus-induced leukocytes.

in·ter·fer·on al·pha (α) 2b (in′tĕr-fēr′on al′fă) A water-soluble protein secreted by cells infected by virus.

in·ter·fer·on be·ta (β) 1b (in′tĕr-fēr′on bā′tă) A purified protein containing 165 amino acids with antiviral and immunomodulatory effects.

in·ter·fer·on gam·ma (γ) (IFN-G, IFN-gamma, INF-gamma) (in′tĕr-fēr′on gam′ă) That elaborated by T lymphocytes in response to either specific antigen or mitogenic stimulation. SYN antigen interferon, immune interferon.

in·ter·fer·on type I (in′tĕr-fēr′on tīp) Antiviral interferons, including interferon-α, and interferon-β.

in·ter·fer·on type II (in′tĕr-fēr′on tīp) Immune interferon.

in·ter·glob·u·lar (in′tĕr-glob′yū-lăr) Between globules.

in·ter·glo·bu·lar den·tin (in′tĕr-glob′ yū-lăr den′tin) Imperfectly calcified matrix of dentin situated between the calcified globules near the dentinal periphery.

in·ter·glu·te·al (in′tĕr-glū′tē-ăl) Between the buttocks.

in·ter·ic·tal (in′tĕr-ik′tăl) The period between convulsions.

in·ter·im den·ture (in′tĕr-im den′chŭr)

A dental prosthesis to be used for a short time for reasons of esthetics, mastication, occlusal support, or convenience. SYN temporary denture.

in·te·ri·or (in-tēr′ē-ŏr) Relating to the inside; situated within.

in·te·ri·or·i·za·tion (in-tēr′ē-ŏr-ī-zā′shŭn) To rationalize external phenomena within one's frame of reference.

in·ter·ki·ne·sis (in′tĕr-ki-nē′sis) Period between the first and second divisions of meiosis.

in·ter·lam·i·nar jel·ly (in′tĕr-lam′i-năr jel′ē) The gelatinous material between ectoderm and endoderm that serves as the substrate on which mesenchymal cells migrate.

in·ter·leu·kin (IL) (in′tĕr-lū′kin) The name given to a group of multifunctional cytokines after their amino acid structure is known. They are synthesized by lymphocytes, monocytes, macrophages, and certain other cells. There are 18 subtypes. SEE ALSO lymphokine, cytokine.

in·ter·lo·bar (in′tĕr-lō′bahr) Between the lobes of an organ or other structure.

in·ter·lo·bar duct (in′tĕr-lō′bahr dŭkt) A duct draining the secretion of the lobe of a gland; formed by the junction of several interlobular ducts.

in·ter·lo·bi·tis (in′tĕr-lō-bī′tis) Inflammation of the pleura separating two pulmonary lobes.

in·ter·lob·u·lar (in′tĕr-lob′yū-lăr) Between the lobules of an organ.

in·ter·lob·u·lar ar·te·ries (in′tĕr-lob′yū-lăr ahr′tĕr-ēz) [TA] Those that pass between lobules of an organ. SYN arteriae interlobulares [TA].

in·ter·lob·u·lar duct (in′tĕr-lob′yū-lăr dŭkt) Any duct leading from a lobule of a gland and formed by the junction of the fine ducts draining the acini.

in·ter·lob·u·lar duc·tules (in′tĕr-lob′yū-lăr dŭk′tyūlz) Bile ductules occupying portal canals between hepatic lobules that open into the biliary ductules. SYN ductuli interlobulares.

in·ter·lob·u·lar em·phy·se·ma (in′tĕr-lob′yū-lăr em′fi-sē′mă) Interstitial emphysema in the connective tissue septa between the pulmonary lobules.

in·ter·lob·u·lar pleu·ri·sy (in′tĕr-lob′yū-lăr plūr′i-sē) Inflammation limited to the pleura in the sulci between the pulmonary lobes.

in·ter·lock·ing gy·ri (in′tĕr-lok′ing jī′rī) Several small gyri in the walls of the central sulcus of the hemisphere; the opposed gyri interlock.

in·ter·max·il·lar·y bone (in′tĕr-mak′si-lar-ē bōn) SYN os incisivum.

in·ter·max·il·lary fix·a·tion (in′tĕr-mak′si-lar-ē fik-sā′shŭn) Fixation of fractures of the mandible or maxilla by applying elastic bands or stainless steel wire between the maxillary and mandibular arch bars or other types of splint. SYN maxillomandibular fixation.

in·ter·max·il·lar·y seg·ment (in′tĕr-mak′si-lar-ē seg′mĕnt) Primordial mass of tissue formed by the merging of the medial nasal prominences of the embryo.

in·ter·max·il·lar·y su·ture (in′tĕr-mak′si-lar-ē sū′chŭr) [TA] The line of union of the two maxillae.

in·ter·me·di·ar·y (in′tĕr-mē′dē-ar-ē) Occurring between.

in·ter·me·di·ar·y me·tab·o·lism (in′tĕr-mē′dē-ar-ē mĕ-tab′ŏ-lizm) Sum of all metabolic reactions between uptake of foodstuffs and formation of excretory products.

in·ter·me·di·ar·y nerve (in′tĕr-mē′dē-ar-ē nĕrv) A root of the facial nerve containing sensory fibers for taste from the anterior two thirds of the tongue. SYN nervus intermedius [TA], intermediate nerve.

in·ter·me·di·ate (in′tĕr-mē′dē-ăt) [TA] **1.** Between two extremes; interposed. **2.** A substance formed in the course of chemical reactions that then proceeds to participate rapidly in further reactions, so that at any given moment it is present in only minute concentrations. **3.** DENTISTRY a cement base. **4.** An element or organ between right and left (or lateral and medial) structures. SYN intermedius.

in·ter·me·di·ate am·pu·ta·tion (in'tĕr-mē'dē-ăt am'pyū-tā'shŭn) An amputation formerly performed during the period between trauma or incipient gangrene and suppuration.

in·ter·me·di·ate ba·sil·ic vein (in'tĕr-mē'dē-ăt bă-sil'ik vān) Medial branch of the median antebrachial vein that joins the basilic vein.

in·ter·me·di·ate care fa·cil·i·ties for the men·tal·ly re·tard·ed (ICF/MR) (in'tĕr-mē'dē-ăt kār fă-sil'i-tēz men'tă-lē rē-tahr'dĕd) A health care provider of therapy that is less highly advanced than that provided in a hospital for patients with learning disabilities.

in·ter·me·di·ate care fa·cil·i·ty (ICF) (in'tĕr-mē'dē-ăt kār fă-sil'i-tē) A residential option for patients who cannot live alone and also need more supervision than in-home services offer but who do not need the level of care found in skilled nursing facilities. SEE nursing facility.

in·ter·me·di·ate den·si·ty lip·o·pro·tein (IDL) (in'tĕr-mē'dē-ăt den'si-tē lip'ō-prō'tēn) Class of lipoproteins formed in degradation of very low density lipoproteins.

in·ter·me·di·ate fil·a·ments (in'tĕr-mē'dē-ăt fil'ă-mĕnts) Class of tough protein filaments (including keratin filaments, neurofilaments, desmin, and vimentin) that make up part of the cytoskeleton of the cytoplasm of most eukaryotic cells.

in·ter·me·di·ate host, in·ter·me·di·ar·y host (in'tĕr-mē'dē-ăt hōst, in'tĕr-mē'dē-ar-ē) **1.** One in which larval or developmental stages occur. **2.** A host through which a microorganism can pass or contains an asexual stage of a parasite.

in·ter·me·di·ate la·mel·la (in'tĕr-mē'dē-ăt lă-mel'ă) SYN interstitial lamella.

in·ter·me·di·ate mass (in'tĕr-mē'dē-ăt mas) SYN interthalamic adhesion.

in·ter·me·di·ate trait (in'tĕr-mē'dē-ăt trāt) A measurable trait in which there is some evidence of the operation of a simple major cause, but in which the variation within the putative categories is such

as to cause overlap and hence ambiguity in classification of any particular reading.

in·ter·me·din (in'tĕr-mē'din) SYN melanotropin.

in·ter·me·di·us (in'tĕr-mē'dē-ŭs) [TA] SYN intermediate.

in·ter·men·stru·al (in'tĕr-men'strū-ăl) Between two consecutive menstrual periods.

in·ter·men·stru·al pain (in'tĕr-men'strū-ăl pān) **1.** Pelvic discomfort occurring approximately at the time of ovulation, usually at the midpoint of the menstrual cycle. **2.** SYN mittelschmerz.

in·ter·mit·tent (in'tĕr-mit'ĕnt) Marked by intervals of complete quietude between two periods of activity.

in·ter·mit·tent a·cute por·phyr·i·a (IAP) (in'tĕr-mit'ĕnt ă-kyūt' pōr-fir'ē-ă) Porphyria caused by hepatic overproduction of δ-aminolevulinic acid, with greatly increased urinary excretion of it and of porphobilinogen, and some increase of uroporphyrin, due to a deficiency of porphobilinogen deaminase. SYN acute intermittent porphyria.

in·ter·mit·tent clau·di·ca·tion (in'tĕr-mit'ĕnt klaw'di-kā'shŭn) A condition caused by ischemia of the muscles; characterized by attacks of lameness and pain, brought on by walking, chiefly in the calf muscles. SYN Charcot syndrome, myasthenia angiosclerotica.

in·ter·mit·tent com·pres·sion (in'tĕr-mit'ĕnt kŏm-presh'ŭn) **1.** A neurodevelopmental treatment technique to facilitate contraction by applying pressure directly to the muscles surrounding a joint requiring better stabilization. **2.** A treatment procedure that employs intermittent external pressure to reduce edema in an extremity.

in·ter·mit·tent ex·plo·sive dis·or·der (in'tĕr-mit'ĕnt eks-plō'siv dis-ōr'dĕr) A disorder that begins in early childhood, characterized by repeated acts of violent, aggressive behavior in otherwise normal people that is markedly out of proportion to the event that provokes it.

in·ter·mit·tent fe·ver (in'tĕr-mit'ănt fē'

in·ter·mit·tent he·mo·di·al·y·sis (IHD) (in'tĕr-mit'ĕnt hē'mō-dī-al'i-sis) Noncontinous therapy to allow kidney function.

in·ter·mit·tent hy·dro·sal·pinx (in'tĕr-mit'ĕnt hī'drō-sal'pingks) Noncontinuous discharge of watery fluid from the oviduct. SYN hydrops tubae profluens.

in·ter·mit·tent man·da·to·ry ven·ti·la·tion (IMV) (in'tĕr-mit'ĕnt man'dă-tōr-ē ven'ti-lā'shŭn) A mode of mechanical ventilation in which the patient can trigger spontaneous breaths between or during preset mandatory breaths.

in·ter·mit·tent per·cus·sive ven·ti·la·tion (IPV) (in'tĕr-mit'ĕnt pĕr-kus'iv ven'ti-lā'shŭn) A ventilatory technique that delivers short high velocity bursts of respiratory gas through a full face mask at a rapid rate (80–650 cycles/min) in addition to a steady flow of gas at a physiologic level.

in·ter·mit·tent pos·i·tive pres·sure breath·ing (IPPB) (in'tĕr-mit'ĕnt poz'i-tiv presh'ŭr brēdh'ing) SYN controlled mechanical ventilation.

in·ter·mit·tent po·si·tive pres·sure ven·ti·la·tion (IPPV) (in'tĕr-mit'ĕnt poz'i-tiv presh'ŭr ven'ti-lā'shŭn) SYN controlled mechanical ventilation.

in·ter·mus·cu·lar (IM) (in'tĕr-mŭs'kyū-lăr) Between the muscles.

in·tern (in'tĕrn) An advanced student or recent graduate undertaking further education by assisting in the medical or surgical care of hospital patients, with supervision and instruction.

in·ter·nal (in-tĕr'năl) [TA] *Often incorrectly used to mean medial.* Away from the surface.

in·ter·nal ad·he·sive pe·ri·car·di·tis (in-tĕr'năl ad-hē'siv per'i-kahr-dī'tis) SYN concretio cordis.

in·ter·nal fis·tu·la (in-tĕr'năl fis'tyū-lă) Passage between hollow viscera.

in·ter·nal fix·a·tion (in-tĕr'năl fik-sā'shŭn) Stabilization of fractured bony parts by direct fixation to one another with surgical wires, screws, pins, or methylmethacrylate.

in·ter·nal hem·or·rhage (in-tĕr'năl hem'ŏr-ăj) Bleeding into organs or cavities of the body.

in·ter·nal her·ni·a (in-tĕr'năl hĕr'nē-ă) Protrusion of an intraperitoneal viscus into a compartment or under band within the abdominal cavity.

in·ter·nal in·ju·ry (in-tĕr'năl in'jŭr-ē) Any trauma that involves organs or cavities of the body.

in·ter·nal·i·za·tion (in-tĕr'năl-ī-zā'shŭn) Adopting the standards and values of another person or of society as one's own.

in·ter·nal med·i·cine (in-tĕr'năl med'i-sin) Medical branch concerned with nonsurgical diseases in adults, but not including diseases limited to the skin or to the nervous system.

in·ter·nal oph·thal·mo·ple·gi·a (in-tĕr'năl of-thal'mō-plē'jē-ă) SYN ophthalmoplegia interna.

in·ter·nal res·pi·ra·tion (in-tĕr'năl res'pir-ā'shŭn) SYN tissue respiration.

in·ter·nal ro·ta·tion (in-tĕr'năl rō-tā'shŭn) Movement of a joint, around its long axis, toward the midline of the body. SYN medial rotation.

in·ter·nal trac·tion (in-tĕr'năl trak'shŭn) A pulling force created by using one of the cranial bones, above the point of fracture, for anchorage.

In·ter·na·tion·al An·a·tom·ic·al Ter·mi·nol·o·gy (FICAT) (in'tĕr-nash'ŭn-ăl an'ă-tom'i-kăl tĕr'mi-nol'ŏ-jē) SEE Terminologia Anatomica.

In·ter·na·tion·al As·so·ci·a·tion of Den·tal Re·search (IADR) (in'tĕr-nash'ŭn-ăl ă-sō'sē-ā'shŭn den'tăl rē'sĕrch) A professional organization that supports programs to promote research and activities related to dentistry and oral health.

In·ter·na·tion·al A·tom·ic En·er·gy A·gen·cy (IAEA) (in'tĕr-nash'ŭn-ăl ă-tom'ik en'ĕr-jē ā'jĕn-sē) Organization headquartered in Vienna, Austria that seeks to control the spread of nuclear weapons and promote peaceful uses of nuclear energy.

In·ter·na·tion·al Clas·si·fi·ca·tion of Dis·eas·es (ICD) (in′tĕr-nash′ŭn-ăl klas′i-fi-kā′shŭn di-zēz′ĕz) The enumeration of specific conditions and groups of conditions determined by an internationally representative expert committee that advises the World Health Organization, which publishes the complete list in a periodically revised book, the *Manual of the International Statistical Classification of Diseases, Injuries and Causes of Death.*

In·ter·na·tion·al Clas·si·fi·ca·tion of Func·tion·ing, Dis·a·bil·i·ty, and Health (in′tĕr-nash′ŭn-ăl klas′i-fi-kā′shŭn fŭngk′shŭn-ing dis′ă-bil′i-tē helth) The World Health Organization's classification.

In·ter·na·tion·al Clas·si·fic·a·tion of Sleep Dis·or·ders (ICSD) (in′tĕr-nash′ŭn-ăl klas′i-fi-kā′shŭn slēp dis-ōr′dĕrz) Coded listing, last revised in 2005, published by the American Academy of Sleep Medicine; used for diagnosis of disorders and disease states related to or active during periods of sleep.

In·ter·na·tion·al Com·mis·sion on Ra·di·o·log·ic·al Pro·tec·tion (ICRP) (in′tĕr-nash′ŭn-ăl kŏ-mish′ŏn rā′dē-ŏ-loj′i′kăl prŏ-tek′shŭn) A nongovernmental organization set up to determine standards of safety for those who work in radiography.

In·ter·na·tion·al Con·fed·e·ra·tion of Mid·wives (ICM) (in′tĕr-nash′ŭn-ăl kŏn-fed′ĕr-ā′shŭn mid′wīvz) A professional organization that seeks to improve the lives of women and infants through strengthening the position and training of the midwife as a valued health care practitioner.

In·ter·na·tion·al Coun·cil of Nurs·es (ICN) (in′tĕr-nash′ŭn-ăl kown′sil nŭr′sĕz) A professional nursing organization; its focus is more on education than on everyday labor issues.

In·ter·na·tion·al Mas·sage As·so·ci·a·tion (IMA) (in′tĕr-nash′ŭn-ăl mă-sazh′ ă-sō′sē-ā′shŭn) Worldwide professional organization of massage therapists.

In·ter·na·tion·al nor·mal·ized ra·ti·o (INR) (in′tĕr-nash′ŭn-ăl nōr′măl-īzd rā′ shē-ō) Prothrombin time ratio that would have been obtained if a standard reagent had been used in a prothrombin time determination.

In·ter·na·tion·al Pho·ne·tic Al·pha·bet (IPA) (in′tĕr-nash′ŭn-ăl fŏ-net′ik al′fă-bet) System of orthographic symbols devised for representing speech sounds; can be used for any language or to represent the sounds of disordered speech.

In·ter·na·tion·al Red Cross So·ci·e·ty (in′tĕr-nash′ŭn-ăl red kraws sŏ-sī′ĕ-tē) A benevolent organization, based in Geneva with aims similar to those of the American Red Cross. It provides humanitarian aid to refugees, prisoners of war, and victims of natural disaster.

In·ter·na·tion·al Sys·tem of U·nits (SI) (in′tĕr-nash′ŭn-ăl sis′tĕm ū′nits) A system of measurements, based on the metric system, adopted in 1960 to cover both the coherent units (basic, supplementary, and derived units) and the decimal multiples and submultiples of these units formed by use of prefixes proposed for general international scientific and technologic use. SI proposes seven basic units: meter (m), kilogram (kg), second (s), ampere (A), Kelvin (K), candela (cd), and mole (mol) for the basic quantities of length, mass, time, electric current, temperature, luminous intensity, and amount of substance; supplementary units proposed include the radian (rad) for plane angle and steradian (sr) for solid angle; derived units (e.g., force, power, frequency) are stated in terms of the basic units (e.g., velocity is in meters per second, m/sec^{-1}). Multiples (prefixes) in descending order are: exa- (E, 10^{18}), peta- (P, 10^{15}), tera- (T, 10^{12}), giga- (G, 10^{9}), mega- (M, 10^{6}), kilo- (k, 10^{3}), hecto- (h, 10^{2}), deca- (da, 10^{1}), deci- (d, 10^{-1}), centi- (c, 10^{-2}), milli- (m, 10^{-3}), micro- (μ, 10^{-6}), nano- (n, 10^{-9}), pico- (p, 10^{-12}), femto- (f, 10^{-15}), atto- (a, 10^{-18}). The prefix zepto (z) has been proposed for 10^{-21}.

in·ter·na·tion·al u·nit (in′tĕr-nash′ŭn-ăl yū′nit) The amount of a substance (e.g., drug, hormone, vitamin, enzyme) that produces a specific effect as defined by an international body and accepted internationally. SYN unit (4).

in·ter·neu·rons (in′tĕr-nūr′onz) Combinations or groups of neurons between sensory and motor neurons that govern coordinated activity. SYN interneurones.

in·tern·ist (in-tĕr′nist) A physician trained in internal medicine.

in·ter·nod·al seg·ment (in′tĕr-nō′dăl seg′mĕnt) The portion of a myelinated nerve fiber between two successive nodes. SYN internode.

in·tern·ship (in′tĕrn-ship) 1. Course of practice-study followed by recent graduates from medical schools in hospitals. 2. Undetermined period when a trainee participates in a given occupation for purposes of learning.

in·ter·nu·cle·ar (in′tĕr-nū′klē-ăr) Between nerve cell groups in the brain or retina.

in·ter·nu·cle·ar oph·thal·mo·ple·gi·a (INO) (in′tĕr-nū′klē-ăr of-thal′mō-plē′jē-ă) Ocular disorder with lesions of the medial longitudinal fasciculus, with failure of adduction in horizontal gaze but with retention of convergence.

in·ter·nun·ci·al (in′tĕr-nun′sē-ăl) 1. Indicating a neuron functionally interposed between two or more other neurons. 2. Acting as a medium of communication between two organs.

in·ter·nus (in-ter′nŭs) [TA] SYN internal.

in·ter·oc·clu·sal (in′tĕr-ŏ-klū′zăl) Between the occlusal surfaces of opposing teeth.

in·ter·oc·clu·sal dis·tance (in′tĕr-ŏ-klū′zăl dis′tăns) The vertical distance between the opposing occlusal surfaces, assuming rest relation unless otherwise designated.

in·ter·oc·clu·sal re·cord, cen·tric in·ter·oc·clu·sal re·cord, ec·cen·tric in·ter·oc·clu·sal re·cord, lat·er·al in·ter·oc·clu·sal re·cord, pro·tru·sive in·ter·oc·clu·sal re·cord (in′tĕr-ŏ-klū′zăl rek′ŏrd, sen′trik, ek-sen′trik, lat′ĕr-ăl, prō-trū′siv) Cast of the positional relationship of the teeth or jaws to each other, recorded by placing a plastic material that hardens (such as plaster of Paris or wax) between the occlusal surfaces of the rims or teeth. SYN checkbite.

in·ter·o·cep·tive (in′tĕr-ō-sep′tiv) Relating to the sensory nerve cells innervating the viscera, their sensory end organs, or the information they convey to the spinal cord and the brain.

in·ter·o·cep·tor (in′tĕr-ō-sep′tŏr) One of the various forms of small sensory end organs (receptors) situated within the walls of the respiratory and gastrointestinal tracts or in other viscera.

in·ter·os·se·ous (in′tĕr-os′ē-ŭs) Lying between or connecting bones; denoting certain muscles and ligaments. SYN interosseal.

in·ter·os·se·ous car·ti·lage (in′tĕr-os′ē-ŭs kahr′ti-lăj) SEE connecting cartilage.

in·ter·pa·ri·e·tal (in′tĕr-pă-rī′ĕ-tăl) Between the walls of a part, or between the parietal bones.

in·ter·par·ox·ys·mal (in′tĕr-par′ok-siz′măl) Occurring between successive paroxysms of a disease.

in·ter·pe·dun·cu·lar (in′tĕr-pe-dŭngk′yū-lăr) Between any two peduncles.

in·ter·per·son·al (in′tĕr-per′sŏn-ăl) Pertaining to relations and social exchanges between people.

in·ter·phase (in′tĕr-fāz) The stage between two successive divisions of a cell nucleus in which the biochemical and physiologic functions of the cell are performed and replication of chromatin occurs. SYN karyostasis.

in·ter·phy·let·ic (in′tĕr-fī-let′ik) Denoting the transitional forms between two kinds of cells during the course of metaplasia.

in·ter·pleu·ral space (in′tĕr-plūr′ăl spās) SYN mediastinum (2).

in·ter·po·lat·ed ex·tra·sy·sto·le (in-tĕr′pŏ-lā′tĕd eks-tră-sis′tŏ-lē) A ventricular extrasystole that, instead of being followed by a compensatory pause, is sandwiched between two consecutive sinus cycles.

in·ter·pre·ta·tion (INTERP) (in-tĕr′prĕ-tā′shŭn) **1.** In psychoanalysis, the characteristic therapeutic intervention of the analyst. **2.** In clinical psychology, drawing inferences and formulating the meaning in terms of the psychological dynamics inherent in a person's responses to psychological tests or during psychotherapy.

in·ter·prox·i·mal (in′tĕr-prok′si-măl) Between adjoining surfaces.

in·ter·prox·i·mal space (in′tĕr-prok′si-măl spās) Gap between adjacent teeth in a dental arch.

in·ter·pu·bic disc (in′tĕr-pyū′bik disk) [TA] The disc of fibrocartilage that unites the pubic bones at the pubic symphysis.

in·ter·rupt·ed su·ture (in′tĕr-ŭp′tĕd sū′chŭr) A single stitch fixed by tying its ends together.

in·ter·scap·u·lo·tho·rac·ic am·pu·ta·tion (in′tĕr-skap′yū-lō-thōr-as′ik amp-yū-tā′shŭn) SYN forequarter amputation.

in·ter·sec·tion (in′tĕr-sek′shŭn) [TA] The site of crossing of two anatomic structures.

in·ter·sec·ti·o ten·din·e·a (in-tĕr-sek′shē-ō ten-din′ē-ă) [TA] SYN tendinous intersection.

in·ter·seg·men·tal vein (in′tĕr-seg-men′tăl vān) A vein receiving blood from adjacent bronchopulmonary segments.

in·ter·sex (in′tĕr-seks) Being between the two sexes anatomically.

in·ter·sex·u·al·i·ty (in′tĕr-sek′shū-al′i-tē) The condition of having both male and female characteristics.

in·ter·space (in′tĕr-spās) Area between two like objects.

in·ter·spi·nal (in′tĕr-spī′năl) Between two spines, such as the spinous processes of the vertebrae. SYN interspinous.

in·ter·spi·nous (in′tĕr-spī′nŭs) SYN interspinal.

in·ter·stice, pl. **in·ter·stic·es** (in′tĕr-

stis, in-tĕr-sti′sēz) *Avoid the mispronunciation in-ter′sti-sēz of the plural of this word.* SYN interstitium.

in·ter·sti·tial (in′tĕr-stish′ăl) **1.** Relating to spaces or interstices in any structure. **2.** Relating to spaces within a tissue or organ, but excluding body cavities or potential space. Cf. intracavitary.

in·ter·sti·tial cells (in′tĕr-stish′ăl selz) **1.** Those between the seminiferous tubules of the testis that secrete testosterone. SYN Leydig cells. **2.** Those derived from the theca interna of atretic follicles of the ovary. **3.** Pineal cells similar to glial cells with long processes.

in·ter·sti·tial cell-stim·u·lat·ing hor·mone (ICSH) (in′tĕr-stish′ăl sel′stim′yū-lā-ting hōr′mŏn) SYN lutropin.

in·ter·sti·tial cys·ti·tis (in′tĕr-stish′ăl sis-tī′tis) A chronic inflammatory condition of unknown etiology involving the mucosa and muscularis of the bladder, resulting in reduced bladder capacity, pain relieved by voiding, and severe bladder irritative symptoms.

in·ter·sti·tial dis·ease (in′tĕr-stish′ăl di-zēz′) A disease chiefly of the connective-tissue framework of an organ.

in·ter·sti·tial em·phy·se·ma (in′tĕr-stish′ăl em′fi-sē′mă) **1.** Presence of air in the pulmonary tissues consequent upon rupture of the air cells. **2.** Presence of air or gas in the connective tissue.

in·ter·sti·tial flu·id (in′tĕr-stish′ăl flū′id) Liquid in spaces between the tissue cells, constituting about 16% of the weight of the human body; closely similar in composition to lymph.

in·ter·sti·tial growth (in′tĕr-stish′ăl grŏth) That from a number of different centers within an area; can occur only when the materials involved are non-rigid.

in·ter·sti·tial her·ni·a (in′tĕr-stish′ăl hĕr′nē-ă) One in which the protrusion is between any two of the layers of the abdominal wall.

in·ter·sti·tial im·plan·ta·tion (in′tĕr-stish′ăl im′plan-tā′shŭn) Form in which the blastocyst lies within the substance of the endometrium.

in·ter·sti·tial in·flam·ma·tion (in′tĕr-stish′ăl in′flă-mā′shŭn) Type in which the inflammatory reaction occurs chiefly in the supportive fibrous connective tissue of an organ.

in·ter·sti·tial ker·a·ti·tis (in′tĕr-stish′ăl ker′ă-tī′tis) An inflammation of the corneal stroma, often with neovascularization.

in·ter·sti·tial la·mel·la (in′tĕr-stish′ăl lă-mel′ă) One of the lamellae of partially resorbed osteons occurring between newer, complete osteons. SYN ground lamella.

in·ter·sti·tial mas·ti·tis (in′tĕr-stish′ăl mas-tī′tis) Inflammation of the connective tissue of the mammary gland.

in·ter·sti·tial neph·ri·tis (in′tĕr-stish′ăl nĕ-frī′tis) A form in which the interstitial connective tissue is most affected.

in·ter·sti·tial plas·ma cell pneu·mo·ni·a (in′tĕr-stish′ăl plaz′mă sel nū-mō′nē-ă) SYN *Pneumocystis jiroveci* pneumonia.

in·ter·sti·tial pneu·mo·ni·a (in′tĕr-stish′ăl nū-mō′nē-ă) SYN giant cell pneumonia.

in·ter·sti·tial preg·nan·cy (in′tĕr-stish′ăl preg′năn-sē) SYN intramural pregnancy.

in·ter·sti·tial tis·sue (in′tĕr-stish′ăl tish′ū) SYN connective tissue.

in·ter·stit·i·um (in′tĕr-stish′ē-ŭm) A small area, space, or gap in the substance of an organ or tissue. SEE ALSO connective tissue. SYN interstice.

in·ter·tar·sal (in′tĕr-tahr′săl) Denoting the articulations of the tarsal bones with each other.

in·ter·tha·lam·ic (in′tĕr-thă-lam′ik) Between the thalami.

in·ter·tha·lam·ic ad·he·sion (in′tĕr-thă-lam′ik ad-hē′zhŭn) [TA] Variable connection between the two thalamic masses across the third ventricle. SYN adhesio interthalamica [TA], massa intermedia, commissura cinerea, commissura grisea (1), intermediate mass.

in·ter·trans·verse (in′tĕr-trans-vĕrs′) Between the transverse processes of the vertebrae.

in·ter·tri·go (in′tĕr-trī′gō) Irritant dermatitis occurring between folds or juxtaposed surfaces of the skin, caused by friction, sweat retention, moisture, warmth, and concomitant overgrowth of resident microorganisms.

in·ter·tro·chan·ter·ic (in′tĕr-trō′kan-ter′ik) Between the two trochanters of the femur.

in·ter·tro·chan·ter·ic frac·ture (in′tĕr-trō′kan-ter′ik frak′shŭr) Fracture of the proximal femur located in the metaphysial bone in the region between the greater and lesser trochanters.

in·ter·tro·chan·ter·ic line (in′tĕr-trō′kan-ter′ik līn) [TA] A rough line that separates the neck and shaft of the femur anteriorly. SYN linea intertrochanterica [TA].

in·ter·u·re·ter·al (in′tĕr-yū-rē′tĕr-ăl) Between the two ureters. SYN interureteric.

in·ter·u·re·ter·ic (in′tĕr-yū′rē-ter′ik) SYN interureteral.

in·ter·va·gi·nal (in′tĕr-vaj′i-năl) 1. Within the vagina. 2. Between any anatomic sheaths.

in·ter·val (in′tĕr-văl) A time or space between two periods or objects; a break in continuity.

in·ter·ve·nous tu·ber·cle (in′tĕr-vē′nŭs tū′bĕr-kĕl) The slight projection on the wall of the right atrium between the orifices of the venae cavae.

in·ter·ven·tion (in′tĕr-ven′shŭn) 1. An action or ministration that produces an effect or that is intended to alter the course of a pathologic process. 2. BIOWARFARE any action, ministration, or device intended to prevent or alter the course of deliberate release of a mass-casualty agent. SYN countermeasure. 3. SEE ALSO absorption.

in·ter·ven·tric·u·lar (IV, I.V.) (in′tĕr-ven-trik′yū-lăr) Between the ventricles.

in·ter·ven·tric·u·lar for·a·men (in′tĕr-ven·trik′yū-lăr fōr-ā′mĕn) [TA] The short, often slitlike passage that, on both the left and right sides, connects the third brain ventricle (of the diencephalon) with the lateral ventricles (of the cerebral hemispheres). SYN Monro foramen, porta (2).

in·ter·ver·te·bral (IV) (in′tĕr-vĕr′tĕ-brăl) *Avoid the mispronunciation in-ter-ver-tĕ′brăl.* Between two vertebrae.

in·ter·ver·te·bral disc (in′tĕr-vĕr′tĕ-brăl disk) A disc interposed between the bodies of adjacent vertebrae; composed of an outer fibrous part that surrounds a central gelatinous mass.

in·ter·ver·te·bral for·a·men (in′tĕr-vĕr′tĕ-brăl fōr-ā′mĕn) [TA] The lateral opening to the vertebral canal that allows for the emergence of spinal nerve roots; composed of inferior and superior vertebral pedicles.

in·ter·view (IV) (in′tĕr-vyū) Interpersonal meeting or consultation for the purpose of obtaining information.

in·ter·vil·lous (in′tĕr-vil′ŭs) Between or among villi.

in·ter·vil·lous cir·cu·la·tion (in′tĕr-vil′ŭs sĭr′kyū-lā′shŭn) Flow of maternal blood through the intervillous space of the placenta; the blood continuously showers the chorionic villi.

in·ter·vil·lous la·cu·na (in′tĕr-vil′ŭs lă-kū′nă) One of the blood spaces in the placenta into which the chorionic villi project.

in·tes·ti·nal ab·sorp·tion (in-tes′ti-năl ăb-sŏrp′shŭn) Movement of nutrients from the small intestine into the blood supply.

in·tes·ti·nal an·gi·na (in-tes′ti-năl an′ji-nă) SYN abdominal angina.

in·tes·ti·nal an·thrax (in-tes′ti-năl an′thraks) Usually fatal form of anthrax marked by chills, high fever, body pain, vomiting, bloody diarrhea, cardiovascular collapse, and frequently hemorrhages from the mucous membranes and in the skin.

in·tes·ti·nal di·ges·tion (in-tes′ti-năl di-jes′chŭn) That part of digestion carried on in the intestine; it affects all cellular nutrients: starches, fats, and proteins.

in·tes·ti·nal em·phy·se·ma (in-tes′ti-năl em′fi-sē′mă) SYN pneumatosis cystoides intestinalis.

in·tes·ti·nal fis·tu·la (in-tes′ti-năl fis′tyū-lă) A tract leading from the lumen of the small intestine to the exterior. SYN fecal fistula.

in·tes·ti·nal flor·a (in-tes′ti-năl flōr′ă) Collective term for those bacteria that normally reside within the intestines and assist in digestion and evacuation.

in·tes·ti·nal fol·li·cles (in-tes′ti-năl fol′i-kĕlz) SYN intestinal glands.

in·tes·ti·nal glands (in-tes′ti-năl glandz) The tubular glands in the mucous membrane of the small and large intestines.

in·tes·ti·nal juice (in-tes′ti-năl jūs) Alkaline straw-colored fluid secreted by the intestinal glands.

in·tes·ti·nal ob·struc·tion (in-tes′ti-năl ŏb-strŭk′shŭn) Partial or complete bowel blockage preventing passage of stool.

in·tes·ti·nal per·fo·ra·tion (in-tes′ti-năl pĕr′fŏr-ā′shŭn) Aperture that extends through large or small intestinal wall.

in·tes·ti·nal pseu·do·ob·struc·tion (IP) (in-tes′ti-năl sū′dō-ŏb-strŭk′shŭn) Clinical manifestations falsely suggesting obstruction of the small intestine.

in·tes·ti·nal schis·to·so·mi·a·sis (in-tes′ti-năl skis′tŏ-sō-mī′ă-sis) SYN schistosomiasis mansoni.

in·tes·ti·nal sta·sis (in-tes′ti-năl stā′sis) SYN enterostasis.

in·tes·ti·nal stran·gu·la·tion (in-tes′ti-năl strang′gyū-lā′shŭn) Disrupted blood flow to bowel that produces swelling and may cause death. SYN intestinal infarction.

in·tes·ti·nal tract (in-tes′ti-năl trakt) Collective term for the small and large intestines and the colon.

in·tes·ti·nal vil·li (in-tes′ti-năl vil′ī) [TA] Projections of the mucous membrane of the intestine.

in·tes·tine (in-tes′tin) [TA] **1.** The digestive tube passing from the stomach to the anus. **2.** Inward; inner. SYN bowel, gut (1).

in·ti·ma, pl. **in·ti·mae** (in′ti-mă, -mē) Innermost. SEE tunica intima.

in·ti·mi·tis (in′ti-mī′tis) Inflammation of an intima, as in endangiitis.

in·tol·er·ance (in-tol′ĕr-ăns) Abnormal metabolism, excretion, or other disposition of a given substance.

in·to·na·tion (in′tō-nā′shŭn) During speech, a pattern of change in voice used to convey linguistic information such as syllabic accent stress or pitch variations to signal interrogation, declaration, or exclamation.

in·tor·sion (in-tōr′shŭn) Conjugate rotation of the upper poles of each cornea inward.

in·tor·tor (in-tōr′tŏr) A muscle that turns a part medialward.

3-in-1 to·tal par·en·ter·al nu·tri·tion (TPN) (tō′tăl par-en′tĕr-ăl nū-trish′-ŭn) Feeding regimen with all three components of nutrition: fats, protein, and dextrose.

in·tox·i·ca·tion (in-tok′si-kā′shŭn) **1.** SYN poisoning. **2.** Temporary acute alcoholism.

intra- Prefix meaning inside; within; opposite of extra-. SEE ALSO endo-, ento-.

in·tra·ar·te·ri·al di·gi·tal sub·trac·tion an·gi·og·ra·phy (in′tră-ahr-tĕr′ē-ăl dij′i-tăl sŭb-trak′shŭn anj′ē-og′ră-fē) Arterial radiograph taken after injection of a dye, which is then compared with radiographs taken before and during the passage of the dye. SYN intravenous digital subtraction angiography.

in·tra·ar·tic·u·lar (IA) (in′tră-ahr-tik′yū-lăr) Within the cavity of a joint.

in·tra·a·tri·al (IA) (in′tră-ā′trē-ăl) Within one or both of the atria of the heart.

in·tra·a·tri·al con·duc·tion (in′tră-ā′trē-ăl kŏn-dŭk′shŭn) Conduction of the cardiac impulse through the atrial myo-

cardium, represented by the P wave in the electrocardiogram.

in·tra·atri·al con·duc·tion time (in′tră-ā′trē-ăl kŏn-dŭk′shŭn tīm) **1.** The total duration of electrical activity of the atria in one cardiac cycle. **2.** The time between right atrial and left atrial activation. SYN interatrial conduction time.

in·tra·bron·chi·al (in′tră-brong′kē-ăl) Within the bronchi or bronchial tubes. SYN endobronchial.

in·tra·can·a·lic·u·lar (in′tră-kan′ă-lik′yū-lăr) Within a canaliculus or canaliculi.

in·tra·cap·su·lar (IC) (in′tră-kap′sŭ-lăr) Within a capsule, especially the capsule of a joint.

in·tra·cap·su·lar an·ky·lo·sis (in′tră-kap′sŭ-lăr ang′ki-lō′sis) Joint stiffness due to the presence of bony or fibrous adhesions between the articular surfaces of the joint.

in·tra·cap·su·lar lig·a·ments (in′tră-kap′sŭ-lăr lig′ă-mĕnts) [TA] Ligaments located within and separate from the articular capsule of a synovial joint. SYN ligamenta intracapsularia [TA].

in·tra·car·di·ac (IC) (in′tră-kahr′dē-ak) Within one of the chambers of the heart. SYN endocardiac (1), endocardial, intracordal.

in·tra·car·di·ac cath·e·ter (in′tră-kahr′dē-ak kath′ĕ-tĕr) One that can be passed into the heart through a vein or artery, to withdraw samples of blood, measure pressures within the heart's chambers or great vessels, and inject contrast media. SYN cardiac catheter.

in·tra·car·di·ac lead (in′tră-kahr′dē-ak lēd) Record obtained when the exploring electrode is placed within one of the heart's chambers, usually by means of cardiac catheterization; used in diagnosis and evaluation of cardiac disorders.

in·tra·car·di·al in·jec·tion (in′tră-kahr′dē-ăl in-jek′shŭn) Introduction of an agent via tube or needle directly into the heart.

in·tra·car·ti·la·gi·nous (in′tră-kahr′ti-laj′i-nŭs) Within a cartilage or cartilaginous tissue. SYN endochondral.

in·tra·cav·i·ta·ry ra·di·a·tion ther·a·py (in′tră-kav′i-tar-ē rā′dē-ā′shŭn thār′ă-pē) Use of sealed radioactive sources placed within a body cavity adjacent to a malignant tumor.

in·tra·cel·lu·lar (in′tră-sel′yū-lăr) Within a cell or cells.

in·tra·cel·lu·lar ca·na·lic·u·lus (in′tră-sel′yū-lăr kan′ă-lik′yū-lŭs) A fine canal formed by invagination of the cell membrane into the cytoplasm of a cell.

in·tra·cel·lu·lar flu·id (ICF) (in′tră-sel′yū-lăr flū′id) The fluid within the tissue cells, constituting about 30–40% of the body weight. SYN intracellular water.

in·tra·cel·lu·lar tox·in (in′tră-sel′yū-lăr tok′sin) SYN endotoxin.

in·tra·ce·re·bral (in′tră-ser′ĕ-brăl) Within the cerebrum.

in·tra·ce·re·bral hem·or·rhage (ICH) (in′tră-ser′ĕ-brăl hem′ŏr-ăj) SYN cerebral hemorrhage.

in·tra·chon·dral os·si·fi·ca·tion (in′tră-kon′drăl os′i-fi-kā′shŭn) SYN endochondral ossification.

in·tra·cis·ter·nal (in′tră-sis-tĕr′năl) Within the cerebral cistern.

in·tra·cor·ne·al im·plants (in′tră-kōr′nē-ăl im′plants) Inserts in corneal pockets to alter the refractive power of the eye.

in·tra·cor·po·re·al (in′tră-kōr-pōr′ē-ăl) 1. Within the body. 2. Within any structure anatomically styled a corpus.

in·tra·cos·tal (in′tră-kos′tăl) On the inner surface of the ribs.

in·tra·cra·ni·al (IC) (in′tră-krā′nē-ăl) Within the cranium, usually meaning within the cranial cavity.

in·tra·cra·ni·al an·eu·rysm (in′tră-krā′nē-ăl an′yūr-izm) Any aneurysm located within the cranium.

in·tra·cra·ni·al pres·sure (ICP) (in′tră-krā′nē-ăl presh′ŭr) Pressure within the cranial cavity, particularly the pressure

of the cerebrospinal fluid as measured by lumbar pressure.

in·tra·crine (in′tră-krin) Denoting self-stimulation through cellular production of a factor that acts within the cell.

in·trac·ta·ble (in-trak′tă-bĕl) 1. SYN refractory (1). 2. SYN obstinate (1).

in·trac·ta·ble pain (in-trak′tă-bĕl pān) That resistant or refractory to ordinary analgesic agents.

in·tra·cu·ta·ne·ous (IC) (in′tră-kyū-tā′nē-ŭs) Within the substance of the skin, particularly the dermis. SYN intradermal, intradermic.

in·tra·cu·ta·ne·ous in·jec·tion (in′tră-kyū-tā′nē-ŭs in-jek′shŭn) Administering a solution between the layers of the skin using a needle and syringe. SYN intradermal injection.

in·tra·cu·ta·ne·ous re·ac·tion, in·tra·der·mal re·ac·tion (in′tră-kyū-tā′nē-ŭs rē-ak′shŭn, in′tră-dĕr′măl) That due to injection of antigen into the skin of a sensitive subject.

in·tra·cys·tic (in′tră-sis′tik) Within a cyst or the urinary bladder.

in·tra·cys·tic pa·pil·lo·ma (in′tră-sis′tik pap′i-lō′mă) Lesion growing within a cystic adenoma, filling the cavity with a mass of branching epithelial processes.

in·tra·cy·to·plas·mic sperm in·jec·tion (in′tră-sī-tō-plaz′mik spĕrm in-jek′shŭn) Treatment for male infertility that places a sperm into an oocyte especially in cases where the donor has sluggish sperms.

in·tra·der·mal, in·tra·der·mic (in′tră-dĕr′măl, -dĕr′mik) SYN intracutaneous.

in·tra·der·mal in·jec·tion (in′tră-dĕr′măl in-jek′shŭn) An injection into the corium, or substance of the skin.

in·tra·der·mal ne·vus (in′tră-dĕr′măl nē′vŭs) A nevus in which nests of melanocytes are found in the dermis, but not at the epidermal-dermal junction; benign pigmented nevi in adults are most commonly intradermal.

in·tra·der·mal test (in′tră-dĕr′măl test) SYN skin test.

in·tra·duc·tal car·ci·no·ma (IDC) (in′tră-dŭk′tăl kahr′si-nō′mă) Carcinoma derived from the epithelial lining of ducts, especially in the breast, where most carcinomas arise from ductal epithelium. SYN ductal carcinoma in situ.

in·tra·duc·tal pap·il·lo·ma (in′tră-dŭk′tăl pap′i-lō′mă) Small, often nonpalpable, benign lesion arising in a lactiferous duct and frequently causing bleeding from the nipple. SYN duct papilloma.

in·tra·du·ral (in′tră-dūr′ăl) Within or enclosed by the dura mater.

in·tra·em·bry·on·ic (in′tră-em′brē-on′ik) Within the embryonic body. Cf. extraembryonic.

in·tra·ep·i·der·mal (in′tră-ep′i-dĕr′măl) Within the top layer of the skin.

in·tra·ep·i·der·mal car·ci·no·ma (in′tră-ep′i-dĕr′măl kahr′si-nō′mă) Carcinoma in situ of the skin.

in·tra·ep·i·the·li·al (IE) (in′tră-ep′i-thē′lē-ăl) Within or among the epithelial cells.

in·tra·fi·lar (in′tră-fī′lăr) Lying within the meshes of a network.

in·tra·fu·sal (in′tră-fyū′zăl) Applied to structures within the muscle spindle.

in·tra·fu·sal fi·bers (in′tră-fyū′zăl fī′bĕrz) Muscle fibers present within a neuromuscular spindle.

in·tra·he·pa·tic duct (IHD) (in′tră-hĕ-pat′ik dŭkt) An anatomic opening within the kidney.

in·tra·lig·a·men·ta·ry (in′tră-lig′ă-mĕn-tar-ē) Within a ligament. SYN intraligamentous.

in·tra·lig·a·men·ta·ry preg·nan·cy (in′tră-lig′ă-men′tar-ē preg′năn-sē) Pregnancy within the broad ligament.

in·tra·lig·a·men·tous (in′tră-lig′ă-men′tŭs) Within a ligament, especially the broad ligament of the uterus.

in·tra·lin·gual in·jec·tion (in′tră-ling′gwăl in-jek′shŭn) Introduction of medication into the tongue with a needle or syringe.

in·tra·lob·u·lar (in′tră-lob′yū-lăr) Within a lobule.

in·tra·lu·mi·nal (in′tră-lū′mi-năl) SYN intratubal.

in·tra·lu·min·al co·ro·na·ry ar·te·ry stent (in′tră-lū′mi-năl kŏr′ŏ-nar-ē ahr′tĕr-ē stent) A metal mesh tube inserted into a cardiac artery after balloon angioplasty to hold the artery open and improve circulation to the cardiac muscle.

in·tra·med·ul·lar·y (IM) (in′tră-med′yŭ-lar-ē) **1.** Within the bone marrow. **2.** Within the spinal cord. **3.** Within the medulla oblongata.

in·tra·mem·bra·nous (in′tră-mem′bră-nŭs) **1.** Within, or between the layers of, a membrane. **2.** Denoting a method of bone formation directly from mesenchymal cells without an intervening cartilage stage.

in·tra·mem·bra·nous os·si·fi·ca·tion (in′tră-mem′bră-nŭs os′i-fi-kā′shŭn) SYN membranous ossification.

in·tra·mu·ral (in′tră-myū′răl) Within the substance of the wall of any cavity or hollow organ. SYN intraparietal (1).

in·tra·mu·ral preg·nan·cy (in′tră-myūr′ăl preg′năn-sē) Implantation and development of the blastocyst in the uterine part of the uterine tube. SYN interstitial pregnancy, tubouterine pregnancy.

in·tra·mus·cu·lar (IM) (in′tră-mŭs′kyū-lăr) Within the substance of a muscle.

in·tra·mus·cu·lar in·jec·tion (IMI) (in′tră-mŭs′kyū-lăr in-jek′shŭn) Injection of fluid into deep muscle.

in·tra·oc·u·lar (in′tră-ok′yū-lăr) Within the eyeball.

in·tra·oc·u·lar lens (IOL) (in′tră-ok′yū-lăr lenz) A mechanical transplant used in ophthalmology to replace the natural lens that has ceased to function due to disease or disruption.

in·tra·oc·u·lar pres·sure (IOP) (in′tră-ok′yū-lăr presh′ŭr) Surface tension of the intraocular fluid, usually measured in millimeters of mercury.

in·tra·op·er·a·tive (in′tră-op′ĕr-ă-tiv) Denotes that which occurs during an operation.

in·tra·op·er·a·tive ra·di·a·tion ther·a·py (IORT) (in′tră-op′ĕr-ă-tiv rā′dē-ā′shŭn thār′ă-pē) Radiation treatment delivered directly to the tumor or tumor bed after the area has been surgically exposed.

in·tra·o·ral (in′tră-ōr′ăl) Inside the mouth.

in·tra·os·se·ous (in′tră-os′ē-ŭs) Route for delivery of fluid, blood, or medication through a needle inserted directly into the marrow of long bones.

in·tra·pa·ri·e·tal (in′tră-pă-rī′ĕ-tăl) **1.** SYN intramural. **2.** Denoting the intraparietal sulcus.

in·tra·par·tum (in′tră-pahr′tŭm) During labor and delivery or childbirth. Cf. antepartum, postpartum.

in·tra·par·tum hem·or·rhage (in′tră-pahr′tŭm hem′ŏr-ăj) Hemorrhage occurring in the course of normal labor and delivery.

in·tra·par·tum pe·ri·od (in′tră-pahr′tŭm pēr′ē-ŏd) In obstetrics, the period from the onset of labor to the end of the third stage of labor.

in·tra·pel·vic (in′tră-pel′vik) Within the pelvis.

in·tra·per·i·to·ne·al (IP, i.p.) (in′tră-per′i-tŏ-nē′ăl) Within the peritoneal cavity.

in·tra·pleu·ral space (in′tră-plūr′ăl spās) Space between the two layers of the pleura.

in·tra·psy·chic (in′tră-sī′kik) Denoting the psychological dynamics that occur inside the mind without reference to the person's exchanges with other persons or events.

in·tra·pul·mo·nar·y (in′tră-pul′mŏ-nar-ē) Within a lung.

in·tra·re·nal (in′tră-rē′năl) Within the kidney.

in·tra·re·nal re·flux (IRR) (in′tră-rē′năl rē′flŭks) Urinary reflux from renal pelvis

and calyces into the collecting ducts. SYN pyelotubular reflux.

in·tra·re·nal veins (in′tră-rē′năl vānz) [TA] Internal veins of the kidney. SYN venae intrenales.

in·tra·seg·men·tal bron·chi (in′tră-seg-ment′ăl brong′kī) [TA] Branches of segmental bronchi to the bronchopulmonary segments of the lungs. SYN bronchi intrasegmentales.

in·tra·spi·nal (in′tră-spī′năl) Within the vertebral canal or spinal cord. SYN intra-rachidian.

in·tra·the·cal (IT, Ith) (in′tră-thē′kăl) **1.** Within a sheath. **2.** Within either the subarachnoid or the subdural space.

in·tra·the·cal in·jec·tion (in′tră-thē′kăl in-jek′shŭn) Introduction of material for diffusion throughout the subarachnoid space by means of lumbar puncture.

in·tra·tho·rac·ic (in′tră-thōr-as′ik) The body region located within the cavity of the chest.

in·tra·tra·che·al (in′tră-trā′kē-ăl) Method of giving medications through the trachea.

in·tra·tub·al (in′tră-tū′băl) Within any tube. SYN intraluminal.

in·tra·tym·pan·ic (in′tră-tim-pan′ik) Within the middle ear or tympanic cavity.

in·tra·u·ter·ine (IU) (in′tră-yū′tĕr-in) Within the uterus.

in·tra·u·ter·ine de·vice, in·tra·u·ter·ine con·tra·cep·tive de·vice (IUD, IUCD) (in′tră-yū′tĕr-in dĕ-vīs′, kon′tră-sep′tiv) Pieces of plastic or metal of various shapes put in the uterus to block conception.

in·tra·u·ter·ine pres·sure cath·e·ter (IUPC) (in′tră-yū′tĕr-in presh′ŭr kath′ĕ-tĕr) Tubular device introduced into the uterus during delivery to measure the increasing strength of contractions.

in·tra·u·ter·ine trans·fu·sion (in′tră-yū′tĕr-in trans-fyū′zhŭn) Rh-negative blood is placed in fetal peritoneal cavity to treat erythroblastosis fetalis.

in·tra·va·sa·tion (in-trav′ă-sā′shŭn) Introduction of foreign matter within a blood vessel.

in·tra·vas·cu·lar (in′tră-vas′kyū-lăr) Within the blood vessels or lymphatics.

in·tra·vas·cu·lar lig·a·ture (in′tră-vas′ kyū-lăr lig′ă-chŭr) Balloon occlusion of the feeding vessels of a cerebral arteriovenous malformation.

in·tra·vas·cu·lar pap·il·lar·y en·do·the·li·al hy·per·pla·si·a (in′tră-vas′ kyū-lăr pap′i-lar-ē en′dō-thē′lē-ăl hī′pĕr-plā′zē-ă) Benign florid papillary endothelial proliferation within the veins of the skin or subcutis.

in·tra·ve·nous (IV) (in′tră-vē′nŭs) Through veins; within a vein.

in·tra·ve·nous a·li·men·ta·tion (in′ tră-vē′nŭs al′i-mĕn-tā′shŭn) SYN parenteral nutrition.

in·tra·ve·nous cath·e·ter (in′tră-vē′nŭs kath′ĕ-tĕr) One surgically introduced into a vein to supply pharmacotherapeutic agents.

in·tra·ve·nous drip (in′tră-vē′nŭs drip) The slow but continuous introduction of solutions intravenously, one drop at a time.

in·tra·ve·nous drug u·ser (IVDU) (in′ tră-vē′nŭs drŭg yū′zĕr) SYN injection drug user.

in·tra·ve·nous in·fu·sion (IV) (in′tră-vē′nŭs in-fyū′zhŭn) Administration of fluids into a vein.

in·tra·ve·nous in·fu·sion fil·ter (in′ tră-vē′nŭs in-fyū′zhŭn fil′tĕr) A device installed in an intravenous line to diminish the possibility of bacteria entering the line.

in·tra·ve·nous in·jec·tion (IVI) (in′tră-vē′nŭs in-jek′shŭn) Injection of fluid directly into a vein; allows larger amounts of fluid to be administered and provides means for rapid absorption of medication.

in·tra·ve·nous push (IVP) (in′tră-vē′ nŭs push) A method of quickly injecting medications into a vein.

in·tra·ve·nous py·el·o·gram, py·el·o·gra·phy (IVP) (in′tră-vē′nŭs pī′ĕ-lō-gram, pī′ĕ-log′ră-fē) SEE intravenous urography.

in·tra·ve·nous re·gion·al an·es·the·si·a (in′tră-vē′nŭs rē′jŭn-ăl an′es-thē′zē-ă) Regional anesthesia by intravenous injection of local anesthetic solution distal to an occlusive tourniquet in an extremity previously exsanguinated by pressure or gravity. SYN Bier method (1).

in·tra·ve·nous trans·fu·sion (IVT) (in′tră-vē′nŭs trans-fyū′zhŭn) Procedure in which a fluid (e.g., medication, nutrient) is introduced into a patient's vein by means of a tube.

in·tra·ve·nous u·rog·ra·phy, ex·cre·to·ry u·rog·ra·phy (in′tră-vē′nŭs yūr-og′ră-fē, eks′krĕ-tōr-ē) Radiography of kidneys, ureters, and bladder following injection of contrast medium into a peripheral vein.

in·tra·ven·tric·u·lar (in′tră-ven-trik′yū-lăr) Within a ventricle of the brain or heart.

in·tra·ven·tric·u·lar block (in′tră-ven-trik′yū-lăr blok) Delayed conduction within the ventricular conducting system or myocardium, including bundle-branch block, periinfarction blocks, fascicular blocks, excitation, and Wolff-Parkinson-White (preexcitation) syndrome; widens QRS duration in electrocardiography.

in·tra·ven·tric·u·lar con·duc·tion de·fects (in′tră-ven-trik′yū-lăr kŏn-dŭk′ shŭn dē′fekts) Failure of the heart to conduct its electrical impulse from the atrioventricular node through the bundle of His, bundle branches, and Purkinje fibers.

in·tra·ven·tric·u·lar hem·or·rhage (IVH) (in′tră-ven-trik′yū-lăr hem′ŏr-ăj) Type of intracranial bleeding primarily affecting premature babies.

in·tra·ven·tric·u·lar pres·sure (in′tră-ven-trik′yū-lăr presh′ŭr) Cardiac pressure, especially in the lower cardiac chambers.

in·tra·ves·i·cal (in′tră-ves′i-kăl) Within a bladder, especially the urinary bladder.

in·tra vi·tam (in′tră vī′tam) Latin phrase meaning during life.

in·trin·sic (in-trin′zik) **1.** Pertaining to the essence or nature of a thing; inherent. **2.** ANATOMY denoting those muscles with an origin and insertion that are both within the structure under consideration. SYN essential (6).

in·trin·sic co·ag·u·la·tion path·way (in-trin′zik kō-ag′yŭ-lā′shŭn path′wā) A part of the coagulation pathway activated by contact of coagulation proteins with negatively charged surfaces.

in·trin·sic dys·men·or·rhe·a (in-trin′zik dis-men′ŏr-ē′ă) SYN primary dysmenorrhea.

in·trin·sic fac·tor (IF) (in-trin′zik fak′tŏr) A relatively small mucoprotein secreted by the neck cell of the gastric glands and required for adequate absorption of vitamin B12.

in·trin·sic re·flex (in-trin′zik rē′fleks) Reflexive muscular contraction elicited by application of a stimulus, usually stretching, to the muscle itself.

in·trin·sic sphinc·ter (in-trin′zik sfingk′tĕr) Thickening of the circular fibers of the muscular coat of an organ.

intro- Prefix meaning inwardly, into; opposite of extra-. Cf. intra-.

in·troi·tus (in-trō′i-tŭs) Entrance of a canal or hollow organ.

in·tro·mis·sion (in′trō-mish′ŭn) Introduction of one body part into another.

in·tron (in′tron) A portion of DNA that lies between two exons, is transcribed into RNA, but does not appear in that RNA after maturation, and so is not expressed (as protein) in protein synthesis.

in·tro·spec·tion (in′trō-spek′shŭn) Looking inward.

in·tro·sus·cep·tion (in′trō-sŭs-sep′shŭn) SYN intussusception.

in·tro·ver·sion (in′trō-vĕr′zhŭn) **1.** The turning of a structure into itself. SEE ALSO intussusception, invagination. **2.** A trait of preoccupation with oneself, as practiced by an introvert. Cf. extraversion.

in·tu·ba·tion (in′tū-bā′shŭn) Insertion of

a tubular device into a canal, hollow organ, or cavity.

in·tu·mes·cen·ti·a (in′tū-mes-sen′shē-ă) [TA] SYN enlargement.

in·tus·sus·cep·tion (in′tŭ-sŭ-sep′shŭn) **1.** The taking up or receiving of one part within another, especially the enfolding of one segment of the intestine within another. SEE ALSO introversion, invagination. **2.** The incorporation of new material in the growth of the cell wall. SYN introsusception.

in·tus·sus·cip·i·ens (in′tŭ-sŭ-sip′ē-ĕnz) The portion of the bowel in intussusception that receives the other portion.

in·u·lin (in′yū-lin) A fructose polysaccharide from the rhizome of *Inula* and other plants. Cf. inulin clearance.

in·u·lin clear·ance (in′yū-lin klēr′ăns) An accurate measure of the rate of filtration through the renal glomeruli, because inulin filters freely with water and is neither excreted nor reabsorbed through tubule walls.

in·unc·tion (in-ŭngk′shŭn) Administration of a drug in ointment form by rubbing to cause absorption of the active ingredient.

in u·ter·o (in yū′tĕr-ō) Within the womb; not yet born.

in vac·u·o (in vak′yū-ō) In a vacuum, e.g., under reduced pressure.

in·vag·i·nate (in-vaj′i-nāt) To ensheathe, infold, or insert a structure within itself or another.

in·vag·i·na·tion (in-vaj′i-nā′shŭn) **1.** The ensheathing, enfolding, or insertion of a structure within itself or another. **2.** The state of being invaginated. SEE ALSO introversion, intussusception.

in·va·sion (in-vā′zhŭn) **1.** The beginning or incursion of a disease. **2.** Local spread of a malignant neoplasm by infiltration or destruction of adjacent tissue; for epithelial neoplasms, invasion signifies infiltration beneath the epithelial basement membrane. **3.** Entrance of foreign cells into a tissue.

in·va·sive (in-vā′siv) **1.** Denoting or characterized by invasion. **2.** Denoting a procedure requiring insertion of an instrument or device into the body through the skin or a body orifice for diagnosis or treatment.

in·va·sive pro·ce·dure (in-vā′siv prŏ-sē′jŭr) Any surgical or exploratory activity in which the body is pierced by a device or instrument or by manual digitation.

in·ven·tor·y (in′vĕn-tōr-ē) A detailed, often descriptive, list of items.

in·verse an·a·phy·lax·is (in-vĕrs′ an′ă-fi-lak′sis) Anaphylactic shock in an animal whose tissues contain Forssman antigen, due to intravenous injection of serum that contains Forssman antibody.

in·verse ra·ti·o ven·ti·la·tion (IRV) (in-vĕrs′ rā′shē-ō ven′ti-lā′shŭn) A mode of mechanical ventilation.

in·verse sym·me·try (in-vĕrs′ sim′ĕ-trē) Correspondence of the right or left side of an asymmetric individual to the left or right side of another.

in·ver·sion (in-vĕr′zhŭn) **1.** A turning inward, upside down, or in any direction contrary to the existing one. **2.** Conversion of a disaccharide or polysaccharide by hydrolysis into a monosaccharide; specifically, the hydrolysis of sucrose to D-glucose and D-fructose; so called because of the change in optical rotation.

in·ver·sion of the u·ter·us (in-vĕr′zhŭn yū′tĕr-ŭs) A turning of the uterus inside out, usually following childbirth.

in·ver·sion trac·tion (in-vĕr′zhŭn trak′shŭn) Low back pain therapy that employs a device to suspend the patient head downward to counter the effects of gravity, thus applying natural traction to the lower back.

in·vert (in-vĕrt′) **1.** In chemistry, subjected to inversion. **2.** To reverse in direction, sequence, or effect.

in·ver·te·brate (in-vĕr′tĕ-brāt, -brăt) **1.** Not possessed of a spinal or vertebral column. **2.** Any animal that has no spinal column.

in·vert·ed fol·lic·u·lar ker·a·to·sis (in-vĕr′tĕd fŏ-lik′yū-lăr ker′ă-tō′sis) Solitary benign epithelial tumor of infundibular hair follicle origin occurring on the face, consisting of a lobulated epidermal downgrowth of keratinizing squamous cells with a pattern of eddies or whorls.

in·vert·ed pap·il·lo·ma (IP) (in-vĕr′tĕd pap′i-lō′mă) Eplithelial tumor of the urinary bladder or nasal cavity in which proliferating epithelium is invaginated beneath the surface.

in·vert sug·ar (in′vĕrt shug′ăr) A mixture of equal parts of D-glucose and D-fructose produced by hydrolysis of sucrose.

in·ves·ti·ga·tion·al new drug (in-ves′ti-gā′shŭn-ăl nū drŭg) A pharmacotherapeutic agent that has not been approved for general use by the U.S. Food and Drug Administration, but is in the course of being tested on humans.

in·vest·ing fas·ci·a (in-vest′ing fash′ē-ă) [TA] Relatively thin fibrous membrane, devoid of fat, which ensheaths a layer of muscles directly on their surfaces, separating individual muscles.

in·vis·ca·tion (in′vis-kā′shŭn) **1.** Smearing with mucilaginous matter. **2.** The mixing of the food, during mastication, with the buccal secretions.

in vi·tro (in vē′trō) In an artificial environment, referring to a process or reaction occurring therein, as in a test tube or culture media. Cf. in vivo.

in vi·tro fer·til·i·za·tion (IVF) (in vē′trō fĕr′til-ī-zā′shŭn) Process whereby (usually multiple) oocytes are placed in a medium to which sperms are added for fertilization, the zygote thus produced then being introduced into the uterus with the objective of full-term development.

in vi·vo (in vē′vō) In the living body, referring to a process or reaction occurring therein. Cf. in vitro.

in vi·vo fer·til·i·za·tion (IVF) (in vē′vō fĕr′til-ī-zā′shŭn) **1.** Aspiration of mature oocytes from ovarian follicles during laparoscopy into a culture medium. **2.** Fertilization of a mature oocyte within the distal uterine tube of a fertile donor female (rather than in an artificial medium), for subsequent nonsurgical transfer to an infertile recipient.

in·vo·lu·crum, pl. **in·vo·lu·cra** (in'vŏ-lū'krŭm, -lū'kră) **1.** An enveloping membrane. **2.** The sheath of new bone that forms around a sequestrum.

in·vol·un·tar·y (in-vol'ŭn-tar-ē) **1.** Independent of the will; not volitional. **2.** Contrary to the will.

in·vol·un·tar·y mus·cles (in-vol'ŭn-tar-ē mŭs'ĕlz) Those not ordinarily under control of the will.

in·vo·lu·tion (in'vŏ-lū'shŭn) **1.** Return of an enlarged organ to normal size. **2.** Turning inward of the edges of a part. **3.** PSYCHIATRY mental decline associated with advanced age.

in·vo·lu·tion·al pto·sis (in-vŏ-lū'shŭn-ăl tō'sis) SYN aponeurotic ptosis.

iod·ic ac·id (ī-od'ik as'id) Crystalline powder, soluble in water; used as an astringent, caustic, and disinfectant.

io·dide (ī'ō-dīd) Negative ion of iodine, I⁻.

io·dide ac·ne (ī'ō-dīd ak'nē) A follicular eruption on the face, trunk, and extremities, due to injection or ingestion of iodide in a hypersensitive person. SEE ALSO iododerma.

io·dine (I) (ī'ŏ-dīn, ī'ō-dēn) A nonmetallic chemical element, atomic no. 53, atomic wt. 126.90447; used as a catalyst, reagent, tracer, constituent of radiographic contrast media, therapy in thyroid disease and other uses.

io·dine de·fi·cien·cy dis·or·der (ī'ō-dīn dĕ-fish'ĕn-sē dis-ōr'dĕr) A lack of iodine that causes growth and development disorders.

io·dine-fast (ī'ŏ-dīn-fast) Denoting hyperthyroidism unresponsive to iodine therapy, which develops frequently in most patients so treated.

io·dine tinc·ture (ī'ŏ-dīn tingk'shŭr) Hydroalcoholic solution containing 2% elemental iodine and 2.4% potassium iodide to facilitate dissolution and 47% alcohol; used as an antiseptic/germicide on the skin surface for cuts and scratches. Has been used as a skin disinfectant before surgery but is now largely replaced by organic forms of iodine.

io·din·o·phil (ī'ō-din'ō-fil) **1.** Staining readily with iodine. SYN iodinophilous. **2.** Any histologic element that stains readily with iodine.

io·din·oph·i·lous (ī'ō-din-of'i-lŭs) SYN iodinophil (1).

io·dism (ī'ŏ-dizm) Disorder marked by acute rhinitis, acneform eruption, weakness, salivation, and foul breath, due to continuous administration of iodine or one of the iodides.

io·dized oil (ī'ŏ-dīzd oyl) An iodine addition product of vegetable oils; a radiopaque medium.

io·dized salt (ī'ŏ-dīzd sawlt) Dietary sodium chloride that has been treated with iodine to prevent goiter. Most commonly available table salt in the United States has been so altered.

io·do·der·ma (ī-ō'dŏ-dĕr'mă) An eruption of follicular papules and pustules, or a granulomatous lesion, caused by iodine toxicity or sensitivity. SEE ALSO iodide acne.

io·do·form gauze (ī-ō'dŏ-fōrm gawz) Sterile strips of gauze impregnated with iodoform; used to pack abscesses to act as a wick to promote drainage.

io·do·hip·pu·rate so·di·um (ī-ō'dŏ-hip'yū-rāt sō'dē-ŭm) A radiopaque compound used intravenously, orally, or for retrograde urography. When tagged with iodine 131, it is used to measure effective renal plasma flow and to image the kidneys for radioisotopic renography.

io·do·met·ric (ī-ō'dŏ-met'rik) Relating to iodometry.

io·do·phil·i·a (ī-ō'dŏ-fil'ē-ă) An affinity for iodine.

io·dop·sin (ī'ō-dop'sin) Any of three visual pigments, composed of 11-*cis*-retinal bound to an opsin, found in the cones of the retina. SYN visual violet.

io·do·qui·nol (ī-ō'dŏ-kwin'ol) An amebicide prepared by the action of iodine monochloride on 8-hydroxyquinoline.

io·hex·ol (ī'ō-heks'ol) A monomeric, nonionic, water-soluble, low osmolar radiographic contrast medium for urography or angiography. Used intrathecally and intravascularly.

ion (ī′on) An atom or group of atoms carrying an electric charge by virtue of having gained or lost one or more electrons.

ion chan·nel dis·or·ders (ī′on chan′ĕl dis-ōr′dĕrz) Those diseases, mostly inherited and episodic in nature, caused by dysfunction of the calcium, chloride, potassium, or sodium channels of nerve or muscle.

ion ex·change chro·ma·tog·ra·phy (ī′on eks-chānj′ krō′mŏ-tog′ră-fē) Process in which cations or anions in the mobile phase are separated by electrostatic interactions with the stationary phase. SEE ALSO cation exchange.

ion·ic bond (i-on′ik bond) A type of chemical bond that forms between metal and non-metal ions through electrostatic attraction; the attraction between oppositely charged ions.

ion·ic med·i·ca·tion (ī-on′ik med′i-kā′shŭn) SYN iontophoresis.

ion·i·za·tion (ī′ŏn-ī-zā′shŭn) 1. Dissociation into ions. 2. Production of ions due to interaction of radiation with matter. 3. SYN iontophoresis.

ion·i·za·tion cham·ber (ī′ŏn-ī-zā′shŭn chăm′bĕr) A chamber for detecting ionization of the enclosed gas; used for determining intensity of ionizing radiation.

ion·to·pho·re·sis (ī-on′tŏ-fŏr-ē′sis) The introduction, by means of electric current, of ions of soluble substances into tissue for therapeutic purposes. SYN ionization (3).

io·pro·mide (ī′ō-prō′mīd) A monomeric, nonionic, water-soluble, low osmolar radiographic contrast medium for intravenous urography or angiography.

io·ta (ι) (ī-ō′tă) 1. The ninth letter in the Greek alphabet. 2. CHEMISTRY denotes the ninth in a series, or the ninth atom from a carboxyl group or other functional group. 3. A minute amount.

iox·ag·late (ī′oks-ag′lāt) A diagnostic radiopaque medium, usually a combination of ioxaglate meglumine and ioxaglate sodium; used in angiography,

aortography, arteriography, venography, and urography.

IP Abbreviation for intraperitoneal; interphalangeal; isoelectric point.

ip·e·cac·uan·ha (ip′ĕ-kak-wahn′ă) The dried root of *Uragoga (Cephaelis) ipecacuanha* (family Rubiaceae), a shrub found in Brazil and other parts of South America; contains emetine, cephaeline, emetamine, ipecacuanhic acid, psychotrine, and methylpsychotrine; has expectorant, emetic, and antidysenteric properties. Source of syrup of ipecac.

ipo·date (ī′pō-dāt) A radiographic contrast medium, given orally for opacification of the gallbladder and central biliary tree.

ipo·me·a (ī-pō-mē′ă) The dried root of *Ipomoea orizabensis* (family Convolvulaceae). SEE ALSO ipomea resin. SYN orizaba jalap root.

ipo·me·a resin (ī-pō-mē′ă rez′in) Resin obtained from the dried root of *Ipomoea orizabensis;* a cathartic.

Ipo·moe·a (ī′pō-mē′ă) A plant genus of the family Convolvulaceae including the morning glory.

ip·ra·tro·pi·um (IPT) (i′prā-trō′pē-ŭm) A synthetic quaternary ammonium compound, chemically related to atropine, which has anticholinergic activity and is a bronchodilator.

♻ **ipsi-** Combining form meaning the same.

ip·si·lat·er·al (ip′si-lat′ĕr-ăl) On the same side, with reference to a given point, e.g., a dilated pupil on the same side as an extradural hematoma.

Ir Symbol for iridium.

♻ **irid-** SEE irido-.

ir·i·dal (ir′i-dăl) Relating to the iris. SYN iridian, iridic.

ir·i·dec·to·my (ir′i-dek′tŏ-mē) 1. Excision of a portion of the iris. 2. The hole in the iris produced by a surgical iridectomy.

ir·i·den·clei·sis (ir′i-den-klī′sis) The incarceration of a portion of the iris by corneoscleral incision in glaucoma to effect filtration between the anterior chamber and subconjunctival space.

irido-, irid- Combining forms meaning the iris.

ir·i·do·a·vul·sion (ir'i-dō-ă-vŭl'shŭn) Avulsion, or tearing away, of the iris.

ir·i·do·cele (ī-rid'ō-sēl) Herniation of a portion of the iris through a corneal defect.

ir·i·do·cho·roid·i·tis (ir'i-dō-kōr'oy-dī'tis) Inflammation of both iris and choroid.

ir·i·do·col·o·bo·ma (ir'i-dō-kol'ŏ-bō'mă) A coloboma or congenital defect of the iris.

ir·i·do·cor·ne·al (ir'i-dō-kōr'nē-ăl) Relating to the iris and the cornea.

ir·i·do·cor·ne·al en·do·the·li·al syn·drome (ir'i-dō-kōr'nē-ăl en'dō-thē'lē-ăl sin'drōm) A congenital disorder comprising glaucoma, iris atrophy, decreased corneal endothelium, anterior peripheral synechia, and multiple iris nodules. SYN Cogan-Reese syndrome, iris-nevus syndrome.

ir·i·do·cy·clec·to·my (ir'i-dō-sī-klek'tō-mē) Removal of the iris and ciliary body for excision of a tumor.

ir·i·do·cy·clo·cho·roid·i·tis (ir'i-dō-sī'klō-kōr'oyd-ī'tis) Inflammation of the iris, involving the ciliary body and the choroid.

ir·i·do·cys·tec·to·my (ir'i-dō-sis-tek'tō-mē) An operation for making an artificial pupil when posterior synechiae follow extracapsular extraction of cataract.

ir·i·do·di·al·y·sis (ir'i-dō-dī-al'i-sis) Separation of the iris root from the scleral; often results from trauma.

ir·i·do·di·la·tor (ir'i-dō-dī'lāt-ŏr) Causing dilation of the pupil; applied to the musculus dilator pupillae.

ir·i·do·do·ne·sis (ir'i-dō-dō-nē'sis) Agitated motion of the iris.

ir·i·do·ker·a·ti·tis (ir'i-dō-ker'ă-tī'tis) Inflammation of the iris and cornea.

ir·i·do·ki·ne·sis, ir·i·do·ki·ne·si·a (ir'i-dō-ki-nē'sis -nē'zē-ă) Contraction and dilation of the pupil as a result of movement of the iris.

ir·i·do·ki·net·ic (ir'i-dō-ki-net'ik) Relating to the movements of the iris. SYN iridomotor.

ir·i·do·lep·tyn·sis (ir'i-dō-lep-tin'sis) Thinning or atrophy of the optic iris.

ir·i·dol·o·gy (ir'i-dol'ŏ-jē) A system of medicine *not based on evidence*, involving examination of the iris, using a chart on which certain areas of the iris are presumed diagnostically specific for particular organs, systems, and structures.

ir·i·do·ma·la·ci·a (ir'i-dō-mă-lā'shē-ă) Degenerative softening of the iris.

ir·i·do·mes·o·di·al·y·sis (ir'i-dō-mes'ō-dī-al'i-sis) Separation of adhesions around the inner margin of the iris.

ir·i·do·mo·tor (ir'i-dō-mō'tŏr) SYN pupillomotor.

ir·i·don·cus (ir'i-dong'kŭs) Swelling of the iris.

ir·i·do·per·i·pha·ki·tis (ir'i-dō-per'i-fa-kī'tis) Inflammation of the capsule of the ocular lens.

ir·i·do·ple·gi·a, ir·i·do·pa·ral·y·sis (ir'i-dō-plē'jē-ă, -păr-al'i-sis) Paralysis of the musculus sphincter iridis. SYN iridoparalysis.

ir·i·dop·to·sis (ir'i-dop-tō'sis) Prolapse of the iris.

ir·i·dor·rhex·is (ir'i-dō-rek'sis) Deliberate, surgical tearing of the iris from the scleral spur to increase the breadth of a coloboma.

ir·i·dos·chi·sis (ir'i-dos'ki-sis) Separation of the anterior layer of the iris from the posterior layer; ruptured anterior fibers float in the aqueous humor.

ir·i·do·scle·rot·o·my (ir'i-dō-skler-ot'ŏ-mē) An incision involving both sclera and iris.

ir·i·do·ste·re·sis (ir'i-do-stĕ-re'sis) The absence of all or part of the iris.

ir·i·do·tas·is (ir′i-dot′ă-sis) Surgically stretching the iris to treat glaucoma.

ir·i·dot·o·my, ir·i·to·my, ir·o·to·my (ir′i-dot′ŏ-mē, i-rit′ŏ-mē, -rot′ŏ-mē) Transverse division of some of the fibers of the iris, forming an artificial pupil.

i·ris, pl. **ir·i·des** (ī′ris, ī′ri-dēz) [TA] The anterior division of the vascular tunic of the eye, a diaphragm, perforated in the center (the pupil), attached peripherally to the scleral spur.

iris-naevus syndrome [Br.] SYN iris-nevus syndrome.

ir·is-ne·vus syn·drome (ī′ris-nē′vŭs sin′drōm) SYN iridocorneal endothelial syndrome, iris-naevus syndrome.

irit·ic (ī-rit′ik) Relating to iritis.

iri·tis (ī-rī′tis) Inflammation of the iris. SEE ALSO iridocyclitis, uveitis.

iron (Fe) (ī′ŏrn) Essential metallic element, atomic no. 26, atomic wt. 55.847, which occurs in the heme of hemoglobin, myoglobin, transferrin, ferritin, and iron-containing porphyrins.

iron-bind·ing ca·pac·i·ty (ī′ŏrn bīnd′ ing kă-pas′i-tē) Ability of iron-binding protein in serum (transferrin) to bind serum iron.

iron de·fi·cien·cy a·ne·mia (IDA) (ī′ ŏrn de-fish′ĕn-sē ă-nē′mē-ă) Hypochromic microcytic anemia characterized by low serum iron, increased serum iron-binding capacity, and decreased serum ferritin and marrow iron stores. SYN hypoferric anemia.

iron lung (ī′ŏrn lŭng) SYN Drinker respirator.

ir·ra·di·a·tion (i-rā′dē-ā′shŭn) **1.** Subjective enlargement of a bright object seen against a dark background. **2.** Exposure to the action of electromagnetic radiation. **3.** Spreading of nervous impulses from one area in the brain or cord, or from a tract, to another tract. SEE ALSO radiation. **4.** Process of preparation in which food is exposed to low doses of radiation to kill bacteria and lengthen shelf life.

ir·re·duc·i·ble (i′rē-dū′si-bĕl) **1.** Not reducible; incapable of being made smaller. **2.** CHEMISTRY incapable of being made simpler, or of being replaced, hydrogenated, or reduced in positive charge.

ir·reg·u·lar a·stig·ma·tism (i-reg′yŭ-lăr ă-stig′mă-tizm) Ocular state in which different parts of the same meridian have different degrees of curvature.

ir·reg·u·lar den·tin, ir·ri·ta·tion den·tin (i-reg′yŭ-lăr den′tin, ir′i-tā′shŭn) SYN tertiary dentin.

ir·re·vers·i·ble (i′rĕ-vĕr′si-bĕl) Permanent.

ir·re·ver·si·ble co·ma (i′rĕ-vĕr′si-bĕl kŏ′mă) Profound unconsciousness that cannot be reversed.

ir·re·vers·i·ble shock (i′rĕ-vĕr′si-bĕl shok) That which has progressed because of cell injury beyond the stage where resuscitation is possible.

ir·ri·ga·tion (ir′i-gā′shŭn) In surgery, washing out a body cavity, space, or wound with a fluid.

ir·ri·ga·tor (ir′i-gā′tŏr) An appliance used in irrigation.

ir·ri·ta·bil·i·ty (ir′i-tă-bil′i-tē) The property inherent in protoplasm of reacting to a stimulus.

ir·ri·ta·ble (ir′i-tă-bĕl) **1.** Capable of reacting to a stimulus. **2.** Tending to react immoderately to a stimulus. Cf. excitable.

ir·ri·ta·ble bow·el syn·drome, ir·ri·ta·ble co·lon (IBS) (ir′i-tă-bĕl bow′ĕl sin′drōm, kŏ′lŏn) A condition characterized by constipation, diarrhea, gas and bloating, without organic pathology. SYN spastic colon.

ir·ri·tant con·tact der·ma·ti·tis (ir′i-tănt kon′takt dĕr′mă-tī′tis) Skin reactions ranging from erythema and scaling to necrotic burns.

ir·ri·ta·tion (ir′i-tā′shŭn) **1.** Inflammatory reaction of the tissues to an injury. **2.** Normal response of nerve or muscle to a stimulus. **3.** Evocation of a normal or exaggerated reaction in the tissues by the application of a stimulus.

Isaac syn·drome, Isaac-Mer·ton syn·

drome (ĭ′zăk sin′drōm, ĭ′zăk mer′tŏn sin′drōm) A disorder due to abnormal, spontaneous muscle activity of neural origin, manifested as continuous muscle stiffness and delayed relaxation after exercise, often accompanied by pain, cramps, fasciculations, hyperhydrosis, and muscle hypertrophy (on electromyogram, manifests as myokymia).

is·aux·e·sis (is′awk-sē′sis) Growth of parts at the same rate as growth of the whole.

ischaemia [Br.] SYN ischemia.

ischaemic heart disease [Br.] SYN ischemic heart disease.

ischaemic hypoxia [Br.] SYN ischemic hypoxia.

is·che·mi·a (is-kē′mē-ă) Local anemia due to mechanical obstruction of blood supply. SYN ischaemia.

is·che·mic heart dis·ease (IHD) (is-kē′mik hahrt di-zēz′) A general term for diseases of the heart caused by insufficient blood supply to myocardium.

is·che·mic hy·pox·i·a (is-kē′mik hī-pok′sē-ă) Tissue hypoxia characterized by tissue oligemia and caused by arterial or arteriolar obstruction or vasoconstriction. SYN ischaemic hypoxia.

is·che·mic lum·ba·go (is-kē′mik lŭm-bā′gō) Backache characterized by a painful muscle cramp in the lumbar region incited by walking or standing; promptly relieved by rest.

is·che·mic neu·rop·a·thy (is-kē′mik nūr-op′ă-thē) Neural disorder resulting from acute or chronic ischemia of the involved nerves.

is·chem·ic pen·um·bra (is-kē′mik pĕ-nŭm′bră) Area peripheral to one of ischemia where metabolism is active but blood flow is diminished.

is·chem·ic pe·ri·car·di·tis (is-kē′mik per′i-kahr-dī′tis) Inflammation of cardiac sac caused by impeded blood flow.

is·chem·ic stroke (is-kē′mik strōk) Thrombosis-induced stroke.

is·chi·ad·ic (is′kē-ad′ik) SYN sciatic (1).

is·chi·al (is′kē-ăl) SYN sciatic (1).

is·chi·al bur·si·tis (is′kē-ăl bŭr-sī′tis) Inflammation of the bursa overlying the ischial tuberosity of the pelvis.

is·chi·al spine (is′kē-ăl spīn) [TA] A pointed process from the posterior border of the ischium on a level with the lower border of the acetabulum.

is·chi·at·ic (is′kē-at′ik) SYN sciatic (1).

is·chi·at·ic her·ni·a (is′kē-at′ik hĕr′nē-ă) One through the sacrosciatic foramen.

ischio- Combining form denoting ischium.

is·chi·o·a·nal (is′kē-ō-ā′năl) Relating to the ischium and anus.

is·chi·o·cap·su·lar (is′kē-ō-kap′sŭ-lăr) Relating to the ischium and the capsule of the hip joint.

is·chi·o·coc·cyg·e·al (is′kē-ō-kok-sij′ē-ăl) Relating to the ischium and the coccyx.

is·chi·o·coc·cyg·e·us (is′kē-ō-kok-sij′ē-ŭs) SEE muscle. SYN coccygeus muscle.

is·chi·o·dyn·i·a (is′kē-ō-din′ē-ă) SYN ischialgia (1).

is·chi·o·ni·tis (is′kē-ō-nī′tis) Inflammation of the ischium.

is·chi·o·pu·bic (is′kē-ō-pyū′bik) Relating to both ischium and pubis.

is·chi·o·rec·tal (is′kē-ō-rek′tăl) Relating to the ischium and rectum.

is·chu·ri·a (is-kyūr′ē-ă) Reduction in the flow of urine from any cause (e.g., dehydration, obstruction).

i·se·thi·o·nate (ĭ′sĕ-thī′ŏ-nāt) A salt or ester of isethionic acid.

is·land (ĭ′lănd) ANATOMY any isolated part, separated from the surrounding tissues by a groove, or marked by a difference in structure. SYN insula (2).

is·land flap (ĭ′lănd flap) A flap in which the pedicle consists solely of the supplying artery and vein(s).

is·land of Lan·ger·hans (ī'lănd lang'er-hahnz) SYN islets of Langerhans.

is·land of Reil (ī'lănd rīl) SYN insula (1).

is·let (ī'lĕt) A small island.

is·let cell tu·mor (ī'lĕt sel tū'mŏr) An endocrine tumor composed of cells equivalent or related to those in the normal islet of Langerhans; may be benign or malignant.

is·lets of Lan·ger·hans (ī'lĕts lang'er-hahnz) Cellular masses varying from a few to hundreds of cells lying in the interstitial tissue of the pancreas; they are the source of insulin and glucagon. SYN island of Langerhans

-ism Suffix meaning **1.** A medical condition or a disease resulting from or involving some specified thing. **2.** A practice, doctrine. Cf. -ia, -ismus.

-ismus L. for -ism; customarily used to imply spasm, contraction.

iso- **1.** Prefix meaning equal, like. **2.** CHEMISTRY prefix indicating ''isomer of'' (isomerism). **3.** IMMUNOLOGY prefix designating similarity with respect to species; in recent years, the meaning has shifted to similarity with respect to genetic constitution of individual people.

iso·ag·glu·ti·nin (ī'sō-ă-glū'ti-nin) An isoantibody that causes agglutination of cells of genetically different members of the same species. SYN isohemagglutinin.

iso·al·lele (ī'sō-ă-lēl') One of a number of alleles that can be distinguished only by special analyses.

iso·am·y·lase (ī'sō-am'il-ās) A hydrolase that cleaves 1,6-α-D-glucosidic branch linkages in glycogen, amylopectin, and their β-limit dextrins.

iso·an·ti·bod·y (ī'sō-an'ti-bod-ē) **1.** An antibody that occurs only in some individuals of a species and reacts specifically with a particular foreign isoantigen. **2.** Sometimes used as a synonym of alloantibody.

iso·an·ti·gen (ī'sō-an'ti-jen) **1.** An antigenic substance that occurs only in some individuals of a species, such as the blood group antigens of humans. **2.** Sometimes used as a synonym of alloantigen.

iso·bar·ic (ī'sō-bar'ik) **1.** Having equal weights or pressures. **2.** With respect to solutions, having the same density as the diluent or medium.

iso·bu·tyl al·co·hol (ī'sō-byū'til al'kŏhol) Synthethic compound formed from carbon monoxide and hydrogen.

iso·cap·nic, iso·cap·ne·ic (ī'sō-kap'nik, -nē'ik) Denotes a constant carbon dioxide level.

iso·cel·lu·lar (ī'sō-sel'yū-lăr) Composed of cells of equal size or of similar character.

iso·chro·mat·ic (ī'sō-krō-mat'ik) **1.** Of uniform color. **2.** Denoting two objects of the same color.

iso·chro·mat·o·phil, i·so·chro·mat·o·phile (ī'sō-krō-mat'ō-fil, -fīl) Having an equal affinity for the same dye; said of cells or tissues.

iso·chro·ni·a (ī'sō-krō'nē-ă) **1.** The state of having the same chronaxie. **2.** Agreement, with respect to time, rate, or frequency, between processes.

iso·chron·ic (ī'sō-kron'ik) Denotes occurring at the same time.

isoch·ro·nous (ī-sok'rŏ-nŭs) Occurring during the same time.

iso·ci·trate (ī'sō-sit'rāt) A salt or ester of isocitric acid.

iso·cit·ric ac·id (ī'sō-sit'rik as'id) An intermediate in the tricarboxylic acid cycle.

iso·co·ri·a (ī'sō-kōr'ē-ă) Equality in the size of the two pupils.

iso·cor·tex (ī'sō-kōr'teks) [TA] The larger part of the mammalian cerebral cortex. SEE ALSO cerebral cortex.

iso·cy·tol·y·sin (ī'sō-sī-tol'i-sin) A cytolysin that reacts with the cells of certain other animals of the same species, but not with the cells of the individual that formed the isocytolysin.

iso·cy·to·sis (ī′sō-sī-tō′sis) Cells of the same size.

iso·dac·tyl·ism (ī′sō-dak′ti-lizm) Condition in which the fingers or toes are all approximately of equal length.

iso·dense (ī′sō-dens) Denoting a tissue having a radiopacity (radiodensity) similar to that of another or adjacent tissue.

iso·dose (ī′sō-dōs) Area of equivalent radiation dose.

iso·dy·nam·ic law (ī′sō-dī-nam′ik law) For energy purposes, different foodstuffs may replace one another in accordance with their caloric values when burned in a calorimeter.

iso·e·lec·tric (ī′sō-e-lek′trik) Of equal electrical potential. Cf. isoelectric point. SYN isopotential.

iso·e·lec·tric fo·cus·ing (IEF) (ī′sō-ĕ-lek′trik fō′kŭs-ing) Electrophoresis of small molecules or macromolecules in a pH gradient.

iso·e·lec·tric point (pI) (ī′sō-ĕ-lek′trik poynt) The pH at which an amphoteric substance is electrically neutral.

iso·en·er·get·ic (ī′sō-en′ĕr-jet′ik) Exerting equal force; equally active.

iso·en·zyme, iso·zyme (ī′sō-en′zīm, ī′sō-zīm) One of a group of enzymes that catalyze the same reaction but may be differentiated by variations in physical properties. SYN isozyme.

iso·e·ryth·rol·y·sis (ī′sō-ĕ-rith-rol′i-sis) Destruction of erythrocytes by isoantibodies.

isog·a·my (ī-sog′ă-mē) Conjugation between two equal gametes or two individual cells alike in all respects.

iso·ge·ne·ic, i·so·gen·ic (ī′sō-jĕ-nē′ik, -jen′ik) SYN syngeneic.

iso·ge·ne·ic an·ti·gen (ī′sō-jen′ik an′ti-jen) Same or similar agent that evokes an immune response.

iso·ge·ne·ic graft (ī′sō-jĕ-nē′ik graft) SYN syngraft, isograft.

iso·gen·e·sis (ī′sō-jen′ĕ-sis) Process whereby something originates from the same tissue or cell.

isog·e·nous (ī-soj′ĕ-nŭs) Of the same origin, as in development from the same tissue or cell.

iso·graft (ī′sō-graft) SYN isogeneic graft, syngraft.

isohaemagglutinin [Br.] SYN isohemagglutinin.

isohaemolysin [Br.] SYN isohemolysin.

isohaemolysis [Br.] SYN isohemolysis.

iso·he·mag·glu·ti·nin (ī′sō-hē′mă-glū′ti-nin) SYN isoagglutinin, isohaemagglutinin.

iso·he·mol·y·sin (ī′sō-hē-mol′i-sin) An isolysin that reacts with red blood cells. SYN isohaemolysin.

iso·he·mol·y·sis (ī′sō-hē-mol′i-sis) Dissolution of red blood cells as a result of the reaction between an isolysin (isohemolysin) and specific antigen in or on the cells. SYN isohaemolysis.

iso·im·mu·ni·za·tion (ī′sō-im′yū-nī-zā′shŭn) Development of a significant titer of specific antibody as a result of antigenic stimulation with material contained on or in the red blood cells of another individual of the same species.

iso·ki·net·ic (ī′sō-ki-net′ik) Maintaining constant muscle tension.

iso·late (ī′sō-lāt, -lăt) **1.** To separate, to set apart; that which is so treated. **2.** To free of chemical contaminants. **3.** PSYCHOANALYSIS to separate experiences or memories from the affects pertaining to them. **4.** GROUP PSYCHOTHERAPY a person to whom others in the group do not respond. **5.** Viable organisms separated on a single occasion from a field sample in experimental hosts, culture systems, or stabilates. **6.** A population that for geographic, linguistic, cultural, social, religious, or other reasons is subject to little or no genetic flow.

iso·la·tion (ī′sō-lā′shŭn) **1.** MICROBIOLOGY separation of an organism from others, usually by making serial cultures. **2.** Separation for the period of communicability of infected people or animals from others to prevent or limit the direct or indirect transmission of the infectious agent from those who are infected to those who are susceptible. Cf. quarantine.

iso·leu·cine (I) (ī'sō-lū'sēn) An L-amino acid found in almost all proteins; a dietary essential amino acid.

isol·o·gous (ī-sol'ŏ-gŭs) SYN syngeneic.

isol·o·gous graft (ī-sol'ŏ-gŭs graft) SYN syngraft.

isol·y·sin (ī-sol'i-sin) An antibody that combines with, sensitizes, and results in complement-fixation and dissolution of cells that contain the specific isoantigen.

isol·y·sis (ī-sol'i-sis) *Avoid the mispronunciation isoly'sis.* Lysis or dissolution of cells as a result of the reaction between an isolysin and specific antigen in or on the cells. SEE ALSO isohemolysis.

iso·malt·ase (ī'sō-mawl'tās) SYN oligo-α-1, 6-glucosidase.

iso·malt·ose (ī'sō-mawl'tōs) A disaccharide in which two glucose molecules are attached by an α1,6 link, rather than an α1,4 link as in maltose.

iso·mer (ī'sō-měr) **1.** One of two or more substances displaying isomerism, e.g., L-glucose and D-glucose or citrate and isocitrate. Cf. stereoisomer. **2.** One of two or more nuclides having the same atomic and mass numbers but differing in energy states for a finite period of time, e.g., ^{99m}Tc and ^{99}Tc.

isom·er·ase (ī-som'ěr-ās) A class of enzymes catalyzing the conversion of a substance to an isomeric form.

isom·er·ism (ī-som'ěr-izm) The existence of a chemical compound in two or more forms that are identical with respect to percentage composition but differ as to the positions of one or more atoms within the molecules, and also in physical and chemical properties.

iso·mer·i·za·tion (ī-som'ěr-ī-zā'shŭn) A process in which one isomer is formed from another.

iso·met·ric (ī'sō-met'rik) **1.** Of equal dimensions. **2.** PHYSIOLOGY denoting the condition when the ends of a contracting muscle are held fixed so that contraction produces increased tension at a constant overall length. Cf. auxotonic, isotonic (3), isovolumic.

iso·met·ric con·trac·tion (ī'sō-met'rik kŏn-trak'shŭn) Force development at constant length. Cf. isotonic contraction.

iso·met·ric ex·er·cise (IME) (ī'sō-met'rik ek'sěr-sīz) That consisting of muscular contractions without movement of the involved parts of the body.

iso·me·tro·pi·a (ī'sō-mě-trō'pē-ă) Equality in refraction in the two eyes.

iso·mor·phic (ī'sō-mōr'fik) SYN isomorphous.

iso·mor·phism (ī'sō-mōr'fizm) Similarity of form between two or more organisms or between parts of the body.

iso·mor·phous (ī'sō-mōr'fŭs) Having the same form or shape, or being morphologically equal. SYN isomorphic.

iso·ni·a·zid (INH) (ī'sō-nī'ă-zid) Most commonly used antituberculosis drug. Organisms rapidly develop resistance against this drug if it is used alone in the treatment of active disease.

isop·a·thy (ī-sop'ă-thē) Treatment of disease with the causal agent or a product of the same disease.

isoph·a·gy (ī-sof'ă-jē) SYN autolysis.

iso·pho·ri·a (ī'sō-for'ē-ă) Equal vertical muscle tension in each eye.

iso·plas·tic (ī'sō-plas'tik) SYN syngeneic.

iso·pre·cip·i·tin (ī'sō-prē-sip'i-tin) An antibody that combines with and precipitates soluble antigenic material in the plasma or serum, or in an extract of the cells, from another member, but not all members, of the same species.

iso·prene (ī'sō-prēn) Unsaturated five-carbon hydrocarbon with a branched chain, which in the plant and animal kingdom is used as the basis for the for-

I

mation of isoprenoids, e.g., terpenes, carotenoids and related pigments, rubber.

iso·pren·oids (ī′sō-prēn′oydz) Polymers with carbon skeletons that consist in whole or in large part of isoprene units joined end to end.

iso·pro·pyl al·co·hol (IPA, IA) (ī′sō-prō′pil al′kŏ-hōl) An isomer of propyl alcohol and a homologue of ethyl alcohol, similar in its properties, when used externally, to the latter, but more toxic when taken internally, used as a rubefacient. SYN dimethylcarbinol, isopropanol.

isop·ter (ī-sop′tĕr) A line of equal retinal sensitivity in the visual field.

iso·sex·u·al (ī′sō-sek′shū-ăl) 1. Relating to the existence of characteristics or feelings of both sexes in one person. 2. Descriptive of an individual's somatic characteristics, or of internal processes, as consonant with the person's sex.

isos·mot·ic (ī′sos-mot′ik) Having the same total osmotic pressure or osmolality as another fluid.

iso·sor·bide (ī′sō-sōr′bīd) A compound with diuretic properties prepared by acid dehydration of D-glucitol.

Isos·po·ra (ī-sos′pŏr-ă) A genus of coccidia chiefly parasitizing mammals.

iso·ther·mal (ī′sō-thĕr′măl) Having the same temperature.

iso·tone (ī′sō-tōn) One of several nuclides having the same number of neutrons in their nuclei.

iso·ton·ic (ī′sō-ton′ik) 1. Relating to isotonicity or isotonia. 2. Having equal tension. 3. In physiology, denoting the condition when a contracting muscle shortens against a constant load, as when lifting a weight. Cf. auxotonic, isometric (2).

iso·ton·ic con·trac·tion (ī′sō-ton′ik kŏn-trak′shŭn) Shortening at constant force development. Cf. isometric contraction.

iso·ton·ic ex·er·cise (ī′sō-ton′ik eks′ĕr-sīz) Exercise in which the muscle contracts against a fixed resistance, without movement. Cf. isometric exercise.

iso·to·nic·i·ty (ī′sō-tŏ-nis′i-tē) 1. The quality of possessing and maintaining a uniform tone or tension. 2. The property of a solution in being isotonic.

iso·tope (ī′sō-tōp) One of two or more nuclides that are chemically identical, having the same number of protons, yet differ in mass number, because their nuclei contain different numbers of neutrons.

iso·trans·plan·ta·tion (ī′sō-trans′plan-tā′shŭn) Transfer of a syngraft.

iso·tro·pic, isot·ro·pous (ī′sō-trō′pik, ī-sot′rŏ-pŭs) Having properties that are the same in all directions.

iso·type (ī′sō-tīp) An antigenic determinant (marker) that occurs in all members of a subclass of an immunoglobulin class.

iso·va·ler·ic ac·id (ī′sō-vă-ler′ik as′id) Metabolic intermediate in oxidative processes; elevated in cases of isovaleric acidemia.

iso·vol·ume pres·sure-flow curve (ī′sō-vol′yūm presh′ŭr-flō′ kŭrv) Relationship between transpulmonary pressure and respiratory air flow.

iso·vol·u·mic (ī′sō-vol-yū′mik) Occurring without an associated alteration in volume, as when, in early ventricular systole, the muscle fibers initially increase their tension without shortening so that ventricular volume remains unaltered. SEE ALSO isometric.

iso·vol·u·mic con·trac·tion (ī′sō-vol-yū′mik kŏn-trak′shŭn) Start of systolic contraction phase of the pumping heart.

iso·zyme (ī′sō-zīm) SYN isoenzyme.

is·sue (ish′ū) Archaic term for a discharge of pus, blood, or other matter.

isth·mec·to·my (is-mek′tŏ-mē) Excision of the midportion of the thyroid.

isth·mic, isth·mi·an (is′mik, -mē-ăn) Denoting an anatomic isthmus.

isth·mo·pa·ral·y·sis (is′mō-păr-al′i-sis) Paralysis of the soft palate and muscles forming the anterior pillars of the fauces. SYN isthmoplegia.

isth·mo·ple·gi·a (is′mō-plē′jē-ă) SYN isthmoparalysis.

isth·mus, pl. **isth·mi,** pl. **isth·mus·es** (is′mŭs, -mī, -mi-sēz) [TA] **1.** A constriction in the embryonic neural tube delineating the anterior portion of the rhombencephalon, the future metencephalon, from the more rostrally located mesencephalon. **2.** SYN rhombencephalic isthmus.

isth·mus of eu·sta·chian tube (is′mŭs yū-stā′shăn tūb) SYN isthmus of pharyngotympanic tube.

itch (ich) **1.** An irritating sensation in the skin that arouses the desire to scratch. SYN pruritus (2). **2.** Common name for scabies (q.v.).

itch·ing (ich′ing) An uncomfortable sensation of irritation of the skin or mucous membranes that causes scratching or rubbing of the affected parts. SYN pruritus (1).

itch mite (ich mīt) General term encompassing several species of minute parasites with biting and sucking mouthparts that cause unpleasant dermatologic reactions.

-ite Suffix meaning **1.** the nature of, resembling. **2.** A salt of an acid that has the termination -ous. **3.** COMPARATIVE ANATOMY denoting an essential portion of the part to the name of which it is attached. SEE ALSO -ites.

iter (ī′tĕr) A passage leading from one anatomic part to another. SEE ALSO canaliculus.

iter·al (ī′tĕr-ăl) Relating to an iter.

-ites Adjectival suffix to nouns, corresponding to L. -alis, -ale, or -inus, -inum, or Eng. -y or -like, or the hyphenated nouns; the adjective so formed is used without the qualified noun. SEE ALSO -ite.

-itic Combining form denoting disorder of.

-itis *Words ending with this suffix form their plurals in -itides. Avoid incorrect singulars in -itide (e.g., arthritide, encephalitide) backformed from such plu-*rals. Suffix denoting inflammation. SEE ALSO -ites.

Ito ne·vus (ē′tō nē′vŭs) Pigmentation of skin innervated by lateral branches of the supraclavicular nerve and the lateral cutaneous nerve of the arm, due to scattered, heavily pigmented, dendritic melanocytes in the dermis.

-ium Combining form usually denoting a natural element (e.g., polonium).

Ives dis·ease (īvz di-zēz′) Increased skin hypersensitivity (''leopard spots''), swelling, and redness seen in old men. Treatment includes avoidance of exposure to sun, systemic adrenocortical steroids, and some other pharmaceuticals.

Ivor Lew·is esoph·a·gec·to·my (ī′vŏr lū′is ĕ-sof′ă-jek′tŏ-mē) Commonly used approach for esophagectomy using laparotomy and right thoracotomy, with intrathoracic anastomosis.

ivo·ry ex·o·sto·sis (ī′vŏr-ē eks′os-tō′sis) Small, rounded, eburnated tumor arising from a bone, usually one of the cranial bones.

IV tub·ing (tū′bing) Modality used to connect the bag of medication to the patient; either gravity driven or forced by a pump calibrated to give the fluids over a longer period.

Ivy meth·od (ī′vē meth′ŏd) A method of testing bleeding time to determine platelet levels.

Ix·o·des (ik-sō′dēz) A genus of hard ticks, many species of which are parasitic in humans and animals.

ix·o·di·a·sis (ik′sō-dī′ă-sis) Skin lesions caused by the bites of ixodid ticks.

ix·od·ic (ik-sod′ik) Relating to or caused by ticks.

ix·o·did (ik′sō-did) Common name for members of the family Ixodidae.

ix·od·i·dae (ik-sod′i-dē) The so-called hard ticks, characterized by rigid body form, presence of a dorsal shield, and an anteriorly projecting capitulum; includes the genera *Ixodes, Hyalomma, Amblyomma,* and others that transmit many important human and animal diseases.

J Abbreviation for joule; electric current density; flux (4).

jack·et (jak′ĕt) **1.** A fixed bandage applied around the body to immobilize the spine. **2.** DENTISTRY an artificial crown composed of fired porcelain or acrylic resin.

jack·knife po·si·tion (jak′nīf pŏ-zish′ŏn) Positioning a patient on her or his stomach, with knees at a 90-degree angle and arms outstretched.

jack·pot syn·drome (jak′pot sin′drōm) Clinical and legal jargon phrase denoting action of a patient who seeks excessive remuneration for what the physician regards as a minor matter.

jack·screw (jak′skrū) A threaded device used in appliances for the separation of approximated teeth or jaws.

jack·so·ni·an sei·zure, jack·so·ni·an ep·i·lep·sy (jak-sō′nē-ăn sē′zhūr, ep′i-lep-sē) One originating in or near the rolandic neocortex, which clinically involves one part of the body; spread is progressive to other parts of the body on the same side; may become generalized.

Ja·cob·son re·flex (jă′kŏb-sŏn rē′fleks) Flexion of the fingers elicited by tapping the flexor tendons over the wrist joint or the lower end of the radius.

jac·ti·ta·tion, jac·ta·tion (jak′ti-tā′shŭn, jak-tā′shŭn) Extreme restlessness or tossing about from side to side.

JADA (ja′dă) Acronym for *Journal of the American Dental Association.*

JAMA (jam′ă) The official name for the journal published by the American Medical Association.

James·town Can·yon vi·rus (JCV) (jāmz′town kan′yŏn vī′rŭs) Member of the California group of arboviruses, which has been associated with a mild febrile illness in humans in North America.

Jane·way le·sion (jān′wā lē′zhŭn) One of the stigmata of infectious endocarditis: irregular, erythematous, flat, painless macules on the palms, soles, thenar and hypothenar eminences of the hands, tips of the fingers, and plantar surfaces of the toes.

Jan·sky-Bi·els·chow·sky dis·ease (yahn′skē by′els-chov′skē di-zēz′) Cerebral sphingolipidosis, early juvenile type.

Jap·a·nese B en·ceph·a·li·tis (JBE) (jap′ă-nēz′ en-sef′ă-lī′tis) Epidemic encephalitis or encephalomyelitis of Japan, Siberian Russia, and other parts of Asia; due to the Japanese B encephalitis virus (genus *Flavivirus*) and transmitted by mosquitoes; can occur as a symptomless, subclinical infection but may cause an acute meningoencephalomyelitis. SYN encephalitis japonica, Russian autumn encephalitis.

Jap·a·nese spot·ted fe·ver (jap′ă-nēz′ spot′ĕd fē′vĕr) A febrile disease caused by the bacterium *Rickettsia japonica* and characterized by headache and exanthema.

jar (jahr) **1.** To jolt or shake. **2.** A jolting or shaking.

jar·gon (jahr′gŏn) **1.** Language or terminology peculiar to a specific field, profession, or group. **2.** Nonsensical speech due to insult or trauma to the brain.

jar·gon a·pha·si·a (jahr′gŏn ă-fā′zē-ă) SYN paragrammatism.

Ja·risch-Herx·hei·mer re·ac·tion (yah′rish herks′hīm-er rē-ak′shŭn) SYN Herxheimer reaction.

Jar·vik ar·ti·fi·cial heart (jahr′vik ahr′ti-fish′ăl hahrt) A pneumatic artificial heart.

jaun·dice (jawn′dis) **1.** A yellowish staining of the integument, sclerae, and deeper tissues and of the excretions with bile pigments, which are increased in plasma. **2.** Symptom of various disorders, including liver disease. SYN icterus.

jaun·dice of the new·born (jawn′dis nū′bōrn) SYN icterus neonatorum.

jaw (jaw) **1.** One of the two bony structures, in which the teeth are set, forming the framework of the mouth. **2.** Common name for either the maxilla or the mandible.

jaw bone (jaw bōn) SYN mandible.

jaw gra·da·tion (jaw grā-dā′shŭn) Controlled vertical mandibular movement during vocalization as a function of length, depth, and amount of muscular contraction.

jaw wink·ing (jaw wingk'ing) A paradoxic movement of eyelids associated with movements of the jaw.

jaw-wink·ing syn·drome (jaw'wingk' ing sin'drōm) An increase in the width of the palpebral fissures during chewing, sometimes with a rhythmic elevation of the upper lid when the mouth is open and ptosis when closed. SYN Gunn syndrome, Marcus Gunn phenomenon, Marcus Gunn syndrome.

JC vi·rus (vī'rŭs) Human polyomavirus of worldwide distribution that produces infections that are usually subclinical in immunocompetent people, but is associated with progressive multifocal leukoencephalopathy in the immunosuppressed.

Jef·fer·son frac·ture (jef'ĕr-sŏn frak' shŭr) Fracture of the atlas, usually due to compressive trauma.

je·ju·nal (jĕ-jū'năl) Relating to the jejunum.

je·ju·nal a·tre·si·a (jĕ-jū'năl ă-trē'zē-ă) Closure or congenital absence of the jejunum portion of the small intestine.

je·ju·nec·to·my (jĕ'jū-nek'tŏ-mē) Excision of all or a part of the jejunum.

jejuno-, jejun- Combining forms meaning the jejunum, jejunal.

je·ju·no·il·e·al by·pass (JIB) (jĕ-jū'nō-il'ē-ăl bī'pas) Union of the upper jejunum to terminal ileum to treat severe obesity. SYN bowel bypass, jejunoileal shunt.

je·ju·no·il·e·al shunt (jĕ-jū'nō-il'ē-ăl shŭnt) SYN jejunoileal bypass.

je·ju·no·il·e·i·tis (jĕ-jū'nō-il'ē-ī'tis) Inflammation of the jejunum and ileum.

je·ju·no·il·e·os·to·my (jĕ-jū'nō-il'ē-os' tŏ-mē) Establishment of a new communication between the jejunum and the ileum.

je·ju·no·je·ju·nos·to·my (jĕ-jū'nō-jĕ' jū-nos'tŏ-mē) An anastomosis between two portions of jejunum.

je·ju·no·plas·ty (jĕ-jū'nō-plas-tē) A corrective surgical procedure on the jejunum.

je·ju·nos·to·my (jĕ'jū-nos'tŏ-mē) Operative establishment of an opening from the abdominal wall into the jejunum, usually with creation of a stoma on the abdominal wall.

je·ju·not·o·my (jĕ'jū-not'ŏ-mē) Incision into the jejunum.

je·ju·num (jĕ-jū'nŭm) [TA] The portion of the small intestine, about 8 feet in length, between the duodenum and the ileum.

jel·ly (jel'ē) *Do not confuse this word with gel.* 1. A semisolid tremulous compound usually containing some form of gelatin in aqueous solution. 2. SYN jellyfish.

jel·ly·fish (jel'ē-fish) Marine coelenterates, including some poisonous species; toxin is injected into the skin by nematocysts on the tentacles, causing linear wheals. SYN jelly.

jerk (jĕrk) 1. A sudden pull. 2. SYN deep reflex.

jerk nys·tag·mus (jĕrk nis-tag'mŭs) Slow drift of the eyes in one direction, followed by a rapid recovery movement, always described in the direction of the recovery movement; it usually arises from labyrinthine or neurologic lesions or stimuli.

jerks (jerks) Chorea or any form of tic.

jet hu·mid·i·fi·er (jet hyū-mid'i-frĕr) Device that adds molecular water to ambient air by means of a jet nozzle apparatus.

jet in·jec·tion (jet in-jek'shŭn) Hypodermic injection of drugs by a jet injection device.

jim·son weed, jim·son·weed (jim'sŏn wēd) SYN *Datura stramonium.*

jock itch (jok ich) SYN tinea cruris.

Jof·froy sign (zhof-rwah' sīn) Disorder of the arithmetical faculty in the early stages of organic brain disease.

jog·ger's heel (jog'ĕrz hēl) SYN plantar fasciitis.

J

joint (joynt) [TA] ANATOMY Place of union, usually more or less movable, between two or more bones. SYN arthrosis (1), articulation (1), junctura (1).

joint cap•sule (joynt kap'sŭl) [TA] Sac enclosing the articulating ends of the bones participating in a synovial joint, formed by an outer fibrous layer and an inner synovial membrane. SYN capsula articularis [TA], articular capsule.

joint chon•dro•ma (joynt kon-drō'mă) A benign cartilaginous tumor that develops in the synovial space of a joint.

Joint Com•mis•sion on Ac•cre•di•ta•tion of Health•care Or•ga•ni•za•tions (JCAHO) (joynt kŏ-mish'ŏn ă-kred-i-tā'shŭn helth'kăr ōr'găn-i-zā' shŭnz) An independent nonprofit organization that evaluates and accredits health care organizations and programs in the United States.

joint ef•fu•sion (joynt ĕ-fyu'zhŭn) Increased fluid in synovial cavity of a joint.

joint ex•ten•sion (joynt eks-ten'shŭn) SYN close-packed position.

joint sense (joynt sens) SYN articular sensibility.

joint sta•bil•i•ty (joynt stă-bil'i-tē) Ability of the kinetic chain (i.e., nervous, skeletal, and muscular systems) to stabilize a joint during movement.

Jones frac•ture (jōnz frak'shŭr) Transverse stress fracture of the proximal shaft of the fifth metatarsal.

Jones test (jōnz test) SYN fluorescein instillation test.

Jou•bert syn•drome (zhū-bār' sin' drŏm) Agenesis of the cerebellar vermis, characterized clinically by attacks of tachypnea or prolonged apnea, abnormal eye movements, ataxia, and mental retardation.

joule (J) (jūl) A unit of energy; the heat generated, or energy expended, by an ampere flowing through an ohm for 1 second; equal to 10^7 ergs and to a newton-meter. It is an approved multiple of the SI fundamental unit of energy, the erg, and is intended to replace the calorie (4.184 J).

Joule e•quiv•a•lent (J) (jūl ĕ-kwiv'ă-lĕnt) Dynamic equivalent of heat; the amount of work converted to heat that will raise the temperature of 1 pound of water 1°F is 778 foot-pounds; in metric units, 1 calorie, which raises 1 g of water 1°C, equals 4.184×10^7 dyne-centimeters, or 4.184 J.

J-pouch (powch) A surgical pouch created at the end of the ileum to retain fecal matter after surgical creation of an ileoanal anastomosis. Surgical resevoir constructed so as to act as an artifical rectum after surgical removal of the large intestine. SEE ALSO ileoanal pouch.

J-tube (tūb) Feeding tube inserted through a jejunostomy.

ju•ga•le (jū-gā'lē) A craniometric point at the union of the temporal and frontal processes of the zygomatic bone. SYN jugal point.

ju•gal point (jū'găl poynt) SYN jugale.

jug•u•lar (jŭg'yū-lăr) **1.** Relating to the throat or neck. **2.** Relating to the jugular veins. **3.** A jugular vein.

jug•u•lar ve•nous pres•sure (jŭg-yū-lăr vē'nŭs presh'ŭr) Blood pressure as measured at the jugular vein.

ju•gum, pl. **ju•ga** (jū'gŭm, -ă) **1.** [TA] A ridge or furrow connecting two points. **2.** A type of forceps.

juice (jūs) **1.** The interstitial fluid of a plant or animal. **2.** A digestive secretion.

juice ther•a•py (jūs thār'ă-pē) The dietary and therapeutic administration of vegetables and fruits that have been mechanically converted to liquids.

ju•men•tous (jū-men'tŭs) Denotes a foul bestial smell.

jump flap (jŭmp flap) A distant flap transferred in stages through an intermediate carrier.

jump•ing dis•ease, jump•er dis•ease (jŭmp'ing di-zēz', jŭm'pĕr) One of the pathologic startle syndromes found in isolated parts of the world, characterized by greatly exaggerated responses, such as jumping, flinging the arms, and yelling, to minimal stimuli. Also called jumping Frenchmen of Maine syndrome.

jump·ing gene (jŭmp'ĭng jēn) One associated with transposable elements. SEE transposon.

junc·ti·o (jŭngk'shē-ō) SYN junction.

junc·tion (jŭngk'shŭn) [TA] The point, line, or surface of union of two parts, mainly bones or cartilages. SYN junctio.

junc·tion·al bi·gem·i·ny (jungk'shŭn-ăl bī-jem'ĭ-nē) Abnormal pairing of heart contractions originating at the atrioventricular junction.

junc·tion·al ep·i·the·li·um (jŭngk'shŭn-ăl ep'i-thē'lē-ŭm) Surface located at the base of the gingival sulcus.

junc·tion·al ex·tra·sys·to·le (jungk'shŭn-ăl eks'tră-sis'tŏ-lē) Premature beat arising from the atrioventricular junction and leading to a simultaneous or almost simultaneous contraction of atria and ventricles. SYN atrioventricular extrasystole.

junc·tion·al pre·ma·ture com·plex (jungk'shŭn-ăl prē'mă-chūr' kom'pleks) Abnormal independent (unitary) heart contraction originating at the atrioventricular junction. SEE ALSO premature ventricular contraction.

junc·tion·al rhythm (jŭngk'shŭn-ăl ridh'ŭm) Rhythms originating anywhere within the atrioventricular junction.

junc·tion·al tach·y·car·di·a (jŭngk'shŭn-ăl tak'i-kahr'dē-ă) Cardiac activation arising from the atrioventricular junction with a ventricular response rate over 100 beats per minute.

junc·tion ne·vus (jŭngk'shŭn nē'vŭs) A nevus consisting of nests of melanocytes in the basal cell zone, at the junction of the epidermis and dermis, appearing as a slightly raised, small, flat, nonhairy pigmented (brown or black) tumor.

junc·tu·ra, pl. **junc·tu·rae** (jŭngk-tyūr'ă, -ē) **1.** [TA] SYN joint. **2.** The point, line, or surface of union of two

parts, mainly bones or cartilages. SYN juncture.

junc·ture (jŭngk'shŭr) **1.** The manner in which syllables are joined together in the context of speech; providing additional differential cues to meaning. **2.** SYN junction.

jun·i·per tar (jū'ni-pĕr tahr) Empyreumatic volatile oil obtained from the woody portion of *Juniperus oxycedrus;* used externally for skin diseases. SYN cade oil.

jur·is·pru·dence, med·i·cal (jūr'is-prū'dĕns) The science of law, its principles and concepts.

Jur·kat cells (yūr'kăt selz) A line of T cells often employed in immunologic research.

ju·ve·nile al·ve·o·lar rhab·do·my·o·sar·co·ma (jū'vĕ-nil al-vē-ō'lăr rab'dō-mī'ō-sahr-kō'mă) A malignant tumor in children and adolescents that develops in striated muscle fibers.

ju·ve·nile ar·thri·tis, ju·ve·nile rheu·ma·toid ar·thri·tis (jū'vĕ-nil ahr-thrī'tis, rū'mă-toyd) Chronic arthritis beginning in childhood, most cases of which are pauciarticular, i.e., affecting few joints. SEE ALSO Still disease.

ju·ve·nile cell (jū'vĕ-nil sel) SYN metamyelocyte.

ju·ve·nile my·o·clon·ic ep·i·lep·sy (jū'vĕ-nil mī'ō-klon'ik ep'i-lep'sē) Inherited syndrome typically beginning in early adolescence, characterized by early morning myoclonic jerks that may progress into a generalized tonic-clonic seizure.

ju·ve·nile pel·vis (jū'vĕ-nil pel'vis) A pelvis justo minor in which the bones are slender.

ju·ve·nile pol·yp (jū'vĕ-nil pol'ip) Smoothly rounded mucosal hamartoma of the large bowel, which may be multiple and cause rectal bleeding, especially in the first decade of life; it is not precancerous. SYN retention polyp.

juxta- Combining form denoting located or situated nearby.

jux·ta·glo·mer·u·lar (jŭks′tă-glō-mer′ yū-lăr) Close to or adjoining a renal glomerulus.

jux·ta·glo·mer·u·lar cells (jŭks′tă-glō-mer′yū-lăr selz) Those located at the vascular pole of the renal corpuscle that secrete renin and form a component of the juxtaglomerular complex.

jux·ta·glo·mer·u·lar com·plex, jux·ta·glo·mer·u·lar ap·pa·ra·tus (jŭks′tă-glō-mer′yū-lăr kom′pleks, ap′ă-rat′ŭs) One consisting of (a) the juxtaglomerular cells, which are modified smooth muscle cells in the wall of the afferent glomerular arteriole and sometimes also the efferent arteriole; (b) extraglomerular mesangium (lacis cells), which are located in the angle between the afferent and efferent glomerular arterioles; (c) the macula densa of the distal tubule; and (d) granular epithelial peripolar cells located at the angle of reflection of the parietal to the visceral capsule of the renal corpuscle; provides feedback control of extracellular fluid volume and glomerular filtration rate by activating the renin-angiotensin system.

jux·ta·med·ul·lar·y (jŭks′tă-med′ŭ-lar-ē) Close to or adjoining the medullary border.

jux·ta·med·ul·lar·y glo·mer·u·lus (jŭks′tă-med′ŭ-lar-ē glō-mer′yū-lŭs) A glomerulus close to the medullary border.

jux·ta·po·si·tion (jŭks′tă-pŏ-zish′ŭn) A position side by side. SEE ALSO apposition, contiguity.

K

kak-, kako- SEE caco-.

kal-, kali- Combining forms indicating potassium.

ka·li·o·pe·ni·a (kā′lē-ō-pē′nē-ă) Insufficiency of potassium in the body.

ka·li·o·pe·nic (kā′lē-ō-pē′nik) Relating to kaliopenia.

ka·li·u·re·sis (kā′lē-yūr-ē′sis) SYN kaluresis.

kal·li·din (kal′i-din) A decapeptide vasodilator consisting of bradykinin with a lysyl group attached to the amino terminus. SYN bradykininogen, kallidin 10, kinin 10, lysyl-bradykinin.

kal·li·kre·ins (kal′i-krē′inz) Enzymes that can convert kininogen by proteolysis to bradykinin or kallidin. SYN kininogenase, kininogenin.

Kall·mann syn·drome (kahl′mahn sin′drōm) SYN hypogonadism with anosmia.

kal·u·re·sis (kal′yūr-ē′sis) Increased urinary excretion of potassium. SYN kaliuresis.

kal·u·ret·ic (kal′yūr-et′ik) Relating to, causing, or characterized by kaluresis. SYN kaliuretic.

ka·o·lin (kā′ō-lin) Hydrated aluminum silicate; when powdered and freed from gritty particles by elution, used as a demulcent and adsorbent. SYN aluminum silicate.

ka·o·lin clot·ting time (KCT) (kā′ō-lin klot′ing tīm) Sensitive test of platelet-poor plasma for detecting lupus anticoagulants in mixtures of plasmas taken from patients and from control groups.

ka·o·lin·o·sis (kā′ō-lin-ō′sis) Pneumonoconiosis caused by the inhalation of clay dust.

Kap·lan-Mei·er anal·y·sis (kap′lăn-mī′ĕr ă-nal′i-sis) Method of calculating survival of a patient population in which the increments are the actual survival times of the patients.

Ka·po·si sar·co·ma (kap′ŏ-zē sahr-kō′mă) Multifocal malignant neoplasm of primitive vasoformative tissue, in skin and sometimes in lymph nodes or viscera, consisting of spindle cells and irregular small vascular spaces frequently infiltrated by hemosiderin-pigmented macrophages and extravasated red blood cells.

Ka·po·si var·i·cel·li·form e·rup·tion (kap′ŏ-zē var′i-sel′i-fŏrm ĕr-ŭp′shŭn) A complication of either herpes simplex or vaccinia superimposed on atopic dermatitis, with generalized vesicles and vesicopapules and high fever.

Kar·nof·sky scale (kahr-nof′skē skāl) A performance scale for rating a person's usual activities; used to evaluate a patient's progress after a therapeutic procedure.

Kar·ta·ge·ner syn·drome (kahr-tag′ĕ-nĕr sin′drōm) Complete situs inversus associated with bronchiectasis and chronic sinusitis associated with ciliary dysmotility and impaired ciliary mucus transport in the respiratory epithelium.

karyo- Combining form meaning nucleus. Cf. nucleo-.

kar·y·o·gam·ic (kar′ē-ō-gam′ik) Relating to or marked by karyogamy.

kar·y·og·a·my (kar′ē-og′ă-mē) Fusion of the nuclei of two cells, as occurs in fertilization or true conjugation.

kar·y·o·gen·ic (kar′ē-ō-jen′ik) Relating to karyogenesis; forming the nucleus.

kar·y·o·kin·e·sis (kar′ē-ō-ki-nē′sis) Cellular and nuclear division.

kar·y·o·lymph (kar′ē-ō-limf) The fluid or gellike substance of the nucleus in which the chromatin material, nucleolus, and other particulate elements of the nucleus are suspended. SYN nuclear hyaloplasm, nuclear sap, nucleochylema, nucleochyme, nucleoplasm.

kar·y·ol·y·sis (kar′ē-ol′i-sis) Destruction of the nucleus of a cell by swelling, with the loss of affinity of its chromatin for basic dyes.

kar·y·o·mere (kar′ē-ō-mēr′) A vesicle

containing only a small part of the typical nucleus, usually following an abnormal mitosis.

kar•y•om•i•tome (kar′ē-om′i-tōm) The nuclear chromatin network.

kar•y•o•mor•phism (kar′ē-ō-mōr′fizm) 1. Development of the nucleus of a cell. 2. Denoting the nuclear shapes of cells, especially leukocytes.

kar•y•o•phage (kar′ē-ō-fāj) An intracellular parasite that feeds on the host nucleus.

kar•y•o•plast (kar′ē-ō-plast) A cell nucleus surrounded by a narrow band of cytoplasm and a plasma membrane.

kar•y•o•pyk•no•sis (kar′ē-ō-pik-nō′sis) Cytologic characteristics of the superficial or cornified cells of stratified squamous epithelium in which there is shrinkage of the nuclei and condensation of the chromatin into structureless masses.

kar•y•or•rhex•is (kar′ē-ō-rek′sis) Fragmentation of the nucleus whereby its chromatin is distributed irregularly throughout the cytoplasm.

kar•y•o•some (kar′ē-ō-sōm) A mass of chromatin often found in the interphase cell nucleus representing a more condensed zone of chromatin filaments.

kar•y•os•ta•sis (kar′ē-os′tă-sis) SYN interphase.

kar•y•o•the•ca (kar′ē-ō-thē′kă) SYN nuclear envelope.

kar•y•o•type (kar′ē-ō-tīp) The chromosome characteristics of an individual cell or of a cell line. SYN idiogram (1).

Kas•a•bach-Mer•ritt syn•drome (kahs′ă-bok-mer′it sin′drōm) Large, progressive vascular malformations in extremities.

Ka•sai op•er•a•tion (kă-sī′ op-er-ā′shŭn) SYN portoenterostomy.

Ka•shin-Bek dis•ease (kah′shin bek di-zēz′) Generalized osteoarthrosis believed due to ingestion of wheat infected with the fungus *Fusarium sporotrichiella*.

kata- Alternative spelling for prefix cata-, meaning down.

kat•al (kat) (kat′ăl) Unit of catalytic activity equal to one mole of product formed (or substrate consumed) per second, as of the amount of enzyme that catalyzes transformation of one mole of substrate per second.

Ka•ta•ya•ma dis•ease (kat′ă-yah′mă di-zēz′) Acute early egg-laying phase of schistosomiasis, a toxemic syndrome in heavy primary infections; considered a form of immune complex disease.

ka•thex•is (kath-eks′is) A disorder characterized by bone marrow retention of myeloid elements leading to severe peripheral neutropenia; neutrophils have a distinctly abnormal appearance. SYN myelokathexis.

Katz in•dex (kats in′deks) Assessment of activities of daily living; correlates with recovery from hip fracture, placement in an assisted-living facility, and mortality rates.

ka•va, ka•va ka•va (kah′vă, kah′vă-kah′vă) Agent derived from *Piper methysticum;* purported antiseizure properties; used to treat anxiety disorders, as a sleep aid, and for its suggested value in therapy for muscle spasms and sexually transmitted diseases. Adverse effects reported include hepatitis, cirrhosis, and parkinsonian syndrome.

Ka•wa•sa•ki dis•ease, Ka•wa•sa•ki syn•drome (kah-wă-sah′kē di-zēz′, sin′drōm) Systemic vasculitis of unknown origin that occurs primarily in children younger than 8 years of age. Symptoms include a fever lasting more than 5 days; polymorphic rash; erythematous, dry, cracking lips; conjunctival injection; swelling of the hands and feet; irritability; adenopathy; and a perineal desquamative rash. SYN mucocutaneous lymph node syndrome.

Keen op•er•a•tion (kēn op-er-ā′shŭn) Removal of sections of the posterior branches of the spinal nerves to the affected muscles, and of the spinal accessory nerve, as a cure for torticollis.

ke•fir (ke-fir′) An enzyme-rich drink made from fermented milk that helps maintain the workings of the gastrointestinal tract.

Keg·el ex·er·cis·es (keg′ĕl eks′ĕr-sīz-ĕz) Alternate contraction and relaxation of perineal muscles for treatment of urinary stress incontinence.

Kell·gren syn·drome (kel′gren sin′drōm) Degenerative joint disease that affects joints of the hands, knees, hips, and back.

Kel·ly clamp (kel′ē klamp) Curved hemostat without teeth, introduced for gynecologic surgery.

Kel·ly op·er·a·tion (kel′ē op-ĕr-ā′shŭn) **1.** Correction of retroversion of the uterus by plication of uterosacral ligaments. **2.** Correction of urinary stress incontinence by vaginally placing sutures beneath the bladder neck.

ke·loid (kē′loyd) A nodular, firm, often linear mass of hyperplastic thickish scar tissue, consisting of irregularly distributed bands of collagen; occurs in the dermis, usually after trauma, surgery, a burn, or severe cutaneous disease.

ke·lo·plas·ty (kē′lō-plas-tē) Surgical removal of a scar or keloid.

kel·vin (K) (kel′vin) A unit of thermodynamic temperature equal to 1/273.16 of the thermodynamic temperature of the triple point of water. SEE ALSO Kelvin scale.

Kel·vin scale (kel′vin skāl) Temperature scale in which the triple point of water is assigned the value of 273.16 K; °C = K − 273.15. SYN absolute scale.

Ken·ne·dy clas·si·fi·ca·tion (ken′ĕ-dē klas′i-fi-kā′shŭn) Listing of several forms of partially edentulous jaws in accordance with the distribution of the missing teeth.

Ken·ne·dy dis·ease (ken′ĕ-dē di-zēz′) An X-linked recessive disorder characterized by progressive spinal and bulbar muscular atrophy; associated features include distal degeneration of sensory axons, and signs of endocrine dysfunction, including diabetes mellitus, gynecomastia, and testicular atrophy.

Ken·ne·dy syn·drome (ken′ĕ-dē sin′drōm) Ipsilateral optic atrophy with central scotoma and contralateral choked disc or papilledema, caused by a meningioma of the ipsilateral optic nerve.

ke·no·pho·bi·a (kē′nō-fō′bē-ă) An irrational fear of large open spaces.

♻ **kerat-** SEE kerato-.

ker·a·tan sul·fate (KS) (ker′ă-tan sŭl′fāt) Sulfated found in cartilage, bone, connective tissue, the cornea, aorta, and in the intervertebral discs.

ker·a·tec·to·my (ker′ă-tek′tŏ-mē) An operation to remove corneal tissue.

ke·rat·ic pre·cip·i·tates (kĕr-at′ik prē-sip′i-tăts) Inflammatory cells on the corneal endothelium.

ker·a·tin (ker′ă-tin) Sulfurous scleroprotein or albuminoid present in hair and nails; sometimes used to coat tablets intended to be dissolved only in the intestine. SYN cytokeratin.

ker·a·tin·as·es (ker′ă-tin-ās′ĕz) Hydrolases catalyzing the hydrolysis of keratin.

ker·a·tin·i·za·tion (ker′ă-tin-ī-zā′shŭn) Development of a horny layer; premature formation of keratin. SYN cornification.

ke·rat·i·no·cyte (kĕ-rat′i-nō-sīt) Cell of living epidermis and some oral epithelium that produces keratin in the process of differentiating into dead and fully keratinized stratum corneum cells.

ker·at·i·noid (kĕ-rat′i-noyd) Resembling keratin or connective tissue.

ke·rat·i·no·phil·ic (kĕ-rat′i-nō-fil′ik) Denoting fungi that use keratin as a substrata, e.g., dermatophytes.

ke·rat·i·nous (kĕ-rat′i-nŭs) Relating to keratin.

ke·rat·i·nous cyst (kĕ-rat′i-nŭs sist) Epithelial lesion containing keratin.

ker·a·ti·tis (ker′ă-tī′tis) Inflammation of the cornea. SEE ALSO keratopathy.

♻ **kerato-, kerat-** Combining forms indicating the cornea; horny tissue or cells. SEE ALSO cerat-, cerato-.

ker·a·to·ac·an·tho·ma (ker′ă-tō-ak′an-

K

thō'mă) Fast-growing, umbilicated tumor, usually on exposed areas of the skin, which invades the dermis but remains localized and usually resolves spontaneously.

ker·a·to·cele (ker'ă-tō-sēl) Hernia of the Descemet membrane through a defect in the outer layers of the cornea.

ker·a·to·con·junc·ti·vi·tis (KC) (ker'ă-tō-kŏn-jŭngk'ti-vī'tis) Inflammation of the conjunctiva and of the cornea.

ker·a·to·con·junc·ti·vi·tis sic·ca (ker'ă-tō-kŏn-jŭngk'ti-vī'tis sik'ă) Chronic mucopurulent conjunctivitis due to deficit of the aqueous component of tears. SYN dry eye syndrome.

ker·a·to·co·nus (KC) (ker'ă-tō-kō'nŭs) A conic protrusion of the cornea caused by thinning of the stroma; usually bilateral. SYN conic cornea.

ker·a·to·cyte (ker'ă-tō-sīt) 1. The fibroblastic stromal cell of the cornea. 2. A variety of poikilocyte that owes its abnormal shape to fragmentation occurring as the cell flows through damaged small vessels. SYN schistocyte.

ker·a·to·der·ma (ker'ă-tō-dĕr'mă) 1. Any horny superficial growth. 2. A generalized thickening of the horny layer of the epidermis.

ker·a·to·der·ma blen·nor·rha·gi·cum (ker'ă-tō-dĕr'mă blen-ō-raj'ĭ-kŭm) Disorder with scattered, thickened hyperkeratotic skin lesions.

ker·a·to·der·ma plan·ta·re sul·ca·tum (ker'ă-tō-dĕr'mă plan-tā'rē sŭl-kā'tŭm) Hyperkeratosis and fissure formation on the soles of the feet. SYN cracked heel.

ker·a·to·gen·e·sis (ker'ă-tō-jen'ĕ-sis) Production of horny cells or tissue.

ker·at·o·gen·ic (ker'ă-tō-jen'ik) Pertaining to the production or growth of thick, hard (horny) tissue.

ker·a·tog·e·nous (ker'ă-toj'ĕ-nŭs) Causing growth of cells that produce keratin and result in formation of horny tissue.

ker·a·tog·e·nous mem·brane (ker-ă-

toj'ĕ-nŭs mem'brān) 1. SYN nail matrix. 2. SYN nail bed.

ker·a·to·glo·bus (ker'ă-tō-glō'bŭs) Congenital anomaly with an enlarged anterior segment of the eye. SYN anterior megalophthalmos, megalocornea.

ker·a·to·hy·a·lin, ker·a·to·hy·a·lin gran·ules (ker'ă-tō-hī'ă-lin, gran'yūlz) The substance in the large basophilic granules of the stratum granulosum of the epidermis.

ker·a·toid ex·an·the·ma (ker'ă-toyd ek'san-thē'mă) A symptom in secondary stage of yaws: patches of fine furfuraceous desquamation, over limbs and trunk.

ker·a·to·i·ri·tis (ker'ă-tō-ī-rī'tis) Inflammation of the iris and the cornea.

ker·a·to·lep·tyn·sis (ker'ă-tō-lep-tin'sis) An operation for removing the surface of the cornea and replacement by bulbar conjunctiva for cosmetic reasons.

ker·a·to·leu·ko·ma (ker'ă-tō-lū-kō'mă) A white corneal opacity.

ker·a·tol·y·sis (ker'ă-tol' i-sis) 1. Separation or loosening of the horny layer of the epidermis. 2. Disease characterized by shedding the epidermis at more or less regular intervals. SYN deciduous skin.

ker·a·to·lyt·ic (ker'ă-tō-lit'ik) Relating to keratolysis.

ker·a·to·ma (ker'ă-tō'mă) 1. SYN callosity. 2. A horny tumor.

ker·a·to·ma·la·ci·a (ker'ă-tō-mă-lā'shē-ă) Dryness with ulceration and corneal perforation in cachectic children; due to severe vitamin A deficiency.

ker·a·tome, ker·at·o·tome (ker'ă-tōm, ker'ă-tō-tōm) A knife used for incising the cornea. SYN keratotome.

ker·a·tom·e·try (ker'ă-tom'ĕ-trē) Measurement of the radii of corneal curvature.

ker·a·to·mi·leu·sis (ker'ă-tō-mī-lū'sis) Correcting refractive error by changing the shape of a deep corneal layer.

ker·a·to·my·co·sis (ker'ă-tō-mī-kō'sis) Fungal infection of the cornea.

ker·a·top·a·thy (ker′ă-top′ă-thē) Any corneal disease, damage, dysfunction, or abnormality. SYN keratopathia.

ker·a·to·phak·i·a (ker′ă-tō-fā′kē-ă) Implantation of a donor cornea or plastic lens within the corneal stroma to modify refractive error.

ker·a·to·plas·ty (ker′ă-tō-plas-tē) Removal of a portion of the cornea and the insertion in its place of a piece of cornea of the same size and shape removed from elsewhere. SYN corneal graft.

ker·a·to·pros·the·sis (ker′ă-tō-pros-thē′sis) Replacement of the central area of an opacified cornea by an artificial lens.

ker·a·to·rhex·is, ker·a·tor·rhex·is (ker′ă-tō-rek′sis) Rupture of the cornea, due to trauma or perforating ulcer.

ker·a·to·scle·ri·tis (ker′ă-tō-skler-ī′tis) Inflammation of both cornea and sclera.

ker·a·to·scope (ker′ă-tō-skōp) An instrument marked with lines or circles by means of which the corneal reflex can be observed. SYN Placido da Costa disc.

ker·a·tos·co·py (ker′ă-tos′kŏ-pē) Examination of the reflections from the anterior surface of the cornea to determine the character and amount of corneal astigmatism.

ker·a·tose (ker′ă-tōs) Keratotic, relating to or marked by keratosis.

ker·a·to·sis, pl. **ker·a·to·ses** (ker′ă-tō′sis, -sēz) Any lesion on the epidermis marked by the presence of circumscribed overgrowths of the horny layer.

ker·a·to·sis fol·lic·u·la·ris (ker′ă-tō′sis fŏ-lik′yū-lā′ris) A familial eruption, beginning usually in childhood, in which keratotic papules originating from both follicles and interfollicular epidermis of the trunk, face, scalp, and axillae encrust; often intensely pruritic. SYN Darier disease, Hailey and Hailey disease.

ker·a·to·sis pi·la·ris (ker-ă-tō′sis pī-lā′ris) Common benign follicular scaly papules; primarily affects extensor surfaces of the arms and thighs.

ker·a·to·sis punc·ta·ta (ker-ă-tō′sis pŭngk-tā′tă) SYN punctate keratoderma.

ker·a·tot·o·my (ker′ă-tot′ŏ-mē) **1.** Any corneal incision. **2.** An operation making a partial thickness corneal incision to flatten it and reduce its refractive power.

ke·ri·on (kē′rē-on) A granulomatous, raised, secondarily infected lesion complicating fungal infection of the hair.

Ker·ley B lines (kĕr′lē līnz) Fine peripheral septal lines.

KERMA (kĕr′mă) Acronym for kinetic energy released in a material.

ker·nic·ter·us (kĕr-nik′tĕr-ŭs) Yellow staining and degenerative lesions in basal ganglia associated with high levels of unconjugated bilirubin in infants; consequences include deafness, cerebral palsy, other sensorineural deficits, and mental retardation. SYN bilirubin encephalopathy, nuclear jaundice.

ket·a·mine (kēt′ă-mēn) A parenterally administered anesthetic that produces catatonia, profound analgesia, increased sympathetic activity, and little relaxation of skeletal muscles.

keto- Combining form denoting a compound containing a ketone group; replaced by oxo- in systematic nomenclature.

ke·to ac·id (kē′tō as′id) An acid containing a ketone group (–CO–) in addition to the acid group(s); α-keto acid refers to a 2-oxo acid (e.g., pyruvic acid); β-keto acid refers to a 3-oxo acid (e.g., acetoacetic acid), etc. SYN oxo acid.

ke·to·ac·i·do·sis (kē′tō-as-i-dō′sis) Acidosis, due to enhanced production of ketone bodies.

ke·to·gen·e·sis (kē′tō-jen′ĕ-sis) Metabolic production of ketones or ketone bodies.

ke·to·gen·ic diet (kē′tō-jen′ik dī′ĕt) A high-fat, low-carbohydrate, and normal protein diet causing ketosis.

α-ke·to·glu·tar·ate (kē′tō-glū-tar′āt) A salt or ester of α-ketoglutaric acid.

ke·to·hep·tose (kē′tō-hep′tōs) A seven-carbon sugar possessing a ketone group.

ke·to·hex·ose (kē′tō-heks′ōs) A six-carbon sugar possessing a ketone group, e.g., fructose. SYN hexulose.

ke•tole (kē′tōl) SYN indole (1).

ketonaemia [Br.] SYN ketonemia.

ke•tone (kē′tōn) A substance with the carbonyl group linking two carbon atoms; the most important in medicine and the simplest in chemistry is dimethyl ketone (acetone).

ke•tone al•co•hol (kē′tōn al′kŏ-hol) A compound containing a carbonyl or ketone group as well as a hydroxyl group, e.g., dihydroxyacetone.

ke•to•ne•mi•a (kē′tō-nē′mē-ă) The presence of recognizable concentrations of ketone bodies in the plasma. SYN ketonaemia.

ke•to•nu•ri•a (kē′tō-nyūr′ē-ă) Enhanced urinary excretion of ketone bodies.

ke•tose (kē′tōs) A carbohydrate containing the characteristic carbonyl group of the ketones.

ke•to•sis (kē-tō′sis) Enhanced production of ketone bodies, as in diabetes mellitus or starvation.

key ridge (kē rij) SYN zygomaxillare.

khat (kot) Local name for tender fresh parts of the shrub *Catha edulis*. SYN African tea, Arabian tea.

ki (kī) SYN chi.

kid•ney (kid′nē) [TA] One of the two bean-shaped organs that excrete urine. SYN ren [TA].

kid•ney fail•ure (kid′nē fāl′yŭr) SYN renal failure.

kid•ney stone (kid′nē stōn) SYN renal calculus.

Kiel clas•si•fi•ca•tion (kēl klas′i-fi-kā′shŭn) Classification of non-Hodgkin lymphoma into low-grade and high-grade forms of malignancy.

Kien•böck dis•ease (kēn′buk di-zēz′) Osteonecrosis of the lunate; bone cause unknown, may occur after trauma. SYN lunatomalacia.

Kies•sel•bach a•re•a (kē′sĕl-bahk ār′ē-ă) Space on the anterior portion of the nasal septum rich in capillaries; often a site of epistaxis. SYN Little area.

killed vac•cine (kild vak-sēn′) One made from dead microorganisms for immunization purposes.

killer cells (kil′ĕr selz) Cytotoxic cells involved in antibody-dependent, cell-mediated immune responses. SYN null cells (1), T-cytotoxic cells.

kilo- (k) Prefix used in the SI and metric system to signify one thousand (10^3).

kil•o•base (kb) (kil′ō-bās) Unit used in designating the length of a nucleic acid sequence; 1 kb equals a sequence of 1000 purine or pyrimidine bases.

kil•o•cal•o•rie (kcal) (kil′ō-kal′ŏr-ē) The quantity of energy required to raise the temperature of 1 kg of water from 14.5–15.5°C; it is 1000 times the value of the small calorie. SYN kilogram calorie, large calorie.

kil•o•gram (kg) (kil′ŏ-gram) The SI unit of mass, 1000 g; equivalent to 15,432.358 gr, 2.2046226 lb. avoirdupois, or 2.6792289 lb. troy.

kil•o•gram cal•o•rie (kcal) (kil′ŏ-gram kal′ŏr-ē) SYN kilocalorie.

kil•o•gram-me•ter (kil′ŏ-gram-mē′tĕr) The energy exerted, or work done, when a mass of 1 kg is raised a height of 1 m; equal to 9.80665 J in the SI system.

kil•o•hertz (kHz) (kil′ŏ-hĕrts) A unit of frequency equal to 10^3 hertz.

kil•o•joule (kil′ŏ-jūl) One thousand joules.

kil•o•li•ter (kil′ŏ-lē′tĕr) One thousand liters.

kil•o•me•ter (ki-lom′ē-tĕr) One thousand meters.

Kim•mel•stiel-Wil•son syn•drome, Kim•mel•stiel-Wil•son dis•ease (kim′ĕl-stēl wil′sŏn sin′drōm, di-zēz′) Nephrotic syndrome and hypertension in diabetic people, associated with diabetic glomerulosclerosis.

kin-, kine- Combining forms denoting movement, motion. SEE ALSO cine-.

kinaesthetic [Br.] SYN kinesthetic.

kinaesthetic sense [Br.] SYN kinesthetic sense.

kin·an·es·the·si·a, cin·an·es·the·si·a (kin′an-es-thē′zē-ă, sin′an-es-thē′zē-ă) Disturbance of deep sensibility with inability to perceive either direction or extent of movement; becomes ataxia. SYN cinanesthesia.

ki·nase (kī′nās) **1.** Enzyme that catalyzes conversion of a proenzyme to an active one; important in salvage and recycling of nucleotides. **2.** Suffix attached to some enzymes to indicate transformation.

kin·e·mat·ic chain (kin′ĕ-mat′ik chān) A combination of several joints linking several limb segments together during a specific movement or posture.

kin·e·mat·ic face-bow (kin′ĕ-mat′ik fās′bō) SYN adjustable axis face-bow.

kin·e·sal·gi·a, ki·ne·si·al·gi·a (kin′ĕ-sal′jē-ă, ki-nē′sē-al′jē-ă) Pain caused by muscular movement.

kinesi-, kinesio-, kineso- Combining forms indicating motion.

ki·ne·si·a (ki-nē′sē-ă) SYN motion sickness.

ki·ne·si·at·rics (ki-nē′sē-at′riks) SYN kinesitherapy.

ki·ne·sics (ki-nē′siks) The study of nonverbal, bodily motion in communication.

ki·ne·si·gen·ic (ki-nē′si-jen′ik) Caused or created by movement.

kin·e·sim·e·ter (kin′ĕ-sim′ĕ-tĕr) An instrument for measuring the extent of a movement. SYN kinesiometer.

kinesio- SEE kinesi-.

ki·ne·si·ol·o·gy (ki-nē′sē-ol′ŏ-jē) The science or the study of movement, and the active and passive structures involved.

kin·es·i·om·e·ter (ki-nē′sē-om′ĕ-tĕr) An instrument used to determine the extent of a bodily movement. SYN kinesimeter.

ki·ne·sis (ki-nē′sis) Motion. As a termination, used to denote movement or activation, particularly the kind induced by a stimulus.

ki·ne·si·ther·a·py (ki-nē′sē-thār′ă-pē) Physical therapy involving motion and range of motion exercises. SEE movement. SYN kinesiatrics.

kineso- SEE kinesi-.

kin·es·the·si·a, kin·es·the·sis (kin′es-thē′zē-ă, -sis) **1.** The sense perception of movement; the muscular sense. **2.** An illusion of moving in space.

kin·es·thet·ic (kin′es-thet′ik) Relating to kinesthesia. SYN kinaesthetic.

kin·es·thet·ic sense (kin′es-thet′ik sens) SYN kinaesthetic sense.

ki·net·ic (KIN) (ki-net′ik) Relating to motion or movement.

ki·net·ic en·er·gy (ki-net′ik en′ĕr-jē) The energy of motion.

ki·net·ics (ki-net′iks) The study of motion, acceleration, or rate of change.

kineto- Combining form indicating motion.

ki·ne·to·chore (ki-nē′tō-kōr) The structural portion of the chromosome to which microtubules attach. Cf. centromere.

ki·ne·to·gen·ic (ki-nē′tō-jen′ik) Causing or producing motion.

ki·ne·to·plasm (ki-nē′tō-plazm) **1.** The most contractile part of a cell. **2.** The cytoplasm of the droplet that covers the sperm head during maturation. SYN cinetoplasm, cinetoplasma, kinoplasm.

kin·e·to·sis (kin′ĕ-tō′sis) Form of motion sickness.

kin·e·to·ther·a·pe·utic bath (kin′ĕ-tō-thār′ă-pyū′tik bath) Immersion that uses underwater exercises to strengthen weak or partially paralyzed muscles.

king·dom (king′dŏm) The highest taxo-

K

nomic category into which living forms are classified.

ki·nin (kī'nin) Polypeptide hormones released from diffuse stores, not from specialized tissue; rapidly inactivated at release site.

ki·nin·o·gen (Kgn) (ki-nin'ō-jen) The globulin precursor of a plasma kinin.

kink·y-hair dis·ease (kingk'ē-hār' di-zēz') An inborn error of copper metabolism with onset within a few weeks of birth; manifested by short, sparse, poorly pigmented kinky hair; failure to thrive; development of seizures; spasticity; and progressive mental deterioration leading to death.

kino- Combining form indicating movement.

kin·o·cil·i·um (kin'ō-sil'ē-ŭm) A cilium, usually motile, having nine peripheral double microtubules and two single central ones.

kin·ship (kin'ship) The state of being genetically related.

Kirk am·pu·ta·tion (kĭrk amp'yū-tā'shŭn) One at the lower end of the femur.

Kirk·land knife (kĕrk'lănd nīf) Heart-shaped knife for gingival surgery.

Kirk·lin stag·ing sys·tem (kĭrk'lin stāj'ing sis'tĕm) A procedure used to determine the potential prognosis of the outcome of colon cancer.

Kirsch·ner ap·pa·ra·tus (kirsh'nĕr ap'ă-rat'ŭs, -rā'tŭs) SYN Kirschner wire.

Kirsch·ner wire (kĭrsh'nĕr wīr) An apparatus for skeletal traction in long bone fracture or for fracture fixation. SYN Kirschner apparatus.

Kleb·si·el·la (kleb-sē-el'ă) A genus of aerobic, facultatively anaerobic, nonmotile, non-spore-forming bacteria containing gram-negative, encapsulated rods that occur singly, in pairs, or in short chains; may or may not be pathogenic in human respiratory, intestinal, and urogenital tracts.

Kleb·si·el·la pneu·mo·ni·ae (kleb-sē-el'ă nū-mō'nē-ē) A bacterial species

found in soil and water, on grain, and in the intestinal tract of humans and other animals; commonly associated with lobar pneumonia among hospitalized patients.

Klei·ger test (klē'gĕr test) Maneuver used to determine stability of the deltoid ligament.

Klieg eye (klēg ī) Reaction to optical exposure to intense light.

Kline·fel·ter syn·drome (klīn'fel-tĕr sin'drŏm) Anomaly in males with chromosome count 47, XXY sex chromosome constitution; usually have seminiferous tubule dysgenesis, elevated urinary gonadotropins, gynecomastia, and eunuchoid habitus. SYN XXY syndrome.

Klip·pel-Feil syn·drome (kli-pĕl' fīl' sin'drŏm) A congenital abnormality of the spine characterized by a reduction in the number of cervical vertebrae and their fusion.

Klump·ke pal·sy, Klump·ke pa·ral·y·sis, Klump·ke-De·jer·ine pal·sy (klump'kĕ pawl'zē, păr-al'i-sis, dĕ-zhĕ-rēn') Obstetric palsy with paralysis of the muscles of the distal forearm and hand caused by a lesion of the lower trunk of the brachial plexus, or of the C8 and T1 cervical roots. SYN Dejerine-Klumpke syndrome.

K_m Symbol for Michaelis constant; Michaelis-Menten constant.

Knapp stri·ae (nap strī'ē) SYN angioid streaks.

knee (nē) [TA] **1.** SYN genu (1). **2.** Any structure of angular shape resembling a flexed knee.

knee-chest po·si·tion (nē-chest' pŏ-zish'ŏn) A prone posture resting on the knees and upper part of the chest, assumed for gynecologic or rectal examination.

knee com·plex (nē kom'pleks) Tibiofemoral joint, the patellofemoral joint, and related musculature and connective tissue.

knee-el·bow po·si·tion (nē-el'bō pŏ-zish'ŏn) Prone position resting on the knees and elbows, assumed for gynecologic or rectal procedures. SYN genu-cubital position.

knee jerk (KJ) (nē jĕrk) SYN patellar reflex.

knee joint (nē joynt) [TA] Compound condylar synovial joint consisting of the joint between the condyles of the femur and the condyles of the tibia. SYN articulatio genus [TA].

knee re·place·ment sur·ger·y (nē rē-plās'mĕnt sŭr'jĕr-ē) Removal of damaged bone and cartilage from thigh bone, shin bone, and kneecap and replacement with an artificial joint.

knife nee·dle (nīf nē'dĕl) Very narrow, needle-pointed knife used in discission of a cataract. SYN cataract needle.

knock-knee (nok'nē) SYN genu valgum.

knock·out mouse (nok'owt mows) A mouse from whose genome a single gene has been artificially deleted.

Knoop hard·ness num·ber (nūp hahrd'nĕs nŭm'bĕr) Method used for measurements of hardness of any materials. Also called Knoop hardness test.

knot (not) ANATOMY, PATHOLOGY a node, ganglion, or circumscribed swelling suggestive of a knot.

knuck·le (nŭk'ĕl) **1.** A joint of a finger when the fist is closed. **2.** A kink or loop of intestine.

knuck·le pads (nŭk'ĕl padz) Thick pads of skin over the proximal phalangeal joints.

Kob·ber·ling-Dun·ni·gan syn·drome (kob'ĕr-ling-dŭn'i-găn sin'drōm) SYN familial partial lipodystrophy.

Koch ba·cil·lus (kōk bă-sil'ŭs) SYN *Mycobacterium tuberculosis.*

Ko·cher sign (kō'kĕr sīn) In Graves disease, on upward gaze, the globe lags behind the movement of the upper eyelid.

Koch pos·tu·lates, Koch law (kok pos'tyū-lăts, law) The four steps that prove a pathogenic microorganism is the cause of a disease. 1) Microorganism must be present in all cases of the disease. 2) It must be isolated from the diseased host and grown in pure culture. 3) This culture must reproduce the disease in a new host. 4) The microorganism must be found and cultured from this new host. SYN Koch law.

Koch-Weeks ba·cil·lus (kōk-wĕks bă-sil'ŭs) SYN *Haemophilus aegyptius.*

Kock pouch (kok powch) A continent ileostomy with a reservoir and valved opening using doubled ileal loops.

Koeb·ner phe·nom·e·non (kerb'ner fĕ-nom'ĕ-non) Heightened susceptibility to the effects of trauma and chemical exposure in those with psoriasis, lichen planus, and other chronic dermatoses.

koi·lo·cyte (koy'lō-sīt) A squamous cell, often binucleated, showing a perinuclear halo.

koi·lo·cy·to·sis (koy'lō-sī-tō'sis) Perinuclear vacuolation. SEE ALSO koilocyte.

koi·lo·nych·i·a (koy'lō-nik'ē-ă) A malformation of the nails in which the outer surface is concave; often associated with iron deficiency or softening by occupational contact with oils.

koi·lo·ster·ni·a (koy'lō-stĕr'nē-ă) SYN pectus excavatum.

kok dis·ease (kōk di-zēz') SYN hyperekplexia.

kolp- SEE colpo-.

kol·y·pep·tic (kō'lē-pep'tik) Impaired or difficult digestion.

ko·lyt·ic (kō-lit'ik) Denoting an inhibitory action.

ko·ni·o·cor·tex (kō'nē-ō-kōr'teks) Regions of the cerebral cortex characterized by a particularly well-developed inner granular layer.

kon·zo (kon'zō) Cyanide-related upper motor neuron disease manifested principally as spastic paraplegia; due to consumption of improperly prepared cassava roots, which contain high concentrations of cyanogenetic glucosides.

Kop·lik spots (kop′lik spots) Small red spots on the buccal mucous membrane; occur early in measles, before the skin eruption; regarded as pathognomonic.

kopro- SEE copro-.

Kor·an·yi sign (kōr′ăn-yē sīn) An increased sound when auscultating the back; indicative of pleural effusion.

Ko·rot·koff sounds (kō-rot′kof sowndz) Sounds originating within the blood passing through a vessel or produced by a vibrating motion of the arterial wall.

Ko·rot·koff test (kō-rot′kof test) Blood pressure in the distal circulation is measured while the artery above an aneurysm is compressed.

Kor·sa·koff syn·drome, Kor·sa·koff psy·cho·sis (kor′sĕ-kawf sin′drŏm, sĭ-kō′sis) An alcohol-related amnestic syndrome characterized by confusion and severe impairment of memory, especially for recent events. SYN amnestic syndrome (1), polyneuritic psychosis.

ko·sher (kō′shĕr) Denotes a diet that follows the laws required in observant Jews; interdicts consumption of some food altogether and requires that dairy and meat items be consumed at different times and on different dishes.

Kras·ke po·si·tion (krahs′kĕ pŏ-zish′ŏn) Lying prone with hips elevated.

Krebs cy·cle (krebz sī′kĕl) SYN tricarboxylic acid cycle.

Krebs-Hen·se·leit cy·cle, Krebs or·ni·thine cy·cle, Krebs u·re·a cy·cle (krebz hen′sĕ-līt sī′kĕl, ŏr′ni-thēn sī′kĕl, yūr-ē′ă) SYN urea cycle.

Krim·sky test (krim′skĕ test) Assessing strabismus by shining a penlight at the eyes.

krin·gle (kring′gĕl) A structural motif or domain seen in certain proteins in which a fold of large loops is stabilized by disulfide bonds.

Kru·ken·berg am·pu·ta·tion (krū′kĕn-berg amp′yū-tā′shŭn) Cineplastic amputation at the carpus with the distal end of the forearm used to create a forklike stump between radius and ulna.

Kru·ken·berg spin·dle (krū′kĕn-berg spin′dĕl) A vertical fusiform area of melanin pigmentation on the posterior surface of the central cornea.

Kru·ken·berg tu·mor (krū′kĕn-berg tū′mŏr) A metastatic carcinoma of the ovary, usually bilateral and secondary to a mucous carcinoma of the stomach, which contains signet-ring cells filled with mucus.

krymo-, kryo- SEE crymo-, cryo-.

kryp·ton (Kr) (krip′ton) One of the noble gases, present in small amounts in the atmosphere; used in studies of cardiac abnormalities.

kryp·ton la·ser (krip′ton lā′zĕr) Device used for ophthalmic procedures, particularly retinal photocoagulation in the presence of vitreous hemorrhage.

KTP la·ser (lā′zĕr) Device in the blue-green to green spectrum, used for hemostasis.

Kuf dis·ease (kūf di-zēz′) A hereditary disease in adults leading to dementia, spastic paralysis, and vision problems.

Küh·ne fi·ber (kĕ′nĕ fī′bĕr) Artificial muscle made by filling the intestine of an insect with a growth of myxomycetes; used to demonstrate the contractility of protoplasm.

Kupf·fer cells (kup′fĕr selz) Phagocytic cells of the mononuclear phagocyte series found on the luminal surface of the hepatic sinusoids.

kur·to·sis (kŭr-tō′sis) The extent to which a unimodal distribution is peaked.

ku·ru (kū′rū) SEE prion, bovine spongiform encephalitis.

Kuss·maul co·ma (kūs′mowl kō′mă) SYN diabetic coma.

Kuss·maul res·pi·ra·tion, Kuss·maul-Kien res·pi·ra·tion (kūs′mowl res′pir-ā′shŭn, kēn) Fast breathing characteristic of diabetic and other types of acidosis.

Kveim test (kvīm test) An intradermal test to detect sarcoidosis, done by injecting Kveim antigen (obtained from spleens of patients with sarcoidosis) and examining skin biopsies after 3 and 6 weeks.

KVO Abbreviation used in charting meaning *keep vein open*.

ky·ma·tism (kī'mǎ-tizm) SYN myokymia.

ky·mo·gram (kī'mō-gram) The graphic curve made by a kymograph.

ky·nu·ren·ic ac·id (KA) (kin'yūr-ē'nik as'id) A product of the metabolism of L-tryptophan; appears in human urine in states of marked pyridoxine deficiency.

ky·nu·ren·ine (kin-yūr'ĕ-nēn) A product of the metabolism of L-tryptophan, excreted in the urine.

ky·phos (kī'fos) A hump, the convex prominence in kyphosis.

ky·pho·sco·li·o·sis (kī'fō-skō-lē-ō'sis) Kyphosis combined with scoliosis; congestive heart failure is a late complication.

ky·pho·sis, hunch·back (kī-fō'sis, hŭnch'bak) **1.** An anteriorly concave curvature of the vertebral column. **2.** Hyperkyphosis; excessive anteriorly concave curvature of a part of the spine.

ky·phot·ic (kī-fot'ik) Relating to or suffering from kyphosis.

Kyr·le dis·ease (kir'lĕ di-zēz') SYN hyperkeratosis follicularis et parafollicularis.

kyr·tor·rhach·ic (kir'tō-rak'ik) Condition where the vertebral body is distorted by a ventrally convex lumbar curvature.

kyte (kīt) Stomach; belly (Scots dialect).

kyto- SEE cyto-.

K

L

L- 1. Abbreviation for levorotatory. Cf. D-. **2.** Prefix indicating a chemical compound to be structurally (sterically) related to L-glyceraldehyde.

La Symbol for lanthanum.

la·bel (lāʹbĕl) **1.** To incorporate into a compound a substance that is readily detected so its metabolism can be followed or its physical distribution detected. **2.** The substance so incorporated.

la·bi·a (lāʹbē-ă) Plural of labium.

la·bi·al (La) (lāʹbē-ăl) **1.** Relating to the lips or any labium. **2.** Toward a lip. **3.** A letter formed using the lips.

la·bi·al bar (lāʹbē-ăl bahr) Major connector labial to the dental arch joining two or more bilateral parts of a mandibular removable partial denture.

la·bi·al flange (lāʹbē-ăl flanj) Portion of the flange of a denture that occupies the labial vestibule of the mouth.

la·bi·al glands (lāʹbē-ăl glandz) [TA] Mucous glands in the submucous tissue of the lips. SYN glandulae labiales [TA].

la·bi·al her·ni·a (lāʹbē-ăl hĕrʹnē-ă) Hernia through the canal of Nuck.

la·bi·al·ly (lāʹbē-ăl-ē) Toward the lips.

la·bi·a mi·no·ra (lāʹbē-ă mi-nōʹră) Plural of labium minus.

la·bi·a o·ris (lāʹbē-ă ōʹris) [TA] SEE lip (1).

la·bile (lāʹbīl) Unstable; unsteady, not fixed.

la·bil·i·ty (lă-bilʹi-tē) The state of being labile.

labio- Combining form denoting lips. SEE ALSO cheilo-.

la·bi·o·cho·re·a (lāʹbē-ō-kōr-ēʹă) A chronic spasm of the lips, interfering with speech.

la·bi·o·cli·na·tion (lāʹbē-ō-kli-nāʹshŭn) Inclination of position more toward the lips than is normal; said of a tooth.

la·bi·o·graph (lāʹbē-ō-graf) Instrument to record the lip movements during speech.

la·bi·o·men·tal (LM) (lāʹbē-ō-menʹtăl) Relating to the lower lip and chin.

la·bi·o·place·ment (lāʹbē-ō-plāsʹmĕnt) Positioning (e.g., of a tooth) more toward the lips than normal.

la·bi·o·ver·sion (lāʹbē-ō-vĕrʹzhŭn) Malposition of an anterior tooth from the normal line of occlusion toward the lips.

la·bi·um, pl. **la·bi·a** (lāʹbē-ŭm, -ă) [TA] **1.** SYN lip. **2.** Any lip-shaped structure.

la·bi·um ma·jus, pl. **la·bi·a ma·jo·ra** (lāʹbē-ŭm māʹjŭs, mă-jōʹră) [TA] One of two rounded folds of integument forming the lateral boundaries of the pudendal cleft.

la·bor, stag·es of la·bor (lāʹbŏr, stāʹjĕz lā bŏr) Three-stage process of expulsion of the fetus and the placenta from the uterus. SYN labour.

la·bor curve (lāʹbŏr kŭrv) SYN partogram, labour curve.

la·bored breath·ing (lāʹbŏrd brēdhʹ ing) SEE dyspnea. Cf. asthma.

la·bor pains (lāʹbŏr pānz) Rhythmic uterine contractions that under normal conditions increase in intensity, frequency, and duration, culminating in vaginal delivery of the infant.

labour [Br.] SYN labor.

la·brum, pl. **la·bra** (lāʹbrŭm, -bră) [TA] **1.** A lip. **2.** A lip-shaped structure. SYN articular labrum, articular lip, labrum articulare.

lab·y·rinth (labʹĭ-rinth) [TA] **1.** The internal or inner ear, composed of the semicircular ducts, vestibule, and cochlea. **2.** Any group of communicating cavities, as in each lateral mass of the ethmoid bone. **3.** A group of communicating culture tubes used for separating motile from nonmotile microorganisms.

lab·y·rin·thec·to·my (labʹĭ-rin-thekʹtŏ-mē) Excision of the labyrinth; a destructive operation to destroy labyrinthine function.

lab•y•rin•thine (lab′ĭ-rin′thēn) Relating to any labyrinth.

lab•y•rin•thine nys•tag•mus (lab′ĭ-rin′thēn nis-tag′mŭs) SYN vestibular nystagmus.

lab•y•rin•thine ver•ti•go (lab′ĭ-rin′thēn vĕr′ti-gō) SYN Ménière disease.

lab•y•rin•thi•tis (lab′ĭ-rin-thī′tis) Inflammation of the labyrinth (the internal ear), sometimes accompanied by vertigo and deafness. SYN otitis interna.

lab•y•rin•thot•o•my (lab′ĭ-rin-thot′ŏ-mē) Incision into the labyrinth.

lac (lak) **1.** SYN milk (1). **2.** Any whitish, milklike liquid.

lac•er•at•ed (las′ĕr-ā-tĕd) Torn; rent; having a ragged edge.

lac•er•a•tion (las′ĕr-ā′shŭn) **1.** A torn or jagged wound caused by blunt trauma; incorrectly applied to a cut. **2.** The process or act of tearing the tissues.

la•cer•tus (lă-sĕr′tŭs) **1.** [TA] A fibrous band, bundle, or slip related to a muscle. **2.** Originally the muscular part of the upper limb from shoulder to elbow.

lac•ri•mal, lach•ry•mal (lak′ri-măl) Relating to the tears, their secretion, the secretory glands, and the drainage apparatus.

lac•ri•mal ap•pa•ra•tus (lak′ri-măl ap′ă-rat′ŭs) [TA] Structures that, with the conjunctival sac, produce and provide drainage for lacrimal fluid (tears), consisting of the lacrimal gland, the lacrimal lake, the lacrimal canaliculi, the lacrimal sac, and the nasolacrimal duct. SYN apparatus lacrimalis [TA].

la•cri•mal duct (lak′ri-măl dŭkt) SYN tear duct.

lac•ri•mal flu•id (lak′ri-măl flū′id) A watery physiologic saline, with a plasmalike consistency, but also contains the bacteriocidal enzyme lysozyme; it moistens the conjunctiva and cornea, providing nutrients and dissolved O_2 to the cornea.

lac•ri•mal gland (lak′ri-măl gland) [TA] The gland that secretes tears.

lac•ri•mal lake (lak′ri-măl lāk) [TA] The small cisternlike area of the conjunctiva at the medial angle of the eye, in which the tears collect after bathing the anterior surface of the eyeball and the conjunctival sac.

lac•ri•mal pa•pil•la (lak′ri-măl pă-pil′ă) [TA] Slight projection from the margin of each eyelid near the medial commissure, in the center of which is the lacrimal punctum (opening of the lacrimal duct). SYN papilla lacrimalis [TA].

lac•ri•mal path•way (lak′ri-măl path′wā) A space between the closed lids and the eyeball through which tears flow to the punctum lacrimale.

lac•ri•mal re•flex (lak′ri-măl rē′fleks) Discharge of tears due to conjunctival irritation.

lac•ri•ma•tion (lak′ri-mā′shŭn) The secretion of tears, especially in excess.

lac•ri•ma•tor (lak′ri-mă-tŏr) An agent that irritates the eyes and produces tears.

lac•ri•ma•to•ry (lak′ri-mă-tōr-ē) Causing lacrimation.

lac•ri•mo•gus•ta•to•ry re•flex (lak′ri-mō-gŭs′tă-tōr-ē rē′fleks) Chewing of food causing secretion of tears.

lac•ri•mot•o•my (lak′ri-mot′ŏ-mē) The operation of incising the lacrimal duct or sac.

lact-, lacti-, lacto- Combining forms for milk. SEE ALSO galacto-.

lac•tac•i•do•sis (lakt-as′i-dō′sis) Acidosis due to increased lactic acid.

lac•ta•gogue (lak′tă-gog) Agent that promotes milk flow.

lac•tal•bu•min (lak′tal-bū′min) The proteinaceous albumin fraction of milk.

lac•tase de•fi•cien•cy (lak′tās dĕ-fish′ĕn-sē) Lack of any lactase in the small intestine, which elicits lactose intolerance.

lac•tate (lak′tāt) **1.** A salt or ester of lactic acid. **2.** To produce milk in the mammary glands.

L

lac·tat·ed Ring·er so·lu·tion (lak′tāt-ĕd ring′ĕr sŏ-lū′shŭn) A solution of sodium lactate and other agents in distilled water used for the same purposes as Ringer used solution. SYN Hartmann solution (1).

lac·tate thresh·old (lak′tāt thresh′ōld) A point, during exercise of increasing intensity, when a measurable increase in venous blood lactate levels occurs in conjunction with an exponential increase in respiratory frequency.

lac·ta·tion (lak-tā′shŭn) **1.** Production of milk. **2.** Period following birth during which milk is secreted in the breasts.

lac·ta·tion a·men·or·rhe·a (lak-tā′shŭn ā-men′ŏr-ē′ă) Physiologic suppression of menses while nursing.

lac·ta·tion hor·mone (lak-tā′shŭn hōr′mōn) SYN prolactin.

lac·ta·tion sup·pres·sion (lak-tā′shŭn sŭ-presh′ŏn) Impeding the production of milk and reducing the chances of breast engorgement after giving birth.

lac·te·al (lak′tē-ăl) *Avoid the mispronunciation lacte′al.* **1.** Relating to or resembling milk; milky. **2.** A lymphatic vessel that conveys chyle. SYN chyle vessel, lacteal vessel.

lac·te·al fis·tu·la (lak′tē-ăl fis′tyū-lă) Fistulous opening into one of the lactiferous ducts. SYN mammary fistula.

♻ **lacti-** Combining form denoting milk. SEE lact-.

lac·tic (lact) (lak′tik) Relating to milk.

lac·tic ac·id (lak′tik as′id) A normal intermediate in the fermentation (oxidation, metabolism) of sugar.

lac·tic ac·i·de·mi·a (lak′tik as′i-dĕ′mē-ă) The presence of dextrorotatory lactic acid in the circulating blood.

lac·tic ac·id fer·men·ta·tion (lak′tik as′id fĕr′men-tā′shŭn) Production of lactic acid in milk due to the presence of a lactic acid bacterium.

lac·tic ac·i·do·sis (lak′tik as′i-dō′sis) Metabolic form caused by accumulation of lactic acid due to tissue hypoxia, drug effect, or unknown etiology.

lac·tif·er·ous (lak-tif′ĕr-ŭs) Yielding milk. SYN lactigerous.

lac·tif·er·ous ducts (lak-tif′ĕr-ŭs dŭkts) [TA] About 20 ducts that drain the lobes of the mammary glands. SYN galactophore, mammillary ducts, milk ducts.

lac·ti·fuge (lak′ti-fyūj) **1.** Causing arrest of the secretion of milk. SYN lactifugal. **2.** An agent having such an effect.

lac·tig·e·nous (lak-tij′ĕ-nŭs) Producing milk.

lac·tig·er·ous (lak-tij′ĕr-ŭs) SYN lactiferous.

Lac·to·ba·cil·lus, pl. *Lac·to·ba·cill·i* (lak′tō-bă-sil′ŭs, -ī) A genus of microaerophilic or anaerobic, non-spore-forming, ordinarily nonmotile bacteria found in dairy products, the effluents of grain and meat products, water, sewage, beer, wine, fruits and fruit juices, pickled vegetables, and in sourdough and mash; part of the normal flora of the mouth, intestinal tract, and vagina of many warm-blooded animals, including humans.

Lac·to·ba·cil·lus ac·i·doph·i·lus (lak′tō-bă-sil′ŭs as′i-dof′i-lŭs) A bacterial species found in the feces of milk-fed infants and also in the feces of older persons on a high milk-, lactose-, or dextrin-containing diet.

lac·to·cele (lak′tō-sēl) SYN galactocele.

lac·to·gen (lak′tō-jen) An agent that stimulates milk production or secretion.

lac·to·gen·ic (lak′tō-jen′ik) Pertaining to lactogenesis.

lac·to·gen·ic hor·mone (lak′tō-jen′ik hōr′mōn) SYN prolactin.

lac·to·glob·u·lin (lak′tō-glob′yŭ-lin) The globulin present in milk; it makes up 50–60% of bovine whey protein.

lac·tone (lak′tōn) An intramolecular organic anhydride formed from a hydroxy-acid by the loss of water between a hydroxyl and a –COOH group; a cyclic ester.

la·cto·o·vo·veg·e·ta·ri·an (lak′tō-ō′vō-vej′i-tar′ē-ăn) A vegetarian who consumes dairy products and eggs but does not eat animal flesh.

lac·to·per·ox·i·dase (lak′tō-per-oks′i-dās) A peroxidase obtained from milk; catalyzes oxidation of iodide to iodine.

lac·tor·rhe·a (lak′tō-rē′ă) SYN galactorrhea, lactorrhoea.

lactorrhoea [Br.] SYN lactorrhea.

lac·tose, lac·tine (LAC) (lak′tōs, -tēn) A reducing disaccharide present in mammalian milk. SYN milk sugar, saccharum lactis.

lac·to·su·ri·a (lak′tō-syūr′ē-ă) Excretion of lactose in urine.

lac·to·troph (lak′tō-trōf) A pituitary cell that produces prolactin.

lac·to·veg·e·tar·i·an (lak′tō-vej-ĕ-tār′ē-ăn) One who lives on a mixed diet of milk and milk products, and vegetables, but eschews meat, eggs, and seafood.

lac·tu·lose (lak′tū-lōs) A synthetic disaccharide used to treat hepatic encephalopathy and chronic constipation.

la·cu·nar (lă-kū′năr) Relating to a lacuna.

la·cu·nar lig·a·ment (lă-kū′năr lig′ă-mĕnt) [TA] A curved fibrous band that passes horizontally backward from the medial end of the inguinal ligament to the pectineal line. SYN ligamentum lacunare [TA].

la·cu·nar state (lă-kū′năr stāt) Presence of cerebral pitting. One of the major factors underlying cerebrovascular disease; high correlation with hypertension and atherosclerosis.

la·cu·nule (lă-kū′nyūl) A very small lacuna.

la·cus, pl. **la·cus** (lā′kŭs) [TA] SYN lake (1).

Ladd band (lad band) Peritoneal attachment of an incompletely rotated cecum, seen in intestinal malrotation.

lad·der splint (lad′ĕr splint) A flexible splint consisting of two stout parallel wires with finer cross wires.

La·ën·nec cir·rho·sis (lah-ĕ-nek′ sir-ō′sis) Hepatic disease in which normal liver lobules are replaced by small regeneration nodules, sometimes containing fat, separated by a fairly regular framework of fine fibrous tissue strands (hobnail liver); usually due to chronic alcoholism.

la·e·trile (lā′ĕ-tril) Unproven antineoplastic drug consisting chiefly of amygdalin derived from apricot pits.

laev- SYN levo-.

laevo- [Br.] SYN levo-.

laevocardia [Br.] SYN levocardia.

laevodopa [Br.] SYN levodopa.

laevorotatory [Br.] SYN levorotatory.

lag (lag) **1.** To move or progress more slowly than normal; to fall behind. **2.** The act or condition of falling behind. **3.** The time interval between a change in one variable and a consequent change in another variable.

-lagnia, -lagny Combining forms denoting an improper sexual predilection.

lag·oph·thal·mos, lag·oph·thal·mi·a, lag·oph·thal·mus (lag′of-thal′mŏs, -thal′mē-ă, -thal′mŭs) A condition in which a complete closure of the eyelids over the eyeball is difficult or impossible. SYN hare's eye.

lake (lāk) **1.** [TA] A small collection of fluid. SYN lacus. **2.** To cause blood plasma to become red as a result of the release of hemoglobin from erythrocytes. SEE ALSO lacuna.

la·ky (lā′kē) Pertaining to the transparent bright red appearance of blood serum or plasma that develops as a result of hemoglobins released from destroyed red blood cells.

-lalia Combining form denoting a speech disorder.

lal-, lalio-, lalo- Combining forms pertaining to speech or speech organs.

lal·ling (lal′ing) A form of stammering in which the speech is almost unintelligible.

la·lo·ple·gi·a (lal′ŏ-plē′jē-ă) Paralysis of the muscles concerned in the mechanism of speech.

La·maze meth·od (lĕ-mahz′ meth′ŏd) A technique of psychoprophylactic preparation for childbirth, designed to minimize the pain of labor.

lamb·doid (lam′doyd) Resembling the Greek letter lambda (λ), as the lambdoid suture does.

lam·bert (L, La) (lam′bĕrt) A unit of brightness; the brightness of a perfectly diffusing surface emitting or reflecting a total luminous flux of 1 lumen/sq cm of surface.

Lam·bert-Ea·ton my·as·then·ic syn·drome (lam′bĕrt-ē′tŏn mī′es-then′ik sin′drōm) A generalized disorder of neuromuscular transmission caused by a defect in the release of acetylcholine quanta from the presynaptic nerve terminals. SYN Eaton-Lambert syndrome.

lam·bli·a·sis (lam-blī′ă-sis) SYN giardiasis.

LAMB syn·drome (lam sin′drōm) Concurrence of lentigines, atrial myxoma, mucocutaneous myxomas, and blue nevi.

la·mel·la (lă-mel′ă), pl. **la·mel·lae** (lă-mel′ă, -ē) [TA] **1.** A thin sheet or layer. **2.** A preparation in the form of a medicated gelatin disc, used to make local applications to the conjunctiva in place of solutions.

lam·el·lar (lă-mel′ăr) **1.** Arranged in thin plates or scales. **2.** Relating to lamellae.

lam·el·lar bone (lă-mel′ăr bōn) The normal type of adult mammalian bone, whether cancellous or compact, composed of parallel lamellae in the former and concentric lamellae in the latter.

lam·el·lar cat·a·ract (lă-mel′ăr kat′ăr-akt) A cataract in which the opacity is limited to the cortex. SYN zonular cataract.

lam·el·lar ich·thy·o·sis (LI) (lă-mel′ăr ik′thē-ō′sis) Dry form of congenital ichthyosiform erythroderma, characterized by ectropion and large, coarse scales over most of the body with thickened palms and soles. SYN ichthyosis congenita.

lam·el·la·ted cor·pus·cles (lam′ĕ-lāt′ĕd kŏr′pŭs-ĕlz) Small oval bodies in the skin of the fingers, in the mesentery, tendons, and elsewhere, formed of concentric layers of connective tissue with a soft core in which the axon of a nerve fiber runs, splitting up into a number of fibrils that terminate in bulbous enlargements; they are sensitive to pressure.

la·mel·li·po·di·um, pl. **la·mel·li·po·di·a** (lă-mel′i-pō′dē-ŭm, -ă) A cytoplasmic veil produced on all sides of migrating polymorphonuclear leukocytes.

lam·i·na, pl. **lam·i·nae** (lam′i-nă, nē) [TA] Thin plate or flat layer. SEE ALSO layer, stratum.

lam·i·na·gram (lam′i-nă-gram) An image made by laminagraphy (q.v.). SEE ALSO tomography.

lam·i·nag·ra·phy, lam·i·nog·ra·phy (lam′i-nag′ră-fē, -nog′ră-fē) Radiographic technique in which the images of tissues above and below the plane of interest are blurred out by reciprocal movement of the x-ray tube and film holder to show a specific area more clearly. SEE ALSO tomography.

lam·i·na·plas·ty, lam·i·no·plas·ty (lam′i-nă-plas′tē, lam′i-nō-) Surgical intervention into the cervical spine to relieve pressure.

lam·i·nar, lam·i·nat·ed (lam′i-năr, -i-nā′tĕd) **1.** Arranged in plates or laminae. **2.** Relating to any lamina.

lam·i·nar flow (lam′i-năr flō) The relative motion of elements of a fluid along smooth parallel paths, which occurs at lower values of Reynolds numbers.

lam·i·na·ri·a (lam′i-nar′ē-ă) Sterile rod made of kelp that is hydrophilic, and, when placed in the cervical canal, absorbs moisture, swells, and gradually dilates the cervix.

lam·i·nat·ed (lam′i-nāt′ĕd) SYN laminar (1).

lam·i·nat·ed clot (lam′i-nā-tĕd klot) One formed in a succession of layers such as occurs in an aneurysm.

lam·i·nat·ed ep·i·the·li·um (lam′i-nă-tĕd ep′i-thē′lē-ŭm) SYN stratified epithelium.

lam·i·nat·ed throm·bus (lam′i-nā-tĕd throm′bŭs) Type formed gradually by clotting of the blood in successive layers.

lam·i·nec·to·my (lam, LAM) (lam′i-nek′tŏ-mē) Excision of a vertebral lamina; commonly used to denote removal of the posterior arch.

lam·i·nin (LN) (lam′i-nin) A large, multimeric glycoprotein component of the basement membrane, particularly the lamina lucida; major protein component of the lamina lucida of the renal glomerulus.

lam·i·ni·tis (lam′i-nī′tis) Inflammation of any lamina.

lam·i·not·o·my (lam′i-not′ŏ-mē) An operation on one or more vertebral laminae. SYN rachiotomy.

lamp (lamp) Illuminating device; source of light. SEE ALSO light.

lance (lans) To incise a part, as an abscess or boil.

Lance·field clas·si·fi·ca·tion (lans′fēld klas′i-fi-kā′shŭn) A serologic classification dividing hemolytic streptococci into groups (A–O) based on precipitation test results for group-specific carbohydrate substances.

lan·cet, lance (lan′sĕt, lans) A surgical knife with a short, wide, sharp-pointed, two-edged blade.

lan·ci·nat·ing (lan′si-nāt-ing) Denoting a sharp cutting or tearing pain.

Lan·ci·si sign (lan-chē′sē sīn) A large systolic jugular venous wave caused by tricuspid regurgitation replacing the normal negative systolic trough (''x'' descent).

Lan·dau-Kleff·ner syn·drome (lan′dow-klef′nĕr sin′drōm) Childhood disorder characterized by generalized and psychomotor seizures associated with acquired aphasia; multifocal spikes and spike and wave discharges in the electroencephalogram. SYN acquired epileptic aphasia.

Lan·dol·fi sign (lan-dol′fē sīn) In aortic insufficiency, systolic contraction and diastolic dilation of the pupil.

Lan·dolt rings (lahn′dōl ringz) A diagnostic instrument for vision testing.

Lan·dry pa·ral·y·sis, Lan·dry syn·drome (lan′drē păr-al′i-sis, sin′drōm) SYN Guillain-Barré syndrome.

Land·ström mus·cle (lahnd′ström mŭs′ĕl) Microscopic muscle fibers in the fascia behind and about the eyeball.

Lan·ger-Gie·di·on syn·drome (lahng′ĕr-gē′dē-ōn sin′drōm) Rare genetic disorder caused by lack of certain chromosomes marked by myriad findings: moderate learning difficulties, facial and skeletal abnormalities, and dental problems.

Lan·ger·hans cells (lahng′er-hahnz selz) 1. Dendritic clear cells in the epidermis, containing distinctive granules that appear rod- or racket-shaped in section; active participants in cutaneous delayed hypersensitivity. SYN interdigitating dendritic cells. 2. Cells seen in eosinophilic granuloma and lymphoma of the lungs.

Lang·er-Sal·din·o syn·drome (lang′ĕr-sal-dē′nō sin′drōm) SYN achondrogenesis type II.

Lang·hans cells (lahng′ahnz selz) 1. Multinucleated giant cells seen in tuberculosis and other granulomatous diseases. 2. SYN cytotrophoblastic cells.

lan·guage de·lay (lang′gwăj dĕ-lā′) In pediatrics and speech-language pathology, denotes a condition in which a child has not developed language skills at an age-appropriate level.

lano- Combining form meaning wool.

lan·o·lin (lan′ŏ-lin) SYN wool fat.

la·nu·gi·nous (lă-nū′ji-nŭs) Covered with lanugo.

la·nu·go (lă-nū′gō) Fine, soft, lightly pigmented fetal hair with minute shafts and large papillae; it appears toward the end of the third month of gestation.

lap·a·rec·to·my (lap′ă-rek′tŏ-mē) Stripping of tissue from the abdominal wall, usually done to correct muscular laxity.

♻ **laparo-** *Avoid the misspelling/mispronunciation lapro-.* Combining form denoting the loins (less properly, the abdomen in general).

lap·a·ro·cele (lap′ă-rō-sēl) SYN abdominal hernia.

lap·a·ro·en·do·scop·ic (lap′ă-rō-en′dŏ-skop′ik) Having to do with the introduction of a laparoscope into the abdominal cavity for a variety of intracavitary procedures.

lap·a·ro·en·ter·os·to·my (lap′ăr-ō-en′tĕr-os′tŏ-mē) Surgical incision to create an artifical opening through the abdominal wall into the intestine.

lap·a·ro·sal·pin·go·o·oph·o·rec·to·my (lap′ă-rō-sal-ping′gō-ō′of-ō-rek′tŏ-mē) Removal of the uterine tube and ovary through an abdominal incision.

lap·a·ro·scope (lap′ă-rō-skōp) An endoscope for examining the peritoneal cavity.

lap·a·ro·scop·ic gas·tric band·ing (lap′ăr-ō-skop′ik gas′trik band′ing) A band surgically placed around the stomach that is used to restrict filling so that the patient will feel full and stop eating.

lap·a·ros·co·py (lap′ă-ros′kŏ-pē) Examination of the contents of the peritoneum with a laparoscope. SEE ALSO peritoneoscopy.

lap·a·rot·o·my (lap′ă-rot′ŏ-mē) **1.** Incision into the loin. **2.** SYN celiotomy.

lap·a·rot·o·my pad (lap′ă-rot′ŏ-mē pad) A compress made from several layers of gauze folded into a rectangular shape; used as a sponge or packing material in surgery. SYN abdominal pad.

lap·i·ni·za·tion (lap′i-nī-zā′shŭn) Serial passage of a virus or vaccine in rabbits.

large cal·o·rie (C) (lahrj kal′ŏr-ē) SYN kilocalorie.

large cell car·ci·no·ma (lahrj sel kahr′si-nō′mă) An anaplastic carcinoma, particularly bronchogenic, composed of cells larger than those in oat cell carcinoma of the lung.

large cell lym·pho·ma (LCL) (lahrj sel lim-fō′mă) Lesion composed of large mononuclear cells of undetermined type.

large in·tes·tine (lahrj in-tes′tin) [TA] The portion of the digestive tube extending from the ileocecal valve to the anus; it comprises the cecum, colon, rectum, and anal canal.

Lar·rey am·pu·ta·tion (lah-rā′ amp′yū-tā′shŭn) Amputation at the shoulder joint.

Lar·sen syn·drome (lahr′sĕn sin′drōm) Disorder characterized by multiple congenital dislocations with osseous anomalies, including characteristic flattened facies and cleft soft palate.

lar·va, pl. **lar·vae** (lahr′vă, -vē) **1.** Developmental stage or stages of an insect or helminth. **2.** The second stage in the life cycle of a tick; the stage in which it hatches from the egg and, following engorgement, molts into the nymph. **3.** The young of fishes or amphibians that often differ in appearance from the adult.

lar·va cur·rens (lahr′vă kŭr′enz) Cutaneous larva migrans caused by rapidly moving larvae of *Strongyloides stercoralis* (up to 10 cm/hour), typically extending from the anal area down the upper thighs and observed as a rapidly progressing linear urticarial trail.

lar·va mi·grans (lahr′vă mī′granz) A larval worm, typically a nematode, which wanders for a period in the host tissues but does not develop to the adult stage; this usually occurs in unusual hosts that inhibit normal development of the parasite.

lar·vate (lahr′vāt) Masked or concealed; applied to a disease with undeveloped, absent, or atypical symptoms.

lar·vi·cide (lahr′vi-sīd) An agent that kills larvae.

♻ **laryng-** SEE laryngo-.

la·ryn·ge·al (lă-rin′jē-ăl) Relating in any way to the larynx.

la·ryn·ge·al a·tre·si·a (lă-rin′jē-ăl ă-trē′zē-ă) Congenital failure of the laryngeal opening to develop, resulting in partial or total obstruction at or just above or below the glottis.

la·ryn·ge·al mask (lă-rin′jē-ăl mask) Oral airway with an inflatable cuff at its lower end that forms a seal above the laryngeal inlet rather than within the larynx. Also called laryngeal mask airway.

la·ryn·ge·al pa·pil·lo·ma·to·sis (lă-rin′jē-ăl pap′i-lō′mă-tō′sis) Multiple squamous papillomas of the larynx in young children.

la·ryn·ge·al pol·yp (lă-rin′jē-ăl pol′ip) Projection from the surface of one of the vocal cords.

la·ryn·ge·al prom·i·nence (lă-rin′jē-ăl prom′i-nĕns) [TA] The projection on the anterior portion of the neck formed by the thyroid cartilage of the larynx.

la·ryn·ge·al re·flex (lă-rin′jē-ăl rē′fleks) SYN cough reflex.

la·ryn·ge·al sten·o·sis (lă-rin′jē-ăl stĕ-nō′sis) Stricture of any or all areas of the larynx; congenital or acquired.

la·ryn·ge·al stri·dor (lă-rin′jē-ăl strī′dŏr) SYN congenital stridor.

la·ryn·ge·al syn·co·pe (lă-rin′jē-ăl sing′kŏ-pē) Paroxysmal neurosis characterized by attacks of coughing, with ticklish sensations in the throat, followed by a brief unconsciousness.

la·ryn·ge·al ver·ti·go (lă-rin′jē-ăl vĕr′ti-gō) SYN cough syncope.

la·ryn·ge·al web (lă-rin′jē-ăl web) Congenital anomaly consisting of mucous membrane–covered connective tissue between the vocal cords located ventrally and extending dorsally for varying distances; it causes airway obstruction and hoarse crying in the newborn.

la·ryn·gec·to·my (lar′in-jek′tŏ-mē) Excision of the larynx.

la·ryn·ges (lă-rin′jēz) Plural of larynx.

la·ryn·gis·mus (lar′in-jiz′mŭs) A spasmodic narrowing or closure of the rima glottidis.

la·ryn·gis·mus stri·du·lus (lar′in-jiz′mŭs strid′yū-lŭs) Spasmodic closure of the glottis, causing noisy inspiration. SYN spasmus glottidis.

la·ryn·gi·tis (lar′in-jī′tis) Inflammation of the mucous membrane of the larynx; accompanied by edema of the vocal cords, which produces hoarseness.

laryngo-, laryng- Combining forms denoting the larynx.

la·ryn·go·cele (lă-ring′gō-sēl) An air sac communicating with the larynx through the ventricle, often bulging outward into the tissue of the neck, especially during coughing.

la·ryn·go·fis·sure (lă-ring′gō-fish′ŭr) Operative opening into the larynx. SYN thyrotomy (2).

lar·yn·gog·ra·phy (lar′ing-gog′ră-fē) Radiography of the larynx after coating mucosal surfaces with contrast material.

la·ryn·gol·o·gist (lar′in-gol′ŏ-jist) A specialist in the study of the diseases and disorders of the voice box.

la·ryn·gol·o·gy (lar′in-gol′ŏ-jē) The branch of medical science concerned with the larynx; the specialty of diseases of the larynx.

la·ryn·go·ma·la·ci·a (lă-ring′gō-mă-lā′shē-ă) The presence of soft laryngeal cartilage, especially of the epiglottis, in infants, resulting in inspiratory stridor.

la·ryn·go·pa·ral·y·sis (lă-ring′gō-păr-al′i-sis) Paralysis of the laryngeal muscles. SYN laryngoplegia.

la·ryn·go·pha·ryn·ge·al re·flux (lă-ring′gō-fă-rin′jē-ăl rē′flŭks) Gastroesophageal reflux disease that produces prominent symptoms and signs in the pharynx and larynx characterized by laryngitis and pharyngitis.

la·ryn·go·phar·yn·gec·to·my (lă-ring′gō-far′in-jek′tŏ-mē) Resection or excision of both larynx and pharynx.

la·ryn·go·phar·ynx (lă-ring′gō-far′ingks) [TA] The part of the pharynx lying below the aperture of the larynx and behind the larynx; it extends from the vestibule of the larynx to the esophagus at the level of the inferior border of the cricoid cartilage. SYN hypopharynx.

la·ryn·go·plas·ty (lă-ring′gō-plas-tē) Reparative or plastic surgery of the larynx.

la·ryn·go·ple·gi·a (lă-ring′gō-plē′jē-ă) SYN laryngoparalysis.

la·ryn·gop·to·sis (lă-ring′gop-tō′sis) An abnormally low position of the larynx, which may be congenital or acquired; does not impair the health of the neonate; also occurs with aging.

lar·yn·gos·co·py (lar′in-gos′kŏ-pē) Inspection of the larynx by means of the laryngoscope.

la·ryn·go·spasm, glot·ti·do·spasm (lă-ring′gō-spazm, glŏ-tī′dō-) Spasmodic closure of the glottic aperture.

la·ryn·go·ste·no·sis (lă-ring′gō-stĕ-nō′sis) Stricture or narrowing of the lumen of the larynx.

la·ryn·gos·to·my (lar′in-gos′tŏ-mē) The establishment of a permanent opening from the neck into the larynx.

la·ryn·got·o·my (lar′in-got′ŏ-mē) A surgical incision of the larynx.

la·ryn·go·tra·che·i·tis (lă-ring′gō-trā′kē-ī′tis) Inflammation of both larynx and trachea.

la·ryn·go·tra·che·o·e·soph·a·ge·al cleft (lă-ring′gō-trā′kē-ō-ē′sŏ-fā′jē-ăl kleft) Absence of fusion of the musculature or cricoid cartilaginous laminae of varying severity: **type 1**, submucous cleft of the interarytenoid muscles; **type 2**, partial cricoid cleft; **type 3**, total cricoid cleft; and **type 4**, extension of the cleft into the esophagus. SYN laryngotracheooesophageal cleft.

laryngotracheo-oesophageal cleft [Br.] SYN laryngotracheoesophageal cleft.

lar·yn·go·tra·che·o·plas·ty (lă-ring′gō-trā′kē-ō-plas′tē) Operation to repair subglottic stenosis.

la·ryn·go·tra·che·ot·o·my (lă-ring′gō-trā′kē-ot′ŏ-mē) A surgical opening made by cutting into the larynx and trachea.

lar·ynx, pl. **la·ryn·ges** (lar′ingks, lă-rin′jēz) [TA] The organ of voice production, which also serves a protective function for the airway; the part of the respiratory tract between the pharynx and the trachea.

La·sègue sign (lah-seg′ sīn) When a subject is supine with hip flexed and knee extended, dorsiflexion of the ankle causing pain or muscle spasm in the posterior thigh indicates lumbar root or sciatic nerve irritation.

la·ser (lā′zĕr) **1.** (noun) Device that concentrates high energies into an intense narrow beam of nondivergent monochromatic electromagnetic radiation; used in microsurgery, cauterization, and diagnostic purposes. **2.** To treat a structure with a laser beam.

la·ser-as·sis·ted ep·i·the·li·al ker·a·to·plas·ty (lā′zĕr ă-sis′tĕd ep′i-thē′lē-ăl ker′ă-tō-plas-tē) Refractive surgery in which the epithelial layer of the cornea is removed.

las·si·tude (las′i-tūd) A sense of weariness.

late au·di·to·ry-e·voked res·ponse (lāt aw′di-tōr-ē-ē-vōkt′ rĕ-spons′) Reaction of the auditory cortex to acoustic stimulation.

late de·cel·er·a·tion (lāt dē-sel′ĕr-ā′shŭn) Any transient fetal bradycardia, with onset of deceleration at the peak of the uterine contraction and nadir as contraction finishes.

late dump·ing syn·drome (lāt dŭmp′ing sin′drōm) Hypoglycemic disorder seen in patients who have had ablation of the pyloric sphincter mechanism; associated with flushing, sweating, dizziness, weakness, and vasomotor collapse 2–3 hours after a meal. SEE ALSO dumping syndrome.

la·ten·cy (lā′tĕn-sē) The state of being latent.

la·ten·cy phase, la·ten·cy pe·ri·od (lā′tĕn-sē fāz, pēr′ē-ŏd) PSYCHIATRY Period of psychosexual development extending from about age 5 to the beginning of adolescence around age 12, during which the apparent cessation of sexual preoccupation stems from a strong, aggressive blockade of libidinal and sexual impulses in an effort to avoid oedipal relationships; during this phase, boys and girls are inclined to choose friends and join groups of their own sex.

la·tent (lā′tĕnt) Not manifest, dormant, but potentially discernible.

la·tent al·ler·gy (lā′tĕnt al′ĕr-jē) One causing no current signs or symptoms but that can be revealed by means of certain immunologic tests with specific allergens.

la·tent car·ri·er (lā′tĕnt kar′ē-ĕr) A person, typically a prospective parent, bearing the appropriate genotype of a trait (homozygous for recessive, homozygous or heterozygous for dominant, hemizygous or homozygous for X-linked) that manifests the trait only under certain conditions.

la·tent con·tent (lā′tĕnt kon′tent) The hidden, unconscious meaning of thoughts or actions, especially in dreams or fantasies.

la·tent en·er·gy (lā′tĕnt en′ĕr-jē) SYN potential energy.

la·tent gout (lā′tĕnt gowt) Hyperuricemia without symptoms of gout; often used synonymously with interval gout.

la·tent heat (lā′tĕnt hēt) Amount of heat that a substance may absorb without an increase in temperature.

la·tent hy·per·o·pi·a (HI) (lā′tent hī′pĕr-ō′pē-ă) The difference between total and manifest hyperopia.

la·tent learn·ing (lā′tĕnt lĕrn′ing) Learning that is not evident to the observer at the time it occurs, but is inferred from later performance in which learning is more rapid than would be expected without the earlier experience.

la·tent nys·tag·mus (lā′tĕnt nis-tag′mŭs) Jerk nystagmus that is brought out by covering one eye. The fast phase is always away from the covered eye.

la·tent pe·ri·od (lā′tĕnt pĕr′ē-ŏd) Duration between application of a stimulus and the response.

la·tent syph·i·lis (lā′tĕnt sif′i-lis) Infec-

tion with *Treponema pallidum*, after the manifestations of primary and secondary syphilis have subsided (or were never noticed), before any manifestations of tertiary syphilis have appeared.

lat·er·al (lat′ĕr-ăl) [TA] **1.** On the side. **2.** Farther from the median or midsagittal plane. **3.** DENTISTRY a position either right or left of the midsagittal plane. **4.** A radiograph made with the film in the sagittal plane; especially, the second view of a chest series.

lat·er·al ab·er·ra·tion (lat′ĕr-ăl ab′ĕr-ā′shŭn) In spheric visual aberration, the distance between paraxial focus of central rays on the optic axis.

lat·er·al ep·i·con·dy·li·tis (lat′ĕr-ăl ep′i-kon′di-lī′tis) Tension stress injury to the lateral epicondyle caused by repeated or forceful contraction of the wrist extensors; often seen in those involved in sports that use racquets. SYN tennis elbow.

lat·er·al her·maph·ro·dit·ism (lat′ĕr-ăl hĕr-maf′rō-dit-izm) A form in which a testis is present on one side and an ovary on the other.

lat·er·a·lis (lat-er-ā′lis) [TA] *This form of the adjective is used with masculine nouns (margo lateralis, plural margines laterales) and feminine nouns (norma lateralis, plural normae laterales). With neuter nouns the form laterale is used (cornu laterale, plural cornua lateralia). The final e of laterale is not silent.* SYN lateral (1), lateral (2), lateral.

lat·er·al·i·ty (lat′ĕr-al′i-tē) Referring to a side of the body or of a structure; specifically, the dominance of one side of the brain or the body.

lat·er·al·i·za·tion (lat′ĕr-ăl-ī-zā′shŭn) The process whereby certain embryologic asymmetries of structure and function are ordained phylogenetically, coded genetically, and realized ontogenetically.

lat·er·al nys·tag·mus (lat′ĕr-ăl nis-tag′mŭs) Ocular disorder characterized by side-to-side oscillation of the eyes.

lat·er·al oc·clu·sion (lat′ĕr-ăl ŏ-klū′zhŭn) Malposition of a tooth or an entire

L

dental arch in a direction away from the midline.

lat·er·al pinch (lat′ĕr-ăl pinch) A grasp pattern in which the object is held between the thumb pads and the radial side of the index finger. (Also referred to as a key grasp).

lat·er·al pro·jec·tion (LC) (lat′ĕr-ăl prŏ-jek′shŭn) Radiographic projection with the x-ray beam in a coronal plane.

lat·er·al re·cum·bent po·si·tion (lat′ĕr-ăl rē-kŭm′bĕnt pŏ-zish′ŏn) SYN Sims position.

lat·er·al re·gion (lat′ĕr-ăl rē′jŏn) SYN flank.

late ric·kets (lāt rik′ĕts) SYN osteomalacia.

latero- Combining form meaning lateral, to one side.

lat·er·o·de·vi·a·tion (lat′ĕr-ō-dē′vē-ā′shŭn) A bending or a displacement to one side.

lat·er·o·duc·tion (lat′ĕr-ō-dŭk′shŭn) A drawing to one side. SYN exduction.

lat·er·o·flex·ion (lat′ĕr-ō-fleks′shŭn) A bending or curvature to one side.

lat·er·o·gnath·ism, lat·er·o·gnath·i·a (lat′ĕr-og-nath′izm, -nath′ē-ă) Asymmetry of the mandible due to retarded growth, fractures, tumors, atrophy, or hypertrophy.

lat·er·o·tor·sion (lat′ĕr-ō-tōr′shŭn) A twisting to one side; denoting rotation of the eyeball around its anteroposterior axis, so that the top part of the cornea turns away from the sagittal plane.

lat·er·o·tru·sion (lat′ĕr-ō-trū′zhŭn) The outward thrust given by the muscles of mastication to the rotating mandibular condyle during movement of the mandible.

lat·er·o·ver·sion (lat′ĕr-ō-vĕr′zhŭn) Version to one side or the other, denoting especially a malposition of the uterus.

late sy·phil·is (lāt sif′i-lis) Involvement of the cardiovascular or central nervous system, or the development of a gumma in any organ, due to infection with *Treponema pallidum;* usually occurs several years to 2–3 decades after the initial infection.

la·tex (lā′teks) **1.** An emulsion or suspension produced by some seed plants; contains suspended microscopic globules of natural rubber. **2.** Colloquially, similar synthetic materials, such as polystyrene and polyvinyl chloride.

la·tex ag·glu·ti·na·tion test (LAT) (lā′teks ă-glū′ti-nā′shŭn test) Passive agglutination test in which antigen is adsorbed onto latex particles which then clump in the presence of antibody specific for the adsorbed antigen. SYN latex fixation test.

la·tex al·ler·gy (lā′teks al′ĕr-jē) Cutaneous hypersensitivity to natural rubber, used in the manufacture of rubber gloves, condoms, and other articles.

la·tex fix·a·tion test (LFT) (lā′teks fiksā′shŭn test) SYN latex agglutination test.

la·tex sen·si·tiv·i·ty (lā′teks sen′si-tiv′i-tē) Hypersensitivity to a specific protein found in processed natural rubber products causing contact dermatitis or anaphylaxis.

la·tis·si·mus (lă-tis′i-mŭs) Latin term denoting great breadth or width.

lat·i·tude (lat) (lat′i-tūd) The range of light or x-ray exposure acceptable with a given photographic emulsion.

La·tro·dec·tus (lat-rō-dek′tŭs) A genus of relatively small spiders, the widow spiders, capable of inflicting highly poisonous, neurotoxic, painful bites; they are responsible for most of the severe reactions from spider envenomation. Medically important species are known from Australia, North and South America, South Africa, and New Zealand.

la·tus, gen. **lat·e·ris,** pl. **lat·e·ra** (lat′ŭs, lă-ter′is, -ă) [TA] The side of the body between the pelvis and the ribs. SYN flank.

Latz·ko ce·sar·e·an sec·tion (lahts′kō sĕ-zar′ē-ăn sek′shŭn) Operation in which the uterus is entered by paravesical blunt dissection without entering the peritoneal cavity.

laugh·ing gas (laf´ing gas) SYN nitrous oxide.

Lau·rence-Moon syn·drome (lawr´ĕns-mūn´ sin´drŏm) Disorder characterized by mental retardation, pigmentary retinopathy, hypogenitalism, and spastic paraplegia.

lau·ric ac·id (law´rik as´id) A fatty acid occurring in spermaceti, in milk, and in laurel, coconut, and palm oils as well as waxes and marine fats. SYN N-dodecanoic acid.

la·vage (lă-vahzh´) The washing out of a hollow cavity or organ by copious injections and rejections of fluid. SEE ALSO gastric lavage.

la·va·tion (lă-vā´shŭn) To wash.

law (law) **1.** A principle or rule. **2.** A statement of a sequence or relation of phenomena that is invariable under the given conditions. SEE ALSO principle, rule, theorem.

law of in·de·pen·dent as·sort·ment (law in´dĕ-pen´dĕnt ă-sŏrt´mĕnt) Different hereditary factors assort independently when the gametes are formed; traits at linked loci are an exception. SYN Mendel second law.

law of re·fer·red pain (law rĕ-fĕrd´ pān) Pain arises only from irritation of nerves that are sensitive to those stimuli that produce pain when applied to the surface of the body.

law of re·frac·tion (law rĕ-frak´shŭn) For two given media, the sine of the angle of incidence bears a constant relation to the sine of the angle of refraction. SYN Descartes law, Snell law.

law of seg·re·ga·tion (law seg´rĕ-gā´shŭn) Factors that affect development retain their individuality from generation to generation, do not become contaminated when mixed in a hybrid, and become sorted out from one another when the next generation of gametes is formed. SYN Mendel first law.

law of sim·i·lars (law sim´i-lărz) SEE similia similibus curantur.

lax·a·tive (lak´să-tiv) Any oral agent that promotes the expulsion of feces, including harsh stimulant forms, saline forms, stool softeners, bulking forms, and lubricants.

lax·i·ty (laks´i-tē) Looseness or freedom of movement in a joint, normal or excessive. SEE ALSO instability.

lay·er (lā´ĕr) [TA] A sheet of one substance lying on another and distinguished from it by a difference in texture or color or by not being continuous with it. SEE ALSO stratum, lamina.

la·zy leu·ko·cyte syn·drome (lā´zē lū´kō-sīt sin´drŏm) Defects in a white blood cell that impede its mobility and keep it from moving to the site of an infection.

LCAT de·fi·cien·cy (dĕ-fish´ĕn-sē) A condition characterized by corneal opacities, hemolytic anemia, proteinuria, renal insufficiency, and premature atherosclerosis, and very low levels of lecithin cholesterol acyltransferase (LCAT) activity; results in accumulation of unesterfied cholesterol in plasma and tissues.

LD$_{50}$ In pharmacology, a dose that proves lethal to 50% of a given population.

L dos·es (dōs´ĕz) A group of terms that indicate the relative activity or potency of diphtheria toxin; different from the minimal lethal dose and minimal reacting dose, inasmuch as the latter two represent the direct effects of toxin, whereas the L doses pertain to the combining power of toxin with specific antitoxin.

lead (Pb) (led) **1.** A metallic element, atomic no. 82, atomic wt. 207.2; occurs in nature as an oxide or one of the salts, but chiefly as the sulfide, or galena; ^{210}Pb (half-life equal to 22.6 years) has been used in the treatment of certain eye conditions. **2.** (lēd) An electrical conductor carrying current or intermittent signals between an organ or tissue and an electrical or electronic device.

lead col·ic (led kol´ik) Severe cramping abdominal pain, with constipation; symptomatic of lead poisoning. SYN Devonshire colic, painter's colic, Poitou colic, saturnine colic.

lead en·ceph·a·lop·a·thy, lead en·ceph·a·li·tis (led en-sef´a-lop´ă-thē, en-sef'ă-lī'tis) A metabolic encephalopathy, caused by ingestion of lead compounds; seen particularly in early childhood; characterized pathologically by extensive cerebral edema, status spongiosus, neurocytolysis, and reactive inflammation; clinical manifestations include convulsions, delirium, and hallucinations. SEE ALSO lead poisoning. SYN lead encephalitis, saturnine encephalopathy.

lead line (led līn) Deposits of lead sulfide in the gingiva in areas of chronic inflammation.

lead-pipe frac·ture (led pīp frak'shŭr) A break in bone that runs along the length of the bone but does not penetrate it completely.

lead-pipe ri·gid·i·ty (led'pīp' ri-jid'i-tē) Increased muscle tone due to an extrapyramidal lesion in which pathologic resistance to passive extension of a joint is constant throughout the range of motion. Should be contrasted with clasp-knife spasticity (q.v.).

lead poi·son·ing (led poy'zŏn-ing) Acute or chronic intoxication by lead or any of its salts; symptoms of **acute lead poisoning** usually are those of acute gastroenteritis in adults or encephalopathy in children; **chronic lead poisoning** is manifested chiefly by anemia, constipation, and many other signs.

leak·age ra·di·a·tion (lēk'ăj rā'dē-ā'shŭn) Radiation that escapes from radiologic equipment when it is in use.

leak point pres·sure (LPP) (lēk poynt presh'ŭr) Storage pressure in the bladder at which leakage occurs passively, usually in people with neuropathic bladder.

lean bod·y mass (lēn bod'ē mas) SYN fat-free body mass.

learn·ing dis·a·bil·i·ty (lĕrn'ing dis'ă-bil'i-tē) A disorder in one or more of the basic cognitive and psychological processes involved in understanding or using written or spoken language; may be manifested in age-related impairment in the ability to read, write, spell, speak, or perform mathematical calculations.

Le·ber he·red·i·tar·y op·tic at·ro·phy (lā'bĕr hĕr-ed'i-tar-ē op'tik at'rŏ-fē) Degeneration of the optic nerve and papillomacular bundle with resulting loss of central vision and blindness, progressive for several weeks, then usually becoming stationary with permanent central scotoma. SYN Leber optic neuropathy.

Le·ber ple·xus (lā'bĕr plek'sŭs) Small venous plexus in the eye between the venous sinuses of the sclera (of Schlemm) and the spaces of the iridocorneal angle (of Fontana).

LE bod·y (bod'ē) Amorphous round body in the cytoplasm of an LE cell.

LE cell (sel) A polymorphonuclear leukocyte containing an amorphous round body; formed in vitro in the blood of patients with systemic lupus erythematosus, or by the action of the patient's serum on normal leukocytes. SYN lupus erythematosus cell.

LE cell test (sel test) The in vitro incubation of the blood or bone marrow of patients with systemic lupus erythematosus, or action of their serum on normal leukocytes; causes formation of characteristic LE cells. SYN lupus erythematosus cell test.

lec·i·thal (les'i-thăl) Having a yolk or pertaining to the yolk of any egg; used especially as a suffix.

lec·i·thin (les'i-thin) Yellowish or brown waxy substances, readily miscible in water, in which they appear under the microscope as irregular elongated particles known as "myelin forms"; found in nervous tissue, especially in the myelin sheaths, in egg yolk, and as essential constituents of animal and vegetable cells.

lec·i·thi·nase (les'i-thi-nās) SYN phospholipase.

lec·i·thin-cho·les·ter·ol a·ce·tyl·trans·fer·ase de·fi·cien·cy (les'i-thin-kō-les'tĕr-ol as'ĕ-til-trans'fĕr-ās dĕ-fish'ĕn-sē) An autosomal-recessive disorder of lipoprotein metabolism.

lec·i·thin-cho·les·ter·ol ac·yl·trans·fer·ase (LCAT) (les'i-thin-kō-les'tĕr-ol as'il-trans'fĕr-ās) An enzyme that reversibly transfers an acyl residue from a lecithin to cholesterol; a deficiency of this enzyme leads to accumulation of unesterified cholesterol in plasma resulting in anemia, proteinuria, renal failure, and corneal opacities. SYN lecithin acyltransferase.

lec·i·thin:sphin·go·my·e·lin ra·ti·o (les'i-thin-sfing'gō-mī'ĕ-lin rā'shē-ō) A ratio used to determine fetal pulmonary maturity, found by testing the amniotic fluid; when the lungs are mature, lecithin exceeds sphingomyelin by 2:1.

lec·i·tho·pro·tein (les'i-thō-prō'tēn) A conjugated protein, with lecithin as the prosthetic group.

leech (lēch) 1. Any bloodsucking aquatic annelid worm; sometimes used in medicine and plastic surgery for local withdrawal of blood. 2. To treat medically by applying leeches.

leech ther·a·py (lēch thār'ă-pē) Application of leeches to body parts that have been reattached or transplanted to prevent a back-up of venous blood or to remove deep areas of infection on the epidermis.

Lee-White meth·od (lē wīt meth'ŏd) Means to determine coagulation time of venous blood in standard bore tubes at body temperature.

Le Fort os·te·o·to·my (lĕ fōrt' os-tē-ot'ŏ-mē) Surgery performed along the classic lines of fracture as described by Le Fort to correct a maxillary skeletal deformity.

left-hand·ed (left-hand'ĕd) Denoting the habitual or more skillful use of the left hand for writing and for most manual functions.

left heart (left hahrt) The left atrium and left ventricle.

left heart by·pass (left hahrt bī'pas) Any procedure that shunts blood returning from the pulmonary circulation to the systemic circulation without passing through the left heart; used during cardiac surgery.

left-sid·ed heart fail·ure (left'sī'dĕd hahrt fāl'yŭr) Inability of the left heart to maintain its circulatory load, with corresponding rise in pressure in the pulmonary circulation usually with pulmonary congestion and ultimately pulmonary edema. SYN left ventricular failure.

left-to-right shunt (left-rīt shŭnt) A diversion of blood from the left side of the heart to right or from the systemic circulation to the pulmonary.

left up·per quad·rant (of ab·do·men) (LUQ) (left ŭp'ĕr kwahd'rănt ab'dōmĕn) Anatomic region used in description for purposes of examination, testing, and diagnosis, as well as charting.

left ven·tric·u·lar fail·ure (left ventrik'yŭ-lăr fāl'yŭr) Congestive heart failure manifested by signs of pulmonary congestion and edema.

left ven·tric·u·lar vol·ume re·duc·tion sur·ger·y (left ven-trik'yŭ-lăr vol' yūm rĕ-dŭk'shŭn sŭr'jĕr-ē) Operation in which the volume of a dilated, nonaneurysmal left ventricle is reduced by myocardial resection in order to improve ventricular geometry and mechanical function and thereby treat end-stage congestive heart failure. SYN partial left ventriculectomy.

leg (leg) [TA] 1. The segment of the inferior limb between the knee and the ankle; commonly used to mean the entire inferior limb. 2. A structure resembling a leg. SYN crus (1) [TA].

le·gal blind·ness (lē'găl blīnd'nĕs) Generally, visual acuity of less than 6/60 or 20/200 using Snellen test types, or visual field restriction to 20° or less in the better eye; the criteria used to define legal blindness vary among different groups.

le·gal med·i·cine (lē'găl med'i-sin) SYN forensic medicine.

Le·gen·dre sign (lĕ-zhahn'drĕ sīn) In facial hemiplegia of central origin, when the examiner raises the lids of the actively closed eyes the resistance is less on the affected side.

Legg-Cal·vé-Per·thes dis·ease, Legg dis·ease, Legg-Per·thes dis·ease (LCPD) (leg'kal-vā'per'tĕz di-zēz', -per' tĕz) Self-limiting pediatric disease of the femoral head caused by poor circulation. The degeneration of the femoral head is followed by regeneration and absorption of bone. The process may take 4 years. Usually found in children aged 4–8 years. SYN coxa plana.

-legia Suffix meaning reading, as distinguished from the G. derivatives, *-lexis* and *-lexy*, which signify speech, from G. *legō*, to say.

Le·gion·el·la (lē-jŏ-nel′lă) A genus of aerobic, motile, non-acid-fast, nonencapsulated, gram-negative bacilli; they dwell in water and are borne by air; pathogenic for humans. The type species is *L. pneumophila*.

Le·gi·o·nel·la mic·da·de·i (lē-jŏ-nel′lă mik-dā′dĕ-ī) A species that causes Pittsburgh pneumonia, a variant of Legionnaire's disease. Accounts for approximately 60% of *Legionella* pneumonias other than those caused by *L. pneumophila*.

Le·gion·el·la pneu·mo·phi·la (LP) (lē-jŏ-nel′ă nū-mō-fil′ă) Bacterial species that is the primary etiologic agent of Legionnaires' disease; believed to grow in plumbing systems or in standing water in ventilation systems. The type species of the genus *Legionella*.

Le·gion·naires' dis·ease, le·gi·o·nel·lo·sis (lē′jŏ-nārz′ di-zēz′, lē′jŏ-nel-ō′sis) An acute infectious disease, caused by various species of *Legionella pneumophila*, with prodromal influenza-like symptoms and a rapidly rising high fever, followed by severe pneumonia and production of usually nonpurulent sputum, and sometimes mental confusion, hepatic fatty changes, and renal tubular degeneration.

Lei·ner dis·ease (lī′nĕr di-zēz′) SYN erythroderma desquamativum.

♻ **leio-** *This combining form is pronounced lī′o, not lē′o.* Smooth.

lei·o·der·mi·a (lī′ō-dĕr′mē-ă) Smooth, glossy skin.

lei·o·my·o·fi·bro·ma (lī′ō-mī′ō-fī-brō′mă) SYN fibroleiomyoma.

lei·o·my·o·ma (lī′ō-mī-ō′mă) A benign neoplasm derived from smooth (nonstriated) muscle.

lei·o·my·o·ma cu·tis (lī′ō-mī-ō′mă kyū′tis) Cutaneous eruption of multiple small painful nodules composed of smooth muscle fibers; derived from arrector muscles of hair. SYN dermatomyoma.

lei·o·my·o·ma·to·sis (lī′ō-mī′ō-mă-tō′sis) The state of having multiple leiomyomas throughout the body.

lei·o·my·o·ma·to·sis per·i·to·ne·al·is dis·sem·i·na·ta (lī′ō-mī′ō-mă-tō′sis per′i-tō-nē-ā′lis di-sem-i-nā′tă) A benign condition characterized by multiple small nodules on abdominal and pelvic peritoneum, grossly mimicking disseminated ovarian cancer but with histologic characteristics of benign myoma; often associated with recent pregnancy.

lei·o·my·o·ma u·te·ri (lī′ō-mī-ō′mă yū′tĕr-ī) A benign smooth-muscle tumor that is located in the uterus.

lei·o·my·o·sar·co·ma (lī′ō-mī′ō-sahr-kō′mă) A malignant neoplasm derived from smooth (nonstriated) muscle; is transmitted through the bloodstream.

Leish·man-Don·o·van bod·y (lēsh′măn don′ŏ-văn bod′ē) The intracytoplasmic, nonflagellated leishmanial form of certain intracellular parasites, such as species of *Leishmania* or the intracellular form of *Trypanosoma cruzi*. SYN amastigote.

Leish·man·i·a (lēsh-man′ē-ă) A genus of digenetic, asexual, protozoan flagellates that occur as amastigotes in the macrophages of vertebrate hosts, and as promastigotes in invertebrate hosts and in cultures.

leish·man·i·a·sis, leish·man·i·o·sis (lēsh′mă-nī′ă-sis, -nē-ō′sis) Infection with a species of *Leishmania* resulting in a clinically ill-defined group of diseases. Transmission is by various sandfly species of the genus *Phlebotomus* or *Lutzomyia*.

leish·man·i·a·sis re·ci·di·vans (LR) (lēsh-mă-nī′ă-sis rē-sid′i-vanz) Partially healing leishmanial lesion caused by *Leishmania tropica*. SYN lupoid leishmaniasis.

leish·ma·nin test (lēsh′mă-nin test) A delayed hypersensitivity test for cutaneous leishmaniasis.

Lem·bert su·ture (lem-bār′ sū′chŭr) An inverting suture for intestinal surgery.

lem·nis·cus, pl. **lem·nis·ci** (lem-nis′kŭs, -kī) [TA] A bundle of nerve fibers ascending from sensory relay nuclei to the thalamus. SYN fillet (1).

Le·nègre syndrome, Le·nègre dis·ease (lĕ-neg′ sin′drŏm′, di-zēz′) Isolated damage of the cardiac conduction system to a sclerodegenerative lesion; characterized ordinarily as idiopathic fibrosis of the atrioventricular nodal, His bundle, or bundle branches with corresponding conduction block(s).

length (length) Linear distance between two points.

length·en·ing re·ac·tion (length′ĕn-ing rē-ak′shŭn) In the decerebrate animal, rather sudden relaxation with lengthening of the extensor muscles when a limb is passively flexed.

Len·nert lym·pho·ma (len′ert lim-fō′mă) Malignant lymphoma with a high proportion of diffusely scattered epithelioid cells, tonsillar involvement, and an unpredictable course.

Len·nox-Gas·taut syn·drome, Len·nox syn·drome (len′ŏks gahs-tō′ sin′drŏm) A generalized myoclonic astatic epilepsy in children, with mental retardation, due to various cerebral afflictions; patients are usually mentally retarded or developmentally delayed.

lens (lenz) [TA] **1.** A transparent material with one or both surfaces having a concave or convex curve; acts on electromagnetic energy to cause convergence or divergence of light rays. **2.** The transparent biconvex cellular refractive structure lying between the iris and the vitreous humor, consisting of a soft outer part (cortex) with a denser part (nucleus), and surrounded by a basement membrane (capsule).

lens cap·sule (lenz kap′sŭl) The capsule enclosing the lens of the eye.

len·ti·co·nus (len′ti-kō′nŭs) Conic projection of the anterior or posterior surface of the ocular lens.

len·tic·u·lar (len-tik′yū′lăr) Relating to or resembling a lens of any kind.

len·tic·u·lar a·stig·ma·tism (len-tik′ yū′lăr ă-stig′mă-tizm) Vision dysfunction due to defect in the curvature, position, or index of refraction of the lens.

len·tic·u·lar loop (len-tik′yū′lăr lūp) The pallidal efferent fibers curving around the medial border of the internal capsule. SYN ansa lenticularis.

len·tic·u·lar nu·cle·us, len·ti·form nu·cle·us (len-tik′yū′lăr nū′klē-ŭs, len′ ti-fŏrm) The large conic mass of gray matter forming the central core of the cerebral hemisphere.

len·tic·u·lar pro·cess of in·cus (len-tik′yū-lăr pros′es ing′kŭs) A knob at the tip of the long limb of the incus, which articulates with the stapes.

len·ti·form (len′ti-fŏrm) Lens-shaped.

len·tig·i·no·sis (len-tij′i-nō′sis) Presence of lentigines in very large numbers or in a distinctive configuration.

len·ti·glo·bus (len′ti-glō′bŭs) Rare congenital anomaly with a spheroid elevation on the posterior surface of the lens of the eye.

len·ti·go, pl. **len·tig·i·nes** (len-tī′gō, len-tij′i-nēz) *The singular form is lentigo, not lentigine.* A benign, acquired brown macule resembling a freckle except that the border is usually regular and microscopic elongation of rete ridges is present, with increased melanocytes and melanin pigment in the basal cell layer. SYN lentigo simplex.

len·ti·go ma·lig·na (len-tī′gō mă-lig′nă) A brown or black mottled, irregularly outlined, slowly enlarging lesion resembling a lentigo with increased numbers of scattered atypical melanocytes in the epidermis, usually occurring on the face of older persons.

Len·ti·vi·rus (len′ti-vī′rŭs) A genus in the family Retroviridae containing five serogroups that reflect the host with which they are associated.

le·on·ti·a·sis (lē′on-tī′ă-sis) A lionlike appearance due to ridges and furrows on the forehead and cheeks of people with advanced lepromatous leprosy. SYN leonine facies.

LEOPARD syn·drome (lep′ărd sin′drŏm) A hereditary syndrome consisting of *l*entigines (multiple), *e*lectrocardiographic abnormalities, *o*cular hypertelorism, *p*ulmonary stenosis, *a*bnormalities

L

of genitalia, *r*etardation of growth, and *deafness* (sensorineural).

Le·o·pold ma·neu·vers (lā′ŏ-pōld mă-nū′věrz) Four maneuvers employed to determine fetal position: 1) determination of what is in the fundus; 2) evaluation of the fetal back and extremities; 3) palpation of the presenting part above the symphysis; and 4) determination of the direction and degree of flexion of the head.

lep·er (lep′ĕr) A person who has leprosy.

le·pid·ic (lĕ-pid′ik) Relating to scales or a scaly covering layer.

lep·re·chaun·ism (lep′rĕ-kawn-izm) Congenital dwarfism characterized by extreme growth retardation, endocrine disorders, and emaciation, with elfin facies and large, low-set ears.

lep·rid (lep′rid) Early cutaneous lesion of leprosy.

le·pro·ma (lĕ-prō′mă) A discrete focus of granulomatous inflammation, caused by *Mycobacterium leprae*.

lep·rom·a·tous (lep-rō′mă-tŭs) Pertaining to, or characterized by, the features of a leproma.

lep·rom·a·tous lep·ro·sy (LL) (lep-rō′mă-tŭs lep′rŏ-sē) Form of leprosy in which nodular cutaneous lesions are infiltrated, have ill-defined borders, and are bacteriologically positive.

lep·ro·sar·i·um, lep·ro·se·ry (lep′rō-sar′ē-ŭm, lep′rō-ser-ē) A hospital especially designed for the care of those suffering from leprosy, especially those who need expert care.

lep·ro·stat·ic (lep′rō-stat′ik) **1.** Inhibiting to the growth of *Mycobacterium leprae*. **2.** An agent having this action.

lep·ro·sy (lep′rŏ-sē) A chronic granulomatous infection caused by *Mycobacterium leprae* affecting the cooler body parts, especially the skin, peripheral nerves, and testes. SYN Hansen disease.

-lepsis, -lepsy Combining forms indicating a seizure.

lepto- A combining form meaning light, thin, frail.

lep·to·cyte (LEPT) (lep′tō-sīt) A target or Mexican hat cell, i.e., an unusually thin or flattened red blood cell with a central rounded area of pigmented material, a middle clear zone that contains no pigment, and an outer pigmented rim at the edge of the cell.

lep·to·men·in·gi·tis (lep′tō-men′in-jī′tis) Inflammation of leptomeninges. SEE ALSO arachnoiditis.

lep·to·men·in·gop·a·thy (lep′tō-men′in-gop′ă-thē) A disease of the arachnoid and pia mater of the meninges.

lep·to·mo·nad (lep′tō-mō′nad) **1.** Common name for a member of the genus *Leptomonas*. **2.** SEE promastigote.

Lep·to·mo·nas (lep′tō-mō′năs) A genus of asexual, monogenetic, parasitic flagellates commonly found in insect hindguts.

lep·to·pel·lic (lep′tō-pel′ik) Denotes having a pelvis that is narrower than the norm.

lep·to·so·mat·ic, lep·to·som·ic (lep′tō-sō-mat′ik, -tō-sōm′ik) Having a slender, light, or thin body.

Lep·to·spi·ra (lep′tō-spī′ră) A genus of aerobic bacteria containing thin, tightly coiled organisms 6–20 mcm in length; seen in icterohemorrhagic fever.

lep·to·spi·ral jaun·dice (lep′tō-spī′răl jawn′dis) Hepatic disease associated with infection by various species of *Leptospira*.

lep·to·spi·ro·sis (lep′tō-spī-rō′sis) An acute infectious disease caused by a spirochete, *Leptospira interrogans;* infection is zoonotic and distributed worldwide.

lep·to·spi·ru·ri·a (lep′tō-spīr-yūr′ē-ă) Urinary presence of species of the genus *Leptospira* due to leptospirosis in the renal tubules.

Lep·to·trich·i·a (lep′tō-trik′ē-ă) A genus of anaerobic, nonmotile bacteria containing gram-negative, straight or slightly curved rods, with one or both ends rounded or pointed. These organisms occur in the human oral cavity. The type species is *Leptotrichia buccalis*.

Lep·to·trom·bid·i·um (lep′tō-trom-bid′ē-ŭm) An important genus of trombiculid mites, which includes all the vectors of scrub typhus (tsutsugamushi disease).

Le·riche op·er·a·tion (lĕ-rēsh′ op-ĕr-ā′shŭn) SYN periarterial sympathectomy.

Le·riche syn·drome (lĕ-rēsh′ sin′drōm) Aortoiliac occlusive disease producing distal ischemic symptoms and signs.

Lé·ri ple·on·o·ste·o·sis (lā-rē′ plē′on-os′tē-ō′sis) SYN dyschondrosteosis.

Lé·ri sign (lĕ-rē′ sīn) Voluntary flexion of the elbow is impossible in a case of hemiplegia when the wrist on that side is passively flexed.

Ler·mo·yez syn·drome (ler-mwah-yā′ sin′drōm) Increasing hearing loss and tinnitus preceding an attack of vertigo, after which the hearing improves.

Ler·ner ho·me·o·sta·sis (ler′nĕr hō′mē-ō-stā′sis) The restorative mechanisms that tend to correct perturbations in the genetic composition of a population. SYN genetic homeostasis.

les·bi·an (lez′bē-ăn) **1.** A female homosexual or a female homosexual lifestyle. **2.** One who practices lesbianism. SEE ALSO gay.

les·bi·an·ism (lez′bē-ăn-izm) Homosexuality involving women. SYN sapphism.

Lesch-Ny·han syn·drome (lesh nī′ăn sin′drōm) Complete inborn deficiency of enzyme hypoxanthine phosphoribosyltransferase in purine metabolism pathway; causes mental retardation, self-mutilation, choreoathetosis, and hyperuricemia. Invariably fatal in childhood.

Le·ser-Tré·lat sign (lā′zā-trā′lah sīn) Sudden appearance and rapid increase in the number and size of seborrheic keratoses with pruritus.

le·sion (lē′zhŭn) **1.** A wound or injury. **2.** A pathologic change in the tissues. **3.** One of the individual points or patches of a multifocal disease.

less·er cir·cu·la·tion (les′ĕr sĭr′kyū-lā′shŭn) SYN pulmonary circulation.

Less·er tri·an·gle (les′ĕr trī′ang-gĕl) The space between the bellies of the digastric muscle and the hypoglossal nerve.

le·thal (lē′thăl) **1.** Pertaining to or causing death; denoting especially the causal agent. **2.** BIOWARFARE an agent that causes death in 10% or more of healthy adults.

le·thal dose (LD) (lē′thăl dōs) Amount of a chemical or biologic preparation of likely to cause death; varies in relation to the type of animal and the route of administration.

le·thal equiv·a·lent (lē′thăl ĕ-kwiv′ă-lĕnt) **1.** Combination of selective effects that on average have the same impact on the composition of the gene pool as one death. **2.** Expression used of the genetic load of recessive genes in heterozygous state that if in homozygous state would cause death or carry a risk of death. The expected number of deaths from all such genes is expressed in lethal equivalent.

le·thal gene (lē′thăl jēn) One that produces a genotype that leads to death of the organism before reproduction is possible or that precludes reproduction; for a recessive gene the homozygous or hemizygous state is lethal.

le·thal·i·ty (lē-thal′i-tē) The quality or state of being lethal.

le·thal mu·ta·tion (lē′thăl myū-tā′shŭn) A trait that leads to a phenotype incompatible with effective reproduction.

let·ter blind·ness (let′ĕr blīnd′nĕs) Visual agnosia for letters, in which letters are seen but not identified.

Let·te·rer-Si·we dis·ease (let′er-er-sē′vē di-zēz′) The acute disseminated form of Langerhans cell histiocytosis. SYN nonlipid histiocytosis.

Leu Abbreviation for leucine; leucyl.

leuc-, leuco- Combining forms meaning white; white blood cell. SEE ALSO leuko-, leuk-.

leucapheresis [Br.] SYN leukapheresis.

leu•cin (lū′sin) A thermostable bactericidal substance extracted from leukocytes. SYN leukin.

leu•cine (lū′sēn) The L-isomer is one of the amino acids of proteins; a nutritionally essential amino acid.

leu•ci•no•sis (lū′si-nō′sis) A condition with an abnormally large proportion of leucine in the tissues and body fluids.

leu•ci•nu•ri•a (lū′si-nyūr′ē-ă) The excretion of leucine in the urine.

leucocidin [Br.] SYN leukocidin.

leucaemia [Br.] SYN leukemia.

leucocyte [Br.] SYN leukocyte.

leucocytic [Br.] SYN leukocytic.

leucocytolysis [Br.] SYN leukocytolysis.

leucocytopenia [Br.] SYN leukopenia.

leucocytosis [Br.] SYN leukocytosis.

leucoderma [Br.] SYN leukoderma.

leucodystrophy [Br.] SYN leukodystrophy.

leucoencephalitis [Br.] SYN leukoencephalitis.

leucoencephalopathy [Br.] SYN leukoencephalopathy.

leucoerythroblastosis [Br.] SYN leukoerythroblastosis.

leucokininase [Br.] SYN leukokininase.

leucoma [Br.] SYN leukoma.

Leu•co•nos•toc (lū′kŏ-nos′tok) A genus of microaerophilic to facultatively anaerobic bacteria containing gram-positive, spheric cells that may, under certain conditions, lengthen and become pointed and even form rods. Lactic and acetic acids are produced by these organisms.

leuconychia [Br.] SYN leukonychia.

leucopenia [Br.] SYN leukopenia.

leucoplakia [Br.] SYN leukoplakia.

leucopoiesis [Br.] SYN leukopoiesis.

leucorrhoea [Br.] SYN leukorrhea.

leucosis [Br.] SYN leukosis.

leucotomy [Br.] SYN leukotomy.

leu•co•vor•in (LV) (lū′kō-vōr′in) SYN folinic acid.

leu•co•vo•rin cal•ci•um (lū′kō-vōr′in kal′sē-ŭm) Calcium salt of folinic acid; used to counteract toxic effects of folic acid antagonists, to treat megaloblastic anemias, and as an adjunct to cyanocobalamin in pernicious anemia. SYN calcium folinate.

♻ **leuk-** SEE leuko-.

leukaemia [Br.] SYN leukemia.

leukaemiacutis [Br.] SYN leukemia cutis.

leukaemic [Br.] SYN leukemia.

leukaemid [Br.] SYN leukemid.

leukaemogen [Br.] SYN leukemogen.

leukaemoid [Br.] SYN leukemoid.

leukaemoid reaction [Br.] SYN leukemoid reaction.

leuk•a•phe•re•sis (lū′kă-fĕr-ē′sis) A procedure, analogous to plasmapheresis, in which leukocytes are removed from the withdrawn blood and the remainder of the blood is retransfused into the donor. SYN leucapheresis.

leu•ke•mi•a (lū-kē′mē-ă) Progressive proliferation of abnormal leukocytes found in hemopoietic tissues, other organs, and usually in the blood in increased numbers. Leukemia is classified by the dominant cell type, and by duration from onset to death, which occurs in acute leukemia within a few months in most cases, and is associated with acute symptoms including severe anemia, hemorrhages, and slight enlargement of lymph nodes or the spleen. The duration of chronic leukemia exceeds 1 year, with a gradual onset of symptoms of anemia or marked enlargement of spleen, liver, or lymph nodes. SYN leucaemia, leukaemia.

leu·ke·mi·a cu·tis (lū-kē′mē-ă kyū′tis) Yellow-brown, red, blue-red, or purple, sometimes nodular lesions associated with diffuse infiltration of leukemic cells in the skin.

leu·ke·mid (lū-kē′mid) Any nonspecific type of cutaneous lesion frequently associated with leukemia, but is not a localized accumulation of leukemic cells.

leu·ke·mo·gen (lū-kē′mō-jen) Any substance or entity considered to be a causal factor in the occurrence of leukemia. SYN leukaemogen.

leu·ke·moid (lū-kē′moyd) Resembling leukemia in various signs and symptoms, especially with reference to changes in circulating blood.

leu·ke·moid re·ac·tion (lū-kē′moyd rē-ak′shŭn) Leukocytosis similar to that occurring in leukemia, but not the result of leukemic disease. Leukemoid reactions are sometimes observed as a feature of infectious disease, intoxication, malignant neoplasms, and acute hemorrhage or hemolysis. SYN leukaemoid reaction.

leu·kin (lū′kin) A thermostable bactericidal substance extracted from leukocytes. SYN leucin.

leuko-, leuk- Combining forms meaning white; white blood cells. For some words beginning this way, see leuc- and leuco-.

leu·ko·ag·glu·ti·nin (lū′kō-ă-glū′ti-nin) An antibody that agglutinates white blood cells.

leu·ko·blas·to·sis (lū′kō-blas-tō′sis) A general term for the abnormal proliferation of leukocytes, especially as occurs in myelocytic and lymphocytic leukemia.

leu·ko·ci·din (lū′kō-sī′din) A heat-labile substance elaborated by many strains of *Staphylococcus aureus*, *Streptococcus pyogenes*, and pneumococci; destructive action on leukocytes, with or without lysis of the cells. SYN leucocidin.

leu·ko·co·ri·a, leu·ko·ko·ri·a (lū′kō-kōr′ē-ă) Reflection from a white mass within the eye giving the appearance of a white pupil.

leu·ko·cyte (lū′kō-sīt) A type of cell formed in the myelopoietic, lymphoid, and reticular portions of the reticuloendothelial system in various parts of the body, and normally present in those sites and in the circulating blood. SYN leucocyte, white blood cell.

leu·ko·cyte es·ter·ase test (lū′kō-sīt es′tĕr-ās test) A chemical assay to determine the presence of lysed or intact white blood cells in urine, performed with a dipstick as part of routine urinalysis.

leu·ko·cyte-func·tion-as·sis·ted an·ti·gen (lū′kō-sīt-fungk′shŭn-ă-sis′tĕd an′ti-jen) Molecule on lymphocytic or endothelial surfaces; acts as adhesion receptor or as receptor for other types of molecules.

leu·ko·cyt·ic (lū′kō-sit′ik) Pertaining to or characterized by leukocytes. SYN leucocytic.

leu·ko·cy·to·gen·e·sis (lū′kō-sī′tō-jen′ĕ-sis) The formation and development of leukocytes.

leu·ko·cy·tol·y·sin (lū′kō-sī-tol′i-sin) Any substance (including lytic antibody) that causes dissolution of leukocytes. SYN leukolysin.

leu·ko·cy·tol·y·sis (lū′kō-sī-tol′i-sis) Dissolution or lysis of leukocytes. SYN leucocytolysis.

leu·ko·cy·to·pe·ni·a (lū′kō-sī′tō-pē′nē-ă) SYN leukopenia.

leu·ko·cy·to·pla·ni·a (lū′kō-sī′tō-plā′nē-ă) Movement of leukocytes from the lumens of blood vessels through serous membranes, or in the tissues.

leu·ko·cy·to·poi·e·sis (lū′kō-sī′tō-poy-ē′sis) SYN leukopoiesis.

leu·ko·cy·to·sis (lū′kō-sī-tō′sis) An actual increase in the total number of leukocytes in the blood. SYN leucocytosis.

leu·ko·cy·to·tax·i·a (lū′kō-sī-tō-tak′sē-ă) **1.** The active ameboid movement of leukocytes, especially the neutrophilic granulocytes, either toward (positive leukocytotaxia) or away from (negative leukocytotaxia) certain microorganisms as well as various substances formed in inflamed tissue. **2.** The property of attracting or repelling leukocytes. SYN leukotaxis.

leu·ko·cy·to·tox·in (lū′kō-sī′tō-tok-sin) Any substance that causes degeneration and necrosis of leukocytes. SYN leukotoxin.

leu·ko·cy·tu·ri·a (lū′kō-sī-tyūr′ē-ă) The presence of leukocytes in urine that is recently voided or collected with a catheter.

leu·ko·der·ma (lū′kō-dĕr′mă) An absence of pigment, partial or total, in the skin. SYN leucoderma, leukopathia, leukopathy.

leu·ko·dys·tro·phy (lū′kō-dis′trŏ-fē) Term for a group of white matter diseases, some familial, characterized by progressive cerebral deterioration usually in early life, and pathologically by primary absence or degeneration of the myelin of the central and peripheral nervous systems with glial reaction. SYN leukodystrophia cerebri progressiva, leukodystrophia, sclerosis of white matter.

leu·ko·e·de·ma (lū′kō-ĕ-dē′mă) A bluish-white opalescence of the buccal mucosa that returns to a normal mucosal color on stretching the tissue; may be considered a normal anatomic variation. SYN leuko-oedema.

leu·ko·en·ceph·a·li·tis (lū′kō-en-sef′ă-lī′tis) Encephalitis restricted to the white matter. SYN leucoencephalitis.

leu·ko·en·ceph·a·lop·a·thy (lū′kō-en-sef′ă-lop′ă-thē) White matter changes first described in children with leukemia, associated with radiation and chemotherapy injury. SYN leucoencephalopathy.

leu·ko·e·ryth·ro·blas·to·sis (lū′kō-ĕ-rith′rō-blas-tō′sis) Any anemic condition resulting from space-occupying lesions in the bone marrow. SYN leucoerythroblastosis, myelophthisic anemia, myelopathic anemia.

leu·ko·ki·nin·ase (lū′kō-kī′ni-nās) An enzyme that cleaves tuftsin to release leukokinin. SYN leucokininase.

leu·ko·krau·ro·sis (lū′kō-kraw-rō′sis) SYN kraurosis vulvae.

leu·kol·y·sin (lū-kol′i-sin) SYN leukocytolysin.

leu·kol·y·sis (lū-kol′i-sis) SYN leukocytolysis.

leu·ko·ma (lū-kō′mă) A dense white opacity of the cornea.

leu·ko·mye·li·tis (lū′kō-mī′ĕ-lī′tis) An inflammatory process involving the white matter of the spinal cord.

leu·ko·ne·cro·sis (lū′kō-nĕ-krō′sis) SYN white gangrene.

leu·ko·nych·i·a (lū′kō-nik′ē-ă) The occurrence of white spots, streaks, or patches under the nails, due to the presence of air bubbles between the nail and its bed. SYN leuconychia.

leuko-oedema [Br.] SYN leukoedema.

leu·ko·path·i·a, leu·kop·a·thy (lū′kō-path′ē-ă, lū-kop′ă-thē) SYN leukoderma.

leu·ko·pe·de·sis (lū′kō-pĕ-dē′sis) Movement of white blood cells (especially polymorphonuclear) through capillary walls and into tissues.

leu·ko·pe·ni·a (lū′kō-pē′nē-ă) Disorder in which the total number of leukocytes in the circulating blood is less than normal. SYN leukocytopenia.

leu·ko·pe·nic (lū′kō-pē′nik) Pertaining to leukopenia.

leu·ko·pe·nic in·dex (lū′kō-pē′nik in′deks) A significant decrease in the white blood cell count after ingestion of food to which a patient is hypersensitive.

leu·ko·phor·e·sis (lū′kō-fŏr-ē′sis) A laboratory procedure that removes white blood cells from the blood and returns remaining blood to the patient.

leu·ko·pla·ki·a (lū′kō-plā′kē-ă) A white patch of oral mucous membrane that cannot be wiped off and diagnosed clinically; associated with pipe smoking. SYN leucoplakia.

leu·ko·pla·ki·a vul·vae (lū′kō-plā′kē-ă vŭl′vē) A clinical term for hyperkeratotic white patches of the vulvar epithelium.

leu·ko·poi·e·sis (lū′kō-poy-ē′sis) Formation and development of the various types of white blood cells. SYN leucopoiesis, leukocytopoiesis.

leu·ko·poi·et·ic (lū′kō-poy-et′ik) Pertaining to or characterized by leukopoiesis, as manifested by portions of the bone marrow and reticuloendothelial and lymphoid tissues, which form (respectively) the granulocytes, monocytes, and lymphocytes.

leu·kor·rhe·a, leu·kor·rha·gi·a (lū′kŏr-ē′ă, lū′kōr-ā′jē-ă) Discharge from the vagina of a white or yellowish viscid fluid. SYN leucorrhoea, leukorrhagia, leukorrhoea.

leukorrhoea [Br.] SYN leukorrhea.

leu·ko·sis (lū-kō′sis) Abnormal proliferation of one or more of the leukopoietic tissues; the term includes myelosis, certain forms of reticuloendotheliosis, and lymphadenosis. SYN leucosis.

leu·ko·tax·is (lū′kō-tak′sis) SYN leukocytotaxia.

leu·kot·ic (lū-kot′ik) Pertaining to, characterized by, or manifesting leukosis.

leu·ko·tome, leu·co·tome (lū′kō-tōm) An instrument for performing leukotomy.

leu·kot·o·my (lū-kot′ŏ-mē) Incision into the white matter of the frontal lobe of the brain. SYN leucotomy.

leu·ko·tox·in (lū′kō-tok′sin) SYN leukocytotoxin.

leu·ko·trich·i·a (lū′kō-trik′ē-ă) Whiteness of the hair.

leu·ko·vi·rus (lū′kō-vī′rŭs) A retrovirus that causes tumors to form.

leu·pro·lide ac·e·tate (LA) (lū′prō-līd as′ĕ-tāt) A synthetic nonapeptide analogue of naturally occurring gonadotropin-releasing hormone.

le·vam·i·sole (lē-vam′i-sōl) Drug that increases immune responses; used adjunctively with fluorouracil to improve response and suppress recurrence.

lev·ar·ter·e·nol (lev′ahr-tēr′ĕ-nol) SYN norepinephrine.

le·va·tor (lĕ-vā′tŏr) [TA] 1. A surgical instrument for prying up the depressed part in a cranial fracture. 2. One of several

muscles the action of which is to raise the part into which it is inserted.

Lev dis·ease (lev di-zēz′) SYN Lev syndrome.

Le·Veen per·i·to·ne·o·ve·nous shunt (lĕ-vēn′ per′i-tŏ-nē′ō-vē′nŭs shŭnt) A surgically implanted tube that is used to drain accumulated fluid from the peritoneal cavity.

lev·el (lev′ĕl) 1. Any rank, position, or status in a graded scale of values. 2. A test for determining such rank or position.

lev·er (lev′ĕr) An instrument used to lift or pry.

lev·i·ta·tion (lev′i-tā′shŭn) Support of the patient on a cushion of air.

♻ **levo-** Combining form meaning left, toward or on the left side. SYN laev-, laevo-.

le·vo·bu·no·lol hy·dro·chlor·ide (lē′vō-byū′nŏ-lol hī′drŏ-klōr′īd) A β-adrenergic blocking agent used primarily as an eye drop in the treatment of chronic open-angle glaucoma and ocular hypertension.

le·vo·car·di·a (lē′vō-kahr′dē-ă) Situs inversus of the other viscera but with the heart normally situated on the left; congenital cardiac lesions are commonly associated. SYN laevocardia.

le·vo·car·ni·tine (lē′vō-kahr′ni-tēn) Used as a supplement for carnitine deficiency.

le·vo·cli·na·tion (lē′vō-kli-nā′shŭn) SYN levotorsion (2).

le·vo·do·pa (L-dopa) (lē′vō-dō′pă) The biologically active form of dopa; an antiparkinsonian agent that is converted to dopamine. SYN laevodopa.

le·vo·ro·ta·to·ry (lē′vō-rō′tă-tōr-ē) Denoting levorotation; or crystals or solutions capable of causing it; as a chemical prefix, usually abbreviated L- or (−). Cf. dextrorotatory. SYN laevorotatory.

le·vo·tor·sion (lē′vō-tōr′shŭn) 1. SYN sinistrorsion. 2. Rotation of the upper pole of the cornea of one or both eyes to the left.

L

le·vo·ver·sion (lĕ′vō-vĕr′zhŭn) **1.** Version toward the left. **2.** Conjugate turning of both eyes to the left.

Lev syn·drome (lev sin′drōm) Bundle branch block in a patient with normal myocardium and normal coronary arteries due to fibrosis and calcification including the conducting system. SYN lev disease.

Lew·is base (lū′is bās) One that is an electron-pair donor. SYN base.

lew·is·ite (L) (lū′i-sīt) A vesicant toxic gas used in warfare.

Le·wy bod·ies (lā′vē bod′ēz) Intracytoplasmic neuronal inclusion; bodies especially noted in pigmented brainstem neurons and seen in parkinsonism, diffuse Lewy body disease, and Alzheimer disease.

♻ **-lexis, -lexy** Combining forms that properly relate to speech, although often confused with -legia (Latin -lego, to read) and thus erroneously employed to relate to reading.

Ley·den neu·ri·tis (lī′dĕn nūr-ī′tis) Fatty degeneration of the fibers of the affected nerve.

Ley·dig cells (lī′dig selz) SYN interstitial cells (1).

Ley·dig cell tu·mor (lī′dig sel tū′mŏr) A testicular and, less commonly, ovarian neoplasm composed of Leydig cells, usually benign but may be malignant; may secrete androgens or estrogens. Causes gynecomastia in adults and precocious sexual development in prepubescents.

Lher·mitte sign (lār-mēt′ sīn) Sudden electriclike shocks extending down the spine on flexing the head.

Li Symbol for lithium.

li·bi·do (li-bē′dō) **1.** Conscious or unconscious sexual desire. **2.** Any passionate interest or form of life force. **3.** In jungian psychology, synonymous with psychic energy.

Lib·man-Sacks en·do·car·di·tis, Libman-Sacks syn·drome (lib′măn saks en′dō-kahr-dī′tis, sin′drōm) Verrucous endocarditis sometimes associated with disseminated lupus erythematosus. SYN atypical verrucous endocarditis, nonbacterial verrucous endocarditis.

lice (līs) Plural of louse.

li·censed prac·ti·cal nurse (LPN) (lī′sĕnst prak′ti-kăl nŭrs) Nurse who has graduated from an accredited school of practical (vocational) nursing, passed the state examination for licensure, and been licensed to practice by a state authority.

li·chen (lī′ken) A discrete flat papule or an aggregate of papules giving a patterned configuration resembling lichen growing on rocks.

li·chen am·y·loi·do·sus (lī′kĕn am′i-loyd-ō′sis) The eruption of darkish papules along the back, shins, and arms.

li·chen·i·fi·ca·tion (lī′ken-i-fi-kā′shŭn) Leathery induration and thickening of the skin with hyperkeratosis, caused by scratching.

li·chen myx·e·de·ma·to·sus (lī′ken miks′ĕ-dē′mă-tō′sŭs) Lichenoid eruption of papules on the upper body of mucinous edema due to deposit of glycosaminoglycans in the skin and fibroblast proliferation, in the absence of endocrine disease. SEE ALSO scleromyxedema. SYN papular mucinosis.

li·chen ni·ti·dus (lī′ken nī′ti-dŭs) Minute asymptomatic whitish or pinkish papules; lesions, which are flat-topped, rarely may coexist with lichen planus, and may involve male genitalia.

li·chen·oid ec·ze·ma (lī′kĕn-oyd ek′sĕ-mă) Thickening of skin with accentuated skin lines in eczema. SYN chronic eczema.

li·chen·oid ker·a·to·sis (LK) (lī′kĕ-noyd ker′ă-tō′sis) Solitary benign papule or plaque, with microscopic features resembling lichen planus. SYN lichen planus-like keratosis.

li·chen pla·nus, li·chen ru·ber pla·nus (lī′ken plā′nŭs, rū′bĕr) Eruption of flat-topped, shiny, violaceous papules on flexor surfaces, male genitalia, and buccal mucosa; of unknown cause.

li·chen scrof·u·lo·so·rum (lī′ken skrof-yū-lō-sō′rŭm) Small asymptomatic papules on the trunk of children with tuberculosis; acid-fast bacilli are not seen in the dermal granulomas. SYN papular tuberculid.

li·chen sim·plex chron·i·cus (LSC) (lī'ken sim'pleks kron'ik-kŭs) Thickened area of itching skin resulting from rubbing and scratching.

li·chen spi·nu·lo·sus (lī'ken spīn-yū-lō'sŭs) Eruption of conical papules, of unknown cause, which have an adherent scaly surface.

li·chen stri·a·tus (lī'ken strī-ā'tŭs) A self-limited papular eruption occurring primarily in children (more commonly in girls); the lesions are arranged in linear groups and usually occur on one extremity.

lic·o·rice (lik'ŏ-ris) SYN glycyrrhiza.

li·do·caine hy·dro·chlor·ide (lī'dō-kān hī'drō-klōr'īd) An amide local anesthetic with antiarrhythmic and anticonvulsant properties; quick action with medium duration.

lie (lī) Relationship of the long axis of the fetus to that of the mother.

Lie·ber·mei·ster rule (lē'ber-mīs'tĕr rūl) In adult febrile tachycardia, about eight pulse beats correspond to an increase of 1°C.

Lie·big the·o·ry (lē'big thē'ŏr-ē) Tenet that the hydrocarbons that oxidize readily and burn are those that produce the greatest quantity of animal heat.

li·en mo·bi·lis (lī'en mō'bi-lis) SYN floating spleen.

li·en·ter·ic di·ar·rhe·a (lī'en-ter'ik dī'ă-rē'ă) Form in which undigested food appears in the stools.

li·en·ter·y (lī'en-ter-ē) Passage of undigested food in stools.

life (līf) 1. Vitality, the essential condition of being alive; the state of existence characterized by such functions as metabolism, growth, reproduction, adaptation, and response to stimuli. 2. Living organisms such as animals and plants.

life cy·cle (līf sī'kĕl) Entire life history of a living organism.

life in·stinct (līf in'stingkt) The tendency of self-preservation and sexual procreation.

Li-Frau·men·i can·cer syn·drome (lē fraw'men-ē kan'sĕr sin'drōm) Familial breast cancer in young women, with soft-tissue sarcomas in children, brain tumors, and other cancers in close relatives.

lig·a·ment (lig'ă-mĕnt) [TA] 1. A band or sheet of fibrous tissue connecting two or more bones, cartilages, or other structures, or serving as support for fascias or muscles. 2. A fold of peritoneum supporting any of the abdominal viscera. 3. Any structure resembling a ligament though not performing the function of such. 4. [TA] The cordlike remains of a fetal vessel or other structure that has lost its original lumen.

lig·and (lī'gand) 1. Any individual atom, group, or molecule attached to a central metal ion by multiple coordinate bonds. 2. An organic molecule attached to a tracer element. 3. A molecule that binds to a macromolecule. 4. The analyte in competitive binding assays. 5. An atom or group covalently attached to a specified carbon atom in an organic molecule.

li·gase (lī'gās) Generic term for enzymes catalyzing the joining of two molecules coupled with the breakdown of a pyrophosphate bond in adenosine triphosphate or a similar compound. SEE ALSO synthetase.

lig·a·ture, li·ga·tion (lig'ă-chŭr, lī-gā'shŭn) 1. A thread, wire, fillet, or the like, tied tightly around a blood vessel, the pedicle of a tumor, or other structure to constrict it. 2. ORTHODONTICS a wire or other material used to secure an orthodontic attachment or tooth to an archwire.

lig·a·ture nee·dle (lig'ă-chŭr nē'dĕl) A surgical needle used to suture a wound or incision.

lig·a·ture wire (lig'ă-chŭr wīr) Soft thin wire of stainless steel used in dentistry to tie an archwire to band attachments or brackets.

light (līt) That portion of electromagnetic radiation to which the retina is sensitive. SEE ALSO lamp.

light ad·ap·ta·tion (līt ad´ap-tā´shŭn) Visual adjustment occurring under increased Illumination in which retinal sensitivity to light is reduced. SYN photopic adapttion.

light bath (līt bath) Therapeutic exposure of the skin to radiant light.

light chain (līt chān) A polypeptide chain with low molecular weight, as the κ or λ chains in immunoglobulin.

light·en·ing (līt´ĕn-ing) Sensation of decreased abdominal distention during the later weeks of pregnancy following the descent of the fetal head into the pelvic inlet.

light mi·cro·scope (līt mī´krŏ-skōp) Class of microscope that forms a magnified image using visible light.

light re·flex (līt rē´fleks) **1.** SYN pupillary reflex. **2.** A red glow reflected from the fundus of the eye when a light is cast on the retina. **3.** SYN red reflex.

light ther·a·py (līt thār´ă-pē) The therapeutic use of ultraviolet, colored, and laser lights to reestablish diurnal rhythms and alleviate pain and depression.

lig·ne·ous (lig´nē-ŭs) Woody; having a woody feeling.

lig·no·cer·ic ac·id (lig´nŏ-ser´ik as´id, -sēr´ik) One present in one type of sphingolipid and in small amounts in triacylglycerols. SYN *N*-tetracosanoic acid.

lil·li·pu·tian hal·lu·ci·na·tion (li´li-pyū´ shŭn hă-lū´si-nā´shŭn) Delusion of reduced size of objects or people.

limb (lim) [TA] **1.** An arm or leg. SYN member. **2.** A segment of any jointed structure. SEE ALSO leg.

limb bud (lim bŭd) Ectodermally covered mesenchymal outgrowth on the embryonic flank giving rise to either the forelimb or hindlimb.

limb-gir·dle mus·cu·lar dys·tro·phy (lim´gĭr´dĕl mŭs´kyū-lăr dis´trŏ-fē) One of the less well-defined types of this disorder, characterized by weakness and wasting, usually symmetric, of the pelvic girdle muscles, the shoulder girdle muscles, or both, but not the facial muscles.

lim·bic (lim´bik) **1.** Relating to a limbus. **2.** Relating to the limbic system.

lim·bic lobe (lim´bik nōd) [TA] The nearly closed ring of the brain structures surrounding the hilus, or margin, of the cerebral hemisphere of mammals. SEE limbic system. SYN lobus limbicus [TA].

lim·bic sys·tem (lim´bik sis´tĕm) Collective term denoting a heterogeneous array of brain structures at or near the medial edge (limbus) of the medial wall of the cerebral hemisphere, in particular the hippocampus, amygdala, and fornicate gyrus.

lim·bus, pl. **lim·bi** (lim´bŭs, -bī) [TA] The edge, border, or fringe of a part.

lime (līm) **1.** An alkaline earth oxide occurring in grayish-white masses (quicklime); on exposure to the atmosphere it becomes converted into calcium hydrate and calcium carbonate (air-slaked lime); direct addition of water to calcium oxide produces calcium hydrate (slaked lime). SYN calx (1). **2.** Fruit of the lime tree, which provides ascorbic acid and acts as an antiscorbutic.

li·men, pl. **lim·i·na** (lī´men, -mi-nă) [TA] Entrance; the external opening of a canal or space, such as the limen insulae. SYN threshold.

lim·i·nal (lim´i-năl) **1.** Pertaining to a threshold. **2.** Pertaining to a stimulus just strong enough to excite a tissue, e.g., nerve or muscle.

lim·i·nom·e·ter (lim´i-nom´ĕ-tĕr) Instrument to measure the strength of a stimulus barely sufficient to produce a reflex response.

lim·it dex·trin (lim´it deks´trin) Polysaccharide fragments remaining at the end (limit) of exhaustive hydrolysis of amylopectin or glycogen by α-1,4-glucan maltohydrolase or β-amylase, which cannot hydrolyze the α-1,6 bonds at branch points. SYN dextrin limit.

limp (limp) A lame walk with a yielding step; asymmetric gait. SEE ALSO claudication.

lin·co·my·cin (L, LM) (lin´kō-mī´sin) An antibacterial substance, composed of substituted pyrrolidine and octapyranose moities, produced by *Streptomyces lincolnensis*.

Lin·dau dis·ease (lin'dow di-zēz') SYN von Hippel-Lindau syndrome.

line (līn) [TA] **1.** A long, narrow mark or a strand of material. **2.** ANATOMY any linear mark or streak distinguished from adjacent tissues by color, texture, or elevation. **3.** A strain of cells or organisms derived from a single ancestor or precursor. **4.** A section of tubing supplying fluid or conducting impulses for monitoring equipment. SYN linea [TA].

lin·e·a, gen. and pl. **lin·e·ae** (lin'ē-ă, -ē) [TA] SYN line.

lin·e·a al·ba (lin'ē-ă al'bă) [TA] A fibrous band running vertically the entire length of the center of the anterior abdominal wall, receiving the attachments of the oblique and transverse abdominal muscles. SYN white line (1).

lin·e·a ar·cu·a·ta (lin'ē-ă ahr-kyū-ā'tă) [TA] SYN arcuate line.

lin·e·a as·pe·ra (lin'ē-ă as'pĕr-ă) [TA] The rough ridge with two pronounced lips running the length of the posterior femur.

lin·e·ae a·tro·ph·i·cae (lin'ē-ē ă-trof'ī-kē) SYN striae cutis distensae.

lin·e·a ep·i·phys·i·a·lis (lin'ē-ă ep'i-fi-sī-ā'lis) [TA] SYN epiphysial line.

line an·gle (līn ang'gĕl) That area formed by the junction of two surfaces of a tooth or two surfaces of a cavity preparation.

lin·e·a nig·ra (lin'ē-ă nī'gră) Linea alba in pregnancy, which then becomes pigmented. SYN black line.

lin·e·ar ab·sorp·tion co·ef·fi·cient (lin'ē-ăr ăb-sōrp'shŭn kō-ĕ-fish'ĕnt) Fraction of ionizing radiation absorbed in a unit thickness of a substance or tissue. SEE ALSO absorption coefficient (3). Cf. attenuation.

line of de·mar·ca·tion (līn dē'mahr-kā'shŭn) Zone of inflammatory reaction separating a gangrenous area from healthy tissue.

lin·er (lī'nĕr) A layer of protective material.

line spread func·tion (līn spred fŭngk'shŭn) Measure of the ability of a system to form sharp images; in radiology, determined by measuring the spatial density distribution on film of the x-ray image of a narrow slit in a dense metal, such as uranium; from this can be calculated the modulation transfer function.

lin·gua, gen. and pl. **lin·guae** (ling'gwă, -gwē) [TA] **1.** SYN tongue (1). **2.** SYN tongue (2).

lin·gua ge·o·gra·ph·i·ca (ling'gwă jē-ō-graf'i-kă) SYN geographic tongue.

lin·gual (ling'gwăl) **1.** Relating to the tongue or any tonguelike part. SYN glossal. **2.** Next to or toward the tongue.

lin·gual arch (ling'gwăl ahrch) Orthodontic arch wire that approximates the lingual surfaces of the teeth.

lin·gual bar (ling'gwăl bahr) Major connector located lingually to a dental arch joining two or more bilateral parts of a mandibular removable partial denture.

lin·gual crib (ling'gwăl krib) Wire orthodontic appliance placed in a position lingual to the maxillary incisors to help a child overcome the habits of thumb sucking and tongue thrusting.

lin·gual fol·li·cles (ling'gwăl fol'i-kĕlz) Collections of lymphoid tissue in the mucosa of the pharyngeal part of the tongue posterior to the terminal sulcus collectively forming the lingual tonsil. SYN folliculi linguales [TA].

lin·gual gin·gi·va (ling'gwăl jin'ji-vă) Portion of gingiva that covers lingual surfaces of teeth and alveolar process.

lin·gual glands (ling'gwăl glandz) [TA] Minor salivary glands of the tongue. SYN glandulae linguales [TA].

lin·gual goi·ter (ling'gwăl goy'tĕr) A tumor of thyroid tissue involving the embryonic rudiment at the base of the tongue.

lin·gual oc·clu·sion (ling'gwăl ŏ-klū'zhŭn) Interdigitation of the teeth as seen from the internal or lingual aspect.

lin·gual pa·pil·la (ling'gwăl pă-pil'ă) **1.** One of numerous variously shaped projections of the mucous membrane of the dorsum of the tongue. **2.** The lingual portion of the gingiva filling the interproximal space between adjacent teeth. SEE ALSO interdental papilla.

lin·gua ni·gra (ling′gwă nī′gră) SYN black tongue.

Lin·guat·u·la (ling-gwat′yū-lă) A genus of endoparasitic bloodsucking arthropods commonly known as tongue worms. Adult worms are found in lungs or air passages of various hosts (e.g., reptiles, birds, carnivores); young worms are found in a great variety of hosts, including humans, but chiefly in animals that serve as prey.

lin·gu·la, gen. and pl. **lin·gu·lae** (ling′gyū-lă, -lē) [TA] **1.** A term applied to several tongue-shaped processes, particularly that of the cerebellum and of the upper lobe of the left lung. **2.** When not qualified, the lingula of the cerebellum.

lin·gu·lec·to·my (ling′gyū-lek′tŏ-mē) **1.** SYN glossectomy. **2.** Excision of lingular portion of upper lobe of left lung.

linguo- Combining form denoting the tongue.

lin·guo·pap·il·li·tis (ling′gwō-pap′i-lī′tis) Small, painful ulcers involving the papillae on the tongue margins.

lin·guo·ver·sion (ling′gwō-věr′zhŭn) Malposition of a tooth lingual to the normal position.

li·ni·tis (li-nī′tis) Inflammation of cellular tissue, specifically of the perivascular tissue of the stomach.

li·ni·tis plas·ti·ca (li-nī′tis plas′ti-kă) Infiltrating scirrhous carcinoma, causing extensive thickening of the wall of the stomach; often called leather-bottle stomach.

link·age (lingk′ăj) **1.** A chemical covalent bond. **2.** The relationship between syntenic loci sufficiently close that the respective alleles are not inherited independently by the offspring; a characteristic of loci, not genes.

link·age dis·e·qui·li·bri·um (lingk′ăj dis-ē′kwi-lib′rē-ŭm) A state involving two loci in which the probability of a joint gamete is not equal to the product of the probabilities of the constituent genes.

link·age group (lingk′ăj grūp) Two or more loci that have been shown by linkage analysis to be physically close in the genome but not yet been assigned to specific chromosomes.

link·age map (lingk′ăj map) Abstract mathematical representation of genetic loci that conserves order of loci, which are spaced in such a way that the distances are algebraically additive.

li·no·le·ate (li-nō′lē-āt) Salt of linoleic acid.

lin·o·le·ic ac·id (LA) (lin′ō-lē′ik as′id) *Do not confuse this word with linolenic acid.* Doubly unsaturated 18-carbon fatty acid, occurring widely in plant glycerides; essential in nutrition in mammals. SYN linolic acid.

lin·o·len·ic ac·id (LNA) (lin′ō-len′ik as′id) *Do not confuse this word with linoleic acid.* An 18-carbon triply unsaturated fatty acid that is essential in the nutrition of mammals.

lip (lip) [TA] **1.** One of the two muscular folds that encircle the mouth anteriorly; each has an outer mucosa with a stratified squamous epithelial surface layer. **2.** Any liplike structure bounding a cavity or groove. SYN labium (1) [TA].

lipaemia [Br.] SYN lipemia.

lipaemia retinalis [Br.] SYN lipemia retinalis.

li·pase (lip′ās) Any fat-splitting or lipolytic enzyme; a carboxylesterase.

li·pase test (lip′ās test, lī′pās) Diagnostic test based on the measurement of lipase in blood and urine as an indicator of pancreatic disease.

lip·ec·to·my (lip-ek′tŏ-mē) Surgical removal of fatty tissue, as in cases of adiposity.

lip·e·de·ma (lip′ĕ-dē′mă) Chronic swelling, usually of the lower extremities, particularly in middle-aged women, caused by the widespread, even distribution of subcutaneous fat and fluid.

li·pe·de·ma·tous al·o·pe·ci·a (lip'ĕ-dē'mă-tŭs al'ō-pē'shē-ă) Condition with itching, soreness, or tenderness of the scalp in black women; the scalp is thickened and soft, subcutaneous fat is increased, and the hair is sparse and short.

li·pe·mi·a (li-pē'mē-ă) The presence of an abnormally high concentration of lipids in the circulating blood. SYN hyperlipidemia, hyperlipoidemia, lipaemia, lipoidemia.

li·pe·mi·a re·ti·na·lis (li-pē'mē-ă ret-i-nā'lis) A creamy appearance of the retinal blood vessels that occurs when the lipids of the blood exceed 5%. SYN lipaemia retinalis.

lip·id (lip'id) ''Fat-soluble,'' an operational term describing a solubility characteristic, not a chemical substance.

lip·id gran·u·lo·ma·to·sis, lip·oid gran·u·lo·ma·to·sis (lip'id gran'yū-lō'mă-tō'sis, lip'oyd) SYN xanthomatosis.

lip·i·do·sis, pl. **lip·i·do·ses** (lip'i-dō'sis, -sēz) Hereditary abnormality of lipid metabolism that results in abnormal amounts of lipid deposition.

lip·id pneu·mo·ni·a, lip·oid pneu·mo·ni·a (lip'id nū-mō'nē-ă, lip'oyd) Pulmonary condition marked by inflammatory and fibrotic changes due to inhalation of various oily or fatty substances, particularly liquid petrolatum, or resulting from accumulation in the lungs of endogenous lipid material, either cholesterol from obstructive pneumonitis or following fracture of a bone. SYN oil pneumonia.

lip·i·du·ri·a (lip'i-dyūr'ē-ă) The presence of fat deposits in the urine.

lipo-, lip- Combining forms meaning fatty, lipid.

lip·o·ar·thri·tis (lip'ō-ahr-thrī'tis) Inflammation of the periarticular fatty tissues of the knee.

lip·o·ate a·ce·tyl·trans·fer·ase (lip'ō-āt ă-sē'til-trans'fĕr-ās) SYN dihydrolipoamide acetyltransferase.

lip·o·a·tro·phic di·a·be·tes (lip'ō-ă-trof'ik dī-ă-bē'tēz) SYN lipoatrophy.

lip·o·at·ro·phy (lip'ō-at'rŏ-fē) Loss of subcutaneous fat. SYN lipoatrophic diabetes.

lip·o·blast (lip'ō-blast) An embryonic fat cell.

lip·o·blas·to·ma (lip'ō-blas-tō'mă) **1.** SYN liposarcoma. **2.** A benign subcutaneous tumor composed of embryonal fat cells separated into distinct lobules, occurring usually in infants.

lip·o·blas·to·ma·to·sis (lip'ō-blas-tō'mă-tō'sis) A diffuse form of lipoblastoma that infiltrates locally but does not metastasize.

lip·o·car·di·ac (lip'ō-kahr'dē-ak) **1.** Relating to fatty heart. **2.** Denoting a person suffering from fatty degeneration of the heart.

lip·o·cer·a·tous (lip'ō-ser'ă-tŭs) SYN adipoceratous.

lip·o·chrome (lip'ō-krōm) A pigmented lipid. SYN chromolipid.

lip·o·cyte (lip'ō-sīt) SYN fat-storing cell.

lip·o·dys·tro·phy, lip·o·dys·tro·phi·a (lip'ō-dis'trŏ-fē, -dis-trō'fē-ă) Defective metabolism of fat.

lip·o·e·de·ma (lip'ō-ĕ-dē'mă) Edema of subcutaneous fat, causing painful swellings, especially in women's legs. SYN cellulite (2), lipo-oedema.

lip·o·fi·bro·ma (lip'ō-fī-brō'mă) A benign neoplasm of fibrous connective tissue, with conspicuous numbers of adipose cells.

lip·o·fus·cin (lip'ō-fyūs'in) Brown pigment granules representing lipid-containing residues of lysosomal digestion and considered one of the aging or ''wear and tear'' pigments; found in the liver, kidney, heart muscle, and elsewhere.

lip·o·fus·ci·no·sis (lip'ō-fyūs'i-nō'sis) Abnormal storage of any one of a group of fatty pigments.

lip·o·gen·e·sis (lip'ō-jen'ĕ-sis) Fat production, either degeneration or infiltration; also applied to the normal deposition of fat or the conversion of carbohydrate or protein to fat. SYN adipogenesis.

lip·o·gen·ic (lip′ō-jen′ik) Relating to lipogenesis. SYN adipogenic, adipogenous, lipogenous.

li·pog·e·nous (li-poj′ĕ-nŭs) SYN lipogenic.

lip·o·gran·u·lo·ma (lip′ō-gran′yŭ-lō′mă) A nodule or focus of granulomatous inflammation (usually of the foreign-body type) in association with lipid material deposited in tissues. SEE ALSO paraffinoma.

lip·o·gran·u·lo·ma·to·sis (lip′ō-gran′ yŭ-lō′mă-tō′sis) **1.** Presence of lipogranulomas. **2.** Local inflammatory reaction to necrosis of adipose tissue.

lip·o·hy·per·tro·phy (lip′ō-hī-pĕr′trŏ-fē) A fat buildup beneath the surface of the skin.

li·po·ic ac·id (li-pō′ik as′id) A bacterial growth factor present in yeast and liver extracts. SYN acetate replacement factor, ovoprotogen, protogen, protogen A, pyruvate oxidation factor, thioctic acid.

lip·oid (lip′oyd) Resembling fat. SYN adipoid.

lipoidaemia [Br.] SYN lipoidemia.

lip·oi·de·mi·a (lip′oy-dē′mē-ă) SYN lipemia.

lip·oid gran·u·lo·ma (lip′oyd gran′yŭ-lō′mă) A lesion characterized by aggregates or accumulations of fairly large mononuclear phagocytes that contain lipid.

lip·oi·do·sis (lip′oy-dō′sis) Presence of anisotropic lipoids in the cells.

li·pol·y·sis (li-pol′i-sis) *Avoid the mispronunciation lipoly′sis.* The splitting up (hydrolysis), or chemical decomposition, of fat. SYN lipoclasis, lipodieresis.

li·po·ma, pl. **li·po·ma·ta** (li-pō′mă, -tă) A benign neoplasm of adipose tissue, composed of mature fat cells. SYN adipose tumor.

lip·o·ma·to·sis (lip′ō-mă-tō′sis) SYN adiposis.

li·po·ma·to·sis do·lor·o·sa (lip′ō-mă-tō′sis dō′lōr-ō′să) A condition in which fatty tissue deposits subcutaneously accumulate in the body; painful to any type of pressure (e.g., touch).

li·po·ma·tous in·fil·tra·tion (li-pō′mă-tŭs in′fil-trā′shŭn) Nonencapsulated adipose tissue forming a lipomalike mass, usually in the cardiac interatrial septum where it may cause arrhythmia and sudden death.

li·po·ma·tous ne·phri·tis (li-pō′mă-tŭs ne-frī′tis) A condition in which fat cells replace renal nephrons, which can result in kidney failure.

li·po·me·nin·go·cele (lip′ō-mĕ-ning′gō-sēl) An intraspinal cauda equinal lipoma associated with a spina bifida.

lipo-oedema [Br.] SYN lipoedema.

lip·o·pe·ni·a (lip′ō-pē′nē-ă) An abnormally small amount, or a deficiency, of lipids in the body.

lip·o·phage (lip′ō-fāj) *Avoid the mispronunciation lip′ō-fahzh.* A cell that ingests fat.

lip·o·pha·gic (lip′ō-fā′jik) Relating to lipophagy.

lip·oph·a·gy (lip-of′ă-jē) Ingestion of fat by a lipophage.

lip·o·phil·ic (lip′ō-fil′ik) Capable of dissolving, of being dissolved in, or of absorbing lipids.

lip·o·pol·y·sac·cha·ride (lip′ō-pol′ē-sak′ă-rīd) A compound or complex of lipid and carbohydrate; endotoxin released from the cell walls of gram-negative organisms that produces septic shock.

lip·o·pro·tein (lip′ō-prō′tēn) Complexes or compounds containing lipid and protein.

lip·o·sar·co·ma (lip′ō-sahr-kō′mă) Malignant neoplasm of adults that occurs in the retroperitoneal tissues and the thigh, usually deep in the intermuscular or periarticular planes. SYN lipoblastoma.

li·po·sis (li-pō′sis) **1.** SYN adiposis. **2.** Fatty infiltration, neutral fats being present in the cells.

lip·o·sol·u·ble (lip′ō-sol′yŭ-bĕl) Fat-soluble.

lip·o·some (lip′ō-sōm) A spheric particle of lipid substance suspended in an aqueous medium within a tissue.

lip·o·suc·tion (lip′ō-sŭk′shŭn) Method of removing unwanted subcutaneous fat using strong percutaneous suction; used in body contouring.

li·pot·ro·phy (li-pot′rŏ-fē) An increase of fat in the body.

lip·o·trop·ic (lip′ō-trō′pik) **1.** Pertaining to substances preventing or correcting hepatic fat deposits. **2.** Relating to lipotrophy.

lip·o·tro·pin (lip′ō-trō′pin) A pituitary hormone mobilizing fat from adipose tissue. SYN lipotropic pituitary hormone.

lip·o·vac·cine (lip′ō-vak-sēn′) A vaccine suspended in vegetable oil as a solvent.

li·pox·y·ge·nase, li·pox·i·dase (li-poks′ē-jĕ-nās, li-poks′i-dās) An enzyme that catalyzes the oxidation of unsaturated fatty acids with oxygen to yield hydroperoxides of the fatty acids. SYN lipoxidase.

lip·ping (lip′ing) The formation of a liplike structure.

lip reading (lip rēd′ing) SYN speech reading.

liq·ue·fa·cient (lik′wĕ-fā′shĕnt) Making liquid; causing a solid to become liquid.

liq·ue·fac·tion (lik′wĕ-fak′shŭn) The act of becoming liquid; change from a solid to a liquid form.

liq·uid par·af·fin (lik′wid par′ă-fin) SYN mineral oil.

li·quor, gen. **li·quor·is,** pl. **li·quo·res** (lik′ŏr, lī′kwŏr-is, -ēz) [TA] **1.** Any liquid or fluid. **2.** The pharmacopeial term for any aqueous solution (not a decoction or infusion) of a nonvolatile substance and for aqueous solutions of gases. SEE ALSO solution.

li·quor cer·e·bro·spi·na·lis (LCS) (lī′kwŏr ser-ĕ-brō-spi-nā′lis) [TA] SYN cerebrospinal fluid.

li·quor fol·lic·u·li (lī′kwŏr fŏ-lik′yū-lī) Fluid within the ovarian follicle antrum.

Lis·franc am·pu·ta·tion (lis-frahngk′ amp′yū-tā′shŭn) Removal of the foot at the tarsometatarsal joint; plantar soft tissues are preserved to make the flap. SYN Lisfranc operation.

Lis·franc tu·ber·cle (lis-frahngk′ tū′bĕr-kĕl) SYN scalene tubercle.

lis·pro in·su·lin (lis′prō in′sŭ-lin) A modified version of natural human insulin, synthesized by a genetically programmed strain of nonpathogenic *Escherichia coli,* in which the amino acids lysine (Lys) and proline (Pro) near the end of the B chain are transposed.

lis·sen·ceph·a·ly, lis·sen·ce·pha·li·a (lis′en-sef′ă-lē, -sĕ-fā′lē-ă) SYN agyria.

***Lis·ter·i·a* (L)** (lis-tēr′ē-ă) A genus of aerobic to microaerophilic, motile, peritrichous bacteria containing small, coccoid, gram-positive rods; found in feces, on vegetation, and in silage; parasitic on poikilothermic and warm-blooded animals, including humans.

***Lis·te·ri·a mon·o·cy·to·ge·nes* (LM)** (lis-tēr′ē-ă mon-ō-sī-toj′ĕ-nēz) Bacterial species causing meningitis, encephalitis, septicemia, endocarditis, abortion, abscesses, and local purulent lesions; often fatal; found in feces, sewage, decaying vegetation, silage, soil, and fertilizer. Sometimes involved in infections in immunocompromised hosts; causes perinatal infections, neonatal sepsis, and septicemia; recently linked to food-borne diseases; especially associated with processed meat and dairy products. Widespread infections reported in Canada in late 2008.

lis·ter·i·o·sis (lis-tēr′ē-ō′sis) A sporadic disease of animals and humans, particularly those immunocompromised or pregnant, caused by *Listeria monocytogenes* (q.v.); very resistant organism (resists salt, acid, heat and nitrite preservatives; can replicate at normally safe refrigerator temperatures (slow growth at 24° F.) SYN listeria meningitis.

Lis·ter meth·od (lis′tĕr meth′ŏd) Antiseptic surgery; the first use of sterile methods in surgery.

li·ter (L) (lē′tĕr) A measure of capacity of 1000 cubic centimeters or 1 cubic decimeter; equivalent to 1.056688 U.S. quarts. SYN litre.

li·thi·a·sis (li-thī′ă-sis) Formation of calculi of any kind.

lith·i·um (Li) (lith′ē-ŭm) An element of the alkali metal group; many of its salts have clinical uses.

lith·i·um car·bon·ate (Li₂CO₃) (lith′ē-ŭm kahr′bŏ-nāt) Agent used to treat depressive, hypomanic, and manic phases of bipolar affective disorders.

litho-, lith- Combining forms denoting stone, calculus, calcification.

lith·o·clast (lith′ō-klast) SYN lithotrite.

lith·o·gen·e·sis, li·thog·e·ny (lith′ō-jen′ĕ-sis, lith-oj′ĕ-nē) Formation of calculi.

li·thol·a·pax·y (li-thol′ă-pak-sē) The technique of crushing a stone in the bladder and washing out the fragments through a catheter.

li·thol·y·sis (li-thol′i-sis) The dissolution of urinary calculi.

lith·o·lyt·ic (lith′ō-lit′ik) 1. Tending to dissolve calculi. 2. An agent having such properties.

lith·o·neph·ri·tis (lith′ō-nĕ-frī′tis) Interstitial nephritis associated with calculus formation.

lith·o·scope (lith′ō-skōp) Surgical instrument for visualizing stones in the bladder.

li·thot·o·my (LITH) (li-thot′ŏ-mē) Cutting operation for the removal of a calculus, especially a vesical type. SYN lithectomy.

li·thot·o·my position (li-thot′ŏ-mē pŏ-zish′ŏn) A supine position with patient's buttocks at the end of the operating table, the hips and knees fully flexed with feet strapped in position.

lith·o·trip·sy, lith·ot·ri·ty (lith′ō-trip-sē, li-thot′ri-tē) The crushing of a stone in the renal pelvis, ureter, or bladder, by mechanical force or sound waves. SYN lithotrity.

lith·o·trip·tic (lith′ō-trip′tik) 1. Relating to lithotripsy. 2. An agent that effects the dissolution of a calculus.

lith·o·trip·tor, lith·o·trip·ter (lith′ō-trip′tŏr, -tĕr) A device used to crush or fragment a calculus in lithotripsy.

lith·o·trip·tos·co·py (lith′ō-trip-tos′kŏ-pē) Crushing of a stone in the bladder under direct vision by use of a lithotriptoscope.

lith·o·trite (lith′ō-trīt) A mechanical instrument used to crush a urinary calculus in lithotripsy. SYN lithoclast.

lith·ur·e·sis (lith′yūr-ē′sis) The passage of gravel in the urine.

lit·mus (lit′mŭs) A blue coloring matter obtained from *Roccella tinctoria*; used as an indicator (reddened by acids and turned blue again by alkalies).

litre [Br.] SYN liter.

lit·ter (lit′ĕr) 1. A stretcher or portable couch for moving the sick or injured. 2. A group of animals of the same parents, born at the same time.

Litz·mann ob·li·qui·ty (lits′măn ō-blik′wi-tē) Inclination of the fetal head so that the biparietal diameter is oblique in relation to the plane of the pelvic brim, the posterior parietal bone presenting to the parturient canal. SYN posterior asynclitism.

li·ve·do (li-vē′dō) Bluish skin discoloration, either limited or generalized.

liv·e·doid (liv′ĕ-doyd) Pertaining to or resembling livedo.

liv·e·doid der·ma·ti·tis (liv′ĕ-doyd dĕr′mă-tī′tis) A reddish-blue mottled condition of the skin due to affection of the cutaneous vascular apparatus.

li·ve·do re·tic·u·la·ris (li-vē′dō re-tik-yū-lā′ris) A persistent purplish network-patterned discoloration of the skin caused by dilation of capillaries and venules due to stasis or changes in underlying blood vessels including hyalinization.

liv·er (liv′ĕr) [TA] Largest gland of the body, lying beneath the diaphragm in the right hypochondrium and upper part of the epigastrium; irregular shape, weighs from 1–2 kg, or about 1/40 the weight of the body; secretes bile; of great importance in both carbohydrate and protein metabolism. SYN hepar [TA].

liv·er breath (liv′ĕr breth) SYN fetor hepaticus.

liver fluke (liv′ĕr flūk) One of many different types of parasitic trematode worms that invade the livers of animals.

liv·er spot (liv′ĕr spot) SYN senile lentigo.

live vac·cine (līv vak-sēn′) Vaccine prepared from living, attenuated organisms.

liv·id (liv′id) Having a black and blue or a leaden or ashy gray color, as in discoloration from a contusion, congestion, or cyanosis.

liv·ing will (liv′ing wil) Legal document used to indicate one's preference to die rather than be sustained artificially if sick or injured beyond the prospect of recovery. SEE advance directive. SYN durable power of attorney (2).

li·vor (lī′vōr) The livid discoloration of the skin on the dependent parts of a corpse.

load·ing (lōd′ing) Administration of a substance for the purpose of testing metabolic function.

load·ing dose (lōd-ing′ dōs) The first dose of a medicine, which is much larger than the following doses, to reach a therapeutic level more rapidly.

lo·bar at·el·ec·ta·sis (lō′bahr at′ĕ-lek′tă-sis) Unventilated or collapsed area of a lobe of the lung.

lo·bar pneu·mo·ni·a (lō′bahr nū-mō′nē-ă) Pulmonary disease affecting one or more lobes, or part of a lobe, in which the consolidation is virtually homogeneous; often due to infection by *Streptococcus pneumoniae;* sputum is scanty and usually of a rusty tint because altered blood is present.

lo·bate (lō′bāt) **1.** Divided into lobes. **2.** Lobe-shaped. SYN lobose, lobous.

lobe (lōb) [TA] **1.** Subdivision of an organ or other part, bounded by fissures, sulci, or other structural demarcations. **2.** A rounded projecting part. SEE ALSO lobule. **3.** One of the larger divisions of the crown of a tooth. SYN lobus [TA].

lo·bec·to·my (lō-bek′tŏ-mē) Excision of a lobe of any organ or gland.

lo·bi cer·e·bri (lō′bī ser′ĕ-brī) Major divisions of the cerebral hemisphere.

lo·bot·o·my (lō-bot′ŏ-mē) **1.** Incision into a lobe. **2.** Division of one or more nerve tracts in a lobe of the cerebrum.

lob·u·lar cap·il·lary he·man·gi·o·ma (lob′yū-lăr kap′i-lar-ē hē-man′jē-ō′mă) SYN pyogenic granuloma.

lob·u·lar car·ci·no·ma (lob′yū-lăr kahr′si-nō′mă) An adenocarcinoma, especially of the breast, where it is less common than ductal carcinoma.

lob·u·lar car·ci·no·ma in si·tu (lob′yū-lăr kahr-si-nō′mă in sit′ū) SYN noninfiltrating lobular carcinoma.

lob·ule (lob′yūl) [TA] A small lobe or subdivision of a lobe. SYN lobulus [TA].

lob·u·lus, gen. and pl. **lob·u·li** (lob′yū-lŭs, -lī) [TA] SYN lobule.

lo·bus, gen. and pl. **lo·bi** (lō′bŭs, -bī) [TA] SYN lobe (1), lobe (3).

lo·cal (lō′kăl) Having reference or confined to a limited part; not general or systemic.

lo·cal an·aph·y·lax·is (lō′kăl an′ă-fi-lak′sis) The immediate, transient kind of response that follows injection of antigen (allergen) into the skin of a sensitized person; limited to the area surrounding inoculation site. SEE ALSO skin test.

lo·cal an·es·the·si·a (lō′kăl an′es-thē′zē-ă) A general term referring to topical, infiltration, field block, or nerve block anesthesia but not usually to spinal or epidural anesthesia.

lo·cal cov·er·age de·ter·mi·na·tion (LCD) (lō′kăl kŭv′ĕr-ăj dē-tĕr′mi-nā′shŭn) Advisories with detailed and updated information about coding and medical necessity of a specific service; used to ensure the accuracy of health care billing.

lo·cal hor·mone (lō′kăl hōr′mōn) Metabolic product secreted by one set of cells that affects the function of nearby cells.

lo·cal im·mu·ni·ty (lō′kăl i-myū′ni-tē) A natural or acquired immunity to some pathogens or infectious agents.

lo·cal·i·za·tion (lō′kăl-ī-zā′shŭn) **1.** Limitation to a definite area. **2.** The reference of a sensation to its point of origin. **3.** The determination of the location of a morbid process.

lo·cal·ized (lō′kăl-īzd) Restricted or limited to a definite part.

lo·cal le·sion (lō′kăl lē′zhŭn) A pathologic change, wound, or injury limited to a single region of the body.

lo·cal stim·u·lant (lō′kăl stim′yŭ-lănt) One with an action confined to the part to which it is applied.

lo·ca·tor (lō′kā-tŏr) An instrument or apparatus for finding the position of a foreign object in tissue.

lo·chi·a (lō′kē-ă) Discharge from the vagina of mucus, blood, and tissue debris, following childbirth.

lo·chi·a al·ba (lō′kē-ă al′bă) The last discharge no longer tinged with blood.

lo·chi·al (lō′kē-ăl) Relating to the lochia.

lo·chi·a ru·bra (lō′kē-ă rū′bră) The initial discharge stained with blood.

lo·chi·a san·gui·no·len·ta (lō′kē-ă sang-gwin-ō-len′tă) Thick, dark red vaginal discharge seen a few days after delivery.

lo·chi·a se·ro·sa (lō′kē-ă ser-ō′să) Thin and watery lochia.

lo·chi·o·me·tra (lō′kē-ō-mē′tră) Distention of the uterus with retained lochia.

lo·chi·or·rhe·a, lo·chi·or·rha·gi·a (lō′kē-ōr-ē′ă, -ā′jē-ă) Profuse flow of the lochia.

lochiorrhoea [Br.] SYN lochiorrhea.

locked-in syn·drome (lokt-in′ sin′drōm) Basis pontis infarct resulting in tetraplegia, horizontal ophthalmoplegia, dysphagia, and facial diplegia with preserved consciousness.

Locke so·lu·tion (lok sŏ-lū′shŭn) A solution used in laboratory experiments to irrigate mammalian heart and other tissues; also used with naturally occurring body substances for culturing animal cells.

lock·ing point (lok′ing poynt) The body's center of gravity; by holding onto it, a health care worker can help patients maintain their balance.

lock·jaw, lock-jaw (lok′jaw) SYN trismus.

lo·co·mo·tion (lō′kŏ-mō′shŭn) Movement of the body.

lo·co·mo·tor a·tax·i·a (lō′kŏ-mō′tŏr ă-tak′sē-ă) Severe gait irregularity seen with tabetic neurosyphilis. Patients walk with feet wide apart, slapping them clumsily to the floor with each step, and depend on visual cues to maintain balance. SEE ALSO tabetic neurosyphilis.

lo·cum ten·ant (lō′kŭm ten′ănt) A temporary substitution of one physician by another. Also called locum tenens.

lo·cus of in·fec·tion (lō′kŭs in-fek′ shŭn) The specific site in or on the body where an infection originates.

Löf·fler en·do·car·di·tis (lĕrf′lĕr en′dō-kahr-dī′tis) Fibroplastic constrictive parietal endocarditis with eosinophilia, characterized by progressive congestive heart failure and multiple systemic emboli.

Löf·fler pa·ri·e·tal fi·bro·plas·tic en·do·car·di·tis (lĕrf′lĕr pa-rī′ĕ-tăl fī′brō-plas′tik en′dō-kahr-dī′tis) Sclerosis of the endocardium in the presence of a high eosinophil count.

Löf·fler stain (lĕrf′lĕr stān) A stain to identify flagella.

log·am·ne·si·a (lawg′am-nē′zē-ă) SYN aphasia.

log·a·pha·si·a (lawg′ă-fā′zē-ă) Aphasia of articulation.

log·as·the·ni·a (lawg′as-thē′nē-ă) SYN aphasia.

-logia Suffix meaning **1.** The study of the subject noted in the body of the word, or a treatise on the same; the English equivalent is -logy, or, with a connecting vowel, -ology. **2.** Collecting or picking. SYN -ology (2).

logo-, log- Combining forms meaning speech, words.

log·o·pe·dics, log·o·pe·di·a (log′ō-pē′diks, -pē′dē-ă) Science of the physiology and pathology of the organs of speech and correction of speech defects.

log·o·ple·gi·a (lawg′ō-plē′jē-ă) Paralysis of the organs of speech.

log·o·spasm (log′ō-spazm) SYN explosive speech.

loin (loyn) The part of the side and back between the ribs and the pelvis. SYN lumbus.

Lom·bard re·flex (lom′bahrd rē′fleks) The increase in vocal intensity when talking over a noisy background.

lo·mus·tine (lō-mŭs′tēn) An antineoplastic agent.

long-act·ing thy·roid stim·u·la·tor (lawng′ak′ting thī′royd stim′yū-lā-tŏr) A substance, found in the blood of some hyperthyroid patients, which exerts a prolonged stimulatory effect on the thyroid gland.

lon·gi·tu·di·nal frac·ture (lon′ji-tū′di-năl frak′shŭr) A break in a bone along the line of its axis.

lon·gi·tu·di·nal stud·y (lon′ji-tū′di-năl stŭd′ē) Research in which the natural course of life or a given disorder in a set of subjects is serially observed over time; no assumptions are made about the stability of the system. SYN diachronic study.

lon·gi·tu·di·nal tear (lon′ji-tū′di-năl tār) Shearing of articular cartilage roughly parallel to the long axis of the bone.

long-term mem·o·ry (lawng′tĕrm mem′ŏ-rē) That phase of the memory process considered the permanent storehouse of information that has been registered, encoded, passed into the short-term memory, coded, rehearsed, and finally transferred and stored for future retrieval; material and information retained there underlies cognitive abilities.

loop (lūp) **1.** A sharp curve or complete bend in a vessel, cord, or other elongate body, forming an oval or circular ring. SEE ALSO ansa. **2.** A wire (usually of platinum or nichrome) fixed into a handle at one end and bent into a circle at the other, rendered sterile by flaming, and used to transfer microorganisms.

loop co·los·to·my (lūp kŏ-los′tŏ-mē) An artificial opening into the colon created by bringing a loop of it through an abdominal wall incision held in place with a plastic rod until healed.

loose bod·y (LB) (lūs bod′ē) Solid tissue fragment lying free in a body cavity.

loos·en·ing of as·so·ci·a·tions (lūs′sĕn-ing ă-sō′sē-ā′shŭnz) Sign of a severe thought disorder characterized by the lack of an obvious connection between one thought and the next, or with the response to a question.

loose skin (lūs skin) SYN dermatochalasis.

lo·phot·ri·chous (lō-fot′ri-kŭs) Referring to a bacterial cell with two or more flagella at one or both poles. SYN lophotrichate.

lor·do·sis (lōr-dō′sis) [TA] An anteriorly convex curvature of the vertebral column. SYN hollow back, saddle back.

lor·dot·ic pel·vis (lōr-dot′ik pel′vis) Pelvic deformity associated with a lordotic curvature of the spine.

lor·dot·ic po·si·tion (lōr-dot′ik pŏ-zish′ŏn) A radiographic position with exaggerated lumbar lordotic curve, allowing x-ray examination of the lung apices without the clavicles being superimposed.

LOS Abbreviation for length of stay.

lo·tion (lō′shŭn) A class of liquid suspensions intended for external application.

Lou Geh·rig dis·ease (lū ger′ig di-zēz′) SYN amyotrophic lateral sclerosis.

loupe (lūp) A magnifying lens.

louse, pl. **lice** (lows, līs) Common name for members of the ectoparasitic insect orders Anoplura (sucking lice) and Mallophaga (biting lice).

low birth weight (LBW) (lō bĭrth wāt) Birth weight less than 2500 g. Can be due to a range of factors, including interference with intrauterine growth or premature birth.

low cho·les·ter·ol (lō kŏ·les′tĕr-ol) A product so labeled contains, by F.D.A. order, less than 20 mg cholesterol per serving and less than 2 g saturated fat per serving.

low den·si·ty li·po·pro·tein-cho·les·ter·ol (LDL-C) (lō den′si-tē li′pō-prō′tēn kŏ-les′tĕr-ol) The so-called bad cholesterol; contains mostly lipids and few proteinaceous elements; ought to be kept to a minimum to improve health.

Lowe dis·ease (lō di-zēz′) X-linked recessive disease characterized by cataracts, mental retardation, and renal problems.

low·er air·way (lō′ĕr ār′wā) Part of the respiratory tract that extends from the subglottis to the terminal bronchioles.

low·er limb (lō′ĕr lim) [TA] The hip, thigh, leg, ankle, and foot. SYN lower extremity.

low·er mo·tor neu·ron dys·arth·ria (lō′ĕr mō′tŏr nūr′on dis-ahr′thrē-ā) Speech disorder due to dysfunction of the motor nuclei and the lower pons or medulla, or other neural connections, central and peripheral to the muscles of articulation.

Low·er tu·ber·cle (lō′wĕr tū′bĕr-kĕl) SYN intervenous tubercle (of right atrium).

low-fat di·et (LFD) (lō-fat′ dī′ĕt) One containing a minimal proportion of fat. Diets are designed to reduce the risk of cardiovascular disease, specifically atherosclerosis. SEE atherosclerosis, free radical.

low-flow ox·y·gen de·li·ver·y sys·tem (lō-flō′ ok′si-jĕn dē-liv′ĕr-ē sis′tĕm) A ventilation system that delivers oxygen at a rate that is lower than the patient's inspiratory needs, thus making up the difference with room air.

low-grade squa·mous in·tra·ep·i·the·li·al le·sion (lō-grād skwā′mŭs in′tră-ep′i-thē′lē-ăl lē′zhŭn) Term used in the Bethesda system for reporting cervical/vaginal cytologic diagnosis to describe a spectrum of noninvasive cervical epithelial abnormalities. SEE ALSO Bethesda system.

low mo·lec·u·lar weight hep·a·rin (LMWH) (lō mō-lek′yū-lăr wāt hep′ăr-in) A form of blood thinner with a longer half life and fewer adverse effects (e.g., thrombocytopenia).

low pur·ine di·et (lō pyūr′ēn dī′ĕt, pyūr′in) Diet low in precursors of purines (e.g., liver, glandular meats) to minimize formation of uric acid. Used to treat patients with gout.

low res·i·due di·et (lō rez′i-dū dī′ĕt) One that leaves minimal unabsorbed components in the intestine to lessen functional colonic stress.

low salt di·et (lō sawlt dī′ĕt) One with restricted amounts of sodium chloride; used to treat some cases of hypertension, heart failure, and other syndromes characterized by fluid retention and/or edema formation.

low salt syn·drome (lō sawlt sin′drōm) Disorder resulting from salt restriction and diuretics; characterized by weakness, drowsiness, and other symptoms. Also seen in cirrhosis with ascites and suprarenal insufficiency.

Lox·o·sce·les (loks-os′ĕ-lēz) A genus of venomous brown spiders, marked by a fiddle-shaped pattern on the cephalothorax and a distinct six-eye pattern, found chiefly in South America. In North America, *L. reclusus*, the brown recluse spider, is the most important.

loz·enge (loz.) (loz′ĕnj) SYN troche.

LPM Abbreviation for liters per minute.

Lr, L_r Symbol for lawrencium.

L se·lec·tin (sĕ-lek′tin) Cell surface receptor produced by leukocytes.

L shell (shell) The next lowest energy

level of electrons in the atom, after the K shell.

L-spine (spīn) Lateral spine.

Lu Symbol for lutetium.

lubb-dupp (lŭb-dŭp´) The onomatopoeic sound that mimics the heartbeat.

lu·cid in·ter·val (lū´sid in´tĕr-văl) In psychoses or delirium, a rational period appearing in the course of the mental disorder.

lu·cid·i·ty (lū-sid´i-tē) The quality or state of being lucid.

Lu·cio lep·ro·sy (lū´syō lep´rŏ-sē) Acute form of pure diffuse lepromatous leprosy. SYN Lucio leprosy phenomenon.

Lu·cio lep·ro·sy phe·nom·e·non (lū´syō lep´rŏ-sē fĕ-nom´ĕ-non) SYN Lucio leprosy.

Lud·wig an·gi·na (LA) (lud´vig an´ji-nă) Cellulitis, usually of odontogenic origin, bilaterally involving the submaxillary, sublingual, and submental spaces, resulting in painful swelling of the floor of the mouth, elevation of the tongue, dysphagia, dysphonia, and (at times) compromise of the airway.

Lu·er sy·ringe (lū´ĕr sir-inj´) A glass syringe with a metal tip and locking device to secure the needle.

lu·es (lū´ēz) A plague or pestilence.

Lukes-Col·lins clas·si·fi·ca·tion (lūks kol´inz klas´i-fi-kā´shŭn) Classification of lymphomas according to the immunologic nature of the cell of origin, based on histologic and clinical data.

lum·ba·go (lŭm-bā´gō) Pain in mid and lower back; a descriptive term not specifying cause.

lum·bar (lŭm´bahr) Relating to the loins, or the part of the back and sides between the ribs and the pelvis.

lum·bar flex·ure (lŭm´bahr flek´shŭr) The normal ventral curve of the vertebral column in the lumbar region.

lum·bar gan·gli·a (lŭm´bahr gang´glē-ă) [TA] Four or more paravertebral sympathetic ganglia on the medial border of the psoas major muscle on either side. SYN ganglia lumbalia [TA].

lum·bar·i·za·tion (lŭm´bahr-ī-zā´shŭn) Congenital anomaly of the lumbosacral junction characterized by development of the first sacral vertebra as a lumbar vertebra resulting in six lumbar vertebrae instead of five.

lum·bar punc·ture (lŭm´bahr pŭngk´ shŭr) A puncture into the subarachnoid space of the lumbar region to obtain spinal fluid for diagnostic or therapeutic purposes. SYN rachiocentesis, spinal tap.

lum·bar rib (lŭm´bahr rib) [TA] An occasional rib articulating with the transverse process of the first lumbar vertebra.

lum·bo·cos·tal (lŭm´bō-kos´tăl) **1.** Relating to the lumbar and the hypochondriac regions. **2.** Relating to the lumbar vertebrae and the ribs.

lum·bo·cos·to·ab·dom·i·nal tri·an·gle (lŭm´bō-kos´tō-ăb-dom´i-năl trī´ang-gĕl) An irregular area bounded by the serratus posterior inferior, obliquus externus, obliquus internus, and erector spinae muscles.

lum·bo·dy·ni·a (lŭm´bō-din´ē-ă) Pain in the lumbar region.

lum·bo·in·gui·nal (lŭm´bō-ing´gwi-năl) Relating to the lumbar and the inguinal regions.

lum·bo·sa·cral (lŭm´bō-sā´krăl) Relating to the lumbar vertebrae and the sacrum. SYN sacrolumbar.

lum·bri·ci·dal (lŭm´bri-sī´dăl) Destructive to lumbricoid (intestinal) worms.

lum·bri·cide (lŭm´bri-sīd) An agent that kills lumbricoid (intestinal) worms.

lum·bri·co·sis (lŭm´bri-kō´sis) Infection with round intestinal worms.

lum·bus, gen. and pl. **lum·bi** (lŭm´bŭs, bī) SYN loin.

lu·men (lm), pl. **lu·mi·na** (lū´mĕn, -mi-nă) **1.** The space in the interior of a tubular structure. **2.** The unit of luminous flux.

lu·mi·nance (lū'mi-năns) The brightness of an object, expressed as the luminous flux per unit of solid angle per unit projected area.

lu·mi·nes·cence (lū'mi-nes'ĕns) Emission of light from a body as a result of a chemical reaction.

lu·mi·nif·er·ous (lū'mi-nif'ĕr-ŭs) Producing or conveying light.

lu·mi·rho·dop·sin (lū'mi-rō-dop'sin) An intermediate between rhodopsin and all-*trans*-retinal plus opsin during bleaching of rhodopsin by light.

lump·ec·to·my (lŭmp-ek'tŏ-mē) Removal of a breast lesion, with preservation of surrounding tissue.

lu·nar (lū'năr) Shaped like the moon when visible only in part. SYN lunate, semilunar.

lu·nate (lū'nāt) [TA] **1.** SYN lunar (2). **2.** Relating to the lunate bone.

lung (lŭng) [TA] One of a pair of viscera occupying the pulmonary cavities of the thorax, the organs of respiration in which aeration of the blood takes place. As a rule, the right lung is slightly larger than the left and is divided into three lobes (an upper, a middle, and a lower or basal), whereas the left has but two lobes (an upper and a lower or basal).

lung ab·scess (lŭng ab'ses) Lesion in the lung parenchyma with cavitation, bronchial communication, and pus.

lung com·pli·ance (lŭng kŏm-plī'ăns) Change in lung volume per unit change in transpulmonary pressure.

lu·poid (lū'poyd) Resembling lupus. SYN lupiform.

lu·poid sy·co·sis (lū'poyd sī-kō'sis) A papular or pustular inflammation of the hair follicles of the beard, followed by punctuate scarring and loss of the hair.

lu·pus (lū'pŭs) A term originally used to depict erosion (as if gnawed) of the skin, now used with modifying terms designating various diseases.

lu·pus band test (lū'pŭs band test) Direct immunofluorescent technique for demonstrating a band of immunoglobulins at the dermal-epidermal junction of the skin of patients with lupus erythematosus.

lu·pus er·y·the·ma·to·sus, ne·o·na·tal, sys·tem·ic, dis·coid (lū'pŭs ĕr-i'thĕ-mă-tō'sŭs, nē'ō-nā'tăl, sis-tem'ik, dis'koyd) An illness characterized either by skin lesions alone or by systemic disorder with antinuclear antibodies and involvement of vital structures.

lu·pus er·y·the·ma·to·sus cell (lū'pŭs ĕr-i'thĕ-mă-tō'sŭs sel) SYN LE cell.

lupus er·y·the·ma·to·sus pro·fun·dus (lū'pŭs ĕr-i'thĕ-mă-tō'sŭs prō-fun'dŭs) A subcutaneous panniculitis with deep-seated, firm, rubbery nodules, usually of the face.

lu·pus mil·i·a·ris dis·se·mi·na·tus fa·ci·ei (LMDF) (lū-pus mil-ē-ar'is dis'sem-i-nā'tus fash'ē-ī) Milletlike papular eruption of the face associated with a tuberculoid perifollicular infiltration but probably due to rosacea rather than tuberculous infection.

lu·pus neph·ri·tis (lū'pŭs nĕ-frī'tis) Glomerulonephritis occurring in some patients with systemic lupus erythematosus, characterized by hematuria and a progressive course culminating in renal failure.

lu·pus per·ni·o (lū'pŭs pĕr'nē-ō) Sarcoid lesions, clinically resembling frostbite and microscopically resembling lupus vulgaris, involving ears, cheeks, nose, hands, and fingers.

lu·pus vul·ga·ris (lū'pŭs vŭl-gā'ris) Cutaneous tuberculosis with characteristic nodular lesions on the face, particularly about the nose and ears.

Lusch·ka ton·sil (lūsh' kah ton'sil) SYN adenoid.

lu·sus na·tur·ae (lū'sŭs nā-tū'rē) Latin for ''freak of nature''; a horribly physically deformed person.

lute (lūt) To seal or fasten with wax or cement.

lu·te·al (lū'tē-ăl) Relating to the corpus luteum (e.g., luteal cells and hormones).

lu·te·al phase (lū'tē-ăl fāz) That portion of the menstrual cycle extending from the time of formation of the corpus luteum to the onset of menses, usually 14 days in length.

lu·te·in (lū'tē-in) **1.** The yellow pigment in the corpus luteum, the yolk of eggs, or any lipochrome. **2.** SYN xanthophyll.

lu·te·in·i·za·tion (lū'tē-in-ī-zā'shŭn) Transformation of the mature ovarian follicle and its theca interna into a corpus luteum after ovulation.

lu·te·i·niz·ing hor·mone (lū'tē-in-ī'zing hŏr'mōn) SYN lutropin.

lu·te·i·niz·ing hor·mone-fol·li·cle stim·u·lat·ing hor·mone-re·leas·ing fac·tor (lū'tē-in-ī'zing hŏr'mōn-fol'i-kĕl-stim'yŭ-lā'ting hŏr'mōn-rĕ-lē'sing fak'tŏr) SYN gonadoliberin (2).

lu·te·i·niz·ing hor·mone-re·leas·ing hor·mone (lū'tē-in-ī'zing hŏr'mōn-rĕ-lē'sing hŏr'mōn) SYN gonadotropin-releasing hormone.

Lu·tem·ba·cher syn·drome (lū'tem-bahk'er sin'drōm) A congenital cardiac abnormality consisting of a defect of the interatrial septum, mitral stenosis, and enlarged right atrium.

lu·te·ol·y·sis (lū'tē-ol'i-sis) *Avoid the mispronunciation luteoly'sis.* Degeneration or destruction of ovarian luteinized tissue.

lu·te·o·ma (lū'tē-ō'mă) An ovarian tumor of granulosa or theca-lutein cell origin, producing progesterone effects on the uterine mucosa. SYN luteinoma.

lu·te·o·tro·pic, lu·te·o·tro·phic (lū'tē-ō-trō'pik, -trōf'ik) Having a stimulating action on the development and function of the corpus luteum.

lu·te·o·tro·pin (lū'tē-ō-trō'pin) Anterior pituitary hormone that acts to maintain the corpus luteum.

lut·ing a·gent (lūt'ing ā'jĕnt) Fastening material or cement used to hold casts to an articulator, or material to hold crowns to teeth.

lu·tro·pin (lū-trō'pin) A glycoprotein hormone that stimulates the final ripening of an ovarian follicle, its secretion of progesterone, its rupture to release the egg, and the conversion of the ruptured follicle into the corpus luteum. SYN interstitial cell-stimulating hormone, luteinizing hormone.

lux (lŭks) A unit of light or illumination; the reception of a luminous flux of 1 lumen per square meter of surface. SYN candle-meter, meter-candle.

lux·a·ted joint (lŭk'sā-tĕd joynt) Dislocated articulation.

lux·a·tion (lŭk-sā'shŭn) **1.** SYN dislocations. **2.** DENTISTRY Dislocation or displacement of the condyle in the temporomandibular fossa.

ly·co·pene (lī'kō-pēn) The red pigment of the tomato.

Ly·ell syn·drome (lī'ĕl sin'drōm) SYN toxic epidermal necrolysis.

Lyme dis·ease, Lyme bor·rel·i·o·sis (līm di-zēz', bŏ-rel-ē-ō'sis) An inflammatory disorder typically contracted during the summer and caused by *Borrelia burgdorferi;* the characteristic skin lesion, erythema chronicum migrans, usually is preceded or accompanied by fever, malaise, fatigue, headache, and stiff neck; neurologic or cardiac manifestations, or arthritis (i.e., Lyme arthritis); other findings possible.

lymph, lym·pha (limf, -ă) [TA] A clear, sometimes faintly yellow and slightly opalescent fluid that is collected from the tissues throughout the body, flows in the lymphatic vessels, and through the lymph nodes, and is eventually added to the venous blood circulation.

lymph- (limf) SEE lympho-.

lym·pha (lim'fă) [TA] SYN lymph.

lym·phad·e·nec·to·my (lim-fad'ĕ-nek'tŏ-mē) Excision of lymph nodes.

lym·phad·e·ni·tis (lim-fad'ĕ-nī'tis) Inflammation of a lymph node or lymph nodes.

lym·phad·e·nog·ra·phy (lim-fad'ĕ-nog'ră-fē) Radiographic visualization of lymph nodes after injection of a contrast medium ; lymphography.

lym·phad·e·noid (lim-fad′ĕ-noyd) Relating to, or resembling, or derived from a lymph node.

lym·phad·e·nop·a·thy (LAN) (lim-fad′ĕ-nop′ă-thē) **1.** Any disease process affecting a lymph node or lymph nodes. **2.** The appearance of enlarged lymph nodes found on a radiologic examination of any kind.

lymphaemia [Br.] SYN lymphemia.

lym·pha·gogue (lim′fă-gog) An agent that increases formation and flow of lymph.

lym·phan·gi·ec·ta·sis, lym·phan·gi·ec·ta·si·a (lim-fan′jē-ek′tă-sis, -ek-tā′zē-a) Dilation of the lymphatic vessels, the basic process that may result in the formation of a lymphangioma.

lym·phan·gi·ec·to·my (lim-fan′jē-ek′tŏ-mē) Excision of a lymph channel.

lym·phan·gi·i·tis (lim-fan′jē-ī′tis) SYN lymphangitis.

♻ **lymphangio-, lymphangi-** Combining forms denoting the lymphatic vessels.

lym·phan·gi·og·ra·phy (LAG) (lim-fan′jē-og′ră-fē) Radiographic demonstration of lymphatics and lymph nodes after injection of a contrast medium.

lym·phan·gi·ol·o·gy (lim-fan′jē-ol′ŏ-jē) The branch of medical science concerned with the lymphatic vessels. SYN lymphology.

lym·phan·gi·o·ma (lim-fan′jē-ō′mă) A well-circumscribed nodule of lymphatic vessels that are usually greatly dilated and lined with normal endothelial cells; occur most frequently in the neck and axilla.

lym·phan·gi·o·ma ca·ver·no·sum (lim-fan′jē-ō′mă kav-ĕr-nō′sŭm) Condition of conspicuous dilation of lymphatic vessels in a fairly circumscribed region, frequently with the formation of cavities or "lakes" filled with lymph. SYN cavernous lymphangiectasis.

lym·phan·gi·o·ma cir·cum·scrip·tum (lim-fan′jē-ō′mă sir-kŭm-skrip′tŭm) Congenital nevoid lesion consisting of a circumscribed group of tense lymph vesicles. SYN lymphangioma simplex.

lym·phan·gi·o·ma sim·plex (lim-fan′jē-ō′mă sim′pleks) Lesion that appears within the skin as a small, lobulated growth filled with clear fluid and sometimes intertriginous low-grade infection. SYN lymphangioma circumscriptum, simple lymphangiectasis.

lym·phan·gi·o·phle·bi·tis (lim-fan′jē-ō-flē-bī′tis) Inflammation of the lymphatic vessels and veins.

lym·phan·gi·o·sar·co·ma (lim-fan′jē-ō-sahr-kō′mă) Malignant neoplasm derived from the endothelial cells of lymphatic vessels.

lym·phan·gi·ot·o·my (lim-fan′jē-ot′ŏ-mē) Incision of lymphatic vessels.

lym·phan·gi·tis, lym·phan·gi·i·tis, lym·phan·ge·i·tis (lim′fan-jī′tis, -an-jē-ī′tis, -an-jē-ī′tis) Inflammation of the lymphatic vessels.

lym·pha·phe·re·sis (lim′fă-fē-rē′sis) SYN lymphocytapheresis.

lym·phat·ic (lim-fat′ik) **1.** Pertaining to lymph. **2.** A vascular channel that transports lymph.

lym·phat·ic fol·li·cles of rec·tum (lim-fat′ik fol′i-kĕlz rek′tŭm) SEE folliculi lymphatici recti.

lym·phat·ic leu·ke·mi·a (lim-fat′ik lū-kē′mē-ă) SYN lymphocytic leukemia.

lym·phat·ic nod·ule (lim-fat′ik nod′yūl) SYN lymphoid nodule.

lym·phat·ic sys·tem (lim-fat′ik sis′tĕm) SYN lymphoid system.

lym·phat·ic tis·sue, lym·phoid tis·sue (lim-fat′ik tish′ū, lim′foyd) A three-dimensional network of reticular fibers and cells with meshes occupied in varying degrees of density with lymphocytes. SYN adenoid tissue.

lym·phat·ic ves·sels (lim-fat′ik ves′ĕlz) [TA] SYN lymph vessels.

lymph cell (limf sel) SYN lymphocyte.

lymph·e·de·ma (lim′fĕ-dē′mă) Swelling

due to obstruction of lymphatic vessels or lymph nodes and the accumulation of large amounts of lymph in the affected region. SYN lymphoedema.

lym·phe·mi·a (lim-fē′mē-ă) Presence of unusually large numbers of lymphocytes or their precursors, or both, in the circulating blood. SYN lymphaemia.

lymph fol·li·cle (limf fol′i-kĕl) One of the spheric masses of lymphoid cells. SYN nodulus lymphaticus.

lymph node (LN) (limf nōd) [TA] One of numerous round, oval, or bean-shaped bodies located along the course of lymphatic vessels, varying greatly in size (1–25 mm in diameter) and usually presenting a depressed area, the hilum, on one side through which blood vessels enter and efferent lymphatic vessels emerge. SYN lymphonodus, lymph gland, lymphaden, lymphoglandula.

lympho-, lymph- Combining forms meaning lymph.

lym·pho·blast (lim′fō-blast) A young immature cell that matures into a lymphocyte and is characterized by more abundant cytoplasm than in a lymphocyte. SYN lymphocytoblast.

lym·pho·blas·tic leu·ke·mi·a (lim′fō-blas′tik lū-kē′mē-ă) Acute lymphocytic leukemia in which the abnormal cells are chiefly (or almost totally) blast forms of the lymphocytic series.

lym·pho·blas·tic lym·pho·ma (lim′fō-blas′tik lim-fō′mă) A diffuse lymphoma in children, with supradiaphragmatic distribution and T lymphocytes with convoluted nuclei.

lym·pho·blas·to·sis (lim′fō-blas-tō′sis) The presence of lymphoblasts in the peripheral blood.

lym·pho·blas·to·ma (lim′fō-blas-tō′mă) A form of malignant lymphoma in which the chief cells are lymphoblasts.

lym·pho·cele (lim′fō-sēl) A cystic mass that contains lymph, usually from diseased or injured lymphatic channels. SYN lymphocyst.

lym·pho·cy·ta·phe·re·sis (lim′fō-sīt′ă-fĕr-ē′sis) Separation and removal of lym-

phocytes from drawn blood, with the remainder of the blood retransfused into the donor. SYN lymphapheresis.

lym·pho·cyte (lim′fō-sīt) A white blood cell formed in lymphatic tissue throughout the body from precursor cells originating in bone marrow and in normal adults making up approximately 22–28% of the total number of leukocytes in the circulating blood.

lym·pho·cyte func·tion as·so·ci·at·ed an·ti·gen (lim′fō-sīt fŭngk′shŭn ă-sō′sē-ā-tĕd an′ti-jen) Member of the integrin family expressed on all leukocytes.

lym·pho·cyte trans·for·mat·ion (lim′fō-sīt trans-fōr-mā′shŭn) Change into large, blastlike forms that occurs when lymphocytes are exposed to histoincompatible antigens or mitogens. SEE ALSO mixed lymphocyte culture test.

lymphocythaemia [Br.] SYN lymphocytosis.

lym·pho·cyt·ic chor·i·o·men·in·gi·tis (lim′fō-sit′ik kōr′ē-ō-men′in-jī′tis) Meningitis that usually occurs in young adults during the fall and winter; due to virus carried by common house mouse.

lym·pho·cyt·ic leu·ke·mi·a (lim′fō-sit′ik lū-kē′mē-ă) Form of hematologic disorder characterized by an uncontrolled proliferation and conspicuous enlargement of lymphoid tissue in various sites and occurrence of increased numbers of cells of the lymphocytic series in blood. SYN lymphatic leukemia.

lym·pho·cyt·ic se·ries, lym·phoid se·ries (lim′fō-sit′ik sēr′ēz, lim′foyd) Cells at various states in the development in lymphoid tissue of the mature lymphocytes.

lym·pho·cy·to·blast (lim′fō-sī′tō-blast) SYN lymphoblast.

lym·pho·cy·to·ma (lim′fō-sī-tō′mă) A circumscribed nodule or mass of mature lymphocytes, grossly resembling a neoplasm.

lym·pho·cy·to·pe·ni·a (lim′fō-sī′tō-pē′nē-ă) SYN lymphopenia.

lym·pho·cy·to·sis (lim′fō-sī-tō′sis) A form of actual or relative leukocytosis

L

with an increased number of lymphocytes. SYN lymphocythemia, lymphocytic leukocytosis.

lym·pho·duct (lim′fō-dŭkt) A lymphatic vessel.

lymphoedema [Br.] SYN lymphedema.

lym·pho·ep·i·the·li·o·ma (lim′fō-ep′i-thē′lē-ō′mă) A poorly differentiated radiosensitive squamous cell carcinoma involving lymphoid tissue in the region of the tonsils and nasopharynx.

lym·pho·gen·e·sis (lim′fō-gen′ĕ-sis) Lymph production.

lym·phog·e·nous (lim-foj′ĕ-nŭs) **1.** Originating from lymph or the lymphatic system. SYN lymphogenic. **2.** Producing lymph.

lym·phog·e·nous me·tas·ta·sis (lim-foj′ĕ-nŭs mĕ-tas′tă-sis) SEE metastasis.

lym·pho·glan·du·la (lim′fō-glan′dyŭ-lă) SYN lymph node.

lym·pho·gran·u·lo·ma (lim′fō-gran′yŭ-lō′mă) Old and nonspecific term used with reference to a few basically dissimilar diseases in which the pathologic processes result in granulomas or granulomalike lesions.

lym·pho·gran·u·lo·ma·to·sis, Hodg·kin dis·ease (lim′fō-gran′yŭ-lō-mă-tō′sis, hoj′kin di-zēz′) Any condition characterized by the occurrence of multiple and widely distributed lymphogranulomas.

lym·pho·gran·u·lo·ma ve·ne·re·um, ve·ne·re·al lymph·o·gran·u·lo·ma (lim′fō-gran-yŭ-lō′mă ve-nē′rē-ŭm, vĕ-nēr′ē-ăl) A sexually transmitted infection usually due to *Chlamydia trachomatis*, characterized by a transient genital ulcer and inguinal adenopathy in the male; in the female, perirectal lymph nodes are involved and rectal stricture is common. SYN tropical bubo.

lym·phog·ra·phy (lim-fog′ră-fē) Visualization of lymphatics, lymph nodes, or both by radiography after intralymphatic injection of a contrast medium.

lym·phoid (lim′foyd) Resembling lymph or lymphatic tissue, or pertaining to the lymphatic system.

lym·phoid in·ter·sti·tial pneu·mo·ni·a (lim′foyd in′tĕr-stish′ăl nū-mō′nē-ă) SYN lymphocytic interstitial pneumonitis.

lym·phoid leu·ke·mi·a (LL) (lim′foyd lū-kē′mē-ă) SYN lymphocytic leukemia.

lym·phoid sys·tem (lim′foyd sis′tĕm) [TA] The lymphatic vessels, nodes, and lymphoid tissue. SYN systema lymphoideum [TA], absorbent system, lymphatic system, systema lymphaticum.

lym·pho·kine (lim′fō-kīn) Hormonelike peptide released by activated lymphocytes that mediates immune response.

lym·pho·kine-ac·ti·va·ted kil·ler cell (LAK) (lim′fō-kīn-ak′ti-vă-tĕd kil′ĕr sel) Leukocytes stimulated by interleukin 2 to make them attack cancerous cells.

lym·pho·ki·ne·sis, lym·pho·ci·ne·sis (lim′fō-ki-nē′sis, -si-nē′sis) **1.** Circulation of lymph in the lymphatic vessels and through the lymph nodes. **2.** Movement of endolymph in the semicircular canals of the inner ear.

lym·pho·lyt·ic (lim′fō-lit′ik) An agent used to break up or dissolve lymphocytes.

lym·pho·ma (lim-fō′mă) Any neoplasm of lymphoid tissue; in colloquial use, synonymous with malignant lymphoma.

lym·pho·ma·toid gran·u·lo·ma·to·sis (LYG) (lim-fō′mă-toyd gran′yŭ-lō-mă-tō′sis) Angiocentric malignant lung lymphoma; upper respiratory tract and other body parts involved. SEE ALSO polymorphic reticulosis.

lym·pho·ma·to·sis (lim′fō-mă-tō′sis) Any condition characterized by the occurrence of multiple, widely distributed sites of involvement with lymphoma.

lym·pho·myx·o·ma (lim′fō-mik-sō′mă) Soft nonmalignant neoplasm that contains lymphoid tissue in a matrix of loose, areolar connective tissue.

lym·pho·no·dus (lim′fō-nō′dŭs) SYN lymph node.

lym·phop·a·thy (lim-fop′ă-thē) Any disease of the lymphatic vessels or lymph nodes.

lym·pho·pe·ni·a, lym·pho·cy·to·pe·ni·a (lim′fō-pē′nē-ă, -sī-tō-pē′nē-ă) A reduction, relative or absolute, in the number of lymphocytes in the circulating blood. SYN lymphocytopenia.

lym·pho·plas·ma·phe·re·sis (lim′fō-plaz′mă-fĕr-ē′sis) Separation and removal of lymphocytes and plasma from the drawn blood, with the remainder of the blood retransfused.

lym·pho·re·tic·u·lo·sis (lim′fō-rĕ-tik′yŭ-lō′sis) Historic term for proliferation of the reticuloendothelial cells (macrophages) of the lymph nodes.

lym·phor·rhe·a, lym·phor·rha·gi·a (lim′fō-rē′ă, -rā′jē-ă) An escape of lymph on the surface from ruptured, torn, or cut lymphatic vessels. SYN lymphorrhoea.

lymphorrhoea [Br.] SYN lymphorrhea.

lym·pho·scin·tig·ra·phy (lim′fō-sin-tig′ră-fē) Scintillation scanning of lymphatics or lymph nodes following intralymphatic or subcutaneous injection of a radionuclide.

lym·phos·ta·sis (lim-fos′tă-sis) Obstruction of the normal flow of lymph.

lym·pho·tax·is (lim′fō-tak′sis) The exertion of an effect that attracts or repels lymphocytes.

lym·pho·tox·ic·i·ty (lim′fō-tok-sis′i-tē) Toxicity to lymphocytes.

lym·pho·tox·in (lim-fō-tok′sin) A lymphokine from T lymphocytes that lyses or damages many cell types.

lym·phot·ro·phy (lim-fot′rō-fē) Nourishment of the tissues by lymph in parts devoid of blood vessels.

lymph space (limf spās) Area in tissue or a vessel, filled with lymph.

lymph va·rix (limf var′iks) Formation of varices or cysts in the lymph nodes in consequence of obstruction in the efferent lymphatics.

lymph ves·sels (limf ves′ĕlz) Those that convey lymph and anastomose with each other. SYN lymphatic vessels

lyo- Combining form denoting dissolution. SEE ALSO lyso-.

ly·on·i·za·tion, Ly·on hy·poth·e·sis (lī′on-ī-zā′shŭn, lī′ŏn hī-poth′ĕ-sis) The normal phenomenon that wherever there are two or more haploid sets of X-linked genes in each cell all but one of the genes are inactivated apparently at random and have no phenotypic expression. SYN X inactivation, X-inactivation.

ly·o·phil·ic (lī′ō-fil′ik) COLLOID CHEMISTRY denoting a dispersed phase with a pronounced affinity for the dispersion medium. SYN lyotropic.

ly·oph·i·li·za·tion (LY) (lī-of′i-lī-zā′shŭn) 1. Isolating a solid substance from solution by freezing the solution and evaporating the ice under vacuum. 2. Imparting lyophilic properties to a substance. SYN freeze-drying.

ly·o·pho·bic (lī′ō-fō′bik) COLLOID CHEMISTRY denoting a dispersed phase having but slight affinity for the dispersion medium.

ly·o·pho·bic col·loid (lī-ō-fō′bik kol′oyd) SYN suspensoid.

ly·o·trop·ic (lī′ō-trō′pik) SYN lyophilic.

ly·pres·sin (lī-pres′in) Vasopressin-containing antidiuretic and vasopressor hormone. SYN 8-lysine vasopressin.

Lys Abbreviation for lysine, or its radicals in peptides.

lys- SEE lyso-.

lyse (līs) To break up, to disintegrate, to effect lysis. SYN lyze.

ly·ser·gic ac·id di·eth·yl·a·mide (LSD) (lī-sĕr′jik as′id dī-eth′il-am′īd) A serotonin antagonist that induces hallucinatory states. SYN lysergide.

ly·ser·gide (lī-sĕr′jīd) SYN lysergic acid diethylamide.

ly·sin (lī′sin) 1. A specific complement-fixing antibody that acts destructively on cells and tissues; the various types are designated in accordance with the form of antigen that stimulates the production of the lysin, e.g., hemolysin, bacteriolysin. **2.** Any substance that causes lysis.

ly·sine (k, Lys) (lī′sēn) A nutritionally essential α-amino acid found in many proteins; distinguished by an ε-amino group.

ly·si·nu·ri·a (lī′si-nyūr′ē-ă) The presence of lysine in the urine.

ly·sis (lī′sis) **1.** Destruction of red blood cells, bacteria, and other structures by a specific lysin, usually referred to by the structure destroyed (e.g., hemolysis, bacteriolysis); may be due to a direct toxin or an immune mechanism **2.** Gradual subsidence of the symptoms of an acute disease; a form of the recovery process.

♻ **lyso-, lys-** Combining forms meaning lysis, dissolution. SEE ALSO lyo-.

ly·so·gen (lī′sō-jen) **1.** That which is capable of inducing lysis. **2.** A bacterium in the state of lysogeny.

ly·so·gen·ic (lī′sō-jen′ik) **1.** Causing or having the power to cause lysis, as the action of certain antibodies and chemical substances. **2.** Pertaining to bacteria in the state of lysogeny.

ly·so·ge·nic·i·ty (lī′sō-jĕ-nis′i-tē) The property of being lysogenic.

ly·so·some (lī′sō-sōm) A cytoplasmic membrane-bound vesicle that contains a wide variety of glycoprotein hydrolytic enzymes active at an acid pH; serves to digest exogenous material, such as bacteria.

ly·so·zyme (lī′sō-zīm) An enzyme that is destructive to cell walls of certain bacteria; present in tears and some other body fluids, in egg white, and in some plant tissues. SYN mucopeptide glycohydrolase, muramidase.

lys·sa (lis′ă) A cartilage in the tongue of the dog.

Lys·sa·vi·rus (lis′ă-vī′rŭs) A genus of viruses (family Rhabdoviridae) that includes the rabies virus group.

Lyt an·ti·gens (an′ti-jenz) Alloantigens present on either T or B murine lymphocytes.

lyt·ic (lit′ik) Pertaining to lysis; used colloquially as an abbreviation for osteolytic.

lyze (līz) SYN lyse.

mac·er·ate (mas′ĕr-āt) To soften by steeping or soaking.

Mac·ew·en sign (măk yū′ĕn sīn) Percussion of the skull gives a cracked-pot sound in cases of hydrocephalus.

ma·chine (mă-shēn′) Any mechanical apparatus or device.

ma·chin·er·y mur·mur (mă-shēn′ĕr-ē mŭr′mŭr) The long ''continuous'' rumbling murmur of patent ductus arteriosus. SYN Gibson murmur.

ma·chis·mo (mah-chēz′mō) A concept of male virility.

macr- SEE macro-.

Mac·ra·can·tho·rhyn·chus (mak′ră-kan′thō-ring′kŭs) A genus of giant thorny-headed worms.

mac·ren·ceph·a·ly, mac·ren·ce·pha·li·a (mak′ren-sef′ă-lē, -sĕ-fā′lē-ă) Hypertrophy of the brain; having a large brain.

macro-, macr- Combining forms meaning large, long. SEE ALSO mega-, megalo-.

mac·ro·ad·e·no·ma (mak′rō-ad′ĕ-nō′mă) A pituitary adenoma larger than 10 mm in diameter.

macroamylasaemia [Br.] SYN macroamylasemia.

mac·ro·am·y·lase (mak′rō-am′i-lās) A form of serum amylase in which the enzyme is joined to a globulin.

mac·ro·am·y·la·se·mi·a (mak′rō-am′i-lā-sē′mē-ă) A form of hyperamylasemia, in which a portion of serum amylase exists as macroamylase. SYN macroamylasaemia.

mac·ro·bi·ot·ic di·et (mak′rō-bī-ot′ik dī′ĕt) One alleged to increase longevity, often by emphasizing whole-grain natural foods and restricting noncereal foods and liquids.

mac·ro·blast (mak′rō-blast) A large erythroblast.

mac·ro·bleph·a·ri·a (mak′rō-blef′ă-rē′ă) Enlarged or swollen eyelids.

mac·ro·car·di·a (mak′rō-kahr′dē-ă) SYN cardiomegaly.

mac·ro·ceph·a·ly, mac·ro·ce·pha·li·a (mak′rō-sef′ă-lē, -sĕ-fā′lē-ă) SYN megacephaly.

mac·ro·chei·li·a, mac·ro·chi·li·a (mak′rō-kī′lē-ă) 1. Abnormally enlarged lips. 2. Cavernous lymphangioma of the lip, a condition of permanent swelling due to the presence of greatly distended lymphatic spaces.

mac·ro·co·lon (mak′rō-kō′lŏn) A sigmoid colon of unusual length; a variety of megacolon.

mac·ro·cyte (mak′rō-sīt) A large erythrocyte (red blood cell), as in pernicious anemia; indicated by an elevated mean corpuscle volume.

mac·ro·cy·the·mi·a (mak′rō-sī-thē′mē-ă) Unusually large numbers of macrocytes in circulating blood. SYN macrocytosis.

mac·ro·cy·to·sis (mak′rō-sī-tō′sis) SYN macrocythemia.

mac·ro·fol·lic·u·lar ad·e·no·ma (mak′rō-fŏ-lik′yū-lăr ad′ĕ-nō′mă) SYN colloid adenoma.

mac·ro·ga·mete (mak′rō-gam′ēt) The female element in anisogamy; larger of the two sex cells, with more reserve material, and usually nonmotile.

mac·ro·ga·me·to·cyte (mak′rō-gă-mē′tō-sīt) The female gametocyte or mother cell producing the female or macrogamete among fungi or protozoa that undergo anisogamy.

ma·crog·li·a (mak-rog′lē-ă) SYN astrocyte.

macroglobulinaemia [Br.] SYN macroglobulinemia.

mac·ro·glob·u·lin·e·mi·a (mak′rō-glob′yū-li-nē′mē-ă) Increased levels of macroglobulins in the blood. SYN macroglobulinaemia.

mac·ro·lide (mak′rō-līd) A natural lactone, with a large atomic ring, several antibiotics (e.g., erythromycin) are macrolides that inhibit protein biosynthesis.

mac·ro·me·li·a (mak′rō-mē′lē-ă) Abnormal size of one or more limbs. SYN megalomelia.

mac·ro·mol·e·cule (mak′rō-mol′ĕ-kyūl) A molecule of colloidal size (e.g., proteins, polynucleic acids).

mac·ro·nor·mo·blast (mak′rō-nōr′mō-blast) 1. A large normoblast. 2. A large, incompletely hemoglobiniferous, nucleated red blood cell with a "cartwheel" nucleus.

mac·ro·nu·cle·us (mak′rō-nū′klē-ŭs) 1. A nucleus that occupies a relatively large portion of the cell, or the larger nucleus where two or more are present in a cell. 2. The larger of the two nuclei in ciliates, which governs vegetative metabolic functions and not reproduction. SEE ALSO micronucleus (2).

mac·ro·nu·tri·ent (mak′rō-nū′trē-ĕnt) Nutrients required in the greatest amount; e.g., carbohydrates, protein, fats.

mac·ro·phage, mac·ro·pha·gus (mak′rō-fāj, mă-krof′ă-gŭs) Any mononuclear, actively phagocytic cell arising from monocytic stem cells in bone marrow; these cells are widely distributed and vary in morphology and motility.

mac·ro·phage ac·ti·va·ting fac·tor (mak′rō-fāj ak′ti-vāt-ing fak′tŏr) Growth factor that induces lymphocytes to prime macrophages to become active against tumor cells.

mac·roph·thal·mi·a (mak′rof-thal′mē-ă) SYN megalophthalmos.

mac·ro·pol·y·cyte (mak′rō-pol′ē-sīt) An unusually large polymorphonuclear neutrophilic leukocyte that contains a multisegmented nucleus (e.g., 8, 10, or more lobes); frequently observed in pernicious anemia and certain other forms of anemia.

ma·crop·si·a (mă-krop′sē-ă) Perception of objects as larger than they are.

mac·ro·scop·ic (mak′rō-skop′ik) 1. Of a size visible with the naked eye or without the use of a microscope. 2. Relating to macroscopy.

mac·ro·scop·ic a·nat·o·my (mak′rō-skop′ik ă-nat′ŏ-mē) SYN gross anatomy.

ma·cro·sis (mă-krō′sis) Increase in length or volume.

mac·u·la, gen. and pl. **mac·u·lae, mac·ules** (mak′yū-lă, mak′yū-lē, mak′yūlz) [TA] 1. A small spot, perceptibly different in color from the surrounding tissue. 2. A small, discolored patch or spot on the skin, neither elevated above nor depressed below the skin's surface. 3. In ocular anatomy, indicates retinal area located within the major vascular arcades, temporal to the optic nerve. SYN spot (1).

mac·u·la ad·he·rens (mak′yū-lă ad-hē′rens) SYN desmosome.

mac·u·la al·bi·da, pl. **mac·u·lae al·bi·dae** (mak′yū-lă al-bī′dă, -ē) Gray-white or white, rounded or irregularly shaped, slightly opaque patches or spots that are sometimes observed postmortem in the epicardium, especially in middle-aged or older people. SYN tache blanche, tache laiteuse (2), tendinous spot, white spot.

mac·u·la cer·u·le·a (mak′yū-lă sĕ-rū′lē-ă) Blue discolorations of skin caused by bites from fleas or lice. SYN blue spot.

mac·u·la den·sa (mak′yū-lă den′să) A closely packed group of densely staining cells in the distal tubular epithelium of a nephron, in direct apposition to the juxtaglomerular cells.

mac·u·lar de·gen·er·a·tion (mak′yū-lăr dĕ-jen′ĕr-ā′shŭn) A progressive deterioration of the macula lutea resulting in the loss of central vision. SYN age-related macular degeneration.

mac·u·lar ret·i·nal dys·tro·phy (mak′yū-lăr ret′i-năl dis′trō-fē) Disorders primarily involving the back of the ocular fundus; due to degeneration in the sensory layer of the retina.

mac·u·lo·ce·re·bral (mak′ū-lō-ser′ĕ-brăl) Relating to the macula lutea and the brain; denoting a type of nervous disease marked by degenerative lesions in both the retina and the brain.

mac·u·lo·pap·u·lar rash (mak′yū-lō-pap′yū-lăr rash) Skin disorder with spots, bumps, and lumps.

mac·u·lop·a·thy (mak′yū-lop′ă-thē)

Any pathologic condition of the macula lutea. SYN macular retinopathy.

mad·a·ro·sis (mad'ă-rō'sis) SYN milphosis.

mad cow dis·ease (mad kow di-zēz') SYN bovine spongiform encephalopathy.

Ma·de·lung de·form·i·ty (mah'dĕ-lūng dĕ-fōrm'i-tē) A distal radioulnar subluxation due to a relative deficiency of axial growth of the medial side of the distal radius, which, as a consequence, is abnormally inclined proximally and ulnarward.

Ma·de·lung neck (mah'dĕ-lūng nek) Multiple symmetric lipomatoses (Madelung disease) confined to the neck.

mad·ness (măd-nĕs) *Avoid this imprecise and meaningless term.* The state of being mentally ill.

Mad·u·ra foot (mă-dū'ră fut) SYN mycetoma.

Mad·u·rel·la (mad'yū-rel'ă) A genus of fungi including a number of species that cause mycetoma.

ma·du·ro·my·co·sis (ma-dū'rō-mī-kō'sis) SYN mycetoma (1).

Maf·fuc·ci syn·drome (mă-fū'chē sin'drŏm) Enchondromas of the limbs in association with venous and lymphaticovenous malformation; propensity to develop other benign or malignant tumors.

mag·al·drate (mag'al-drāt) An antacid with aluminum hydroxide and magnesium hydroxide.

mag·got (mag'ŏt) A fly larva or grub.

mag·ic·al think·ing (maj'i-kăl thingk'ing) Irrational belief that one can bring about a circumstance or event by thinking about it or wishing for it; normal in preschool children, it also occurs in schizophrenia.

mag·ma (mag'mă) **1.** A soft mass left after extraction of the active principles. **2.** A salve or thick paste.

mag·ne·si·um (Mg) (mag-nē'zē-ŭm) An alkaline earth element that oxidizes to magnesia; a bioelement; many salts have clinical applications.

mag·ne·si·um cit·rate (mag-nē'zē-ŭm sit'rāt, sī'trāt) Laxative usually administered as an effervescent flavored beverage.

mag·ne·si·um ox·ide (mag-nē'zē-ŭm ok'sīd) An antacid and laxative. SYN calcined magnesia, magnesia.

mag·ne·si·um sa·lic·y·late (mag-nē'zē-ŭm să-lis'i-lāt) Sodium-free salicylate derivative with antiinflammatory, analgesic, and antipyretic actions; used for relief of mild to moderate pain.

mag·ne·si·um sul·fate ($MgSO_4$) (mag-nē'zē-ŭm sŭl'fāt) Active ingredient of most natural laxative waters; used as a fast-acting cathartic in certain poisonings. SYN Epsom salts.

mag·ne·si·um tri·sil·i·cate (mag-nē'zē-ŭm trī-sil'i-kāt) Compound of magnesium oxide and silicon dioxide with varying proportions of water; a gastric antacid.

mag·net·ic field (H) (mag-net'ik fēld) The sphere of influence of a magnet.

mag·net·ic res·o·nance an·gi·og·ra·phy (mag-net'ik rez'ŏ-năns an'jē-og'ră-fē) Method of visualizing vessels that contain flowing nuclei by producing a contrast between them and the stationary nuclei.

mag·net·ic res·o·nance im·a·ging (MRI) (mag-net'ik rez'ŏ-năns im'ăj-ing) A diagnostic modality in which the magnetic nuclei (especially protons) of a patient are aligned in a strong, uniform magnetic field, absorb energy from tuned radiofrequency pulses, and emit radiofrequency signals as their excitation decays.

mag·ni·fi·ca·tion (mag'ni-fi-kā'shŭn) **1.** The seeming increase in size of an object viewed under the microscope. **2.** The increased amplitude of a tracing, caused by the use of a lever with a long writing arm.

Ma·haim fi·ber (mă-hām' fī'bĕr) Area of cardiac electrical conductivity between the atrioventricular node and the septum. SYN nodoventricular fibers.

main·te·nance (mān'těn-ăns) The extent to which the patient continues good heath practices without supervision, incorporating them into a general lifestyle. Cf. compliance.

main·te·nance drug ther·a·py (mān'tě-nǎns drŭg thār'ă-pē) In chemotherapy, systematic dosage at a level that maintains protection against exacerbation.

main·te·nance of wake·ful·ness test (mān'tě-nǎns wāk'fŭl-něs test) Assessment that lasts up to 8 hours in which a patient is studied during naps and wakefulness in a sleep-inducing environment.

ma·jor (mā'jŏr) *This form of the adjective is used with masculine nouns (sulcus major, plural sulci majores) and feminine nouns (pelvis major, plural pelves majores). With neuter nouns the form majus is used (omentum majus, plural omenta majora).* Larger or greater in size of two similar structures.

ma·jor ag·glu·ti·nin (mā'jŏr ă-glū'ti-nin) Immune agglutinin present in greatest quantity in an antiserum and evoked by the most dominant of a mosaic of antigens. SYN chief agglutinin.

ma·jor con·nec·tor (mā'jŏr kŏ-nek'tŏr) Plate or bar used to unite partial denture bases.

ma·jor de·pres·sion, ma·jor de·pres·sive dis·or·der (MD) (mā'jŏr dě-presh'ŏn, dě-pres'iv dis-ŏr'děr) Mental illness characterized by sustained depression of mood, anhedonia, sleep and appetite disturbances, and feelings of worthlessness, guilt, and hopelessness. SYN clinical depression.

ma·jor for·ceps (mā'jŏr fŏr'seps) Occipital radiation of the corpus callosum. SYN forceps major.

ma·jor his·to·com·pat·i·bil·i·ty com·plex (mā'jŏr his'tō-kŏm-pat'i-bil'i-tē kom'pleks) Linked loci, collectively termed HLA complex in humans, which codes for cell-surface histocompatibility antigens and is the principal determinant of tissue type and transplant compatibility. SEE ALSO human leukocyte antigens.

mal (mahl) A disease or disorder.

ma·la (mā'lă) **1.** SYN cheek.

mal·ab·sorp·tion (mal'ăb-sōrp'shŭn) Imperfect, inadequate, or otherwise disordered gastrointestinal absorption.

mal·ab·sorp·tion syn·drome (mal'ăb-sōrp'shŭn sin'drŏm) A state characterized by diverse features (e.g., diarrhea, weakness, edema) due to any of several conditions with ineffective absorption of nutrients (e.g., sprue, gluten-induced enteropathy).

-malacia Combining form indicating softening of a structure.

ma·la·ci·a (mă-lā'shē-ă) Softening or loss of consistency and contiguity in any of the organs or tissues. SYN mollities (2), malacosis.

mal·a·co·sis (mal'ă-kō'sis) SYN malacia.

mal·ad·ap·tion (mal'ă-dap'shŭn) Having difficulty dealing with change or adjusting to a new environment.

mal·ad·just·ment (mal'ăd-jŭst'měnt) PSYCHOLOGY/PSYCHIATRY an inability to cope with the problems and challenges of everyday living.

mal·a·dy (mal'ă-dē) A disease or illness.

ma·laise (mă-lāz') A feeling of general discomfort or uneasiness, often the first indication of disease.

mal·a·lign·ment (mal'ă-līn'měnt) Displacement of a tooth or teeth from a normal position in the dental arch.

ma·lar (mā'lăr) Relating to the mala, the cheek or cheek bones.

ma·lar·i·a (mă-lar'ē-ă) A disease caused by the presence of the sporozoan *Plasmodium* in the erythrocyte phase, usually transmitted by the bite of an infected female mosquito of the genus *Anopheles.* Characterized by episodic severe chills and high fever, prostration, and occasionally death or immunologically mediated sequelae. SEE ALSO *Plasmodium.* SYN swamp fever (2).

Ma·las·se·zi·a (mal'ă-sē'zē-ă) A genus of fungi of low pathogenicity that lack the ability to synthesize medium- and long-chain fatty acids and require an exogenous supply of these lipids for growth.

mal·ate (mal´āt) A salt or ester of malic acid.

mal·ax·a·tion (mal´ak-sā´shŭn) **1.** Formation of ingredients into a mass for pills and plasters. **2.** A kneading process in massage.

mal de Me·le·da (mahl dĕ mā-lā´dă) An autosomal recessive skin disorder affecting the palms of the hand and the soles of the feet.

male (māl) **1.** ZOOLOGY denoting the sex to which those belong that produce spermatozoa; an individual of that sex. **2.** SYN masculine.

ma·le·ic ac·id (mă-lē´ik as´id) Butenedioic acid; used for preparing maleate salts. SYN toxilic acid.

male pat·tern al·o·pe·ci·a, male pat·tern bald·ness (māl pat´ĕrn al´ŏ-pē´shē-ă, bawld´nĕs) Most common form of androgenic alopecia, seen in men as receding frontal and bilateral triangular temple hair lines, and a balding patch on the vertex; may progress to complete alopecia.

mal·for·ma·tion (mal´fōr-mā´shŭn) Failure of proper or normal development; a primary structural defect due to a localized error of morphogenesis.

mal·func·tion (mal-fŭngk´shŭn) Disordered, inadequate, or abnormal function.

mal·ic ac·id (mal´ik as´id) Hydroxysuccinic acid; found in apples and various other tart fruits.

ma·lig·nan·cy (mă-lig´năn-sē) The property or condition of being malignant.

ma·lig·nant (mă-lig´nănt) **1.** Resistant to treatment; occurring in severe form, and frequently fatal; tending to become worse and leading to an ingravescent course. **2.** In reference to a neoplasm, having the property of locally invasive and destructive growth and metastasis. **3.** Cancerous.

ma·lig·nant a·troph·ic pap·u·lo·sis (MAP) (mă-lig´nănt ā-trō´fik pap´yū-

lō´sis) Cutaneovisceral syndrome characterized by pathognomonic umbilicated porcelain-white papules with elevated telangiectatic anular borders, followed by the development of intestinal ulcers that perforate, causing peritonitis. SYN Degos disease, Degos syndrome.

ma·lig·nant en·do·car·di·tis (mă-lig´nănt en´dō-kahr-dī´tis) Acute bacterial endocarditis, usually secondary to suppuration elsewhere. SYN septic endocarditis.

ma·lig·nant fi·brous his·ti·o·cy·to·ma (mă-lig´nănt fī´brŭs his´tē-ō-sī-tō´mă) A deeply situated tumor, especially on the extremities of adults, frequently recurring after surgery and metastasizing to the lungs.

ma·lig·nant hep·a·to·ma (mă-lig´nănt hep´ă-tō´mă) Cancer derived from parenchymal cells of the liver. SYN hepatocarcinoma.

ma·lig·nant hy·per·py·rex·i·a (mă-lig´nănt hī´pĕr-pī-rek´sē-ă) SYN heatstroke.

ma·lig·nant hy·per·ten·sion (mă-lig´nănt hī´pĕr-ten´shŭn) Severe hypertension that runs a rapid course, causing necrosis of arteriolar walls in kidney and retina, hemorrhages, and death; most frequently due to uremia or rupture of a cerebral vessel.

ma·lig·nant hy·per·ther·mi·a (mă-lig´nănt hī´pĕr-thĕr´mē-ă) Rapid onset of extremely high fever with muscle rigidity, precipitated by exogenous agents in susceptible people.

ma·lig·nant lym·pho·ma (mă-lig´nănt lim-fō´mă) General term for neoplasms of lymphoid and reticuloendothelial tissues that present as solid tumors composed of cells that appear primitive or resemble lymphocytes, plasma cells, or histiocytes. Hodgkin disease and Burkitt lymphoma are specific forms.

ma·lig·nant my·o·pi·a (mă-lig´nănt mī-ō´pē-ă) SYN pathologic myopia.

ma·lig·nant tu·mor (mă-lig´nănt tū´mŏr) Lesion that invades surrounding tissues, is usually capable of producing metastases, may recur after attempted removal,

M

and is likely to kill the host unless adequately treated. SEE ALSO cancer.

ma·lin·ger·ing (mă-ling′gĕr-ing) Feigning illness or inability to work due to an ulterior motive.

mal·le·a·ble (mal′ē-ă-bĕl) Capable of being shaped by being beaten or by pressure (e.g., gold, silver).

mal·let fin·ger (mal′ĕt fing′gĕr) Avulsion, partial or complete, of the long finger extensor from the base of the distal phalanx, resulting in the inability to fully extend the distal interphalangeal joint actively. SYN baseball finger, drop finger, hammer finger.

Mal·lo·ry bod·ies (mal′ŏr-ē bod′ēz) Large, poorly defined accumulations of eosinophilic material in the cytoplasm of damaged hepatic cells in cirrhosis and marked fatty change especially due to alcoholism.

mal·nu·tri·tion (mal′nū-trish′ŭn) Faulty nutrition resulting from malabsorption, poor diet, or overeating.

mal·oc·clu·sion (mal′ŏ-klū′zhŭn) **1.** Any deviation from a physiologically acceptable contact of opposing dentitions. **2.** Any deviation from a normal occlusion.

mal·pi·ghi·an cor·pus·cles (mal-pig′ē-ăn kōr′pŭs-ĕlz) **1.** SYN renal corpuscle. **2.** SYN splenic lymph follicles.

mal·pi·ghi·an lay·er (mal-pig′ē-ăn lā′ĕr) SYN malpighian stratum.

mal·pi·ghi·an re·te (mal-pig′ē-ăn rē′tē) SYN malpighian stratum.

mal·pigh·i·an strat·um (mahl-pig′ē-ăn strā′tŭm) Epidermal layer including the stratum basale, stratum spimosum, and stratum granulosum. SYN malpighian layer.

mal·po·si·tion (mal′pŏ-zish′ŭn) SYN dystopia.

mal·prac·tice (mal-prak′tis) Mistreatment of a patient through ignorance, carelessness, neglect, or criminal intent.

mal·pre·sen·ta·tion (mal′prez-ĕn-tā′shŭn) Faulty presentation of the fetus; presentation of any part other than the occiput.

MALT·o·ma (mawl-tō′-mă) B-cell lymphoma of *m*ucosa-*a*ssociated *l*ymphoid *t*issue. SYN extranodal marginal zone lymphoma.

mal·tose (mawl′tōs) A disaccharide formed in the hydrolysis of starch and consisting of two D-glucose residues.

ma·lum (mā′lŭm) A disease.

mal·un·ion (mal-yūn′yŭn) Faulty union of the ends of a broken bone resulting in a deformity or a crooked limb. SYN vicious union.

mam·ma, gen. and pl. **mam·mae** (mam′ă, -ē) [TA] SEE ALSO mammary gland. SYN breast.

mam·mal (mam′ăl) An animal of the class Mammalia.

mam·mal·gi·a (mă-mal′jē-ă) SYN mastodynia.

Mam·ma·li·a (mă-mā′lē-ă) The highest class of living organisms; includes all vertebrate animals (monotremes, marsupials, and placentals) that suckle their young, possess hair, and (except for the egg-laying monotremes) bring forth living young rather than eggs.

mam·ma·plas·ty, mam·mo·plas·ty, mas·to·plas·ty (mam′ă-plas-tē, mam′ō-, mas′tō-) Surgical procedure of the breast to alter its shape, size, or position, or all of these. SYN mammoplasty, mastoplasty.

mam·ma·ry (măm′ă-rē) Relating to the breasts.

mam·ma·ry duct ec·ta·si·a (măm′ă-rē dŭkt ek-tā′zē-ă) Dilation of mammary ducts by lipid and cellular debris in older women; rupture of ducts may result in granulomatous inflammation and infiltration by plasma cells. SEE ALSO plasma cell mastitis.

mam·ma·ry gland (măm′ă-rē gland) [TA] Potential and active compound, alveolar, mostly merocrine (with possible apocrine components) milk-secreting gland lying within the breast. SEE ALSO breast (2). SYN glandula mammaria [TA], lactiferous gland, milk gland.

mam·ma·ry neu·ral·gi·a (mam´ăr-ē nŭr-al´gē-ă) Neuralgia of the intercostal nerve or nerves supplying the breast.

mam·ma·ry souf·fle (mam´ăr-ē sū´fĕl) Blowing murmur heard late in pregnancy and during lactation at the medial border of the breast, sometimes only systolic and sometimes continuous.

mam·mec·to·my (mă-mek´tŏ-mē) SYN mastectomy.

mam·mi·form (mam´i-fŏrm) Resembling a breast. SYN mammose (1).

mammil-, mammilli- Combining forms indicating the mammillae.

mam·mil·la, mamil·la, pl. **mam·mil·lae** (mă-mil´ă, -ē) **1.** A small rounded elevation resembling the female breast. **2.** SYN nipple.

mam·mil·la·plas·ty (mă-mil´ă-plas-tē) Plastic surgery of the nipple and areola.

mam·mil·la·re (mam´i-lar-ē) [TA] SYN mammillary.

mam·mil·lar·i·a (mam´i-lar´ē-ă) SEE mammillary body.

mam·mil·lary (mam´i-lar-ē) Nipplelike. SYN mammillare.

mam·mil·lar·y bod·y (mam´i-lar-ē bod´ē) [TA] A small, round, paired cell group that protrudes into the interpeduncular fossa from the inferior aspect of the hypothalamus. SYN corpus mammillare [TA].

mam·mil·lar·y ducts (mam´i-lar-ē dŭkts) SYN lactiferous ducts.

mam·mil·la·tion (mam´i-lā´shŭn) A nipplelike projection.

mam·mil·li·tis (mam´i-lī´tis) Inflammation of the nipple.

mammo- Combining form indicating the breasts.

mam·mo·gram (mam´ō-gram) The record produced by mammography.

mam·mog·ra·phy (mă-mog´ră-fē) Im-

aging examination of the breast by means of x-rays; used for screening and diagnosis of breast disease.

Mam·mo·mon·o·ga·mus (mam´ō-mon-og´ă-mus) Genus of syngamid trematodes found in the respiratory system of ruminants and occasionally reported in humans.

mam·mo·plas·ty (mam´ō-plas-tē) SYN mammaplasty.

mam·mose (mam´ōs) **1.** SYN mammiform. **2.** Having large breasts.

mam·mot·o·my (ma-mot´ŏ-mē) SYN mastotomy.

mam·mot·ro·pic, mam·mo·tro·phic (mam´ō-trō´pik, -trō´fik) Having a stimulating effect on the development, growth, or function of the mammary glands.

man·aged care (man´ăjd kār) System in the U.S. whereby a third-party payer (e.g., insurance company, government) mediates between physicians and patients, negotiating fees for service and overseeing treatment given.

man·da·to·ry breath (man´dă-tōr-ē breth) A breath for which either the timing or size is controlled by a ventilator; the machine starts or ends the breath.

man·di·ble (man´di-bĕl) [TA] A U-shaped bone, forming the lower jaw, articulating by its upturned extremities with the temporal bone on either side. SYN jaw bone, mandibula.

man·dib·u·la, pl. **man·dib·u·lae** (man-dib´yū-lă, -lē) [TA] SYN mandible.

man·dib·u·lar (man-dib´yū-lăr) Relating to the lower jaw. SYN inframaxillary.

man·dib·u·lar arch (man-dib´yū-lăr ahrch) The first pharyngeal or postoral arch in the pharyngeal (branchial *in fish*) arch series.

man·dib·u·lar block (man-dib´yū-lăr blok) A nerve block injection used in dentistry.

man·dib·u·lo·fa·cial dys·o·sto·sis (man-dib´yū-lō-fā´shăl dis´os-tō´sis) SYN Treacher Collins syndrome.

man·dib·u·lo·oc·u·lo·fa·cial (man-dib´

M

yū-lō-ok′yū-lō-fā′shăl) Relating to the mandible and the facial orbit.

man·drel, man·dril (man′drĕl, man′dril) **1.** The shaft or spindle to which a tool is attached and by means of which it is rotated. **2.** SYN mandrin. **3.** DENTISTRY an instrument used in a handpiece to hold a disc, stone, or cup used for grinding, smoothing, or finishing.

man·drin (man′drin) A stiff wire or stylet inserted into the lumen of a soft catheter to give it shape and firmness while passing through a hollow tubular structure. SYN mandrel (2), mandril.

man·ga·nese (Mn) (mang′gă-nēz) A metallic element resembling and often associated, in ores, with iron; its salts are sometimes used in medicine.

♻ **-mania** Suffix indicating an abnormal love for, or morbid impulse toward, some specific object, place, or action.

man·ic episode, ma·ni·a (ME) (man′ik ep′i-sōd, mā′nē-ă) Manifestation of major mood disorder involving enduring periods of persistent and significant elevated, expansive, or irritable mood, and associated symptoms including decreased sleep, psychomotor speeding, racing thoughts, flight of ideas, grandiosity, and poor judgment leading to behavior that may later be regretted. SEE bipolar disorder.

man·i·fes·ta·tion (man′i-fes-tā′shŭn) The display or disclosure of characteristic signs or symptoms of an illness.

man·i·fest con·tent (man′i-fest kon′tent) Those elements of fantasy and dreams that are consciously available and reportable.

man·i·fest hy·per·o·pi·a (man′i-fest hī′pĕr-ō′pē-ă) Part of a disorder of optic long-sightedness that cannot be corrected by a physiologic response of the ciliary muscle.

man·i·fest·ing het·er·o·zy·gote (man′i-fest′ing het′ĕr-ō-zī′gōt) An organism heterozygous for what is ordinarily a recessive condition, which, as a result of special mechanisms (e.g., lyonization), has phenotypic manifestations.

man·i·kin, man·ni·kin, man·ne·quin

(man′i-kin) A model, especially one with movable pieces, of the human body or any of its parts. SEE ALSO phantom (2).

man·ip·u·la·tion (mă-nip′yū-lā′shŭn) **1.** Skillful manual exploration of an object or person. SEE ALSO mobilization. **2.** A passive therapeutic intervention associated with small-amplitude high-velocity movement at the end of a subject's available range of motion in a joint.

man-made death (man′mād deth) **1.** SYN euthanasia. **2.** SYN slow code.

man·nose (man′ōs) An aldohexose obtained from various plant sources (i.e., from mannans).

man·no·si·do·sis (man′ō-si-dō′sis) Congenital deficiency of α-mannosidase and mannose in tissues; associated with coarse facial features, enlarged tongue, mental retardation, kyphosis, radiographic skeletal abnormalities, and vacuolated lymphocytes.

ma·nom·e·ter (mă-nom′ĕ-tĕr) *Avoid the misspelling/mispronunciation monometer.* An instrument for indicating the pressure of any fluid or the difference in pressure between two fluids, whether gas or liquid.

ma·nom·e·try (mă-nom′ĕ-trē) *Avoid the misspelling/mispronunciation monometry.* Measurement of the pressure of gases or fluids by means of a manometer. SYN manoscopy.

Man·so·ni·a (man-sō′nē-ă) A genus of brown or black medium-sized mosquitoes, distributed worldwide and, in the tropics, are important vectors of *Brugia malayi.*

Man·so·ni schis·to·so·mi·a·sis (man-sō′nī skis′tō-sŏ-mī′ă-sis) SYN schistosomiasis mansoni.

man·tle (man′tĕl) A covering layer.

man·tle cell lym·pho·ma (man′tĕl sel lim-fō′mă) A clinically and biologically distinct B-cell neoplasm with a recurring acquired genetic abnormality, and a heterogeneous histologic appearance that may lead to confusion with reactive or other neoplastic lymphoproliferative disorders.

man·tle ra·di·o·ther·a·py (man'těl rā'dē-ō-thār'ă-pē) Radiotherapy with protection of uninvolved radiosensitive structures or organs.

Man·toux test (mahn-tū' test) SEE tuberculin test.

man·u·al air·way ma·neu·ver (man'yū-ăl ār'wā mă-nū'vĕr) SYN head-tilt/chin-lift maneuver.

man·u·al lymph drain·age (man'yū-ăl limf drān'ăj) Massage technique to promote absorption of interstitial fluid by stimulating flow in lymphatic channels. SYN lymph drainage.

man·u·al mus·cle test·ing (MMT) (man'yū-ăl mŭs'ĕl test'ing) Assessment modality for the strength of a muscle through manual evaluation. Rating is done by moving the involved part through its full-range of motion against gravity and then against gravity with resistance.

ma·nu·bri·um, pl. **ma·nu·bri·a** (mă-nū'brē-ŭm, -ă) [TA] The portion of the sternum or of the malleus that represents the handle.

man·u·dy·na·mom·e·ter (man'yū-dī'nă-mom'ĕ-tĕr) In dentistry, a device for measuring the force exerted by the thrust of an instrument.

ma·nus (mā'nŭs) [TA] SYN hand.

map (map) A representation of a region or structure; e.g., of a stretch of DNA.

ma·ple syr·up u·rine dis·ease (mā'pĕl sir'ŭp yūr'in di-zēz') Inborn error of metabolism caused by defective oxidative decarboxylation of α-keto acids of leucine, isoleucine, and valine; manifestations include feeding difficulties, physical and mental retardation, and a urine odor similar to that of maple syrup; neonatal death is common. SYN branched chain ketoaciduria, branched chain ketonuria, ketoacidemia.

map·ping (map'ing) The process of identifying the relative position of sites or elements.

Ma·ra·ñón sign (mahr-ahn-yōn' sīn) In Graves disease, a vasomotor reaction following stimulation of the skin over the throat.

ma·ras·moid (mă-raz'moyd) Resembling marasmus.

ma·ras·mus (mă-raz'mŭs) Cachexia, especially in young children, primarily due to prolonged dietary deficiency of protein and calories. SYN Parrot disease (2).

mar·ble bones (mahr'bĕl bōnz) SYN osteopetrosis.

Mar·burg dis·ease, Mar·burg vi·rus dis·ease (mahr'bŭrg di-zēz', vī'rŭs) Infection caused by a virus of the genus *Marburg*. The virus is "pantropic" and affects most organ systems. The disease is characterized by a prominent rash and hemorrhages in many organs and often fatal. Some person-to-person spread has been observed.

march frac·ture (mahrch frak'shŭr) A stress fracture in the shaft of a metatarsal bone, most often at the first metatarsal due to prolonged running or walking in military recruits unaccustomed to such activity.

march he·mo·glob·i·nu·ri·a (mahrch hē'mŏ-glō'bi-nyūr'ē-ă) Blood disorder occurring after marathon races, protracted marching, or heavy physical exercise.

Mar·chi·a·fa·va-Big·na·mi dis·ease (mahr-kē-ă-fah'vah-bēn-yah'mē di-zēz') A disorder characterized by demyelination of the corpus callosum and cortical laminar necrosis involving the frontal and temporal lobes; predominantly in chronic alcoholics, particularly wine drinkers.

Mar·cus Gunn phe·nom·e·non, Mar·cus Gunn syn·drome (mahr'kŭs gŭn fē-nom'ĕ-non, sin'drōm) SYN jaw-winking syndrome.

Mar·fan syn·drome (mahr-fahn' sin'drōm) A connective tissue multisystemic disorder characterized by skeletal changes (arachnodactyly, long limbs, joint laxity, pectus excavatum), cardiovascular defects (aortic aneurysm, which may dissect, mitral valve prolapse), and ectopia lentis.

mar·gin (mahr'jin) [TA] A boundary, edge, or border, as of a surface or structure. SEE ALSO border. SYN margo [TA].

mar·gi·nal bleph·a·ri·tis (mahr´ji-năl blef´ăr-ī´tis) SYN blepharitis marginalis.

mar·gi·nal zone lym·pho·ma (mahr´ji-năl zōn lim-fō´mă) A heterogeneous group of neoplasms originating from the B-cell-rich zones of the lymph nodes, spleen, or extranodal lymphoid tissue. Those tumors originating from mucosa-associated lymphoid tissue (MALT), most often in the stomach, intestines, salivary glands, and lungs, are called MALTomas.

mar·gin·a·tion (mahr´ji-nā´shŭn) A phenomenon that occurs during the relatively early phases of inflammation; as a result of dilation of capillaries and slowing of the bloodstream, leukocytes tend to occupy the periphery of the cross-sectional lumen and adhere to the endothelial cells that line the vessels.

mar·gi·no·plas·ty (mahr´ji-nō-plas-tē) Plastic surgery of the tarsal border of an eyelid.

mar·go, gen. **mar·gi·nis** (mahr´gō, -ji-nis) [TA] SYN margin, border.

Ma·rie hy·per·tro·phy (mah-rē´ hī-pĕr´trō-fē) Enlargement of the joints due to a chronic periostitis.

mar·i·jua·na, mar·i·hu·a·na (mahr´i-hwahn´ă) Popular name for the dried flowering leaves of *Cannabis sativa,* which are smoked as cigarettes, "joints," or "blunts." In the U.S., marijuana includes any part of, or any extracts from, the female plant. SEE ALSO cannabis.

Ma·rine-Len·hart syn·drome (mah´rēn-len´hahrt sin´drōm) Toxic multinodular goiter.

mark·er (mahrk´ĕr) **1.** A device used to make a mark or to indicate measurement. **2.** A characteristic or factor by which a cell or molecule can be recognized or identified. **3.** A locus containing two or more alleles that, being harmless, are common and therefore yield high frequencies of heterozygotes that facilitate linkage analysis.

mark·er trait (mahr´kĕr trāt) A trait that may be of little importance in itself but which by association, linkage, or other means facilitates the detection, anticipation, or understanding of a disease or (for genetic diseases) the localization of the causative gene on the karyotype.

mar·riage ther·a·py, mari·i·tal ther·a·py (măr´ij thār´ă-pē, mar´i-tăl) Family therapy that involves both husband and wife and focuses on a relationship as it affects the individual personalities, behaviors, and psychopathologies of the partners.

mar·row (mar´ō) [TA] A highly cellular hematopoietic connective tissue filling the medullary cavities and spongy epiphyses of bones that becomes predominantly fatty with age, particularly in the long bones of the limbs.

mar·row-mes·en·chyme con·nec·tions (mar´ō-mez´ĕn´kīm kŏ-nek´shŭnz) Uninterrupted continuations between bone marrow and mesenchyme of fetal and newborn middle ears.

Mar·seilles fe·ver (mahr-sā´ fē´vĕr) SYN Mediterranean spotted fever.

Mar·shall-Mar·chet·ti-Krantz op·er·a·tion, Mar·shall-Mar·chet·ti op·er·a·tion (mahr´shăl mahr-chet´ē krants op-ĕr-ā´shŭn) Surgery for urinary stress incontinence, performed retropubically.

mar·su·pi·al·i·za·tion (mahr-sū´pē-ăl-ī-zā´shŭn) Exteriorization of a cyst or other such enclosed cavity by resecting the anterior wall and suturing the cut edges of the remaining wall to adjacent edges of the skin, thereby creating a pouch.

Mar·ti·not·ti cell (mahr-ti-nawt´tē sel) A small multipolar nerve cell with short branching dendrites scattered through various layers of the cerebral cortex.

mas·cu·line (mas´kyū-lin) Relating to or marked by the characteristics of the male sex or gender. SYN male (2).

mas·cu·lin·i·za·tion (mas´kyū-lin-ī-zā´shŭn) Condition marked by attainment of male characteristics, such as facial hair, either physiologically as part of male maturation, or pathologically by individuals of either sex.

mask (mask) **1.** Any disease state producing alteration or discoloration of the skin of the face. **2.** The expressionless appearance seen in certain diseases (e.g., Parkinson facies). **3.** A facial bandage. **4.** A shield designed to cover the mouth and nose for maintenance of aseptic conditions.

mask·ed (maskt) **1.** Concealed. **2.** SYN blind.

mask·ed gout (maskt gowt) SYN latent gout.

mask·ed vi·rus (maskt vī'rŭs) One ordinarily occurring in the host in a noninfective state, but which may be activated and demonstrated by special procedures such as blind passage in experimental animals.

mask·ing (mask'ing) **1.** The use of noise of any kind to interfere with the audibility of another sound. **2.** AUDIOLOGY application of a noise applied to one ear while testing the hearing acuity of the other ear.

mask of preg·nan·cy (mask preg'năn-sē) SYN melasma.

mas·och·ism (mas'ŏ-kizm) Passive algolagnia; a form of perversion, often sexual in nature, in which a person experiences pleasure in being abused, humiliated, or maltreated. Cf. sadism.

ma·son's lung (mā'sŏnz lŭng) Silicosis occurring in stone masons.

mass, mas·sa (mas, mas'ă) **1.** A lump or aggregation of coherent material. **2.** PHARMACY a soft but solid preparation containing an active medicinal agent, of such consistency that it can be divided into small pieces and rolled into pills. **3.** One of the seven fundamental quantities in the Système International d'Unitès; its unit is the kilogram (kg).

mas·sage (mă-sahzh') Body manipulation using by rubbing, pinching, kneading, or tapping.

mas·sage the·ra·py, mas·so·ther·a·py (mă-sahzh' thăr'ă-pē, mas'ō-thār'ă-pē) A collection of modalities intended to improve health through manipulation of the body through human touch and the manipulation of soft tissues using rubbing, pinching, kneading, or tapping to increase circulation, improve muscle tone, and ameliorate the relaxation of the patient or client. SEE ALSO Swedish massage, reflexology, manual lymph drainage, craniosacral therapy, polarity therapy, shiatsu, acupressure, proprioceptive neuromuscular facilitation, bodywork.

mas·seur, mas·seuse (mă-sur', mă-suz') A person who massages.

mass me·di·an ae·ro·dy·nam·ic di·am·e·ter (mas mē'dē-ăn ār'ō-dī-nam'ik dī-am'ĕ-tĕr) The geometric mean of the aerodynamic diameters of a given sample of inhaled particles.

mass num·ber (A) (mas nŭm'bĕr) Atomic mass of a particular isotope relative to hydrogen-1 (or to 1/12 the mass of carbon 12); generally very close to the whole number represented by the sum of the protons and neutrons in the atomic nucleus of the isotope (indicated in the name or symbol of the isotope, e.g., oxygen-16, ^{16}O); not to be confused with the atomic weight of an element, which may include a number of isotopes in their natural proportion.

mass per·i·stal·sis (mas per'i-stal'sis) Forcible peristaltic movements of short duration, occurring only three or four times a day, which move the contents of the large intestine from one division to the next, as from the ascending to the transverse colon. SYN mass movement.

mass re·flex (mas rē'fleks) In gross spinal cord injury, as the stage of reflex activity follows the primary flaccidity of the shock, a condition arises in which a strong stimulus to any part of one of the paralyzed limbs will be followed by contraction of the hip, knee, and ankle of the same side.

mass spec·trom·e·try (MS) (mas spek-trom'ĕ-trē) The analysis obtained using a mass spectrograph.

mast- SEE masto-.

mas·tad·e·ni·tis (mast'ad-ĕ-nī'tis) SYN mastitis.

Mas·tad·e·no·vi·rus (mast-ad'ĕ-nō-vī'rŭs) A genus of the family Adenoviridae, including adenoviruses that infect mammals, with over 40 antigenic types (species) being infective for humans. They cause respiratory infections in children, epidemic acute respiratory disease in military recruits, acute follicular conjunctivitis in adults, epidemic keratocon-

M

junctivitis and gastroenteritis; many infections are inapparent.

mas·tat·ro·phy, mas·ta·tro·phi·a (mastat′rŏ-fē, -ă-trō′fē-ă) Atrophy or wasting of the breasts.

mast cell (MC) (mast sel) A connective tissue cell that contains coarse, basophilic, metachromatic granules; secretes heparin and histamine. SYN mastocyte.

mast cell leu·ke·mi·a (mast sel lūkē′mē-ă) SYN basophilic leukemia.

mas·tec·to·my (mas-tek′tŏ-mē) Excision of the breast. SYN mammectomy.

Mas·ter of Sci·ence in Nur·sing (MSN) (mas′tĕr sī′ĕns nŭrs′ing) A degree granted after a prescribed graduate program of nursing education.

Mas·ter two-step ex·er·cise test (mas′tĕr tū′step eks′ĕr-sīz test) Simple cardiac stress test; the patient is instructed to step up and down a single step or wooden block repeatedly.

mas·ti·cate (mas′ti-kāt) To chew.

mas·ti·ca·tion (mas′ti-kā′shŭn) Chewing food in preparation for deglutition and digestion.

mas·ti·ca·to·ry sys·tem (mas′ti-kă-tōrē sis′tĕm) Organs and structures primarily functioning in chewing: the jaws, teeth with their supporting structures, temporomandibular joint, muscles of mastication, tongue, lips, cheeks, and oral mucosa. SYN dental apparatus.

mas·ti·tis (mas-tī′tis) Inflammation of the breast. SYN mastadenitis.

mas·ti·tis ne·o·na·to·rum (mas-tī′tis nē′ō-nā-tō′rŭm) Inflammation in the secreting breast tissue of the newborn, usually staphylococcal.

mast leu·ko·cyte (mast lū′kō-sīt) SYN basophilic leukocyte.

♻ **masto-, mast-** Combining forms denoting the breast; the mastoid.

mas·to·cyte (mas′tō-sīt) SYN mast cell.

mas·to·cy·to·sis (mas′tō-sī-tō′sis) Abnormal proliferation of mast cells in a variety of tissues; may be systemic, involving a variety of organs, or cutaneous (urticaria pigmentosa).

mas·to·dyn·i·a (mas′tō-din′ē-ă) Pain in the breast. SYN mammalgia.

mas·toid (mast) (mas′toyd) **1.** Resembling a mamma; breast-shaped. **2.** Relating to the mastoid process. SYN mastoidal.

mas·toid cells (mas′toyd selz) [TA] Numerous small intercommunicating cavities in the mastoid process of the temporal bone that empty into the mastoid or tympanic antrum. SYN cellulae mastoideae [TA], mastoid air cells, mastoid sinuses.

mas·toi·dec·to·my (mas′toy-dek′tŏ-mē) Hollowing out of the mastoid process by curretting, gouging, drilling, or otherwise removing the bony partitions forming the mastoid cells.

mas·toi·di·tis (mas′toy-dī′tis) Inflammation of any part of the mastoid process.

mas·ton·cus (mas-tongk′ŭs) A tumor or swelling of the breasts.

mas·to·oc·cip·i·tal (mas′tō-ok-sip′i-tăl) Relating to the mastoid portion of the temporal bone and to the occipital bone, denoting the suture uniting them.

mas·top·a·thy (mas-top′ă-thē) Any disease of the breasts.

mas·to·pex·y (mas′tō-pek-sē) Surgical procedure to affix sagging breasts in a more elevated and normal position, often with some improvement in shape.

mas·to·pla·si·a, ma·zo·pla·si·a (mas′tō-plā′zē-ă, mā′zō-) Enlargement of the breast.

mas·to·plas·ty (mas′tō-plas-tē) SYN mammaplasty.

mas·top·to·sis (mas′top-tō′sis) Ptosis or sagging of the breast.

mas·tor·rha·gi·a (mas′tōr-ā′jē-ă) Hemorrhage from a breast.

mas·to·squa·mous (mas′tō-skwā′mŭs)

Relating to the mastoid and the squamous portion of the temporal bone.

mas·tot·o·my (mas-tot′ŏ-mē) Incision of the breast. SYN mammotomy.

mas·tur·ba·tion (mas′tŭr-bā′shŭn) Self-stimulation of the genitals for erotic pleasure, often resulting in orgasm.

match·ing (mach′ing) Process of making a study group and a comparison group in an epidemiologic study comparable with respect to extraneous or confounding factors (e.g., age, sex).

ma·te·ri·a (mă-tē′rē-ă) Substance or matter.

ma·te·ri·a al·ba (mă-tē′rē-ă al′bă) Accumulation or aggregation of microorganisms, desquamated epithelial cells, blood cells, and food debris loosely adherent to surfaces of plaques, teeth, gingiva, or dental appliances.

Ma·te·ri·al Safe·ty Da·ta Sheet (MSDS) (mă-tē′rē-ăl sāf′tē dā′tă shēt) Information sheets generally prepared by manufacturers listing ingredients by generic name, toxic properties, recommendations for safe use, and other important information.

ma·te·ri·a med·i·ca (mă-tē′rē-ă med′i-kă) Aspect of medical science concerned with the origin and preparation of drugs, their doses, and their mode of administration. SEE ALSO pharmacognosy, pharmacology.

ma·ter·nal (mă-tĕr′năl) Relating to or derived from the mother.

ma·ter·nal death (mă-tĕr′năl deth) Demise of a woman while pregnant or within 42 days after the termination of gestation, irrespective of the duration and site of pregnancy and the cause of death.

ma·ter·nal dep·ri·va·tion syn·drome (mă-tĕr′năl dep′ri-vā′shŭn) Failure to thrive seen in infants and young children exhibited as a constellation of physical signs, symptoms, and behaviors, usually associated with maternal loss, absence or neglect, and characterized by lack of responsiveness to the environment and often depression.

ma·ter·nal im·mu·ni·ty (mă-tĕr′năl i-myū′ni-tē) That acquired by a fetus because of maternal immunoglobulin G that passes through the placenta.

ma·ter·nal in·her·i·tance (mă-tĕr′năl in-her′i-tăns) Transmission of characters dependent on properties of the egg cytoplasm produced by nuclear genes or by mitochondrial genes or both.

ma·trix, pl. **ma·tri·ces** (mā′triks, -tri-sēz) [TA] **1.** Formative portion of a tooth or a nail. **2.** Intercellular substance of a tissue. **3.** Surrounding substance within which something is contained or embedded. **4.** A mold in which anything is cast or swaged. **5.** Rectangular array of numbers or symbol quantities that simplify the execution of linear operations of tedious complexity.

ma·trix band (mā′triks band) A metal or plastic band secured around the crown of a tooth to confine restorative material to be adapted into a prepared cavity.

ma·trix re·tain·er (mā′triks rē-tā′nĕr) Mechanical device designed to hold a matrix around a tooth during restorative procedures.

ma·trix un·guis (mā′triks ŭng′gwis) [TA] SYN nail matrix.

ma·trix ves·i·cles (mā′triks ves′i-kĕlz) Hydroxyapatite-containing, membrane-enclosed vesicles secreted by odontoblasts, osteoblasts, and some chondrocytes; believed to serve as nucleation centers for the mineralization process in dentin and bone.

mat·ter (mat′ĕr) SYN substance.

mat·tress su·ture (mat′trĕs sū′chŭr) Ligature using a double stitch that forms a loop about the tissue on both sides of a wound. SYN quilted suture.

mat·u·ra·tion (mach′ūr-ā′shŭn) **1.** Achievement of full development or growth. **2.** Developmental changes that lead to maturity. **3.** Processing of a macromolecule.

mat·u·ra·tion ar·rest (mach′ūr-ā′shŭn ă-rest′) Cessation of complete differentiation of cells at an immature stage.

ma·ture (mă-chūr′) **1.** Ripe; fully developed. **2.** To ripen; to become fully developed.

M

ma·ture cat·a·ract (mă-chūr′ kat′ăr-akt) A cataract in which both the nucleus and cortex are opaque.

ma·ture on·set di·a·bet·es of youth (MODY) (mă-chūr′ on′set dī′ă-bē′tēz yūth) SEE Type 2 diabetes.

Mau·rer dots (mow′rer dots) Finely granular precipitates or irregular cytoplasmic particles that usually occur diffusely in red blood cells infected with the trophozoites of *Plasmodium falciparum*, occasionally those of *P. malariae*.

Mauth·ner sheath (mowt′ner shēth) SYN axolemma.

max·il·la, gen. and pl. **max·il·lae** (mak-sil′ă, ē) [TA] An irregularly shaped pneumatized bone, supporting the superior teeth and taking part in the formation of the orbit, hard palate, and nasal cavity and containing the maxillary sinus. SYN upper jaw bone, upper jaw.

max·il·lar·y pro·trac·tion (mak′si-lar-ē prō-trak′shŭn) Facial anomaly in which the subnasion lies anterior to the orbital plane.

max·il·lo·fa·cial (mak-sil′ō-fā′shăl) Pertaining to the jaws and face.

max·il·lo·man·dib·u·lar (mak-sil′ō-man-dib′yū-lăr) Relating to the upper and lower jaws.

max·il·lo·man·dib·u·lar fix·a·tion (mak′si-lō-man-dib′yū-lăr fik-sā′shŭn) SYN intermaxillary fixation.

max·il·lot·o·my (mak′si-lot′ŏ-mē) Surgical sectioning of the maxilla to allow movement of all or a part of the maxilla into the desired position.

max·i·mal ex·pi·ra·to·ry pres·sure (mak′si-măl ek-spīr′ă-tōr-ē presh′ŭr) Measure of the maximal static expiratory pressure attainable by a patient attempting to exhale into a closed system.

max·i·mal ox·y·gen con·sump·tion (mak′si-măl ok′si-jĕn kŏn-sŭmp′shŭn) Highest amount of oxygen someone can consume during maximal exercise of several minutes' duration.

max·i·mum (mak′si-mŭm) The greatest amount, value, or degree attained or attainable.

max·i·mum ex·pi·ra·to·ry pres·sure (mak′si-mŭm eks-pīr′ă-tōr-ē presh′ŭr) The greatest pressure within the alveoli that occurs during a forceful expiration; the measurement is made when the lungs are full of air.

max·i·mum in·spi·ra·to·ry pres·sure (MIP) (mak′si-mŭm in-spīr′ă-tōr-ē presh′ŭr) The greatest pressure within the alveoli that occurs during inspiration; the measurement of MIP provides a global assessment of inspiratory muscle function.

max·i·mum per·mis·si·ble dose (mak′si-mŭm per-mis′i-bĕl dōs) Defined by the International Commission on Radiological Protection as the largest dose of radiation that, in the light of present knowledge, is not expected to cause detectable bodily injury to a person at any time during his or her lifetime.

max·i·mum vol·un·tar·y con·trac·tion (mak′si-mŭm vol′ŭn-tar-ē kŏn-trak′shŭn) The greatest amount of tension a muscle can generate and hold, however briefly.

max·i·mum vol·un·tar·y ven·ti·la·tion (mak′si-mŭm vol′ŭn-tar-ē ven′ti-lā′shŭn) The volume of air breathed when an individual breathes as deeply and as quickly as possible for a given time.

May-Hegg·lin a·nom·a·ly (mī heg′lin ă-nŏm′ă-lē) SYN Hegglin anomaly.

May·neord fac·tor (mā′nōrd fak′tŏr) An application of the inverse square law in radiation therapy.

Mayo op·er·a·tion (mā′ō op-ĕr-ā′shŭn) Procedure for the radical surgical cure of umbilical hernia.

maze (māz) Labyrinth; used to study higher functions of the nervous system in rats.

mazo- Combining form indicating the breast. SEE ALSO masto-.

Mc·Bur·ney point (mik-bŭr′nē poynt) A site one third the distance from the anterior superior iliac spine to the umbilicus that with deep palpation produces rebound tenderness indicating appendicitis. SEE ALSO appendicitis.

Mc·Cune-Al·bright syn·drome (mik-kyūn′awl′brīt sin′drōm) Polyostotic fibrous dysplasia with irregular brown patches of cutaneous pigmentation and endocrine dysfunction, especially precocious puberty in girls. SEE ALSO pseudohypoparathyroidism. SYN Albright disease.

mcg Abbreviation for microgram.

Mc·Mur·ray test (mik-mŭr′ē test) Rotation of the tibia on the femur to determine injury to meniscal structures.

Mc·Vay op·er·a·tion (mik-vā′ op-ĕr-ā′shŭn) Repair of inguinal and femoral hernias by suture of the transversus abdominis muscle and its associated fasciae to the pectineal ligament.

Md Symbol for mendelevium.

Me Symbol for methyl.

mead·ow der·ma·ti·tis, mead·ow grass der·ma·ti·tis (mĕd′ō dĕr′mă-tī′tis, gras) Photoallergic skin reaction to contact with a plant containing furocoumarin.

mean (mēn) A statistical measurement of central tendency or average of a set of values, usually assumed to be the arithmetic mean unless otherwise specified.

mean ar·te·ri·al pres·sure (mēn ahr-tēr′ē-ăl presh′ŭr) Average of the systolic and diastolic blood pressure.

mean cor·pus·cu·lar he·mo·glo·bin (mēn kōr-pŭs′kyū-lăr hē′mŏ-glō-bin) Hemoglobin content of the average red blood cell (RBC), calculated from the hemoglobin therein and the RBC count, in RBC indices.

mean cor·pus·cu·lar he·mo·glo·bin con·cen·tra·tion (mēn kōr-pŭs′kyū-lăr hē′mŏ-glō′bin kon′sĕn-trā′shŭn) The average hemoglobin concentration in a given volume of packed red blood cells, calculated from the hemoglobin therein and the hematocrit, in erythrocyte indices.

mea·sles (mē′zĕlz) Acute exanthematous disease caused by measles virus; marked by fever, catarrhal inflammation of the respiratory mucous membranes, and reddish maculopapular eruptions. SYN morbilli.

mea·sles, mumps, and ru·bel·la vac·cine (mē′zĕlz mŭmps rū-bel′ă vak-sēn′) Combination of live attenuated forms of these viruses in an aqueous suspension.

mea·sles vi·rus (mē′zĕlz vī′rŭs) Ribonucleic acid virus of the genus *Morbillivirus* that causes measles and is transmitted through the respiratory tract. SYN rubeola virus.

mea·sure (mezh′ŭr) **1.** To determine the magnitude or quantity of a substance by comparing it against some accepted standard. **2.** A specified magnitude of a physical quantity.

meato- Combining form indicating meatus.

me·a·to·plas·ty (mē-at′ō-plas-tē) Enlargement or other surgical reconfiguring of a meatus or canal.

me·a·tos·co·py (mē-ă-tos′kŏ-pē) Inspection, usually instrumental, of any meatus, especially of the meatus of the urethra.

me·a·tot·o·my (mē′ă-tot′ŏ-mē) An incision made to enlarge a meatus.

me·a·tus, pl. **me·a·tus** (mē-ā′tŭs) [TA] A passage or channel.

mec·a·myl·a·mine hy·dro·chlor·ide (mek′ă-mil′ă-mēn hī-drŏ-klōr′īd) A secondary amine that blocks transmission of impulses at autonomic ganglia.

me·chan·i·cal an·ti·dote (mĕ-kan′i-kăl an′ti-dōt) A substance that prevents the absorption of a poison.

me·chan·ic·al dead air·space (mĕ-kan′i-kăl ded ār′spās) Volume of gas rebreathed through a mechanical ventilator.

me·chan·i·cal il·e·us (mĕ-kan′i-kăl il′ē-ŭs) Bowel obstruction due to some mechanical cause.

me·chan·i·cal jaun·dice (mĕ-kan′i-kăl jawn′dis) SYN obstructive jaundice.

M

me·chan·i·cal vec·tor (mĕ-kan'i-kăl vek'tŏr) Agent that conveys pathogens to a susceptible individual without essential biologic development of the pathogens in the vector.

me·chan·i·cal ven·ti·la·tion (mĕ-kan' i-kăl ven'ti-lā'shŭn) The use of an automatic mechanical device to perform all or part of the work of breathing. SEE ALSO ventilator.

me·chan·ics (mĕ-kan'iks) The science of the action of forces in promoting motion or equilibrium.

mech·a·nism (mek'ă-nizm) **1.** Arrangement or grouping of the parts of anything that has a definite action. **2.** The means by which an effect is obtained. **3.** Chain of events in a particular process. **4.** Detailed description of a reaction pathway.

mech·a·no·re·cep·tor (mek'ă-nō-rē-sep'tŏr) A receptor that responds to mechanical pressure or distortion.

me·chlor·eth·a·mine (mek'lŏr-eth'ă-mēn) SEE nitrogen mustards.

Mec·kel di·ver·ti·cu·lum (mek'el dī'vĕr-tik'yū-lŭm) The remains of the yolk stalk of the embryo; may be attached to the umbilicus and, if the lining includes gastric mucosa, peptic ulceration and bleeding can occur. SYN ileal diverticulum.

Mec·kel space (mek'ĕl spās) SYN trigeminal cave.

me·co·ni·um (mĕ-kō'nē-ŭm) The greenish first intestinal discharges of the newborn, consisting of epithelial cells, mucus, and bile.

me·co·ni·um as·pi·ra·tion (mĕ-kō'nē-ŭm as'pir-ā'shŭn) Intrauterine fetal inhalation of amniotic fluid contaminated by meconium due to fetal hypoxic distress.

me·co·ni·um as·pi·ra·tion syn·drome (mĕ-kō'nē-ŭm as'pir-ā'shŭn sin'drōm) SYN fetal aspiration syndrome.

me·co·ni·um il·e·us (mĕ-kō'nē-ŭm il'ē-ŭs) Intestinal obstruction in the fetus and newborn following inspissation of meconium; caused by lack of trypsin.

me·co·ni·um plug (mĕ-kō'nē-ŭm plŭg)

A plug of thick, inspissated meconium that may cause intestinal obstruction.

me·di·a (mē'dē-ă) **1.** SYN tunica media. **2.** Plural of medium.

me·di·al (mē'dē-ăl) [TA] Relating to the middle or center; nearer to the median or midsagittal plane. SYN medialis.

me·di·al fore·brain bun·dle (mē'dē-ăl fōr'brān bŭn'dĕl) [TA] A fiber system coursing longitudinally through the lateral zone of the hypothalamus, connecting the latter reciprocally with the midbrain tegmentum and with various components of the limbic system.

me·di·a·lis (mē'dē-ā'lis) [TA] *This form of the adjective is used with masculine nouns (meniscus medialis, plural menisci mediales). With feminine nouns the form mediana is used (fissura mediana, plural fissurae medianae), and with neuter nouns the form medianum (septum medianum, plural septa mediana). Avoid confusing this word with medianus 'median' or medius 'middle.'* SYN medial.

med·i·al·i·za·tion (mē'dē-ăl-ī-zā'shŭn) An operation to move a part toward the midline.

me·di·al ro·ta·tion (mē'dē-ăl rō-tā'shŭn) SYN internal rotation.

me·di·an (mē'dē-ăn) **1.** Central; middle; lying in the midline. SYN medianus. **2.** The middle value in a set of measurements.

me·di·an ef·fec·tive dose (ED$_{50}$) (mē'dē-ăn e-fek'tiv dōs) SEE effective dose.

median ep·i·si·ot·o·my (mē'dē-ăn ĕ-piz'ē-ot'ŏ-mē) SYN midline episiotomy.

me·di·an la·ryn·go·to·my (mē'dē-ăn lar'in-got'ŏ-mē) SYN laryngofissure.

me·di·an le·thal dose (mē'dē-ăn lē'thăl dōs) The amount of a substance that will kill half the organisms it encounters.

me·di·an lin·gual swell·ing (mē'dē-ăn ling'gwăl swel'ing) A smooth swelling in the midline of the floor of the primordial mouth between the first and second pharyngeal arches. SYN median tongue bud, tuberculum impar.

me·di·an pa·la·tal cyst (mē'dē-ăn pal'

ă-tăl sist) Developmental lesion located in the midline of the hard palate.

me·di·an plane (mē′dē-ăn plān) [TA] Vertical area in the anatomic position, through the midline of the body that divides the body into right and left halves. SYN planum medianum [TA].

me·di·an rhom·boid glos·si·tis (mē′dē-ăn rom′boyd glos-ī′tis) An asymptomatic, ovoid or rhomboid, macular or mammillated, erythematous lesion with papillary atrophy on the dorsum of the tongue just anterior to the circumvallate papillae.

me·di·an ster·not·o·my (MS) (mē′dē-ăn stĕr-not′ŏ-mē) Incision through the midline of the sternum, used to gain access to the heart.

me·di·an um·bil·ical fold (mē′dē-ăn ŭm-bil′ĭ-kăl fōld) Peritoneal fold on the anterior wall of the abdomen covering the urachus.

me·di·a·nus (mē′dē-ā′nŭs) SYN median (1).

me·di·as·ti·nal (mē′dē-ă-stī′năl) Relating to the mediastinum.

me·di·as·ti·nal em·phy·se·ma (mē′dē-ă-stī′năl em′fi-sē′mă) Deflection of air, usually from a ruptured emphysematous bleb in the lung, into the mediastinal tissue.

me·di·as·ti·nal fi·bro·sis (mē′dē-ă-stī′năl fī-brō′sis) Fibrosis that may obstruct the superior vena cava, pulmonary arteries, veins, or bronchi.

me·di·as·ti·nal space (mē′dē-ă-stī′năl spās) SYN mediastinum (2).

me·di·as·ti·ni·tis (mē′dē-as′ti-nī′tis) Inflammation of the cellular tissue of the mediastinum.

me·di·as·ti·nog·ra·phy (mē′dē-as′ti-nog′ră-fē) Radiography of the mediastinum.

me·di·as·tin·o·per·i·car·di·tis (mē′dē-ă-stī′nō-per′i-kahr-dī′tis) Inflammation of the pericardium and of the surrounding mediastinal cellular tissue.

me·di·as·ti·nos·co·py (mē′dē-as′ti-nos′

kŏ-pē) Exploration of the mediastinum through a suprasternal incision.

me·di·as·ti·num (mē′dē-ă-stī′nŭm) [TA] **1.** A septum between two parts of an organ or a cavity. **2.** The median partition of the thoracic cavity, covered by the mediastinal part of the parietal pleura and containing all the thoracic viscera and structures except the lungs. SYN mediastinal space.

me·di·a·sti·num tes·tis (mē′dē-ă-stī′nŭm tes′tis) [TA] Mass of fibrous tissue continuous with the tunica albuginea. SYN Highmore body.

me·di·ate (mē′dē-ăt, -āt) **1.** Situated between; intermediate. **2.** To effect something by means of an intermediary substance, as in complement-mediated phagocytosis.

me·di·at·ed trans·port (mē′dē-ă-tĕd trans′pōrt) Movement of a solution across a membrane with the aid of a transport agent.

me·di·ate per·cus·sion (mē′dē-ăt pĕr-kŭsh′ŭn) That effected by the intervention of a finger or a plessimeter between the striking finger or plessor and the part percussed.

me·di·ate trans·fu·sion (mē′dē-ăt trans-fyū′zhŭn) SYN indirect transfusion.

med·i·ca·ble (med′i-kă-bĕl) Treatable, with hope of a cure.

med·i·cal (med′i-kăl) **1.** Relating to medicine or the practice of medicine. SYN medicinal (2). **2.** SYN medicinal (1).

med·i·cal as·sis·tant (med′i-kăl ă-sis′tănt) A person who supports a physician or other health care provider by performing administrative and clinical tasks.

med·i·cal care (med′i-kăl kār) Portion of care under a physician's direction.

med·ic·al cas·tra·tion (med′i-kăl kas-trā′shŭn) SYN functional castration.

med·i·cal er·ror (med′i-kăl er′ŏr) In nursing usage, any failure to implement a planned action as intended or the implementation of the wrong nursing plan.

med·i·cal ex·am·i·ner (ME) (med′i-kăl

M

eg-zam'in-ĕr) **1.** Physician who examines someone and reports findings to the company or individual at whose request the examination was made. **2.** In jurisdictions where the office of coroner has been abolished, a physician appointed to investigate all cases of sudden, violent, or suspicious death.

med·i·cal ge·net·ics (med'i-kăl jĕ-net' iks) Study of the etiology, pathogenesis, and natural history of human diseases at least partially genetic in origin.

med·i·cal in·ten·sive care u·nit (med'i-kăl in-ten'siv kār yū'nit) Hospital area designated for care of critically ill patients with nonsurgical conditions.

med·i·cal ju·ris·pru·dence (med'i-kăl jŭr'is-prū'dĕns) SYN forensic medicine.

med·i·cal la·bo·ra·to·ry tech·ni·cian (MLT) (med'i-kăl lab'ŏr-ă-tōr-ē tek-nish'ăn) A trained health care professional who performs clinical testing on bodily substances in a laboratory setting.

Med·i·cal Lit·er·a·ture A·nal·y·sis and Re·trie·val Sys·tem (MED-LARS) (med'i-kăl lit'ĕr-ă-chŭr ă-nal'i-sis rē-trē'văl sis'tĕm) A computerized system of databases and databanks maintained by the U.S. National Library of Medicine.

med·i·cal path·ol·o·gy (med'i-kăl pă-thol'ŏ-jē) That pertaining to various diseases not suitable for treatment by surgery.

med·i·cal re·view of·fi·cer (MRO) (med'i-kal rĕ-vyū' awf'i-sĕr) A physician trained and certified to review and analyze substance abuse testing results.

med·i·cal staff (med'i-kăl staf) Professional medical personnel who have been granted permission to practice their discipline in a health care facility.

med·i·cal tran·scrip·tion·ist (med'i-kăl tran-skrip'shŭn'ist) A person who performs machine transcription of physician-dictated medical records; a certified medical transcriptionist (CMT) has satisfied the requirements for certification by the American Association for Medical Transcription (AAMT).

med·i·ca·men·to·sus (med'i-kă-men-tō'sŭs) *This form of the adjective is used only with masculine nouns (lupus erythematosus medicamentosus). With feminine nouns the form medicamentosa is used (rhinitis medicamentosa), and with neuter nouns, medicamentosum (exanthema medicamentosum).* Relating to a drug or drug eruption.

Med·i·care (med'i-kār) **1.** A U.S. national health insurance plan that covers Social Security and Railroad Retirement beneficiaries age 65 years and older, people who have been entitled for at least 24 months to receive Social Security or Railroad Retirement disability benefits, and certain people with end-stage renal disease; established in 1965 by an amendment to the Social Security Act. **2.** The universal public health insurance system of Canada, administered by the provincial governments under guidelines set by the Canadian federal government; initiated under the Canada Health Act. **3.** A national public health insurance system in Australia; provides for free care in public hospitals, and free or subsidized care in clinical settings for certain conditions; established in 1984.

Med·i·care Part A (med'i-kār pahrt) The portion of the U.S. Medicare Program that covers inpatient hospital stays, skilled nursing facility care, hospice care, and some home health care.

Med·i·care Part B (med'i-kār pahrt) The portion of the U.S. Medicare Program that helps pay for physician services, outpatient hospital care, durable medical equipment, and some services not covered by Medicare Part A.

me·dic·i·nal (me-dis'i-năl) **1.** Relating to medicine having curative properties. SYN medical (2). **2.** SYN medical (1).

me·di·ci·nal soft soap (mĕ-dis'i-năl sawft sōp) One made with vegetable oils and other ingredients; used as a cleansing agent and stimulant in chronic skin disease. SYN green soap.

med·i·cine (med'i-sin) **1.** A drug. **2.** Preventing, diagnosing, and treating disease. **3.** The study and treatment of general diseases or those affecting the internal parts of the body.

med·i·co·le·gal (med'i-kō-lē'găl) Relating to both medicine and the law. SEE ALSO forensic medicine.

medio-, medi- Combining forms meaning middle, median.

me·di·o·car·pal (mē′dē-ō-kahr′păl) SYN midcarpal.

me·di·o·dor·sal (mē′dē-ō-dōr′săl) Relating to the median plane and the dorsal plane.

me·di·o·lat·er·al (ML, M/L) (mē′dē-ō-lat′ĕr-ăl) Relating to the median plane and one side.

me·di·o·ne·cro·sis (mē′dē-ō-nĕ-krō′sis) Necrosis of a tunica media.

med·i·ta·tion (med′i-tā′shŭn) Any mental activity intended to keep the practitioner's attention in the present; sometimes employed as part of overall therapy for diverse medical conditions (e.g., providing pain relief).

Med·i·ter·ra·ne·an di·et (med′i-tĕr-ā′nē-ăn dī′ĕt) One high in grains, fruits, vegetables, and olive oil with small amounts of meat and poultry.

Med·i·ter·ra·ne·an spot·ted fe·ver (med′i-tĕr-ā′nē-ăn spot′ĕd fē′vĕr) Tickborne infection by *Rickettsia conorii*; has various names based on locale where found; usually involves dermatologic findings. SYN eruptive fever.

me·di·um, pl. **me·di·a** (mē′dē-ŭm, -ă) **1.** A means. **2.** A substance through which impulses or impressions are transmitted. **3.** SYN culture medium. **4.** The liquid holding a substance in solution or suspension.

me·di·um-chain ac·yl-CoA de·hy·dro·gen·ase (MCAD) (mē′dē-ŭm chān as′il dē′hī-droj′ĕn-ās) SEE acyl-CoA dehydrogenase (NADPH).

me·di·us (mē′dē-ŭs) *This form of the adjective is used only with masculine nouns (truncus medius, plural trunci medii). With feminine nouns the form media is used (tunica media, plural tunicae mediae), and with neuter nouns the form medium (ganglion medium, plural ganglia media). Avoid confusing this word with medialis 'medial' or medianus 'median'.* SYN middle.

me·dul·la, gen. and pl. **me·dul·lae** (me-dŭl′ă, -ē) [TA] Any soft marrowlike structure, especially in the center of a part. SEE ALSO medulla oblongata. SYN substantia medullaris (1).

me·dul·la os·si·um (me-dŭl′ă os′ē-ŭm) [TA] SYN bone marrow.

me·dul·lar (med′ŭ-lăr) Related to a medulla. SYN medullary.

med·ul·lar·y (med′ŭ-lar′ē) Relating to the medulla or marrow. SYN medullar.

med·ul·lar·y car·ci·no·ma (MC) (med′ŭ-lar′ē kahr′si-nō′mă) Malignant neoplasm, comparatively soft, which consists of neoplastic epithelial cells.

med·ul·lar·y mem·brane (med′ŭ-lar′ē mem′brān) SYN endosteum.

med·ul·lar·y sheath (med′ŭ-lar′ē shēth) SYN myelin sheath.

med·ul·lar·y space (med′ŭ-lar′ē spās) Marrow-filled central cavity and cellular intervals between osseous trabeculae.

med·ul·lar·y sponge kid·ney (med′ŭ-lar′ē spŏnj kid′nē) Cystic disease of the renal pyramids associated with calculus formation and hematuria.

med·ul·lar·y sub·stance (med′ŭ-lar′ē sŭb′stăns) **1.** The lipid material present in the myelin sheath of nerve fibers. **2.** Medulla of bones and other organs. SYN substantia medullaris (2).

me·dul·la spi·na·lis (me-dŭl′ă spī-nā′lis) [TA] SYN spinal cord.

med·ul·lat·ed (med′ŭ-lā-tĕd) **1.** Having a medulla or medullary substance. **2.** SYN myelinated.

med·ul·lec·to·my (med′ŭl-ek′tō-mē) Excision of any medullary substance.

med·ul·li·za·tion (med′ŭ-lī-zā′shŭn) Enlargement of the medullary spaces in rarefying osteitis.

medullo- Combining form indicating the medulla. Cf. myel-.

me·dul·lo·blas·to·ma (me-dŭl′ō-blas-tō′mă) A tumor consisting of neoplastic cells that resemble the undifferentiated cells of the primitive medullary tube;

usually located in the vermis of the cerebellum.

me·dul·lo·ep·i·the·li·o·ma (mĕd'ŭ-lō-ep'ĭ-thē'lē-ō'mă) A rare, primitive, rapidly growing intracranial neoplasm thought to originate from the cells of the embryonic medullary canal.

mega- 1. Combining form meaning large, oversize; opposite of micro-. SEE ALSO macro-, megalo-. **2.** Prefix used in the SI and metric system to signify one million (10^6).

meg·a·car·y·o·cyte (meg'ă-kar'ē-ō-sīt') SYN megakaryocyte.

meg·a·ce·pha·li·a (meg'ă-se-fā'lē-ă) SYN megacephaly.

meg·a·ce·phal·ic (meg'ă-se-fal'ik) Denotes a brain of abnormal largeness. SYN megacephalous.

meg·a·ceph·a·lous (meg'ă-sef'ă-lŭs) SYN megacephalic.

meg·a·ceph·a·ly (meg'ă-sef'ă-lē) Condition involving an abnormally large brain.

meg·a·cins (meg'ă-sinz) Antibacterial proteins produced by strains of *Bacillus megaterium.*

meg·a·cys·tis (meg'ă-sis'tis) Pathologically large bladder in children. SYN megabladder, megalocystis.

meg·a·dyne (Mdyn) (meg'ă-dīn) One million dynes.

meg·a·e·soph·a·gus (meg'ă-ĕ-sof'ă-gŭs) Great enlargement of the lower portion of the esophagus. SYN mega-oesophagus.

meg·a·kar·y·o·blast, meg·a·car·y·o·blast (meg'ă-kar'ē-ō-blast) The precursor of a megakaryocyte. SYN megacaryoblast.

meg·a·kar·y·o·cyte, meg·a·car·y·o·cyte (meg'ă-kar'ē-ō-sīt) A large cell with a multilobed nucleus; normally present in bone marrow, not in the circulating blood. SYN megalokaryocyte.

meg·a·kar·y·o·cyte growth and de·

ve·lop·ment fac·tor (meg'ă-kar'ē-ō-sīt grōth dĕ-vel'ŏp-mĕnt fak'tŏr) SYN thrombopoietin.

meg·a·kar·y·o·cyt·ic leu·ke·mi·a (meg'ă-kar'ē-ō-sit'ik lū-kē'mē-ă) Unusual form of myelopoietic disease characterized by a seemingly uncontrolled proliferation of megakaryocytes in the bone marrow, and sometimes by the presence of a considerable number of megakaryocytes in the circulating blood.

meg·al·gi·a (meg-al'jē-ă) Very severe pain.

megalo-, megal- Combining forms meaning large; opposite of micro-. SEE ALSO macro-, mega-.

meg·a·lo·blast (meg'ă-lō-blast) A large, nucleated, embryonic type of cell that is a precursor of erythrocytes in an abnormal erythropoietic process observed in pernicious anemia. SEE ALSO erythroblast.

meg·a·lo·blas·tic a·ne·mi·a (MA) (meg'ă-lō-blast'ik ă-nē'mē-ă) Disorder with a predominant number of megaloblastic erythroblasts, and relatively few normoblasts, among the hyperplastic erythroid cells in the bone marrow.

meg·a·lo·ceph·a·ly, meg·a·lo·ce·pha·li·a (meg'ă-lō-sef'ă-lē, -sĕ-fā'lē-ă) SYN megacephaly.

meg·a·lo·cor·ne·a (meg'ă-lō-kōr'ō-nar-ē) SYN keratoglobus.

meg·a·lo·cyte (meg'ă-lō-sīt) A large (i.e., 10–20 mcm) nonnucleated red blood cell.

meg·a·lo·en·ter·on (meg'ă-lō-en'tĕr-on) Abnormal largeness of the intestine. SYN enteromegaly, enteromegalia.

meg·a·lo·gas·tri·a (meg'ă-lō-gas'trē-ă) Abnormally large stomach. SYN macrogastria.

meg·a·lo·he·pat·i·a (meg'ă-lō-hĕ-pat'ē-ă) SYN hepatomegaly.

meg·a·lo·kar·y·o·cyte (meg'ă-lō-kar'ē-ō-sīt) SYN megakaryocyte.

meg·a·lo·ma·ni·a (meg'ă-lō-mā'nē-ă) **1.** A type of delusion in which the afflicted person considers himself or herself possessed of greatness. lawyer, physician, clergyman. **2.** Morbid verbalized over-evaluation of oneself or of some aspect of oneself.

meg·a·lo·ma·ni·ac, me·ga·lo·ma·ni·a·cal (meg'ă-lō-mā'nē-ak, -mă-nī'ă-kăl) A person exhibiting megalomania.

meg·a·lo·mel·ia (meg'ă-lō-mē'lē-ă) Abnormal largeness of one of more limbs. SYN macromelia.

meg·a·loph·thal·mos (meg'ă-lof-thal'mŏs) Congenital large eyeball or globe. SYN macrophthalmia, megophthalmus.

meg·a·lo·pi·a (meg'ă-lō'pē-ă) Perception of objects appearing larger than they are in reality.

meg·a·lo·syn·dac·ty·ly, meg·a·lo·syn·dac·tyl·i·a (meg'ă-lō-sin-dak'ti-lē, -sin'dak-til'ē-ă) Condition of webbed or fused fingers or toes that are of large size.

meg·a·lo·u·re·ter, meg·a·ur·e·ter (meg'ă-lō-yūr'ĕ-tĕr, meg'ă-yūr'ĕ-tĕr) An enlarged, dilated ureter.

meg·a·lo·u·re·thra (meg'ă-lō-yūr-ē'thră) Congenital dilation of the urethra.

-megaly Suffix meaning large.

mega-oesophagus [Br.] SYN megaesophagus.

meg·a·volt (MV, MeV) (meg'ă-vōlt) One million volts.

meg·a·volt·age (meg'ă-vōl'tăj) In radiation therapy, a term for voltage above one million volts.

meg·ohm (MΩ) (meg'ōm) One million ohms.

mei·bo·mi·an cyst (mī-bō'mē-ăn sist) SYN chalazion.

mei·o·sis (mī-ō'sis) *Do not confuse this word with miosis.* Special process of cell division comprising two nuclear divisions in rapid succession that result in four gametocytes. SYN meiotic division.

mei·ot·ic (mī-ot'ik) Pertaining to meiosis.

Meiss·ner plex·us (mīs'ner pleks'ŭs) SYN submucosal (nerve) plexus.

mel (mel) **1.** SYN honey. **2.** Unit of pitch; a pitch of 1000 mels results from a simple tone of frequency 1000 Hz at 40 dB above the normal threshold of audibility.

me·lal·gi·a (mel-al'jē-ă) Pain in a limb.

melan-, melano- Combining forms meaning black, extreme darkness of hue.

mel·an·cho·li·a (mel'ăn-kō'lē-ă) Severe depression marked by anhedonia, insomnia, and guilt. SYN melancholy.

mel·an·e·de·ma (mel'ăn-ĕ-dē'mă) SYN melanoedema.

mel·a·nin (MELAN) (mel'ă-nin) Any of the dark brown to black polymers that normally occur in the skin, hair, pigmented coat of the retina, and inconstantly in the medulla and zona reticularis of the suprarenal gland. SYN melanotic pigment.

mel·a·nism (mel'ă-nizm) Unusually marked, diffuse melanin pigmentation of body hair and skin (usually not affecting the iris). SEE ALSO melanosis.

melano- SEE melan-.

mel·a·no·am·e·lo·blas·to·ma (mel'ă-nō-am'ĕ-lō-blas-tō'mă) SYN melanotic neuroectodermal tumor of infancy.

mel·a·no·blast (mel'ă-nō-blast) A cell derived from the neural crest, which matures into a melanocyte.

mel·a·no·cyte (mel'ă-nō-sīt) A pigment-producing cell located in the basal layer of the epidermis with branching processes by means of which melanosomes are transferred to epidermal cells, resulting in pigmentation of the epidermis.

mel·a·no·cyte-stim·u·lat·ing hor·mone (MSH) (mel'ă-nō-sīt-stim'yū-lā-ting hōr'mōn) SYN melanotropin, bioregulator.

mel·a·no·cyt·ic ne·vus (mel'ă-nō-sit'ik nē'vŭs) SYN mole.

mel·a·no·cy·to·ma (mel'ă-nō-sī-tō'mă) **1.** A pigmented tumor of the uveal

M

stroma. **2.** Usually benign melanoma of the optic disc, appearing as a small deeply pigmented tumor at the edge of the disc, sometimes extending into the retina and choroid.

mel·a·no·der·ma (mel′ă-nō-dĕr′mă) Abnormal darkening of skin by deposition of excess melanin or deposition of dark metallic substances, such as silver and iron.

mel·a·no·der·ma·ti·tis (mel′ă-nō-dĕr′mă-tī′tis) Excessive deposit of melanin in an area of dermatitis.

melanoedema [Br.] SYN melanedema.

me·la·no·gen (mĕ-lan′ŏ-jen) A colorless substance that may be converted into melanin.

mel·a·no·gen·e·sis (mel′ă-nō-jen′ĕ-sis) Formation of melanin.

mel·a·no·glos·si·a (mel′ă-nō-glos′ē-ă) SYN black tongue.

mel·a·noid (mel′ă-noyd) A dark pigment, resembling melanin, formed from glucosamines in chitin.

mel·a·no·leu·ko·der·ma (mel′ă-nō-lū′kō-dĕr′mă) Marbled, or marmorated, skin.

mel·a·no·leu·ko·der·ma col·li (mel′ă-nō-lū′kō-dĕr′mă kol′ī) SYN syphilitic leukoderma.

mel·a·no·lib·er·in (mel′ă-nō-lib′ĕr-in) Hexapeptide similar to oxytocin; stimulates release of of melanotropin. SYN melanotropin-releasing factor.

mel·a·no·ma (mel′ă-nō′mă) A malignant neoplasm, derived from cells that are capable of forming melanin, arising most commonly in the skin or in the eye, and, rarely, in the mucous membranes of the genitalia, anus, oral cavity, or other sites.

mel·a·no·nych·i·a (mel′ă-nō-nik′ē-ă) Black pigmentation of the nails.

mel·a·no·phage (mel′ă-nō-fāj) A histiocyte that has phagocytized melanin.

mel·a·no·phore (mel′ă-nō-fōr′) Nonhuman dermal pigment cell that does not secrete its pigment granules but participates in rapid color changes by intracellular aggregation and dispersal of melanosomes.

mel·a·no·pla·ki·a (mel′ă-nō-plā′kē-ă) The occurrence of pigmented patches on the tongue and buccal mucous membrane.

mel·a·no·sis (mel′ă-nō′sis) Abnormal dark brown or brown-black pigmentation of various tissues or organs due to melanin or other substances that resemble melanin to varying degrees.

mel·a·no·sis co·li (mel′ă-nō′sis kō′lī) Melanosis of the large intestinal mucosa due to accumulation of pigment of uncertain composition within macrophages in the lamina propria.

mel·a·no·some (mel′ă-nō-sōm) Oval pigment granule produced by melanocytes. SYN eumelanosome.

mel·an·o·sta·tin (mel′ă-nō-stat′in) Inhibits synthesis and release of melanotropin; neuropeptide Y. SYN melanotropin release-inhibiting hormone.

mel·a·not·ic (mel′ă-not′ik) **1.** Pertaining to the presence, normal or pathologic, of melanin. **2.** Relating to melanosis.

mel·a·no·troph (mel′ă-nō-trōf) A cell of the intermediate lobe of the hypophysis that produces melanotropin.

mel·a·no·tro·pin (mel′ă-nō-trō′pin) Polypeptide hormone secreted by the intermediate lobe of the hypophysis in humans. SYN intermedin.

mel·a·no·tro·pin-re·leas·ing fac·tor, mel·a·no·tro·pin-re·leas·ing hor·mone (mel′ă-nō-trō′pin rĕ′lēs′ing fak′tŏr, hōr′mōn) SYN melanoliberin.

mel·a·nu·ria (mel′ă-nyū′rē-ă) Excretion of dark-colored urine, due to melanin or action of phenol.

MELAS (mel′as) Acronym for a constellation of findings that includes *m*itochondrial myopathy, *e*ncephalopathy, *l*actic *a*cidosis, and *s*trokelike episodes.

me·las·ma (mĕ-laz′mă) A patchy pigmentation of sun-exposed skin.

me·las·ma grav·i·da·rum (mĕ-laz′mă grav′i-dā′rŭm) Chloasma occurring in pregnancy.

mel·a·to·nin (mel′ă-tō′nin) A substance formed by the pineal gland that appears to depress gonadal function. Cf. bioregulator.

me·le·na ne·o·na·to·rum (MN) (mĕ-lē′nă nē-ō-nā-tō′rŭm) Melena of the newborn.

mel·i·oi·do·sis (mel′ē-oy-dō′sis) An infectious disease of rodents in India and Southeast Asia caused by *Pseudomonas pseudomallei* that is communicable to humans. SYN pseudoglanders, Whitmore disease.

Mel·kers·son-Ro·sen·thal syn·drome (mel′kĕr-sŏn rō′zen-thahl sin′drōm) Disorder involving cheilitis granulomatosa, fissured tongue, and recurrent facial nerve paralysis.

mel·on-seed bod·y (mel′ŏn-sēd bod′ē) Small fibrous loose body in a joint or tendon sheath.

mel·o·plas·ty, mel·o·no·plas·ty (mel′ō-plas-tē, mel′ă-nō-) Surgical repair of the cheek.

mel·o·rhe·os·to·sis (mel′ō-rē′os-tō′sis) Rheostosis confined to the long bones.

melt·ing point (melt′ing poynt) Temperature at which a solid becomes a liquid.

mem·ber (mem′bĕr) SYN limb (1).

mem·bra·na vi·tel·li·na (mem-brā′nă vit-ĕ-lī′nă) Tissue layer enveloping the yolk.

mem·brane (mem′brān) **1.** A thin sheet or layer of pliable tissue, serving as a covering or envelope, the lining of a cavity, a partition or septum, or a connection between two structures. SYN membrana [TA]. **2.** SYN biomembrane.

mem·brane po·ten·tial (mem′brān pŏ-ten′shăl) The potential inside a cell membrane, measured relative to the fluid just outside; it is negative under resting conditions and becomes positive during an action potential.

mem·bran·i·form (mem-bran′i-fōrm) Resembling a membrane in some way. SYN membranoid.

mem·bra·no·car·ti·lag·i·nous (mem′brǎ-nō-kahr′ti-laj′i-nŭs) **1.** Partly membranous and partly cartilaginous. **2.** Derived from both a mesenchymal membrane and cartilage.

mem·bra·noid (mem′brǎ-noyd) SYN membraniform.

mem·bra·nous (mem′brǎ-nŭs) Relating to or of the form of a membrane.

mem·bra·nous cat·a·ract (mem′brăn-ŭs kat′ăr-akt) A secondary cataract composed of the remains of the thickened capsule and degenerated lens fibers.

mem·bra·nous dys·men·or·rhe·a (mem′brǎ-nŭs dis-men′ŏ-rē′ă) Menstrual disorder accompanied by exfoliation of the menstrual decidua.

mem·bra·nous os·si·fi·ca·tion (mem′brǎ-nŭs os′i-fi-kā′shŭn) Development of bony tissue that occurs in mesenchymal tissue with prior formation of cartilage. SYN intramembranous ossification.

mem·bra·nous pha·ryn·gi·tis (mem′brăn-ŭs far′in-jī′tis) Inflammation accompanied by a fibrinous exudate, which forms a nondiphtheritic false membrane.

mem·bra·nous u·re·thra (mem′brăn-ŭs yūr-ē′thră) SYN intermediate part of male urethra.

mem·brum, pl. **mem·bra** (mem′brŭm, -bră) A limb; a member.

mem·o·ry (mem′ŏ-rē) **1.** Generally, recollection of that which was once experienced or learned. **2.** The mental information processing system that receives (registers), modifies, stores, and retrieves informational stimuli; composed of three stages: encoding, storage, and retrieval.

mem·o·ry B cells (mĕm′ŏ-rē selz) B lymphocytes that mediate immunologic memory.

mem·o·ry T cells (mĕm′ŏ-rē selz) T lymphoctyes that mediate immunologic memory.

me·nac·me (me-nak′mē) The period of menstrual activity in a woman's life.

M

men·a·qui·none (men´ă-kwin´ōn) Dietary supplement made from putrified fish meal. SYN vitamin K2.

me·nar·che (men-ahr´kē) *Avoid the mispronunciation men´arche.* Establishment of the menstrual function; the time of the first menstrual period.

Men·del-Bech·te·rew re·flex (men´děl bek-těr´yev rē´fleks) SYN Bechterew-Mendel reflex.

men·de·le·vi·um (Md) (men´dě-lě´vē-ŭm) An element, atomic no. 101, atomic wt. 258.1, prepared in 1955 by bombardment of einsteinium with alpha particles.

men·del·i·an in·her·i·tance (men-dē´lē-ăn in-her´i-tăns) Inheritance in which stable and undecomposable characters controlled entirely or overwhelmingly by a single genetic locus are transmitted over many generations. SYN alternative inheritance.

Men·del·i·an In·her·i·tance in Man (MIM) (men-dē´lē-ăn in-her´i-tăns man) A standard, comprehensive, regularly updated reference source for traits in humans that have been shown to be mendelian or that are thought on reasonable grounds to be so. Each entry has a six-digit catalog number.

men·del·ism (men´del-izm) Hereditary principles of single gene traits derived from work of Gregor Mendel.

Men·del·sohn ma·neu·ver (men´děl-sŏn mă-nū´věr) Therapeutic technique for management of swallowing disorders.

Mé·né·tri·er dis·ease, Mé·né·tri·er syn·drome (mā-nā-trē-ā´ di-zēz´, sin´drŏm) Gastric mucosal hyperplasia, either mucoid or glandular.

Mé·ni·ère dis·ease, Mé·ni·ère syn·drome (men-yār´ di-zēz´, sin´drŏm) An affliction characterized clinically by vertigo, nausea, vomiting, tinnitus, and progressive hearing loss due to hydrops of the endolymphatic duct. SYN endolymphatic hydrops, labyrinthine vertigo.

me·nin·ge·al (mě-nin´jē-ăl) Relating to the meninges.

me·nin·ge·al car·ci·no·ma (mě-nin´jē-ăl kahr´si-nō´mă) Infiltration of cancerous cells in the arachnoid and subarachnoid space; may be primary or secondary. SYN leptomeningeal carcinoma, leptomeningeal carcinomatosis, meningeal carcinomatosis.

me·nin·ge·o·cor·ti·cal (mě-nin´jē-ō-kōr´ti-kăl) SYN meningocortical.

me·nin·ge·or·rha·phy (mě-nin´jē-ōr´ă-fē) Suture of the cranial or spinal meninges or of any membrane.

me·nin·gi·o·ma (mě-nin´jē-ō´mă) A benign, encapsulated neoplasm of arachnoidal origin, occurring most frequently in adults.

me·nin·gism (men´in-jizm) A condition in which the symptoms simulate meningitis, but without actual inflammation of these membranes.

men·in·git·ic streak (men´in-jit´ik strēk) A red line resulting from drawing a point across the skin. SYN Trousseau spot.

men·in·gi·tis, pl. **men·in·git·i·des** (men´in-jī´tis, -jit´ti-dēz) Inflammation of the membranes of the brain or spinal cord. SEE ALSO arachnoiditis, leptomeningitis. SYN cerebrospinal meningitis.

me·nin·go·cele (mě-ning´gō-sēl) Protrusion of the membranes of the brain or spinal cord through a defect in the cranium or vertebral column.

meningococcaemia [Br.] SYN meningococcemia.

me·nin·go·coc·cal me·nin·gi·tis (mě-ning´gō-kok´ăl men-in-jī´tis) Acute infectious disease of children and young adults, caused by *Neisseria meningitidis* and characterized by fever, headache, photophobia, vomiting, nuchal rigidity, seizures, coma, and a purpuric eruption. SYN cerebrospinal fever, epidemic cerebrospinal meningitis.

me·nin·go·coc·ce·mi·a (mě-ning´gō-kok-sē´mē-ă) Presence of meningococci in the circulating blood.

me·nin·go·coc·cus, pl. **me·nin·go·coc·ci** (mě-ning-gō-kok´ŭs, -kok´sī) SYN *Neisseria meningitidis*.

me·nin·go·cor·ti·cal, me·nin·ge·o·cor·ti·cal (mĕ-ning′gō-kōr′ti-kăl, -jē-ō-kōr′ti-kăl) Relating to the meninges and the cortex of the brain.

me·nin·go·cyte (mĕ-ning′gō-sīt) A mesenchymal epithelial cell of the subarachnoid space; it may become a macrophage.

me·nin·go·en·ceph·a·li·tis (mĕ-ning′gō-en-sef′ăl-ī′tis) An inflammation of the brain and its membranes. SYN cerebromeningitis, encephalomeningitis.

me·nin·go·en·ceph·a·lo·cele (mĕ-ning′gō-en-sef′ă-lō-sēl) A protrusion of the meninges and brain through a congenital cranial defect in the cranium. SYN encephalomeningocele.

me·nin·go·en·ceph·a·lo·my·e·li·tis (mĕ-ning′gō-en-sef′ă-lō-mī-ă-lī′tis) Inflammation of the brain, spinal cord, and their membranes.

me·nin·go·en·ceph·a·lop·a·thy (mĕ-ning′gō-en-sef′ă-lop′ă-thē) Disorder affecting the meninges and the brain. SYN encephalomeningopathy.

me·nin·go·ma·la·ci·a (mĕ-ning′gō-mă-lā′shē-ă) Softening of a portion of the meninges.

me·nin·go·my·e·li·tis (mĕ-ning′gō-mī-ă-lī′tis) Inflammation of the spinal cord and of its enveloping arachnoid and pia mater.

me·nin·go·my·e·lo·cele (mĕ-ning′gō-mī′ĕ-lō-sēl) Protrusion of the meninges and spinal cord through a defect in the vertebral column. SYN myelocystomeningocele, myelomeningocele.

me·nin·go·os·te·o·phle·bi·tis (mĕ-ning′gō-os′tē-ō-flĕ-bī′tis) Inflammation of the veins of the periosteum.

me·nin·go·ra·dic·u·lar (mĕ-ning′gō-ră-dik′yū-lăr) Relating to the meninges covering cranial or spinal nerve roots.

me·nin·gor·rha·gi·a (mĕ-ning′gō-rā′jē-ă) Hemorrhage into or beneath the cerebral or spinal meninges.

men·in·go·sis (men′in-gō′sis) Membranous union of bones.

me·ninx, gen. **me·nin·gis**, pl. **me·nin·ges** (mē′ningks, mĕ-nin′jis, -jēz) [TA] Any membrane; specifically, one of the membranous coverings of the brain and spinal cord. SEE ALSO dura mater, pia mater.

men·is·cec·to·my (men′i-sek′tŏ-mē) Excision of a meniscus, usually from the knee joint.

men·is·ci·tis (men′i-sī′tis) Inflammation of a fibrocartilaginous meniscus.

me·nis·co·cyte (mĕ-nis′kō-sīt) SYN sickle cell.

me·nis·cus, pl. **me·nis·ci** (mĕ-nis′kŭs, -shī) [TA] 1. SYN meniscus lens. 2. [TA] Any crescent-shaped structure. 3. A crescent-shaped fibrocartilaginous structure of the knee. 4. The crescentic curvature of the surface of a liquid standing in a narrow vessel (e.g., pipette, burette).

me·nis·cus lens (mĕ-nis′kŭs lenz) A lens having a spheric concave curve on one side and a spheric convex curve on the other. SYN meniscus (1).

meno- Combining form indicating the menses, menstruation.

men·o·me·tror·rha·gi·a (men′ō-mē′trō-rā′jē-ă) Irregular or excessive bleeding during menstruation and between menstrual periods.

men·o·pause (men′ŏ-pawz) Permanent cessation of the menses.

men·or·rha·gi·a (men′ŏ-rā′jē-ă) SYN hypermenorrhea.

men·or·rhal·gi·a (men′ŏ-ral′jē-ă) SYN dysmenorrhea.

men·or·rhea (men′ō-rē′ă) The monthly flow of blood from a woman's uterus.

me·nos·che·sis (me-nos′kĕ-sis) Suppression of menstruation.

men·o·stax·is (men′ŏ-stak′sis) SYN hypermenorrhea.

men·o·tro·pins (men′ŏ-trō′pinz) Extract of postmenopausal urine that primarily contains the follicle-stimulating hormone. SEE ALSO human menopausal gonadotropin, urofollitropin.

M

men·o·xe·ni·a (men'ō-zē'nē-ă) Any abnormality of menstruation.

men·ses (men'sēz) A periodic physiologic hemorrhage, which occurs at approximately 4-week intervals, its source is the uterine mucous membrane; usually the bleeding is preceded by ovulation and predecidual changes in the endometrium. SEE ALSO menstrual cycle. SYN emmenia, menstrual period.

men·stru·al age (MA) (men'strū-ăl āj) Age of the conceptus computed from the start of the mother's last menstrual period.

men·stru·al col·ic (men'strū-ăl kol'ik) intermittent cramplike lower abdominal pains associated with menstruation.

men·stru·al cy·cle (men'strū-ăl sī'kĕl) The period in which an oocyte or ovum matures, is ovulated, and enters the uterine lumen through the uterine tube; ovarian hormonal secretions effect endometrial changes such that, if fertilization occurs, nidation will be possible; in the absence of fertilization, ovarian secretions wane, the endometrium sloughs, and menstruation begins; this cycle lasts an average of 28 days, with day 1 of the cycle designated as that day on which menstrual flow begins.

men·stru·al pe·ri·od (men'strū-ăl pēr'ē-ŏd) SYN menses.

men·stru·al phase (men'strū-ăl fāz) The first day of menstruation indicates the beginning of the endometrial menstrual cycle; the phase lasts 4–5 days and coincides with the bleeding and shedding of degenerated endometrium from the previous menstrual cycle.

men·stru·a·tion (men'strū-ā'shŭn) Cyclic endometrial shedding and discharge of a bloody fluid from the uterus during the menstrual cycle. SEE menstruate.

men·su·ra·tion (men'sŭr-ā'shŭn) The act or process of measuring.

men·tal (men'tăl) **1.** Relating to the mind. **2.** Relating to the chin. SYN genial, genian.

men·tal ab·er·ra·tion (men'tăl ab'ĕr-ā'shŭn) Disturbed loosening of association, ambivalence, hallucination, or behavior that connotes psychological or psychiatric impairment. SEE delusion.

men·tal age (MA) (men'tăl āj) Measure, expressed in years and months, of a child's intelligence relative to age norms as determined by testing with the Stanford-Binet intelligence scale.

men·tal dis·or·der (men'tăl dis-ōr'dĕr) A psychological syndrome or behavioral pattern associated with either subjective distress or objective impairment. SEE ALSO mental illness, behavior disorder.

men·tal ill·ness (men'tăl il'nĕs) **1.** A broadly inclusive term, generally denoting either or both a disease of the brain, with predominant behavioral symptoms; a disease of the "mind" or personality, evidenced by abnormal behavior, as in hysteria or schizophrenia. **2.** Any psychiatric illness listed in *Current Medical Information and Terminology* of the American Medical Association or in the *Diagnostic and Statistical Manual of Mental Disorders* of the American Psychiatric Association. SEE ALSO behavior disorder.

men·tal pro·tu·ber·ance (men'tăl prō-tū'bĕr-ăns) [TA] Prominence of the chin at the anterior part of the mandible. SYN protuberantia mentalis [TA], mental process.

men·tal re·tar·da·tion (men'tăl rē'tahr-dā'shŭn) Subaverage general intellectual functioning that originates during the developmental period and is associated with impairment in adaptive behavior. Mental retardation classification requires assignment of an index for performance relative to a person's peers on two interrelated criteria: measured intelligence (IQ) and overall socioadaptive behavior. In general, an IQ of 70 or lower indicates mental retardation. Some clinicians and laypeople suggest this term may be offensive in some contexts.

men·tal stat·us ex·am·i·na·tion (men'tăl stat'ŭs eg-zam'mi-nā'shŭn) Detailed examination of a patient's mental functioning, through a series of tests or questions designed to determine level of consciousness, orientation to the environment, and higher cognitive function.

men·ta·tion (men-tā'shŭn) The process of reasoning and thinking.

Men·tha (men'thă) A genus of plants of the family Labiatae. *Mentha piperita* is peppermint; *Mentha pulegium*, pennyroyal; *Mentha viridis*, spearmint. SYN mint.

men·thol (men'thol) A waxy, crystalline substance, useful as a local anesthetic, antipruritic, and counterirritant; also available as a dietary supplement in the form of peppermint oil.

men·to·la·bi·al furrow (men'tō-lā'bē-ăl fŭr'ō) SYN mentolabial sulcus.

men·to·la·bi·al sul·cus (men'tō-lā'bē-ăl sŭl'kŭs) The indistinct line separating the lower lip from the chin. SYN mentolabial furrow.

men·ton (Me) (men'tŏn) In cephalometrics, lowest point in the symphysial shadow as seen on a lateral jaw projection.

men·to·plas·ty (men'tō-plas-tē) Surgical repair of the chin. SYN genioplasty.

men·to·trans·verse po·si·tion (men'tō-tranz-vĕrs' pŏ-zish'ŏn) A cephalic presentation of the fetus with its chin pointing to the right (right mentotranverse, RMT) or to the left (left mentotransverse, LMT) iliac fossa of the mother.

men·tum, gen. **men·ti,** pl. **men·ta** (men'tŭm, -tī, -tă) [TA] SYN chin.

me·per·i·dine hy·dro·chlor·ide (mĕ-per'i-dēn hī'drŏ-klōr'īd) A widely used narcotic analgesic. SYN pethidine.

me·phit·ic (mĕ-fit'ik) Foul, poisonous, or noxious.

me·pro·ba·mate (MPB) (mĕ-prō'bă-māt) *Avoid the misspelling/mispronunciation meprobromate.* An oral anxiolytic with potential for dependency and addiction.

mEq/L Abbreviation for milliequivalents per liter.

me·ral·gi·a (mĕr-al'jē-ă) Pain in the thigh.

me·ral·gia par·es·thet·i·ca (mĕr-al'jē-ă par'es-thet'i-kă) Burning pain, tingling, pruritus, or formication along the lateral aspect of the thigh in the distribution of the lateral femoral cutaneous nerve due to entrapment of that nerve. SYN Bernhardt disease, Bernhardt-Roth syndrome.

mer·cap·tan (mĕr-kap'tan) **1.** A class of substances in which the oxygen of an alcohol has been replaced by sulfur. SYN thioalcohol. **2.** In dentistry, a class of elastic impression compounds sometimes referred to as rubber base materials.

6-mer·cap·to·pu·rine (mer-kap'tō-pyūr'ēn) An analogue of hypoxanthine and of adenine; an antineoplastic agent.

Mer·ci·er bar (mer-sē-ā' bahr) SYN interureteric crest.

mer·cu·ri·al (mĕr-kyūr'ē-ăl) **1.** Relating to mercury. **2.** Any salt of mercury used medicinally. **3.** Having the characteristic of rapidly changing moods.

mer·cu·ric (mĕr-kyūr'ik) Denoting a salt of mercury in which the ion of the metal is bivalent.

mer·cu·ric chlo·ride (mĕr-kyūr'ik klōr'īd) A topical antiseptic and disinfectant for inanimate objects. SYN mercury bichloride, mercury perchloride, corrosive mercury chloride.

mer·cu·rous (mĕr-kyūr'ŭs) Denoting a salt of mercury in which the ion of the metal is univalent.

mer·cu·ry (Hg) (mĕr'kyūr-ē) A dense, liquid metallic element, used in thermometers, and other scientific instruments; some salts and organic mercurials are used medicinally.

mer·cu·ry bi·chlo·ride, mer·cu·ry per·chlo·ride, cor·ro·sive mer·cu·ry chlo·ride (mĕr'kyūr-ē bī-klōr'īd, pĕr-klōr'īd, kŏr-ō'siv) SYN mercuric chloride.

mer·cu·ry va·por lamp (mĕr'kyūr-ē vā'pŏr lamp) Light fixture in which the electric arc is in an ionized mercury vapor atmosphere; produces ultraviolet light that can be used therapeutically or for diagnosis.

mere-, mero- Combining forms meaning part; also indicating one of a series of similar parts.

me·rid·i·an (mĕr-id′ē-an) **1.** A line encircling a globular body at right angles to its equator and touching both poles, or the half of such a circle extending from pole to pole. **2.** ACUPUNCTURE the lines connecting different anatomic sites.

me·rid·i·a·nus, pl. **me·rid·i·a·ni** (mĕr-id′ē-ā′nŭs, -nī) [TA] SYN meridian (1).

Mer·kel cell car·ci·no·ma (mĕr′kĕl sel kahr′si-nō′mă) Rare and highly aggressive skin cancer; lesions develop on or just below the skin on sun-exposed body areas; appear as painless, firm nodules or tumors; metastasize quickly.

mer·o·an·en·ceph·a·ly (mer′ō-an′en-sef′ă-lē) Congenital absence of the calvaria and most of the brain, usually the forebrain and midbrain. SYN anencephalia, anencephaly.

mer·o·blast·ic (mer′ō-blas′tik) An incomplete separation of the egg from the ovary due to an overly large yolk.

mer·o·crine (mer′ŏ-krin, -krīn, -krĕn) SEE merocrine gland.

mer·o·crine gland (mer′ŏ-krin gland) One that releases only an acellular secretory product.

mer·o·en·ceph·a·ly (mĕr′ō-en-sef′ă-lē) Congenital defective development of the brain in which the brain and cranium are present in rudimentary form. SYN anencephaly.

mer·o·gen·e·sis (mer′ō-jen′ē-sis) **1.** Reproduction by segmentation. **2.** Cleavage of an oocyte.

mer·o·ge·net·ic, mer·o·gen·ic (mer′ō-jĕ-net′ik, -jen′ik) Relating to merogenesis.

me·rog·o·ny (mĕ-rog′ŏ-nē) The incomplete development of an ovum or oocyte that has been disorganized.

mer·o·me·li·a (mer′ō-mē′lē-ă) Partial absence of part of a limb (exclusive of girdle); e.g., hemimelia, phocomelia.

mer·o·ra·chis·chi·sis, mer·or·rha·chis·chi·sis (mer′ō-ră-kis′ki-sis) Fissure of a portion of the spinal cord. SYN rachischisis partialis.

me·rot·o·my (mĕ-rot′ŏ-mē) Clinical procedure of cutting into parts.

mer·o·zo·ite (mer′ō-zō′īt) The motile infective stage of sporozoan protozoa that results from schizogony or a similar type of asexual reproduction.

Mer·ri·field knife (mer′i-fēld nīf) Long, narrow, triangular knife used in gingival surgery.

mes-, meso-1. Combining forms meaning middle, mean, intermediate. **2.** Combining forms indicating a mesentery, mesenterylike structure. **3.** Combining forms denoting a compound, containing more than one chiral center, having an internal plane of symmetry.

me·sad (mē′zad, mē′sad) Passing or extending toward the median plane of the body or of a part. SYN mesiad.

mes·an·gi·al ne·phri·tis (mes-an′jē-ăl nĕ-frī′tis) Glomerulonephritis with an increase in glomerular mesangial cells or matrix, or mesangial deposits.

mes·an·gi·al pro·lif·er·a·tive glo·mer·u·lo·ne·phri·tis (mes-an′jē-ăl prŏ-lif′ĕr-ă-tiv glō-mer′yū-lō-nĕ-frī′tis) Disorder characterized clinically by the nephrotic syndrome and histologically by diffuse glomerular increases in endocapillary and mesangial cells and in mesangial matrix; in some cases, there are mesangial deposits of IgM and complement.

mes·a·or·ti·tis (mes′ā-ōr-tī′tis) Inflammation of the middle or muscular coat of the aorta.

mes·ax·on (mes-ak′son) Plasma membrane of the neurolemma that is folded in to surround a nerve axon.

mes·ca·line (mes′kă-lin) Naturally occurring psychedelic drug in long use, especially in Native American religious ceremonies; produces visual hallucinations and radically altered states of consciousness. Schedule I hallucinogen; considered a poisonous alkaloid, also called peyote.

me·sec·to·derm (mes-ek′tō-dĕrm) **1.** Cells in the area around the dorsal lip of the blastopore where mesoderm and ectoderm undergo a process of separation. **2.** That part of the mesenchyme derived from ectoderm, especially from the neural crest in the cephalic region in very young embryos.

mes·en·ce·phal·ic flex·ure (mes′en-sĕ-fal′ik flek′shŭr) SYN cephalic flexure.

mes·en·ceph·a·lon (mes′en-sef′ă-lon) [TA] That part of the brainstem developing from the middle of the three primary cerebral vesicles of the embryo. SYN midbrain.

mes·en·ceph·a·lot·o·my (mes′en-sef′ ă-lot′ŏ-mē) **1.** Sectioning of any structure in the midbrain, especially of the spinothalamic tracts to relieve intractable pain or the cerebral peduncle for dyskinesias. **2.** A mesencephalic spinothalamic tractotomy.

mes·en·chyme, mes·en·chy·ma (mes′ eng-kīm, mes-engk′i-mă) **1.** An aggregation of mesenchymal or fibroblastlike cells. **2.** Primordial embryonic connective tissue of mesenchymal cells, usually stellate, supported in interlaminar jelly.

mes·en·ter·ic, mes·a·ra·ic, mes·a·re·ic (mes′ĕn-ter′ik, mes′ă-rā′ik, -rē′ik) Relating to the mesentery.

mes·en·ter·ic ad·e·ni·tis (mes′en-ter′ ik ad′ĕ-nī′tis) Illness with abdominal pain and fever due to enlargement and inflammation of the mesenteric lymph nodes; often mistaken for appendicitis.

mes·en·ter·i·o·pex·y (mes′ĕn-ter′ē-ŏ-pek′sē) Fixation or attachment of a torn or incised mesentery. SYN mesopexy.

mes·en·ter·i·or·rha·phy (mes′en-ter′ē-ōr′ă-fē) Suture of the mesentery. SYN mesorrhaphy.

mes·en·ter·i·pli·ca·tion (mes′ĕn-ter′i-pli-kā′shŭn) Reducing redundancy of a mesentery by making one or more tucks in it.

mes·en·ter·on (mes-en′ter-on) The midportion of the insect alimentary canal and site of digestion.

me·si·ad (mē′zē-ad) SYN mesad.

me·si·al (mē′zē-ăl) Toward the median plane following the curvature of the dental arch. SYN proximal (2).

me·si·o·buc·co·oc·clu·sal (mē′zē-ō-bŭk′ō-ŏ-klū′zăl) Relating to the angle formed by the junction of the mesial, buccal, and occlusal surfaces of a bicuspid or molar tooth.

me·si·oc·clu·sion (mē′zē-ŏ-klū′zhŭn) A malocclusion in which the mandibular arch articulates with the maxillary arch in a position mesial to normal.

me·si·o·dens, me·di·o·dens (mē′zē-ō-denz, -dē-ō-denz) Supernumerary tooth located in the midline of the anterior maxillae between the maxillary central incisor teeth.

me·si·o·lin·guo·oc·clu·sal (mē′zē-ō-ling′gwō-ŏ-klū′zăl) Denoting angle formed by junction of the mesial, lingual, and occlusal surfaces of a bicuspid or molar tooth.

me·si·o·oc·clu·sal (mē′zē-ō-ŏ-klū′zăl) Denoting the angle formed by the junction of the mesial and occlusal surfaces of a premolar or molar tooth.

me·si·o·ver·sion (mē′zē-ō-vĕr′zhŭn) Malposition of a tooth mesial to normal, in an anterior direction following the curvature of the dental arch.

mes·mer·ism (mez′mĕr-izm) A system of therapeutics from which were developed hypnotism and therapeutic suggestion.

meso-, mes- Combining forms denoting **1.** Middle, mean, intermediacy. **2.** A mesentery. **3.** A compound, containing more than one chiral center, having an internal plane of symmetry.

mes·o·bi·lane (mez′ō-bī′lān) A reduced mesobilirubin with no double bonds between the pyrrole rings and, consequently, colorless. SYN mesobilirubin.

mes·o·bil·i·ru·bin·o·gen (mez′ō-bil′i-rū-bin′ō-jen) SYN mesobilane.

mes·o·blas·te·ma (mez′ō-blas-tē′mă) All those cells taken collectively that constitute the early undifferentiated mesoderm.

mes·o·blas·tem·ic (mez′ō-blas-tē′mik)

M

Relating to or derived from the mesoblastema.

mes·o·blas·tic (mez′ō-blas′tik) Relating to or derived from the mesoderm.

mes·o·blas·tic neph·ro·ma (mez-ō-blas′tik ne-frō′mă) Spindle cell neoplasm of the infant and, rarely, adult kidney with entrapped renal tubules.

mesocaecum [Br.] SYN mesocecum.

mes·o·ce·cum (mez′ō-sē′kŭm) Part of the mesocolon, supporting the cecum, which occasionally persists when the ascending colon becomes retroperitoneal during fetal life. SYN mesocaecum.

mes·o·col·ic node (mez′ō-kol′ik nōd) Nodes located near the colon and along the arteries supplying blood to the colon.

mes·o·co·lon (mez′ō-kō′lŏn) [TA] The fold of peritoneum attaching the colon to the posterior abdominal wall.

mes·o·co·lo·pex·y (mez′ō-kō′lō-pek-sē) An operation to shorten the mesocolon to correct undue mobility and ptosis. SYN mesocoloplication.

mes·o·co·lo·pli·ca·tion (mez′ō-kō′lō-pli-kā′shŭn) SYN mesocolopexy.

mes·o·du·o·de·num (mez′ō-dū′ō-dē′nŭm) The mesentery of the duodenum.

mes·o·ep·i·did·y·mis (mez′ō-ep-i-did′i-mis) An occasional fold of the tunica vaginalis binding the epididymis to the testis.

mes·o·gen·ic (mez′ō-jen′ik) Denoting the virulence of a virus capable of inducing lethal infection in embryonic hosts, after a short incubation period, and an inapparent infection in immature and adult hosts.

me·so·gli·a (me-sog′lē-ă) Neuroglial cells of mesodermal origin. SYN mesoglial cells.

me·sog·li·al cells (mě-sog′lē-ăl selz) SYN mesoglia.

mes·o·glu·te·al (mez′ō-glū′tē-ăl) Relating to the musculus gluteus medius.

mes·o·il·e·um (mez′ō-il′ē-ŭm) The mesentery of the ileum.

mes·o·je·ju·num (mez′ō-jĕ-jū′nŭm) The mesentery of the jejunum.

mes·o·lym·pho·cyte (mez′ō-lim′fō-sīt) A mononuclear leukocyte of medium size, probably a lymphocyte, with a deeply staining nucleus of large size but relatively smaller than that in most lymphocytes.

me·som·er·ism (mě-som′ĕr-izm) Displacement or delocalization of electrons within a molecule so as to create fractional charges on different molecular parts.

mes·o·me·tri·um (mez′ō-mē′trē-ŭm) [TA] The broad ligament of the uterus, below the mesosalpinx.

mes·o·morph (mez′ō-mōrf) A constitutional body type or build (biotype or somatotype) in which tissues that originate from the mesoderm prevail; morphologically, a balance exists between trunk and limbs.

mes·o·mor·phic (mez′ō-mōrf′ik) Relating to mesomorphs.

me·son (mez′on) An elementary particle having a rest mass intermediate in value between the mass of an electron and that of a proton.

mes·o·neph·ric tu·bule (mez-ō-nef′rik tū′byūl) Excretory tubule of the mesonephros. SYN segmental tubule.

mes·o·ne·phro·ma of sal·i·var·y glands (mez′ō-nef-rō′mă sal′i-vār-ē glandz) A malignant tumor, comprising several subtypes such as clear cell oncocytoma, hyalinizing clear cell carcinoma, and epithelial-myoepithelial (intercalated duct) carcinoma.

mes·o·neu·ri·tis (mez′ō-nūr-ī′tis) Inflammation of a nerve or of its connective tissue without involvement of its sheath.

mes·o·phil·ic (mez′ō-fil′ik) Pertaining to a mesophil.

mes·o·phle·bi·tis (mez′ō-flĕ-bī′tis) Inflammation of the middle coat of a vein.

mes·oph·ry·on (mez-of′rē-on) SYN glabella (2).

mes·or·chi·al (mez-ōr′kē-ăl) Relating to the mesorchium.

mes·or·chi·um (mez-ōr′kē-ŭm) **1.** In the fetus, a fold of tunica vaginalis testis supporting the mesonephros and the developing testis. **2.** In the adult, a fold of tunica vaginalis testis between the testis and epididymis.

mes·or·rha·phy (mez-ōr′ă-fē) SYN mesenteriorrhaphy.

mes·o·sal·pinx (mez′ō-sal′pingks) [TA] Part of the broad ligament investing the uterine tube.

mes·o·sig·moid (mez′ō-sig′moyd) Sigmoid mesocolon. SEE mesocolon.

mes·o·sig·moid·o·pex·y (mez′ō-sig-moy′dō-pek-sē) Surgical fixation of the mesosigmoid.

mes·o·the·li·o·ma (mez′ō-thē-lē-ō′mă) A rare malignant neoplasm, derived from the lining cells of the pleura and peritoneum, which grows as a thick sheet covering the viscera.

mes·o·the·li·um, pl. **mes·o·the·li·a** (mez′ō-thē′lē-ŭm, -ă) A single layer of flattened cells forming an epithelium that lines serous cavities.

mes·o·tym·pan·um (mez′-ō-tim′pă-nŭm) The portion of the middle ear medial to the tympanic membrane.

mes·o·va·ri·um, pl. **mes·o·va·ri·a** (mez′ō-vā′rē-ŭm, -ă) [TA] A short peritoneal fold connecting the anterior border of the ovary with the posterior layer of the broad ligament of the uterus.

mes·sen·ger (mes′ĕn-jĕr) **1.** That which carries a message. **2.** Having message-carrying properties.

mes·sen·ger RNA (mRNA) (mes′ĕn-jĕr) **1.** Ribonucleic acid (RNA) reflecting the exact nucleoside sequence of genetically active deoxyribonucleic acid (DNA) and carrying the "message" of the latter, coded in its sequence, to the cytoplasmic areas where protein is made in amino acid sequences specified by mRNA, and hence primarily by DNA. SYN informational RNA, template RNA. **2.** SEE ribonucleic acid.

meta- (m-) 1. Combining form denoting after, subsequent to, behind, or hindmost. Cf. post-. **2.** CHEMISTRY an italicized prefix denoting joint, action sharing. **3.** CHEMISTRY an italicized prefix denoting compound formed by two substitutions in the benzene ring separated by one carbon atom (i.e., linked to the first and third, second and fourth) carbon atoms of the ring. SYN m-.

met·a·bi·o·sis (met′ă-bī-ō′sis) Dependence of one organism on another for its existence. SEE ALSO commensalism, mutualism, parasitism.

met·a·bol·ic ac·id·o·sis (met′ă-bol′ik as′i-dō′sis) Decreased pH and bicarbonate concentration in body fluids caused either by accumulation of acids or abnormal losses of fixed base from the body.

met·a·bol·ic al·ka·lo·sis (met′ă-bol′ik al′kă-lō′sis) A disorder associated with an increased arterial bicarbonate concentration, due to an excessive intake of alkaline materials or an excessive loss of acid in the urine or through persistent vomiting. SEE ALSO compensated alkalosis.

met·a·bol·ic bal·ance (met′ă-bol′ik bal′ăns) Equipoise that exists between the amount of energy consumed and used.

met·a·bol·ic burst (met′ă-bol′ik bŭrst) A transient increase in oxygen consumption by a neutrophil immediately after phagocytosis.

met·a·bol·ic cir·rho·sis (met′ă-bol′ik sir-ō′sis) Cirrhosis due to a metabolic disorder that causes the deposition of minerals in the liver.

met·a·bol·ic co·ma (met′ă-bol′ik kō′mă) State due to diffuse failure of neuronal metabolism, caused by such abnormalities as intrinsic disorders of neuron or glial cell metabolism.

met·a·bol·ic cra·ni·op·a·thy (met′ă-bol′ik krā′nē-op′ă-thē) SYN Morgagni syndrome.

met·a·bol·ic dis·ease (met-ă-bol′ik di-zēz′) Generic term for disease caused by an abnormal metabolic process; can be congenital, due to inherited enzyme abnormality, or acquired, due to disease of

M

an endocrine organ or failure of function of a metabolic important organ.

met·a·bol·ic path·way (met′ă-bol′ik path′wā) Intercellular chemical reactions catalyzed by enzymes; principal chemical reactions, mostly enzyme-dependent, which an organism needs to maintain homeostasis and to break down or build up molecules.

met·a·bol·ic syn·drome (met′ă-bol′ik sin′drōm) A group of health risks that increase the chances of developing heart disease, stroke, and diabetes. SYN insulin-resistance syndrome, multiple metabolic syndrome, syndrome X.

me·tab·o·lism (mĕ-tab′ŏ-lizm) The sum of the chemical and physical changes occurring in tissue, consisting of anabolism, those reactions that convert small molecules into large, and catabolism, those reactions that convert large molecules into small, including both endogenous large molecules as well as biodegradation of xenobiotics.

me·tab·o·lite (mĕ-tab′ŏ-līt) Any product or substrate of metabolism, especially of catabolism. SYN metabolin.

met·a·car·pal (met′ă-kahr′păl) **1.** Relating to the metacarpus. **2.** Any one of the metacarpal bones (I–V).

met·a·car·po·pha·lan·ge·al (met′ă-kahr′pō-fă-lan′jē-ăl) Relating to the metacarpus and the phalanges.

met·a·car·pus, pl. **met·a·car·pi** (met′ă-kahr′pŭs, -pī) [TA] The five bones of the hand between the carpus and the phalanges.

met·a·cen·tric (met′ă-sen′trik) Having the centromere about equidistant from the extremities.

met·a·cer·car·i·a, pl. **met·a·cer·ca·ri·ae** (met′ă-sĕr-kar′ē-ă, -ē) That postcercarial encysted stage in the life history of a fluke, before transfer to the definitive host.

met·a·chro·ma·si·a (met′ă-krō-mā′zē-ă) The condition in which a cell or tissue component takes on a color different from the dye solution with which it is stained. SYN metachromatism (2).

met·a·chro·mat·ic (met′ă-krō-mat′ik) Denoting cells or dyes that exhibit metachromasia. SYN metachromophil, metachromophile.

met·a·chro·mat·ic leu·ko·dys·tro·phy (met′ă-krō-mat′ik lū′kō-dis′trŏ-fē) A metabolic disorder, usually of infancy, characterized by myelin loss, accumulation of metachromatic lipids (galactosyl sulfatidates) in the white matter of the central and peripheral nervous systems, progressive paralysis, and mental retardation; psychosis and dementia are seen in adults.

met·a·chro·mo·phil, met·a·chro·mo·phile (met′ă-krō′mŏ-fil, -fīl) SYN metachromatic.

met·a·cone (met′ă-kōn) **1.** The distobuccal cusp of human upper molars. **2.** A cusp derived from the protocone in the evolutionary history of the molars.

met·a·co·nid (met′ă-kon′id) The mesiolingual cusp of human lower molars.

Met·a·gon·i·mus (met′ă-gon′i-mŭs) A genus of flukes that encyst on fish and infect various fish-eating animals, including humans.

me·tal·lo·en·zyme (mĕ-tal′ō-en′zīm) An enzyme containing a metal (ion) as an integral part of its active structure.

me·tal·lo·por·phy·rin (mĕ-tal′ō-pōr′fi-rin) A combination of a porphyrin with a metal.

me·tal·lo·pro·tein (mĕ-tal′ō-prō′tēn) A protein with a tightly bound metal ion or ions; e.g., hemoglobin.

met·a·mere (met′ă-mēr) One of a series of homologous body segments. SEE ALSO somite.

met·a·mer·ic ner·vous sys·tem (met′ă-mer′ik nĕr′vŭs sis′tĕm) That part of the nervous system that innervates body structures developed in ontogeny from the segmentally arranged somites or, in the head region, pharyngeal arches.

met·a·mor·pho·sis (met′ă-mōr′fŏ-sis) **1.** A change in form, structure, or function. **2.** Transition from one developmental stage to another. SYN transformation (1).

met•a•mor•phot•ic (met′ă-mōr-fot′ik) Relating to or marked by metamorphosis.

met•a•my•e•lo•cyte (met′ă-mī′ĕ-lō-sīt) A transitional form of myelocyte with nuclear construction intermediate between the mature myelocyte and the two-lobed granular leukocyte. SYN juvenile cell.

met•a•neph•ric (met′ă-nef′rik) Of or pertaining to the metanephros.

met•a•neph•rine (MN) (met′ă-nef′rin) A catabolite of epinephrine found in the serum, urine and in some tissues.

met•a•neph•ro•gen•ic, met•a•ne•phrog•e•nous (met′ă-nef-rō-jen′ik, -nĕ-froj′ĕ-nŭs) Applied to the more caudal part of the intermediate mesoderm, which, under the inductive action of the metanephric diverticulum, has the potency to form metanephric tubules.

met•a•phy•si•al, met•a•phy•se•al (met′ă-fiz′ē-ăl) *Avoid the mispronunciation* metaphysi′al. Relating to a metaphysis.

met•a•phy•si•al dys•pla•si•a (met′ă-fiz′ē-ăl dis-plā′zē-ă) An abnormality that occurs when new bone at the metaphyses of long bones fails to undergo remodeling to the normal tubular structure.

me•taph•y•sis, pl. **me•taph•y•ses** (mĕ-taf′i-sis, -sēz) [TA] A conic segment between the epiphysis and diaphysis of a long bone.

met•a•pla•si•a (met′ă-plā′zē-ă) Abnormal transformation of adult, fully differentiated tissue of one kind into another kind.

met•a•plasm (met′ă-plazm) SYN cell inclusions (1).

met•a•ru•bri•cyte (met′ă-rū′bri-sīt) Orthochromatic normoblast (q.v.); the oldest type of nucleated red cell.

me•tas•ta•sis (mĕ-tas′tă-sis, -sēz) **1.** The shifting of a disease or its local manifestations, from one part of the body to another. **2.** The spread of a disease process from one part of the body to another, as in the appearance of neoplasms in parts of the body remote from the site of the primary tumor. **3.** Transportation of bacteria from one part of the body to another, through the bloodstream or lymph channels.

me•tas•ta•size (mĕ-tas′tă-sīz) To pass into or invade by metastasis.

met•a•tar•sal (met′ă-tahr′săl) Relating to the metatarsus or to one of the metatarsal bones.

met•a•tar•sal•gi•a (met′ă-tahr-sal′jē-ă) Pain in the forefoot near the metatarsal heads.

met•a•tar•so•pha•lan•ge•al (met′ă-tahr′sō-fă-lan′jē-ăl) Relating to the metatarsal bones and the phalanges.

met•a•tar•sus, pl. **me•ta•tar•si** (met′ă-tahr′sŭs, -sī) The part of the foot between the tarsus and the toes, having as its skeleton the five long bones (metatarsal bones).

met•a•thal•a•mus (met′ă-thal′ă-mŭs) [TA] The most caudal and ventral part of the thalamus, composed of the medial and lateral geniculate bodies.

me•tath•e•sis (me-tath′ĕ-sis) Transfer of a pathologic product from one place to another where it causes less inconvenience or injury, when it is not possible or expedient to remove it from the body.

met•a•troph•ic (met′ă-trō′fik) Denoting the ability to undertake anabolism or to obtain nourishment from varied sources.

Met•a•zo•a (met′ă-zō′ă) A subkingdom of the kingdom Animalia, including all multicellular animal organisms in which the cells are differentiated and form tissues.

met•en•ceph•a•lon (met′en-sef′ă-lon) [TA] The anterior of the two major subdivisions of the rhombencephalon, composed of the pons and the cerebellum.

me•te•or•ism (mē′tē-ŏ-rizm) SYN tympanites.

me•ter (mē′tĕr) **1.** The fundamental unit of length in both the SI and metric system, equivalent to 39.37007874 inches. Defined to be the length of path traveled by light in a vacuum in $1/299792458$ sec. **2.** A device for measuring the quantity of that which passes through it. SYN metre.

M

me·tered-dose in·hal·er (mĕ'tĕrd-dōs' in-hāl'ĕr) SYN inhaler.

meth-, metho- Chemical prefixes usually denoting a methyl or methoxy group.

meth·a·cho·line chal·lenge (meth'ă-kō'lēn chal'ĕnj) A breathing test involving having the patient breathe successively higher doses of methacholine between breathing measurements for diagnostic purposes.

meth·a·cryl·ic ac·id (meth'ă-kril'ik as'id) A chemical in oil from Roman camomile; used in the manufacture of methacrylate resins and plastics. SYN methylacrylic acid.

meth·a·done hy·dro·chlor·ide (meth'ă-dōn hī'drŏ-klōr'īd) A synthetic narcotic; an orally effective analgesic similar in action to morphine but with slightly greater potency and longer duration. It produces psychic and physical dependence, as does morphine, but withdrawal symptoms are somewhat milder; used as a replacement (oral route) for morphine and heroin.

methaemalbumin [Br.] SYN methemalbumin.

methaemoglobin [Br.] SYN methemoglobin.

meth·ane (meth'ān) An odorless gas produced by the decomposition of organic matter; explosive when mixed with 7 or 8 volumes of air, constituting in such cases the firedamp in coal mines.

meth·an·o·gen (meth-an'ō-jen) Any methane-producing bacterium of the family Methanobacteriaceae.

meth·a·nol, wood al·co·hol (meth'ă-nol, wud al'kŏ-hol) SYN methyl alcohol.

met·hem·al·bu·min (met-hēm'al-bū'min) An abnormal compound formed in the blood as a result of heme combining with plasma albumin. SYN methaemalbumin.

met·he·mo·glo·bin (metHb) (met-hē'mŏ-glō'bin) A transformation product of oxyhemoglobin; useless for respiration; found in bloody effusions and in the circulating blood after poisoning with various other substances. SYN hemiglobin, methaemoglobin.

meth·en·a·mine (me-then'ă-mēn) A condensation product obtained by the action of ammonia on formaldehyde; in acidic urine, it decomposes to yield formaldehyde, a urinary antiseptic. SYN hexamine.

me·thi·o·nine (me-thī'ŏ-nēn) A nutritionally essential amino acid and the most important natural source of ''active methyl'' groups in the body.

meth·od (meth'ŏd) SEE ALSO operation, procedure, stain, technique.

meth·o·dol·o·gy (meth'ŏ-dol'ŏ-jē) **1.** A body of methods rules, and postulates employed by a discipline; a particular procedure or set of procedures. **2.** Analysis of the principles or procedures of inquiry in a particular field.

meth·o·trex·ate (meth'ŏ-trek'sāt) A folic acid antagonist used as an antineoplastic agent and to treat psoriasis and rheumatoid arthritis. SYN amethopterin.

meth·yl al·co·hol (meth'il al'kŏ-hol) A flammable, toxic, mobile liquid, used as an industrial solvent and antifreeze, and to manufacture chemicals. SYN methanol.

meth·yl·ate (meth'i-lāt) **1.** To mix with methanol. **2.** To introduce a methyl group. **3.** A compound in which a metal ion methyl replaces the alcoholic hydrogen of alcohol.

meth·yl·cel·lu·lose (meth'il-sel'yū-lōs) A methyl ester of cellulose that forms a colorless viscous liquid when dissolved in water, alcohol, or ether; used to increase bulk of the intestinal contents, to relieve constipation, or of the gastric contents, to reduce appetite in obesity.

meth·yl·di·chlor·o·ar·sine (meth'il-dī-klōr'ŏ-ahr'sēn) A vesicant; irritating to the respiratory tract; produces lung and eye injury; has been used in certain military operations.

meth·yl·glu·ca·mine (meth'il-glū'kă-mēn) Cation commonly used in water-soluble iodinated radiographic contrast media. SYN N-methylglucamine.

meth·yl·ma·lon·ic ac·id (meth'il-mă-lon'ik as'id) An important intermediate in fatty acid metabolism; seen in elevated levels in cases of vitamin B12 deficiency. SYN isosuccinic acid.

meth·yl meth·ac·ry·late (meth´il meth-ă-kril´āt) Thermoplastic material used for denture bases.

meth·yl sa·lic·y·late (meth´il să-lis´il-āt) The methyl ester of salicylic acid; used externally and internally for the treatment of various forms of rheumatism. SYN checkerberry oil, gaultheria oil, sweet birch oil, wintergreen oil.

meth·yl·tes·tos·ter·one (meth´il-tes-tos´těr-ōn) A methyl derivative of testosterone that is active when given orally or sublingually. Used in the treatment of hypogenitalism. SYN 17α-methyltestosterone.

meth·yl·trans·fer·ase (meth´il-trans´fěr-ās) Any enzyme transferring methyl groups from one compound to another. SYN transmethylase.

met·my·o·glo·bin (met-mī´ō-glō´bin) Myoglobin in which the ferrous ion of the heme prosthetic group is oxidized to ferric ion; ferrimyoglobin.

me·top·ic (mē-top´ik) Relating to the forehead or anterior portion of the cranium.

me·to·pi·on (me-tō´pē-on) *Avoid the misspelling/mispronunciation metropion.* A craniometric point midway between the frontal eminences. SYN metopic point.

me·tox·e·nous (me-tok´sě-nŭs) SYN heterecious.

metr-, metra-, metro- Combining forms denoting the uterus. SEE ALSO hystero-(1), utero-.

me·tra (mē´tră) SYN uterus.

me·tra·to·ni·a (mē´tră-tō´nē-ă) Atony of the uterine walls after childbirth.

metre [Br.] SYN meter.

metred-dose inhaler [Br.] SYN metered-dose inhaler.

met·ric (met´rik) Quantitative; relating to measurement. SEE metric system.

met·ric sys·tem (met´rik sis´těm) A system of weights and measures, universal for scientific use, based on the meter, the gram, and the liter.

me·tri·tis (mē-trī´tis) Inflammation of the uterus.

me·triz·a·mide (mě-triz´ă-mīd) SYN metrizoate sodium.

me·tri·zo·ate so·di·um (met´ri-zō´āt sō´dē-ŭm) A diagnostic radiopaque medium. SYN metrizamide.

metro- SEE metr-.

me·tro·fi·bro·ma (mē´trō-fī-brō´mă) A fibroma of the uterus.

me·tro·pa·ral·y·sis (mē´trō-pă-ral´i-sis) Flaccidity or paralysis of the uterine muscle during or immediately after childbirth.

me·trop·a·thy, me·tro·path·i·a (mē-trop´ă-the, mē´trō-path´ē-ă) Any disease of the uterus.

me·tro·per·i·to·ni·tis (mē´trō-per´i-tō-nī´tis) SYN perimetritis.

me·tro·phle·bi·tis (mē´trō-flě-bī´tis) Inflammation of the uterine veins usually following childbirth.

met·ro·plas·ty (mē´trō-plas-tē) SYN uteroplasty.

me·tror·rha·gi·a (mē´trō-rā´jē-ă) Any irregular, acyclic bleeding from the uterus between menstrual periods.

me·tror·rhe·a (mē´trō-rē´ă) Discharge of mucus or pus from the uterus. SYN metrorrhoea.

metrorrhoea [Br.] SYN metrorrhea.

me·tro·stax·is (mē´trō-stak´sis) Small but continuous hemorrhage of the uterine mucous membrane.

me·tro·ste·no·sis (mē´trō-stě-nō´sis) A narrowing of the uterine cavity.

-metry Combining form indicating measurement of some physiologic parameter.

me·tyr·a·pone (me-tir´ă-pōn) Inhibitor of adrenocortical steroid C-11 β-hydroxylation, administered orally or intravenously to determine the ability of the pituitary gland to increase its secretion of corticotropin. SYN mepyrapone.

me·ty·ro·sine (mĕ-tī′rō-sin, -sēn) An inhibitor of tyrosine hydroxylase and therefore a powerful inhibitor of catecholamine synthesis; used for controlling the manifestations of pheochromocytoma and in preoperative preparation.

Mg Symbol for magnesium.

mg Abbreviation for milligram.

MHz Abbreviation for megahertz.

mi·as·ma (mī-az′mă) A smoky or vaporous environment; fog.

Mi·bel·li dis·ease (mē-bel′ē di-zēz′) SYN porokeratosis.

Mi·chae·lis con·stant (mi-kā′lis kon′stänt) The true dissociation constant for the enzyme-substrate binary complex in a single-substrate rapid equilibrium enzyme-catalyzed reaction.

-micin Combining form used to form names for aminoglycoside antibiotics.

mi·cren·ceph·a·ly, mi·cren·ce·ph·a·li·a, mi·cro·en·ceph·a·ly (mī′kren-sef′ă-lē, -sĕ-fā lē-ă, mī′krō-en-sef′ă-lē) Abnormal smallness of the brain.

micro-, micr- 1. Combining forms denoting smallness. 2. In the SI and metric system used to signify one millionth (10^{-6}) of such unit. 3. CHEMISTRY terms denoting chemical procedures or analyses that use minimal quantities of substance to be examined; specimen materials and reagents.

mi·cro·ad·e·no·ma (mī′krō-ad-ĕ-nō′mă) A pituitary adenoma less than 10 mm in diameter.

mi·cro·aer·o·phil (mī′krō-ār′ō-fil, -fīl) 1. An aerobic bacterium that requires oxygen, but less than is present in the air, and grows best under modified atmospheric conditions. 2. Relating to such an organism. SYN microaerophilic.

mi·cro·aer·o·phil·ic (mī′krō-ār′ō-fil′ik) SYN microaerophil (2).

mi·cro·aer·o·to·nom·e·ter (mī′krō-ār′ō-tō-nom′ĕ-tĕr) An instrument to assist in determining the amount of gases dissolved in blood.

mi·cro·ag·gre·gate (mī′krō-ag′rĕ-gāt) A small loose mass of fibrin, degenerating platelets, white blood cells, or cellular debris that forms in blood stored in the refrigerator five days or longer.

mi·cro·al·bu·mi·nu·ria (mī′krō-al-bū′min-yūr′ē-ă) A slight increase in urinary albumin excretion that can be detected using immunoassays but not with conventional urine protein measurements.

mi·cro·a·nal·y·sis (mī′krō-ă-nal′i-sis) Analytic techniques involving unusually small samples.

mi·cro·a·nat·o·my (mī′krō-ă-nat′ŏ-mē) SYN histology.

mi·cro·an·eu·rysm (mī′krō-an′yūr-izm) Focal dilation of retinal capillaries in diabetes mellitus, retinal vein obstruction, and absolute glaucoma.

mi·cro·an·gi·og·ra·phy (mī′krō-an-jē-og′ră-fē) Radiography of the finer organ vessels after injection of a contrast medium.

mi·cro·an·gi·o·path·ic he·mo·lyt·ic a·ne·mi·a (mī′krō-an-jē-ō-path′ik hē′mō-lit′ik ă-nē′mē-ă) Hemolysis attributed to narrowing or obstruction of small blood vessels usually due to inflammation.

mi·cro·an·gi·op·a·thy (mī′krō-an′jē-op′ă-thē) SYN capillaropathy.

mi·crobe (mī′krōb) Any minute organism, including both microscopic and ultramicroscopic organisms (spirochetes, bacteria, rickettsiae, and viruses). These organisms are considered to form a biologically distinctive group, in that the genetic material is not surrounded by a nuclear membrane and mitosis does not occur during replication.

mi·cro·bi·ci·dal (mī-krō′bi-sī′dăl) Destructive to microbes. SYN microbicide (1).

mi·cro·bi·cide (mī-krō′bi-sīd) 1. SYN microbicidal. 2. An agent destructive to microbes; a germicide; an antiseptic.

mi·cro·bi·ol·o·gist (mī′krō-bī-ol′ŏ-jist) One who specializes in the science of microbiology.

mi·cro·bi·ol·o·gy (mī′krō-bī-ol′ŏ-jē) The science concerned with microorganisms, including fungi, protozoa, bacteria, and viruses.

mi·cro·blast (mī′krō-blast) A small, nucleated red blood cell.

mi·cro·bod·y (mī′krō-bod′ē) A cytoplasmic organelle, bounded by a single membrane and containing oxidative enzymes. Microbodies include peroxisomes and glyoxysomes.

mi·cro·ceph·a·ly, mi·cro·ceph·a·li·a (mī′krō-sef′ă-lē, -sĕ-fă′lē-ă) Abnormal smallness of the head; usually associated with mental retardation.

mi·cro·chem·is·try (mī′krō-kem′is-trē) The use of chemical procedures involving minute quantities or reactions not visible to the unaided eye.

mi·cro·cin·e·ma·tog·ra·phy (mī′krō-sin′ĕ-mă-tog′ră-fē) The application of moving pictures taken through magnifying lenses to the study of an organ or system in motion.

mi·cro·cir·cu·la·tion (mī′krō-sīr′kyū-lā′shŭn) Passage of blood in the smallest vessels, namely arterioles, capillaries, and venules.

Mi·cro·coc·cus (mī′krō-kok′ŭs) A genus of bacteria containing gram-positive, spheric cells that occur in irregular masses. These organisms are saprophytic, facultatively parasitic, or parasitic but are not truly pathogenic. The type species is *M. luteus.*

mi·cro·cu·rie (mCi) (mī′krō-kyūr′ē) One millionth of a curie; a quantity of any radionuclide with 3.7×10^4 disintegrations per second.

mi·cro·cyte (mī′krō-sīt) A small (i.e., 5 mcm or less) nonnucleated red blood cell; with decreased mean corpuscular volume. SYN microerythrocyte.

microcythaemia [Br.] SYN microcythemia.

mi·cro·cy·the·mi·a (mī′krō-sī-thē′mē-ă) The presence of many microcytes in the circulating blood. SYN microcythaemia, microcytosis.

mi·cro·cyt·ic (mī′krō-sit′ik) Denotes presence of a cell smaller than 5 mcm.

mi·cro·cyt·ic hy·po·chrom·ic a·ne·mi·a (mī′krō-sit′ik hī′pō-krō′mik ă-nē′mē-ă) Any anemia with microcytes that are reduced in size and in hemoglobin content; the most common type is iron deficiency anemia.

mi·cro·dac·ty·ly, mi·cro·dac·ty·li·a (mī′krō-dak′ti-lē, -dak-til′ē-ă) Smallness or shortness of the fingers or toes.

mi·cro·di·al·y·sis (mī′krō-dī-al′i-sis) Study of extracellular fluid composition and response to exogenous agents, with a tiny tubular probe with a dialysis membrane and fluid flow rates of 1–3 mcL/min, inserted into tissues.

mi·cro·dis·sec·tion (mī′krō-di-sek′shŭn) Dissection of tissues under a microscope or magnifying glass, usually done by teasing the tissues apart by means of needles.

mi·cro·e·lec·trode (mī′krō-ĕ-lek′trōd) An electrode of very fine caliber consisting usually of a fine wire or a glass tube of capillary diameter drawn to a fine point and filled with saline or a metal; used in physiologic experiments to stimulate or to record action currents of extracellular or intracellular origin.

mi·cro·e·ryth·ro·cyte (mī′krō-ĕ-rith′rō-sīt) SYN microcyte.

mi·cro·fi·bril (mī′krō-fī′bril) A very small fibril having an average diameter of 13 nm; it may be a bundle of still smaller elements, the microfilaments.

mi·cro·fil·a·ment (mī′krō-fil′ă-mĕnt) The finest filamentous element of the cytoskeleton, having a diameter of about 5 nm and consisting primarily of actin. SEE ALSO actin filament.

microfilaraemia [Br.] SYN microfilaremia.

mi·cro·fil·a·re·mi·a (mī′krō-fil′ă-rē′mē-ă) Infection of the blood with microfilariae.

M

mi·cro·fi·lar·i·a, pl. **mi·cro·fi·lar·i·ae** (mī′krō-fi-lar′ē-ă, -ē) Term for embryos of filarial nematodes in the family Onchocercidae.

mi·cro·film (mī′krō-film) **1.** A photographic film bearing greatly reduced images of printed records. **2.** To record on microfilm.

mi·cro·flo·ra (mī′krō-flōr′ă) The bacteria and fungi that inhabit an area.

mi·cro·ga·mete (mī′krō-gam′ēt) The male element in anisogamy, or conjugation of cells of unequal size.

mi·cro·ga·me·to·cyte (mī′krō-gă-mē′tō-sīt) The mother cell producing the microgametes, or male elements of sexual reproduction in sporozoan protozoans and fungi.

mi·crog·li·a (mī-krog′lē-ă) Small neuroglial cells, which may become phagocytic, in areas of inflammation. SYN Hortega cells.

mi·cro·glob·u·lin (mī′krō-glob′yū-lin) **1.** Any serum or urinary globulin with a molecular mass less than about 40 kD. **2.** On occasion, a term used to refer to 7S immunoglobins (e.g., IgG).

mi·cro·gna·thi·a (mī′krog-nath′ē-ă) *In the diphthong gn, the g is silent only at the beginning of a word.* Abnormal smallness of the jaws, especially of the mandible.

mi·cro·gram (mcg) (mī′krō-gram) One millionth of a gram.

mi·cro·graph (mī′krō-graf) SYN photomicrograph.

mi·cro·gy·ri·a (mī′krō-ji′rē-ă) Abnormal narrowness of the cerebral convolutions.

mi·cro·he·ma·to·crit con·cen·tra·tion (mī′krō-hĕ-mat′ŏ-krit kon′sĕn-trā′shŭn) Centrifugation of whole anticoagulated blood using microhematocrit tubes to obtain a buffy coat layer containing white blood cells.

mi·cro·he·pat·i·a (mī′krō-he-pā′shē-ă) Abnormal smallness of the liver.

mi·cro·in·ci·sion (mī′krō-in-sizh′ŭn) An incision made with the aid of a microscope.

mi·cro·in·jec·tor (mī′krō-in-jek′tŏr) An instrument for infusion of very small amounts of fluids or drugs.

mi·cro·in·va·sion (mī′krō-in-vă′zhŭn) Invasion of tissue immediately adjacent to a carcinoma in situ, the earliest stage of malignant neoplastic invasion.

mi·cro·in·va·sive car·ci·no·ma (mī′krō-in-vă′siv kahr′si-nō′mă) Lesion seen most frequently in the uterine cervix, in which carcinoma in situ of squamous epithelium, on the surface or replacing the lining of glands, is accompanied by small collections of abnormal epithelial cells that infiltrate a very short distance into the stroma.

mi·cro·li·ter (mcL, mcl) (mī′krō-lē-tĕr) One millionth of a liter. SYN microlitre.

mi·cro·li·thi·a·sis (mī′krō-li-thī′ă-sis) The formation, presence, or discharge of minute concretions, or gravel.

microlitre [Br.] SYN microliter.

mi·cro·ma·nip·u·la·tion (mī′krō-mă-nip′yū-lā′shŭn) Dissection, stimulation, and other mechanical operations performed on minute structures under a microscope.

mi·cro·ma·nip·u·la·tor (mī′krō-mă-nip′yū-lā′tŏr) An instrument used in micromanipulation, whereby microdissection, microinjection, and other maneuvers are performed, usually with the aid of a microscope.

mi·cro·mere (mī′krō-mēr) A small blastomere.

mi·cro·me·tas·ta·sis, mi·cro·me·tas·ta·ses (mī′krō-mĕ-tas′tă-sis, -sēz) A stage of metastasis when the secondary tumors are too small to be clinically detected, as in micrometastatic disease.

mi·cro·met·a·stat·ic (mī′krō-met′ă-stat′ik) Denoting or characterized by micrometastasis.

mi·crom·e·ter (mcm) (mī-krom′ĕ-tĕr) **1.** One millionth of a meter; formerly called micron. **2.** A device for measuring various objects in an accurate and precise manner.

mi·cro·my·e·lo·blast (mī′krō-mī′ĕl-ō-blast) A small myeloblast, often the predominating cell in myeloblastic leukemia.

mi·cro·my·el·o·blas·tic leu·ke·mi·a (mī′krō-mī′ĕl-ō-blast′ik lū-kē′mē-ă) A form of myelocytic leukemia in which relatively large proportions of micromyeloblasts are found in circulating blood and in bone marrow and other tissues.

mi·cro·nee·dle (mī′krō-nē′dĕl) A small glass needle used in microsurgical manipulation.

mi·cro·nod·u·lar (mī′krō-nod′yū-lăr) Characterized by presence of minute nodules; has a coarser appearance than that of a granular tissue or substance.

mi·cro·nu·cle·us (mī′krō-nū′klē-ŭs) A small nucleus in a large cell, or the smaller nuclei in cells that have two or more such structures.

mi·cro·nu·tri·ents (mī′krō-nū′trē-ĕnts) Essential food factors required in only small quantities by the body; e.g., vitamins, trace minerals.

mi·cro·or·gan·ism (mī′krō-ōr′găn-izm) A microscopic organism (plant or animal).

mi·cro·phage (mī′krō-fāj) A phagocytic (q.v.) polymorphonuclear leukocyte.

mi·cro·pleth·ys·mog·ra·phy (mī′krō-pleth′iz-mog′ră-fē) The technique of measuring minute changes in the volume of a part as a result of blood flow into or out of it.

mi·crop·si·a, mi·crop·sy (mī-krop′sē-ă, mī′krop-sē) Perception of objects as smaller than they are.

mi·cro·ra·di·og·ra·phy (mī′krō-rā′dē-og′ră-fē) Making radiographs of histologic sections of tissue for enlargement.

mi·cro·re·frac·tom·e·ter (mī′krō-rē-frak-tom′ĕ-tĕr) A refractometer used in the study of blood cells.

mi·cro·res·pi·rom·e·ter (mī′krō-res-pi-rom′ĕ-tĕr) An apparatus for measuring the use of oxygen by small particles of isolated tissues or cells or particles of cells.

mi·cro·scope (mī′krō-skōp) An instrument that gives an enlarged image of an object or substance that is minute or not visible with the naked eye; usually denotes a compound microscope; for low magnifications the term ''simple microscope,'' or ''magnifying glass,'' is used.

mi·cro·scop·ic, mi·cro·scop·i·cal (mī′krō-skop′ik, -skop′i-kăl) **1.** Of minute size; visible only with the aid of the microscope. **2.** Relating to a microscope.

mi·cro·scop·ic a·nat·o·my (mī′krō-skop′ik ă-nat′ō-mē) Branch of anatomy in which the structure of cells, tissues, and organs is studied with the light microscope. SEE histology.

mi·cros·co·py (mī-kros′kŏ-pē) Investigation of minute objects by means of a microscope. SEE ALSO microscope.

mi·cro·some (mī′krō-sōm) One of the small spheric vesicles derived from the endoplasmic reticulum after disruption of cells and ultracentrifugation.

mi·cro·spec·tro·scope (mī′krō-spek′trō-skōp) An instrument to observe a spectrum of microscopic objects.

mi·cro·sphe·ro·cy·to·sis (mī′krō-sfēr′ō-sī-tō′sis) A condition of the blood seen in hemolytic icterus in which small spherocytes are predominant; the red blood cells are smaller and more globular than normal.

mi·cro·spor·id·i·o·sis, mi·cro·spor·id·i·a·sis (mī′krō-spō-rid′ē-ō′sis, -spōr′i-dī′a-sis) Infection with a member of the phylum Microspora, the microsporidians.

Mi·cros·po·rum (mī′krō-spō′rŭm) A genus of pathogenic fungi causing dermatophytosis.

mi·cro·sur·ger·y (mī′krō-sŭr′jĕr-ē) Surgical procedures performed under the magnification of a surgical microscope.

mi·cro·su·ture (mī′krō-sū′chŭr) Small caliber suture material, often 9-0 or 10-0, with an attached needle of corresponding size, for use in microsurgery.

M

mi·cro·sy·ringe (mī′krō-si-rinj′) A hypodermic syringe that has a micrometer screw attached to the piston, whereby accurately measured minute quantities of fluid may be injected.

mi·cro·ther·my (mī′krō-thĕr′mē) Radiating heat used in physical therapy.

mi·cro·throm·bus (mī′krō-throm′bŭs) A very small cardiovascular clot.

mi·cro·ti·a (mī-krō′shē-ă) Abnormal smallness of the auricle of the acoustic external ear with a blind or absent external auditory meatus.

mi·cro·tome (mī′krō-tōm) An instrument for making sections of biologic tissue for examination under the microscope. SYN histotome.

mi·crot·o·my (mī-krot′ŏ-mē) The making of thin sections of tissues for examination under the microscope. SYN histotomy.

mi·cro·tu·bule (mī′krō-tū′byūl) A cylindric cytoplasmic element that occurs widely in the cytoskeleton of plant and animal cells.

mi·cro·vil·lus (MV), gen. and pl. **mi·cro·vil·li** (mī′krō-vil′ŭs, -ī) One of the minute projections of cell membranes greatly increasing surface area.

mi·cro·volt (mcV) (mī′krō-vōlt) One millionth of a volt.

mi·cro·zo·on (mī′krō-zō′on) A microscopic form of the animal kingdom; a protozoon.

mic·tion (mik′shŭn) SYN urination.

mic·tu·rate (mik′chŭr-āt) SYN urinate.

mic·tu·ri·tion (mik-chŭr-ish′ŭn) **1.** SYN urination. **2.** The desire to urinate. **3.** Frequency of urination.

mic·tu·ri·tion re·flex (mik′chŭr-ish′ŭn rē′fleks) Contraction of bladder walls and relaxation of the trigone and urethral sphincter in response to a rise in pressure within the bladder. SYN bladder reflex, urinary reflex, vesical reflex.

mic·tu·ri·tion syn·co·pe (mik′chŭr-ish′ŭn sin′kŏ-pē) Loss of consciousness in association with the act of emptying the bladder.

mid- Combining form meaning middle.

mid·car·pal (mid-kahr′păl) **1.** Relating to the central part of the carpus. **2.** Denoting the articulation between the two rows of carpal bones. SYN mediocarpal.

mid·dle (mid′ĕl) Denoting an anatomic structure that is between two other similar structures or that is midway in position.

mid·dle ear (mid′ĕl ēr) SEE ear. SEE ALSO tympanic cavity.

mid·dle fos·sa ap·proach (mid′ĕl fos′ă ă-prōch′) Surgical path to the cerebellopontine angle through that portion of the floor of the middle cranial fossa that is the anterior surface of the petrous pyramid of the temporal bone.

mid·dle kid·ney (mid′ĕl kid′nē) SEE mesonephros.

mid·dle lobe syn·drome (mid′ĕl lōb sin′drōm) Atelectasis with chronic pneumonitis of the middle lobe of the (right) lung, due to compression of the middle lobe bronchus, usually by enlarged lymph nodes, which may be tuberculous; chief symptoms are chronic cough, wheezing, recurrent respiratory infections, hemoptysis, chest pain, malaise, easy fatigability, and loss of weight. SYN Brock syndrome.

mid·dle me·di·as·ti·num (mid′ĕl mē′dē-ă-stī′nŭm) [TA] Large central portion of the inferior mediastinum, which includes the pericardium and the contained heart, as well as the phrenic nerves and cardiacophrenic vessels. SYN mediastinum medium [TA].

mid·dle na·sal con·cha (mid′ĕl nā′zăl kong′kă) [TA] The middle thin, spongy, bony plate with curved margins, part of the ethmoidal labyrinth, projecting from the lateral wall of the nasal cavity and separating the superior meatus from the middle meatus.

mid·gut (mid′gŭt) **1.** The central portion of the digestive tube; the distal duodenum, small intestine, and proximal colon. **2.** The portion of the embryonic gut between the foregut and the hindgut that originally is open to the yolk sac.

mid·gut loop (mid′gŭt lūp) The U-shaped part of the embryonic midgut that herniates into the extraembryonic celom in the proximal part of the umbilical cord when the embryonic celom temporarily becomes too small to contain the intestinal loops. SYN umbilical intestinal loop.

mid·line epi·si·ot·o·my (mid′līn ĕ-piz′ē-ot′ŏ-mē) Incision of the perineum in the midline during childbirth to ease delivery. SYN median episiotomy.

mid·line le·thal gran·u·lo·ma (mid′līn lē′thăl gran′yū-lō′mă) Destruction of the nasal septum, hard palate, lateral nasal walls, paranasal sinuses, skin of the face, orbit, and nasopharynx by an inflammatory infiltrate with atypical lymphocytic and histiocytic cells. The prognosis is poor, despite radiotherapy.

mid·line my·e·lot·o·my (mid′līn mī-ĕ-lot′ŏ-mē) Section of the midline transverse fibers of the spinal cord for the treatment of intractable pain. SYN commissurotomy (2).

mid·oc·cip·i·tal (mid′ok-sip′i-tăl) Relating to the central portion of the occiput. SYN medioccipital.

mid-spec·trum a·gent (mid-spek′trŭm ā′jĕnt) A term increasingly used to refer to toxins, synthetic viruses, and genocidal agents as mass-casualty agents having features of both chemical-warfare agents and biological-warfare agents.

mid-stream ur·ine spe·ci·men (mid-strēm yūr′in spes′i-mĕn) A urine sample collected from the middle flow of urine after cleansing of the external genitalia. Used to identify infective agents and test antibiotic sensitivity.

mid·wife (mid′wīf) A person qualified to practice midwifery, having received specialized training in obstetrics and child care.

mid·wife·ry (mid-wif′ĕ-rē) SEE ALSO doula.

mi·fe·pris·tone (RU-486) (mif′ĕ-pris-tōn) Synthetic chemical compound with antiprogesterone properties used for early pregnancy termination.

mi·graine (mī′grān) A symptom complex occurring periodically and characterized by pain in the head (usually unilateral), vertigo, nausea and vomiting, photophobia, and scintillating appearances of light. SYN hemicrania (1), sick headache.

mi·graine-re·lat·ed ves·tib·u·lop·a·thy (mī′grān′ rē-lā′tĕd ves-tib′yū-lŏp′ă-thē) A disorder characterized by movement-associated disequilibrium, unsteadiness, space and motion discomfort, and vertigo before onset of headache.

mi·gra·tion (mī-grā′shŭn) **1.** Passage from one part to another. **2.** SYN diapedesis. **3.** Movement of a tooth or teeth out of normal position. **4.** Movement of molecules during electrophoresis. **5.** Geographic spread of disease-causing agents, rectors, or populations.

mi·gra·tion in·hib·i·tor·y fac·tor test (mī-grā′shŭn in-hib′ī-tŏ-rē fak′tŏr test) Assessment to measure the presence of migration inhibitory factor, a 25-kD lymphokine. SYN macrophage migration inhibition test, migration inhibition test.

Mi·ku·licz dis·ease (mē′kū-lich di-zēz′) Benign swelling of the lacrimal, and usually also of the salivary, glands due to infiltration of and replacement of the normal gland structure by lymphoid tissue. SEE ALSO Sjögren syndrome.

mil·i·a·ri·a (mil′ē-ā′rē-ă) An eruption of minute vesicles and papules due to retention of fluid at the orifices of sweat glands.

mil·i·a·ri·a ru·bra (mil′-ē-ā′rē-ă rū′bră) An eruption of papules and vesicles at the orifices of sweat glands, accompanied by redness and inflammatory reaction of the skin. SYN heat rash, prickly heat, lichen tropicus.

mil·i·a·ry (mil′ē-ār′-ē) **1.** Resembling a millet seed in size. **2.** Marked by the presence of nodules of millet seed size on any surface.

mil·i·ary an·eur·ysm (mil′ē-ār-ē an′yŭr-izm) Dilation in the diameter of small arteries and arterioles secondary to lipohyalinosis from long-standing hyper-

M

tension; associated with intracerebral hematomas.

mil·i·a·ry car·ci·no·sis (mil′ē-ār′-ē kahr′si-nō′sis) Collection of small cancerous nodules.

mil·i·a·ry em·bo·lism (mil′ē-ār′-ē em′bŏ-lizm) One occurring simultaneously in a number of capillaries.

mil·i·a·ry tu·ber·cu·lo·sis (mil′ē-ār′-ē tū-bĕr′kyū-lō′sis) General dissemination of tubercle bacilli in the blood, resulting in the formation of miliary tubercles in various organs and tissues, and occasionally producing symptoms of profound toxemia. SYN generalized tuberculosis.

mil·ieu in·té·ri·eur, mil·ieu in·ter·ne (mēl-yu′ an[h]-ter-ē-ur′, in-tārn) **1.** Internal environment. **2.** The fluids bathing the tissue cells of multicellular animals.

Mil·i·ta·ry Health Ser·vic·es Sys·tem (MHSS) (mil′i-tar-rē helth sĕr′vis-ez sis′tĕm) The network of hospitals and clinics that comprise the health care system of the U.S. Department of Defense. Although its primary function is to maintain the health of members of the U.S. Armed Forces, it also provides health care if space and services are available to dependents, retirees, and other participants in TRICARE, the U.S. military health benefit plan.

mil·i·um, pl. **mil·i·a** (mil′ē-ŭm, -ă) A small subepidermal keratin cyst, usually multiple and therefore commonly referred to in the plural. SYN whitehead (1).

milk (milk) **1.** A white liquid, containing nutrients and other substances (e.g., proteins, sugar, and lipids), secreted by the mammary glands after birth, and serving to nourish the infant or young animal. **2.** Any whitish, milky fluid; e.g., the juice of the coconut or a suspension of various metallic oxides. **3.** A pharmacopeial preparation that is a suspension of insoluble drugs in a water medium; distinguished from gels mainly in that the suspended particles of milk are larger. **4.** SYN strip (1).

milk-al·ka·li syn·drome (milk-al′kă-lī sin′drōm) A chronic disorder of the kidneys, reversible in its early stages, induced by taking large doses of calcium

and alkali in to relieve pains from a peptic ulcer; can progress to renal failure. SYN Burnett syndrome.

milk crust (milk krŭst) SYN crusta lactea.

milk fe·ver (milk fē′vĕr) A slight elevation of temperature following childbirth, due to establishment of milk secretion, but probably the same as absorption fever.

milk·ing (milk′ing) A procedure used to express the contents of a tube or duct to obtain a specimen or to test for tenderness.

Milk·man syn·drome (milk′man sin′drōm) Osteomalacia with multiple pseudofractures, usually bilateral and symmetric; true pathologic fractures may also develop.

milk of mag·ne·si·a (MOM) (milk mag-nē′zē-ă) Aqueous solution of magnesium hydroxide; used as an antacid and laxative. SYN magnesia magma.

milk sick·ness (milk sik′nĕs) Human disease caused by ingesting contaminated milk from cows suffering from trembles; clinical manifestations include severe vomiting, labored breathing, delirium, convulsions, coma, and death; recovery from nonlethal illness is slow. SYN lactimorbus.

Mil·ler-Ab·bott tube (mil′ĕr ab′ŏt tūb) Tube with two lumens, one ending in asmall collapsible balloon and the other in a metallic tip with numerous perforations; used for intestinal decompression. SYN Abbott tube.

milli- Combining form for one thousandth.

mil·li·am·pere (ma, mA) (mil′ē-am′pēr) One thousandth of an ampere.

mil·li·cu·rie (mc, mCi) (mil′i-kyūr′ē) A unit of radioactivity equivalent to 3.7×10^7 disintegrations per second.

mil·li·e·quiv·a·lent (mEq, meq) (mil′ē-ē-kwiv′ă-lĕnt) One thousandth equivalent; 10^{-3} mole divided by valence.

mil·li·gram (mg) (mil′i-gram) One thousandth of a gram.

mil·li·li·ter (mL, ml) (mil′i-lē′tĕr) One thousandth of a liter.

mil·li·me·ter (mm) (mil′ĭ-mē′tĕr) One thousandth of a meter.

mil·li·mole (mmol) (mil′ĭ-mōl) One thousandth of a gram-molecule.

mil·li·pede (mil′ĭ-pēd) A venomous arthropod, characterized by two pairs of legs per leg-bearing segment. The venom is purely defensive, oozed or squirted from pores along the body, producing irritation to the skin or severe inflammation if it reaches the eyes.

mil·li·rad (mrad) (mil′ĭ-rad) One-thousandth of a.

mil·li·sec·ond (msec) (mil′ĭ-sek′ŏnd) One thousandth of a second.

mil·li·volt (mV) (mil′ĭ-vōlt) One thousandth of a volt.

mil·pho·sis (mil-fō′sis) Loss of eyelashes.

Mil·wau·kee brace (mil-waw′kē brās) A back brace used to correct scoliosis, lordosis, or kyphosis.

mi·me·sis (mi-mē′sis) **1.** Hysteric simulation of organic disease. **2.** The symptomatic imitation of one organic disease by another.

mind (mīnd) **1.** Seat of consciousness and higher functions of the human brain (e.g., cognition, reasoning). **2.** Organized totality of all mental processes and psychic activities, with emphasis on relatedness of phenomena.

mind blind·ness (mīnd blīnd′nĕs) Visual agnosia for objects, in which objects are seen but not identified; caused by a lesion in Brodmann area 18 of the occipital cortex.

min·er·al (min′ĕr-ăl) Any homogeneous inorganic material usually found in the earth's crust.

min·er·al·i·za·tion (min′ĕr-ăl-ī-zā′shŭn) Introduction of minerals into a structure, as in the normal mineralization of bones and teeth or pathologic mineralization of tissues.

min·er·al·o·cor·ti·coid (min′ĕr-ăl-ō-kōr′ti-koyd) One of the steroids of the cortex of the suprarenal gland that influ-

ence salt (sodium and potassium) metabolism.

min·er·al oil (min′ĕr-ăl oyl) A mixture of liquid hydrocarbons obtained from petroleum, used as a vehicle in pharmaceutical preparations, and as an intestinal lubricant. SYN heavy liquid petrolatum, liquid paraffin, liquid petroleum.

min·er's lung (mī′nĕrz lŭng) SYN black lung.

Mi·ner·va cast (mi-nĕr′vă kast) A cast applied around the neck and trunk of the body; used postsurgery on the neck or back.

min·i·mal brain dys·func·tion (min′ĭ-măl brān dis-fŭngk′shŭn) SEE attention deficit disorder.

min·i·mal in·hib·i·tor·y con·cen·tra·tion (min′ĭ-măl in-hib′ĭ-tōr-ē kon′sĕn-trā′shŭn) Lowest concentration of antibiotic sufficient to inhibit bacterial growth when tested in vitro.

mi·ni·mal·ly in·va·sive di·rec·ted cor·o·na·ry ar·te·ry by·pass graft (min′ĭ-mă-lē in-vā′siv dĭ-rĕk′tĕd kōr′ŏ-nar-y ahr′tĕr-ē bī′pas graft) Graft performed through a left anterior thoracotomy without cardiopulmonary bypass.

min·i·mal·ly in·va·sive sur·ge·ry (min′ĭ-mă-lē in-vā′siv sŭr′jĕr-ē) Operation using the smallest possible incision or no incision at all; includes laparoscopic, thoracoscopic, and endoscopic procedures.

min·i·mum leak tech·nique (min′ĭ-mŭm lēk tek-nēk′) In respiratory therapy, a form of mechanical ventilation often used in association with tracheotomy. An invasive procedure; carries a substantial risk of patients' aspirating of fluids.

mi·ni·plate (min′ē-plāt) Metal prosthesis for surgical fracture fixation of a minimal quantity of material formed into a strip or lattice.

Min·ne·so·ta Mul·ti·pha·sic Per·son·al·i·ty In·ven·to·ry (min-ĕ-sō′tă mŭl′tē-fā′zik pĕr′sŏn-al′i-tē in′vĕn-tōr-ē) A questionnaire for ages 16 years and older, with 550 true-false statements coded in 4 validity and 10 personality

M

scales; administered in either an individual or group format.

mi·nor (mī′nŏr) Smaller; lesser; denoting the smaller of two similar structures.

mi·nor ag·glu·ti·nin (mī′nŏr ă-glū′ti-nin) Immune agglutinin in an antiserum in lesser concentration than the major agglutinin. SYN partial agglutinin.

mi·nor for·ceps (mī′nŏr fōr′seps) Frontal radiation of the corpus callosum. SYN forceps minor.

mi·nor his·to·com·pat·i·bil·i·ty com·plex (MHC) (mī′nŏr his′tō-kŏm-pat′i-bil′i-tē kom′pleks) Genes outside the MHC present on various chromosomes that encode antigens contributing to graft rejection.

mi·nor op·er·a·tion (mī′nŏr op-ĕr-ā′shŭn) A relatively slight surgical procedure not in itself hazardous to life.

mint (mint) SYN *Mentha*.

min·ute vol·ume (min′ŭt vol′yūm) The amount of any gas or fluid moved in 1 minute (e.g., cardiac output or the respiratory minute volume). Also called minute ventilation.

mio- Combining form meaning less.

mi·o·sis (mī-ō′sis) *Do not confuse this word with meiosis.* Contraction of the pupil.

mi·o·sphyg·mi·a (mī′ō-sfig′mē-ă) Condition in which pulse beats are fewer than heart beats.

mi·ot·ic (mī-ot′ik) **1.** Related to constriction of the pupil. **2.** An agent that causes the pupil to constrict.

mire (mēr) A test object in the ophthalmometer; its image (also called a mire), mirrored on the corneal surface, is measured to determine the radii of corneal curvature.

mir·ror (mir′ŏr) A polished surface reflecting the rays of light reflected from objects in front of it.

mir·ror speech (mir′ŏr spēch) A reversal of the order of syllables in a word, analogous to mirror writing.

mis- Combining form denoting not, opposite, incorrect, improper.

mis·car·riage (mis′kar-ăj) Spontaneous expulsion of products of pregnancy before mid-second trimester.

mis·ci·ble (mis′i-bĕl) Capable of being and staying mixed after the mixing process.

mis·o·pe·di·a, mis·op·e·dy (mis′ō-pē′dē-ă, mis·op′-ĕ-dē) Aversion to or hatred of children.

mi·so·pros·tol (mī′sō-prost′ol) **1.** Prostaglandin analogue used to prevent gastric and duodenal ulcers. **2.** A component of the mifepristone regimen for early termination of pregnancy.

missed la·bor (mist lā′bŏr) Brief uterine contractions that do not lead to labor and expulsion of the infant, but cease, resulting in the indefinite retention of the fetus (usually lifeless) either in utero or in the abdominal cavity.

missed pe·ri·od (mist pēr′ē-ŏd) Failure of menstruation to occur in any month at the expected time.

mis·sense mu·ta·tion (mis′sens myū-tā′shŭn) Mutation in which a base change or substitution results in a codon that causes insertion of a different amino acid into the growing polypeptide chain.

mite (mīt) A minute arthropod of the order Acarina; a vast assemblage of parasitic and (primarily) free-living organisms.

mith·ra·my·cin (MTF) (mith′ră-mī′sin) An antineoplastic antibiotic produced by *Streptomyces argillaceus* and *S. tanashiensis*. SYN aureolic acid, mitramycin.

mi·ti·ci·dal (mī′ti-sī′dăl) Destructive to mites.

mi·ti·cide (mī′ti-sīd) An agent destructive to mites.

mi·to·chon·dri·al chro·mo·some (mī′tō-kon′drē-ăl krō′mŏ-sōm) The DNA component of mitochondria, the chief function of which is synthesis of adenosine triphosphate and the management of cellular energy.

mi·to·chon·dri·al dis·or·ders (mī′-tō-kon′drē-ăl dis-ōr′dĕrz) A group of diverse hereditary disorders caused by genetic mutation of mitochondrial DNA; includes: ragged red fiber myopathy; progressive external ophthalmoplegia; Leigh syndrome; myoclonic epilepsy with ragged red fiber myopathy (MERRF); mitochondrial myopathy, encephalopathy, lactacidosis, and stroke (MELAS); and Lieber optic neuropathy.

mi·to·chon·dri·al DNA (mī′tō-kon′drē-ăl) Species of deoxyribonucleic acid (DNA) present in mitochondria, where it participates in energy metabolism, rather than in the nucleus.

mi·to·chon·dri·al mem·brane (mī′tō-kon′drē-ăl mem′brān) Mitochondrion has two membranes: the inner where the electron transport system is located and the outer, which acts as a gatekeeper and allows only certain molecules to enter.

mi·to·chon·dri·al my·op·a·thy (mī′tō-kon′drē-ăl mī-op′ă-thē) Weakness and hypotonia of muscles, primarily those of the neck, shoulder, and pelvic girdles, with onset in infancy or childhood.

mi·to·chon·dri·on, pl. **mi·to·chon·dri·a** (mī′tō-kon′drē-ŏn, -ă) An organelle of the cell cytoplasm consisting of two sets of membranes, a smooth continuous outer coat and an inner membrane arranged in tubules or more often in folds that form platelike double membranes called cristae.

mi·to·gen (mī′tō-jen) A substance that stimulates mitosis and lymphocyte transformation.

mi·to·gen·e·sis (mī′tō-jen′ĕ-sis) The induction of mitosis in a cell.

mi·to·ge·net·ic (mī′tō-jĕ-net′ik) Pertaining to the factor or factors promoting cell mitosis.

mi·to·my·cin (mī′tō-mī′sin) Antibiotic family produced by *Streptomyces caespitosus*; mitomycin C is an antineoplastic and bacteriocide; inhibits DNA synthesis.

mi·to·sis, pl. **mi·to·ses** (mī-tō′sis, -sēz) Usual somatic reproduction of cells consisting of a sequence of modifications of the nucleus that result in formation of two daughter cells with exactly the same chromosome and DNA content as that of the original cell. SEE ALSO cell cycle. SYN indirect nuclear division.

mi·tot·ic in·dex (MI) (mī-tot′ik in′deks) Ratio of cells in a tissue that are undergoing mitosis.

mi·tot·ic pe·ri·od (mī-tot′ik pēr′ē-ŏd) The proportion of cells in a tissue that are undergoing mitosis, expressed as a mitotic index or, roughly, as the number of cells in mitosis in each microscopic high-power field in tissue sections. SYN M phase

mi·tot·ic rate (mī-tot′ik rāt) Proportion of cells in a tissue that are undergoing mitosis, expressed as a mitotic index.

mi·tot·ic spin·dle (mī-tot′ik spin′dĕl) The fusiform figure characteristic of a dividing cell. SYN nuclear spindle.

mi·tral (mī′trăl) Relating to the mitral or bicuspid valve.

mi·tral a·tre·si·a (mī′trăl ă-trē′zē-ă) Congenital absence of the mitral valve between the left atrium and left ventricle.

mi·tral in·suf·fi·cien·cy (mī′trăl in′sŭ-fish′ĕn-sē) SEE valvular regurgitation.

mi·tral·i·za·tion (mī′trăl′ī-zā′shŭn) Straightening the left heart border on a chest radiograph due to prominence of the left atrial appendage or the pulmonary outflow tract.

mi·tral re·gur·gi·ta·tion (mī′trăl rē-gŭr′ji-tā′shŭn) SEE valvular regurgitation.

mi·tral ste·no·sis (MS) (mī′trăl stĕ-nō′sis) Pathologic narrowing of the orifice of the mitral valve.

mi·tral valve (mī′trăl valv) [TA] The valve closing the orifice between the left atrium and left ventricle of the heart; its two cusps are called anterior and posterior. SYN bicuspid valve.

mi·tral valve pro·lapse (MVP) (mī′trăl valv prō′laps) Excessive retrograde movement of one or both mitral valve leaflets into the left atrium during left ventricular systole, often allowing mitral regurgitation.

M

mi·tral valve pro·lapse syn·drome (MVPS) (mī′trăl valv prō′laps sin′drōm) Clinical constellation of findings with or without symptoms due to prolapse of the mitral valve. Symptoms are nonspecific and may include vague chest pains and dyspnea on exertion. SYN billowing mitral valve syndrome.

mit·tel·schmerz (mit′el-schmārts) Abdominal pain occurring at the time of ovulation, resulting from irritation of the peritoneum by bleeding from the ovulation site. SYN intermenstrual pain (2).

mix·ed a·pha·si·a (mikst ă-fā′zē-ă) SYN global aphasia.

mix·ed a·stig·ma·tism (mikst ă-stig′mă-tizm) A vision defect in which one meridian is hyperopic while the one at a right angle to it is myopic.

mix·ed dust pneu·mo·co·ni·o·sis (mikst dŭst nū′mō-kō′nē-ō′sis) Pulmonary disorder caused by inhaling a variety of dust particles.

mix·ed ep·i·sode (mikst ep′i-sōd) Sign of a major mood disorder involving simultaneous symptoms of manic and a major depressive episodes. SEE bipolar disorder, manic episode.

mix·ed gli·o·ma (mikst glī-ō′mă) Lesion composed of two or more malignant elements, most frequently astrocytoma and oligodendroglioma.

mix·ed hear·ing loss (mikst hēr′ing laws) Combination of conductive and sensorineural hearing loss.

mix·ed in·fec·tion (mikst in-fek′shŭn) Infection by more than one variety of pathogenic microorganisms.

mix·ed leu·ke·mi·a, mix·ed cell leu·ke·mi·a (mikst lū-kē′mē-ă, mikst sel) Granulocytic leukemia with occurrence in the blood of increased numbers of cells in the myeloid series.

mix·ed lym·pho·cyte cul·ture test (mikst lim′fō-sīt kŭl′chŭr test) An assay for histocompatibility of human leukocyte antigens in which donor and recipient lymphocytes are mixed in culture; the degree of incompatibility is indicated by the number of cells that have undergone transformation and mitosis, or by the uptake of radioactive isotope-labeled thymidine.

mix·ed mid·ex·pi·ra·to·ry flow rate (mikst mid-eks-pīr′ă-tōr-ē flō rāt) Using spirometry, a measurement of the force of air exhaled from the lungs.

mix·ed nerve (mikst nĕrv) [TA] One with both afferent and efferent fibers.

mix·ed pa·ral·y·sis (mikst păr-al′i-sis) Combined motor and sensory paralysis.

mix·ed tu·mor (mikst tū′mŏr) Lesion with two or more varieties of tissue.

-mixis, -mixia, -mixy, mixo- Combining word forms, meaning ''related to reproduction.''

mix·ture (miks′chŭr) A mutual incorporation of two or more substances, without chemical union, and with the physical characteristics of each of the components being retained.

Mi·ya·ga·wa·nel·la (mē′yă-gah-wă-nel′ă) SEE *Chlamydia*.

mmHg Abbreviation for millimeters of mercury. SEE ALSO torr.

MMR Abbreviation for measles, mumps, rubella; usually used with reference to the vaccine.

Mn Symbol for manganese.

mo·bile arm sup·port (mō′bil ahrm sŭ-pōrt′) Orthopedic device that supports patients with diminished strength in the upper body.

mo·bi·li·za·tion (mō′bi-lī-zā′shŭn) **1.** Restoring the power of motion in a joint. **2.** The act or the result of the act of mobilizing.

mo·dal·i·ty (mō-dal′i-tē) **1.** A form of application or employment of a therapeutic agent or regimen. **2.** Various forms of sensation.

mode (mōd) In a set of measurements, that value which appears most frequently.

mod·el (mod′ĕl) **1.** A representation of something, often idealized or modified to make it conceptually easier to understand. **2.** Something to be imitated. **3.**

DENTISTRY a cast. **4.** A mathematical representation of a particular phenomenon.

mod·i·fi·ca·tion (mod′i-fi-kā′shŭn) Nonhereditary change in an organism; e.g., one that is acquired from its own activity or environment.

mod·if·ied bar·i·um swal·low (mod′i-fīd bar′ē-ŭm swah′lō) Radiologic test to assess the structure and function of the oropharynx, pharynx, larynx, and upper esophagus before, during, and after the swallow.

mod·i·fied milk (mod′i-fīd milk) Cow's milk altered, by increasing the fat and reducing the amount of protein, to resemble human milk in composition.

mod·i·fied rad·i·cal mas·tec·to·my (MRM) (mod′i-fīd rad′i-kăl mas-tek′tŏmē) Excision of the entire breast including the nipple, areola, and overlying skin, and lymph bearing axillary tissue to preserve the pectoral muscles.

mod·if·ied rad·i·cal mas·toid·ec·to·my (mod′i-fīd rad′i-kăl mas′toy-dek′tŏmē) Surgery to manage cholesteatoma that lies lateral to the remnant of the tympanic membrane and middle-ear ossicles.

mod·if·ied tri·chrome stain (mod′i-fīd trī′krōm stān) A reformulation of the Gomori trichrome stain with a tenfold increase of chromotype 2R dye, adapted for detection of microsporidian spores.

mod·i·fi·er (mod′i-fī′ĕr) That which alters or limits.

mod·u·la·tion (mod′yŭ-lā′shŭn) **1.** Functional and morphologic fluctuation of cells in response to changing environmental conditions. **2.** Systematic variation in a characteristic of a sustained oscillation to code additional information. **3.** A change in the kinetics of an enzyme or metabolic pathway.

mod·u·la·tion trans·fer func·tion (MTF) (mod′yū-lā′shŭn trans′fĕr fŭngk′shŭn) In testing radionuclide detectors or radiographic systems, the efficiency, at each spatial frequency, of reproducing the variation (contrast) in the object density or signal in the image.

mod·u·la·tor (mod′yū-lā′tŏr) That which regulates or adjusts.

Moel·ler glos·si·tis (mĕrl′ĕr glos-ī′tis) Lingual inflammation that indicates sensitivity to spicy food.

Mohs fresh tis·sue che·mo·sur·ger·y tech·nique (mōz fresh tish′ū kē′mō-sŭr′jĕr-ē tek-nēk′) Chemosurgery in which superficial cancers are excised after fixation in vivo.

moi·e·ty (moy′i-tē) **1.** Originally indicated half; now, less precisely, a portion of something. **2.** Functional group.

moist rale (moyst rahl) A bubbling rale caused by air mixing with a fluid exudate in the bronchial tubes or a body cavity.

mo·lal (mō′lăl) Denoting 1 mol of solute dissolved in 1000 g of solvent; such solutions provide a definite ratio of solute to solvent molecules. Cf. molar (4).

mo·lal·i·ty (m) (mō-lal′i-tē) Moles of solute per kilogram of solvent. Cf. molarity.

mo·lar (mō′lăr) **1.** Denoting a grinding, abrading, or wearing away. **2.** SYN molar tooth. **3.** Denoting a concentration of 1 gram-molecular weight (1 mol) of solute per liter of solution, the common unit of concentration in chemistry. Cf. molal.

mo·lar·i·ty (m) (mō-lar′i-tē) Moles per liter of solution (mol/L). Cf. molality.

mo·lar preg·nan·cy (mō′lăr preg′năn-sē) Condition marked by a neoplasm within the uterus.

mo·lar tooth (mō′lăr tūth) [TA] A tooth having a somewhat quadrangular crown with four or five cusps on the grinding surface. SYN dens molaris [TA], molar (2).

mold (mōld) **1.** A filamentous fungus, generally a circular colony that may be cottony, wooly, or glabrous, but with filaments not organized into large fruiting bodies. **2.** A shaped receptacle into which wax is pressed or fluid plaster is poured in making a cast. **3.** To shape a mass of plastic material according to a definite pattern. **4.** To change in shape; denoting especially the adaptation of the fetal head to the pelvic canal.

mold·ing (mōld′ing) Shaping by means of a mold.

mole (mol) (mōl) **1.** SYN nevus (2). **2.** SYN nevus pigmentosus. **3.** An intrauterine mass formed by the degeneration of the partly developed products of conception. **4.** In the SI, the unit of amount of substance. SEE ALSO Avogadro number.

mo·lec·u·lar dis·ease (mŏ-lek'yū-lăr di-zēz') Disorder in which the manifestations are due to alterations in molecular structure and function.

mo·lec·u·lar ep·i·de·mi·ol·o·gy (mŏ-lek'yū-lăr ep'i-dē-mē-ol'ŏ-jē) Use in epidemiologic studies of techniques of molecular biology such as deoxyribonucleic acid typing.

mo·lec·u·lar for·mu·la (mŏ-lek'yū-lăr fōrm'yū-lă) SYN empiric formula.

mo·lec·u·lar ge·net·ics (mŏ-lek'yū-lăr jĕ-net'iks) Molecular biology applied to genetics.

mo·lec·u·lar mass (mŏ-lek'yū-lăr mas) SYN molecular weight.

mo·lec·u·lar path·ol·o·gy (mŏ-lek'yū-lăr pă-thol'ŏ-jē) Study of biochemical and biophysical cellular mechanisms as the basic factors in disease.

mo·lec·u·lar sieve (mŏ-lek'yū-lăr siv) Gellike material with pore sized to exclude molecules above certain sizes.

mo·lec·u·lar weight (MW) (mŏ-lek'yū-lăr wāt) The sum of the atomic weights of all the atoms constituting a molecule. SEE ALSO atomic weight. SYN molecular mass, molecular weight ratio, relative molecular mass.

mol·e·cule (mol'ĕ-kyūl) The smallest possible quantity of a di-, tri-, or polyatomic substance that retains the chemical properties of the substance.

mo·li·men, pl. **mo·lim·i·na** (mō-lī'men, -lim'i-nă) An effort; laborious performance of a normal function.

mol·li·ti·es (mō-lish'ē-ēz) **1.** Characterized by a soft consistency. **2.** SYN malacia.

Mol·lusc·i·pox·vi·rus (mo-lusk'i-poks-vī'rŭs) Viral genus that causes localized wartlike skin lesions.

mol·lus·cum (mo-lŭs'kŭm) A benign viral disease marked by the occurrence of soft rounded tumors of the skin.

mol·lus·cum con·ta·gi·o·sum (mo-lŭs'kŭm kon-tă'jē-ō'sŭm) A contagious skin disease due to intranuclear proliferation of a virus characterized by the appearance of small, pearly, umbilicated papular epidermal growths. In adults it typically occurs on or near the genitals and is sexually transmitted.

mo·lyb·de·num (Mo) (mō-lib'dē-nŭm) A silvery white metallic bioelement found in a number of proteins (e.g., xanthine oxidase).

mon·ad (mō'nad) **1.** A univalent element or radical. **2.** A unicellular organism. **3.** In meiosis, the single chromosome derived from a tetrad after the first and second maturation divisions.

monaesthetic [Br.] SYN monesthetic.

Mo·na·kow syn·drome (mō-nah'kof sin' drōm) Contralateral hemiplegia, hemianesthesia, and homonomous hemianopsia due to occlusion of the anterior choroidal artery.

mon·am·ide (mon-am'id) SYN monoamide.

mon·am·ine (mon-am'in) SYN monoamine.

mon·ar·thric (mon-ahr'thrik) SYN monarticular.

mon·ar·thri·tis (mon'ahr-thrī'tis) Arthritis of a single joint.

mon·ar·tic·u·lar (mon'ahr-tik'yū-lăr) Relating to a single joint. SYN monarthric.

mon·as·ter (mon-as'tĕr) The single star figure at the end of prophase in mitosis.

mon·ath·e·to·sis (mon'ath-ĕ-tō'sis) Motor disorder affecting one hand or foot.

mon·a·tom·ic (mon'ă-tom'ik) **1.** Relating to or containing a single atom. **2.** SYN monovalent (1).

mon·au·ral (mon-aw'răl) Pertaining to one ear.

Mön·ck·e·berg ar·te·ri·o·scle·ro·sis, Mön·cke·berg cal·cif·i·ca·tion, Mön·cke·berg scle·ro·sis (merng´kĕ-bĕrg ahr-tēr´ĕ-ō-skle-rō´sis, kal´si-fi-kā-shŭn, skle-rō´sis) Arterial sclerosis involving the peripheral arteries with deposition of calcium in the medial coat but little or no luminal encroachment.

Mo·ne·ra (mō-nē´ră) The prokaryotes; the blue-green algae and bacteria.

mon·es·thet·ic (mon´es-thet´ik) Relating to a single sense or sensation. SYN monaesthetic.

mon·go·li·an spot (mong-gō´lē-ăn spot) Congenital dark-bluish or mulberry-colored rounded or oval spots on the skin in the sacral region due to the ectopic presence of scattered melanocytes in the dermis; frequent in black, Native American, and Asian children from 2–12 years of age after which time they gradually recede. SYN blue spot (2).

mo·nil·e·thrix (mō-nil´ĕ-thriks) An inherited trichodystrophy in which brittle hairs show a series of constrictions. SYN beaded hair, moniliform hair.

Mo·nil·i·a (mō-nil´ē-ă) Generic term for a group of fungi commonly known as fruit molds.

mo·nil·i·form (mō-nil´i-fōrm) Shaped like a string of beads or beaded necklace.

mo·nil·i·form hair (mō-nil´i-fōrm hār) SYN monilethrix.

mon·i·tor (mon´i-tŏr) **1.** A device that displays or records specified data for a given series of events, operations, or circumstances. **2.** To assess a function of the body on a close constant basis.

mono-, mon- Combining forms indicating the participation or involvement of a single element or part. Cf. uni-.

mon·o·am·ine, mon·a·mine (mon´ō-ă-mēn´, mon-am´īn) A molecule containing one amine group.

mon·o·a·mine ox·i·dase in·hib·it·or (MAOI) (mon´ō-ă-mēn´ ok´si-dās in-hib´i-tŏr) An antidepressant that inhibits enzymatic breakdown of monoamine neurotransmitters of the sympathetic/adrenergic system; not used as first-line therapy because of the risk of hypertensive crisis after consumption of foods or beverages containing pressor amines, including cheese, chocolate, beer, and wine.

mon·o·am·i·ner·gic (mon´ō-am´i-něr´jik) Referring to nerve cells or fibers that transmit nervous impulses by the medium of a catecholamine or indolamine.

mon·o·am·ni·ot·ic (mon´ō-am´nē-ot´ik) Denoting two or more progeny of a multiple pregnancy sharing a common amniotic sac.

mon·o·bac·tam (mon´ō-bak´tam) Antibiotic that has a monocyclic β-lactam nucleus and is structurally different from other β-lactams.

mon·o·ba·sic (mon´ō-bā´sik) Denoting an acid with only one replaceable hydrogen atom or one replaced hydrogen atom.

mon·o·ba·sic acid (mon´ō-bā´sik as´id) One containing one ionizable atom of hydrogen in the molecule. SEE acid (1).

mon·o·blast (mon´ō-blast) An immature cell that develops into a monocyte.

mon·o·cho·re·a (mon´ō-kō-rē´ă) Chorea affecting the head alone or only one extremity.

mon·o·chro·mat·ic (mon´ō-krō-mat´ik) **1.** Having but one color. **2.** Indicating a light of a single wavelength. **3.** Relating to or characterized by monochromatism.

mon·o·chro·ma·tism (mon´ō-krō´mă-tizm) **1.** The state of having or exhibiting only one color. **2.** SYN achromatopsia.

mon·o·chro·mat·o·phil, mon·o·chro·mato·phile (mon´ō-krō-mat´ō-fil, -fīl) **1.** Taking only one stain. **2.** A cell or any histologic element staining with only one kind of dye.

mon·o·clo·nal (mon´ō-klōn´ăl) IMMUNOCHEMISTRY pertaining to a protein from a single clone of cells, all molecules of which are the same.

mon·o·clo·nal im·mu·no·glob·u·lin (mon´ō-klōn´ăl im´yū-nō-glob´yū-lin) Homogeneous immunoglobulin due to proliferation of a single clone of plasma cells that during electrophoresis of serum, appears as a narrow band or "spike." SYN paraprotein (2).

mon•o•crot•ic (mon'ō-krot'ik) Denoting a pulse with a curve that has no notch or subsidiary wave in its descending line.

mon•oc•ro•tism (mon-ok'rŏ-tizm) The state in which the pulse is monocrotic.

mon•oc•u•lar (mon-ok'yū-lăr) Relating to, affecting, or visible by one eye only.

mo•noc•u•lar di•plo•pi•a (mon-ok'yū-lăr dip-lō'pē-ă) A double image or an extra ghost image produced in one eye.

mon•o•cyte (mon'ō-sīt) Large mononuclear leukocyte; normally constitute 3–7% of the leukocytes of circulating blood; normally found in lymph nodes, spleen, bone marrow, and loose connective tissue.

mon•o•cyt•ic leu•ke•mi•a (mon'ō-sit'i-k lū-kē'mē-ă) A form of leukemia characterized by large numbers of cells that can be definitely identified as monocytes, in addition to larger, apparently related cells formed from the uncontrolled proliferation of the reticuloendothelial tissue; acute or subacute course in older people; characterized by swelling of gums, bleeding in skin or mucous membranes, secondary infection, and splenomegaly.

mon•o•cy•toid cell (mon'ō-sī'toyd sel) A cell that resembles a monocyte but is nonphagocytic.

mon•o•cy•to•pe•ni•a (mon'ō-sī-tō-pē'nē-ă) A decrease in the number of monocytes in the circulating blood.

mon•o•fix•a•tion syn•drome (mon'ō-fik-sā'shŭn sin'drōm) A small-angle strabismus (less than 10 prism diopters) with central fixation by the preferred eye, central suppression of the deviating eye, and binocular fusion of peripheral vision.

mon•o•ga•met•ic (mon'ō-gă-met'ik) SYN homogametic.

mon•o•gen•e•sis (mon'ō-jen'ĕ-sis) **1.** The production of similar organisms in each generation. **2.** The production of young by one parent only, as in nonsexual generation and parthenogenesis. **3.** The process of parasitizing a single host, in which the life cycle of the parasite is passed.

mon•o•ge•net•ic (mon'ō-jĕ-net'ik) Relating to monogenesis.

mon•o•gen•ic (mon'ō-jen'ik) Relating to a hereditary disease or syndrome, or to an inherited characteristic.

mo•nog•e•nous (mŏ-noj'ĕ-nŭs) Asexually produced, as by fission, gemmation, or sporulation.

mon•o•kine (mon'ō-kīn) Cytokines secreted by both monocytes and macrophages. SEE cytokine.

mon•o•loc•u•lar (mon'ō-lok'yū-lăr) Having one cavity or chamber. SYN unicameral, unicamerate.

mon•o•ma•ni•a (mon'ō-mā'nē-ă) An obsession for a single idea or subject.

mon•o•mer (mon'ō-mĕr) **1.** The molecular unit that, by repetition, constitutes a large structure or polymer. **2.** The protein structural unit of a virion capsid. SEE virion.

mon•o•mer•ic (mon'ō-mer'ik) **1.** Consisting of a single component. **2.** In genetics, relating to a hereditary disease or characteristic controlled by genes at a single locus. **3.** Consisting of monomers.

mon•o•mo•lec•u•lar (mon'ō-mŏ-lek'yū-lăr) **1.** SYN unimolecular. **2.** Relating to a singular molecular entity.

mon•o•mor•phic (mon'ō-mōr'fik) Of one shape; unchangeable in shape.

mon•o•mor•phic ad•e•no•ma (MA) (mon'ō-mōr'fik ad'ĕ-nō'mă) Benign ductal neoplasm of the salivary glands, with a uniform epithelial pattern and lacking the chondromyxoid stroma of a pleomorphic adenoma.

mon•o•neu•ral, mon•o•neu•ric (mon'ō-nūr'ăl, -ik) **1.** Having only one neuron. **2.** Supplied by a single nerve.

mon•o•neu•ral•gi•a (mon'ō-nūr-al'jē-ă) Pain along the course of one nerve.

mon•o•neu•ri•tis (mon'ō-nūr-ī'tis) Inflammation of a single nerve.

mon·o·neu·rop·a·thy (mon′ō-nūr-op′ă-thē) Disorder involving a single nerve.

mon·o·neu·rop·a·thy mul·ti·plex (mon′ō-nūr-op′ă-thē mŭl′tē-pleks) Nontraumatic involvement of two or more portions of the peripheral nervous system, usually sequentially and in different areas of the body; most often due to vasculitis.

mon·o·nu·cle·ar (MN) (mon′ō-nū′klē-ăr) Having one nucleus; used in reference to phagocytic cells.

mon·o·nu·cle·ar leu·ko·cyte (MNL) (mon′ō-nū′klē-ăr lū′kō-sīt) A white blood cell with a single nucleus that is indented or shaped like a horseshoe.

mon·o·nu·cle·ar phag·o·cyte sys·tem (mon′ō-nū′klē-ăr fag′ō-sīt sis′tĕm) A widely distributed phagocytic family of both free and fixed macrophages derived from bone marrow precursor cells by way of monocytes.

mon·o·nu·cle·o·sis (mon′ō-nū-klē-ō′sis) Presence of abnormally large numbers of mononuclear leukocytes in the circulating blood, especially with reference to forms that are not normal.

mon·o·oc·ta·no·in (mon′ō-ok′tā-nō′in) Semisynthetic esterified glycerol used as a solubilizing agent for radiolucent gallstones in the biliary tract after cholecystectomy.

monoparaesthesia [Br.] SYN monoparesthesia.

mon·o·par·es·the·si·a (mon′ō-par′es-thē′zē-ă) Paresthesia affecting a single region only. SYN monoparaesthesia.

mon·o·path·ic (mon′ō-path′ik) Relating to a monopathy.

mon·oph·thal·mos (mon′of-thal′mŏs) Failure of outgrowth of a primary optic vesicle with absence of ocular tissues.

mon·o·phy·let·ic (mon′ō-fi-let′ik) Having a single cell type of origin; derived from one line of descent.

mon·o·ple·gi·a (mon′ō-plē′jē-ă) Paralysis of one limb.

mon·o·ploid (mon′ō-ployd) SYN haploid.

mon·o·po·di·a (mon′ō-pō′dē-ă) Malformation in which sirenomelia is accompanied by fusion of the feet into a single structure.

mon·o·po·lar cau·te·ry (mon′ō-pō′lăr kaw′tĕr-ē) Electrocautery by high frequency electrical current passed from a single electrode, where the cauterization occurs, with the patient's body serving as a ground.

mon·o·pty·chi·al (mon′ŏp-tī′kē-ăl) Arranged in a single but folded layer, as the cells in the epithelium of the gallbladder or certain glands.

mon·or·chid·ic, mon·or·chid (mon′ōr-kid′ik, mon-ōr′kid) **1.** Having only one testis. **2.** Having apparently only one testis, the other being absent or undescended.

mon·or·chism, mon·or·chid·ism (mon′ōr-kizm, mon-ōr′ki-dizm) A condition in which only one testis is apparent, the other being absent or undescended.

mon·o·sac·cha·ride (mon′ō-sak′ă-rīd) A carbohydrate that cannot form any simpler sugar by simple hydrolysis.

mon·o·so·di·um glu·ta·mate (MSG) (mon′ō-sō′dē-ŭm glū′tă-māt) The monosodium salt; used as a flavor enhancer that is a cause or contributing factor to ''Chinese restaurant'' syndrome.

mon·o·so·my (mon′ō-sō′mē) Absence of one chromosome of a pair of homologous chromosomes.

mon·o·spasm (mon′ō-spazm) Spasm affecting only one muscle or group of muscles or a single extremity.

mon·o·sper·my (mon′ō-spĕr′mē) Fertilization by a single sperm into the oocyte.

mon·o·stra·tal (mon′ō-strā′tăl) Composed of a single layer.

mon·o·sy·nap·tic (mon′ō-si-nap′tik) Referring to direct neural connections not involving an intermediary neuron.

mon·o·ther·mi·a (mon′ō-thĕr′mē-ă) Evenness of bodily temperature; absence of an evening rise in body temperature.

mon·o·va·lence, mon·o·va·len·cy

M

(mon′ō-vā′lĕns, -sē) A combining power (valence) equal to that of a hydrogen atom. SYN univalence, univalency.

mon·o·va·lent (mon′ō-vā′lĕnt) **1.** Having combining power of a hydrogen atom. SYN monatomic (2), univalent. **2.** Pertaining to a monovalent antiserum to a single antigen or organism.

mon·ox·e·nic cul·ture (mon′ō-zē′nik kŭl′chŭr) Culture containing a single known species.

mon·o·zy·got·ic twins (mon′ō-zī-got′ik twinz) Twins resulting from a single zygote that at an early stage of development separate into independently growing cell aggregations creating two individuals of the same sex and identical genetic constitution. SYN enzygotic twins, identical twins.

mons, gen. **mon·tis,** pl. **mon·tes** (monz, mon′tis, -tēz) [TA] An anatomic prominence above the general surface level.

Mon·sel so·lu·tion (mon-sel′ sŏ-lū′ shŭn) Ferric subsulfate solution used to coagulate superficial bleeding such as that following skin biopsy.

mons pu·bis (monz pyū′bis) [TA] The prominence caused by a pad of fatty tissue over the symphysis pubis in the female.

mon·ster (mon′stĕr) *This word is best avoided in medical speech and writing because of its objectionable lay connotations.* Outmoded and inappropriate term for a malformed embryo, fetus, or individual. SEE ALSO teras.

Mon·te·zu·ma's re·venge (mon′tĕ-zū′ măz rĕ-venj′) A colloquial term for traveler's diarrhea contracted in Mexico; caused by *Escherichia coli*, *Shigella*, and *Campylobacter jejuni*. SYN turista.

mon·tic·u·lus, pl. **mon·tic·u·li** (montik′yū-lŭs, -lī) Any slight rounded projection above a surface.

mood (mūd) The pervasive feeling, tone, and internal emotional state that, when impaired, can markedly influence virtually all aspects of a person's behavior or perception of external events.

mood-con·gru·ent hal·lu·ci·na·tion

(mūd-kŏn-grū′ĕnt hă-lū′si-nā′shŭn) One in which the content is mood appropriate.

mood dis·or·ders (mūd dis-ōr′dĕrz) Mental illness involving a disturbance of mood, accompanied by either a full or partial manic or depressive syndrome that is not due to any other mental disorder.

mood-in·con·gru·ent hal·lu·ci·na·tion (mūd′in-kŏn-grū′ĕnt hă-lū′si-nā′ shŭn) Delusional idea not consistent with external stimuli.

mood swing (mūd swing) Oscillation of a person's emotional feeling between euphoria and depression.

moon face (mūn fās) Round, usually red face, with large jowls, seen in Cushing disease.

Moon mo·lars (mūn mōl′ărz) Small dome-shaped first molar teeth occurring in congenital syphilis.

Moore light·ning streaks (mūr līt′ning strēks) Photopsia manifested by vertical flashes of light, seen usually on the temporal side of the affected eye, caused by the involutional shrinkage of vitreous humor.

Moore meth·od (mūr meth′ŏd) Treatment of aneurysm by the introduction of silver or zinc wire into the sac to induce fibrin deposition.

Moo·ren ul·cer (mō′rĕn ŭl′sĕr) Chronic inflammation of the peripheral cornea that slowly progresses centrally with corneal thinning and sometimes perforation.

MOPP (mop) Acronym for mission-oriented protective posture.

Mor·ax·el·la (mōr′ak-sel′ă) A genus of obligately aerobic nonmotile bacteria containing gram-negative coccoids or short rods; do not produce acid from carbohydrates, are oxidase positive, penicillin susceptible, and infect the mucous membranes of humans and other mammals.

Mor·ax·el·la ca·tar·rha·lis **(MC)** (mōr-ak-sel′ă kă-tahr-ră′lis) Bacterial species that causes upper respiratory tract infections, particularly in immunocompromised hosts.

Mor·ax·el·la la·cu·na·ta (mōr-ak-sel´ ă lak-yū-nā′tă) Bacterial species causing conjunctivitis in humans.

mor·bid (mōr′bid) **1.** Diseased or pathologic. **2.** In psychology, abnormal or deviant.

mor·bid·i·ty (mōr-bid′i-tē) **1.** A disease state. **2.** The ratio of sick-to-well people in a community.

mor·bid·i·ty rate (mōr-bid′i-tē rāt) Proportion of patients with a given disease during a given year per given unit of population.

mor·bid o·be·si·ty (mōr′bid ō-bē′si-tē) Being sufficiently overweight so as to prevent normal activity or physiologic function or to cause the onset of a pathologic disorder.

mor·bif·ic (mōr-bif′ik) SYN pathogenic.

mor·bil·li (mōr-bil′ī) SYN measles (1).

mor·bil·li·form (mōr-bil′i-fōrm) Resembling measles (1).

Mor·bil·li·vi·rus (mōr-bil′i-vī′rŭs) A genus in the family Paramyxoviridae, including measles and canine distemper.

mor·bus (mōr′bŭs) SYN disease (1).

mor·cel·la·ted ne·phrec·to·my (mōr′ se-lā′tĕd nĕ-frek′tŏ-mē) Removal of a kidney in pieces.

mor·cel·la·tion, mor·celle·ment (mōr′ sĕ-lā′shŭn, mōr-sel-mōwn[h]′) Division into and removal of small pieces, as of a tumor.

Mor·ga·gni cat·a·ract (mōr-gahn′yē kat′ăr-akt) Hypermature type in which the nucleus gravitates within the capsule.

Mor·ga·gni for·a·men her·ni·a (mōr-gahn′yē fŏr-ā′mĕn hĕr′nē-ă) SYN retrosternal hernia, parasternal hernia.

Mor·ga·gni glands (mōr-gahn′yē glandz) Mucus-secreting glands lining the urethral lumen in males.

Mor·ga·gni glob·ules (mōr-gahn′yē glob′ yūlz) Vesicles beneath the capsule and between lens fibers in early cataract.

Mor·ga·gni pro·lapse (mōr-gahn′yē prō′ laps) Chronic inflammation of laryngeal ventricle.

Mor·ga·gni syn·drome (mōr-gahn′yē sin′drōm) Hyperostosis frontalis interna in elderly women, with obesity and neuropsychiatric disorders of uncertain cause. SYN metabolic craniopathy, Stewart-Morel syndrome.

Mor·gan lens (mōr′găn lenz) Contact lens-like device for ocular irrigation.

morgue (mōrg) **1.** A building where unidentified cadavers are kept pending identification before burial. **2.** A building or room in a hospital or other facility where the dead are kept pending autopsy, burial, or cremation; often includes a laboratory to perform autopsies.

mor·i·bund (mōr′i-bŭnd) Dying; at the point of death.

morn·ing af·ter pill (mōr′ning af′tĕr pil) An oral medication, consisting of two pills taken 12 hours apart that, when taken by a woman within 2–3 days after intercourse, reduces the probability that she will become pregnant. SYN emergency contraceptive, emergency hormonal contraception, postcoital contraception.

morn·ing sick·ness (mōr′ning sik′nĕs) The nausea and vomiting of early pregnancy. SYN nausea gravidarum.

Mo·ro re·flex (MR) (mō′rō rē′fleks) SYN startle reflex.

mor·phe·a (mōr-fē′ă) Cutaneous lesion(s) characterized by indurated, slightly depressed plaques of thickened dermal fibrous tissue. SYN localized scleroderma, morphoea.

-morphia, -morphy Combining forms meaning "a condition or form."

mor·phine (mōr′fēn) The major phenanthrene alkaloid of opium; produces a combination of depression and excitation in the central nervous system and some peripheral tissues; repeated administration leads to the development of tolerance, physical dependence, and (in instances of abuse) psychic dependence. Used as an

M

mor·pho-, morph- Combining forms meaning shape, structure.

mor·pho·gen (mōr'fō-jen) A soluble molecule secreted at a distance from the target cells that specifies the fates of cells.

mor·pho·gen·e·sis (mōr'fō-jen'ĕ-sis) The ability of a molecule or group of molecules (particularly macromolecules) to assume a certain shape.

mor·pho·ge·net·ic (mōr'fō-jĕ-net'ik) Relating to morphogenesis.

mor·phol·o·gy (mōr-fol'ŏ-jē) Science concerned with the structure of animals and plants.

mor·pho·sis (mōr-fō'sis) Mode of development of a part.

Mor·qui·o syn·drome (mōr'kyō sin'drōm) Disorder characterized by severe skeletal defects with short stature, severe deformity of spine and thorax, long bones with irregular epiphyses but with shafts of normal length, enlarged joints, flaccid ligaments, and waddling gait. SYN Brailsford-Morquio disease, Morquio disease, Morquio-Ullrich disease, mucopolysaccharidosis type IVA, IVB.

mor·tal·i·ty (mōr-tal'i-tē) 1. The state of being mortal. 2. SYN death rate. 3. A fatal outcome.

mor·tal·i·ty rate (MR) (mōr-tal'i-tē rāt) SYN death rate.

mor·tar (mōr'tăr) A vessel with a rounded interior in which crude drugs and other substances are crushed or bruised by means of a pestle.

mor·ti·fi·ca·tion (mōr'ti-fi-kā'shŭn) SYN gangrene (1).

Mor·ton neu·ral·gi·a (mōr'tŏn nūr-al'jē-ă) Neuralgia of an interdigital nerve due to compression of the nerve by the metatarsophalangeal joint.

Mor·ton neu·ro·ma (mōr'tŏn nūr-ō'mă) Metatarsal pain caused by compression of sensory nerves by the metatarsal heads, sometimes with neuroma formation.

analgesic, sedative, and anxiolytic. Classified as a U.S. Schedule II controlled medication.

Mor·ton toe (mōr'tŏn tō) Anatomic anomaly wherein the second toe is longer than the great toe; causes metatarsalgia.

Mor·van cho·re·a (mōr-vah[n]' kōr-ē'ă) SYN myokymia.

mo·sa·ic (mō-zā'ik) 1. Inlaid; resembling inlaid work. 2. The juxtaposition in an organism of genetically different tissues.

mo·sa·ic in·her·i·tance (mō-zā'ik inher'i-tăns) That form in which the paternal influence is dominant in one group of cells and the maternal in another. Cf. lyonization.

mo·sa·i·cism (mō-zā'i-sizm) Condition of being mosaic.

mo·sa·ic pat·tern (mō-zā'ik pat'ĕrn) On high-resolution CT scans of the lungs, a pattern of brighter and darker regions corresponding to differences in perfusion or aeration; found in some cases of chronic thromboembolism or of bronchiolitis obliterans. Cf. oligemia.

mo·sa·ic wart (mō-zā'ik wōrt) Plantar growth of numerous closely aggregated warts forming a mosaic appearance, frequently caused by human papillomavirus type 2.

mos·qui·to, pl. **mos·qui·toes** (mŏs-kē'tō, -tōz) A blood-sucking dipterous insect; *Aedes, Anopheles, Culex, Mansonia,* and *Stegomyia* are genera containing most species involved in the transmission of protozoan and other disease-producing parasites.

mos·qui·to clamp (mŏs-kē'tō klamp) A small hemostat, straight or curved, with or without teeth; used to hold delicate tissue or for hemostasis.

Moss tube (maws tūb) 1. A triple-lumen, nasogastric, feeding-decompression tube that uses a gastric balloon to occlude the cardioesophageal junction, with simultaneous esophageal aspiration and intragastric feeding. 2. A double-lumen, gastric lavage tube that provides continuous delivery of saline through a small bore, with simultaneous aspiration of fluid and some particles through a large bore.

moth·er cell (mŏdh'ĕr sel) A cell that, by division, gives rise to two or more daughter cells. SYN metrocyte.

moth·er cyst (mŏdh'ĕr sist) A hydatid cyst from the inner layer, from which secondary cysts containing daughter cysts are developed; most frequent in the liver. SYN parent cyst.

moth·er yaw (mŏdh'ĕr yaw) Large granulomatous lesion, considered to be the initial lesion in yaws, most commonly on the hand, leg, or foot. SYN buba madre, frambesioma.

mo·tile (mō'til) **1.** Having the power of spontaneous movement. **2.** Denoting the type of mental imagery in which one learns and recalls most readily that which has been felt.

mo·til·in (mō-til'in) A 22-amino acid polypeptide occurring in duodenal mucosa as a controller of normal gastrointestinal motor activity.

mo·til·i·ty (mō-til'i-tē) The power of spontaneous movement.

mo·tion sick·ness (mō'shŭn sik'nĕs) The syndrome of pallor, nausea, weakness, and malaise, which may progress to vomiting and incapacitation, due to stimulation of the semicircular canals during travel or motion. SYN kinesia.

motoneurone [Br.] SYN motor neuron.

mo·tor (mō'tŏr) **1.** ANATOMY, PHYSIOLOGY denoting those neural structures that, by the impulses generated and transmitted by them cause muscle fibers or pigment cells to contract, or glands to secrete. SEE ALSO motor cortex, motor neuron. **2.** PSYCHOLOGY denoting the overt reaction of an organism to a stimulus (motor response). **3.** Pertaining to a set of skills involving movement or motion.

mo·tor a·pha·si·a (mō'tŏr ă-fā'zē-ă) SYN expressive aphasia, Broca aphasia (1).

mo·tor a·prax·i·a (mō'tŏr ă-prak'sē-ă) An inability to make movements or to use objects for the purpose intended.

mo·tor a·tax·i·a (mō'tŏr ă-tak'sē-ă) That developing on attempting to perform coordinated muscular movements. SYN kinetic ataxia.

mo·tor con·trol (mō'tŏr kŏn-trōl') The process of initiating, directing, and grading purposeful voluntary movement.

mo·tor cor·tex (mō'tŏr kōr'teks) Region of the cerebral cortex most nearly immediately influencing movements of the face, neck and trunk, and upper and lower extremities. SYN excitable area, Rolando area.

mo·tor fi·bers (mō'tŏr fī'bĕrz) Nerve fibers that transmit impulses that activate effector cells.

mo·tor im·age (mō'tŏr im'ăj) The image of body movements.

mo·tor nerve (mō'tŏr nĕrv) [TA] An efferent nerve conveying an impulse that excites muscular contraction.

mo·tor neu·ron, mo·to·neu·ron (mō'tŏr nūr'on, mō'tō-) Nerve cell in the spinal cord, rhombencephalon, or mesencephalon characterized by having an axon that leaves the central nervous system to establish a functional connection with an effector (muscle or glandular) tissue. SYN anterior horn cell, motoneuron.

mo·tor neu·ron dis·ease (mō'tŏr nūr'on di-zēz') A general term comprising progressive spinal muscular atrophy, amyotrophic lateral sclerosis, progressive bulbar paralysis, and primary lateral sclerosis.

mo·tor pa·ral·y·sis (mō'tŏr păr-al'i-sis) Loss of the power of muscular contraction.

mo·tor u·nit (mō'tŏr yū'nit) A single somatic motor neuron and the group of muscle fibers innervated by it.

MOTT (mot) Acronym used to describe mycobacteria other than *Mycobacterium tuberculosis* (q.v.), *M. bovis* (q.v.), and *M. africanus* (*M. tuberculosis* complex).

mot·tle (mot'tĕl) Fine inhomogeneity of an area of generally uniform opacity on a photograph or radiograph; noise.

mot·tled e·nam·el (mŏt'ĕld ĕ-nam'ĕl) Alterations in dental enamel structure often due to excessive fluoride ingestion during tooth formation; may also be caused by tetracycline in women during the first half of pregnancy or in children whose teeth are still developing.

mot·tling (mot'ĕ-ling) An area of skin

M

composed of macular lesions of varying shades or colors.

mound·ing (mownd′ing) SYN myoedema.

mount (mownt) **1.** To prepare for microscopic examination. **2.** To climb on for purposes of copulation. **3.** To organize and present, as a fever, an immunologic response.

mouth (mowth) **1.** SYN oral cavity. **2.** The opening, usually the external opening, of a cavity or canal. SEE os (2), ostium, orifice, stoma (2).

mouth breath·ing (mowth brēdh′ing) Habitual respiration through the mouth instead of the nose, usually due to obstructed nasal airways.

mouth guard (mowth gahrd) A pliable plastic device, adapted to cover the maxillary teeth, which is worn to reduce potential injury to oral structures during participation in contact sports.

mouth mir·ror (mowth mir′ŏr) Small mirror on a handle used to facilitate visualization in the examination of the teeth.

mouth·stick (mowth′stik) Prosthetic device held in the teeth to perform functions such as painting, reading, and pressing buttons or keys.

mouth-to-mouth res·pi·ra·tion (mowth-mowth res′pir-ā′shŭn) A method of artificial ventilation involving an overlap of the patient's mouth (and nose in small children) with the rescuer's mouth to inflate the patient's lungs by blowing, followed by an unassisted expiratory phase brought about by elastic recoil of the patient's chest and lungs.

mov·a·ble spleen (mūv-ă′bĕl splēn) SYN floating spleen, moveable spleen.

move·ment (mūv′mĕnt) **1.** Active change of position or location; said of the entire body or of one or more of its members or parts. **2.** SYN stool. **3.** SYN defecation.

Mow·ry col·loi·dal i·ron stain (mow′rē kol-oyd′ăl ī′ŏrn stān) A stain used for demonstrating acid mucopolysaccharides.

mox·a (mok′să) A cone of cotton wool or other material, placed on the skin and ignited to produce counterirritation. SEE ALSO moxibustion.

mox·a·lac·tam (MOX) (moks′a-lak′tam) A third-generation cephalosporin with a broad spectrum of antibacterial action; causes bleeding disorders, which limit its use.

mox·i·bus·tion (mok′si-bŭs′chŭn) Burning of herbal agents, such as moxa, on the skin as a counterirritant in the treatment of disease; a component of traditional Chinese and Japanese medicine.

M phase (fāz) SYN mitotic period.

M_r Symbol for molecular weight ratio or relative molecular mass.

MRSA Abbreviation for methicillin-resistant *Staphylococcus aureus*. SEE multidrug-resistant organisms.

MTCC Abbreviation for medical transcription certification commission.

muci- Combining form indicating mucous, mucin. SEE ALSO muco-.

mu·ci·form (myū′si-fōrm) Resembling mucus. SYN blennoid, mucoid (2).

mu·ci·lage (muc) (myū′si-lăj) A pharmacopeial preparation consisting of a solution in water of the mucilaginous principles of vegetable substances; used as a soothing application to the mucous membranes.

mu·cin (myū′sin) A secretion containing carbohydrate-rich glycoproteins such as that from the goblet cells of the intestine, the submaxillary glands, and other mucous glandular cells.

mu·ci·noid (myū′si-noyd) **1.** SYN mucoid (1). **2.** Resembling mucin.

mu·ci·nous (myū′si-nŭs) Relating to or containing mucin. SYN mucoid (3).

mu·ci·nous car·ci·no·ma (myū′si-nŭs kahr′si-nō′mă) An adenocarcinoma in which the neoplastic cells secrete conspicuous quantities of mucin; so the neoplasm is likely to be glistening, sticky, and gelatinoid. SYN colloid cancer, colloid carcinoma.

mu·ci·nu·ri·a (myū′si-nyū′rē-ă) The presence of mucin in the urine.

mu·cip·a·rous (myū-sip′ă-rŭs) Producing or secreting mucus. SYN blennogenic, blennogenous, mucid, mucigenous, mucilaginous (2).

muco- Combining form denoting mucus, mucous (mucous membrane). SEE ALSO muci-, myxo-.

mu·co·cele (myū′kō-sēl) A retention cyst of the salivary gland, lacrimal sac, paranasal sinuses, appendix, or gallbladder.

mu·co·cil·i·ar·y (myū′kō-sil′ē-ar-ē) Pertaining to ciliated columnar epithelium found in the bronchial tree to the level of the terminal bronchioles, and in the uterine tubes. SEE ciliary.

mu·co·cil·i·ar·y clear·ance (myū′kō-sil′ē-ar-ē klēr′ăns) The movement of the mucous covering of the respiratory epithelium by the beating of cilia: rapid, forward (effective) stroke and slow, return (recovery) stroke.

mu·co·cu·ta·ne·ous (myū′kō-kyū-tā′nē-ŭs) Relating to mucous membrane and skin. SYN cutaneomucosal.

mu·co·cu·ta·ne·ous leish·man·i·a·sis (myū′kō-kyū-tā′nēŭs lēsh′mă-nī′ă-sis) SEE ALSO espundia. SYN New World leishmaniasis.

mu·co·cu·ta·ne·ous lymph node syn·drome (myū′kō-kyū-tā′nē-ŭs limf nōd sin′drōm) SYN Kawasaki disease.

mu·co·en·ter·i·tis (myū′kō-en′tĕr-ī′tis) 1. Inflammation of the intestinal mucous membrane. 2. SYN mucomembranous enteritis.

mu·co·ep·i·der·moid (myū′kō-ep′i-dĕr′moyd) Denoting a mixture of mucus-secreting and epithelial cells.

mu·co·ep·i·der·moid car·ci·no·ma (MEC) (myū′kō-ep′i-dĕr′moyd kahr′si-nō′mă) Most commonly a salivary gland carcinoma of low-grade malignancy composed of mucous, epidermoid, and intermediate cells, with mucous cells abundant only in low-grade carcinoma; recurrence is frequent. SYN mucoepidermoid tumor.

mu·coid (myū′koyd) 1. General term for a mucin, mucoprotein, or glycoprotein. SYN mucinoid (1). 2. SYN muciform. 3. SYN mucinous.

mu·coid de·gen·er·a·tion (myū′koyd dē-jen′ĕr-ā′shŭn) Conversion of any connective tissues into a gelatinous or mucoid substance. SYN myxoid degeneration, myxomatous degeneration, myxomatosis (1).

mu·co·lip·i·do·sis, pl. **mu·co·lip·i·do·ses** (myū′kō-lip′i-dō′sis, -sēz) Any of a group of lysosomal storage diseases in which symptoms of visceral and mesenchymal mucopolysaccharide, glycoprotein, oligosaccharide, or glycolipid storage are present.

mu·co·lyt·ic (myū′kō-lit′ik) Capable of dissolving, digesting, or liquefying mucus.

mu·co·mem·bra·nous (myū′kō-mem′bră-nŭs) Relating to a mucous membrane.

mu·co·mem·bra·nous en·ter·i·tis (myū′kō-mem′bră-nŭs en′tĕ-rī′tis) A disorder of the intestinal mucous membrane characterized by constipation or diarrhea (sometimes alternating), colic, and the passage of pseudomembranous shreds or incomplete casts of the intestine. SYN mucoenteritis (2).

mu·co·per·i·os·te·um (myū′kō-per′ē-os′tē-ŭm) Mucous membrane and periosteum so intimately united as to form practically a single membrane, as that covering the hard palate.

mu·co·pol·y·sac·cha·ride (myū′kō-pol′ē-sak′ă-rīd) General term for a protein-polysaccharide complex obtained from proteoglycans and containing as much as 95% polysaccharide; includes the blood group substances. A more modern term is glycosaminoglycan.

mu·co·pol·y·sac·cha·ri·do·sis, pl. **mu·co·pol·y·sac·cha·ri·do·ses** (myū′kō-pol′ē-sak′ă-ri-dōs′is, -sēz) Any of a group of lysosomal storage diseases that have in common a disorder in metabolism of mucopolysaccharides with resulting various defects of bone, cartilage, connective tissue, and other organs.

mu·co·pro·tein (myū′kō-prō′tēn) General term for a protein-polysaccharide complex.

mu·co·pu·ru·lent (myū′kō-pyūr′yŭ-lĕnt) Pertaining to an exudate containing pus and conspicuous proportions of mucous material.

mu·co·pus (myū′kō-pŭs) A mucopurulent discharge; a mixture of mucous material and pus. SYN mycopus.

Mu·cor (myū′kōr) A genus of fungi, most species of which are saprobic; several are pathogenic in humans.

Mu·cor·al·es (myū′kō-rā′lēz) An order of the fungal class Zygomycetes that contains all the species causing zygomycosis in humans.

mu·cor·my·co·sis (myū′kōr-mī-kō′sis) SYN zygomycosis.

mu·co·sa, gen. and pl. **mu·co·sae** (myū-kō′să, -ē) [TA] A mucous tissue lining various tubular structures, consisting of epithelium, lamina propria, and, in the digestive tract, a layer of smooth muscle. SYN mucous membrane.

mu·co·sal re·lief ra·di·og·ra·phy (myū-kō′zăl rĕ-lēf′ rā′dē-og′ră-fē) Technique showing fine detail of gastrointestinal mucosa after coating it with a barium suspension and distending the organ with air or gas released from an ingested powder.

mu·co·sec·to·my (myū′kō-sek′tŏ-mē) Excision of the mucosa.

mu·co·si·tis (myū′kō-sī′tis) Inflammation of a mucous membrane.

mu·cous (myū′kŭs) Relating to mucus or a mucous membrane.

mu·cous co·li·tis (myū′kŭs kō-lī′tis) An affliction of the colonic mucous membrane characterized by colicky pain, constipation, diarrhea, and passage of slimy pseudomembranous shreds and patches.

mu·cous con·nec·tive tis·sue (myū′kŭs kŏ-nek′tiv tish′ū) A type of connective tissue little differentiated beyond the mesenchymal stage; its ground substance of glycoproteins is abundant and contains fine collagenous fibers and fibroblasts; in its most characteristic form, it

appears in the umbilical cord as Wharton jelly. SYN gelatinous tissue.

mu·cous cyst (myū′kŭs sist) A retention cyst resulting from obstruction in the duct of a mucous gland.

mu·cous mem·brane (myū′kŭs mem′brān) SYN mucosa.

mu·cous plug (myū′kŭs plŭg) **1.** A mass of mucus and cells filling the cervical canal between periods or during pregnancy. **2.** A mass of mucous occluding a main or lobar bronchus.

mu·co·vis·ci·do·sis (myū′kō-vis′i-dō′sis) SYN cystic fibrosis.

mu·cus (myū′kŭs) The clear viscid secretion of the mucous membranes, consisting of mucin, epithelial cells, leukocytes, and various inorganic salts suspended in water.

Muel·ler-Hin·ton me·di·um (myū′lĕr hin′tŏn mē′dē-ŭm) The standard agar-based medium for antibacterial susceptibility tests for the most common aerobic and facultatively anaerobic bacteria.

Mules op·er·a·tion (myūlz op-ĕr-ā′shŭn) Evisceration of the eyeball followed by the insertion within the sclera of a spheric prosthesis to support an artificial eye.

mule-spin·ner's can·cer (myūl spin′ĕrz kan′sĕr) Carcinoma of the scrotum or adjacent skin exposed to oil, observed in some workers in cotton spinning mills.

mu·li·brey nan·ism (mŭ′li-brā nan′izm) *Because mulibrey is not a proper noun, it is spelled with a lowercase m.* Disorder with defects of liver, brain, muscle, and eyes.

mu·li·e·bri·a (mŭ′lē-ē′brē-ă) The female genital organs.

Mül·ler fix·a·tive (mēl′er fisk′ă-tiv) A hardening agent composed of potassium dichromate, sodium sulfate, and distilled water, similar to Regaud fixative.

Mül·ler law (mēl′er law) Each type of sensory nerve ending, however stimulated (electrically, mechanically), gives rise to its own specific sensation.

Mül·ler sign (mēl′er sīn) In aortic insufficiency, rhythmic pulsatory movements of the uvula, synchronous with cardiac contractions.

multi- Combining form meaning many. SEE ALSO pluri-. Cf. poly-.

mul·ti·ar·tic·u·lar (mŭl'tē-ahr-tik'yū-lăr) Relating to or involving many joints. SYN polyarticular.

mul·ti·ax·i·al joint (mŭl'tē-aks'ē-ăl joynt) One in which movement occurs in a number of axes. SEE ball-and-socket joint.

mul·ti·bac·il·lar·y (mŭl'tē-bas'i-lar'ē) Made up of, or denoting the presence of, many bacilli.

mul·ti·cel·lu·lar (mŭl'tē-sel'yū-lăr) Composed of many cells.

mul·ti·cen·tric re·tic·u·lo·his·ti·o·cy·to·sis (mŭl'tē-sen'trik rĕ-tik'yū-lō-his-tē-ō'sis) Rare disease in which cutaneous papules composed of histiocytes containing glycolipids are associated with polyarthritis.

mul·ti·drug re·sis·tance (MDR) (mŭl'tē-drŭg rē-zis'tăns) Insensitivity of various tumors to chemically related anticancer drugs; mediated by a process of inactivating the drug or removing it from the target tumor cells.

mul·ti·drug-re·sis·tant or·gan·isms (mŭl'tē'drŭg-rē-zis'tănt ōr'găn-izmz) Bacteria and other microorganisms resistant to many antimicrobial drugs (e.g., methicillin-resistant *Staphylococcus aureus*, vancomycin-resistant enterococci, and penicillin-resistant *Streptococcus pneumoniae*).

mul·ti·fo·cal (mŭl'tē-fō'kăl) Relating to or arising from many foci.

mul·ti·fo·cal a·tri·al tach·y·car·di·a (MAT) (mŭl'tē-fō'kăl ā'trē-ăl tak'i-kahr'dē-ă) SYN atrial chaotic tachycardia.

mul·ti·form (mŭl'tē-fōrm) SYN polymorphic.

mul·ti·grav·i·da (mŭl'tē-grav'i-dă) A pregnant woman who has been pregnant one or more times previously.

mul·ti·in·farct de·men·ti·a (mŭl'tē-in-fahrkt dĕ-men'shē-ă) SYN vascular dementia.

mul·ti·in·fec·tion (mŭl'tē-in-fek'shŭn) Mixed infection with two or more varieties of microorganisms developing simultaneously.

mul·ti·lo·bar, mul·ti·lo·bate, mul·ti·lobed (mŭl'tē-lō'bahr, -lō'bāt, -lōbd') Having several lobes.

mul·ti·loc·u·lar (mŭl'tē-lok'yū-lăr) Many-celled; having many compartments or loculi.

mul·ti·loc·u·lar cyst (mŭl'tē-lok'yū-lăr sist) Lesion with compartments formed by membranous septa. SYN compound cyst.

mul·ti·nod·u·lar, mul·ti·nod·u·late (mŭl'tē-nod'yū-lăr, -yū-lăt) Having many nodules.

mul·ti·nod·u·lar goi·ter (mŭl'tē-nod' yū-lăr goy'tĕr) Adenomatous goiter with several colloid nodules.

mul·ti·nu·cle·ar (mŭl'tē-nū'klē-ăr) Having two or more nuclei.

mul·tip·a·ra (mŭl-tip'ă-ră) A woman who has given birth at least twice to an infant, liveborn or not, weighing 500 g or more, or having an estimated length of gestation of at least 20 weeks.

mul·ti·par·i·ty (mŭl'tē-par'i-tē) Condition of being a multipara.

mul·tip·a·rous (mŭl-tip'ă-rŭs) Relating to a multipara.

mul·ti·pen·nate mus·cle (mŭl'tē-pen'āt mŭs'ĕl) [TA] One with several central tendons toward which the muscle fibers converge like the barbs of feathers. SYN musculus multipennatus [TA].

mul·ti·pha·sic screen·ing (MPS) (mŭl'tē-fā'zik skrēn'ing) Routine use of multiple tests to detect disease at a preventable or curable stage.

mul·ti·ple en·do·crine ne·o·pla·si·a 1 (MEN1) (mŭl'ti-pĕl en'dō-krin nē'ō-plā'zē-ă) Syndrome characterized by tumors of the pituitary gland, pancreatic islet cells, and parathyroid glands.

M

mul·ti·ple en·do·crine ne·o·pla·si·a 2 (MEN2) (mŭl'ti-pĕl en'dō-krin nē'ō-plā'zē-ă) Syndrome associated with pheochromocytoma, parathyroid adenoma, and medullary thyroid carcinoma.

mul·ti·ple en·do·crine ne·o·pla·si·a 3 (MEN3) (mŭl'ti-pĕl en'dō-krin nē'ō-plā'zē-ă) Syndrome characterized by tumors found in MEN2, tall, thin habitus, prominent lips, and neuromas of the tongue and eyelids. Also called multiple endocrine neoplasia 2B.

mul·ti·ple ep·i·phys·i·al dys·pla·si·a (mŭl'ti-pĕl ep'i-fiz'ē-ăl dis-plā'zē-ă) Abnormality of epiphyses characterized by difficulty in walking, pain and stiffness of joints, stubby fingers, and often dwarfism of short-limb type. SYN dysplasia epiphysialis multiplex.

mul·ti·ple-ga·ted ac·qui·si·tion scan (MUGA) (mŭl'ti-pĕl-gāt'ĕd ak'wi-zi'shŭn skan) A nuclear medicine cardiac blood pool study collected by multiple-gated acquisition; used for ejection fraction and wall motion assessment.

mul·ti·ple in·tes·ti·nal pol·y·po·sis (mŭl'ti-pĕl in-tes'ti-năl pol'i-pō'sis) **1.** A disorder that usually begins in late childhood; polyps increase in numbers, causing symptoms of chronic colitis, and carcinoma of the colon almost invariably develops in untreated cases. **2.** Hamartomatous polyposis of the small or large intestine.

mul·ti·ple mark·er screen (mŭl'ti-pĕl mahr'kĕr skrēn) Use of two or more markers in the maternal serum to determine the relative risk of an abnormal fetus. SEE ALSO triple screen.

mul·ti·ple me·ta·bo·lic syn·drome (mŭl'ti-pĕl met'ă-bol'ik sin'drōm) SYN metabolic syndrome.

mul·ti·ple my·e·lo·ma, my·e·lo·ma mul·ti·plex (mŭl'ti-pĕl mī-ĕ-lō'mă, mī-ĕ-lō'mă mŭl'tē-pleks) An uncommon disease that occurs more frequently in men and is associated with anemia, hemorrhage, recurrent infections, and weakness. SEE ALSO plasma cell myeloma. SYN plasma cell myeloma (1).

mul·ti·ple my·o·si·tis (mŭl'ti-pĕl mī'ō-sī'tis) The occurrence of multiple foci of acute inflammation in the muscular tissue and overlying skin in various parts of the body, accompanied by fever and other signs of systemic infection. SEE ALSO dermatomyositis.

mul·ti·ple preg·nan·cy (mŭl'ti-pĕl preg'năn-sē) Bearing two or more fetuses simultaneously.

mul·ti·ple scle·ro·sis (MS) (mŭl'ti-pĕl skler-ō'sis) Common demyelinating disorder of the central nervous system, causing patches of sclerosis (plaques) in the brain and spinal cord; occurs primarily in young adults.

mul·ti·ple stain (mŭl'ti-pĕl stān) A mixture of several dyes each having an independent selective action on one or more portions of the tissue.

mul·ti·ple sul·fa·tase de·fi·cien·cy (MSD) (mŭl'ti-pĕl sŭl'fă-tās dĕ-fish'ĕn-sē) Inherited disorder with failure to hydrolyze sulfatides and sulfated mucopolysaccharides leading to accumulation in neural and extraneural tissues.

mul·ti·ple sym·met·ric lip·o·ma·to·sis (mŭl'ti-pĕl si-met'rik lip'ō-mă-tō'sis) Accumulation and progressive enlargement of collections of adipose tissue in the subcutaneous tissue of the head, neck, upper trunk, and upper portions of the upper extremities; seen primarily in adult males and of unknown cause. SYN Madelung disease.

mul·ti·ple-sys·tem at·ro·phy (mŭl'ti-pĕl sis'tĕm at'rŏ-fē) Nonhereditary, neurodegenerative disease of unknown cause, characterized clinically by the development of parkinsonism, ataxia, autonomic failure, or pyramidal tract signs, in various combinations.

mul·ti·plex pol·y·mer·ase chain re·ac·tion (PCR) (mŭl'tē-pleks pŏ-lim'ĕr-ās chān rē-ak'shŭn) Method that uses two primer sets in the same tube. Each primer set is specific for a different target.

mul·ti·po·lar mi·to·sis (mŭl'tē-pō'lăr mī-tō'sis) Pathologic form in which the spindle has three or more poles, resulting in the formation of a corresponding number of nuclei.

mul·ti·va·lent (mŭl'tē-vā'lĕnt) **1.** CHEMISTRY having a combining power (valence) of more than one hydrogen atom. **2.** Efficacious in more than one direction. **3.** Antisera specific for more than one antigen or organism. SYN polyvalent (1).

mum·mi·fi·ca·tion (mŭm′i-fi-kā′shŭn) **1.** SYN dry gangrene. **2.** Shriveling of a dead retained fetus. **3.** DENTISTRY treatment of inflamed dental pulp with fixative drugs to retain teeth so treated for relatively short periods.

mumps (mŭmps) An acute infectious and contagious disease caused by a mumps virus of the genus *Rubulavirus* and characterized by fever, inflammation and swelling of the parotid gland. SYN epidemic parotitis.

mumps skin test an·ti·gen (MSTA) (mŭmps skin test an′ti-jen) Sterile suspension of killed mumps virus in isotonic sodium chloride solution; used to determine susceptibility to mumps or to confirm previous exposure.

Munch·hau·sen syn·drome (mūn′ chow-zĕn sin′drōm) Repeated fabrication of clinically convincing simulations of disease to get medical attention. SEE factitious disorder.

Munch·hau·sen syn·drome by proxy (mūn′chow-zĕn sin′drōm prok′sē) Child abuse inflicted by a caretaker (usually the mother) with fabrications of symptoms and/or induction of signs of disease, leading to unnecessary investigations and interventions, with occasional serious health consequences, including death of the child. SYN factitious illness by proxy.

Mun·ro mi·cro·ab·scess (mŭn-rō′ mī′ krō-ab′ses) Microscopic collection of polymorphonuclear leukocytes found in the stratum corneum in psoriasis.

Mun·ro point (mŭn-rō′ poynt) A point at the right edge of the rectus abdominis muscle, between the umbilicus and the anterior superior spine of the ilium, where pressure elicits tenderness in appendicitis.

mu·ral (myū′răl) Relating to the wall of any cavity.

mu·ral en·do·car·di·tis (myū′răl en′dō-kahr-dī′tis) Inflammation of the endocardium involving the walls of the chambers of the heart.

mu·ral preg·nan·cy (myūr′ăl preg′năn-sē) Pregnancy in uterine muscular wall.

mu·ral throm·bo·sis (myū′răl throm-bō′sis) The formation of a thrombus in contact with the endocardial lining of a cardiac chamber, or a large blood vessel, if not occlusive.

mu·ral throm·bus (myū′răl throm′bŭs) Clot formed on and attached to a diseased patch of endocardium. SEE ALSO parietal thrombus.

mu·ri·at·ic ac·id (myūr′ē-at′ik as′id) SYN hydrochloric acid.

mur·ine (myūr-ēn′) Relating to mice.

mu·rine ty·phus (myūr-ēn′ tī′fŭs) A milder form of epidemic typhus caused by *Rickettsia typhi* and transmitted to humans by fleas from rats or mice. SYN endemic typhus.

mur·mur (mŭr′mŭr) An abnormal, usually periodic sound heard on auscultation of the heart or blood vessels.

Mus (mŭs) A genus of the family Muridae that includes about 16 species of mice; domesticated strains are numerous and genetically well defined.

Mus·ca (mŭs′kă) A genus of flies that includes the common housefly, *Musca domestica;* breeds in filth and organic waste; involved in transfer of numerous pathogens.

mus·cae vol·i·tan·tes (mŭs′kē vol-i-tan′tēz) Floaters; moving spots appearing before the eyes.

mus·ca·rine (mŭs′kă-rēn) A toxin with neurologic effects, first isolated from *Amanita muscaria* and also present in some species of *Hebeloma* and *Inocybe*; pharmalogic effects include cardiac inhibition, vasodilation, salivation, and lacrimation.

mus·ca·rin·ic (mŭs′kă-rin′ik) Having a muscarinelike action, i.e., producing effects that resemble postganglionic parasympathetic stimulation.

mus·ca·rin·ic re·cep·tors (mŭs-kăr-in′ik rē-sep′tŏrz) Membrane-bound proteins with an extracellular domain that

M

contains a recognition site for acetylcholine.

mus·cle (mŭs'ĕl) [TA] A primary tissue, consisting predominantly of highly specialized contractile cells, which may be classified as skeletal muscle, cardiac muscle, or smooth muscle. SYN musculus.

mus·cle con·trac·tion head·ache (mŭs'ĕl kŏn-trak'shŭn hed'āk) SYN tension headache.

mus·cle en·er·gy tech·nique (MET) (mŭs'ĕl en'ĕr-jē tek-nēk') A massage therapy modality that works to adjust proprioceptive activity and levels of resting tension through stretches and muscle contraction with resistance. SEE ALSO proprioceptive neuromuscular facilitation. SYN strain-counterstrain.

mus·cle fi·ber (mŭs'ĕl fī'bĕr) Muscle is classified as fiber based on contractile and metabolic characteristics.

mus·cle he·mo·glo·bin (mŭs'ĕl hē'mŏ-glō-bin) SYN myoglobin.

mus·cle plate (mŭs'ĕl plāt) SYN myotome (2).

mus·cle re·lax·ant (MR) (mŭs'ĕl rē-laks'ănt) Drug able to reduce muscle tone; may be either a peripherally or centrally acting muscle relaxant.

mus·cle-spar·i·ng tho·ra·cot·o·my (mŭs'ĕl-spăr'ing thŏr'ă-kot'ŏ-mē) Any type of thoracic surgery that does not involve significant division of the latissimus dorsi and serratus anterior muscles.

mus·cle tone (mŭs'ĕl tōn) **1.** The internal state of muscle-fiber tension within individual muscles and muscle groups. **2.** Degree of muscle tension or resistance during rest or in response to stretching. SEE ALSO hypotonia (3).

mus·cu·lar (mŭs'kyū-lăr) **1.** Relating to a muscle or the muscles. **2.** Having well-developed musculature.

mus·cu·lar ar·te·ry (mŭs'kyū-lăr ahr'tĕr-ē) An artery with a tunica media composed principally of circularly arranged smooth muscle. SYN distributing artery.

mus·cu·lar as·the·no·pi·a (mŭs'kyū-lăr as'thĕ-nō'pē-ă) Ocular disorder due to imbalance of the extrinsic ocular muscles.

mus·cu·lar at·ro·phy (mŭs'kyū-lăr at'rŏ-fē) Wasting of muscular tissue.

mus·cu·lar dys·tro·phy (mŭs'kyū-lăr dis'trŏ-fē) General term for hereditary progressive degenerative disorders affecting skeletal muscles. SYN myodystrophia.

mus·cu·lar hy·per·es·the·si·a (mŭs'kyū-lăr hī'pĕr-es-thē'zē-ă) Sensitiveness of the muscles to pressure.

mus·cu·lar in·com·pe·tence (mŭs'kyū-lăr in-kom'pĕ-tĕns) Imperfect closure of an anatomically normal cardiac valve.

mus·cu·la·ris (mŭs-kyū-lā'ris) Muscular coat of a hollow organ or tubular structure.

mus·cu·lar lay·er (mŭs'kyū-lăr lā'ĕr) The muscular, usually middle, layer of a tubular structure; for most of the gastrointestinal tract, it consists of an outer longitudinal layer of muscle and an inner circular layer.

mus·cu·lar rheu·ma·tism (mŭs'kyū-lăr rū'mă-tizm) SYN fibrositis (2).

mus·cu·lar sys·tem (mŭs'kyū-lăr sis'tĕm) [TA] All the muscles of the body collectively. SYN systema musculare [TA].

mus·cu·lar tis·sue (mŭs'kyū-lăr tish'ū) A tissue characterized by the ability to contract upon stimulation; its three varieties are skeletal, cardiac, and smooth. SEE muscle. SYN flesh (2).

mus·cu·la·ture (mŭs'kyū-lă-chŭr) The arrangement of the muscles in a part or in the body as a whole.

mus·cu·lo·ap·o·neu·rot·ic (mŭs'kyū-lō-ap'ŏ-nūr-ot'ik) Relating to muscular tissue and an aponeurosis of origin or insertion.

mus·cu·lo·cu·ta·ne·ous (MC) (mŭs'kyū-lō-kyū-tā'nē-ŭs) Relating to both muscle and skin. SYN myocutaneous, myodermal.

mus·cu·lo·cu·ta·ne·ous flap (mŭs′kyū-lō-kyū-tā′nē-ŭs flap) A pedicled skin flap, often an island flap, with attached subjacent muscle, investing fascia, and blood supply. SYN myocutaneous flap.

mus·cu·lo·phren·ic (mŭs′kyū-lō-fren′ik) Relating to the muscular portion of the diaphragm.

mus·cu·lo·skel·e·tal (mŭs′kyū-lō-skel′ĕ-tăl) Relating to muscles and to the skeleton.

mus·cu·lo·spi·ral (mŭs′kū-lō-spī′răl) Denoting the musculospiral nerve. SEE radial nerve.

mus·cu·lo·spi·ral pa·ral·y·sis (mŭs′kyū-lō-spī′răl păr-al′i-sis) Paralysis of the muscles of the forearm due to injury of the radial nerve.

mus·cu·lo·ten·di·nous (mŭs′kyū-lō-ten′di-nŭs) Relating to both muscular and tendinous tissues.

mus·cu·lo·ten·di·nous cuff (mŭs′kyū-lō-ten′di-nŭs kŭf) SYN rotator cuff of shoulder.

mus·cu·lus, gen. and pl. **mus·cu·li** (mŭs′kyū-lŭs, -lī) [TA] SYN muscle.

mush·room poi·son·ing (mŭsh′rūm poy′zŏn-ing) SEE mycetism.

mu·si·cal a·lex·i·a (myū′zi-kăl ă-lek′sē-ă) Loss of the power to read musical notation.

mu·si·cal mur·mur (myū′zi-kăl mŭr′mŭr) Cardiac or vascular sound with a high-pitched musical character.

mu·si·cian's ear·plugs (myū-zish′ănz ēr′plŭgz) Custom-fitted earplugs that attenuate all frequencies evenly in relation to normal hearing sensitivity.

music ther·a·py, mu·si·co·ther·a·py (myū′zik thār′ă-pē, myū′zik-ō-thār′ă-pē) An adjunctive treatment of mental disorders by means of music.

mus·si·ta·tion (mŭs′i-tā′shŭn) Movements of the lips as if speaking, but without sound; observed in delirium and in semicoma.

Mus·tard op·er·a·tion (mŭs′tărd op-ĕr-ā′shŭn) Atrial correction of hemodynamic abnormality due to transposition of the great arteries by an intraatrial baffle to direct pulmonary venous blood through the tricuspid orifice into the right ventricle and the systemic venous blood through the mitral valve into the left ventricle.

mu·ta·cism (myū′tă-sizm) SYN mytacism.

mu·ta·gen (myū′tă-jen) Any agent that promotes a mutation or causes an increase in the rate of mutational events.

mu·ta·gen·e·sis (myū-tă-jen′ĕ-sis) **1.** Production of a mutation. **2.** Production of genetic alteration through use of chemicals or radiation.

mu·tant (myū′tănt) **1.** A phenotype in which a mutation is manifested. **2.** A gene that is rare and usually harmful, in contrast to a wild-type gene, not necessarily generated recently.

mu·tant gene (myū′tănt jēn) A gene that has been changed from an ancestral type, not necessarily in the current generation.

mu·ta·ro·tase (myū′tă-rō-tās) SYN aldose 1L-epimerase.

mu·ta·ro·ta·tion (myū′tă-rō-tā′shŭn) Changing specific rotation at a given wavelength. SYN birotation, multirotation.

mu·tase (myū′tās) Any enzyme that catalyzes the apparent migration of groups within one molecule.

mu·ta·tion (myū-tā′shŭn) **1.** A change in the chemistry of a gene that is perpetuated in subsequent divisions of the cell in which it occurs; a change in the sequence of base pairs in the chromosomal molecule. **2.** The sudden production of a species, as distinguished from variation.

mu·ta·tion·al fal·set·to (myū-tā′shŭn-ăl fawl-set′ō) Habitual use of an abnormally high-pitched voice that persists after puberty. SYN puberphonia.

mu·ta·tion rate (myū-tā′shŭn rāt) The probability (or proportion) of progeny genes with a particular component of the

M

genome not present in either biologic parent.

mute (myūt) **1.** Unable or unwilling to speak. **2.** A person who does not have the faculty of speech.

mu·tein (myū′tēn) A protein arising as a result of a mutation.

mu·ti·lat·ing ker·a·to·der·ma (myū′ti-lāt′ing ker′ă-tō-dĕr′mă) Diffuse skin disease of the limbs.

mu·ti·la·tion (myū-ti-lā′shŭn) Disfigurement or injury by removal or destruction of any conspicuous or essential part of the body.

mut·ism (myū′tizm) **1.** The state of being silent. **2.** Organic or functional absence of the faculty of speech.

mu·ton (myū′ton) GENETICS the smallest unit of a chromosome in which alteration can cause a mutation.

mu·tu·al·ism (myū′chyū-ăl-izm) Symbiotic relationship from which both species derive benefit. Cf. commensalism, metabiosis, parasitism.

my·al·gi·a (mī-al′jē-ă) Muscular pain. SYN myodynia.

my·al·gic as·the·ni·a (mī-al′jik as-the′nē-ă) A condition associated with muscle pain and/or tenderness, generalized weakness, and loss of strength.

my·as·the·ni·a (mī′as-thē′nē-ă) Muscular weakness.

my·as·the·ni·a gra·vis (mī′as-thē′nē-ă gra′vis) Disorder of neuromuscular transmission, marked by fluctuating weakness, especially of the oculofacial muscles and the proximal limb muscles. SYN Goldflam disease.

my·as·then·ic cri·sis (mī-as-then′ik krī′sis) Severe, life-threatening exacerbation of the manifestations of myasthenia gravis requiring intensive treatment.

my·a·to·ni·a, my·at·o·ny (mī′ă-tō′nē-ă, mī-at′ŏ-nē) Abnormal extensibility of a muscle.

my·at·ro·phy (mī-at′rŏ-fē) SYN muscular atrophy.

my·ce·li·um, pl. **my·ce·li·a** (mī-sē′lē-ŭm, -a) The mass of hyphae making up a colony of fungi.

mycet-, myceto-, myco- Combining forms denoting fungus.

my·cete (mī′sēt) A fungus.

my·ce·tism (mī′sē-tizm) Poisoning by certain species of mushrooms.

my·ce·to·ma (mī′sĕ-tō′mă) **1.** Chronic infection involving the feet characterized by formation of localized lesions with tumefactions and multiple draining sinuses. SYN Madura boil, maduromycosis. **2.** Any tumor with draining sinuses produced by filamentous fungi.

My·co·bac·te·ri·a·ce·ae (mī′kō-bak-tē′rē-ā′sē-ē) A family of aerobic bacteria containing gram-positive, spheric to rod-shaped cells usually acid fast; occur in soil and dairy products and as parasites on humans and other animals.

My·co·bac·te·ri·um (mī′kō-bak-tēr′ē-ŭm) A genus of aerobic, nonmotile bacteria (family Mycobacteriaceae) containing gram-positive, acid-fast, slender, straight or slightly curved rods; several species are associated with infections in immunocompromised people, especially those with AIDS.

My·co·bac·te·ri·um a·vi· um (mī′kō-bak-tēr′ē-ŭm ā′vī-ŭm) A bacterial species causing tuberculosis in fowl and other birds; linked to opportunistic infections in humans. SYN tubercle bacillus (3).

My·co·bac·te·ri·um tu·ber·cu·lo·sis (mī′kō-bak-tēr′ē-ŭm tū-bĕr′kyū-lō′sis) A bacterial species that causes tuberculosis in humans. It is the type species of the genus *Mycobacterium*. SYN Koch bacillus, tubercle bacillus (1).

my·col·o·gy (mī-kol′ŏ-jē) The study of fungi including pathogenicity.

My·co·plas·ma (mī′kō-plaz′mă) A genus of aerobic to facultatively anaerobic bacteria containing gram-negative cells that do not possess a true cell wall but are bounded by a three-layered membrane; found in humans and other animals and are parasitic to pathogenic.

my·co·plas·mal pneu·mo·ni·a (mī′

kō-plaz′măl nū-mō′nē-ă) SYN primary atypical pneumonia.

My·co·plas·ma pneu·mo·ni·ae (mī′ kō-plaz′mă nū-mō′nē-ē) A bacterial species causing primary atypical pneumonia in human beings.

my·co·sis (mī-kō′sis) Any disease caused by a fungus (filamentous or yeast).

my·co·sis fun·goi·des (mī-kō′sis fŭng-goyd′ēz) A chronic progressive dermal lymphoma that initially simulates eczema; in advanced cases, ulcerated tumors and infiltrations of lymph nodes may occur.

my·cot·ic (mī-kot′ik) Relating to or caused by a fungus.

my·cot·ic an·eu·rysm (mī-kot′ik an′ yūr-izm) One caused by the growth of fungi within the vascular wall, usually following impaction of a septic embolus; also used to refer to the growth of bacteria within the vascular wall of an aneurysm.

my·co·tox·i·co·sis (mī′kō-tok′si-kō′sis) Poisoning due to the ingestion of preformed substances produced by the action of certain fungi on particular foodstuffs or by ingestion of the fungi themselves; e.g., ergotism.

my·co·tox·in (mī′kō-tok′sin) Toxic compound produced by certain fungi; some are used for medicinal purposes.

my·dri·a·sis (mi-drī′ă-sis) Dilation of the pupil.

myd·ri·at·ic (mid′rē-at′ik) 1. Causing mydriasis or dilation of the pupil. 2. An agent that dilates the pupil.

my·ec·to·my (mī-ek′tŏ-mē) Excision of all or part of a muscle.

myel-, myelo- Combining forms indicating bone; spinal cord and medulla oblongata; myelin sheath of nerve fibers. Cf. medullo-.

my·el·a·ceph·a·lus (mī′ăl-ā-sef′ă-lŭs) A fetus that is severely malformed and attached to its monozygotic twin.

my·el·ap·o·plex·y (mī′el-ap′ŏ-plek-sē) SYN hematomyelia.

my·el·aux·e (mī′ĕl-awk′sē) Hypertrophy of the spinal cord.

my·e·lin (mī′ĕ-lin) The lipoproteinaceous material of the myelin sheath, composed of alternating membranes of lipid and protein.

my·e·lin·a·ted (mī′ĕ-li-nāt-ĕd) Having a myelin sheath. SYN medullated (2).

my·e·li·nat·ed nerve (mī′ĕ-li-nā-tĕd nĕrv) Peripheral nerve with axons surrounded by layers of Schwann cell membranes that form the myelin sheath; also called medullated nerve.

my·e·li·na·tion, my·e·li·ni·za·tion (mī′ ĕ-li-nā′shŭn, -lin-ī-zā′shŭn) The acquisition, development, or formation of a myelin sheath around a nerve fiber. SYN medullation (2), myelinization, myelinogenesis.

my·e·lin·o·ly·sis (mī′ĕ-li-nol′i-sis) Dissolution of the myelin sheaths of nerve fibers.

my·e·lin sheath (mī′ĕ-lin shēth) Lipoproteinaceous envelope in vertebrates surrounding most axons larger than 0.5-mcm diameter. SYN medullary sheath.

my·e·li·tis (mī′ĕ-lī′tis) 1. Spinal cord inflammation. 2. Bone marrow inflammation.

my·e·lo·blas·tic leu·ke·mi·a (mī′ĕ-lō-blas′tik lū-kē′mē-ă) A form of granulocytic leukemia in which there are large numbers of myeloblasts in various tissues and in the blood. Used synonymously for acute granulocytic leukemia.

my·e·lo·blas·to·ma (mī′ĕ-lō-blas-tō′ mă) A nodular focus or fairly well-circumscribed accumulation of myeloblasts.

my·e·lo·cele (mī′ĕ-lō-sēl) 1. Protrusion of the spinal cord in spina bifida. 2. The central canal of the spinal cord.

my·e·lo·clast (mī′ĕ-lō-klast) A cell type that destroys the myelin sheaths of nerve cells.

my·e·lo·cyst (mī′ĕ-lō-sist) Any cyst that develops from a rudimentary central canal in the central nervous system.

my·e·lo·cys·to·cele (mī′ĕ-lō-sis′tō-sēl) Spina bifida containing spinal cord substance.

my·e·lo·cys·to·me·nin·go·cele (mī′ĕ-lō-sis′tō-mĕ-ning′gō-sēl) SYN meningomyelocele.

my·e·lo·cyte (mī′ĕ-lō-sīt) **1.** A young cell of the granulocytic series, occurring normally in bone marrow, but not in circulating blood. **2.** A nerve cell of the gray matter of the brain or spinal cord.

my·e·lo·cyt·ic leu·ke·mi·a, my·e·lo·gen·ic leu·ke·mi·a, my·e·log·e·nous leu·ke·mi·a, my·e·loid leu·ke·mi·a (mī′ĕ-lō-sit′ik lū-kē′mē-ă, mī′ĕ-lō-jen′ik, mī′ĕ-loj′ĕ-nŭs, mī′ĕ-loyd) SYN granulocytic leukemia.

my·e·lo·cy·to·ma (mī′ĕ-lō-sī-tō′mă) A nodular focus or fairly well-circumscribed, relatively dense accumulation of myelocytes.

my·e·lo·cy·to·sis (mī′ĕ-lō-sī-tō′sis) The occurrence of abnormally large numbers of myelocytes in the circulating blood, or tissues, or both.

my·e·lo·dys·pla·si·a (mī′ĕ-lō-dis-plā′zē-ă) **1.** An abnormality in development of the spinal cord, especially the lower part. **2.** Bone marrow disorder, characterized by proliferation of abnormal stem cells, which have the potential of developing into leukemia.

my·e·lo·dys·plas·tic syn·drome (mī′ĕ-lō-dis-plast′ik sin′drōm) A progressive, primary, neoplastic, pluripotential stem cell disorder characterized by peripheral blood cytopenias and prominent maturation abnormalities in the bone marrow.

my·e·lo·fi·bro·sis (mī′ĕ-lō-fī-brō′sis) Fibrosis of the bone marrow, especially generalized, associated with myeloid metaplasia of the spleen and other organs, leukoerythroblastic anemia, and thrombocytopenia. SYN myelosclerosis.

my·e·lo·gen·e·sis (mī′ĕ-lō-jen′ĕ-sis) **1.** Development of bone marrow. **2.** Development of the central nervous system. **3.** Formation of myelin around an axon.

my·e·lo·gen·ic (mī′ĕ-lō-jen′ik) Related to myelogenesis. SYN myelogenous.

my·e·log·e·nous (mī-ĕ-loj′ĕ-nŭs) SYN myelogenetic (2).

my·e·log·ra·phy (mī′ĕ-log′ră-fē) Radiography of the spinal cord and nerve roots after the injection of a contrast medium into the spinal subarachnoid space.

my·e·loid (mī′ĕ-loyd) **1.** Pertaining to, derived from, or manifesting certain features of the bone marrow. **2.** Pertaining to certain characteristics of myelocytic forms, but not necessarily implying origin in the bone marrow.

my·e·loid met·a·pla·si·a (mī′ĕ-loyd met′ă-plā′zē-ă) A syndrome characterized by anemia, enlargement of the spleen, nucleated red blood cells and immature granulocytes in the blood, and foci of extramedullary hemopoiesis in the spleen and liver.

my·e·loi·do·sis (mī′ĕ-loy-dō′sis) General hyperplasia of myeloid tissue.

my·e·loid tis·sue (mī′ĕ-loyd tish′ū) Bone marrow consisting of the developmental and adult stages of erythrocytes, granulocytes, and megakaryocytes in a stroma of reticular cells and fibers, with sinusoidal vascular channels.

my·e·lo·li·po·ma (mī′ĕ-lō-li-pō′mă) Nodular accumulations of cells derived from localized proliferation of reticuloendothelial tissue in the blood sinuses of the suprarenal glands.

my·e·lo·ma (mī′ĕ-lō′mă) **1.** A tumor composed of cells derived from hemopoietic tissues of the bone marrow. **2.** A plasma cell tumor.

my·e·lo·ma·la·ci·a (mī′ĕ-lō-mă-lā′shē-ă) Softening of the spinal cord.

my·e·lo·ma·to·sis (mī′ĕ-lō-mă-tō′sis) A disease characterized by the occurrence of myeloma in various sites.

my·e·lo·me·nin·go·cele (mī′ĕ-lō-mĕ-ning′gō-sēl) SYN meningomyelocele.

my·e·lo·mere (mī′ĕ-lō-mēr) Neuromere of the brain or spinal cord.

my·e·lop·a·thy (mī′ĕ-lop′ă-thē) **1.** Disorder of the spinal cord. **2.** A disease of the myelopoietic tissues.

my·e·lop·e·tal (mī′ĕ-lop′ĕ-tăl) Proceeding in a direction toward the spinal cord; said of different nerve impulses.

my·e·lo·phthis·ic a·ne·mi·a, my·e·lo·path·ic a·ne·mi·a (mī′ĕ-lof-thiz′tik ă-nē′mē-ă, -path′ik) SYN leukoerythroblastosis.

my·e·loph·thi·sis (mī′ĕ-lof′thi-sis) **1.** Wasting or atrophy of the spinal cord. **2.** Replacement of hematopoietic tissue in the bone marrow by abnormal tissue, usually fibrous tissue or malignant tumors that are most commonly metastatic carcinomas.

my·e·lo·plast (mī′ĕ-lō-plast) Any leukocytic series of cells in the bone marrow.

my·e·lo·poi·e·sis (mī′ĕ-lō-poy-ē′sis) Formation of the tissue elements of bone marrow, or any of the types of blood cells derived from bone marrow; or both.

my·e·lo·pro·lif·er·a·tive (mī′ĕ-lō-prō-lif′ĕr-ă-tiv) Pertaining to or characterized by unusual proliferation of myelopoietic tissue.

my·e·lo·pro·lif·er·a·tive syn·dromes (mī′ĕ-lō-prō-lif′ĕr-ă-tiv sin′drōmz) Conditions due to a disorder in the rate of formation of cells of the bone marrow, including chronic granulocytic leukemia, erythremia, myelosclerosis, panmyelosis, and erythremic myelosis and erythroleukemia.

my·e·lo·ra·dic·u·li·tis (mī′ĕ-lō-ră-dik′yū-lī′tis) Inflammation of the spinal cord and nerve roots.

my·e·lo·ra·dic·u·lo·dys·pla·si·a (mī′ĕ-lō-ră-dik′yū-lō-dis-plā′zē-ă) Congenital maldevelopment of the spinal cord and spinal nerve roots.

my·e·lo·ra·dic·u·lop·a·thy (mī′ĕ-lō-ră-dik′yū-lop′ă-thē) Disease involving the spinal cord and nerve roots. SYN radiculomyelopathy.

my·e·lor·rha·gi·a (mī′ĕ-lō-rā′jē-ă) SYN hematomyelia.

my·e·lo·sar·co·ma (mī′ă-lō-sahr-kō′mă) Cancer originating in the bone marrow.

my·e·los·chi·sis (mī′ĕ-los′ki-sis) Cleft spinal cord due to failure of the neural folds to close normally in the formation of the neural tube.

my·e·lo·scle·ro·sis (mī′ĕ-lō-skle-rō′sis) SYN myelofibrosis.

my·e·lo·sis (mī′ĕ-lō′sis) **1.** A condition characterized by abnormal proliferation of tissue or cellular elements of bone marrow. **2.** A condition with abnormal proliferation of medullary tissue in the spinal cord.

my·e·lo·spon·gi·um (mī′ĕ-lō-spŭn′jē-ŭm) Fibrocellular meshwork in the spinal cord of the embryo, from which the neuroglia is developed.

my·e·lo·sup·pres·sion (mī′ĕ-lō-sŭ-presh′ŭn) A reduction in the ability of the bone marrow to produce blood cells: platelets, red blood cells, and white blood cells. Typically caused by cancer chemotherapy and radiation therapy.

my·e·lo·tox·ic (mī′ĕ-lō-tok′sik) **1.** Inhibitory, depressant, or destructive to one or more of the components of bone marrow. **2.** Pertaining to, derived from, or manifesting the features of diseased bone marrow.

my·lo·hy·oid (mī′lō-hī′oyd) Relating to the molar teeth, or posterior portion of the lower jaw, and to the hyoid bone.

my·lo·hy·oid (mus·cle) (mī′lō-hī′oyd mŭs′ĕl) *Origin*, mylohyoid line of mandible; *insertion*, upper border of hyoid bone and raphe separating muscle from its fellow; *action*, elevates floor of mouth and the tongue, depresses jaw when hyoid is fixed; *nerve supply*, nerve to mylohyoid from mandibular division of trigeminal.

myo- Combining form meaning muscle.

my·o·ar·chi·tec·ton·ic (mī′ō-ahr-ki-tek-ton′ik) Relating to the structural arrangement of muscle or of fibers in general.

my·o·at·ro·phy (mī′ō-at′rŏ-fē) SYN muscular atrophy.

my·o·blast (mī′ō-blast) A primordial muscle cell with the potentiality of developing into a muscle fiber. SYN sarcoblast.

my•o•blas•to•ma (mī′ō-blas-tō′mă) A tumor of immature muscle cells.

my•o•car•di•al, my•o•car•di•ac (mī′ō-kahr′dē-ăl, -ē-ak) Relating to the myocardium.

my•o•car•di•al de•pres•sant fac•tor (mī′ō-kahr′dē-ăl dĕ-pres′ănt fak′tŏr) Toxic factor (e.g., peptide) in shock that impairs cardiac contractility.

my•o•car•di•al in•farc•tion (MI) (mī′ō-kahr′dē-ăl in-fahrk′shŭn) Infarction of an area of the heart muscle. SYN heart attack, infarctus myocardii.

my•o•car•di•al in•suf•fi•cien•cy (mī′ō-kahr′dē-ăl in′sŭ-fish′ĕn-sē) SYN heart failure (1).

my•o•car•di•al is•che•mi•a (M Isch, MI) (mī′ō-kahr′dē-ăl is-kē′mē-ă) Inadequate circulation of blood to the myocardium. SEE ALSO angina pectoris, myocardial infarction.

my•o•car•di•o•graph (mī′ō-kahr′dē-ō-graf) An instrument composed of a tambour with recording lever attachment, by means of which a tracing is made of the movements of the heart muscle.

my•o•car•di•op•a•thy (mī′ō-kahr′dē-op′ă-thē) SYN cardiomyopathy.

my•o•car•di•tis (mī′ō-kahr-dī′tis) Inflammation of the muscular walls of the heart.

my•o•car•di•um, pl. **my•o•car•di•a** (mī′ō-kahr′dē-ŭm, -ă) [TA] The middle layer of the heart, consisting of cardiac muscle.

my•o•cele (mī′ō-sēl) **1.** Protrusion of muscle substance through a tear in its sheath. **2.** The small cavity that appears in somites.

my•o•clon•ic sei•zure (mī′ō-klon′ik sē′zhŭr) One characterized by sudden, brief contractions of muscle fibers, muscles, or groups of muscles of variable topography.

my•oc•lo•nus (mī′ok′lŏ-nŭs) One or a series of shocklike contractions of a group of muscles, of variable regularity, synchrony, and symmetry, generally due to a central nervous system lesion.

my•oc•lo•nus ep•i•lep•sy (mī′ok′lŏ-nŭs ep′i-lep′sē) Clinically diverse group of epilepsy syndromes, some benign, some progressive. SYN localization-related epilepsy (1).

my•o•cu•ta•ne•ous (mī′ō-kyū-tā′nē-ŭs) SYN musculocutaneous.

my•o•cyte (mī′ō-sīt) A muscle cell.

my•o•cy•tol•y•sis (mī′ō-sī-tol′i-sis) Dissolution of muscle fiber.

my•o•cy•to•ma (mī′ō-sī-tō′mă) A benign neoplasm derived from muscle.

my•o•de•mi•a (mī′ō-dē′mē-ă) Fatty degeneration of muscle.

my•o•di•as•ta•sis (mī′ō-dī-as′tă-sis) Separation of muscle.

my•o•dyn•i•a (mī′ō-din′ē-ă) SYN myalgia.

my•o•dys•to•ny (mī′ō-dis′tŏ-nē) A condition of slow relaxation, interrupted by a succession of slight contractions, following electrical stimulation of a muscle.

my•o•e•de•ma (mī′ō-ĕ-dē′mă) A localized contraction of a degenerating muscle at the point of a sharp blow. SYN idiomuscular contraction, mounding, myo-oedema.

my•o•e•las•tic (mī′ō-ĕ-las′tik) Pertaining to closely associated smooth muscle fibers and elastic connective tissue.

my•o•e•lec•tric (mī′ō-ĕ-lek′trik) Relating to the electrical properties of muscle.

my•o•ep•i•the•li•al (mī′ō-ep′i-thē′lē-ăl) Relating to myoepithelium.

my•o•ep•i•the•li•o•ma (mī′ō-ep′i-thē-lē-ō′mă) A benign tumor of myoepithelial cells.

my•o•ep•i•the•li•um (mī′ō-ep′i-thē′lē-ŭm) Spindle-shaped, contractile, smooth musclelike cells of epithelial origin arranged longitudinally or obliquely around sweat glands and the secretory alveoli of the mammary gland. SYN muscle epithelium.

my•o•fas•ci•al (mī′ō-fash′ē-ăl) Of or relating to the fascia surrounding and separating muscle tissue.

my·o·fas·ci·al pain-dys·func·tion syn·drome (mī′ō-fash′ē-ăl pān-dis-fŭngk′shŭn sin′drōm) A condition involving the development of regional trigger points that create pain, weakness, limited range of motion, and general dysfunction.

my·o·fas·ci·tis (mī′ō-fash-ī′tis) SYN myositis fibrosa.

my·o·fi·bril (mī′ō-fī′bril) Fine longitudinal fibril in skeletal or cardiac muscle fiber consisting of many regularly overlapped ultramicroscopic thick and thin myofilaments.

my·o·fi·bro·blast (mī′ō-fī′brō-blast) A cell thought to be responsible for contracture of wounds and eruption of the teeth.

my·o·fi·bro·ma (mī′ō-fī-brō′mă) A benign neoplasm that consists chiefly of fibrous connective tissue, with variable numbers of muscle cells forming portions of the neoplasm.

my·o·fi·bro·sis (mī′ō-fī-brō′sis) Chronic myositis with diffuse hyperplasia of the interstitial connective tissue pressing on and causing atrophy of the muscular tissue.

my·o·fi·bro·si·tis (mī′ō-fī-brō-sī′tis) Inflammation of the perimysium.

my·o·fil·a·ments (mī′ō-fil′ă-mĕnts) The ultramicroscopic threads of filamentous proteins making up myofibrils in striated muscle.

my·o·gen·e·sis (mī′ō-jen′ĕ-sis) Embryonic formation of muscle cells or fibers.

my·o·ge·net·ic, my·o·gen·ic (mī′ō-jĕ-net′ik, -jen′ik) 1. Originating in or starting from muscle. 2. Relating to the origin of muscle cells or fibers. SYN myogenous.

my·o·glo·bin (mī′ō-glō′bin) The oxygen-transporting and storage protein of muscle, resembling blood hemoglobin in function but with a molecular weight approximately one quarter that of hemoglobin. SEE ALSO oxymyoglobin. SYN muscle hemoglobin.

my·o·glob·u·lin (Mgb) (mī′ō-glob′yū-lin) Globulin present in muscle tissue.

my·o·graph (mī′ō-graf) A recording instrument with which tracings are made of muscular contractions.

my·og·ra·phy (mī-og′ră-fē) 1. The recording of muscular movements by the myograph. 2. A description of or treatise on the muscles. SYN descriptive myology.

my·oid (mī′oyd) 1. Resembling muscle. 2. One of the fine, contractile, threadlike protoplasmic elements found in certain epithelial cells in lower animals.

my·oid cells (mī′oyd selz) Flattened smooth musclelike cells of mesodermal origin that lie just outside the basal lamina of the seminiferous tubule. SYN peritubular contractile cells.

my·o·ki·nase (mī′ō-kī′nās) SYN adenylate kinase.

my·o·ky·mi·a (mī′ō-kī′mē-ă) Continuous involuntary quivering or rippling of muscles at rest, caused by spontaneous, repetitive firing of groups of motor unit potentials. SYN kymatism, Morvan chorea.

my·ol·o·gy (mī-ol′ŏ-jē) The branch of science concerned with the muscles and their accessory parts, tendons, aponeuroses, bursae, and fasciae.

my·o·ma (mī-ō′mă) A benign neoplasm of muscular tissue. SEE ALSO leiomyoma.

my·o·ma·la·ci·a (mī′ō-mă-lā′shē-ă) Pathologic softening of muscular tissue.

my·o·ma·tous (mī-ō′mă-tŭs) Pertaining to or characterized by the features of a myoma.

my·o·mel·a·no·sis (mī′ō-mel-ă-nō′sis) Abnormal dark pigmentation of muscular tissue. SEE ALSO melanosis.

my·o·mere (mī′ō-mēr) SYN myotome (4).

my·om·e·ter (mī-om′ĕ-tĕr) An instrument for measuring the extent of a muscular contraction.

M

my·o·me·tri·al (mī′ō-mē′trē-ăl) Relating to the myometrium.

my·o·me·tri·tis (mī′ō-mē-trī′tis) Inflammation of uterine muscular wall.

my·o·me·tri·um (mī′ō-mē′trē-ŭm) [TA] The muscular wall of the uterus.

my·o·neme (mī′ō-nēm) **1.** A muscle fibril. **2.** One of the contractile fibrils of certain protozoans.

my·o·neu·ral (mī′ō-nūr′ăl) Relating to both muscle and nerve. SEE ALSO neuromuscular.

myo·oedema [Br.] SYN myoedema.

my·o·pal·mus (mī′ō-pal′mŭs) Muscle twitching.

my·o·pa·ral·y·sis (mī′ō-pă-ral′i-sis) Muscular paralysis.

my·o·pa·re·sis (mī′ō-pă-rē′sis) Slight muscular paralysis.

my·op·a·thy (mī-op′ă-thē) Any abnormal condition or disease of the muscular tissues; commonly designates a disorder involving skeletal muscle.

my·ope (mī′ōp) A nearsighted person.

my·o·per·i·car·di·tis (mī′ō-per′i-kahr-dī′tis) Inflammation of the muscular cardiac wall and enveloping pericardium.

my·o·phos·phor·y·lase (mī′ō-fos-fōr′i-lās) Muscle phosphorylase.

my·o·pi·a (mī-ō′pē-ă) That optic condition in which parallel light rays are brought by the ocular media to focus in front of the retina. SYN nearsightedness, shortsightedness.

my·o·pic a·stig·ma·tism (mī-op′ik ă-stig′mă-tizm) Form of astigmatism in which one meridian is myopic and the one at right angle to it is without refractive error. SYN simple myopic astigmatism.

my·o·pic cres·cent (mī-op′ik kres′ěnt) A white or grayish white crescentic area in the fundus of the eye located on the temporal side of the optic disc.

my·o·plasm (mī′ō-plazm) The contractile portion of the muscle cell, as distinguished from the sarcoplasm.

my·o·plas·tic (mī′ō-plas′tik) Relating to plastic or reconstructive muscle surgery.

my·o·plas·ty (mī′ō-plas-tē) Plastic or reconstructive surgery of muscular tissue.

my·or·rhex·is (mī′ō-rek′sis) Tearing of a muscle.

my·o·sal·pinx (mī′ō-sal′pingks) The muscular tunic of the uterine tube.

my·o·sar·co·ma (mī′ō-sahr-kō′mă) A general term for a malignant neoplasm derived from muscular tissue. SEE ALSO leiomyosarcoma, rhabdomyosarcoma.

my·o·scle·ro·sis (mī′ō-skle-rō′sis) Chronic myositis with hyperplasia of the interstitial connective tissue.

my·o·sin (mī′ō-sin) A globular protein present in muscle and in nonmuscle cells that has an adenosine triphosphatase activity; forms the thick filaments in muscle.

my·o·sin fil·a·ment (mī′ō-sin fil′ă-měnt) Contractile element in skeletal, cardiac, and smooth muscle fibers.

my·o·sit·ic (mī′ō-sit′ik) Relating to myositis.

my·o·si·tis (mī′ō-sī′tis) Inflammation of a muscle. SYN initis (2).

my·o·si·tis fi·bro·sa (mī′ō-sī′tis fī-brō′să) Induration of a muscle through an interstitial growth of fibrous tissue. SYN myofascitis.

my·o·si·tis os·sif·i·cans (MO) (mī′ō-sī′tis os-if′i-kanz) Deposit of bone in muscle with fibrosis, causing pain and swelling in muscles.

my·o·spasm, my·o·spas·mus (mī′ō-spazm, mī-ō-spaz′mŭs) Spasmodic muscular contraction.

my·o·stro·ma (mī′ō-strō′mă) Supporting connective framework of muscular tissue.

my·o·tac·tic (mī′ō-tak′tik) Relating to the muscular sense.

my·o·tac·tic re·flex (mī′ō-tak′ik rē′fleks) Tonic contraction of the muscles in response to a stretching force, due to stimulation of muscle proprioceptors. SYN muscle spindle reflex, stretch reflex.

my·ot·a·sis (mī-ot′ă-sis) Stretching of a muscle.

my·o·tat·ic con·trac·tion (mī′ō-tat′ik kŏn-trak′shŭn) Reflex contraction of skeletal muscle that occurs due to stimulation of the stretch receptors in the muscle.

my·o·tat·ic ir·ri·ta·bil·i·ty (mī′ō-tat′ik ir′i-tă-bil′i-tē) The ability of a muscle to contract in response to the stimulus produced by a sudden stretching.

my·o·tat·ic re·flex (mī′ō-tat′ik rē′fleks) Tonic contraction of the muscles in response to a stretching force, due to stimulation of muscle proprioceptors. SYN Liddell-Sherrington reflex, muscular reflex, stretch reflex.

my·o·ten·o·si·tis (mī′ō-ten-ō-sī′tis) Inflammation of a muscle with its tendon.

my·o·tome (mī′ō-tōm) **1.** A knife for dividing muscle. **2.** In embryos, that part of the somite that develops into skeletal muscle. SYN muscle plate. **3.** All muscles derived from one somite and innervated by one segmental spinal nerve.

my·o·to·ni·a (mī′ō-tō′nē-ă) Delayed relaxation of a muscle after a strong contraction, or prolonged contraction after mechanical stimulation or brief electrical stimulation.

my·o·to·ni·a con·gen·i·ta (mī′ō-tō′nē-ă kŏn-jen′i-tă) Uncommon muscle disorder, with onset in infancy or early childhood, characterized by muscle hypertrophy, myotonia, and a nonprogressive course.

my·o·ton·ic chon·dro·dys·tro·phy (mī′ō-ton′ik kon′drō-dis′trŏ-fē) Rare congenital disease that causes myotonia, muscular hypertrophy, joint and long bone abnormalities, and weakness. SYN Schwartz-Jampel disease.

my·o·ton·ic dys·tro·phy (mī′ō-tōn′ik dis′trŏ-fē) Most common adult muscular dystrophy, characterized by progressive muscle weakness and wasting of some of the cranial innervated muscles, as well as the distal limb muscles. SYN Steinert disease.

my·o·ton·ic re·sponse (mī-ō-ton′ik rĕ-spons′) Failure of muscle relaxation caused by repetitive discharge of muscle fiber action potentials.

my·ot·o·noid (mī-ot′ō-noyd) Denoting a muscular reaction, naturally or electrically excited, characterized by slow contraction and, especially, slow relaxation.

my·ot·o·nus (mī-ot′ō-nŭs) A tonic spasm or temporary rigidity of a muscle or group of muscles.

my·ot·o·ny, my·ot·one (mī-ot′ŏ-nē, mī′ō-tōn) Muscular tonus or tension. SYN myotone.

my·ot·ro·phy (mī-ot′rŏ-fē) Nutrition of muscular tissue.

my·o·tube (mī′ō-tūb) A skeletal muscle fiber formed by the fusion of myoblasts during a developmental stage.

my·o·tu·bule (mī′ō-tū′byūl) Former term for myotube.

My·Pyr·a·mid (mī ′pir′ă-mid) SYN Food Guide Pyramid.

my·rin·gec·to·my, my·rin·go·dec·to·my (mir′in-jek′tŏ-mē, mi-ring′gō-dek′tŏ-mē) Excision of the tympanic membrane.

my·rin·gi·tis (mir′in-jī′tis) Inflammation of the tympanic membrane. SYN tympanitis.

myringo-, myring- Combining forms indicating the membrana tympani.

my·rin·go·my·co·sis (mir-ing′gō-mī-kō′sis) Inflammation of the eardrum caused by a fungus.

my·rin·go·scle·ro·sis (mi-ring′gō-skler-ō′sis) Formation of dense connective tissue in the tympanic membrane, usually not associated with hearing loss.

my·rin·go·sta·pe·di·o·pex·y (mi-ring′gō-stā-pē′dē-ō-pek′sē) A technique of tympanoplasty in which the drum

M

membrane or grafted drum membrane is brought into functional connection with the stapes.

my·rin·got·o·my (mir'in-got'ŏ-mē) Paracentesis of the tympanic membrane. SYN tympanostomy, tympanotomy.

my·ris·tic ac·id (mi-ris'tik as'id) A saturated fatty acid present as an acylglycerol in milk, vegetable fats, and cod liver oil. SYN tetradecanoic acid.

my·so·phil·i·a (mī'sō-fil'ē-ă) Sexual interest in excretions.

my·so·pho·bi·a (mī'sō-fō'bē-ă) Morbid fear of dirt or defilement from touching familiar objects.

my·ta·cism (mī'tă-sizm) A form of stammering in which the letter *m* is frequently substituted for other consonants. SYN mutacism.

♻ **myx-, myxo-** Combining forms relating to mucus (e.g., myxocyte).

myx·ad·e·no·ma (miks'ad-ĕ-nō'mă) A benign neoplasm derived from glandular epithelial tissue.

myx·as·the·ni·a (miks'as-thē'nē-ă) Faulty secretion of mucus.

myx·e·de·ma (miks'ĕ-dē'mă) Hypothyroidism characterized by a relatively hard edema of subcutaneous tissue.

myx·e·de·ma·toid (miks'ĕ-dem'ă-toyd) Resembling myxedema. SYN myxoedematoid.

myx·e·dem·a·tous (miks'ĕ-dem'ă-tŭs) Relating to myxedema. SYN myxoedematous.

myx·o·chon·dro·fi·bro·sar·co·ma (miks'ō-kon'drō-fī'brō-sahr-kō'mă) A malignant neoplasm derived from fibrous connective tissue, with intimately associated foci of cartilaginous and myxomatous tissue.

myx·o·chon·dro·ma (miks'ō-kon-drō'mă) A benign neoplasm of cartilaginous tissue, where the stroma resembles relatively primitive mesenchymal tissue. SYN myxoma enchondromatosum.

myx·o·cyte (mik'sō-sīt) One of the stellate or polyhedral cells present in mucous tissue.

myxoedema [Br.] SYN myxedema.

myxoedematoid [Br.] SYN myxedematoid.

myxoedematous [Br.] SYN myxedematous.

myx·o·fi·bro·ma (mik'sō-fī-brō'mă) Benign neoplasm of fibrous connective tissue that resembles primitive mesenchymal tissue.

myx·o·fi·bro·sar·co·ma (mik'sō-fī'brō-sahr-kō'mă) A malignant fibrous histiocytoma with a predominance of myxoid areas that resemble primitive mesenchymal tissue.

myx·oid (mik'soyd) Resembling mucus.

myx·oid cyst (mik'soyd sist) SYN ganglion (2).

myx·o·li·po·ma (mik'sō-li-pō'mă) A benign neoplasm of adipose tissue in which portions of the tumor resemble mucoid mesenchymal tissue.

myx·o·ma (mik-sō'mă) A benign neoplasm derived from connective tissue.

myx·o·ma·to·sis (mik'sō-mă-tō'sis) 1. SYN mucoid degeneration. 2. Multiple myxomas.

myx·o·ma·tous (mik-sō'mă-tŭs) 1. Pertaining to or characterized by the features of a myxoma. 2. Said of tissue that resembles primitive mesenchymal tissue.

myx·o·sar·co·ma (mik'sō-sahr-kō'mă) A sarcoma, usually a liposarcoma or malignant fibrous histiocytoma, with an abundant component of myxoid tissue resembling primitive mesenchyme containing connective tissue mucin.

myx·o·vi·rus (mik'sō-vī'rŭs) Term formerly used for viruses with an affinity for mucins, now included in the families Orthomyxoviridae and Paramyxoviridae. The myxoviruses included influenza virus, parainfluenza virus, respiratory syncytial virus, measles virus, and mumps virus.

N

N$_A$ Abbreviation for Avogadro number.

Na Symbol for sodium.

na·cre·ous (nā′krē-ŭs) Lustrous, like mother-of-pearl.

na·dir (nā′dēr) The lowest value of blood counts after chemotherapy.

naevoid [Br.] SYN nevoid.

naevose [Br.] SYN nevose.

naevus [Br.] SYN nevus.

naevus cell [Br.] SYN nevus cell.

naevus comedonicus [Br.] SYN nevus comedonicus.

naevus flammeus [Br.] SYN nevus flammeus.

naevus pigmentosus [Br.] SYN nevus pigmentosus.

naevus pilosus [Br.] SYN nevus pilosus.

naevus spilus [Br.] SYN nevus spilus.

naevus unius lateris [Br.] SYN nevus unius lateris.

naevus vascularis [Br.] SYN nevus vascularis.

Nä·ge·le ob·li·qui·ty (nah′gĕ-lĕ ŏ′blik-wi-tē) Inclination of fetal head in cases of flat pelvis. SYN anterior asynclitism.

Nä·ge·le pel·vis (nah′gĕ-lĕ pel′vis) An obliquely contracted or unilateral synostotic pelvis.

Nä·ge·le rule (nah′gĕ-lĕ rūl) Determination of the estimated delivery date by adding 7 days to the first day of the last normal menstrual period, counting back 3 months, and adding 1 year.

nail (nāl) **1.** One of the thin, horny, translucent plates covering the dorsal surface of the distal end of each terminal phalanx of fingers and toes. **2.** A slender rod of metal, bone, or other solid substance, used to attach divided extremities of a broken bone surgically. SYN onyx.

nail bed (nāl bed) The area of the corium on which the nail rests. SYN keratogenous membrane (2), matrix unguis.

nail fold (nāl fōld) The fold of skin overlapping the lateral and proximal margins of the nail.

nail mat·rix (nāl mā′triks) [TA] Sensitive area of the corium on which the nail rests. SYN matrix unguis [TA], keratogenous membrane, nail bed, onychostroma.

nail pits (nāl pits) Small punctate depressions on nail plate surface due to defective nail formation.

nail wall (nāl wawl) [TA] Skin fold overlapping the lateral and proximal margins of the nail. SYN vallum unguis [TA].

Na·le·buff arth·ro·de·sis (nāl′bŭf ahr-throd′ĕ-sis) Use of a device with a Steinmann pin passing through the bone to surgically immobilize the wrist.

nal·i·dix·ic ac·id (NA) (nal′i-dik′sik as′id) Oral antibacterial agent used to treat of genitourinary tract infections.

nal·or·phine (nal-ōr′fēn) An early antagonist of most depressant and stimulatory effects of morphine and related narcotic analgesics. SYN *N*-allylnormorphine.

nal·ox·one hy·dro·chlor·ide (nal-ok′sōn hī′drŏ-klōr′īd) A synthetic congener used to treat opiate overdose and to reverse coma and respiratory depression.

nal·trex·one (NTX) (nal-treks′ōn) Orally active narcotic antagonist; devoid of pharmacologic action when administered without narcotics.

NAME syn·drome (nām sin′drōm) Concurrence of *n*evi, *a*trial myxoma, *m*yxoid neurofibromas, and *e*philides.

nano- (n) 1. Prefix meaning dwarfism (nanism). **2.** Prefix used in the SI and metric system to signify one billionth (10^{-9}).

nan·o·gram (ng) (nan′ō-gram) One billionth of a gram (10^{-9} g).

na·nom·e·ter (nm, NM) (nan′ō-mē-tĕr) One billionth of a meter (10^{-9} m).

nanometre [Br.] SYN nanometer.

nan·o·sec·ond (nan′ō-sek-ŏnd) One bil-lionth of a second.

nape (nāp) SYN nucha.

naph·tha (naf′thă) SYN petroleum ben-zin.

nar·cis·sis·tic per·son·al·i·ty dis·or·der (NPD) (nahr′si-sis′tik pĕr-sŏ-nal′i-tē dis-ŏr′dĕr) Pervasive pattern in adult-hood of self-centeredness, self-impor-tance, lack of empathy, sense of entitle-ment, and viewing others largely as ob-jects to meet one's needs, manifested in a variety of contexts.

narco- Prefix meaning stupor, narcosis.

nar·co·hyp·ni·a (nahr′kō-hip′nē-ă) A general numbness sometimes experi-enced when waking.

nar·co·hyp·no·sis (nahr′kō-hip-nō′sis) Stupor or deep sleep induced by hyp-nosis.

nar·co·lep·sy (nahr′kō-lep-sē) A sleep disorder that usually appears in young adulthood, consisting of recurring epi-sodes of sleep during the day and often disrupted nocturnal sleep. SYN Gélineau syndrome, paroxysmal sleep.

nar·co·lep·tic (nar′kō-lep′tik) **1.** A sleep-inducing drug. **2.** A person with narcolepsy.

nar·co·sis (nahr-kō′sis) General and non-specific reversible depression of neu-ronal excitability, produced by various physical and chemical agents.

nar·co·ther·a·py (nahr′kō-thār′ă-pē) Psychotherapy conducted with a sedated patient.

nar·cot·ic (nahr-kot′ik) **1.** Any drug de-rived from opioids with potent analgesic effects associated with both significant alteration of mood and behavior and potential for dependence and tolerance. **2.** Any drug, synthetic or naturally occur-ring, with effects similar to those of opium and opium derivatives.

nar·cot·ic block·ade (nahr-kot′ik blok-ād′) The use of drugs to inhibit the effects of narcotic substances, as with naloxone.

nar·cot·ic re·ver·sal (nahr-kot′ik rē-

vĕr′săl) The use of narcotic antagonists to terminate the action of narcotics.

na·ris, pl. **na·res** (nā′ris, -rēs) [TA] SYN nostril.

na·sal (nā′zăl) Relating to the nose. SYN rhinal.

na·sal cav·i·ty (nā′zăl kav′i-tē) [TA] Space on either side of the nasal septum, lined with ciliated respiratory mucosa, extending from the naris anteriorly to the choana posteriorly, and communicating with the paranasal sinuses through their orifices in the lateral wall. SYN cavitas nasi [TA], cavum nasi.

na·sal crest (nā′zăl krest) [TA] The mid-line ridge in the nasal cavity floor formed by union of the paired maxillae and pala-tine bones.

na·sal fin (nā′zăl fin) A platelike fin be-tween the lateral and medial nasal promi-nences that disappears as the nose forms.

na·sal gli·o·ma (nā′zăl glī-ō′mă) Lesion that is probably not a true neoplasm, but a teratoma consisting of glial tissue with reactive astrocytes, ganglionic neurons, and ependymal cells in small nodules at the nasal dorsum, often with intracranial connections.

na·sal pol·yp (NP) (nā′zăl pol′ip) In-flammatory or allergic polyp, arising from the ostium or cavity of one of the paranasal sinuses, which projects into the nasal cavity.

nas·cent (nā′sĕnt) **1.** Beginning; being born or produced. **2.** Denoting the state of a chemical element at the moment it is set free from one of its compounds.

na·si·on (nā′zē-on) [TA] Cranial point corresponding to the medial nasofrontal suture. SYN nasal point.

naso- Combining form meaning the nose.

na·so·al·ve·o·lar cyst (nā′zō-al-vē′ŏ-lăr sist) Soft tissue lesion located near the attachment of the ala over the max-illa. SYN Klestadt cyst, nasolabial cyst.

na·so·an·tral (nā′zō-an′trăl) Relating to the nose and the maxillary sinus.

na·so·bas·i·lar line (nā′zō-bas′i-lăr līn) SYN basinasal line.

na·so·cil·i·ar·y (nā′zō-sil′ē-ar-ē) Relating to the nose and eyelids. SEE nasociliary nerve.

na·so·fron·tal (nā′zō-frŭn′tăl) Relating to the nose and forehead, or to the nasal cavity and frontal sinuses.

na·so·fron·tal vein (nā′zō-frŭn′tăl vān) [TA] Located in the anterior medial part of the orbit that connects the superior ophthalmic vein with the angular vein.

na·so·gas·tric (nā′zō-gas′trik) Pertaining to or involving the nasal passages and the stomach, as in nasogastric intubation.

na·so·gas·tric tube (nā′zō-gas′trik tūb) A tube used for feeding or suctioning stomach contents; inserted through the nose and down the esophagus into the stomach.

na·so·la·bi·al (nā′zō-lā′bē-ăl) Relating to the nose and upper lip.

na·so·la·bi·al lymph node (nā′zō-lā′bē-ăl limf nōd) [TA] A facial lymph node located near junction of superior labial and facial arteries. SYN nodus lymphoideus nasolabialis [TA], nasolabial node.

nasolachrymal [Br.] SYN nasolacrimal.

na·so·lac·ri·mal (NL) (nā′zō-lak′ri-măl) Relating to the nasal and lacrimal bones, or to nasal cavity and lacrimal ducts.

na·so·man·dib·u·lar fix·a·tion (nā′zō-man-dib′yū-lăr fik-sā′shŭn) Mandibular immobilization, with maxillomandibular splints, especially for toothless jaws.

na·so·men·tal ref·lex (nā′zō-men′tăl rē′fleks) Contraction of the mentalis muscle after a tap on the side of the nose.

na·so·o·ral (nā′zō-ōr′ăl) Relating to the nose and mouth.

na·so·pal·a·tine (nā′zō-pal′ă-tīn) Relating to the nose and the palate.

na·so·pha·ryn·ge·al (nā′zō-fă-rin′jē-ăl) Relating to the nose or nasal cavity and the pharynx.

na·so·pha·ryn·ge·al car·ci·no·ma (nā′zō-fă-rin′jē-ăl kahr′si-nō′mă) A squamous cell lesion arising from the surface epithelium of the nasopharynx.

na·so·pha·ryn·ge·al cul·ture (nā′zō-fă-rin′jē-ăl kŭl′chŭr) Microbial culture of a specimen obtained with a swab inserted through the nose into the nasopharynx.

na·so·pha·ryn·go·la·ryn·go·scope (nā′zō-fă-ring′gō-lă-ring′gŏ-skōp) An instrument, often of fiberoptic type, used to visualize the upper airways and pharynx.

na·so·phar·ynx (nā′zō-far′ingks) [TA] Part of the pharynx that lies above the soft palate. SYN epipharynx.

na·so·si·nu·si·tis (nā′zō-sī-nŭ-sī′tis) Inflammation of the nasal cavities and of the accessory sinuses.

na·so·tra·che·al (nā′zō-trā′kē-ăl) Pertaining to the nose and the trachea. Pertaining to the nose and trachea.

na·so·tra·che·al tube (nā′zō-trā′kē-ăl tūb) A tracheal tube inserted through the nasal passages.

na·sus (nā′sŭs) 1. SYN external nose. 2. SYN nose.

na·tal (nā′tăl) 1. Relating to birth. 2. Relating to the buttocks or nates.

na·tal tooth (nā′tăl tūth) A deciduous tooth that is in the oral cavity at birth.

na·ta·my·cin (nā′tă-mī′sin) SYN pimaricin.

na·tes (nā′tēz) [TA] SYN buttocks.

na·ti·mor·tal·i·ty (nā′ti-mōr-tal′i-tē) The perinatal death rate.

Na·tion·al Black Nurs·es As·so·ci·a·tion (NBNA) (nash′ŏ-năl blak nŭr′sĕz ă-sō′sē-ā′shŭn) Professional health care organization, founded in 1971 with headquarters in Silver Spring, Maryland, which is focused on the special needs of African Americans.

Na·tion·al Cen·ter for Com·ple·men·tar·y and Al·ter·nat·ive Med·i·cine (NCCAM) (nash′ŏ-năl sen′tĕr kom′plĕ-ment′ă-rē awl-tĕr′nă-tiv med′i-sin) A federal program established to support development and research of complementary and alternative medicines for public safety.

Na·tion·al Cor·rect Cod·ing I·ni·tia·tive (NCCI) (nash´ŏ-năl kŏr-ekt´ kōd´ing in-ish´ă-tiv) Software used by health care providers and insurers in the Medicare system to prevent overpayment for procedures.

Na·tion·al Counc·il Li·cen·sure Ex·am·in·a·tion–Prac·ti·cal Nurse (NCLEX-PN) (nash´ŏ-năl kown´sil lĭ´sĕn-shŭr eg-zam´in-ā´shŭn prak´tik-ăl nŭrs) A standardized computer-administered examination taken by new applicants for state licensure; offered in all states by the National Council of State Boards of Nursing. A passing standard is set to determine the applicant's minimum competence for safe practice.

Na·tion·al Coun·cil Li·cen·sure Ex·am·i·na·tion–Reg·is·tered Nurse (NCLEX-RN) (nash´ŏ-năl kown´sil lĭ´sĕn-shŭr eg-zam´in-ā´shŭn rej´is-tĕrd nŭrs) A standardized computer administered examination that is taken by new applicants for state licensure. The test is offered in all states by the National Council of State Boards of Nursing. A passing standard is set to determine the applicant's minimum competence for safe practice.

Na·tion·al For·mu·lar·y (NF) (nash´ŏ-năl fōr´myŭ-lar-ē) An official compendium formerly issued by the American Pharmaceutical Association but now published by the United States Pharmacopeial Convention to provide standards and specifications that can be used to evaluate the quality of pharmaceuticals and therapeutic agents.

Na·tion·al In·sti·tute for Oc·cu·pa·tion·al Safe·ty and Health (NIOSH) (nash´ŏ-năl in´sti-tūt ok´yŭ-pā´shŭn-ăl sāf´tē helth) U.S. federal agency established to perform epidemiologic and laboratory research into the causes of occupational diseases and injuries and methods of preventing them.

Na·tion·al In·sti·tutes of Health (nash´ŏ-năl in´sti-tūts helth) A nonregulatory U.S. federal agency that oversees research activities funded by the Institute.

Na·tion·al League of Nurs·ing (NLN) (nash´ŏ-năl lēg nŭrs´ing) An international federation of about 120 national professional organizations; based in Geneva, Switzerland; promotes nursing educational standards.

Na·tion·al Li·brar·y of Med·i·cine (nash´ŏ-năl lī´brar-ē med´i-sin) World's largest medical library. Web site that provides access to multiple types of health care information.

Na·tion·al Pro·vi·der I·den·ti·fi·er (NPI) (nash´ŏ-năl prŏ-vī´dĕr ī-den-ti-fī´ĕr) A standard and unique identification number created by the U.S. Department of Health and Human Services for each provider of health care services, supplies, and equipment.

Na·tion·al Stu·dent Nurs·es As·so·ci·a·tion (nash´ŏ-năl stū´dĕnt nŭrs´ĕz ă-sō´sē-ā´shŭn) A nonprofit organization, founded in 1952, for students enrolled in all generic nursing programs as well as generic graduate nursing programs.

Na·tive Amer·i·can med·i·cine (nā´tiv ă-mer´i-kăn med´i-sin) Therapy based on a spiritual view of life. Methods of healing include prayer, chanting, music, smudging (burning sage or aromatic woods), herbs, laying-on of hands, massage, and other modalities.

natraemia [Br.] SYN natremia.

na·tre·mi·a, na·tri·e·mi·a (nā-trē´mē-ă, -trē-ē´mē-ă) The presence of sodium in the blood. SYN natraemia.

na·tri·u·re·sis (nā´trē-yū-rē´sis) Urinary excretion of sodium.

na·tri·u·ret·ic (nā´trē-yū-ret´ik) **1.** Pertaining to or characterized by natriuresis. **2.** A substance that increases urinary excretion of sodium, usually as a result of decreased tubular reabsorption of sodium ions from glomerular filtrate.

nat·u·ral kil·ler cells (NK) (nach´ŭr-ăl kil´ĕr selz) Large granular lymphocytes that do not express markers of either T- or B-cell lineage. These cells possess Fc receptors for IgG and can kill target cells using antibody-dependent cell-mediated cytotoxicity. SYN NK cells.

nat·u·ral se·lec·tion (nach´ŭr-ăl sĕ-lek´shŭn) Colloquially, "survival of the fittest," the principle that in nature those individuals best able to adapt to their environment will survive and reproduce, whereas those less able will die without progeny, and the genes carried by the survivors will increase in frequency.

na•tur•o•path•ic med•i•cine (nach′ŭr-ŏ-path′ik med′i-sin) A branch of health care based on recognition of the healing power of nature. It supplements conventional medical theory and practice with emphasis on understanding and treating the whole patient, avoiding potentially harmful therapies, adding education for self-care, and aiding nature to restore health and equilibrium.

na•tur•op•a•thy (nach′ŭr-op′ă-thē) Therapeutics based on natural (nonmedicinal) forces to prevent disease and restore function.

nau•se•a (naw′zē-ă) Being sick to the stomach; an inclination to vomit.

nau•se•a grav•i•da•r•um (naw′zē-ă grav-i-dā′rŭm) SYN morning sickness.

nau•se•ant (naw′zē-ănt) **1.** Nauseating; causing nausea. **2.** An agent that causes nausea.

nau•se•ate (naw′zē-āt) To cause an inclination to vomit.

nau•seous (naw′shŭs) Causing nausea.

na•vel (nā′vĕl) SYN umbilicus.

na•vic•u•la (nă-vik′yū-lă) A small boat-shaped structure.

na•vic•u•lar (nă-vik′yū-lăr) [TA] SYN scaphoid.

NCLEX-PN Abbreviation for National Council Licensure Examination–Practical Nurse.

NCLEX-RN Abbreviation for National Council Licensure Examination–Registered Nurse.

ND Abbreviation for Doctor of Naturopathic Medicine.

near point (nēr poynt) Position in conjugate focus with the retina when the eye exerts maximal accommodation. SYN punctum proximum.

near•sight•ed•ness (nēr-sīt′ĕd-nĕs) SYN myopia.

ne•ar•thro•sis, ne•o•ar•thro•sis (nē-ahr-thrō′sis, nē′ō-) A new joint (e.g., a pseudarthrosis arising in an ununited fracture, or an artificial joint resulting from a total joint replacement operation). SYN neoarthrosis.

neb•u•la, pl. **neb•u•lae** (neb′yū-lă, -lē) **1.** A translucent foglike opacity of the cornea. **2.** A spray.

neb•u•li•za•tion (neb′yū-lī-zā′shŭn) Spraying or vaporization.

neb•u•lize (neb′yū-līz) To break up a liquid into a fine spray or vapor; to vaporize.

neb•u•liz•er (neb′yū-lī-zĕr) A device used to disperse liquid medicine in a mist of extremely fine particles. SEE ALSO atomizer, vaporizer.

Ne•ca•tor (nĕ-kā′tŏr) A genus of nematode hookworms with species that include *N. americanus,* the New World hookworm; suck intestinal blood; cause abdominal discomfort, diarrhea and cramps; and hypochromic microcytic anemia. SEE ALSO *Ancylostoma.*

neck (nek) [TA] **1.** Part of body by which the head is connected to the trunk: it extends from the base of the cranium to the top of the shoulders. **2.** In anatomy, any constricted portion having a fancied resemblance to the neck of an animal. **3.** The germinative portion of an adult tapeworm that develops the segments or proglottids; the region of cestode segmentation behind the scolex. SYN cervix (1) [TA], collum.

neck•lace (nek′lăs) Term used to describe a rash that encircles the neck.

neck re•flex•es (nek rē′flek-sĕz) Head change positions cause alterations in tone of the neck muscles through stimulation of proprioceptors in the labyrinth that bring the head into its correct position in space.

ne•crec•to•my (nĕ-krek′tŏ-mē) Operative removal of any necrosed tissue.

nec•ro•bac•il•lo•sis (nek′rō-bas-il-ō′sis) Any disease associated with *Fusobacterium necrophorum.*

nec•ro•bi•o•sis (nek′rō-bī-ō′sis) Physiologic or normal death of cells or tissues due to changes associated with development or aging. SYN bionecrosis.

nec·ro·bi·o·sis li·poi·di·ca, nec·ro·bi·o·sis li·poi·di·ca di·a·be·ti·co·rum (nek′rō-bī-ō′sis li-poyd′i-kă, dī-ă-bet′i-kōr′ŭm) A condition often associated with diabetes, in which one or more yellow, atrophic lesions develop on the legs.

nec·ro·cy·to·sis (nek′rō-sī-tō′sis) Abnormal death of cells

nec·ro·gen·ic (nek′rō-jen′ik) Relating to, living in, or having origin in dead matter.

nec·ro·gen·ic wart (nek′rō-jen′ik wŏrt) SYN postmortem wart.

ne·crog·e·nous (nĕ-kroj′ĕ-nŭs) SYN necrogenic.

ne·crol·o·gy (nĕ-krol′ŏ-jē) The science of the collection, classification, and interpretation of mortality statistics.

ne·crol·y·sis (nĕ-krol′i-sis) Necrosis and loosening of tissue.

nec·ro·ma·ni·a (nek′rō-mā′nē-ă) **1.** A morbid tendency to dwell with longing on death. **2.** A morbid attraction to dead bodies.

ne·croph·a·gous (nĕ-krof′ă-gŭs) **1.** Living on carrion. **2.** SYN necrophilous.

nec·ro·phil·i·a, nec·roph·i·lism, nec·roph·i·ly (nek′rō-fil′ē-ă, nĕ-krof′i-lizm, -lē) **1.** A morbid fondness for being in the presence of dead bodies. **2.** The impulse to have sexual contact, or the act of such contact, with a dead body, usually of males with female corpses.

ne·croph·i·lous (nĕ-krof′i-lŭs) Having a preference for dead tissue; denoting certain bacteria. SYN necrophagous (2).

nec·ro·pho·bi·a (nek′rō-fō′bē-ă) Morbid fear of corpses.

nec·rop·sy, nec·ro·sco·py (nek′rop-sē, nek′rō-skop-ē) SYN autopsy.

ne·crose (nek′rōs) **1.** To cause necrosis. **2.** To become the site of necrosis.

ne·cro·sis, pl. **ne·cro·ses** (nĕ-krō′sis, -sēz) Pathologic death of one or more cells, or of a portion of tissue or organ, resulting from irreversible damage.

nec·ro·sper·mi·a (nek′rō-spĕr′mē-ă) A condition with dead or immobile sperms in semen.

nec·ro·tax·is (nek′rō-tak′sis) Movement of white blood cells toward dead or dying cells.

ne·crot·ic (nĕ-krot′ik) Pertaining to or affected by necrosis.

ne·crot·ic in·flam·ma·tion, nec·ro·tiz·ing in·flam·ma·tion (nĕ-krot′ik in′flă-mā′shŭn, nek′rō-tīz-ing) Acute inflammatory reaction in which the predominant histologic change is fairly rapid necrosis that occurs extensively in relatively large foci throughout the affected tissue.

ne·crot·ic pulp (nĕ-krot′ik pŭlp) Necrosis of the dental pulp that clinically does not respond to thermal stimulation. SYN dead pulp, nonvital pulp.

nec·ro·tiz·ing (nek′rō-tīz-ing) That which causes the death of tissues or organisms. SEE necrosis.

nec·ro·tiz·ing ar·te·ri·o·li·tis (nek′rō-tīz-ing ahr-tēr′ē-ō-lī′tis) Necrosis in the media of arterioles, characteristic of malignant hypertension. SYN arteriolonecrosis.

nec·ro·tiz·ing en·te·ro·co·li·tis (nek′rō-tīz-ing en′tĕr-ō-kō-lī′tis) Extensive ulceration and necrosis of the ileum and colon in premature infants.

nec·ro·tiz·ing ker·a·ti·tis (nek′rō-tīz-ing ker′ă-tī′tis) Severe inflammation and destruction of corneal tissue that may be seen in response to herpes infection.

nec·ro·tiz·ing si·a·lo·met·a·pla·si·a (nek′rō-tīz-ing sī′ă-lō-met-ă-plā′zē-ă) Squamous cell metaplasia of the salivary gland ducts and lobules.

nec·ro·tiz·ing ul·cer·a·tive gin·gi·vi·tis (nek′rō-tīz-ing ŭl′sĕr-ă-tiv jin′ji-vī′tis) An acute or recurrent gingivitis of young and middle-aged adults characterized clinically by gingival erythema and pain, fetid odor, and necrosis and sloughing of interdental papillae and marginal gingiva that give rise to a gray pseudo-membrane. SYN fusospirochetal gingivitis, ulceromembranous gingivitis, Vincent disease, Vincent infection.

ne·crot·o·my (ně-krot′ŏ-mē) **1.** SYN dissection. **2.** Operation for the removal of a necrotic portion of bone (sequestrum).

ne·do·cro·mil (ně-dok′rŏ-mil) A nonbronchodilator, antiinflammatory, antiasthmatic drug that acts on the mast cells to inhibit the release of histamine.

nee·dle (nē′děl) **1.** A slender, solid, usually sharp-pointed instrument used for puncturing tissues, suturing, or passing a ligature around or through a vessel. **2.** A hollow needle used for injection, aspiration, biopsy, or to guide introduction of a catheter into a vessel or other space. **3.** To perform discission of a cataract by means of a knife needle.

nee·dle bi·op·sy (nē′děl bī′op-sē) Any method in which the specimen for biopsy is removed by aspirating it through an appropriate needle or trocar that pierces the skin or the external surface of an organ. SYN aspiration biopsy.

nee·dle cri·co·thy·rot·o·my (nē′děl krī′kō-thī-rot′ŏ-mē) Cricothyrotomy performed by passing a large-bore needle percutaneously through the cricothyroid membrane into the trachea. Used as an emergency airway procedure when surgical cricothyrotomy is not possible.

nee·dle·stick (nē′děl-stik) Accidental puncture of a health care worker's skin with a contaminated needle.

need·ling (nēd′ling) Discission of a soft or secondary cataract or opening of a blocked glaucoma filtering bleb with a needle puncture.

neg·a·tive (neg′ă-tiv) **1.** Not positive. **2.** MATHEMATICS amount less than zero. **3.** PHYSICS, CHEMISTRY having an electric charge due to a gain or overabundance of electrons. **4.** MEDICINE denoting a response to a diagnostic maneuver or laboratory study that indicates the absence of the disease or condition tested for.

neg·a·tive ac·com·mo·da·tion (neg′ă-tiv ă-kom′ŏ-dā′shŭn) The decrease of accommodation that occurs when shifting from near vision to distance vision.

neg·a·tive con·ver·gence (neg′ă-tiv kŏn-věr′jěns) Slight divergence of the visual axes when convergence is at rest.

neg·a·tive feed·back (neg′ă-tiv fēd′bak) That which occurs if the sign or sense of the returned signal results in reduced amplification.

neg·a·tive pres·sure (neg′ă-tiv presh′ŭr) Pressure less than that of the ambient atmosphere.

neg·a·tive pres·sure ven·ti·la·tion (neg′ă-tiv presh′ŭr ven′ti-lā′shŭn) Mechanical respiration in which a positive transrespiratory pressure is generated by decreasing body surface pressure below the pressure at the airway opening.

neg·a·tive sco·to·ma (neg′ă-tiv skō-tō′mă) Ocular condition that is not ordinarily perceived and is detected only on examination of the visual field.

neg·a·tiv·ism (neg′ă-tiv-izm) A tendency to do the opposite of what one is requested to do; seen in catatonic states and in toddlers.

ne·glect (ně-glekt′) **1.** To disregard or ignore; to fail to perform a duty or to give due attention or care. **2.** Lack of proper attention or care.

Neil-Ro·bert·son lit·ter (nēl-rob′ěrt-sŏn lit′ěr) A backboard used for transporting patients with spinal injuries.

Neis·se·ri·a (nī-sē′rē-ă) A genus of aerobic parasitic bacteria containing gram-negative cocci that occur in pairs with the adjacent sides flattened.

Neis·se·ri·a gon·or·rhoe·ae (nī-sē′rē-ă gon-ō-rē′ē) A bacterial species that causes gonorrhea and other infections in humans. It is the type species of the genus *Neisseria*. SYN gonococcus.

Neis·se·ri·a me·nin·gi·ti·dis (nī-sēr′ē-ă men-in-jit′i-dis) A species found in the nasopharynx; the causative agent of meningococcal meningitis. SYN meningococcus.

Neis·se·ri·a sic·ca (nī-sēr′ē-ă sik′ă) Gram-negative diplococci characterized

N

by dry grayish or slimy white or yellow colonies; part of the normal flora of the human nasopharynx, saliva, and sputum.

NEJM Common abbreviation for *New England Journal of Medicine*.

nem (nem) A nutritional unit defined as 1 g breast milk of specific nutritional components having a caloric value equivalent to 2/3 calorie.

nem·a·line my·op·a·thy (nem´ă-līn mī-op´ă-thē) Congenital, nonprogressive muscle weakness most evident in the proximal muscles. SYN rod myopathy.

Nem·a·thel·min·thes (nem´ă-thel-min´thēz) Formerly considered a phylum to incorporate the pseudocelomate organisms, which now are divided into the distinct phyla Acanthocephala, Entoprocta, Rotifera, Gastrotricha, Kinorhyncha, Nematoda, and Nematomorpha.

Nem·a·to·da (nem-ă-tō´dă) The roundworms: helminths parasitic in humans. Parasitic nematodes include intestinal roundworms and filarial roundworms of the blood, lymphatic tissues, and viscera and some subcutaneous and migratory roundworms.

nem·a·toid (nem´ă-toyd) Relating to nematodes.

♻ **neo-** Prefix meaning new, recent.

ne·o·ad·ju·vant (nē´ō-ad´jū-vănt) Chemotherapy or radiation given before cancer surgery or other phase of treatment.

ne·o·an·ti·gens (nē´ō-an´ti-jenz) SYN tumor antigens.

ne·o·blad·der (nē´ō-blad´ĕr) Surgically constructed replacement for urinary bladder, usually using stomach or intestine.

ne·o·blas·tic (nē´ō-blas´tik) Developing in or characteristic of new tissue.

ne·o·cer·e·bel·lum (nē´ō-ser-ĕ-bel´ŭm) [TA] The larger lateral portion of the cerebellar hemisphere, receiving its dominant input from the pontine nuclei that, in turn, are dominated by afferent nerves from the cerebral cortex.

ne·o·cor·tex (nē´ō-kōr´teks) [TA] The newest part of the cerebral cortex, involved in higher functions such as sensory perception, generation of motor commands, conscious thought, and in humans, language; consists of gray matter surrounding the deeper white matter of the cerebrum. SYN neopallium.

ne·o·dym·i·um (Nd) (nē´ō-dim´ē-ŭm) One of the rare earth elements; atomic no. 60, atomic wt. 144.24.

ne·o·gen·e·sis (nē´ō-jen´ĕ-sis) SYN regeneration (1).

ne·o·glot·tis (nē´ō-glot´is) Surgically replacing the tongue with a structure to restore ability to speak after laryngectomy.

ne·ol·o·gism (nē-ol´ŏ-jizm) A new word or phrase of the patient's own making often seen in schizophrenia or an existing word used in a new sense.

ne·o·mem·brane (nē´ō-mem´brān) SYN false membrane.

ne·o·my·cin sul·fate (nē´ō-mī´sin sŭl´fāt) The sulfate of an antibacterial antibiotic substance produced by the growth of *Streptomyces fradiae*, active against a variety of gram-positive and gram-negative bacteria.

ne·on (Ne) (nē´on) An inert gaseous element in the atmosphere; atomic no. 10, atomic wt. 20.1797.

ne·o·na·tal (nē´ō-nā´tăl) Relating to the period immediately after birth through the first 28 days of life. SYN newborn.

ne·o·na·tal con·junc·ti·vi·tis (nē´ō-nā´tăl kŏn-jungk´ti-vī´tis) SEE ophthalmia neonatorum.

ne·o·na·tal di·ag·no·sis (nē´ō-nā´tăl dī-ăg-nō´sis) Systematic evaluation of the newborn for evidence of disease or malformations, and the conclusion reached.

ne·o·na·tal mor·tal·i·ty rate (nē´ō-nā´tăl mōr-tal´i-tē rāt) The number of deaths in the first 28 days of life divided by the number of live births occurring in the same population during the same period of time.

ne·o·na·tal pe·ri·od (nē´ō-nā´tăl pēr´ē-ŏd) The time elapsed between birth and 28 days of age. The first 24 hours of life are the most vulnerable time for the neonate because major physiologic adjustments are needed for extrauterine life.

ne·o·na·tal tet·a·ny (nē′ō-nā′tăl tet′ă-nē) Hypocalcemic tetany in neonates or young infants, due to transient functional hypoparathyroidism in consumption of cow's milk. SYN tetanism.

ne·o·nate (nē′ō-nāt) An infant aged 1 month or younger. SYN newborn.

ne·o·na·tol·o·gy (nē′ō-nā-tol′ŏ-jē) The pediatric subspecialty concerned with disorders of the neonate. SYN neonatal medicine.

ne·o·pal·li·um (nē′ō-pal′ē-ŭm) SYN isocortex.

ne·o·pla·si·a (nē′ō-plā′zē-ă) The pathologic process that results in the formation and growth of a neoplasm.

ne·o·plasm (nē′ō-plazm) An abnormal tissue that grows by cellular proliferation more rapidly than normal and continues to grow after the stimuli that initiated the new growth cease. SYN tumor (2).

ne·o·plas·tic (nē′ō-plas′tik) Pertaining to or characterized by neoplasia, or containing a neoplasm.

ne·o·prene sleeve (nē′ō-prēn′ slēv) A sheath of synthetic rubber used to provide warmth and minor support to an upper or lower limb.

ne·op·ter·in (nē-op′tĕr-in) A pteridine present in body fluids; elevated levels result from immune system activation, malignant disease, allograft rejection, and viral infections (especially as in AIDS).

Ne·o·ri·ckett·si·a (nē′ō-ri-ket′sē-ă) Bacterial genus of the proteobacter group; medically significant species within the genus include the agent that produces Potomac horse fever.

ne·o·thal·a·mus (nē′ō-thal′ă-mŭs) The portion of the thalamus projecting to the neocortex.

ne·o·vas·cu·lar·i·za·tion (nē′ō-vas′kyū-lăr-ī-zā′shŭn) Proliferation of blood vessels in tissue not normally containing them, or proliferation of blood vessels of a different kind than usual in tissue.

ne·per (Np) (nē′pĕr) A unit for comparing the magnitude of two powers, usually in electricity or acoustics. SYN napier.

neph·e·lom·e·ter (nef′ĕ-lom′ĕ-tĕr) An instrument used in nephelometry.

ne·phrec·to·my (ne-frek′tŏ-mē) Removal of a kidney.

neph·rel·co·sis (nef-rel-kō′sis) Ulceration of the mucous membrane of the pelvis or calyces of the kidney.

-nephric Suffix meaning kidneys (e.g., cardionephric).

neph·ric (nef′rik) Relating to the kidney. SYN renal.

neph·ric duct (nef′rik dŭkt) The duct of the pronephros.

ne·phrit·ic (nĕ-frit′ik) Relating to or suffering from nephritis.

ne·phrit·ic gin·gi·vi·tis (ne-frit′ik jin′ji-vi′tis) Membranous gingivitis and stomatitis associated with renal failure.

ne·phri·tis (nĕ-frī′tis) Inflammation of the kidneys.

ne·phrit·o·gen·ic (ne-fri′tō-jen′ik) Causing nephritis; said of conditions or agents.

nephro-, nephr- Combining forms meaning the kidney. SEE ALSO reno-.

neph·ro·cal·ci·no·sis (nef′rō-kal-si-nō′sis) Renal lithiasis characterized by diffusely scattered foci of calcification in the renal parenchyma.

neph·ro·cele (nef′rō-sēl) 1. Hernial displacement of a kidney. 2. In lower vertebrates, the developmental cavity connecting the myocele with the celom.

neph·ro·gen·ic cord (nef′rō-jen′ik kōrd) Longitudinal dorsolateral tract of intermediate mesoderm.

neph·ro·gen·ic di·a·bet·es in·sip·i·dus (nef′rō-jen′ik dī-ă-bē′tēz in-sip′i-dŭs) Condition due to inability of the kidney tubules to respond to antidiuretic hormone. SYN vasopressin-resistant diabetes.

N

ne·phrog·e·nous (nĕ-froj'ĕ-nŭs) Developing from kidney tissue.

neph·roid (nef'royd) Kidney-shaped; resembling a kidney. SYN reniform.

neph·ro·lith (nef'rō-lith) SYN renal calculus.

neph·ro·li·thi·a·sis (nef'rō-li-thī'ă-sis) Presence of renal calculi.

neph·ro·li·thot·o·my (nef'rō-li-thot'ŏ-mē) Incision into the kidney for the removal of a renal calculus.

ne·phrol·o·gy (nĕ-frol'ŏ-jē) Medical science concerned with diseases of the kidneys.

ne·phrol·y·sis (nĕ-frol'i-sis) **1.** Freeing of the kidney from inflammatory adhesions, with preservation of the capsule. **2.** Destruction of renal cells.

ne·phro·ma (nĕ-frō'mă) A tumor arising from renal tissue.

neph·ro·meg·a·ly (nef'rō-meg'ă-lē) Extreme hypertrophy of one or both kidneys.

neph·ron (nef'ron) A long convoluted tubular structure in the kidney, consisting of the renal corpuscle, the proximal convoluted tubule, the nephronic loop, and the distal convoluted tubule.

neph·ron loop (nef'ron lūp) The U-shaped part of the nephron, extending from the proximal to the distal convoluted tubules, consisting of descending and ascending limbs, located in the renal medulla and medullary ray. SYN Henle loop.

neph·ro·pa·ral·y·sis (nef'rō-păr-al'i-sis) Paralysis of the kidneys that causes them to stop functioning.

ne·phrop·a·thy, neph·ro·pa·thi·a (nĕ-frop'ă-thē, nef'rō-path'ē-ă) Any disease of the kidney including inflammatory and degenerative conditions. SYN nephropathia, nephrosis (1).

neph·ro·pex·y (nef'rō-pek-sē) Operative fixation of a floating or mobile kidney.

neph·rop·to·sis, neph·rop·to·si·a (nef'rop-tō'sis, -tō'sē-ă) Prolapse of the kidney.

neph·ro·py·o·sis (nef'rō-pī-ō'sis) SYN pyonephrosis.

neph·ror·rha·phy (nef-rōr'ă-fē) Nephropexy by suturing the kidney.

neph·ro·scle·ro·sis (nef'rō-skle-rō'sis) Induration of the kidney from overgrowth and contraction of the interstitial connective tissue.

neph·ro·scope (nef'rō-skōp) An endoscope passed into the renal pelvis to view it. Route of access may be percutaneous or retrograde through the ureter.

ne·phro·sis (nef'rō'sis) **1.** SYN nephropathy. **2.** Degeneration of renal tubular epithelium.

ne·phros·to·ma, neph·ro·stome (nef'fros'tō-mă, nef'rō-stōm) One of the ciliated funnel-shaped openings by which pronephric and some primordial mesonephric tubules communicate with the celom.

ne·phros·to·my (nef'ros'tŏ-mē) Establishment of an opening in the pelvis of the kidney through its cortex to the exterior of the body.

ne·phros·to·my tube (nef'ros'tŏ-mē tūb) A tube placed in the renal collecting system for drainage, diagnostic tests, or removal of calculi.

neph·rot·ic (nef-rot'ik) Relating to, caused by, or similar to nephrosis.

neph·ro·to·mo·gram (nef-rō-tō'mŏ-gram) A tomographic examination of the kidneys after intravenous administration of water-soluble iodinated contrast material.

ne·phrot·o·my (ne-frot'ŏ-mē) Incision into the kidney.

neph·ro·tox·ic (nef'rō-tok'sik) Pertaining to nephrotoxin; toxic to renal cells.

neph·ro·tox·ic·i·ty (nef'rō-tok-sis'i-tē) The quality or state of being toxic to kidney cells.

neph·ro·u·re·ter·ec·to·my (nef'rō-yūr-ē'tĕr-ek'tŏ-mē) Surgical removal of a kidney and its ureter. SYN ureteronephrectomy.

nerve (nĕrv) [TA] A whitish cordlike structure composed of one or more bundles (fascicles) of myelinated or unmyelinated nerve fibers, or more often mixtures of both, coursing outside of the central nervous system. SYN nervus [TA].

nerve block (nĕrv blok) Interruption of conduction of impulses in peripheral nerves or nerve trunks by injection of local anesthetic solution.

nerve cell (nĕrv sel) SEE neuron.

nerve deaf·ness, neu·ral deaf·ness (ND) (nĕrv def'nĕs, nūr'ăl) Older terms for sensorineural hearing loss.

nerve de·com·pres·sion (nĕrv dē'kŏm-presh'ŭn) Release of pressure on a nerve trunk by the surgical excision of constricting bands or widening of a bony canal.

nerve fi·ber (nĕrv fī'bĕr) Axon of a nerve cell, ensheathed by oligodendroglial cells in brain and spinal cord and by Schwann cells in peripheral nerves.

nerve graft (nĕrv graft) A nerve, or part of a nerve transplanted elsewhere in the body.

nerve plex·us (nĕrv pleks'ŭs) [TA] A plexus formed by the interlacing of nerves with numerous communicating branches.

ner·vi·mo·tor, neu·ri·mo·tor (nĕr'vi-mō'tŏr, nūr'i-) Relating to a motor nerve. SYN neurimotor.

ner·vine (nĕr-vēn') A natural substance, such as an herb, which is calming to the nervous system.

ner·von·ic ac·id (nĕr-von'ik as'id) A 24-carbon straight-chain fatty acid unsaturated between C-15 and C-16.

ner·vous (nĕrv) (nĕr'vŭs) **1.** Relating to a nerve or the nerves. **2.** Easily excited or agitated; suffering from mental or emotional instability; tense or anxious.

ner·vous dys·pep·sia (nĕr'vŭs dis-pep'sē-ă) Indigestion caused by emotional

upset or stress. SYN functional dyspepsia.

ner·vous sys·tem (nĕr'vŭs sis'tĕm) [TA] The entire neural apparatus, composed of a central part, the brain and spinal cord, and a peripheral part, the cranial and spinal nerves, autonomic ganglia, and plexuses.

ner·vous tis·sue (nĕr'vŭs tish'ū) Highly differentiated tissue composed of nerve cells, nerve fibers, dendrites, and supporting tissue.

ner·vus, gen. and pl. **ner·vi** (nĕr'vŭs, -vī) [TA] SYN nerve.

ne·sid·i·ec·to·my (nē-sid'ē-ek'tŏ-mē) Excision of islet tissue of the pancreas.

ne·sid·i·o·blast (nē-sid'ē-ō-blast) A pancreatic islet-forming cell.

nest (nest) A group or collection of similar objects. SEE ALSO nidus.

nest·ed pol·y·mer·ase chain re·ac·tion (PCR) (nest'ĕd pŏ-lim'ĕr-ās chān rē-ak'shŭn) Use of serial PCR in series, so that a specified piece of deoxyribonucleic acid (DNA) is amplified, and then a portion contained within the first piece is amplified further; used where extremely low amounts of DNA are present.

net·tle rash (net'ĕl rash) Red itchy swelling of skin contacted by a stinging nettle plant.

net·work (net'wŏrk) **1.** A structure bearing a resemblance to a woven fabric. A network of nerve fibers or small vessels. SYN rete (1) [TA], net. **2.** The people in a patient's environment, especially as significant for the course of the illness. SEE ALSO reticulum.

net·work mod·el HMO (net'wŏrk mod'ĕl) Arrangement by which an HMO contracts with group practice physicians to be providers for HMO subscribers, with the physicians retaining the option to see other patients.

neur-, neuri-, neuro- Combining forms meaning nerve, nerve tissue, the nervous system.

neu·ral (nūr'ăl) **1.** Relating to any structure composed of nerve cells or their processes. **2.** Referring to the dorsal side of the vertebral bodies or their precursors, where the spinal cord is located, as opposed to hemal (2).

neu·ral canal (nūr′ăl kă-nal′) The ependyma-lined lumen (cavity) of the neural tube, the cerebral part of which remains patent to form the ventricles of the brain, while the spinal part forms the central canal of the spinal cord, which in the adult is often reduced to a solid strand of modified ependyma. SYN syringocele (1).

neu·ral crest (nūr′ăl krest) A band of neuroectodermal cells along either side of the line of closure of the embryonic neural groove.

neu·ral·gi·a (nūr-al′jē-ă) Pain of a severe, throbbing, or stabbing character in the course or distribution of a nerve.

neu·ral·gic a·my·o·tro·phy (nūr-al′jik ā′mī-ot′rŏ-fē) A neurologic disorder of unknown cause, characterized by the sudden onset of severe pain, usually about the shoulder and often beginning at night, soon followed by weakness and wasting of various forequarter muscles, particularly shoulder girdle muscles. SYN shoulder-girdle syndrome.

neu·ral spine (nūr′ăl spīn) The middle point of the neural arch of the typical vertebra, represented by the spinous process.

neu·ral tube de·fect (nūr′ăl tūb dē′fekt) A birth defect that may be caused by a deficiency of folate early in pregnancy, characterized by incomplete midline fusion of the embryonic central nervous system.

neu·ran·a·gen·e·sis (nūr′an-ă-jen′ĕ-sis) Regeneration of a nerve.

neu·ra·prax·i·a (nūr′ă-prak′sē-ă) *Avoid the misspelling/mispronunciation neuropraxia. Avoid the jargonistic use of 'this word in the general sense of nerve lesion.'* Mildest type of focal nerve lesion that produces clinical deficits; localized loss of conduction along a nerve without axon degeneration.

neu·ras·then·ic (nūr′as-then′ik) Relating to, or suffering from, neurasthenia.

neu·rec·to·my, neu·ro·ec·to·my (nūr-

ek′tŏ-mē, nūr′ō-) Excision of a segment of a nerve.

neu·rec·to·pi·a, neur·ec·to·py (nūr′ek-tō′pē-ă, nūr-ek′tŏ-pē) A condition in which a nerve follows an anomalous course.

neu·ren·ter·ic ca·nal (nūr′en-ter′ik kă-nal′) Transitory communication between the neural tube, notochordal canal, and gut endoderm in vertebrate embryos.

neu·rer·gic (nūr-ĕr′jik) Relating to the activity of a nerve.

neu·ri·lem·ma (nūr′i-lem′ă) A cell that enfolds one or more axons of the peripheral nervous system; in myelinated fibers its plasma membrane forms the lamellae of myelin.

neu·ri·lem·mo·ma, neu·ro·lem·mo·ma (nūr′i-lē-mō′mă, nūr′ō-) *Despite etymologic arguments in favor of the alternative spellings neurilenoma and neurolemmoma, by far the most usual spelling is neurilemmoma.* SYN schwannoma.

neu·ri·tis, pl. **neu·ri·ti·des** (nūr-ī′tis, -it′i-dēz) **1.** Inflammation of a nerve. **2.** SYN neuropathy.

neu·ro·an·as·to·mo·sis (nūr′ō-ă-nas′tŏ-mō′sis) Surgical formation of a junction between nerves.

neu·ro·a·nat·o·my (nūr′ō-ă-nat′ŏ-mē) The anatomy of the nervous system, usually specific to the central nervous system.

neu·ro·ar·throp·a·thy (nūr′ō-ahr-throp′ă-thē) A joint disorder caused by loss of joint sensation.

neu·ro·as·tro·cy·to·ma (nūr′ō-as′trō-sī-tō′mă) A glioma found in the ventricle and temporal lobes of the brain.

neu·ro·be·ha·vior·al (nūr′ō-bē-hāv′yŏr-ăl) Activity based on neural stimuli or disorders.

neu·ro·bi·ol·o·gy (nū′rō-bī-ol′ŏ-jē) The biology of the nervous system.

neu·ro·blast (NB) (nūr′ō-blast) An embryonic nerve cell.

neu·ro·blas·to·ma (nūr′ō-blas-tō′mă) A

malignant neoplasm characterized by immature nerve cells of embryonic type (e.g., neuroblasts).

neu·ro·car·di·ac (nūr′ō-kahr′dē-ak) **1.** Relating to the nerve supply of the heart. **2.** Relating to a cardiac neurosis.

neu·ro·cen·tral joint (nūr′ō-sen′trăl joynt) SYN neurocentral synchondrosis.

neu·ro·chem·is·try (nūr′ō-kem′is-trē) The science concerned with the chemical aspects of nervous system structure and function.

neu·ro·cho·ri·o·ret·i·ni·tis (nūr′ō-kōr′ ē-ō-ret′in-ī′tis) Inflammation of the choroid, the retina, and the optic nerve.

neu·ro·cho·roi·di·tis (nūr′ō-kōr′oyd-ī′ tis) Inflammation of the choroid and the optic nerve.

neu·ro·cir·cu·la·to·ry (nūr′ō-sĭr′kyū-lă-tōr-ē) Pertaining to neural and circulatory functions.

neu·ro·coele (nūr′ō-sēl) The central tunnels of the spinal cord and brain. One or more cavities containing the brain and spinal cord.

neu·ro·cra·ni·um (nūr′ō-krā′nē-ŭm) [TA] Cranial bones enclosing the brain, as distinguished from the bones of the face. SYN brain box, braincase.

neu·ro·cris·top·a·thy (nūr′ō-kris-top′ă-thē) Congenital anomaly due to abnormal neural crest development.

neu·ro·cu·ta·ne·ous mel·a·no·sis (nūr′ō-kyū-tā′nē-ŭs mel′ă-nō′sis) Cutaneous giant pigmented nevi associated with melanosis of the leptomeninges.

neu·ro·cy·tol·y·sin (nūr′ō-sī-tol′i-sin) A toxic substance in the venom of some snakes (e.g., cobras, coral snakes) that causes the lysis of nerve cells.

neu·ro·cy·to·ma (nūr′ō-sī-tō′mă) Tumor of neuronal differentiation, usually intraventricular, consisting of sheets of cells with uniform nuclei and occasional perivascular pseudorosette formation.

neu·ro·ef·fec·tor (nūr′ō-e-fek′tŏr) Pertaining to neural and effector organ tissue, as in neuroeffector junction.

neu·ro·en·ceph·a·lo·my·e·lop·a·thy (nūr′ō-en-sef′ă-lō-mī-ĕ-lop′ă-thē) Disease of the brain, spinal cord, and nerves.

neu·ro·en·do·crin·ol·o·gy (nūr′ō-en′dō-krin-ol′ŏ-jē) The specialty concerned with the anatomic and functional relationships between the nervous system and the endocrine apparatus.

neu·ro·ep·i·the·li·um, neu·rep·i·the·li·um (nūr′ō-ep-i-thē′lē-ŭm, nūr′ep-) Epithelial cells specialized for the reception of external stimuli.

neu·ro·fi·bril (nūr′ō-fī′bril) A filamentous structure seen with the light microscope in the body, dendrites, axons, and sometimes synaptic endings of a nerve cell.

neu·ro·fi·bro·ma (nūr′ō-fī-brō′mă) A benign, encapsulated tumor resulting from proliferation of Schwann cells. SYN fibroneuroma.

neu·ro·fi·bro·ma·to·sis (nūr′ō-fī-brō-mă-tō′sis) Two distinct major hereditary disorders: **Type 1 (peripheral) neurofibromatosis**, by far the more common, is characterized by café-au-lait spots and both cutaneous and subcutaneous tumors. If a hamartoma is found in the iris of affected patients, the disease is called. **Type 2 (central) neurofibromatosis** has few cutaneous manifestations, and consists primarily of acoustic neuromas that can cause deafness, often accompanied by other intracranial/paraspinal neoplasms. SYN elephant man disease (2).

neu·ro·fil·a·ment (nūr′ō-fil′ă-mĕnt) A class of intermediate filaments found in neurons.

neu·ro·gen·e·sis (nūr′ō-jen′ĕ-sis) Formation of the nervous system or formation of neurons within the adult brain.

neu·ro·gen·ic, neu·ro·ge·net·ic, neu·ro·ge·nous (nūr′ō-jen′ik, -jĕ-net′ik, nūr-oj′ĕ-nŭs) **1.** Originating in, starting from, or caused by, the nervous system or nerve impulses. SYN neurogenous. **2.** Relating to neurogenesis.

neu·ro·gen·ic blad·der (nūr′ō-jen′ik blad′ĕr) SYN neuropathic bladder.

neu·ro·gen·ic clau·di·ca·tion (nūr′ō-jen′ik klaw′di-kā′shŭn) Claudication with neurologic injury, usually in association with lumbar spinal stenosis.

neu·rog·e·nous (nūr-oj′ĕ-nŭs) SYN neurogenic (1).

neu·rog·li·a, neu·rog·li·a cells (nūr-og′lē-ă, sĕlz) [TA] Nonneuronal cellular elements of the central and peripheral nervous systems: oligodendroglia cells, astrocytes, ependymal cells, and microglia cells. SYN glia, reticulum (2).

neu·ro·gli·o·ma (nūr′ō-glī-ō′mă) General term for a tumor of the neuroglia (q.v.).

neu·ro·gli·o·sis (nūr′ō-glī-ō′sis) SYN gliomatosis.

neu·ro·gly·co·pe·ni·a (nū′rō-glī-kō-pē′nē-ă) Neurologic sequelae of low serum glucose levels, including seizures and coma.

neu·rog·ra·phy (nū-rog′ră-fē) A method of depicting the state of a peripheral nerve (e.g., electrical recording).

neu·ro·his·tol·o·gy (nūr′ō-his-tol′ŏ-jē) The microscopic anatomy of the nervous system. SYN histoneurology.

neu·ro·hor·mone (nūr′ō-hōr′mōn) A hormone (e.g., norepinephrine) formed by neurosecretory cells and liberated by nerve impulses.

neu·ro·hy·po·phys·i·al hor·mones (nūr′ō-hī-pō-fiz′ē-ăl hōr′mōnz) Those produced in the hypothalamus; e.g., oxytocin, vasopressin.

neu·ro·hy·poph·y·sis (nūr′ō-hī-pof′i-sis) [TA] A neuroendocrine structure suspended from the base of the hypothalamus. SEE ALSO hypophysis. SYN lobus posterior hypophyseos [TA], posterior lobe of hypophysis.

neu·ro·ker·a·tin (nū′rō-ker′ă-tin) 1. The proteinaceous network that remains of the myelin sheath of axons after fixation and the removal of the fatty material. 2. The insoluble protein matter of brain remaining after extraction with solvents after proteolytic digestion; it is unrelated to the keratins. SYN neurochitin.

neu·ro·lept·an·al·ge·si·a (nūr′ō-lept-an-ăl-jē′zē-ă) An intense analgesic and amnesic state produced by administration of narcotic analgesics and neuroleptic drugs.

neu·ro·lep·tic (nūr′ō-lep′tik) 1. Denotes class of psychotropic drugs used to treast psychosis, particularly schizophrenia. 2. Denoting a condition similar to that produced by such an agent. SEE ALSO antipsychotic agent.

neu·ro·log·ic (nūr′ō-loj′ik) Pertaining to the nervous system or to the study of the nervous system.

neu·ro·log·ic as·ses·sment (nūr′ō-loj′ik ă-ses′mĕnt) The appraisal of the nervous system by a health care provider.

neu·ro·log·ic sta·tus (nūr′ō-loj′ik stat′ŭs) Assessment of overall condition of nervous system function.

neu·rol·o·gist (nūr-ol′ŏ-jist) A specialist in the diagnosis and treatment of disorders of the neuromuscular system: the central, peripheral, and autonomic nervous systems, the neuromuscular junction, and muscle.

neu·rol·o·gy (nūr-ol′ŏ-jē) Branch of medical science concerned with the various nervous systems.

neu·rol·y·sin (nūr-ol′i-sin) Antibody that destroys ganglion and cortical cells. SYN neurotoxin (1).

neu·rol·y·sis (nūr-ol′i-sis) 1. Destruction of nerve tissue. 2. Freeing of a nerve from inflammatory adhesions.

neu·ro·ma, neu·ri·no·ma, pl. **neu· ro·ma·ta,** pl. **neu·ro·mas** (nūr-ō′mă, nūr′i-nō-mă, -tă, -rō′măz) General term for any neoplasm derived from cells of the nervous system.

neu·ro·ma cu·tis (nūr-ō′mă kyū′tis) Dermal neurofibroma.

neu·ro·ma·la·ci·a (nūr′ō-mă-lā′shē-ă) Pathologic softening of nervous tissue.

neu·ro·ma tel·an·gi·ec·to·des (nūr-ō′mă tel-an′jē-ek-tō′dēz) A neurofibroma with a conspicuous number of blood vessels, some of which have unusually large lumens.

neu·ro·ma·to·sis (nūr'ō-mă-tō'sis) The presence of multiple neuromas, as in neurofibromatosis.

neu·ro·mere (nūr'ō-mēr) Elevations in the wall of the developing neural tube that divide the developing spinal cord into portions to which the dorsal and ventral roots are attached. SYN encephalomere, neural segment, neurotome (2).

neu·ro·mi·met·ic (nū'rō-mi-met'ik) Relating to drug action that mimics response of an effector organ to nerve impulses.

neu·ro·mod·u·lat·ion (nūr'ō-mod-yū-lā'shŭn) Therapeutic alteration of activity in the central, peripheral, or autonomic nervous systems with implanted devices.

neu·ro·mo·tor (nūr'ō-mō'tŏr) Pertaining to the muscular and nervous systems and the impulses between them.

neu·ro·mus·cu·lar (nūr'ō-mŭs'kyū-lăr) Referring to the relationship between nerves and muscles. SEE ALSO myoneural.

neu·ro·mus·cu·lar block·ade (nūr'ō-mŭs'kyū-lăr blok-ād') The blockage of transmission through the myoneural junction at nicotinic receptors, decreasing skeletal muscle tone and resulting in muscle weakness and/or paralysis.

neu·ro·my·e·li·tis (nūr'ō-mī-ĕ-lī'tis) Neuritis combined with spinal cord inflammation. SYN myeloneuritis.

neu·ro·my·op·a·thy (nūr'ō-mī-op'ă-thē) 1. A disorder of muscle due to impairment of its nerve supply. 2. Simultaneous disorders of nerve and muscles.

neu·ro·my·o·to·ni·a (nūr'ō-mī'ō-tō'nē-ă) Spasm or contraction of muscle due to neural stimulation.

neu·ro·ne·vus (nūr'ō-nē'vŭs) A variety of intradermal nevus in adults in which nests of atrophic nevus cells in the lower dermis are hyalinized and resemble nerve bundles.

neu·ron·i·tis (nūr'ō-nī'tis) Inflammatory disorder of the neuron.

neu·ro·nop·a·thy (nūr'ō-nop'ă-thē) Disorder, often toxic, of the neuron (1).

neu·ro·oph·thal·mol·o·gy (nūr'ō-of'thăl-mol'ŏ-jē) Study of the nerves of the eyes and vision.

neu·ro·o·tol·o·gy (nūr'ō-ō-tol'ŏ-jē) The branch of medicine concerned with the nervous system related to the auditory and vestibular systems.

neu·ro·par·a·lyt·ic (nūr'ō-par-ă-lit'ik) Denoting or characterized by neuroparalysis.

neu·ro·path·ic (nūr'ō-path'ik) Relating in any way to neuropathy.

neu·ro·path·ic blad·der (nūr'ō-path'ik blad'ĕr) Any defective functioning of bladder due to impaired innervation. SYN neurogenic bladder.

neu·ro·path·ic joint (nūr'ō-path'ik joynt) Destructive joint disease caused by diminished proprioceptive sensation, with gradual destruction of the joint by repeated subliminal injury, commonly associated with tabes dorsalis, diabetic neuropathy, or syringomyelia.

neu·ro·path·ic pain (nūr'ō-path'ik pān) Pain that results from neurologic disease.

neu·ro·path·o·ge·ni·ci·ty (nūr'ō-path'ō-jĕ-nis'i-tē) Process of eliciting pathologic changes in nerve tissue.

neu·ro·pa·thol·o·gy (nūr'ō-pă-thol'ŏ-jē) 1. Pathology of the nervous system. 2. That branch of pathology concerned with the nervous system.

neu·rop·a·thy (nūr'ŏp'ă-thē) 1. Any disorder affecting the nervous system. 2. Disease involving the cranial nerves, or the peripheral or autonomic nervous systems. SYN neuritis (2), neuropathia.

neu·ro·pep·tide (nūr'ō-pep'tīd) Any of a variety of peptides found in neural tissue.

neu·ro·phar·ma·col·o·gy (nūr'ō-fahr'mă-kol'ŏ-jē) The study of drugs that affect neuronal tissue.

neu·ro·phys·i·ol·o·gy (nūr'ō-fiz-ē-ol'ŏ-jē) Physiology of the nervous system.

neu·ro·pil, neu·ro·pile (nūr'ō-pil, -pīl) The complex, feltlike net of axonal, den-

N

dritic, and glial arborizations that forms most of the gray matter of the central nervous system, in which the nerve cell bodies lie embedded.

neu·ro·plasm (nūr´ō-plazm) The protoplasm of a nerve cell.

neu·ro·plas·ty (nūr´ō-plas-tē) Surgical repair of the nerves.

neu·ro·ple·gi·a (nūr´ō-plē´jē-ă) Condition of paralysis that originates from disorders of the nervous system.

neu·ro·ple·gic (nūr´ō-plē´jik) Pertaining to paralysis due to nervous system disease.

neu·ro·po·di·a (nūr´ō-pō´dē-ă) SYN axon terminals.

neu·ro·pore (nūr´ō-pōr) An opening in the embryo leading from the neural canal of the neural tube to the exterior of the tube.

neu·ro·psy·chi·a·trist (nūr´ō-sī-kī´ă-trist) A doctor who treats neurologic and psychiatric conditions.

neu·ro·psy·chi·a·try (NP) (nūr´ō-sī-kī´ă-trē) Medical specialty dealing with both organic and psychic disorders of the nervous system.

neu·ro·psy·chol·o·gy (nū´rō-sī-kol´ō-jē) A specialty of psychology concerned with the study of the relationships between the brain and behavior.

neu·ro·psy·chop·a·thy (nūr´ō-sī-kop´ă-thē) An emotional illness of neurologic and/or functional origin.

neu·ro·ra·di·og·ra·phy (nūr´ō-rā´dē-og´ră-fē) The use of radiologic images to study the nervous system.

neu·ro·ra·di·ol·o·gy (nūr´rō-rā-dē-ol´ō-jē) The clinical subspecialty concerned with the diagnostic radiology of diseases of the central nervous system, head, and neck.

neu·ro·reg·u·la·tor (nūr´ō-reg´yū-lā-tŏr) A chemical factor that exerts a modulatory effect on a neuron.

neu·ro·ret·i·ni·tis (nūr´ō-ret-i-nī´tis) Inflammation affecting the optic nerve head and the posterior pole of the retina, with cells in the nearby vitreous. SYN papilloretinitis.

neu·ro·ret·i·nop·a·thy (nūr´ō-ret´i-nop´ă-thē) Study of the retina and nervous system.

neu·ror·rha·phy (nūr-ōr´ă-fē) Joining together, usually by suture, of the two parts of a divided nerve. SYN neurosuture.

neu·ro·sar·co·clei·sis (nūr´ō-sahr-kō-klī´sis) Operation to relieve neuralgia, consisting of resection of one of the walls of an osseous canal traversed by the nerve and transposition of the nerve into the soft tissues.

neu·ro·sar·co·ma (nū´rō-sahr´kō´mă) Sarcoma with neuromatous elements; includes neurofibrosarcoma, neurogenic sarcoma, and malignant schwannoma.

neu·ro·sci·ence (nūr´ō-sī´ĕns) The scientific discipline concerned with the development, structure, function, chemistry, pharmacology, clinical assessments, and pathology of the nervous system.

neu·ro·se·cre·tion (nūr´ō-sē-krē´shŭn) Release of a secretory substance from the axon terminals of certain nerve cells in the brain into the circulating blood.

neu·ro·sis, pl. **neu·ro·ses** (nūr-ō´sis, -sēz) **1.** A psychological or behavioral disorder in which anxiety is the primary characteristic. **2.** A functional nervous disease, or one for which there is no evident lesion. **3.** A peculiar state of tension or irritability of the nervous system. SYN neurotic disorder, psychoneurosis.

neu·ro·skel·e·ton (nūr´ō-skel´ĕ-tŏn) Those parts of the skeleton that protect the brain and spinal cord.

neu·ro·spasm (nūr´o-spazm) Sudden contraction of a muscle due to a muscular motorneuron disorder.

neu·ro·sur·geon (nūr´ō-sŭr´jŭn) A surgeon specializing in operations on the nervous system.

neu·ro·su·ture (nūr´ō-sū´chūr) SYN neurorrhaphy.

neu·ro·syph·i·lis (nūr′ō-sif′i-lis) Infection of the central nervous system by *Treponema pallidum*.

neu·ro·ten·di·nous (nūr′ō-ten′di-nŭs) Relating to both nerves and tendons.

neu·ro·the·ke·o·ma (nūr′ō-thē′kē-ō′mă) A benign myxoma of cutaneous nerve sheath origin.

neu·rot·ic (nūr-ot′ik) Relating to or suffering from a neurosis. SEE neurosis.

neu·rot·ic dis·or·der (nūr-ot′ik dis-ōr′dĕr) SYN neurosis.

neu·rot·i·za·tion (nūr′ō-tī-zā′shŭn) The acquisition of nervous substance; the regeneration of a nerve.

neu·rot·me·sis (nūr′ot-mē′sis) Axon loss lesion due to focal peripheral nerve injury in which, at the lesion site, the nerve stroma is damaged to varying degrees, as well as the axon and myelin, which degenerate from that point distally. SEE neurapraxia.

neu·ro·tome (nū′rō-tōm) 1. A very slender knife or needle, used for teasing apart nerve fibers in microdissection. 2. SYN neuromere.

neu·rot·o·my (nūr-ot′ŏ-mē) Operative division of a nerve.

neu·ro·ton·ic (nūr′ō-ton′ik) 1. Strengthening or stimulating impaired nervous action. 2. An agent that improves the tone or force of the nervous system.

neu·rot·o·ny (nū-rot′ŏ-nē) Stretching of a nerve to help palliate pain.

neu·ro·tox·i·ci·ty (nūr′ō-tok-sis′i-tē) Process of poisoning or damaging nervous tissue.

neu·ro·tox·in (nūr′ō-tok′sin) 1. SYN neurolysin. 2. Any toxin that acts specifically on nervous tissue.

neu·ro·trans·mit·ter (nūr′ō-trans′mit-ĕr) Any specific chemical agent released by a presynaptic cell, on excitation, which crosses the synapse to stimulate or inhibit the postsynaptic cell.

neu·ro·trau·ma (nū′rō-traw′mă) 1. Trauma of the nervous system. 2. Trauma to a nerve. SYN neurotrosis.

neu·ro·troph·ic ker·a·ti·tis (nūr′ō-trō′fik ker′ă-tī′tis) Inflammation or decreased corneal sensation of the cornea after corneal anesthesia.

neu·ro·trop·ic vi·rus (nūr′ō-trō′pik vī′rŭs) One with an affinity for nervous tissue.

neu·rot·ro·py, neu·rot·ro·pism (nū-rot′rŏ-pē, -pizm) 1. Affinity of basic dyes for nervous tissue. 2. Attraction of certain pathogenic microorganisms, poisons, and nutritive substances toward the nerve centers.

neu·ro·tro·sis (nū′rō-trō′sis) Trauma or wounding of a nerve.

neu·ro·tu·bule (nūr′ō-tūb′yūl) A microtubule occurring in the cell body, dendrites, axon, and synaptic endings of neurons.

neu·ro·vac·cine (nūr′ō-vak-sēn′) A fixed or standardized vaccine virus of definite strength, obtained by continued passage through the brains of rabbits.

neu·ro·vas·cu·lar (nūr′ō-vas′kyū-lăr) Relating to both nervous and vascular systems; relating to the vasomotor nerves that supply the walls of the blood vessels.

neu·ro·vi·rus (nūr′ō-vī′rŭs) Vaccine virus modified by means of passage into and growth in nervous tissue.

neu·ro·vis·cer·al (nūr′ō-vis′ĕr-ăl) Referring to the innervation of the internal organs by the autonomic nervous system.

neu·ter (nū′tĕr) To sterilize a male or female animal surgically.

neu·tral (neut) (nū′trăl) 1. Exhibiting no positive properties; indifferent. 2. CHEMISTRY neither acid nor alkaline, e.g., $[OH^-] = [H^+]$. 3. Having the same number of positive and negative charges.

neu·tral fat (nū′trăl fat) Triester of fatty acids and glycerol (i.e., triacylglycerol).

neu·tral·i·za·tion (nū′trăl-ī-zā′shŭn)

1. The change in reaction of a solution from acid or alkaline to neutral by the addition of a just sufficient amount of an alkaline or of an acid substance, respectively. **2.** The rendering ineffective of any action, process, or potential.

neu·tral·i·za·tion plate (nū′trăl-ī-zā′shŭn plāt) A metal plate used for the internal fixation of a long bone fracture to neutralize the forces producing displacement.

neu·tral mu·ta·tion (nū′trăl myū-tā′shŭn) A mutation with a negligible impact on genetic fitness.

neu·tral oc·clu·sion (nū′trăl ŏ-klū′zhŭn) **1.** An arrangement of teeth such that the maxillary and mandibular first permanent molars are in normal anteroposterior relation. SYN normal occlusion (2). **2.** SYN neutroclusion.

neu·tro·clu·sion (nū′trō-klū′zhŭn) Malocclusion with a normal anteroposterior relationship between the maxilla and mandible. SYN neutral occlusion (2).

neu·tron (nū′tron) An electrically neutral particle in the nuclei of all atoms (except hydrogen-1) with a mass slightly larger than that of a proton.

neu·tro·pe·ni·a (nū′trō-pē′nē-ă) Abnormally small numbers of neutrophils in the circulating blood. SYN neutrophilic leukopenia, neutrophilopenia.

neu·tro·phil, neu·tro·phile (nū′trō-fil, -fīl) **1.** A mature white blood cell in the granulocytic series, formed by bone marrow and released into the circulating blood, where neutrophils normally represent from 54 to 65% of the total number of leukocytes in a differential. SEE ALSO leukocyte, leukocytosis. **2.** Any cell or tissue that manifests no special affinity for acid or basic dyes.

neu·tro·phil·i·a (nū′trō-fil′ē-ă) An increase of neutrophilic leukocytes in blood or tissues. SYN neutrophilic leukocytosis.

neu·tro·phil·ic (nū′trō-fil′ik) **1.** Pertaining to or characterized by neutrophils. **2.** Characterized by a lack of affinity for acid or basic dyes. SYN neutrophilous.

neu·tro·phil·ic leu·ko·cyte (nū′trō-fil′ik lū′kō-sīt) A neutrophilic granulocyte, the most frequent of the polymorphonuclear leukocytes, and also the most active phagocyte among the various types of white blood cells.

neu·tro·phil·ic leu·ko·cy·to·sis (nū′trō-fil′ik lū′kō-sī-tō′sis) SYN neutrophilia.

neu·tro·tax·is (nū′trō-tak′sis) A phenomenon in which neutrophilic leukocytes are stimulated by a substance in such a manner that they are either attracted and move toward it or they are repelled and move away from it.

ne·vo·cyte (nē′vō-sīt) SYN nevus cell.

ne·void (nē′voyd) Resembling a nevus. SYN naevoid, nevose (2), nevous.

ne·vose, ne·vous (nē′vōs, -vŭs) **1.** Marked with nevi. **2.** SYN nevoid. SYN naevose.

ne·vus, gen. and pl. **ne·vi** (nē′vŭs, -vī) **1.** A circumscribed malformation of the skin, especially one colored by hyperpigmentation or increased vascularity. **2.** A benign localized overgrowth of melanin-forming cells of the skin at birth or appearing early in life. SYN mole (1). SYN naevus.

ne·vus cell (nē′vŭs sel) The cell of a pigmented cutaneous nevus that differs from a normal melanocyte in that it lacks dendrites. SYN naevus cell.

ne·vus co·me·do·n·i·cus, com·e·do ne·vus (nē′vŭs kom′ĕ-dō-nik′ŭs, kom′ĕ-dō) Congenital or childhood linear keratinous cystic invaginations of the epidermis, with failure of development of normal pilosebaceous follicles. SYN naevus comedonicus.

ne·vus flam·me·us, flame ne·vus (nē′vŭs flam′ē-ŭs, flām) A large purplish congenital vascular nevus; usually found on the head and neck that persists throughout life. SYN naevus flammeus, port-wine mark, port-wine stain.

ne·vus pig·men·to·sus (nē′vŭs pig-men-tō′sŭs) A benign pigmented melanocytic proliferation; raised or level with the skin, present at birth or arising early in life. SYN mole (2), naevus pigmentosus.

ne·vus pi·lo·sus (nē′vŭs pī-lō′sŭs) A mole covered with an abundant growth of hair. SYN hairy mole, naevus pilosus.

ne·vus spi·lus (nē′vŭs spī′lŭs) A form of (flat) nevus pigmentosus. SYN naevus spilus.

ne·vus u·ni·us la·te·ris (nē′vŭs ū-nī′ŭs lat′ĕr-is) A congenital systematized linear nevus limited to one side of the body or to portions of the limbs on one side; lesions are often extensive, forming wavelike bands on the trunk and spiraling streaks on the limbs. SYN naevus unius lateris.

ne·vus vas·cu·la·ris, ne·vus vas·cu·lo·sus (nē′vŭs vas-kū-lā′ris, -lō′sŭs) SYN capillary hemangioma, naevus vascularis.

new·born (nb, NB) (nū′bŏrn) SYN neonatal, neonate.

new·ton (N) (nū′tŏn) Derived unit of force in the SI, expressed as meters-kilograms per second squared (m·kg s^{-2}); equivalent to 10^5 dynes in the CGS system.

New York Heart As·so·ci·a·tion clas·si·fi·ca·tion (nū yŏrk hahrt ă-sō′sē-ā′shŭn klas′i-fi-kā′shŭn) A functional classification to assess cardiovascular disability. Class I: cardiac disease without limitation of physical activity. Class II: cardiac disease with slight limitation of activity. Class III: cardiac disease producing marked limitation of activity. Class IV: cardiac disease resulting in inability to carry on any physical activity without discomfort.

New York vi·rus (NYV) (nū yŏrk vī′rŭs) Species of *Hantavirus* in the United States that causes a pulmonary syndrome.

nex·ins (neks′inz) Proteins that bridge adjacent microtubule doublets of the axoneme of cilia and flagella.

nex·us, pl. **nex·us** (neks′ŭs) SYN gap junction.

Ni Symbol for nickel.

ni·a·cin (nī′ă-sin) SYN nicotinic acid.

ni·a·cin·am·ide (nī′ă-sin′ă-mīd) SYN nicotinamide.

NIC (nik) Acronym for Nursing Interventions Classification.

niche (nich, nēsh) An ecologic term for the position occupied by a species in a biotic community, particularly its relationships to various other competitor, predator, prey, and parasite species.

nick·el (Ni) (nik′ĕl) Metallic bioelement; closely resembles cobalt and often associated with it. Protects ribosome structure against heat denaturation.

nick·el der·ma·ti·tis (nik′ĕl dĕr′mă-tī′tis) Allergic reaction due to contact with, or in some cases ingestion of, nickel or other metals containing nickel.

Ni·co·las-Fav·re dis·ease (nē-kō-lah′ fahv′ di-zēz′) SYN venereal lymphogranuloma.

nic·o·tin·a·mide (NA, N) (nik′ō-tin′ă-mīd) The biologically active amide of nicotinic acid, used in the prevention and treatment of pellagra. SYN niacinamide, nicotinic acid amide.

nic·o·tin·a·mide ad·e·nine di·nu·cle·o·tide (nik′ō-tin′ă-mīd ad′ĕ-nēn dī-nū′klē-ō-tīd) Ribosylnicotinamide 5′-phosphate (NMN) and adenosine 5′-phosphate (AMP) linked by phosphoanhydride linkage between the two phosphoric groups; binds as a coenzyme to proteins, serves in respiratory metabolism (hydrogen acceptor and donor) through alternate oxidation and reduction (NAD$^+$ ⇌ NADH).

nic·o·tin·a·mide ad·e·nine di·nu·cle·o·tide phos·phate (nik′ō-tin′ă-mīd ad′ĕ-nēn dī-nū′klē-ō-tīd fos′fāt) A coenzyme of many oxidases, in which the reaction NADP$^+$ + 2H ⇌ NADPH + H$^+$ takes place; the third phosphoric group esterifies the 2′-hydroxyl of the adenosine moiety of NAD$^+$.

nic·o·tin·a·mide mon·o·nu·cle·o·tide (nik′ō-tin′ă-mīd mon′ō-nū′klē-ō-tīd) Condensation product of nicotinamide and ribose 5-phosphate, precursor in synthesis of nicotinamide adenine dinucleotide.

nic·o·tine (nik′ō-tēn′) A poisonous volatile alkaloid derived from tobacco and responsible for many of the effects of tobacco; it first stimulates (small doses), then depresses (large doses) at autonomic ganglia and myoneural junctions.

nic·o·tine pol·a·cri·lex (nik´ō-tēn pol´ă-kril´ex) Active ingredient in nicotine gum to help people stop smoking.

nic·o·tin·ic ac·id (NA) (nik´ō-tin´ik as´id) Part of the vitamin B complex; used to prevent and treat pellagra and as a vasodilator. SYN antiblack-tongue factor, antipellagra factor, niacin, pellagra-preventing factor, vitamin PP.

nic·o·tin·ic re·cep·tors (nik´ō-tin´ik rē-sep´tŏrz) Cholinergic receptors on skeletal muscle cells linked to ion channels in the cell membrane.

ni·dus, gen. and pl. **ni·di** (nī´dŭs, -dī) **1.** A nest. **2.** The nucleus or central point of origin of a nerve. **3.** A focus of infection. **4.** The coalescence of molecules or small particles that is the beginning of a crystal or similar solid deposit. **5.** The focus of reduced density at the center of an osteoid osteoma, on bone radiographs.

night blind·ness (XN) (nīt blīnd´nĕs) SYN nyctalopia.

night guard (nīt gahrd) A removable acrylic appliance intended to relieve temporomandibular joint pain and other effects due to grinding the teeth. SYN occlusal guard.

night·mare (nīt´mār) A terrifying dream, as in which one is unable to cry for help or to escape from a seemingly impending evil.

night·shade (nīt´shād) Plants of the genus *Solanum* or *Atropa*, many of which have medicinal or toxic properties.

night sight (nīt sīt) SYN hemeralopia.

night soil (nīt soyl) Human feces used for fertilizer.

night sweat (nīt swet) Perspiration that occurs during sleep; may be a symptom of disease.

night ter·rors (nīt ter´ŏrz) A childhood disorder in which a child awakes screaming with fright, the distress persisting for a time during a state of semiconsciousness. SYN sleep terror.

night vi·sion (nīt vizh´ŭn) SYN scotopic vision.

ni·gri·ti·es (nī-grish´ē-ēz) A black pigmentation.

ni·gro·sin, ni·gro·sine (nī´grō-sin, -sēn) [C.I. 50420] A variable mixture of blue-black aniline dyes; used as a histologic stain for nervous tissue and as a negative stain for studying bacteria and spirochetes.

ni·gro·stri·a·tal (nī´grō-strī-ā´tăl) Referring to the efferent connection of the substantia nigra (especially its compact part) with the striatum. SEE substantia nigra.

ni·hil·ism (nī´i-lizm) **1.** PSYCHIATRY the delusion of the nonexistence of everything, especially of the self or part of the self. **2.** Engagement in acts that are totally destructive to one's own purposes and those of one's group.

ni·hil·is·tic de·lu·sion (nī-i-lis´tik dĕ-lū´zhŭn) SYN delusion of negation.

Ni·kol·sky sign (ni-kol´skē sīn) Peculiar skin vulnerability in pemphigus vulgaris; apparently normal epidermis may be separated at the basal layer and rubbed off when pressed with a sliding motion.

nil per os (NPO, n.p.o.) (nil per os) [L.] Latin for nothing by mouth; instruction often included in dietary orders for patients scheduled for surgery.

NIOSH (nī´osh) Acronym for U.S. National Institute for Occupational Safety and Health.

nip·ple (nip´ĕl) [TA] A blunt conic projection at the apex of the breast on the surface of which the lactiferous ducts open; it is surrounded by a circular pigmented area, the areola. SYN mammilla (2), teat (1), thelium (3).

nip·ple shield (nip´ĕl shēld) A cap or dome placed over the nipple to protect it during nursing.

Nis·sen fun·dop·li·ca·tion (nis´ĕn fŭn´dō-pli-kā´shŭn) 360° fundoplication; can be done through abdominal or thoracic approach; currently most often performed laparoscopically.

nit (nit) **1.** The ovum of a body, head, or

crab louse; attaches to human hair or clothing by a layer of chitin. **2.** A unit of luminance; a luminous intensity of 1 candela per square meter of orthogonally projected surface.

Ni·ta·buch mem·brane, Ni·ta·buch stri·a, Ni·ta·buch lay·er (nē′tă-bŭk mem′brăn, strī′ă, lā′ĕr) A layer of fibrin between the boundary zone of the compact endometrium and the cytotrophoblastic shell in the placenta.

ni·trate (nī′trāt) A salt of nitric acid.

ni·tric ac·id (nī′trik as′id) A strong acid; an oxidant and corrosive.

ni·tric ox·ide (NO) (nī′trik ok′sīd) A colorless, free-radical gas.

ni·tri·da·tion (nī′tri-dā′shŭn) Formation of nitrogen compounds through action of ammonia.

ni·tride (nī′trīd) A compound of nitrogen and one other element; e.g., magnesium nitride, Mg_3N_2.

ni·tri·fi·ca·tion (nī′tri-fi-kā′shŭn) **1.** Bacterial conversion of nitrogenous matter into nitrates. **2.** Treatment of a material with nitric acid.

ni·trite (nī′trīt) A salt of nitrous acid.

ni·tri·toid re·ac·tion (nī′troyd rē-ak′shŭn) Severe reaction resembling that following administration of nitrites, sometimes following intravenous administration of arsphenamine or other drugs; consists of flushing of the face, edema of the tongue and lips, other symptoms, and sometimes death.

ni·tri·tu·ri·a (nī′tri-tyūr′ē-ă) The presence of nitrites in the urine.

ni·tro·cel·lu·lose (NC) (nī′trō-sel′yū-lōs) SYN pyroxylin.

ni·tro·fu·ran·to·in (nī′trō-fyūr-an′tō-in) A urinary antibacterial agent with a wide range of activity against both gram-positive and gram-negative organisms.

ni·tro·gen (nī′trŏ-jĕn) **1.** A gaseous element. **2.** The molecular form of nitrogen, N_2. **3.** Pharmaceutical grade N_2, containing not less than 99.0% by volume of N_2; used as a diluent for medicinal gases, and

for air replacement in pharmaceutical preparations.

ni·tro·gen 13 (^{13}N) (nī′trŏ-jĕn) A cyclotron-produced, positron-emitting radioisotope of nitrogen with a half-life of 9.97 minutes; used in protein metabolism studies and in positron-emission tomography.

ni·tro·ge·nase (nī-troj′ĕ-nās) A term for enzyme systems that catalyze the reduction of molecular nitrogen to ammonia in nitrogen-fixing bacteria with reduced ferredoxin and adenosine triphosphate.

ni·tro·gen bal·ance (nī′trŏ-jĕn bal′ăns) The difference between the total nitrogen intake by an organism and total nitrogen loss. A normal, healthy adult has a zero nitrogen balance.

ni·tro·gen cy·cle (nī′trŏ-jĕn sī′kĕl) The series of events in which the nitrogen of the atmosphere is fixed, thus made available for plant and animal life, and is then returned to the atmosphere.

ni·tro·gen dis·tri·bu·tion (nī′trŏ-jĕn dis′tri-byū′shŭn) SYN nitrogen partition.

ni·tro·gen e·quiv·a·lent (nī′trŏ-jĕn ĕ-kwiv′ă-lĕnt) The nitrogen content of protein; used in calculating the protein breakdown in the body from the nitrogen excreted in the urine.

ni·tro·gen fix·a·tion (nī′trŏ-jen fik-sā′shŭn) Process in which atmospheric nitrogen is converted to ammonia.

ni·tro·gen group (nī′trŏ-jĕn grŭp) Five trivalent or quinquivalent elements with basic hydrogen compounds and oxyacids that vary from monobasic to tetrabasic: nitrogen, phosphorus, arsenic, antimony, and bismuth.

ni·tro·gen lag (nī′trŏ-jĕn lag) The length of time after the ingestion of a given protein before the amount of nitrogen equal to that in the protein has been excreted in the urine.

ni·trog·e·nous (nī-troj′ĕ-nŭs) Relating to or containing nitrogen.

ni·tro·gen par·ti·tion (nī′trŏ-jĕn pahr-ti′shŭn) Determination of the distribution of nitrogen in the urine among the var-

N

ious constituents. SYN nitrogen distribution.

ni·tro·glyc·er·in (nī′trō-glis′ĕr-in) An explosive, yellowish, oily fluid formed by the action of sulfuric and nitric acids on glycerin; used as a vasodilator. SYN 1, 2, 3-propanetriol trinitrate, glyceryl trinitrate, trinitroglycerin.

ni·tro·glyc·er·in tab·lets (nī′trō-glis′ĕr-in tab′lĕts) Medication used in angina pectoris to dilate blood vessels and relieve chest pain.

ni·tro·prus·side (NP) (nī′trō-prŭs′īd) Agent used as an intravenous vasodilator.

S-ni·tro·so·he·mo·glo·bin (nī-trō′sō-hē′mŏ-glō′bin) Nitric oxide bound with hemoglobin.

ni·tro·so·ur·e·a (nī-trō′sō-yūr′ē-ă) Alkylating agent used in the treatment of many neoplasms.

ni·tro·syl (nī′trō-sil) A univalent radical or atom group, $-N=O$, forming the nitroso compounds.

ni·trous (nī′trŭs) Denoting a nitrogen compound containing one less atom of oxygen than the nitric compounds.

ni·trous ac·id (nī′trŭs as′id) A standard biologic and clinical laboratory reagent.

ni·trous ox·ide (NO) (nī′trŭs ok′sīd) A nonflammable, nonexplosive gas widely used as a rapidly acting, rapidly reversible, nondepressant, and nontoxic inhalation analgesic to supplement other anesthetics and analgesics. SYN laughing gas.

ni·tryl (nī′tril) The radical $-NO_2$ of the nitro compounds.

NK cells (selz) SYN natural killer cells.

no·bel·i·um (No) (nō-bel′ē-ŭm) An unstable transuranium element; atomic no. 102; atomic wt. 259.1009; prepared by bombardment of curium with carbon-12 nuclei and similar heavy ions on other elements of the transuranium series.

no·ble gas·es (nō′bĕl gas′ĕz) Elements in the zero group in the periodic series:

helium, neon, argon, krypton, xenon, and radon. SYN inert gases.

NOC (nok) Acronym for Nursing Outcomes Classification.

No·car·di·a (nō-kahr′dē-ă) A genus of aerobic higher bacteria, containing weakly acid-fast, slender rods or filaments; may be a cause of mycetoma or nocardiosis.

No·car·di·a as·ter·oi·des (nō-kahr′dē-ă as-tē-roy′dēz) A bacterial species of aerobic, gram-positive, partially acid-fast, branching organisms causing nocardiosis and possibly mycetoma in humans.

No·car·di·a bra·sil·i·en·sis (nō-kahr′dē-ă bră-sil-ē-en′sis) A partially acid-fast bacterial species associated with subcutaneous skin infections.

No·car·di·a ca·vi·ae (nō-kahr′dē-ă kā′vē-ē) A bacterial species that causes mycetoma in humans.

No·car·di·a·ce·ae (nō-kahr′dē-ā′sē-ē) A family of acid-fast, gram-positive, aerobic bacteria that includes the genus *Nocardia*.

No·car·di·a med·i·ter·ra·ne·i (nō-kahr′dē-ă med′i-tĕr-ā′nē-ī) A bacterial species that produces rifamycin.

No·car·di·a or·i·en·ta·lis (nō-kahr′dē-ă ōr-ē-en-tā′lis) A bacterial species that produces vancomycin.

No·car·di·a o·ti·ti·dis·ca·vi·a·rum (nō-kahr′dē-ă ō-tī-ū-dis-kav-ī-ā′rŭm) Higher bacterium living in soil; a cause of nocardiosis and actinomycetoma.

No·car·di·a trans·va·len·sis (nō-kahr′dē-ă trans-vā-len′sis) A bacterial aerobic actinomycete; a cause of nocardiosis.

No·car·di·op·sis (nō-kahr′dē-op′sis) A genus of higher bacteria living in soil that causes subacute or chronic pneumonia, subcutaneous infection, or disseminated disease.

No·car·di·op·sis das·son·vil·le·i (nō-kahr′dē-op′sis das′ŏn-vil′-ē-ī) An aerobic bacterial actinomycete, formerly *Nocardia dassonvillei;* a cause of actinomycetoma.

no•car•di•o•sis (nō-kahr′dē-ō′sis) Generalized disease in humans and other animals caused by *Nocardia asteroides* and *N. brasiliensis;* characterized by primary pulmonary lesions that may be subclinical or chronic with hematogenous spread, and usually with involvement of the central nervous system.

no•ce•bo (nō-sē′bō) An unpleasant side effect attributable to administration of a placebo.

noci- Prefix meaning hurt, pain, injury.

no•ci•cep•tor (nō′si-sep′tŏr) A peripheral nerve organ or mechanism for the reception and transmission of painful or injurious stimuli.

no•ci•fen•sor (nō′si-fen′sŏr) Mechanisms that act to protect the body from injury; nervous system that reacts to adjacent injury by causing vasodilation.

no•ci•per•cep•tion (nō′si-pĕr-sep′shŭn) Perception of injurious influences in nerve centers.

no code (nō kōd) Statement that indicates that the patient has refused cardiopulmonary resuscitation if breathing stops and heart failure occurs.

noc•te (nok′tē) At night.

noc•tu•ri•a, nyc•tu•ri•a (nok-tyūr′ē-ă, nik-) Frequent urination at night.

noc•tur•nal (noc) (nok-tŭr′năl) Pertaining to the hours of darkness; opposite of diurnal (1).

noc•tur•nal am•bly•o•pi•a (nok-tŭr′năl am′blē-ō′pē-ă) SYN nyctalopia.

noc•tur•nal e•mis•sion (nok-tŭr′năl ē-mish′ŭn) Seminal discharge during sleep.

noc•tur•nal en•u•re•sis (nok-tŭr′năl en-yūr-ē′sis) Urinary incontinence during sleep. SYN bed-wetting.

noc•tur•nal my•o•clo•nus (nok-tŭr′năl mī-ok′lŏ-nŭs) Frequently repeated muscular jerks at the moment of dropping off to sleep.

no•dal rhythm (nō′dăl ridthm) SYN atrioventricular junctional rhythm.

nod•ding spasm (nod′ing spazm) **1.** In infants, a drop of the head on the chest due to loss of tone in the neck muscles as in epilepsia nutans, or to tonic spasm of anterior neck muscles as in West syndrome. **2.** In adults, a nodding of the head from clonic spasms of the sternomastoid muscles.

node (nōd) [TA] **1.** A knob; a circumscribed swelling. **2.** ANATOMY a circumscribed mass of differentiated tissue. SYN nodus.

node of Clo•quet (nōd klō-kā′) One of the deep inguinal lymph nodes located in or adjacent to the femoral canal; sometimes mistaken for a femoral hernia when enlarged.

node of Ran•vi•er (nōd rahn-vē-ā′) SYN Ranvier node.

no•dose (nō′dōs) Having nodes or knotlike swellings. SYN nodular, nodulate, nodulated, nodulous.

no•dose rheu•ma•tism (nō′dōs rū′mă-tizm) **1.** SYN rheumatoid arthritis. **2.** An acute or subacute articular rheumatism, accompanied by the formation of nodules on the tendons, ligaments, and periosteum in the neighborhood of the affected joints.

no•dos•i•ty (nō-dos′i-tē) **1.** A node; a knoblike or knotty swelling. **2.** The condition of being nodose.

nod•u•lar amy•loid•o•sis (nod′yū-lăr am′i-loy-dō′sis) Localized form in which amyloid occurs as hard masses or nodules beneath the skin or mucous membranes; may be associated with plasma cell dyscrasia or systemic amyloidosis. SYN amyloid tumor, focal amyloidosis.

nod•u•lar fas•ci•i•tis (nod′yū-lăr fash′ē-ī′tis) Fast-growing tumorlike proliferation of fibroblasts, not thought to be neoplastic, with mild inflammatory exudation in fascia; may infiltrate surrounding tissue but does not progress indefinitely nor metastasize.

nod•u•lar lym•pho•ma (nod′yū-lăr lim-fō′mă) Malignant lymphoma arising from small or large lymphoid follicular B cells, growing in a nodular pattern. SYN follicular lymphoma.

nod·u·lar mel·a·no·ma (NM) (nod′yū-lăr mel′ă-nō′mă) Primary cutaneous lesion that presents as rapidly growing smoothly spheroid or ulcerated nodules in which tumor cells microscopically invade the dermis beneath all the lateral epidermal margins of involvement.

nod·u·la·tion (nod′yū-lā′shŭn) The formation or the presence of nodules.

nod·ule (nod′yūl) [TA] A small node. SYN nodulus (1).

nod·u·lus, pl. **no·du·li** (nod′yū-lŭs, -lī) [TA] **1.** SYN nodule. **2.** The posterior extremity of the inferior vermis of the cerebellum, forming with the posterior medullary velum the central portion of the flocculonodular lobe.

nod·u·lus lym·pha·ti·cus (nod′yū-lŭs lim-fat′ik-ŭs) SYN lymph follicle.

no·dus, pl. **no·di** (nō′dŭs, -dī) [TA] SYN node.

noise pol·lu·tion (noyz pŏ-lū′shŭn) Damaging environmental noise levels, as from automobile engines, industrial machinery, or amplified music.

no·ma (nō′mă) Gangrenous stomatitis with conspicuous necrosis and sloughing of tissue. SYN stomatonecrosis.

no·men·cla·ture (nō′měn-klā-chŭr) A system of names, as of anatomic structures, molecular entities, or organisms, used in any science.

nom·i·nal (nom′i-năl) Minimal, limited.

nom·i·nal a·pha·si·a (nom′i-năl ă-fā′zē-ă) SYN anomic aphasia.

nom·o·gram (nō′mō-gram) Line chart showing scales for variables involved in a particular formula so that corresponding values for each variable lie in a straight line intersecting all the scales.

no·mo·top·ic (nō′mō-top′ik) Relating to, or occurring at, the usual or normal place.

non- A prefix meaning the reverse of something; opposite; negative.

non-A-E hep·a·ti·tis (hep′ă-tī′tis) Acute liver disease not caused by any identified viral agents A through E.

non-A, non-B hep·a·ti·tis, non-B hep·a·ti·tis (NANB) (hep′ă-tī′tis) Liver disease caused by infectious agents not detectable by methods that reveal hepatitis viruses A and B.

non·a·vail·a·bil·i·ty state·ment (non′ ă-vāl′ă-bil′i-tē stāt′měnt) A statement issued by the base commander to a patient that allows such patient or dependent to go off base for treatment even though less than 40 miles from a military treatment facility.

non·bac·te·ri·al throm·bot·ic en·do·car·di·tis (non′bak-tēr′ē-ăl throm-bot′ ik en′dō-kahr-dī′tis) Verrucous endocardial lesions occurring in the terminal stages of many chronic infectious and wasting diseases. SYN abacterial thrombotic endocarditis, cachectic endocarditis, terminal endocarditis, thromboendocarditis.

non·bac·te·ri·al ver·ru·cous en·do·car·di·tis (non′bak-tēr′ē-ăl věr-ū′kŭs en′dō-kahr-dī′tis) SYN Libman-Sacks endocarditis.

non·chro·mo·ge·nic (non′krō-mō-jen′ ik) Nonphotoreactive; pertains to lack of pigment production when colonies are exposed to light.

non·com·pli·ance (non′kŏm-plī′ăns) State of a patient who fails to follow health care direction given by a professional (e.g., failure to exercise, not taking medicine as prescribed).

non com·pos men·tis (non kom′pŏs men′tis) Not of sound mind; mentally incapable of managing one's affairs.

non·con·ju·ga·tive plas·mid (non-kon′jū-gă-tiv plaz′mid) A plasmid that cannot effect conjugation and self-transfer to another bacterium (bacterial strain); transfer depends on mediation of another (and conjugative) plasmid.

non·con·tained disc her·ni·a·tion (non′kŏn-tānd′ disk hěr′nē-ā′shŭn) Herniated disc material that comes directly in contact with the anterior epidural space through a complete defect in the posterior anulus fibrosus and posterior longitudinal ligament.

non·co·va·lent bond (non′kō-vā′lĕnt bond) Bond in which electrons are not shared between atoms.

non·dis·junc·tion (non′dis-jŭngk′shŭn) Failure of one or more pairs of chromosomes to separate at the meiotic stage of karyokinesis, with the result that both chromosomes are carried to one daughter cell and none to the other.

non·e·lec·tro·lyte (non′ĕ-lek′trō-līt) A substance with molecules that do not, in solution, dissociate to ions and, therefore, do not carry an electric current.

non·es·sen·tial ami·no ac·ids (non′ĕ-sen′shăl ă-mē′nō as′idz) Those amino acids that may be synthesized by an organism and are thus not required as such in its diet.

non·fea·sance (non-fē′zăns) Negligent; failure by a health care professional to do something required or by acting outside established norms of care.

non·gon·o·coc·cal u·re·thri·tis (non′gon-ō-kok′ăl yūr′ĕth-rī′tis) Form not resulting from gonococcal infection; venereally transmitted *Chlamydia trachomatis* is the most common causative agent.

non·gran·u·lar leu·ko·cyte (non-gran′yū-lăr lū′kō-sīt) General, nonspecific term frequently used with reference to lymphocytes, monocytes, and plasma cells. SEE ALSO leukocyte.

non-Hodg·kin lym·pho·ma (non-hoj′kin lim-fō′mă) A lymphoma other than Hodgkin disease, classified into a nodular or diffuse tumor pattern and by cell type.

non·im·mune se·rum (non′i-myūn′ sēr′ŭm) A serum from a subject that is not immune; one free of antibodies to a given antigen.

non·in·fil·tra·ting lob·u·lar car·ci·no·ma (non-in′fil-trāt-ing lob′yū-lăr kahr′si-nō′mă) Carcinoma of the breast in which small tumor cells fill preexisting acini within lobules, without invading the surrounding stroma. SYN lobular carcinoma in situ.

non·in·su·lin-de·pen·dent di·a·be·tes mel·li·tus (non-in′sŭ-lin dĕ-pen′dĕnt dī-ă-bē′tēz mel′i-tŭs) SYN Type 2 diabetes.

non·in·va·sive (non′in-vā′siv) Denoting a procedure that does not require insertion of an instrument or device through the skin or a body orifice for diagnosis or treatment.

non·i·on·ic (non′ī-on′ik) Radiographic contrast media that do not ionize in solution, decreasing effective osmolarity and toxicity.

non·i·so·lat·ed pro·tein·u·ri·a (non-ī′sō-lā-tĕd prō′tē-nyūr′ē-ă) The urinary disorder, when associated with other abnormalities.

non·ke·tot·ic hy·per·gly·ci·ne·mi·a (non′kē-tot′ik hī′pĕr-glī-sē′mē-ă) Inborn error of glycine metabolism, due to a deficiency of glycine dicarboxylase P protein (GCSP), a component of glycine cleavage system.

non·la·mel·lar bone (non′lă-mel′ăr bōn) SYN woven bone.

non·le·thal a·gent (non-lē′thăl ā′jĕnt) A common but incorrect term for incapacitation chemical agent.

non·lip·id his·ti·o·cy·to·sis (non-lip′id his′tē-ō-sī-tō′sis) SYN Letterer-Siwe disease.

non·ma·lef·i·cence (non′mă-lef′i-sĕns) Ethical principle of doing no harm.

non·med·ul·lat·ed fi·bers (non-med′ŭ-lăt-ĕd fī′bĕrz) SYN unmyelinated fibers.

non·neu·ro·gen·ic neu·ro·gen·ic blad·der (non-nūr′ō-jen′ik nūr′ō-jen′ik blad′ĕr) Detrusor-sphincter incoordination with urinary incontinence, constipation, urinary tract infection, upper tract changes. SYN Hinman syndrome.

non·nu·cle·o·side re·verse tran·scrip·tase in·hib·i·tors (NNRTI) (non-nū′klē-ō-sīd rē-vĕrs′ trans-krip′tās in-hib′i-tŏrz) Class of medications to treat HIV infection.

non·os·si·fy·ing fi·bro·ma (non-os′i-fī-ing fī-brō′mă) Loculated osteolytic focus of cellular fibrous tissue, which slightly expands a bone, usually near the end of a long bone in older children.

non·os·te·o·gen·ic fib·ro·ma (non-os′

tē-ō-jen'ik fī-brō'mă) SYN fibrous cortical defect.

no·nox·y·nol 9 (non-oks'i-nol) Compounds that are surface-acting agents used in spermicidal preparations.

non·par·ous (non-par'ŭs) SYN nulliparous.

non·par·ti·ci·pat·ing phy·si·cian (non' par-tis'i-pāt-ing fi-zish'ŭn) In the U.S. Medicare program, a physician who does not accept assignment on all Medicare claims.

non·path·o·gen·ic (non-path'ŏ-jen'ik) Not causing disease.

non·pen·e·trat·ing wound (non-pen'ĕ-trāt-ing wūnd) Injury, especially within the thorax or abdomen, produced without disruption of the surface of the body.

non·pit·ting edema (non-pit'ing ĕ-dē'mă) Swelling of subcutaneous tissues that cannot be indented easily by compression; usually due to metabolic abnormality, such as increased glycosaminoglycan content, like that which occurs in Graves disease (pretibial myxedema) or in early phase of scleroderma. SYN brawny edema.

non·pre·scrip·tion drug (non'prĕ-skrip'shŭn drŭg) A pharmaceutical that may be obtained without a physician's prescription. SYN over-the-counter medication.

non·pro·duc·tive cough (non'prŏ-dŭk'tiv kawf) Cough in which the patient is unable to bring up or get rid of excretions.

non·pro·pri·e·tar·y name (non'prŏ-prī'ĕ-tar-ē nām) A short name (often called a generic name) of a chemical, drug, or other substance that is not subject to trademark rights but is, in contrast to a trivial name (q.v.), recognized or recommended by government agencies and by quasiofficial organizations for general public use. Cf. systematic name.

non·pro·tein ni·tro·gen (non-prō'tēn nī'trŏ-jĕn) The nitrogen content of other than protein bodies.

non·re·as·su·ring fe·tal sta·tus (non-rē'ă-shŭr'ing fē'tăl stat'ŭs) Abnormal

fetal heart rate or rhythm on electronic monitoring, suggesting fetal ischemia.

non·rig·id con·nec·tor (non-rij'id kŏ-nek'tŏr) Connector or joint that is not rigid or solid. SYN stress-broken connector, stress-broken joint.

non·se·cre·tor (non'sĕ-krē'tŏr) A person whose saliva does not contain antigens of the ABO blood group. SEE ALSO secretor.

non·sense mu·ta·tion (non'sens myū-tā'shŭn) SYN suppressor mutation.

non·sex·u·al gen·er·a·tion (non-sek'shū-ăl jen'ĕr-ā'shŭn) SYN asexual generation.

non·shi·ver·ing ther·mo·gen·e·sis (NST) (non-shiv'ĕr-ing thĕr'mō-jen'ĕ-sis) Form due to the effects of the sympathetic nervous system neurotransmitters, epinephrine, and norepinephrine, acting to increase the cellular metabolic rate in skeletal muscle and other tissues, thereby increasing heat production.

non-small cell car·ci·no·ma (non' smawl' sel kahr'si-nō'mă) SYN bronchogenic carcinoma.

non·spe·cif·ic build·ing-re·la·ted ill·ness·es (non'spĕ-sif'ik bild'ing-rē-lāt'ĕd il'nĕs-ĕz) A heterogeneous group of work- or domicile-related symptoms without clear objective physical or laboratory findings.

non·spe·ci·fic im·mu·ni·ty (non'spĕ-sif'ik i-myū'ni-tē) Resistance manifested by a species (or by races, families, and individuals in a species) that has not been immunized (sensitized, allergized) by previous infection or vaccination; much of it results from body mechanisms that are poorly understood but differ from those responsible for the altered reactivity associated with the specific nature of acquired immunity; in general, innate immunity is nonspecific and is not stimulated by specific antigens. SYN innate immunity

non·spe·cif·ic pro·tein (non'spĕ-sif'ik prō'tēn) A protein substance that elicits a response not mediated by specific antigen-antibody reaction.

non·spe·cif·ic ur·e·thri·tis (non-spĕ-sif´ik yūr´ĕth-rī´tis) Form not resulting from gonococcal, chlamydial, or other specific infectious agents. SYN simple urethritis.

non·ste·roi·dal an·ti·in·flam·ma·to·ry drug (NSAID) (non´ster-oy´dăl an´tē-in-flam´ă-tŏr-ē drŭg) Any one of a group of pharmacotherapeutic agents exerting antiinflammatory (and also usually analgesic and antipyretic) actions (e.g., aspirin).

non·stress test (non´stres´ test) Assessment to evaluate fetal well-being by evaluating fetal heart rate response to fetal movement.

non·sup·pur·a·tive os·te·o·my·e·li·tis (non-sŭp´yŭr-ă-tiv os´tē-ō-mī´ĕ-lī´tis) Inflammation of the bone that does not produce pus or purulent drainage.

non·throm·bo·cy·to·pe·nic pur·pu·ra (non-throm´bō-sī´tō-pē´nik pŭr´pyŭr-ă) SYN purpura simplex.

non·tox·ic (non-tok´sik) Denotes a substance that is not poisonous.

non·tox·ic goi·ter (non´toks´ik goy´tĕr) Goiter not accompanied by hyperthyroidism.

non·un·ion (non-yūn´yŭn) Failure of normal healing of a fractured bone.

non·va·lent (non-vā´lĕnt) Having no valency; not capable of entering into chemical composition.

non·ve·ne·re·al syph·i·lis (non´vĕ-nēr´ē-ăl sif´i-lis) The disease caused by organisms closely related to *Treponema pallidum;* spread by personal, although not necessarily venereal, contact; usually acquired in childhood, most common in areas of poverty and overcrowding; rare in the U.S.; includes yaws, pinta, and bejel. SYN endemic syphilis.

non·vi·a·ble (non-vī´ă-bĕl) 1. Incapable of independent existence. 2. Denoting a microorganism or parasite incapable of metabolic or reproductive activity.

non·vi·su·al re·ti·na (non-vizh´ū-ăl ret´i-nă) An anterior continuation of the pigment layer of the retina not sensitive to light.

non-weight-bear·ing ex·er·cise (non-wāt´bār-ing ek´sĕr-sīz) Exercise performed with one's body weight artificially supported (e.g., stationary cycling). SYN weight-supported exercise.

no·o·trop·ic (nō´ō-trop´ik) Denotes an agent having an effect on memory.

nor- 1. Chemical prefix denoting 1) elimination of one methylene group from a chain, the highest permissible locant being used; 2) contraction of a (steroid) ring by one CH_2 unit, the locant being the capital letter identifying the ring. Elimination of two methylene groups is denoted by the prefix dinor-; three groups, by trinor-. **2.** Chemical prefix denoting ''normal,''i.e., unbranched chain of carbon atoms in aliphatic compounds; a branched chain with the same number of carbon atoms.

nor·ep·i·neph·rine (nŏr´ep-i-nef´rin) A catecholamine hormone, acting on α- and β-receptors; it is stored in chromaffin granules in the medulla of suprenal gland in much smaller amounts than epinephrine and secreted in response to hypotension and physical stress; used pharmacologically as a vasopressor. SYN noradrenaline.

norm (nōrm) **1.** The usual value. **2.** The desirable value or behavior.

nor·mal (nōr´măl) **1.** Typical; usual; according to the rule or standard. **2.** BACTERIOLOGY nonimmune; untreated; denoting an animal, or the serum or substance contained therein, which has not been experimentally immunized against any microorganism or its products. **3.** Denoting a solution containing one equivalent of replaceable hydrogen or hydroxyl per liter. **4.** PSYCHIATRY, PSYCHOLOGY denoting a level of effective functioning that is satisfactory to both the patient and the patient's social milieu.

nor·mal an·ti·tox·in (nŏr´măl an´tē-tok´sin) Serum capable of neutralizing an equivalent quantity of a normal toxin.

nor·mal con·cen·tra·tion (n) (nŏr´măl kon´sĕn-trā´shŭn) SEE normal (3).

nor·mal dis·tri·bu·tion (nŏr´măl dis´tri-byū´shŭn) SYN gaussian distribution.

nor·mal flor·a (nŏr´măl flōr´ă) Microor-

N

ganisms that normally reside at a given site and under normal circumstances do not cause disease.

nor·mal hu·man plas·ma (nōr′măl hyū′măn plaz′mă) Sterile plasma obtained by pooling approximately equal amounts of the liquid portion of anticoagulated whole blood from eight or more adult humans who have been certified as free from any disease tranmissible by transfusion, and treating it with ultraviolet irradiation to destroy possible bacterial and viral contaminants.

nor·mal hu·man se·rum al·bu·min (nōr′măl hyū′măn sēr′ŭm al-bū′min) A sterile preparation obtained by fractionating blood plasma proteins from healthy people.

nor·mal oc·clu·sion (nōr′măl ŏ-klū′zhŭn) **1.** Arrangement of teeth and their supporting structure usually found in health. **2.** SYN neutral occlusion (1).

nor·mal op·so·nin (nōr′măl op′sŏ-nin) One normally present in the blood; is relatively thermolabile and reacts with various organisms. SYN common opsonin, thermolabile opsonin.

nor·mal range (nōr′măl rānj) SYN reference range.

nor·mal res·pir·a·tor·y se·cre·tions (nōr′măl res′pir-ă-tōr-ē sĕ-krē′shŭnz) Clear, colorless, or white sputum.

nor·mal sa·line so·lu·tion (nōr′măl sā′lĕn sŏ-lū′shŭn) A sterile solution of 0.9% w/v (grams of solute per mL of solution) sodium chloride in water, considered to be isotonic with blood; used intravenous for dehydrated patients who cannot take fluids orally. SYN normal saline.

nor·mal se·rum (nōr′măl sēr′ŭm) A nonimmune serum, usually with reference to a serum obtained before immunization.

nor·mal si·nus rhythm (nōr′măl sī′nŭs ridh′ŭm) Beating of the heart that falls within the range of what is considered to indicate good health.

nor·mal so·lu·tion (nōr′măl sŏ-lū′shŭn) SEE normal (3).

nor·mal tem·per·a·ture (nōr′măl temp′ĕr-ă-chūr) Body temperature of 98.6 degrees F or 37 degrees C.

nor·mal val·ues (nōr′măl val′yūz) Laboratory test values used to characterize apparently healthy people; replaced by reference values.

normo- Prefix meaning normal, usual.

nor·mo·blast (nōr′mō-blast) A nucleated red blood cell, the immediate precursor of a normal erythrocyte in humans. SEE ALSO erythroblast.

nor·mo·blas·to·sis (nōr′mō-blas-tō′sis) Excessive production of normoblasts by the bone marrow.

nor·mo·cap·ni·a (nōr′mō-kap′nē-ă) A state in which the arterial carbon dioxide pressure is normal, about 40 mmHg.

nor·mo·chro·mi·a (nōr′mō-krō′mē-ă) Normal color; referring to blood in which the amount of hemoglobin in the red blood cells is normal.

nor·mo·cyte (nōr′mō-sīt) A red blood cell of normal size, shape, and color. Cf. macrocyte, microcyte.

nor·mo·cyt·ic a·ne·mi·a (nōr′mō-sit′ik ă-nē′mē-ă) Type in which the erythrocytes are of normal size.

nor·mo·cy·to·sis (nōr′mō-sī-tō′sis) A normal state of the blood cell with regard to its component formed elements.

nor·mo·ka·le·mi·a, nor·mo·ka·li·e·mi·a (nōr′mō-kă-lē′mē-ă, -kă-lē-ē′mē-ă) A normal level of potassium in the blood.

nor·mo·ka·le·mic per·i·od·ic pa·ral·y·sis (nōr′mō-kă-lē′mik pēr′ē-od′ik păr-al′i-sis) Periodic paralysis in which the serum potassium level is within normal limits during attacks; onset usually occurs between the ages of 2 and 5 years. SYN sodium-responsive periodic paralysis.

nor·mo·ten·sive (NT) (nōr′mō-ten′siv) Indicating a normal arterial blood pressure. SYN normotonic (2).

nor·mo·ther·mi·a (nōr′mō-thĕr′mē-ă) Environmental temperature that does not increase or depress cellular activity.

nor·mo·ton·ic (nōr′mō-ton′ik) **1.** Relating to or characterized by normal muscular tone. SYN eutonic. **2.** SYN normotensive.

nor·mo·tri·gly·cer·i·dem·ic a·be·ta·lip·o·pro·tein·e·mi·a (nōr´mō-trī-glis-ĕr-i-dē´mik ă-bā´tă-lip´ō-prō-tē-nē´mē-ă) Form with normal levels of triglycerides.

normovolaemia [Br.] SYN normovolemia.

nor·mo·vol·e·mi·a (nōr´mō-vō-lē´mē-ă) A normal blood volume. SYN normovolaemia.

nor·mox·i·a (nōr-mok´sē-ă) A state in which the partial pressure of oxygen in the inspired gas is equal to that of air at sea level.

norm-ref·er·enced (nōrm-ref´ĕr-ĕnst) A psychometric property of a standardized test that compares a person's performance with those of the general population.

Nor·ris cor·pus·cle (nōr´is kōr´pŭs-ĕl) Decolorized red blood cell invisible or almost invisible in the blood plasma, unless appropriately stained.

North A·mer·i·can blas·to·my·co·sis (nōrth ă-mer´i-kăn blas´tō-mī-kō´sis) SEE blastomycosis.

North A·mer·i·can Nurs·ing Di·ag·no·sis As·so·ci·a·tion (NANDA) (nōrth ă-mer´i-kăn nŭrs´ing dī-ăg-nō´sis ă-sō´sē-ā´shŭn) NURSING organization for development and classification of nursing diagnoses.

North·ern blot an·al·y·sis (nōr´thĕrn blŏt ă-nal´i-sis) A procedure similar to the Southern blot analysis, used mostly to separate and identify RNA fragments. SYN blot.

Nor·walk gas·tro·en·ter·i·tis (nōr´wawk gas´trō-en´tĕr-ī´tis) Potentially serious vomiting and diarrhea caused by a Norwalk virus.

Nor·we·gian sca·bies (nōr-wē´jăn skā´bēz) Severe form of scabies with innumerable mites in thickened stratum corneum; has been linked with cellular immune deficiencies, including AIDS. SYN crusted scabies, Norway itch.

nose (nōz) That portion of the respiratory pathway above the hard palate; includes both the external nose and the nasal cavity. SYN nasus (2).

nose·bleed (nōz´blēd) SYN epistaxis.

No·se·ma (nō-sē´mă) A protozoan genus with species pathogenic for invertebrates of economic importance (bees, silkworms); others are being studied as possible agents of biologic control of pest insects or other target invertebrates.

noso- Combining form meaning disease.

no·so·ac·u·sis (nō´sō-ă-kyū´sis) Hearing loss due to disease, as opposed to aging.

nos·o·co·mi·al (nos´ō-kō´mē-ăl) 1. Relating to a hospital. 2. Denoting a new disorder (not the patient's original condition) associated with being treated in a hospital, such as a hospital-acquired infection.

no·sol·o·gy (nō-sol´ō-jē) 1. The science of classification of diseases. 2. Classification of sick people into groups, whatever the criteria for the classification, and agreement as to the boundaries of the groups. SYN nosonomy, nosotaxy.

no·son·o·my (nō-son´ō-mē) SYN nosology.

nos·o·phil·i·a (nos´ō-fil´ē-ă) A morbid desire to be sick.

nos·o·pho·bi·a (nos´ō-fō´bē-ă) An inordinate dread and fear of disease.

nos·o·poi·et·ic (nos´ō-poy-et´ik) SYN pathogenic.

Nos·o·psyl·lus (nos´ō-sil´ŭs) A flea genus commonly found on rodents. *N. fasciatus*, the northern rat flea, infrequently transmits plague bacillus to humans.

nos·tril (nos´tril) Anterior opening to either side of the nasal cavity. SYN naris, prenaris.

nos·trum (nos´trŭm) General term for a therapeutic agent, sometimes patented but usually of secret composition, offered to the general public as a specific remedy for any disease or class of diseases.

no·tal·gi·a (nō-tal´jē-ă) General term for any sort of back pain.

notch (noch) [TA] 1. An indentation at

the edge of any structure. **2.** Any short, narrow, V-shaped deviation, whether positive or negative, in a linear tracing. SYN incisura [TA], incisure.

No·tice of Pri·va·cy Prac·ti·ces (nō′tis prī′vă-sē prak′tis-ĕz) Printed advisory given to patients that explains the health care office's use of the patient's protected health information (PHI).

no·ti·fi·a·ble dis·ease (nō′ti-fī′ă-bĕl di-zēz′) Disorder that, by statutory requirements, must be reported to public health or veterinary authorities or to law enforcement agencies. SYN reportable disease.

nox·ious (nok′shŭs) Injurious; harmful.

NPH in·su·lin (in′sŭ-lin) Modified form of insulin composed of insulin, protamine, and zinc; an intermediate acting preparation used for the treatment of diabetes mellitus. SYN isophane insulin.

N ω-phos·pho·no·cre·a·tine (fos′fō-nō-krē′ă-tēn) SYN phosphocreatine.

NPO, npo, n.p.o. Abbreviation for L. *nil per os,* nothing by mouth.

NSAID (en′sād) Acronym for nonsteroidal antiinflammatory drug.

nu (nū) Thirteenth letter of the Greek alphabet, *ν.*

nu·cha (nū′kă) The back of the neck. SYN nape.

nu·chal arm (nū′kăl ahrm) Situation in vaginal breech delivery during which one or both fetal arms are found around the back of the neck, interfering with delivery.

nu·chal plane (nū′kăl plān) The external surface of the squamous part of the occipital bone below the superior nuchal line, giving attachment to the muscles of the back of the neck.

♻ **nucl-** SEE nucleo-.

nu·cle·ar (nū′klē-ăr) *Avoid mispronunciation nucular.* Relating to a nucleus, either cellular or atomic.

nu·cle·ar ag·gre·ga·tion (nū′klē-ăr ag′rĕ-gā′shŭn) SYN syncytial knot.

nu·cle·ar cat·a·ract (nū′klē-ăr kat′ăr-akt) A cataract involving the nucleus of the lens.

nu·cle·ar:cy·to·plas·mic (N:C) ra·ti·o (nū′klē-ăr-sī′tō-plaz′mik rā′shē-ō) The ratio of the volume of the cell's nucleus to the volume of the cytoplasm.

nu·cle·ar en·er·gy (nū′klē-ăr en′ĕr-jē) That given off in the course of a nuclear reaction or stored in the formation of an atomic nucleus.

nu·cle·ar en·vel·ope (nū′klē-ăr en′vĕ-lōp) The double membrane at the boundary of the nucleoplasm. SYN nuclear membrane.

nu·cle·ar fac·tor-κB (NF-κB) (nū′klē-ăr fak′tŏr) Evolutionarily conserved eukaryotic transcription factor system that contributes to the mounting of an effective immune response but also plays an important role in many other cellular processes.

nu·cle·ar hy·a·lo·plasm (nū′klē-ăr hī′ă-lō-plazm) SYN karyolymph.

nu·cle·ar in·clu·sion bod·ies (nū′klē-ăr in-klū′zhŭn bod′ēz) SEE inclusion bodies.

nu·cle·ar jaun·dice (nū′klē-ăr jawn′dis) SYN kernicterus.

nu·cle·ar lam·i·na (nū′klē-ăr lam′i-nă) Protein-rich layer lining the inner surface of the nuclear membrane in interphase cells.

nu·cle·ar mag·net·ic res·o·nance (NMR) (nū′klē-ăr mag-net′ik rez′ŏ-năns) The phenomenon in which certain atomic nuclei possessing a magnetic moment will precess around the axis of a strong external magnetic field, the frequency of precession being specific for each nucleus and the strength of the magnetic field; used to identify covalent bonds.

nu·cle·ar med·i·cine (nū′klē-ăr med′i-sin) Clinical discipline concerned with diagnostic and therapeutic uses of radionuclides, excluding therapeutic use of sealed radiation sources.

nu·cle·ar mem·brane (nū′klē-ăr mem′brăn) SYN nuclear envelope.

nu·cle·ar oph·thal·mo·ple·gi·a (nū′klē-ăr of-thal′mō-plē′jē-ă) Ophthalmoplegia due to a lesion of the nuclei of origin of the motor nerves of the eye.

nuc·le·ar ra·di·ol·o·gy (nū-klē-ăr rā′dē-ol′ŏ-jē) Science or study of the use of radioactive materials in diagnosis or therapy.

Nu·cle·ar Reg·u·la·tor·y Com·mis·sion (NRC) (nū′klē-ăr reg′yū-lă-tōr′ē kŏ-mish′ŭn) The U.S. federal commission supervising the use of radioactive by-product material for commercial and medical purposes.

nuc·le·ar scan·ning (nū′klē-ăr skan′ing) A scan or test that uses radioactive isotopes to make the assessment.

nu·cle·ar spin·dle (nū′klē-ăr spin′dĕl) SYN mitotic spindle.

nu·cle·ase (nū′klē-ās) General term for enzymes that catalyze the hydrolysis of nucleic acid into nucleotides or oligonucleotides. Cf. exonuclease, endonuclease.

nu·cle·at·ed (nū′klē-āt-ĕd) Provided with a nucleus, a characteristic of all true cells.

nu·cle·ic ac·id (nū-klē′ik as′id) A family of macromolecules found in the chromosomes, nucleoli, mitochondria, and cytoplasm of all cells, and in viruses; in complexes with proteins, they are called nucleoproteins.

nu·cle·i·form (nū′klē-i-fōrm) Shaped like or having the appearance of a nucleus. SYN nucleoid (1).

nu·cle·i of or·i·gin (nū′klē-ī ōr′i-jin) Collections of motor neurons (forming a continuous column in the spinal cord, discontinuous in the medulla and pons) giving origin to the spinal and cranial motor nerves. SYN nucleus originis [TA], motor nuclei.

nucleo-, nucl- Combining forms meaning nucleus, nuclear. SEE ALSO karyo-, caryo-.

nu·cle·o·chy·le·ma (nū′klē-ō-kī-lē′mă) SYN karyolymph.

nu·cle·o·fu·gal (nū′klē-ō-f′yū-găl) 1. Moving within the cell body in a direction away from the nucleus. 2. Moving away from a nerve nucleus.

nu·cle·o·his·tone (nū′klē-ō-his′tōn) A complex of histone and deoxyribonucleic acid, the form in which the latter is usually found in the nuclei of cells.

nu·cle·oid (nū′klē-oyd) 1. SYN nucleiform. 2. A nuclear inclusion body. 3. SYN nucleus (2).

nu·cle·o·lar or·gan·i·zer (nū′klē-ō′lăr ōr′gă-nī-zĕr) Region of the satellites on the acrocentric chromosomes that is active in nucleolus formation. SYN nucleolar zone, nucleolus organizer.

nu·cle·o·li·form (nū′klē-ō′li-fōrm) Resembling a nucleolus. SYN nucleoloid.

nu·cle·o·loid (nū′klē-ō-loyd) SYN nucleoliform.

nu·cle·o·lo·ne·ma (nū′klē-ō′lŏ-nē′mă) The irregular network or rows of fine ribonucleoprotein granules or microfilaments forming most of the nucleolus.

nu·cle·o·lus, pl. **nu·cle·o·li** (nū-klē′ŏ-lŭs, -lī) *Avoid the mispronunciation nucleo′lus.* 1. A small, rounded mass within the cell nucleus where ribosomal ribonucleoprotein is produced. 2. A more-or-less central body in the vesicular nucleus of certain protozoa in which an endosome is lacking but one or more Feulgen-positive (deoxyribonucleic acid+) nucleoli are present.

nu·cle·on (nū′klē-on) 1. One of the subatomic particles of the atomic nucleus; i.e., either a proton or a neutron. 2. Slang term for specialist in nuclear medicine.

nu·cle·o·pe·tal (nū′klē-op′ĕ-tăl) 1. Moving in the cell body in a direction toward the nucleus. 2. Moving in a direction toward a nerve nucleus; said of a nervous impulse.

nu·cle·o·phil (nū′klē-ō-fil) The electron pair donor atom in a chemical reaction in which a pair of electrons is picked up by an electrophil. SYN nucleophilic (1).

nu·cle·o·phil·ic (nū′klē-ō-fil′ik) 1. SYN nucleophil (2). 2. A reaction involving a nucleophile.

nu·cle·o·plasm (nū′klē-ō-plazm) The protoplasm of the nucleus of a cell.

nu·cle·o·plas·min (nū′klē-ō-plas′min) Contents of resting (interphase) nucleus.

N

nu·cle·o·pro·tein (nū′klē-ō-prō′tēn) A complex of protein and nucleic acid.

nu·cle·or·rhex·is (nū′klē-ō-rek′sis) Fragmentation of a cell nucleus.

nu·cle·o·si·das·es (nū′klē-ō-sī′dās-ĕz) Enzymes that catalyze the hydrolysis or phosphorolysis of nucleosides, releasing the purine or pyrimidine base.

nu·cle·o·side (Nuc, N) (nū′klē-ō-sīd) A compound of a sugar with a purine or pyrimidine base by way of an *N*glycosyl link.

nu·cle·o·some (nū′klē-ō-sōm) A localized aggregation of histone and DNA that is evident when chromatin is in the uncondensed stage. SYN nu body.

nu·cle·o·ti·das·es (nū′klē-ō-tī′dās-ĕz) Enzymes that catalyze the hydrolysis of nucleotides into phosphoric acid and nucleosides.

nu·cle·o·tide (nū′klē-ō-tīd) A combination of a (nucleic acid) purine or pyrimidine, one sugar (usually ribose or deoxyribose), and a phosphoric group.

nu·cle·o·tid·yl·trans·fer·as·es (nū′klē-ō-tī′dil-trans′fĕr-ās-ĕz) Enzymes transferring nucleotide residues (nucleotidyls) from nucleoside di- or triphosphates into dimer or polymer forms.

nu·cle·o·tox·in (nū′klē-ō-tok′sin) A toxin acting on the cell nuclei.

nu·cle·us, gen. and pl. **nu·cle·i**, pl. **nu·cle·us·es** (nū′klē-ŭs, -ī, -ŭs-ĕz) [TA] **1.** CYTOLOGY typically a rounded or oval mass of protoplasm within the cytoplasm of a plant or animal cell; it is surrounded by a nuclear envelope, which encloses euchromatin, heterochromatin, and one or more nucleoli and undergoes mitosis during cell division. **2.** By extension, because of similar function, the genome of microorganisms (microbes), which is relatively simple in structure, lacks a nuclear membrane and does not undergo mitosis during replication. SYN nucleoid (3). **3.** NEUROANATOMY a group of nerve cell bodies in the brain or spinal cord that can be demarcated from neighboring groups on the basis of either differences in cell type or the presence of a surrounding zone of nerve fibers or cell-poor neuropil. **4.** Any substance around which a urinary or other calculus is formed. **5.** The central portion of an atom (composed of protons and neutrons) where most of the mass and all of the positive charge are concentrated. **6.** A particle on which a crystal, droplet, or bubble forms. **7.** A characteristic arrangement of atoms in a series of molecules. SEE ALSO virion.

nu·clide (nū′klīd) A particular (atomic) nuclear species with defined atomic mass and number. SEE ALSO isotope.

null-cell ad·e·no·ma (nŭl′sel′ ad′ĕ-nō′mă) Hypophysial lesion composed of cells for which there is no overt evidence of hormone production, but which usually produces hypopituitarism and visual disturbances by compression of adjacent structures. SYN undifferentiated cell adenoma.

null cells (nŭl selz) **1.** SYN killer cells. **2.** Large granular lymphocytes that lack surface markers or membrane-associated proteins of either B or T lymphocytes.

null hy·po·the·sis (nŭl hī-poth′ĕ-sis) The statistical hypothesis that one variable has no association with another, or that experimental results do not differ from those that might be expected by the operation of chance alone.

nul·li·grav·i·da (nŭl′i-grav′i-dă) A woman who has never conceived a child.

nul·lip·a·ra (nŭ-lip′ă-ră) A woman who has never borne children.

nul·li·par·i·ty (nŭl′i-par′i-tē) Condition of having borne no children.

nul·lip·a·rous (nŭl-ip′ă-rŭs) Having never borne children.

null-, nulli- Combining forms meaning no, none, missing or absence of.

numb (nŭm) Denotes absence of feeling or sensation.

num·ber (nŭm′bĕr) **1.** A symbol expressive of a certain value or of a specific quantity determined by count. **2.** The place of any unit in a series.

numb·ness (nŭm′nĕs) Imprecise term for abnormal sensation, including absent or reduced sensory perception as well as paresthesias.

nu·mer·ic pain scale (nū-mer´ik păn skāl) A method by which patients may self-rate their level of pain with 0 as no pain and a 10 being the worst pain; some come as printed samples so that patients may point to the level of pain for a health care worker.

nu·mer·ic tax·on·o·my (nū-mer´ik taks-on´ŏ-mē) Approach to the classification of organisms that strives for objectivity, wherein characteristics of organisms are given equal weight and the relationships of the organisms are numerically determined, usually by computer.

num·mu·lar (nŭm´yū-lăr) 1. Discoid or coin-shaped. 2. Arranged like stacks of coins, denoting the lining up of the red blood cells into rouleaux formation.

num·mu·lar ec·ze·ma, num·mu·lar der·ma·ti·tis (nŭm´yū-lăr ek´sĕ-mă, dĕr´mă-tī-tis) Discrete, coin-shaped patches of eczema.

num·mu·lar spu·tum (nŭm´yū-lăr spyūt´ŭm) A thick, coherent mass expectorated in globular shape that does not run at the bottom of the cup but forms a discoid coin-shaped mass.

nurse (nŭrs) 1. To breast-feed; suckle. 2. To provide care of the sick. 3. One who is educated in the scientific basis of nursing under defined standards of education and is concerned with the diagnosis and treatment of human responses to actual or potential health problems.

nurse an·es·the·tist (nŭrs ă-nes´thĕ-tist) A registered nurse qualified to administer anesthesia, in both inpatient and outpatient settings; in the U.S., the title "certified registered nurse anesthetist" (CRNA) is conferred on registered nurses with at least 1 year of acute care experience who complete a graduate program recognized by the American Association of Nurse Anesthetists and pass a national certification examination.

nurse cells (nŭrs selz) SYN Sertoli cells.

nurse-cli·ent re·la·tion·ship (nŭrs klī´ent rĕ-lā´shŭn-ship) A professional relationship between a patient and a nurse based on therapeutic communication. Not a social relationship.

nurse ep·i·de·mi·ol·o·gist (nŭrs ep´ĭ-dē´mē-ol´ŏ-jist) A registered nurse with additional education in the monitoring and prevention of nosocomial infections in the client population in an agency. SYN infection control nurse.

nurse-mid·wife (nŭrs-mid´wīf) A nurse with specialized training in delivering babies.

nurse prac·tice act (nŭrs prak´tis akt) Legal provisions in each U.S. state regulating nursing practice; intent is to protect public and enforce acceptable standards of practice.

nurse prac·ti·tion·er (NP) (nŭrs prak-tish´ŭn-ĕr) A registered nurse with advanced education in the primary care of particular groups of patients; who provides services, within the scope of nursing practice, in the areas of health promotion, disease prevention, therapy, rehabilitation, and support.

nurs·ing (nŭrs´ing) 1. A discipline, profession, and area of practice. As a discipline, nursing is centered on knowledge development. Emphasis is placed on discovering, describing, extending, and modifying knowledge for professional nursing practice. As a profession, nursing has a social mandate to be responsible and accountable to the public it serves. Nursing is an integral part of the health care system, and as such encompasses the promotion of health, prevention of illness, and care of physically ill, mentally ill, and disabled people of all ages, in all health care settings and other community contexts. 2. Feeding an infant at the breast; tending and caring for a young child.

nurs·ing au·dit (nŭrs´ing aw´dit) A method of evaluating nursing practice by reviewing records that document the care provided to patients.

nurs·ing care plan (nŭrs´ing kār plan) Care plan created by a nurse for patients as a result of assessment of patient needs; focused on nursing interventions, not medical interventions.

nurs·ing con·cep·tu·al frame·work (nŭrs´ing kŏn-sep´shū´ăl frām´wŏrk) A grouping of related concepts and theories that are of importance to nurses to guide nursing practice, education, and research. SYN nursing model.

nurs·ing di·ag·no·sis (nŭrs'ing dī'ăg-nō'sis) The process of assessing potential or actual health problems, including those pertaining to an individual patient, a family or community, which fall within the scope of nursing practice. SEE ALSO diagnosis.

nurs·ing ed·u·ca·tion pro·gram (nŭrs'ing ed'yŭ-kā'shŭn prō'gram) Planned curriculum usually with clinical practice experiences to prepare nurses; includes diploma (hospital school of nursing), at associate, baccalaureate (bachelor's), master's, and doctoral levels; also includes certificate, continuing education, and in-service programs.

nurs·ing his·to·ry (nŭrs'ing his'tŏr-ē) Comprehensive set of information about a patient's medical history, including the history of the present illness, as well as the person's psychosocial and spiritual history.

nurs·ing home (nŭrs'ing hōm) SYN extended-care facility.

nurs·ing in·for·ma·tics (nŭrs'ing in'fōr-mat'iks) 1. Nursing specialty surrounding the use of computer technology to support nursing practice, management, research, and education. 2. Integration of data to support patient care, nurses, and other providers.

nurs·ing in·ter·ven·tion (nŭrs'ing in'tĕr-ven'shŭn) Treatments that nurses perform in all settings and in all specialties; activities nurses perform; nursing care measures.

Nurs·ing In·ter·ven·tions Clas·si·fi·ca·tion (NIC) (nŭrs'ing in'tĕr-ven'shŭnz klas'i-fi-kā'shŭn) Standardized classification of patient outcomes for evaluating effects of nursing interventions.

Nurs·ing Min·i·mum Da·ta Set (nŭrs'ing min'i-mŭm dā'tă set) 1. Standardized set of nursing data developed to describe nursing care applicable across diverse clinical practice settings. 2. Smallest amount of information necessary to define cost and quality of nursing care.

Nurs·ing Out·comes Clas·si·fi·ca·tion (NOC) (nŭrs'ing owt'kŭmz klas'i-fi-kā'shŭn) Standardized classification of

patient outcomes for evaluating effects of nursing interventions.

nurs·ing pro·cess (nŭrs'ing pros'es) Structured, organized, and systematic approach to developing and delivering patient care including assessment, diagnosis, planning, implementation, and evaluation. Nursing theories and conceptual frameworks guide each step of the nursing process.

nurs·ing the·o·ry (nŭrs'ing thē'ŏr-ē) Set of concepts, definitions, and propositions that present a systematic view of various phenomena related to nursing's unique role.

nur·ture (nŭr'chŭr) 1. To train or bring up. 2. To help someone by giving them encouragement.

nu·ta·tion (nū-tā'shŭn) CHIROPRACTIC the backward rotation of the ilium on the sacrum. USAGE NOTE this concept is not shared by some medical practitioners.

nu·tra·ceu·ti·cal, nu·tri·ceu·ti·cal (nū'tră-sū'ti-kăl, nū'tri-) A product derived from a food marketed in the form of medicine and demonstrated to have a physiologic benefit. Cf. functional food.

nu·tra·ge·nom·ics (nū'tră-jē-nō'miks) SYN nutrigenomics.

nu·tri·ent (nū'trē-ĕnt) A constituent of food necessary for normal physiologic function.

nu·tri·ent ar·te·ry (nū'trē-ĕnt ahr'tĕr-ē) [TA] Blood vessel of variable origin that supplies the medullary cavity of a long bone. SYN arteria nutricia [TA], nutrient vessel.

nu·tri·ent en·e·ma (nū'trē-ĕnt en'ĕ-mă) Rectal injection of predigested food.

nu·tri·ent for·a·men (nū'trē-ĕnt fōr-ā'mĕn) [TA] External opening for the entrance of blood vessels in a bone. SYN foramen nutricium [TA].

nu·tri·ent sup·ple·ments (nū'trē-ĕnt sŭp'lĕ-mĕnts) Herbal remedies, minerals, and vitamins that are taken daily to provide items lacking in the diet (e.g., calcium).

nu·tri·ge·nom·ics (nū'tri-jē-nō'miks)

The study of how diet influences gene expression, and thus, health. SYN nutragenomics, nutritional genomics.

nu·tri·tion (nū-trish'ŭn) 1. A function of living plants and animals, consisting in the taking in and metabolism of food material whereby tissue is built up and energy liberated. 2. The study of the food and liquid requirements of human beings or animals for normal physiologic function.

nu·trit·ion·al am·bly·o·pi·a (nū-trish'ŏn-ăl am'blē-ō'pē-ă) Ocular condition resulting from lack of vitamin-B-complex constituents.

nu·trit·ion·al a·ne·mi·a (nū-trish'ŏn-ăl ă-nē'mē-ă) Any blood disorder resulting from a dietary deficiency of materials essential to red blood cell formation, e.g., iron, vitamins, protein. SYN deficiency anemia.

nu·tri·tion·ist (nū-trish'ŏn-ist) A health care specialist who concentrates on the body's requirements for particular foods, liquids, and nutrients to keep it in homeostasis.

nu·tri·tion ther·a·py (nū-trish'ŏn thār'ă-pē) Health care specialty area based on attaining better health through diet.

nu·tri·ti·ous (nū-trish'ŭs) Denotes a food or liquid good for your body.

nu·tri·tive (nū'tri-tiv) 1. Pertaining to nutrition. 2. Capable of nourishing.

nu·tri·ture (nū'tri-chŭr) State of the body with regard to nourishment.

nyc·tal·gi·a (nik-tal'jē-ă) Denoting especially the osteocopic pains of syphilis occurring at night.

nyc·ta·lo·pi·a (nik'tă-lō'pē-ă) Decreased ability to see in reduced illumination. SYN night blindness.

nyc·ter·ine (nik'tĕr-ēn) 1. By night. 2. Dark or obscure.

nycto-, nyct- Combining forms meaning night, nocturnal.

nyc·to·phil·i·a (nik'tō-fil'ē-ă) Preference for the night or darkness. SYN scotophilia.

nyc·tu·ri·a (nik-tyū'rē-ă) SYN nocturia.

nymph (nimf) 1. The earliest series of stages in metamorphosis following hatching in the development of hemimetabolous insects. 2. The third stage in the life cycle of a tick, between the larva and the adult.

nym·pha, pl. **nym·phae** (nim'fă, -fē) One of the labia minora.

nym·phec·to·my (nim-fek'tŏ-mē) Surgical removal of hypertrophied labia minora.

nym·phi·tis (nim-fī'tis) Inflammation of the labia minora.

nympho-, nymph- Combining forms indicating the nymphae (labia minora).

nym·pho·ma·ni·a (nim'fō-mā'nē-ă) An insatiable impulse to engage in sexual behavior in a female.

nym·phon·cus (nim-fongk'ŭs) Swelling or hypertrophy of one or both labia minora.

nym·phot·o·my (nim-fot'ŏ-mē) Incision into the labia minora or the clitoris.

nys·tag·mic (nis-tag'mik) Relating to or suffering from nystagmus.

nys·tag·mo·graph (nis-tag'mō-graf) An apparatus for measuring the amplitude, periodicity, and velocity of ocular movements in nystagmus, by measuring the change in the resting potential of the eye as the eye moves.

nys·tag·moid (nis-tag'moyd) Resembling nystagmus. SYN nystagmiform.

nys·tag·mus (nyst) (nis-tag'mŭs) Involuntary rhythmic oscillation of the eyeballs, either pendular or with a slow and fast component.

ny·stat·in (NY) (nī-stat'in) An antibiotic substance effective in the treatment of all forms of candidiasis, particularly in the intestine, skin, and mucous membranes.

Ny·sten law (nē-stan[h]' law) That rigor mortis affects first the muscles of the head and spreads toward the feet.

nyx·is (nik'sis) A pricking; paracentesis.

N

O

O ag·glu·ti·nin (ă-glū′ti-nin) One formed as the result of stimulation by, and that reacts with, the relatively thermostable antigen(s) in the cell bodies of microorganisms.

O an·ti·gen (an′ti-jen) Somatic antigen of enteric gram-negative bacteria.

oat cell car·ci·no·ma (ōt sel kahr′si-nō′mă) An anaplastic, highly malignant, and usually bronchogenic carcinoma composed of small ovoid cells with very scanty cytoplasm. SYN small cell carcinoma (2).

ob·dor·mi·tion (ob′dōr-mi′shŭn) Numbness of an extremity, due to pressure on the sensory nerve.

o·be·li·on (ō-bē′lē-on) A craniometric point on the sagittal suture between the parietal foramina near the lambdoid suture.

O·ber·stei·ner-Red·lich zone (ō′bĕr-stī′-nĕr red′lik zōn) Narrow line along the course of a nerve (or nerve root) where the Schwann cells and connective tissue that support its axons are replaced by glia cells. The zone marks the true boundary between the central and the peripheral nervous system.

o·bese (ō-bēs′) *Negative or pejorative connotations of this word may render it offensive in some contexts.* Excessively fat.

o·be·si·ty (ō-bē′si-tē) An excessive accumulation of fat in the body. SYN adiposity (1), corpulency.

o·be·si·ty-hy·po·ven·ti·la·tion syn·drome (ō-bē′si-tē hī′pō-ven′ti-lā′shŭn sin′drŏm) Constellation of findings consisting of obesity, hypoxemia, hypercapnia, erythrocytosis, and lethargy.

ob·fus·ca·tion (ob′fŭs-kā′shŭn) 1. Rendering something dark or obscure. 2. A deliberate attempt to confuse or to prevent understanding.

OB/GYN (ob-gīn′) Acronym and abbreviation for obstetrics and gynecology. SEE obstetrics; gynecology.

ob·ject choice (ob′jekt choys) In psychoanalysis, the object (usually a person) on which psychic energy is centered.

ob·ject con·stan·cy (ob′jekt kon′stăn-sē) 1. Tendency for objects to be perceived as unchanging despite variations in the positions in and conditions under which the objects are observed. 2. In psychoanalysis, relatively enduring emotional investment in another person.

ob·jec·tive (ŏb-jek′tiv) 1. The lens or lenses in the object end of the body tube of a microscope, by means of which the rays coming from the object examined are brought to a focus. SYN object glass. 2. Viewing events or phenomena as they exist in the external world, impersonally, or in an unprejudiced way; open to observation by oneself and by others. Cf. subjective.

ob·jec·tive as·sess·ment da·ta (ŏb-jek′tiv ă-ses′mĕnt dā′tă) Information about a patient that is observable and measurable by the nurse.

ob·jec·tive sen·sa·tion (ŏb-jek′tiv sen-sā′shŭn) A sensation caused by a verifiable stimulus.

ob·jec·tive sign (ŏb-jek′tiv sīn) Finding that is evident to the examiner.

ob·jec·tive symp·tom (ŏb-jek′tiv simp′tŏm) A symptom that is evident to the observer.

ob·ject per·ma·nence (ob′jekt pĕr′mă-nĕns) Developmental term for a child's ability to understand that objects still exist even when out of sight. Infants 8 months old or younger rarely have this ability.

ob·ject re·la·tion·ship (ob′jekt rĕ-lā′shŭn-ship) BEHAVIORAL SCIENCES the emotional bond between an individual and another person (or between two groups), as opposed to the individual's or group's interest in self.

ob·li·gate (ob′li-găt) Without an alternative system or pathway.

ob·li·gate aer·obe (ob′li-găt ār′ōb) An organism that cannot live or grow in the absence of oxygen.

ob·li·gate an·aer·obe (ob′li-găt an′ār-ōb) An anaerobe that will grow only in the absence of free oxygen.

ob·li·gate pa·ra·site (ob′li-găt par′ă-sīt)

A parasite that cannot lead an independent nonparasitic existence.

ob·lique (ō-blēk′) **1.** Slanting; deviating from the perpendicular, horizontal, sagittal, or coronal plane of the body. **2.** RADIOGRAPHY a projection that is neither frontal nor lateral.

ob·lique am·pu·ta·tion (ō-blēk′ amp′yū-tā′shŭn) Surgery in which the line of section through an extremity is at other than a right angle.

ob·lique band·age (ō-blēk′ ban′dăj) Dressing in which successive turns proceed obliquely up or down a limb, in a slanting or sloping pattern.

ob·lique di·am·e·ter (ō-blēk′ dī-am′ĕ-tĕr) [TA] Measurement across the pelvic inlet from the sacroiliac joint of one side to the opposite iliopectineal eminence. SYN diameter obliqua [TA].

ob·lique frac·ture (ō-blēk′ frak′shŭr) A break along the line that runs obliquely to the axis of the bone.

ob·lique pres·en·ta·tion (ō-blēk′ prez′ĕn-tā′shŭn) A fetal presentation in which the long axis of the fetus is oblique (i.e., slanted) with respect to the long axis of the mother. Also called oblique lie.

ob·lique ridge (ō-blēk′ rij) Crest on the upper molar occlusal surfaces comprising the distal cusp ridge of the mesiolingual cusp and the triangular ridge of the distobuccal cusp.

ob·lit·er·a·tion (ob-lit′ĕr-ā′shŭn) **1.** Blotting out. **2.** RADIOLOGY disappearance of the contour of an organ when the adjacent tissue has the same x-ray absorption.

o·blit·er·a·tive bron·chi·tis, bron·chi·tis ob·li·te·rans (ŏ-blit′ĕr-ā′tiv brongk′ī-tis, ŏb-lit′ĕr-anz) Fibrinous bronchitis in which the exudate is not expectorated but becomes organized, obliterating the affected portion of the bronchial tubes with consequent permanent collapse of affected portions of the lung.

ob·ses·sion (ŏb-sesh′ŭn) A recurrent and persistent idea, thought, or impulse to carry out an act that is ego dystonic, which is experienced as senseless or repugnant, but that the person cannot voluntarily suppress.

ob·ses·sive-com·pul·sive dis·or·der (OCD) (ŏb-ses′iv-kŏm-pŭl′siv dis-ōr′dĕr) Anxiety disorder the essential features of which include recurrent obsessions, persistent intrusive ideas, thoughts, impulses or images, or compulsions (repetitive, purposeful, and intentional behaviors performed to decrease anxiety in response to an obsession) sufficiently severe to cause marked distress, be time consuming, or significantly interfere with the person's normal routine, occupational functioning, or usual social activities or relationships with others. SEE ALSO obsessive-compulsive personality disorder.

ob·ses·sive-com·pul·sive per·son·al·i·ty dis·or·der (OCPD) (ŏb-ses′iv-kŏm-pŭl′siv pĕr′sŏ-nal′i-tē dis-ōr′dĕr) Pervasive pattern in adulthood characterized by unattainable perfectionism; preoccupation with rules, details, and orderliness; unreasonable attempts to control others; excessive devotion to work; and rumination to the point of indecisiveness, all at the expense of flexiblity, openness, and efficiency. SYN compulsive personality.

ob·so·les·cence (ob′sŏ-les′ĕns) Falling into disuse; denoting abolition of a function.

ob·stet·ric, ob·stet·ri·cal (ob-stet′rik, -ri-kăl) Relating to obstetrics.

ob·stet·ric bind·er (ob-stet′rik bīn′dĕr) A supporting garment covering the abdomen from the ribs to the trochanters, tightly pinned at the back, affording support after childbirth or, rarely, during childbirth.

ob·stet·ric con·ju·gate (ob-stet′rik kon′jŭ-găt) The shortest diameter through which the fetal head must pass in descending into the superior strait.

ob·stet·ric for·ceps (ob-stet′rik fōr′seps) Forceps used for grasping and applying traction to or for rotation of the fetal head.

ob·stet·rics (OB) (ob-stet′riks) The specialty of medicine concerned with the care of women during pregnancy, parturition, and the puerperium.

O

ob·sti·nate (ob'sti-năt) **1.** Firmly adhering to one's own purpose or opinion, even when wrong. SYN intractable (2), refractory (2). **2.** SYN refractory (1).

ob·sti·pa·tion (ob'sti-pā'shŭn) Intestinal obstruction; severe constipation.

ob·struc·tion (ŏb-strŭk'shŭn) Blockage or clogging, e.g., by occlusion or stenosis.

ob·struc·tive air·ways dis·ease (ŏb-strŭk'tiv ār'wāz di-zēz') Respiratory disorder that affects the airway by constricting it completely or partially.

ob·struc·tive ap·pen·di·ci·tis (ŏb-strŭk'tiv ă-pen'di-sī'tis) Acute form due to infection of retained secretions behind an obstructed lumen by a fecalith or some other cause, including cancer.

ob·struc·tive hy·dro·ceph·a·lus (ŏb-strŭk'tiv hī'drō-sef'ă-lŭs) Form secondary to a block in cerebrospinal fluid flow in the ventricular system or between the ventricular system and spinal canal.

ob·struc·tive jaun·dice (ŏb-strŭk'tiv jawn'dis) Hepatic disorder resulting from obstruction to the flow of bile into the duodenum, whether intra- or extrahepatic. SYN mechanical jaundice.

ob·struc·tive mur·mur (ŏb-strŭk'tiv mŭr'mŭr) Second caused by narrowing of one of the valvular orifices.

ob·struc·tive sleep ap·ne·a (OSA) (ŏb-strŭk'tiv slēp ap'nē-ă) A disorder characterized by recurrent interruptions of breathing during sleep due to temporary obstruction of the airway by lax, excessively bulky, or malformed pharyngeal tissues with resultant hypoxemia and chronic lethargy.

ob·struc·tive u·rop·a·thy (ŏb-strŭk'tiv yūr-op'ă-thē) Any pathologic condition, anatomic or functional, of the urinary tract caused by obstruction.

ob·tun·da·tion (ob'tŭn-dā'shŭn) A condition in which the senses have been dulled by trauma, mistreatment, or psychological stress.

ob·tu·ra·tor (ob'tŭr-ā-tŏr) **1.** Any structure that occludes an opening. **2.** Denoting the obturator foramen, the obturator

membrane, or any of several parts in relation to this foramen. **3.** A prosthesis used to close an opening in the hard palate, usually in a cleft palate. **4.** The stylus or removable plug used during the insertion of many tubular instruments.

ob·tu·ra·tor her·ni·a (ob'tŭr-ā-tŏr hĕr'nē-ă) Hernia through the obturator foramen.

ob·tu·sion (ŏb-tū'zhŭn) **1.** Dullness of sensibility. **2.** A dulling or deadening of sensibility.

oc·cip·i·tal (ok-sip'i-tăl) Relating to the occiput; referring to the occipital bone or to the back of the head.

oc·cip·i·tal an·chor·age (ok-sip'i-tăl ang'kŏr-ăj) Form in which the top and back of the head are used for resistance by means of a piece of headgear.

oc·cip·i·tal horn syn·drome (ok-sip'i-tăl hōrn sin'drōm) Disorder with defective biliary excretion of copper, resulting in a lysyl oxidase deficiency causing skin and joint laxity.

oc·cip·i·tal·i·za·tion (ok-sip'i-tăl-ī-zā'shŭn) Bony ankylosis between the atlas and occipital bone.

oc·cip·i·tal lobe of cer·e·brum (ok-sip'i-tăl lōb ser'ĕ-brŭm) [TA] The posterior, somewhat pyramidal part of each cerebral hemisphere, demarcated by no distinct surface markings on the lateral convexity of the hemisphere from the parietal and temporal lobes, but sharply delineated from the parietal lobe by the parieto-occipital sulcus on the medial surface. At times called simply occipital lobe.

oc·cip·i·tal plane (ok-sip'i-tăl plān) [TA] External surface of the occipital bone above the superior nuchal line. SYN planum occipitale [TA].

oc·cip·i·tal si·nus (ok-sip'i-tăl sī'nŭs) [TA] An unpaired dural venous sinus commencing at the confluence of the sinuses and passing downward in the base of the falx cerebelli to the foramen magnum.

oc·cip·i·tal tri·an·gle (ok-sip'i-tăl trī'ang-gĕl) Area of the neck bounded by the trapezius, the sternocleidomastoid, and the omohyoid muscles. SEE ALSO inferior occipital triangle.

oc·cip·i·to·breg·mat·ic (ok-sip′i-tō-breg-mat′ik) Relating to the occiput and bregma; denoting a measurement in craniometry.

oc·cip·i·to·cer·vi·cal (ok-sip′i-tō-sĕr′vi-kăl) Denotes involvement of both the back of the head and the neck.

oc·cip·i·to·fron·tal (ok-sip′i-tō-frŏn′tăl) **1.** Relating to the occiput and forehead. **2.** Relating to the occipital and frontal lobe of the cerebral cortex and association pathways them.

oc·cip·i·to·mas·toid (ok-sip′i-tō-mas′toyd) Relating to the occipital bone and mastoid process.

oc·cip·i·to·men·tal (OM) (ok-sip′i-tō-men′tăl) Relating to the occiput and chin.

oc·cip·i·to·pa·ri·e·tal (OP) (ok-sip′i-tō-pă-rī′ĕ-tăl) Relating to the occipital and parietal bones.

oc·cip·i·to·pos·te·ri·or po·si·tion (ok-sip′i-tō-pos-tēr′ē-ōr pŏ-zish′ŏn) A cephalic presentation of the fetus with its occiput turned toward the right or left sacroiliac joint of the mother.

oc·cip·i·to·tem·po·ral (ok-sip′i-tō-tem′pŏ-răl) Relating to the occiput and temple, or the occipital and temporal bones.

oc·cip·i·to·tha·lam·ic (ok-sip′i-tō-thă-lam′ik) Relating to the nerve fibers leading from the occipital lobe of the cerebral cortex to the thalamus.

oc·cip·i·to·trans·verse po·si·tion (ok-sip′i-tō-trans-vĕrs′ pŏ-zish′ŏn) A cephalic presentation of the fetus with its occiput turned toward the right or left iliac fossa of the mother.

oc·ci·put, gen. **oc·cip·i·tis** (ok′si-put, ok-sip′i-tis) [TA] The back of the head.

oc·clude (ŏ-klūd′) **1.** To close, plug, obstruct, or bring together. **2.** To enclose. SEE occlusion.

oc·clu·ding throm·bus (ŏ-klūd′ing throm′bŭs) A clot that completely blocks the interior of a blood vessel.

oc·clu·sal (ŏ-klū′zăl) **1.** Pertaining to occlusion or closure. **2.** In dentistry, pertaining to the contacting surfaces of opposing occlusal units (teeth or occlusion rims) or the masticating surfaces of the posterior teeth.

oc·clu·sal a·nal·ysis (ŏ-klū′zăl ă-nal′i-sis) A study of the relations of the occlusal surfaces of opposing teeth and their effect on related structures. SYN bite analysis.

oc·clu·sal form (ŏ-klū′zăl fōrm) Shape of the occlusal surface of a tooth or a row of teeth. SYN occlusal pattern.

oc·clu·sal har·mo·ny (ŏ-klū′zăl hahr′mŏ-nē) Occlusion without deflective or interceptive occlusal contacts in centric jaw relation as well as eccentric movements.

oc·clu·sal plane, plane of oc·clu·sion (ŏ-klū′zăl plān, ŏ-klū′zhŭn) Imaginary surface related anatomically to the cranium and theoretically touches the incisal edges of the incisors and the tips of the occluding surfaces of the posterior teeth. SEE ALSO curve of occlusion. SYN bite plane.

oc·clu·sal ra·di·o·graph (ŏ-klū′zăl rā′dē-ō-graf) Intraoral section film positioned on the occlusal plane used in visualizing entire sections of the jaw.

oc·clu·sal rest (ŏ-klū′zăl rest) Rigid extension of a removable partial denture onto the occlusal surface of a posterior tooth for support of the prosthesis.

oc·clu·sal trau·ma (ŏ-klū′zăl traw′mă) Abnormal occlusal stresses capable of producing or that have produced pathologic changes in the tooth and its surrounding structures.

oc·clu·sion (ŏ-klū′zhŭn) **1.** The act of closing or the state of being closed. **2.** In chemistry, the absorption of a gas by a metal or the inclusion of one substance within another. **3.** Any contact between the incising or masticating surfaces of the upper and lower teeth. **4.** The relationship between the occlusal surfaces of the maxillary and mandibular teeth when in contact.

oc·clu·sion rim (ŏ-klū′zhŭn rim) Occluding surfaces built on temporary or permanent denture bases to make maxil-lomandibular relation records and arrange teeth. SYN bite rim, occlusal rim, record rim.

oc·clu·sive (ŏ-klū′siv) Serving to close; denoting a bandage or dressing that closes a wound and excludes it from the air.

oc·clu·sive dress·ing (ŏ-klū′siv dres′ ing) A dressing that hermetically seals a wound.

oc·clu·sive il·e·us (ŏ-klū′siv il′ē-ŭs) Complete mechanical blocking of the intestinal lumen.

oc·clu·sive men·in·gi·tis (ŏ-klū′siv men′ in-jī′tis) Leptomeningitis causing occlusion of the spinal fluid pathways.

oc·cult (ŏ-kŭlt′) 1. Hidden; concealed; not manifest. 2. Denoting a concealed hemorrhage, the blood being inapparent or localized to a site where it is not visible. SEE occult blood. 3. In oncology, a clinically unidentified primary tumor with recognized metastases.

oc·cult blood (ŏ-kŭlt′ blŭd) Blood in the feces in amounts too small to be seen by the naked eye but detectable by chemical tests.

oc·cult car·ci·no·ma (ŏ-kŭlt′ kahr′si-nō′mă) Small lesion, either asymptomatic or giving rise to metastases without symptoms due to the primary carcinoma.

oc·cult frac·ture (ŏ-kŭlt′ frak′shŭr) A condition with clinical signs of fracture but no radiologic evidence.

oc·cult PEEP (ŏ-kŭlt′ pēp) SEE auto-positive-end-expiratory-pressure.

oc·cu·pa·tion·al per·for·mance (ok′ yū-pā′shŭn-ăl pĕr-fōr′măns) Broadly, engagement in purposeful activity; such behavior has an organizing and integrating effect on psychological and social functioning; it is employed in occupational therapy to restore or maintain interest and self-confidence, overcome disability, or combat various features of physical or mental illness.

oc·cu·pa·tion·al role (ok′yū-pā′shŭn-ăl rōl) Behaviors connected to social norms that allow someone to organize and allo-cate time for self-care activities, work, play, social activities, leisure, and rest.

Oc·cu·pa·tion·al Safe·ty and Health Ad·min·i·stra·tion (OSHA) (ok′yū-pā′shŭn-ăl sāf′tē helth ad-min′i-strā′ shŭn) A division of the U.S. Department of Labor, responsible for establishing and enforcing safety and health standards in the workplace.

oc·cu·pa·tion·al ther·a·pist (ok′yū-pā′shŭn-ăl thār′ă-pist) A degree conferred on completion of a 2-year professional course pursued by the holder of a B.A. or B.Sc. degree. Practitioners use their skills to help patients regain or continue living a normal life after illness or injury.

oc·cu·pa·tion·al ther·a·py (ok′yū-pā′shŭn-ăl thār′ă-pē) Therapeutic use of self-care, work, and recreational activities to increase independent function, enhance development, prevent disability, and achieve optimal quality of life.

O·chro·bac·trum (ō-krō-bak′trŭm) A gram-negative bacterial genus found in environmental and water sources; isolated from clinical facilities where it may cause of nosocomial bacteremia.

o·chrom·e·ter (ō-krom′ĕ-tĕr) An instrument for determining the capillary blood pressure.

o·chron·o·sis (ō′kron-ō′sis) A condition observed in people with alkaptonuria, characterized by pigmentation of the cartilages; also may affect the sclerae, mucous membrane of the lips, and skin of the ears, face, and hands.

o·chron·ot·ic (ō′kron-ot′ik) Relating to or characterized by ochronosis.

oct-, octi-, octo-, octa- Combining forms meaning eight.

oc·ta·fluor·o·pro·pane (ok′tă-flōr′ō-prō′ pān) A drug used for contrast enhancement during ultrasound imaging.

oc·tan (ok′tan) Applied to fever, the paroxysms of which recur every eighth day, the day of a paroxysm being counted as the first in the computation.

oc·to·pa·mine (ok-tō′pă-mēn) A sympathomimetic amine. SYN norsympatol, norsynephrine.

oc·tre·o·tide (OCT) (ok′trē-ō-tīd) Somatostatin analogue used to treat secretory diarrheal states and gastrointestinal bleeding.

oc·u·lar (ok′yū-lăr) **1.** SYN ophthalmic. **2.** The eyepiece of a microscope, the lens or lenses at the observer end of a microscope, by means of which the image focused by the objective is viewed.

oc·u·lar al·bin·ism 1 (ok′yū-lăr al′bin-izm) Visual disorder characterized by depigmentation of the fundus and prominent choroidal vessels, nystagmus, and titubation; vision is usually impaired. SYN Nettleshop-Falls albinism.

oc·u·lar al·bin·ism 2 (ok′yū-lăr al′bin-izm) Visual disorder characterized by hypoplasia of the fovea, marked impairment of vision, nystagmus, myopia, astigmatism, and protanomalous color blindness, in addition to albinism of the fundus. SYN Forsius-Eriksson albinism.

oc·u·lar al·bin·ism 3 (ok′yū-lăr al′bin-izm) Visual disorder characterized by impaired vision, translucent irides, congenital nystagmus, photophobia, albinotic fundi with hyperplasia of the fovea, and strabismus.

oc·u·lar bob·bing (ok′yū-lăr bob′ing) Sudden conjugate downward deviation of the eyes with a slow return to the normal position.

oc·u·lar cic·a·tri·cial pem·phi·goid (ok′yū-lăr sik′ă-trish′ăl pem′fi-goyd) A chronic disease that produces adhesions and progressive cicatrization and shrinkage of the conjunctival, oral, and vaginal mucous membranes.

oc·u·lar dys·met·ri·a (ok′yū-lăr dis-mē′trē-ă) Abnormality of ocular movements in which the eyes overshoot on attempting to fixate an object.

oc·u·lar hu·mor (ok′yū-lăr hyū′mŏr) One of two humors of the eye: aqueous and vitreous.

oc·u·lar·ist (ok′yū-lăr-ist) One skilled in the design, fabrication, and fitting of artificial eyes and the making of prostheses

associated with the appearance or function of the eyes.

oc·u·lar lar·va mi·grans (ok′yū-lăr lahr′vă mī′granz) Visceral larva migrans involving the eyes, primarily of older children; clinical symptoms include decreased visual acuity and strabismus.

oc·u·lar lar·va mi·grans gran·u·loma (ok′yū-lăr lahr′vă mī′granz gran′yū-lō′mă) Eosinophilic granulomata found surrounding dead worms (generally, *Toxocara* spp.) in the eye.

oc·u·lar mi·graine (ok′yū-lăr mī′grān) A form of migraine with transient monocular vision loss, typically in young adults, which may or may not be associated with headache around the eye.

oc·u·lar mus·cles (ok′yū-lăr mŭs′ĕlz) SYN extraocular muscles.

oc·u·lar ten·sion (Tn) (ok′yū-lăr ten′shŭn) Resistance of ocular tunics to deformation. Ocular pressure is measured in increased mmHg levels with a tonometer (q.v.).

oc·u·lar ver·ti·go (ok′yū-lăr vĕr′ti-gō) Dizziness attributed to refractive errors or imbalance of the extrinsic muscles.

oculo- Combining form meaning the eye, ocular. SEE ALSO ophthalmo-.

oc·u·lo·car·di·ac re·flex (ok′yū-lō-kahr′dē-ak rē′fleks) Decreased pulse rate associated with traction on extraocular muscles or compression of the eyeball. SYN Aschner phenomenon, Aschner reflex, Aschner-Dagnini reflex.

oc·u·lo·cu·ta·ne·ous (ok′yū-lō-kyū-tā′nē-ŭs) Relating to the eyes and the skin.

oc·u·lo·cu·ta·ne·ous al·bin·ism (ok′yū-lō-kyū-tā′nē-ŭs al′bi-nizm) Disorder characterized by deficiency of pigment in skin, hair, and eyes, photophobia, nystagmus, and decreased visual acuity.

oc·u·lo·dyn·i·a (ok′yū-lō-din′ē-ă) Pain in the eyeball. SYN ophthalmalgia.

oc·u·lo·fa·cial (ok′yū-lō-fā′shăl) Relating to the eyes and the face.

oc·u·log·ra·phy (ok′yū-log′ră-fē) A method of recording eye position and movements.

oc·u·lo·gy·ri·a (ok'yū-lō-jī'rē-ă) The limits of rotation of the eyeballs.

oc·u·lo·gy·ric (ok'yū-lō-jī'rik) Referring to rotation of the eyeballs; characterized by oculogyria.

oc·u·lo·man·dib·u·lo·dys·ceph·a·ly (OMD) (ok'yū-lō-man-dib'yū-lō-dis-sef'ă-lē) SYN dyscephalia mandibulooculofacialis.

oc·u·lo·mo·tor (ok'yū-lō-mō'tŏr) Pertaining to the oculomotor cranial nerve.

oc·u·lo·mo·tor nu·cle·us (ok'yū-lō-mō'tŏr nū'klē-ŭs) The composite group of motor neurons innervating all of the external eye muscles except the musculus rectus lateralis and musculus obliquus superior, and including the musculus levator palpebrae superioris.

oc·u·lo·my·co·sis (ok'yū-lō-mī-kō'sis) A fungal disease of the eyes.

oc·u·lo·na·sal (ok'yū-lō-nā'zăl) Relating to the eyes and the nose.

oc·u·lo·pha·ryn·ge·al dys·tro·phy (ok'yū-lō-fă-rin'jē-ăl dis'trŏ-fē) Chronic progressive external ophthalmoplegia usually presenting in middle life or old age with chronic ptosis and difficulty swallowing; many sufferers have Québecois ancestry.

oc·u·lo·pneu·mo·pleth·ys·mog·ra·phy (ok'yū-lō-nū'mō-pleth-iz-mog'ră-fē) A method of bilateral measurement of ophthalmic artery pressure that reflects pressure and flow in the internal carotid artery. SEE oculoplethysmography.

oc·u·lo·pu·pil·lar·y (ok'yū-lō-pyū'pil-ar-ē) Pertaining to the pupil of the eye.

oc·u·lo·sym·pa·thet·ic (ok'yū-lō-sim-pă-thet'ik) Pertaining to the sympathetic pathway to the eye, damage to which produces Horner syndrome.

oc·u·lo·zy·go·mat·ic (ok'yū-lō-zī-gō-mat'ik) Relating to the orbit or its margin and the zygomatic bone.

oc·u·lus, pl. **oc·u·li** (ok'yū-lŭs, -lī) [TA] SYN eye (1).

o·dax·et·ic (ō'dak-set'ik) Denotes causing formication or itching.

odont-, odonto- Combining forms meaning a tooth, teeth.

o·don·tal·gic (ō'don-tal'jik) Relating to or marked by toothache.

o·don·ti·a·sis (ō'don-tī'ă-sis) Teething.

o·don·tic (ō-don'tik) Denotes something pertaining to the teeth.

o·don·ti·tis (ō'don-tī'tis) SYN pulpitis.

o·don·to·blas·to·ma (ō-don'tō-blas-tō'mă) A tumor composed of neoplastic epithelial and mesenchymal cells that may differentiate into cells able to produce calcified tooth substances.

o·don·to·clast (ō-don'tō-klast) Osteoclastic cells believed to produce root resorption in deciduous teeth.

o·don·to·dys·pla·si·a (ō-don'tō-dis-plā'zē-ă) Developmental disturbance of one or of several adjacent teeth, of unknown etiology, characterized by deficient formation of enamel and dentin. SYN odontogenesis imperfecta, odontogenic dysplasia.

o·don·to·gen·e·sis (ō-don'tō-jen'ĕ-sis) Development of teeth. SYN odontogeny, odontosis.

o·don·to·gen·ic cyst (ō-don'tō-jen'ik sist) Lesion derived from odontogenic epithelium.

o·don·to·gen·ic ker·a·to·cyst (ō-don'tō-jen'ik ker'ă-tō-sist) A cyst originating in the dental lamina with a high recurrence rate, a corrugated parakeratin surface, uniformly thin epithelium, and a palisaded basal layer.

o·don·to·gen·ic myx·o·ma (ō-don'tō-jen'ik mik-sō'mă) Benign, expansile, multilocular radiolucent neoplasm of the jaws consisting of myxomatous fibrous connective tissue; presumably derived from the mesenchymal components of the odontogenic apparatus.

o·don·tog·e·ny (ō'don-toj'ĕ-nē) SYN odontogenesis.

o·don·toid (ō-don'toyd) **1.** Shaped like a

tooth. **2.** Relating to the toothlike odontoid process of the second cervical vertebra.

o·don·toid pro·cess (ō-don′toyd pros′es) SYN dens (2).

o·don·toid pro·cess of ep·i·stro·phe·us (ō-don′toyd pros′es ep′i-strō′fē-ŭs) SYN dens (2).

o·don·toid ver·te·bra (ō-don′toyd věr′tě-bră) SYN axis (4).

o·don·tol·o·gy (ō′don-tol′ŏ-jē) SYN dentistry.

o·don·tol·y·sis (ō′don-tol′i-sis) SYN erosion (3).

o·don·to·ma (ō′don-tō′mă) A tumor of odontogenic origin.

o·don·to·neu·ral·gi·a (ō-don′tō-nū-ral′jē-ă) Facial neuralgia caused by a carious tooth.

o·don·top·a·thy (ō′don-top′ă-thē) Any disease of the teeth or of their sockets.

o·don·tot·o·my (ō′don-tot′ŏ-mē) Cutting into the crown of a tooth.

o·dor (ō′dŏr) Emanation from any substance that stimulates the olfactory cells in the organ of smell.

o·dor·ant (ō′dŏr-ănt) A substance with an odor.

o·dor·if·er·ous, o·dor·ous (ō′dōr-if′ĕr-ŭs, ō′dōr-ŭs) Having a scent, perfume, or odor.

o·dyn·a·cu·sis (ō-din′ă-kyū′sis) Hypersensitivity of the organ of hearing, so that noises cause actual pain.

-odynia Combining form pertaining to pain.

o·dy·nom·e·ter (ō′di-nom′ě-těr) SYN algesiometer.

o·dyn·o·pha·gi·a (ō-din′ō-fā′jē-ă) Pain on swallowing.

oe- For words so beginning and not found here, see e-.

oedema [Br.] SYN edema.

oed·i·pal phase (ed′i-păl fāz) PSYCHO-ANALYSIS a stage in the psychosexual development of the child, characterized by erotic attachment to the parent of the opposite sex, repressed because of fear of the parent of the same sex; usually seen in children aged 3–6 years.

oesophageal [Br.] SYN esophageal.

oesophageal achalasia [Br.] SYN esophageal achalasia.

oesophageal hiatus [Br.] SYN esophageal hiatus.

oesophageal speech [Br.] SYN esophageal speech.

oesophageal veins [Br.] SYN esophageal veins.

oesophagectasis [Br.] SYN esophagectasis.

oesophagitis [Br.] SYN esophagitis.

oesophagocardioplasty [Br.] SYN esophagocardioplasty.

oesophagocele [Br.] SYN esophagocele.

oesophagoduodenostomy [Br.] SYN esophagoduodenostomy.

oesophagoenterostomy [Br.] SYN esophagoenterostomy.

oesophagogastrectomy [Br.] SYN esophagogastrectomy.

oesophagogastric junction [Br.] SYN esophagogastric junction.

oesophagogastroduodenoscopy [Br.] SYN esophagogastroduodenoscopy.

oesophagogastroplasty [Br.] SYN esophagogastroplasty.

oesophagogastrostomy [Br.] SYN esophagogastrostomy.

oesophagogram [Br.] SYN esophagogram.

oesophagomalacia [Br.] SYN esophagomalacia.

oesophagomyotomy [Br.] SYN esophagomyotomy.

oesophagoplasty [Br.] SYN esophagoplasty.

oesophagoplication [Br.] SYN esophagoplication.

oesophagoptosis [Br.] SYN esophagoptosis.

oesophagoscope [Br.] SYN esophagoscope.

oesophagoscopy [Br.] SYN esophagoscopy.

oesophagostenosis [Br.] SYN esophagostenosis.

oesophagotomy [Br.] SYN esophagotomy.

oesophagus [Br.] SYN esophagus.

oestradiol [Br.] SYN estradiol.

oes·tra·di·ol (es'tră-dī'ol) SYN estradiol.

oestrogen [Br.] SYN estrogen.

oestrogenic [Br.] SYN estrogenic.

oestrogen receptor [Br.] SYN estrogen receptor.

oestrogen replacement therapy [Br.] SYN estrogen replacement therapy.

oestrone [Br.] SYN estrone.

oestruation [Br.] SYN estruation.

oestrus [Br.] SYN estrus.

of·fice hy·per·ten·sion (awf'is hī'pĕr-ten'shŭn) SYN white coat hypertension.

Of·fice of In·spec·tor Gen·er·al (OIG) (aw'fis in-spek'tŏr jen'ĕr-ăl) Government (federal, state) agency that investigates and prosecutes fraud in government health care programs.

of·fi·cial for·mu·la (ŏ-fish'ăl fōrm'yū-lă) A formula contained in the Pharmacopeia or the National Formulary.

of·fic·i·nal (ŏ-fis'i-năl) Denoting a chemical or pharmaceutical preparation kept in stock, in contrast to magistral (pre-pared extemporaneously according to a physician's prescription).

off-la·bel in·di·ca·tion (awf-lā'bĕl in'di-kā'shŭn) Use of a medication for a purpose other than those approved by the U.S. Food and Drug Administration.

off-site tran·scrip·tion (awf'sīt tran-skrip'shŭn) System in which medical transcription is done outside of the health care facility. SYN remote transcription.

O·gu·chi dis·ease (ō-gū'chē di-zēz') Rare congenital nonprogressive night blindness with diffuse yellow or gray coloration of fundus.

ohm (Ω) (ōm) The practical unit of electrical resistance.

Ohm law (ōm law) In an electric current passing through a wire, the intensity of the current (I) in amperes equals the electromotive force (E) in volts divided by the resistance (R) in ohms: $I = E/R$.

ohm·me·ter (ōm'mē-tĕr) An instrument for determining the resistance, in ohms, of a conductor.

oh·ne Hauch (ō'nĕ howk[h]) Term used to designate the nonspreading growth of nonflagellated bacteria on agar media. SEE ALSO O antigen.

-oid Combining form meaning resemblance to, joined properly to words formed from Greek roots; equivalent to English -form.

o·id·i·o·my·cin (ō-id'ē-ō-mī'sin) An antigen used to demonstrate cutaneous hypersensitivity in patients infected with *Candida*.

oil (oyl) An inflammable liquid of fatty consistency and slippery feel that is insoluble in water, soluble or insoluble in alcohol, and freely soluble in ether.

oil of clove (oyl klōv) Volatile oil used in dentistry as a local anesthetic and component of temporary fillings of the teeth. Also used to flavor foods; strong, pungent odor. SYN clove oil.

oil re·ten·tion en·e·ma (oyl rĕ-ten'shŭn

en′ĕ-mă) Oil-based fluid, prescribed to soften a hardened fecal mass and ease its passage through the anal canal, after being retained by the patient for at least 30 minutes. SYN emollient enema, lubricating enema.

oint·ment (oynt′mĕnt) Semisolid preparation of containing medicinal substances intended for external application. SYN salve, unguent.

oint·ment base (oynt′mĕnt bās) Vehicle into which active ingredients may be incorporated (e.g., petrolatum).

OKT cells (selz) Cells recognized by monoclonal antibodies to T lymphocyte antigens. Current usage favors cluster of differentiation (CD) designations.

-ol Combining form denoting that a substance is an alcohol or a phenol.

ol·a·mine (ōl′ă-mēn) USAN-approved contraction for ethanolamine.

o·le·ag·i·nous (ō′lē-aj′i-nŭs) Oily or greasy.

o·le·ate (ō′lē-āt) **1.** A salt of oleic acid. **2.** A pharmacopeial preparation consisting of a combination or solution of an alkaloid or metallic base in oleic acid, used as an inunction.

o·le·cran·ar·thri·tis (ō-lek′ran-ahr-thrī′tis) Inflammation of the elbow.

o·lec·ra·non (ō-lek′ră-non) [TA] The prominent curved proximal extremity of the ulna. SYN elbow bone, point of elbow.

o·le·ic ac·id (OA) (ō-lē′ik as′id) Unsaturated fatty acid that is the most widely distributed and abundant found in nature; used as a pharmaceutical solvent.

o·le·in (ō′lē-in) A triacylglycerol, solely containing oleoyl moieties, found in fats and oils. SYN triolein.

oleo- Combining form meaning oil. SEE ALSO eleo-.

o·le·o·res·in (ō′lē-ō-rez′in) **1.** A compound of an essential oil and resin, present in some plants. **2.** A pharmaceutical preparation. **3.** SYN balsam.

ol·fac·tion (ōl-fak′shŭn) The sense of smell. SYN osmesis, osphresis.

ol·fac·tol·o·gy (ōl′fak-tol′ŏ-jē) Study of the sense of smell.

ol·fac·tom·e·ter (ōl′fak-tom′ĕ-tĕr) A device for estimating the sensitivity to odorants.

ol·fac·to·ry (ōl-fak′tŏr-ē) Relating to the sense of smell. SEE olfaction.

ol·fac·to·ry ag·no·si·a (ōl-fak′tŏr-ē ag-nō′zē-ă) Inability to classify or identify an odorant, although the ability to distinguish between or recognize odorants may be normal.

ol·fac·to·ry au·ra (ōl-fak′tŏr-ē awr′ă) Epileptic aura characterized by illusions or smell. SEE ALSO aura (1).

ol·fac·to·ry bulb (ōl-fak′tŏr-ē bŭlb) [TA] The grayish expanded rostral extremity of the olfactory tract, lying on the cribriform plate of the ethmoid and receiving the olfactory filaments. SYN bulbus olfactorius [TA].

ol·fac·to·ry cen·ter (ōl-fak′tŏr-ē sen′tĕr) Area of the brain that controls the sense of smell.

ol·fac·to·ry ep·i·the·li·um (ōl-fak′tŏr-ē ep′i-thē′lē-ŭm) A pseudostratified epithelium that contains olfactory, receptor, and nerve cells extend to brain's olfactory bulb.

ol·fac·to·ry for·a·men (ōl-fak′tŏr-ē fōr-ă′mĕn) An opening in the cribriform plate of the ethmoid bone, transmitting the olfactory nerves.

ol·fac·to·ry glands (ōl-fak′tŏr-ē glandz) [TA] Branched tubuloalveolar serous secreting glands (of Bowman) in the mucous membrane of the olfactory region of the nasal cavity.

ol·fac·to·ry glo·me·ru·lus (ōl-fak′tŏr-ē glō-mer′yū-lŭs) One of the small spheric territories in the olfactory bulb in which dendrites of mitral and tufted cells connect with axons of olfactory receptor cells.

ol·fac·to·ry hal·lu·ci·na·tion (ōl-fak′tŏr-ē hă-lū′si-nā′shŭn) False perception related to smell.

ol·fac·to·ry mem·brane (ōl-fak′tŏr-ē mem′brān) Part of nasal mucosa with olfactory receptor cells and glands of Bowman.

ol·fac·tory neu·ro·ep·i·the·li·um (ōl-fak′tŏr-ē nūr′ō-ep-i-thē′lē-ŭm) The olfactory organ is composed of receptor and supporting cells and olfactory glands of Bowman, located in the superior part of the nasal cavities.

ol·fac·to·ry re·cep·tor cells (ōl-fak′ tŏr-ē rĕ-sep′tŏr selz) Very slender nerve cells, with large nuclei surmounted by six to eight long, sensitive cilia in the olfactory epithelium at the roof of the nose; receptors for sense of smell. Sometimes called olfactory cells.

ol·fac·to·ry tri·gone (ōl-fak′tŏr-ē trī′ gōn) [TA] Grayish triangular area corresponding to the attachment of the olfactory peduncle (''olfactory nerve'' or olfactory tract) to the base of the brain. SYN trigonum olfactorium [TA].

ol·fac·to·ry ves·i·cle (ōl-fak′tŏr-ē ves′i̇-kĕl) Vesicle in the embryo that develops into the olfactory bulb and tract.

o·lib·a·num (ō-lib′ă-nŭm) A gum used as a stimulant expectorant in bronchitis, for fumigations, and as incense. SYN frankincense, thus.

oligaemia [Br.] SYN oligemia.

oligaemic [Br.] SYN oligemic.

ol·i·gam·ni·os (ol′i-gam′nē-os) SYN oligohydramnios.

ol·i·ge·mi·a (ol′i-jē′mē-ă) Blood deficiency anywhere in the body. SYN oligaemia.

ol·i·ge·mic (ol′i-jē′mik) Pertaining to or characterized by oligemia. SYN oligaemic.

♻ **oligo-, olig- 1.** Combining forms meaning a few, a little. **2.** CHEMISTRY used in contrast to ''poly-'' in describing polymers (e.g., oligosaccharide).

ol·i·go·am·ni·os, ol·i·gam·ni·os (ol′i-gō-am′nē-os, ol′i-gam′nē-os) SYN oligohydramnios.

ol·i·go·as·the·no·sper·mi·a (ol′i-gō-

as-thē′nŏ-spĕr′mē-ă) Loss of sperm motility or production of scanty inactive sperm.

ol·i·go·cys·tic (ol′i-gō-sis′tik) Consisting of only a few cysts.

ol·i·go·dac·ty·ly, ol·i·go·dac·tyl·i·a (ol′i-gō-dak′ti-lē, -dak-til′ē-ă) SYN hypodactyly.

ol·i·go·den·dro·cyte (ol′i-gō-den′drō-sīt) A cell of the oligodendroglia.

ol·i·go·den·drog·li·a (ol′i-gō-den-drog′ lē-ă) One of three types of glia cells (the other two being macroglia or astrocytes, and microglia) that, together with nerve cells, compose the tissue of the central nervous system. SYN oligodendria.

ol·i·go·dip·si·a (ol′i-gō-dip′sē-ă) Abnormal lack of thirst. SEE ALSO hypodipsia.

ol·i·go·don·ti·a (ol′i-gō-don′shē-ă) SYN hypodontia.

ol·i·go·dy·nam·ic (ol′i-gō-dī-nam′ik) Active in very small quantity.

ol·i·go·ga·lac·ti·a (ol′i-gō-gă-lak′shē-ă) Slight or scant secretion of milk.

ol·i·go·hy·dram·ni·os (ol′i-gō-hī-dram′nē-os) The presence of an insufficient amount of amniotic fluid. SYN hypamnion, hypamnios, oligamnios, oligoamnios.

ol·i·go·men·or·rhe·a (ol′i-gō-men′ōr-ē′ă) *Do not confuse this word with hypomenorrhea.* Scanty menstruation.

oligomenorrhoea [Br.] SYN oligomenorrhea.

ol·i·go·mer (ol′i-gō-mĕr) A polymer containing fewer than 20 repeating units.

o·li·go·mer·i·za·tion (ol′i-gō-mĕr-ī-zā′ shŭn) Formation of oligomers from larger or smaller molecules.

ol·i·go·mor·phic (ol′-i-gō-mōr′fik) Presenting few changes of form; not polymorphic.

ol·i·go·nu·cle·o·tide (ol′i-gō-nū′klē-ō-tīd) A compound made up of the condensation of a small number. Cf. polynucleotide.

ol·i·go·pep·tide (ol′i-gō-pep′tīd) A peptide with the molecule which contains that amino acid residues up to about 20.

ol·i·gop·ne·a (ol′i-gop-nē′ă) SYN hypopnea.

ol·i·go·pty·a·lism (ol′i-gop-tī′ă-lizm) A scanty secretion of saliva.

ol·i·go·sac·cha·ride (ol′i-gō-sak′ă-rīd) A compound made up of the condensation of a small number of monosaccharide units. Cf. polysaccharide.

ol·i·go·sper·mi·a, ol·i·go·sper·ma·tism (ol′i-gō-spĕrm′ē-ă, -mă-tizm) A subnormal concentration of sperms in the penile ejaculate. SYN oligozoospermia.

ol·i·go·sy·nap·tic (ol′i-gō-si-nap′tik) Referring to neural conduction pathways that are interrupted by only a few synaptic junctions.

ol·i·go·tro·phi·a, ol·i·got·ro·phy (ol′i-gō-trō′fē-ă, -got′rŏ-fē) Deficient nutrition.

ol·i·gu·ri·a, ol·i·gu·re·sis, ol·i·gu·re·si·a (ol′i-gyūr′ē-ă, -gyūr-ē′sis, -ē′zē-ă) Scanty urine production (i.e., less than 500 mL in 24 hours); results in inefficient excretion of the products of metabolism.

o·lis·thy (o-lis′thē) The slippage of bone(s) from the normal anatomic site.

ol·i·var·y (ol′i-var-ē) **1.** Relating to the oliva. **2.** Relating to or shaped like an olive.

ol·ive oil (ol′iv oyl) **1.** The expressed oil of the fruit of *Olea europaea;* used as a cholagogue, laxative, and emollient, and in the preparation of liniments and foods. **2.** SEE oil.

ol·i·vif·u·gal (ol′i-vif′yū-găl) In a direction away from the olive. **2.** SEE UNDER oil.

ol·i·vip·e·tal (ol′i-vip′ĕ-tăl) In a direction toward the oliva.

ol·i·vo·pon·to·cer·e·bel·lar a·tro·phy (ol′i-vō-pon′tō-ser-ĕ-bel′ăr at′rŏ-fē) Group of genetically distinct neurologic diseases characterized by loss of neurons in the cerebellar cortex, basis pontis, and inferior olivary nuclei; results in ataxia, tremor, involuntary movement, and dysarthria.

Ol·li·er the·o·ry (ō-lē-ā′ thē′ŏr-ē) A theory of compensatory osseous growth.

-oma, -omata Combining forms denoting tumor or neoplasm.

o·me·ga (ω)-3 fat·ty ac·ids (ō-māg′ă fat′ē as′idz) A series of dietary polyunsaturated fatty acids; reportedly, they play a role in lowering cholesterol and levels of low-density lipoprofeins.

o·me·ga-ox·i·da·tion, ω-ox·i·da·tion (ō-māg′ă-ok′si-dā′shŭn) Oxidation at the carbon atom farthest removed (ω-carbon) from the carboxyl group (carbon 1).

o·me·ga-ox·i·da·tion the·o·ry (ō-māg′ă ok′si-dā′shŭn thē′ŏr-ē) That the oxidation of fatty acids commences at the CH_3 group.

O·menn syn·drome (ō′men sin′drŏm) A rapidly fatal immunodeficiency disease characterized by erythroderma, diarrhea, repeated infections, hepatosplenomegaly, and leukocytosis with eosinophilia.

omen·tec·to·my (ō′men-tek′tŏ-mē) Resection or excision of the omentum.

omen·ti·tis (ō′men-tī′tis) Peritonitis involving the omentum.

omen·to·pex·y, omen·to·fix·a·tion (ō-men′tō-pek-sē, -fiks-ā′shŭn) **1.** Suture of the greater omentum to the abdominal wall to induce collateral portal circulation. **2.** Suture of the omentum to another organ to increase arterial circulation. SYN omentofixation.

omen·tor·rha·phy (ō′men-tōr′ă-fē) Suture of an opening in the omentum.

omen·tum, pl. **o·men·ta** (ō-men′tŭm, -tă) [TA] A fold of peritoneum passing from the stomach to another abdominal organ.

omen·tum ma·jus (ō-men′tŭm mī′ŭs) [TA] SYN greater omentum.

O

o·mis·sion (ō-mish′ŭn) PHARMACY drug error in which the requisite dose is erroneously missed.

om·ni·fo·cal lens (om′nē-fō′kăl lenz) A lens for near and distant vision in which the reading portion is a continuously variable curve.

om·niv·o·rous (om-niv′ŏ-rŭs) Living on food of all kinds, on both animal and vegetable food.

o·mo·cla·vic·u·lar (ō′mō-klă-vik′yū-lăr) Relating to the shoulder and clavicle.

o·mo·hy·oid mus·cle (ō′mō-hī′oyd mŭs′ĕl) Formed of two bellies attached to intermediate tendon; *origin*, by inferior belly from upper border of scapula between superior angle and notch; *insertion*, by superior belly into hyoid bone; *action*, depresses hyoid; *nerve supply*, upper cervical spinal nerves through ansa cervicalis. SYN musculus omohyoideus [TA].

o·mo·pha·gi·a (ō′mō-fā′jē-ă) The consumption of raw flesh.

om·pha·lec·to·my (om′fă-lek′tŏ-mē) Excision of the umbilicus or of a neoplasm connected with it.

om·phal·el·co·sis (om′fal-el-kō′sis) Ulceration at the umbilicus.

om·phal·ic (om-fal′ik) SYN umbilical.

om·pha·li·tis (om′fă-lī′tis) Inflammation of the umbilicus and surrounding parts.

om·phal·o·cele (om-fal′ŏ-sēl) Congenital herniation of viscera into the base of the umbilical cord, with a covering membranous sac of peritoneum-amnion. SEE ALSO umbilical hernia. SYN exomphalos (3), exumbilication (3).

om·pha·lo·en·ter·ic (om′fă-lō-en-ter′ik) Relating to the umbilicus and intestine.

om·pha·lo·phle·bi·tis (om′fă-lō-flĕ-bī′tis) Inflammation of the umbilical veins.

om·pha·lor·rha·gi·a (om′fă-lō-rā′jē-ă) Bleeding from the umbilicus.

om·pha·lor·rhe·a (om′fă-lōr-ē′ă) A serous discharge from the umbilicus. SYN omphalorrhoea.

om·pha·lor·rhex·is (om′fă-lōr-ek′sis) Umbilical cord rupture at birth.

omphalorrhoea [Br.] SYN omphalorrhea.

om·pha·lo·site (om′fă-lō-sīt) Underdeveloped twin of allantoid angiopagous twins; joined by umbilical vessels. SYN placental parasitic twin.

om·pha·lo·spi·nous (om′fă-lō-spī′nŭs) Denoting a line connecting the umbilicus and the anterior superior spine of the ilium, on which lies McBurney point.

om·pha·lot·o·my (om′fă-lot′ŏ-mē) Cutting of the umbilical cord at birth.

o·nan·ism (ō′năn-izm) **1.** Withdrawal of the penis before ejaculation, to prevent conception. **2.** Incorrectly, but commonly, masturbation.

On·cho·cer·ca (ong′kō-ser′kă) A genus of elongated filariform nematodes that inhabit the connective tissue of their hosts. SYN Oncocerca.

♻ **onco-, oncho-** Combining forms indicating a tumor.

on·co·cyte (ong′kō-sīt) A large, granular, acidophilic tumor cell containing numerous mitochondria; a neoplastic oxyphil cell.

on·co·cyt·ic car·ci·no·ma (ong′kō-sit′ik kahr′si-nō′mă) SYN Hürthle cell carcinoma.

on·co·cyt·ic he·pa·to·cel·lu·lar tu·mor (ong′kō-sit′ik hĕ-pat′ō-sel′yū′lăr tū′mŏr) SYN fibrolamellar liver cell carcinoma.

on·co·cy·to·ma (ong′kō-sī-tō′mă) A glandular tumor composed of large cells with cytoplasm that is granular and eosinophilic because of the presence of abundant mitochondria.

on·co·cy·to·sis (ong′kō-sī-tō′sis) Spectrum of changes in the kidneys harboring oncocytomas.

on·co·fe·tal (ong′kō-fē′tăl) Relating to

tumor-associated substances present in fetal tissue, as oncofetal antigens.

on·co·fe·tal an·ti·gens (ong′kō-fē′tăl an′ti-jenz) Tumor-associated antigens present in fetal tissue but not in normal adult tissue, including α-fetoprotein and carcinoembryonic antigen.

on·co·gene (ong′kō-jēn) Any of a family of genes, which under normal circumstances, code for proteins involved in cell growth or regulation but may foster malignant processes if mutated or activated by contact with retroviruses. SEE antioncogene.

on·co·gen·e·sis (ong′-kō-jen′ĕ-sis) Origin and growth of a neoplasm.

on·co·gen·ic vi·rus (ong′kō-jen′ik vī′rŭs) A virus of one of the two groups that induce tumors; the ribonucleic acid tumor viruses, which are well defined and rather homogeneous, or the deoxyribunucleid acid viruses, which are more diverse. SYN tumor virus.

on·cog·en·ous, on·co·gen·ic (ong-koj′ĕ-nŭs, -kō-jen′ik) Causing, inducing, or being suitable for the formation and development of a neoplasm. SYN oncogenic.

on·co·log·ic e·mer·gen·cies (ong′kō-loj′ik ē-měr′jĕn-sēz) Life-threatening medical emergencies that result from cancer or cancer therapies; can be obstructive, metabolic, or infiltrative.

on·col·o·gist (ong-kol′ŏ-jist) A specialist in oncology.

on·col·o·gy (ong-kol′ŏ-jē) The study or science dealing with the physical, chemical, and biologic properties and features of neoplasms, including causation, pathogenesis, and treatment.

on·col·o·gy cer·ti·fied nurse (OCN) (ong-kol′ŏ-jē sĕr′ti-fīd nŭrs) One who specializes in treatment of patients with cancer and has passed a certification examination, developed and administered by the Oncology Nursing Certification Corporation (ONCC).

on·col·y·sis (ong-kol′i-sis) Destruction of a neoplasm; sometimes used with reference to the reduction of any swelling or mass.

on·co·lyt·ic (ong′kō-lit′ik) Pertaining to, characterized by, or causing oncolysis.

on·co·sphere (ong′kō-sfēr) SYN hexacanth.

on·cot·ic (ong-kot′ik) Relating to or caused by edema or any swelling (oncosis).

on·cot·ic pres·sure (ong-kot′ik presh′ŭr) The osmotic pressure attributed to proteins and other macromolecules.

on·co·trop·ic (ong′kō-trō′pik) Manifesting a special affinity for neoplasms or neoplastic cells.

o·nei·ric, on·ir·ic (ō-nī′rik) 1. Pertaining to dreams. 2. Pertaining to the clinical state of oneirophrenia (q.v.).

o·nei·rism (ō-nī′rizm) A waking dream state.

on·go·ing as·sess·ment (on′gō-ing ă-ses′mĕnt) Repeat of the focused or rapid emergency department assessment of a prehospital patient to detect changes in condition and to judge the effectiveness of treatment before or during transport.

on·lay (on′lā) 1. A metal cast restoration of the occlusal surface of a posterior tooth or the lingual surface of an anterior tooth, the entire surface of which is in dentin without side walls. 2. A graft applied on the exterior of a bone, or the surface of an organ or structure.

on·set of ac·tion (on′set ak′shŭn) The time from drug administration until the drug exerts an observable specific effect or response.

on-site mas·sage (on-sīt mă-sahzh′) SYN seated massage.

on·to·gen·e·sis (on′tō-jen′ĕ-sis) SYN ontogeny.

on·to·ge·net·ic, on·to·gen·ic (on′tō-jĕ-net′ik, -jen′ik) Relating to ontogeny.

on·tog·e·ny (on-toj′ĕ-nē) Development of the individual, as distinguished from phylogeny, which is evolutionary development of the species. SYN ontogenesis.

on·y·chal·gi·a (on′i-kal′jē-ă) Pain in the nails.

on·y·cha·tro·phi·a, on·y·cha·tro·phy (on′i-kă-trō′fē-ă, on′i-kat′rō-fē) Atrophy of the nails.

on·y·chaux·is (on′i-kawk′sis) Marked overgrowth of the fingernails or toenails.

on·y·chec·to·my (on′i-kek′tŏ-mē) Ablation of a toenail or fingernail.

o·nych·i·a, on·y·chi·tis (ō-nik′ē-ă, on′i-kī′tis) Inflammation of the matrix of the nail. SYN onychitis.

♻ **onycho-, onych-** Combining forms denoting a fingernail or a toenail.

on·y·choc·la·sis (on′i-kok′lă-sis) Breaking of the nails.

on·y·cho·cryp·to·sis (on′i-kō-krip-tō′sis) SYN ingrown nail.

on·y·cho·dys·tro·phy (on′i-kō-dis′trŏ-fē) Dystrophic changes in the nails occurring as a congenital defect or due to any illness or injury that may cause a malformed nail.

on·y·cho·graph (on′i-kō-graf) An instrument for recording the capillary blood pressure as shown by the circulation under the nail.

on·y·cho·gry·po·sis (on′i-kō-gri-pō′sis) Enlargement with increased thickening and curvature of the fingernails or toenails.

on·y·cho·het·er·o·to·pi·a (on′i-kō-het′ĕr-ō-tō′pē-ă) Abnormal placement of nails.

on·y·choid (on′i-koyd) Resembling a fingernail in structure or form.

on·y·chol·y·sis (on′i-kol′i-sis) Loosening of the nails, beginning at the free border, and usually incomplete.

on·y·cho·ma·de·sis (on′i-kō-mă-dē′sis) Complete shedding of the nails, usually associated with systemic disease.

on·y·cho·ma·la·ci·a (on′i-kō-mă-lā′shē-ă) Abnormal softness of the nails.

on·y·cho·my·co·sis (on′i-kō-mī-kō′sis) Very common fungus infections of the nails, causing thickening, roughness, and splitting. SYN ringworm of nails.

on·y·cho·path·ic (on′i-kō-path′ik) Relating to or suffering from any disease of the nails.

on·y·chop·a·thy (on′i-kop′ă-thē) Any disease of the nails.

on·y·cho·plas·ty (on′i-kō-plas-tē) A corrective or surgical operation on the nail matrix.

on·y·chor·rhex·is (on′i-kō-rek′sis) Abnormal brittleness of the nails with splitting of the free edge.

on·y·chot·o·my (on′i-kot′ŏ-mē) Incision into a toenail or fingernail.

on·yx (on′iks) SYN nail.

♻ **oo-** Prefix meaning egg, ovary. SEE ALSO oophor-, ovario-, ovi-, ovo-.

o·o·cyst (ō′ŏ-sist) The encysted form of the fertilized macrogamete, or zygote, in coccidian Sporozoea in which sporogonic multiplication occurs.

o·o·cyte (ō′ŏ-sīt) Female gamete or sex cell. When fertilized by a sperm, an oocyte is capable of developing into a new individual of the same species. SEE ALSO egg, ovum. SYN ovocyte.

o·o·gen·e·sis (ō′ŏ-jen′ĕ-sis) Process of formation and development of the oocyte. SYN ovigenesis.

o·o·ge·net·ic (ō′ŏ-jĕ-net′ik) Producing oocytes (ova). SYN ovigenetic, ovigenic.

o·o·go·ni·um, pl. **o·o·go·ni·a** (ō′ŏ-gō′nē-ŭm, -nē-ă) Primordial germ cells. In fungi, female gametangium bearing one or more oospores.

o·o·ki·ne·sis, o·o·ki·ne·si·a (ō′ŏ-ki-nē′sis, -nē′zē-ă) Chromosomal movements of the oocyte during maturation and fertilization.

o·o·lem·ma (ō′ŏ-lem′ă) Plasma membrane of the oocyte.

♻ **oophor-, oophoro-** Combining forms meaning the ovary. SEE ALSO oo-, ovario-.

o·oph·or·al·gi·a (ō-of′ŏr-al′jē-ă) SYN ovarialgia.

o·oph·or·ec·to·my (ō′of-ŏr-ek′tŏ-mē) SYN ovariectomy.

o·oph·or·i·tis (ō′of-ŏr-ī′tis) Inflammation of an ovary.

o·oph·or·o·cys·tec·to·my (ō-of′ŏr-ō-sis-tek′tŏ-mē) Excision of an ovarian cyst.

o·oph·or·o·cys·to·sis (ō-of′ŏr-ō-sis-tō′sis) Ovarian cyst formation.

o·oph·or·o·hys·ter·ec·to·my (ō-of′ŏr-ō-his-tĕr-ek′tŏ-mē) SYN ovariohysterectomy.

o·oph·or·o·pex·y (ō-of′ŏr-ō-pek′sē) Surgical fixation or suspension of an ovary.

o·oph·or·o·plas·ty (ō-of′ŏr-ō-plas-tē) Surgical repair on an ovary.

o·oph·or·o·sal·pin·gec·to·my (ō-of′ŏr-ō-sal′pin-jek′tŏ-mē) The surgical removal of one or both ovaries, along with the corresponding uterine tube(s).

o·oph·or·o·sal·pin·gi·tis (ō-of′ŏr-ō-sal′pin-jī′tis) Inflammation that involves the ovary and uterine tube. SYN ovariosalpingitis.

o·oph·or·os·to·my (ō-of′ŏr-os′tŏ-mē) SYN ovariostomy.

o·oph·or·ot·o·my (ō-of′ŏr-ot′ŏ-mē) SYN ovariotomy.

o·oph·or·rha·gi·a (ō-of′ŏr-rā′jē-ă) Ovarian hemorrhage.

o·o·plasm (ō′ō-plazm) Protoplasmic portion of the oocyte.

o·pac·i·fi·ca·tion (ō-pas′i-fi-kā′shŭn) **1.** The process of making opaque. **2.** The formation of opacities.

o·pal cod·on (ō′păl kō′don) SYN umber codon.

o·pa·les·cent den·tin (ō′pă-les′ĕnt den′tin) That associated with dentinogenesis imperfecta; gives an unusual opalescent or translucent appearance to the teeth.

o·pen am·pu·ta·tion (ō′pĕn amp′yū-tā′shŭn) An amputation that leaves the stump unsutured (without skin flap closure) for several weeks while débridement and antibiotic therapy are carried out.

o·pen-an·gle glau·co·ma (ō′pĕn-ang′gĕl glaw-kō′mă) Primary glaucoma in which the aqueous humor has free access to the trabecular meshwork. SYN chronic glaucoma, compensated glaucoma, simple glaucoma, glaucoma simplex.

o·pen bite (ō′pĕn bīt) **1.** SYN large interarch distance. **2.** SYN apertognathia.

o·pen chain com·pound (ō′pĕn chān kom′pownd) SYN acyclic compound.

o·pen chest mas·sage (ō′pĕn chest mă-sahzh′) Rhythmic manual compression of the ventricles of the heart with the hand inside the thoracic cavity.

o·pen-cir·cuit meth·od (ō′pĕn-sïr′kŭt meth′ŏd) A process for measuring oxygen consumption and carbon dioxide production by collecting the expired gas over a known period of time and measuring its volume and composition.

open-cir·cuit ni·tro·gen wash-out (ō′pĕn-sïr′kŭt nī′trŏ-jĕn wawsh′owt) A gas-dilution technique for measuring the functional residual capacity; the patient breathes 100% oxygen to wash out the nitrogen.

o·pen com·e·do (ō′pĕn kom′ĕ-dō) A blackhead with a wide opening on the skin surface capped with a melanin-containing blackened mass of epithelial debris.

o·pen dis·lo·ca·tion (ō′pĕn dis′lō-kā′shŭn) One complicated by a wound opening from the surface down to the affected joint.

o·pen drain·age (ō′pĕn drān′ăj) Drainage allowing air to enter.

o·pen flap (ō′pĕn flap) SYN flat flap.

o·pen heart sur·ge·ry (ō′pĕn hahrt sŭr′jĕr-ē) Operative procedure(s) performed on or within the exposed heart.

o·pen·ing (ō′pĕn-ing) [TA] A gap in or entrance to an organ, tube, or cavity. SEE ALSO aperture, fossa, ostium, orifice, pore.

O

o·pen·ing snap (OS) (ōʹpĕn-ing snap) Sharp, high-pitched click in early diastole, usually best heard between the cardiac apex and the lower left sternal border, related to opening of the abnormal valve in cases of mitral stenosis.

o·pen-pack·ed po·si·tion (ōʹpĕn-pakt pŏ-zishʹŏn) **1.** Joint position in which contact between the articulating structures is minimal. **2.** SYN flexion.

o·pen pneu·mo·tho·rax (ōʹpĕn nū'mō-thōrʹaks) A free communication between the atmosphere and the pleural space either through the lung or through the chest wall. SYN sucking chest wound, sucking wound.

o·pen re·duc·tion of frac·tures (ōʹpĕn rē-dukʹshŭn frakʹshŭrz) Reduction by manipulation of bone, after incision in skin and muscle over the site of the fracture.

o·pen sys·tem (ōʹpĕn sisʹtĕm) One with continual exchange of material, energy, and information with the environment.

o·pen tu·ber·cu·lo·sis (ōʹpĕn tū-bĕrʹkyū-lōʹsis) Pulmonary tuberculosis, tuberculous ulceration, or other form in which the tubercle bacilli are present in the excretions or secretions.

o·pen wound (ōʹpĕn wūnd) Trauma in which tissues are exposed to the air.

op·er·a·ble (opʹĕr-ă-bĕl) Denoting a patient or condition on which a surgical procedure can be performed with a reasonable expectation of cure or relief.

op·er·ant (opʹĕr-ănt) In conditioning, any behavior or specific response chosen by the experimenter; its frequency is intended to increase or decrease by the judicious pairing with it of a reinforcer when it occurs. SYN target response.

op·er·ant con·di·tion·ing (opʹĕr-ănt kŏn-dishʹŭn-ing) Experiment in which an experimenter waits for the target response (head scratching) to be conditioned to occur (emitted) spontaneously, immediately after which the organism is given a reinforcer reward. SYN skinnerian conditioning.

op·er·ate (opʹĕr-āt) To perform a therapeutic procedure on the body with the hands or with instruments.

op·er·at·ing mi·cro·scope (opʹĕr-āʹting mīʹkrŏ-skōp) SYN surgical microscope.

op·er·at·ing room tech·ni·cian (opʹĕr-āt-ing rūm tek-nishʹŭn) The member of the surgical team who assists in preparing the operating room for surgery and performing other tasks. Training lasts 1–2 years. Students must pass an examination by the Association of Surgical Technologists to become certified. SYN surgical technician, surgical technologist.

op·er·a·tion (opʹĕr-āʹshŭn) **1.** Any surgical procedure. **2.** The act, manner, or process of functioning. SEE ALSO method, procedure, technique.

op·er·a·tive cho·lan·gi·o·graphy (opʹĕr-ă-tiv kō-lanʹjē-ogʹră-fē) Radiographic examination of the bile ducts with contrast medium during surgery to detect residual biliary calculi.

op·er·a·tive den·tis·try (opʹĕr-ă-tiv denʹtis-trē) Individual restoration of teeth with metallic or nonmetallic materials. SYN restorative dentistry.

op·er·a·tor gene (opʹĕr-ā-tŏr jēn) A gene with the function of activating the production of messenger RNA by one or more adjacent structural loci.

o·per·cu·lar (ō-pĕrʹkyū-lăr) Relating to an operculum.

o·per·cu·li·tis (ō-per'kyū-līʹtis) A pericoronitis originating under an operculum.

o·per·cu·lum, gen. **o·per·cu·li,** pl. **o·per·cu·la** (ō-pĕrʹkyū-lŭm, -lī, -lă) [TA] Anything resembling a lid or cover.

op·er·on (opʹĕr-on) A genetic functional unit that controls production of a messenger ribonucleic acid.

ophi·a·sis (ō-fīʹă-sis) A form of alopecia areata in which the loss of hair occurs in bands along the scalp margin, partially or completely encircling the head.

oph·ri·tis (of-rīʹtis) Dermatitis in the region of the eyebrows.

oph·ry·o·sis (ofʹrē-ōʹsis) Spasmodic twitching of the upper portion of the orbicularis palpebrarum muscle causing eyebrow wrinkling.

oph·thal·ma·gra (of'thăl-mag'ră) Sharp, sudden ocular pain.

oph·thal·mal·gi·a (of'thăl-mal'jē-ă) Ocular pain.

oph·thal·mec·to·my (of'thăl-mek'tŏ-mē) Surgical removal of an eye.

oph·thal·mi·a (of-thal'mē-ă) 1. Severe, often purulent, conjunctivitis. 2. Inflammation of the deeper structures of the eye.

oph·thal·mi·a ne·o·na·to·rum (of-thal'mē-ă nē-ō'nă-tō'rŭm) Conjunctival inflammation occurring within the first 10 days of life. SYN blennorrhea neonatorum, infantile purulent conjunctivitis, neonatal conjunctivitis.

oph·thal·mic (of-thal'mik) Relating to the eye. SYN ocular (1).

oph·thal·mic so·lu·tion (of-thal'mik sŏ-lū'shŭn) Sterile solution, free from foreign particles and suitably compounded and dispensed for instillation into the eye.

oph·thal·mi·tis (of'thal-mi'tis) Ocular inflammation.

ophthalmo-, ophthalm- Combining forms indicating a relationship to the eye. SEE ALSO oculo-.

oph·thal·mo·dy·na·mom·e·ter (of-thal'mō-dī'nă-mom'ĕ-tĕr) An instrument to measure the blood pressure in the retinal vessels.

oph·thal·mo·dy·na·mom·e·try (of-thal'mō-dī'nă-mom'ĕ-trē) The measurement of blood pressure in the retinal vessels by means of an ophthalmodynamometer.

oph·thal·mo·dyn·ia (of-thal'mō-din'ē-ă) Ocular pain.

oph·thal·mol·o·gy (of'thăl-mol'ŏ-jē) The medical specialty concerned with the eye, its diseases, and refractive errors.

oph·thal·mo·ma·la·ci·a (of-thal'mō-mă-lā'shē-ă) Abnormal softening of the eyeball.

oph·thal·mo·my·co·sis (of-thal'mō-mī-kō'sis) Any disease of the eye or its appendages caused by a fungus.

oph·thal·mo·my·ot·o·my (of-thal'mō-mī-ot'ŏ-mē) Surgical cutting into the muscle of the eye.

oph·thal·mo·neu·ri·tis (of-thal'mō-nūr-ī'tis) Inflammation of the optic nerve.

oph·thal·mop·a·thy (of'thal-mop'ă-thē) Any disease of the eyes. SYN oculopathy.

oph·thal·mo·plas·ty (of-thal'mō-plas'tē) Surgical repair of the eye.

oph·thal·mo·ple·gi·a (of-thal'mō-plē'jē-ă) Paralysis of one or more of the ocular muscles.

oph·thal·mo·ple·gi·a ex·ter·na (of-thal'mō-plē'jē-ă eks-tĕr'nă) Paralysis affecting one or more of the extrinsic eye muscles. SYN external ophthalmoplegia.

oph·thal·mo·ple·gi·a in·ter·na (of-thal'mō-plē'jē-ă in-tĕr'nă) Paralysis affecting only the sphincter muscle of the pupil and the ciliary muscle. SYN internal ophthalmoplegia.

oph·thal·mo·ple·gic mi·graine (of-thal'mō-plē'jik mī'grān) Form of migraine associated with paralysis of the extraocular muscles.

oph·thal·mor·rha·gi·a (of-thal'mō-rā'jē-ă) Ocular hemorrhage.

oph·thal·mor·rhe·a (of-thal'mō-rē'ă) An ocular discharge.

oph·thal·mor·rhex·is (of-thăl'mō-rek'sis) Rupture of an eye, usually due to trauma.

oph·thal·mo·scope (of-thal'mō-skōp) A device for studying the interior of the eyeball through the pupil. SYN funduscope.

oph·thal·mo·scop·ic (of'thăl-mŏ-skop'ik) Relating to examination of the interior of the eye.

oph·thal·mos·co·py (of'thăl-mos'kŏ-pē) Examination of the fundus of the eye by means of the ophthalmoscope.

oph·thal·mo·vas·cu·lar (of-thal'mō-vas' kyū-lăr) Relating to the blood vessels of the eye.

o·pi·ate (ō'pē-ăt) Any preparation or derivative of opium.

o·pi·ate re·cep·tors (ō'pē-ăt rĕ-sep'tŏrz) Regions of the brain that have the capacity to bind morphine.

opi·oid (ō'pē-oyd) A narcotic substance, either natural or synthetic.

o·pi·oid ant·ag·on·ist (ō'pē-oyd an-tag'ŏ-nist) These drugs block the effects of exogenously administered opioids or of endogenously released endorphins and enkephalins.

o·pis·the·nar (ō-pis'thē-năr) Dorsum of the hand.

o·pis·thi·on (ō-pis'thē-on) [TA] The middle point on the posterior margin of the foramen magnum, opposite the basion.

♻ **opistho-** Combining form meaning backward, behind, dorsal.

o·pis·thot·on·ic (ō-pis-thot'ŏ-nik) Relating to or characterized by opisthotonos.

o·pis·thot·o·nos, o·pis·thot·o·nus (ō-pis-thot'ŏ-nos, -nŭs) A tetanic spasm in which the spine and extremities are bent with convexity forward, the body resting on the head and the heels.

o·pi·um (O) (ō'pē-ŭm) The air-dried milky exudation obtained by incising the unripe capsules of *Papaver somniferum*. Contains some 20 alkaloids, including morphine, noscapine, codeine, papaverine, and thebaine. Used as an analgesic, hypnotic, and diaphoretic, and for diarrhea and spasmodic conditions. SYN gum opium, meconium (2).

op·por·tu·nis·tic (op'ŏr-tū-nis'tik) Denoting an organism capable of causing disease only in a host with lowered resistance.

op·por·tu·nis·tic path·o·gen (op'ŏr-tū-nis'tik path'ŏ-jen) Organism capable of causing disease only when the host's resistance is lowered by other diseases or drugs.

op·po·si·tion·al de·fi·ant dis·or·der (op'pŏ-zish'ŭn-ăl dĕ-fī'ănt dis-ŏr'dĕr) A disorder of childhood or adolescence characterized by a recurrent pattern of negativistic, hostile, and disobedient behavior toward authority figures.

op·pres·sion (ŏ-pres'shŭn) NURSING acts of subjugation or coercion related to decisions about health care.

♻ **ops-, opto-, opti-, optico-** Combining forms meaning the eye or vision.

op·sin (op'sin) The protein portion of the rhodopsin molecule; at least three separate opsins are located in cone cells.

op·sin·o·gen (op-sin'ō-jen) A substance that stimulates the formation of opsonin. SYN opsogen.

op·si·u·ri·a (op'sē-yūr'ē-ă) A more rapid excretion of urine during fasting than after a full meal.

op·so·clo·nus, op·so·clo·ni·a (op'sō-klō'nus, -nē-ă) Repetitive irregular multidirectional ocular movement associated with cerebellar or brainstem disorders.

op·son·ic in·dex (op-son'ik in'deks) A value that indicates the relative content of opsonin in the blood of a person with an infectious disease.

op·so·nin (op'sŏ-nin) A substance that binds to antigens, enhancing phagocytosis (q.v.).

op·son·i·za·tion (op'sŏ-nī-zā'shŭn) The process by which bacteria and other cells are altered in such a manner that they are more readily engulfed by phagocytes.

op·so·nize (op'sŏn-īz) To prepare microorganisms for phagocytosis and ultimate destruction.

op·so·nom·e·try (op'sŏ-nom'ĕ-trē) Determination of the opsonic index or the opsonocytophagic activity.

op·ti·c ac·ti·vi·ty (op'tik ak-tiv'i-tē) The ability of a compound in solution to rotate the plane of polarized light.

op·tic ax·is (op'tik ak'sis) [TA] The axis of the eye connecting the anterior and posterior poles.

op•tic disc (op′tik disk) [TA] An oval area of the ocular fundus devoid of light receptors where the axons of the retinal ganglion cells converge to form the optic nerve head. SYN discus nervi optici [TA], blind spot (3), optic papilla.

op•ti•cian (opt.) (op-tish′ăn) *Do not confuse this word with ophthalmologist or optometrist.* One who practices opticianry.

op•ti•cian•ry (op-tish′ăn-rē) The professional practice of filling prescriptions for ophthalmic lenses, dispensing spectacles, and making and fitting contact lenses.

op•tic il•lu•sion (op′tik i-lū′zhŭn) False evaluation of the color, form, size, or movement of a visual sensation.

op•tic ker•a•to•plas•ty (op′tik ker′ă-tō-plas′tē) Transplantation of transparent corneal tissue to replace a leukoma or scar that impairs vision.

op•tic neu•ri•tis (op′tik nūr-ī′tis) Optic nerve inflammation. SEE ALSO retrobulbar neuritis, papillitis.

op•tic neu•rop•a•thy (op′tik nūr-op′ă-thē) Pathologic injury to the optic nerve, usually involves only one eye.

op•ti•co•ki•net•ic nys•tag•mus (op′ti-kō-ki-net′ik nis-tag′mŭs) SYN optokinetic nystagmus.

op•ti•co•pu•pil•lar•y (op′ti-kō-pyū′pi-lar-ē) Relating to the optic nerve and the pupil.

op•tic pa•pil•la (op′tik pă-pil′ă) SYN optic disc.

op•tic ra•di•a•tion (op′tik rā′dē-ā′shŭn) [TA] The massive, fanlike fiber system passing from the lateral geniculate body of the thalamus to the visual cortex. SYN radiatio optica.

op•tics (op′tiks) The science concerned with the properties of light, its refraction and absorption, and the refracting media of the eye in that relation.

op•tic tract (op′tik trakt) [TA] The continuation of the optic nerve fibers beyond their hemidecussation in the optic chiasm. SYN tractus opticus [TA].

op•ti•mal dose (op′ti-măl dōs) Amount of a drug or radiation that will produce the desired effect with least likelihood of undesirable symptoms.

op•ti•mal pitch (op′ti-măl pich) The frequency of vocal fold movement that allows optimal resonance with least vocal effort. SEE ALSO fundamental frequency. SYN natural pitch.

opto-, optico- Combining forms meaning optic; ocular.

op•to•ki•net•ic nys•tag•mus (op′tō-ki-net′ik nis-tag′mŭs) nystagmus induced by looking at moving visual stimuli. SYN opticokinetic nystagmus, railroad nystagmus.

op•tom•e•ter (op-tom′ĕ-tĕr) An instrument for determining the refraction of the eye.

op•tom•e•trist (op-tom′ĕ-trist) One who practices optometry.

op•tom•e•try (op-tom′ĕ-trē) **1.** The profession concerned with the examination of the eyes and related structures to determine the presence of vision problems and eye disorders and with the prescription and adaptation of lenses and other optical aids or the use of visual training for maximum visual efficiency. **2.** The use of an optometer.

op•to•my•om•e•ter (op′tō-mī-om′ĕ-tĕr) An instrument for determining the relative power of the extrinsic muscles of the eye.

o•ra, pl. **o•rae** (ō′ră, -rē) An edge or a margin. Plural of L. *os,* the mouth.

or•ad (ōr′ad) **1.** In a direction toward the mouth. **2.** Situated nearer the mouth in relation to a specific reference point; opposite of aborad.

or•al (ōr′ăl) Relating to the mouth.

or•al and max•il•lo•fa•cial sur•ge•ry (ōr′al mak′sil-ō-fā′shăl sŭr′jĕr-ē) The dental specialty that includes the surgical correction of injuries and malformations of the midface, jaws, and dentition.

or•al can•di•di•a•sis (ōr′ăl kan′di-dī′ă-sis) SYN thrush.

or·al ca·vi·ty (ōr'ăl kav'i-tē) [TA] The region consisting of the vestibulum oris, the narrow cleft between the lips and cheeks and the teeth and gums, and the cavitas oris propria. SYN mouth (1).

or·al con·tra·cep·tive (ōr'ăl kon'tră-sep'tiv) A medication taken by mouth designed to prevent conception.

or·al hy·giene (ōr'ăl hī'jēn) Cleaning the mouth by brushing, flossing, irrigating, massaging, or the use of other devices.

or·al pa·thol·o·gy (ōr'ăl pă-thol'ŏ-jē) The branch of dentistry concerned with the etiology, pathogenesis, and clinical, gross, and microscopic aspects of oral and paraoral disease.

or·al po·li·o·vi·rus vac·cine (ōr'-ăl pō'lē-ō-vī'rŭs vak-sēn') SEE poliovirus vaccines (2).

or·ange (awr'ănj) **1.** The fruit of the orange tree. **2.** A color between red and yellow in the spectrum.

or·ange-top tube (awr'ănj-top tūb) A tube of this color indicates the container has been treated with lithium heparin.

ora ser·ra·ta re·ti·nae (ōr'ă ser-ā'tă ret'i-nē) The serrated extremity of the optic part of the retina, located a little behind the ciliary body.

or·bic·u·lar (ōr-bik'yū-lăr) Circular; round.

or·bic·u·lar bone (ōr-bik'yū-lăr bōn) SYN lenticular process of incus.

or·bic·u·la·re (ōr-bik'yū-lā'rē) SYN lenticular process of incus.

or·bic·u·la·ris oc·u·li re·flex (ōr-bik'yū-lā'ris ok'yū-lī rē'fleks) Contraction of orbicularis oculi muscles on tapping the margin of the orbit, or the bridge or tip of the nose. SYN nose-bridge-lid reflex, nose-eye reflex.

or·bic·u·lar mus·cle (ōr-bik'yū-lăr mŭs'ĕl) [TA] Sphincterlike sheet of muscle that encircles an orifice such as the mouth or the palpebral fissures. SYN musculus orbicularis [TA], orbicularis muscle, orbicularis (2).

or·bic·u·lus (ōr-bik'yū-lŭs) Any muscle surrounding an orifice.

or·bic·u·lus ciliaris (ōr-bik'yū-lŭs sil'ē-ăr'is) The darkly pigmented posterior zone of the ciliary body continuous with the retina at the ora serrata.

or·bit (ōr'bit) [TA] Bony cavity containing the eyeball and its adnexa. SYN orbita [TA], orbital cavity.

or·bi·ta, gen. and pl. **or·bi·tae** (ōr'bi-tă, -tē) [TA] SYN orbit.

or·bi·ta·le (ōr-bi-tā'lē) In cephalometrics, the lowermost point in the lower margin of the bony orbit that may be palpated under the skin.

or·bi·tog·ra·phy (ōr'bi-tog'ră-fē) Radiographic evaluation of the orbit.

or·bi·to·me·a·tal line (ōr'bi-tō-mē-ā'tăl līn) SYN baseline.

or·bi·to·na·sal (ōr'bi-tō-nā'zăl) Relating to the orbit and the nose or nasal cavity.

or·bi·to·nom·e·ter (ōr'bi-tō-nom'ĕ-tĕr) An instrument that measures the resistance offered to pressing the eyeball backward into its socket.

or·bi·to·nom·e·try (ōr'bi-tō-nom'ĕ-trē) Measurement by means of the orbitonometer.

or·bi·top·a·thy (ōr'bi-top'ă-thē) Disease of the orbit and its contents.

or·bi·tot·o·my (ōr-bi-tot'ŏ-mē) Surgical incision into the orbit.

Or·bi·vi·rus (ōr'bī-vī'rŭs) A genus of viruses of vertebrates that multiply in insects, including human Colorado tick fever virus.

or·chec·to·my (ōr-kek'tŏ-mē) SYN orchiectomy.

♻ **orchi-, orchido-, orchio-** Combining forms meaning the testes.

or·chi·al·gi·a, orch·al·gia, or·chi·o·neu·ral·gi·a, or·chi·dal·gi·a (ōr-kē-al'jē-ă, ōr-kal'jē-ă, ōr'kē-ō-nūr-al'jē-ă, ōr'ki-dal'jē-ă) Pain in the testis.

or·chid·ic (ōr-kid'ik) Relating to the testis.

orchido- SEE orchi-.

or·chi·dom·e·ter, or·chi·om·e·ter (ōr′ki-dom′ĕ-tĕr, ōr′kē-om′ĕ-tĕr) **1.** A caliper device used to measure the size of testes. **2.** A set of sized models of testes for comparison of testicular development.

or·chi·ec·to·my, or·chi·dec·to·my, or·chec·to·my (ōr′kē-ek′tŏ-mē, -ki-dek′tŏ-mē, -kek′tŏ-mē) Removal of one or both testes. SYN testectomy.

or·chi·ep·i·did·y·mi·tis (ōr′kē-ep′i-did′i-mī′tis) Inflammation of the testis and epididymis.

or·chi·op·a·thy (ōr′kē-op′ă-thē) Disease of a testis.

or·chi·o·pex·y, or·chi·do·pex·y, or·chi·dor·rha·phy (ōr′kē-ō-pek′sē, -kid′ō-pek-sē, -ki-dōr′ă-fē) Surgical treatment of an undescended testicle by freeing it and implanting it into the scrotum. SYN cryptorchidopexy.

or·chi·o·plas·ty (ōr′kē-ō-plas-tē) Surgical reconstruction of the testis.

or·chi·ot·o·my, or·chot·o·my, or·chi·dot·o·my (ōr′kē-ot′ŏ-mē, -kot′ŏ-mē, -ki-dot′ŏ-mē) Incision into a testis.

or·chit·ic (ōr-kit′ik) Denoting orchitis.

or·chi·tis, or·chi·di·tis, tes·ti·tis (ōr-kī′tis, -ki-dī′tis, tes-tī′tis) Inflammation of the testis.

or·der (ōr′dĕr) **1.** In biologic classification, the division just below the class (or subclass) and above the family. **2.** In a reaction, order is the sum of the exponents of all the concentration terms in that reaction's rate expression. Cf. molecularity. **3.** The sequence of residues in a heteropolymer.

or·der of draw (ōr′dĕr draw) Recommended sequence in which blood specimens should be drawn so as to minimize interference in testing caused by carryover of additives in tubes.

or·di·nate (ōr′di-năt) In a cartesian plane coordinate system, the vertical axis (y).

Or·e·gon grape (ōr′ĕ-gon grāp) SYN barberry.

O·rem self-care de·fi·cit the·o·ry (ōr′em self-kār′ def′i-sit thē′ŏr-ē) Theory that the focus of nursing is teaching patients self-care.

-orexia Combining form meaning (condition of the) appetite, e.g., anorexia.

o·rex·i·gen·ic (ŏ-rek′si-jen′ik) Appetite-stimulating.

or·gan (ōr′găn) [TA] A differentiated structure or part of a system of the body; composed of tissues and cells; exercises a specific function. SYN organum [TA], organon.

or·gan·elle (ōr′gă-nel′) One of the specialized parts of a protozoan or tissue cell. SYN organoid (3).

or·gan·ic (ōr-gan′ik) **1.** Relating to an organ. **2.** Relating to or formed by an organism. **3.** Organized; structural. **4.** SEE organic compound. **5.** Denotes agricultural production of a more ecologically beneficial type.

or·gan·ic acid (ōr-gan′ik as′id) An acid composed of molecules containing organic radicals; e.g., acetic acid, citric acid, which contain the ionizable —COOH group.

or·gan·ic brain syn·drome (ōr-gan′ik brān sin′drōm) A constellation of behavioral or psychological signs and symptoms including problems with attention, concentration, memory, confusion, anxiety, and depression caused by transient or permanent dysfunction of the brain.

or·gan·ic chem·is·try (ōr-gan′ik kem′is-trē) Branch concerned with covalently linked atoms, centering around carbon compounds of this type; chemistry of natural products.

or·gan·ic compound (ōr-gan′ik kom′pownd) A compound composed of atoms (some of which are carbon) held together by covalent (shared electron) bonds. Cf. inorganic compound.

or·gan·ic de·lu·sions (ōr-gan′ik dĕ-lū′zhŭnz) False beliefs experienced in the delirium associated with injury to the brain, organic change as in Alzheimer syndrome, or drug induced.

or·gan·ic dis·ease (ōr-gan′ik di-zēz′)

Disorder with anatomic or pathophysiologic changes in some bodily tissue or organ, in contrast to a disorder of psychogenic origin.

or·gan·ic head·ache (ōr-gan´ik hed´āk) That due to intracranial disease.

or·gan·ic hear·ing im·pair·ment (ōr-gan´ik hēr´ing im-pār´měnt) Deafness due to a pathologic process or an organic cause, as opposed to psychogenic hearing impairment.

or·gan·ic mood syn·drome (ōr-gan´ik mūd sin´drōm) Syndrome attributed to an organic factor characterized by either depressive or manic mood. SEE ALSO bipolar disorder.

or·gan·ic mur·mur (ōr-gan´ik mŭr´mŭr) Sound caused by structural change.

or·gan·ic ver·ti·go (ōr-gan´ik věr´ti-gō) The dizziness-related disorder due to brain damage.

or·gan·i·fi·ca·tion (ōr-gan´i-fi-kā´shŭn) Addition of thyroidal inorganic iodine ot tyrosine residues by thyroid peroxidase.

or·gan·ism (ōr´gă-nizm) Any living individual, whether plant or animal, considered as a whole.

or·gan·i·za·tion (ōr´găn-ī-zā´shŭn) 1. An arrangement of distinct but mutually dependent parts. 2. A facility that provides health care. 3. Conversion of coagulated blood, exudate, or dead tissue into fibrous tissue.

or·gan·iz·er (ōr´găn-ī-zěr) Any group of cells having such a controlling influence, the effects being brought about through the action of an evocator.

♻ **organo-** Prefix meaning organ; organic.

or·gan of Cor·ti (ōr´găn kōr´tē) SYN spiral organ.

or·ga·no·gen·e·sis, or·ga·nog·e·ny (ōr´gă-nō-jen´ě-sis, ōr´găn-oj´ě-nē) Formation of organs during development.

or·ga·noid (ōr´gă-noyd) 1. Resembling in superficial appearance or in structure any of the organs or glands of the body. 2. Composed of glandular or organic elements and not of a single tissue. SEE ALSO histoid. 3. SYN organelle.

or·ga·noid tu·mor (ōr´gă-noyd tū´mŏr) A tumor of complex structure, glandular in origin, containing epithelium and connective tissue.

or·gan·o·mer·cu·ri·al (ōr´gă-nō-měr-kyūr´ē-ăl) Any organic mercurial compound (e.g., merbromin, thimerosal).

or·ga·no·me·tal·lic (ōr´gă-nō-mě-tal´ik) Denoting an organic compound containing metallic atoms in its structure.

or·ga·no·ther·a·py (ōr´gă-nō-thār´ă-pē) Treatment of disease by preparations made from animal organs; now frequently synthetic not natural glandular extracts of a gland.

or·ga·no·troph·ic (ōr´gă-nō-trō´fik) 1. Pertaining to the nourishment of an organ. 2. Pertaining to a microorganism that uses organic sources as a reducing power.

or·ga·no·trop·ic (ōr´gă-nō-trō´pik) Pertaining to or characterized by organotropism.

or·ga·no·tro·pism (ōr´gă-nō-trō´pizm) The special affinity of certain drugs, pathogens, or metastatic tumors for particular organs or their component parts. Cf. parasitotropism.

or·gans of Zuc·ker·kan·dl (ōr´gănz tsuk´ěr-kahn-děl) SYN para-aortic bodies.

or·gan-spe·cif·ic an·ti·gen (ōr´găn-spě-sif´ik an´ti-jen) A heterogenetic antigen with organ specificity; e.g., in addition to species-specific antigen, a kidney of one species contains antigen that is identical to that in a kidney of another species. SYN tissue-specific antigen.

or·gasm (ōr´gazm) The peak state of excitement in the sexual act. SYN climax (2).

or·gas·mic dis·or·ders (ōr-gaz´mik dis-ōr´děrz) Physical or psychological impairment that interferes with the ability to have an sexual orgasm.

or·i·en·ta·tion (ōr´ē-ěn-tā´shŭn) 1. The recognition of one's temporal, spatial, and personal relationships and environment. **2.** The relative position of an atom with respect to another atom to which it is connected.

O·ri·en·ti·a (ōr-ē-en'shă) A genus of the bacterial family Rickettsiaceae.

Or·i·en·ti·a tsu·tsu·ga·mu·shi (ōr-ē-en'shă tsū-tsū-gă-mū'shē) A bacterial species that causes tsutsugamushi disease and scrub typhus; transmitted by trombiculid mites; formerly known as *Rickettsia tsutsugamushi*.

or·i·ent·ing ref·lex, or·i·ent·ing re·sponse (ōr'ē-en-ting rē'fleks, rĕ-spons') An aspect of attending in which an organism's initial response to a change or to a novel stimulus is such that the organism becomes more sensitive to the stimulation; e.g., dilation of the pupil of the eye in response to dim light. SYN investigatory reflex.

or·i·fice (ōr'i-fis) [TA] Any aperture or opening. SYN orificium.

or·i·gin (ōr'i-jin) **1.** The less movable of two sites of attachment of a muscle; that which is attached to the more fixed part of the skeleton. **2.** The starting point of a cranial or spinal nerve. The former have two origins: the ental origin, deep origin, or real origin, the cell group in the brain or medulla whence the fibers of the nerve begin, and the ectal origin, superficial origin, or apparent origin, the point where the nerve emerges from the brain.

or·li·stat (ōr'li-stat) A lipase inhibitor that works in the gastrointestinal tract to reduce the body's absorption of fat.

or·ni·thine (Orn) (ōr'ni-thēn) The amino acid formed when L-arginine is hydrolyzed by arginase; an important intermediate in the urea cycle; elevated levels seen in certain defects of the urea cycle.

or·ni·thi·ne·mi·a (ōr'ni-thi-nē'mē-ă) A toxic condition occasionally producing localized cerebral swelling, caused by abnormal amounts of ornithine in the blood.

or·ni·thi·nu·ri·a (ōr'ni-thi-nyūr'ē-ă) Excretion of excessive amounts of ornithine in urine.

Or·ni·thod·o·ros (ōr'ni-thod'ŏ-ros) A genus of soft ticks, some of which are vectors of pathogens of various relapsing fevers.

or·ni·tho·sis (ōr'ni-thō'sis) SYN psittacosis.

or·o·fa·cial (ōr'ō-fā'shăl) Relating to the mouth and face.

or·o·lin·gual (ōr'ō-ling'gwăl) Relating to the mouth and tongue.

or·o·na·sal (ōr'ō-nā'zăl) Relating to the mouth and nose.

or·o·pha·ryn·ge·al (ōr'ō-fă-rin'jē-ăl) Relating to the oropharynx.

or·o·phar·ynx (ōr'ō-far'ingks) [TA] The portion of the pharynx that lies posterior to the mouth. SYN pars oralis pharyngis [TA], oral part of pharynx, oral pharynx.

Oro·pou·che fe·ver (ōr'ō-pū'shĕ fē'vĕr) Acute febrile illness caused by a species of *Bunyavirus*.

or·o·tate (Oro) (ōr'ŏ-tāt) A salt or ester of orotic acid.

o·rot·ic ac·id (Oro, OA) (ōr-ot'ik as'id) 6-Carboxyuracil; an important intermediate in the formation of the pyrimidine nucleotides. SYN uracil-6-carboxylic acid.

or·o·tra·cheal (ōr'ō-trā'kē-ăl) Pertaining to the passage between the mouth and the trachea.

or·o·tra·che·al tube (ōr'ō-trā'kē-ăl tūb) A tracheal tube inserted through the mouth.

or·phan dis·ease (ōr'făn di-zēz') Disorder for which no treatment has been developed because its rarity. SEE ALSO orphan products.

or·phan pro·ducts (ōr'făn prod'ŭkts) Drugs, biologicals, and medical devices (including diagnostic in vitro tests) that might treat rare diseases but are not considered commercially viable.

or·phan re·cep·tor (ōr'făn rĕ-sep'tŏr) A nuclear receptor for which no ligand has yet been identified.

✿ -orrhagia, -rrhagia, -rrhage Combining forms meaning excessive flow.

-orrhea, -rrhea Combining forms meaning discharge or flow.

-orrhexis, -rrhexis Combining forms meaning to rupture.

or·thet·ics (ōr-thet'iks) SYN orthotics.

ortho-, orth- 1. Combining forms meaning straight, normal, in proper order. 2. CHEMISTRY italicized prefix denoting that a compound has two substitutions on adjacent carbon atoms in a benzene ring.

or·tho·cho·re·a (ōr'thō-kŏr-ē'ă) A form of chorea with spasms that occur only or chiefly in upright patients.

or·tho·chro·mat·ic (ōr'thō-krō-mat'ik) Denoting any tissue or cell that stains the color of the dye used.

or·tho·de·ox·i·a (ōr'thō-dē-oks'ē-ă) Fall in arterial blood oxygen on assuming the upright posture.

or·tho·don·tic ap·pli·ance (ōr'thō-don'tik ă-plī'ăns) Mechanism for the application of force to the teeth and their supporting tissues to produce changes in the relationship of the teeth and/or the related osseous structures.

or·tho·don·tic band (ōr'thō-don'tik band) Thin strip of metal or plastic closely adapted to the crown of a tooth to which wires may be attached for tooth movement.

or·tho·don·tics (ōr'thō-don'tiks) Branch of dentistry concerned with the correction and prevention of irregularities and malocclusion of the teeth.

or·tho·dont·ist (ōr'thō-don'tist) A dental specialist who practices orthodontics.

or·tho·dro·mic (ōr'thō-drō'mik) Denoting the propagation of an impulse along an axon in the normal direction. Cf. antidromic.

or·tho·gen·e·sis (ōr'thō-jen'ĕ-sis) The doctrine that evolution is governed by intrinsic factors and occurs in predictable directions.

or·tho·gen·ic (ōr'thō-jen'ik) Relating to orthogenesis.

or·tho·gnath·i·a, or·tho·gnath·ism (ōr'thog-nath'ē-ă, -izm) The study of the causes and treatment of conditions related to malposition of the bones of the jaws.

or·tho·gnath·ic, or·thog·na·thous (ōr'thōg-nath'ik, -thog'nă-thŭs) 1. Relating to orthognathia. 2. Having a face without a projecting jaw, that is, one with a gnathic index less than 98. 3. Having a normal relationship of the jaws.

or·tho·grade (ōr'thō-grād) Walking or standing erect; as with human beings.

or·tho·ker·a·tol·o·gy (ōr'thō-ker'ă-tol'ŏ-jē) A method of molding the cornea with contact lenses to improve unaided vision.

or·tho·ker·a·to·sis (ōr'thō-ker'ă-tō'sis) Formation of an anuclear keratin layer, as in the normal epidermis.

or·tho·ki·net·ics (ōr'thō-ki-net'iks) A method advocated for the treatment of hypertrophic osteoarthritis in which an attempt is made to change muscular action from one group of muscles to another set of muscles to protect the diseased joint.

or·tho·me·chan·i·cal (ōr'thō-mĕ-kan'i-kăl) Pertaining to braces, prostheses, and appliances.

or·tho·mo·lec·u·lar (ōr'thō-mŏ-lek'yū-lăr) A therapeutic approach designed to provide an optimal molecular environment for body functions, especially of optimal concentrations of substances normally present in the body.

or·tho·mo·lec·u·lar ther·a·py, or·tho·mol·e·cu·lar med·i·cine (ōr'thō-mŏ-lek'yū-lăr thār'ă-pē, med'i-sin) Treatment designed to remedy deficiencies in any of the normal chemical constituents of the body.

Or·tho·myx·o·vir·i·dae (ōr'thō-mik'sō-vir'i-dē) The family of viruses that comprises the three groups of influenza viruses, types A, B, and C.

or·tho·pae·dic [Br.] SYN orthopedic.

orthopedic (ōr'thō-pē'dik) Relating to orthopedics.

or·tho·pe·dics, or·tho·pae·dics (ōr'

thŏ-pē'diks) *Although this is the correct U.S. spelling according to rule and precedent, the American Academy of Orthopaedic Surgeons has officially adopted the spelling orthopaedics.* Medical specialty concerned with the preservation, restoration, and development of form and function of the musculoskeletal system, extremities, spine, and associated structures by medical, surgical, and physical methods.

or·tho·pe·dic sur·ger·y (ORS, OS) (ōr'thŏ-pē'dik sŭr'jĕr-ē) Surgery that embraces treatment of acute and chronic disorders of the musculoskeletal system, including injuries, diseases, dysfunction, and deformities in the extremities and spine.

or·tho·per·cus·sion (ōr'thŏ-pĕr-kŭsh'ŭn) Very light percussion of the chest, used to determine the size of the heart.

or·tho·phor·i·a (ōr'thŏ-fōr'ē-ă) Absence of heterophoria; the condition of binocular fixation in which the lines of sight meet at a distant or near point of reference in the absence of a fusion stimulus.

or·thop·ne·a (ōr-thop'nē'ă) Discomfort in breathing that is brought on or aggravated by lying flat. Cf. platypnea.

or·thop·ne·ic po·si·tion (ōr-thop-nē'ik pŏ-zish'ŏn) Placement assumed by patients with orthopnea, namely sitting propped up in bed by several pillows. SYN orthopnea position.

or·tho·psy·chi·a·try (ōr'thŏ-sī-kī'ă-trē) A cross-disciplinary science combining child psychiatry, developmental psychology, pediatrics, and family care devoted to the discovery, prevention, and treatment of mental and psychological disorders in children and adolescents.

or·thop·tic (ōr-thop'tik) Relating to orthoptics.

or·thop·tics (ōr-thop'tiks) The study and treatment of defective binocular vision, of defects in the action of the ocular muscles, or of faulty visual habits.

or·thop·tist (ōr-thop'tist) One skilled in orthoptics.

or·tho·sis, pl. **or·tho·ses** (ōr-thō'sis, -sēz) An external orthopedic appliance that prevents or assists movement of the spine or limbs.

or·tho·stat·ic (ōr'thō-stat'ik) Relating to an erect posture or position.

orth·o·sta·tic con·ges·tion (ōr'thō-stat'ik kŏn-jes'chŭn) Pooling of blood in lower parts of the body due to upright posture.

or·tho·stat·ic de·con·di·tion·ing (ōr'thō-stat'ik dē'kŏn-dish'ŏn-ing) Negative effects of prolonged bed rest or of space flight at minimal gravity, resulting in tachycardia and hypotension in the upright position.

or·tho·stat·ic hy·po·ten·sion (ōr'thō-stat'ik hī'pō-ten'shŭn) A form of low blood pressure that occurs in a standing patient. SYN postural hypotension.

or·tho·stat·ic in·tol·er·ance (ōr'thō-stat'ik in-tol'ĕr-ăns) Decreased venous return in the upright position typically experienced by astronauts after returning to an environment subject to gravity.

or·tho·stat·ic pro·tein·u·ri·a, pos·tur·al pro·tein·u·ri·a (OP) (ōr'thō-stat'ik prō'tē-nūr'ē-ă, pos'chŭr-ăl) SYN orthostatic albuminuria.

or·tho·tic (ōr-thot'ik) **1.** Pertaining to orthotics. **2.** An orthotic appliance.

or·thot·ics (ōr-thot'iks) The science concerned with the making and fitting of orthopedic appliances. SYN orthetics.

or·tho·tist (ōr-thot'ist) A maker and fitter of orthopedic appliances.

or·thot·o·nos, or·thot·o·nus (ōr-thot'ŏ-nos, -nŭs) A form of tetanic spasm in which the neck, limbs, and body are held fixed in a straight line.

or·tho·top·ic (ōr'thō-tō'pik) In the normal or usual position.

or·tho·top·ic ur·e·ter·o·cele (ōr'thō-tō'pik yū-rē'tĕr-ō-sēl) A ureterocele entirely within the bladder.

or·tho·trop·ic (ōr'thō-trō'pik) Extending in a straight especially vertical, direction.

or·tho·vol·tage (ōr'thŏ-vōl'tăj) In radiation therapy, a term for voltage between 400 and 600 kV.

Orth stain (orth stān) A lithium carmine stain for nerve cells and their processes.

Os (os) Symbol for osmium.

os (os) [TA] **1.** gen. **o•ris,** pl. **o•ra** [TA] The mouth. **2.** gen. **o•ris,** gen. **os•sis,** pl. **os•sa** (os, ōr′is, -ă, os′is, os′ă) Bone. **3.** Term applied sometimes to an opening into a hollow organ or canal, especially one with thick or fleshy edges. SYN bone.

♲ **osche-, oscheo-** Combining forms meaning the scrotum.

os•che•i•tis (os′kē-ī′tis) Inflammation of the scrotum.

os•che•o•hy•dro•cele (os′kē-ō-hī′drō-sēl) Scrotal hydrocele.

os•che•o•plas•ty (os′kē-ō-plas-tē) SYN scrotoplasty.

os•cil•lat•ing vi•sion (os′il-āt′ing vizh′ŭn) SYN oscillopsia.

os•cil•la•tion (os′il-ā′shŭn) **1.** A to-and-fro movement. **2.** A stage in inflammation in which the accumulation of leukocytes in small vessels arrests the passage of blood and there is a to-and-fro movement at each cardiac contraction.

os•cil•lop•si•a (os′i-lop′sē-ă) The subjective sensation of oscillation of objects viewed. SYN oscillating vision.

os•cil•lo•scope (ŏ-sil′ŏ-skōp) An oscillograph in which the record of oscillations is continuously visible.

os•cu•lum, pl. **os•cu•la** (os′kyū-lŭm, -lă) A pore or minute opening.

♲ **-ose 1.** CHEMISTRY a suffix usually indicating a carbohydrate. **2.** Suffix appended to some Latin stems, with significance of the more common suffix, -ous (2). **3.** Suffix meaning full of, having much of.

Os•good-Schlat•ter dis•ease (oz′gud shlaht′er di-zēz′) Inflammation or partial avulsion of the tibial apophysis due to traction forces. SYN Schlatter disease, Schlatter-Osgood disease.

os in•ci•si•vum (os in′si-sī′vŭm) The anterior and inner portion of the maxilla, which in the fetus and sometimes in the adult is a separate bone; the incisive suture runs from the incisive canal between the lateral incisor and the canine tooth. SYN intermaxillary bone.

♲ **-osis** Combining form meaning a process, condition, or state, usually abnormal or diseased; production of an abnormal substance, increase of a normal substance, or parasitic infestation.

os•mate (oz′māt) A salt of osmic acid.

os•mat•ic (oz-mat′ik) SYN olfactory.

os•mic ac•id (oz′mik as′id) A volatile caustic and strong oxidizing agent; colorless crystals, poorly soluble in water, but soluble in organic solvents; the aqueous solution is a fat and myelin stain and a general fixative for electron microscopy.

os•mics (oz′miks) The science of olfaction.

os•mi•dro•sis (oz′mī-drō′sis) SYN bromidrosis.

os•mi•um (Os) (oz′mē-ŭm) A metallic element, atomic no. 76, atomic wt. 190.2.

♲ **osmo- 1.** Prefix meaning osmosis. **2.** Prefix meaning smell, odor.

os•mo•lal•i•ty (os′mō-lal′i-tē) The concentration of a solution expressed in osmoles of solute particles per kilogram of solvent.

os•mo•lar•i•ty (os′mō-lar′i-tē) *Do not confuse this word with osmolality.* The osmotic concentration of an osmotically active substance in solution, expressed as osmoles of solute particles per liter of solution.

os•mole (os′mōl) The molecular weight of a solute, in grams, divided by the number of ions or particles into which it dissociates in solution.

os•mol•o•gy (oz-mol′ŏ-jē) **1.** The study of odors, their production, and their effects. SYN osphresiology. **2.** The study of osmosis.

os•mom•e•ter (os-mom′ĕ-tĕr) Instrument used to determine concentration of free particles in solution; usually by freezing point depression or vapor pressure. SEE ALSO osmolality.

os·mom·e·try (os-mom′ĕ-trē) Technique used to determine the number of solute particles in solution by measuring changes in a colligative property.

os·mo·phore (oz′mō-fōr) The group of atoms in the molecule of a compound that is responsible for the compound's characteristic odor.

os·mo·sis (os-mō′sis) The process by which solvent tends to move through a semipermeable membrane from a solution of lower to a solution of higher osmolal concentration of the solutes to which the membrane is relatively impermeable.

os·mot·ic di·u·re·sis (os-mot′ik dī′yūr-ē′sis) Type due to a high concentration of osmotically active substances in the renal tubules that limit the reabsorption of water.

os·mot·ic di·u·ret·ics (os-mot′ik dī′yūr-et′iks) Drugs that by their osmotic effects promote the elimination of water and electrolytes in the urine.

os·mot·ic fra·gil·i·ty (os-mot′ik frǎ-jil′i-tē) The susceptibility of erythrocytes to hemolyze when exposed to increasingly hypotonic saline solutions. SYN fragility of the blood.

os·mot·ic pres·sure (II) (os-mot′ik presh′ŭr) The pressure that must be applied to a solution to prevent the passage into it of solvent when solution and pure solvent are separated by a membrane permeable only to the solvent.

osphresio- Prefix denoting odor; sense of smell.

os·sa (os′ă) Plural of L. *os*, bone.

os·se·in, os·se·ine (os′ē-in, -īn) SYN collagen.

osseo- Combining form meaning bony. SEE ALSO ossi-, osteo-.

os·se·o·car·ti·lag·i·nous (os′ē-ō-kahr′ti-laj′i-nŭs) Relating to, or composed of,

both bone and cartilage. SYN osteocartilaginous.

os·se·o·in·te·gra·tion (os′ē-ō-in′tĕ-grā′shŭn) The direct attachment to bone of an inert, alloplastic material without intervening connective tissue, as with dental implants.

os·se·o·mu·cin (os′ē-ō-myū′sin) The ground substance of bony tissue.

os·se·ous, os·te·al (os′ē-ŭs, -tē-ăl) Bony; of bonelike consistency or structure.

os·se·ous la·cu·na (os′ē-ŭs lǎ-kū′nǎ) A cavity in bony tissue occupied by an osteocyte.

os·se·ous tis·sue (os′ē-ŭs tish′ū) A connective tissue with matrix that consists of collagen fibers and ground substance and with deposits of calcium salts in the form of an apatite.

ossi- Combining form denoting bone. SEE ALSO osseo-, osteo-.

os·si·cle (os′i-kĕl) [TA] A small bone; specifically, one of the bones of the tympanic cavity or middle ear. SYN bonelet, ossiculum.

os·sic·u·lec·to·my (os′i-kyū-lek′tŏ-mē) Removal of one or more of the ossicles of the middle ear.

os·sic·u·lot·o·my (os′i-kyū-lot′ŏ-mē) Division of one of the ossicles of the middle ear.

os·sic·u·lum, pl. **os·sic·u·la** (ŏ-sik′yū-lŭm, -lǎ) [TA] SYN ossicle.

os·sif·er·ous (ŏ-sif′ĕr-ŭs) Containing or producing bone.

os·sif·ic (ŏ-sif′ik) Relating to a change into, or formation of, bone.

os·si·fi·ca·tion, os·to·sis (os′i-fi-kā′shŭn, os-tō′sis) **1.** The formation of bone. **2.** A change into bone.

os·si·fy (os′i-fī) To form bone or convert into bone.

os·te·al·gi·a (os′tē-al′jē-ă) Pain in a bone. SYN osteodynia.

os·te·al·gic (os′tē-al′jik) Relating to or marked by bone pain.

os·tec·to·my, os·te·o·ec·to·my (os-tek′tŏ-mē, os-tē′ŏ-ek-tŏ-mē) **1.** Surgical removal of bone. **2.** DENTISTRY resection of osseous structures to eliminate peri-odontal pockets.

os·te·ec·to·pi·a (os′tē-ek-tō′pē-ă) Os-seous displacement.

os·te·i·tis (os′tē-ī′tis) Inflammation of bone. SYN ostitis.

os·te·i·tis de·for·mans (os′tē-ī′tis dĕ-fōr′manz) SYN Paget disease (1).

os·te·i·tis fi·bro·sa cys·ti·ca (os′tē-ī′tis fī-brō′să sis′ti-kă) Increased osteo-clastic resorption of calcified bone with replacement by fibrous tissue. SYN Recklinghausen disease of bone.

os·te·mi·a (os-tē′mē-ă) **1.** Congestion of blood in a bone. **2.** Hyperemia of a bone.

os·tem·py·e·sis (os′tem-pī-ē′sis) Sup-puration in bone.

♻ **osteo-, ost-, oste-** Combining forms de-noting bone. SEE ALSO osseo-, ossi-. Combining form denoting bone.

os·te·o·an·a·gen·e·sis (os′tē-ō-an-ă-jen′ĕ-sis) Regeneration of bone.

os·te·o·ar·thri·tis (os′tē-ō-ahr-thrī′tis) Arthritis characterized by erosion of ar-ticular cartilage, which becomes soft, frayed, and thinned with eburnation of subchondral bone and outgrowths of marginal osteophytes; pain and loss of function result; mainly affects weight-bearing joints, is more common in women, the overweight, and in older people. SYN degenerative joint disease, hypertrophic arthritis, osteoarthrosis.

os·te·o·ar·throp·a·thy (os′tē-ō-ahr-throp′ă-thē) A disorder affecting bones and joints.

os·te·o·ar·throt·o·my (os′tē-ō-ahr-throt′ŏ-mē) Surgical incision into a joint.

os·te·o·blast (os′tē-ō-blast) A bone-forming cell that is derived from mesen-chymal progenitor cells and forms an os-seous matrix in which it becomes en-closed as an osteocyte.

os·te·o·blas·to·ma (os′tē-ō-blas-tō′mă) An uncommon benign tumor of osteo-blasts with areas of osteoid and calcified tissue, occurring most frequently in the spine of a young person. SYN giant oste-oid osteoma.

os·te·o·chon·dri·tis (os′tē-ō-kon-drī′tis) Inflammation of a bone and its overlying articular cartilage.

os·te·o·chon·dri·tis dis·se·cans (os′tē-ō-kon-drī′tis dis′sĕ-kanz) Complete or incomplete separation of a portion of joint cartilage and underlying bone, usu-ally involving the knee, associated with epiphysial aseptic necrosis.

os·te·o·chon·dro·ma (os′tē-ō-kon-drō′mă) A benign cartilaginous neoplasm that consists of a pedicle of normal bone covered with a rim of proliferating carti-lage cells; multiple osteochondromas are inherited and referred to as hereditary multiple exostoses.

os·te·o·chon·dro·sar·co·ma (os′tē-ō-kon′drō-sahr-kō′mă) Chondrosarcoma arising in bone. Sarcomas in bone con-taining foci of neoplastic cartilage as well as bone are classified as osteogenic sarcomas.

os·te·o·chon·dro·sis (os′tē-ō-kon-drō′sis) Any of a group of disorders of one or more ossification centers in children, characterized by degeneration or aseptic necrosis followed by reossification; in-cludes the various forms of epiphysial aseptic necrosis.

os·te·oc·la·sis, os·te·o·cla·si·a (os′tē-ok′lă-sis, -ō-klā′zē-ă) Intentional frac-ture of a bone to correct deformity.

os·te·o·clast (os′tē-ō-klast) **1.** A large multinucleated cell, possibly of mono-cytic origin, with abundant acidophilic cytoplasm, functioning in the absorption and removal of osseous tissue. SYN os-teophage. **2.** An instrument used to frac-ture a bone to correct a deformity.

os·te·o·clast ac·ti·vat·ing fac·tor (os′tē-ō-klast ak′ti-vāt-ing fak′tŏr) A lym-phokine that stimulates bone resorption and inhibits bone-collagen synthesis.

os·te·o·clas·tic (os′tē-ō-klas′tik) Per-taining to osteoclasts, especially with ref-erence to their activity in the absorption and removal of osseous tissue.

os·te·o·clas·to·ma (os'tē-ō-klas-tō'mǎ) SYN giant cell tumor of bone.

os·te·o·cra·ni·um (os'tē-ō-krā'nē-ŭm) The cranium of the fetus after ossification of the membranous cranium has made it firm.

os·te·o·cys·to·ma (os'tē-ō-sis-tō'mǎ) SYN solitary bone cyst.

os·te·o·cyte (os'tē-ō-sīt) A cell of osseous tissue that occupies a lacuna and has cytoplasmic processes that extend into canaliculi and make contact with the processes of other osteocytes.

os·te·o·den·si·tom·e·ter (os'tē-ō-den'si-tom'ĕ-tĕr) Device used to measure the bone density.

os·te·o·den·tin (os'tē-ō-den'tin) Rapidly formed tertiary dentin that contains entrapped fibroblasts or odontoblasts and occasionally displays dentinal tubules; it thus superficially resembles bone.

os·te·o·der·mi·a (os'tē-ō-dĕrm'ē-ǎ) SYN osteoma cutis.

os·te·o·di·as·ta·sis (os'tē-ō-dī-as'tǎ-sis) Separation of two adjacent bones.

os·te·o·dyn·i·a (os'tē-ō-din'ē-ǎ) SYN ostealgia.

os·te·o·dys·tro·phy, os·te·o·dys·tro·phi·a (os'tē-ō-dis'trŏ-fē, -dis-trō'fē-ǎ) Defective formation of bone. SYN osteodystrophia.

os·te·o·e·piph·y·sis (os'tē-ō-e-pif'i-sis) An epiphysis of a bone.

os·te·o·fi·bro·ma (os'tē-ō-fī-brō'mǎ) A benign lesion of bone, probably not a true neoplasm, consisting chiefly of fairly dense, moderately cellular, fibrous connective tissue with small foci of osteogenesis.

os·te·o·gen (os'tē-ō-jen) A bone matrix-producing tissue or layer.

os·te·o·gen·e·sis (os'tē-ō-jen'ĕ-sis) The formation of bone. SYN osteogeny, osteosis (2), ostosis (2).

os·te·o·gen·e·sis im·per·fec·ta, os·te·o·gen·e·sis im·per·fec·ta con·gen·i·ta, os·te·o·gen·e·sis im·per·fec·ta tar·da (OI) (os'tē-ō-jen'ĕ-sis im-pĕr-fek'tǎ, kŏn-jen'ĭ-tǎ, tahr'dǎ) Abnormal fragility and plasticity of bone, with recurring fractures on trivial trauma; variable associated features include deformity of long bones, blueness of sclerae, laxity of ligaments, and otosclerosis. SYN brittle bones.

os·te·o·ge·net·ic fi·bers (os'tē-ō-jĕ-net'ik fī'bĕrz) The fibers in the osteogenetic layer of the periosteum.

os·te·o·gen·ic, os·te·o·ge·net·ic (os'tē-ō-jen'ik, -jĕ-net'ik) Relating to osteogenesis. SYN osteogenous.

os·te·o·gen·ic sar·co·ma (os'tē-ō-jen'ik sahr-kō'mǎ) Most common and malignant of bone sarcomas.

os·te·o·ha·lis·ter·e·sis (os'tē-ō-ha-lis'tĕr-ē'sis) Softening of the bones through absorption or insufficient supply of the mineral portion.

os·te·oid (os'tē-oyd) **1.** Relating to or resembling bone. **2.** Newly formed organic bone matrix before calcification.

os·te·oid os·te·o·ma (os'tē-oyd os'tē-ō'mǎ) A painful benign neoplasm that usually originates in one of the bones of the lower extremities, especially in adolescents and young adults.

os·te·o·lip·o·chon·dro·ma (os'tē-ō-lip'ō-kon-drō'mǎ) A benign neoplasm of cartilaginous tissue, in which metaplasia occurs and foci of adipose cells and osseous tissue are formed.

os·te·ol·o·gy (os'tē-ol'ŏ-jē) Anatomy of the bones; the science concerned with the bones and their structure.

os·te·ol·y·sis (os'tē-ol'i-sis) *Avoid mispronunciation osteoly'sis.* Softening, absorption, and destruction of bony tissue.

os·te·o·ma (os'tē-ō'mǎ) A benign slow-growing mass of mature, predominantly lamellar bone, usually arising from the skull or mandible.

os·te·o·ma cu·tis (os'tē-ō'mǎ kyū'tis) Cutaneous ossification in foci of degeneration in tumors or inflammatory lesions. SYN osteodermia, osteosis cutis.

os·te·o·ma·la·ci·a (os'tē-ō-mă-lā'shē-ă) A disease characterized by a gradual softening and bending of the bones with varying severity of pain. SYN adult rickets, late rickets.

os·te·o·ma·lac·ic pel·vis (os'tē-ō-mă-lā'sik pel'vis) A pelvic deformity in osteomalacia. SYN beaked pelvis.

os·te·o·ma spon·gi·o·sum (os'tē-ō'mă spŭn'jē-ō'sŭm) One that consists chiefly of cancellous bone tissue.

os·te·o·my·e·li·tis (os'tē-ō-mī-ĕ-lī'tis) Inflammation of the bone marrow and adjacent bone. SYN central osteitis (1).

os·te·o·my·e·lo·dys·pla·si·a (os'tē-ō-mī'ĕ-lō-dis-plā'zē-ă) A disease characterized by enlargement of the marrow cavities of the bones, thinning of the osseous tissue, leukopenia, and irregular fever.

os·te·on, os·te·one (os'tē-on, -ōn) A central canal containing blood capillaries and the concentric osseous lamellae around it. SYN haversian system.

os·te·o·ne·cro·sis (os'tē-ō-nĕ-krō'sis) The extensive death of bone.

os·te·o·neu·ral·gi·a (os'tē-ō-nūr-al'jē-ă) A general name for osseous pain.

os·te·o·pa·thi·a stri·a·ta (os'tē-ō-path'ē-ă strī-ā'tă) Linear striations seen radiographically in the metaphyses of long bones and also flat bones. SYN Voorhoeve disease.

os·te·o·pa·thol·o·gy (os'tē-ō-pă-thol'ō-jē) Study of diseases of bone.

os·te·op·a·thy (os'tē-op'ă-thē) 1. Any disease of bone. 2. A school of medicine based on a concept of the normal body as a vital machine capable, when in correct adjustment, of making its own remedies against infections and other toxic conditions; practitioners use conventional medicine in addition to manipulative measures. SYN osteopathic medicine.

os·te·o·pe·ni·a (os'tē-ō-pē'nē-ă) 1. Decreased calcification or density of bone. 2. Reduced bone mass due to inadequate osteoid synthesis.

os·te·o·per·i·os·te·al graft (os'tē-ō-per-ē-os'tē-ăl graft) Bone graft of bone with its attached periosteum.

os·te·o·per·i·os·ti·tis (os'tē-ō-per'ē-os-tī'tis) Inflammation of the periosteum and of the underlying bone.

os·te·o·pe·tro·sis (os'tē-ō-pĕ-trō'sis) Excessive formation of dense trabecular bone and calcified cartilage. SYN Albers-Schönberg disease.

os·te·o·phle·bi·tis (os'tē-ō-flĕ-bī'tis) Inflammation of the veins of a bone.

os·te·o·phyte, os·te·o·phy·ma (os'tē-ō-fīt, -fī'mă) A bony outgrowth or protuberance.

os·te·o·plas·ty (os'tē-ō-plas-tē) 1. Bone grafting; reparative or plastic surgery of bones. 2. In dentistry, resection of osseous structures to achieve acceptable gingival contour.

os·te·o·po·ro·sis (os'tē-ō-pŏr-ō'sis) Reduction in the quantity of bone or atrophy of skeletal tissue in postmenopausal women and older men.

os·te·o·po·rot·ic (os'tē-ō-pŏr-ot'ik) Pertaining to, characterized by, or causing a porous condition of the bones.

os·te·o·ra·di·o·ne·cro·sis (os'tē-ō-rā'dē-ō-ne-krō'sis) Bone death produced by ionizing radiation; may be planned or unplanned.

os·te·or·rha·phy (os'tē-ōr'ă-fē) Wiring together the fragments of a broken bone.

os·te·o·scle·ro·sis (os'tē-ō-skle-rō'sis) Abnormal osseous hardening or eburnation.

os·te·o·sis (os'tē-ō'sis) 1. A morbid process in bone. 2. SYN osteogenesis.

os·te·o·sy·no·vi·tis (os'tē-ō-sin'ō-vī'tis) Inflammation of synovial membranes and surrounding bones.

os·te·o·syn·the·sis (os'tē-ō-sin'thĕ-sis) Internal fixation of a fracture by means of a mechanical device.

os·te·o·throm·bo·sis (os'tē-ō-throm-bō'sis) Thrombosis in one or more of the veins of a bone.

os·te·o·tome (os′tē-ō-tōm) An instrument for use in cutting bone.

os·te·ot·o·my (os′tē-ot′ō-mē) Cutting a bone, usually by means of a saw or chisel.

os·ti·tis (os-tī′tis) SYN osteitis.

os·ti·um (os′tē-ŭm) [TA] A small opening, especially one of entrance into a hollow organ or canal.

os·to·mate (os′tō-māt) Term for one who has an ostomy.

-ostomy Combining form for surgical creation of a new opening.

os·to·my (os′tō-mē) **1.** An artificial stoma or opening into the urinary or gastrointestinal canal, or the trachea. **2.** Any operation by which a permanent opening is created between two hollow organs or between a hollow viscus and the skin externally, as in tracheostomy.

os tri·go·num (os trī-gō′nŭm) [TA] Independent ossicle sometimes present in the tarsus.

os ve·sa·li·a·num (os ve-sā′lē-ā′nŭm) The tuberosity of the fifth metatarsal bone sometimes existing as a separate bone.

O·ta ne·vus (ō′tah nē′vŭs) SYN oculodermal melanosis.

O·thel·lo syn·drome (ō-thel′ō sin′drōm) Delusional belief in the infidelity of one's spouse.

o·tic (ō′tik) Relating to the ear.

o·tic cap·sule (ō′tik kap′sŭl) The cartilage that, in the embryo, surrounds the developing otic vesicle and develops into the bony labyrinth of the internal ear. SYN auditory capsule.

o·tic ves·i·cle (ō′tik ves′i-kĕl) A paired sac of invaginated ectoderm that develops into the membranous labyrinth of the internal ear. SYN acoustic vesicle, auditory vesicle.

o·tit·ic (ō-tit′ik) Relating to otitis.

o·tit·ic hy·dro·ceph·a·lus (ō-tit′ik hī′drō-sef′ă-lŭs) Form associated with otitis media and thrombosis of one or both sigmoid sinuses of the dura.

o·tit·ic men·in·gi·tis (ō-tit′ik men′in-jī′tis) Infection of the meninges secondary to mastoiditis or otitis media.

o·ti·tis (ō-tī′tis) Inflammation of the ear.

o·ti·tis ex·ter·na (ō-tī′tis eks-tĕr′nă) Inflammation of the external auditory canal.

o·ti·tis in·ter·na (ō-tī′tis in-tĕr′nă) SYN labyrinthitis.

o·ti·tis mas·toi·de·a (ō-tī′tis mas-toy′dē-ă) Inflammation of the middle ear that involves the mastoid space. SEE ALSO ear.

o·ti·tis me·di·a (OM) (ō-tī′tis mē′dē-ă) Inflammation of the middle ear, or tympanum.

oto- Combining form denoting the ear. SEE ALSO auri-.

o·to·ceph·a·ly (ō′tō-sef′ă-lē) Malformation characterized by markedly defective development of the lower jaw and the union or close approach of the ears on the front of the neck.

o·to·cra·ni·um (ō′tō-krā′nē-ŭm) The bony case of the internal and middle ear, consisting of the petrous portion of the temporal bone.

oto·dyn·ia (ō′tō-din′ē-ă) Pain in the ear.

o·to·en·ceph·a·li·tis (ō′tō-en-sef′ă-lī′tis) Inflammation of the brain by extension of the process from the middle ear and mastoid cells.

o·to·gen·ic, o·tog·e·nous (ō′-tō-jen′ik, ō-toj′ĕ-nŭs) Of otic origin; originating within the ear, especially from inflammation of the ear.

o·to·lar·yn·gol·o·gy (ō′tō-lar-in-gol′ŏ-jē) The combined specialties of diseases of the ear and larynx, often including upper respiratory tract and many diseases of the head and neck, tracheobronchial tree, and esophagus.

o·to·lith·ic crisis (ō′tō-lith′ik krī′sis) A

sudden drop attack without loss of consciousness, vertigo, auditory disturbances, or autonomic manifestations.

o·to·liths, o·to·lites (ō′tō-līths, -līts) [TA] Crystalline particles of calcium carbonate and a protein adhering to the gelatinous membrane of the maculae of the utricle and saccule.

o·tol·o·gist (ō-tol′ŏ-jist) A specialist in otology.

o·tol·o·gy (ō-tol′ŏ-jē) The branch of medical science concerned with the study, diagnosis, and treatment of diseases of the ear and related structures.

o·to·mu·cor·my·co·sis (ō′tō-myū′kōr-mī-kō′sis) Mucormycosis of the ear.

♻ **-otomy** SEE -tomy.

o·to·my·co·sis (ō′tō-mī-kō′sis) Fungal infection in the external auditory canal, with scaling, itching, and pain as the primary symptoms.

o·to·neu·ral·gi·a (ō′tō-nū-ral′jē-ă) Noninflammatory earache of neuralgic origin.

o·to·neu·rol·o·gy (ō′tō-nūr-ol′ŏ-jē) SYN neurootology.

o·top·a·thy (ō-top′ă-thē) Any disease of the ear.

o·to·pha·ryn·ge·al (ō′tō-fă-rin′jē-ăl) Relating to the middle ear and the pharynx.

o·to·plas·ty (ō′tō-plas-tē) Reparative surgery of the auricle of the ear.

o·to·py·or·rhe·a (ō′tō-pī′ŏ-rē′ă) Discharge of pus from the ears.

o·to·py·osis (ō′tō-pī-ō′sis) Presence of pus in the ear.

o·to·rhi·no·lar·yn·gol·o·gy (ō′tō-rī′nō-lar′in-gol′ŏ-jē) The combined specialties of diseases of the ear, nose, and larynx; including diseases of related structures of the head and neck. SEE ALSO otolaryngology.

o·to·rhi·nol·o·gy (ō′tō-rī-nol′ŏ-jē) Study of diseases of the ears and nose.

o·tor·rhe·a (ō′tō-rē′ă) A discharge from the ear. SYN otorrhoea.

otorrhoea [Br.] SYN otorrhea.

o·to·scle·ro·sis (ō′tō-skle-rō′sis) A new formation of spongy bone about the stapes and fenestra vestibuli, resulting in progressively increasing deafness, without signs of disease in the auditory tube or tympanic membrane.

o·to·scope (ō′tō-skōp) An instrument for examining the drum membrane or auscultating the ear.

o·tos·co·py (ō-tos′kŏ-pē) Inspection of the ear, especially of the drum membrane.

o·to·spon·dy·lo·me·ga·epi·phy·si·al dys·pla·si·a (ō′tō-spon′di-lō-meg′ă-ep′i-fiz′ē-ăl dis-plā′zē-ă) SYN chondrodystrophy with sensorineural deafness.

o·to·spon·gi·o·sis (ō′tō-spŭn-jē-ō′sis) A condition involving pathologic changes in otosclerosis.

o·tos·te·al (ō-tos′tē-ăl) Relating to the ossicles of the ear.

o·to·tox·ic (ō′tō-tok′sik) Having a poisonous action on the ear.

o·to·tox·ic·i·ty (ō′tō-tok-sis′i-tē) The property of being poisonous to the ear.

♻ **-ous 1.** Chemical suffix attached to the name of an element in one of its lower valencies. Cf. -ic (1). **2.** Combining form meaning having much of.

Out·come and As·sess·ment In·for·ma·tion Set (OASIS) (owt′kŭm ă-ses′mĕnt in′fŏr-mā′shŭn set) Standard system used in home health care to measure service and patient satisfaction; mandated by the U.S. Department of Health and Human Services.

out·let (owt′lĕt) [TA] An exit or opening of a passageway. SEE ALSO aperture.

out·let for·ceps de·li·ver·y (owt′lĕt fōr′seps dĕ-liv′ĕr-ē) Delivery by forceps applied to the fetal head when it has reached the perineal floor and is visible between contractions.

out·li·er (owt′lī-ĕr) **1.** Deviant values or figures that are obviously from a different population than those from the rest of the sample; identified and eliminated because it distorts analysis of the entire sample. **2.** Additions to an estimated cost of delivered services when exceeding a fixed loss threshold.

out of bed (OOB) (owt bed) Charting notation indicating that a patient has become ambulatory.

out-of-bod·y ex·pe·ri·ence (owt bod´ē ek-spēr´ē-ĕns) Perception of one's self, including mind and sensation, existing extracorporeally; reported as a near-death phenomenon.

out of phase (owt fāz) Moving in opposite directions at the same time; 180° out of line; possible characteristic of two simultaneous oscillations of similar frequency.

out·pa·tient (owt´pā´shĕnt) A patient treated in a hospital dispensary or clinic instead of in a room or ward.

out·pa·tient de·part·ment (owt´pā´shĕnt dĕ-pahrt´mĕnt) Hospital medical unit where nonurgent ambulatory medical care is provided.

out·put (owt´put) The quantity produced, ejected, or excreted of a specific entity in a specified period of time or per unit time.

out·stand·ing ear (owt-stand´ing ēr) Excessive protrusion of the auricle of the external ear from the head, usually due to failure of the antihelical fold to develop. SYN protruding ear.

o·va·le ma·la·ri·a, o·va·le ter·tian ma·la·ri·a (ō-vā´lē mǎ-lar´ē-ǎ, tĕr´shē-ǎn) Form caused by *Plasmodium ovale.*

o·var·i·an (ō-var´ē-ǎn) Relating to the ovary.

o·var·i·an can·cer (ō-var´ē-ǎn kan´sĕr) A malignancy that arises from the female reproductive organ; one of the most common gynecologic malignancies and one of the most frequent causes of cancer death in women, with 50% of all cases occurring in women older than age 65.

o·var·i·an cy·cle (ō-var´ē-ǎn sī´kĕl) The normal sex cycle that includes development of an ovarian follicle, rupture of the follicle with discharge of the oocyte or ovum, and formation and regression of a corpus luteum.

o·var·i·an cyst (ō-var´ē-ǎn sist) Tumor of the ovary, either nonneoplastic or neoplastic.

o·var·i·an fim·bri·a (ō-var´ē-ǎn fim´brē-ǎ) [TA] Longest of the fimbriae of the uterine tube; extends from the infundibulum to the ovary. SYN infundibuloovarian ligament.

o·var·i·an fol·li·cle (ō-var´ē-ǎn fol´i-kĕl) One of the spheroidal cell aggregations in the ovary containing an oocyte.

o·var·i·an fos·sa (ō-var´ē-ǎn fos´ǎ) [TA] Depression in the pelvic parietal peritoneum; bounded in front by the obliterated umbilical artery, and behind by the ureter and the uterine vessels; it lodges in the ovary.

o·var·i·an preg·nan·cy (ō-var´ē-ǎn preg´nǎn-sē) Implantation and development of a blastocyst in the ovary. SYN ovariocyesis.

o·var·i·an va·ri·co·cele (ō-var´ē-ǎn var´i-kō-sēl) Varicosity of the pampiniform plexus in the broad ligament of the uterus. SYN tuboovarian varicocele, utero-ovarian varicocele.

o·var·i·ec·to·my (ō´var-ē-ek´tŏ-mē) Excision of one or both ovaries. SYN oophorectomy.

ovario-, ovari- Combining forms meaning ovary. SEE ALSO oo-, oophor-.

o·var·i·o·cele (ō-var´ē-ō-sēl) Hernia of an ovary.

o·var·i·o·cen·te·sis (ō-var´ē-ō-sen-tē´sis) Puncture of an ovary or an ovarian cyst.

o·var·i·o·hys·ter·ec·to·my (ō-var´ē-ō-his-tĕr-ek´tŏ-mē) Removal of ovaries and uterus. SYN oophorohysterectomy.

o·var·i·o·pexy (ō-var´ē-ō-pek´sē) Surgical fixation of the ovary to the abdominal wall.

o·var·i·or·rhex·is (ō-var´ē-ō-rek´sis) Rupture of an ovary.

o·var·i·o·sal·pin·gec·to·my (ō-var´ē-ō-sal-pin-jek´tŏ-mē) Operative removal of an ovary and the corresponding oviduct.

O

o·var·i·os·to·my (ō′var-ē-os′tŏ-mē) Establishment of a temporary fistula for drainage of a cyst of the ovary. SYN oophorostomy.

o·var·i·ot·o·my (ō′var-ē-ot′ŏ-mē) An incision into an ovary, e.g., a biopsy or a wedge excision. SYN oophorotomy.

o·va·ry, o·var·i·um (ō′vă-rē, ō-var′ē-ŭm) [TA] One of the paired female reproductive glands containing the oocytes (ova) or germ cells; its stroma is a vascular connective tissue containing ovarian follicles, each enclosing an oocyte. SYN oophoron.

o·ver·bite (ō′vĕr-bīt) SYN vertical overlap.

o·ver·clo·sure (ō′vĕr-klō′zhŭr) A decrease in occlusal vertical dimension.

o·ver·com·pen·sa·tion (ō′vĕr-kom′pĕn-sā′shŭn) 1. Exaggeration of personal capacity by which one overcomes a real or imagined inferiority. 2. Process in which a psychological deficiency inspires exaggerated correction. SEE compensation.

o·ver·de·ter·mi·na·tion (o′vĕr-dĕ-tĕr′min-ā′shŭn) PSYCHOANALYSIS ascribing the cause of a single behavioral or emotional reaction, mental symptom, or dream to the operation of two or more forces.

o·ver·e·rup·tion (ō′vĕr-ē-rŭp′shŭn) Occlusal projection of a tooth beyond the line of occlusion.

o·ver·flow in·con·ti·nence (ō′vĕr-flō in-kon′ti-nĕns) Involuntary urine loss associated with overdistention of the bladder, with or without a detrusor contraction. SYN paradoxical incontinence, passive incontinence.

o·ver·graft·ing (ō′vĕr-graft′ing) Placing additional grafts over a previously healed graft from which the epithelium has been removed by excision, dermabrasion, or laser, to strengthen and thicken a previously grafted area.

o·ver·hang (ō′vĕr-hang) Excess of dental filling material beyond the cavity margin or normal tooth contour.

o·ver·lap (ō′vĕr-lap) Suturing of one layer of tissue above or under another to gain strength.

o·ver·lay (ō′vĕr-lā) An addition to an already existing condition.

o·ver·lay den·ture, o·ver·den·ture (ō′vĕr-lā den′chŭr, ō′vĕr-den′chŭr) A complete denture that is supported by both soft tissue and natural teeth that have been altered to permit the denture to fit over them. SYN overdenture.

o·ver·load prin·ci·ple (ō′vĕr-lōd prin′si-pĕl) EXERCISE SCIENCE fundamental principle of training stating that exercise at an intensity above that normally attained will induce highly specific adaptations, enabling the body to function more efficiently.

o·ver·sens·ing (ō′vĕr-sens′ing) Sensing of electrical or magnetic signals, which normally should not be sensed by a pacemaker, but result in inappropriate inhibition of the pacemaker's output.

o·ver·shoot (ō′vĕr-shūt) 1. Any response to a step change in some factor that is greater than the steady-state response to the new level of that factor. 2. Momentary reversal of the membrane potential of a cell during an action potential.

o·ver the coun·ter (OTC) (ō′vĕr kown′tĕr) Denotes drugs or therapeutic aids sold to the consumer without the necessity of prescription provided by a health care professional.

o·ver·tone (ō′vĕr-tōn) Any of the tones, other than the lowest or fundamental tone, of which a complex sound is composed.

o·ver·train·ing syn·drome (ō′vĕr-trān′ing sin′drōm) A group of symptoms resulting from excessive physical training; includes fatigue, poor exercise performance, frequent upper-respiratory tract infections, altered mood, general malaise, weight loss, muscle stiffness and soreness, and loss of interest in high-level training. SYN staleness.

o·ver·use syn·drome (ō′vĕr-yūs sin′drōm) Injury caused by accumulated microtraumatic stress placed on a structure or body area.

o·ver·ven·ti·la·tion (ō′vĕr-ven′ti-lā′shŭn) SYN hyperventilation.

o·ver·weight (ō′vĕr-wāt′) Classification

of body weight, greater than normal but less than obese; a body mass index between 25 and 30 kg/m².

o·ver·win·ter·ing (ō′vĕr-win′tĕr-ing) Persistence of an infectious agent in its vector for extended periods, during which the vector has no opportunity to be reinfected or to infect another host.

ovi- Prefix meaning egg or oocyte. SEE ALSO oo-, ovo-.

o·vi·ci·dal (ō′vi-sī′dăl) Causing death of the egg or oocyte.

o·vif·er·ous (ō-vif′ĕr-ŭs) Carrying, containing, or producing oocytes (ova).

o·vi·gen·e·sis (ō′vi-jen′ĕ-sis) SYN oogenesis.

o·vip·a·rous (ō-vip′ă-rŭs) Egg-laying; the young develop in eggs outside the maternal body.

o·vi·po·si·tion (ō′vi-pō-zi′shŭn) Act of laying or depositing eggs by insects.

o·vi·pos·i·tor (ō′vi-poz′i-tŏr, -tōr) A specialized female organ especially well developed in insects for laying or depositing eggs.

ovo- Prefix meaning oocyte or egg. SEE ALSO oo-, ovi-.

o·vo·fla·vin (ō′vō-flā′vin) Riboflavin found in eggs.

o·vo·glob·u·lin (ō′vō-glob′yū-lin) Globulin in egg white.

o·void (ō′voyd) An oval or egg-shaped form. SYN oviform.

o·vo·lac·to·ve·ge·tar·i·an (ō′vō-lakt′ō-vej-ĕ-tar′ē-ăn) One whose diet contains vegetables, eggs, and dairy products. SEE ALSO vegetarian, vegan.

o·vo·mu·cin (ō′vō-myū′sin) A glycoprotein in egg white.

o·vo·mu·coid (ō′vō-myū′koyd) A mucoprotein obtained from egg white.

o·vo·plasm (ō′vō-plazm) Protoplasm of an unfertilized oocyte (ovum).

ovo-veg·e·ta·ri·an (ō′vō-vej′i-tar′ē-ăn) A vegetarian who consumes eggs but not dairy products nor animal flesh.

o·vo·vi·vip·ar·ous (ō′vō-vi-vip′ă-rŭs) Denoting those fish, amphibians, and reptiles that produce eggs that hatch within the body of the parent.

ov·u·lar (ov′yū-lăr) Relating to an ovule.

ov·u·lar mem·brane (ov′yū-lăr mem′brăn) SYN membrana vitellina (1).

ov·u·la·tion (ov′yū-lā′shŭn) Release of an oocyte from the ovarian follicle.

ov·u·la·to·ry (ov′yū-lă-tōr-ē) Relating to ovulation.

ov·ule (ov′yūl) **1.** The oocyte of a mammal. **2.** A small beadlike structure bearing a resemblance to an ovule. SYN ovulum.

o·vum, gen. **o·vi**, pl. **o·va** (ō′vŭm, -vī, -vă) SYN oocyte.

ox·a·late (ok′să-lāt) A salt of oxalic acid.

ox·a·late cal·cu·lus (ok′să-lāt kal′kyū-lŭs) A urinary calculus of calcium oxalate.

ox·a·le·mi·a (ok′să-lĕ′mē-ă) The presence of an abnormally large amount of oxalate in the blood.

ox·a·lo·a·ce·tic ac·id (ok′să-lō-ă-sē′tik as′id) A ketodicarboxylic acid and important intermediate in the tricarboxylic acid cycle.

ox·a·lo·sis (ok′să-lō′sis) Widespread deposition of calcium oxalate crystals in the kidneys, bones, arterial media, and myocardium, with increased urinary excretion of oxalate.

ox·a·zol·i·di·none (oks-ā′zō-lī′di-nōn) Member of a class of antibiotics that works by inhibiting protein synthesis.

ox·i·dant (ok′si-dănt) A reduced substance that oxidizes the other component of an oxidation-reduction system.

ox·i·dase (ok′si-dās) One of a group of enzymes that bring about organic reactions in which oxygen acts as an acceptor (of hydrogen or of electrons).

ox·i·da·tion (ok′si-dā′shŭn) **1.** Combination with oxygen. **2.** BACTERIOLOGY aerobic dissimilation of substrates with the production of energy and water.

ox·i·da·tion-re·duc·tion (ok′si-dā′shŭn rē-dŭk′shŭn) Any chemical oxidation or reduction reaction, which must, in toto, comprise both oxidation and reduction; often shortened to ''redox.''

ox·ide (ok′sīd) A compound of oxygen with another element or a radical.

ox·i·dize (ok′si-dīz) To combine or cause an element or radical to combine with oxygen or to lose electrons.

ox·i·do·re·duc·tase (ok′si-dō-rē-dŭk′tās) An enzyme catalyzing an oxidation-reduction reaction. SEE ALSO oxidase.

ox·ime (ok′sēm) A compound resulting from the action of hydroxylamine, NH_2OH, on a ketone or an aldehyde to yield the group $=N–OH$ attached to the former carbonyl carbon atom.

ox·im·e·ter (ok-sim′ĕ-tĕr) A laboratory instrument capable of measuring the concentration of oxyhemoglobin, reduced hemoglobin, carboxyhemoglobin, and methemoglobin in a sample of blood. SYN cooximeter, hemoximeter.

ox·im·e·try (ok-sim′ă-trē) Measurement with an oximeter of the oxygen saturation of hemoglobin in a sample of blood.

oxo- Combining form denoting addition of oxygen; used in place of keto- in systematic nomenclature. SEE ALSO hydroxy-, oxy-.

oxy- 1. Combining form meaning shrill; sharp, pointed; quick (incorrectly used for ocy-, from G. *ōkys*, swift). **2.** CHEMISTRY combining form denoting the presence of oxygen, either added or substituted, in a substance. SEE ALSO hydroxy-, oxa-, oxo-.

ox·y·cal·o·rim·e·ter (ok′sē-kal′ō-rim′ĕ-tĕr) Device measuring energy content of substances in terms of oxygen consumed.

ox·y·ceph·a·ly, ox·y·ceph·a·li·a (ok′sē-sef′ă-lē, -se-fā′lē-ă) A type of craniosynostosis in which premature closure of the lambdoid and coronal sutures, resulting in an abnormally high, peaked, or conical cranium. SYN acrocephalia,

acrocephaly, hypsicephaly, hypsocephaly, oxycephalia, steeple skull, tower skull, turricephaly.

ox·y·co·done (ok′sē-kō′dōn) A narcotic analgesic often prepared with aspirin or acetaminophen.

ox·y·gen (O) (ok′si-jĕn) **1.** Abundant and widely distributed gaseous chemical element, which combines with most other elements to form oxides and essential to animal and plant life. **2.** The molecular form of oxygen, O_2.

ox·y·gen-af·fin·i·ty hy·pox·i·a (ok′si-jĕn ă-fin′i-tē hī-pok′sē-ă) Form due to a reduced capacity of hemoglobin to release oxygen.

ox·y·ge·nase (ok′si-jĕ-nās) One of a group of enzymes catalyzing direct incorporation of oxygen into substrates. Cf. dioxygenase, monooxygenases.

ox·y·ge·nate (ok′si-jĕ-nāt) To accomplish oxygenation.

ox·y·ge·na·tion (ok′si-jĕ-nā′shŭn) Addition of oxygen to any chemical or physical system.

ox·y·gen con·cen·tra·tor (ok′si-jĕn kon′sĕn-trā′tŏr) An electrically powered device for oxygen delivery in the home; it uses a filtering mechanism to separate oxygen from room air.

ox·y·gen con·sump·tion ($\dot{V}O_2$) (ok′si-jĕn kŏn-sŭmp′shŭn) The volume of oxygen consumed by the body in 1 minute.

ox·y·gen con·tent (ok′si-jĕn kon′tent) The total amount of oxygen carried in the blood; equal to the amount of oxygen carried by the hemoglobin in the red blood cells plus the amount of oxygen dissolved in the plasma.

ox·y·gen debt (ok′si-jĕn det) The extra oxygen, taken in by the body during recovery from exercise, beyond the resting needs of the body.

ox·y·gen de·fi·cit (ok′si-jĕn def′i-sit) The difference between oxygen uptake of the body during early stages of exercise and during a similar duration in a steady state of exercise.

ox·y·gen de·sa·tu·ra·tion (ok′si-jĕn dē-sach′ŭr-ā′shŭn) Decrease in oxygen concentration in the blood due to any condition that affects the exchange of carbon dioxide and oxygen. SEE ALSO oxygen debt, oxygen deficit.

ox•y•gen di•lu•tion meth•od (ok'si-jen di-lū'shŭn meth'ŏd) A technique using 100% oxygen when assessing residual lung volume.

ox•y•gen ex•trac•tion (ok'si-jĕn ekstrak'shŭn) Amount of oxygen removed from the blood as it passes through capillaries.

ox•y•gen pulse ($\dot{V}O_2$ **HR**) (ok'si-jĕn pŭls) Volume of oxygen consumed by the body per heartbeat.

ox•y•gen sat•u•ra•tion (SaO_2) (ok-si'jĕn sach'ŭr-ā'shŭn) The percentage of oxygen-binding sites in blood that are combined with oxygen.

ox•y•gen sa•tu•ra•tion test (SaO_2 **test**) (ok-si-jĕn sach'ŭr-ā'shŭn tĕst) Noninvasive measurement of blood oxygen saturation by differential absorption of red and infrared light beams with an oximeter applied to the skin.

ox•y•gen tent (ok'si-jĕn tent) Transparent enclosure, suspended over the bed and enclosing the patient; used to supply a high concentration of oxygen.

ox•y•gen ther•a•py (oks'i-jĕn thār'ă-pē) Treatment in which an increased concentration of oxygen is made available for breathing, through a nasal catheter, tent, chamber, or mask.

ox•y•gen tox•i•ci•ty (ok'si-jĕn tok-sis'i-tē) A body disturbance resulting from breathing high partial pressures of oxygen.

ox•y•geu•si•a (ok'sē-gū'sē-ă) SYN hypergeusia.

oxyhaemoglobin [Br.] SYN oxyhemoglobin.

ox•y•he•mo•glo•bin (ok'sē-hē'mŏ-glō'bin) Hemoglobin in combination with oxygen; the form of hemoglobin present in arterial blood, scarlet or bright red when dissolved in water. SYN oxyhaemoglobin.

ox•y•my•o•glo•bin (MbO_2) (ok'sē-mī'ŏ-glō'bin) Myoglobin in its oxygenated form, analogous in structure to oxyhemoglobin.

ox•y•phil cell (ok'sē-fil sel) Cell of the parathyroid gland that increases in number with age. Sometimes called oxyphil.

ox•y•phil•ic (ok'sē-fil'ik) Having an affinity for acid dyes; denoting certain cell or tissue elements.

ox•yt•a•lan (ok-sit'ă-lan) A type of connective tissue fiber found in the periodontal ligaments of animals with the same ultrastructural features as immature elastin.

ox•y•to•ci•a (ok'sē-tō'shē-ă) Rapid parturition.

ox•y•to•cic (ok'sē-tō'sik) Hastening childbirth.

ox•y•to•cin (ok'sē-tō'sin) A nonapeptide neurohypophysial hormone that causes myometrial contractions at term and promotes milk release during lactation produced in the posterior pituitary gland.

ox•y•to•cin chal•lenge test (ok'sē-tō'sin chal'ĕnj test) A contraction stress test accomplished by administration of intravenous dilute oxytocin solution to stimulate contractions. SYN contraction stress test.

ox•y•ur•i•a•sis (ok'sē-yūr-ī'ă-sis) Infection with nematode parasites of the genus *Oxyuris*.

ox•y•ur•i•cide (ok'sē-yūr'i-sīd) An agent that destroys pinworms.

ox•yu•rid (ok-sē-yū'rid) Common name for members of the family Oxyuridae.

-oyl Suffix denoting an acyl radical; -yl replaces -ic in acid names.

ozaena [Br.] SYN ozena.

o•ze•na (ō-zē'nă) A disease characterized by intranasal crusting, atrophy, and fetid odor. SYN ozaena.

o•zone (O_3) (ō'zōn) Powerful oxidizing agent; air containing a perceptible amount of O_3 formed by an electric discharge or by the slow combustion of phosphorus; smells like chlorine.

pace·fol·low·er (pās'fol'ō-ĕr) Any cell in excitable tissue that responds to stimuli from a pacemaker.

pace·mak·er, pa·cer (pās'mă-kĕr, pā' sĕr) 1. Biologically, any rhythmic center that establishes a pace of activity. 2. An artificial regulator of rate activity. 3. CHEMISTRY the substance with a rate of reaction that sets the pace for a series of chain reactions.

pace·mak·er lead (pās'mă-kĕr lēd) A wire transmitting impulses from an artificial pacemaker to the heart.

pace·mak·er rule (pās'mă-kĕr rūl) That the site with the fastest rate will control the heart.

pace·mak·er syn·drome (pās'mă-kĕr sin'drōm) A complex of signs and symptoms that occur when atrioventricular (AV) synchrony is lost during pacing and relieved when AV synchrony is restored. Symptoms may include vertigo, syncope, dyspnea, weakness, orthopnea, and postural hypotension.

♻ **pachy-** Combining form meaning thick.

pach·y·bleph·a·ron (pak'ē-blef'ă-ron) Thickening of the tarsal border of the eyelid.

pach·y·ce·phal·ic, pach·y·ceph·a·lous (pak'ē-se-fal'ik, -sef'ă-lŭs) Relating to or marked by pachycephaly.

pach·y·ceph·a·ly (pak'ē-sef'ă-lē) Abnormal thickness of the skull. SYN pachycephalia.

pach·y·chei·li·a, pach·y·chi·li·a (pak' ē-kī'lē-ă) Swelling or abnormal thickness of the lips.

pach·y·cho·li·a (pak'ē-kō'lē-ă) An increased thickening of bile.

pach·y·chro·mat·ic (pak'ē-krō-mat'ik) Having a coarse chromatin reticulum.

pach·y·chy·mi·a (pak'ē-kī'mē-ă) Inspissation of chyme.

pach·y·dac·ty·ly (pak'ē-dak'ti-lē) Enlargement of the fingers or toes, especially extremities. SYN pachydactylia.

pach·y·der·ma (pak'ē-dĕr'mă) Abnormally thick skin. SYN pachydermatosis.

pach·y·der·ma la·ryn·gis (pak'ē-dĕr' mă lă-rinj'is) A circumscribed connective tissue hyperplasia at the posterior commissure of the larynx.

pach·y·der·mat·o·cele (pak'ē-dĕr-mat' ō-sēl) SYN dermatochalasis.

pach·y·der·ma·tous (pak'ē-dĕr'mă-tŭs) Denotes having very thick skin.

pach·y·der·ma ve·si·cae (pak'ē-dĕr' mă ves'i-sē) Elephantiasis with nodules composed of lymph vesicles on the skin surface.

pach·y·der·mo·per·i·os·to·sis (pak' ē-dĕr'mō-per'ē-os-tō'sis) A syndrome of clubbing of the digits, periosteal new bone formation, and coarsening of the facial features with thickening, furrowing, and oiliness of the skin of the face and forehead. SYN acropachyderma.

pach·y·glos·si·a (pak'ē-glos'ē-ă) An enlarged, thick tongue.

pach·y·gna·thy (pă-kig'năth-ē) Condition of having a thick or large jaw.

pach·y·lep·to·men·in·gi·tis (pak'ē-lep' tō-men-in-jī'tis) Inflammation of all membranes of the brain or spinal cord.

pach·y·me·ni·a (pak'ē-mē'nē-ă) Thickening of the skin or other membranes.

pach·y·men·in·gi·tis (pak'ē-men-in-jī' tis) Inflammation of the dura mater. SYN perimeningitis.

pach·y·men·in·gop·a·thy (pak'ē-men-in-gop'ă-thē) Disease of the dura mater.

pach·y·me·ninx (pak'ē-mē'ningks) [TA] The dura mater.

pach·y·o·nych·i·a con·gen·i·ta (pak' ē-ō-nik'ē-ă kŏn-jen'i-tă) Syndrome of ectodermal dysplasia of abnormal thickness and elevation of nail plates with palmar and plantar hyperkeratosis; the tongue is whitish and glazed owing to papillary atrophy. SYN Jadassohn-Lewandowski syndrome.

pach·y·per·i·os·ti·tis (pak'ē-per'ē-ōs-tī'tis) Proliferative thickening of the periosteum caused by inflammation.

pach·y·sal·pin·go·o·va·ri·tis (pak'ē-sal·ping'gō-ō'vă-rī'tis) Chronic parenchymatous inflammation of the ovary and uterine (fallopian) tube.

pach·y·so·mi·a (pak'ē-sō'mē-ă) Pathologic thickening of the soft parts of the body.

pach·y·tene, pach·y·ne·ma (pak'i-tēn, -nē'mĕ-ă) The stage of prophase in meiosis in which pairing of homologous chromosomes is complete.

pa·ci·fi·er (pas'i-fī-ĕr) An object, usually of hard plastic or some other material permitting sterilization, which is sucked by a nursing infant for solace.

pac·ing cath·e·ter (pās'ing kath'ĕ-tĕr) A cardiac catheter with one or more electrodes at its tip that can be used to artificially pace the heart; usually inserted into a patient's right ventricle.

pack (pak) **1.** To fill, stuff, or tampon. **2.** To enwrap or envelop the body in a sheet, blanket, or other covering. **3.** To apply a dressing or covering to a surgical site. **4.** Prepackaged organized container for medications.

pack·age in·sert (pak'ăj in'sĕrt) Printed materials available in the legal pharmacologic description of a drug, subject to detailed regulatory specifications, including approved chemical and proprietary names, description and classification, clinical pharmacology, approved indications and usage, contraindications, warnings, precautions, adverse reactions, drug abuse and dependence information, overdosage discussion, dosage and administration, formulations, and appropriate references; in the U.S., such materials are negotiated between the drug's manufacturer(s) and the U.S. Food and Drug Administration. SEE ALSO label (3).

pack·ed cells (pakt selz) A blood product consisting of concentrated cells, most of the plasma having been removed. Also called packed red blood cells.

pack·ing (pak'ing) **1.** Filling a natural cavity, a wound, or a mold with some material. **2.** The material so used.

pack years (pak yērz) Person's cigarette consumption calculated as the packs of cigarettes smoked per day, multiplied by the length of consumption in years (e.g., 1.5 packs of cigarettes smoked per day for 20 years is 30 pack years).

pac·li·tax·el (PTX) (pak'li-taks'ĕl) Antitumor agent that promotes microtubule assembly by preventing depolymerization; used in salvage therapy for ovarian metastatic carcinoma.

pad (pad) **1.** A thin cushion of resilient or absorbent material applied to relieve pressure or absorb fluid. **2.** A more or less encapsulated body of fat or some other tissue that fills a space or acts as a cushion in the body.

paed- SEE ped-.

paederasty [Br.] SYN pederasty.

-paedia [Br.] SYN -pedia.

paediatric dentistry [Br.] SYN pediatric dentistry.

paediatrician [Br.] SYN pediatrician.

paediatrics [Br.] SYN pediatrics.

paedodontia [Br.] SYN pedodontia.

paedodontics [Br.] SYN pedodontics.

paedomorphism [Br.] SYN pedomorphism.

paedophilia [Br.] SYN pedophilia.

Pa·get dis·ease (paj'ĕt di-zēz') **1.** A generalized skeletal disease, frequently familial, of older people in which bone resorption and formation are both increased, leading to thickening and softening of bones and bending of weight-bearing bones; SYN osteitis deformans. **2.** A disease of elderly women, characterized by an infiltrated, somewhat eczematous lesion surrounding and involving the nipple and areola, and associated with subjacent intraductal cancer of the breast and infiltration of the lower epidermis by malignant cells.

pag·et·oid (paj'ĕ-toyd) Resembling or characteristic of Paget disease.

-pagus Suffix indicating conjoined twins, the first element of the word denoting the parts fused. SEE ALSO -didymus, -dymus.

pain (pān) An unpleasant sensation associated with actual or potential tissue damage, and mediated by specific nerve fibers to the brain, where its conscious appreciation may be modified by various factors.

pain as·sess·ment (pān ă-ses'mĕnt) Method of clinically evaluating the intensity of pain experienced by patients.

pain·ful arc sign (pān'fŭl ahrk sīn) Pain elicited during active abduction of the upper extremity between 60 and 120 degrees.

pain·ful heel (pān'fŭl hēl) A condition in which bearing weight on the heel causes pain of varying severity. SYN calcaneodynia, calcodynia.

pain-spasm-pain cy·cle (pān'spazm-pān' sī'kĕl) A self-perpetuating cycle in which skeletal muscle spasm causes local ischemia and pain, which exacerbates the spasm, which in turn exacerbates the pain. Also called pain-spasm ischemia cycle. SEE ALSO myofascial pain-dysfunction syndrome, trigger point.

PA in·ter·val (in'tĕr-văl) The time from onset of the P wave to the initial rapid deflection of the A wave in the His bundle electrogram.

pain thresh·old (pān thresh'ōld) Lowest intensity of a painful stimulus at which the subject perceives pain.

pair (Pr) (pār) Two objects considered together because of similarity, for a common purpose, or because of some attracting force between them.

pal·a·ta·ble (pal'ă-tă-bĕl) Agreeable or pleasant (e.g., usually thought of in taste and smell).

pal·a·tal, pal·a·tine (pal'ă-tăl, -tīn) Relating to the palate or the palate bone.

pal·a·tal lift (pal'ă-tăl lift) A prosthetic device designed to fit against the hard palate, anchored by the teeth, with an extension along the soft palate to occlude part of the velopharyngeal opening.

pal·a·tal my·o·clo·nus (pal'ă-tăl mī-ok'lŏ-nŭs) Tinnitus that may be elicited by contractions of the soft palate.

pal·a·tal re·flex, pal·a·tine re·flex (pal'ă-tăl rē'fleks, pal'ă-tīn) Swallowing reflex induced by stimulation of the palate.

pal·ate (pal'ăt) [TA] Bony, muscular partition between the oral and nasal cavities.

pal·ate hook (pal'ăt huk) Instrument for pulling forward the soft palate to facilitate posterior rhinoscopy.

pal·a·tine bone (pal'ă-tīn bōn) [TA] An irregularly shaped bone posterior to the maxilla, which enters into the formation of the nasal cavity, the orbit, and the hard palate.

pal·a·ti·tis (pal'ă-tī'tis) Inflammation of the palate.

palato- Combining form meaning palate.

pal·a·to·glos·sal (pal'ă-tō-glos'ăl) Relating to the palate and the tongue, or to the palatoglossus muscle.

pal·a·to·glos·sal arch (pal'ă-tō-glos'ăl ahrch) [TA] One of a pair of ridges or folds of mucous membrane passing from the soft palate to the side of the tongue.

pal·a·tog·na·thous (pal'ă-tog'nă-thŭs) Having a cleft palate.

pal·a·to·graph (pal'ă-tō-graf) An instrument used in recording the movements of the soft palate in speaking and during respiration. SYN palate myograph, palatomyograph.

pal·a·to·max·il·lar·y (pal'ă-tō-mak'si-lar-ē) Relating to the palate and the maxilla.

pal·a·to·na·sal (pal'ă-tō-nā'zăl) Relating to the palate and the nasal cavity.

pal·a·to·pha·ryn·ge·al (pal'ă-tō-fă-rin'jē-ăl) Relating to palate and pharynx.

pal·a·to·pha·ryn·go·plas·ty (PPP) (pal'ă-tō-fă-rin'gō-plas'tē) Surgical resection of unnecessary palatal and oropharyngeal tissue in selected cases of snoring, with or without sleep apnea. SYN uvulopalatopharyngoplasty.

pal·a·to·phar·yn·gor·rha·phy (pal′ă-tō-far′in-gōr′ă-fē) SYN staphylopharyngorrhaphy.

pal·a·to·plas·ty (pal′ă-tō-plas-tē) Surgery of the palate to restore form and function. SYN uranoplasty.

pal·a·to·ple·gi·a (pal′ă-tō-plē′jē-ă) Paralysis of the muscles of the soft palate.

pal·a·tor·rha·phy (pal′ă-tōr′ă-fē) The surgical repair of a cleft palate. SYN uranorrhaphy.

pal·a·tos·chi·sis (pal′ă-tos′ki-sis) SYN cleft palate.

paleo-, pale- Combining forms meaning old, primordial, primary, early.

pa·le·o·cer·e·bel·lum (pā′lē-ō-ser′ĕ-bel′ŭm) [TA] Phylogenetic term referring to the portion of the cerebellum including most of the vermis and the adjacent zones of the cerebellar hemispheres rostral to the primary fissure.

pa·le·o·cor·tex (pā′lē-ō-kōr′teks) [TA] The oldest part phylogenetically of the cortical mantle of the cerebral hemisphere, represented by the olfactory cortex.

pa·le·o·ki·net·ic (pā′lē-ō-ki-net′ik) Denoting the primitive motor mechanisms underlying muscular reflexes and automatic, stereotyped movements.

pa·le·o·pa·thol·o·gy (pā′lē-ō-pă-thol′ŏ-jē) The science of disease in prehistoric times as revealed in bones, mummies, and archaeologic artifacts.

pal·i·ki·ne·si·a, pal·i·ci·ne·si·a (pal′i-ki-nē′zē-ă, -si-nē′zē-ă) Involuntary repetition of movements.

pal·in·drome (pal′in-drōm) MOLECULAR BIOLOGY a self-complementary nucleic acid sequence.

pal·in·dro·mi·a (pal′in-drō′mē-ă) A relapse or recurrence of a disease.

pal·in·dro·mic rheu·ma·tism (pal′in-drō′mik rū′mă-tizm) Intermittent joint pain and swelling, which may resolve spontaneously but then recur.

pal·in·gen·e·sis (pal′in-jen′ĕ-sis) Surgical restoration of a lost body part.

pa·li·nop·si·a (pal′i-nop′sē-ă) Abnormal recurring visual hallucinations.

pal·i·phra·si·a (pal′i-frā′zē-ă) In speech, involuntary repetition of words or sentences. Also called palilalia. SEE ALSO echolalia.

pallaesthesia [Br.] SYN pallesthesia.

pallaesthetic [Br.] SYN pallesthetic.

pallanaesthesia [Br.] SYN pallanesthesia.

pal·lan·es·the·si·a (pal′an-es-thē′zē-ă) Absence of pallesthesia. SYN pallanaesthesia.

pal·les·the·si·a (pal′es-thē′zē-ă) Appreciation of vibration, a form of pressure sense. SYN pallaesthesia.

pal·les·thet·ic (pal′es-thet′ik) Pertaining to pallesthesia. SYN pallaesthetic.

pal·li·al (pal′ē-ăl) Relating to the pallium.

pal·li·ate (pal′ē-āt) To reduce the severity of. SYN mitigate.

pal·li·a·tive (pal′ē-ă-tiv) Reducing the severity of.

pal·li·a·tive treat·ment (pal′ē-ă-tiv trēt′mĕnt) Therapy that alleviates symptoms but does not cure the disease.

pal·lid (pal′id) Pale, faint, or deficient in color.

pal·li·dec·to·my (pal′i-dek′tŏ-mē) Excision or destruction of the globus pallidus, usually by stereotaxy.

pal·li·do·an·sot·o·my (pal′i-dō-an-sot′ŏ-mē) Production of lesions in the globus pallidus and ansa lenticularis.

pal·lor (pal′ŏr) Paleness, as of the skin.

palm (pahlm) [TA] The flat anterior of the hand. SYN palma [TA].

pal·ma, pl. **pal·mae** (pahl′mă, -mē) [TA] SYN palm.

pal·mar (pahl′măr) [TA] Pertaining to the palm of the hand or the caudal aspect of the carpus on the forelimb of an animal.

pal·mar ap·o·neu·ro·sis (pahl′măr ap′ ŏ-nūr-ō′sis) [TA] Thickened, central portion of the deep palmar fascia. SYN aponeurosispalmaris [TA], Dupuytren fascia.

pal·mar er·yth·e·ma (pahl′măr er′i-thē′ mă) Reddening of the palms, associated with various physiologic as well as pathologic changes, the principal one of which is portal hypertension.

pal·mar fi·bro·ma·to·sis (pahl′mar fī-brō′mă-tō′sis) Nodular fibroplastic proliferation in the palmar fascia of one or both hands, preceding or associated with Dupuytren contracture (q.v.).

pal·mar·is (pal-mā′ris) [TA] *This form of the adjective is used with masculine nouns (ramus palmaris, plural rami palmares) and feminine nouns (aponeurosis palmaris, plural aponeuroses palmares). With neuter nouns the form palmare is used (ligamentum palmare), plural ligamenta palmaria). The final e of palmare is not silent.* SYN palmar.

pal·mar pinch (pahl′măr pinch) OCCUPATIONAL THERAPY pinch between the pad of the thumb and the pads of the index and middle fingers. SEE ALSO pinch.

pal·mar re·flex (pahl′măr rē′fleks) Flexion of the fingers due to tickling of the palm.

Pal·mer den·tal no·men·cla·ture (pahl′ mĕr den′tăl nŏ′mĕn-klā-chŭr) 1. A system of identifying permanent teeth by the use of a number indicating the sequential position of a tooth distally from the midline; the number is bracketed with a right angle to identify the tooth's dental quadrant. 2. A system for deciduous teeth analogous to the permanent tooth with letters substituted for numbers (A through E or a through e). SEE ALSO F.D.I. dental nomenclature. SYN Zsigmondy dental nomenclature.

pal·mi·tin (pal′mi-tin) The triglyceride of palmitic acid occurring in palm oil. SYN tripalmitin.

pal·mo·men·tal re·flex (pal′mō-men′tăl rē′fleks) Unilateral (sometimes bilateral) contraction of the mentalis and orbicularis oris muscles caused by a brisk scratch made on the palm of the ipsilateral hand. SYN palm-chin reflex.

pal·mo·plan·tar ker·a·to·der·ma (pal′ mō-plan′tăr ker′ă-tō-dĕr′mă) Occurrence of symmetric diffuse or patchy areas of hypertrophy of the horny layer of the epidermis on the palms and soles. SYN ichthyosis palmaris et plantaris, keratoderma palmare et plantare, keratoderma symmetrica, keratoma plantare sulcatum, keratosis palmaris et plantaris, tylosis palmaris et plantaris.

pal·pa·ble (pal′pă-bĕl) 1. Perceptible to touch; capable of being palpated. 2. Evident; plain. SEE palpation.

pal·pate (pal′pāt) To examine by feeling and pressing with the palms of the hands and the fingers.

pal·pa·tion (pal-pā′shŭn) Examination with the hands, feeling for organs, masses, or infiltration of a part of the body, feeling the heart or pulse beat, vibrations in the chest, and other diagnostic functions.

pal·pa·to·ry per·cus·sion (pal′pă-tōr′ē pĕr-kŭsh′ŭn) Finger percussion in which attention is focused on the resistance and reverberation of the tissues under the finger as well as on the sound elicited.

pal·pe·bra, pl. **pal·pe·brae** (pal-pē′bră, -brē) [TA] SYN eyelid.

pal·pe·bral fis·sure (pal′pĕ-brăl fish′ŭr) [TA] SYN rima palpebrarum.

pal·pe·brate (pal′pĕ-brăt, -brāt) 1. Having eyelids. 2. To wink.

pal·pe·bri·tis (pal′pĕ-brī′tis) Inflammation of an eyelid.

pal·pi·tate (pal′pi-tāt) 1. To beat or throb with excessive rapidity. 2. To move with a slight tremulous motion.

pal·pi·ta·tion (pal′pi-tā′shŭn) *Do not confuse this word with palpation. Avoid the colloquial and jargonistic use of the plural of this abstract noun in the sense of 'strong or irregular heartbeats'.* Forcible or irregular pulsation of the heart, perceptible to the patient, usually with an increase in frequency or force, with or without irregularity in rhythm. SYN trepidatio cordis.

pal·sy (pawl′zē) Paralysis or paresis.

pam·pin·i·form (pam-pin′i-fōrm) Having the shape of a tendril; denoting a vinelike structure.

pan- Prefix meaning all, entire (properly affixed to words derived from Greek roots). SEE ALSO pant-.

pan·a·ce·a (pan′ă-sē′ă) A cure-all; a remedy claimed to be curative of all diseases.

pan·ac·i·nar em·phy·se·ma (pan-as′i-năr em′fi-sē′mă) SYN panlobular emphysema.

panaesthesia [Br.] SYN panesthesia.

pan·ag·glu·ti·na·ble (pan′ă-glū′ti-nă-bĕl) Agglutinable with all types of human serum.

pan·ag·glu·ti·nins (pan′ă-glū′ti-ninz) Agglutinins that react with all human erythrocytes.

pan·an·gi·i·tis (pan′an-jē-ī′tis) Inflammation of all layers of a blood vessel.

pan·ar·ter·i·tis (pan′ahr-tĕr-ī′tis) An inflammatory disorder of the arteries characterized by involvement of all structural layers of the vessels. SYN endoperiarteritis.

pan·ar·thri·tis (pan′ahr-thrī′tis) **1.** Inflammation involving all joint tissues. **2.** Inflammation of all the joints of the body.

pan·at·ro·phy (pan-at′rŏ-fē) **1.** Atrophy of all the parts of a structure. **2.** General atrophy of the body.

pan·bron·chi·o·li·tis (pan′brong-kē-ō-lī′tis) Idiopathic inflammation and obstruction of bronchioles, eventually accompanied by bronchiectasis. SYN diffuse panbronchiolitis.

pan·cake kid·ney (pan′kāk kid′nē) A disc-shaped organ produced by fusion of both poles of the contralateral kidney primordia. SYN disc kidney.

pan·car·di·tis (pan′kahr-dī′tis) Inflammation of all the structures of the heart.

pan·cre·as, pl. **pan·cre·a·ta** (pan′krē-ăs, -ā′tă) [TA] An elongated lobulated retroperitoneal gland extending from the duodenum to the spleen.

pancreat-, pancreatico-, pancreato-, pancreo- Combining forms denoting involving the pancreas.

pan·cre·a·tec·to·my, pan·cre·ec·to·my (pan′krē-ă-tek′tŏ-mē, -krē-ek′tŏ-mē) Excision of the pancreas.

pan·cre·at·em·phrax·is (pan′krē-ăt-em-frak′sis) Obstruction in the pancreatic duct, causing swelling of the gland.

pan·cre·at·ic (pan′krē-at′ik) Relating to the pancreas.

pan·cre·at·ic ab·scess (pan′krē-at′ik ab′ses) Lesion in the pancreatic or peripancreatic area usually related to pancreatitis.

pan·cre·at·ic cyst·o·du·od·e·nos·to·my (pan′krē-at′ik sis′tō-dū′ō-dĕ-nos′tŏ-mē) Surgical or endoscopic drainage of a pancreatic pseudocyst into the duodenum. SYN duodenocystostomy (3).

pan·cre·at·ic di·a·be·tes (pan′krē-at′ik dī-ă-bē′tēz) **1.** Diabetes mellitus demonstrably dependent on a pancreatic lesion. **2.** Diabetes following removal of the pancreas in an animal.

pan·cre·at·ic di·ges·tion (pan′krē-at′ik di-jes′chŭn) Digestion in the intestine by the enzymes of the pancreatic juice.

pan·cre·at·ic duct (pan′krē-at′ik dŭkt) [TA] The excretory duct of the pancreas. SYN Wirsung canal, Wirsung duct.

pan·cre·at·ic juice (pan′krē-at′ik jūs) External secretion of the pancreas; a clear alkaline fluid containing several enzymes.

pan·cre·at·i·co·du·o·de·nal, pan·cre·at·o·du·o·de·nal (pan′krē-at′i-kō-dū′ō-dē′năl, pan′krē-at′ō-) Relating to the pancreas and the duodenum.

pan·cre·at·i·co·du·od·en·ec·to·my (pan′krē-at′i-kō-dū′ō-dĕ-nek′tŏ-mē) SYN pancreatoduodenectomy.

P

pan·cre·at·ic·o·du·od·e·nos·to·my, pan·cre·at·i·o·du·o·de·nos·to·my (pan´krē-at´i-kō-dū´ō-dĕ-nos´tŏ-mē, -at´ē-ō-dū´ō-dĕ-nos´tŏ-mē) Surgical anastomosis of a pancreatic duct, cyst, or fistula to the duodenum.

pan·cre·at·ic·o·en·ter·os·to·my, pan·cre·at·o·en·ter·os·to·my (pan´krē-at´ik-ō-en´tĕr-os´tŏ-mē, pan´krē-at´ō-) Surgical creation of a new opening between the pancreas and the small intestine.

pan·cre·at·ic·o·gas·tros·to·my (pan´krē-at´ik-ō-gas-tros´tŏ-mē) Surgical creation of a new opening between the pancreas and the stomach.

pan·cre·at·ic·o·je·ju·nos·to·my (pan´krē-at´ik-ō-jĕ-jū-nos´tŏ-mē) Creation of a new opening between the pancreas and the jejunum.

pan·cre·a·tin (pan´krē-ă-tin) A mixture of the enzymes from the pancreas of the ox or hog, used internally as a digestive, and also as a peptonizing agent in preparing predigested foods.

pan·cre·a·ti·tis (pan´krē-ă-tī´tis) Inflammation of the pancreas.

pan·cre·at·o·du·o·de·nec·to·my, pan·cre·at·i·co·duo·den·ec·to·my (pan´krē-at´ō-dū´ō-dĕ-nek´tŏ-mē, -at´i-kō-dū´ō-dĕ-nek´ŏ-mē) Excision of all or part of the pancreas together with the duodenum and usually the distal stomach. SYN Whipple operation.

pan·cre·at·o·gas·tros·to·my, pan·cre·at·ic·o·gas·tros·to·my (pan´krē-at´ō-gas-tros´tŏ-mē, -at´i-kō-gas-tros´tŏ-mē) Surgical anastomosis of a pancreatic cyst or fistula to the stomach.

pan·cre·at·o·gen·ic, pan·cre·at·og·e·nous (pan´krē-at´ō-jen´ik, -toj´ĕ-nŭs) Of pancreatic origin; formed in the pancreas.

pan·cre·a·tog·ra·phy (pan´krē-ă-tog´ră-fē) Radiographic demonstration of the pancreatic ducts, after retrograde injection of radiopaque material into the distal duct.

pan·cre·a·to·je·ju·nos·to·my, pan·cre·at·ic·o·je·ju·nos·to·my (pan´krē-ă-tō-jĕ´jūn-os´tŏ-mē, -at´i-kō-jĕ´jū-nos´tŏ-mē) The surgical formation of an artificial opening between the jejunum and a pancreatic duct, cyst, or fistula.

pan·cre·at·o·li·thi·a·sis (pan´krē-at´ō-li-thī´ă-sis) Stones in the pancreas, usually found in the pancreatic duct system.

pan·cre·at·o·li·thot·o·my, pan·cre·at·o·lith·ec·to·my (pan´krē-at´ō-li-thot´ō-mē, -li-thek´tŏ-mē) Removal of a pancreatic concretion.

pan·cre·a·tol·y·sis, pan·cre·ol·y·sis (pan´krē-ă-tol´i-sis, -krē-ol´i-sis) Destruction of the pancreas.

pan·cre·a·to·meg·a·ly (pan´krē-ă-tō-meg´ă-lē) Abnormal pancreatic enlargement.

pan·cre·a·top·a·thy, pan·cre·op·a·thy (pan´krē-ă-top´ă-thē, -krē-op´ă-thē) Pancreatic disease.

pan·cre·at·o·re·nal syn·drome (pan´krē-ă-tō-rē´năl sin´drōm) Acute renal failure occurring in a patient with severe acute pancreatitis; the mortality rate is high.

pan·cre·a·tot·o·my, pan·cre·at·o·my (pan´krē-ă-tot´ŏ-mē, -krē-at´ŏ-mē) Incision of the pancreas.

pan·cre·at·o·tro·pic (pan´krē-at´ik-ō-trō´pik) Denotes something that has an effect on the pancreas.

pan·cre·a·trop·ic (pan´krē-ă-trō´pik) Exerting an action on the pancreas.

pan·cre·ec·to·my (pan´krē-ek´tŏ-mē) SYN pancreatectomy.

pan·cre·li·pase (pan´krē-lip´ās) A concentrate of pancreatic enzymes standardized for lipase content.

pancreo- SEE pancreat-.

pan·cre·o·zy·min (pan´krē-ō-zī´min) SYN cholecystokinin.

pan·cu·ro·ni·um bro·mide (pan´kyū-rō´nē-ŭm brō´mīd) A nondepolarizing steroidal neuromuscular blocking agent resembling curare.

pan·cy·to·pe·ni·a (pan´sī-tō-pē´nē-ă)

Pronounced reduction in the number of erythrocytes, leukocytes, and blood platelets in the circulating blood.

pan·dem·ic (pan-dem′ik) Denoting a disease affecting or attacking the population of an extensive region, country, continent; extensively epidemic.

pan·di·a·stol·ic (pan′dī-ă-stol′ik) SYN holodiastolic.

pan·en·ceph·a·li·tis (pan′en-sef′ă-lī′tis) A diffuse inflammation of the brain.

pan·en·do·scope (pan-en′dŏ-skōp) An illuminated instrument for inspection of the interior of the urethra as well as the bladder.

pan·es·the·si·a (pan′es-thē′zē-ă) The sum of all the sensations experienced by a person at one time. SEE ALSO cenesthesia. SYN panaesthesia.

pang (pang) A sudden sharp, brief pain.

pan·hys·te·ro·sal·pin·gec·to·my (pan-his′tĕr-ō-sal′pin-jek′ŏ-mē) Surgical removal of the uterus, cervix, and the uterine tubes.

pan·hys·te·ro·sal·pin·go·o·o·pho·rec·to·my (pan-his′tĕr-ō-sal-ping′gō-ō-of′ŏr-ek′tŏ-mē) Surgical removal of the uterus, cervix, ovaries, and the uterine tubes.

pan·ic at·tack, pan·ic dis·or·der (pan′ik ă-tak′, dis-ōr′dĕr) Sudden onset of intense apprehension, fear, terror, or sense of impending doom accompanied by increased autonomic nervous system activity and by various constitutional disturbances.

pan·i·dro·sis, pan·hi·dro·sis (pan′i-drō′sis, -hi-drō′sis) Sweating of the entire surface of the body.

pan·im·mu·ni·ty (pan′i-myū′ni-tē) A general immunity to all infectious diseases.

pan·lo·bar (pan′lō′bahr) Pertaining to all of the lung lobe.

pan·lob·u·lar em·phy·se·ma (pan-lōb′yū-lăr em′fi-sē′mă) Emphysema affecting all parts of the lobules, in part, or usually the whole, of the lungs, and usu-

ally associated with α_1-antiprotease deficiency emphysema.

pan·my·e·lo·sis (pan′mī-ĕ-lō′sis) Myeloid metaplasia with abnormal immature blood cells in the spleen and liver.

pan·nic·u·lar her·ni·a (pă-nik′yū-lăr hĕr′nē-ă) The escape of subcutaneous fat through a gap in a fascia or an aponeurosis. SYN fatty hernia.

pan·nic·u·lec·to·my (pă-nik′yū-lek′tŏ-mē) Surgical excision of redundant paniculus adiposus, usually of the abdomen.

pan·nic·u·li·tis (pă-nik′yū-lī′tis) Inflammation of subcutaneous adipose tissue.

pan·nic·u·lus, gen. and pl. **pan·nic·u·li** (pă-nik′yū-lŭs, -lī) [TA] A sheet or layer of tissue.

pan·ning (pan′ing) Use of plastic plates or surfaces coated with either antigen or antibody to separate or concentrate specific cells with appropriate receptors.

pan·nus, gen. and pl. **pan·ni** (pan′ŭs, -ī) A membrane of granulation tissue covering a normal surface.

pan·oph·thal·mi·tis (pan′of-thal-mī′tis) Purulent inflammation of all ocular layers.

pan·op·tic (pan-op′tik) All revealing, denoting the effect of multiple or differential staining.

pan·o·ram·ic ra·di·o·graph (pan′ŏ-ram′ik rā′dē-ō-graf) Radiographic view of the maxillae and mandible from the left to the right glenoid fossae. SYN panoramic x-ray film.

pan·o·ram·ic x-ray film (pan′ŏ-ram′ik eks′rā film) In dentistry, a radiograph taken to give a panoramic view of the entire upper and lower dental arch as well as the temporomandibular joints.

pan·o·ti·tis (pan′ō-tī′tis) General inflammation of all parts of the ear.

pan·scle·ro·sis (pan′skle-rō′sis) Universal sclerosis of an organ or part.

pan·sys·tol·ic (pan′sis-tol′ik) Lasting throughout systole, extending from first to second heart sound. SYN holosystolic.

pan·sys·tol·ic mur·mur (pan'sis-tol'ik mŭr'mŭr) Sound occupying the entire systolic interval, from first to second heart sounds.

♻ **pant-, panto-** Combining forms meaning entire. SEE ALSO pan-.

pan·tal·gi·a (pan-tal'jē-ă) Pain involving the entire body.

pan·te·the·ine (pan'tĕ-thē'in) *Avoid the mispronunciation pan'te-thēn.* Condensation product of pantothenic acid and aminoethanethiol. SYN *Lactobacillus bulgaricus* factor.

Pan·to·e·a ag·glom·er·ans (pan-tō-ē'ă ă-glom'ĕ-ranz) Formerly *Enterobacter agglomerans*, member of the family Enterobacteriaceae; associated with infections acquired from contaminated intravenous fluids.

pan·to·mo·graph (pan'tō'mŏ-graf) A panoramic radiographic instrument that permits visualization of the entire dentition, alveolar bone, and contiguous structures on a single extraoral film.

pan·to·mog·ra·phy (pan'tŏ-mog'ră-fē) Radiography by which a radiograph of the maxillary and mandibular dental arches and their contiguous structures may be obtained on a single film.

Pan·ton-Val·en·tine leu·ko·ci·din (pan'tŏn-val'ĕn-tīn lū'kŏ-sī'din) A staphylococcal cytolytic toxin that can act on polymorphonuclear leukocytes.

pan·to·scop·ic (pan'tŏ-skop'ik) Designed for observing objects at all distances; denoting bifocal lenses.

pan·to·scop·ic tilt (pan'tŏ-skop'ik tilt) Oblique astigmatism caused by slanting a spheric lens so that light rays strike the lens at a nonperpendicular angle, altering the spheric and cylindric refractive power of the lens.

pan·to·then·ic ac·id (pan'tŏ-then'ik as'id) A growth substance widely distributed in plant and animal tissues; essential for growth of a number of organisms.

Pa·num a·re·a (pah'nŭm ār'ē-ă) Space

surrounding the empiric horopter where single binocular vision is observed despite stimulation of noncorresponding retinal points.

pap (pap) A soft food, (e.g., breadcrumbs soaked in milk or water).

Pa·pa·ni·co·laou (Pap) smear (pa-pă-ni'kō-low pap smēr) A smear of vaginal or cervical cells obtained for cytologic study.

Pa·pa·ni·co·laou (Pap) stain (pa-pă-ni'kō-low pap stān) A multichromatic stain used on exfoliated cytologic specimens and based on aqueous hematoxylin with multiple counterstaining dyes in 95% ethyl alcohol, giving great transparency and delicacy of detail; important in cancer screening, especially of gynecologic smears.

Pa·pa·ni·co·laou (Pap) test (pa-pă-ni' kō-low pap test) Microscopic examination of cells exfoliated or scraped from a mucosal surface after staining with Papanicolaou stain; used especially for detection of cancer of the uterine cervix.

pa·pav·er·ine (pă-pav'ĕr-ēn) A nonnarcotic benzylisoquinoline alkaloid of opium that has mild analgesic action and is a powerful spasmolytic.

pa·per (pā'pĕr) A square of paper folded over so as to form an envelope containing a dose of any medicinal powder.

pa·per chrom·a·tog·ra·phy (pā'pĕr krō'mă-tog'ră-fē) Partition chromatography in which the moving phase is a liquid and the stationary phase is paper.

pa·pil·la, gen. and pl. **pa·pil·lae** (pă-pil'ă, -ē) [TA] Any small, nipplelike process. SEE ALSO dental papilla. SYN teat (3).

pa·pil·la pi·li (pă-pil'ă pī'lī) A knoblike indentation of the bottom of the hair follicle, on which the hair bulb fits like a cap. SYN hair papilla.

pap·il·lar·y, pap·il·late (pap'i-lar-ē, -i-lāt) Relating to, resembling, or provided with papillae.

pap·il·lar·y ad·e·no·car·ci·no·ma (pap'i-lar-ē ad'ĕ-nō-kahr'si-nō'mă) Lesion with fingerlike processes of vascular connective tissue covered by neoplastic epithelium, projecting into cysts or the cavities of glands or follicles.

pap·il·lar·y car·ci·no·ma (pap'i-lar-ē kahr'si-nō'mă) A malignant neoplasm characterized by the formation of numerous irregular fingerlike projections of fibrous stroma covered with a layer of neoplastic epithelial cells.

pap·il·lar·y cys·tic ad·e·no·ma (pap'i-lar-ē sis'tik ad'ĕ-nō'mă) Lesion in which the lumens of the acini are frequently distended by fluid; neoplastic epithelial elements tend to form irregular, fingerlike projections.

pap·il·lar·y mus·cle (pap'i-lar-ē mŭs'ĕl) [TA] One of the group of myocardial bundles that terminate in the chordae tendineae that attach to the cusps of the atrioventricular valves. SYN musculus papillaris [TA].

pap·il·lar·y tu·mor (pap'i-lar-ē tū'mŏr) SYN papilloma.

pap·il·lec·to·my (pap-i-lek'tŏ-mē) Surgical removal of any papilla.

pa·pil·le·de·ma (pap'il-ĕ-dē'mă) Edema of the optic disc, often due to increased intracranial pressure. SYN choked disc.

pa·pil·li·form (pă-pil'i-fŏrm) Resembling or shaped like a papilla.

pap·il·li·tis (pap'i-lī'tis) 1. Optic neuritis with swelling of the optic disc. 2. Inflammation of the renal papilla.

papillo- Combining form meaning a papilla, papillary.

pap·il·lo·ad·e·no·cys·to·ma (pap'i-lō-ad'ĕ-nō-sis-tō'mă) A benign epithelial neoplasm characterized by glands or glandlike structures, formation of cysts, and fingerlike projections of neoplastic cells.

pap·il·lo·car·ci·no·ma (pap'i-lō-kahr'si-nō'mă) 1. Malignant papilloma. 2. Carcinoma characterized by papillary, fingerlike projections of neoplastic cells in association with cores of fibrous stroma as a supporting structure.

papilloedema [Br.] SYN papilledema.

pap·il·lo·ma (pap'i-lō'mă) A circumscribed benign epithelial tumor projecting from the surrounding surface consisting of villous or arborescent outgrowths of fibrovascular stroma covered by neoplastic cells. SYN papillary tumor, villoma.

pap·il·lo·ma·to·sis (pap'i-lō-mă-tō'sis) 1. The development of numerous papillomas. 2. Papillary projections of the epidermis forming a microscopically undulating surface.

Pap·il·lo·ma·vi·rus (pap'i-lō'mă-vī'rŭs) A genus of viruses containing DNA and including the papilloma viruses and wart viruses of humans and other animals, some of which are associated with induction of carcinoma.

pap·il·lo·ret·i·ni·tis (pap'i-lō-ret'i-nī'tis) SYN neuroretinitis.

pap·il·lot·o·my (pap'i-lot'ŏ-mē) An incision into the major duodenal papilla.

Pap·pen·hei·mer bod·ies (pahp'ĕn-hī'mĕr bod'ēz) Phagosomes, containing ferruginous granules, found in red blood cells in some diseases.

pap·pus (pap'ŭs) The first downy growth of beard.

PA pro·jec·tion (prŏ-jek'shŭn) A radiographic study in which x-rays travel from posterior to anterior. SYN posteroanterior projection.

pap·u·lar (pap'yū-lăr) Relating to papules.

pap·u·lar ac·ro·der·ma·ti·tis of child·hood (pap'yū-lăr ak'rō-dĕr-mă-tī'tis chīld'hud) SYN Gianotti-Crosti syndrome.

pap·u·lar ur·ti·ca·ri·a (pap'yū-lăr ŭr'ti-kar'ē-ă) A sensitivity reaction to insect bites, especially human and pet fleas, seen mostly in young children. SYN lichen urticatus.

pap·u·la·tion (pap'yū-lā'shŭn) The formation of papules.

pap·ule (pap'yūl) A small, circumscribed, solid elevation on the skin.

papulo- Prefix meaning papule.

pap·u·lo·er·y·them·a·tous (pap′yū-lō-er′i-them′ă-tŭs) Denoting an eruption of papules on an erythematous surface.

pap·u·lo·ne·crot·ic tu·ber·cu·lid (pap′yū-lō-nĕ-krot′ik tū-bĕr′kyū-lid) Dusky-red papules followed by crusting and ulceration primarily on the extremities and predominantly in young adults with a deep focus of tuberculosis or with a history of preceding infection.

pap·u·lo·pus·tu·lar (pap′yū-lō-pŭs′chyŭ-lăr) Denoting an eruption composed of papules and pustules.

pa·pu·lo·sis (pap′yū-lō′sis) The occurrence of numerous widespread papules.

pap·u·lo·squa·mous (pap′yū-lō-skwā′mŭs) Denoting an eruption composed of both papules and scales.

pap·u·lo·ve·sic·u·lar (pap′yū-lō-ve-sik′yū-lăr) Denoting an eruption composed of papules and vesicles.

pap·y·ra·ceous (pap′i-rā′shŭs) Like parchment or paper.

par (pahr) A pair; specifically a pair of cranial nerves, e.g., par nonum, ninth pair, glossopharyngeal, or par vagum, the vagus or tenth pair.

par·a (par′ă) A woman who has given birth to one or more infants. Para followed by a roman numeral or preceded by a Latin prefix (primi-, secundi-, terti-, quadri-, etc.) designates the number of times a pregnancy has culminated in a single or multiple birth; e.g., **para I**, primipara; a woman who has given birth for the first time; **para II**, secundipara; a woman who has given birth for the second time to one or more infants. Cf. gravida.

♻ **para-** 1. Prefix denoting a departure from the normal. 2. Prefix denoting involvement of two like parts or a pair. 3. Prefix denoting adjacent, beside, near.

par·ac·an·tho·ma (par′ak-an-thō′mă) A neoplasm arising from abnormal hyperplasia of the prickle cell layer of the skin.

par·a·ca·se·in (par′ă-kā′sē-in) The compound produced by the action of rennin on κ-casein, which precipitates with calcium ion as the insoluble curd.

par·a·cel·lu·lar trans·port (par′ă-sel′yū-lăr trans′pōrt) Solvent movement across an epithelial cell layer through the tight junctions between cells. Cf. transcellular transport.

par·a·cel·si·an meth·od (par′ă-sel′sē-ăn meth′ŏd) Older term for the treatment of disease using only chemical agents.

paracenaesthesia [Br.] SYN paracenesthesia.

par·a·ce·nes·the·si·a (par′ă-sē′nes-thē′zē-ă) Deterioration in one's sense of bodily well-being (i.e., of the normal functioning of one's organs). SYN paracenaesthesia.

par·a·cen·te·sis (par′ă-sen-tē′sis) Passage into a cavity of a trocar, cannula, needle, or other hollow instrument to remove fluid; variously designated according to the cavity punctured. SYN tapping (2).

par·a·cen·tral (par′ă-sen′trăl) Close to or beside the center or some structure designated "central."

par·a·cer·vi·cal (par′ă-sĕr′vi-kăl) Connective tissue adjacent to the uterine cervix.

par·a·chol·er·a (par′ă-kol′ĕr-ă) A disease resembling Asiatic cholera due to a vibrio species but not *Vibrio cholerae*.

par·a·chor·dal (par′ă-kōr′dăl) Alongside the anterior portion of the notochord in the embryo; designating the bilateral cartilaginous bars that enter into the formation of the base of the cranium.

par·a·chute re·flex (par′ă-shūt rē′fleks) SYN startle reflex (1).

par·a·ci·ca·tri·cial em·phy·se·ma (par′ă-sik′ă-trish′ăl em′fi-sē′mă) Dilated terminal air spaces adjacent to a scar in the lung.

par·ac·me (par-ak′mē) 1. The stage of subsidence of a fever. 2. The period of life beyond the prime; the decline or stage of involution of an organism. SYN paracmasis.

par·a·co·li·tis (par′ă-kō-lī′tis) Inflammation of the peritoneal coat of the colon.

par·a·col·pi·um (par′ă-kol′pē-ŭm) The tissues alongside the vagina.

par·a·cor·tex (par′ă-kōr′teks) Area of a lymph node between the subcapsular cortex and medullary cords; consists of long-lived lymphocytes (T cells) derived from the thymus. SYN deep cortex, tertiary cortex, thymus-dependent zone.

par·a·crine (par′ă-krin) Relating to a kind of hormone function in which the effects of the hormone are restricted to the local environment. Cf. endocrine.

par·a·cu·sis, par·a·cu·si·a, par·a·cou·sis (par′ă-kyū′sis, -zē-ă, par′ă-kyū′sis) 1. Impaired hearing. 2. Auditory illusions or hallucinations.

par·a·cyst·ic (par′ă-sis′tik) Beside or near a bladder, specifically the urinary bladder.

par·a·cys·ti·tis (par′ă-sis-tī′tis) Inflammation of the connective tissue and other structures about the urinary bladder.

par·a·digm (par′ă-dīm) Conceptual model or construct that develops from examples.

par·a·dip·si·a (par′ă-dip′sē-ă) An abnormal desire to consume fluids, without regard to bodily need.

par·a·dox (par′ă-doks) That which is apparently, although not actually, inconsistent with or opposed to the known facts in any case.

par·a·dox·ic con·trac·tion (par′ă-dok′sik kŏn-trak′shŭn) Tonic contraction of the anterior tibial muscles when a sudden passive dorsal flexion of the foot is made.

par·a·dox·ic di·a·phragm phe·nom·e·non (par′ă-doks′ik dī′ă-fram fē-nom′ĕ-non) In pyopneumothorax, hydropneumothorax, and some injuries, the diaphragm on the affected side rises during inspiration and falls during expiration.

par·a·dox·ic ef·fect (par′ă-dok′sik e-fekt′) As related to minimal bactericidal concentration testing, decreased bactericidal activity of an antimicrobial agent at higher concentrations.

par·a·dox·ic em·bo·lism (par′ă-dok′sik em′bŏ-lizm) 1. Obstruction of a systemic artery by an embolus originating in the venous system that passes through a septal defect, patent foramen ovale, or other shunt to the arterial system. 2. Obstruction by a minute clot that passes through the pulmonary capillaries from the venous to the arterial system. SYN crossed embolism.

par·a·dox·ic ex·ten·sor re·flex (par′ă-doks′ik eks-ten′sŏr rē′fleks) SYN Babinski sign (1).

par·a·dox·i·c pulse (par′ă-doks′ik pŭls) Reversal of the normal variation in the pulse volume with respiration, the pulse becoming weaker with inspiration and stronger with expiration.

par·a·dox·ic pu·pil·lar·y re·flex (par′ă-doks′ik pyū′pi-lar-ē rē′fleks) Constriction of pupils in darkness, the reverse of that expected.

par·a·dox·ic re·flex (par′ă-doks′ik rē′fleks) Any reflex in which the usual response is reversed or does not conform to the pattern characteristic of the particular reflex.

par·a·dox·i·c vo·cal cord move·ment (par′ă-doks′ik vō′kăl kōrd mūv′mĕnt) Adduction of the vocal cords on inspiration, resulting in stridor and airway obstruction.

par·a·du·o·de·nal her·ni·a (par′ă-dū-ō-dē′năl hĕr′nē-ă) Internal hernia resulting from abnormal or incomplete midgut rotation that involves one of several paraduodenal spaces.

par·a·e·soph·a·ge·al her·ni·a (par′ă-ĕ-sof-ă-jē′ăl hĕr′nē-ă) Herniation through or adjacent to the esophageal hiatus of the diaphragm in which the esophagogastric junction remains below the diaphragm and the stomach rolls up into the chest.

par·a·es·the·si·a (par′es-thē′zē-ă) SYN paresthesia.

paraesthesia [Br.] SYN paresthesia.

par·af·fin (par′ă-fin) 1. One of the methane series of acyclic hydrocarbons. 2. SYN hard paraffin.

par·af·fin bait tech·nique (par′ă-fin bāt

tek-nēk′) Technique used to recover *Nocardia* spp. and aerobic actinomycetes from contaminated samples.

par·af·fin bath (par′ă-fin bath) Warmed paraffin wax and mineral oil mixture used to coat a body part, causing heat to penetrate into the tissues; used to treat joint inflammation.

par·af·fi·no·ma (par′ă-fi-nō′mă) A tumefaction, usually a granuloma, caused by the prosthetic or therapeutic injection of paraffin into the tissues. SEE ALSO lipogranuloma.

par·a·func·tion (par′ă-fŭngk′shŭn) **1.** Disordered function. **2.** DENTISTRY movements of the mandible that are outside normal function.

par·a·geu·si·a (par′ă-gū′sē-ă) Disordered or abnormal sense of taste.

par·a·gon·i·mi·a·sis (par′ă-gon′i-mī′ă-sis) Infection with a worm of the genus *Paragonimus*, especially *P. westermani*. SYN pulmonary distomiasis.

Par·a·gon·i·mus (par′ă-gon′i-mŭs) A genus of lung flukes, parasitic in humans and a wide variety of mammals that feed on crustacea carrying the metacercariae.

par·a·gram·ma·tism (par′ă-gram′ă-tizm) Speech that is fluent but consists mainly of semantic and phonetic errors (paraphasias), so that grammatic structure and meaning cannot be determined. SYN jargon aphasia.

par·a·graph·i·a (par′ă-graf′ē-ă) **1.** Loss of the power of writing from dictation, although the words are heard and comprehended. **2.** Writing one word when another is intended.

par·a·hor·mone (par′ă-hōr′mōn) A product of ordinary metabolism, not produced for a specific purpose, which acts like a hormone in modifying the activity of some distant organ.

par·a·in·flu·en·za vi·rus·es (par′ă-in-flū-en′ză vī′rŭs-ĕz) Viruses of the genus *Paramyxovirus*.

par·a·ker·a·to·sis (par′ă-ker′ă-tō′sis) Retention of nuclei in the cells of the stratum corneum of the epidermis, observed in many scaling dermatoses.

par·a·ki·ne·si·a, par·a·ki·ne·sis, par·a·ci·ne·sia, par·a·ci·ne·sis (par′ă-ki-nē′zē-ă, -sis, -si-nē′zē-ă, -si-nē′sis) Any motor abnormality.

par·a·la·li·a (par′ă-lā′lē-ă) Any speech defect; especially one in which one letter is habitually substituted for another.

par·al·de·hyde (par-al′dĕ-hīd) A cyclic polymer of acetaldehyde; a potent hypnotic and sedative; its offensive odor limits its use. SYN paracetaldehyde.

par·a·lex·i·a (par′ă-lek′sē-ă) Misapprehension of written or printed words, other meaningless words being substituted for them in reading.

par·al·ge·si·a (par′al-jē′zē-ă) Painful paresthesia; any disorder or abnormality of the sense of pain.

par·al·lac·tic (par′ă-lak′tik) Relating to a parallax.

par·al·lax (par′ă-laks) The apparent displacement of an object that follows a change in the position from which it is viewed.

par·al·lax test (par′ă-laks test) Measurement of the deviation in strabismus by the alternate cover test combined with neutralization of the deviation using prisms.

pa·ral·lel play (par′ă-lel plā) A developmental psychology concept in which toddlers (ages 2–3 years) play alongside each other, in similar activities, without obvious communication or interaction.

par·al·ler·gic (par′ă-lĕr′jik) Denoting an allergic state in which the body becomes predisposed to nonspecific stimuli following original sensitization with a specific allergen.

par·a·lo·gi·a, pa·ral·o·gism, pa·ral·o·gy (par′ă-lō′jē-ă, pă-ral′ŏ-jizm, -jē) False reasoning, involving self-deception.

pa·ral·y·sis, pl. **pa·ral·y·ses** (păr-al′i-sis, -sēz) **1.** Loss of power of voluntary movement in a muscle through injury to or disease of its nerve supply. **2.** Loss of any function.

par·a·lyt·ic (par′ă-lit′ik) Relating to paralysis or suffering from paralysis.

par·a·lyt·ic in·con·ti·nence (par'ă-lit'ik in-kon'tĕ-nĕns) Urinary incontinence symptomatic of neurogenic disorders involving damage to the brain or the spinal cord. SYN reflex bladder.

par·a·ly·zant (pă-ral'i-zănt) 1. Causing paralysis. 2. Any agent, such as curare, which causes paralysis.

par·a·lyze (par'ă-līz) To render incapable of movement.

par·a·mas·ti·tis (par'ă-mas-tī'tis) Inflammation around the breasts.

Par·a·me·ci·um (par'ă-mē'sē-ŭm) An abundant genus of freshwater holotrichous ciliates, characteristically slipper shaped and often large enough to be visible to the naked eye.

par·a·me·di·an in·ci·sion (par'ă-mē'dē-ăn in-sizh'ŭn) An incision lateral to the midline.

par·a·med·ic (par'ă-med'ik) SYN prehospital provider.

par·a·me·ni·a (par'ă-mē'nē-ă) Any disorder or irregularity of menstruation.

pa·ram·e·ter (pă-ram'ĕ-tĕr) One of many dimensions or ways of measuring or describing an object or evaluating a subject.

par·a·met·ric, par·a·me·trit·ic (par'ă-met'rik, -mĕ-trit'ik) Relating to the parametrium, or structures near the uterus.

par·a·me·tri·tis (par'ă-mē-trī'tis) Inflammation of the tissue adjacent to the uterus, particularly in the broad ligament. SYN pelvic cellulitis.

par·a·mim·i·a (par'ă-mim'ē-ă) Gestures unsuited to the words that they accompany.

par·am·ne·si·a (par'am-nē'zē-ă) False recollection, as of events that have never occurred.

par·am·y·loi·do·sis (par-am'i-loy-dō'sis) 1. Deposition in tissues of an amyloid like protein in primary amyloidosis or in atypical amyloidosis of multiple myeloma. 2. Various hereditary amyloidoses characterized by progressive hypertrophic polyneuritis with sensory changes, ataxia, paresis, and muscle atrophy due to amyloid deposits in peripheral and visceral nerves.

par·a·my·o·to·ni·a (par'ă-mī'ō-tō'nē-ă) An atypical form of myotonia.

Par·a·myx·o·vir·i·dae (par'ă-mik'sō-vir'i-dē) Viruses containing ribonucleic acid about twice the size of the influenza viruses (*Orthomyxoviridae*) but similar to them in morphology. Diseases associated with these viruses include croup and other upper respiratory infections, measles, mumps, and pneumonia.

Par·a·myx·o·vi·rus (par'ă-mik'sō-vī'rŭs) A genus of viruses that includes Newcastle disease, mumps, and the parainfluenza viruses (types 1–4).

paranaesthesia [Br.] SYN paranesthesia.

par·a·na·sal (par'ă-nā'zăl) Adjacent to the nasal cavities.

par·a·na·sal si·nus·es (par'ă-nā'zăl sī'nŭs-ĕz) [TA] Paired air-filled cavities in facial bones lined by mucous membrane continuous with that of the nasal cavity. SYN sinus paranasales [TA].

par·a·ne·o·pla·si·a (par'ă-nē-ō-plā'zē-ă) Hormonal, neurologic, hematologic, and other clinical and biochemical disturbances associated with malignant neoplasms but they are not directly related to invasion by the primary tumor or its metastases.

par·a·ne·o·plas·tic (par'ă-nē-ō-plas'tik) Relating to or characteristic of paraneoplasia.

par·a·ne·o·plas·tic en·ceph·a·lo·my·e·lop·a·thy (par'ă-nē-ō-plas'tik en-sef'ă-lō-mī-ĕ-lop'ă-thē) Encephalomyelopathy as a remote effect of carcinoma, most often oat cell carcinoma of the lung.

par·a·neph·ric (par'ă-nef'rik) 1. Relating to the suprarenal gland (i.e., paranephros). 2. SYN pararenal.

par·a·neph·ric fat (par'ă-nef'rik fat) Perirenal fat.

par·a·ne·phri·tis (par'ă-nef-rī'tis) 1. Inflammation of the suprarenal gland. **2.** Inflammation of tissue near the kidney.

par·a·neph·ros, pl. **par·a·neph·roi** (par'ă-nef'ros, -roy) SYN suprarenal gland.

par·an·es·the·si·a (par'an-es-thē'zē-ă) Anesthesia of the lower half of the body.

par·a·noi·a (par'ă-noy'ă) A disorder characterized by the presence of systematized delusions, often of a persecutory character involving being followed, poisoned, or harmed by other means, in an otherwise intact personality. SEE ALSO paranoid personality.

par·a·noi·ac (par'ă-noy'ăk) **1.** Relating to or affected with paranoia. **2.** One who is suffering from paranoia.

par·a·noid (par'ă-noyd) **1.** Relating to or characterized by paranoia. **2.** Having delusions of persecution.

par·a·noid per·son·al·i·ty (par'ă-noyd pĕr-sŏn-al'i-tē) A personality disorder characterized by hypersensitivity, rigidity, unwarranted suspicion, jealousy, and a tendency to blame others and ascribe evil motives to them.

par·a·noid per·son·al·i·ty dis·or·der (par'ă-noyd pĕr-sŏ-nal'i-tē dis-ōr'dĕr) Disease less debilitating than paranoid or delusional paranoid disorder; essential feature is a pervasive and unwarranted tendency, beginning in early adulthood and present in a variety of contexts, to misinterpret the actions of others as deliberately exploitive or harmful.

par·a·noid schiz·o·phre·ni·a (par'ă-noyd skits'ŏ-frē'nē-ă) A form of that mental disorder characterized predominantly by delusions of persecution and megalomania.

par·a·nu·cle·ar (par'ă-nū'klē-ăr) Outside, but near the nucleus.

par·a·nu·cle·us (par'ă-nū'klē-ŭs) An accessory nucleus or small mass of chromatin lying outside, though near, the nucleus.

par·a·op·er·a·tive (par'ă-op'ĕr-ă-tiv) SYN perioperative.

par·a·o·ral (par'ă-ōr'ăl) Near or adjacent to the mouth.

par·a·pa·re·sis (par'ă-pă-rē'sis) Weakness affecting the lower extremities.

par·a·pe·de·sis (par'ă-pĕ-dē'sis) Excretion or secretion through an abnormal channel.

par·a·per·i·to·ne·al (par'ă-per'i-tō-nē'ăl) Outside the peritoneum.

par·a·per·i·to·ne·al her·ni·a (per'ă-per'i-tō-nē'ăl hĕr'nē-ă) Vesical hernia in which only a part of the protruded organ is covered by the peritoneum of the sac.

par·a·pha·si·a, par·a·phra·si·a (par'ă-fā'zē-ă, -frā'zē-ă) Aphasia with loss of ability to speak correctly. SYN paragrammatism.

par·a·phi·a, par·ap·si·a (pă-rā'fē-ă, -rap'sē-ă) Any disorder of the sense of touch. SYN pseudesthesia (1), pseudoesthesia (1).

par·a·phil·i·a (par'ă-fil'ē-ă) **1.** A condition, in either men or women, of compulsive responsivity and obligatory dependence on an unusual or socially unacceptable external stimulus or internal fantasy for sexual arousal or orgasm. **2.** In law, perversion or deviancy.

par·a·phi·mo·sis (par'ă-fī-mō'sis) Painful constriction of the glans penis by a phimotic foreskin that has been retracted behind the corona.

par·a·ple·gi·a (par'ă-plē'jē-ă) Paralysis of both lower limbs and, generally, the lower trunk.

par·a·ple·gic, par·a·plec·tic (par'ă-plē'jik, -plek'tik) *Avoid the mispronunciation par-ă-pă-lē'jik.* Relating to or suffering from paraplegia.

par·a·prax·i·a (par'ă-prak'sē-ă) A condition analogous to paraphasia and paragraphia with defective performance of purposive acts.

par·a·proc·ti·tis (par'ă-prok-tī'tis) Inflammation of the cellular tissue surrounding the rectum.

par·a·pro·tein (par'ă-prō'tēn) **1.** Monoclonal immunoglobulin of blood plasma, produced by a clone of plasma cells arising from the abnormal rapid multiplication of a single cell; may be seen in serum in various malignant, benign, or nonneoplastic diseases. **2.** SYN monoclonal immunoglobulin.

par·a·pro·tein·e·mi·a (par′ă-prō-tēn-ē′mē-ă) The presence of abnormal proteins in the blood.

pa·rap·si·a (pă-rap′sē-ă) SYN paraphia.

par·a·pso·ri·a·sis (par′ă-sō-rī′ă-sis) Heterogenous group of skin disorders including pityriasis lichenoides.

par·a·quat (par′ă-kwaht) A weedkiller that produces delayed toxic effects on the liver, kidneys, and lungs when ingested.

par·a·re·flex·i·a (par′ă-rē-flek′sē-ă) A condition characterized by abnormal reflexes.

par·a·re·nal (par′ă-rē′năl) Near or adjacent to the kidneys. SYN paranephric (2).

par·ar·rhyth·mi·a (par′ă-ridh′mē-ă) A cardiac dysrhythmia in which two independent rhythms coexist, but not as a result of atrioventricular block.

par·a·sac·ral (par′ă-sā′krăl) Adjacent to the sacrum.

par·a·sal·pin·gi·tis (par′ă-sal′pin-jī′tis) Inflammation of the tissues surrounding the uterine or the pharyngotympanic (auditory) tube.

par·a·sep·tal em·phy·se·ma (par′ă-sep′tăl em′fi-sē′mă) Lung disorder involving the periphery of the pulmonary lobules. SYN distal acinar emphysema

par·a·si·noi·dal (par′ă-sī-noy′dăl) Near a sinus.

par·a·site (par′ă-sīt) An organism that lives on or in another and draws its nourishment therefrom.

par·a·si·te·mi·a (păr′ă-sī-tē′mē-ă) Presence of parasites in circulating blood.

par·a·sit·ic cyst (par′ă-sit′ik sist) Lesion formed by the larva of a metazoan parasite, such as a hydatid or trichinal cyst.

par·a·sit·i·cide (par′ă-sīt′i-sīd) An agent that destroys parasites.

par·a·sit·ic mel·a·no·der·ma (par′ă-sit′ik mel′ă-nō-dĕr′mă) Excoriations and melanoderma caused by scratching the bites of the body louse, *Pediculus corporis*. SYN vagabond's disease, vagrant's disease.

par·a·si·tism (par′ă-sīt-izm) A symbiotic relationship in which one species (the parasite) benefits at the expense of the other (the host). Cf. mutualism, commensalism, symbiosis, metabiosis.

par·a·si·to·gen·ic (par′ă-sī′tō-jen′ik) **1.** Caused by certain parasites. **2.** Favoring parasitism.

par·a·si·tol·o·gy (par′ă-sī-tol′ŏ-jē) Science concerned with all aspects of parasitism.

par·a·si·to·sis (par′ă-sī-tō′sis) Infestation or infection with parasites.

par·a·si·to·trop·ic (par′ă-sī′tō-trō′pik) Pertaining to or characterized by parasitotropism.

par·a·sit·ot·ro·pism (par′ă-sī-tot′rŏ-pizm) The special affinity of particular drugs or other agents for parasites rather than for their hosts, including microparasites that infect a larger parasite.

par·a·som·ni·a (par′ă-som′nē-ă) Any dysfunction associated with sleep.

par·a·sta·sis (par′ă-stā′sis) **1.** A reciprocal relationship among causal mechanisms that can compensate for, or mask defects in, each other. **2.** GENETICS a relationship between nonalleles (classified by some as a form of epistasis).

par·a·ster·nal (par′ă-stĕr′năl) Adjacent to the sternum.

par·a·ster·nal her·ni·a (par′ă-stĕr′năl hĕr′nē-ă) SYN Morgagni foramen hernia.

par·a·sym·pa·thet·ic (par′ă-sim′pă-thet′ik) Pertaining to a division of the autonomic nervous system. SEE autonomic division of nervous system.

par·a·sym·pa·thet·ic ner·vous sys·tem (par′ă-sim′pă-thet′ik nĕr′vŭs sis′tĕm) The branch of the autonomic nervous system that sends motor signals to glandular smooth muscle, and cardiac tissue, during recovery from threat. Cf. sympathetic nervous system.

par·a·sym·pa·thet·ic re·sponse (par′ă-sim′pă-thet′ik rĕ-spons′) Action of glandular, smooth muscle, and cardiac tissue during relief from threat or stress.

par·a·sym·path·o·lyt·ic (par′ă-sim′pă-thō-lit′ik) Relating to an agent that annuls or antagonizes the effects of the parasympathetic nervous system (e.g., atropine).

par·a·sym·path·o·mi·met·ic drug (par′ă-sim′pă-thō-mi-met′ik drŭg) A drug that acts by stimulating or mimicking the parasympathetic nervous system.

par·a·sy·nap·sis (par′ă-si-nap′sis) Union of chromosomes side to side in the process of reduction.

par·a·sy·no·vi·tis (par′ă-sin′ō-vī′tis) Inflammation of the tissues immediately adjacent to a joint.

par·a·tax·ic dis·tor·tion (par′ă-taks′ik dis-tōr′shŭn) An attitude toward another person based on a distorted evaluation, usually because of too close an identification of that person with other emotionally significant figures in the patient's past life.

par·a·ten·ic host (par′ă-ten′ik hōst) Intermediate host with no parasitic development, although its presence may be an essential link in completion of the parasite's life cycle. SYN transport host.

par·a·ten·on (par′ă-ten′on) The tissue, fatty or synovial, between a tendon and its sheath.

par·a·thi·on (par′ă-thī′on) An organic phosphate insecticide, highly toxic to animals and humans, which is an irreversible inhibitor of cholinesterases.

par·a·thor·mone (par′ă-thōr′mōn) SYN parathyroid hormone.

par·a·thy·mi·a (par′ă-thī′mē-ă) Misdirection of the emotional faculties; disordered mood.

par·a·thy·roid (par′ă-thī′royd) Adjacent to the thyroid gland.

par·a·thy·roid·ec·to·my (par′ă-thī-roy-dek′tŏ-mē) Excision of the parathyroid glands.

par·a·thy·roid hor·mone (par′ă-thī′royd hōr′mōn) A peptide hormone formed by the parathyroid glands; maintains serum calcium level by promoting intestinal absorption and renal tubular reabsorption of calcium, and release of calcium from bone to extracellular fluid. Cf. bioregulator.

par·a·thy·roid hor·mone test (par′ă-thī′royd hōr′mōn test) A venous blood assessment performed to determine the serum levels of a hormone secreted by the parathyroid gland in response to low blood calcium levels.

par·a·thy·roid tet·a·ny, par·a·thy·ro·pri·val tet·a·ny (par′ă-thī′royd tet′ă-nē, par′ă-thī-rō-prī′văl) Disorder due to a lack of parathyroid function, spontaneously or following excision of the parathyroid glands.

par·a·thy·ro·trop·ic, par·a·thy·ro·tro·phic (par′ă-thī′rō-trō′pik, -trō′fik) Influencing the growth or activity of the parathyroid glands.

par·a·tope (par′ă-tōp) That part of an antibody molecule composed of the variable regions of both the light and heavy chains that combine with the antigen. SYN antibody-combining site, antigen-binding site.

par·a·tri·cho·sis (par′ă-tri-kō′sis) Any disorder in the growth of the hair, with particular reference to quantity.

par·a·typh·li·tis (par′ă-tif-lī′tis) Inflammation of the connective tissue adjacent to the cecum.

par·a·ty·phoid fe·ver (par′ă-tī′foyd fē′vĕr) An acute infectious disease with symptoms and lesions resembling those of typhoid fever, although milder.

par·a·u·re·thral (par′ă-yū-rē′thrăl) Adjacent to the urethra.

par·a·vag·i·ni·tis (par′ă-vaj-i-nī′tis) Inflammation of the connective tissue alongside the vagina.

par·a·ver·te·bral (par′ă-vĕr′tĕ-brăl) Beside or near the vertebral column.

par·a·ves·i·cal (par′ă-ves′i-kăl) SYN paracystic.

par·ax·i·al (par-ak′sē-ăl) By the side of the axis of any body or part.

par·ax·on (par-ak′son) A collateral branch of an axon.

parch·ment skin (pahrch′mĕnt skin) Parchmentlike appearance of the skin caused by loss of underlying connective and elastic tissue, or by rapid and persistent water loss from the horny layer.

par·e·gor·ic (PG) (par′ĕ-gōr′ik) Camphorated opium tincture, an antiperistaltic agent containing powdered opium, anise oil, benzoic acid, camphor, glycerin, and diluted alcohol.

par·en·ceph·a·li·tis (par′en-sef′ă-lī′tis) Inflammation of the cerebellum.

par·en·ceph·a·lo·cele (par′en-sef′ă-lō-sēl) Protrusion of the cerebellum through a defect in the cranium.

pa·ren·chy·ma, pa·ren·chy·mal cell (pă-rengk′i-mă, -măl sel) [TA] 1. The distinguishing or specific cells of a gland or organ, contained in and supported by the connective tissue framework, or stroma. 2. The endoplasm of a protozoan cell.

pa·ren·chy·ma·ti·tis (par′ĕn-kim′ă-tī′tis) Inflammation of the parenchyma or differentiated substance of a gland or organ.

par·en·chym·a·tous, par·en·chy·mal (par′ĕn-kim′ă-tŭs, păr-eng′ki-măl) *Avoid the mispronunciation par′eng-kī′mă-tŭs.* Relating to the parenchyma.

par·en·chym·a·tous de·gen·er·a·tion (par′ĕn-kim′ă-tŭs dĕ-jen′ĕr-ā′shŭn) SYN cloudy swelling.

par·en·chym·a·tous goi·ter (par′ĕn-kim′ă-tŭs goy′tĕr) Form with a great increase in the follicles with proliferation of the epithelium. SYN follicular goiter.

par·en·chym·a·tous hem·or·rhage (par′ĕn-kim′ă-tŭs hem′ŏr-ăj) Bleeding into the substance of an organ.

par·en·chym·a·tous neu·ri·tis (par′ĕn-kim′ă-tŭs nūr-ī′tis) Inflammation of the

nervous substance proper, the axons, and myelin.

par·ent (par′ĕnt) 1. An individual that produced at least one offspring through sexual reproduction. 2. Any source or basis.

pa·ren·tal gen·er·a·tion (P1) (pă-ren′tăl jen′ĕr-ā′shŭn) The parents of a mating, commonly experimental, involving contrasting genotypes.

par·ent cyst (par′ĕnt sist) SYN mother cyst.

pa·ren·ter·al (pă-ren′tĕr-ăl) Nutrition by some other means than through the gastrointestinal tract; referring particularly to the introduction of substances into an organism by intravenous, subcutaneous, intramuscular, or intramedullary injection.

pa·ren·ter·al ab·sorp·tion (pă-ren′tĕr-ăl ăb-sōrp′shŭn) That by any route other than through the alimentary canal.

pa·ren·ter·al hy·per·al·i·men·ta·tion (pă-ren′tĕr-ăl hī′pĕr-al-i-mĕn-tā′shŭn) Overconsumption of nutrients through a central venous catheter in patients who cannot consume adequate nutrition by the enteral route.

pa·ren·ter·al nu·tri·tion (pă-ren′tĕr-ăl nū-trish′ŭn) Providing the body with nutrition intravenously.

par·en·ter·ic fe·ver (par′en-ter′ik fē′vĕr) Fever clinically resembling typhoid and paratyphoid A and B, but caused by bacteria differing specifically from those of either of these diseases.

pa·re·sis (pă-rē′sis) *Although the classically correct pronunciation of this word is with stress on the first syllable, the second syllable is commonly stresed in the U.S.* Partial or incomplete paralysis.

par·es·the·si·a (par′es-thē′zē-ă) A subjective report of any abnormal sensation, could be experienced as numbness, tingling, or what is colloquially called ''pins and needles.'' SYN paraesthesia.

pa·ret·ic (pă-ret′ik) Relating to or suffering from paresis.

pa·ret′ic neu·ro·syph·i·lis (pă-ret′ik nūr′ō-sif′i-lis) Form of later tertiary syphilis, clinically manifested by progressive dementia (often with delusional systems), seizures, Argyll-Robertson pupils, dysarthria, myoclonic jerks, action tremors, generalized hyperreflexia, and Babinski signs. SYN general paresis.

par·fo·cal (pahr-fō′kăl) Describes a microscope with interchangeable objectives that do not require refocus.

par·i·es, gen. **par·i·e·tis** (par′ē-ēz, -ē′tis, tēz) [TA] SYN wall.

pa·ri·e·tal (pă-rī′ĕ-tăl) **1.** Relating to the wall of any cavity. **2.** SYN somatic (1). **3.** SYN somatic (2). **4.** Relating to the parietal bone.

pa·ri·e·tal cell (pă-rī′ĕ-tăl sel) One of the cells of the gastric glands; it lies on the basement membrane, is covered by the chief cells, and secretes hydrochloric acid that reaches the lumen of the gland through fine intracellular and intercellular canals (canaliculi). SYN acid cell.

pa·ri·e·tal fistula (pă-rī′ĕ-tăl fis′tyū-lă) A fistula, either blind or complete, opening on the wall of the thorax or abdomen.

pa·ri·e·tal her·nia (pă-rī′ĕ-tăl hĕr′nē-ă) A hernia in which only a portion of the wall of the intestine is engaged.

pa·ri·e·tal per·i·to·ne·um (pă-rī′ĕ-tăl per′ī-tŏ-nē′ŭm) [TA] Layer of peritoneum lining the abdominal walls. SYN peritoneum parietale [TA].

pa·ri·e·tal throm·bus (pă-rī′ĕ-tăl throm′bŭs) Arterial clot adhering to one side of the wall of the vessel. SEE ALSO mural thrombus.

pa·ri·e·tal wall (pă-rī′ĕ-tăl wawl) The body wall or the somatopleure from which it is formed.

parieto- Combining form denoting wall or a parietal bone.

pa·ri·e·to·fron·tal (pă-rī′ĕ-tō-frŭn′tăl) Relating to the parietal and the frontal bones or the parts of the cerebral cortex corresponding thereto.

pa·ri·e·to·oc·cip·i·tal (pă-rī′ĕ-tō-ok-sip′i-tăl) Relating to the parietal and occipital bones or to the parts of the cerebral cortex corresponding thereto.

pa·ri·e·to·tem·po·ral (pă-rī′ĕ-tō-tem′pŏr-ăl) Relating to the parietal and the temporal bones.

pa·ri·e·to·vis·cer·al (pă-rī′ĕ-tō-vis′ĕr-ăl) Relating to the wall of a cavity and to the contained viscera. SYN parietosplanchnic.

Pa·ri·naud con·junc·ti·vi·tis (pah-rinō′ kŏn-jŭngk′ti-vī′tis) A chronic necrotic inflammation of the conjunctiva characterized by large, irregular, reddish follicles and regional lymphadenopathy.

Pa·ri·naud oc·u·lo·glan·du·lar syn·drome (pah-ri-nō′ ok′yū-lō-glan′dyū-lăr sin′drōm) Unilateral conjunctival granuloma with preauricular adenopathy in tularemia, chancre, tuberculosis, and catscratch disease.

Pa·ri·naud syn·drome, Pa·ri·naud oph·thal·mo·ple·gi·a (pah-ri-nō′ sin′ drōm, of-thal′mō-plē′jē-ă) Paralysis of conjugate upward gaze with a lesion at the level of the superior colliculi. SYN dorsal midbrain syndrome.

par·ish nurs·ing (par′ish nŭrs′ing) Nursing care and spiritual counseling provided by visiting nurses to members of a spiritual community.

par·i·ty (par′i-tē) The condition of having given birth to an infant or infants, alive or dead.

Park an·eur·ysm (pahrk an′yūr-izm) An arteriovenous aneurysm in which the brachial artery communicates with the brachial and median basilic veins.

Par·kin·son fa·ci·es (pahr′kin-sŏn fā′shē-ēz) The expressionless or masklike facies characteristic of parkinsonism (1). SYN masklike face.

par·kin·so·ni·an (pahr′kin-sō′nē-ăn) Relating to or the suffering from parkinsonism (1).

par·kin·so·ni·an dys·arth·ri·a (pahr′ kin-sō′nē-ăn dis-ahr′thrē-ă) Hypokinetic dysarthria associated with parkinsonism, characterized by rigidity and reduced range of articulatory movements, monotony of pitch and loudness, reduced loudness, short rushes of speech, and rapid rate. SEE parkinsonism.

par·kin·son·ism, Par·kin·son dis·ease (PKN) (pahr′kin-sŏn-izm, pahr′kin-son di-zēz′) A neurologic syndrome usually due to a deficiency of the neurotransmitter dopamine as the consequence of degenerative, vascular, or inflammatory changes in the basal ganglia.

par lev·el (PAR) (pahr lev′ĕl) The minimum quantity of an item stocked, which will be automatically reordered, should the level fall below a preset level.

par·oc·cip·i·tal (par′ok-sip′i-tăl) Near or beside the occipital bone or the occiput.

pa·role (pă-rōl′) In psychiatry, conditional release of a formally committed patient from a mental hospital before formal discharge, so that the patient may be returned to the hospital if necessary without fresh legal action.

par·om·phal·o·cele (par′om-fal′ŏ-sēl) **1.** A tumor near the umbilicus. **2.** A hernia through a defect in the abdominal wall near the umbilicus.

par·o·nych·i·a (par′ō-nik′ē-ă) Suppurative inflammation of the nail fold surrounding the nail plate.

par·o·nych·i·al (par′ō-nik′ē-ăl) Relating to paronychia.

par·o·oph·o·ri·tis (par′ō-of′ō-rī′tis) Inflammation of tissues adjacent to the ovaries.

par·o·rex·i·a (par′ō-rek′sē-ă) An abnormal or disordered appetite.

par·os·mi·a (par-oz′mē-ă) Any disorder of the sense of smell.

par·os·te·al (păr-os′tē-ăl) Relating to the tissues immediately adjacent to the periosteum of a bone.

pa·ros·te·al os·te·o·sar·co·ma (păr-os′tē-ăl os′tē-ō-sahr-kō′mă) Low-grade lesion arising on the surface of bone without involvement of the underlying marrow.

par·os·te·i·tis (păr-os′tē-ī′tis) Inflammation of the tissues immediately adjacent to a bone. SYN parostitis.

par·os·te·o·sis, par·os·to·sis (păr-os′tē-ō′sis, -os-tō′sis) **1.** Development of

bone in an unusual location. **2.** Abnormal or defective ossification.

pa·rot·ic (pă-rot′ik) Near or beside the ear.

pa·rot·id (pă-rot′id) Situated near the ear.

pa·rot·id ab·scess (pă-rot′id ab′ses) Suppuration in the parotid gland; an often rapidly progressing complication of parotitis.

pa·rot·i·di·tis, pa·rot·i·tis (pă-rot′-i-dī′tis, par′ō-tī′tis) Inflammation of the parotid gland.

par·o·var·i·an (par′ō-var′ē-ăn) **1.** Relating to the paroophoron. **2.** Beside or in the neighborhood of the ovary.

par·ox·ysm (par′ok-sizm) **1.** A sharp spasm or convulsion. **2.** A sudden onset of a symptom or disease, especially one with recurrent manifestations such as the chills and rigor of malaria.

par·ox·ys·mal cold he·mo·glo·bi·nu·ri·a (PCH) (par′ok-siz′măl kōld hē′mō-glō-bi-nyūr′ē-ă) Rare disorder in which acute severe hemolysis follows exposure to cold.

par·ox·ys·mal cough (par′ok-siz′măl kawf) Cough that occurs often and without warning.

par·ox·ys·mal hy·per·ten·sion (pă-rok-siz′măl hī′pĕr-ten′shŭn) SYN episodic hypertension.

par·ox·ys·mal noc·tur·nal dysp·ne·a (PND) (pă-rok-siz′măl nok-tŭr′năl disp′nē-ă) Acute dyspnea appearing suddenly at night, usually waking the patient from sleep; caused by pulmonary congestion with or without pulmonary edema.

par·ox·ys·mal noc·tur·nal he·mo·glo·bi·ne·mi·a (pă-rok-siz′măl nok-tŭr′năl hē′mō-glō-bi-nē′mē-ă) An acquired hematopoietic stem cell disorder characterized by formation of defective platelets, granulocytes, erythrocytes, and possibly lymphocytes.

par·ox·ys·mal noc·tur·nal he·mo·glo·bi·nu·ri·a (PNH) (pă-rok-siz′măl nok-tŭr′năl hē′mō-glō′bi-nyūr′ē-ă) Infrequent disorder with insidious onset (usually in the third or fourth decade) and

P

chronic course, characterized by episodes of hemolytic anemia, hemoglobinuria (chiefly at night), pallor, icterus or bronzing of the skin, a moderate degree of splenomegaly, and sometimes hepatomegaly. SYN Marchiafava-Micheli anemia, Marchiafava-Micheli syndrome.

par·ox·ys·mal tach·y·car·di·a (păr-ok-siz′măl tak′i-kahr′dē-ă) Recurrent attacks of tachycardia, usually with abrupt onset and often also abrupt termination.

par·rot beak tear (par′ŏt bēk tār) An injury to articular cartilage resulting in the separation of a narrow, curved wedge resembling a parrot's beak.

Par·rot dis·ease (par′ŏt di-zēz′) Pseudoparalysis in infants, due to syphilitic osteochondritis.

pars, pl. **par·tes** (pahrz, pahr′tēz) [TA] SYN part.

part (pahrt) A portion. SYN pars [TA].

part. aeq. Abbreviation for L. partes aequales, in equal parts (amounts).

par·the·no·gen·e·sis (pahr′thĕ-nō-jen′ĕ-sis) Nonsexual reproduction, or agamogenesis, in which the female reproduces its kind without male fecundation. SYN apogamia, apogamy, apomixia, virgin generation.

par·tial ag·glu·tin·in (pahr′shăl ă-glū′ti-nin) SYN minor agglutinin.

par·tial an·ti·gen (pahr′shăl an′ti-jen) SYN hapten.

par·tial cri·coid cleft (pahr′shăl krī′koyd kleft) SEE laryngotracheoesophageal cleft.

par·tial den·ture, dis·tal ex·ten·sion (pahr′shăl den′chŭr, dis′tăl ek-sten′shŭn) A dental prosthesis that restores one or more, but not all, of the natural teeth or associated parts and is supported by the teeth or the mucosa; it may be removable or fixed. SYN bridgework.

par·tial il·e·al by·pass (pahr′shăl il′ē-ăl bī′pas) Removal of lower third of the small intestine and anastomosis of the remainder to the cecum.

par·tial left ven·tric·u·lec·to·my (pahr′shăl left ven-trik′yū-lek′tō-mē) SYN left ventricular volume reduction surgery.

par·tial pres·sure (pahr′shăl presh′ŭr) The pressure exerted by a single component of a mixture of gases, commonly expressed in mmHg or torr.

par·tial re·breath·ing mask (pahr′shăl rē-brēdh′ing mask) A face mask and a reservoir bag permitting a portion of exhaled gas to enter the bag for mixing with source gas.

par·tial seiz·ure (pahr′shăl sē′zhŭr) Attack characterized by localized cerebral ictal onset, symptoms depend the cortical area of ictal onset or seizure spread.

par·tial-thick·ness burn (pahr′shăl thik′nĕs bŭrn) A burn involving the epidermis and dermis that usually forms blisters. SYN second-degree burn.

par·tial throm·bo·plas·tin time (PTT) (pahr′shăl throm′bō-plas′tin tīm) SEE activated partial thromboplastin time.

par·ti·cle (pahr′ti-kĕl) **1.** A small portion of anything. **2.** An elementary particle.

par·tic·u·late (pahr-tik′yū-lăt) Relating to or occurring in the form of fine particles.

par·ti·tion chrom·a·tog·ra·phy (pahr-tish′ŭn krō′mă-tog′ră-fē) The separation of similar substances by repeated divisions between two immiscible liquids, so that the substances, in effect, cross the partition between the liquids in opposite directions.

par·to·gram (pahr′tō-gram) Graph of labor parameters of time and dilation with alert and action lines to prompt intervention if the curve deviates from expected. SYN labor curve.

par·tu·ri·ent (pahr-chŭr′ē-ĕnt) Relating to or in the process of childbirth.

par·tu·ri·om·e·ter (pahr-chŭr′ē-om′ĕ-tĕr) Device for determining the force of the uterine contractions in childbirth.

par·tu·ri·tion (pahr′chŭr-ish′ŭn) SYN childbirth.

par·u·re·sis (par′yū-rē′sis) Inhibited urination, especially in the presence of strangers. SYN shy bladder syndrome.

Par•vo•vir•i•dae (pahr′vō-vir′i-dē) A family of small viruses containing single-stranded DNA. Three genera are recognized: *Parvovirus, Densovirus,* and *Dependovirus,* which includes the adeno-associated satellite virus.

Par•vo•vi•rus B19 (pahr′vō-vī′rŭs) Virus that causes erythema infectiosum (fifth disease) and aplastic crises.

par•vule (pahr′vyūl) A very small pill.

pas•cal (Pa) (pas-kahl′) A derived unit of pressure or stress in the SI system, expressed in newtons per square meter.

Pas•cal law (pahs-kahl′ law) Fluids at rest transmit pressure equally in every direction.

pas•sage (pas′ăj) **1.** The act of passing. **2.** A bodily discharge. **3.** Inoculation of a series of animals with the same strain of a pathogenic microorganism whereby the virulence usually is increased, but is sometimes diminished. **4.** A channel, duct, pore, or opening.

pas•sive (pas′iv) Not active; submissive.

pas•sive-ag•gres•sive per•son•al•i•ty (pas′iv-ă-gres′siv pěr′sŏn-al′i-tē) A personality disorder in which aggressive feelings are shown in passive ways, especially through mild obstructionism and stubbornness.

pas•sive a•tel•ec•ta•sis (pas′iv at′ĕ-lek′tă-sis) Pulmonary collapse that occurs due to a space-occupying intrathoracic process such as pneumothorax or hydrothorax.

pas•sive clot (pas′iv klot) A clot formed in an aneurysmal sac consequent to cessation or slowing of circulation.

pas•sive con•ges•tion (pas′iv kŏn-jes′chŭn) Fluid build-up due to obstruction or slowing of the venous drainage, resulting in partial stagnation of blood in the capillaries and venules.

pas•sive eu•tha•na•si•a (pas′iv yū′thă-nā′zē-ă) Mode of ending life in which a physician is given an option not to pre-

scribe futile treatments for the hopelessly ill patient.

pas•sive ex•er•cise (pas′iv ek′sĕr-sīz) Exercise done by the therapist without the assistance of the patient, usually to improve mobility and increase range of motion.

pas•sive he•mag•glu•ti•na•tion (pas′iv hē′mă-glū-ti-nā′shŭn) Agglutination in which erythrocytes, usually modified by treatment with chemicals, adsorb soluble antigen and then agglutinate in the presence of antiserum specific for the adsorbed antigen. SYN indirect hemagglutination test.

pas•sive hy•per•e•mi•a (pas′iv hī′pĕr-ē′mē-ă) Blood build-up due to an obstruction in the flow of blood from the affected part.

pas•sive im•mu•ni•za•tion (pas′iv im′yū-nī-zā′shŭn) Production of passive immunity.

pas•sive in•con•ti•nence (pas′iv in-kon′ti-něns) SYN overflow incontinence.

pas•sive move•ment (pas′iv mūv′měnt) Movement imparted to an organism or any of its parts by external agency.

pas•sive range of mo•tion (PROM) (păs-iv′ rănj mō′shŭn) Amount of motion at a given joint when the joint is moved by an external force or therapist.

pas•sive stretch•ing (pas′iv strech′ing) Stretching muscles to improve flexibility and relieve muscular spasms and pain without the assistance of the patient.

pas•sive trans•port (pas′iv trans′pōrt) The movement of particles or ions across a semipermeable membrane without the expenditure of energy; influenced by chemical or electrical gradients.

paste (pāst) A soft semisolid of firmer consistency than pap but soft enough to flow slowly and not retain its shape.

Pas•teur ef•fect (pahs-tur′ e-fekt′) The inhibition of fermentation by oxygen.

Pas•teu•rel•la (pas-tur-el′ă) A genus of aerobic to facultatively anaerobic, nonmotile bacteria containing small, gram-negative cocci or ellipsoidal to elongated

P

rods that, with special methods, may show bipolar staining; parasites of humans and other animals.

pas·teur·el·lo·sis (pas′tur-ĕ-lō′sis) Infection with bacteria of the genus *Pasteurella*.

pasteurisation [Br.] SYN pasteurization.

pas·teur·i·za·tion (pas′tyūr-ī-zā′shŭn) The heating of milk, wines, fruit juices, etc., for about 30 minutes at 68°C (154.4°F) whereby living bacteria are destroyed, but the flavor or bouquet is preserved; the liquid is then chilled to 10°C (50°F) or colder. SEE ALSO sterilization.

Pas·ti·a sign (pahs′tē-ah sīn) The presence of pink or red transverse lines at the bend of the elbow in the preeruptive stage of scarlatina; they persist through the eruptive stage and remain as pigmented lines after desquamation. SYN Thomson sign.

pas·tille, pas·til (pas-tēl′, pas′til) **1.** A small mass of benzoin and other aromatic substances to be burned for fumigation. **2.** SYN troche.

patch (pach) **1.** A small, circumscribed area differing in color or structure from the surrounding surface. **2.** DERMATOLOGY a flat area larger than 1.0 cm in diameter. **3.** An intermediate stage in the formation of a cap on the surface of a cell.

patch test (pach test) A test of skin sensitiveness: a small piece of paper, tape, or a cup, wet with a dilute solution or suspension of test material, is applied to skin of the upper back or upper outer arm, and after 48 hours the area previously covered is compared with the uncovered surface; an erythematous reaction with vesicles occurs if the substance causes contact allergy. SEE ALSO photo-patch test.

pa·tel·lar (pă-tel′ăr) Relating to the patella.

pa·tel·lar ap·pre·hen·sion sign, pa·tel·la ap·pre·hen·sion test (pă-tel′ ăr ap-prē-hen′shŭn sīn, test) A physical finding in which forced lateral displacement of the patella produces anxiety and resistance in patients with a history of lateral patellar instability. SYN patella apprehension test.

pa·tel·lar re·flex (pă-tel′ăr rē′fleks) Sudden contraction of the anterior muscles of the thigh, caused by a smart tap on the patellar tendon while the leg hangs loosely at a right angle with the thigh. SYN knee jerk, knee reflex, knee-jerk reflex, patellar tendon reflex, quadriceps reflex.

pat·el·lec·to·my (pat-ĕ-lek′tŏ-mē) Excision of the patella.

pa·tel·lo·fem·o·ral syn·drome (pă-tel′ō-fem′ŏ-răl sin′drōm) Degenerative condition affecting the articular cartilage of the patella caused by abnormal compression or shearing forces at the knee joint; may cause patellalgia. Also called patellofemor stress syndrome.

pa·ten·cy (pā′tĕn-sē) The state of being freely open or exposed.

pa·tent med·i·cine (pa′tĕnt med′i-sin) Antiquated term for a nonprescription medication or over-the-counter medical product marketed to the public, rather than physicians.

pa·ter·ni·ty test (pă-tĕr′ni-tē test) Blood test to determine the father of a child.

path (path) The route or course along which something travels.

♻ **path-, -pathy, patho-, path·ic** Combining forms denoting disease.

♻ **-pathic, -pathetical** Combining forms meaning emotions.

pa·thet·ic (pă-thet′ik) **1.** Denoting cranial nerve IV (pathetic nerve), the trochlear nerve. **2.** Denoting that which arouses sorrow or pity.

path·find·er (path′fīnd-ĕr) A filiform bougie for introduction into a narrow stricture as a guide for passage of a larger sound or catheter.

♻ **-pathic** Combining form meaning disease or suffering.

path·o·bi·ol·o·gy (path′ō-bī-ol′ŏ-jē) Pathology with emphasis more on the biologic than on the medical aspects.

path·o·clis·is (path′ŏ-klis′is) Specific tendency to sensitivity to special toxins.

path·o·gen (path′ŏ-jĕn) Any virus, microorganism, or other substance that causes disease.

path·o·gen·e·sis (path′ŏ-jen′ĕ-sis) The pathologic, physiologic, or biochemical mechanism resulting in the development of a disease or morbid process. Cf. etiology.

path·o·gen·ic, path·o·ge·net·ic (path′ŏ-jen′ik, -jĕ-net′ik) Causing disease or abnormality. SYN morbific, morbigenous, nosopoietic.

path·o·ge·nic·i·ty (path′ŏ-jĕ-nis′i-tē) The condition or quality of being pathogenic, or the ability to cause disease.

path·o·gen·ic oc·clu·sion (path′ŏ-jen′ik ŏ-klū′zhŭn) An occlusal relationship capable of producing pathologic changes in supporting tissues.

path·og·no·mon·ic, path·og·nom·ic (path′og-nō-mon′ik, path′og-nom′ik) Characteristic or indicative of a given disease.

path·o·log·ic, path·o·log·i·cal (path′ŏ-loj′ik, -i-kăl) **1.** Pertaining to the essential nature of disease and to the physical, functional, biochemical, and immunologic changes induced by illness. **2.** Morbid or diseased; resulting from disease.

path·o·log·ic ab·sorp·tion (path′ŏ-loj′ik ăb-sōrp′shŭn) Parenteral absorption of any excremental or pathologic material into the bloodstream (e.g., pus, urine, bile).

path·o·log·ic a·men·or·rhe·a (path′ŏ-loj′ik ă-men′ŏ-rē′ă) Cessation of menses due to organic disease; e.g., ovarian or pituitary failure.

path·o·log·ic di·ag·no·sis (path′ŏ-loj′ik dī′ag-nō′sis) Determination of disease, sometimes postmortem, made from an anatomic or histologic study of the lesions present.

path·o·log·ic frac·ture (path′ŏ-loj′ik frak′shŭr) Break at a bony site weakened by preexisting disease, especially neoplasm or necrosis, of the bone.

path·o·log·ic my·o·pi·a (path′ŏ-loj′ik mī-ŏ′pē-ă) Progressive nearsightedness marked by fundus changes, posterior staphyloma, and subnormal corrected acuity.

path·o·log·ic phys·i·ol·o·gy (path′ŏ-loj′ik fiz′ē-ol′ŏ-jē) Science concerned with disordered function, as distinguished from anatomic lesions. SYN physiopathology.

path·o·log·ic re·trac·tion ring (path′ŏ-loj′ik rĕ-trak′shŭn ring) A constriction located at the junction of the thinned lower uterine segment with the thick retracted upper uterine segment, resulting from obstructed labor. SYN Bandl ring.

pa·thol·o·gist (pă-thol′ŏ-jist) Physician who performs, interprets, or supervises diagnostic tests, using materials removed from living or dead patients, and functions as a laboratory consultant to clinicians, or who conducts experiments or other investigations to determine the causes or nature of disease changes.

pa·thol·o·gy (pă-thol′ŏ-jē) The medical science, and specialty practice, concerned with all aspects of disease but with special reference to the essential nature, causes, and development of abnormal conditions, as well as the structural and functional changes that result from the disease processes.

path·o·mi·me·sis (path′ŏ-mi-mē′sis) Mimicry of a disease or dysfunction, whether intentional or unconscious.

path·o·mor·phism (path′ŏ-mōr′fizm) Abnormal morphology.

path·o·phys·i·ol·o·gy (path′ŏ-fiz-ē-ol′ŏ-jē) **1.** The study of structural and functional changes in tissue and organs that lead to disease. **2.** Derangement of function seen in disease; alteration in function as distinguished from structural defects.

path·way (path′wā) A collection of axons establishing a conduction route for nerve impulses from one group of nerve cells to another group or to an effector organ composed of muscle or gland cells.

pa·tient care tech·ni·cian (pā′shĕnt kār tek-nish′ŭn) A health care worker who uses both nursing and medical assisting skills to provide patient care in a hospital setting.

pa·tient-con·trolled an·al·ge·si·a, pa·tient-con·trolled an·es·the·si·a (pā'shĕnt kŏn-trōld' an'ăl-jē'zē-ă, an'es-thē'zē-ă) Pain control based on use of a pump for the constant intravenous or, less frequently, epidural infusion of a dilute narcotic that includes a mechanism for self-administration at predetermined intervals of a predetermined amount of the narcotic if the infusion fails to relieve pain.

Pa·tient's Bill of Rights (pā'shĕnts bil rīts) Developed by the American Hospital Association to affirm patients' rights. Key elements are the right to respectful and considerate care, privacy, information about treatment and prognosis, and the right to refuse treatment.

pat·ri·lin·e·al (pat'ri-lin'ē-ăl) Related to descent through the male line; inheritance of the Y chromosome is exclusively patrilineal.

pat·tern dis·tor·tion am·bly·o·pi·a (pat'ĕrn dis-tōr'shŭn am'blē-ŏ'pē-ă) Visual impairment due to a blurred retinal image during the amblyogenic period of visual development.

pat·tern ret·i·nal dys·tro·phy (pat'ĕrn ret'i-năl dis'trŏ-fē) A spectrum of autosomal dominant diseases affecting the retinal pigment epithelium, leading to mild to moderate vision loss.

pat·tern-sen·si·tive ep·i·lep·sy (pat'ĕrn-sen'si-tiv ep'i-lep'sē) A form of reflex epilepsy precipitated by viewing certain patterns.

pau·ci·ar·tic·u·lar (paw'sē-ahr-tik'yū-lăr) Joint condition in which only a few joints are involved.

pau·ci·bac·il·lar·y (paw'sē-bas'i-lar-ē) Made up of, or denoting the presence of, few bacilli.

Pau·li ex·clu·sion prin·ci·ple (pawl'ē eks-klū'zhŭn prin'si-pĕl) The theory limiting the number of electrons in the orbit or shell of an atom.

pause sig·nal (pawz sig'năl) A DNA sequence that causes pausing of RNA polymerase transcription.

Pau·tri·er mi·cro·ab·scess (pō-trē-ā' mī'krō-ab'ses) Microscopic lesion in the epidermis. SYN Pautrier abscess.

Payne op·er·a·tion (pān op-ĕr-ā'shŭn) A jejunoileal bypass for morbid obesity utilizing end-to-side anastomosis of the upper jejunum to the terminal ileum, with closure of the proximal end of the bypassed intestine.

Payr clamp (pīr klamp) A large, slightly curved clamp used in gastrectomy or enterectomy.

Payr sign (pīr sīn) Pain on pressure over the sole of the foot.

PCO_2, pCO_2 Abbreviation for partial pressure (tension) of carbon dioxide. SEE partial pressure.

peak and trough spe·ci·mens (pēk trawf spes'i-mĕnz) A serum sample collected to determine the changing levels of an antibiotic or other medication in the blood.

peak ex·pi·ra·to·ry flow rate (pēk ek-spīr'ă-tōr-ē flō rāt) The maximum flow at the outset of forced expiration, which is reduced in proportion to the severity of airway obstruction, as in asthma.

peak flow me·ter (pēk flō mē'tĕr) Hand-held device that measures peak expiratory flow.

peak lev·el (pēk lev'ĕl) The highest concentration reached by a drug, as determined by therapeutic drug monitoring.

pea·nut oil (pē'nŭt oyl) Oil extracted from the kernels of one or more cultivated varieties of *Arachis hypogaea*; used as a solvent for intramuscular injections and in food preparation. SYN arachis oil.

pearl (pĕrl) **1.** A concretion formed around a grain of sand or other foreign body within the shell of certain mollusks. **2.** A number of small, tough masses (e.g., mucus occurring in the sputum in asthma).

pearl bar·ley (pĕrl bahr'lē) SYN barley.

Pearl in·dex (pĕrl in'deks) The number of failures of a contraceptive method per 100 woman years of exposure.

peau d'or·ange (pō dŏ-rōnzh′) A swollen, pitted skin surface overlying carcinoma of the breast with both stromal infiltration and lymphatic obstruction with edema.

pec·ten (pek′těn) **1.** A structure with comblike processes or projections. **2.** SYN anal pecten.

pec·ten an·a·lis (pek′těn ā-nā′lis) [TA] SYN anal pecten.

pec·ten·i·tis (pek′ten-ī′tis) Inflammation of the anal sphincter.

pec·ten·o·sis (pek′ten-ō′sis) Exaggerated enlargement of the pecten band.

pec·ten pu·bis, pec·ten os·sis pu·bis (pek′těn pyū′bis, os′is) [TA] The continuation on the superior ramus pubis of the linea terminalis, forming a sharp ridge.

pec·tin (pek′tin) *Do not confuse this word with pecten.* **1.** Broad generic term for what are now more correctly called pectic substances or materials. **2.** Commercial pectins, sometimes called pectinic acids, are whitish, soluble powders prepared from the rinds of citrus fruits; used to make jams, jellies, and similar food products where they increase viscosity; therapeutically, used to control diarrhea, as a plasma expander, and as a protectant.

pec·ti·nate (pek′ti-nāt) Combed; comb-shaped. Also called pectiniform.

pec·tin·e·al, pec·ti·ne·us (pek-tin′ē-ăl, -ŭs) Ridged; relating to the os pubis or to any comblike structure.

pector- Combining form meaning breast.

pec·to·ral (pek′tŏr-ăl) Relating to the chest.

pec·to·ral·gi·a (pek′tŏr-al′jē-ă) Pain in the chest.

pec·to·ral gir·dle (pek′tŏr-ăl gǐr′děl) [TA] SYN shoulder girdle.

pec·to·ral region (pek′tŏr-ăl rē′jŭn) [TA] Chest area demarcated by the outline of the pectoralis major muscle. SEE ALSO regions of chest.

pec·to·ral veins (pek′tŏr-ăl vānz) [TA] Veins that drain the pectoral muscles and empty directly into the subclavian vein.

pec·to·ril·o·quy (pek′tō-ril′ŏ-kwē) Increased transmission of the voice sound through the pulmonary structures, so that it is clearly audible on auscultation of the chest.

pec·tus, gen. **pec·to·ris,** pl. **pec·to·ra** (pek′tŭs, pek-tō′ris, -ră) [TA] SYN chest.

pec·tus ca·ri·na·tum (pek′tŭs kar′i-nă′tŭm) Flattening of the thorax (chest) on either side with forward projection of the sternum resembling the keel of a boat.

pec·tus ex·ca·va·tum (pek′tŭs eks-kă-vā′tŭm) *Avoid using the simple word pectus in the special sense of pectus excavatum. Avoid the incorrect phrase pectus excavatus.* A hollow at the lower part of the chest caused by a backward displacement of the xiphoid cartilage. SYN foveated chest, funnel chest, funnel breast, koilosternia, pectus recurvatum, trichterbrust.

ped-, pedi-, pedo- 1. Combining forms denoting child. **2.** Combining forms denoting foot, feet. SYN paed-.

ped·al (ped′ăl) *Avoid the mispronunciation pē′dal. Avoid the redundant phrase foot pedal.* Relating to the feet, or to any structure called pes.

ped·er·as·ty (ped′ĕr-as-tē) Sexual relations between a man and a boy. SYN paederasty.

Pe·der·son spec·u·lum (pē′děr-sŏn spek′yŭ-lŭm) A narrow, flat probe used to examine a vagina with a narrow introitus.

-pedia Combining form meaning to educate or indicating a full list/inventory of knowledge (e.g., pharmacopedia). SYN -paedia.

pedia-, pedo- Combining forms meaning child.

pe·di·at·ric den·tis·try (pē′dē-at′rik den′tis-trē) SYN pedodontics.

pe·di·a·tric·ian (pē′dē-ă-trish′ăn) A specialist in pediatrics. SYN pediatrist.

pe·di·a·tric in·ten·sive care u·nit

(PICU) (pĕ'dē-at'rik in-ten'siv kār yū' nit) Hospital unit designated for care of critically ill children.

pe·di·at·rics (pē'dē-at'riks) The medical specialty concerned with the study and treatment of children in health and disease from birth through adolescence. SYN paediatrics.

ped·i·cle (ped'i-kĕl) [TA] **1.** A constricted portion or stalk. SYN pediculus (1). **2.** A stalk by which a nonsessile tumor is attached to normal tissue. SYN pedunculus. **3.** A stalk through which a flap receives nourishment until its transfer to another site results in the nourishment coming from that site.

pe·dic·u·li·cide (pĕ-dik'yū-li-sīd) A chemical agent used to kill lice.

pe·dic·u·lo·sis (pĕ'dik'yū-lō'sis) Lice infestation.

pe·dic·u·lous (pĕ-dik'yū-lŭs) Infested with lice.

Pe·dic·u·lus (pĕ-dik'yū-lŭs) A genus of parasitic lice that live in the hair and feed periodically on blood.

pe·dic·u·lus, pl. **pe·dic·u·li** (pĕ-dik'yū-lŭs, -lī) [TA] **1.** SYN pedicle (1). **2.** A louse. SEE *Pediculus.*

ped·i·cure (ped'i-kyūr) Care and treatment of the feet.

pe·do·don·ti·a (pē'dō-don'shē-ă) SYN pediatric dentistry, paedodontia.

pe·do·don·tics (pē'dō-don'tiks) Dentistry concerned with the dental care of children. SYN pediatric dentistry, pedodontia.

ped·o·dy·na·mom·e·ter (ped'ō-dī-nă-mom'ĕ-tĕr) An instrument for measuring the strength of the leg muscles.

pe·do·gen·e·sis (pē'dō-jen'ĕ-sis) Permanent larval stage with sexual development. Cf. neoteny.

pe·dom·e·ter (pĕ-dom'ĕ-tĕr) Portable device usually attached to clothing at waist level, which mechanically registers hip elevations during walking or running; also measures steps taken, although some models can be calibrated to estimate distance and energy cost of walking.

pe·do·mor·phism (pē'dō-mōr'fizm) Description of adult behavior in terms appropriate to child behavior. SYN paedomorphism.

pe·do·phil·i·a (pē'dō-fil'ē-ă) In psychiatry, an abnormal attraction to children by an adult for sexual purposes.

ped·orth·ics (ped-ōr'thiks) Foot and ankle support products to help alleviate foot problems and pain.

pe·dun·cu·lar (pĕ-dŭngk'yū-lăr) Relating to a pedicle.

pe·dun·cu·lot·o·my (pĕ-dŭngk'yū-lot'ŏ-mē) **1.** A total or partial section of a cerebral peduncle. **2.** A mesencephalic pyramidal tractotomy.

peel·ing (pēl'ing) A stripping off or loss of epidermis, as follows burns or therapeutic exfoliations.

peer re·view (pēr rĕ-vyū') Assessment of research proposals, manuscripts submitted for publication, or a physician's clinical practice by other physicians or scientists in the same field.

peg (peg) A cylindric projection.

peg·ged tooth (pegd tūth) A conic tooth with sides that converge from the cervical to the incisal region.

Pel-Eb·stein fe·ver, Pel-Eb·stein dis·ease (pel eb'stīn fē'vĕr, di-zēz') Remittent fever common in Hodgkin disease.

pe·li·o·sis (pel'ē-ō'sis) SYN purpura.

pe·li·o·sis hep·a·tis (pel'ē-ō'sis hē-pā'tis) The presence throughout the liver of blood-filled cavities that may become lined by endothelium or become organized. Also called peliosis hepatitis.

Pe·li·zae·us-Merz·bach·er dis·ease (pā-lē-tsā'ŭs merts'bah-kĕr di-zēz') Leukodystrophy with a tiger-striped appearance of the myelin resulting from patchy demyelination. SYN Merzbacher-Pelizaeus disease.

pel·lag·ra (pĕ-lag'ră) An affliction characterized by diarrhea, dermatitis, and dementia due to dietary deficiency of nicotinic acid (niacin).

pel·lag·ra si·ne pel·lag·ra (pĕ-lag´rǎ sī´nē pĕ-lag´rǎ) Disease without characteristic skin lesions.

Pel·le·gri·ni dis·ease (pel-ĕ-grē´nē di-zēz´) Calcific density in the medial collateral ligament and/or bony growth on the medial aspect of the medial condyle of the femur. Also called Pellegrini-Stieda disease.

pel·let (pel´ĕt) **1.** A pilule, or very small pill. **2.** A small, rod-shaped dosage form composed essentially of pure steroid hormones in compressed form, intended for subcutaneous implantation in body tissues.

pel·li·cle (pel´i-kĕl) **1.** Literally and nonspecifically, a thin skin. **2.** A film or scum on the surface of a liquid.

pel·lu·cid (pĕ-lū´sid) Allowing the passage of light.

pel·lu·cid mar·gin·al cor·ne·al de·gen·er·a·tion (pĕ-lū´sid mahr´ji-nǎl kōr´nē-ǎl dē-jen´ĕr-ā´shŭn) Bilateral opacification and vascularization of the periphery of the cornea, progressing to formation of a gutter and ectasia. SYN ectatic marginal degeneration of cornea.

pel·lu·cid zone (pĕ-lū´sid zōn) SYN zona pellucida.

pel·ta·tion (pel-tā´shŭn) Protection provided by inoculation with an antiserum or with a vaccine.

pelvi-, pelvio-, pelvo- Combining forms denoting the pelvis. Cf. pyelo-, pelyco-.

pel·vic (pel´vik) Relating to the pelvis.

pel·vic ab·scess (pel´vik ab´ses) Lesion in the pelvic peritoneal cavity, developing as a complication of peritonitis or of localized peritonitis associated with abdominal or pelvic inflammatory disease; pus frequently collects in the rectovesical or rectouterine pouch.

pel·vic cell·u·li·tis (pel´vik sel´yū-lī´tis) SYN parametritis.

pel·vic di·a·phragm, di·a·phragm of

pel·vis (pel´vik dī´ǎ-fram, pel´vis) [TA] The paired levator ani and coccygeus muscles together with the fascia above and below them.

pel·vi·ceph·a·lom·e·try (pel´vi-sef´ǎ-lom´ĕ-trē) Measurement of the female pelvic diameters in relation to the fetal head.

pel·vic ex·en·ter·a·tion (pel´vik eks´en-tĕr-ā´shŭn) Removal of all organs and adjacent structures of the pelvis; usually performed to surgically ablate cancer involving urinary bladder, uterine cervix, and rectum.

pel·vic hem·a·to·cele (pel´vik hē´mǎ-tō-sēl) Intraperitoneal pelvic blood effusion.

pel·vic in·clin·a·tion (pel´vik in´kli-nā´shŭn) [TA] Angle that the plane of the superior pelvic aperture makes with the horizontal plane. SYN inclinatio pelvis [TA], inclination of pelvis.

pel·vic in·flam·ma·to·ry dis·ease (pel´vik in-flam´ǎ-tōr-ē di-zēz´) Acute or chronic inflammation in the organs of the female pelvic cavity, in particular suppurative lesions of the upper genital tract; most commonly due to infection by *Chlamydia trachomatis* or *Neisseria gonorrhoeae*, which have ascended into the uterus, uterine tubes, or ovaries from the lower genital tract as a result of childbirth or surgical procedures.

pel·vic kid·ney (pel´vik kid´nē) Congenital abnormality with the kidney in the pelvis.

pel·vic limb (pel´vik lim) SYN lower limb.

pel·vic per·i·to·ni·tis (pel´vik per´i-tŏ-nī´tis) Generalized inflammation of the peritoneum surrounding the uterus and uterine tubes. SYN pelviperitonitis.

pel·vic plane of great·est di·men·sions (pel´vik plān grāt´ĕst di-men´shŭnz) The plane that extends from the middle of the posterior surface of the pubic symphysis to the junction of the second and third sacral vertebrae.

pel·vic plane of least di·men·sions (pel´vik plān lēst di-men´shŭnz) The plane that extends from the end of the sacrum to the inferior border of the pubic symphysis.

pel·vic pole (pel′vik pōl) The breech end of the fetus.

pel·vic pre·sen·ta·tion (pel′vik prez′ĕn-tā′shŭn) SYN breech presentation.

pel·vic tilt (pel′vik tilt) An exercise that strengthens abdominal muscles, relieves backache, and improves posture; most commonly recommended prenatal exercise for back pain.

pel·vic ver·sion (pel′vik vĕr′zhŭn) Version (q.v.) by means of which a transverse or oblique presentation is converted into a pelvic presentation by manipulating the buttocks of the fetus.

pel·vi·fix·a·tion (pel′vi-fik-sā′shŭn) Surgical attachment of a floating pelvic organ to the wall of the pelvic cavity.

pel·vi·li·thot·o·my (pel′vi-li-thot′ŏ-mē) SYN pyelolithotomy.

pel·vim·e·ter (pel-vim′ĕ-tĕr) Calipers for measuring the diameters of the pelvis.

pel·vim·e·try (pel-vim′ĕ-trē) Measurement of the diameters of the pelvis. SYN radiocephalpelvimetry.

pel·vi·ot·o·my, pel·vit·o·my (pel′vē-ot′ŏ-mē, pel-vit′ŏ-mē) 1. SYN symphysiotomy. 2. SYN pubiotomy. 3. SYN pyelotomy.

pel·vis, pl. **pel·ves** (pel′vis, -vēz) [TA] 1. The massive, cup-shaped ring of bone, with its ligaments, at the lower end of the trunk, formed of the hip bone (the pubic bone, ilium, and ischium) on either side and in front, and of the sacrum and the coccyx posteriorly. 2. Any basinlike or cup-shaped cavity.

pel·vi·sa·cral (pel′vi-sā′krăl) Relating to both the pelvis, or hip bones, and the sacrum.

pel·vi·ver·te·bral an·gle (pel′vi-vĕr′tĕ-brăl ang′gĕl) The angle made by the pelvis as defined by the plane of the superior pelvic aperture with the general axis of the trunk or vertebral column.

pel·vo·cal·i·ec·ta·sis (pel′vō-kal′ē-ek-tā′sis) SYN hydronephrosis.

pel·vo·spon·dy·li·tis (pel′vō-spon′di-lī′tis) Inflammation of the pelvic portion of the spine.

pel·vo·spon·dy·li·tis os·sif·i·cans (pel′vō-spon′di-lī′tis os-if′i-kanz) Deposit of bony substance between the vertebrae of the sacrum.

pem·phi·goid (pem′fi-goyd) 1. Resembling pemphigus. 2. Disease resembling pemphigus but significantly distinguishable histologically and clinically.

pem·phi·gus (pem′fi-gŭs) 1. Autoimmune bullous diseases with acantholysis: pemphigus vulgaris, pemphigus foliaceus, pemphigus erythematosus, or pemphigus vegetans. 2. A nonspecific term for blistering skin diseases.

pem·phi·gus er·y·the·ma·to·sus (pem′fi-gŭs er′i-thē′mă-tō′sŭs) An eruption involving sun-exposed skin, especially the face; the lesions are scaling erythematous macules and blebs.

pem·phi·gus fo·li·a·ce·us (pem′fi-gŭs fō-lī-ā′shē-ŭs) A generally chronic form of pemphigus in which extensive exfoliative dermatitis may be present in addition to the bullae.

pem·phi·gus veg·e·tans (pem′fi-gŭs vej′ĕ-tanz) 1. Rare, verrucous form of pemphigus vulgaris in which vegetation develops on the eroded surfaces left by ruptured bullae; new bullae continue to form. SYN Neumann disease. 2. Chronic benign vegetating form of pemphigus, with lesions commonly in the axillae and perineum. SYN Hallopeau disease.

pem·phi·gus vul·ga·ris (pem′fi-gŭs vŭl-gā′ris) A serious form of pemphigus, occurring in middle age, in which cutaneous bullae and oral erosions may be localized a few months before becoming generalized; blisters break easily and are slow to heal.

pen·du·lar nys·tag·mus (pen′dyū-lăr nis-tag′mŭs) Ocular condition that, in most positions of gaze, has oscillations equal in speed and amplitude, usually arising from a visual disturbance.

pen·du·lous (pen′dyū-lŭs) Like a pendulum, hanging, swinging.

pen·du·lum rhythm (pen´dyū-lŭm ridhm) SYN embryocardia.

pe·nec·to·my (pē-nek´tŏ-mē) SYN phallectomy.

pen·e·trate (pen´ĕ-trāt) To pierce; to pass into the deeper tissues or into a cavity.

pen·e·trat·ing wound (pen´ĕ-trā´ting wŭnd) Trauma with disruption of the body surface that extends into underlying tissue or into a body cavity.

pen·e·tra·tion (pen´ĕ-trā´shŭn) 1. A piercing or entering. 2. Mental acumen.

-penia Suffix meaning deficiency.

pen·i·cil·la·mine (PCA) (pen´i-sil´ă-mēn) A degradation product of penicillin; a chelating agent used to treat lead poisoning, hepatolenticular degeneration, and cystinuria. SYN β, β-dimethylcysteine.

pen·i·cil·lic ac·id (pen´i-sil´ik as´id) An antibiotic produced by *Penicillium puberulum*, a mold found on corn; active against gram-positive and gram-negative bacteria but toxic to animal tissues.

pen·i·cil·lin (pen´i-sil´in) 1. Originally, an antibiotic substance obtained from cultures of the molds *Penicillium notatum* or *P. chrysogenum*; interferes with cell wall synthesis in bacteria. 2. One of a family of natural or synthetic variants of penicillic acid. They are mainly bactericidal, are especially active against gram-positive organisms, and, with the exception of hypersensitivity reactions, show a particularly low toxic action on animal tissue.

pen·i·cil·li·nase (pen´i-sil´i-nās) 1. SYN β-lactamase. 2. A purified enzyme preparation obtained from cultures of a strain of *Bacillus cereus*.

pen·i·cil·lin G (pen´i-sil´in) An antibiotic obtained from the mold *Penicillium chrysogenum* used orally and parenterally; primarily active against gram-positive staphylococci and streptococci; destroyed by bacterial β-lactamase. SYN benzyl penicillin, benzylpenicillin.

pen·i·cil·li·o·sis (pen´i-sil´ē-ō´sis) Invasive infection by a species of *Penicillium*.

Pen·i·cil·li·um (pen´i-sil´ē-ŭm) A genus of fungi, some species of which yield various antibiotic substances and biologicals. SEE penicillin.

pen·i·cil·lo·yl pol·y·ly·sine (pen´i-sil´ō-il pol´ē-lī´sēn) A preparation of polylysine and a penicillic acid, used intradermally in the diagnosis of penicillin sensitivity.

pen·i·cil·lus, gen. and pl. **pe·ni·cil·li** (pen-i-sil´ŭs, -ī) [TA] 1. A tuft formed by the repeated subdivision of the minute arterial twigs in the spleen. 2. In fungi, one of the branched conidiophores bearing chains of conidia in *Penicillium* species.

pe·nile, pe·ni·al (pē´nīl, pē´nē-ăl) Relating to the penis.

pe·nile imp·lant (pē´nīl im´plant) Rigid, flexible, or inflatable device surgically placed in the corpora cavernosa to produce an erection.

pe·nile pros·the·sis (pē´nīl pros-thē´sis) Device placed inside the penis to correct erectile failure.

pe·nis, pl. **pe·ni·ses**, pl. **pe·nes** (pē´nis, -ni-sĕz, pē´nēz) [TA] The organ of copulation and urination in the male; formed of three columns of erectile tissue, two arranged laterally on the dorsum (corpora cavernosa penis) and one median ventrally (corpus spongiosum penis). SYN intromittent organ, membrum virile, phallus (2), priapus, virga.

pe·nis en·vy (pē´nis en´vē) Psychoanalytic concept that a female envies male characteristics or capabilities, especially the possession of a penis.

pe·ni·tis (pē-nī´tis) Inflammation of the penis.

pen·nate (pen´āt) Feathered; resembling a feather.

pe·no·plas·ty (pē´nō-plas´tē) Surgical repair of the penis.

pe·no·scro·tal trans·po·sit·ion (pē´nō-skrō´tăl trans´pŏ-zish´ŭn) Developmental error, seen with hypospadias, whereby hemiscrotal units are separated and lie lateral to the penile shaft or even cranial to it.

P

Pen·rose drain (pen'rōz drān) Soft, tubular, rubbery drain.

penta- Combining form meaning five.

pen·tad (pen'tad) **1.** A collection of five things in some way related. **2.** In chemistry, a pentavalent element.

pen·ta·dac·tyl, pen·ta·dac·tyle (pen'tă-dak'til, -tīl) Having five fingers or toes on each hand or foot. SYN quinquedigitate.

pen·ta·gas·trin test (pent'ă-gas'trin test) Alternative to histamine for stimulation of acid secretion in gastric analysis.

pen·taz·o·cine (pen-taz'ō-sēn) An opioid agonist-antagonist analgesic with some possibility for addiction but only rarely involved in withdrawal syndrome and tolerance.

pen·tet·ic ac·id (pen-tet'ik as'id) A pentaacetic acid triamine used as the calcium sodium chelate to treat iron-storage disease and poisoning from heavy metals and radioactive metals. SEE ALSO ethylenediaminetetraacetic acid.

pen·to·san (pen'tō-san) A poly- or oligosaccharide of a pentose.

pen·tose (pen'tōs) A monosaccharide containing five carbon atoms in the molecule.

pen·tose phos·phate path·way (pen'tōs fos'fāt path'wā) A secondary pathway for the oxidation of D-glucose, generating reducing power in the cytoplasm outside the mitochondria and synthesizing pentoses and a few other sugars. SYN Dickens shunt.

pen·to·su·ri·a (pen'-tō-syūr'ē-ă) Urinary excretion of pentoses.

pen·tyl (pen'til) **1.** SYN amyl. **2.** The $CH_3(CH_2)_3CH_2-$ moiety.

pep·lo·mer (pep'lō-měr) A part or knob-like subunit of the peplos of a virion, the assemblage of which produces the complete peplos.

pep·los (pep'lōs) Coat or envelope of lipoprotein material that surrounds some virions.

pep·per·mint (pep'ěr-mint) Dried leaves and flowering tops of *Mentha piperita* (family Labiatae); a carminative and antiemetic.

pep pills (pep pilz) Colloquialism for tablets containing a central nervous system stimulant, especially amphetamine.

pep·sin (pep'sin) The enzyme produced by the stomach for the digestion of protein.

pep·sin·o·gen (pep-sin'ō-jen) A proenzyme formed and secreted by the chief cells of the gastric mucosa. SYN propepsin.

pep·si·nu·ri·a (pep'si-nyu'rē-ă) Primary excretion of pepsin in the urine.

pep·tic, pep·sic (pep'tik, -sik) Relating to the stomach, to gastric digestion, or to pepsin A.

pep·tic ul·cer (pep'tik ŭl'sěr) Lesion of the alimentary mucosa, usually in the stomach or duodenum, which has been exposed to acid gastric secretion.

pep·ti·dase (pep'ti-dās) Any enzyme capable of hydrolyzing a peptide bond of a peptide. SYN peptide hydrolase.

pep·tide (pep'tīd) A compound of two or more amino acids in which a carboxyl group of one is united with an amino group of another, with the elimination of a molecule of water, thus forming a peptide bond, $-CO-NH-$; i.e., a substituted amide. Cf. bioregulator.

pep·tide bond (pep'tīd bond) The common link ($—CO—NH—$) between amino acids in proteins, formed by elimination of H_2O between the $—COOH$ of one amino acid and the $H_2N—$ of another.

pep·ti·der·gic (pep'-ti-děr'jik) Referring to nerve cells or fibers that are believed to employ small peptide molecules as their neurotransmitter.

pep·ti·do·gly·can (pep'ti-dō-glī'kan) A compound containing amino acids linked to sugars, with the latter preponderant. Cf. glycopeptide.

Pep·to·coc·cus (pep-tō-kok'ŭs) A genus of nonmotile, anaerobic, chemoorganotrophic bacteria containing gram-positive, spheric cells that occur singly, in pairs, tetrads, or irregular masses, more rarely in short chains; frequently found in association with pathologic conditions.

pep·to·gen·ic, pep·tog·e·nous (pep'tō-jen'ik, pep-toj'ĕ-nŭs) **1.** Producing peptones. **2.** Promoting digestion.

pep·tol·y·sis (pep-tol'ī-sis) The hydrolysis of peptones.

pep·to·lyt·ic (pep'tō-lit'ik) **1.** Pertaining to peptolysis. **2.** Denoting an enzyme or other agent that hydrolyses peptones.

pep·tone (pep'tōn) Descriptive term applied to intermediate polypeptide products, formed in partial hydrolysis of proteins; soluble in water, diffusible, and not coagulable by heat.

pep·ton·ic (pep-ton'ik) Relating to or containing peptone.

pep·ton·i·za·tion (pep'tōn-ī-zā'shŭn) Conversion by enzymic action of native protein into soluble peptone.

Pep·to·strep·to·coc·cus (pep'tō-strep-tō-kok'ŭs) Bacteria found in normal and pathologic female genital tracts and blood in puerperal fever, in respiratory and intestinal tracts of healthy humans and other animals, in the oral cavity, and in pyogenic infections, putrefactive war wounds, and appendicitis; may be pathogenic.

Pep·to·strep·to·coc·cus an·aer·o·bi·us (pep'tō-strep-tō-kok'ŭs an-er-ō'bē-ŭs) Bacterial species found in the mouth, intestinal and respiratory tracts, and cavities, especially the vagina, of humans and other animals.

per- 1. Prefix meaning through; denoting intensity. **2.** CHEMISTRY more or most, with respect to the amount of a given element or radical contained in a compound; the degree of substitution for hydrogen, as in peroxides, peroxy acids (e.g., hydrogen peroxide, peroxyformic acid). SEE ALSO peroxy-.

per·a·cute (per'ă-kyūt') Very acute; said of a disease.

per an·um (pĕr ā'nŭm) By or through the anus.

per·cep·tiv·i·ty (pĕr'sep-tiv'i-tē) The power of perception.

per·cep·tu·al nar·row·ing (pĕr-sep'shū-ăl nar'ō-ing) Tendency of an individual to narrow the attentional focus and miss certain types of information in the environment as the level of arousal increases.

per·cep·tu·al pro·ces·sing (pĕr-sep'shū-ăl prō'ses-ing) The organization of sensory input into meaningful patterns.

per·co·la·tion (pĕr'kō-lā'shŭn) **1.** SYN filtration. **2.** Extraction of the soluble portion of a solid mixture by passing a solvent liquid through it. **3.** Passage of saliva or other fluids into the interface between tooth structure and restoration.

per con·tin·u·um (pĕr kŏn-tin'yū-ŭm) In continuity. Also called per contiguum.

per·cus·sion (pĕr-kŭsh'ŭn) **1.** A diagnostic procedure designed to determine the density of a part by the sound produced by tapping the surface with the finger or a plessor. **2.** A form of massage, consisting of repeated blows or taps of varying force.

per·cus·sion sound (pĕr-kŭsh'ŭn sownd) That elicited on percussing one of the cavities of the body.

per·cu·ta·ne·ous (pĕr'kyū-tā'nē-ŭs) Denoting the passage of substances through unbroken skin; passage through the skin by needle puncture.

per·cu·ta·ne·ous co·ro·nar·y in·ter·ven·tion (pĕr'kyū-tā'nē-ŭs kōr'ŏ-nar'ē in'tĕr-ven'shŭn) Treatment used during cardiac catheterization to reduce or remove occlusion within the coronary arteries and increase perfusion to the myocardium. SYN intracoronary stenting.

per·cu·ta·ne·ous en·do·scop·ic gas·tros·to·my (PEG) (pĕr'kyū-tā'nē-ŭs en'dō-skop'ik gas-tros'tŏ-mē) Surgery performed without opening the abdominal cavity; usually involves gastroscopy, insufflation of the stomach, and puncture of stomach and abdominal wall, followed by tube placement.

per·cu·ta·ne·ous en·do·scop·ic gas·tros·to·my tube (PEG tube) (pĕr'kyū-tā'nē-ŭs en'dō-skop'ik găs-tros'tŏ-

P

mē tūb) Tube placed through the abdominal wall with the aid of an endoscope into the stomach; used to feed patients unable to swallow. SYN G-tube, gastrostomy tube.

per·cu·ta·ne·ous trans·he·pa·tic chol·an·gi·og·ra·phy (pĕr′kyū-tā′nē-ŭs trans′hē-pat′ik kō-lan′jē-og′ră-fē) Contrast radiographic examination of the biliary system performed by injection through a percutaneously placed needle inserted into an intrahepatic bile duct.

per·cu·ta·ne·ous trans·lu·mi·nal an·gi·o·plas·ty (pĕr′kyū-tā′nē-ŭs trans-lū′mĕn-ăl an′jē-ō-plas-tē) An operation to enlarge a narrowed vascular lumen by inflating and withdrawing a balloon on the tip of an angiographic catheter through the stenotic region.

per·cu·ta·ne·ous trans·lu·mi·nal cor·o·nar·y an·gi·o·plas·ty (pĕr′kyū-tā′nē-ŭs trans-lū′mi-năl kōr′ŏ-nar-ē an′jē-ō-plas′tē) Operation for enlarging the narrowed lumen of a coronary artery by inflating and withdrawing through the stenotic region a balloon on the tip of an angiographic catheter.

pe·ren·ni·al rhi·ni·tis (pĕr-en′ē-ăl rī-nī′tis) Inflammation of the nose, usually causing clear discharge, due to something that occurs around the same time each year (e.g., ragweed).

per·fect fun·gus (pĕr′fĕkt fŭng′gŭs) One possessing both sexual and asexual means of reproduction, and in which both mating forms are recognized.

per·fect stage (pĕr′fĕkt stāj) MYCOLOGY Sexual fungal life cycle phase in which spores form after nuclear fusion.

per·fla·tion (per-flā′shŭn) Blowing air into or through a cavity or canal to force apart its walls or to expel any contained material.

per·fo·rans (per′fōr-anz) A term applied to several muscles and nerves that, in their course, perforate other structures.

per·for·ate (pĕr′fōr-āt) To make holes or punctures.

per·fo·rat·ed (pĕr′fōr-āt-ĕd) Pierced with one or more holes.

per·fo·rat·ed space (pĕr′fōr-ā-tĕd spās) SEE anterior perforated substance, posterior perforated substance.

per·fo·rat·ed ul·cer (pĕr′fōr-āt-ĕd ŭl′sĕr) Lesion extending through the wall of an organ.

per·for·at·ing ab·scess (pĕr′fōr-āt-ing ab′ses) An abscess that breaks down tissue barriers to enter adjacent areas.

per·fo·rat·ing wound (pĕr′fōr-āt-ing wūnd) Any wound with entrance and exit openings.

per·fo·ra·tion (pĕr′fōr-ā′shŭn) Abnormal opening in a hollow organ or viscus. SEE ALSO perforated. SYN tresis.

per·for·mance ar·e·as, per·for·mance pat·terns (pĕr-fōr′măns ār′ē-ăz, pat′ĕrnz) Activities of daily living, work or other productive activity, play, and leisure that determine a person's functional abilities and define human activity.

per·for·mance com·po·nents (pĕr-fōr′măns kŏm-pō′nĕnts) Sensorimotor, cognitive, psychosocial, and psychological elements of performance required for successful engagement in performance areas.

per·for·mance con·text (pĕr-fōr′măns kon′tekst) A set of conditions, both internal and external, which mediate, support, and influence someone's performance of human activities.

per·form·ance in·ten·si·ty (pĕr-fōr′măns in-ten′si-tē) The improvement in recognition of spoken words that occurs with increasing intensity of sound.

per·fus·ate (per′fyūz′āt) The fluid used for perfusion.

per·fuse (pĕr-fyūz′) To force blood or other fluid to flow from the artery through the vascular bed of a tissue or through the lumen of a hollow structure.

per·fu·sion (pĕr-fyū′zhŭn) 1. The act of perfusing. 2. The flow of blood or other perfusate per unit volume of tissue, as in ventilation:perfusion ratio.

per·fu·sion·ist (pĕr-fyū′zhŭn-ist) The operator of an oxygenator.

peri- Prefix denoting around, about, near. Cf. circum-.

per·i·ac·i·nal, per·i·ac·i·nous (per'ē-as'i-năl, -i-nŭs) Surrounding an acinus.

per·i·ad·e·ni·tis (per'ē-ad-ĕ-nī'tis) Inflammation of the tissues surrounding a gland.

per·i·ad·e·ni·tis mu·co·sa ne·cro·ti·ca re·cur·rens (per'ē-ad-ĕ-nī'tis myū-kō'să ne-krot'i-kă rē-kŭr'enz) SYN aphthae major.

per·i·a·nal (per'ē-ā'năl) Pertaining to the area around the anus.

per·i·a·nal ab·scess (per'ē-ā'năl ab'ses) An infection of the soft tissues surrounding the anal canal, with formation of a discrete abscess cavity.

per·i·an·gi·tis (per'ē-an-jī'tis) Inflammation of the adventitia of a blood vessel or of the tissues surrounding it or a lymphatic vessel. SEE ALSO periarteritis, periphlebitis, perilymphangitis.

per·i·a·or·tic (per'ē-ā-ōr'tik) Surrounding or adjacent to the aorta.

per·i·a·or·ti·tis (per'ē-ā-ōr-tī'tis) Inflammation of the adventitia of the aorta and of the tissues surrounding it.

per·i·ap·i·cal (per'ē-ā'pi-kăl) **1.** At or around the apex of a root of a tooth. **2.** Denoting the periapex.

per·i·ap·i·cal ab·scess (per'-ē-ā'pi-kăl ab'ses) Alveolar lesion localized around the apex of a tooth root. SYN apical abscess, apical periodontal abscess.

per·i·ap·i·cal cu·ret·tage (per'ē-ā'pi-kăl kūr'ē-tahzh') **1.** Removal of a cyst or granuloma from its pathologic bony crypt, using a curette. **2.** Removal of tooth fragments and debris from sockets at the time of extraction or subsequent removal of bone sequestra.

per·i·ap·i·cal film (per'ē-ā'pi-kăl film) Intraoral radiographic projection taken to include tooth apices and surrounding alveolar bone. Also called periapical radiograph.

per·i·ap·ic·al gran·u·lo·ma (per'ē-ā'pi-kăl gran'yū-lō'mă) A proliferation of granulation tissue surrounding the apex of a nonvital tooth and arising in response to pulpal necrosis. SYN apical granuloma.

per·i·ap·pen·di·ci·tis (per'ē-ă-pen'di-sī'tis) Inflammation of the tissue surrounding the vermiform appendix.

per·i·ap·pen·dic·u·lar (per'ē-ap'ĕn-dik'yū-lăr) Surrounding an appendix, especially the vermiform appendix.

per·i·ar·te·ri·al (per'ē-ahr-tē'rē-ăl) Surrounding an artery.

per·i·ar·te·ri·al sym·pa·thec·to·my (per'ē-ahr-tēr'ē-ăl sim'pă-thek'tŏ-mē) Sympathetic denervation by arterial decortication. SYN histonectomy, Leriche operation.

per·i·ar·te·ri·tis (per'ē-ahr-tĕr-ī'tis) Inflammation of the adventitia of an artery.

per·i·ar·te·ri·tis no·do·sa (per'ē-ahr-tĕr-ī'tis nō-dō'să) SYN polyarteritis nodosa.

per·i·ar·thri·tis (per'ē-ahr-thrī'tis) Inflammation of the parts surrounding a joint.

per·i·ar·tic·u·lar ab·scess (per'ē-ahr-tik'yū-lăr ab'ses) An abscess surrounding a joint, but not necessarily involving it.

per·i·ax·i·al (per'ē-ak'sē-ăl) Surrounding an axis.

per·i·bron·chi·al (per'i-brong'kē-ăl) Surrounding a bronchus or the bronchi.

per·i·bron·chi·ol·i·tis (per'i-brong'kē-ō-lī'tis) Inflammation of the tissues surrounding the bronchioles.

per·i·bron·chi·tis (per'i-brong-kī'tis) Inflammation of the tissues surrounding the bronchi or bronchial tubes.

per·i·car·di·ac, per·i·car·di·al (per'i-kahr'dē-ak, -ăl) **1.** Surrounding the heart. **2.** Relating to the pericardium.

per·i·car·di·al de·comp·res·sion (per'i-kahr'dē-ăl dē'kŏm-presh'ŭn) SYN cardiac decompression.

per·i·car·di·al ef·fu·sion (per'i-kahr'dē-ăl ĕ-fyū'zhŭn) Increased amounts of fluid within the pericardial sac.

per·i·car·di·al frem·i·tus (per'i-kahr'dē-ăl frem'i-tŭs) Vibration in the chest wall produced by friction of opposing roughened surfaces of the pericardium. SEE ALSO pericardial rub.

per·i·car·di·al mur·mur (per'i-kahr'dē-ăl mŭr'mŭr) A friction sound heard in some cases of pericarditis.

per·i·car·di·ec·to·my (per'i-kahr'dē-ek'tŏ-mē) Excision of a portion of the pericardium.

per·i·car·di·o·cen·te·sis, per·i·car·di·cen·te·sis (per'i-kahr'dē-ō-sen-tē'sis, -di-sen-tē'sis) Needle or catheter drainage of the pericardium. SYN pericardial tap, pericardicentesis.

per·i·car·di·ol·o·gy (per'i-kahr'dē-ol'ŏ-jē) The science or study of the pericardium, its physiology, and diseases.

per·i·car·di·o·phren·ic (per'i-kahr'dē-ō-fren'ik) Relating to the pericardium and the diaphragm.

per·i·car·di·or·rha·phy (per'i-kahr'dē-ōr'ă-fē) Suture of the pericardium.

per·i·car·di·os·to·my (per'i-kahr'dē-os'tŏ-mē) Establishment of an opening into the pericardium.

per·i·car·di·ot·o·my, per·i·car·dot·o·my (per'i-kahr'dē-ot'ŏ-mē, -kahr-dot'ŏ-mē) Incision into the pericardium for drainage.

per·i·car·di·tis (per'i-kahr-dī'tis) Inflammation of the pericardium.

per·i·car·di·tis ob·li·te·rans (per'i-kahr-dī'tis ob-lit'ĕr-anz) Inflammation of the pericardium leading to adhesion of the two layers, obliterating the sac. SEE ALSO adhesive pericarditis.

per·i·car·di·tis with ef·fu·sion (per'i-kahr-dī'tis ĕ-fyū'zhŭn) Pericardial inflammation producing excess pericardial fluid.

per·i·chon·dri·tis (per'i-kon-drī'tis) Inflammation of the perichondrium.

per·i·chon·dri·um (per'i-kon'drē-ŭm) [TA] The dense irregular connective tissue membrane around cartilage.

per·i·chor·dal (per'i-kōr'dăl) Relating to the perichord.

per·i·cho·roi·dal, per·i·cho·ri·oid·al (per'i-kŏ-roy'dăl, -ē-oy'dăl) Surrounding the choroid coat of the eye.

per·i·chrome (per'i-krōm) Denoting a nerve cell in which the chromophil substance, or stainable material, is scattered throughout the cytoplasm.

per·i·co·li·tis, per·i·co·lon·i·tis (per'i-kō-lī'tis, -lon-ī'tis) Inflammation of the connective tissue or peritoneum surrounding the colon.

per·i·col·pi·tis (per'i-kol-pī'tis) SYN perivaginitis.

per·i·cor·ne·al (per'i-kōr'nē-ăl) Inflammation around the crown of a tooth, usually a partially emerged one; it is commonly seen in the eruption of a third molar.

per·i·cor·o·nal (per'i-kōr'ŏ-năl) Around the crown of a tooth.

per·i·cor·o·ni·tis (per'i-kōr'ŏ-nī'tis) Inflammation around the crown of a tooth; commonly seen in the eruption of a third molar.

per·i·cra·ni·tis (per'i-krā-nī'tis) Inflammation of the pericranium.

per·i·cra·ni·um (per'i-krā'nē-ŭm) [TA] The periosteum of the skull.

per·i·cys·tic (per'i-sis'tik) 1. Surrounding the urinary bladder. 2. Surrounding the gallbladder.

per·i·derm, per·i·der·ma (per'i-dĕrm, -dĕr'mă) The outermost layer of the epidermis of the embryo and fetus up to the sixth month of intrauterine life. SYN epitrichium.

per·i·des·mi·tis (per'i-dez-mī'tis) Inflammation of the connective tissue surrounding a ligament.

per·i·des·mi·um (per'i-dez'mē-ŭm) The connective tissue membrane surrounding a ligament.

per·i·did·y·mi·tis (per'i-did'i-mī'tis) Inflammation of the perididymis.

per·i·di·ver·tic·u·li·tis (per'i-dī'vĕr-tik' yū-lī'tis) Inflammation of the tissues around an intestinal diverticulum.

per·i·duc·tal (per'i-dŭk'tăl) Pertaining to the area around a duct.

per·i·du·o·de·ni·tis (per'i-dū'ō-dĕ-nī'tis) Inflammation around the duodenum.

per·i·du·ral an·es·the·si·a (per'i-dūr' ăl an'es-thē'zē-ă) SYN epidural anesthesia.

per·i·en·ceph·a·li·tis (per'ē-en-sef'ă-lī' tis) Inflammation of the cerebral membranes or of the pia mater with involvement of the underlying cortex.

per·i·en·ter·i·tis (per'ē-en'tĕr-ī'tis) Inflammation of the peritoneal coat of the intestine. SYN seroenteritis.

per·i·e·soph·a·gi·tis (per'ē-ē-sof'ă-jī' tis) Inflammation of the tissues surrounding the esophagus.

per·i·fo·cal (per'i-fō'kăl) Surrounding a focus; denoting tissues, or the blood that they contain, in the vicinity of an infective focus.

per·i·fol·lic·u·lar (per'i-fō-lik'yū-lăr) Surrounding a hair follicle; usually used to describe the histopathologic appearance of the infiltrate surrounding a hair follicle.

per·i·fol·lic·u·li·tis (per'i-fō-lik'yū-lī'tis) The presence of an inflammatory infiltrate surrounding hair follicles.

per·i·fol·lic·u·li·tis ab·sce·dens et suf·fo·di·ens (per'i-fō-lik'yū-lī'tis ab-sē'denz et sŭf-ō'dē-enz) Chronic dissecting folliculitis of the scalp.

per·i·gas·tri·tis (per'i-gas-trī'tis) Inflammation of the peritoneal coat of the stomach.

per·i·glot·tic (per'i-glot'ik) Around the tongue, especially around the base of the tongue and the epiglottis, or around the glottis, the rima glottidis.

per·i·hep·a·ti·tis (per'i-hep'ă-tī'tis) Inflammation of the serous, or peritoneal, covering of the liver. SYN hepatic capsulitis, hepatitis externa, hepatoperitonitis.

per·i·je·ju·ni·tis (per'i-jĕ-jū-nī'tis) Inflammation around the jejunum.

per·i·kar·y·on, pl. **per·i·kar·y·a** (per'i-kar'ē-on, -ă) 1. The cytoplasm around the nucleus. 2. The body of the odontoblast, excluding the odontoblastic process. 3. The cell body of the nerve cell.

per·i·lab·y·rin·thi·tis (per'i-lab'i-rin-thī'tis) Inflammation of the parts about the labyrinth.

per·i·len·tic·u·lar (per'i-len-tik'yū-lăr) Surrounding the lens of the eye. SYN circumlental.

per·i·lymph, per·i·lym·pha (per'i-limf, -lim'fă) [TA] The fluid contained within the osseous labyrinth, surrounding and protecting the membranous labyrinth.

per·i·lym·phan·gi·tis (per'i-lim-fan-jī' tis) Inflammation of the tissues surrounding a lymphatic vessel.

per·i·lym·phat·ic space (per'i-lim-fat' ik spās) [TA] Space between the bony and membranous portions of the labyrinth.

per·i·men·in·gi·tis (per'i-men-in'jī'tis) SYN pachymeningitis.

per·i·men·o·pause (per'i-men'ŏ-pawz) The 3- to 5-year period before menopause when estrogen levels begin to drop.

pe·rim·e·ter (pĕ-rim'ĕ-tĕr) 1. A circumference, edge, or border. 2. An instrument, usually half a circle or sphere, used to measure the field of vision.

per·i·met·ric (per'i-met'rik) 1. Surrounding the uterus; relating to the perimetrium. SYN periuterine. 2. Relating to the circumference of any part or area. 3. Relating to perimetry.

per·i·me·tri·tis (per'i-me-trī'tis) Inflammation of the uterus involving the perimetrial covering. SYN metroperitonitis.

per·i·me·tri·um, pl. **per·i·me·tri·a** (per'i-mē'trē-ŭm, -ă) [TA] The serous (peritoneal) coat of the uterus.

pe·rim·e·try (pĕr-im'ĕ-trē) 1. The determination of the limits of the visual field.

P

2. The mapping of the sensitivity contours of the visual field.

per·i·mol·y·sis, per·i·my·lo·ly·sis (per′i-mol′i-sis, -mī-lol′i-sis) Decalcification of the teeth from exposure to gastric acid in people with chronic vomiting.

per·i·my·e·li·tis (per′i-mī′ĕ-lī′tis) SYN endosteitis.

per·i·my·o·si·tis (per′i-mī′ō-sī′tis) Inflammation of the loose cellular tissue surrounding a muscle. SYN perimysiitis (2), perimysitis.

per·i·mys·i·al (per′i-mis′ē-ăl) Relating to the perimysium; surrounding a muscle.

per·i·mys·i·i·tis, per·i·my·si·tis (per′i-mis′ē-ī′tis, -mī-sī′tis) **1.** Inflammation of the perimysium. **2.** SYN perimyositis.

per·i·na·tal (per′i-nā′tăl) Occurring during, or pertaining to, the periods before, during, or after the time of birth.

per·i·na·tal mor·tal·i·ty (PM, PNM) (per′i-nā′tăl mōr-tal′i-tē) Death around the time of birth, conventionally limited to the period from 28 weeks' gestation to 1 week postnatally.

per·i·na·tol·o·gy, per·i·na·tal med·i·cine (per′i-nā-tol′ŏ-jē, per′i-nā′tăl med′i-sin) A subspeciality of obstetrics concerned with care of the mother and fetus during pregnancy, labor, and delivery.

per·i·ne·al (per′i-nē′ăl) Relating to the perineum.

per·i·ne·al her·ni·a (per′i-nē′ăl hĕr′nē-ă) A hernia protruding through the pelvic diaphragm.

per·i·ne·al re·gion (per′i-nē′ăl rē′jŏn) [TA] Area at the lower end of the trunk, anterior to the sacral region and posterior to the pubic region between the thighs. SYN regio perinealis [TA].

per·i·ne·al sec·tion (per′i-nē′ăl sek′shŭn) Any cutting through the perineum.

perineo- Combining form indicating the perineum.

per·i·ne·o·cele (per′i-nē′ō-sēl) Hernia in the perineal region.

per·i·ne·o·plas·ty (per′i-nē′ō-plas-tē) Plastic surgery of the perineum.

per·i·ne·or·rha·phy (per′i-nē-ōr′ă-fē) Suture of the perineum, performed in perineoplasty.

per·i·ne·os·to·my (per′i-nē-os′tŏ-mē) Urethrostomy through the perineum.

per·i·ne·ot·o·my (per′i-nē-ot′ŏ-mē) Incision into the perineum to facilitate childbirth. SEE ALSO episiotomy.

per·i·ne·o·vag·i·nal (per′i-nē′ō-vaj′i-năl) Relating to the perineum and the vagina.

per·i·neph·ri·al (per′i-nef′rē-ăl) Relating to the perinephrium.

per·i·neph·ric (per′i-nef′rik) Surrounding the kidney in whole or part. SYN circumrenal, perirenal.

per·i·neph·ric ab·scess (per′i-nef′rik ab′ses) An abscess within the Gerota fascia but outside the renal capsule.

per·i·ne·phri·tis (per′i-nĕ-frī′tis) Inflammation of perinephric tissue.

per·i·neph·ri·um (per′i-nef′rē-ŭm) The connective tissue and fat surrounding the kidney.

per·i·ne·um (per′i-nē′ŭm, -ă) [TA] Surface area between the thighs extending from the coccyx to the pubis that includes the anus posteriorly and the external genitalia anteriorly.

per·i·neu·ral an·es·the·si·a (per′i-nūr′ăl an′es-thē′zē-ă) Anesthesia produced by injection of an anesthetic agent around a nerve.

per·i·neu·ri·al (per′i-nūr′ē-ăl) Relating to the perineurium.

per·i·neu·ri·tis (per′i-nūr-ī′tis) Inflammation of the perineurium. SEE ALSO adventitial neuritis.

per·i·neu·ri·um, pl. **per·i·neu·ri·a** (per′i-nūr′ē-ŭm, -ă) [TA] A supporting structure of peripheral nerve trunks, consisting of layers of flattened cells and collagenous connective tissue, which surround the nerve fasciculi and form the major diffusion barrier within the nerve.

per·i·nu·cle·ar (per'i-nū'klē-ăr) Surrounding a nucleus. SYN circumnuclear.

per·i·od (pēr'ē-ŏd) **1.** A certain duration or division of time. **2.** One of the stages of a disease. SEE ALSO stage, phase. **3.** Colloquialism for menses. **4.** Any of the horizontal rows of chemical elements in the periodic table.

per·i·o·dic·i·ty (per'ē-ō-dis'i-tē) Tendency to recurrence at regular intervals.

per·i·od·ic limb move·ments dis·or·der (pēr'ē-od'ik lim mūv'mĕnts dis-ōr'dĕr) SEE restless legs syndrome.

per·i·od·ic neu·tro·pe·ni·a (pēr'ē-od'ik nū'trō-pē'nē-ă) Neutropenia that recurs at regular intervals, in association with various types of infectious diseases.

per·i·od·ic pa·ral·y·sis (pēr'ē-od'ik păr-al'i-sis) Term for a group of diseases characterized by recurring episodes of muscular weakness or flaccid paralysis without loss of consciousness, speech, or sensation. SEE hyperkalemic periodic paralysis, hypokalemic periodic paralysis, normokalemic periodic paralysis.

pe·ri·od·ic table (pēr'ē-od'ik tā'bĕl) A graphic arrangement of chemical elements by atomic number and chemical properties.

per·i·o·di·za·tion (pēr'ē-ŏd-ī-zā'shŭn) Sequenced strength-training program that varies training volume and intensity to optimize physiologic functional capacity and exercise performance by structuring training into time blocks of different duration. The goal is to prevent staleness while peaking physiologically for competition.

per·i·o·don·tal (per'ē-ŏ-don'tăl) Around a tooth.

per·i·o·don·tal ab·scess (per'ē-ō-don'tăl ab'ses) An alveolar abscess or a lateral periodontal abscess.

Per·i·o·don·tal In·dex (PI) (per'ē-ŏ-don'tăl in'deks) An index for the epidemiologic classification of periodontal disease.

per·i·o·don·tal pock·et (per'ē-ŏ-don'tăl pok'ĕt) Pathologically deepened gingival sulcus.

per·i·o·don·tal probe (per'ē-ŏ-don'tăl prōb) Calibrated instrument used to measure the depth and topography of periodontal pockets.

Per·i·o·don·tal Screen·ing and Re·cord·ing (per'ē-ŏ-don'tăl skrēn'ing rĕ-kōr'ding) An early detection system of the American Dental Association for periodontal disease.

per·i·o·don·tics (per'ē-ŏ-don'tiks) Branch of dentistry concerned with the study of the normal tissues and the treatment of abnormal conditions of the tissues immediately about the teeth.

per·i·o·don·ti·tis (per'ē-ŏ-don-tī'tis) **1.** Inflammation of the periodontium. **2.** A chronic inflammatory disease of the periodontium occurring in response to bacterial plaque on the adjacent teeth.

per·i·o·don·to·cla·si·a, per·i·o·don·to·ly·sis (per'ē-ō-don'tō-klā'zē-ă, -don-tol'i-sis) Destruction of periodontal tissues, gingiva, pericementum, alveolar bone, and cementum.

per·i·o·oph·o·ri·tis (per'ē-ō-of'ōr-ī'tis) Inflammation of the peritoneal covering of the ovary. SYN periovaritis.

per·i·o·oph·o·ro·sal·pin·gi·tis (per'ē-ō-of'ōr-ō-sal'pin-jī'tis) Inflammation of the peritoneum and other tissues around the ovary and oviduct.

per·i·op·er·a·tive (per'ē-op'ĕr-ă-tiv) Around the time of operation. SYN paraoperative.

per·i·o·ral (per'ē-ō'răl) Around the mouth. SYN circumoral, peristomatous.

per·i·or·bi·ta, per·i·or·bit (per'ē-ōr'bi-tă, -ōr'bit) [TA] The periosteum of the orbit.

per·i·or·bi·tal (per'ē-ōr'bi-tăl) **1.** Relating to the periorbita. **2.** SYN circumorbital.

per·i·or·bit·i·tis (per'ē-ōr-bi-tī'tis) Inflammation of the area around the eye socket.

per·i·or·chi·tis (per'ē-ōr-kī'tis) Inflammation of the tunica vaginalis testis.

per·i·os·te·al (per'ē-os'tē-ăl) Relating to the periosteum.

per·i·os·te·al bud (per'ē-os'tē-ăl bŭd) Vascular connective tissue bud from the perichondrium that invades the ossification center of the cartilaginous model of a developing long bone.

per·i·os·te·al el·e·va·tor (per'ē-os'tē-ăl el'ĕ-vā-tŏr) An instrument used for separating the periosteum from the bone. SYN rugine (1).

per·i·os·te·al graft (per'ē-os'tē-ăl graft) A graft of periosteum, usually placed on bare bone.

per·i·os·te·al os·te·o·sar·co·ma (per' ē-os'tē-ăl graft) Chondroblastic osteosarcoma occurring on the surface of bones without involvement of the marrow.

♻ **periosteo-** Combining form indicating the periosteum.

per·i·os·te·o·ma, per·i·os·te·o·phyte (per'ē-os'tē-ō'mă, -os'tē-ō-fīt) A neoplasm derived from the periosteum. SYN periostoma.

per·i·os·te·o·my·e·li·tis (per'ē-os'tē-ō-mī-ĕ-lī'tis) Inflammation of the entire bone, with the periosteum and marrow.

per·i·os·te·o·plas·tic am·pu·ta·tion (per'ē-os'tē-ō-plas'tik amp'yū-tā'shŭn) SYN subperiosteal amputation.

per·i·os·te·o·sis (per'ē-os'tē-ō'sis) The formation of a periosteoma. SYN periostosis.

per·i·os·te·ot·o·my (per'ē-os'tē-ot'ō-mē) The operation of cutting through the periosteum to the bone.

per·i·os·te·um, pl. **per·i·os·te·a** (per' ē-os'tē-ŭm, -ă) [TA] The thick, fibrous membrane covering the entire surface of a bone except its articular cartilage. SEE ALSO perichondral bone.

per·i·os·ti·tis, per·i·os·te·i·tis (per'ē-os-tī'tis, -tē-ī'tis) Inflammation of the periosteum.

per·i·o·tic (per'ē-ō'tik, -ot'ik) Surrounding the internal ear.

per·i·o·va·ri·tis (per'ē-ō'văr-ī'tis) SYN periophoritis.

per·i·o·vu·lar (per'ē-ov'yū-lăr) Surrounding the ovum.

per·i·pach·y·men·in·gi·tis (per'i-pak' ē-men-in-jī'tis) Inflammation of the area between the dura and bony covering of the central nervous system.

per·i·pan·cre·a·ti·tis (per'i-pan'krē-ă-tī'tis) Inflammation of the peritoneal coat of the pancreas.

per·i·pap·il·lar·y (per'i-pap'i-lar'ē) Surrounding a papilla.

per·i·pa·tet·ic (per'i-pă-tet'ik) **1.** Walking around. **2.** Relating to a disease imported to a nonendemic area by a host clinically unaffected during the transport phase.

pe·riph·er·ad (pĕr-if'ĕr-ad) In a direction toward the periphery.

pe·riph·er·al (pĕr-if'ĕr-ăl) [TA] **1.** Relating to or situated at the periphery. **2.** Situated nearer the periphery of an organ or part of the body in relation to a specific reference point; opposite of central (centralis). SYN eccentric (3).

pe·riph·er·al ar·te·ri·o·scler·o·sis (pĕr-if'ĕr-ăl ahr-tēr'ē-ō-sker-ō'sis) Disorder in any of the vessels beyond the aorta; most often refers to the lower limbs.

pe·riph·er·al·ly in·sert·ed cen·tral cath·e·ter (pĕr-if'ĕr-ăl-ē in-sĕr'tĕd sĕn'trăl kath'ĕ-tĕr) Tube inserted into the superior vena cava through a peripheral vein.

pe·riph·er·al ner·vous sys·tem (PNS) (pĕr-if'ĕr-ăl nĕr'vŭs sis'tĕm) [TA] The part of the nervous system external to the brain and spinal cord from their roots to their peripheral terminations.

pe·riph·er·al os·si·fy·ing fi·bro·ma (pĕr-if'ĕr-ăl os'i-fī-ing fī-brō'mă) A reactive focal gingival overgrowth derived histogenetically from cells of the periodontal ligament and usually developing in response to local irritants on associated teeth.

pe·riph·er·al re·sis·tance (pĕr-if′ĕr-ăl rĕ-zis′tăns) Resistance to blood flow through arterioles and capillaries.

pe·riph·er·al sco·to·ma (pĕr-if′ĕr-ăl skō-tō′mă) A scotoma outside of the central 30 degrees of the visual field.

pe·ri·pher·al vas·cu·lar dis·ease (PVD) (pĕr-if′ĕr-ăl vas′kyū-lăr di-zēz′) Noncardiac-centered disease of blood vessels, often in extremities; spider veins are one sign of such disease.

pe·riph·er·al vi·sion (pĕr-if′ĕr-ăl vizh′ŭn) Vision resulting from retinal stimulation beyond the macula. SYN indirect vision.

pe·riph·e·ry (pĕr-if′ĕr-ē) 1. The part of a body away from the center; the outer part or surface. 2. SYN denture border.

per·i·phle·bi·tis (per′i-flĕ-bī′tis) Inflammation of the outer coat of a vein or of the tissues surrounding it.

Per·i·pla·ne·ta (per′i-plă-nē′tă) A genus of large cockroaches including several household pests found wherever food is available, especially in moist protected areas.

per·i·por·i·tis (per′i-pŏr-ī′tis) Miliary papules and papulovesicles with staphylococcic infection.

per·i·proc·ti·tis (per′i-prok-tī′tis) Inflammation of the areolar tissue about the rectum. SYN perirectitis.

per·i·py·le·phle·bi·tis (per′i-pī′lĕ-flĕ-bī′tis) Inflammation of the tissues around the portal vein.

per·i·rec·tal (per′i-rek′tăl) Surrounding the rectum.

per·i·rec·ti·tis (per′i-rek-tī′tis) SYN periproctitis.

per·i·re·nal (per′i-rē′năl) SYN perinephric.

per·i·rhi·zo·cla·si·a (per′i-rī-zō-klă′zē-ă) Inflammatory destruction of tissues immediately around the root of a tooth.

per·i·sal·pin·gi·tis (per′i-sal′pin-jī′tis) Inflammation of the peritoneum covering the uterine tube.

per·i·scop·ic (per′i-skop′ik) Denoting that which gives the ability to see objects to one side as well as in the direct axis of vision.

per·i·sig·moid·i·tis (per′i-sig′moy-dī′tis) Inflammation of the connective tissues surrounding the sigmoid flexure, giving rise to symptoms, referable to the left iliac fossa, similar to those of perityphlitis in the right iliac fossa. SYN pericolitis sinistra.

per·i·splanch·ni·tis (per′i-splangk-nī′tis) Inflammation surrounding any viscus or viscera.

per·i·sple·ni·tis (per′i-splē-nī′tis) Inflammation of the peritoneum covering the spleen.

per·i·spon·dy·li·tis (per′i-spond′i-lī′tis) Inflammation of the tissues about a vertebra.

per·i·stal·sis (per′i-stal′sis) Movement of the intestine or other tubular structure, characterized by waves of alternate circular contraction and relaxation of the tube by which the contents are propelled onward. SYN vermicular movement.

per·i·stal·tic (per′i-stal′tik) Relating to peristalsis.

pe·ris·to·le (pĕr-is′tŏ-lē) The tonic activity of the walls of the stomach whereby the organ contracts about its contents.

per·i·tec·to·my (per′i-tek′tŏ-mē) 1. The removal of a paracorneal strip of the conjunctiva for the relief of corneal disease. 2. SYN circumcision (2).

pe·ri·ten·din·e·um, pl. **pe·ri·ten·di·ne·a** (per′i-ten-din′ē-ŭm, -ă) One of the fibrous sheaths surrounding the primary bundles of fibers in a tendon.

per·i·ten·di·ni·tis, per·i·ten·on·ti·tis (per′i-ten′di-nī′tis, -ŏ-nī′tis) Inflammation of the sheath of a tendon. SYN peritenonitis.

per·i·the·li·um, pl. **per·i·the·li·a** (per'i-thē'lē-ŭm, -ă) Connective tissue that surrounds small vessels and capillaries.

per·i·thy·roid·i·tis (per'i-thī'royd-ī'tis) Inflammation of the capsule or tissues surrounding the thyroid gland.

pe·rit·o·my (pĕr-it'ŏ-mē) **1.** A circumcorneal incision through the conjunctiva. **2.** SYN circumcision (1).

per·i·to·ne·al (per'i-tŏ-nē'ăl) Relating to the peritoneum.

per·i·to·ne·al cav·i·ty (per'i-tŏ-nē'ăl kav'i-tē) [TA] The interior of the peritoneal sac, normally only a potential space between the parietal and visceral layers of the peritoneum.

♻ **peritoneo-** Combining form denoting the peritoneum.

per·i·to·ne·o·cen·te·sis (per'i-tŏ-nē'ō-sen-tē'sis) Paracentesis of the abdomen.

per·i·to·ne·oc·ly·sis (per'i-tŏ-nē-ok'li-sis) Irrigation of the abdominal cavity.

per·i·to·ne·o·pex·y (per'i-tŏ-nē'ō-pek-sē) A suspension or fixation of the peritoneum.

per·i·to·ne·o·plas·ty (per'i-tŏ-nē'ō-plas-tē) Loosening adhesions and covering the raw surfaces with peritoneum to prevent reformation.

per·i·to·ne·os·co·py (per'i-tŏ-nē-os'kŏ-pē) Examination of the contents of the peritoneum with a peritoneoscope passed through the abdominal wall. SEE ALSO laparoscopy. SYN celioscopy, ventroscopy, abdominoscopy.

per·i·to·ne·ot·o·my (per'i-tŏ'nē-ot'ŏ-mē) Incision of the peritoneum.

per·i·to·ne·um, pl. **per·i·to·nea** (per'i-tŏ-nē'ŭm, -ă) [TA] The serous membrane, consisting of mesothelium and connective tissue, which lines the abdominal cavity and covers most of the viscera contained therein.

per·i·to·ni·tis (per'i-tŏ-nī'tis) Inflammation of the peritoneum.

per·i·ton·sil·lar (per'i-ton'si-lăr) Denotes around a tonsil or the tonsils.

per·i·ton·sil·li·tis (per'i-ton'si-lī'tis) Inflammation of the connective tissue above and behind the tonsil.

per·i·tu·bu·lar con·trac·tile cells (per'i-tū'byū-lăr kŏn-trak'tīl selz) SYN myoid cells.

per·i·um·bil·i·cal (per'ē-ŭm-bil'i-kăl) Around or near the umbilicus. SYN periomphalic.

per·i·un·gual (per'ē-ŭng'gwăl) Surrounding a nail; involving the nail folds.

per·i·un·gual fi·bro·ma (per'ē-ung'gwăl fī-brō'mă) Multiple smooth firm nodules formed at the nail folds.

per·i·u·re·ter·i·tis (per'ē-yū-rē'tĕr-ī'tis) Inflammation of the tissues about a ureter.

per·i·u·re·thri·tis (per'ē-yū-rē-thrī'tis) Inflammation of the tissues about the urethra.

per·i·vag·i·ni·tis (per'i-vaj-i-nī'tis) Inflammation of the connective tissue around the vagina. SYN pericolpitis.

per·i·vas·cu·lar (per'i-vas'kyū-lăr) Surrounding a blood or lymph vessel. SYN circumvascular.

per·i·ver·te·bral (per'i-vĕr'tĕ-brăl) Around a vertebra or vertebrae. SYN perispondylic.

per·i·ves·ic·u·li·tis (per'i-vĕ-sik'yū-lī'tis) Inflammation of tissue surrounding the seminal vesicles.

per·i·vis·cer·i·tis (per'i-vis'ĕr-ī'tis) Inflammation surrounding any viscus or viscera.

per·i·vi·tel·line (per'i-vi-tel'in, -īn) Surrounding the vitellus or yolk.

per·i·vi·tel·line space (per'i-vi-tel'in spās) Area between the embryonic vitelline membrane and the zona pellucida.

PERLA (pĕr'lă) Acronym for pupils equal and reactive to light and accommodation.

per·lin·gual (per-ling'gwăl) Through or by way of the tongue.

per·ma·nent den·ti·tion (pĕr'mă-nĕnt den-tish'ŭn) The adult dentition of 32 teeth. SEE ALSO permanent tooth.

per·ma·nent thresh·old shift (PTS) (pĕr'mă-nĕnt thresh'ōld shift) Irreversible hearing loss due to exposure to intense impulse or continuous sound.

per·ma·nent tooth (pĕr'mă-nĕnt tūth) [TA] One of the 32 teeth belonging to the second, or permanent, dentition. SYN dens permanens [TA], second tooth, secondary dentition.

per·me·a·bil·i·ty (P) (pĕr'mē-ă-bil'i-tē) The property of being permeable.

per·me·a·bil·i·ty co·ef·fi·cient (pĕr'mē-ă-bil'i-tē kō'ĕ-fi'shĕnt) A coefficient associated with simple diffusion through a membrane proportional to the partition coefficient and the diffusion coefficient.

per·me·a·bil·i·ty con·stant (pĕr'mē-ă-bil'i-tē kon'stănt) A measure of the ease with which an ion can cross a unit area of membrane driven by a 1.0 M difference in concentration.

per·me·a·ble (pĕr'mē-ă-bĕl) Permitting the passage of substances (e.g., liquids, gases), as through a membrane or other structure. SYN pervious.

per·me·ate (pĕr'mē-āt, -ăt) **1.** To pass through a membrane or other structure. **2.** That which can so pass.

per mem·ber per month (pĕr mem'bĕr pĕr mŭnth) SYN capitation.

per·ni·cious (pĕr-nish'ŭs) Destructive; harmful; denoting a disease of severe character and usually fatal without appropriate treatment.

per·ni·cious a·ne·mi·a (pĕr-nish'ŭs ă-nē'mē-ă) Chronic progressive anemia of older adults due to failure of absorption of vitamin B12. SYN Addison anemia, malignant anemia.

pero- Combining form meaning maimed, malformed.

pe·ro·bra·chi·us (pē'rŏ-brā'kē-ŭs) A person with a congenital malformation of one or both forearms and hands.

pe·ro·chi·rus (pē'rŏ-kī'rŭs) A person with a congenital malformation of one or both hands.

pe·ro·dac·ty·lus (pēr'ŏ-dak'ti-lŭs) Congenital deformity of fingers or toes, which may include absent digits.

pe·ro·dac·ty·ly, pe·ro·dac·tyl·i·a (pē-rŏ-dak'ti-lē, -dak'til'ē-ă) Congenitally malformed fingers or toes.

pe·ro·me·li·a, pe·rom·e·ly (pē'rŏ-mē'lē-ă, pĕ-rom'ĕ-lē) Severe congenital malformations of limbs, including absence of hand or foot.

per·o·ne·al (pĕr'ŏ-nē'ăl) *Do not confuse this word with perineal.* SYN fibular (1).

per·o·ne·al mus·cu·lar at·ro·phy (pĕr'ŏ-nē'ăl mŭs'kyŭ-lăr at'rŏ-fē) A group of familial peripheral neuromuscular disorders, sharing the common feature of marked wasting of the distal parts of the extremities. SYN Charcot-Marie-Tooth disease.

per·o·ral (per-ōr'ăl) Through the mouth, denoting a method of medication or an approach.

per os (PO, p.o.) (per os) By or through the mouth, denoting a method of delivering medication.

pe·ro·splanch·ni·a (pē'rō-splangk'nē-ă) Congenital malformation of the viscera.

per·ox·i·dase (PX, POD) (pĕ-rok'si-dās) Hydrogen peroxide–reducing oxidoreductase.

pe·rox·i·some (pĕr-ok'si-sōm) A membrane-bound organelle found in nearly all eukaryotic cells. SYN microbody.

peroxy- Prefix denoting the presence of an extra O atom, as in peroxides and peroxy acids.

per·phe·na·zine (PPZ) (pĕr-fen'ă-zēn) An antipsychotic of the phenothiazine type.

per pri·mam in·ten·ti·o·nem (per prī'mam in-ten-shē-ō'nem) By first intention. SEE healing by first intention.

per rec·tum (PR) (per rek'tŭm) By or through the rectum.

P

per·salt (pĕr′sawlt) CHEMISTRY any salt that contains the greatest possible amount of the acid radical.

per·sev·er·a·tion (pĕr-sĕv′ĕr-ā′shŭn) The constant repetition of a meaningless word or phrase.

per·sis·tence (pĕr-sis′tĕns) **1.** Obstinate continuation of characteristic behavior. **2.** Survival despite adverse environmental conditions.

per·sis·tent a·gent (pĕr-sis′tĕnt ā′jĕnt) A chemical agent that under given conditions of temperature, pressure, wind, and other variables remains in the environment for longer than 1 day.

per·sis·tent chron·ic hep·a·ti·tis (pĕr-sis′tĕnt kron′ik hep′ă-tī′tis) A benign chronic liver disease that may follow acute viral hepatitis B or C infection or complicated bowel diseases.

per·sis·tent clo·a·ca (pĕr-sis′tent klō-ā′kă) A condition in which the urorectal septum has failed to divide the cloaca of the embryo into rectal and urogenital portions.

per·sis·tent trem·or (pĕr-sis′tĕnt trem′ŏr) A tremor that is constant, whether the subject is at rest or moving. SYN continuous tremor.

per·sis·tent trun·cus ar·te·ri·o·sus (pĕr-sis′tĕnt trungk′ŭs ahr-tē-rē-ō′sŭs) A congenital cardiovascular anomaly due to failure of development of the spiral septum and consisting of a common arterial trunk opening out of both ventricles.

per·sis·tent ve·ge·ta·tive state (PVS) (pĕr-sis′tĕnt vej′ĕ-tā-tiv stāt) Vegetative state of prolonged duration (defined in different sources as duration of longer than 1 month, 1 year, or 2 years); usually permanent. SEE ALSO vegetative.

per·son·al e·qua·tion (pĕr′sŏn-ăl ĕ-kwā′zhŭn) Slight error in judgment, perceptual response, or action peculiar to the individual and so constant that it is usually possible to allow for it in accepting the person's statements or conclusions, thus arriving at approximate exactness.

per·son·al·i·ty dis·or·der (pĕr′sŏn-al′i-tē dis-ōr′dĕr) General term for a group of behavioral disorders characterized by usually lifelong, ingrained, maladaptive patterns of deviant behavior, lifestyle, and/or social adjustment that are different in quality from psychotic and neurotic symptoms. SEE ALSO antisocial personality disorder.

per·son·al·i·ty pro·file (pĕr′sŏn-al′i-tē prō′fīl) A method by which the results of psychological testing are presented in graphic form.

per·son·al·i·ty test (pĕr′sŏn-al′i-tē test) Psychological assessment designed to test the characteristics of the personality, emotional status, or mental disorder.

per·son·al pro·tec·tive e·quip·ment (pĕr′sŏn-ăl prŏ-tek′tiv ĕ-kwip′mĕnt) Specialized clothing or equipment used by workers (e.g., emergency medical services personnel) to protect themselves from direct exposure to blood or other potentially hazardous materials to avoid injury or disease.

per·son·al space (pĕr′sŏn-ăl spās) Physical area immediately surrounding a person who is in proximity to one or more others, whether known or unknown; serves as a body buffer zone in such interpersonal transactions. Measure of space determined as appropriate varies widely among ethnic groups and cultures.

per·son·al un·con·scious (pĕr′sŏn-ăl ŭn-kon′shŭs) More superficial layer of the unconscious in which complexes reside. SEE ALSO collective unconscious, complex (3).

pers·pi·ra·tion (pĕrs′pir-ā′shŭn) **1.** The excretion of fluid by the sweat glands of the skin. SYN diaphoresis, sudation, sweating. **2.** All fluid loss through normal skin. **3.** The fluid excreted by the sweat glands; it consists of water containing sodium chloride and phosphate and other waste products. SEE ALSO sweat (2), sweat (1).

Per·thes test (pār′tĕs test) Measure for patency of the deep femoral vein.

Per·tik di·ver·tic·u·lum (per′tik dī′vĕr-tik′yū-lŭm) An abnormally deep recessus pharyngeus.

per tu·bam (per tū′băm) Through a tube.

per·tus·sis, whoop·ing cough (pĕr-tŭs´is, hūp´ing kawf) An acute infectious inflammation of the larynx, trachea, and bronchi caused by *Bordetella pertussis*; characterized by recurrent bouts of spasmodic coughing that continues until the breath is exhausted, then ends in a noisy inspiratory stridor (the ''whoop'').

per·tus·sis im·mune glob·u·lin (pĕr-tŭs´is i-myūn´ glob´yū-lin) Sterile solution of globulins derived from the plasma of adult human donors who have been immunized with pertussis vaccine. SYN pertussis immunoglobulin.

per·tus·sis vac·cine (pĕr-tŭs´is vak-sēn´) SEE diphtheria toxoid.

per·va·sive de·vel·op·men·tal dis·or·der (pĕr-vā´siv dĕ´vel-ŏp-men´tăl dis-ōr´dĕr) Mental disorder of infancy, childhood, or adolescence characterized by distortions in the development of the multiple basic psychological functions involved in the development of social skills and language.

per·ver·sion (pĕr-ver´zhŭn) *Negative and pejorative connotations of this word may render it offensive in some contexts.* A deviation from the norm, especially concerning sexual interests or behavior.

per·vi·ous (pĕr´vē-ŭs) SYN permeable.

pes, gen. **pe·dis,** pl. **pe·des** (pes, pē´dis, -dēz) [TA] **1.** SYN foot (1). **2.** Any foot-like or basal structure or part. **3.** Talipes; in this sense, pes is always qualified by a word expressing the specific type.

pes ca·vus (pes kā´vŭs) Condition characterized by increased height of the foot's medial longitudinal arch. SYN claw foot.

pes e·qui·nus (pes ē-kwī´nŭs) SYN talipes equinus.

pes pla·nus (pes plā´nŭs) SYN talipes planus.

pes·sa·ry (pes´ă-rē) **1.** An appliance of varied form, introduced into the vagina to support the uterus or to correct any displacement. **2.** A medicated vaginal suppository.

pes·ti·lence (pes´ti-lĕns) **1.** SYN plague

(2). **2.** A virulent outbreak of any disease.

pes·tle (pes´ĕl) Rod-like instrument with one rounded and weighted extremity, used to break, grind, and mix substances in a mortar (q.v.).

pes val·gus (pes val´gŭs) SYN talipes valgus.

peta- (P) Prefix used in SI and the metric system to signify multiples of one quadrillion (10^{15}).

-petal Suffix meaning seeking; movement toward the part indicated by the main portion of the word.

pe·te·chi·ae (pĕ-tē´kē-ē) Minute hemorrhagic spots, of pinpoint to pinhead size, in the skin, which are not blanched by diascopy.

pet·i·o·late, pet·i·o·lat·ed (pet´ē-ō-lāt, -ĕd) Having a stem or pedicle. SYN petioled.

pe·ti·o·lus, pet·i·ole (pĕ-tī´ō-lŭs, pē´tē-ōl) A stem or pedicle.

Pe·tit her·ni·a (pĕ-tē´ hĕr´nē-ă) Lumbar hernia, occurring in inferior lumbar triangle.

Pe·tit her·ni·ot·o·my (pĕ-tē´ her´nē-ot´ŏ-mē) Herniotomy without incision into the sac.

pe·tit mal (pĕ-tē´ mahl) Type of seizure.

pe·tit mal ep·i·lep·sy (pĕ-tē´ mahl ep´i-lep-sē) SYN childhood absence epilepsy.

Pe·tri dish (pē´trē dish) Small, shallow, circular dish made of thin glass or clear plastic with a loosely fitting, overlapping cover used in microbiology; frequently called a plate.

Pe·tri dish cul·ture (pē´trē dish kŭl´chŭr) Combination of filter paper, fecal specimen, and tap water placed in a Petri dish; provides an environment in which nematode eggs may hatch and larvae develop.

pet·ri·fac·tion (pet´ri-fak´shŭn) Fossilization, as in conversion into stone.

P

pé·tris·sage (pā-trē-sahzh′) A movement in massage that involves the lifting of tissues away from underlying structures, with the intention of improving elasticity and stimulating blood and lymph circulation.

pe·tro·la·tum, pe·tro·le·um jel·ly (pet-rō-lā′tŭm, pĕ-trō′lē-ŭm jel′ē) A yellowish mixture of the softer members of the paraffin or methane series of hydrocarbons used as a soothing application to burns and abrasions of the skin. SYN petroleum jelly, yellow soft paraffin.

pet·ro·mas·toid (pet′rō-mas′toyd) Relating to the petrous and the squamous portions of the temporal bone.

pet·ro·oc·cip·i·tal (pet′rō-ok-sip′i-tăl) Denoting the cranial suture between the occipital bone and the petrous portion of the temporal.

pe·tro·sal (pĕ-trō′săl) Relating to the petrosa. SYN petrous (2).

pet·ro·si·tis (pet′rō-sī′tis) An inflammation involving the petrous portion of the temporal bone and its air cells.

pet·ro·sphe·noid (pet′rō-sfē′noyd) Relating to the petrous portion of the temporal bone and to the sphenoid bone.

pet·rous (pet′rŭs) **1.** Of stony hardness. **2.** SYN petrosal.

Petz·val sur·face (pets′vahl sŭr′făs) The curved image plane on which any extended linear object is focused by a lens. SEE ALSO barrel distortion, pincushion distortion.

Peutz-Jeg·hers syn·drome (puts jā′gĕrz sin′drōm) Generalized hamartomatous multiple polyposis of the intestinal tract, consistently involving the jejunum, associated with melanin spots of the lips, buccal mucosa, and fingers. SYN Jeghers-Peutz syndrome.

pex·is (pek′sis) Fixation of substances in the tissues.

-pexy Combining form meaning fixation, usually surgical.

Pey·er glands (pī′ĕr glandz) SYN Aggregated lymphoid nodules of the small intestine.

Pey·er patch·es (pī′ĕr pach′ĕz) Collections of many lymphoid follicles closely packed together, forming oblong elevations on the mucous membrane of the small intestine.

pe·yo·te, pe·yo·tl (P) (pā-yō′tē, pā-yō′tĕl) Aztec name for *Lophophora williamsii,* a small cactus indigenous to Mexico and the southwestern U.S. used in Native American tribal ceremonies to induce trances and hallucinations. SYN pellote.

Pey·ro·nie dis·ease (pā-rō-nē′ di-zēz′) Disorder in which plaques or strands of dense fibrous tissue surrounding the corpus cavernosum of the penis cause penile bending and pain on erection; sometimes associated with Dupuytren contracture. SYN penile fibromatosis, van Buren disease.

Pey·rot tho·rax (pā-rō′ thōr′aks) An obliquely oval deformity of the chest in cases of a very large pleural effusion.

Pfeif·fer ba·cil·lus (fī′fĕr bă-sil′ŭs) SYN *Haemophilus influenzae.*

pg Abbreviation for picogram.

P-gly·co·pro·tein (Pgp, P-170, P-gp) (glī′kō-prō′tēn) Protein associated with tumor multidrug resistance. SYN P-170.

Ph Abbreviation for phenyl.

pH Symbol for the negative logarithm of the H^+ ion concentration (measured in moles per liter); a solution with pH 7.00 is neutral at 22°C, one with a pH of more than 7.0 is alkaline, and one with a pH lower than 7.00 is acid.

phaco- Combining form meaning (1) lens-shaped, relating to a lens. (2) birthmark; as in phacomatosis.

pha·co·an·a·phy·lax·is, pha·ko·an·aph·y·lax·is (fak′ō-an-ă-fi-lak′sis) Hypersensitivity to protein of the ocular lens.

phac·o·cele (fak′ō-sēl) Hernia of the lens of the eye through the sclera.

phac·o·e·mul·si·fi·ca·tion, phak·o·e·mul·si·fi·ca·tion (fak′ō-ē-mŭl-si-fi-kā′shŭn) A method of emulsifying and aspirating a cataract with a low-frequency ultrasonic needle.

phac·o·er·y·sis (fak′ō-er′i-sis) Extraction of the ocular lens with a suction cup called the erysophake.

pha·col·y·sis (fă-kol′i-sis) Operative breaking down and removal of the lens.

pha·co·lyt·ic, pha·ko·lyt·ic (fak′ō-lit′ik) Characterized by or referring to phacolysis.

pha·co·ma (fa-kō′mă) A hamartoma found in phacomatosis; often refers to a retinal hamartoma in tuberous sclerosis. SYN phakoma.

pha·co·ma·la·ci·a, pha·ko·ma·la·ci·a (fak′ō-mă-lā′shē-ă) Softening of the ocular lens.

pha·co·ma·to·sis, pha·ko·ma·to·sis (fak′ō-mă-tō′sis) A generic term for hereditary diseases characterized by hamartomas involving multiple tissues. SYN phakomatosis.

phac·o·mor·phic glau·co·ma (fak′ō-mōr′fik glaw-kō′mă) Secondary glaucoma caused by either excessive size or spheric shape of the lens.

phac·o·scope (fak′ō-skōp) An instrument in the form of a dark chamber for observing the changes in the lens during accommodation.

phaeo- SEE pheo-.

phaeo- [Br.] SYN pheo-.

phaeochromocyte [Br.] SYN pheochromocyte.

phae·o·hy·pho·my·co·sis (fē′ō-hī′fō-mī-kō′sis) A group of superficial and deep infections caused by fungi that form pigmented hyphae and yeastlike cells in tissue.

-phage, -phagia, -phagy Combining forms meaning eating, devouring.

phage (fāj) SYN bacteriophage.

phago- Prefix meaning eating, devouring.

phag·o·cyte (fag′ō-sīt) A cell possessing the property of ingesting bacteria, foreign particles, and other cells. Phagocytes are divided into two general classes: microphages and macrophages.

phag·o·cy·tol·y·sis (fag′ō-sī-tol′i-sis) **1.** Destruction of phagocytes, or leukocytes, occurring in the process of blood coagulation or due to introduction of certain antagonistic foreign substances into the body. **2.** Spontaneous breakdown of phagocytes.

phag·o·cy·to·sis (făg′ō-sī-tō′sis) The process of ingestion and digestion by cells of solid substances. SEE ALSO endocytosis.

phag·o·ly·so·some (fag′ō-lī′sō-sōm) A body formed by union of a phagosome or ingested particle with a lysosome having hydrolytic enzymes.

phag·o·some (fag′ō-sōm) A vesicle that forms around a particle (bacterial or other) within the phagocyte that engulfed it, separates from the cell membrane, and then fuses with and receives the contents of cytoplasmic granules (lysosomes).

phag·o·type (fag′ō-tīp) MICROBIOLOGY Subdivision of a species distinguished from other strains therein by sensitivity to a certain bacteriophage or set of bacteriophages.

pha·kic eye (fak′ik ī) An eye containing the natural lens.

phako- For words so beginning and not listed here, SEE phaco-.

pha·ko·ma (fă-kō′mă) SYN phacoma.

phak·o·ma·to·sis (fă-kō′mă-tō′sis) SYN phacomatosis.

pha·lan·ge·al (fă-lan′jē-ăl) *Avoid the mispronunciation phalange′al.* Relating to a phalanx.

phal·an·gec·to·my (fal′ăn-jek′tŏ-mē) Excision of one or more of the phalanges of hand or foot.

phal·an·gi·tis (fal′an-jī′tis) Inflammation of one or more phalanges.

phall-, phalli-, phallo- Combining forms meaning the penis.

phal·lec·to·my (fal-ek'tŏ-mē) Surgical removal of the penis.

phal·lic (fal'ik) **1.** Relating to the penis. **2.** PSYCHOANALYSIS relating to the penis, especially during the phases of infantile psychosexuality. SEE ALSO phallic phase.

phal·lic phase (fal'ik fāz) Stage in psychosexual development, occurring when a child is 2–6 years old, during which interest and pleasurable experiences are centered around the penis in boys and the clitoris in girls. SEE genital phase.

phal·li·tis (fal-ī'tis) Inflammation of the penis.

phal·lo·dyn·i·a (fal'ō-din'ē-ă) Pain in the penis.

phal·loi·din (fă-loy'din) Best known of the toxic cyclic peptides produced by the poisonous mushroom, *Amanita phalloides*.

phal·lo·plas·ty (fal'ō-plas-tē) Surgical reconstruction of the penis.

phal·lot·o·my (fal-ot'ŏ-mē) Surgical incision into the penis.

phal·lus, pl. **phal·li** (fal'ŭs, -ī) The primordium of the penis or clitoris that develops from the embryonic genital tubercle.

phan·er·o·sis (fan'ĕr-ō'sis) The act or process of becoming visible.

phan·ta·si·a (fan-tā'zē-ă) SYN fantasy.

phan·tom (fan'tŏm) RADIOLOGY a mechanical or computer-generated model for predicting irradiation dosage deep in the body.

phan·tom limb, phan·tom limb pain (fan'tŏm lim, pān) The sensation that an amputated limb is still present, often associated with painful paresthesia. SYN phantom limb, pseudesthesia (3), pseudoesthesia (3), stump hallucination.

phan·tom tu·mor (fan'tŏm tū'mŏr) **1.** Accumulation of fluid in the interlobar spaces of the lung, secondary to congestive heart failure. **2.** A muscle contraction or gaseous distortion of the intestines.

Phar.D. Abbreviation for Doctor of Pharmacy.

phar·ma·ceu·tic, phar·ma·ceu·ti·cal (fahr'-mă-sū'tik, -ăl) Relating to pharmacy or to pharmaceutics. SYN pharmacal.

phar·ma·ceu·ti·cal care (fahr'mă-sū'ti-kăl kār) The responsible provision of drug therapy to get definite outcomes that improve a patient's quality of life.

phar·ma·cist (PHAR) (fahr'mă-sist) One licensed to prepare and dispense drugs and is knowledgeable concerning their properties. SYN pharmaceutist.

pharmaco- Combining form meaning drugs.

phar·ma·co·di·ag·no·sis (fahr'mă-kō-dī'ag-nō'sis) Use of drugs in diagnosis.

phar·ma·co·dy·nam·ics (fahr'mă-kō-dī-nam'iks) The study of uptake, movement, binding, and interactions of pharmacologically active molecules at their tissue site(s) of action.

phar·ma·co·ge·net·ics, phar·ma·co·ge·no·mics (fahr'mă-kō-jĕ-net'iks, -nō'miks) The study of genetically determined variations in responses to drugs in humans or in laboratory organisms.

phar·ma·cog·no·sy (fahr'mă-kog'nō-sē) A branch of pharmacology concerned with the physical characteristics and botanic and animal sources of crude drugs.

phar·ma·co·ki·net·ics (fahr'mă-kō-ki-net'iks) Study of the movement of drugs within biologic systems, as affected by absorption, distribution, metabolism, and excretion.

phar·ma·co·log·ic, phar·ma·co·log·i·cal (fahr'mă-kŏ-loj'ik, -i-kăl) Relating to pharmacology or to the composition, properties, and actions of drugs.

phar·ma·co·log·ic stress test (fahr'mă-kō-loj'ik stres test) An assessment of cardiovascular fitness, and especially of coronary perfusion.

phar·ma·col·o·gist (fahr'mă-kol'ŏ-jist) A specialist in pharmacology.

phar·ma·col·o·gy (PC) (fahr'mă-kol'ŏ-jē) The science concerned with drugs, their sources, appearance, chemistry, actions, and uses.

phar·ma·co·ther·a·py (fahr′mă-kō-thār′ă-pē) Treatment of disease with drugs.

phar·ma·cy (fahr′mă-sē) **1.** The practice of preparing and dispensing drugs and the delivery of pharmaceutic care. **2.** A facility licensed to dispense medications to the public.

pha·ryn·gal·gi·a (far′ing-gal′jē-ă) Pain in the pharynx; sore throat.

pha·ryn·ge·al (făr-in′jē-ăl) *Avoid the mispronunciation pharynge′al.* Relating to the pharynx. SYN pharyngeus.

pha·ryn·ge·al fis·tu·la (fă-rin′jē-ăl fish′tyū-lă) A congenital fistula in the neck resulting from incomplete closure of a pharyngeal groove or cleft. SYN branchial fistula.

pha·ryn·ge·al groove (făr-in′jē-ăl grūv) The ectodermal groove between two pharyngeal arches in the human embryo. SYN branchial cleft, pharyngeal cleft.

pha·ryn·ge·al hy·poph·y·sis (fă-rin′jē-ăl hī-pof′i-sis) Residual tissue derived from the hypophysial diverticulum that lies in the lamina propria of the nasopharynx. SYN hypophysis pharyngealis [TA], pars pharyngea hypophyseos.

pha·ryn·ge·al la·cu·na (făr-in′jē-ăl lă-kū′nă) Depression near the pharyngeal opening of the pharyngotympanic (auditory) tube.

pha·ryn·ge·al lym·phat·ic ring (făr-in′jē-ăl lim-fat′ik ring) A broken ring of lymphoid tissue, formed by the lingual, faucial, and pharyngeal tonsils.

pha·ryn·ge·al mus·cles (fă-rin′jē-ăl mŭs′ĕlz) [TA] Muscular layer of the pharyngeal wall. SYN muscular layer of pharynx [TA], tunica muscularis pharyngis [TA], muscle layer of pharynx, muscular coat of pharynx.

pha·ryn·ge·al re·flex (făr-in′jē-ăl rē′fleks) **1.** SYN swallowing reflex. **2.** SYN vomiting reflex.

pha·ryn·ge·al tra·che·al lu·men air·way (făr-in′jē-ăl trā′kē-ăl lū′mĕn ār′wā) SYN pharyngeal tracheal multiple balloon system.

pha·ryn·ge·al tra·che·al mul·ti·ple bal·loon sys·tem (făr-in′jē-ăl trā′kē-ăl mŭl′ti-pĕl bă-lūn′ sis′tĕm) Airway management adjunct that consists of two tubes, endotracheal and esophageal. The device is inserted blindly into the oropharynx and passes either into the trachea or the esophagus. SYN esophageal tracheal airway, pharyngeal tracheal lumen airway.

phar·yn·gec·to·my (far′in-jek′tŏ-mē) Resection of the pharynx.

phar·yn·gis·mus (far′in-jiz′mŭs) Spasm of the muscles of the pharynx. SYN pharyngospasm.

phar·yn·git·ic (far′in-jit′ik) Relating to pharyngitis.

phar·yn·gi·tis (far′in-jī′tis) Inflammation of the mucous membrane and underlying parts of the pharynx.

pharyngo-, pharyng- Combining form denoting pharynx.

pha·ryn·go·cele (fă-ring′gō-sēl) A diverticulum from the pharynx.

pha·ryn·go·con·junc·ti·val fe·ver (fă-ring′gō-kŏn-jŭngk′ti-văl fē′vĕr) Adenoviral disease characterized by fever, pharyngitis, and conjunctivitis.

pha·ryn·go·e·soph·a·ge·al (fă-ring′gō-ĕ-sof′ă-jē′ăl) Relating to the pharynx and the esophagus. SYN pharyngo-oesophageal.

pha·ryn·go·e·soph·a·ge·al con·stric·tion (fă-ring′gō-ĕ-sof′ă-jē′ăl kŏn-strik′shŭn) [TA] Normal narrowing of the alimentary tract, demonstrated radiographically after a barium swallow, at the junction of the pharynx with the esophagus (C5 vertebral level) caused by the tonic or active contraction of the cricopharyngeal part of the inferior constrictor of the pharynx (upper esophageal sphincter). SYN constrictio pharyngoesophagealis [TA], upper esophageal constriction.

pha·ryn·go·e·soph·a·ge·al di·ver·tic·u·lum (fă-ring′gō-ĕ-sof′ă-jē′ăl dī-vĕr-tik′yū-lŭm) Most common diverticulum of the esophagus; arises between the inferior pharyngeal constrictor and the cricopharyngeus muscle; also known as Zenker diverticulum.

P

pha·ryn·go·my·co·sis (fă-ring′gō-mī-kō′sis) Invasion of the mucous membrane of the pharynx by fungi.

pharyngo-oesophageal [Br.] SYN pharyngoesophageal.

pha·ryn·go·ple·gi·a (fă-ring′gō-plē′jē-ă) Paralysis of the muscles of the pharynx.

pha·ryn·go·scope (fă-ring′gŏ-skōp) An instrument like a laryngoscope, used to inspect the mucous membrane of the pharynx.

pha·ryn·go·spasm (fă-ring′gō-spazm) SYN pharyngismus.

pha·ryn·go·ste·no·sis (fă-ring′gō-stĕ-nō′sis) Stricture of the pharynx.

phar·yn·got·o·my (far′ing-got′ŏ-mē) Any cutting operation on the pharynx either from without or from within.

pha·ryn·go·ton·sil·li·tis (fă-ring′gō-ton′si-lī′tis) Inflammation of the pharynx and tonsils.

phar·ynx, gen. **pha·ryn·gis**, pl. **pha·ryn·ges** (far′ingks, fă-rin′jis, -jēz) [TA] The upper expanded portion of the digestive tube, between the esophagus below and the mouth and nasal cavities above and in front.

phase (fāz) **1.** A stage in the course of change or development. **2.** A homogeneous, physically distinct, and separable portion of a heterogeneous system. **3.** The time relationship between two or more events. **4.** A particular part of a recurring time pattern or wave form. SEE ALSO stage, period.

phase I block (fāz blok) Inhibition of nerve impulse transmission across the myoneural junction associated with depolarization of the motor endplate.

phase II block (fāz blok) Inhibition of nerve impulse transmission across the myoneural junction unaccompanied by depolarization of the motor endplate.

phase im·age (fāz im′ăj) A magnetic resonance image showing only phase shift information, to detect motion.

phase mi·cro·scope, phase-con·

trast mi·cro·scope (fāz mī′krŏ-skōp, fāz-kon′trast) A specially constructed microscope that has a special condenser and objective containing a phase-shifting ring whereby small differences in index of refraction are made visible as intensity or contrast differences in the image.

pha·sic bite pat·tern (fā′zik bīt pat′ĕrn) A reflexive response seen in 5–6-month-old infants; appears as a jaw opening and closing; not a functional bite.

phas·mid (faz′mid) **1.** One of a pair of caudal chemoreceptors seen in nematodes of the class Secernentasida. **2.** Common name for a member of the class Phasmidia, now called Secernentasida.

PH con·duc·tion time (kŏn-dŭk′shŭn tīm) SEE atrioventricular conduction.

Phe Symbol for phenylalanine or phenylalanyl.

Phem·is·ter graft (fem′is-tĕr graft) An autogenous onlay bone graft used in treating delayed union of fractures.

♻ **phen-, pheno-** **1.** Combining forms meaning appearance. **2.** CHEMISTRY combining forms denoting derivation from benzene (phenyl-).

phen·cy·cli·dine (PCP) (fen-sī′kli-dēn) A substance of abuse, used for its hallucinogenic properties; its hydrochloride has analgesic and anesthetic properties.

phe·no·bar·bi·tal (fē′nō-bahr′ bi-tahl) A long-acting oral or parenteral sedative, anticonvulsant, and hypnotic. SYN phenylethylbarbituric acid, phenylethylmalonylurea.

phe·no·cop·y (fē′nō-kop-ē) **1.** A set of clinical and laboratory characteristics that would ordinarily warrant the diagnosis of a specific genetic abnormality, but are of environmental rather than genetic etiology. **2.** A condition of environmental etiology that mimics one usually of genetic etiology.

phe·nol (fē′nol) Hydroxybenzene; an antiseptic, anesthetic, and disinfectant. SYN carbolic acid, phenyl alcohol.

phe·no·lu·ri·a (fē′nol-yūr′ē-ă) The excretion of phenols in the urine.

phe·nom·e·non, pl. **phe·nom·e·na** (fĕ-nom'ĕ-non, -ă) **1.** An occurrence or object as perceived by the senses, whether ordinary or extraordinary, in relation to a disease. **2.** Any unusual fact or occurrence.

phe·no·thi·a·zine (fē'nō-thī'ă-zēn) A compound formerly used extensively for the treatment of intestinal nematodes in animals. SYN thiodiphenylamine.

phe·no·type (fē'nō-tīp) Manifestation of a genotype or the combined manifestation of several different genotypes.

phen·pro·pi·o·nate (fen-prō'pē-ŏ-nāt') USAN-approved contraction for 3-phenylpropionate.

phen·yl (Ph, Φ) (fen'il) The univalent radical, C_6H_5-, of benzene.

phen·yl·a·ce·tic ac·id (fen'il-ă-sē'tik as'id) An abnormal product of phenylalanine catabolism, appearing in the urine of people with phenylketonuria.

phen·yl·al·a·nine (F) (fen'il-al'ă-nēn) One of the common amino acids in proteins; a nutritionally essential amino acid.

phen·yl·eph·rine hy·dro·chlor·ide (fen'il-ef'rin hī'drŏ-klōr'īd) A powerful vasoconstrictor, used as a nasal decongestant and mydriatic.

phen·yl·eth·yl al·co·hol (fen'il-eth'il al'kŏ-hol) A natural constituent of some volatile oils; used as an antibacterial agent in ophthalmic solutions. SYN benzyl carbinol, phenethyl alcohol.

phe·nyl·ke·to·nu·ri·a (fen'il-kē'tō-nyūr'ē-ă) Congenital deficiency of phenylalanine 4-monooxygenase that can cause severe mental retardation, often with seizures, other neurologic abnormalities such as retarded myelination, and deficient melanin formation leading to hypopigmentation of the skin and eczema. SYN Folling disease.

phen·yl sa·lic·y·late (fen'il să-lis'i-lāt) Phenylic ester of salicylic acid; an intestinal analgesic and antipyretic; used as an enteric coating for tablets. SYN salol.

phen·yl·thi·o·u·re·a (fen'il-thī'ō-yūr-ē'ă) A substance that tastes bitter to some

people but is tasteless to others. SEE taste deficiency. SYN phenylthiocarbamide.

phen·y·to·in (PHT, PT) (fĕ-nit'ŏ-in) Anticonvulsant used to treat generalized tonic clonic and complex partial epilepsy. SYN 5, 5-diphenylhydantoin.

pheo- **1.** Prefix denoting the same substituents on a phorbin or phorbide (porphyrin) residue as are present in chlorophyll, excluding any ester residues and magnesium. **2.** Combining form meaning gray, dark colored.

phe·o·chro·mo·blast (fē'ŏ-krō'mŏ-blast) A primordial chromaffin cell that, with sympathetoblasts, enters into the formation of the suprarenal gland.

phe·o·chro·mo·cyte (fē'ŏ-krō'mŏ-sīt) Chromaffin cell of a sympathetic paraganglion, medulla of a suprarenal gland, or of a pheochromocytoma. SYN phaeochromocyte.

phe·re·sis (fĕ-rē'sis) *Do not confuse this word with phoresis.* Procedure in which blood is removed from a donor, separated, and a portion retained; the remainder is returned to the donor.

pher·o·mone (fer'ŏ-mōn) An ectohormone secreted by an individual and perceived by a second individual of the same or similar species, thereby changing the sexual or social behavior of that individual.

phi (φ, Φ) (fī) **1.** The 21st letter of the Greek alphabet (φ). **2.** Phenyl; potential energy; magnetic flux (Φ). **3.** Plane angle; volume fraction; quantum yield; the dihedral angle of rotation about the $N-C_\alpha$ bond associated with a peptide bond (φ).

Phi·a·loph·o·ra (fī-ă-lof'ŏ-ră) Fungal genus of which at least two species cause chromoblastomycosis.

-phil, -phile, -philic, -philia Combining forms denoting affinity for, craving for.

Phil·a·del·phi·a chro·mo·some (fil'ă-del'fē-ă krō'mŏ-sōm) An abnormal minute chromosome; found in cultured leukocytes of many patients with chronic granulocytic leukemia.

Phi·la·del·phi·a col·lar (fil'ă-del'fē-ă kol'ăr) Commonly used Styrofoam neck collar used for immobilization.

♻ **-philia, -phily, -philous** Combining forms meaning that which has an attraction to or is stained by.

phil·trum, pl. **phil·tra** (fil'trŭm, -tră) [TA] **1.** A philter or love potion. **2.** [NA] The infranasal depression; the groove in the midline of the upper lip.

phi·mo·sis, gen. and pl. **phi·mo·ses** (fī-mō'sis, -sēz) Narrowness of the opening of the prepuce, preventing its being drawn back over the glans.

♻ **phleb-** SEE phlebo-.

phleb·an·gi·o·ma (fleb-an'jē-ō'mă) An aneurysm that develops in a vein.

phleb·ar·te·ri·ec·ta·si·a (fleb'ahr-tēr-ē-ek-tā'zē-ă) Disordered dilation of veins and arteries.

phleb·ec·ta·si·a (fleb'ek-tā'zē-ă) Dilation of vein(s). SYN venectasia.

phle·bec·to·my (flĕ-bek'tŏ-mē) Excision of a segment of a vein, sometimes performed to cure varicose veins. SEE ALSO strip (2). SYN venectomy.

phleb·em·phrax·is (fleb'em-frak'sis) Blockage of a vein by a clot.

phleb·is·mus (fleb-iz'mŭs) Obstruction that causes veins to swell.

phle·bi·tis (flĕ-bī'tis) Inflammation of a vein.

♻ **phlebo-, phleb-** Combining forms meaning vein

phleb·o·cly·sis (fleb'ō-klī'sis) Intravenous injection of an isotonic solution of dextrose or other substances in quantity. SYN venoclysis.

phleb·o·gram (fleb'ō-gram) A tracing of the jugular or other venous pulse. SYN venogram (2).

phleb·o·graph (fleb'ŏ-graf) An instrument for making a tracing of the venous pulse.

phleb·og·ra·phy (flĕ-bog'ră-fē) **1.** Re-

cording the venous pulse. **2.** SYN venography.

phleb·o·li·thi·a·sis (fleb'ō-li-thī'ă-sis) The formation of phleboliths (stones within veins).

phleb·o·ma·nom·e·ter (fleb'ō-mă-nom'ĕ-tĕr) A manometer for measuring venous blood pressure.

phleb·o·phle·bos·to·my (fleb'ō-flĕ-bos'tŏ-mē) SYN venovenostomy.

phle·bor·rha·phy (fle-bōr'ă-fē) Suture of a vein.

phleb·o·scle·ro·sis (fleb'ō-skler-ō'sis) Fibrous hardening of the walls of the veins.

phleb·o·sta·sis (flĕ-bos'tă-sis) **1.** Abnormally slow motion of blood in veins, usually with venous distention. **2.** Treatment of congestive heart failure by compressing proximal veins of the extremities with tourniquets.

phleb·o·throm·bo·sis (fleb'ō-throm-bō'sis) Venous thrombosis, without primary inflammation.

phle·bot·o·mist (flĕ-bot'ŏ-mist) One trained and skilled in phlebotomy.

phle·bot·o·mize (flĕ-bot'ō-mīz) **1.** To draw blood from. **2.** To achieve iron overload reduction by repeated removal of blood, as in hemochromatosis.

phle·bot·o·my (fle-bot'ŏ-mē) Incision into a vein to draw blood. SYN venesection, venotomy.

phle·bot·o·my: ar·te·ri·al blood sam·ple (fleb-ot'ŏ-mē ahr-tēr'ē-ăl blŭd samp'ĕl) Surgical incision to draw blood from an artery.

phle·bot·o·my: blood u·nit ac·qui·si·tion (fleb-ot'ŏ-mē blŭd yū'nit ak'wi-zish'ŭn) Surgical incision to obtain blood for storage or donation.

phle·bot·o·my: ve·nous blood sam·ple (fleb-ot'ŏ-mē vē'nŭs blŭd samp'ĕl) Surgical incision to draw blood for medical testing from a vein.

phlegm (flem) **1.** Abnormal amounts of

mucus, especially as expectorated from the mouth. **2.** One of the four humors of the body, according to the ancient Greek humoral doctrine.

phleg·ma·si·a ce·ru·le·a do·lens (fleg-mā'zē-ă cer-ū'lē-ă dō'lenz) Thrombosis of the veins of a limb, with sudden severe pain with swelling, cyanosis, and edema of the part, followed by circulatory collapse and shock.

phleg·mat·ic (fleg-mat'ik) Relating to the heaviest of four ancient Greek humors, phlegm: therefore calm, apathetic, unexcitable.

phleg·mon·ous (fleg'mŏn-ŭs) Term denoting phlegmon, an inflammatory state.

phlyc·te·na, pl. **phlyc·te·nae, phlyc·ten·ule** (flik-tē'nă, -nē, -ten'yūl) A small vesicle.

phlyc·ten·u·lar (flik-ten'yū-lăr) Relating to a phlyctenula.

phlyc·ten·u·lar con·junc·ti·vi·tis, phlyc·ten·u·lar oph·thal·mi·a (flik-ten'yū-lăr kŏn-jŭngk'ti-vī'tis, of-thal-mē'ă) Circumscribed ocular disorder with formation of small red nodules of lymphoid tissue on the conjunctiva. SYN phlyctenular ophthalmia.

phlyc·ten·u·lar ker·a·ti·tis (flik-ten'yū-lăr ker'ă-tī'tis) Inflammation of the corneal conjunctiva with formation of small red nodules of lymphoid tissue near the corneoscleral limbus.

-phobia Combining form for fear.

pho·bi·a (fō'bē-ă) Any objectively unfounded morbid dread or fear that arouses a state of panic.

pho·bic (fō'bik) Pertaining to or characterized by phobia.

pho·bic de·sen·si·ti·za·tion (fō'bik dē-sen'si-tī-zā'shŭn) Clinical method to treat irrational fears or phobias by exposing the person to the dreaded object and using talk therapy to help the patient tolerate it by increasing exposure to it.

pho·nal (fō'năl) Relating to the voice or to sound.

phon·as·the·ni·a (fō'nas-thē'nē-ă) Difficult or abnormal voice production, the enunciation being too high, too loud, or too hard.

pho·na·tion (fō-nā'shŭn) The utterance of sounds by means of vocal folds.

pho·na·tor·y (fō'nă-tōr'ē) Relating to phonation.

pho·neme (fō'nēm) The smallest sound unit that, in terms of the phonetic sequences of sound, controls meaning.

pho·net·ic bal·ance (fō-net'ik bal'ăns) That property by which a group of words used to measure hearing has the various phonemes occurring at approximately the same frequency at which they occur in ordinary conversation in that language; phonetically balanced word lists are used in determining the discrimination score.

pho·net·ics (fō-net'iks) The science of speech and of pronunciation.

pho·ni·at·rics (fō'-nē-at'riks) The study of speech; the science of speech.

phon·ic (fon'ik) Relating to sound or to the voice.

phono-, phon- Combining forms meaning sound, speech, or voice sounds.

pho·no·an·gi·og·ra·phy (fō'nō-an'-jē-og'ră-fē) Recording and analysis of the frequency-intensity components of the bruit of turbulent arterial blood flow through a stenotic lesion.

pho·no·car·di·o·graph (fō'nō-kahr'dē-ō-graf) An instrument, using microphones, amplifiers, and filters, to graphically record heart sounds, and display them with an oscilloscope.

pho·no·cath·e·ter (fō'nō-kath'ĕ-tĕr) A cardiac catheter with a diminutive microphone housed in its tip, to record sounds from the heart and great vessels.

pho·no·gram (fō'nŏ-gram) A graphic curve depicting the duration and intensity of a sound.

pho·nom·e·ter (fō-nom'ĕ-tĕr) An instrument for measuring the pitch and intensity of sounds.

P

pho·no·my·oc·lo·nus (fō'nō-mī-ok'lŏ-nŭs) Clonic spasms of muscles in response to aural stimuli.

pho·no·my·og·ra·phy (fō'nō-mī-og'ră-fē) The recording of the varying sounds made by contracting muscular tissue.

pho·nop·a·thy (fō-nop'ă-thē) Any disease of the vocal organs affecting speech.

pho·no·pho·re·sis (fō'nō-fōr-ē'sĭs) Introducing anti-inflammatory drugs through the skin with ultrasound. SEE ALSO iontophoresis.

pho·no·pho·tog·ra·phy (fō'nō-fō-tog'ră-fē) Recording on a moving photographic plate movements imparted to a diaphragm by sound waves.

pho·no·re·cep·tor (fō'nō-rē-sep'tŏr) A receptor for sound stimuli.

pho·no·sur·ger·y (fō'nō-sŭr'jĕr-ē) A group of operations designed to improve or alter the voice.

phor·bol (fōr'bol) Parent alcohol of the cocarcinogens, which are 12,13(9,9a) diesters of phorbol found in croton oil; hydrocarbon skeleton is a cyclopropabenzazulene; its esters mimic 1,2-diacylglycerol as activators of protein kinase C.

-phore Combining form meaning carrier.

-phoresis Combining form meaning condition of being a carrier or assisting transmission of.

phor·i·a (fōr'ē-ă) The relative directions assumed by the eyes during binocular fixation of a given object in the absence of an adequate fusion stimulus.

phoro-, phor- Combining forms for carrying, bearing; a carrier, a bearer; phobia.

phos- Prefix meaning light.

phose (fōz) A subjective visual sensation, such as the perception of a flash of light or color.

phosph-, phospho-, phosphor-, phosphoro- Combining forms indicating the presence of phosphorus in a compound.

phos·pha·gen (fos'fă-jen) Energy-rich guanidinium or amidine phosphate, serving as an energy store in muscle and brain.

phosphataemia [Br.] SYN phosphatemia.

phos·pha·tase (fos'fă-tās) Any of a group of enzymes that liberate inorganic phosphate from phosphoric esters.

phos·phate (fos'fāt) A salt or ester (especially inorganic) of phosphoric acid.

phos·pha·te·mi·a (fos'fă-tē'mē-ă) An abnormally high concentration of inorganic phosphates in the blood. SYN phosphataemia.

phos·pha·tide (fos'fă-tīd) Former name for 1) phosphatidic acid and 2) phosphatidate.

phos·pha·tid·ic ac·id (fos'fă-tid'ik as'id) Derivative of glycerophosphoric acid in which the two remaining hydroxyl groups of the glycerol are esterified with fatty acids.

phos·pha·tu·ri·a (fos'fă-tyūr'ē-ă) Excessive excretion of phosphates in the urine.

phos·phene (fos'fēn) Sensation of light produced by stimulation of the peripheral or central optic pathway of the nervous system.

phospho- Prefix for *O*-phosphono-, which may replace the suffix phosphate; for instance, glucose phosphate is *O*-phosphonoglucose or phosphoglucose.

phos·pho·cre·a·tine (PCr) (fos'fō-krē'ă-tēn) Compound of creatine with phosphoric acid; a source of energy in the contraction of muscle in vertebrates. SYN creatine phosphate, N^{ω}-phosphonocreatine.

phos·pho·glyc·er·ate ki·nase (fos'fō-glis'ĕr-āt kī'nās) An enzyme that is a part of the glycolytic pathway; a deficiency of it results in impaired glycolysis in most cells.

phos·pho·in·o·si·tide (fos'fō-in-ō'si-tīd) SYN phosphatidylinositol.

phos·pho·lip·ase (fos'fō-lip'ās) An enzyme that catalyzes the hydrolysis of a phospholipid. SYN lecithinase.

phos·pho·lip·id (fos′fō-lip′id) Fatty substance containing phosphorus, thus including the lecithins and other phosphatidyl derivatives, sphingomyelin, and plasmalogens.

phos·pho·pro·tein (fos′fō-prō′tēn) A protein containing phosphoryl groups attached directly to the side chains of some of its constituent amino acids.

phos·phor·ic ac·id (fos-fōr′ik as′id) Strong acid of industrial importance; dilute solutions have been used as urinary acidifiers and as dressings to remove necrotic debris. In dentistry, it constitutes about 60% of the liquid used in zinc phosphate and silicate cements.

phos·phor·ism (fos′fŏr-izm) Chronic poisoning with phosphorus.

phos·phor·ous ac·id (fos′fŏr-ŭs as′id) H_3PO_3; its salts are phosphites.

phos·phor·us (fos′fŏr-ŭs) A nonmetallic chemical element, occurring extensively in nature, always in chemical combination; elemental form is extremely poisonous, causing intense inflammation and fatty degeneration; repeated inhalation of fumes may cause jaw necrosis.

phos·phor·us 32 (fos′fŏr-ŭs) Radioactive phosphorus isotope; used as tracer in metabolic studies and to treat certain diseases of the osseous and hematopoietic systems.

phos·phor·y·lase (fos-fōr′i-lās) A phosphorylated enzyme cleaving poly(1,4-α-D-glucosyl)$_n$ with inorganic phosphate to form poly(1,4-α- D-glucosyl)$_{n-1}$ and α-D-glucose 1-phosphate.

phos·phor·y·lase ki·nase (fos-fōr′i-lās kī′nās) Enzyme that uses adenosine triphosphate to phosphorylate phosphorylase b and thus reform phosphorylase a, active form of phosphorylase.

phos·phor·y·la·tion (fos′fŏr-i-lā′shŭn) Addition of phosphate to an organic compound, through the action of a phosphotransferase (phosphorylase) or kinase.

phot (fōt) A unit of illumination.

pho·tal·gi·a (fō-tal′jē-ă) Light-induced pain, especially affecting the eyes.

pho·tic (fō′tik) Relating to light.

pho·tic driv·ing (fō′tik drīv′ing) Electroencephalographic phenomenon whereby the frequency of the activity recorded over the parietooccipital regions is time locked to the flash frequency during photic stimulation.

pho·tic ep·i·lep·sy (fō′tik ep′i-lep-sē) Seizures that are caused by flashing lights.

pho·tism (fō′tizm) Production of a sensation of light or color by a stimulus to another sense organ (e.g., hearing, taste, or touch).

photo-, phot- Combining forms meaning light.

pho·to·ab·la·tion (fō′tō-ă-blā′shŭn) The process of photoablative decomposition of tissue by laser light.

pho·to·ac·tive (fō′tō-ak′tiv) The body's chemical reaction to sunlight or ultraviolet rays.

pho·to·ag·ing (fō′tō-āj′ing) Damage from years of sun exposure, particularly wrinkling of skin.

pho·to·al·ler·gen (fō′tō-al′ĕr-jen) An agent that produces an allergic reaction (response) to light.

pho·to·al·ler·gic (fō′tō-ă-lĕr′jik) Pertaining to producing photoallergy.

pho·to·al·ler·gy (fō′tō-al′ĕr-jē) SEE photosensitization.

pho·to·bi·ol·o·gy (fō′tō-bī-ol′ŏ-jē) The study of the effects of light upon plants and animals.

pho·to·bi·ot·ic (fō′tō-bī-ot′ik) Living or flourishing only in the light.

pho·to·cat·a·lyst (fō′tō-kat′ă-list) A substance that helps bring about a light-catalyzed reaction, e.g., chlorophyll.

pho·to·chem·i·cal (fō′tō-kem′i-kăl) Denoting chemical changes caused by or involving light.

P

pho·to·chem·is·try (fō'tō-kem'is-trē) Form of chemistry concerned with light-induced chemical changes.

pho·to·che·mo·ther·a·py (fō'tō-kē'mō-thār'ă-pē) SYN photoradiation.

pho·to·co·ag·u·la·tion (PC) (fō'tō-kō-ag'yū-lā'shŭn) A method by which a beam of electromagnetic energy is directed to a desired tissue under visual control.

pho·to·co·ag·u·la·tor (fō'tō-kō-ag'yū-lā-tŏr) The apparatus used in photocoagulation.

pho·to·der·ma·ti·tis (fō'tō-dĕr'mă-tī'tis) Skin condition due to sun exposure; may be phototoxic or photoallergic, and can result from topical application, or injection of mediating phototoxic or photoallergic material. SEE ALSO photosensitization. SYN actinic dermatitis, actinodermatitis.

pho·to·dis·tri·bu·tion (fō'tō-dis'tri-byū'shŭn) Areas on the skin that receive the greatest amount of exposure to sunlight and those that are involved in eruptions due to photosensitivity.

pho·to·dy·nam·ic (fō'tō-dī-nam'ik) Relating to the energy or force exerted by light.

pho·to·dy·nam·ic ther·a·py (fō'tō-dī-nam'ik thār'ă-pē) A surgical laser-assisted procedure to correct wet macular degeneration.

pho·to·e·lec·tric (fō'tō-ĕ-lek'trik) Denoting electronic or electric effects produced by the action of light.

pho·to·e·lec·tron (fō'tō-ĕ-lek'tron) An electron freed by the action of light.

pho·to·flu·o·rog·ra·phy (fō'tō-flōr-og'ră-fē) Miniature radiographs made by contact photography of a fluoroscopic screen. SYN fluorography.

pho·to·gas·tro·scope (fō'tō-gas'trŏ-skōp) An instrument for taking photographs of the interior of the stomach.

pho·to·gen·ic, pho·tog·e·nous (fō'tō-jen'ik, fō-toj'ĕ-nŭs) Denoting or capable of photogenesis.

pho·to·gen·ic e·pi·lep·sy (fō'tō-jen'ik ep'i-lep'sē) A form of reflex epilepsy precipitated by light.

pho·to·in·ac·ti·va·tion (fō'tō-in-ak'ti-vā'shŭn) **1.** Acute sensitivity to light. **2.** Inactivation by light (e.g., treating herpes simplex by application of a photoactive dye then exposure to a fluorescent lamp).

pho·to·ki·net·ic (fō'tō-ki-net'ik) **1.** Pertaining to photokinesis. **2.** Pertaining to photokinetics.

pho·to·lu·mi·nes·cent (fō'tō-lū'mi-nes'ĕnt) Having the ability to become luminescent on exposure to visible light.

pho·tol·y·sis (fō-tol'i-sis) Decomposition of a chemical compound by the action of light.

pho·to·lyt·ic (fō'tō-lit'ik) Pertaining to photolysis.

pho·tom·e·ter (PHA) (fō-tom'ĕ-tĕr) An instrument designed to measure the intensity of light or to determine the light threshold.

pho·tom·e·try (fō-tom'ĕ-trē) The measurement of the intensity of light.

pho·to·mi·cro·graph (fō'tō-mī'krō-graf) An enlarged photograph of an object viewed with a microscope, as distinguished from microphotograph. SYN micrograph (2).

pho·to·mi·crog·ra·phy (fō'tō-mī-krog'ră-fē) The production of a photomicrograph. SYN micrography (3).

pho·ton (fō'ton) PHYSICS a corpuscle of energy or particle of light; a quantum of light or other electromagnetic radiation.

pho·to·patch test (fō'tō pach test) A test of contact photosensitization.

pho·to·per·cep·tive (fō'tō-pĕr-sep'tiv) Capable of both receiving and perceiving light.

pho·toph·thal·mi·a (fō'tof-thal'mē-ă) Keratoconjunctivitis caused by ultraviolet energy, as in snow blindness, exposure to an ultraviolet lamp, arc welding, or the short circuit of a high-tension electric current.

pho·top·ic vi·sion (fō-top'ik vizh'ŭn) Sight when the eye is adapted to light. SEE light-adapted eye.

pho·top·si·a, pho·top·sy (fō-top'sē-ă, fō'top-sē) Subjective sense of lights, sparks, or colors due to electrical or mechanical ocular stimulation. SEE ALSO Moore lightning streaks.

pho·top·sin (fō-top'sin) The protein moiety (opsin) of the pigment (iodopsin) in the cones of the retina.

pho·to·ra·di·a·tion, pho·to·ra·di·a·tion ther·a·py (fō'tō-rā'dē-ā'shŭn, thār'ă-pē) Cancer treatment by intravenous injection of a photosensitizing agent, followed by exposure to visible light of superficial tumors or of deep tumors by a fiberoptic probe. SYN photochemotherapy.

pho·to·re·ac·tion (fō'tō-rē-ak'shŭn) One caused or affected by light.

pho·to·re·ac·ti·va·tion (fō'tō-rē-ak'ti-vā'shŭn) Activation by light of something or of some process previously inactive or inactivated.

pho·to·re·cep·tive (fō'tō-rē-sep'tiv) Functioning as a photoreceptor.

pho·to·re·cep·tor (fō'tō-rē-sep'tŏr) A light-sensitive receptor (e.g., a retinal rod or cone).

pho·to·re·frac·tive ker·a·tec·to·my (fō'tō-rē-frak'tiv ker'ă-tek'tō-mē) Removal of part of the cornea with a laser to change its shape, and thus to modify the refractive error of the eye (reduce its myopia, for example).

pho·to·ret·i·nop·a·thy, pho·to·ret·i·ni·tis (fō'tō-ret'i-nop'ă-thē, -nī'tis) A macular burn from excessive exposure to sunlight or other intense light (e.g., the flash of a short circuit); characterized subjectively by reduced visual acuity.

pho·to·sen·si·tive (fō'tō-sen'si-tiv) 1. An abnormally heightened reactivity of the skin to sunlight. 2. Responding to light.

pho·to·sen·si·tiv·i·ty (PS) (fō'tō-sen'si-tiv'i-tē) Abnormal sensitivity to light, especially the eyes.

pho·to·sen·si·ti·za·tion (fō'tō-sen'si-ti-zā'shŭn) 1. Sensitization of the skin to light, usually due to the action of certain drugs, plants, or other substances. 2. SYN photosensitisation.

pho·to·sta·ble (fō'tō-stā'bĕl) Not subject to change on exposure to light.

pho·to·steth·o·scope (fō'tō-steth'ō-skōp) Device that converts sound into flashes of light; used for continuous observation of the fetal heart.

pho·to·stim·u·la·ble phos·phor (fō'tō-stim'yū-lă-bĕl fos'fŏr) Chemical that coats the phosphor plate in a computed radiography system.

pho·to·syn·the·sis (fō'tō-sin'thĕ-sis) 1. Compounding or building up of chemical substances under the influence of light. 2. The process by which green plants, using chlorophyll and the energy of sunlight, produce carbohydrates from water and carbon dioxide.

pho·to·tax·is (fō'tō-tak'sis) Reaction of living protoplasm to light, involving bodily motion of the whole organism toward or away from it. Cf. phototropism.

pho·to·ther·a·peu·tic ker·a·tec·to·my (PTK) (fō'tō-thār'ă-pyū'tik ker'ă-tek'tŏ-mē) Ablation of diseased corneal tissue using an excimer laser.

pho·to·ther·a·py (fō'tō-thār'ă-pē) Treatment of disease by means of light rays. SYN light treatment.

pho·to·ther·a·py in the new·born (fō'tō-thār'ă-pē nū'bōrn) Light-based treatment of neonatal hyperbilirubinemia.

pho·to·tox·ic (fō'tō-tok'sik) Relating to, characterized by, or causing phototoxicity.

pho·to·tox·ic·i·ty (fō'tō-tok-sis'i-tē) Condition due to overexposure to ultraviolet light. SEE ALSO photosensitization.

pho·tot·ro·pism (fō-tot'rŏ-pizm) Movement of a part of an organism toward or away from light. Cf. phototaxis.

pho·tu·ri·a (fō-tyūr'ē-ă) Passage of phosphorescent urine.

phren (fren) **1.** SYN diaphragm (1). **2.** The mind.

phre·nec·to·my (frĕ-nek'tŏ-mē) SYN phrenicectomy.

phre·net·ic (frĕ-net'ik) Frenzied; maniacal.

phreni- SEE phreno-.

-phrenia Combining form denoting **1.** The diaphragm. **2.** The mind.

phren·ic (fren'ik) **1.** SYN diaphragmatic. **2.** Relating to the mind.

phren·ic am·pul·la (fren'ik am-pul'ă) Physiologic localized dilatation of the distal esophagus, commonly demonstrated by esophagography.

phren·i·cec·to·my, phren·ec·to·my, phren·i·co·ex·er·e·sis, phren·i·co·neu·rec·tomy (fren'i-sek'tŏ-mē, -ek'tŏ-mē, -i-kō-ek-ser'ĕ-sis, -i-kō-nūr-ek'tŏ-mē) Exsection of a portion of the phrenic nerve, to prevent reunion such as may follow phrenicotomy. SYN phrenicoexeresis.

phren·i·co·col·ic, phren·o·col·ic (fren'i-kō-kol'ik, -ō-kol'ik) Relating to the diaphragm and the colon.

phren·i·co·gas·tric, phren·o·gas·tric (fren'i-kō-gas'trik, -ō-gas'trik) Relating to the diaphragm and the stomach.

phren·i·co·he·pa·tic, phre·no·he·pat·ic (fren'i-kō-hĕ-pat'ik) Relating to the diaphragm and the liver.

phren·i·cot·o·my (fren'i-kot'ŏ-mē) Surgery on the phrenic nerve to induce unilateral paralysis of the diaphragm, which is then pushed up by the abdominal viscera to compress a diseased lung.

phreno-, phren-, phreni-, phrenico- Combining forms denoting **1.** The diaphragm. **2.** The mind. **3.** The phrenic nerve.

phren·o·car·di·a (fren'ō-kahr'dē-ă) Precordial pain and dyspnea of psychogenic origin, often a symptom of anxiety neurosis. SEE cardiac neurosis.

phren·o·he·pat·ic (fren'ō-hĕ-pat'ik) SYN phrenicohepatic.

phren·o·ple·gi·a (fren'ō-plē'jē-ă) Paralysis of the diaphragm.

phren·op·to·si·a, phren·op·to·sis (fren'op-tō'sē-ă, -ō'sis) Abnormal diaphragmatic sinking.

phren·o·trop·ic (fren'ō-trō'pik) Affecting or working through the mind or brain.

phryn·o·der·ma (frin'ō-dĕr'mă) A follicular hyperkeratotic eruption thought to be due to deficiency of vitamin A. SYN toad skin.

phthi·ri·a·sis (thī-rī'ă-sis) Eyelid infection caused by infestation of crab lice.

phyl·lo·quin·one (fil'ō-kwin'ōn) Compound isolated from alfalfa; also prepared synthetically; major form of vitamin K found in plants. SYN vitamin K1.

phylo- Combining form meaning tribe, race; a taxonomic phylum.

phy·lo·gen·e·sis (fī'lō-jen'ĕ-sis) SYN phylogeny.

phy·lo·ge·net·ic, phy·lo·gen·ic (fī'lō-jĕ-net'ik, -jen'ik) Relating to phylogenesis.

phy·log·e·ny, phy·lo·gen·e·sis (fī-loj'ĕ-nē, fī'lō-jen'ĕ-sis) The evolutionary development of species, as distinguished from ontogeny, development of the individual. SYN phylogenesis.

phy·lum, pl. **phy·la** (fī'lŭm, -ă) A taxonomic division below the kingdom and above the class.

phy·ma (fī'mă) Nonspecific term for a benign circumscribed nodular tumor, usually cutaneous.

phy·ma·to·sis (fī'mă-tō'sis) The growth or the presence of phymas or small nodules in the skin.

physi- SEE physio-.

phys·i·at·rics (fiz'ē-at'riks) **1.** Old term for physical therapy. **2.** Rehabilitation management.

phys·i·a·trist (fiz-ī'ă-trist, fiz'ī-ă-trist, fiz-ē-at'rist) A physician who specializes in the areas of physical medicine and rehabilitation.

phys·i·a·try (fǐ-zīʹă-trē) SYN physical medicine.

phys·i·cal (fĭzʹi-kăl) Relating to the body, as distinguished from the mind.

phys·i·cal ac·tiv·i·ty (fĭzʹi-kăl ak-tivʹi-tē) Any body movement produced by muscles that results in energy expenditure. SEE exercise.

phys·i·cal ac·tiv·i·ty pyr·a·mid (fĭzʹi-kăl ak-tivʹi-tē pirʹă-mid) A visual representation demonstrating how to increase physical activity until it becomes a part of daily routine.

phys·i·cal a·gent (fĭzʹi-kăl āʹjĕnt) Acoustic, aqueous, electrical, mechanical, thermal, or light energy applied to living tissues to alter physiologic processes for therapeutic purposes. SEE ALSO modality.

phys·i·cal al·ler·gy (fĭzʹi-kăl alʹĕr-jē) Excessive response to factors in the environment such as heat or cold.

phys·i·cal con·di·tion·ing (fĭzʹi-kăl kŏn-dĭʹshŭn-ing) Systematic use of regular physical activity to induce functional and structural adaptations that enhance energy capacity and exercise performance.

phys·i·cal ex·am·i·na·tion (fĭzi-kăl eg-zam-i-nāʹshŭn) One using visual inspection, palpation, percussion, and auscultation to collect information for diagnosis.

phys·i·cal fit·ness (fĭzʹi-kăl fitʹnĕs) A set of attributes relating to one's ability to perform physical activity.

phys·i·cal med·i·cine (fĭzʹi-kăl medʹi-sin) The study and treatment of disease by mechanical and other physical methods. SYN physiatry.

phys·i·cal sign (fĭzʹi-kăl sīn) A finding evident on inspection or elicited by auscultation, percussion, or palpation.

phys·i·cal ther·a·pist (fĭzʹi-kăl thārʹă-pist) A practitioner of physical therapy.

phys·i·cal ther·a·pist as·sis·tant (fĭzʹi-kăl thārʹă-pist ă-sisʹtănt) A paraprofessional who assists and works under the direction of a physical therapist.

phys·i·cal ther·a·py (PT) (fĭzʹi-kăl thārʹă-pē) **1.** Treatment of pain, disease, or injury by physical means. **2.** The health profession concerned with promotion of health, with prevention of physical disabilities, with evaluation and rehabilitation of people disabled by pain, disease, or injury, and with treatment by physical therapeutic measures.

phy·si·cian (fi-zishʹŭn) **1.** A doctor; a person who has been educated, trained, and licensed to practice the art and science of medicine. **2.** A practitioner of medicine, as contrasted with a surgeon.

phy·si·cian as·sis·tant (fi-zishʹŭn ă-sisʹtănt) Someone certified to provide basic medical services under the supervision of a licensed medical physician.

phy·si·cian-as·sist·ed su·i·cide (fi-zishʹŭn ă-sistʹĕd sūʹi-sīd) Voluntary termination of one's own life by administration of a lethal substance with the direct or indirect assistance of a physician. SEE ALSO end-of-life care, advance directive.

phy·si·cian ex·tend·er (fi-zishʹŭn eks-tenʹdĕr) A specially trained and licensed person who performs tasks that might otherwise be performed by physicians themselves, under the direction of a supervising physician. Examples include nurse practitioners and physician assistants.

phy·si·cian of·fice lab·or·a·to·ry (fi-zishʹŭn awfʹis labʹŏr-ă-tōr-ē) Clinical laboratory located in a physician's office for on-site testing of specimens from patients seen by the physician.

phys·i·co·chem·i·cal (fĭzʹi-kō-kemʹi-kăl) Relating to the field of physical chemistry.

phys·ics (fĭzʹiks) The branch of science concerned with the phenomena of matter and energy and their interactions.

physio-, physi- Combining forms meaning physical, physiologic; natural, relating to physics.

phys·i·o·gen·ic (fĭzʹē-ō-jenʹik) Related to or caused by physiologic activity.

phys·i·og·no·my (fiz´ē-og´nŏ-mē) The physical appearance of one's face, especially regarded as an indication of character.

phys·i·o·log·ic, phys·i·o·log·ic·al (fiz´ē-ō-loj´ik, -i-kăl) **1.** Relating to physiology. **2.** Normal, as opposed to pathologic; denoting the various vital processes. **3.** Denoting something apparent by its functional effects rather than its anatomic structure. **4.** Denoting a dose of a hormone, neurotransmitter, or other naturally occurring agent within the range of natural concentrations. Cf. homeopathic (2), pharmacologic (2).

phys·i·o·log·ic age (fiz´ē-ō-loj´ik āj) Age estimated in terms of function.

phys·i·o·log·ic al·bu·mi·nu·ri·a (fiz´ē-ō-loj´ik al´būm´i-nyūr´ē-ă) **1.** Slight traces of protein in otherwise normal urine. **2.** SYN functional albuminuria.

phys·i·o·log·ic a·men·or·rhe·a (fiz´ē-ō-loj´ik ă-men´ŏr-ē´ă) Menstrual disorder of pregnancy or menopause, not associated with an organic disorder.

phys·i·o·log·ic an·ti·dote (fiz´ē-ō-loj´ik an´ti-dōt) Agent that produces systemic effects contrary to those of a given poison.

phys·i·o·log·ic dead space (fiz´ē-ō-loj´ik ded spās) Sum of anatomic and alveolar dead space; calculated when the carbon dioxide pressure in systemic arterial blood is used instead of that of alveolar gas in the Bohr equation.

phys·i·o·log·i·c drives (fiz´ē-ō-loj´ik drīvz) Needs such as hunger and thirst that stem from the biology of an organism. SYN primary drives.

phys·i·o·log·i·c ho·me·o·sta·sis (fiz´ē-ō-loj´ik hŏ´mē-ō-stā´sis) SYN Bernard-Cannon homeostasis.

phys·i·o·log·ic hy·per·tro·phy (fiz´ē-ō-loj´ik hī-pĕr´trō-fē) Temporary increase in organ size to provide for a natural increase of function. SYN functional hypertrophy.

phys·i·o·log·ic jaun·dice (fiz´ē-ō-loj´ik jawn´dis) Form observed frequently in newborn infants in the first 1–2 weeks of life. SYN icterus neonatorum, jaundice of the newborn, neonatal jaundice.

phys·i·o·log·ic leu·ko·cy·to·sis (fiz´ē-ō-loj´ik lū´kō-sī-tō´sis) Any form associated with apparently normal situations and not directly related to pathology.

phys·i·o·log·ic oc·clu·sion (fiz´ē-ō-loj´ik ŏ-klū´zhŭn) Occlusion in harmony with functions of the masticatory system.

phys·i·o·log·ic rest po·sit·ion (fiz´ē-ō-loj´ik rest pŏ-zish´ŭn) SYN rest position.

phys·i·o·log·ic sco·to·ma (fiz´ē-ō-loj´ik skō-tō´mă) The negative scotoma in the visual field, corresponding to the optic disc. SYN blind spot (1).

phys·i·o·log·ic trem·or (fiz´ē-ō-loj´ik trem´ŏr) Fine tremor, 8–13 Hz frequency, which is a normal phenomenon.

phys·i·o·log·ic u·nit (fiz´ē-ō-loj´ik yū´nit) The smallest division of an organ that will perform its function, e.g., the uriniferous tubule.

phys·i·ol·o·gy (fiz´ē-ol´ŏ-jē) The science concerned with the normal vital processes of animal and vegetable organisms.

phys·i·o·path·o·log·ic, phys·i·o·path·o·log·ic·al (fiz´ē-ō-path´ō-loj´ik, -i-kăl) Relating to pathologic physiology.

phys·i·o·ther·a·peu·tic (fiz´ē-ō-thār´ă-pyū´tik) Pertaining to physical therapy.

phy·sique (fi-zēk´) Constitutional type; the physical or bodily structure; one's "build."

physo- Combining form denoting **1.** Tendency to swell or inflate. **2.** Relation to air or gas.

phy·so·me·tra (fī´sō-mē´tră) Distention of the uterine cavity with air or gas. SYN uterine tympanites.

phyto-, phyt- Combining forms meaning plants.

phy·to·be·zoar (fī´tō-bē´zōr) A gastric concretion formed of vegetable fibers, with the seeds and skins of fruits, and sometimes starch granules and fat globules. SYN food ball.

phy·to·chem·i·cal (fī′tō-kem′i-kăl) A biologically active but nonnutrient substance found in plants; includes antioxidants and phytosterols. SYN bioactive nonnutrient, phytoprotectant.

phy·to·der·ma·ti·tis (fī′tō-děr-mă-tī′tis) Dermatitis caused by mechanical and chemical injury, allergy, or photosensitization at skin sites previously exposed to plants.

phy·to·es·tro·gen (fī-tō-es′trō-jen) A plant constituent with a structure similar to that of estrogen.

phytohaemagglutinin [Br.] SYN phytohemagglutinin.

phy·to·hem·ag·glu·ti·nin (fī′tō-hē′mă-glū′ti-nin) A phytomitogen from plants that agglutinates red blood cells used specifically to refer to lectin obtained from the red kidney bean, which is also a mitogen that stimulates T lymphocytes more vigorously than B lymphocytes. SYN phytolectin.

phy·toid (fī′toyd) Resembling a plant; denoting an animal having many of the biologic characteristics of a vegetable.

phy·tol (fī′tol) An unsaturated primary alcohol derived from the hydrolysis of chlorophyll. SYN phytyl alcohol.

phy·to·med·i·cine (fī′tō-med′i-sin) Herbal-based traditional therapy that uses various plant materials in ways considered both preventive and therapeutic.

phy·to·mi·to·gen (fī′tō-mī′tō-jen) A mitogenic lectin causing lymphocyte transformation accompanied by mitotic proliferation of the resulting blast cells identical to that produced by antigenic stimulation.

phy·to·path·o·gen·ic (fī′tō-path′ŏ-jen′ik) Denotes production of disease in plants.

phy·to·path·ol·o·gy (fī′tō-pă-thol′ŏ-jē) Study of plant disease.

phy·to·pho·to·der·ma·ti·tis (fī′tō-fō′tō-děr′mă-tī′tis) Phytodermatitis resulting from photosensitization.

phy·to·pro·tec·tant (fī′tō-prō-tek′tănt) SYN phytochemical.

phy·to·sis (fī-tō′sis) A disease process caused by infection with a vegetable organism, such as a fungus.

phy·to·te·ro·le·mi·a (fī′tō-tě′rō-lē′mē-ă) An inherited disorder in which hyperabsorption of phytosterols and shellfish sterols results in tendon and tuberous xanthomata.

phy·to·tox·ic (fī′tō-tok′sik) 1. Poisonous to plant life. 2. Pertaining to a phytotoxin.

phy·to·tox·in (fī′tō-tok′sin) Any toxin produced by a plant.

pi, π (π, Π) (pī) 1. The 16th letter of the Greek alphabet. 2. (Π). Symbol for osmotic pressure; in mathematics, symbol for the product of a series. 3. (π). Symbol for the ratio of the circumference of a circle to its diameter (approximately 3.14159).

pi·a mat·er (pī′ă mā′těr) [TA] A delicate, vasculated fibrous membrane firmly adherent to the glial capsule of the brain and spinal cord. Also called pia.

pi·a·no key sign (pē-an′ō kē sīn) A maneuver used to determine injury to the coracoclavicular ligament, whereby a downward pressure is applied on the distal end of the clavicle.

pi·ca (pī′kă) A perverted appetite for substances not fit as food or of no nutritional value; e.g., clay, dried paint, starch.

Pic·chi·ni syn·drome (pī-kē′nē sin′drōm) A form of polyserositis involving the three great serosae in contact with the diaphragm, sometimes also the meninges, tunica vaginalis testis, synovial sheaths, and bursae, caused by a trypanosome.

Pick dis·ease (pik di-zēz′) Progressive circumscribed cerebral atrophy.

Pick·les chart (pik′ĕlz chahrt) Day-by-day plots of new cases of infectious disease used to demonstrate the progress of an epidemic in a small, relatively isolated population.

pico- (p) 1. Prefix meaning small. **2.** Prefix used in the SI and the metric system to signify one trillionth (10^{-12}). SYN bicro-.

pi·co·gram (pg) (pī′kō-gram) One trillionth of a gram.

pi·co·kat·al (pkat) (pī′kō-kat′ăl) One trillionth of a katal.

pi·co·me·ter (pm) (pī′kō-mē′tĕr) One trillionth of a meter. SYN bicron, picometre.

picometre [Br.] SYN picometer.

pi·co·mo·lar (pM) (pī′kō-mō′lăr, pē′kō-mō′lăr) Denotes one trillionth of a mole.

pi·co·mole (pmol) (pī′kō-mōl) One trillionth of a mole.

pi·cor·na·vi·rus (PV) (pi-kōr′nă-vī′rŭs) A virus of the family Picornaviridae.

pic·ric ac·id (pik′rik as′id) Agent used as an application in burns, eczema, erysipelas, and pruritus. SYN carbazotic acid, nitroxanthic acid.

Pid·gin Sign Eng·lish (PSE) (pij′in sīn ing′glish) A system of communication that is a manual representation of English in which American Sign Language signs are used in English word order; there are no inflectional signs, and finger spelling is used for proper names.

pie·bald eye·lash (pī′bawld ī′lash) An isolated bundle of white eyelashes among normally pigmented eyelashes.

pie·bald·ness, pie·bald·ism (pī′bawld-nĕs, -izm) Patchy absence of the pigment of scalp hair, giving a streaked appearance.

Pi·erre Rob·in syn·drome (pē-yār′ rō-ban[h]′ sin′drōm) A complex of congenital anomalies including micrognathia and abnormal smallness of the tongue, often with cleft palate, severe myopia, congenital glaucoma, and retinal detachment. SYN Robin syndrome.

pi·e·sim·e·ter, pi·e·som·e·ter, pi·e·

zom·e·ter (pī′ē-sim′ĕ-ter, -som′ĕ-ter, -zom′ĕ-tĕr) An instrument for measuring the pressure of a gas or a fluid.

pi·e·zo·chem·is·try (pē-ā′zō-kem′is-trē) The study of the effect of high pressures on chemical reactions.

pi·e·zo·e·lec·tric ef·fect (pē-ā′ē-zō-ĕ-lek′trik e-fekt′) Property of certain crystalline or ceramic materials to emit electricity when deformed and to deform when an electric current is passed across them, a mechanism of interconverting electrical and acoustic energy.

pi·e·zo·e·lec·tric ul·tra·son·ic de·vice (pē-ā′zō-ĕ-lek′trik ŭl′tră-son′ik dĕ-vīs′) An electronic tool that uses the rapid energy vibrations of a powered instrument tip to fracture dental.

pi·geon chest, pi·geon breast (pij′ŏn chest, brest) An abnormality of the thoracic cage that gives a convex appearance to the anterior chest.

pi·geon toe (pij′ŏn tō) Disorder of feet in which the toes turn inward.

pig·ment (pig′mĕnt) Any coloring matter, as, for example, that of the red blood cells, hair, or iris, or the stains used in histologic or bacteriologic work, or that in paints.

pig·men·tar·y re·ti·nop·a·thy (pig′mĕn-tar-ē ret′i-nop′ă-thē) Photoreceptor degeneration associated with pigmentary changes in the retina and choroid. SEE ALSO retinitis pigmentosa.

pig·men·ta·tion (pig′mĕn-tā′shŭn) Coloration, either normal or pathologic, of the skin or tissues resulting from a deposit of pigment.

pig·ment cell (pig′mĕnt sel) One containing pigment granules.

pig·men·ted (pig-men′tĕd) Colored as the result of a deposit of pigment.

pig·men·ted vil·lo·nod·u·lar sy·no·vi·tis (pig-men′tĕd vil′ō-nod′yū-lăr sin′ō-vī′tis) Diffuse outgrowths of synovial membrane of a joint, composed of synovial villi and fibrous nodules infiltrated by hemosiderin- and lipid-containing macrophages and multinucleated giant cells; may be inflammatory; recurrence likely with incomplete removal.

pig·tail cath·e·ter (pig′tāl kath′ĕ-tĕr) One with a tightly curled end and multiple side holes to reduce the impact of the injectant on the vessel wall or to remain in space for drainage.

pi·lar, pi·la·ry (pī′lăr, pil′ă-rē) SYN hairy.

pi·lar cyst (pī′lăr sist) Common skin lesion that contains sebum and keratin.

pile (pīl) 1. A series of plates of two different metals imposed alternately one on the other, separated by a sheet of material moistened with a dilute acid solution, used to produce a current of electricity. 2. An individual hemorrhoidal tumor. SEE hemorrhoids.

pi·lif·er·ous cyst (pī-lif′ĕr-ŭs sist) Dermoid lesion containing hair.

pi·li tor·ti (pī′lī tōr′tī) A condition in which many hair shafts are twisted on the long axis. SYN twisted hairs.

pill (pil) 1. A small, globular mass of soluble material containing a medicinal substance to be swallowed; colloquially, any solid dosage form of oral medicine, including tablets and capsules. 2. "The pill"; colloquial term for an oral contraceptive.

pil·lar (pil′ăr) Any structure resembling a column or pillar.

pill e·soph·a·gi·tis (pil ĕ-sof′ă-jī′tis) Mucosal injury due to swallowed medicine in solid form retained in the esophagus.

pil·low splint (pil′ō splint) One that is inflatable or made from unusually bulky fabric.

pill-roll·ing trem·or (pil′rōl-ing trem′ŏr) A rhythmic circular movement of the opposed tips of the thumb and index finger, a form of tremor noted in parkinsonism, tardive dyskinesia, and other extrapyramidal syndromes.

pilo- Combining form meaning hair.

pi·lo·car·pine (pī′lō-kahr′pēn) An alkaloid obtained from the leaves of *Pilocar-*

pus microphyllus or *P. jaborandi*, shrubs of the West Indies and tropical America; a parasympathomimetic agent used experimentally to induce seizures externally as a miotic and in the treatment of glaucoma.

pi·lo·car·pine i·on·to·phor·e·sis sweat chlo·ride test (pī′lō-kahr′pēn ī′ŏn-tō-fōr-ē′sis swet klōr′īd test) Definitive procedure to confirm diagnosis of cystic fibrosis.

pi·lo·cys·tic (pi′lō-sis′tik) Denoting a dermoid cyst containing hair.

pi·lo·e·rec·tion (pī′lō-ĕ-rek′shŭn) Erection of hair due to action of arrectores pilorum muscles.

pi·loid (pī′loyd) Hairlike; resembling hair.

pi·lo·jec·tion (pī′lō-jek′shŭn) Process of shooting shafts of stiff mammalian hair into a saccular aneurysm in the brain to produce thrombosis.

pi·lo·ma·trix·o·ma (pī′lō-mā′trik-sō′mă) A benign solitary hair follicle tumor, often starting in childhood, containing cells resembling basal cell carcinoma and areas of epithelial necrosis. SYN Malherbe calcifying epithelioma.

pi·lo·mo·tor (pī′lō-mō′tŏr) Moving the hair; denoting the arrectores pilorum muscles of the skin and the postganglionic sympathetic nerve fibers innervating these small, smooth muscles.

pi·lo·ni·dal (pī′lō-nī′dăl) Denoting presence of hair in a dermoid cyst or in a sinus opening on the skin.

pi·lo·ni·dal si·nus, pi·lo·ni·dal cyst, pi·lo·ni·dal fis·tu·la (pī′lō-nī′dăl sī′nŭs, sist, fish′tyū-lă) Fistula or pit in the sacral region, communicating with the exterior, containing hair, which may act as a foreign body producing chronic inflammation. SYN pilonidal fistula.

pi·lo·se·ba·ceous (pī′lō-sĕ-bā′shŭs) Relating to the hair follicles and sebaceous glands.

pi·lus, pl. **pi·li** (pī′lŭs, -lī) [TA] One of the fine, keratinized, filamentous epidermal growths arising from the skin of the body of mammals except the palms, soles, and flexor surfaces of the joints; the full length and texture of the hair varies markedly in different body sites.

pi·mar·i·cin (pi-mar'i-sin) Topical antifungal antibiotic. SYN natamycin.

pi·me·li·tis (pi'mĕ-lī'tis) Inflammation of fatty tissue.

pimelo- Prefix meaning fat, fatty.

pim·ple (pim'pĕl) A papule or small pustule; usually meant to denote an inflammatory lesion of acne.

pin (pin) Rod used in surgical treatment of bone fractures. SEE ALSO nail.

Pi·nard ma·neu·ver (pē-nahr' mă-nū'vĕr) In management of a frank breech presentation, pressure on the popliteal space is made by the index finger while the other three fingers flex the leg while sliding it along the other thigh as the foot of the flexed leg is brought down and out.

pince·ment (pans-mahn[h]') A pinching manipulation in massage.

pin·cer grasp (pin'sĕr grasp) A grasp pattern emerging in the 10th–12th month whereby a small object is held between the distal pads of the opposed thumb and index or middle finger.

pinch (pinch) OCCUPATIONAL THERAPY a grip between the fingers at the most distal joints. SEE ALSO lateral pinch, pad-to-pad pinch, palmar pinch, tip pinch.

pinch graft (pinch graft) Small bits of skin, of partial or full thickness, removed from a healthy area and seeded in a site to be covered.

pin·cush·ion dis·tor·tion (pin'kŭsh-ŭn dis-tōr'shŭn) Irregular image produced when axial magnification is greater than peripheral magnification. SEE Petzval surface.

pin·do·lol (pin'dō-lol) A β-adrenergic blocking agent used to treat hypertension.

pin·e·al (pin'ē-ăl) **1.** Shaped like a pine cone. SYN piniform. **2.** Pertaining to the pineal body.

pin·e·al·ec·to·my (pin'ē-ă-lek'tŏ-mē) Removal of the pineal body.

pin·e·a·lo·cyte (pin'ē-al'ō-sīt) Pineal body cell with long processes ending in bulbous expansions; direct innervation from sympathetic neurons that form recognizable synapses.

Pi·nel sys·tem (pē-nel' sis'tĕm) The abolition of forcible restraint in the treatment of the mental hospital patient.

pine tar (PT) (pīn tahr) Substance obtained by destructive distillation of the wood of *Pinus palustris*; used internally as an expectorant and externally treat skin diseases. SYN liquid pitch.

ping-pong frac·ture (ping'pawng frak'shŭr) SEE derby hat fracture.

pin·guec·u·la, pin·guic·u·la, pl. **pin·gue·cu·lae** (ping-gwek'yū-lă, -gwik'yū-lă, -gwek'yū-lē) A yellowish accumulation of protein on the conjunctiva.

pin·hole pu·pil (pin'hōl pyū'pil) An extremely constricted pupil.

pink dis·ease (pingk di-zēz') SYN acrodynia (2).

pink·eye (pingk'ī) SYN acute viral conjunctivitis.

pink-top tube (pingk-top tūb) A tube of this color indicates the container has been treated with ethylenediaminetetraacetic acid as an anticoagulant.

pin·na, pl. **pin·nae** (pin'ă, -ē) **1.** SYN auricle (1). **2.** A feather, wing, or fin.

pin·nal (pin'ăl) Relating to the pinna.

pin·o·cyte (pin'ō-sīt) A cell that exhibits pinocytosis.

pin·o·cy·to·sis (pin'ō-sī-tō'sis) The cellular process of actively engulfing liquid, a phenomenon in which minute incuppings or invaginations are formed in the surface of the cell membrane and then close to form fluid-filled vesicles. Cf. phagocytosis.

pin·o·some (pin'ō-sōm) A fluid-filled vacuole formed by pinocytosis.

Pins sign (pinz sīn) SYN Ewart sign.

pint (pīnt) A measure of quantity (U.S. liquid), containing 16 fluid ounces, 28.875 cubic inches, 473.1765 cubic centimeters. An imperial pint contains 20 British fluid ounces, 34.67743 cubic inches, 568.2615 cubic centimeters.

pin·worm (pin′wŏrm) A member of the nematode genus *Enterobius* causing intestinal parasitism in a large variety of vertebrates, including humans.

pip·e·cur·o·ni·um (pip′ĕ-kyūr-ō′nē-ŭm) A nondepolarizing steroid muscle relaxant structurally related to pancuronium and characterized by long duration of action.

Pi·per for·ceps (pī′pĕr fŏr′seps) Obstetric forceps used to facilitate delivery of the fetal head in breech presentation.

pi·pette, pi·pet (pī-pet′) A graduated tube (marked in mL) used to transport a definite volume of a gas or liquid in laboratory work.

pir·i·form, pyr·i·form (pir′i-fōrm) Pear-shaped.

Pi·ro·goff am·pu·ta·tion (pĕr′ō-gof amp′ yū-tā′shŭn) Surgical removal of the foot.

Pir·quet test (pēr-kvet′ test) Cutaneous tuberculin test (q.v.). Also called Pirquet reaction.

pis·i·form (pis′i-fōrm) [TA] In the shape or size of a pea.

pis·tol-shot sound (pis′tŏl-shot sownd) Noise created by lightly compressing an artery during aortic regurgitation.

pit (pit) **1.** Any natural depression on the surface of the body. Cf. dimple. **2.** SYN pockmark. **3.** A depression in the enamel surface of a tooth due to faulty or incomplete calcification or formed at the confluent point of two or more lobes of enamel. **4.** To indent or become indented.

pitch (pich) Auditory perception of tone on a scale ranging from low to high, based on the frequency of vibration of the object emitting the tone. For the human voice, pitch relates to frequency of vibration of the vocal folds. SEE voice, frequency.

pith·e·coid (pith′ĕ-koyd) Resembling an ape.

Pi·tres sign (pē′trĕ sīn) **1.** SYN haphalgesia. **2.** Diminished sensation in the testes and scrotum in tabes dorsalis.

pit·ted ker·a·tol·y·sis (pit′tĕd ker′ă-tol′ i-sis) Noninflammatory gram-positive bacterial infection of the plantar surfaces producing small depressions in the stratum corneum; associated with humidity and hyperhidrosis.

pit·ting (pit′ing) DENTISTRY Formation of well-defined, relatively deep depressions in a surface, usually used to describe surface defects; it may arise from a variety of causes, although clinical occurrence often associated with corrosion. SEE ALSO pitting edema, nail pits.

pit·ting e·de·ma (pit′ing ĕ-dē′mă) Swelling that retains for a time the indentation produced by pressure.

Pitts·burgh pneu·mo·ni·a (pits′bŭrg nū-mō′nē-ă) A variant of Legionnaire's disease caused by *Legionella micdadei*.

pi·tu·i·tar·ism (pi-tū′i-tăr-izm) Pituitary dysfunction.

pi·tu·i·tar·y (pi-tū′i-tar-ē) Relating to the pituitary gland (hypophysis).

pi·tu·i·tar·y ad·e·no·ma (PA) (pi-tū′i-tar-ē ad-ĕ-nō′mă) Benign neoplasm of the pituitary generally arising in the adenohypophysis.

pi·tui·ta·ry dy·sto·pi·a (pi-tū′i-tar-ē dis-tō′pē-ă) Failure of union of neurohypophysis and adenohypophysis.

pi·tu·i·tar·y gi·gan·tism (pi-tū′i-tar-ē jī-gant′izm) Overgrowth due to hypersecretion of pituitary growth hormone; commonly the result of a pituitary adenoma.

pi·tu·i·tar·y gland (pi-tū′i-tar-ē gland) [TA] SYN hypophysis.

pi·tu·i·tar·y myx·e·de·ma (pi-tū′i-tar-ē mik′sĕ-dē′mă) A form of hypothyroidism due to inadequate secretion of the thyrotropic hormone.

pi·tu·i·tar·y stalk (pi-tū′i-tar-ē stawk) A process comprising the tuberal part in-

P

vesting the infundibular stem that attaches the hypophysis to the tuber cinereum at the base of the brain.

pit·y·ri·a·sis (pit'i-rī'ă-sis) A dermatosis marked by branny desquamation.

pi·ty·ri·as·is al·ba (pit'i-rī'ă-sis al'bă) Patchy hypopigmentation of the skin resulting from mild dermatitis.

pi·tyr·i·a·sis li·che·noi·des (pit-i-rī'ă-sis lī-ken-oy'dēz) Self-limited skin disorder of children and adults. SYN parapsoriasis guttata.

pit·y·ri·a·sis li·chen·oid·es et va·ri·o·li·for·mis a·cu·ta (pit'i-rī'ă-sis lī'kĕ-noy'dēz et var'rē-ō-li-fōr'mis ă-kyū'tă) An acute dermatitis affecting children and young adults that runs a relatively mild course and is self limited, although persistence of lesions and recurrence of attacks are not uncommon.

pi·tyr·i·a·sis ro·se·a (PR) (pit'i-rī'ă-sis rō'sē'ă) *Avoid the mispronunciation rose'a.* A self-limited eruption of macules or papules involving the trunk and, less frequently, limbs, scalp, and face.

pi·tyr·i·a·sis ru·bra pi·la·ris (pit'i-rī'ă-sis rū'bră pī-lā'ris) An uncommon chronic pruritic eruption of the hair follicles, which become firm, red, surmounted with a horny plug, and often confluent to form scaly plaques.

pi·tyr·i·a·sis ver·si·col·or (pit'i-rī'ă-sis ver'si-kŏl-ŏr) SYN tinea versicolor.

pit·y·roid (pit'i-royd) SYN furfuraceous.

Pit·y·ros·po·rum (pit'i-rō-spō'rŭm) A genus of fungi found in dandruff and seborrheic dermatitis.

piv·ot joint (piv'ŏt joynt) [TA] A synovial joint in which a section of a cylinder of one bone fits into a corresponding cavity on the other. SYN rotatory joint, trochoid joint.

pla·ce·bo (plă-sē'bō) **1.** A medicinally inactive substance given as a medicine for its suggestive effect. **2.** An inert compound identical in appearance to material being tested in experimental research, which may or may not be known to the physician or patient, administered to distinguish between drug action and suggestive effect of the material under study.

pla·cen·ta (plă-sen'tă) Fetomaternal organ of metabolic interchange between embryo or fetus and mother.

pla·cen·ta ac·cre·ta (plă-sen'tă ă-krē'tă) The abnormal adherence of the chorionic villi to the myometrium, associated with partial or complete absence of the decidua basalis and, in particular, the stratum spongiosum.

pla·cen·ta cir·cum·val·la·ta (plă-sen'tă sĕr-kŭm-val-ā'tă) Cup-shaped placenta with raised edges and a thick, round, white, opaque ring around its periphery.

pla·cen·ta fe·nes·tra·ta (plă-sen'tă fĕnes-trā'tă) A placenta with areas of thinning where placental tissue is absent.

pla·cen·ta in·cre·ta (plă-sen'tă in-krē'tă) A placenta in which the chorionic villi invade the myometrium.

pla·cen·tal (plă-sen'tăl) Relating to the placenta.

pla·cen·tal ab·rup·tion (plă-sen'tăl ăb-rŭp'shŭn) Premature separation of a normally situated placenta from the uterine wall after the 20th week of gestation.

pla·cen·tal bar·ri·er (plă-sen'tăl bar'ē-ĕr) SYN placental membrane.

pla·cen·tal cir·cu·la·tion (plă-sen'tăl sĭr'kyū-lā'shŭn) The movement of fetal blood through the placenta during intrauterine life, serving the needs of the fetus for aeration, absorption, and excretion.

pla·cen·tal dys·to·ci·a (plă-sen'tăl distō'sē-ă) Retention or difficult delivery of the placenta.

pla·cen·tal mem·brane (plă-sen'tăl mem'brān) Semipermeable layer of fetal tissue separating the maternal from the fetal blood in the placenta. SYN placental barrier.

pla·cen·tal pre·sen·ta·tion (plă-sen'tăl prez'ĕn-tā'shŭn) SYN placenta previa.

pla·cen·tal throm·bo·sis (plă-sen'tăl throm-bō'sis) Clotting of the veins of the uterus at the placental site.

pla·cen·tal trans·fu·sion (plă-sen′tăl trans-fyū′zhŭn) Return to the newborn through the umbilical vessels of some of the fetal placental blood.

pla·cen·ta mar·gi·na·ta (plă-sen′tă mahr-ji-nā′tă) A placenta with raised edges, less pronounced than in placenta circumvallata. SEE ALSO placenta reflexa.

pla·cen·ta mem·bra·na·ce·a (plă-sen′ tă mĕm′bră-nā′shē-ă) An abnormally thin placenta covering an unusually large area of the decidua basalis (uterine lining).

pla·cen·ta per·cre·ta (plă-sen′tăl pĕr-krē′tă) Denotes state when the villi have invaded the full thickness of myometrium to or through the serosa of the uterus, causing incomplete or complete uterine rupture, respectively. SEE ALSO placenta accreta.

pla·cen·ta pre·vi·a (plă-sen′tă prev′ē-ă) The condition in which the placenta is implanted in the lower segment of the uterus, extending to the margin of the internal os of the cervix or obstructing it. SYN placental presentation.

pla·cen·ta prev·i·a cen·tra·lis (plă-sen′tă prev′ē-ă sen-trā′lis) Form of placenta previa in which the placenta entirely covers the internal os of the uterus.

pla·cen·ta pre·vi·a par·ti·a·lis (plă-sen′tă prev′ē-ă pahr-shē-ā′lis) State in which the internal os of the uterus is partially covered by placental tissue.

pla·cen·ta re·flex·a (plă-sen′tă rē-fleks′ă) Placental anomaly in which the thickened margin seems to turn back on itself. SEE ALSO placenta marginata.

pla·cen·ta spu·ri·a (plă-sen′tă spū′rē-ă) A mass of placental tissue that has no vascular connection with the main placenta.

plac·en·ta·tion (plas′en-tā′shŭn) The structural organization and mode of attachment of fetal to maternal tissues in the formation of the placenta.

plac·en·ti·tis (plas′en-tī′tis) Inflammation of the placenta.

pla·fond (plă-fond′) A ceiling, especially the ceiling of the ankle joint.

plagio- Combining form meaning oblique, slanting.

plague (plāg) **1.** Disease of wide prevalence or excessive mortality. **2.** Acute infectious disease caused by *Yersinia pestis* marked by high fever, toxemia, prostration, a petechial eruption, lymph node enlargement, and pneumonia, or hemorrhage from the mucous membranes; primarily a disease of rodents, transmitted to humans by fleas that have bitten infected animals. In humans, the disease takes one of four clinical forms: bubonic plague, septicemic plague, pneumonic plague, or ambulant plague. SYN pestilence (1). SEE ALSO black death.

plague vac·cine (plāg vak-sēn′) One licensed for use in the U.S. prepared from cultures of *Yersinia pestis.*

plain film (plān film) A radiograph made without use of a contrast medium.

-plakia Combining form denoting a plate or flat plane, usually on a mucous membrane.

plane (plān) [TA] **1.** A flat surface. SEE ALSO planum. **2.** Imaginary surface formed by extension through any axis or two definite points, in pelvimetry and craniometry.

plane joint (plān joynt) [TA] A synovial joint in which the opposing surfaces are nearly planes and in which there is only a slight, gliding motion, as in the intermetacarpal joints. SYN arthrodial joint, gliding joint.

plane su·ture (plān sū′chŭr) [TA] A simple, firm apposition of two smooth surfaces of bones, without overlap, as seen in the lacrimomaxillary suture. SYN harmonic suture.

plano-, plan-, plani- Combining forms denoting **1.** A plane; flat, level. **2.** Wandering.

pla·no·cel·lu·lar (plă′nō-sel′yū-lăr) Relating to or composed of flat cells.

pla·no·con·cave (plă′nō-kon′kāv) Flat on one side and concave on the other; denoting a lens of that shape.

pla·no·con·vex (plă′nō-kon′veks) Flat

P

on one side and convex on the other; denoting a lens of that shape.

pla·nog·ra·phy (plă-nog'ră-fē) SYN tomography.

plan·ta, gen. and pl. **plan·tae** (plan'tă, -tē) [TA] SYN sole.

plan·tal·gi·a (plan-tal'jē-ă) Pain on the plantar surface of the foot over the plantar fascia.

plan·tar (plan'tahr) [TA] Relating to the sole of the foot or the caudal aspect of the tarsus on the hind limb of an animal.

plan·tar ap·o·neu·ro·sis (plan'tahr ap'ō-nūr-ō'sis) [TA] Thick, central portion of the fascia investing the plantar muscles. SYN aponeurosis plantaris [TA].

plan·tar arch (plan'tahr ahrch) **1.** The arterial arch formed by the lateral plantar artery running across the bases of the metatarsal bones and anastomosing with the dorsalis pedis artery. **2.** Either of two bony arches of the foot, the longitudinal arch or transverse arch.

plan·tar fas·ci·i·tis (plan'tahr fash'ē-ī'tis) Inflammation of the fascia of the plantar surface of the foot, usually at the calcaneal attachment.

plan·tar fi·bro·ma·to·sis (plan'tahr fī'brō-mă-tō'sis) Nodular fibroblastic proliferation in plantar fascia of one or both feet. SYN Dupuytren disease of the foot.

plan·tar flex·i·on (PF) (plan'tahr flek'shŭn) Bending the foot or toes toward the plantar surface.

plan·tar·is (plan-tā'ris) [TA] SYN plantar.

plan·tar neu·ro·ma (plan'tahr nūr-ō'mă) Tumor composed of nerve tissue on the plantar (bottom) surface of the foot.

plan·tar re·flex (plan'tahr rē'fleks) The response to tactile stimulation of the ball of the foot, normally plantar flexion of the toes; the pathologic response is the Babinski sign (1).

plan·tar ul·cer (plan'tahr ŭl'sĕr) A breakdown of the skin of the sole (bottom) of the foot that results in a pitted lesion.

plan·tar wart (plan'tahr wŏrt) An often painful wart on the sole; usually caused by human papillomavirus type 1. SYN verruca plantaris.

plan·ti·grade (plan'ti-grād) Walking with the entire sole and heel of the foot on the ground, as humans and bears do.

plant tox·in (plant tok'sin) SYN phytotoxin.

plan·u·la, pl. **plan·u·lae** (plan'yū-lă, -ē) A coelenterate embryo that has only two primary germ layers, the ectoderm and endoderm.

pla·num, pl. **pla·na** (plā'nŭm, -nă) [TA] A plane or flat surface. SEE ALSO plane.

plaque, placque (plak) **1.** A patch or small, differentiated area on a body surface or on the cut surface of an organ (e.g., brain). **2.** An area of clearing in a flat, confluent growth of bacteria or tissue cells. **3.** A sharply defined zone of demyelination characteristic of multiple sclerosis. **4.** SEE dental plaque.

-plasia Suffix denoting formation (especially of cells). SEE plasma-.

plas·ma, plasm (plaz'mă, plazm) **1.** Fluid portion of the circulating blood, as distinguished from the serum obtained after coagulation. SYN blood plasma. **2.** The fluid portion of the lymph.

plasma-, plasmat-, plasmato-, plasmo- Combining forms meaning formative; organized; plasma.

plas·ma·blast (plaz'mă-blast) Precursor of the plasma cell.

plas·ma cell (plaz'mă sel) An ovoid cell with an eccentric nucleus having chromatin arranged like a clock face or spokes of a wheel; derived from B lymphocytes and are active in the formation of antibodies.

plas·ma cell leu·ke·mi·a (plaz'mă sel lū-kē'mē-ă) An unusual disease characterized by leukocytosis and other signs and symptoms that are suggestive of leukemia, in association with diffuse infiltrations and aggregates of plasma cells in the spleen, liver, bone marrow, and lymph nodes, and plasma cells in the blood.

plas·ma cell mas·ti·tis (plaz′mă sel mas-tī′tis) A condition of the breasts characterized by tumorlike indurated masses containing numerous plasma cells, usually resulting from mammary duct ectasia.

plas·ma cell my·e·lo·ma (plaz′mă sel mī-ĕ-lō′mă) **1.** SYN multiple myeloma. **2.** Plasmacytoma of bone, which is usually a solitary lesion and not associated with the occurrence of Bence Jones protein or other disturbances in the metabolism of protein (as observed in multiple myeloma).

plas·ma·crit test (plaz′mă-krit test) A serologic screening method for syphilis.

plas·ma·cy·to·ma (plaz′mă-sī-tō′mă) A discrete, presumably solitary mass of neoplastic plasma cells in bone or in one of various extramedullary sites.

plas·ma·cy·to·sis (plaz′mă-sī-tō′sis) The presence of plasma cells in the circulating blood or in unusually large proportions in tissues or exudates.

plas·ma·gene (plaz′mă-jēn) A group of highly active oligopeptides found in sera that act on smooth muscle of blood vessels, uterus, bronchi, etc., e.g., bradykinin, kallidin.

plas·ma·phe·re·sis (plaz′mă-fĕr-ē′sis) Removal of whole blood from the body, separation of its cellular elements by centrifugation, and reinfusion of these elements in a suspension of saline or some other plasma substitute, thus depleting the body's own plasma without depleting its cells.

plas·ma pro·teins (plaz′mă prō′tēnz) Dissolved proteins of blood plasma, mainly albumins and globulins.

plas·ma re·nin ac·tiv·i·ty (plaz′mă rē′nin ak-tiv′i-tē) Estimation of renin in plasma by measurement of the rate of formation of angiotensin I or II.

plas·ma vol·ume ex·tend·er (plaz′mă vol′yūm ek-stend′ĕr) A liquid compound that is administered after major blood loss to help the remaining plasma work more effectively.

plas·mid (plaz′mid) A genetic particle physically separate from the chromosome of the host cell that can stably function and replicate. SYN extrachromosomal element, extrachromosomal genetic element.

plas·min (plaz′min) A serine proteinase catalyzing the hydrolysis of peptides and of esters of L-arginine and L-lysine and converting fibrin to soluble products. SYN fibrinase (2), fibrinolysin.

plas·min·o·gen (plaz-min′ŏ-jen) A precursor of plasmin; deficiency may promote thrombosis. SEE ALSO plasmin.

plas·min·o·gen ac·ti·va·tor (PA) (plaz-min′ŏ-jen ak′ti-vā-tŏr) Proteinase converting plasminogen to plasmin by cleavage of an Arg-Val bond in the former.

plas·min·o·gen ac·tiv·a·tor in·hi·bi·tor (plaz-min′ŏ-jen ak′ti-vā-tŏr in-hib′i-tŏr) Plasma protein active in thrombus turnover; with tissue plasminogen activator and lipoprotein, was found to increase in patients with angiographically verified coronary artery disease.

plas·min·o·gen ac·ti·va·tor in·hib·i·tor-1 (plaz-min′ŏ-jen ak′ti-vā-tŏr in-hib′it-tŏr) Peptide adipokine produced by visceral adipose tissue; has a regulatory role in fibrinolysis and thrombus formation.

Plas·mo·di·um (plaz-mō′dē-ŭm) Protozoan blood parasites of vertebrates; includes the causal agents of malaria.

plas·mo·di·um, pl. **plas·mo·di·a** (plaz-mō′dē-ŭm, -ă) Protoplasmic mass with several nuclei, due to multiplication of the nucleus with cell division.

plas·mog·a·my (plaz-mog′ă-mē) Union of two or more cells with preservation of the individual nuclei; formation of a plasmodium.

plas·mol·y·sis (plaz-mol′i-sis) **1.** Dissolution of cellular components. **2.** Shrinking of plant cells by osmotic loss of cytoplasmic water.

plas·mor·rhex·is (plaz′mō-rek′sis) The splitting open of a cell from the pressure of the protoplasm.

plas·mos·chi·sis (plaz-mos′ki-sis) The splitting of protoplasm into fragments.

P

plas·ter (plas′tĕr) A solid preparation that can be spread when heated and becomes adhesive at body temperature; used to keep the edges of a wound in apposition, to protect raw surfaces, or to apply medicine topically for local or systemic effects.

plas·ter ban·dage (plas′tĕr ban′dăj) A roller bandage impregnated with plaster of Paris and applied moist; used to make a rigid dressing for a fracture or diseased joint.

plas·tic (plas′tik) 1. Capable of being formed or molded. 2. A material that can be shaped by pressure or heat to the form of a cavity or mold.

plas·tic en·ve·lope cul·ture (plas′tik en′vĕ-lōp kŭl′chŭr) Simplified method for transport and culture of specimens to diagnose infection with *Trichomonas vaginalis*.

plas·tic·i·ty (plas-tis′i-tē) The capability of being formed or molded; the quality of being plastic.

plas·tic sur·ge·ry (plas′tik sŭr′jĕr-ē) Surgical specialty concerned with the restoration, construction, reconstruction, or improvement in the form, function, and appearance of body structures that are missing, defective, damaged, or misshapen. Encompasses both reconstructive and aesthetic surgery.

plas·tid (plas′tid) Differentiated structure in cytoplasm of plant cells where photosynthesis or other cellular processes are carried on; contain DNA and are self-replicating. SYN trophoplast.

♻ **-plasty** Combining form denoting a molding or shaping of a defect to restore form and function to a body part.

plate (plāt) [TA] 1. ANATOMY a thin, relatively flat structure. 2. A metal bar, perforated for screws, applied to a fractured bone to maintain the ends in apposition.

pla·teau pres·sure (pla-tō′ presh′ŭr) The equilibrium pressure between airways and alveoli in a patient-ventilator system; considered to be an approximation of alveolar pressure.

pla·teau pulse (pla-tō′ pŭls) A slow, sustained pulse.

plate·let (plāt′lĕt) An irregularly shaped, disclike, cytoplasmic fragment of a megakaryocyte shed in the marrow sinus and subsequently found in the peripheral blood, where it functions in clotting. SYN blood disc, thromboplastid (1).

plate·let-ag·gre·gat·ing fact·or (plāt′lĕt ag′rĕ-gā′ting fak′tŏr) Phospholipid mediator of platelet aggregation, inflammation, and anaphylaxis; produced in response to specific stimuli by a variety of cell types, including neutrophils, basophils, platelets, and endothelial cells. SYN platelet-activating factor.

plate·let ag·gre·ga·tion (plāt′lĕt ag′rĕ-gā′shŭn) Clumping together of platelets in the blood; part of the sequence leading to the formation of a clot or hemostatic plug.

plate·let ag·gre·ga·tion test (plāt′lĕt ag′rĕ-gā′shŭn test) A test of the ability of platelets to adhere to each other and hence form a hemostatic plug to prevent bleeding; failure to aggregate occurs in several conditions, e.g., thrombasthenia, Von Willebrand disease, and following administration of aspirin, phenylbutazone, and indomethacin.

plate·let-de·rived growth fac·tor (PDGF) (plāt′lĕt grōth fak′tŏr) Factor that is mitogenic for cells at the site of a wound, e.g., causing endothelial proliferation.

plate·let neut·ral·i·za·tion pro·ce·dure (plāt′lĕt nū′trăl-ī-zā′shŭn prŏ-sē′jŭr) Technique based on the ability of platelets to bypass the effect of a lupus anticoagulant by correcting prolonged coagulation times in various phospholipid-dependent test systems.

plate·let·phe·re·sis (plāt′lĕt-fĕr-ē′sis) Removal of blood from a donor with replacement of all blood components except platelets.

♻ **-platin** Combining form meaning a chemotherapeutic agent that is platinum based.

plat·i·num (Pt) (plat′i-nŭm) A metallic element, used for making small parts for chemical apparatus because of its resistance to acids. A derivative, cisplatin, is used as an antineoplastic agent.

platy- Prefix meaning width; flatness.

plat·y·ba·si·a (plat'i-bā'sē-ă) A developmental anomaly of the cranium or an acquired softening of the cranial bones that allows the floor of the posterior cranial fossa to bulge upward around the foramen magnum.

plat·y·hel·minth (plat'i-hel'minth) Common name for any flatworm of the phylum Platyhelminthes; any cestode (tapeworm) or trematode (fluke).

Plat·y·hel·min·thes (plat'i-hel-min'thēz) A phylum of flatworms that are bilaterally symmetric, flattened, and acelomate.

plat·y·pel·lic pel·vis (plat'i-pel'ik pel'vis) Flat, oval pelvis, in which the transverse diameter is more than 3 cm longer than the anteroposterior diameter.

plat·y·pel·loid pel·vis (plat'i-pel'oyd pel'vis) One with an inlet with a transverse diameter that exceeds the anteroposterior diameter, the inlet thus appearing as a flat oval. SYN platypellic pelvis.

pla·typ·ne·a (plă-tip'nē-ă) Difficulty in breathing when upright; relieved by recumbency. Cf. orthopnea.

play (plā) **1.** To perform or participate in an activity for recreation or amusement. **2.** General term for individual or group activities engaged in for fun or recreation.

play ther·a·py (plā thār'ă-pē) Child therapy in which they can express or reveal their problems and fantasies by playing with dolls or other toys, drawing, or other indirect means.

pled·get (plej'ĕt) A tuft of wool, cotton, or lint.

-plegia Suffix meaning paralysis.

plei·o·trop·ic gene (plī'ō-trō'pik jēn) A gene that has multiple, apparently unrelated, phenotypic manifestations. SYN polyphenic gene.

plei·ot·ro·py, plei·o·tro·pi·a (plī-ot'rŏ-pē, plī'ŏ-trō'pē-ă) Production by a single mutant gene of apparently unrelated multiple effects at the clinical or phenotypic level.

pleo- Prefix meaning more.

ple·o·cy·to·sis (plē'ō-sī-tō'sis) Presence of more cells than normal, often denoting leukocytosis and especially lymphocytosis or round cell infiltration.

ple·o·mor·phic ad·e·no·ma (plē'ō-mōr'fik ad'ĕ-nō'mă) Benign neoplasm composed of salivary gland epithelial and mesodermal elements. SYN mixed tumor of salivary gland.

ple·o·mor·phous (plē'ō-mōr'fŭs) SYN polymorphic.

ple·on·os·te·o·sis (plē'on-os-tē-ō'sis) Superabundance of bone formation.

ple·ro·cer·coid (plē'rō-ser'koyd) A stage in the development of a tapeworm following the procercoid stage, which develops in an animal serving as the second or subsequent intermediate host.

pless-, plessi- Combining forms meaning a striking, especially percussion.

ples·ses·the·si·a (ples'es-thē'zē-ă) Historic term for palpatory percussion.

ples·sim·e·ter (ple-sim'ĕ-tĕr) Historic term for an oblong flexible plate used in mediate percussion by being placed against the surface and struck with the plessor. SYN plexometer.

ples·sor (ples'ŏr) A small hammer, usually with a soft rubber head, used to tap the body part directly, or with a plessimeter, in percussion of the chest or other part. SYN plexor.

pleth·o·ra (pleth'ŏr-ă) **1.** SYN hypervolemia. **2.** An excess, especially of any of the body fluids. SYN repletion (2).

ple·thor·ic (plĕ-thōr'ik) Relating to plethora. SYN sanguine (1), sanguineous (2).

pleth·ys·mo·graph (plĕ-thiz'mŏ-graf) A device for measuring and recording changes in volume of a part, organ, or whole body.

pleth·ys·mog·ra·phy (pleth'iz-mog'ră-fē) Measuring and recording changes in volume of an organ or other part of the body by a plethysmograph.

pleth·ys·mom·e·try (pleth'iz-mom'ĕ-trē) Measuring the fullness of a hollow organ or vessel, as of the pulse.

♻ **pleur-, pleura-, pleuro-** Combining forms denoting rib, side, pleura.

pleur·a, gen. and pl. **pleu·rae** (plūr′ă, -ē) [TA] The serous membrane enveloping the lungs and lining the walls of the pleural cavity.

pleur·a·cen·te·sis (plūr′ă-sen-tē′sis) SYN thoracentesis.

pleu·ra·cot·o·my (plūr′ă-kot′ŏ-mē) Surgical incision into the pleura, which is the tissue covering over the lungs.

pleur·al cav·i·ty (plūr′ăl kav′i-tē) [TA] The potential space between the parietal and visceral layers of the pleura.

pleur·al ef·fu·sion (plūr′ăl ĕ-fyū′zhŭn) Increased amounts of fluid within the pleural cavity, usually due to inflammation.

pleur·al rub (plūr′ăl rŭb) Friction sound caused by the rubbing together of the roughened surfaces of the costal and visceral pleurae. SYN pleural rale.

pleur·al tap (plūr′ăl tap) SYN thoracentesis.

pleur·ec·to·my (plūr-ek′tŏ-mē) Excision of pleura, usually parietal.

pleur·i·sy, pleu·ri·tis (plūr′i-sē, plūr-ī′tis) Inflammation of the pleura. SYN pleuritis.

pleur·i·sy with ef·fu·sion (plūr′i-sē ĕ-fyū′zhŭn) The inflammatory disorder accompanied by serous exudation.

pleu·rit·ic pneu·mo·ni·a (plūr-it′ik nū-mō′nē-ă) Pneumonia associated with inflammation of the overlying pleura.

pleur·o·cen·te·sis, pleur·a·cen·te·sis (plūr′ō-sen-tē′sis, -ă-sen-tē′sis) SYN thoracentesis.

pleur·o·dyn·i·a (plūr′ō-din′ē-ă) **1.** Pleuritic pain in the chest. **2.** A painful affection of the tendinous attachments of the thoracic muscles. SYN costalgia.

pleur·o·gen·ic (plūr′ō-jen′ik) Of pleural origin. SYN pleurogenous (1).

pleur·og·e·nous (plūr-oj′ĕ-nŭs) **1.** SYN pleurogenic. **2.** In fungi, denoting spores or conidia developed on the sides of a conidiophore or hypha.

pleur·og·ra·phy (plūr-og′ră-fē) Radiography of the pleural cavity after injection of contrast medium.

pleur·o·hep·a·ti·tis (plūr′ō-hep-ă-tī′tis) Liver disease with extension of the inflammation to the neighboring portion of the pleura.

pleu·rol·y·sis (plūr-ol′i-sis) Locating pleural adhesions by the aid of an endoscope and then dividing them with the electric cautery.

pleur·o·per·i·car·di·al rub (plūr′ō-per′i-kahr′dē-ăl rŭb) Friction between the surfaces of the pleura and pericardium.

pleur·o·per·i·car·di·tis (plūr′ō-per′i-kahr-dī′tis) Combined inflammation of the pericardium and of the pleura.

pleur·o·per·i·to·ne·al (plūr′ō-per′i-tō-nē′ăl) Relating to both pleura and peritoneum.

pleur·o·per·i·to·ne·al cav·i·ty (plūr′ō-per′i-tō-nē′ăl kav′i-tē) That part of the embryonic celom later partitioned to give rise to the pleural and peritoneal cavities.

pleur·o·per·i·to·ne·al shunt (plūr′ō-per′i-tō-nē′ăl shŭnt) Surgically implanted catheter for transport of fluid from a pleural space into the peritoneal cavity, where it is absorbed; used mainly for treatment of malignant pleural effusions.

pleur·o·pneu·mo·nec·to·my (plūr′ō-nū′mō-nek′tŏ-mē) Surgical resection of an entire lung along with the parietal pleura; a method of treating malignant mesothelioma.

pleur·o·pneu·mo·ni·a (plūr′ō-nū-mō′nē-ă) Pleurisy accompanied by pneumonia.

pleu·ro·pneu·mo·ni·a·like or·gan·isms (plūr′ō-nū-mō′nē-ă-līk ōr′gă-nizms) The original name given to a group of bacteria that do not possess cell walls, as isolated from humans and other animals, soil, and sewage.

plex·ect·o·my (plek-sek′tŏ-mē) Surgical excision of a plexus.

plex·i·form (plek′si-fōrm) Weblike, or resembling or forming a plexus.

plex·i·form neu·ro·fi·bro·ma (plek′si-fōrm nūr′ō-fī-brō′mă) A type of neurofibroma, representing an anomaly rather than a true neoplasm, in which the proliferation of Schwann cells occurs from the inner aspect of the nerve sheath; seen most frequently in neurofibromatosis. SYN plexiform neuroma.

plex·i·form neu·ro·ma (plek′si-fōrm nūr-ō′mă) SYN plexiform neurofibroma.

plex·i·tis (plek-sī′tis) Inflammation of a plexus.

plex·o·gen·ic (plek′sō-jen′ik) Giving rise to weblike or plexiform structures.

plex·or (plek′sŏr) SYN plessor.

plex·us, pl. **plex·us,** pl. **plex·us·es** (plek′sŭs, -ĕz) [TA] A network or interjoining of nerves and blood vessels or of lymphatic vessels.

-plexy Combining form meaning stroke or seizure.

plic- Combining form meaning a fold or ridge.

pli·ca, gen. and pl. **pli·cae** (plī′kă, -kē) [TA] **1.** [TA] One of several anatomic structures in which there is a folding over of the parts. **2.** SYN false membrane. SEE ALSO fold.

pli·cate (plī′kāt) Folded; pleated; tucked.

pli·ca·tion (plī-kā′shŭn) A folding or putting together in pleats.

pli·cot·o·my (plī-kot′ŏ-mē) Division of the posterior malleolar fold.

-ploid Combining form meaning multiple in form; its combinations are used both adjectivally and substantively of a (specified) multiple of chromosomes.

ploi·dy (ploy′dē) The number of haploid sets in a cell. Gametes normally contain one; somatic cells two. SEE ALSO polyploidy.

plug (plŭg) Any mass filling a hole or closing an orifice.

plug·ger (plŭg′ĕr) A dental instrument used for condensing gold (foil), amalgam, or any plastic material in a tooth cavity, operated by hand or by mechanical means.

Plum·mer dis·ease (plŭm′ĕr di-zēz′) Eponym sometimes applied to hyperthyroidism resulting from a nodular toxic goiter, usually not accompanied by exophthalmos.

Plum·mer-Vin·son syn·drome (plŭm′ĕr vin′sŏn sin′drōm) Iron deficiency anemia, dysphagia, esophageal web, and atrophic glossitis.

pluri- Prefix meaning several, more. SEE ALSO multi-, poly-.

plur·i·glan·du·lar (plūr′i-glan′dyū-lăr) Denoting several glands or their secretions.

PLWH Abbreviation for person(s) living with HIV.

ply·o·met·ric train·ing (plī′ō-met′rik trān′ing) Exercise training that exploits the stretch-recoil characteristics of skeletal muscle and neurologic modulation.

pm Abbreviation for picometer.

-pnea Combining form denoting breath, respiration.

pneo- Combining form denoting breath or respiration. SEE ALSO pneum-, pneumo-.

pneum-, pneuma-, pneumat-, pneumato- Combining forms denoting presence of air or gas, the lungs, or breathing. SEE ALSO pneo-, pneumo-.

pneum·ar·throg·ra·phy (nū′mahr-throg′ră-fē) Radiographic examination of a joint following the introduction of air, with or without another contrast medium.

pneum·ar·thro·sis (nū′mahr-thrō′sis) Presence of air in a joint.

pneu·mat·ic (nū-mat′ik) **1.** Relating to air or gas, or to a structure filled with air. **2.** Relating to respiration.

P

pneu·mat·ic an·ti·shock gar·ment (nū-mat′ik an′tē-shock′ gahr′ment) An inflatable suit used to apply pressure to the peripheral circulation, thus reducing blood flow and fluid exudation into tissues, to maintain central blood flow in the presence of shock.

pneu·mat·ic bone (nū-mat′ik bōn) One that is hollow or contains many air cells. SYN hollow bone.

pneu·mat·ic space (nū-mat′ik spās) Any one of the paranasal sinuses.

pneu·mat·ic ton·om·e·ter (nū-mat′ik tō-nom′ĕ-tĕr) A recording applanation tonometer operated by compressed gas.

pneu·ma·ti·za·tion (nū′mă-tī-zā′shŭn) Development of air cells (e.g., mastoid bones).

pneu·mat·o·cele (nū-mat′ō-sēl) 1. An emphysematous or gaseous swelling. 2. SYN pneumonocele. 3. A thin-walled cavity within the lung, one of the characteristic sequelae of staphylococcal pneumonia and *Pneumocystis jiroveci* pneumonia.

pneu·ma·to·sis (nū′mă-tō′sis) Abnormal accumulation of gas in any tissue or part of the body.

pneu·ma·to·sis cys·toi·des in·tes·ti·na·lis (nū′mă-tō′sis sis-toyd′ēz in-tes-ti-nā′lis) Condition of unknown cause characterized by the occurrence of gas cysts in the intestinal mucous membrane. SYN intestinal emphysema.

pneu·ma·tu·ri·a, pneu·ma·ti·nu·ria (nū′mă-tyūr′ē-ă, -ti-nyūr′ē-ă) Passage of gas or air from the urethra during or after urination, due to decomposition of bladder urine or from an intestinal fistula.

♻ **pneumo-, pneumon-, pneumono-** Combining forms meaning the lungs, air or gas, respiration, or pneumonia.

pneu·mo·ceph·a·lus (nū′mō-sef′ă-lŭs) Presence of air or gas within the cranial cavity.

pneumococcaemia [Br.] SYN pneumococcemia.

pneu·mo·coc·cal (nū′mō-kok′ăl) Pertaining to or containing the pneumococcus.

pneu·mo·coc·cal vac·cine (nū′mō-kok′ăl vak-sēn′) One composed of purified capsular polysaccharide antigen from 23 types of *Streptococcus pneumoniae*; some have been conjugated with protein to make them antigenic for children younger than 2 years of age.

pneu·mo·coc·ce·mi·a (nū′mō-kok-sē′mē-ă) Presence of pneumococci in the blood. SYN pneumococcaemia.

pneu·mo·coc·ci·dal (nū′mō-kok-sī′dăl) Destructive to pneumococci.

pneu·mo·coc·co·su·ri·a (nū′mō-kok-ō-syūr′ē-ă) The presence of pneumococci or their specific capsular substance in the urine.

pneu·mo·co·ni·o·sis, pneu·mo·no·co·ni·o·sis, pneu·mo·ko·ni·o·sis, pl. **pneu·mo·co·ni·o·ses** (nū′mō-kōnē-ō′sis, nū-mō′nō-, -sēz) Inflammatory disorder commonly leading to fibrosis of the lungs caused by the inhalation of dust incident to various occupations. SYN anthracotic tuberculosis, pneumonokoniosis.

pneu·mo·cra·ni·um (nū′mō-krā′nē-ŭm) Air present between the cranium and the dura mater; commonly used to indicate extradural or subdural air.

pneu·mo·cys·ti·a·sis (nū′mō-sis-tī′a-sis) Interstitial cell pneumonia.

Pneu·mo·cys·tis (nū′mō-sis′tis) A fungus of the Ascomycetes class that has morphologic similarities to the protozoa.

***Pneu·mo·cys·tis ca·rin·i·i* (PC)** (nū-mō-sis′tis kă-rī′nē-ī) Former name for *Pneumocystis jiroveci* (q.v.).

Pneu·mo·cys·tis jir·o·ve·ci (nū′mō-sis′tis jī-rō-vē′chē) Revised name for *Pneumocystis carinii*, the microorganism that causes interstitial plasma cell pneumonia in immunodeficient people.

pneu·mo·cys·tog·ra·phy (nū′mō-sis-tog′ră-fē) Radiography of the bladder following injection of air.

pneu·mo·der·ma (nū′mō-dĕr′mă) SYN subcutaneous emphysema.

pneu·mo·dy·nam·ics (nū′mō-dī-nam′ iks) The mechanics of respiration.

pneu·mo·en·ceph·a·log·ra·phy (nū′ mō-en-sef′ă-log′ră-fē) Radiographic visualization of cerebral ventricles and subarachnoid spaces by use of gas such as air; no longer used.

pneu·mo·en·te·ri·tis (nū′mō-en′tĕr-ī′ tis) Inflammation of the lung(s) and intestine(s).

pneu·mo·gram, pneu·mat·o·gram (nū′ mō-gram, -mat-ō-gram) **1.** The record or tracing made by a pneumograph. **2.** Radiographic record of pneumography.

pneu·mog·ra·phy, pneu·mat·o·gra·phy (nū-mog′ră-fē, -mă-tog′ră-fē) **1.** Examination with a pneumograph. **2.** A general term indicating radiography after injection of air. SYN pneumoroentgenography.

pneu·mo·he·mo·per·i·car·di·um (nū′ mō-hē′mō-per-i-kahr′dē-ŭm) SYN pneumohaemopericardium.

pneu·mo·hy·dro·me·tra (nū′mō-hī′drŏ-mē′tră) The presence of gas and serum in the uterine cavity.

pneu·mo·hy·dro·per·i·car·di·um (nū′ mō-hī′drŏ-per-i-kahr′dē-ŭm) SYN hydropneumopericardium.

pneu·mo·me·di·as·ti·num (nū′mō-mē′ dē-ă-stī′nŭm) Abnormal presence of air in mediastinal tissues; multiple causes include pulmonary interstitial emphysema, ruptured bleb, and perforated abdominal viscus. SYN mediastinal emphysema.

pneu·mo·nec·to·my (nū′mō-nek′tŏ-mē) Removal of all pulmonary lobes from a lung in one operation.

pneu·mo·ni·a (nū-mō′nē-ă) Inflammation of the lung parenchyma characterized by consolidation of the affected part, the alveolar air spaces being filled with exudate, inflammatory cells, and fibrin. SEE ALSO pneumonitis.

pneu·mon·ic plague (nū-mon′ik plāg) A rapidly progressive and frequently fatal form of plague with areas of pulmonary consolidation, with chills, pain in the side, bloody expectoration, and high fever. SEE ALSO *Yersinia pestis.*

pneu·mo·ni·tis (nū′mō-nī′tis) Inflammation of the lungs. SEE ALSO pneumonia.

♻ **pneumono-** SEE pneumo-.

pneu·mon·o·cele (nū-mon′ō-sēl) Protrusion of a portion of the lung through a defect in the chest wall. SYN pneumatocele (2), pneumocele.

pneu·mo·nop·a·thy (nū′mō-nop′ă-thē) Disease of the lung.

pneu·mo·no·pex·y (nū-mō′nō-pek-sē) Fixation of the lung by suturing the costal and pulmonary pleurae or otherwise causing adhesion of the two layers.

pneu·mo·no·nor·rha·phy (nū′mō-nōr′ă-fē) Suture of the lung.

pneu·mo·no·ther·a·py (nū′mō-nō-thār′ ă-pē) Medical treatment of lung disorders.

pneu·mo·not·o·my, pneu·mot·o·my (nū′mō-not′ŏ-mē, nū-mot′ŏ-mē) Incision of the lung.

pneu·mo·or·bi·tog·ra·phy (nū′mō-ōr′ bi-tog′ră-fē) Radiographic visualization of the orbital contents following injection of a gas, usually air.

pneu·mo·per·i·car·di·um (nū′mō-per′ i-kahr′dē-ŭm) Presence of gas in the pericardial sac.

pneu·mo·per·i·to·ne·um (nū′mō-per′i-tō-nē′ŭm) Presence of air or gas in the peritoneal cavity due to disease, or produced artificially in the abdomen to achieve exposure during laparoscopy and laporoscopic surgery for treatment of pulmonary or intestinal tuberculosis, bronchiectasis, tuberculous empyema, and certain other conditions.

pneu·mo·per·i·to·ni·tis (nū′mō-per′i-tō-nī′tis) Inflammation of the peritoneum with an accumulation of gas in the peritoneal cavity.

pneu·mo·pleu·ri·tis (nū′mō-plūr-ī′tis) Pleurisy with air or gas in the pleural cavity.

P

pneu·mo·py·o·per·i·car·di·um (nū′ mō-pī′ō-per′i-kahr′dē-ŭm) Presence of air or gas and pus in the pericardium.

pneu·mo·ret·ro·per·i·to·ne·um (nū′ mō-ret′rō-per′i-tō-nē′ŭm) Pathologic presence of air in the retroperitoneal tissues.

pneu·mo·thor·ax, pl. **pneu·mo·tho·ra·ces** (nū′mō-thōr′aks, -ēz) The presence of air or gas in the pleural cavity.

Pneu·mo·vi·rus (nū′mō-vī′rŭs) A genus of viruses including respiratory syncytial virus, which causes severe lower respiratory tract disease in infants.

Po Symbol for polonium.

pock (pok) The specific pustular cutaneous lesion of smallpox.

pock·et (pok′ĕt) **1.** A cul-de-sac or pouchlike cavity. **2.** A diseased gingival attachment. **3.** To enclose within a confined space. **4.** A collection of pus in a nearly closed sac. **5.** To approach the surface at a localized spot.

pock·et do·si·me·ter (pok′ĕt dō-sim′ĕ-tĕr) Small ionization chamber that provides an immediate reading of radiation exposure. SEE ALSO film badge.

pock·mark (pok′mahrk) The small depressed scar left after the healing of the smallpox pustule.

pod-, podo- Combining forms denoting foot, foot-shaped. Cf. ped-.

po·dag·ra (pŏ-dag′ră) Severe pain in the foot.

po·dal·gi·a (pō-dal′jē-ă) Pain in the foot. SYN pododynia, tarsalgia.

po·dal·ic ver·sion (pō-dal′ik vĕr′zhŭn) A manual obstetric procedure that results in a feet-first extraction.

pod·ar·thri·tis (pod′ahr-thrī′tis) Inflammation of any of the tarsal or metatarsal joints.

po·di·a·tric (pō′dē-at′rik) Relating to podiatry.

po·di·a·try (pŏ-dī′ă-trē) The health care specialty concerned with the diagnosis or medical, surgical, mechanical, physical, and adjunct treatment of the diseases, injuries, and defects of the human foot. SYN chiropody, podiatric medicine.

pod·o·dy·na·mom·e·ter (pod′ō-dī′nă-mom′ĕ-tĕr) An instrument for measuring the strength of the muscles of the foot or leg.

pod·o·dyn·i·a (pod′ō-din′ē-ă) SYN podalgia.

po·do·fil·ox (pō-dof′il-oks) An antimitotic agent used to treat external genital and perianal warts.

pod·o·gram (pod′ō-gram) An imprint of the sole of the foot, showing the contour and the condition of the arch, or an outline tracing.

po·dol·o·gy (pŏ-dol′ŏ-jē) SYN podiatry.

pod·o·mech·a·no·ther·a·py (pod′ō-mek′ă-nō-thār′ă-pē) Treatment of foot conditions with mechanical devices, e.g., arch supports, orthoses.

pod·o·phyl·lin (pod′ō-fil′in) SYN podophyllum.

pod·o·phyl·lo·tox·in (pod′ō-fil′ō-tok′sin) A toxic polycyclic substance with cathartic properties present in podophyllum; has antineoplastic action.

POEMS syn·drome (pō′ĕmz sin′drōm) A condition characterized by *p*olyneuropathy, *o*rganomegaly, *e*ndocrinopathy, *m*onoclonal gammopathy, and *s*kin changes. SYN Crow-Fukase syndrome.

pOH The negative logarithm of the OH^- concentration (in moles per liter).

-poiesis Suffix meaning production; producing.

-poietin Combining form meaning the root agent has a role in formation or production of something (e.g., erythropoietin).

poikilo- Combining form meaning irregular, varied.

poi·ki·lo·blast (poy′ki-lō-blast) A nucleated red blood cell of irregular shape.

poi·ki·lo·cyte (poy′ki-lō-sīt) A red blood cell of irregular shape.

poi·ki·lo·cy·the·mi·a (poy′ki-lō-sī-thē′ mē-ă) SYN poikilocytosis, poikilocythaemia.

poi·ki·lo·cy·to·sis (poy′ki-lō-sī-tō′sis) The presence of poikilocytes in the peripheral blood. SYN poikilocythemia.

poi·ki·lo·der·ma (poy′ki-lō-děr′mă) A variegated hyperpigmentation and telangiectasia of the skin, followed by atrophy.

poi·ki·lo·der·ma of Ci·vatte (poy′ki-lō-děr′mă sē-vaht′) Reticulated pigmentation and telangiectasia of the sides of the cheeks and neck; common in middle-aged women.

poi·ki·lo·ther·mic (poy′ki-lō-thěr′mik) 1. Varying in temperature according to the temperature of the surrounding medium; denoting the so-called cold-blooded animals, such as the reptiles and amphibians, and plants. SYN cold-blooded. 2. Capable of existence and growth in media of varying temperature.

point (poynt) 1. SYN punctum. 2. A sharp end or apex. 3. A slight projection. 4. A stage or condition reached. 5. To become ready to open, referring to an abscess or boil, the wall of which is becoming thin and is about to break. 6. In mathematics, a dimensionless geometric element. 7. A location or position on a graph, plot, or diagram.

point ep·i·dem·ic (poynt ep′i-dem′ik) An epidemic in which a pronounced clustering of cases of disease occurs within a short time due to exposure of persons or animals to a common source of infection such as food or water.

poin·til·lage (pwahn-tē-ahzh′) A massage manipulation with the tips of the fingers.

point of fix·a·tion (poynt fik-sā′shŭn) Retinal area at which the rays coming from an object seen directly are focused.

point-of-ser·vice plan (poynt sěr′vis plan) Managed care program that allows members to see contracted providers at a discounted rate without a referral from a primary care provider.

poise (poyz, pwahz) The unit of viscosity

equal to 1 dyne-second per square centimeter and to 0.1 pascal-second.

Poi·seu·il·le vis·cos·i·ty co·ef·fi·cient (pwah-soy′ vis-kos′i-tē kŏ′ĕ-fish′ ĕnt) An expression of viscosity as determined by the capillary tube method.

poi·son (P, pois) (poy′zŏn) 1. Any substance, either taken internally or applied externally, injurious to health or dangerous to life. 2. A substance that inhibits a chemical reaction or inactivates a catalyst.

poi·son con·trol cen·ter (poy′zŏn kŏn-trōl′ sen′tĕr) A facility staffed 24 hours a day to answer calls about people exposed to substances that might be harmful.

poi·son·ing (poy′zŏn-ing) 1. The administering of poison. 2. The state of being poisoned. SYN intoxication (1).

poi·son i·vy, poi·son oak, poi·son su·mac (Pl) (poy′zŏn ī′vē, ōk, sū′mak) 1. SEE *Toxicodendron*. 2. Common name for the cutaneous eruption caused by contact with these species of *Toxicodendron*.

pok·er spine (pō′kĕr spīn) Stiff spine due to widespread joint immobility or overwhelming muscle spasm as might occur in osteomyelitis of a vertebra or a rheumatoid spondylitis.

Po·land syn·drome (pō′lănd sin′drōm) An anomaly consisting of absence of the pectoralis major and minor muscles, ipsilateral breast hypoplasia, two to four rib segments.

po·lar (pō′lăr) 1. Relating to a pole. 2. Having poles; said of certain nerve cells having one or more processes.

po·lar a·ne·mi·a (pō′lăr ă-nē′mē-ă) Form sometimes observed in former residents of temperate climates when they migrate to the Arctic or Antarctic regions.

po·lar bod·y (pō′lăr bod′ē) One of two small cells formed by the first and second meiotic division of oocytes; the first is usually released just before ovulation, the second not until discharge of the oocyte from the ovary.

P

po·lar cat·a·ract (pō′lăr kat′ăr-akt) A capsular cataract limited to an area of the anterior or posterior pole of the lens.

po·lar·im·e·try (pō′lăr-im′ĕ-trē) Measurement by polarimeter.

po·lar·i·ty (pō-lar′i-tē) **1.** The property of having two opposite poles, as that possessed by a magnet. **2.** The possession of opposite properties or characteristics. **3.** The direction or orientation of positivity relative to negativity. **4.** The direction along a polynucleotide chain, or any biopolymer, or macro structure (e.g., microtubules).

po·lar·i·za·tion (P) (pō′lăr-ī-zā′shŭn) **1.** In electricity, coating of an electrode with a thick layer of hydrogen bubbles, with the result that the flow of current is weakened or arrested. **2.** A change effected in a ray of light passing through certain media, whereby the transverse vibrations occur in one plane only, instead of in all planes as in an ordinary light ray.

po·lar·ized light (pō′lăr-īzd līt) Light in which, as a result of reflection or transmission through certain media, the vibrations are all in one plane, transverse to the ray, instead of in all planes.

pole (pōl) [TA] **1.** One of two points at axial extremities of any organ. **2.** Either of the two points on a sphere at the greatest distance from the equator. **3.** One of the two points in a magnet or an electric battery or cell having extremes of opposite properties; the negative pole is a cathode, the positive pole an anode. **4.** Either end of a spindle. **5.** Either of the differentiated zones at opposite ends of an axis in a cell, organ, or organism. SYN polus [TA].

po·lice·man (pŏ-lēs′măn) An instrument, usually a rubber-tipped rod, for removing solid particles from a glass container.

po·lio (pō′lē-ō) Shortened common form of poliomyelitis.

♻ **polio-** Prefix meaning gray; gray matter (substantia grisea).

po·li·o·clas·tic (pō′lē-ō-klas′tik) Destructive to gray matter of the nervous system.

po·li·o·dys·tro·phi·a ce·re·bri pro·gres·si·va in·fan·ti·lis (pō′lē-ō-dis-trō′fē-ă ser′ă-brī prŏ-gres-ī′vă in-fan-tā′lis) Progressive spastic paresis of extremities with progressive mental deterioration, with development of seizures, blindness, and deafness, beginning during the first year of life, with destruction and disorganization of nerve cells of the cerebral cortex. SYN Alpers disease, Christensen-Krabbe disease, progressive cerebral poliodystrophy.

po·li·o·dys·tro·phy (pō′lē-ō-dis′trŏ-fē) Wasting of the gray matter of the nervous system.

po·li·o·en·ceph·a·li·tis (pō′lē-ō-en-sef′ă-lī′tis) Inflammation of the gray matter of the brain, either of the cortex or of the central nuclei; in contrast to inflammation of the white matter.

po·li·o·en·ceph·a·lo·my·e·li·tis (pō′lē-ō-en-sef′ă-lō-mī′ĕ-lī′tis) SYN poliomyeloencephalitis.

po·li·o·en·ceph·a·lop·a·thy (pō′lē-ō-en-sef′ă-lop′ă-thē) Any disease of the gray matter of the brain.

po·li·o·my·e·li·tis (pō′lē-ō-mī′ĕ-lī′tis) An inflammatory process involving the gray matter of the spinal cord.

po·li·o·my·e·lop·a·thy (pō′lē-ō-mī′ĕ-lop′ă-thē) Any disease of the gray matter of the spinal cord.

po·li·o·sis (pō′lē-ō′sis) A patchy absence or lessening of melanin in hair of the scalp, brows, or lashes, due to lack of pigment in the epidermis; hereditary, but also may be caused by inflammation or infection.

po·li·o·vi·rus (pō′lē-ō-vī′rŭs) An enterovirus in the family Picornaviridae. There are three distinct serotypes, with Type 1 responsible for 85% of the cases of paralytic polio and most epidemics.

po·li·o·vi·rus vac·cine (pō′lē-ō-vī′rŭs vak-sēn′) **1.** Inactivated poliovirus vaccine (IPV), an aqueous suspension of inactivated strains of poliomyelitis virus used by injection. **2.** Oral poliovirus vaccine (OPV), an aqueous suspension of live, attenuated strains of poliomyelitis virus for active immunization against poliomyelitis.

pol·ish·ing (pol′ish-ing) In dentistry, the act or process of making a restoration smooth and glossy.

pol·itz·er·i·za·tion (pol′it-zĕr-ī-zā′shŭn) Inflation of the pharyngotympanic (auditory) tube and middle ear by the Politzer method.

pol·len (pol′ĕn) Microspores of seed plants carried by wind or insects prior to fertilization; important in the etiology of hay fever and other allergies.

pol·len al·ler·gen (pol′ĕn al′ĕr-jen) Plant microspores that produce an allergic reaction.

pol·le·no·sis (pol′ē-nō′sis) SYN pollinosis.

pol·lex, gen. **pol·li·cis**, pl. **pol·li·ces** (pol′eks, pol′i-sis, -sēz) [TA] SYN thumb.

pol·li·no·sis, pol·le·no·sis (pol′i-nō′sis, -lē-nō′sis) Hay fever excited by the pollen of various plants.

pol·lu·tant (pŏ-lū′tănt) An undesired contaminant that results in pollution.

po·lo·ni·um (Po) (pŏ-lō′nē-ŭm) A radioactive element, atomic no. 84, isolated from pitchblende.

po·lox·a·mer (pō-loks′a-mĕr) A surfactant derived from natural gas and oil.

po·lus, pl. **po·li** (pō′lŭs, lī) [TA] SYN pole.

poly- 1. Prefix meaning many; multiplicity. Cf. multi-, pluri-. 2. CHEMISTRY prefix meaning "polymer of," as in polypeptide, polysaccharide, polynucleotide.

pol·y·ad·e·ni·tis, pol·y·ad·e·no·sis (pol′ē-ad′ĕ-nī′tis, -nō′sis) Inflammation of many lymph nodes, especially with reference to the cervical group.

pol·y·ad·e·nop·a·thy (pol′ē-ad′ĕ-nop′ă-thē) Adenopathy affecting many lymph nodes. SYN polyadenosis.

polyaesthesia [Br.] SYN polyesthesia.

Pól·ya gas·trec·to·my, Pól·ya op·er·a·tion (pōl′yah gas-trek′tŏ-mē, op-ĕr-ā′shŭn) Surgery to remove a portion of the stomach when a retrocolic gastrojejunostomy is constructed.

pol·y·am·ine (pol′ē-am′ēn) *Although this word is correctly stressed on the second-last syllable, U.S. usage often stresses it on the last syllable.* Many arise from bacterial action on protein; others are normally occurring body constituents of wide distribution or are essential growth factors for microorganisms.

pol·y·an·gi·i·tis (pol′ē-an′jē-ī′tis) Inflammation of multiple blood vessels involving more than one type of vessel.

pol·y·ar·ter·i·tis (pol′ē-ahr′tĕr-ī′tis) Simultaneous inflammation of a number of arteries.

pol·y·ar·te·ri·tis no·do·sa (pol′ē-ahr′tĕr-ī′tis nō-dō′să) Segmental inflammation, with infiltration by eosinophils, and necrosis of medium or small arteries; more common in males. SYN periarteritis nodosa.

pol·y·ar·thral·gia (pol′ē-ahr-thral′jē-ă) Pain in multiple joints.

pol·y·ar·thri·tis (pol′ē-ahr-thrī′tis) Simultaneous inflammation of several joints.

pol·y·ba·sic (pol′ē-bā′sik) Having more than one replaceable hydrogen atom; denoting an acid with a basicity over 1.

pol·y·car·box·y·late ce·ment (pol′ē-kahr-bok′si-lāt sĕ-ment′) Powder containing primarily zinc oxide mixed with a liquid containing polyacrylic acid that reacts to form a hard crystalline mass on standing.

pol·y·cen·tric (PC) (pol′ē-sen′trik) Having several centers.

pol·y·chlo·rin·at·ed bi·phe·nyl (pol′ē-klōr′i-nā-tĕd bī-fen′il) Agent in which some or all of the hydrogen atoms attached to ring carbons are replaced by chlorine atoms; possible human carcinogen and teratogen.

pol·y·chon·dri·tis (pol′ē-kon-drī′tis) A widespread disease of cartilage.

pol·y·chro·mat·ic (pol′ē-krō-mat′ik) Multicolored.

pol·y·chro·mat·ic ra·di·at·ion (pol′ē-krō-mat′ik rā′dē-ā′shŭn) That containing gamma rays.

pol·y·chro·mat·o·phil, pol·y·chro·ma·to·phile (pol′ē-krō-mat′ŏ-fil, -fīl) 1. Staining readily with acid, neutral, and basic dyes; denoting certain cells, especially certain red blood cells. SYN polychromatophilic. 2. A young or degenerating erythrocyte that manifests acidic and basic staining affinities.

pol·y·chro·ma·to·phil·i·a (pol′ē-krō′mă-tō-fil′ē-ă) Condition characterized by the presence of many red blood cells that have an affinity for acid, basic, or neutral stains.

pol·y·clin·ic (pol′ē-klin′ik) A dispensary for the treatment and study of diseases of all kinds.

pol·y·clo·nal (pol′ē-klō′năl) In immunochemistry, pertaining to proteins (i.e., antibodies) from more than a single clone of cells, in contradistinction to monoclonal.

pol·y·crot·ic (pol′ē-krot′ik) Relating to or marked by polycrotism.

pol·y·cys·tic kid·ney, pol·y·cys·tic dis·ease of kid·neys (pol′ē-sis′tik kid′nē, di-zēz′ kid′nēz) Progressive disease characterized by formation of multiple cysts of varying size scattered diffusely throughout both kidneys, resulting in compression and destruction of kidney parenchyma, usually with hypertension.

pol·y·cys·tic o·va·ry (pol′ē-sis′tik ō′văr-ē) An enlarged pearl-white, cystic ovary, with thickened tunica albuginea. SEE ALSO polycystic ovary syndrome.

pol·y·cys·tic o·va·ry syn·drome (pol′ē-sis′tik ō′văr-ē sin′drōm) A condition commonly characterized by signs of masculinization such as hirsutism, as well as obesity, menstrual abnormalities, infertility, and enlarged ovaries. SEE ALSO polycystic ovary.

pol·y·cy·the·mi·a (pol′ē-sī-thē′mē-ă) Abnormal increase in number of red blood cells. SYN erythrocythemia, polycythaemia.

pol·y·cy·the·mi·a ru·bra (pol′ē-sī-thē′ mē-ă rū′bră) SYN polycythemia vera, polycythaemia rubra.

pol·y·cy·the·mi·a ru·bra ve·ra (pol′ē-sī-thē′mē-ă rū′bră ver′ă) SYN polycythemia vera.

pol·y·cy·the·mi·a ve·ra (pol′ē-sī-thē′ mē-ă ver′ă) Chronic form of polycythemia of unknown cause; characterized by bone marrow hyperplasia, blood cell anomalies, redness of the skin, and splenomegaly. SYN erythremia, polycythemia rubra, Vaquez disease.

pol·y·dac·ty·ly, pol·y·dac·tyl·ism (pol′ē-dak′ti-lē, -til-izm) Presence of more than five fingers or toes on hand or foot.

pol·y·dip·si·a (pol′ē-dip′sē-ă) Excessive thirst that is relatively prolonged.

pol·y·dys·pla·si·a (pol′ē-dis-plā′zē-ă) Tissue development abnormal in several respects.

pol·y·em·bry·o·ny (pol′ē-em′brē-ō-nē) Condition of a zygote's giving rise to two or more embryos.

pol·y·en·do·crin·op·athy (pol′ē-en′dō-kri-nop′ă-thē) A disease usually caused by insufficiency of multiple endocrine glands. SEE ALSO multiple endocrine deficiency syndrome.

pol·y·es·the·si·a (pol′ē-es-thē′zē-ă) A disorder of sensation in which a single touch or other stimulus is felt as several. SYN polyaesthesia.

pol·y·ga·lac·ti·a (pol′ē-gă-lak′shē-ă) Excessive secretion of breast milk, especially during weaning.

pol·y·gen·ic (pol′ē-jen′ik) Relating to a hereditary disease or normal characteristic controlled by the added effects of genes at multiple loci.

pol·y·graph (pol′ē-graf) 1. An instrument for obtaining simultaneous tracings from several different sources. An electrocardiogram is nearly always included for timing. 2. An instrument for recording changes in respiration, blood pressure, galvanic skin response, and other physiologic changes while the subject is interviewed or asked to give associations to relevant and irrelevant words; physiologic changes are presumed to be emotional reactions, and thus indicative of whether the subject is telling the truth.

pol·y·hy·brid (pol'ē-hī'brid) The off-spring of parents differing from each other in more than three characters.

pol·y·hy·dram·ni·os (pol'ē-hī-dram'nē-os) Excess amount of amniotic fluid.

pol·y·hy·dric (pol'ē-hī'drik) Containing more than one hydroxyl group, as in polyhydric alcohols and polyhydric acids.

pol·y·lep·tic (pol'ē-lep'tik) Denoting a disease with many paroxysms, e.g., malaria.

pol·y·lep·tic fe·ver (pol'ē-lep'tik fē'vĕr) That occurring in two or more paroxysms; e.g., smallpox, relapsing fever.

pol·y·mas·ti·gote (pol'ē-mas'ti-gōt) A mastigote having several grouped flagella.

pol·y·me·li·a (pol'ē-mē'lē-ă) Developmental defect with supernumerary limbs or parts of limbs.

pol·y·men·or·rhe·a (pol'ē-men'ŏr-ē'ă) Occurrence of menstrual cycles of greater than usual frequency.

pol·ym·er·ase chain re·ac·tion (PCR) (pŏ-lim'ĕr-ās chān rē-ăk'shŭn) An enzymatic method for the repeated copying and amplification of the two strands of DNA of a particular gene sequence.

po·lym·er·i·za·tion (pŏ-lim'ĕr-ī-zā' shŭn) A reaction in which a high molecular weight product is produced by successive additions to or condensations of a simpler compound.

pol·y·mi·cro·bi·al (pol'ē-mī-krō'bē-ăl) Denotes disease state involving multiple species of microorganisms.

pol·y·mor·phic (pol'ē-mōr'fik) Occurring in more than one morphologic form. SYN multiform, pleomorphic (1), pleomorphous, polymorphous.

pol·y·mor·phic re·tic·u·lo·sis (pol' ē-mōr'fik re-tik'yū-lō'sis) Necrotizing lymphoproliferative lesion with a predilection for the upper respiratory tract.

pol·y·mor·pho·cel·lu·lar (pol'ē-mōr' fō-sel'yū-lăr) Relating to or formed of cells of several different kinds.

pol·y·mor·pho·cyt·ic leu·ke·mi·a (pol' ē-mōr'fō-sit'ik lū-kē'mē-ă) Granulocytic form, especially a variety in which the predominant cells are mature, segmented granulocytes.

pol·y·mor·pho·nu·cle·ar (pol'ē-mōr' fō-nū'klē-ăr) Having nuclei of varied forms; denoting a variety of leukocyte.

pol·y·mor·pho·nu·cle·ar leu·ko·cyte, pol·y·nu·cle·ar leu·ko·cyte (pol'ē-mōr'fō-nū'klē-ăr lū'kō-sīt, pol'ē-nū'klē-ăr) Common term for granulocyte or granulocytic white blood cell includes basophilic, eosinophilic, and neutrophilic leukocytes.

pol·y·mor·phous light e·rup·tion (pol' ē-mōr'fŭs līt ĕr-ŭp'shŭn) A common pruritic papular outbreak appearing in a few hours and lasting up to several days on skin exposed to shortwave ultraviolet light.

pol·y·mor·phous low-grade car·ci·no·ma of sal·i·var·y glands (pol'ē-mōr'fus lō-grād kahr'si-nō'mă sal'i-var-ē glandz) A low-grade malignant tumor of salivary glands showing several histologic patterns, such as cribriform, ductal, and papillary growth.

pol·y·my·al·gi·a (pol'ē-mī-al'jē-ă) Pain in several muscle groups.

pol·y·my·al·gi·a rheu·ma·ti·ca (pol'ē-mī-al'jē-ă rū-mat'i-kă) Syndrome within the group of collagen diseases different from spondylarthritis or from humeral scapular periarthritis by the presence of an elevated sedimentation rate; much commoner in women than in men.

pol·y·my·oc·lo·nus (pol'ē-mī-ok'lŏ-nŭs) SYN myoclonus multiplex.

pol·y·my·op·a·thy (pol'ē-mī-op'ă-thē) Disease afftecting many muscles.

pol·y·my·o·si·tis (pol'ē-mī'ō-sī'tis) Inflammation of a number of voluntary muscles simultaneously.

pol·y·my·xin (P) (pol'ē-mik'sin) A mixture of antibiotic substances obtained from cultures of *Bacillus polymyxa*, an

P

organism found in water and soils and obtainable as a crystalline hydrochloride. SEE ALSO colistimethate sodium.

pol·y·ne·sic (pol′ē-nē′sik) Occurring in many separate foci.

pol·y·neu·ral·gi·a (pol′ē-nūr-al′jē-ă) Neuralgia of several nerves simultaneously.

pol·y·neu·rop·a·thy (pol′ē-nūr-op′ă-thē) **1.** A disease process involving a number of peripheral nerves (literal sense). **2.** A nontraumatic generalized disorder of peripheral nerves, affecting the distal fibers most severely, with proximal shading (e.g., the feet are affected sooner or more severely than the hands), and typically symmetrically. **3.** SYN acrodynia (2). SYN multiple neuritis.

pol·y·nu·cle·o·tide (pol′ē-nū′klē-ō-tīd) A linear polymer containing an indefinite (usually large) number of nucleotides, linked from one ribose (or deoxyribose) to another via phosphoric residues. Cf. oligonucleotide.

pol·y·o·don·ti·a, pol·y·den·ti·a (pol′ē-ō-don′shē-ă, -den′shē-ă) Presence of extra teeth.

pol·y·o·pi·a, pol·y·op·si·a (pol′ē-ō′pē-ă, -op′sē-ă) The perception of several images of the same object.

pol·y·os·tot·ic, pol·y·stot·ic (pol′ē-os-tot′ik, pol′ē-stot′ik) Involving more than one bone.

pol·y·ov·u·lar (pol′ē-ov′yū-lăr) Containing more than one oocyte (ovum).

pol·y·ov·u·la·tor·y (pol′ē-ov′yū-lă-tōr-ē) Discharging several oocytes (ova) in one ovulatory cycle.

pol·yp (pol′ip) A general descriptive term used with reference to any mass of tissue that bulges or projects outward or upward from the normal surface level, thereby being macroscopically visible as a hemispheroid, spheroid, or irregular moundlike structure growing from a relatively broad base or a slender stalk; polyps may be neoplasms, foci of inflammation, degenerative lesions, or malformations.

pol·y·pep·tide (PP) (pol′ē-pep′tīd) A

peptide formed by the union of an indefinite (usually large) number of amino acids by peptide links (–NH–CO–).

pol·y·phy·let·ic (pol′ē-fī-let′ik) **1.** Derived from more than one source, or having several lines of descent, in contrast to monophyletic. **2.** HEMATOLOGY relating to polyphyletism.

pol·y·plas·tic (pol′ē-plas′tik) **1.** Formed of several different structures. **2.** Capable of assuming several forms.

pol·y·ploi·dy (pol′ē-ploy′dē) The state of a cell nucleus containing three or more haploid sets.

pol·y·poid, pol·yp·i·form (pol′i-poyd, po-lip′i-fōrm) Resembling a polyp in gross features.

pol·y·po·sis (pol′i-pō′sis) Presence of several polyps.

pol·y·pous (pol′i-pŭs) Manifesting the gross features of, or characterized by the presence of a polyp or polyps.

pol·y·pous gas·tri·tis (pol′i-pŭs gas-trī′tis) Chronic gastritis form, with irregular atrophy of the mucous membrane with cystic glands giving rise to a knobby surface appearance.

pol·yp·tych·i·al (pol′ip-tik′ē-ăl) Folded or arranged so as to form more than one layer.

pol·y·ra·dic·u·lo·neu·rop·a·thy (pol′ē-ra-dik′yū-lō-nūr-op′ă-thē) Coexisting polyradiculopathy and polyneuropathy.

pol·y·sac·char·ide (pol′ē-sak′ă-rīd) A carbohydrate containing a large number of saccharide groups (e.g., starch). Cf. oligosaccharide. SYN glycan.

pol·y·sac·char·ide con·ju·gated vac·cine (pol′ē-sak′ă-rīd kon′jū-gā-těd vak-sēn′) One made from the capsular polysaccharide of the microorganism conjugated with a protein.

pol·y·ser·o·si·tis (pol′ē-sēr′ō-sī′tis) Chronic inflammation with effusions in several serous cavities resulting in fibrous thickening of the serosa and constrictive pericarditis. SYN Bamberger disease (2), Concato disease.

pol·y·som·no·gra·phy (pol′ē-som-nog′ră-fē) Simultaneous and continuous monitoring of relevant normal and abnormal physiologic activity during sleep.

pol·y·so·my (pol′ē-sō′mē) State of a cell nucleus with a specific chromosome is represented more than twice. Cf. polyploidy.

pol·y·sper·mi·a, pol·y·sper·mism, pol·y·sperm·y (pol′ē-spĕr′mē-ă, -mizm, -mē) An abnormally profuse spermatic secretion.

pol·y·sple·ni·a (pol′ē-splē′nē-ă) A condition in which splenic tissue is divided into nearly equal masses or totally absent.

pol·y·syn·ap·tic (pol′ē-sin-ap′tik) Referring to neural pathways formed by a chain of a large number of synaptically connected nerve cells.

pol·y·tene (pol′i-tēn) Consisting of many filaments of chromatin as the result of repeated division of chromonemata without separation of filaments.

poly·ten·o·syn·o·vi·tis (pol′ē-ten′ō-sin′ō-vī′tis) Inflammation of several tendons and of synovial fluid.

pol·y·the·li·a (pol′ē-thē′lē-ă) Presence of supernumerary nipples, either on the breast or elsewhere on the body. SYN hyperthelia.

pol·y·un·sa·tu·ra·ted fat (pol′ē-ŭn-sach′ŭr-ā-tĕd fat) A type of unsaturated fat used to lower cholesterol levels.

pol·y·u·ri·a (pol′ē-yūr′ē-ă) Excessive excretion of urine resulting in profuse micturition; causes include diabetes and hypercalcemia, but sometimes due to overhydration.

pol·y·va·lent (pol′ē-vā′lĕnt) **1.** SYN multivalent. **2.** SEE polyvalent serum.

pol·y·va·lent vac·cine (pol′ē-vā′lĕnt vak-sēn′) One prepared from cultures of two or more strains of the same species or microorganism.

pol·y·vi·nyl chlo·ride (PVC) (pol′ē-vī′nil klōr′īd) A polymer plastic used as a rubber substitute in many industrial applications; suspected of being carcino-

genic in humans. SYN chlorethene homopolymer.

po·made ac·ne (pom-ād′ ak′nē) That caused by repeated application of hair creams containing oils that block release of sebum from hair follicles; most commonly seen on forehead and temples in young African Americans.

pons, pl. **pon·tes** (ponz, pon′tēz) [TA] **1.** [TA] In neuroanatomy, the pons varolii or pons cerebelli; that part of the brainstem between the medulla oblongata caudally and the mesencephalon rostrally, composed of the basilar part of pons and the tegmentum of pons. **2.** Any bridge-like formation connecting two more-or-less disjoined parts of the same structure or organ.

pons hep·a·tis (ponz hē-pā′tis) Bridge of liver tissue that sometimes overlaps the fossa of the inferior vena cava. SYN ponticulus hepatis.

pon·tic (pon′tik) An artificial tooth on a fixed or removable partial denture; it replaces the lost natural tooth and restores its functions.

pon·ti·cu·lus (pon-tik′yū-lŭs) A vertical ridge on the eminentia conchae giving insertion to the auricularis posterior muscle.

pon·tine flex·ure (pon′tēn flek′shŭr) The dorsally concave curvature of the rhombencephalon in the embryo. SYN basicranial flexure, transverse rhombencephalic flexure.

pool (pūl) **1.** A collection of blood or other fluid in any region of the body; results from dilation and retardation of the circulation in the capillaries and veins. **2.** A combination of resources.

pool·ed se·rum, pool·ed blood se·rum (pūld sēr′ŭm, blŭd) Mixed serum from a number of people.

Pool phe·nom·e·non (pūl fĕ-nom′ĕ-non) **1.** In tetany, spasm of both the quadriceps and calf muscles when the extended leg is flexed at the hip. SYN Schlesinger sign. **2.** In tetany, contraction of the arm muscles following the stretching of the brachial plexus by elevation of the arm above the head with the forearm extended.

poor·ly dif·fer·en·ti·at·ed lym·pho·cyt·ic lym·pho·ma (pōr′lē dif′er-en′shē-āt-ĕd lim′fō-sit′ik lim-fō′mă) A B-cell lymphoma with nodular or diffuse lymph node or bone marrow involvement by large lymphoid cells.

pop·u·la·tion (pop′yū-lā′shŭn) Statistical term denoting all the objects, events, or subjects in a particular class. Cf. sample.

pop·u·la·tion ge·net·ics (pop′yū-lā′shŭn jĕ-net′iks) The study of genetic influences on the components of cause and effect in the somatic characteristics of populations.

por·ce·lain (pōr′sĕ-lin) A powder composed of a clay, silica, and a flux that, when mixed with water, forms a paste that is molded to form artificial teeth, inlays, jacket crowns, and dentures. When heated, the materials fuse to form a ceramic.

por·cine (pōr′sīn, -sin) Relating to pigs.

pore, po·rus (pōr, pōr′ŭs) 1. An opening, hole, perforation, or foramen. 2. SYN sweat pore.

por·en·ceph·a·li·tis (pōr′en-sef′ă-lī′tis) Chronic inflammation of the brain, with the formation of cavities.

por·en·ceph·a·ly, por·en·ceph·a·li·a (pōr′en-sef′ă-lē, -sĕ-fā′lē-ă) The occurrence of cavities in the brain substance, communicating usually with the lateral ventricles. SYN spelencephaly.

por·i·o·ma·ni·a (pōr′ē-ō-mā′nē-ă) A morbid impulse to wander or journey away from home.

por·i·on, pl. **po·ri·a** (pōr′ē-on, -ă) The central point on the upper margin of the external auditory meatus.

po·ro·ker·a·to·sis (pōr′ō-ker′ă-tō′sis) A rare dermatosis with thickening of the stratum corneum with an anular keratotic rim or coronoid lamella surrounding progressive centrifugal atrophy. SYN Mibelli disease.

po·ro·ma (pōr-ō′mă) 1. SYN callosity. 2. SYN exostosis. 3. Induration after a phlegmon. 4. Tumor cells lining the skin openings of sweat glands.

po·ro·sis, pl. **po·ro·ses, po·ros·i·ty** (pōr-ō′sis, -sēz, pōr-os′i-tē) A porous condition. SYN porosity (1).

po·rous (pōr′ŭs) Having openings that pass directly or indirectly through the substance.

por·phin, por·phine (pōr′fin, pōr′fēn) The unsubstituted cyclic tetrapyrrole nucleus that is the basis of the porphyrins. Cf. chlorin, corrin. SYN porphyrin.

por·phyr·i·a (pōr-fir′ē-ă) Disorders involving heme biosynthesis, characterized by excessive excretion of porphyrins or their precursors; may be acquired or inherited.

por·phy·ri·a cu·ta·ne·a tar·da (pōr-fir′ē-ă kyū-tā′nē-ă tahr′dă) Familial or sporadic porphyria characterized by liver dysfunction and photosensitive cutaneous lesions, with hyperpigmentation and sclerodermalike changes in the skin and increased excretion of uroporphyrin. SYN symptomatic porphyria.

por·phy·rin (pōr′fi-rin) SYN porphin.

por·phyr·i·nu·ri·a, por·phy·rur·i·a (pōr′fir-i-nyūr′ē-ă, -ryūr′ē-ă) Excretion of porphyrins and related compounds in the urine. SYN purpurinuria.

por·ta·ca·val, por·to·ca·val (pōr′tă-kā′văl, pōr′tō-) Concerning the portal vein and the inferior vena cava.

por·ta·ca·val shunt (pōr′tă-kā′văl shŭnt) 1. Surgical anastomosis between portal and systemic veins. 2. Surgical anastomosis between the portal vein and the vena cava.

por·ta hep·a·tis (pōr′tă hē-pā′tis) [TA] A transverse fissure on the visceral surface of the liver between the caudate and quadrate lobes. SYN caudal transverse fissure, portal fissure.

por·tal (pōr′tăl) 1. Relating to any porta or hilum. 2. The point of entry into the body of a pathogenic microorganism. SYN port.

por·tal cir·cu·la·tion (pōr′tăl sĭr′kyū-lā′shŭn) 1. Circulation of blood to the liver from the small intestine, the right half of the colon, and the spleen through the portal vein. 2. More generally, any part of the systemic circulation in which blood draining from the capillary bed of one structure flows through a larger vessel(s) to supply the capillary bed of another structure before returning to the heart.

por·tal hy·per·ten·sion (pōr′tăl hĭ′pĕr-ten′shŭn) Elevation of pressure in the hepatic portal circulation due to cirrhosis or other fibrotic change in liver tissue.

por·tal hy·po·phy·si·al circulation (pōr′tăl hĭ′pō-fĭz′ē-ăl sĭr′kyū-lā′shŭn) A capillary network that carries hormones from the hypothalamus to their sites of action in the anterior hypophysis. SYN hypophysioportal system.

por·tal of en·try (pōr′tăl en′trē) Refers to the process whereby a pathogen enters the body, gains access to susceptible tissues, and causes disease or infection.

por·tal sys·tem (pōr′tăl sis′tĕm) A system of vessels in which blood, after passing through one capillary bed, is conveyed through a second capillary network.

por·tal-sys·tem·ic en·ceph·a·lop·a·thy (pōr′tăl sis-tem′ik en-sef′a-lop′ă-thē) Brain disorder associated with cirrhosis of the liver, attributed to the passage of toxic nitrogenous substances from the portal to the systemic circulation; cerebral manifestations may include coma. SYN hepatic encephalopathy (1).

Por·ter-Sil·ber re·ac·tion (pōr′tĕr sil′bĕr rē-ak′shŭn) Basis of the 17-hydroxy-corticosteroid test.

por·ti·o, pl. **por·ti·o·nes** (pōr′shē-ō, -ō′nēz) [TA] *Avoid using the simple word portio in the special sense of portio vaginalis cervicis.* A part.

porto- Prefix meaning portal.

por·to·en·ter·os·to·my (pōr′tō-en′tĕr-os′tŏ-mē) An operation for biliary atresia in which a Roux-en-Y loop of jejunum is anastomosed to the hepatic end of the divided extravascular portal structures. SYN Kasai operation.

por·tog·ra·phy (pōr-tog′ră-fē) Delineation of portal circulation by radiographs, using radiopaque material, introduced

into the spleen or portal vein at operation.

por·to·sys·tem·ic, por·tal-sys·tem·ic (pōr′tō-sis-tem′ik, pōr′tăl-) Relating to connections between the portal and systemic venous systems.

port-wine mark, port-wine stain (pōrt-wīn mahrk, stān) SYN nevus flammeus.

po·rus, pl. **po·ri** (pō′rŭs, -rī) **1.** [TA] SYN pore. **2.** SYN sweat pore.

-posia Combining form meaning intake of fluid or drinking.

po·si·tion (pŏ-zish′ŏn) **1.** An attitude, posture, or placement. **2.** A posture or attitude assumed by a patient for comfort and to facilitate diagnostic, surgical, or therapeutic procedures. **3.** OBSTETRICS the relation of an arbitrarily chosen portion of the fetus to the right or left side of the mother. Cf. presentation.

po·si·tion·al nys·tag·mus (pŏ-zish′ŏn-ăl nis-tag′mŭs) Form occurring only when the head is in a particular position.

po·si·tion·al ver·ti·go (pŏ-zish′ŏn-ăl vĕr′ti-gō) Whirling sensation occurring with a change in body position.

po·si·tion ef·fect (pŏ-zish′ŏn e-fekt′) A change in the phenotypic expression of one or more genes due to a change in physical location with respect to other genes.

po·si·tion·er (pŏ-zish′ŏn-ĕr) A resilient elastoplastic or rubber removable appliance fitting over the occlusal surface of the teeth to limit tooth movement or provide stabilization.

po·si·tion sense (pŏ-zish′ŏn sens) SYN posture sense.

pos·i·tive (poz′i-tiv) **1.** Affirmative; definite; not negative. **2.** MATHEMATICS having a value more than zero. **3.** PHYSICS, CHEMISTRY having an electric charge resulting from a loss or deficit of electrons, hence able to attract or gain electrons. **4.** MEDICINE denoting a response to a diagnostic maneuver or laboratory study that indicates the presence of the disease or condition tested for.

pos·i·tive ac·com·mo·da·tion (poz′i-tiv ă-kom′ŏ-dā′shŭn) Increased refractivity of the eye that occurs when shifting from the distance to a near object.

pos·i·tive con·ver·gence (poz′i-tiv kŏn-vĕr′jĕns) Inward deviation of the visual axes even when convergence is at rest.

pos·i·tive end-ex·pi·ra·to·ry pres·sure (PEEP) (poz′i-tiv end-eks-pīr′ă-tōr-ē presh′ŭr) A technique used in respiratory therapy in which airway pressure exceeding atmospheric pressure is achieved at the end of exhalation by introduction of a mechanical impedance to exhalation.

pos·i·tive en·er·gy bal·ance (poz′i-tiv en′ĕr-jē bal′ăns) When energy output is less than energy consumption and results in increased body weight.

pos·i·tive feed·back (poz′i-tiv fēd′bak) That found when the sign or sense of the returned signal results in increased amplification or leads to instability.

pos·i·tive-neg·a·tive pres·sure breath·ing (poz′i-tiv-neg′ă-tiv presh′ŭr brēdh′ing) Inflation of the lungs with positive pressure and deflation with negative pressure by a ventilator.

pos·i·tive ni·tro·gen bal·ance (poz′i-tiv nī′trŏ-jen bal′ăns) Nitrogen intake exceeds the sum of all nitrogen excretion.

pos·i·tive pre·dic·tive val·ue (PPV) (poz′i-tiv prē-dik′tiv val′yū) The probability that a positive result accurately indicates that the analyte or the specific disease is present.

pos·i·tive pres·sure ven·ti·la·tion (PPV) (poz′i-tiv presh′ŭr ven′ti-lā′shŭn) Mechanical ventilation in which a positive transrespiratory pressure is generated by increasing airway opening pressure above body surface pressure.

pos·i·tive sco·to·ma (poz′i-tiv skŏ-tō′mă) Vision disorder that is perceived as a white spot within the field of vision.

pos·i·tive stain (poz′i-tiv stān) Direct binding of a dye with a tissue component to produce contrast.

pos·i·tive symp·tom (poz′i-tiv simp′tŏm) One of the acute or florid symptoms of schizophrenia, including hallucinations, delusions, thought disorders, loose associations, ambivalence, or affective lability.

pos·i·tron (β+) (poz′i-tron) A subatomic particle of mass and charge equal to the electron but of opposite (i.e., positive) charge.

pos·i·tron e·mis·sion tom·og·ra·phy (PET) (poz′i-tron ĕ-mish′ŭn tŏ-mog′ră-fē) Tomographic images formed by computer analysis of photons detected from annihilation of positrons emitted by radionuclides incorporated into biochemical substances.

post- Prefix meaning after, behind, posterior; opposite of anti-. Cf. meta-.

post·a·nal gut (pōst-ā′năl gŭt) Extension of the hindgut caudal to the point at which the anal opening forms. SYN postcloacal gut, tailgut.

post·an·es·the·si·a care u·nit (PACU) (pōst′an-es-thē′zē-ă kār yū′nit) Department with special personnel and equipment designated for recovery of patients after administration of anesthesia. SYN recovery room.

post·an·ti·bi·ot·ic ef·fect (PAE) (pōst′an′ti-bī-ot′ik e-fekt′) Continual inhibition of bacterial growth after exposure to an antimicrobial agent; the time for the organism to recover from the effects of antimicrobial exposure.

post·ax·i·al (pōst-ak′sē-ăl) **1.** Posterior to the axis of the body or any limb, the latter being in the anatomic position. **2.** Denoting the portion of a limb bud that lies caudal to the axis of the limb.

post·bra·chi·al (pōst-brā′kē-ăl) Denotes on or in the posterior part of the upper arm.

post·cen·tral (pōst-sen′trăl) Referring to the cerebral convolution forming the posterior bank of the central sulcus: the postcentral gyrus.

post·cen·tral gy·rus (pōst-sen′trăl jī′rŭs) [TA] The anterior convolution of the parietal lobe, bounded in front by the central sulcus and posteriorly by the interparietal sulcus.

post·co·i·tal head·ache (pōst-kō´i-tăl hed´āk) Headache that occurs after sexual intercourse.

post·co·i·tal test (pōst-kō´i-tăl test) A test on cervical mucus about time of ovulation to evaluate its receptivity to sperms.

post·date preg·nan·cy (pōst´dāt preg´năn-sē) A pregnancy exceeding 294 days or 42 completed weeks.

post·di·a·stol·ic (pōst´dī-ă-stol´ik) Following diastole.

post·di·crot·ic (pōst´dī-krot´ik) Following the dicrotic wave in a sphygmogram; denoting an additional variation in the descending line of the pulse tracing.

pos·te·ri·or (pos-tēr´ē-ŏr) **1.** After, in relation to time or space. **2.** HUMAN ANATOMY denoting the back surface of the body. SYN dorsal (2). **3.** Near the tail or caudal end of certain embryos. **4.** A substitute for caudal in quadrupeds; in veterinary anatomy, posterior is used only to denote some structures of the head.

pos·te·ri·or em·bry·o·tox·on (pos-tēr´ē-ŏr em´brē-ō-tok´son) A developmental abnormality marked by a prominent white ring of Schwalbe and iris strands that partially obscure the chamber angle.

pos·te·ri·or pal·a·tal seal a·re·a (pos-tēr´ē-ŏr pal´ă-tăl sēl ār´ē-ă) Soft tissues along the junction of the hard and soft palates on which pressure within the physiologic limits of the tissues can be applied by a denture to aid in the retention of the denture. SYN post dam area, postpalatal seal area.

pos·te·ri·or spi·no·cer·e·bel·lar tract (pos-tēr´ē-ŏr spī´nō-ser´ĕ-bel´ăr trakt) [TA] Compact bundle of heavily myelinated, thick fibers at the periphery of the posterior half of the lateral funiculus of the spinal cord, originating in the ipsilateral thoracic nucleus and entering the cerebellum by way of the inferior cerebellar peduncle. SYN tractus spinocerebellaris posterior [TA], dorsal spinocerebellar tract, Flechsig tract.

pos·te·ri·or tooth (pos-tēr´ē-ŏr tūth) Any premolar or molar tooth.

pos·te·ri·or u·ve·i·tis (pos-tēr´ē-ŏr yū´vē-ī´tis) SYN choroiditis.

pos·te·ri·or vein of left ven·tri·cle (pos-tēr´ē-ŏr vān left ven´tri-kĕl) Arises on the diaphragmatic surface of the heart near the apex, runs to the left and parallel to the posterior interventricular sulcus, and empties in the coronary sinus.

pos·te·ri·or walk·er (pos-tē´ē-ŏr wawk´ĕr) Ambulatory assistive device oriented with the open aspect of the device in front of the user.

postero- Prefix meaning posterior; at the back of.

pos·ter·o·an·te·ri·or (PA) (pos´tĕr-ō-an-tēr´ē-ŏr) A term denoting the direction of view or progression, from posterior to anterior, through a part.

pos·ter·o·clu·sion (pos´tĕr-ō-klū´zhŭn) SYN posterior occlusion.

pos·ter·o·lat·er·al, pos·ter·o·ex·tern·al (pos´tĕr-ō-lat´ĕr-ăl, -eks-tĕr´nal) Behind and to one side, specifically to the outer side.

pos·ter·o·lat·er·al tho·ra·cot·o·my (pos´tĕr-ō-lat´ĕr-ăl thōr´ă-kot´ŏ-mē) Chest surgery involving division of the latissimus dorsi muscle and the serratus anterior muscle.

pos·ter·o·me·di·al (pos´tĕr-ō-mē´dē-ăl) Behind and to the inner side. SYN posterointernal.

pos·ter·o·me·di·an (pos´tĕr-ō-mē´dē-ăn) Occupying a central position posteriorly.

pos·ter·o·pa·ri·e·tal (pos´tĕr-ō-pă-rī´ĕ-tăl) Relating to the posterior portion of the parietal lobe of the cerebrum.

pos·ter·o·su·per·i·or (pos´tĕr-ō-sŭ-pēr´ē-ŏr) Situated behind and at the upper part.

post·gan·gli·on·ic (pōst´gang-glē-on´ik) Distal to or beyond a ganglion.

post·gas·trec·to·my syn·drome (pōst´gas-trek´tŏ-mē sin´drōm) SYN dumping syndrome.

post·hep·a·tit·ic cir·rho·sis (pōst-hep′ă-tit′ik sir-ō′sis) SYN chronic active hepatitis.

post·her·pet·ic neu·ral·gi·a (pōst-hĕr-pet′ik nūr-al′jē-ă) Causalgia and hyperesthesia in the dermatome served by a spinal nerve infected by herpes zoster, persisting after resolution of the skin eruption.

pos·thi·o·plas·ty (pos′thē-ō-plas-tē) Surgical reconstruction of the prepuce.

pos·thi·tis (pos-thī′tis) Inflammation of the prepuce.

post·hu·mous (pos′tyū-mŭs) Denotes occurring after a person's death.

post·hyp·not·ic (pōst′hip-not′ik) Following hypnotism.

post·hyp·not·ic sug·ges·tion (pōst′ hip-not′ik sŭg-jes′chŭn) SYN hypnotic suggestion.

post·ic·tal (pōst-ik′tăl) Following a seizure (e.g., epileptic).

post·ma·la·ri·a neu·ro·log·ic syn·drome (pōst′mă-lar′ē-ă nūr′ō-loj′ik sin′ drŏm) A self-limited central nervous system disorder that develops soon after recovery from a severe bout of falciparum malaria.

post·ma·ture, post·ma·ture in·fant, post·term in·fant (pōst′mă-chŭr′, in′ fănt, pōst-tĕrm′) Fetus that remains in the uterus longer than the normal gestational period, i.e., longer than 42 weeks (288 days) in humans.

post·men·o·pau·sal (pōst′men-ŏ-paw′ zăl) Relating to the period following the menopause.

post·mor·tem (pōst-mōr′tĕm) 1. Pertaining to or occurring during the period after death. 2. Colloquialism for autopsy (1). Also called 'post.'

post·mor·tem clot (pōst-mōr′tĕm klot) Blockage in the heart or great vessels after death.

post·mor·tem de·li·ver·y (pōst-mōr′ tĕm dĕ-liv′ĕr-ē) Extraction of a fetus after the death of its mother. SYN perimortem delivery.

post·mor·tem li·ve·do, post·mor·tem li·vid·i·ty (pōst-mōr′tĕm li-vē′dō, li-vid′i-tē) Purple discoloration of dependent parts, except in areas of contact pressure, appearing within 30 minutes to 2 hours after death. SYN postmortem hypostasis, postmortem suggillation.

post·mor·tem ri·gi·di·ty (pōst-mōr′tĕm ri-jid′i-tē) SYN rigor mortis.

post·mor·tem wart (pōst-mōr′tĕm wŏrt) Tuberculous warty growth on the hand of one who performs postmortem examinations. SYN anatomic tubercle, anatomic wart.

post·na·sal (pōst-nā′zăl) 1. Posterior to the nasal cavity. 2. Relating to the posterior portion of the nasal cavity.

post·na·sal drip (pōst-nā′zăl drip) Sensation of mucoid discharge from the nose into the pharynx.

post·na·tal (pōst-nā′tăl) Occurring after birth.

post·ne·crot·ic cir·rho·sis (pōst′ nĕ-krot′ik sir-ō′sis) Hepatic disorder characterized by necrosis involving whole hepatic lobules, with collapse of the reticular framework to form large scars; regeneration nodules are also large. SYN necrotic cirrhosis.

post·op·er·a·tive (pōst-op′ĕr-ă-tiv) Following an operation.

post·o·ral (pōst-ōr′ăl) In the posterior part of, or posterior to, the mouth.

post·par·a·lyt·ic (pōst′par-ă-lit′ik) Following or consequent to paralysis.

post·par·tum (pōst-pahr′tŭm) After childbirth. Cf. antepartum, intrapartum.

post·par·tum al·o·pe·cia (pōst-pahr′ tŭm al′ō-pē′shē-ă) Temporary diffuse telogen loss of scalp hair at the termination of pregnancy. SYN telogen effluvium.

post·par·tum blues (pōst-pahr′tŭm blūz) Mood disturbance (including insomnia, depression, anxiety, and irritability) experienced by up to 50% of women the first week after birth; precipitated by progesterone withdrawal. Cf. postpartum psychosis.

post·par·tum hem·or·rhage (pōst-pahr′tŭm hem′ŏr-ăj) Hemorrhage from the birth canal in excess of 500 mL after a vaginal delivery or 1000 mL after a cesarean delivery during the first 24 hours after birth.

post·par·tum psy·cho·sis (pōst-pahr′tŭm sī-kō′sis) Acute maternal mental disorder with depression after childbirth.

post·per·fu·sion syn·drome (pōst-pĕr-fyū′zhŭn sin′drōm) Organ dysfunction observed in patients after cardiopulmonary bypass surgery.

post·per·i·car·di·ot·o·my per·i·car·di·tis (pōst-per′i-kahr′dē-ot′ŏ-mē per′i-kahr-dī′tis) A syndrome characterized by fever, substernal chest pain, and pericardial rub following cardiac surgery.

post·po·li·o syn·drome (PPS) (pōst-pō′lē-ō sin′drōm) Progressive muscular weakness and deterioration in a person previously affected by poliomyelitis; usually affects the muscles most heavily disordered by the disease, but may also affect others. SYN postpoliomyelitis syndrome.

post·pran·di·al glu·cose test (pōst-pran′dē-ăl glū′kōs test) Assessment of blood sugar levels after a meal (usually 2 hours).

post·pu·ber·ty (pōst-pyū′bĕr-tē) The period after puberty.

post·pu·bes·cent, post·pu·ber·tal (pōst′pyū-bes′ĕnt, -bĕr-tăl) Subsequent to the period of puberty.

post·ro·tar·y nys·tag·mus (pōst-rō′tă-rē ni-stag′mŭs) **1.** Reflexive movements of the eyes that occur after elicitation from a quick rotational movement (e.g., spinning) used to determine vestibular dysfunction. **2.** Involuntary oscillation of the eyes as a result of being rotated after stimulation of the vestibular system by spinning activities.

post·stead·y state (pōst-sted′ē stāt) Any period of time, particularly in an enzyme-catalyzed reaction, after the steady-state interval, e.g., when the rate of product formation is declining in an enzyme-catalyzed reaction.

post·syn·ap·tic (pōst′sin-ap′tik) Pertaining to the area on the distal side of a synaptic cleft.

post·term in·fant (pōst-tĕrm in′fănt) Infant with a gestational age of 42 completed weeks or more (294 days or more).

post·trau·mat·ic (pōst′traw-mat′ik) Occurring after trauma, and, by implication, caused by it.

post·trau·mat·ic de·lir·i·um (pōst′traw-mat′ik dĕ-lir′ē-ŭm) Delirium caused by a structural traumatic brain injury.

post·trau·mat·ic de·men·ti·a (pōst′traw-mat′ik dĕ-men′shē-ă) Dementia caused by traumatic brain injury.

post·trau·mat·ic ep·i·lep·sy (pōst′traw-mat′ik ep′i-lep′sē) A convulsive state following and causally related to head injury, with brain damage either manifested clinically or ascertained by special examinations such as computed tomography.

post·trau·mat·ic stress dis·or·der (PTSD) (pōst′traw-mat′ik stres dis-ōr′dĕr) Anxiety disorder with a syndrome of responses to extremely disturbing, often life-threatening events such as combat, natural disaster, torture, maltreatment, or rape.

post·trau·mat·ic syn·drome (pōst′traw-mat′ik sin′drōm) A clinical disorder that often follows head injury, characterized by headache, dizziness, neurasthenia, hypersensitivity to stimuli, and diminished concentration.

post·trau·mat·ic ver·ti·go (pōst′traw-mat′ik vĕr′ti-gō) Sense of imbalance that follows trauma, most commonly occurring when an irritable labyrinthine focus develops during the weeks and months after the incident.

post·treat·ment mor·bid·i·ty (pōst-trēt′mĕnt mōr-bid′i-tē) Denotes the untoward signs and symptoms resulting from a treatment procedure such as surgery or chemotherapy.

pos·tur·al con·trac·tion (pos′chŭr-ăl kŏn-trak′shŭn) Maintenance of muscular tension (usually isometric) sufficient to maintain posture.

P

pos·tur·al drain·age (pos'chŭr-ăl drān' ăj) Procedure to remove liquid in bronchiectasis and lung abscess.

pos·tur·al hy·po·ten·sion (pos'chŭr-ăl hī'pō-tĕn'shŭn) SYN orthostatic hypotension.

pos·tur·al in·se·cu·ri·ty (pos'chŭr-ăl in'sĕ-kyŭr'i-tē) SYN gravitational insecurity.

pos·tur·al po·si·tion, pos·tur·al rest·ing po·si·tion (pos'chŭr-ăl pŏ-zish'ŏn, rest'ing) SYN rest position.

pos·tur·al re·flex (pos'chŭr-ăl rē'fleks) Responses that control the position of the trunk and extremities. SEE righting reflexes. SYN static reflexes (1).

pos·tu·ral sway re·sponse (pos'chŭr-ăl swā rĕ-spons') The body sway induced by vestibular stimulation.

pos·tur·al syn·co·pe (pos'chŭr-ăl sing'kŏ-pē) Syncope on assuming an upright position; caused by failure of normal vasoconstrictive mechanisms.

pos·tur·al trem·or (pos'chŭr-ăl trem'ŏr) Tremor present when the limbs or trunk are kept in certain positions and when they are moved actively, usually due to near-synchronous rhythmic bursts in opposing muscle groups.

pos·tur·al ver·ti·go (pos'chŭr-ăl vĕr'ti-gō) **1.** SYN benign positional vertigo. **2.** Light-headedness that appears particularly in elderly people with change of position, usually from lying or sitting to standing; due to orthostatic hypotension.

pos·ture (pos'chŭr) Position of limbs or carriage of the body as a whole.

pos·ture sense (pos'chŭr sens) The ability to recognize the position in which a limb is passively placed, with the eyes closed. SYN position sense.

post·vac·ci·nal en·ceph·a·lo·my·e·li·tis, post·vac·ci·nal en·ceph·a·li·tis (pōst-vak'sĕ-năl en-sef'a-lō-mī'ĕ-lī-tis, en-sef'ă-lī'tis) A severe type of encephalomyelitis that can follow a rabies vaccination.

post·val·var, post·val·vu·lar (pōst-val'văr, -val'vyū-lăr) Relating to a posi-

tion distal to the pulmonary or aortic valves.

po·ta·ble (pō'tă-bĕl) Drinkable; fit to drink.

Po·tain sign (pō-tan[h]' sīn) In dilation of the aorta, dullness on percussion extending from the manubrium sterni toward the second intercostal space and the third costal cartilage on the right.

po·tas·si·um (K) (pŏ-tas'ē-ŭm) An alkaline metallic element, occurring abundantly in nature but always in combination; its salts are used medicinally.

po·tas·si·um 39 (pŏ-tas'ē-ŭm) Most abundant, nonradioactive isotope of potassium; accounts for 93.1% of natural potassium.

po·tas·si·um bi·tar·trate (pŏ-tas'ē-ŭm bī-tahr'trāt) A diuretic and laxative. SYN cream of tartar, potassium acid tartrate.

po·tas·si·um chlo·ride (KCl) (pŏ-tas'ē-ŭm klōr'īd) Agent used to correct potassium deficiency.

po·tas·si·um cit·rate (pŏ-tas'ē-ŭm sit'rāt) Deliquescent powder, soluble in water; used as a diuretic, diaphoretic, expectorant, and systemic and urinary alkalizer. SYN Rivière salt.

po·tas·si·um ni·trate (pŏ-tas'ē-ŭm nīt'rāt) Agent sometimes used as a diuretic and diaphoretic; formerly it was included in asthmatic powders containing stramonium leaves.

po·tas·si·um per·man·ga·nate (pŏ-tas'ē-ŭm pĕr-mang'gă-nāt) Strong oxidizing agent used in solution as an antiseptic and deodorizing application for malodorous lesions; also used as a fixative.

po·tas·si·um phos·phate (pŏ-tas'ē-ŭm fos'fāt) Mild saline cathartic and diuretic. SYN dibasic potassium phosphate, dipotassium phosphate.

po·tas·si·um-spar·ing di·u·ret·ics (pŏ-tas'ē-ŭm spār'ing dī'yūr-et'iks) Agents that retain potassium; used to treat hypertension and congestive heart failure.

po·ten·cy (pō'tĕn-sē) **1.** Power, force, or

po·tent (pō'tĕnt) **1.** Possessing force, power, strength. **2.** Specifically, sexual potency. **3.** In therapeutics, the relative pharmacologic activity of a dose of a compound compared with the dose of a different agent producing the same effects.

po·tent (pō'tĕnt) **1.** Possessing force, power, strength. **2.** Indicating the ability of a primordial cell to differentiate. **3.** Possessing sexual potency.

po·ten·tial (pŏ-ten'shăl) **1.** Capable of doing or being, although not yet doing or being. **2.** A state of tension in an electric source enabling it to do work under suitable conditions.

po·ten·tial a·cu·i·ty me·ter (pŏ-ten'shăl ă-kyū'i-tē mē'tĕr) Instrument used to project an image such as Snellen test types through a cataractous lens onto the retina to predict likely visual function if the cataract were removed.

po·ten·ti·al di·ag·no·sis (pŏ-ten'shăl dī'ăg-nō'sis) NURSING health problem that may occur because of presence of certain risk factors.

po·ten·tial en·er·gy (pŏ-ten'shăl en'ĕr-jē) The energy, existing in a body by virtue of its position or state of existence, which is not being exerted at the time.

po·ten·ti·a·tion (pŏ-ten'shē-ā'shŭn) Interaction between two or more drugs or agents resulting in a pharmacologic response greater than the sum of individual responses.

po·ten·ti·om·e·ter (pŏ-ten'shē-om'ĕ-tĕr) **1.** An instrument used for measuring small differences in electrical potential. **2.** An electrical resistor of fixed total resistance between two terminals, but with a third terminal attached to a slider that can make contact at any desired point along the resistance.

po·tion (pō'shŭn) A draft or large dose of liquid medicine.

Pott ab·scess (pot ab'ses) Tuberculous abscess of the spine.

Pot·ter fa·cies (pot'ĕr fash'ēz) Characteristic facies seen in bilateral renal agenesis and other severe renal malformations, exhibiting ocular hypertelorism, low-set ears, receding chin, and flattening of the nose.

Pot·ter syn·drome (pot'ĕr sin'drōm) Renal agenesis with hypoplastic lungs and associated neonatal respiratory distress, hemodynamic instability, acidosis, cyanosis, edema, and characteristic (Potter) facies; death usually occurs from respiratory insufficiency, which develops before uremia.

Pott frac·ture (pot frak'shŭr) Break in the lower part of the fibula and of the malleolus of the tibia, with lateral displacement of the foot.

Pott pa·ra·ple·gi·a (pot par'ă-plē'jē-ă) Paralysis of the lower part of the body and the extremities, due to pressure on the spinal cord as the result of tuberculous spondylitis.

Potts clamp (pots klamp) A fine-toothed, multiple-point, vascular fixation clamp that imparts limited trauma to the vessel while securely holding it.

Potts op·er·a·tion (pots op-ĕr-ā'shŭn) Direct side-to-side anastomosis between aorta and pulmonary artery as a palliative procedure in congenital malformation of the heart.

pouch cul·ture (powch kŭl'chŭr) Plastic culture system used for transport of specimens for the isolation, growth, and detection of *Trichomonas vaginalis*.

pouch·i·tis (powch-ī'tis) Acute inflammation of the mucosa of an ileal reservoir or pouch that has been surgically created, usually following total colectomy for inflammatory bowel disease or multiple polyposis.

pouch of Doug·las (POD) (dŭg'lăs powch) SYN rectouterine pouch.

pou·drage (pū-drahzh') Powdering.

poul·tice (pōl'tis) A soft magma or mush prepared by wetting various powders or other absorbent substances with oily or watery fluids, sometimes medicated, and usually applied hot to the surface.

pound (pownd) A unit of weight, containing 12 ounces (apothecaries' weight) or 16 ounces (avoirdupois).

po·vi·done (pō'vi-dōn) A synthetic polymer used as a dispersing and suspending agent. SYN polyvidone, polyvinylpyr-rolidone.

po·vi·done i·o·dine (pō′vi-dōn ī′ō-dīn) A water complex of iodine with polyvinylpyrrolidone. Applied as an antiseptic in the form of solutions or ointments, it releases iodine. Used in cleaning and disinfecting the skin, preparing the skin preoperatively, and treating infections susceptible to iodine. SYN polyvinylpyrrolidone-iodine complex.

pox (poks) An eruptive disease, usually qualified by a descriptive prefix; e.g., smallpox, cowpox, chickenpox.

Pox·vir·i·dae (poks-vir′i-dē) A family of large complex viruses, with a marked affinity for skin tissue, which are pathogenic for humans and other animals.

pox·vi·rus (poks′vī-rŭs) Any virus of the family Poxviridae.

ppm Abbreviation for parts per million.

PPPPPP A mnemonic designating the symptom complex of acute arterial occlusion (*p*ain, *p*allor, *p*araesthesia, *p*ulselessness, *p*aralysis, *p*rostration).

prac·tice (prak′tis) **1.** Direct professional involvement in health care services. **2.** Rehearsal of a task or skill with the goal of achieving proficiency.

prac·ti·tion·er (prak-tish′ŭn-ĕr) A person who practices medicine or one of the allied health care professions.

Pra·der-Wil·li syn·drome (prah′dĕr-vē′lē sin′drōm) A congenital syndrome characterized by severe obesity, mental retardation, small hands and feet, and small genitalia.

♻ **prae-** SEE pre-.

praecordia [Br.] SYN precordia.

praecordial [Br.] SYN precordial.

praecordial leads [Br.] SYN precordial leads.

praecordium [Br.] SYN precordium.

praenaris [Br.] SYN prenaris.

praenasal [Br.] SYN prenasal.

prag·mat·ics (prag-mat′iks) **1.** LINGUISTICS the set of rules that govern the use of language in context, including social conventions. **2.** The effects of social setting and environment on language.

prag·ma·tism (prag′mă-tizm) Philosophy emphasizing practical applications and consequences of beliefs and theories, that the meaning of ideas is determined by the testability of the idea in real life.

Prague ma·neu·ver (prahg mă-nū′vĕr) A technique for delivery of the fetus in breech position when the fetal occiput is posterior.

pran·di·al (pran′dē-ăl) Relating to a meal.

prax·i·ol·o·gy (prak′sē-ol′ŏ-jē) The study of behavior; excludes the study of consciousness and nonobjective metaphysical concepts.

prax·is (prak′sis) OCCUPATIONAL THERAPY conception and planning of a motor act in response to an environmental demand.

♻ **pre-** Combining form denoting anterior; before (in time or space). SEE ALSO ante-, pro- (1).

pre·ag·o·nal (prē-ag′ŏ-năl) Immediately preceding death.

pre·a·nal (prē-ā′năl) Anterior to the anus.

pre·au·ric·u·lar (prē′aw-rik′yū-lăr) Anterior to the auricle of the ear; denoting lymphatic nodes so situated.

pre·ax·i·al (prē-ak′sē-ăl) **1.** Anterior to the axis of the body or a limb. **2.** Denoting the portion of a limb bud that lies cranial to the axis of the limb.

pre·bi·ot·ics (prē′bī-ot′iks) Nondigestible food ingredients that select targeted groups of the human colonic microflora.

pre·can·cer·ous (prē-kan′sĕr-ŭs) Pertaining to any lesion that is interpreted as precancer. SYN premalignant.

pre·car·di·ac (prē-kahr′dē-ak) Anterior to the heart.

pre·cen·tral (prē-sen′trăl) Referring to the cerebral convolution immediately anterior to the central sulcus.

pre·cer·ti·fi·ca·tion (prē-sĕr'ti-fi-kā'shŭn) Verification of a procedure as a covered benefit for a third-party payer before a health care service is performed. It does not guarantee coverage.

pre·ces·sion (prē-sesh'ŭn) The secondary spin of magnetic movements around the main magnetic field.

pre·chor·dal, pro·chor·dal (prē-kōr'dăl, prō-) Located cephalic to the notochord. SYN prochordal.

pre·cip·i·tant (prē-sip'i-tănt) Anything causing a precipitation from a solution.

pre·cip·i·tate (prē-sip'i-tāt, -tăt) 1. To cause a substance in solution to separate as a solid. 2. A solid separated from a solution or suspension; a clump. 3. Accumulation of inflammatory cells on the corneal endothelium in uveitis.

pre·cip·i·tat·ed sul·fur (prē-sip'i-tā-tĕd sŭl'fŭr) Sulfur boiled with lime water, the lime being removed from the precipitate by washing with diluted hydrochloric acid; used in preparing sulfur ointment and in skin disorders. SYN lac sulfuris, milk of sulfur.

pre·cip·i·tate la·bor (prē-sip'i-tăt lā'bŏr) Very rapid labor ending in delivery of the fetus.

pre·cip·i·ta·tion (prē-sip'i-tā'shŭn) 1. The process of formation of a solid previously held in solution or suspension in a liquid. 2. The phenomenon of clumping of proteins in serum produced by the addition of a specific precipitin. SEE ALSO precipitate.

pre·cip·i·tin (P) (prē-sip'i-tin) An antibody that under suitable conditions combines with and causes its specific and soluble antigen to precipitate from solution. SYN precipitating antibody.

pre·cip·i·tin·o·gen, pre·cip·i·to·gen (prē-sip'i-tin'ō-jen, -sip'i-tō-jen) 1. An antigen that stimulates the formation of specific precipitin when injected into an animal body. 2. A precipitable soluble antigen.

pre·cip·i·tin test (prē-sip'i-tin test) An in vitro procedure in which antigen is in soluble form and precipitates when it combines with added specific antibody in the presence of an electrolyte. SEE ALSO gel diffusion precipitin tests.

pre·ci·sion at·tach·ment (prē-si'zhŭn ă-tach'mĕnt) 1. Frictional or mechanically retained unit used in fixed or removable prosthodontics. 2. Attachment that may be rigid in function or may incorporate a movable stress control unit to reduce the torque on the abutment. SYN frictional attachment, internal attachment, key attachment, keyway attachment, parallel attachment, slotted attachment.

pre·clin·i·cal (prē-klin'i-kăl) 1. Before the onset of disease. 2. A period in medical education before the student becomes involved with patients and clinical work.

pre·co·cious (prē-kō'shŭs) Developing unusually early or rapidly.

pre·co·cious pseu·do·pu·ber·ty (prē-kō'shŭs sū'dō-pyū'bĕr-tē) Development of pseudopuberty in very young children; commonly characterized by secretion of gonadal hormones, without stimulation of gametogenesis.

pre·co·cious pu·ber·ty (prē-kō'shŭs pyū'bĕr-tē) Condition in which pubertal changes begin at an unexpectedly early age.

pre·cog·ni·tion (prē'kog-nish'ŭn) Advance knowledge, by means other than the normal senses, of a future event; a form of extrasensory perception.

pre·con·cep·tu·al stage (prē'kŏn-sĕp'shū-ăl stāj) In psychology, stage of development in an infant's life, before actual conceptual thinking begins, in which sensorimotor activity predominates.

pre·con·scious (prē-kon'shŭs) PSYCHOANALYSIS one of the three divisions of the psyche, the other two being the conscious and unconscious; includes all ideas, thoughts, past experiences, and other memory impressions that with effort can be consciously recalled.

pre·con·vul·sive (prē'kŏn-vŭl'siv) Denoting the stage in an epileptic paroxysm preceding convulsions (e.g., aura).

pre·cor·di·a (prē-kōr'dē-ă) The epigastrium and anterior surface of the lower part of the thorax. SYN praecordia.

P

pre·cor·di·al (PC) (prē-kōr′dē-ăl) Relating to the precordia.

pre·cor·di·al leads (prē-kōr′dē-ăl lēdz) SYN chest leads, praecordial leads.

pre·cor·di·um (prē-kōr′dē-ŭm) Singular of precordia. SYN praecordium.

pre·cos·tal (prē-kos′tăl) Before the ribs.

pre·cur·sor (prē′kŭrs-ŏr) That which precedes another or from which another is derived.

pre·Des·ce·met cor·ne·al dys·tro·phy (prē′des-ĕ-mā′ kōr′nē-ăl dis′trŏ-fē) Opacification with primary involvement of the posterior stroma of the cornea.

pre·di·a·be·tes (prē′dī-ă-bē′tēz) A state of potential diabetes mellitus, with normal glucose tolerance but with an increased risk of developing Type 2 diabetes.

pre·di·as·to·le (prē′dī-as′tŏ-lē) The interval in the cardiac rhythm immediately preceding diastole. SYN late systole.

pre·di·crot·ic (prē′dī-krot′ĭk) Preceding the dicrotic notch.

pre·dic·tive va·li·di·ty (prē-dik′tiv vă-lid′ĭ-tē) Criterion-related standard used to predict performance in a real-life task at a future time. SEE construct validity.

pre·di·ges·tion (prē′dī-jes′chŭn) The artificial initiation of digestion of proteins (proteolysis) and starches (amylolysis) before they are eaten.

pre·dis·pos·ing cause (prē′dis-pōz′ing kawz) Anything that produces a disposition to a condition without actually eliciting it.

pre·dis·po·si·tion (prē′dis′pō-zish′ŭn) A condition of special susceptibility to a disease.

pred·nis·o·lone (pred-nis′ŏ-lōn) A dehydrogenated glucocorticoid analogue of cortisol with the same actions and uses.

pred·ni·sone (pred′ni-sōn) A dehydrogenated analogue of cortisone with the same actions and uses; must be converted to prednisolone before active; inhibits proliferation of lymphocytes.

pre·do·na·ted au·tol·o·gous blood (prē-dō′nā-tĕd aw-tol′ŏ-gŭs blŭd) That donated before a surgical procedure that might involve blood loss by the patient who is going to undergo the procedure.

pre·e·clamp·si·a (prē′ĕ-klamp′sē-ă) Development of hypertension with proteinuria or edema, or both, due to pregnancy or the influence of a recent pregnancy.

pre·ex·ci·ta·tion (prē′ek-sī-tā′shŭn) Premature activation of part of the ventricular myocardium by an impulse that travels by an anomalous path and so avoids physiologic delay in the atrioventricular junction.

pre·ex·ci·ta·tion synd·rome (prē′ek-sī-tā′shŭn sin′drōm) SYN Wolff-Parkinson-White syndrome.

pre·ex·is·ting con·di·tion (prē′eg-zist′ing kŏn-dish′ŭn) A health problem that existed or for which treatment was received before the effective date of a policy from new insurance company.

pre·fer·red pro·vid·er or·gan·i·za·tion (PPO) (prē-fĕrd′ prŏ-vī′dĕr ōr′găn-ī-zā′shŭn) A U.S. health care organization that negotiates set rates of reimbursement with participating health care providers for services to insured clients. SEE ALSO health maintenance organization.

pre·fron·tal (prē-frŏn′tăl) 1. Denoting the anterior portion of the frontal lobe of the cerebrum. 2. Denoting the granular frontal cortex rostral to the premotor area.

pre·fron·tal lo·bo·to·my (prē-frŭn′tăl lō-bot′ŏ-mē) Division of one or more nerve tracts in the prefrontal area of the brain for surgical treatment of pain and emotional disorder. SYN prefrontal leukotomy.

pre·gan·gli·on·ic (prē′gang-glē-on′ĭk) Situated proximal to or preceding a ganglion.

preg·nan·cy (preg′năn-sē) The state of a female after conception and until the termination of the gestation. SYN gestation.

preg·nane (preg′nān) Parent hydrocarbon of the progesterones, pregnane alcohols, ketones, and several adrenocortical hormones.

preg·nane·di·ol (preg′năn-dī′ol) Chief steroid metabolite of progesterone that is biologically inactive and occurs as pregnanediol glucuronate in the urine.

preg·nane·tri·ol (preg′năn-trī′ol) A urinary metabolite of 17-hydroxyprogesterone and a precursor in the biosynthesis of cortisol; its excretion is enhanced in certain diseases of the cortex of the suprarenal gland and following administration of corticotropin.

preg·nant (preg′nănt) Denoting a gestating female. SYN gravid.

preg·nen·o·lone (Pg, Pe) (preg-nēn′ō-lōn) A steroid that serves as an intermediate in the biosynthesis of numerous hormones, including progesterone.

pre·hal·lux (prē-hal′ŭks) A supernumerary digit, usually only partial, attached to the medial border of the great toe.

pre·hen·sile (prē-hen′sil) Adapted for taking hold of or grasping.

pre·hen·sion (prē-hen′shŭn) The act of grasping, or taking hold of.

pre·hor·mone (prē-hōr′mōn) A glandular secretory product, having little or no inherent biologic potency, which is converted peripherally to an active hormone. Cf. prohormone.

pre·hos·pi·tal care (prē-hos′pi-tăl kār) Assessment, stabilization, and care of a medical emergency or trauma victim, including transport to the appropriate receiving facility.

pre·hos·pi·tal care re·port (prē-hos′pi-tăl kār rĕ-pōrt′) An electronic or written report completed by a prehospital provider that contains demographic and medical information as well as a record of the treatment and transport of a patient. A copy of the prehospital care report often is left at the receiving facility as a medical reference and for inclusion in the patient's medical record.

pre·hy·per·ten·sion (prē-hī′pĕr-ten′-shŭn) Classification from *The Seventh Report of the Joint National Committee on Prevention, Detection, Evaluation, and Treatment of High Blood Pressure* for blood pressure systolic reading of 120–139 mmHg and diastolic reading of 80–89 mmHg. Blood pressure in this range warrants management to prevent progression to hypertension.

pre·ic·tal (prē-ik′tăl) Occurring before a seizure or stroke.

pre·in·duc·tion (prē′in-dŭk′shŭn) A modification in the third generation due to environmental action on the germ cells of one or both individuals of the grandparental generation.

pre·in·va·sive (prē′in-vā′siv) Denotes to a stage of cancer when the cells have not spread beyond their original location.

pre·kal·li·kre·in (prē′kal-i-krē′in) A plasma glycoprotein that in complex with kininogen serves as a cofactor in the activation of factor XII. Prekallikrein also serves as the proenzyme for plasma kallikrein. SYN Fletcher factor.

pre·lim·bic (prē-lim′bik) Anterior to the limbus of the fossa ovalis.

pre·load (prē′lōd) The load to which a muscle is subjected before shortening.

pre·log·i·cal think·ing (prē-loj′ik-ăl thingk′ing) A concrete type of thinking, characteristic of children and primitives, to which schizophrenic people sometimes regress.

pre·ma·lig·nant (prē′mă-lig′nănt) SYN precancerous.

pre·ma·ture (prē′mă-chūr) 1. Occurring before the usual or expected time. 2. Denoting an infant born less than 37 weeks (8-1/2 months) after conception.

pre·ma·ture alo·pe·ci·a, alo·pe·ci·a pre·ma·tu·ra (prē′mă-chūr′ al′ō-pē′shē-ă, pre-mă-tū′răˇ) Male pattern baldness appearing at an unusually early age.

pre·ma·ture a·tri·al con·trac·tion (prē′mă-chūr′ ā′trē-ăl kŏn-trak′shŭn) A premature cardiac beat arising from an ectopic atrial focus.

pre·ma·ture birth, pre·ma·ture de·liv·er·y (prē′mă-chūr′ bĭrth, dĕ-liv′er-ē) Birth of an infant after viability has been achieved with gestation of at least 20 weeks or birth weight of at least 500 g, but before 37 weeks.

pre·ma·ture e·jac·u·la·tion (prē′mă-chŭr′ ē-jak′yū-lā′shŭn) During sexual intercourse, too rapid achievement of climax and ejaculation in the male relative to his own or his partner's wishes.

pre·ma·ture junc·tion·al con·trac·tion (prē′mă-chŭr′ jungk′shŭn-ăl kŏn-trak′shŭn) A premature cardiac beat arising from the atrioventricular junction, accompanied by normal or abnormal QRS complexes.

pre·ma·ture la·bor (prē′mă-chŭr′ lā′bŏr) Onset of labor after 20 weeks' gestation and before the 37th completed week of pregnancy dated from the last normal menstrual period.

pre·ma·ture mem·brane rup·ture (prē′mă-chŭr′ mem′brān rŭp′chŭr) Break in membranes before onset of labor.

pre·ma·ture men·o·pause (prē′mă-chŭr′ men′ŏ-pawz) Failure of cyclic ovarian function before age 40.

pre·ma·ture rup·ture of mem·branes (prē′mă-chŭr′ rŭp′chŭr mem′brănz) Rupture of the amnionic sac before onset of labor.

pre·ma·ture ven·tri·cu·lar con·trac·tion (prē′mă-chŭr′ ven-trik′yū-lăr kŏn-trak′shŭn) Compression within the lower cardiac chambers.

pre·ma·tu·ri·ty (prē′mă-chŭr′i-tē) 1. The state of being premature. 2. DENTISTRY deflective occlusal contact.

pre·max·il·la (prē′mak-sil′ă) Central isolated bony part in a complete bilateral cleft of the lip.

pre·max·il·lar·y (pre-mak′si-lar′ē) 1. Anterior to the maxilla. 2. Denoting the premaxilla.

pre·med·i·ca·tion (prē′med-i-kā′shŭn) Administration of drugs before induction of general anesthesia to allay apprehension, produce sedation, and facilitate administration of anesthetic.

pre·men·ar·chal (prē′men-ahr′kăl) Denotes the time period before the onset of menstrual cycles.

pre·men·o·pau·sal (prē-men′ŏ-paw′zăl) Pertaining to the time prior to onset of menopause, sometimes called perimenopause.

pre·men·stru·al (prē-men′strū-ăl) Relating to the period of time preceding menstruation.

pre·men·stru·al dys·phor·ic dis·or·der (prē-men′strū-ăl dis-fōr′ik dis-ōr′dĕr) A pervasive pattern occurring during the last week of the luteal phase in most menstrual cycles for at least a year and remitting within a few days of the onset of the follicular phase, with some combination of depressed mood, mood lability, marked anxiety, or irritability; various specific physical symptoms; and significant functional impairment; the symptoms are comparable in severity to those seen in a major depressive episode, distinguishing this disorder from the far more common premenstrual syndrome. SEE ALSO premenstrual syndrome.

pre·men·stru·al syn·drome (PMS) (prē-men′strū-ăl sin′drōm) In some women of reproductive age, the regular monthly experience of physiologic and emotional distress, usually during the several days preceding menses; characterized by nervousness, depression, fluid retention, and weight gain. SYN late luteal phase dysphoria, menstrual molimina, premenstrual tension.

pre·mo·lar (prē-mō′lăr) 1. Anterior to a molar tooth. 2. Denotes permanent teeth that replace the deciduous molars.

pre·mo·lar tooth (prē-mō′lăr tūth) [TA] A tooth usually having two tubercles or cusps on the grinding surface and a flattened root, single in the lower jaw and upper second premolar, and furrowed in the upper first premolar. There are four premolars in each jaw. SYN dens premolaris [TA], bicuspid tooth, dens bicuspidus.

pre·mo·ni·tion (prem′ŏ-nish′ŭn) A feeling about impending event, generally of dire significance.

pre·mon·o·cyte (prē-mon′ō-sīt) An immature monocyte normally not seen in the circulating blood.

pre·mor·bid (prē-mōr′bid) Preceding the occurrence of disease.

pre·mo·tor a·re·a (prē-mō′tŏr ăr′ē-ă) SYN premotor cortex.

pre·mo·tor cortex (pre-mō′tŏr kōr′teks) Somewhat vague term usually referring to the agranular cortex of Brodmann area 6. SYN premotor area.

pre·mu·ni·tion (prē′myū-nish′ŭn) Extant resistance of a host to infection or reinfection with a parasite.

pre·my·e·lo·blast (prē-mī′ĕ-lō-blast) The earliest recognizable precursor of the myeloblast.

pre·na·ris, pl. **pre·na·res** (prē-nā′ris, -rēz) SYN nostril, praenaris.

pre·na·sal (prē-nā′zăl) In front of the nose. SYN praenasal.

pre·na·tal (prē-nā′tăl) Preceding birth.

pre·na·tal di·ag·no·sis (prē-nā′tăl dī′ăg-nō′sis) That using procedures available for the recognition of diseases and malformations in utero, and the conclusion reached.

pre·ne·o·plas·tic (prē-nē′ō-plas′tik) Preceding the formation of any neoplasm, benign or malignant.

pre·op·tic (prē-op′tik) Referring to the preoptic region.

pre·ox·y·gen·a·tion (prē′ok-si-jĕ-nā′shŭn) Denitrogenation with 100% oxygen before induction of general anesthesia or endotracheal intubation.

pre·pa·tel·lar (prē′pă-tel′ăr) Anterior to the patella.

pre·pa·tel·lar bur·si·tis (prē-pă-tel′ăr bŭr-sī′tis) SYN housemaid's knee.

pre·pa·tent pe·ri·od (prē-pā′tĕnt pēr′ē-ŏd) PARASITOLOGY the interval to the incubation period of microbial infections; it varies biologically, however, because the parasite undergoes developmental stages in the host.

pre·per·i·to·ne·al (prē′per-i-tŏ-nē′ăl) Denoting a fatty layer between the peritoneum and the transversalis fascia in the lower anterior abdominal wall.

pre·pran·di·al (prē-pran′dē-ăl) Before eating.

pre·pro·in·su·lin (prē′prō-in′sŭ-lin) The precursor protein to proinsulin. SEE preprotein.

pre·pro·tein (prē′prō-prō′tēn) A precursor to an inactive secretory proprotein.

pre·psy·chot·ic (prē′sī-kot′ik) **1.** Relating to the period before the onset of psychosis. **2.** Denoting potential for an imminent psychotic episode.

pre·pu·ber·al, pre·pu·ber·tal (prē-pyū′bĕr-ăl, -bĕr-tăl) Before puberty.

pre·pu·bes·cent (prē-pyū-bes′ĕnt) Immediately before the commencement of puberty.

pre·puce (prē′pyūs) [TA] The free fold of skin that covers the glans penis more or less completely. SYN preputium [TA], foreskin.

pre·pu·ti·al (prē-pyū′shē-ăl) Relating to the prepuce.

pre·pu·ti·ot·o·my (prē-pyū′shē-ot′ŏ-mē) Incision of prepuce.

pre·pu·ti·um (prē-pyū′shē-ŭm) [TA] SYN prepuce.

pre·py·lor·ic (prē′pī-lōr′ik) Anterior to or preceding the pylorus; denoting a temporary constriction of the wall of the stomach separating the fundus from the antrum during digestion.

pre·re·nal (prē-rē′năl) Anterior to a kidney.

pre·sa·cral (prē-sā′krăl) Anterior to or preceding the sacrum.

pre·sa·cral neu·rec·to·my, pre·sa·cral sym·pa·thec·to·my (prē-sā′krăl nŭr-ek′tŏ-mē, sim′pă-thek′tŏ-mē) Cutting the presacral nerve to relieve severe dysmenorrhea. SYN Cotte operation, presacral sympathectomy.

presby-, presbyo- Combining forms denoting old age. SEE ALSO gero-.

pres·by·car·di·a (prez′bē-kahr′dē-ă) Abnormal cardiac condition due to old age, hallmarked by decreased functional capacity.

pres·by·cu·sis (prez′bē-kyū′sis) SYN presbyacusis.

pres·by·o·pi·a (Pr) (prez′bē-ō′pē-ă) The physiologic loss of accommodation in the eyes in advancing age, said to begin when the near point has receded beyond 22 cm (9 inches).

pres·by·op·ic (prez′bē-op′ik) Relating to or suffering from presbyopia.

pre·scribe (prĕ-skrīb′) To give directions, either orally or in writing, for the preparation and administration of a remedy to be used to treat a disease.

pre·scrip·tion (prĕ-skrip′shŭn) **1.** A written formula for the preparation and administration of any remedy. **2.** A medicinal preparation compounded according to formulated directions, consisting of four parts: 1) superscription, consisting of the word *recipe*, take, or its sign, ℞; 2) inscription, the main part of the prescription, containing the names and amounts of the drugs ordered; 3) subscription, directions for mixing the ingredients and designation of the form (pill, powder, solution) in which the drug is to be made; 4) signature, directions to the patient regarding the dose and times of taking the remedy. SEE prescribe.

pre·se·nile de·men·ti·a, de·men·ti·a pre·se·ni·lis (PSD) (prē-sen′il dĕ-men′shē-ă, prē-sē-nā′lis) **1.** Dementia of Alzheimer disease developing before age 65. **2.** SYN Alzheimer disease.

pre·se·nil·i·ty (prē′sĕ-nil′i-tē) Premature old age; condition of someone, not old in years, who displays physical and mental characteristics of old age but not senility.

pre·sen·ta·tion (prez′ĕn-tā′shŭn) That part of the fetus presenting at the superior aperture of the maternal pelvis. SEE ALSO position (3).

pre·sent·ing symp·tom (prē-zent′ing simp′tŏm) Complaint offered by the patient as the main reason for seeking medical care; usually synonymous with chief complaint.

pre·sep·tal cel·lu·li·tis (prē-sep′tăl sel′yū-lī′tis) Infection involving the superficial tissue and periocular layers anterior to the orbital septum.

pre·ser·va·tive (prē-zĕr′vă-tiv) A substance added to food products to prevent chemical change or bacterial action.

pre·sphe·noid (prē-sfē′noyd) In front of the sphenoid bone or cartilage.

pres·sor (pres′ŏr) Exciting to vasomotor activity; producing increased blood pressure; denoting afferent nerve fibers that, when stimulated, excite vasoconstrictors, which increase peripheral resistance. SYN hypertensor.

pres·so·re·cep·tive (pres′ō-rĕ-sep′tiv) Capable of detecting or responding to changes in pressure, especially changes of blood pressure.

pres·sor fi·bers (pres′ŏr fī′bĕrz) Sensory nerve fibers with stimulation that causes vasoconstriction and raises blood pressure.

pres·sor nerve (pres′ŏr nĕrv) Afferent nerve, developing a reflex vasoconstriction, during stimulation; raises blood pressure.

pres·sure (presh′ŭr) **1.** A stress or force acting in any direction against resistance. **2.** PHYSICS, PHYSIOLOGY the force per unit area exerted by a gas or liquid against the walls of its container or that would be exerted on a wall immersed at that spot in the middle of a body of fluid.

pres·sure con·trolled ven·ti·la·tion (presh′ŭr kŏn-trōld′ ven′ti-la′shŭn) A mode of mechanical ventilation in which the ventilator delivers a preset pressure waveform.

pres·sure dres·sing (presh′ŭr dres′ing) A bandage that exerts pressure on the area covered to prevent the collection of fluids in the underlying tissues.

pres·sure e·qual·i·za·tion tube (presh′ŭr ē′kwăl-ī-zā′shŭn tūb) A grommet placed through the tympanic membrane to provide continuous middle ear ventilation.

pres·sure pa·ral·y·sis (presh′ŭr păr-al′i-sis) Paralysis due to compression of a nerve, nerve trunk, or spinal cord.

pres·sure point (presh′ŭr poynt) Cutaneous locus with pressure-sensitive elements that, when compressed, produce a sensation of pressure.

pres·sure pulse dif·fer·en·ti·a·tion (presh'ŭr pŭls dif'ĕr-en'shē-ā'shŭn) The processing of a pressure pulse signal so that the output depends on the rate of change of the input.

pres·sure-reg·u·la·ted vol·ume con·trol (presh'ŭr-reg'yū-lā-tĕd vol'yūm kŏn-trōl') A mode of mechanical ventilation.

pres·sure re·ver·sal (presh'ŭr rĕ-vĕr'săl) Cessation of anesthesia by hyperbaric pressure.

pres·sure sense (presh'ŭr sens) The faculty of discriminating various degrees of pressure on the surface. SYN piesesthesia.

pres·sure sore (presh'ŭr sōr) SYN decubitus ulcer.

pres·sure sta·sis (presh'ŭr stā'sis) SYN traumatic asphyxia.

pres·sure sup·port ven·ti·la·tion (presh'ŭr sŭ-pōrt' ven'ti-lā'shŭn) A mode of mechanical ventilation in which pressure is limited and flow cycled.

pres·sure time in·dex (PTI) (presh'ŭr tīm in'deks) Calculation of the area under the diastolic component of the arterial blood pressure curve, used to determine left ventricular mass index and ventricular load in diastolic hypertension and chronic obstructive pulmonary disease.

pres·sure ul·cer (DECUB) (presh'ŭr ŭl'sĕr) SYN decubitus ulcer.

pres·sure ven·ti·la·tor (presh'ŭr ven'ti-lā-tŏr) A device designed to deliver pressure-controlled ventilation.

pres·sure-vol·ume in·dex (presh'ŭr-vol'yūm in'deks) Method of evaluating the cerebrospinal fluid hydrodynamics.

pre·sumed oc·u·lar his·to·plas·mo·sis (POH) (prē-zūmd' ok'yū-lăr his'tō-plaz-mō'sis) Subretinal neovascularization in the macular region associated with chorioretinal atrophy and pigment proliferation adjacent to the optic disc and peripheral chorioretinal atrophy ("histo-spots").

pre·sump·tive signs of preg·nan·cy (prē-zŭmp'tiv sīnz preg'năn-sē) Signs and symptoms suggestive of pregnancy that may also indicate another condition; occur early and are more subjective; presumptive signs are amenorrhea, nausea and vomiting, frequent urination, and fatigue.

pre·syn·ap·tic (prē'si-nap'tik) Pertaining to the area on the proximal side of a synaptic cleft.

pre·sys·tol·ic (prē'sis-tol'ik) Late diastolic, relating to the interval immediately preceding systole.

pre·term in·fant, pre·term new·born (prē'tĕrm in'fănt, nū'bōrn) One with gestational age of more than 20 weeks and less than 37 completed weeks (259 completed days).

pre·term mem·brane rup·ture (prē'tĕrm mem'brān rŭp'chūr) Break in fetal membranes before term (less than 37 weeks' gestation).

pre·thy·roid, pre·thy·roi·de·al, pre·thy·roi·de·an (prē-thī'royd, -thī-roy'dē-ăl, -dē-ăn) Anterior to or preceding the thyroid gland or cartilage.

pre·tib·i·al (prē-tib'ē-ăl) Relating to the anterior portion of the leg; denoting especially certain muscles.

pre·tib·i·al fe·ver (prē-tib'ē-ăl fē'vĕr) A mild disease first observed among U.S. military personnel at Fort Bragg, NC, characterized by fever, moderate prostration, splenomegaly, and a rash on the anterior aspects of the legs. SYN Fort Bragg fever.

pre·treat·ment mor·bid·i·ty (prē-trēt'mĕnt mōr-bid'i-tē) The state of an illness and the degree of symptoms present immediately before the initiation of treatment.

prev·a·lence (prev'ă-lĕns) *Do not confuse this word with incidence.* The number of cases of a disease existing in a given population at a specific period of time (*period prevalence*) or at a particular moment in time (*point prevalence*).

pre·ver·te·bral (prē-ver'tĕ-brăl) Anterior to the body of a vertebra or of the vertebral column.

P

pre·ves·i·cal (prē-ves′i-kăl) Anterior to the bladder; denoting especially the retropubic space.

pre·vil·lous em·bry·o (prē-vil′ŭs em′ brē-ō) That of a placental mammal prior to the formation of chorionic villi.

pri·a·pism (prī′ă-pizm) Persistent erection of the penis, accompanied by pain and tenderness, resulting from a pathologic condition rather than sexual desire.

pri·a·pi·tis (prī′ă-pī′tis) Inflammation of the penis.

Price-Jones curve (prīs-jōnz kŭrv) A distribution curve of the measured diameters of red blood cells.

prick·le cell (prik′ĕl sel) One of the cells of the stratum spinosum of the epidermis.

prick·ly heat (prik′lē hēt) SYN miliaria rubra.

♻ **prim-, primi-** Combining forms meaning first.

pri·mal scene (prī′măl sēn) PSYCHOANALYSIS The actual or fantasized observation by a child of sexual intercourse, particularly between the child's parents.

pri·ma·quine phos·phate (prī′mă-kwin fos′fāt) An antimalarial agent especially effective against *Plasmodium vivax*; usually administered with chloroquine.

pri·mar·y (prī′mar-ē) 1. First or foremost, as a disease to which others may be secondary or complications. 2. Relating to the first stage of growth or development. SEE ALSO primordial.

pri·mar·y ad·he·sion (prī′mar-ē ad-hē′zhŭn) SYN healing by first intention.

pri·mar·y a·dre·no·cor·ti·cal in·suf·fi·cien·cy (prī′mar-ē ă-drē′nō-kōr′ti-kăl in′sŭ-fish′ĕn-sē) Adrenocortical insufficiency caused by disease, destruction, or surgical removal of the cortices of the suprarenal gland.

pri·mar·y al·dos·te·ron·ism (prī′mar-ē al-dos′tĕr-ōn-izm) An adrenocortical disorder caused by excessive secretion of aldosterone and characterized by head-aches, nocturia, polyuria, and other symptoms; may be associated with small, benign adrenocortical adenomas. SYN Conn syndrome, idiopathic aldosteronism.

pri·mar·y a·me·bic men·in·go·en·ceph·a·li·tis (prī′mar-ē ă-mē′bik mĕ-ning′gō-en-sef-ă-lī′tis) Invasive, rapidly fatal cerebral infection by soil amebae, chiefly *Naegleria fowleri*, found in humans and other primates and experimentally in rodents; characterized by a high fever, neck rigidity, and symptoms associated with upper respiratory infection such as cough and nausea; death usually occurs 2–3 days after onset of symptoms.

pri·mar·y a·men·or·rhe·a (prī′mar-ē ă-men′ŏr-ē′ă) Amenorrhea in which menses has never occurred.

pri·mar·y amyl·oi·do·sis (prī′mar-ē am′i-loy-dō′sis) Amyloidosis not associated with other recognized disease; tends to involve arterial walls and mesenchymal tissues in the tongue, lungs, intestinal tract, skin, skeletal muscle, and myocardium.

pri·mar·y an·es·thet·ic (prī′mar-ē an′es-thet′ik) Compound that contributes most to loss of sensation when a mixture of anesthetics is administered.

pri·mar·y at·e·lec·ta·sis (prī′mar-ē at′ĕ-lek′tă-sis) Nonexpansion of the lungs after birth, found in all stillborn infants and liveborn infants who die before respiration begins.

pri·mar·y a·typ·i·cal pneu·mo·ni·a (prī′mar-ē ā-tip′i-kăl nū-mō′nē-ă) An acute systemic disease with involvement of the lungs, caused by *Mycoplasma pneumoniae* marked by high fever, cough, and scattered densities on x-rays. SYN atypical pneumonia, mycoplasmal pneumonia.

pri·mar·y bil·i·ar·y cir·rho·sis (PBC) (prī′mar-ē bil′ē-ar-ē sir-ō′sis) Disease in middle-aged women, characterized by cholestasis with hyperlipemia, pruritus, and hyperpigmentation of the skin; serum antimitochondrial antibodies are present in 85–90% of patients. SYN Hanot cirrhosis.

pri·mar·y blast in·ju·ry (prī′mar-ē blast

in′jŭr-ē) Trauma largely to hollow and fluid-filled organs, caused by impact of an overpressure wave from a high-grade explosive.

pri·mar·y bron·chus (prī′mär-ē brong′kŭs) Main bronchus arising at the tracheal bifurcation extending into the developing embryonic.

pri·mar·y car·ci·no·ma (prī′mär-ē kahr′si-nō′mă) Cancer at the site of origin, with local invasion in that organ.

pri·mar·y care (prī′mar-ē kār) Continuing, comprehensive, and preventive health care services that are the first point of health care for a patient in an ambulatory setting.

pri·mar·y care phy·si·cian (prī′mar-ē kār fi-zish′ŭn) A physician in family practice, internal medicine, obstetrics/gynecology, or pediatrics who is a patient's first contact for health care in an ambulatory setting. SEE ALSO health care provider.

pri·ma·ry cil·i·ar·y dys·ki·ne·si·a (PCD) (prī′mar-ē sil′ē-ar-ē dis-ki-nē′zē-ă) Disorder in which mucus clearance is sluggish and bronchiectasis is prevalent and intractable. SYN dyskinesia syndrome.

pri·mar·y coc·cid·i·oi·do·my·co·sis (prī′mar-ē kok-sid′ē-oyd′ō-mī-kō′sis) A disease caused by inhalation of the arthroconidia of *Coccidioides immitis;* acute onset of respiratory symptoms accompanied by fever, aches, malaise, arthralgia, headache, and occasionally an early erythematous or papular eruption. SYN desert fever, San Joaquin Valley disease, San Joaquin Valley fever, valley fever.

pri·mar·y com·plex (prī′mar-ē kom′pleks) The typical lesions of primary pulmonary tuberculosis, consisting of a small peripheral focus of infection, with hilar or paratracheal lymph node involvement.

pri·ma·ry cur·va·ture of ver·te·bral col·umn (prī′mar-ē kŭr′vă-chŭr vĕr′tĕ-brăl kol′ŭm) [TA] Ventrally concave curve of the fetal vertebral column, retained in the thoracic and sacral regions as thoracic and sacral kyphoses. SEE

ALSO kyphosis. SYN curvatura primaria columnae vertebralis [TA].

pri·mar·y den·tin (prī′mar-ē den′tin) Dentin that forms until the root is completed.

pri·mar·y den·ti·tion (prī′mar-ē den′tish′ŭn) SYN deciduous tooth.

pri·mar·y de·vi·a·tion (prī′mar-ē dē′vē-ā′shŭn) The ocular deviation seen in paralysis of an ocular muscle when the nonparalyzed eye is used for fixation.

pri·mar·y di·ges·tion (prī′mar-ē di-jes′chŭn) Digestion in the alimentary tract.

pri·mar·y dis·ease (prī′mar-ē di-zēz′) A disorder that arises spontaneously and not associated with or caused by a previous disease, or event; may lead to secondary disease.

pri·mar·y dys·men·or·rhe·a (prī′mar-ē dis-men′ŏr-ē′ă) Condition due to a functional disturbance and not inflammation, new growth, or anatomic factors. SYN essential dysmenorrhea, functional dysmenorrhea, intrinsic dysmenorrhea.

pri·mar·y fis·sure of cer·e·bel·lum (prī′mar-ē fish′ŭr ser′ĕ-bel′ŭm) [TA] The deepest fissure of the cerebellum.

pri·mar·y gain (prī′mar-ē gān) Interpersonal or financial advantages from conversion of emotional stress directly into demonstrably organic illness. Cf. secondary gain.

pri·mar·y hem·or·rhage (prī′mar-ē hem′ŏr-ăj) Bleeding immediately after injury or operation.

pri·mar·y im·mune re·sponse (prī′mar-ē i-myūn′ rĕ-spons′) SEE immune response.

pri·mar·y lat·er·al scle·ro·sis (prī′mar-ē lat′ĕr-ăl skler-ō′sis) Considered by many to be a subtype of motor neuron disease; a slowly progressive degenerative disorder of the motor neurons of the cerebral cortex, resulting in widespread weakness on an upper motor neuron basis.

pri·mar·y nurs·ing (prī′mar-ē nŭrs′ing) A method of providing nursing services to inpatients whereby one nurse plans the

P

care of specific patients for a period of 24 hours; provides direct care to those patients when working; responsible for directing and supervising their care in collaboration with other health care team members.

pri·mar·y o·o·cyte (prī′mar-ē ō′ō-sīt) One during its growth phase before it completes the first meiotic division.

pri·mar·y or·gan·i·zer (prī′mār-ē ōr′gă-nī-zĕr) One situated on the dorsal lip of the blastopore.

pri·mar·y pre·ven·tion (prī′mār-ē prē-ven′shŭn) Avoidance of disease.

pri·mar·y pro·gres·sive a·pha·si·a (PPA) (prī′mar-ē prŏ-gres′iv ă-fāz′ē-ă) A degenerative disorder of which the early major symptom is an aphasia that increases in severity and (usually) eventually includes dementia.

pri·mar·y re·nin·ism (prī′mar-ē re′nin-izm) Overproduction of renin by juxtaglomerular cells in the absence of a stimulus; leads to hyperaldosteronism, hypertension, hypokalemia, and edema.

pri·mar·y scle·ro·sing chol·an·gi·tis (PSC) (prī′mar-ē sker-ŏs′ing kō-lan-jī′tis) Idiopathic chronic hepatobiliary disease characterized by diffuse inflammation and fibrosis of the extrahepatic biliary system resulting in patchy, irregular stricturing of the bile ducts.

pri·mar·y sen·sa·tion (prī′mar-ē sen-sā′shŭn) Perception that is the direct result of a stimulus.

pri·mar·y se·ques·trum (prī′mar-ē sē-kwes′trŭm) Completely detached necrotic tissue.

pri·mar·y sex char·ac·ter (prī′mar-ē seks kar′ăk-tĕr) Sex glands, testes or ovaries, and the accessory sex organs. SYN primary sex characteristic.

pri·mar·y shock (prī′mar-ē shok) A shock mainly nervous, from pain and anxiety, which ensues almost immediately on receipt of a severe injury.

pri·mar·y sper·ma·to·cyte (prī′mar-ē spĕr-mat′ŏ-sīt) One derived by a growth phase from a spermatogonium, and undergoes first division of meiosis.

pri·mar·y syph·i·lis (prī′mar-ē sif′i-lis) The first stage of syphilis. SEE ALSO syphilis.

pri·mar·y tu·ber·cu·lo·sis (prī′mar-ē tū-bĕr′kyū-lō′sis) First infection by *Mycobacterium tuberculosis*, typically seen in children but also in adults, characterized in the lungs by formation of a primary complex consisting of small peripheral pulmonary focus with spread to hilar or paratracheal lymph nodes. SYN childhood type tuberculosis.

prim·er (prī′mĕr) **1.** A molecule, which may be a small polymer, which initiates synthesis of a larger structure. SYN starter. **2.** A pheromone that causes a long-term physiologic change.

pri·mi·grav·i·da (prī′mi-grav′i-dă) SEE gravida.

pri·mip·a·ra (prī-mip′ă-ră) SEE para.

prim·i·tive groove (prim′i-tiv grūv) The median depression in the primitive streak flanked by primitive ridges.

prim·i·tive neu·ro·ec·to·der·mal tu·mor (PNET) (prim′i-tiv nūr′ō-ek-tō-dĕr′măl tū′mŏr) Designation used to refer to a group of morphologically similar embryonal neoplasms that arise in intracranial and peripheral sites of the nervous system.

prim·i·tive re·flex (prim-i′tiv rē′fleks) Any of a group of reflexes seen during gestation and infancy that typically become integrated by an early age (most by 6 months).

pri·mor·di·al (prī-mōr′dē-ăl) **1.** Relating to a primordium. **2.** Relating to a structure in its first or earliest stage of development. SYN primal (2), primitive.

pri·mor·di·al germ cell (PGC) (prī-mōr′dē-ăl jĕrm sel) Earliest undifferentiated sex cell, found initially outside the gonad. SYN gonocyte.

pri·mor·di·al gut (prī-mōr′dē-ăl gŭt) A flat sheet of intraembryonic endoderm that changes into a tubular gut due to the folding of embryonic body. SYN primitive gut.

pri·mor·di·um, pl. **pri·mor·di·a** (prī-mōr′dē-ŭm, -ă) An aggregation of cells in the embryo indicating the first trace of an organ or structure. SYN anlage (1).

prin·ceps, pl. **prin·ci·pes** (prin'seps, -si-pēz) Principal.

prin·ci·pal di·ag·no·sis (prin'si-păl dī'ăg-nō'sis) Determination, after testing and study, of the main reason for the patient's need for health care services.

prin·ci·pal op·tic ax·is (prin'si-păl op'tik ak'sis) A line passing through the center of the lens of a refracting system at right angles to its surface.

prin·ci·pal point (prin'si-păl poynt) One of two points on an optic axis so related that an object at one is exactly imaged at the other without magnification, minification, or inversion.

prin·ci·ple (prin'si-pěl) **1.** A fundamental doctrine or tenet. SEE ALSO law, rule, theorem. **2.** Essential ingredient in a substance, especially what gives it its distinctive quality or effect.

Prinz·met·al an·gi·na (prints'met-ăl an'ji-nă) A form characterized by pain that is not precipitated by cardiac work, is of longer duration, is usually more severe, and is associated with unusual electrocardiographic manifestations including elevated ST segments in leads that are ordinarily depressed in typical angina. Treatment includes nitroglycerine or beta-blocker medications. SYN angina inversa, variant angina.

pri·on, pri·on pro·tein (prī'on, prō'tēn) Small, infectious proteinaceous particle, of nonnucleic acid composition; the causative agent of four spongiform encephalopathies in humans: kuru, Creutzfeldt-Jakob disease, Gerstmann-Straüssler-Scheinker syndrome, and fatal familial insomnia.

prism (prizm) A transparent solid, with sides that converge at an angle, which deflects a ray of light toward the thickest portion and splits white light into its component colors.

prism bar (prizm bahr) A graduated series of prisms mounted on a frame and used in ocular diagnosis.

prism di·op·ter (Δ) (prizm dī-op'těr) Unit of measurement of deviation of light in passing through a prism, being a deflection of 1 cm at a distance of 1 m.

pri·vate du·ty nurse (prī'văt dū'tē nŭrs) **1.** A nurse who is not a member of a hospital staff but is hired on a fee-for-service basis to care for a patient. **2.** A nurse who specializes in the care of patients with diseases of a particular type.

pri·vate hos·pi·tal (prī'văt hos'pi-tăl) **1.** A hospital similar to a group hospital except that it is controlled by a single practitioner or by the practitioner and the associates in his or her office. **2.** A hospital operated for profit.

pri·vi·leged com·mu·ni·ca·tion (priv'ě-lějd kŏ-myū'ni-kā'shŭn) Confidential information given to a health care professional.

Pro Symbol for proline or prolyl.

pro- 1. Prefix denoting before, forward. SEE ALSO ante-, pre-. **2.** In chemistry, prefix indicating precursor of. SEE ALSO -gen.

pro·ac·cel·er·in (prō'ak-sel'ěr-in) SYN factor V.

pro·ac·ti·va·tor (prō-ak'ti-vā-tŏr) A substance that, when chemically split, yields a fragment (activator) capable of rendering another substance enzymatically active.

prob·a·bil·i·ty (prob'ă-bil'i-tē) **1.** A measure, ranging from 0–1, of the degree of belief in a hypothesis or statement. **2.** The limit of the relative frequency of an event in a sequence of N random trials as N approaches infinity.

prob·a·ble signs of preg·nan·cy (prob'ă-běl sīnz preg'năn-sē) More certain than presumptive signs but are not definitive; include basal body temperature, breast tenderness and swelling, chloasma, linea nigra, and others.

pro·bac·te·ri·o·phage (prō'bak-tēr'ē-ō-fāj) The stage of a temperate bacteriophage in which the genome is incorporated into the genetic apparatus of the bacterial host. SYN prophage.

pro·band (prō'band) HUMAN GENETICS the patient or member of the family that brings a family under study.

P

pro·bang (prō-bang′) A flexible rod with some soft material at the distal end used injudiciously to try to advance or retrieve foreign bodies from the esophagus; a practice condemned as dangerous.

probe (prōb) **1.** A slender rod of flexible material, with blunt bulbous tip, used for exploring sinuses, fistulae, other cavities, or wounds. **2.** A device or agent used to detect or explore a substance.

probe sy·ringe (prōb sir-inj′) A syringe with an olive-shaped tip, used in treatment of diseases of the lacrimal passages.

prob·lem (prob) (prob′lĕm) In the mental health professions, a term often used to denote the difficulties or challenges of life.

prob·lem-o·ri·ent·ed med·i·cal re·cord (POR, POMR) (prob′lĕm-ōr′ē-en-tĕd med′i-kăl rek′ōrd) A medical record model designed to organize patient information by the presenting problem. The record includes the patient database, problem list, plan of care, and progress notes in an accessible format.

pro·cain·a·mide hy·dro·chlor·ide (prō-kān′ă-mīd hī′drŏ-klōr′īd) Potent antiarrhythmic agent to treat cardiac disorders.

pro·caine hy·dro·chlor·ide (prō′kān hī′drŏ-klōr′īd) Local anesthetic for infiltration and spinal use, although it lacks activity when used topically.

pro·car·ba·zine hy·dro·chlor·ide (prō-kahr′bă-zēn hī′drŏ-klōr′īd) An antineoplastic agent.

pro·car·box·y·pep·ti·dase (prō′kahr-boks′ē-pep′ti-dās) Inactive precursor of a carboxypeptidase.

Pro·car·y·o·tae (prō′kar-ē-ō′tē) SYN Prokaryotae.

pro·ce·du·ral mem·o·ry (prō-sē′jŭr-ăl mem′ŏr-ē) Knowledge needed to perform the procedures composing a given task.

pro·ce·dure (prŏ-sē′jŭr) Act or conduct of diagnosis, treatment, or operation. SEE ALSO method, operation, technique.

pro·ce·dure code (prō-sē′jĕr kōd) Numbers that identify health care services provided to a patient.

pro·cen·tri·ole (prō-sen′trē-ōl) Early phase in de novo development of centrioles or basal bodies from the centrosphere.

pro·ce·phal·ic (prō-sĕ-fal′ik) Relating to the anterior part of the head.

pro·cer·coid (prō′sĕr-koyd) The first stage in the aquatic life cycle of certain tapeworms, such as the pseudophyllideans.

pro·cess (pros′es) **1.** ANATOMY A projection or outgrowth. **2.** A method or mode of action used to get a result. **3.** A natural progression, development, or sequence of events. SEE ALSO processus. **4.** A pathologic condition or disease. **5.** DENTISTRY Operations that convert a wax pattern into a solid denture base of another material.

pro·ces·sor (pros′es-sŏr) A device that converts one form of energy into another or one form of material into another.

pro·cess skills (pros′es skilz) Skills used to manage and modify actions in the completing of daily living tasks.

pro·ces·sus va·gi·na·lis pe·ri·to·ne·i (prō-ses′ŭs vaj-i-nā′lis per-i-tō′nē-ī) SYN processus vaginalis of peritoneum.

pro·chon·dral (prō-kon′drăl) Denoting a developmental stage before formation of cartilage.

pro·chy·mo·sin (prō-kī′mō-sin) The precursor of chymosin. SYN prorenin.

pro·ci·den·ti·a (pros′i-den′shē-ă) A sinking down or prolapse of any organ or part.

pro·col·la·gen (prō-kol′ă-jen) Soluble precursor of collagen formed by fibroblasts and other cells in the process of collagen synthesis.

pro·con·ver·tin (prō′kŏn-vĕr′tin) SYN factor VII.

pro·cre·ate (prō′krē-āt′) To beget; to produce by the sexual act.

pro·cre·a·tion (prō′krē-ā′shŭn) SYN reproduction (1).

proc·tal·gi·a (prok-tal′jē-ă) Pain around the anus, or in the rectum. SYN proctodynia, rectalgia.

proc·tec·to·my (prok-tek′tŏ-mē) Surgical resection of the rectum.

proc·ti·tis (prok-tī′tis) Inflammation of the mucous membrane of the rectum.

procto-, proct- Combining form denoting the anus or rectum.

proc·to·cele (prok′tŏ-sēl) Prolapse or herniation of the rectum.

proc·to·co·lec·to·my (prok′tō-kŏ-lek′tŏ-mē) Surgical removal of the rectum together with part or all of the colon.

proc·to·co·lo·nos·co·py (prok′tō-kō-lŏn-os′kŏ-pē) Inspection of the interior of the rectum and colon.

proc·to·col·po·plas·ty (prok′tō-kol′pŏ-plas-tē) Surgical closure of a rectovaginal fistula.

proc·to·cys·tot·o·my (prok′tō-sis-tot′ŏ-mē) Incision into the bladder from the rectum.

proc·to·de·um, pl. **proc·to·de·a** (prok′tō-dē′ŭm, -ă) SYN proctodaeum.

proc·tol·o·gy (prok-tol′ŏ-jē) Specialty concerned with diseases of the anus and rectum.

proc·to·pa·ral·y·sis (prok′tō-păr-al′i-sis) Paralysis of the anus, leading to incontinence of feces.

proc·to·pex·y (prok′tō-pek-sē) Surgical fixation of a prolapsing rectum.

proc·to·plas·ty (prok′tō-plas-tē) Surgical repair of the anus or rectum.

proc·to·ple·gi·a (prok′tō-plē′jē-ă) Paralysis of the anus and rectum occurring with paraplegia.

proc·tor·rha·phy (prok-tōr′ă-fē) Repair by suture of a lacerated rectum or anus.

proc·tor·rhe·a (prok′tōr-ē′ă) A mucoserous discharge from the rectum.

proc·tos·co·py (prok-tos′kŏ-pē) Visual examination of the rectum and anus, as with a rectoscope.

proc·to·sig·moi·dec·to·my (prok′tō-sig′moyd-ek′tŏ-mē) Excision of the rectum and sigmoid colon.

proc·to·sig·moi·di·tis (prok′tō-sig′moyd-ī′tis) Inflammation of the sigmoid colon and rectum.

proc·to·sig·moi·dos·co·py (prok′tō-sig′moyd-os′kŏ-pē) Direct inspection through a sigmoidoscope of the rectum and sigmoid colon.

proc·to·ste·no·sis (prok′tō-stĕ-nō′sis) Stricture of the rectum or anus. SYN rectostenosis.

proc·tos·to·my (prok-tos′tŏ-mē) The formation of an artificial opening into the rectum. SYN rectostomy.

proc·tot·o·my (prok-tot′ŏ-mē) An incision into the rectum. SYN rectotomy.

proc·to·val·vot·o·my (prok′tō-val-vot′ŏ-mē) Incision of rectal valves.

pro·cur·sive ep·i·lep·sy (prō-kŭr′siv ep′i-lep′sē) A psychomotor attack initiated by whirling or running.

pro·dro·mal, pro·drom·ik, pro·drom·ous (prō-drō′măl, -drōm′ik, -ŭs) Relating to a prodrome.

pro·dro·mal labor (prō-drō′măl lā′bŏr) Early phase of labor that does not progress normally: contractions do not strengthen and dilatation is minimal. Cf. active labor.

pro·dro·mal stage (prō-drō′măl stāj) SYN incubation period (1).

pro·drome, pro·dro·mus (prō′drōm, prod′rŏ-mŭs) An early or premonitory symptom of a disease.

pro·drug (prō′drŭg) A class of drugs with a pharmacologic action due to conversion by metabolic processes within the body.

prod·uct (P, prod.) (prod′ŭkt) Anything produced or made, either naturally or artificially.

P

pro·duc·tive (prŏ-dŭk'tiv) Producing or capable of producing.

pro·duct·ive cough (prŏ-dŭk'tiv kawf) A cough accompanied by expectoration.

pro·duc·tive in·flam·ma·tion (prŏ-dŭk'tiv in-flă-mā'shŭn) Vague term ordinarily used with reference to proliferative inflammation, with or without an exudate or with any inflammation grossly visible exudate.

pro·en·zyme (prō-en'zīm) The precursor of an enzyme, requiring some change to render it active. SYN zymogen.

pro·e·ryth·ro·blast (prō'ĕ-rith'rō-blast) SYN pronormoblast.

pro·es·tro·gen (prō-es'trŏ-jen) A substance that acts as an estrogen only after it has been metabolized in the body to an active compound. SYN pro-oestrogen.

pro·file (prō'fīl) 1. An outline or contour, especially one representing a side view of the human head. SYN norma. 2. A summary or brief account. 3. BIOWARFARE set of suspected characteristics linked to a person or group allegedly responsible for terrorist activity involving use of biologic weapons.

pro·fun·da (prō-fŭn'dă) Deep; a term applied to structures that lie deep in the tissues, especially when contrasted with a similar, more superficial (sublimis) structure.

pro·gas·trin (prō-gas'trin) Precursor of gastric secretion in the mucous membrane of the stomach.

pro·gen·i·tor (prō-jen'i-tŏr) A precursor, ancestor; one who begets.

prog·e·ny (proj'ĕ-nē) Offspring; descendants.

pro·ge·ri·a (prō-jēr'ē-ă) A condition of precocious aging with onset at birth or early childhood; characterized by growth retardation, a senile appearance with dry wrinkled skin, total alopecia, and birdlike facies. SYN Hutchinson-Gilford disease, Hutchinson-Gilford syndrome, premature senility syndrome.

pro·ges·ta·tion·al (prō'jes-tā'shŭn-ăl) 1. Favoring pregnancy; conducive to gestation. 2. Referring to progesterone, or to a drug with progesteronelike properties.

pro·ges·ter·one (prō-jes'tĕr-ōn) An antiestrogenic steroid used to correct abnormalities of the menstrual cycle, as a contraceptive, and to control habitual abortion. SYN luteohormone, progestational hormone.

pro·ges·tin (prō-jes'tin) 1. A hormone of the corpus luteum. 2. Generic term for any substance, natural or synthetic, which effects some or all of the biologic changes produced by progesterone.

pro·ges·to·gen (prō-jes'tō-jen) 1. Any agent capable of producing biologic effects similar to those of progesterone. 2. A synthetic derivative from testosterone or progesterone with some of the physiologic activity and pharmacologic effects of progesterone.

pro·glos·sis (prō-glos'is) The anterior portion, or tip, of the tongue.

pro·glot·tid (prō-glot'id) A tapeworm segment, containing the reproductive organs. SYN proglottis.

prog·na·thism, prog·na·thi·a (prog'nă-thizm, prog-nā'thē-ă) Having an abnormal forward projection of one or of both jaws beyond the established normal relationship with the cranial base. SYN progenia.

prog·no·sis (prog-nō'sis) A forecast of the probable course and/or outcome of a disease.

prog·nos·ti·cate (prog-nos'ti-kāt) To give a prognosis.

pro·gram·ma·ble hear·ing aid (prō-gram'ă-bĕl hēr'ing ād) Multichannel hearing aid that can use more than one level-dependent frequency response strategy.

pro·gres·sive (prō-gres'iv) Advancing; denoting the course of a disease, especially, when unqualified, an unfavorable course.

pro·gres·sive bul·bar pal·sy (PBP) (prō-gres'iv bŭl'bahr pawl'zē) Subgroup of motor neuron disease; a progressive degenerative disorder of the motor neurons of primarily the brainstem, manifested as weakness of the various bulbar muscles, resulting in dysarthria and dysphagia.

SYN bulbar paralysis, Erb disease, glosso-labiolaryngeal paralysis, glossolabiopharyngeal paralysis, glossopalatolabial paralysis, glossopharyngeolabial paralysis, progressive bulbar paralysis.

pro·gres·sive bul·bar pa·ral·y·sis (prŏ-gres'iv bŭl'bahr păr-al'i-sis) Progressive weakness and atrophy of the muscles of the tongue, lips, palate, pharynx, and larynx; most often caused by motor neuron disease. SYN bulbar paralysis.

pro·gres·sive mul·ti·fo·cal leu·ko·en·ceph·a·lop·a·thy (PML) (prŏ-gres'iv mŭl'tē-fō'kăl lū'kō-en-sef'ă-lop'ă-thē) Rare, subacute, afebrile disease characterized by areas of demyelinization surrounded by markedly altered neuroglia, including inclusion bodies in glial cells; occurs usually in people with AIDS, leukemia, lymphoma, or other debilitating diseases, or in those who have been receiving immunosuppressive treatment.

pro·gres·sive my·o·pi·a (prŏ-gres'iv mī-ō'pē-ă) Nearsightedness that worsens over time.

pro·gres·sive os·se·ous het·er·o·pla·si·a (POH) (prŏ-gres'iv os'ē-ŭs het'ĕr-ō-plā'zē-ă) Genetic disease linked to GNAS1 mutation.

pro·gres·sive out·er ret·i·nal ne·cro·sis (PORN) (prŏ-gres'iv owt'ĕr ret'i-năl nĕ-krō'sis) A viral syndrome occurring in AIDS patients, caused by herpesvirus and characterized by destruction of peripheral retina.

pro·gres·sive pig·men·tar·y der·ma·to·sis (prŏ-gres'iv pig'mĕn-tar-ē dĕr'mă-tō'sis) Chronic purpura, especially of the legs in men, spreading to form red-brown patches and puncta described as cayenne pepper spots; associated microscopically with perivascular lymphocytic infiltration, diapedesis, and hemosiderosis. SYN Schamberg fever.

pro·gres·sive-re·sis·tance ex·er·cise (PRE) (prŏ-gres'iv-rĕ-zis'tăns ek'sĕr-sīz) The practical application of the overload principle to improve muscular strength and size.

pro·gres·sive stain·ing (prŏ-gres'iv stān'ing) A procedure in which staining is continued until the desired intensity of coloring of tissue elements is attained.

pro·gres·sive su·pra·nu·cle·ar pal·sy (PSNP, PSP) (prŏ-gres'iv sū'pră-nū'klē-ăr pawl'zē) Slowly progressive, ultimately fatal neurologic disorder with onset after age of 40. SYN Steele-Richardson-Olszewski disease, Steele-Richardson-Olszewski syndrome.

pro·gress notes (prog'res nōts) Records kept by health care workers that indicate the course of the patient during care.

pro·in·su·lin (PI) (prō-in'sŭ-lin) A single-chain precursor of insulin.

pro·jec·tile vom·i·ting (PV) (prŏ-jek'tīl vom'it-ing) Expulsion of the contents of the stomach with great propulsive force.

pro·jec·tion (prŏ-jek'shŭn) **1.** A pushing out; an outgrowth or protuberance. **2.** The referring of a sensation to the object producing it. **3.** PSYCHOLOGY/PSYCHIATRY A defense mechanism by which a repressed complex in the patient is denied and conceived as belonging to another person. **4.** The conception by the consciousness of a mental occurrence belonging to the self as of external origin. **5.** Localization of visual impressions in space. **6.** NEUROANATOMY the system of nerve fibers by which a group of nerve cells discharges its nerve impulses to one or more other cell groups. **7.** Plane image of a three-dimensional object. **8.** RADIOGRAPHY a standard x-ray study, named by body part, position, direction of the x-ray beam through the body part, or eponym.

pro·jec·tive i·den·ti·fi·ca·tion (prŏ-jek'tiv ī-den'ti-fi-kā'shŭn) A defensive attribution of one's own psychic processes to another person.

pro·jec·tive test (prŏ-jek'tiv test) Loosely structured psychological assessment containing ambiguous stimuli that require the subject to reveal feelings, personality, or psychopathology in response.

pro·kar·y·ote, pro·car·y·ote (prō-kar'ē-ōt) Organism consisting of a single cell, or a precellular organism, which lacks a nuclear membrane or paired organized chromosomes. SEE ALSO eukaryote.

pro·la·bi·um (prō-lā'bē-ŭm) The exposed carmine margin of the lip.

P

pro·lac·tin (PRL) (prō-lak′tin) Protein hormone of the hypophysial anterior lobe that stimulates secretion of breast milk. SYN lactogenic hormone.

pro·lac·tin-pro·duc·ing ad·e·no·ma (prō-lak′tin-prō-dūs′ing ad′ĕ-nō′mă) A pituitary adenoma composed of prolactin-producing cells; it gives rise to symptoms of nonpuerperal amenorrhea and galactorrhea (Forbes-Albright syndrome) in women and to impotence in men.

pro·lac·to·lib·er·in (prō-lak′tō-lib′ĕr-in) A substance of hypothalamic origin that stimulates the release of prolactin.

pro·lac·to·stat·in (prō-lak′tō-stat′in) A substance of hypothalamic origin capable of inhibiting the synthesis and release of prolactin.

pro·lapse (prō′laps) **1.** To sink down; said of an organ or other part. **2.** A sinking of an organ or other part, especially its appearance at a natural or artificial orifice. SEE ALSO procidentia, ptosis.

pro·lapse of um·bil·i·cal cord (prō′laps ŭm-bil′i-kăl kōrd) Presentation of part of the umbilical cord ahead of the fetus; may cause fetal death due to compression of the cord between the presenting part of the fetus and the maternal pelvis.

pro·lapse of u·ter·us (prō′laps yū′tĕr-ŭs) Downward uterine movement due to laxity and atony of the muscular and fascial structures of the pelvic floor, usually resulting from injuries of childbirth or advanced age.

pro·lep·sis (prō-lep′sis) Recurrence of the paroxysm of a periodical disease at regularly shortening intervals.

pro·lif·er·ate (prō-lif′ĕr-āt) To grow and increase in number by means of reproduction of similar forms.

pro·lif·er·a·tion (prō-lif′ĕr-ā′shŭn) Growth and reproduction of similar cells.

pro·lif·er·a·tive glo·mer·u·lo·neph·ri·tis (PGN) (prō-lif′ĕr-ă-tiv glō-mer′yū-lō-nĕ-frī′tis) Form with hypercellularity of glomeruli due to proliferation of endothelial or mesangial cells.

pro·lif·er·a·tive my·o·si·tis (prō-lif′ĕr-ă-tiv mī′ō-sī′tis) Rapidly growing benign infiltrating fibrous nodule in skeletal muscle.

pro·lif·er·a·tive re·ti·nop·a·thy (prō-lif′ĕr-ă-tiv ret′i-nop′ă-thē) Neovascularization of the retina extending into the vitreous humor.

pro·lif·ic (prō-lif′ik) Fruitful; bearing many children or offspring.

pro·line (Pro, P) (prō′lēn) Pyrrolidine-2-carboxylic acid; the L-isomer is found in proteins, especially the collagens. SYN pyrrolidine-2-carboxylate.

pro·line di·pep·ti·dase (prō′lēn dī-pep′ti-dās) An enzyme cleaving aminoacyl-L-proline bonds in dipeptides containing a C-terminal prolyl residue.

pro·lo·ther·a·py (prō′lō-thār′ă-pē) A technique to assist the rebuilding of damaged connective tissue structures through the injection of various substances designed to stimulate collagen proliferation.

pro·lyl di·pep·ti·dase (prō′lil dī-pep′ti-dās) An enzyme cleaving L-prolyl-amino acid bonds in dipeptides containing N-terminal prolyl residues.

pro·meg·a·lo·blast (prō-meg′ă-lō-blast) The earliest of four maturation stages of the megaloblast. SEE erythroblast.

pro·me·thi·um (Pm) (prō-mē′thē-ŭm) A radioactive element of the rare earth series, atomic no. 61; first chemically identified in 1945.

prom·i·nence (prom′i-nĕns) [TA] ANATOMY A tissue or part that projects beyond a surface. SYN prominentia.

prom·on·to·ry, prom·on·to·ri·um (prom′ŏn-tōr′ē, -ŭm) [TA] An eminence or projection.

pro·mo·ter (prō-mō′tĕr) **1.** CHEMISTRY a substance that increases catalytic activity. **2.** MOLECULAR BIOLOGY DNA sequence at which RNA polymerase binds and initiates transcription.

prompt in·su·lin zinc sus·pen·sion (prompt in′sŭ-lin zingk sŭs-pen′shŭn) Sterile suspension of insulin in buffered water for injection. SYN amorphous insulin zinc suspension, semilente insulin.

pro·my·e·lo·cyte (prō-mī′ĕ-lō-sīt) Developmental stage of a granular leukocyte between myeloblasts and myelocytes, when a few specific granules appear in addition to azurophilic ones.

pro·nate (prō′nāt) To assume a prone position.

pro·na·tion (prō-nā′shŭn) [TA] **1.** The condition of being prone. **2.** Transverse plane motion at the radioulnar joint or transverse tarsal joint.

pro·na·tor syn·drome (prō′nāt-ĕr sin′drōm) Condition where trapping of the median nerve by the pronator teres results in pain in the forearm.

prone (PR) (prōn) *Do not confuse this word with supine.* **1.** The body when lying face downward. **2.** Pronation of the forearm or foot.

pro·neph·ric tubule (prō-nef′rik tū′byūl) Excretory unit of the pronephros, present only in vestigial form in human embryos.

pro·nor·mo·blast (prō-nōr′mō-blast) The earliest of four stages in development of the normoblast. SEE ALSO erythroblast. SYN proerythroblast, rubriblast.

pro-oestrogen [Br.] SYN proestrogen.

pro·o·pi·o·mel·a·no·cor·tin (POMC) (prō-ō′pē-ō-mel′ă-nō-kōr′tin) A large molecule found in the anterior and intermediate lobes of the pituitary gland, the hypothalamus, and other parts of the brain as well as in the lungs, gastrointestinal tract, and placenta; the precursor of adrenocorticotropic hormone, corticotropinlike intermediate (lobe peptide), β-lipotropin, β-melanocyte-stimulating hormone, and β-endorphin.

prop·a·ga·tion (prop′ă-gā′shŭn) The act of propagating.

pro·per·din (P) (prō′pĕr-din) A control protein for the alternate complement cascade; stabilizes the C_3 convertase enzyme, a deficiency of which increases susceptibility to systemic meningococcal infections. SEE ALSO factor P.

pro·per·i·to·ne·al (prō′per′i-tŏ-nē′ăl) In front of the peritoneum.

pro·phage (prō′fāj) SYN probacteriophage.

pro·phase (prō′fāz) The first stage of mitosis or meiosis, consisting of linear contraction and increased chromosomal thickness accompanied by migration of the two daughter centrioles and their asters toward the cell poles.

pro·phy·lac·tic (prō′fi-lak′tik) **1.** Preventing disease. **2.** An agent that acts to prevent a disease.

pro·phy·lac·tic treat·ment (prō′fi-lak′tik trēt′mĕnt) Measures designed to protect a person from a disease to which he or she has been, or is liable to be, exposed.

pro·phy·lax·is, pl. **pro·phy·lax·es** (prō′fi-lak′sis, -sēz) Prevention of disease or of a process that can lead to disease.

pro·pi·o·nate (prō′pē-ŏ-nāt) A salt or ester of propionic acid.

Pro·pi·on·i·bac·te·ri·um (prō′pē-on-i-bak-tēr′ē-ŭm) A genus of nonmotile, non-spore-forming, anaerobic to aerotolerant bacteria containing gram-positive rods that are usually pleomorphic, diphtheroid, or club-shaped, with one end rounded, the other tapered or pointed; occur in dairy products, on human skin, and in the intestinal tracts of humans and other animals. They may be pathogenic.

pro·pi·on·ic ac·id (PA) (prō′pē-on′ik as′id) Methylacetic acid; found in sweat; elevated in cases of ketotic hyperglycemia and biotin deficiency.

pro·po·fol (prō′pō-fōl) Hypnotic agent with rapid onset and short duration of action; used intravenously to induce and maintain general anesthesia. SYN 2, 6-diisopropyl phenol.

pro·por·tion·al as·sist ven·ti·la·tion (PAV) (prŏ-pōr′shŭn-ăl ă-sist′ ven′ti-lā′shŭn) Mechanical form of ventilation in which the patient controls the flow of oxygen by the amount of effort expended in breathing.

pro·pos·i·tus, pl. **pro·po·si·ti** (prō-poz′i-tŭs, -tī) **1.** Sexual proband. **2.** A premise.

pro·pran·o·lol hy·dro·chlor·ide (prō-pran′ō-lōl hī′drō-klōr′īd) An adrenergic β-receptor blocking agent; used to treat angina pectoris, hypertension, and other conditions.

pro·pri·e·tar·y med·i·cine (prō-prī′ĕ-tar′ē med′i-sin) A medicinal compound for which the formula and mode of manufacture are the property of the maker.

pro·pri·e·tar·y name (prō-prī′ĕ-tar-ē nām) The protected brand name or trademark, registered with the U.S. Patent Office, under which a manufacturer markets its product; written with a initial capital letter and often further distinguished by ®. Cf. generic name, nonproprietary name.

pro·pri·o·cep·tion (prō′prē-ō-sep′shŭn) A sense or perception, usually at a subconscious level, of the movements and position of the body and especially its limbs, independent of vision.

pro·pri·o·cep·tive (prō′prē-ō-sep′tiv) Capable of receiving stimuli originating in muscles, tendons, and other internal tissues.

pro·pri·o·cep·tive neu·ro·mus·cu·lar fa·cil·i·ta·tion (PNF) (prō′prē-ō-sep′tiv nūr′ō-mŭs′kyū-lăr fă-sil′i-tā′shŭn) Technique to improve range of joint motion by stimulating proprioceptors in muscles, joints, and tendons before joint extension.

pro·pri·o·cep·tor (prō′prē-ō-sep′tŏr) One of a variety of sensory end organs in muscles, tendons, and joint capsules that sense position or state of contraction.

pro·pul·sion (prō-pŭl′shŭn) The tendency to fall forward; responsible for the festination in paralysis agitans.

pro·pyl (Pr) (prō′pil) The alkyl radical of propane, $CH_3CH_2CH_2-$.

pro·py·lene (prō′pi-lēn) Methylethylene; a gaseous olefinic hydrocarbon.

prop·y·lene gly·col (PG) (prō′pi-lēn glī′kol) Solvent for several water-insoluble drugs intended for parenteral administration; used in part to prepare injectable solutions of diazepam, phenytoin, and drugs.

pro·pyl·thi·o·u·ra·cil (PTU, PT) (prō′pil-thī′ō-yū′ră-sil) An antithyroid agent that inhibits synthesis of thyroid hormones; used to treat hyperthyroidism.

pro re na·ta (PRN, p.r.n.) (prō rē nā′tă) Latin phrase meaning as the occasion arises, as necessary.

pro·ru·bri·cyte (prō-rū′bri-sīt) Basophilic normoblast. SEE ALSO erythroblast.

pro·se·cre·tin (prō′se-krē′tin) Unactivated secretin.

pro·sec·tor (prō′sek-tŏr) One who prepares the material for a demonstration of anatomy before a class.

pros·en·ceph·a·lon, pro·en·ceph·a·lon (pros′en-sef′ă-lon, prō′) [TA] The anterior primordial cerebral vesicle and most rostral of the three primary brain vesicles of the embryonic neural tube. SYN forebrain.

pro·se·rum pro·throm·bin con·ver·sion ac·cel·er·a·tor (PPCA) (prō-sēr′ŭm prō-throm′bin kŏn-vĕr′zhŭn ak-sel′ĕr-ā-tŏr) SEE factor VIII.

pros·o·dem·ic (pros′ō-dem′ik) Denoting disease transmitted directly from person to person.

pros·o·pag·no·si·a (pros′ō-pag-nō′zē-ă) Difficulty in recognizing familiar faces.

pros·o·pla·si·a (pros′ō-plā′zē-ă) Progressive transformation or development. SEE ALSO cytomorphosis.

prosopo-, prosop- Combining forms denoting the face. SEE ALSO facio-.

pros·o·po·ple·gi·a (pros′ō-pō-plē′jē-ă) SYN facial paralysis.

pros·o·pos·chi·sis (pros′ō-pos′ki-sis) Congenital facial cleft from mouth to the medial canthus of the eye.

pros·o·po·spasm (pros′ō-pō-spazm) SYN facial tic.

pros·o·po·thor·a·cop·a·gus (pros′ō-pō-thōr′ă-kop′ă-gŭs) Conjoined twins attached by the face and thorax.

pros·pec·tive   pay·ment   sys·tem (PPS) (prŏ-spek′tiv pā′mĕnt sis′tĕm) Arrangement mandated by the U.S. Tax Equity and Fiscal Responsibility Act of 1982 (TEFRA) to control Medicare costs.

pros·ta·cy·clin (PGI₂) (pros′tă-sī′klin) A potent natural inhibitor of platelet aggregation and a powerful vasodilator. SYN epoprostenol, epoprostenol sodium.

pros·ta·glan·din (PG) (pros′tă-glan′ din) Physiologically active substance present in many tissues, with effects such as vasodilation, vasoconstriction, stimulation of intestinal or bronchial smooth muscle, uterine stimulation, and antagonism to hormones influencing lipid metabolism.

pros·ta·glan·din   en·do·per·ox·ide syn·thase (pros′tă-glan′din en′dŏ-pĕr-ok′sīd sin′thās) Protein complex that catalyzes two steps in prostaglandin biosynthesis. SYN cyclooxygenase.

pros·ta·noid (pros′tă-noyd) Denoting having properties of prostaglandins.

pros·tate, pros·tate gland (pros′tāt gland) [TA] A chestnut-shaped body, surrounding the beginning of the urethra in the male, which consists of two lateral lobes connected anteriorly by an isthmus and posteriorly by a middle lobe lying above and between the ejaculatory ducts. The secretion of the glands is a milky fluid that is discharged by excretory ducts into the prostatic urethra at the time of the emission of semen. SYN prostata [TA].

pros·ta·tec·to·my (pros′tă-tek′tŏ-mē) Removal of part or all of the prostate.

pros·tate-spe·cif·ic an·ti·gen (PSA) (pros′tāt-spĕ-sif′ik an′ti-jen) A single-chain, 31-kD glycoprotein with 240 amino acid residues and 4 carbohydrate side-chains. Elevations of serum PSA are highly organ-specific but occur in both cancer and benign disease.

pros·tat·ic (pros) (pros-tat′ik) Relating to the prostate.

pros·tat·ic cal·cu·lus (pros-tat′ik kal′ kyū-lŭs) A concretion formed in the prostate gland.

pros·tat·ic flu·id (pros-tat′ik flū′id) Succus prostaticus; a whitish secretion that is one of the constituents of semen.

pros·tat·ic in·tra·ep·i·the·li·al ne·o·pla·si·a (PIN) (pros-tat′ik in-tra-ep′i-thē′lē-ăl nē′ō-plā′zē-ă) Dysplastic changes involving glands and ducts of the prostate that may be a precursor of adenocarcinoma.

pros·tat·ic mas·sage (pros-tat′ik mă-sahzh′) 1. Manual expression of prostatic secretions by digital rectal technique. 2. Emptying of prostatic sinuses and ducts by repeated downward compression maneuvers; used to treat various congestive and inflammatory prostatic conditions.

pros·ta·tism (pros′tă-tizm) A syndrome, occurring mostly in older men, usually caused by enlargement of the prostate gland and manifested by irritative symptoms (e.g., nocturia, frequency, and urgency incontinence) and obstructive symptoms.

pros·ta·ti·tis (pros′tă-tī′tis) Inflammation of the prostate.

pros·ta·to·cys·ti·tis (pros′tă-tō-sis-tī′ tis) Inflammation of the prostate and the bladder; cystitis by extension of inflammation from the prostatic urethra.

pros·ta·to·li·thot·o·my (pros′tă-tō-li-thot′ŏ-mē) Incision of the prostate for removal of a calculus.

pros·ta·to·meg·a·ly (pros′tă-tō-meg′ă-lē) Enlargement of the prostate gland.

pros·ta·tor·rhe·a (pros′tă-tō-rē′ă) Abnormal discharge of prostatic fluid. SYN prostatorrhoea.

prostatorrhoea [Br.] SYN prostatorrhea.

pros·ta·tot·o·my, pros·ta·to·my (pros′tă-tot′ŏ-mē, pros-tat′ŏ-mē) An incision into the prostate.

pros·ta·to·ve·sic·u·lec·to·my (pros′tă-tō-vĕ-sik′yū-lek′tŏ-mē) Surgical removal of the prostate gland and seminal vesicles.

P

pros·ta·to·ve·sic·u·li·tis (pros'tă-tō-vĕ-sik'yū-lī'tis) Inflammation of the prostate gland and seminal vesicles.

pros·the·sis, pl. **pros·the·ses** (pros-thē'sis, -sēz) Fabricated substitute for a diseased or missing part of the body.

pros·thet·ic group (pros-thet'ik grūp) A nonamino acid compound attached to a protein, often reversibly, which confers new properties on the conjugated protein thus produced. SEE ALSO coenzyme.

pros·thet·ics (pros-thet'iks) The art and science of making and adjusting artificial parts of the human body.

pros·the·tist (pros'thē-tist) One skilled in constructing and fitting prostheses.

pros·thi·on (pros'thē-on) The most anterior point on the maxillary alveolar process in the midline. SYN alveolar point.

pros·tho·don·tics, pros·thet·ic den·tis·try (pros'thŏ-don'tiks, pros-thet'ik den'tis-trē) Science and art of providing suitable substitutes for the coronal portions of teeth, or for one or more lost or missing teeth and their associated parts.

pros·tra·tion (pros-trā'shŭn) A marked loss of strength, as in exhaustion.

♲ **prot-** SEE proteo-, proto-.

pro·ac·tin·i·um (Pa) (prō'tak-tin'ē-ŭm) A radioactive element, atomic no. 91, atomic wt. 231.03588, formed in the decay of uranium and thorium.

pro·ta·nom·a·ly (prō'tă-nom'ă-lē) A deficiency of color perception in which the red-sensitive pigment in cones is decreased.

pro·ta·no·pi·a, pro·ta·nop·si·a (prō'tă-nō'pē-ă, -tă-nop'sē-ă) A form of dichromatism characterized by absence of the red-sensitive pigment in cones, decreased luminosity for long wavelengths of light, and confusion in recognition of red and green.

pro·te·ase (PR) (prō'tē-ās) Enzymes, both endopeptidases and exopeptidases; enzymes that hydrolyze (break) polypeptide chains.

pro·te·ase in·hib·i·tor (prō'tē-ās in-hib'i-tŏr) Synthetic drugs used to treat HIV infection.

pro·tec·ted health in·for·ma·tion (prŏ-tek'tĕd helth in'fŏr-mā'shŭn) An umbrella term embracing all data collected and stored in any medium relating to the health of the individual patient. This legal construct forbids giving such information to a third party without express permission.

pro·tec·tion test (prŏ-tek'shŭn test) A procedure to determine the antimicrobial activity of a serum by inoculating a susceptible animal with a mixture of the serum and the virus or other microbe being tested.

pro·tein (prō'tēn) Macromolecules consisting of long sequences of α-amino acids [$H_2N–CHR–COOH$] in peptide (amide) linkage (elimination of H_2O between the α-NH_2 and α-COOH of successive residues). Cf. bioregulator.

pro·tein·a·ceous (prō'tē-nā'shŭs) Resembling a protein.

pro·tein-bound i·o·dine (PBI) (prō'tēn-bownd ī'ŏ-dīn) Thyroid hormone in its circulating form, consisting of one or more of the iodothyronines bound to one or more of the serum proteins.

pro·tein C (prō'tēn) Vitamin-K-dependent glycoprotein that inhibits coagulation by enzymatic cleavage of the activated forms of factors V and VIII, and thus interferes with the regulation of intravascular clot formation.

pro·tein ef·fi·cien·cy ra·ti·o (PER) (prō'tēn ĕ-fish'ĕn-sē rā'shē-ō) Weight gain in grams divided by protein intake in grams.

pro·tein en·er·gy mal·nu·tri·tion (PEM) (prō'tēn en'ĕr-jē mal'nū-trish'ŭn) A deficiency of protein, energy, or both that includes marasmus (or chronic PEM) and kwashiorkor (typically, acute PEM).

pro·tein hy·drol·y·sate (prō'tēn hī-drol'i-sāt) A sterile solution of amino acids and soft-chain peptides used intravenously to maintain nitrogen balance in severe illness, and after alimentary tract surgery.

pro·tein in·duced by vit·a·min K ab·sence (PIVKA) (prō'tēn in-dūst' vī'tǎ-min ab'sěns) Nonfunctional protein precursors of the prothrombin group of coagulation factors synthesized in the liver in the absence of vitamin K.

pro·tein K·cal·o·rie mal·nu·tri·tion (PCM) (prō'tēn kal'ŏr-ē mal'nū-trish'ŭn) SYN protein energy malnutrition.

pro·tein me·ta·bo·lism (prō'tēn mě-tab'ŏ-lizm) Decomposition and synthesis of protein in the tissues.

pro·tein·o·sis (prō'tēn-nō'sis) Condition characterized by disordered protein formation and distribution.

pro·tein S (prō'tēn) A vitamin-K-dependent antithrombotic protein that functions as a cofactor with activated protein C.

pro·tein·u·ri·a (prō'tē-nyūr'ē-ǎ) **1.** Presence of urinary protein in concentrations greater than 0.3 g in a 24-hour urine collection; specimens must be clean-voided midstream or obtained by catheterization. **2.** SYN albuminuria.

proteo-, prot- *Do not confuse this combining form with the prefix proto-.* Combining form meaning protein.

pro·te·o·gly·can (PG) (prō'tē-ō-glī'kan) Glycoaminoglycans bound to protein chains in covalent complexes; found in extracellular matrix of connective tissue.

pro·te·ol·y·sis (prō'tē-ol'i-sis) Decomposition of protein.

pro·te·o·lyt·ic (prō'tē-ō-lit'ik) Relating to or effecting proteolysis. SYN proteoclastic.

Pro·te·us (prō'tē-ŭs) A genus of motile, peritrichous, non-spore-forming, aerobic to facultatively anaerobic bacteria containing gram-negative rods; found in fecal matter and in putrefying materials.

Pro·te·us mi·ra·bi·lis (prō'tē-ŭs mi-rab'i-lis) A bacterial species widely recognized as a human pathogen commonly recovered from urinary, traumatic, and bacteremic infections.

Pro·te·us syn·drome (prō'tē-ŭs sin'drŏm) A sporadic disorder with a variable and changing phenotype characterized by gigantism of the hands and feet, distorted abnormal growth, pigmented nevi, thickening of the palms and soles, and subcutaneous lipomas. SYN elephant man disease (1).

Pro·te·us vul·ga·ris (prō'tē-ŭs vŭlgā'ris) Bacterium found in putrefying materials; associated with nosocomial infections of the respiratory and urinary tracts, and decubitus ulcers, and abscesses.

pro·throm·bin (pro) (prō-throm'bin) A glycoprotein formed and stored in the parenchymal cells of the liver and present in blood in a concentration of approximately 20 mg/100 mL. SYN serozyme, thrombinogen, thrombogen.

pro·throm·bin test (prō-throm'bin test) A quantitative test for prothrombin in blood based on clotting time of oxalated blood plasma in the presence of thromboplastin and calcium chloride. SEE ALSO prothrombin time.

pro·throm·bin time (PT) (prō-throm' bin tīm) Duration required for clotting after thromboplastin and calcium are added in optimal amounts to blood of normal fibrinogen content. SEE ALSO prothrombin test.

Pro·tis·ta (prō-tis'tǎ) A kingdom of both plantlike and animallike eukaryotic unicellular organisms, either in the form of solitary organisms, e.g., protozoa, or colonies of cells lacking true tissues.

proto-, prot- Combining forms meaning the first in a series; the highest in rank.

pro·to·col (prō'tŏ-kawl) A precise and detailed plan for the study of a biomedical problem or for a regimen of therapy.

pro·to·du·o·de·num (prō'tō-dū'ō-dē'nŭm, dū-od'ē-nŭm) The first part of the duodenum, which extends from the pylorus to the major duodenal papilla and develops from the caudal foregut of the embryo.

pro·ton (prō'ton) Positively charged unit of the nuclear mass; protons form part of the nucleus of the atom around which the negative electrons revolve.

pro·ton pump (prō'ton pŭmp) Molecular mechanism for the net transport of protons across a membrane; usually in-

P

volves the activity of adenosine triphosphatase.

pro·ton pump in·hib·i·tor (prō'ton pŭmp in-hib'i-tŏr) Agent that blocks transport of hydrogen ions into the stomach; used to treat hyperacidity.

pro·to·path·ic (prō'tō-path'ik) Denoting a supposedly primitive set or system of peripheral sensory nerve fibers conducting a low order of pain and poorly localized temperature sensibility.

pro·to·plasm (prō'tō-plazm) 1. Living matter, the substance of which animal and vegetable cells are formed. 2. The total cell material, including cell organelles. SYN plasmogen.

pro·to·plast (prō'tō-plast) A bacterial cell from which the rigid cell wall has been completely removed; the bacterium loses its characteristic form.

pro·to·por·phyr·i·a (prō'tō-pōr-fir'ē-ă) Enhanced fecal excretion of protoporphyrin.

pro·to·troph (prō'tō-trōf) Bacterial strain with the same nutritional requirements as the wild-type strain from which it comes.

pro·to·type (prō'tō-tīp) The primitive form; the first form to which subsequent individuals of the class or species conform.

pro·to·ver·te·bra (prō'tō-vĕr'tĕ-bră) The caudal half of each sclerotomal concentration, which is the primordium of the centrum of a vertebra.

Pro·to·zo·a (prō'tō-zō'ă) Formerly considered a phylum, now regarded as a subkingdom of the animal kingdom, including all of the so-called acellular or unicellular forms. They consist of a single functional cell unit or aggregation of nondifferentiated cells, loosely held together and not forming tissues.

pro·to·zo·an, pro·to·zo·al (prō'tō-zō'ăn, -zō'ăl) Relating to protozoa.

pro·trac·tion (prō-trak'shŭn) Forward movement of the scapula. 1. DENTISTRY the extension of teeth or other maxillary or mandibular structures into a position anterior to normal. SEE ALSO protractor. 2. Forward movement of the scapula.

pro·trac·tor (prō-trak'tŏr) A muscle drawing a part forward.

pro·trud·ed disc (prō-trūd'ĕd disk) SYN herniated disc.

pro·trud·ing ear (prō-trū'ding ēr) SYN outstanding ear.

pro·tru·sion (prō-trū'zhŭn) 1. The state of being thrust forward or projected. 2. DENTISTRY a position of the mandible forward from centric relation.

pro·tru·sive oc·clu·sion (prō-trū'siv ŏ-klū'zhŭn) Occlusion that results when the mandible is protruded forward from centric position.

pro·tu·ber·ance (prō-tū'bĕr-ăns) [TA] A swelling, protruding, or knoblike outgrowth or part. SYN protuberantia.

pro·tu·ber·ant ab·do·men (prō-tū'bĕr-ănt ab'dŏ-mĕn) Unusual or prominent convexity of the abdomen, due to excessive subcutaneous fat, poor muscle tone, or an increase in intraabdominal content.

pro·tu·ber·an·ti·a (prō-tū'bĕr-an'shē-ă) [TA] SYN protuberance.

proud flesh (prowd flesh) Exuberant granulation tissue on the surface of a wound.

pro·ur·o·ki·nase (prō'yūr-ō-kī'nās) The precursor of an activator of plasminogen, urokinase.

Prov·i·den·ci·a (prov-i-den'sē-ă) A genus of motile, peritrichous, non-spore-forming, aerobic, or facultatively anaerobic bacteria containing gram-negative rods; found in urinary tract infections and in cases of diarrheal disease.

pro·vid·er (prō-vī'dĕr) A person or agency that supplies goods or services, particularly medical or paramedical services.

pro·vid·er i·den·ti·fi·ca·tion num·ber (PIN) (prō-vī'dĕr ī-den'ti-fi-kā'shŭn nŭm'bĕr) Method used to identify a health care provider as regards a specific insurance company.

pro·vi·rus (prō-vī'rŭs) The precursor of an animal virus.

pro·vi·ta·min (prō'vī'tă-min) A substance that can be converted into a vitamin; e.g., β-carotene.

pro·vi·ta·min A (prō-vī'tă-min) Trivial name for carotenoids exhibiting qualitatively the biologic activity of β-carotene.

pro·vi·ta·min D$_2$ (prō-vī'tă-min) Substance that can give rise to ergocalciferol (vitamin D$_2$); e.g., ergosterol.

pro·vi·ta·min D$_3$ (prō-vī'tă-min) SYN 7-dehydrocholesterol.

prox·em·ics (prok-sē'miks) Scientific discipline concerned with the various aspects of urban overcrowding.

prox·i·mad (prok'si-mad) In a direction toward a proximal part, or toward the center; not distad.

prox·i·mal (prok'si-măl) [TA] 1. Nearest the trunk or the point of origin; said of part of a limb, of an artery or a nerve, so situated. 2. SYN mesial. 3. DENTAL ANATOMY denoting the surface of a tooth in relation to a neighboring or adjacent tooth.

prox·i·mal con·tact, prox·i·mate con·tact (prok'si-măl kon'takt, prok'si-măt) Area where the surfaces of two adjacent teeth in the same arch touch.

prox·i·mal in·ter·pha·lan·ge·al joints (PIP) (proks'i-măl in'těr-fă-lan'jē-ăl joynts) The synovial joints between the proximal and middle phalanges of the fingers and of the toes.

prox·i·mate (prok'si-măt) Immediate; next; proximal.

prox·i·mate cause (prok'si-măt kawz) Immediate trigger that precipitates a condition.

prox·i·mo·buc·cal (prok'si-mō-bŭk'ăl) Relating to the proximal and buccal surfaces of a tooth; denoting the angle formed by their junction.

pro·zone (prō'zōn) A phenomenon in which visible agglutination and precipitation do not occur in mixtures of specific antigen and antibody because of antibody excess.

pru·ri·go (prū-rī'gō) A chronic disease of the skin marked by a persistent eruption of papules that itch intensely.

pru·ri·go mi·tis (prū-rī'gō mī'tis) A mild form of a chronic dermatitis characterized by recurring, intensely itching papules and nodules, probably atopic.

pru·ri·go sim·plex (prū-rī'gō sim'pleks) Mild form of prurigo having a pronounced tendency to relapse.

pru·rit·ic ur·ti·car·i·al pap·ules and plaques of preg·nan·cy (PUPPP) (prūr-it'ik ŭr'ti-kar'ē-ăl pap'yūlz plaks preg'năn-sē) Intensely pruritic papulovesicles that begin on the abdomen in the third trimester and spread peripherally, resolve rapidly after delivery, and do not affect the fetus.

pru·ri·tus (prū-rī'tŭs) 1. SYN itching. 2. SYN itch (1).

pru·ri·tus a·ni (prū-rī'tŭs ā'nī) Anal itching; may be associated with seborrheic dermatitis, candidosis, external hemorrhoids, or systemic disease.

pru·ri·tus se·ni·lis, se·nile pru·ri·tus (prū-rī'tŭs sĕ-nil'is, sen'il) Itching associated with dry skin in the aged.

pru·ri·tus vul·vae (prū-rī'tŭs vŭl'vē) Itching in external female genitalia, due to seborrheic dermatitis, allergy, senile vulvar atrophy, or systemic disease.

psammo- Combining form denoting sand.

psam·mo·ma bod·ies (sa-mō'mă bod'ēz) Mineralized bodies in the meninges, choroid plexus, and in some meningiomas.

psam·mo·ma·tous (sa-mō'mă-tŭs) Possessing or characterized by the presence of psammoma bodies.

psam·mo·ma·tous men·in·gi·o·ma (sa-mō'mă-tŭs mĕ-nin'jē-ō'mă) A firm cellular neoplasm derived from fibrous tissue of the meninges, choroid plexus, and certain other structures associated with the brain, and characterized by the formation of multiple, discrete, concentrically laminated, calcareous bodies (psammoma bodies). SYN Virchow psammoma.

PSA ve·loc·i·ty (vĕ-los'i-tē) A measure of the rapidity of change in a person's level of prostate-specific antigen (PSA).

pseud·al·les·che·ri·a·sis (sūd´ăl-es-kĕ-rī´ă-sis) Clinical diseases due to infection with *Pseudallescheria boydii*.

pseu·dar·thro·sis, pseu·do·ar·thro·sis (sūd´ahr-thrō´sis, -sū´dō-) A new, false joint at the site of an ununited fracture. SYN false joint, pseudoarthrosis.

pseud·es·the·si·a, pseu·do·es·the·si·a (sūd´es-thē´zē-ă, sū´dō-) 1. SYN paraphia. 2. A subjective sensation not arising from an external stimulus. 3. SYN phantom limb.

♻ **pseudo-, pseud-** Combining forms meaning false.

pseu·do·ac·an·tho·sis ni·gri·cans (sū´dō-ak´an-thō´sis nī´gri-kanz) Acanthosis nigricans due to skin maceration from excessive sweating, or in obese and dark-complexioned adults.

pseu·do·an·eu·rysm (PA, PSA) (sū´dō-an´yū-rizm) 1. Pulsating, encapsulated hematoma in communication with the lumen of a ruptured vessel. 2. Ventricular pseudoaneurysm, a cardiac rupture contained and loculated by pericardium, which forms its external wall. SYN communicating hematoma, false aneurysm, pulsatile hematoma.

pseu·do·an·o·don·ti·a (sū´dō-an´ō-don´shē-ă) Clinical absence of teeth due to a failure in eruption.

pseu·do·bul·bar (sū´dō-bŭl´bahr) Denoting a supranuclear paralysis of the bulbar nerves.

pseu·do·bul·bar pa·ral·y·sis (sū´dō-bŭl´bahr păr-al´i-sis) Paralysis of the lips and tongue, simulating progressive bulbar paralysis but due to supranuclear lesions with bilateral involvement of the upper motor neurons.

pseu·do·ceph·a·lo·cele (sū´dō-sef´ă-lō-sēl) Acquired herniation of intracranial tissues caused by injury or disease.

pseu·do·chan·cre (sū´dō-shang´kĕr) A nonspecific indurated sore, usually penile, resembling a chancre.

pseu·do·chro·mi·dro·sis, pseu·do·chrom·hi·dro·sis (sū´dō-krō´mi-drō´sis, -hi-drō´sis) Skin pigmentation associated with sweating, but due to the local action of pigment-forming bacteria and not to excretion of colored sweat.

pseu·do·chy·lous as·cit·es (sū´dō-kī´lŭs ă-sī´tēz) Peritoneal presence of an opalescent or cloudy fluid that does not contain fat.

pseu·do·co·arc·ta·tion (sū´dō-kō´ahrk-tā´shŭn) Distortion, often with slight narrowing, of the aortic arch at the level of insertion of the ligamentum arteriosum. SYN buckled aorta, kinked aorta.

pseu·do·col·loid (sū´dō-kol´oyd) A colloidlike or mucoid substance found in ovarian cysts and elsewhere.

pseu·do·cow·pox vi·rus (sū´dō-kow´poks vī´rŭs) Virus of the genus *Parapoxvirus* that causes pseudocowpox in humans and cattle.

pseu·do·cox·al·gi·a (sū´dō-koks-al´jē-ă) SYN Legg-Calvé-Perthes disease.

pseu·do·cri·sis (sū´dō-krī´sis) Temporary drop in temperature in a disease usually ending by crisis; not a true crisis.

pseu·do·cyl·in·droid (sū´dō-sil´in-droyd) A shred of mucus or other substance resembling a renal cast in the urine.

pseu·do·cyst (sū´dō-sist) 1. Fluid accumulation in a cystlike loculus, but without an epithelial or other membranous lining. 2. A cyst with a wall formed by a host cell and not by a parasite. 3. A mass of 50 or more *Toxoplasma* bradyzoites, found within a host cell, frequently in the brain.

pseu·do·de·men·ti·a (sū´dō-dĕ-men´shē-ă) A condition resembling dementia but usually due to a depressive disorder rather than brain dysfunction.

pseu·do·e·phed·rine hy·dro·chlor·ide (sū´dō-e-fed´rin hī´drō-klōr´īd) Naturally occurring isomer of ephedrine with similar actions and uses.

pseu·do·fol·lic·u·li·tis (sū´dō-fŏ-lik´yū-lī´tis) Erythematous follicular papules or, less commonly, pustules due to close shaving of curly hair; tips of growing hairs reenter the skin, producing ingrown hairs.

pseu·do·frac·ture (sū´dō-frak´shŭr) A condition in which a radiograph shows formation of new bone with thickening of periosteum at the site of an injury to bone.

pseu·do·fu·sion beat (sū′dō-fyū′zhŭn bēt) Electrocardiographic representation of a cardiac depolarization produced by superimposition of an ineffectual electronic pacemaker spike on a QRS-complex originating from a spontaneous focus within the heart.

pseu·do·gene (sū′dō-jēn) **1.** Nucleotide sequence that is not transcribed and has no phenotypic effect. **2.** Inactive DNA segment that arose by a mutation of a parental active gene.

pseu·do·gli·o·ma (sū′dō-glī-ō′mă) Any intraocular opacity liable to be mistaken for retinoblastoma.

pseu·do·gout (sū′dō-gowt) Acute episodes of synovitis caused by deposits of calcium pyrophosphate crystals rather than urate crystals as in true gout.

pseu·do-Grae·fe sign (sū′dō-grā′fĕ sīn) Lid retraction similar to Graefe sign, but due to aberrant regeneration of fibers of the oculomotor nerve into the upper lid levator.

pseu·do·gy·ne·co·mas·ti·a (sū′dō-gī′nĕ-kō-mas′tē-ă) Fatty enlargement of the male breast with no increase in breast tissue.

pseu·do·he·ma·tu·ri·a (sū′dō-hē′mă-tyūr′ē-ă) Reddish urine caused by foods or drugs, and thus not actually hematuria. SYN false hematuria, pseudohaematuria.

pseu·do·her·maph·ro·dit·ism (sū′dō-hĕr-maf′rō-di-tizm) A state in which the person is of an unambiguous gonadal sex but has ambiguous external genitalia. SYN false hermaphroditism.

pseu·do·her·ni·a (sū′dō-her′nē-ă) Scrotal tissue inflammation or of an inguinal gland, simulating strangulated hernia.

pseu·do·hy·per·ka·le·mi·a (sū′dō-hī′pĕr-kă-lē′mē-ă) A spurious elevation of the serum concentration of potassium, occurring when potassium is released in vitro from cells in a blood sample collected for a potassium measurement.

pseu·do·hy·per·par·a·thy·roid·ism (sū′dō-hī′pĕr-par-ă-thī′roy-dizm) Hypercalcemia in a patient with a malignant neoplasm in the absence of skeletal metastases or primary hyperparathyroidism.

pseu·do·hy·per·ten·sion (sū′dō-hī′pĕr-ten′shŭn) Elevated blood pressure readings secondary to noncompressible vessels.

pseu·do·hy·per·troph·ic mus·cu·lar dys·tro·phy (PHMD) (sū′dō-hī-pĕr-trō′fik mŭs′kyū-lăr dis′trō-fē) SYN Duchenne dystrophy.

pseu·do·hy·per·tro·phy (sū′dō-hī-pĕr′trĕ-fē) Increased size of an organ or a part, due not to increase in size or number of specific functional elements but to other tissue.

pseu·do·hy·po·na·tre·mi·a (sū′dō-hī′pō-nă-trē′mē-ă) A low serum sodium concentration due to volume displacement by massive hyperlipidemia or hyperproteinemia.

pseu·do·hy·po·par·a·thy·roid·ism (sū′dō-hī′pō-par′ă-thī′royd-izm) A disorder resembling hypoparathyroidism, due to lack of end-organ responsiveness to parathyroid hormone.

pseu·do·ic·ter·us (sū′dō-ik′tĕr-ŭs) A yellowish discoloration of the skin resembling jaundice but due to some substance other than bile pigments.

pseu·do·il·e·us (sū′dō-il′ē-ŭs) Absolute obstipation, stimulating ileus, due to paralysis of the intestinal wall.

pseu·do·i·so·chro·mat·ic (sū′dō-ī′sō-krō-mat′ik) Apparently of the same color; denoting certain charts containing colored spots mixed with figures printed in confusion colors; used in testing for color vision deficiency.

pseu·do·lym·pho·ma (sū′dō-lim-fō′mă) A benign infiltration of lymphoid cells or histiocytes that microscopically resembles a malignant lymphoma.

pseu·do·ma·ni·a (sū′dō-mā′nē-ă) **1.** Factitious mental disorder. **2.** Mental disorder in which the patient falsely claims to have committed a crime. **3.** Morbid impulse to lie.

pseu·do·meg·a·col·on (sū′dō-meg′ă-kō′lŏn) Distal colon enlargement with sluggish muscular function without the neurologic abnormalities of congenital megacolon.

P

pseu·do·mel·a·no·sis (sū′dō-mel′ă-nō′sis) Dark greenish or blackish post-mortem discoloration of the abdominal viscera, due to the action of sulfureted hydrogen on disintegrated hemoglobin iron.

pseu·do·mem·bra·nous (sū′dō-mem′-brǎ-nŭs) Relating to or marked by the presence of a false membrane.

pseu·do·mem·bra·nous en·ter·o·co·li·tis, pseu·do·mem·bra·nous co·lit·is (sū′dō-mem′brǎ-nŭs en′tĕr-ō-kō-lī′tis, kō-lī′tis) Intestinal inflammation with the formation and passage of pseudomembranous material, due to infection by *Clostridium difficile*. SYN pseudomembranous enteritis.

pseu·do·mem·bra·nous gas·tri·tis (sū′dō-mem′brǎ-nŭs gas-trī′tis) Gastritis due to the formation of a false membrane.

pseu·do·men·stru·a·tion (sū′dō-men′strū-ā′shŭn) Blood-tinged mucoid vaginal discharge occurring during the first week of life due to withdrawal of maternal estrogen.

Pseu·do·mo·nas (sū′dō-mō′năz) A genus of motile, polar-flagellate, non-spore-forming, strictly aerobic bacteria; common in soil and in freshwater and marine environments; some species involved in human infections.

Pseu·do·mo·nas ae·ru·gi·no·sa (sū′dō-mō′năz ē-rū-ji-nō′să) Bacterial species found in soil, water, and commonly in clinical specimens (wound infections, infected burn lesions, urinary tract infections); causes blue pus. SYN blue pus bacillus.

pseu·do·my·o·pi·a (sū′dō-mī-ō′pē-ă) A condition simulating myopia due to spasm of the ciliary muscle.

pseu·do·myx·o·ma (sū′dō-miks-ō′mă) A gelatinous mass resembling a myxoma but composed of mucus.

pseu·do·myx·oma pe·ri·to·ne·i (sū′dō-miks-ō′mă per′i-tō′nē-ī) Accumulation of large quantities of mucoid or mucinous material in the peritoneal cavity.

pseu·do·pap·il·le·de·ma (sū′dō-pap′il-ĕ-dē′mă) Anomalous elevation of the optic disc; seen in severe hyperopia and optic nerve drusen. SYN pseudopapilloedema.

pseudopapilloedema [Br.] SYN pseudopapilledema.

pseu·do·pa·ral·y·sis (sū′dō-păr-al′i-sis) Apparent paralysis due to voluntary inhibition of motion because of pain, to incoordination, or other cause, without actual paralysis. SYN pseudoparesis (1).

pseu·do·pa·re·sis (sū′dō-păr-ē′sis) **1.** SYN pseudoparalysis. **2.** Condition marked by the pupillary changes, tremors, and speech disturbances suggestive of early paresis.

pseu·do·pe·lade (sū′dō-pĕ-lahd′) Scarring alopecia; usually occurs in scattered, irregular patches.

pseu·do·per·i·car·di·tis (sū′dō-per′i-kahr-dī′tis) An artifact of auscultation resembling a friction rub, but due to movement of the tissue in the intercostal space when the diaphragm of the stethoscope is placed over the apex beat.

pseu·do·phak·i·a (sū′dō-fak′ē-ă) An eye in which the natural lens is replaced with an intraocular lens.

Pseu·do·phyl·lid·e·a (sū′dō-fi-lid′ē-ă) Order of tapeworms with an aquatic life cycle, developing into adults in fish, marine mammals, or fish-eating mammals.

pseu·do·po·di·um, pl. **pseu·do·po·di·a** (sū′dō-pō′dē-ŭm, -ă) A temporary protoplasmic process, put forth by an ameboid stage or amebic protozoan for locomotion or for prehension of food.

pseu·do·pol·yp (sū′dō-pol′ip) A projecting mass of granulation tissue, large numbers of which may develop in ulcerative colitis; may become covered by regenerating epithelium.

pseu·do·prog·na·thism (sū′dō-prog′nă-thizm) *In the diphthong gn, the g is silent only at the beginning of a word.* An acquired projection of the mandible due to occlusal disharmonies that force the mandible forward.

pseu·do·pter·yg·i·um (sū′dō-tĕr-ij′ē-ŭm) Adhesion of the conjunctiva to the cornea, occurring after injury.

pseu·dop·to·sis (sū′dō-tō′sis) Condition resembling an inability to elevate the eyelid, due to blepharophimosis, blepharochalasis, or some other affliction. SYN false blepharoptosis.

pseu·do·pu·ber·ty (sū′dō-pyū′bĕr-tē) Condition characterized by the precocious development of a varying number of the somatic and functional changes typical of puberty; commonly due to hormonal secretions of an ovarian, testicular, or adrenocortical tumor.

pseu·do·re·ac·tion (sū′dō-rē-ak′shŭn) A false reaction; one not due to specific causes in a given test.

pseu·do·ret·i·ni·tis pig·men·to·sa (sū′dō-ret′i-nī′tis pig′men-tō′să) Widespread pigmentary retinal mottling that may follow severe eye trauma, especially a penetrating injury.

pseu·do·sar·co·ma (sū′dō-sahr-kō′mă) A bulky polyploid malignant tumor of the esophagus, composed of spindle cells with a focus of squamous cell carcinoma.

pseu·do·scar·la·ti·na (sū′dō-skahr′lă-tē′nă) Erythema with fever, due to causes other than *Streptococcus pyogenes*.

pseu·do·scle·ro·sis (sū′dō-skle-rō′sis) Inflammatory induration or fatty or other infiltration simulating fibrous thickening.

pseu·dos·to·ma (sū-dos′tō-mă) An apparent opening in a cell, membrane, or other tissue, due to a defect in staining or other cause.

pseu·do·stra·bis·mus (sū′dō-stră-biz′mŭs) The appearance of strabismus when the eyes are straight, caused by epicanthal folds, abnormality in interorbital distance, or corneal light reflex not corresponding to the center of the pupil.

pseu·do·strat·i·fied ep·i·the·li·um (sū′dō-strat′i-fīd ep′i-thē′lē-ŭm) One that gives a superficial appearance of being stratified because the cell nuclei are at different levels, but in which all cells reach the basement membrane.

pseu·do·ta·bes (sū′dō-tā′bēz) A syndrome with characteristics of tabetic neurosyphilis but not due to syphilis. SYN Leyden ataxia.

pseu·do·trun·cus ar·te·ri·o·sus (sū′dō-trŭng′kŭs ahr-tēr′ē-ō′sŭs) Congenital cardiovascular malformation with pulmonic valve atresia and absence of the main pulmonary artery.

pseu·do·tu·ber·cle (sū′dō-tū′bĕr-kĕl) Nodule histologically similar to a tuberculous granuloma, but due to infection by some microorganism other than *Mycobacterium tuberculosis*.

pseu·do·tu·ber·cu·lo·sis (sū′dō-tū-bĕr′kyū-lō′sis) A disease of a wide variety of animal species due to *Yersinia pseudotuberculosis*. Epizootics of pseudotuberculosis are commonly seen in birds and rodents, often with high case-fatality rates. SYN pseudotubercular yersiniosis.

pseu·do·tu·mor ce·re·bri (PTC) (sū′dō-tū-mŏr ser′ĕ-brī) Disorder most common in obese young women, unknown etiology; characterized clinically by headache, blurred vision, and visual obscurations. SYN idiopathic intracranial hypertension.

pseu·do·u·ri·dine (υ, Q) (sū′dō-yŭr′i-dēn) A naturally occurring isomer of uridine found in transfer ribonucleic acids; unique in that the ribosyl is attached to carbon (C-5) rather than to nitrogen; excreted in urine.

pseu·do·vi·ta·min (sū′dō-vī′tă-min) A substance having a chemical structure similar to that of a given vitamin, but lacking the usual physiologic action.

psi (sī) The 23rd letter of the Greek alphabet (ψ).

psi·lo·cy·bin (sī′lō-sī′bin) Fungal agent used as a hallucinogen (and by native Mexicans to induce trances). SYN indocybin.

psit·ta·co·sis (sit′ă-kō′sis) Infectious flulike disease in psittacine birds and humans caused by the bacterium *Chlamydia psittaci*. SYN ornithosis, Parrot disease (3), parrot fever.

psor·a·len (PSOR, P) (sōr′ă-len) A phototoxic drug used topically or orally to treat vitiligo and psoriasis.

pso·rel·co·sis (sōr′el-kō′sis) Cutaneous ulceration resulting from scabies.

psor·en·ter·i·tis (sōr'en-tĕr-ī'tis) In-flammatory swelling of the solitary lymphatic follicles of the intestine.

pso·ri·a·sis (sōr-ī'ă-sis) A common inherited condition characterized by the eruption of reddish, silvery-scaled maculopapules, predominantly on the elbows, knees, scalp, and trunk.

psy·chal·gi·a, psy·chal·ga·li·a (sī-kal'jē-ă, sī'kal-gā'lē-ă) *Do not confuse this word with psychroalgia.* **1.** Distress attending a mental effort. SYN phrenalgia (1). **2.** SYN psychogenic pain.

psy·cha·tax·i·a (sī'kă-tak'sē-ă) Mental confusion; inability to fix one's attention or to make any continued mental effort.

psy·che (sī'kē) Term for the subjective aspects of the mind, self, soul; the psychological or spiritual as distinct from the bodily nature of people.

psy·che·del·ic (sī'kĕ-del'ik) Pertaining to a rather imprecise category of drugs with mainly central nervous system action, and with effects said to be the expansion or heightening of consciousness, e.g., lysergic acid diethylamide (LSD), hashish, psilocybin.

psy·chi·at·ric (sī'kē-at'rik) Relating to psychiatry.

psy·chi·a·tric re·hab·i·li·ta·tion (sī'kē-at'rik rē'hă-bil'i-tā'shŭn) Service and support provided, with limited professional intervention, to people with long-term psychiatric disabilities to assist them in the performance of self-directed, self-satisfying functional life tasks.

psy·chi·a·try, psy·chi·at·rics (sī-kī'ă-trē, sī'kē-at'riks) The medical specialty concerned with the diagnosis and treatment of mental disorders.

psy·chic, psy·chic·al (sī'kik, -ki-kăl) Relating to the phenomena of consciousness, mind, or soul.

psy·chic en·er·gy (sī'kik en'ĕr-jē) In psychoanalysis, a hypothetic mental force, analogous to the physical concept of energy, which enables and vitalizes a person's psychological activity. SEE ALSO libido. SYN psychic force.

psy·chic im·po·tence (sī'kik im'pŏ-tens) Erectile failure due to psychological factors.

psy·chic trau·ma (sī'kik traw'mă) Upsetting experience precipitating or aggravating an emotional or mental disorder.

psycho-, psych-, psyche- Combining forms denoting the mind; mental; psychological.

psy·cho·a·cous·tics (sī'kō-ă-kūs'tiks) A discipline combining experimental psychology and physics that deals with the physical features of sound as related to audition and the physiology and psychology of sound receptor processes.

psy·cho·ac·tive (sī'kō-ak'tiv) Possessing the ability to alter mood, anxiety, or mental state; usually applied to pharmacologic agents.

psy·cho·a·nal·y·sis (sī'kō-ă-nal'i-sis) Form of psychotherapy, designed to bring preconscious and unconscious material to consciousness primarily through the analysis of transference and resistance. SEE ALSO freudian psychoanalysis. SYN psychoanalytic therapy.

psy·cho·an·a·lyst (sī'kō-an'ă-list) A psychotherapist, usually a psychiatrist or clinical psychologist, trained in psychoanalysis and employing its methods in the treatment of emotional disorders.

psy·cho·an·a·lyt·ic, psy·cho·an·a·lyt·ic·al (sī'kō-an'ă-lit'ik, i-kăl) Pertaining to psychoanalysis.

psy·cho·an·a·lyt·ic psy·chi·a·try (sī'kō-an'ă-lit'ik sī-kī'ă-trē) Psychiatric theory and practice emphasizing the principles of psychoanalysis. SYN dynamic psychiatry.

psy·cho·an·a·lyt·ic ther·a·py (sī'kō-an'ă-lit'ik thār'ă-pē) SYN psychoanalysis.

psy·cho·bi·ol·o·gy (sī'kō-bī-ol'ŏ-jē) The study of the interrelationships of biology and psychology in cognitive functioning, including intellectual, memory, and related neurocognitive processes.

psy·cho·di·ag·no·sis (sī'kō-dī'ăg-nō'sis) **1.** Any method used to discover the factors that underlie behavior, especially maladjusted or abnormal. **2.** A subspecialty within clinical psychology that emphasizes the use of psychological tests and techniques for assessing psychopathology.

psy·cho·dra·ma (sī′kō-drah′mă) Psychotherapy in which patients act out their personal problems by spontaneously enacting without rehearsal diagnostically specific roles in dramatic performances put on before their patient peers.

psy·cho·dy·nam·ics (sī′kō-dī-nam′iks) Systematized study and theory of the psychological forces that underlie human behavior, emphasizing the interplay between unconscious and conscious motivation.

psy·cho·en·do·cri·nol·o·gy (sī′kō-en′ dō-kri-nol′ŏ-jē) Study of the interrelationships between endocrine function and mental states, incorporating the idea that variation in physiologic hormonal response to stress is related to psychological variables. SEE relaxation response.

psy·cho·gal·van·ic (sī′kō-gal-van′ik) Relating to changes in electric properties of the skin.

psy·cho·gen·der (sī′kō-jen′dĕr) The attitudes adopted by a person related to his or her identification as either a male or a female.

psy·cho·gen·e·sis (sī′kō-jen′ĕ-sis) The origin and development of the psychic processes, including mental, behavioral, emotional, personality, and related psychological processes.

psy·cho·gen·e·tic (sī-kō-gĕ-net′ik) Refers to the interplay between genetic variability and psychological and psychiatric phenomena. SEE ALSO psychogenic.

psy·cho·gen·ic (sī′kō-jen′ik) **1.** Of mental origin or causation. SEE ALSO psychogenetic. **2.** Relating to emotional and related psychological development or to psychogenesis.

psy·cho·gen·ic pain (sī′kō-jen′ik pān) Somatoform pain, that associated with or correlated with a psychological, emotional, or behavioral stimulus. SYN psychalgia (2).

psy·cho·gen·ic pain dis·or·der (sī′ kō-jen′ik pān dis-ŏr′dĕr) One in which the principal complaint is pain out of proportion to objective findings.

psy·cho·gen·ic vom·it·ing (sī′kō-jen′ ik vom′it-ing) Emesis associated with emotional distress and anxiety.

psy·cho·geu·sic (sī′kō-gyū′sik) Denoting mental perception and interpretation of taste.

psy·cho·ki·ne·sis, psy·cho·ki·ne·sia (sī′kō-ki-nē′sis, -nē′zē-ă) **1.** The influence of mind on matter. **2.** Impulsive behavior.

psy·cho·lin·guis·tics (sī′kō-ling-gwis′ tiks) Study of a host of psychological factors associated with speech, including voice, attitudes, emotions, and grammatical rules.

psy·cho·log·i·cal (sī′kō-loj′i-ăl) **1.** Relating to psychology. **2.** Relating to the mind and its processes. SEE ALSO psychology.

psy·chol·o·gist (sī-kol′ŏ-jist) A specialist in psychology licensed to practice professional psychology, qualified to teach psychology as a scholarly discipline, or whose scientific specialty is a subfield of psychology.

psy·chol·o·gy (sī-kol′ŏ-jē) Study of the behavior of humans and animals, and related mental and physiologic processes.

psy·chom·e·try, psy·cho·met·rics (sī′ kom′ĕ-trē, sī′kō-met′riks) Discipline of psychological and mental testing, and quantitative analysis of a person's psychological traits or attitudes or mental processes. SYN psychometrics.

psy·cho·mo·tor (sī′kō-mō′tŏr) **1.** Relating to the psychological processes associated with muscular movement and to the production of voluntary movements. **2.** Relating to the combination of psychic and motor events, including disturbances.

psy·cho·mo·tor ep·il·ep·sy (sī′kō-mō′tŏr ep′i-lep′sē) Attacks with elaborate and multiple sensory, motor, and psychic components, the common feature being a clouding or loss of consciousness and amnesia for the event. SEE ALSO procursive epilepsy.

psy·cho·mo·tor re·tar·da·tion (PMR) (sī′kō-mō′tŏr rē-tahr-dā′shŭn) Slowed psychic activity or motor activity, or both.

psy·cho·neu·ro·im·mu·nol·o·gy (sī′ kō-nū′rō-im′yū-nol′ŏ-jē) An area of study that focuses on emotional and other psychological states that affect the immune system, rendering the patient less or more susceptible to disease or the course of a disease.

psy·cho·neu·ro·sis (sī′kō-nūr-ō′sis) A mental or behavioral disorder of mild or moderate severity.

psy·cho·neu·rot·ic (sī′kō-nūr-ot′ik) Pertaining to or suffering from psychoneurosis.

psy·cho·on·col·o·gy (sī′kō-on-kol′ŏ-jē) Psychological aspects of the treatment and management of the patient with cancer; it combines elements of psychiatry, psychology, and medicine.

psy·cho·path (sī′kō-path) Former designation for a person with an antisocial type of personality disorder. SEE ALSO antisocial personality disorder, sociopath.

psy·cho·path·ic (sī′kō-path′ik) Relating to or characteristic of psychopathy.

psy·cho·pa·thol·o·gy (sī′kō-pă-thol′ŏ-jē) **1.** Science of pathology of the mind and behavior. **2.** Science of mental and behavioral disorders.

psy·cho·phar·ma·ceu·ti·cals (sī′kō-fahr′mă-sū′ti-kălz) Drugs used in the treatment of emotional disorders.

psy·cho·phar·ma·col·o·gy (sī′kō-fahr′mă-kol′ŏ-jē) **1.** The use of drugs to treat mental and psychological disorders. **2.** The science of drug-behavior relationships.

psy·cho·phys·i·cal (sī′kō-fiz′i-kăl) **1.** Relating to the mental perception of physical stimuli. SEE ALSO psychophysics. **2.** SYN psychosomatic.

psy·cho·phys·i·ol·o·gy (sī′kō-fiz′ē-ol′ŏ-jē) The science of the relationship between psychological and physiologic processes.

psy·cho·sen·so·ry, psy·cho·sen·so·ri·al (sī′kō-sen′sŏr-ē, -sen-sōr′ē-ăl) **1.** Denoting the mental perception and interpretation of sensory stimuli. **2.** Denoting a hallucination that, with effort, the mind is able to distinguish from reality.

psy·cho·sex·u·al (sī′kō-sek′shū-ăl) Pertaining to relationships among the emotional, mental, physiologic, and behavioral components of sex or sexual development.

psy·cho·sex·u·al de·vel·op·ment (sī′kō-sek′shū-ăl dĕ-vel′ŏp-mĕnt) Maturation and development of the psychic and behavioral phases of sexuality from birth to adult life through the oral, anal, phallic, latency, and genital phases.

psy·cho·sex·u·al dys·func·tion, sex·u·al dys·func·tion (sī′kō-sek′shū-ăl dis-fŭngk′shŭn, sek′shū-ăl) A disturbance in sexual function (e.g., impotence, premature ejaculation, anorgasmia) presumed to be from psychological rather than physical causes.

psy·cho·sis, pl. **psy·cho·ses** (sī-kō′sis, -sēz) A mental and behavioral disorder causing gross distortion or disorganization of a person's mentation.

psy·cho·so·cial (sī′kō-sō′shăl) Involving both psychological and social aspects.

psy·cho·so·mat·ic (sī′kō-sŏ-mat′ik) Pertaining to the influence of the mind or higher functions of the brain on body functions. SYN psychophysical (2).

psy·cho·so·mat·ic dis·or·der, psy·cho·phys·i·o·log·ic dis·or·der (sī′kō-sŏ-mat′ik dis-ōr′dĕr, sī′kō-fiz′ē-ŏ-loj′ik dis-or′dĕr) Condition characterized by physical symptoms of psychic origin, usually involving a single organ system innervated by the autonomic nervous system.

psy·cho·so·mat·ic med·i·cine (sī′kō-sŏ-mat′ik med′i-sin) The study and treatment of diseases, disorders, or abnormal states in which psychological processes resulting in physiologic reactions are believed to play a prominent role.

psy·cho·stim·u·lant (sī′kō-stim′yū-lănt) An pharmacotherapeutic agent with antidepressant properties.

psy·cho·sur·ger·y (sī′kō-sŭr′jĕr-ē) The treatment of mental disorders by surgery on the brain (e.g., lobotomy).

psy·cho·ther·a·pist (sī′kō-thār′ă-pist) A person, usually a psychiatrist or clinical psychologist, professionally trained and engaged in psychotherapy.

psy·cho·ther·a·py (sī′kō-thār′ă-pē) Treatment of emotional, behavioral, personality, and psychiatric disorders based primarily on verbal or nonverbal communication and interventions with the patient. SEE ALSO psychoanalysis, psychiatry, psychology, therapy.

psy·chot·ic (sī-kot′ik) Relating to or affected by psychosis.

psy·chot·o·gen·ic (sī-kot′ō-jen′ik) Little-used term meaning capable of inducing psychosis.

psy·chot·o·mi·met·ic (sī-kot′ō-mi-met′ik) A drug or substance that produces psychological and behavioral changes resembling those of psychosis.

psy·cho·tro·pic (sī′kō-trō′pik) Capable of affecting the mind, emotions, and behavior; denoting drugs used in the treatment of mental illnesses.

psychro- Combining form denoting cold. SEE ALSO cryo-, crymo-.

psy·chro·al·gi·a (sī′krō-al′jē-ă) A painful sensation of cold.

psy·chrom·e·try (sī-krom′ĕ-trē) The calculation of relative humidity and water vapor pressures from wet and dry bulb temperatures and barometric pressure. SYN hygrometry.

psy·chro·phil·ic (sī′krō-fil′ik) Pertaining to a preference for cold.

psy·chro·phore (sī′krō-fōr) A double catheter through which cold water is circulated to apply cold to the urethra or another canal or cavity.

psyl·li·um (sil′ē-ŭm) The husk of the psyllium seed used to relieve constipation and treat some other gastrointestinal problems.

Pt Symbol for platinum.

pter-, ptero- Combining forms denoting wing; feather.

pte·ryg·i·um (tĕr-ij′ē-ŭm) **1.** A triangular patch of hypertrophied bulbar subconjunctival tissue. **2.** Forward growth of the cuticle over the nail plate. **3.** An abnormal skin web.

pter·y·goid (ter′i-goyd) Wing-shaped; resembling a wing.

pter·y·go·man·dib·u·lar (ter′i-gō-man-dib′yū-lăr) Relating to the pterygoid process and the mandible.

pter·y·go·max·il·lar·y (ter′i-gō-mak′si-lar-ē) Relating to the pterygoid process and the maxilla.

pter·y·go·pal·a·tine (ter′i-gō-pal′ă-tīn) Relating to the pterygoid process and the palatine bone.

Pthir·us (thir′ŭs) A genus of lice; main species is *P. pubis*, the crab or pubic louse, a parasite that infests the pubes and adjacent hairy parts of the body.

pto·maine (tō′mān) An indefinite term applied to poisonous substances formed in the decomposition of protein by the decarboxylation of amino acids by bacterial action.

-ptosis Suffix meaning a sinking down or prolapse of an organ.

pto·sis, pl. **pto·ses** (tō′sis, -sēz) **1.** A sinking down or prolapse of an organ. **2.** SYN blepharoptosis.

ptyal-, ptyalo- Combining forms denoting the salivary glands, saliva. SEE ALSO sialo-.

pu·bar·che (pyū′bahr-kē) Onset of puberty, particularly as manifested by the growth of pubic hair.

pu·ber·ty (pyu′bĕr-tē) Sequence of events by which a child becomes a young adult, characterized by the beginning of gonadotropin secretion, gametogenesis, secretion of gonadal hormones, development of secondary sexual characteristics and reproductive functions. Ethnic and geographic factors may influence the time at which various events typical of puberty occur.

pu·bes (pyū′bēz) [TA] **1.** [TA] The area above the external genitals where hair growth signals puberty. **2.** One of the pubic hairs; the hair of the pubic region. USAGE NOTE Often incorrectly called pubis.

pu·bic (pyū′bik) Relating to the pubes or to the pubic bone.

P

pu·bic hair (PH) (pyŭ′bik hār) [TA] SYN pubes (1) [TA].

pu·bic reg·ion (pyŭ′bik rē′jŭn) [TA] The lower central region of the abdomen below the umbilical region.

pu·bi·ot·o·my (pyŭ-bē-ot′ŏ-mē) Severance of the pubic bone a few centimeters lateral to the symphysis, to increase the capacity of a contracted pelvis sufficiently to permit the passage of a living child. SYN pelviotomy (2), pelvitomy.

pu·bis, pl. **pu·bes** (pyŭ′bis, -bēz) Official alternate term for os pubis, the pubic bone.

pub·lic health (pŭb′lik helth) The art and science of community health, concerned with statistics, epidemiology, hygiene, and the prevention and eradication of epidemic diseases.

pub·lic health nurse (pŭb′lik helth nŭrs) One who provides care to individual patients or groups in a community outside of institutions, usually through government aegis. SYN community health nurse, community nurse.

pu·bo·pros·tat·ic (pyŭ′bō-pros-tat′ik) Relating to the pubic bone and the prostate.

pu·bo·ves·i·cal (pyŭ′bō-ves′i-kăl) Relating to the pubic bone and the bladder.

pu·den·dal (pyū-den′dăl) Relating to the external genitals.

pu·den·dum, pl. **pu·den·da** (pyū-den′dŭm, -dă) The external genitals, especially the female genitals (vulva).

pu·er·per·a, pl. **pu·er·per·ae** (pyū-er′pĕr-ă, -ē) A woman who has just given birth.

pu·er·per·al (pyū-er′pĕr-ăl) Relating to the puerperium, or period after childbirth. SYN puerperant (1).

pu·er·per·al ec·lamp·sia (pyū-er′pĕr-ăl ĕ-klamp′sē-ă) Convulsions and coma associated with hypertension, edema, and proteinuria occurring in a woman after delivery of a child.

pu·er·per·al fe·ver, pu·er·per·al sep·sis (pyū-er′pĕr-ăl fē′vĕr, sep′sis) Postpartum sepsis with a rise in fever after the first 24 hours following delivery, but before the eleventh postpartum day. SYN childbed fever.

pu·er·per·al mas·ti·tis (pyū-er′pĕr-ăl mas-tī′tis) Breast inflammation, usually suppurative, occurring in the later part of the puerperium. SYN lactational mastitis.

pu·er·per·al sep·ti·ce·mi·a (pyū-er′pĕr-ăl sep′ti-sē′mē-ă) A severe bloodstream infection resulting from an obstetric delivery or procedure.

pu·er·pe·ri·um (pyū′er-pēr′ē-ŭm, -ă) Period from the termination of labor to complete involution of the uterus, usually defined as 42 days.

Pul·frich phe·nom·e·non (pŭl′frik fĕ-nom′ĕ-non) Binocular perception that an small target oscillating in the frontal plane is moving elliptically when one eye is covered by a filter or in unilateral optic neuropathy.

pu·lic·i·cide, pu·li·cide (pyŭ′lis′i-sīd, pyŭ′li-sīd) A chemical agent that kills fleas.

pulmo-, pulmon-, pulmono- Combining forms meaning the lungs. SEE ALSO pneum-, pneumo-.

pul·mo·a·or·tic (pul′mō-ā-ōr′tik) Relating to the pulmonary artery and the aorta.

pul·mo·nar·y, pul·mon·ic (pul′mŏ-nar-ē, pul-mon′ik) Relating to the lungs, to the pulmonary artery, or to the aperture leading from the right ventricle into the pulmonary artery. SYN pneumonic (1), pulmonic.

pul·mo·nar·y aci·nus (pul′mŏ-nar-ē as′i-nŭs) That part of the airway consisting of a respiratory bronchiole and all of its branches. SYN primary pulmonary lobule.

pul·mo·nar·y al·ve·o·lar mi·cro·lith·i·a·sis (pul′mŏ-nar-ē al-vē′ŏ-lăr mī′krō-li-thī′ă-sis) Microscopic granules of calcium or bone disseminated throughout the lungs.

pul·mo·nar·y al·ve·o·lar pro·tein·o·sis (PAP) (pul′mŏ-nar-ē al-vē′ŏ-lăr prō′tē-nō′sis) Chronic progressive lung disease of adults, characterized by alveolar accumulation of fatty granular proteinaceous material with little inflammatory cellular exudate; cause unknown.

pul·mo·nar·y am·e·bi·a·sis (pul´mŏ-nar-ē ă´mē-bī´ă-sis) Amebiatic lung infection; usually indicates extension of *Entamoeba histolytica* infection from a liver abscess, penetrating through the diaphragm into the lung.

pul·mo·nar·y an·thrax (pul´mŏ-nar-ē an´thraks) Anthrax acquired by inhalation of dust containing *Bacillus anthracis.*

pul·mo·nar·y a·tre·si·a (PA) (pul´mŏ-nar-ē ă-trē´zē-ă) Congenital absence of the pulmonary valve orifice.

pul·mo·nar·y cap·il·lar·y wedge pres·sure (PCWP) (pul´mŏ-nar-ē kap´i-lar-ē wej presh´ŭr) The pressure obtained when a catheter is passed from the right side of the heart into pulmonary artery as far as it will go and ''wedged'' into an end artery.

pul·mo·nar·y cir·cu·la·tion (PC) (pul´mŏ-nar-ē sĭr´kyū-lā´shŭn) Passage of blood from the right ventricle through the pulmonary artery to the lungs and back through the pulmonary veins to the left atrium. SYN lesser circulation.

pul·mo·nar·y col·lapse (pul´mŏ-nar-ē kŏ-laps´) Secondary atelectasis due to bronchial obstruction, pleural effusion or pneumothorax, or enlargement of other adjacent structures.

pul·mo·nar·y dys·ma·tu·ri·ty syn·drome (pul´mŏ-nar-ē dis´mă-chŭr´i-tē sin´drŏm) Respiratory disorder in small, premature infants incapable of normal pulmonary ventilation who often die of hypoxia after an illness lasting 6–8 weeks. SYN Wilson-Mikity syndrome.

pul·mo·nar·y e·de·ma (pul´mŏ-nar-ē ĕ-dē´mă) Accumulation of extravascular fluid in lung tissues and alveoli usually resulting from mitral stenosis or left ventricular failure.

pul·mo·nar·y em·bo·lism (PE) (pul´mŏ-nar-ē em´bŏ-lizm) Obstruction of pulmonary arteries, most frequently by detached fragments of thrombus from a leg or pelvic vein.

pul·mo·nar·y func·tion test (PFT) (pul´mŏ-nar-ē fŭnk´shŭn test) An assessment of the respiratory system that provides information about ventilation, airflow, lung volumes and capacity, and the diffusion of gas.

pul·mo·nar·y groove (pul´mŏ-nar-ē grūv) A deep vertical recess formed on either side of the thoracic cage by the posterior curvature of the ribs and containing the posterior portions of the lung.

pul·mo·nar·y hy·per·ten·sion (pul´mŏ-nar-ē hī´pĕr-ten´shŭn) Hypertension in the pulmonary circuit; may be primary or secondary to pulmonary or cardiac disease.

pul·mo·nar·y in·suf·fi·cien·cy (pul´mŏ-nar-ē in´sŭ-fish´ĕn-sē) SEE valvular regurgitation.

pul·mo·nar·y in·ter·sti·tial em·phy·se·ma (PIE) (pŭl´mŏ-nar-ē in´tĕr-stish´ăl em´fă-sē´mă) The presence of air in interstitial lung tissue due to excessive ventilatory pressure.

pul·mo·nar·y ste·no·sis (pul´mŏ-nar-ē stĕ-nō´sis) Narrowing of the opening into the pulmonary artery from the right ventricle.

pul·mo·nar·y toi·let (pul´mŏ-nar-ē toy´lĕt) Cleansing of the trachea and bronchial tree.

pul·mo·nar·y tu·ber·cu·lo·sis (PT, PTB) (pul´mŏ-nar-ē tū-bĕr´kyū-lō´sis) Tuberculosis of the lungs.

pul·mo·nar·y tu·la·re·mi·a (pul´mŏ-nar-ē tū-lă-rē´mē-ă) Tularemia affecting the lungs; tularemic pneumonia. SYN pulmonic tularemia.

pul·mo·nar·y vas·cu·lar re·sis·tance (pul´mŏ-nar-ē vas´kyū-lăr rĕ-zis´tăns) The resistance to blood flow through the pulmonary circulation.

pul·mo·nar·y veins (pul´mŏ-nar-ē vānz) [TA] Four veins, two on each side, conveying oxygenated blood from the lungs to the left atrium of the heart. SYN venae pulmonales [TA].

pul·mo·nar·y ven·ti·la·tion (pul´mŏ-nar-ē ven´ti-lā´shŭn) Respiratory minute volume, i.e., the total volume of gas per

P

minute inspired (V_I) or expired (V_E) expressed in liters per minute.

pul·mon·ic re·gur·gi·ta·tion (PR) (pul-mon´ik rē-gŭr´ji-tā´shŭn) Incompetence of the pulmonic valve permitting retrograde flow.

pulp, pulp·a (pŭlp, pŭl´pă) **1.** A soft, moist, coherent solid. **2.** SYN dental pulp. **3.** SYN chyme.

pulp ab·scess (pŭlp ab´ses) Lesion involving soft tissue within the pulp chamber of a tooth.

pul·pal (pŭl´păl) Relating to the pulp.

pulp ca·nal (pŭlp kă-nal´) SYN root canal of tooth.

pulp cav·i·ty (pŭlp kav´i-tē) [TA] The central hollow of a tooth consisting of the crown cavity and the root canal.

pulp cham·ber (pŭlp chăm´bĕr) The portion of the pulp cavity contained in the crown or body of the tooth.

pulp·ec·to·my (pŭl-pek´tŏ-mē) Removal of the entire pulp structure of a tooth.

pul·pi·fac·tion (pŭlp´i-fak´shŭn) Reduction to a pulpy condition.

pul·pi·tis (pŭl-pī´tis) Inflammation of the pulp of a tooth.

pulp·less tooth (pŭlp´les tūth) One with a nonvital or necrotic pulp, or one from which the pulp has been extirpated.

pulp·ot·o·my (pŭl-pot´ŏ-mē) Removal of a portion of the pulp structure of a tooth, usually the coronal portion.

pulp·y (pŭl´pē) In the condition of a soft, moist solid.

pul·sate (pŭl´sāt) To throb rhythmically; said of the heart or an artery.

pul·sa·tile (pŭl´să-til) Throbbing or beating.

pul·sa·til·i·ty in·dex (PI) (pŭls´ă-til´i-tē in´deks) Calculation of Doppler measurements of systolic and diastolic velocities in the uterine, umbilical, or fetal circulations.

pul·sa·tion (pŭl-sā´shŭn) Rhythmic beating, as of the pulse or the heart.

pulse (pŭls) Palpable rhythmic expansion of an artery, produced by the increased volume of blood pushed or forced into the vessel by the contraction of the heart.

pulse def·i·cit (pŭls def´i-sit) Absence of palpable pulse waves in a peripheral artery for one or more heart beats.

pulsed la·ser (pŭlst lā´zĕr) A laser with rhythmic energy output.

pulse gen·er·a·tor (pŭls jen´ĕr-ā-tŏr) Device that produces an electrical discharge with a regular or rhythmic waveform in which the electromotive force varies in a specific pattern in relation to time.

pulse height an·a·ly·zer (pŭls hīt an´ă-līz-ĕr) Electronic circuitry that determines the energy of scintillations recorded by a detector.

pulse ox·i·me·ter (pŭls oks-im´ĕ-tĕr) A spectrophotometric device that noninvasively estimates saturation of arterial oxyhemoglobin by use of selected wavelengths of light.

pulse pres·sure (pŭls presh´ŭr) Variation in blood pressure occurring in an artery during the cardiac cycle.

pulse rate (PR, P-R) (pŭls rāt) Rate of the pulse as observed in an artery; recorded as beats per minute.

pulse se·quence (pŭls sē´kwĕns) MAGNETIC RESONANCE IMAGING a series of changes in the induced magnetic field, which includes the phase and frequency-encoding gradients and read-out functions.

pulse wave (PW) (pŭls wāv) Progressive expansion of the arteries occurring with each contraction of the left ventricle of the heart.

pul·sion (pŭl´shŭn) A pushing outward or swelling.

pul·sus bis·fe·ri·ens (pŭl´sŭs bis-fer´ē-enz) SYN bisferious pulse.

pul·sus dif·fer·ens (pŭl´sŭs dif´ĕr-enz) A condition in which the pulses in the two radial or other corresponding arteries differ in strength.

pul·sus tar·dus (pŭl'sŭs tahr'dŭs) A pulse with pathologically gradual up-stroke typical of severe aortic stenosis. SEE ALSO plateau pulse.

pul·ta·ceous (pŭl-tā'shŭs) Macerated; pulpy.

pul·vi·nar (pŭl'vī-năr) [TA] The expanded posterior extremity of the thalamus that forms a cushionlike prominence overlying the geniculate bodies.

pump (pŭmp) **1.** An apparatus for forcing a gas or liquid from or to any part. **2.** Any mechanism for using metabolic energy to accomplish active transport of a substance.

pump-ox·y·gen·a·tor (pŭmp-ok'si-jĕ-nā'tŏr) A mechanical device that can substitute for both the heart (pump) and the lungs (oxygenator) during open heart surgery.

punch bi·op·sy (pŭnch bī'op-sē) Any method that removes a small cylindric specimen with a special instrument that pierces the organ directly or through the skin or a small incision in the skin.

punch-drunk syn·drome, punch·drunk (pŭnch'drŭngk sin'drōm) A condition seen in prizefighters, often years after retirement; presumably caused by repeated cerebral injury, characterized by weakness in the lower limbs, slowness of movements, tremors, and slow cerebration.

punch grafts (pŭnch grafs) Small, full-thickness hirsute grafts, removed with a circular punch and transplanted to a bald area to grow hair on it.

punc·tate (pŭngk'tāt) Marked with points differentiated from the surrounding surface by color, elevation, or texture.

punc·tate ker·a·to·der·ma (pŭngk'tāt ker'ă-tō-dĕr'mă) Horny papules over the palms, soles, and digits that develop central plugs; seen commonly in blacks; autosomal dominant inheritance. SYN keratosis punctata.

punc·ti·form (pŭngk'ti-fŏrm) Very small but not microscopic, having a diameter of less than 1 mm.

punc·tum, gen. **punc·ti,** pl. **punc·ta** (pŭngk'tŭm, -ti, -tă) [TA] **1.** Tip of a sharp process. **2.** Minute round spot differing in color or otherwise from surrounding tissues. **3.** Opening into the lacrimal drainage system in the upper and lower eyelids. SYN point (1).

punc·ture (pungk'shŭr) **1.** To make a hole with a small pointed object. **2.** A prick or small hole made with a pointed instrument.

punc·ture wound (pungk'shŭr wūnd) A wound in which the opening is relatively small with the depth.

pu·pil (p) (pyū'pil) [TA] The circular orifice in the center of the iris, through which light rays enter the eye.

pu·pil·la·ry (pyū'pi-lar-ē) Relating to the pupil.

pu·pil·la·ry re·flex (pyū'pi-lar-ē rē'fleks) Change in diameter of the pupil as a reflex response to any type of stimulus. SYN light reflex (1).

pu·pil·la·ry ruff (pyū'pi-lar-ē rŭf) Dark-brown, wrinkled rim of the normal pupil, which is the posterior pigment epithelium of the iris.

pu·pil·lar·y skin re·flex (pyū'pi-lar'ē-skin rē'fleks) Dilation of the pupil following scratching of the skin of the neck. SYN ciliospinal reflex.

♻ **pupillo-** Prefix indicating the pupils.

pu·pil·lom·e·ter (pyū'pi-lom'ĕ-tĕr) An instrument for measuring and recording the diameter of the pupil.

pu·pil·lom·e·try (pyū'pi-lom'ĕ-trē) Measurement of the pupil.

pu·pil·lo·mo·tor (pyū'pi-lō-mō'tŏr) Relating to the autonomic nerve fibers that supply the smooth muscle of the iris.

pu·pil·lo·sta·tom·e·ter (pyū'pi-lō-stă-tom'ĕ-tĕr) An instrument for measuring the distance between the centers of the pupils.

pu·pil re·ac·tion (pyū'pil rē-ak'shun) Constriction of the pupil in response to light rays.

PUPPP Abbreviation for *p*ruritic *u*rticarial *p*apules and *p*laques of *p*regnancy; intensely pruritic, occasionally vesicular, eruption of the trunk and arms appearing in the third trimester of pregnancy.

pure autonomic failure (pyūr aw'tō-nom'ik fāl'yŭr) A degenerative, sporadic neurologic disorder of adult onset, manifested principally as orthostatic hypotension and syncope, with no neurologic defects other than autonomic nervous system dysfunction evident. SYN Bradbury-Eggleston syndrome.

pure col·or (pyūr kŏl'ŏr) Visual sensation produced by light of a specific wavelength.

pure cul·ture (pyūr kŭl'chŭr) In the ordinary bacteriologic sense, a culture consisting of the descendants of a single cell.

pure tone av·er·age (pyūr tōn av'răj) The usual hearing threshold level for the pure tone frequencies of 500 Hz, 1 kHz, and 2 kHz; referred to as speech frequencies because many English phonemes are within this frequency range.

pur·ga·tive (pŭr'gă-tiv) An agent used for purging the bowels. SEE ALSO cathartic (2).

purge (pŭrj) **1.** To cause a copious evacuation of the bowels. **2.** A cathartic remedy.

pu·ri·fied cot·ton (pyūr'i-fīd kot'ŏn) Absorbent cotton in which the hairs of the seed of *Gossypium* are freed from impurities, deprived of fatty matter, bleached, and sterilized.

Pur·kin·je cell lay·er (pŭr-kin'jē sel lā'yĕr) The layer of large neuron cell bodies located at the interface of molecular and granular layers in the cerebellar cortex. Also called Purkinje cells, Purkinje corpuscles.

Pur·kin·je net·work (pŭr-kin'jē net' wŏrk) The network formed by Purkinje fibers beneath the endocardium.

Pur·kin·je sys·tem (pŭr-kin'jē sis'tĕm) SYN subendocardial conducting system of heart.

pur·pu·ra (pŭr'pyūr-ă) A condition characterized by hemorrhage into the skin. SYN peliosis.

pur·pu·ra ful·mi·nans (pŭr'pyūr-ă ful' mi-nanz) Severe and rapidly fatal form of purpura hemorrhagica, especially in children, with hypotension, fever, and disseminated intravascular coagulation.

pur·pu·ra se·ni·lis (pŭr'pyūr-ă sĕ-nil'is) Petechiae and ecchymoses on the atrophic skin of the legs in aged and debilitated patients.

pur·pu·ra sim·plex (pŭr'pyū-ră sim' pleks) The eruption of petechiae or larger ecchymoses, not associated with systemic illness. SYN nonthrombocytopenic purpura.

pur·pu·ric (pŭr-pyūr'ik) Relating to or affected with purpura.

pursed-lip breath·ing (pŭrst lip brēdh' ing) Respirations characterized by a prolonged expiratory maneuver in which a person exhales through puckered lips.

purse-string su·ture (pŭrs'string sū'chŭr) Continuous circular suture either for inversion or closure.

pu·ru·lence, pu·ru·len·cy (pyūr'ŭ-lĕns, -lĕn-sē) The condition of containing or forming pus.

pur·u·lent con·junc·ti·vi·tis (pyūr'ŭ-lĕnt kŏn-jŭngk'ti-vī'tis) Violently acute inflammation of the conjunctiva, with copious pus and a marked tendency for corneal involvement.

pur·u·lent in·flam·ma·tion (pyūr'ŭ-lĕnt in'flă-mā'shŭn) An acute exudative inflammation in which the accumulation of polymorphonuclear leukocytes is sufficiently great that their enzymes cause liquefaction of the affected tissues; the purulent exudate is frequently termed pus.

pur·u·lent oph·thal·mi·a (pyūr'ŭ-lĕnt of-thal'mē-ă) Purulent conjunctivitis, usually of gonorrheal origin.

pur·u·lent pleu·ri·sy (pyūr'ŭ-lĕnt plūr'i-sē) Inflammation of pleura with empyema.

pu·ru·loid (pyū'rū-loyd) Resembling pus.

pus (pŭs) A fluid product of inflammation containing leukocytes and the debris of dead cells and tissue elements.

pus cell (pŭs sel) SYN pus corpuscle.

pus cor·pus·cle (pŭs kōr'pŭs-ĕl) One of the polymorphonuclear leukocytes that comprise the chief portion of the formed elements in pus. SYN pus cell.

pus·tu·lar (pŭs'tyū-lăr) Relating to or marked by pustules.

pus·tule (pŭs'tyūl) A small, circumscribed elevation of the skin, containing purulent material.

pus·tu·lo·sis (pŭs'tyū-lō'sis) 1. An eruption of pustules. 2. Term occasionally used to designate acropustulosis.

pus·tu·lo·sis pal·ma·ris et plan·ta·ris (pŭs'tyū-lō'sis pahl'mahr-is et plan-tahr'is) A sterile pustular eruption of the fingers and toes. SYN acrodermatitis perstans.

pu·tre·fac·tion (pyū'trĕ-fak'shŭn) Decomposition or rotting; the breakdown of organic matter, characterized usually by the presence of toxic or malodorous products. SYN decay (2), decomposition.

pu·tre·fac·tive (pyū'trĕ-fak'tiv) Relating to or causing putrefaction.

pu·tre·fy (pyū'trĕ-fī) To cause to become, or to become, putrid.

pu·tres·cence (pyū-tres'ĕns) The state of putrefaction.

pu·tres·cine (pyū-tres'ēn) Poisonous polyamine formed from arginine during putrefaction; found in urine and feces.

pu·trid (pyū'trid) 1. In a state of putrefaction. 2. Denoting putrefaction.

PUVA (pū'vă) Acronym for oral administration of *p*soralen and subsequent exposure to long wavelength *u*ltraviolet light (*uv-a*); used to treat psoriasis.

P wave (wāv) Waveform in an electrocardiographic tracing representing atrial depolarization.

pyaemia [Br.] SYN pyemia.

pyaemic embolism [Br.] SYN pyemic embolism.

py·ar·thro·sis (pī'ahr-thrō'sis) Suppurative pus within a joint cavity.

pycno- SEE pykno-.

pycnodysostosis [Br.] SYN pyknodysostosis.

pycnometer [Br.] SYN pyknometer.

py·e·lec·ta·sis, py·e·lec·ta·si·a (pī'ĕ-lek'tă-sis, -lek-tā'zē-ă) Dilation of the pelvis of the kidney.

py·e·li·tis (pī'ĕ-lī'tis) Inflammation of the renal pelvis.

pyelo-, pyel- Combining forms meaning pelvis, usually the renal pelvis.

py·e·lo·cys·ti·tis (pī'ĕ-lō-sis-tī'tis) Inflammation of the renal pelvis and the bladder.

py·e·lo·flu·o·ros·co·py (pī'ĕ-lō-flōr-os'kŏ-pē) Fluoroscopic examination of the renal pelves and ureters, following administration of contrast medium.

py·el·o·gram, py·e·lo·u·re·ter·o·gram (pī'el-ō-gram, -yūr-ē'tĕr-ō-gram) A radiograph of the renal pelvis and ureter, following injection of contrast medium.

py·e·log·ra·phy, pel·vi·u·re·te·ro·ra·di·og·ra·phy, py·e·lo·ur·e·ter·og·ra·phy, ur·e·ter·o·py·e·log·ra·phy (pī'ĕ-log'ră-fē, pel'vē-yūr-ē'tĕr-ō-rā-dē-og'ră-fē, pī'ĕ-lō-yūr-ē'tĕr-og'ră-fē, yūr-ē'tĕr-ō-pī-ă-log'ră-fē) Radiologic study of the kidney, ureters, and usually the bladder, performed with the aid of a contrast agent.

py·e·lo·li·thot·o·my, pel·vi·lith·ot·o·my (pī'ĕ-lō-li-thot'ŏ-mē, pel'vi-) Operative removal of renal calculus through an incision in the renal pelvis. SYN pelvilithotomy.

py·e·lo·ne·phri·tis (pī'ĕ-lō-nĕ-frī'tis) Inflammation of the renal parenchyma, calyces, and pelvis, particularly due to local bacterial infection.

py·e·lo·plas·ty, pel·vi·o·plas·ty (pī'ĕ-lō-plas-tē, pel'vē-ō-) Surgical reconstruction of the kidney pelvis to correct an obstruction. SYN pelvioplasty (2).

py·e·los·co·py (pī'ĕ-los'kŏ-pē) Fluoroscopic observation of the pelvis and calyces of the kidney, and the ureter, after the injection through the ureter of a radiopaque solution.

P

py·e·los·to·my (pī'ĕ-los'tŏ-mē) Formation of an opening into the kidney pelvis to establish urinary drainage.

py·e·lot·o·my (pī'ĕ-lot'ŏ-mē) Incision into the pelvis of the kidney. SYN pelviotomy (3), pelvitomy.

py·e·lo·ve·nous (pī'ĕ-lō-vē'nŭs) Relating to the renal pelvis and renal veins.

py·em·e·sis (pī-em'ĕ-sis) The vomiting of pus.

py·e·mi·a (pī-ē'mē-ă) Septicemia due to pyogenic organisms causing multiple abscesses. SYN pyaemia.

py·e·mic em·bo·lism (pī-ē'mik em'bŏ-lizm) Plugging of an artery by an embolus detached from a suppurating thrombus. SYN infective embolism, pyaemic embolism.

pyk·nic (pik'nik) Denoting a constitutional body type characterized by well-rounded external contours and ample body cavities.

♲ **pykno-, pyk-** Combining forms meaning thick, dense, compact.

pyk·no·dys·os·to·sis (pik'nō-dis'os-tō'sis) [TA] A familial dysmorphism characterized by short stature, delayed closure of the fontanelles, and hypoplasia of the terminal phalanges. SYN pycnodysostosis.

pyk·nom·e·ter (pik-nom'ĕ-tĕr) A flask of standard volume, used to determine the specific gravity of fluids by weighing. SYN pycnometer.

pyk·no·sis (pik-nō'sis) A thickening or condensation.

py·le·phle·bi·tis (pī'lĕ-flĕ-bī'tis) Inflammation of the portal vein or any of its branches.

py·le·throm·bo·phle·bi·tis (pī'lĕ-throm'bō-flĕ-bī'tis) Inflammation of the portal vein with the formation of a thrombus.

py·lo·rec·to·my (pī'lōr-ek'tŏ-mē) Excision of the pylorus. SYN gastropylorectomy, pylorogastrectomy.

py·lor·ic (pī-lōr'ik) Relating to the pylorus.

py·lor·ic con·stric·tion (pī-lōr'ik kŏn-strik'shŭn) A prominent fold of mucous membrane at the gastroduodenal junction overlying the pyloric sphincter.

py·lor·ic ste·no·sis (pī-lōr'ik stĕ-nō'sis) Narrowing of the gastric pylorus. SEE ALSO hypertrophic pyloric stenosis.

py·lo·ri·ste·no·sis, py·lo·ro·ste·no·sis (pī-lōr'i-stĕ-nō'sis, pī-lōr'ŏ-) Stricture or narrowing of the orifice of the pylorus. SYN pylorostenosis.

♲ **pyloro-, pylor-** Combining forms indicating the pylorus.

py·lo·ro·du·o·de·ni·tis (pī-lōr'ŏ-dū-od'ĕ-nī'tis) Inflammation involving the pyloric outlet of the stomach and the duodenum.

py·lo·ro·gas·trec·to·my (pī-lōr'ŏ-gas-trek'tŏ-mē) SYN pylorectomy.

py·lo·ro·my·ot·o·my (pī-lōr'ŏ-mī-ot'ŏ-mē) Longitudinal incision through the anterior wall of the pyloric canal to the level of the submucosa, to treat hypertrophic pyloric stenosis. SYN Fredet-Ramstedt operation, Ramstedt operation.

py·lo·ro·plas·ty (pī-lōr'ŏ-plas-tē) Widening of the pyloric canal and any adjacent duodenal stricture with a longitudinal incision closed transversely.

py·lo·ro·spasm (pī-lōr'ŏ-spazm) Spasmodic contraction of the pylorus.

py·lo·ros·to·my (pī'lō-ros'tŏ-mē) Establishment of a fistula from the abdominal surface into the stomach near the pylorus.

py·lo·rot·o·my (pī'lō-rot'ŏ-mē) Incision of the pylorus.

py·lo·rus, gen. and pl. **py·lo·ri** (pī-lōr'ŭs, -ī) [TA] 1. The muscular tissue surrounding and controlling the aboral outlet of the stomach. 2. A muscular or myovascular device to open and to close an orifice or the lumen.

♲ **pyo-** Combining form meaning suppuration, accumulation of pus.

py·o·cele (pī'ŏ-sēl) An accumulation of pus in the scrotum.

py·o·che·zi·a (pī'ō-kē'zē-ă) A discharge of pus from the bowel.

py·o·col·po·cele (pī'ō-kol'pŏ-sēl) A vaginal tumor or cyst containing pus.

py·o·col·pos (pī'ō-kol'pos) Accumulation of pus in the vagina.

py·o·cy·an·ic (pī'ō-sī-an'ik) Relating to blue pus or the organism that causes blue pus, *Pseudomonas aeruginosa*.

py·o·cyst (pī'ō-sist) A cyst with purulent contents.

py·o·der·ma (pī'ō-dĕr'mă) Any pyogenic infection of the skin.

py·o·der·ma gan·gre·no·sum (pī'ō-dĕr'mă gang-grĕ-nō'sŭm) A chronic, noninfective eruption of spreading, undermined ulcers showing central healing.

py·o·gen·e·sis (pī'ō-jen'ĕ-sis) SYN suppuration.

py·o·gen·ic, py·o·ge·net·ic, py·og·e·nous (pī'ō-jen'ik, -jĕ-net'ik, pī-oj'ĕ-nŭs) Pus-forming; relating to pus formation.

py·o·gen·ic gran·u·lo·ma, gran·u·lo·ma py·o·gen·i·cum (pī'ō-jen'ik gran'yū-lō'mă, pī'ō-jen'i-kŭm) An acquired small, rounded mass of highly vascular granulation tissue, projecting from the skin or mucosa. SYN lobular capillary hemangioma.

py·o·he·mo·tho·rax (pī'ō-hē'mŏ-thōr'aks) Presence of pus and blood in the pleural cavity.

py·oid (pī'oyd) Resembling pus.

py·o·me·tri·tis (pī'ō-mē-trī'tis) Inflammation of uterine musculature associated with pus in the uterine cavity.

py·o·my·o·si·tis (pī'ō-mī'ō-sī'tis) Abscesses, carbuncles, or infected sinuses lying deep in muscles.

py·o·ne·phri·tis (pī'ō-nĕ-frī'tis) Suppurative inflammation of the kidney.

py·o·neph·ro·li·thi·a·sis (pī'ō-nef'rō-li-thī'ă-sis) Presence in the kidney of pus and calculi.

py·o·ne·phro·sis, ne·phro·py·o·sis (pī'ō-nĕ-frō'sis, nef'rō-pī-ō'sis) Distension of the pelvis and calyces of the kidney with pus, usually associated with obstruction. SYN nephropyosis.

py·o·per·i·car·di·um (pī'ō-per'i-kahr'dē-ŭm) An accumulation of pus in the pericardial sac.

py·o·per·i·to·ne·um (pī'ō-per'i-tŏ-nē'ŭm) An accumulation of pus in the peritoneal cavity.

py·o·phy·so·me·tra (pī'ō-fī'sō-mē'tră) Presence of pus and gas in the uterine cavity.

py·o·pneu·mo·cho·le·cys·ti·tis (pī'ō-nū'mō-kō'lē-sis-tī'tis) Combination of pus and gas in an inflamed gallbladder.

py·o·pneu·mo·hep·a·ti·tis (pī'ō-nū'mō-hep'ă-tī'tis) Combination of pus and gas in the liver.

py·o·pneu·mo·per·i·car·di·um (pī'ō-nū'mō-per'i-kahr'dē-ŭm) Presence of pus and gas in the pericardial sac.

py·o·pneu·mo·per·i·to·ni·tis (pī'ō-nū'mō-per'i-tŏ-nī'tis) Peritonitis with gas-forming organisms or with gas introduced from a ruptured bowel.

py·o·pneu·mo·tho·rax (pī'ō-nū'mō-thōr'aks) Presence of gas with a purulent effusion in the pleural cavity.

py·o·py·e·lec·ta·sis (pī'ō-pī'ĕ-lek'tă-sis) Dilation of the renal pelvis with pus-producing inflammation.

py·or·rhe·a (pī'ō-rē'ă) A purulent discharge.

py·o·sal·pin·gi·tis (pi'ō-sal'pin-jī'tis) Suppurative inflammation of the uterine tube.

py·o·sal·pin·go·o·oph·o·ri·tis (pī'ō-sal-ping'gō-ō-of'ŏ-rī'tis) Suppurative inflammation of the uterine tube and the ovary.

py·o·sal·pinx (pī'ō-sal'pingks) Distention of a uterine tube with pus.

py·o·tho·rax (pī'ō-thōr'aks) Empyema in a pleural cavity.

py·o·u·re·ter (pī'ō-yŭr'ĕ-tĕr) Distention of a ureter with pus.

P

py·ram·i·dal de·cus·sa·tion (pir-am′i-dăl dē′kŭs-ā′shŭn) The intercrossing of the bundles of the pyramidal tracts at the lower border region of the medulla oblongata. SYN decussatio pyramidum [TA], motor decussation.

py·ram·i·dal ra·di·a·tion (pir-am′i-dăl rā′dē-ā′shŭn) Corticospinal fibers passing from the cortex into the pyramid. SYN radiatio pyramidalis.

pyr·a·nose (pīr′ă-nōs) A cyclic form of a sugar in which the oxygen bridge forms a pyran.

py·ret·ic (pī-ret′ik) SYN febrile.

♻ **pyreto-** Combining form denoting fever. SEE ALSO pyro- (1).

py·re·to·ther·a·py (pī′rĕ-tō-thār′ă-pē) Treatment of fever.

py·rex·i·a (pī-rek′sē-ă) SYN fever.

py·rex·i·a of un·known or·i·gin (pī-rek′sē-ă ŭn′nōn ōr′i-jin) SYN fever of unknown origin.

py·ri·do·stig·mine bro·mide (PB) (pir′i-dō-stig′mēn brō′mīd) The bromide salt of a carbamate compound; used as a preexposure antidotal enhancer against the nerve agent soman. SYN 2-PAM chloride.

pyr·i·dox·a·mine (pir′i-dok′să-mēn) Amine of pyridoxine (q.v.) with a similar physiologic action.

pyr·i·dox·ine (pir′i-dok′sēn) The original vitamin B6; a term that now includes pyridoxal and pyridoxamine; deficiency may result in increased irritability, convulsions, and peripheral neuritis.

pyr·i·form (pir′i-fōrm) *Although the combining form pyr- usually refers to fire or heat, in this word it is derived from a medieval respelling of Latin pirum 'pear.'* SYN piriform.

py·rim·i·dine (pir-im′i-dēn) A heterocyclic substance, the formal parent of several "bases" present in nucleic acids (uracil, thymine, cytosine) as well as of the barbiturates.

♻ **pyro-** **1.** Combining form denoting fire, heat, or fever. SEE ALSO pyreto-. **2.** CHEMISTRY combining form denoting derivatives formed by removal of water (usually by heat) to form anhydrides.

py·ro·cat·e·chol (pī′rō-kat′ĕ-kol) A constituent of the catecholamines, epinephrine and norepinephrine, and dopa; used externally as an antiseptic. SYN catechol (1).

py·ro·gen (pī′rō-jen) A fever-inducing agent; produced by bacteria, molds, viruses, and yeasts.

py·ro·gen·ic (pī′rō-jen′ik) Causing fever.

py·rol·y·sis (pī-rol′i-sis) Decomposition of a substance by heat.

py·ro·ma·ni·a (pī′rō-mā′nē-ă) A morbid impulse to set fires.

py·ro·phos·phate (PP) (pī′rō-fos′fāt) A salt of pyrophosphoric acid; accumulates in cases of hypophosphatasia.

py·ro·sis (pī-rō′sis) A substernal pain or burning sensation, usually associated with regurgitation of acid and peptic gastric juice into the esophagus. SYN heartburn.

py·rox·y·lin (pi-rok′si-lin) Consists chiefly of cellulose tetranitrate, obtained by the action of nitric and sulfuric acids on cotton; used in the preparation of collodion. SYN nitrocellulose.

pyr·rol·i·dine (pir-ol′i-dēn) **1.** Pyrrole to which four H atoms have been added; the structural basis of proline and hydroxyproline. **2.** A class of alkaloids containing a pyrrolidine (1) moiety or a pyrrolidine derivative.

py·ru·vate (pī′rū-vāt) A salt or ester of pyruvic acid.

py·ru·vate ki·nase def·i·cien·cy (pī′rū-vāt kī′nās dē-fish′ĕn-sē) Disorder with a deficiency of pyruvate kinase in red blood cells.

py·ru·vic ac·id (pī-rū′vik as′id) An intermediate compound in the metabolism of carbohydrates. SEE ALSO phosphoenolpyruvic acid.

py·ur·i·a (pī-yūr′ē-ă) Presence of pus in the urine.

Q 1. Abbreviation for coulomb; quantity; quaternary; glutamine; glutaminyl; pseudouridine; coenzyme Q; electric charge. **2.** The second product formed in an enzyme-catalyzed reaction.

q 1. CYTOGENETICS long arm of a chromosome (in contrast to p for the short arm). **2.** Abbreviation for Latin *quodque*, each, every. **3.** Symbol for heat.

Q fe•ver (fē′vĕr) A febrile disease characterized by headache, myalgia, and sometimes pneumonitis or hepatitis; caused by *Coxiella burnetii*.

q.h. Abbreviation for L. quaque hora, every hour.

QH$_2$ Symbol for ubiquinol.

qi (kī) SYN chi (4).

q.i.d. Abbreviation for L. quater in die, four times a day.

Q-probes (prōbz) An external peer comparison program sponsored by the College of American Pathologists that addresses process, outcome, and structure-oriented quality assurance issues.

quack (kwak) SYN charlatan.

quack•er•y (kwak′ĕr-ē) SYN charlatanism.

quadr-, quadri- Combining forms meaning four.

quad•rant (quad) (kwahd′rănt) One quarter of a circle, especially anatomic.

quad•ran•ta•no•pia (kwahd-ran′tă-nō-pē-ă) Loss of 25% of vision in one or both eyes.

quad•rate (kwahd′rāt) Having four equal sides; square.

quad•rate mus•cle (kwahd′rāt mŭs′ĕl) [TA] One that is approximately square or four sided. SYN musculus quadratus [TA], quadratus muscle.

quadri- Prefix meaning four.

quad•ri•ceps, pl. **qua•dri•ceps,** pl. **quad•ri•cep•ses** (kwahd′ri-seps, -ĕz) Having four heads; denoting a muscle of the thigh, quadriceps femoris muscle, and one of the calf, quadriceps surae muscle.

quad•ri•ceps re•flex (kwahd′ri-seps rē′fleks) SYN patellar reflex.

quad•ri•gem•i•nal (kwahd′ri-jem′i-năl) Fourfold.

quad•ri•gem•i•nal rhythm (kwahd′ri-jem′i-năl ridh′ŭm) Cardiac arrhythmia in which the heartbeats are grouped in fours. SYN quadrigeminy.

quad•ri•ge•mi•ny (kwahd′ri-jem′i-nē) A cardiac arrhythmia in which every fourth beat is a premature contraction.

quad•ri•pe•dal ex•ten•sor re•flex (kwah′dri-ped′ăl eks-ten′sŏr rē′fleks) Extension of the arm of a hemiplegic patient when turned prone as if on all fours.

quad•ri•ple•gi•a (kwahd′ri-plē′jē-ă) Paralysis of all four limbs.

quad•ri•ple•gic (kwahd′ri-plē′jik) Pertaining to or afflicted with quadriplegia.

quad•ri•tu•ber•cu•lar (kwahd′ri-tū-bĕr′kyū-lăr) Having four tubercles or cusps, as a molar tooth.

quad•ri•va•lent (kwahd′ri-vā′lĕnt) Having the combining power (valency) of four.

quad•ru•ped (kwahd′rū-ped) A four-footed animal.

quad•ru•ple rhythm (kwahd-rū′pĕl ridh′ŭm) Quadruple cadence to the heart sounds due to the easy audibility of both third and fourth heart sounds. SYN trainwheel rhythm.

quad•rup•let (kwahd-rŭp′let) One of four children born at one birth.

qual•i•fied clin•i•cal so•cial work•er (QCSW) (kwah′li-fīd klin′i-kăl sō′shăl wŏrk′ĕr) A clinician trained in advanced classes to deal with patients with psychiatric problems.

qual•i•ta•tive a•nal•y•sis (kwahl′i-tā′tiv ă-nal′i-sis) Determination of the nature, as opposed to the quantity, of each of the elements composing a substance.

qual·i·ty of life (Q.O.L.) (kwah'li-tē līf) An overall assessment of a person's well-being, which may include physical, emotional, and social dimensions, as well as stress level, sexual function, and self-perceived health status.

quan·ti·ta·tive a·nal·y·sis (kwahn'ti-tā'tiv ă-nal'i-sis) Determination of the amount, as well as the nature, of each of the elements composing a substance.

quan·ti·ty not suf·fi·cient (QNS) (kwahn'ti-tē not sŭf-fish'ĕnt) Charting notation indicating that the amount of specimen submitted to a laboratory is determined to be inadequate to perform test(s) requested.

quan·ti·ty suf·fi·ci·ent to make (q.s. ad) (kwahn'ti-tē sŭ-fish'ĕnt māk) Adding enough of an ingredient to achieve a specific final volume or total weight.

Quant sign (kwahnt sīn) A T-shaped depression in the occipital bone seen in many patients with rickets, especially in infants lying constantly in bed with pressure on the occiput.

quan·tum, pl. **quan·ta** (kwahn'tŭm, -tă) **1.** A unit of radiant energy (ε) varying according to the frequency (ν) of the radiation. **2.** A certain definite amount.

quan·tum the·o·ry (kwahn'tŭm thē'ŏr-ē) That energy can be emitted, transmitted, and absorbed only in discrete quantities (quanta), so that atoms and subatomic particles can exist only in certain energy states.

quar·an·tine (kwŏr'ăn-tēn') **1.** The isolation of a person with a known or possible contagious disease. **2.** A period (originally 40 days) of detention of vessels and their passengers coming from an area where an infectious disease prevails.

quart (kwōrt) **1.** A measure of fluid capacity; the fourth part of a gallon; the equivalent of 0.9468 liter. **2.** A dry measure holding a little more than the fluid measure.

quar·tan (kwōr'tăn) Recurring every fourth day.

quartz (kwōrts) A crystalline form of sili-

con dioxide used in chemical apparatus and in optic and electrical instruments.

qua·si·con·tin·u·ous wave la·ser (kwā'zī-kŏn-tin'yū-ŭs wāv lā'zĕr) Laser, with output that can be controlled in milliseconds or similarly small increments by electronic control.

qua·ter·nar·y (Q) (kwah'tĕr-nar-ē) **1.** Denoting a chemical compound containing four elements. **2.** Fourth in a series.

qua·ter·nar·y blast in·ju·ry (kwah'tĕr-nar-ē blast in'jŭr-ē) An injury or other condition (including burns and crush-type injury) caused by an explosion but not categorized as primary, secondary, or tertiary blast injury.

Queck·en·stedt-Stook·ey test (kvek'en-shtet stūk'ē test) Compression of the jugular vein in a healthy person causes an increase in the pressure of the spinal fluid in the lumbar region within 10–12 seconds.

quench·ing (kwench'ing) **1.** The process of extinguishing a physical property. **2.** Process of stopping a chemical or enzymatic reaction.

quer·ce·tin (kwer'sĕ-tin) An aglycon of quercitrin, rutin, and other glycosides used to treat abnormal capillary fragility. SYN meletin, sophoretin.

quick·en·ing (kwik'ĕn-ing) Signs of life felt by the mother as a result of fetal movements, usually appearing 16–20 weeks into pregnancy.

qui·et lung (kwī'ĕt lŭng) Lung collapse during thoracic operations undertaken to facilitate surgical procedure through absence of lung movement.

Quin·cke dis·ease (kving'kĕ di-zēz') Well-localized edematous disorder that may variably involve the deeper skin layers and subcutaneous tissues as well as mucosal surfaces of the upper respiratory and gastrointestinal tracts. SYN angioedema (2), angioneurotic edema (2).

Quin·cke pulse (kving'kĕ pŭls) Capillary pulse as appreciated in the fingernails and toenails during aortic regurgitation. SYN Quincke sign.

quin·i·dine (kwin'i-dēn, -din) A cinchona

alkaloid; used as an antimalarial and to treat atrial fibrillation and flutter. SYN conquinine.

qui·nine (kwī'nīn) The most important of the alkaloids derived from cinchona; an antimalarial effective against the asexual and erythrocytic forms of the parasite, but having no effect on the exoerythrocytic forms.

quin·o·line (kwin'ō-lēn, -lin) A volatile nitrogenous base obtained by the distillation of coal tar, bones, alkaloids, and other substances; also used as an antimalarial. SYN chinoleine, leucoline.

quin·o·lone-re·sis·tant *Ne·is·se·ria gon·or·rho·e·ae* (kwin´ō-lōn-rē-zis´ tănt nī-sēr´ē-ă gon´ō-rē´ē) Bacterial sexually transmitted infection that does not respond to a quinolone (e.g., ciprofloxacin).

quint- Combining form meaning fifth or fivefold.

quin·tan (kwin'tăn) Recurring every fifth day.

quin·tu·plet (kwin-tŭp'lĕt) One of five children born at one birth.

3-quin·u·cli·di·nyl ben·zi·late (kwi-nū'kli-din'il ben'zi-lāt) An anticholinergic compound developed for use as an incapacitating chemical-warfare agent.

quo·tid·i·an (kwō-tid'ē-ăn) Daily; occurring every day.

quo·tid·i·an ma·la·ri·a (kwō-tid'ē-ăn mă-lar'ē-ă) Disorder in which the paroxysms occur daily; usually a double tertian malaria, in which there is an infection by two distinct groups of *Plasmodium vivax* parasites sporulating alternately every 48 hours.

quo·tient (Q) (kwō'shĕnt) The number of times one amount is contained in another. SEE ALSO index (2), ratio.

Q

R

R$_f$, R$_F$ Symbol denoting movement of a substance in paper or thin layer chromatography; equal to the migration distance of a substance divided by the migration distance of the solvent front.

Ra Symbol for radium.

rab·id (rab'id) Relating to or suffering from rabies.

ra·bies (rā'bēz) Highly fatal infectious disease transmitted by the bite of infected animals; caused by a neurotropic lyssavirus that replicates in the central nervous system and the salivary glands. The symptoms are excitement, aggressiveness, and madness, followed by paralysis and death. SYN hydrophobia.

ra·bies vac·cine, Flu·ry strain egg·pas·sage (rā'bēz vak-sēn', flūr'ē strān eg'pas-ăj) Vaccine introduced by Pasteur as a method of treatment for the bite of a rabid animal.

ra·bies vi·rus, Ke·lev strain, Flu·ry strain (rā'bēz vī'rŭs, kel'ev strān, flūr'ē) A large, bullet-shaped virus of the genus *Lyssavirus*; the causative agent of rabies.

♻ **rac-** Prefix meaning racemic.

ra·ce·mase (rā'sĕ-mās) An enzyme capable of catalyzing racemization.

ra·ce·mate (rā'sĕ-māt) A racemic compound, or the salt or ester of such a compound. SEE ALSO racemic.

ra·ce·mic (r, R, rad) (rā-sē'mik) Denoting a mixture of optically active compounds that is itself optically inactive, being composed of an equal number of dextrorotatory and levorotatory substances, which are separable.

ra·ce·mi·za·tion (rā'sĕ-mī-zā'shŭn) Partial conversion of one enantiomorph into another (as an L-amino acid to the corresponding D-amino acid) so that the specific optic rotation is decreased, or even reduced to zero, in the resulting mixture.

rac·e·mose (ras'ĕ-mōs) Branching, with nodular terminations; resembling a bunch of grapes.

rac·e·mose an·eu·rysm (ras'ĕ-mōs an'yūr-izm) SYN cirsoid aneurysm.

♻ **rachi-, rachio-** Combining forms meaning the spine.

ra·chi·al·gi·a (rā'kē-al'jē-ă) Pain in the vertebral column.

ra·chi·graph (rā'kē-graf) A graph for recording curves of the vertebrae.

ra·chil·y·sis (ră-kil'i-sis) Forcible correction of lateral curvature of the spine by lateral pressure against the convexity of the curve.

ra·chi·om·e·ter (rā'kē-om'ĕ-tĕr) An instrument for measuring the curvature of the spine, natural or pathologic, or of the spinal column.

ra·chi·op·a·gus, rac·hip·a·gus (rā'kē-op'ă-gŭs, ră-kip') Conjoined twins united back to back with union of their spinal columns. SEE conjoined twins. SYN rachipagus.

ra·chi·ot·o·my, ra·chit·o·my (rā'kē-ot'ŏ-mē, ră-kit') SYN laminotomy.

ra·chis, pl. **rach·i·des,** pl. **ra·chis·es** (rā'kis, -ki-dēz, rā'ki-sēz) SYN vertebral column.

ra·chis·chi·sis (ră-kis'ki-sis) 1. Embryologic failure of fusion of neural arches and neural tube with consequent exposure of neural tissue at the surface. 2. Spinal dysraphism.

ra·chit·ic (ră-kit'ik) Relating to or suffering from rickets (rachitis).

ra·chit·ic pel·vis (ră-kit'ik pel'vis) Contracted and deformed pelvis.

ra·chit·ic ro·sa·ry (ră-kit'ik rō'zăr-ē) Row of beading at the junction of the ribs with their cartilages. SYN beading of the ribs.

ra·chi·tis (ră-kī'tis) SYN rickets.

ra·chit·o·gen·ic (ră-kit'ō-jen'ik) Producing or causing rickets.

rack·et am·pu·ta·tion (rak'ĕt amp'yū-tā'shŭn) A circular or slightly oval amputation, in which a long incision is made in the axis of the limb.

rack·et nail (rak'ĕt nāl) Broad flat thumbnail resulting from a congenital shorter and wider distal phalanx of the thumb.

ra·dec·to·my (rā-dek′tŏ-mē) SYN root amputation.

Rad·ford no·mo·gram (rad′fŏrd nō′mō-gram) Graph used to predict necessary tidal volume for artificial respiration on the basis of respiratory rate, body weight, and gender.

ra·di·ad (rā′dē-ad) In a direction toward the radial side.

ra·di·al (rā′dē-ăl) **1.** Relating to the radius (bone of the forearm), to any structures named from it, or to the radial or lateral aspect of the upper limb as compared with the ulnar or medial aspect. **2.** Relating to any radius. **3.** Radiating; diverging in all directions from any given center. SYN brachio- (2).

ra·di·al de·vi·a·tion (rā′dē-ăl dē′vē-ā′shŭn) Movement of the wrist toward the thumb side of the forearm.

ra·di·al ker·a·tot·o·my (rā′dē-ăl ker′ă-tot′ŏ-mē) A form of refractive keratoplasty used in the treatment of myopia.

ra·di·al re·flex (rā′dē-ăl rē′fleks) On tapping the lower end of the radius, flexion of the forearm occurs, and sometimes, on strong percussion, flexion of the fingers.

ra·di·ant (rā′dē-ănt) **1.** Giving out rays. **2.** A point from which light radiates to the eye.

ra·di·ant en·er·gy (Q) (rā′dē-ănt en′ĕr-jē) That contained in light rays or any other form of radiation.

ra·di·ant heat (RH) (rā′dē-ănt hēt) Warmth given off from any body in the form of infrared waves.

ra·di·ate lig·a·ment (rā′dē-ăt lig′ă-mĕnt) SYN radiate ligament of head of rib.

ra·di·ate lig·a·ment of head of rib (rā′dē-ăt lig′ă-mĕnt hed rib) The radiate, stellate, or anterior costovertebral ligament connecting the head of each rib to the bodies of the two vertebrae with which it articulates. SYN radiate ligament.

ra·di·a·ti·o, pl. **ra·di·a·ti·o·nes** (rā-dē-ā′shē-ō, ō′nēz) [TA] In neuroanatomy, a term applied to any one of the thalamocortical fiber systems that together compose the corona radiata of the cerebral hemisphere's white matter. SYN radiation (3).

ra·di·a·tion (rā′dē-ā′shŭn) **1.** The act or condition of diverging in all directions from a center. **2.** The sending forth of light, short radio waves, ultraviolet or x-rays, or any other rays for treatment or diagnosis or for other purpose. Cf. irradiation (2). **3.** SYN radiatio. **4.** A ray. **5.** Radiant energy or a radiant beam.

ra·di·a·tion bi·ol·o·gy (rā′dē-ā′shŭn bī-ol′ŏ-jē) Science that studies the biologic effects of ionizing radiation.

ra·di·a·tion cat·a·ract (rā-dē-ā′shŭn kat′ăr-akt) One caused by excessive or prolonged exposure to ultraviolet rays, x-rays, radium, gamma rays, heat, or radioactive isotopes.

ra·di·a·tion ne·cro·sis (rā′dē-ā′shŭn nĕ-krō′sis) Death of cells or tissues resulting from the effects of radiation exposure.

ra·di·a·tion of cor·pus cal·lo·sum (rā′dē-ā′shŭn kōr′pŭs kă-lō′sŭm) [TA] The spreading out of the fibers of the corpus callosum in the centrum semiovale of each cerebral hemisphere. SYN radiatio corporis callosi [TA].

ra·di·a·tion sick·ness (rā′dē-ā′shŭn sik′nĕs) Systemic condition caused by substantial whole-body irradiation, seen after nuclear explosions or accidents, rarely after radiotherapy. SYN radiation poisoning.

ra·di·a·tion ther·a·py, ra·di·o·ther·a·py (rā′dē-ā′shŭn thār′ă-pē, rā′dē-ō-thār′ă-pē) Treatment with x-rays or radionuclides.

ra·di·a·tion tol·er·ance dose (rā′dē-ā′shŭn tol′ĕr-ăns dōs) The amount of radiation exposure that normal tissue can tolerate and still function properly.

rad·i·cal (rad′i-kăl) **1.** CHEMISTRY a group of elements or atoms usually passing intact from one compound to another, but usually incapable of prolonged existence in a free state. **2.** Thorough or extensive. **3.** Denoting treatment by extreme, dras-

R

tic, or innovative, as opposed to conservative, measures. **4. SYN** free radical.

rad·i·cal hys·ter·ec·to·my (RH) (radʹi-kăl hisʹtĕr-ek'tŏ-me) Complete removal of the uterus, upper vagina, and parametrium.

rad·i·cal mas·tec·to·my (radʹi-kăl mas-tek'tŏ-me) Excision of the entire breast, as well as the pectoral muscles, lymphatic-bearing tissue in the axilla, and various other neighboring tissues. **SYN** Halsted operation (2).

rad·i·cal mas·toi·dec·to·my (radʹi-kăl mas'toyd-ek'tŏ-me) An operation for the management of extensive cholesteatoma. **SYN** tympanomastoidectomy.

rad·i·cle (radʹi-kĕl) *Do not confuse this word with radical.* Smallest branch of a vessel or nerve.

ra·dic·u·lal·gia (ră-dik'yū-lal'jē-ă) Neuralgia due to irritation of the sensory root of a spinal nerve.

ra·dic·u·lar (ră-dik'yū-lăr) **1.** Relating to a radicle. **2.** Pertaining to the root of a tooth.

ra·dic·u·lo·gang·li·on·i·tis (ră-dik'yū-lō-gang'glē-ŏ-nīʹtis) Involvement of roots and ganglia.

ra·dic·u·lo·my·e·lop·a·thy (ră-dik'yū-lō-mī'ĕ-lop'ă-thē) **SYN** myeloradiculopathy.

ra·dic·u·lo·neu·rop·a·thy (ră-dik'yū-lō-nūr-op'ă-thē) Disease of the spinal nerve roots and nerves.

ra·dic·u·lop·a·thy (ră-dik'yū-lop'ă-thē) Disorder of the spinal nerve roots.

radio- Combining form denoting radiation, chiefly (in medicine) gamma ray or x-ray.

ra·di·o·ac·tive i·o·dine (RAI) (rāʹdē-ō-ak'tiv īʹŏ-dīn) Iodine radioisotopes ^{131}I, ^{125}I, or ^{123}I used as tracers in biology and medicine.

ra·di·o·ac·tiv·i·ty (rāʹdē-ō-ak-tiv'i-tē) The property of some atomic nuclei of spontaneously emitting gamma rays or subatomic particles (α and β rays) by the process of nuclear disintegration and

measured in disintegrations per second (dps).

ra·di·o·al·ler·go·sor·bent test (rāʹdē-ō-al'ĕr-gō-sōrʹbĕnt test) A radioimmunoassay-based procedure to detect immunoglobulin-E-bound allergens responsible for tissue hypersensitivity.

ra·di·o·bi·cip·i·tal (rāʹdē-ō-bī-sip'i-tăl) Relating to the radius and the biceps muscle.

ra·di·o·bi·ol·o·gy (rāʹdē-ō-bī-ol'ŏ-jē) The study of the biologic effects of ionizing radiation on living tissue. Cf. radiopathology.

ra·di·o·car·di·o·gram (rāʹdē-ō-kahrʹdē-ō-gram) A graphic record of the concentration of injected radioisotope within the cardiac chambers.

ra·di·o·car·di·og·ra·phy (rāʹdē-ō-kahrʹdē-og'ră-fē) The technique of recording or interpreting radiocardiograms.

ra·di·o·car·pal (rāʹdē-ō-kahrʹpăl) **1.** Relating to the radius and the bones of the carpus. **2.** On the radial or lateral side of the carpus.

ra·di·o·car·pal ar·tic·u·la·tion (rāʹdē-ō-kahrʹpăl ahr-tik'yū-lā'shŭn) **SYN** wrist joint.

ra·di·o·chem·is·try (rāʹdē-ō-kem'is-trē) **1.** The science of using radionuclides to synthesize labeled compounds for biochemical or biologic research, or radiopharmaceuticals for clinical diagnostic studies. **2.** The study of methods of labeling compounds with radionuclides.

ra·di·o·den·si·ty (rāʹdē-ō-den'si-tē) **SYN** radiopacity.

ra·di·o·der·ma·ti·tis (rāʹdē-ō-dĕrʹmă-tīʹtis) Dermatitis due to exposure to x-rays or gamma rays causing ionization of tissue water with acute changes resembling thermal injury.

ra·di·o·di·ag·no·sis (rāʹdē-ō-dīʹăg-nōʹsis) Diagnosis using x-rays; or, more broadly, diagnostic imaging, including radiology, ultrasound, and magnetic resonance.

ra·di·o·graph, ra·di·o·gram (rāʹdē-ō-graf, -gram) A negative image on photographic film made by exposure to x-rays that have passed through matter or tissue.

ra·di·o·gra·phic den·si·ty (rā′dē-ō-graf′ik den′si-tē) The amount of blackening on an x-ray film produced by the interaction of silver halide crystals with developing agents.

ra·di·og·ra·phy (rā′dē-og′ră-fē) Examination of any part of the body for diagnostic purposes by means of x-rays with the record of the findings usually impressed on a photographic film.

ra·di·o·hu·mer·al (rā′dē-ō-hyū′měr-ăl) Relating to the radius and the humerus.

ra·di·o·im·mu·ni·ty (rā′dē-ō-i-myū′nitē) Lessened sensitivity to radiation.

ra·di·o·im·mu·no·as·say (RIA) (rā′dē-ō-im′yū-nō-as′sā) Any method for detecting or quantitating antigens or antibodies using radiolabeled reactants.

ra·di·o·im·mu·no·dif·fu·sion (rā′dē-ō-im′yū-nō-di-fyū′zhŭn) A method for the study of antigen-antibody reactions by gel diffusion using radioisotope-labeled antigen or antibody.

ra·di·o·im·mun·o·sor·bent test (rā′dē-ō-im′yū′nō-sōr′bĕnt test) A competition assessment, performed in vitro, used to measure immunoglobulin E specific for a particular antigen.

ra·di·o·i·o·dine (RAI) (rā′dē-ō-ī′ō-dīn) A radioactive isotope of iodine.

ra·di·o·i·so·tope (RI) (rā′dē-ō-ī′sŏ-tōp) An isotope that changes to a more stable state by emitting radiation.

ra·di·o·li·gand (rā′dē-ō-lī′gand) A molecule with a radionuclide tracer attached.

ra·di·ol·o·gy (rā′dē-ol′ŏ-jē) Science of high-energy radiation and of the chemical, physical, and biologic effects of such radiation; the term usually refers to the diagnosis and treatment of disease.

ra·di·o·lu·cent (rā′dē-ō-lū′sĕnt) Relatively penetrable by x-rays or other forms of radiation. Cf. radiopaque.

ra·di·om·e·ter (rā′dē-om′ĕ-tĕr) A device

for determining the penetrative power of x-rays.

ra·di·o·ne·cro·sis (rā′dē-ō-nĕ-krō′sis) Cell death due to radiation.

ra·di·o·neu·ri·tis (rā′dē-ō-nūr-ī′tis) Neuritis caused by prolonged or repeated exposure to x-rays or radium.

ra·di·o·nu·clide (rā′dē-ō-nū′klīd) An isotope of artificial or natural origin that exhibits radioactivity. Radionuclides are used in diagnostic imaging and cancer therapy.

ra·di·o·nu·clide an·gi·o·car·di·og·ra·phy, ra·di·o·nu·clide ven·tric·u·log·ra·phy (rā′dē-ō-nū′klīd an′jē-ō-kahr′dē-og′ră-fē, ven-trik′yū-log′ră-fē) The display, by means of a stationary scintillation camera device, of the passage of a bolus of a rapidly injected radiopharmaceutical.

ra·di·o·pac·i·ty (rā′dē-ō-pas′i-tē) State of being radiopaque. SYN radiodensity.

ra·di·o·pa·thol·o·gy (rā′dē-ō-pă-thol′ŏ-jē) A branch of radiology or pathology concerned with the effects of radiation on cells and tissues. Cf. radiobiology.

ra·di·o·phar·ma·ceu·ti·cal (rā′dē-ō-fahr′mă-sū′ti-kăl) A therapeutic agent chemically bound to a radionuclide.

ra·di·o·re·cep·tor (rā′dē-ō-rē-sep′tŏr) **1.** A receptor that normally responds to radiant energy. **2.** A receptor used as a binding agent for unlabeled and radiolabeled analyte in a radioreceptor assay.

ra·di·o·sen·si·tiv·i·ty (rā′dē-ō-sen′si-tiv′i-tē) The condition of being readily affected by radiant energy.

ra·di·o·te·lem·e·try (rā′dē-ō-tĕ-lem′ĕ-trē) SEE telemetry.

ra·di·o·ther·a·peu·tic (rā′dē-ō-thār-ă-pyū′tik) Relating to radiotherapy or to radiotherapeutics.

ra·di·o·ther·a·py (rā′dē-ō-thār′ă-pē) Medical specialty that uses electromagnetic or particulate radiation to treat disease.

ra·di·o·ther·my (rā′dē-ō-thĕr′mē) Diathermy effected by heat from radiant sources.

R

radiotoxaemia [Br.] SYN radiotoxemia.

ra·di·o·tox·e·mi·a (rā′dē-ō-tok-sē′mē-ă) Radiation sickness caused by the products of disintegration produced by the action of x-rays or other forms of radioactivity. SYN radiotoxaemia.

ra·di·o·trac·er (rā′dē-ō-trā′sĕr) A radionuclide or radiolabeled chemical.

ra·di·o·trans·par·ent (rā′dē-ō-transpar′ĕnt) Allowing relatively free transmission of radiant energy.

ra·di·o·trop·ic (rā′dē-ō-trō′pik) Affected by radiation.

ra·di·o·ul·nar (RU) (rā′dē-ō-ŭl′năr) Relating to both radius and ulna.

ra·di·um (Ra) (rā′dē-ŭm) Alkaline earth metal with properties similar to those of barium; therapeutic action similar to that of x-rays.

ra·di·us, gen. and pl. **ra·di·i** (rā′dē-ŭs, -ī) **1.** [TA] Lateral and shorter of the two bones of the forearm. **2.** A straight line passing from a circle's center to its periphery.

ra·dix (rā′diks) **1.** [TA] SYN root (1). **2.** SYN root of tooth. **3.** The hypothetical size of the birth cohort in a life table, commonly 1,000 or 100,000.

ra·don (Rn) (rā′don) A gaseous radioactive element, resulting from the breakdown of radium; used to treat certain malignancies. Homes in some parts of the country have accumulated a dangerous amount of naturally occurring radon gas.

rale (rahl) An extraneous sound heard on auscultation of breath sounds; used by some to denote rhonchus and by others for crepitation.

ral·ox·i·fene (răl-ox′i-fēn) A selective estrogen receptor modulator with estrogen-agonistic effects on bone and lipid metabolism but estrogen antagonistic effects on breast and uterus.

ra·mal (rā′măl) Relating to a ramus.

Ram·fjord In·dex Teeth (ram′fyōrd in′deks tēth) Specific teeth used for epidemiologic studies of periodontal diseases.

ram·i·fi·ca·tion (ram′i-fi-kā′shŭn) The process of dividing into a branchlike pattern.

ram·i·fy (ram′i-fī) To split into a branchlike pattern.

ram·i·sec·tion (ram′i-sek′shŭn) Section of the rami communicantes of the sympathetic nervous system. SYN ramicotomy.

ram·i·tis (ram-ī′tis) Inflammation of a ramus.

ra·mose, ra·mous (rā′mōs, -mŭs) SYN branching.

ramp test (ramp test) A form of graded exercise test in which treadmill speed is kept constant but grade increases each minute between 1 and 4% until volitional exhaustion or other test termination criteria are achieved (e.g., Harbor protocol).

ram·u·lus, pl. **ram·u·li** (ram′yū-lŭs, -lī) **1.** A small branch or twig. **2.** A terminal division of a ramus.

ra·mus, gen. and pl. **ra·mi** (rā′mŭs, -mī) **1.** [TA] SYN branch. **2.** One of the primary divisions of a nerve or blood vessel. SEE ALSO artery, nerve. **3.** A part of an irregularly shaped bone that forms an angle with the main body. **4.** Primary division of a cerebral sulcus.

ra·mus com·mu·ni·cans, pl. **ra·mi com·mu·ni·can·tes** (rā′mŭs kŏ-myū′ni-kanz, rā′mī kŏ-myū′ni-kan′tēz) [TA] SYN communicating branch.

ra·mus of man·di·ble (rā′mŭs man′di-bĕl) [TA] Upturned perpendicular extremity of the mandible; gives attachment on its lateral surface to the masseter muscle. SYN ramus mandibulae [TA].

Ran·cho Los A·mi·gos Lev·els of Cog·ni·tive Func·tion·ing Scale (ranch′ō lōs ah-mē′gōs lev′ĕlz kog′ni-tiv fŭngk′shŭn-ing skāl) A measure used to gauge the level of cognitive function of people with head injury by close observation of behavioral signs.

ran·cid·i·ty (ran-sid′i-tē) The state of being decomposition with a foul sour odor.

ran·dom am·pli·fied pol·y·mor·phic

de·ox·y·ri·bo·nu·cle·ic acid (ran′dŏm amp′li-fīd pol′ē-mōr′fik dē-ok′sē-rī′bō-nū-klē′ik as′id) An strain-typing procedure that uses primers with random sequences that anneal to random chromosomal DNA sequences of the strain of interest.

ran·dom·i·za·tion (ran′dŏm-ī-zā′shŭn) Assignment of the subjects of experimental research to groups by chance.

ran·dom mat·ing (ran′dŏm māt′ing) A practice of mating in a population in which at some specified locus mating patterns occur with expected frequencies predicted by the product of the frequencies of the genotypes in the population.

range (rānj) Statistical measure of the variation of values determined by the endpoint values themselves or the difference between them.

range of mo·tion (ROM) (rānj mō′shŭn) **1.** The measured beginning and terminal angles, as well as the total degrees of motion, traversed by a joint moved by active muscle contraction or by passive movement. **2.** Joint movement carried out to assess the arc of joint motion.

range-of-mo·tion (ROM) ex·er·cise (rānj mō′shŭn eks′ĕr-sīz) A passive, assistive, or active exercise used to increase the range of movement in a joint or to prevent its contracture.

ra·nine (rā′nīn) **1.** Relating to the frog. **2.** Relating to the undersurface of the tongue.

Ran·kin clamp (rang′kin klamp) Three-bladed clamp used in resection of colon.

Ran·kine scale (rang′kin skāl) Thermometer scale in which each degree Rankine (°Rank) is equal to the Fahrenheit but applied to the absolute temperature scale with its zero point at absolute zero; °Rank = °F + 459.67.

Ran·so·hoff sign (ran′sŏ-hof sīn) Yellow pigmentation in the umbilical region in rupture of the common bile duct.

ran·u·la (ran′yū-lă) **1.** Hypoglottis. **2.** Any cystic tumor of the undersurface of the tongue or floor of the mouth, especially one of the floor of the mouth. SYN ranine tumor, sublingual cyst.

Ran·vi·er node (rahn-vē-ā′ nōd) A short interval in the myelin sheath of a nerve fiber, occurring between segments of the myelin sheath. SYN node of Ranvier.

Ra·oult law (rah-ūl′ law) Vapor pressure of a solution of a nonvolatile nonelectrolyte is that of the pure solvent multiplied by the mole-fraction of the solvent in the solution.

rape (rāp) **1.** Sexual intercourse by force, duress, intimidation, or without legal consent (as with a minor). **2.** The performance of such an act.

ra·phe, rha·phe (rā′fē) [TA] The line of union of two contiguous, bilaterally symmetric structures.

ra·phe nu·cle·i (rā′fē nū′klē-ī) [TA] Collective term denoting a variety of nerve cell groups in and along the median plane of the medulla oblongata. SYN nuclei raphes [TA].

rap·id eye move·ment (REM) sleep (rap′id ī mūv′mĕnt slēp) Deep sleep in which rapid eye movements, alert electroencephalographic pattern, and dreaming occur. SEE ALSO paradoxic sleep.

rap·id plas·ma re·a·gin test (RPR) (rap′id plaz′mă rē-ā′jin test) Serologic tests for syphilis in which unheated serum or plasma is reacted with a standard test antigen containing charcoal particles; positive tests yield a flocculation. SYN RPR test.

ra·pid se·quence in·tu·ba·tion (RSI) (rap′id sĕ′kwĕns in′tū-bā′shŭn) Endotracheal intubation performed on a patient to whom a paralytic drug has been administered.

ra·pid trau·ma as·sess·ment (rap′id traw′mă ă-ses′mĕnt) Quick head-to-toe physical examination of an unresponsive prehospital trauma patient for the purpose of discovering and assessing injuries before transport.

Ra·po·port-Leu·ber·ing shunt (rap′ŏ-pōrt-loy′ber-ing shŭnt) A shunt of the glycolytic pathway helping to enhance release of oxygen from hemoglobin to the tissues.

Ra·po·port test (rap′ŏ-pōrt test) Differential ureteral catheterization assessment used to evaluate suspected renovascular hypertension.

rap·port (rap-ōr′) A conscious feeling of harmonious accord, trust, empathy, and mutual responsiveness between two or more people (e.g., physician and patient) that fosters the therapeutic process.

rar·e·fac·tion (rār′ĕ-fak′shŭn) Process of becoming light or less dense.

ras·pa·to·ry (ras′pă-tōr-ē) A surgical instrument used to smooth the edges of a divided bone.

rasp·ber·ry tongue (raz′ber-ē tŭng) Dark red tongue associated with scarlatina.

Ras·tel·li op·er·a·tion (rahs-tel′ē op-ĕr-ā′shŭn) Surgery for "anatomic" repair of transposition of the great arteries with ventricular septal defect.

rat-bite fe·ver (rat′bīt fē′vĕr) Designation for two bacterial diseases associated with rat bites, one caused by *Streptobacillus moniliformis*, the other by *Spirillum minus*. SYN rat-bite disease, sokosho.

rate (rāt) **1.** A measurement of an event or process in terms of its relation to some fixed standard. **2.** A measure of the frequency of an event in a defined population.

rate of per·ceived ex·er·tion (RPE) (rāt pĕr-sēvd′ eg-zĕr′shŭn) Scale used to measure a person's perception of the intensity of an exercise.

ra·ti·o (rā′shē-ō) An expression of the relation of one quantity to another (e.g., of a proportion or rate). SEE ALSO index (2), quotient.

ra·tion·al (rash′ŭn-ăl) **1.** Pertaining to reasoning or to the higher thought processes; based on objective or scientific knowledge. **2.** Influenced by reason rather than by emotion. **3.** Having the faculty of reason.

rat·tle·snake (rat′ĕl-snāk) A member of the crotalid genera *Crotalus* and *Sistrurus*, characterized by possession of cuticular warning rattles on the tail.

Rau·wol·fi·a ser·pen·ti·na (row-wūl′fē-ă sĕr-pen-tī′nă) A genus of tropical trees and shrubs; has alkaloids that produce a sedative-antihypertensive-bradycardiac action.

ray (rā) **1.** A beam of light, heat, or other form of radiation. **2.** A part or branch that extends radially from a structure. **3.** One of the grooves of the embryonic hand and foot indicating where the digital rays will develop.

rayl (rāl) Unit of acoustic impedance. 1 rayl = $1 \text{ kg} \times \text{m}^{-2} \times \text{sec}^{-1}$.

Ray·naud syn·drome, Ray·naud phe·nom·e·non (rā-nō′ sin′drŏm, fē-nom′ĕ-non) Bilateral arterial and arteriolar cyanosis of the fingers due to vasoconstriction of uncertain cause; may be brought on by low temperatures or emotional stress. SEE ALSO Raynaud phenomenon.

Rb Symbol for rubidium.

R-band·ing stain (band′ing stān) Reverse Giemsa chromosome banding method that produces bands complementary to G-bands; induced by treatment with high temperature, low pH, or acridine orange staining.

Re Symbol for rhenium.

re- Prefix meaning again or backward.

re·ac·tance (X) (rē-ak′tăns) The weakening of an alternating electric current by passage through a coil of wire.

re·ac·tant (rē-ak′tănt) A substance taking part in a chemical reaction.

re·ac·tion (rē-ak′shŭn) **1.** The response of a muscle or other living tissue or organism to a stimulus. **2.** The color change effected in litmus and certain other organic pigments by contact with substances such as acids or alkalis. **3.** CHEMISTRY the intermolecular action of two or more substances on each other, whereby these substances are made to disappear and new ones are formed in their place. **4.** IMMUNOLOGY action of an antibody on a specific antigen in vivo or in vitro, with or without the involvement of complement or other components of the immunologic system.

re·ac·tion for·ma·tion (rē-ak′shŭn fōr-mā′shŭn) PSYCHOANALYSIS postulated defense mechanism in which attitudes and behaviors that are adopted are the opposites of that which the person would ordinarily be expected to express and actually feel at an unconscious level.

re·ac·tion of de·gen·er·a·tion (DR) (rē-ak′shŭn dĕ-jen′ĕr-ā′shŭn) Electrical reaction in a degenerated nerve and the muscles supplied by it.

re·ac·tion time (RT) (rē-ak′shŭn tīm) Interval between presentation of a stimulus and response to it.

re·ac·ti·va·tion (rē′ak-ti-vā′shŭn) **1.** Restoration of the lytic activity of an inactivated serum by adding complement. **2.** Restoration of activity in an inactivated enzyme.

re·ac·tive ar·thri·tis (ReA, RA) (rē-ak′tiv ahr-thrī′tis) Sterile, usually transient polyarthropathy following various infectious diseases.

re·ac·tive at·tach·ment dis·or·der (RAD) (rē-ak′tiv ă-tach′mĕnt dis-ōr′dĕr) Mental disorder of infancy or early childhood characterized by disturbed social relatedness; thought to be caused by grossly poor care.

re·ac·tive de·pres·sion (rē-ak′tiv dĕ-presh′ŭn) A psychological state occasioned directly by an intensely sad external situation relieved by the removal of that situation.

re·ac·tive hy·per·e·mi·a (rē-ak′tiv hī′pĕr-ē′mē-ă) Hyperemia following the arrest and subsequent restoration of the blood supply to a part.

re·ac·tive schiz·o·phre·ni·a (rē-ak′tiv skit′sō-frē′nē-ă) Forms of severe schizophrenic disorders distinguished from process schizophrenia by their more acute onset, greater relation to environmental stress, and better prognosis.

re·ac·tive sys·tem·ic am·y·loi·do·sis (rē-ak′tiv sis-tem′ik am′i-loyd-ō′sis) SYN secondary amyloidosis.

read·ing (rēd′ing) **1.** The perception and understanding of the meaning of visual symbols by the scanning of writing or print with the eyes. **2.** Any of several alternative ways of interpreting symbols,

such as Braille or the close observation of a speaker's facial movements.

re·a·gent (rē-ā′jĕnt) Any substance added to a solution of another substance to participate in a chemical reaction.

re·a·gin (rē-ā′jin) **1.** Wolff-Eisner term for antibody. **2.** Antibody that mediates immediate hypersensitivity reactions. **3.** SYN homocytotropic antibody.

REAL clas·si·fi·ca·tion (rēl klas′i-fi-kā′shŭn) A classification of lymphoma based on the correlation of clinical features with their histopathology and immunophenotype and genotype of neoplastic cells.

real im·age (rēl im′ăj) That formed by the convergence of the actual rays of light from an object. SYN inverted image.

re·al·i·ty (rē-al′i-tē) That which exists objectively and in fact, and can be consensually validated.

ream·er (rē′mĕr) A dental rotating drill used to shape or enlarge a hole.

re·at·tach·ment (rē′ă-tach′mĕnt) New epithelial or connective tissue attachment to the surface of a tooth that was surgically detached and not exposed to oral environment.

re·base (rē′bās) In dentistry, to refit a denture by replacing the denture base material without changing the occlusal relationship of the teeth. SEE ALSO reline.

re·bound (rē′bownd) Act or condition of recovery or improvement in a patient.

re·bound ten·der·ness (rē′bownd ten′dĕr-nĕs) Sensitivity experienced when pressure, particularly abdominal, is suddenly released.

re·breath·ing an·es·the·si·a (rē-brēdh′ing an′es-thē′zē-ă) Inhalation anesthesia method in which some or all exhaled gases are subsequently inhaled after carbon dioxide has been absorbed.

re·breath·ing tech·nique (rē-brēdh′ing tek-nēk′) Use of a respiration circuit in which exhaled air is subsequently in-

R

haled either with or without absorption of carbon dioxide from the exhaled air.

Ré·ca·mi·er op·er·a·tion (rā-kahm-ē-ā′ op-ĕr-ā′shŭn) Curettage of the uterus.

re·ca·nal·i·za·tion (rē-kan′ăl-ī-zā′shŭn) **1.** Restoration of a lumen in a blood vessel following thrombotic occlusion, by organization of the thrombus with formation of new channels. **2.** Spontaneous restoration of the continuity of the lumen of any occluded duct or tube, as with postvasectomy recanalization.

re·ca·pit·u·la·tion the·o·ry (rē′kă-pich′yū-lā′shŭn thē′ŏr-ē) Tenet that people during their embryonic development pass through stages similar in general structural plan to the stages their species passed through in its evolution. SYN biogenetic law, law of biogenesis, Haeckel law, law of recapitulation.

re·ceiv·er (rē-sē′vĕr) In chemistry, a vessel attached to a condenser to receive the product of distillation.

re·ceiv·er op·er·at·ing char·ac·ter·is·tic (ROC) (rē-sē′vĕr op′ĕr-āt-ing kar′ăk-tĕr-is′tik) Plot of the sensitivity of a diagnostic test as a function of nonspecificity (one minus the specificity). The ROC curve indicates the intrinsic properties of a test's diagnostic performance and can be used to compare the relative merits of competing procedures.

re·cep·tac·u·lum, pl. **re·cep·tac·u·la** (rē-sĕp-tak′yū-lŭm, -lă) A receptacle.

re·cep·tive (rē-sep′tiv) Sensitive or responsive to stimulus.

re·cep·tive a·pha·si·a (rē-sĕp′tiv ă-fā′zē-ă) A condition including impairment in the comprehension of spoken and written words, associated with effortless, articulated, but paraphasic speech and writing; malformed words, substitute words, and neologisms are characteristic. When severe, and speech is incomprehensible, it is called jargon aphasia. SYN fluent aphasia, Wernicke aphasia.

re·cep·tor (rē-sep′tŏr) **1.** A structural protein molecule on the cell surface or within the cytoplasm that binds to a specific factor. **2.** Any one of the various sensory nerve endings in the skin, deep tissues, viscera, and special sense organs.

re·cep·tor pro·tein (rē-sep′tŏr prō′tēn) Intracellular protein that has a high specific affinity for binding a known stimulus to cellular activity.

re·cep·tor site (rē-sep′tŏr sīt) Point of attachment to cell membranes for viruses, hormones, or other activators.

re·cess (rē′ses) [TA] A small hollow or indentation. SYN recessus [TA].

re·ces·sive (rē-ses′iv) **1.** Drawing away; receding. **2.** GENETICS denoting a trait due to a particular allele that does not manifest itself in the presence of other alleles that generate traits dominant to it.

re·ces·sive char·ac·ter (rē-ses′iv kar′ăk-tĕr) An inherited character expressed in the homozygous state only.

re·ces·sus, pl. **re·ces·sus** (rē-ses′ŭs) [TA] SYN recess.

re·cid·i·va·tion (rē-sid′i-vā′shŭn) Relapse of a disease, a symptom, or a behavioral pattern such as an illegal activity for which one was previously imprisoned.

re·cid·i·vism, re·cid·i·vi·ty (rē-sid′i-vizm, -vid-i-tē) A tendency toward recidivation.

rec·i·pe (Rx) (res′i-pē) **1.** The superscription of a prescription, usually indicated by the sign ℞. **2.** A prescription or formula.

re·cip·i·ent (recip) (rē-sip′ē-ĕnt) One who receives, as in blood transfusion or tissue or organ transplant.

re·cip·ro·cal beat (rē-sip′rŏ-kăl bēt) SEE reciprocal rhythm.

re·cip·ro·cal gait or·thot·ic (RGO) (rē-sip′rŏ-kăl gāt ŏr-thot′ik) A hip-knee-ankle-foot orthotic that incorporates a cable system to activate hip extension and opposite hip flexion during ambulation, reducing the energy required when compared with traditional knee-ankle-foot orthotics.

re·cip·ro·cal rhythm (rē-sip′rŏ-kăl ridhm) Cardiac arrhythmia in which the impulse arising in the atrioventricular junction descends to and activates the ventricles on one intrajunctional pathway and simultaneously ascends toward the atria in parallel pathways.

re·cip·ro·cal trans·fu·sion (rĕ-sip′rŏ-kăl trans-fyū′zhŭn) An attempt to confer immunity by transfusing blood taken from a donor into a receiver suffering from the same affection, the balance being maintained by transfusing an equal amount from the receiver to the donor.

re·cip·ro·cal trans·lo·ca·tion (rĕ-sip′rŏ-kăl tranz′lō-kā′shŭn) Transposition without demonstrable loss of genetic material.

re·cip·ro·ca·tion (rĕ-sip′rŏ-kā′shŭn) In prosthodontics, the means by which one part of an appliance is made to counter the effect created by another part.

rec·luse spi·der (rek′lūs spī′dĕr) The (brown) recluse spider is a venomous arachnid, *Loxosceles reclusa*, native to the United States from the southern Midwest south to the Gulf of Mexico. Most bites are minor with no necrosis, but some are worse.

rec·og·ni·tion fac·tors (rek′ŏg-nish′ŭn fak′tŏrz) Determinants that affect "recognition" of target antigens by polymorphonuclear leukocytes.

re·com·bi·nant (rē-kom′bi-nănt) **1.** A progeny that has received chromosomal parts from different parental strains due to uncorrected crossing over. **2.** Pertaining to or denoting such organisms. **3.** In linkage analysis, the change of coupling phase at two loci during meiosis.

re·com·bi·nant de·ox·y·ri·bo·nu·cle·ic ac·id (rē-kom′bi-nănt dē-ok′sē-rī′bō-nū-kle′ik as′id) Altered DNA due to insertion into the chain, by chemical, enzymatic, or biologic means, of a sequence (a whole or partial chain of DNA) not originally present in that chain.

re·com·bi·nant vec·tor (rē-kom′bi-nănt vek′tŏr) A vector into which foreign DNA has been inserted. SYN vector (5).

re·com·bi·na·tion (rē-kom′bi-nā′shŭn) **1.** Process of reuniting separated parts. **2.** The reversal of coupling phase in meiosis as gauged by the resulting phenotype. SEE ALSO recombinant. **3.** Formation of new genetic combinations.

re·con·struc·tion (rē′kŏn-strŭk′shŭn) Computed synthesis of one or more two-dimensional images from a series of x-ray projections in tomography, or from a large number of measurements in magnetic resonance imaging.

re·con·struc·tive mam·ma·plas·ty (rē′kŏn-strŭk′tiv mam′ă-plas-tē) The making of a simulated breast by plastic surgery, to reproduce the appearance of one that has been removed.

rec·ord (rek′ŏrd) **1.** A chronologic written account that includes a patient's initial complaint(s) and medical history, the physician's physical findings, the results of diagnostic tests and procedures, and any therapeutic medications or procedures. Cf. health record. **2.** DENTISTRY registration of desired jaw relations in a plastic material or on a device to permit these relationships to be transferred to an articulator.

re·cov·er·y room (rĕ-kŏv′ĕr-ē rūm) Area adjacent to the operating suite used for the recovery of patients following surgery.

rec·re·a·tion·al drug (rek′rē-ā′shŭn-ăl drŭg) SYN street drug.

re·cru·des·cence (rē′krū-des′ĕns) Resumption of a morbid process or its symptoms after remission.

re·cru·des·cent ty·phus (rē′krū-des′ĕnt tī′fŭs) SYN Brill-Zinsser disease.

re·cruit·ment (rĕ-krūt′mĕnt) **1.** AUDIOLOGY unequal reaction of the ear to equal steps of increasing intensity, measured in decibels, with greater than normal increment in perceived loudness. **2.** Bringing additional motor neurons into action, causing greater activity in response to increased duration of the stimulus applied to a given receptor or afferent nerve. SEE ALSO irradiation. **3.** Adding parallel channels of flow in any system.

rec·tal (rek′tăl) Relating to the rectum.

rec·tal al·i·men·ta·tion (rek′tăl al′i-men-tā′shŭn) Nourishment provided by retention enemas.

rec·tal am·pul·la (rek′tăl am-pul′lă) [TA] A dilated portion of the rectum just above the anal canal.

R

rec·tal·gi·a (rek-tal′jē-ă) SYN proctalgia.

rec·tal re·flex (rek′tăl rē′fleks) Entrance of fecal matter into the rectum from the sigmoid colon causes an impulse to defecate.

rec·ti·fi·er (rek′ti-fī′ěr) Electronic device to convert alternating voltage to direct.

rec·to·ab·dom·i·nal (rek′tō-ab-dom′i-năl) Relating to the rectum and the abdomen.

rec·to·sig·moid (rek′tō-sig′moyd) The rectum and sigmoid colon considered as a unit.

rec·tos·to·my (rek-tos′tŏ-mē) SYN proctostomy.

rec·to·u·re·thral (RU) (rek′ō-yūr-ē′thrăl) Relating to the rectum and the urethra.

rec·to·u·ter·ine (rek′tō-yū′těr-in) Relating to the rectum and the uterus.

rec·to·u·ter·ine pouch (rek′tō-yū′těr-in powch) [TA] Pocket formed by peritoneal deflection from the rectum to the uterus. SYN excavatio rectouterina [TA], cul-de-sac (2).

rec·to·vag·i·nal (RV) (rek′tō-vaj′i-năl) Relating to the rectum and the vagina.

rec·to·vag·i·nal fis·tu·la (rek′tō-vaj′i-năl fis′tyū-lă) Fistulous passage connecting the rectum and the vagina.

rec·to·ves·i·cal (rek′tō-ves′i-kăl) Relating to the rectum and the bladder.

rec·tum, pl. **rec·tums,** pl. **rec·ta** (rek′tŭm, -tŭmz, -tă) [TA] The terminal portion of the digestive tube, extending from the rectosigmoid junction to the anal canal.

re·cum·bent (rě-kŭm′běnt) Leaning; reclining; lying down.

re·cu·per·a·tion (rě-kū′pěr-ā′shŭn) Recovery of or restoration to the normal state of health and function.

re·cur·rence (rě-kŭr′ěns) **1.** A return of the symptoms in the course of a disease, following improvement or remission. **2.**

SYN relapse. **3.** Appearance of a genetic trait in a relative of a proband.

re·cur·rent (rě-kŭr′ěnt) **1.** ANATOMY turning back on itself. **2.** Denoting symptoms or lesions reappearing after a remission.

re·cur·rent aph·thous sto·ma·ti·tis (RAS) (rě-kŭr′ěnt af′thŭs ŭl′sěr) SYN aphtha (2).

re·cur·rent fe·ver (rě-kŭr′ěnt fē′věr) SYN relapsing fever.

re·cur·va·tion (rē′kŭr-vā′shŭn) A backward bending or flexure.

red (red) One of the primary colors, produced by the longest waves of the visible spectrum, with violet at the other end.

red blood cell (rbc, RBC) (red blŭd sel) SYN erythrocyte.

red blood cell count (red blŭd sel kownt) The concentration of erythrocytes in a specimen of whole blood. SYN erythrocyte count.

red blood count (RBC) (red blŭd kownt) SEE blood count.

red cell (red sel) SYN erythrocyte.

red cor·pus·cle (RC) (red kōr′pŭs-ěl) SYN erythrocyte.

red in·dur·a·tion (red in′dŭr-ā′shŭn) Pulmonary condition involving advanced degree of acute passive congestion, acute pneumonitis (sometimes termed interstitial pneumonia), or a similar pathologic process.

red nu·cle·us (red nū′klē-ŭs) A large, well-defined, somewhat elongated cell mass, of reddish-gray hue in the fresh brain, located in the rostral mesencephalic tegmentum.

red oil (red oyl) A weakly acid diazo oil-soluble dye, used in histologic demonstration of neutral fats.

re·dox (rē′doks) Contraction of reduction-oxidation.

red pulp (red pŭlp) Splenic pulp seen grossly as a reddish-brown substance, due to its abundance of red blood cells, consisting of splenic sinuses and the tissue intervening between them.

red straw·ber·ry tongue (red staw´ber-ē tŭng) Clinical manifestation of Kawasaki disease.

re·duce (rĕ-dūs´) **1.** To perform reduction (1). **2.** CHEMISTRY to initiate reduction (2).

re·duced he·mo·glo·bin (rĕ-dūst´ hē´mō-glō-bin) The form of hemoglobin in red blood cells after the oxygen of oxyhemoglobin is released in the tissues.

re·duc·i·ble (rĕ-dūs´i-bĕl) Capable of being reduced.

re·duc·i·ble her·ni·a (rĕ-dūs´i-bĕl hĕr´nē-ă) One in which the sac's contents can be returned to their normal location.

re·duc·tant (rĕ-dŭk´tănt) The substance that is oxidized in the course of reduction.

re·duc·tase (rĕ-dŭk´tās) An enzyme that catalyzes a reduction. SYN reducing enzyme.

re·duc·tion (rĕ-dŭk´shŭn) **1.** The restoration, by surgical or manipulative procedures, of a part to its normal anatomic relation. SYN repositioning. **2.** CHEMISTRY a reaction involving a gain of one or more electrons by a substance. **3.** Surgical procedure to reduce size.

re·duc·tion de·for·mi·ty (rĕ-dŭk´shŭn dĕ-fōrm´i-tē) Congenital absence or attenuation of one or more body parts.

re·duc·tion of chro·mo·somes (rĕ-dŭk´shŭn krō´mŏ-sōmz) The process during meiosis whereby one member of each homologous pair of chromosomes is distributed to a sperm or ovum (oocyte); the diploid set of chromosomes (46 in humans) is thus reduced to the haploid set in each gamete; union of the sperm and ovum (oocyte) restores the diploid or somatic number in the one-cell zygote.

re·du·pli·ca·tion (rē-dū´pli-kā´shŭn) **1.** A redoubling. **2.** A duplication or doubling. **3.** A fold or duplicature.

red, white, and blue sign (red wīt blū sīn) The contemporaneous occurrence of erythema, ischemia, and necrosis in a wound, as in loxoscelism.

Reed-Frost mod·el (rēd-frawst mod´ĕl) Mathematical model of infectious disease transmission and group immunity.

reef·ing (rēf´ing) Surgically reducing the extent of a tissue by folding it and securing with sutures, as in plication.

re·en·trant mech·a·nism (rē-en´trănt mek´ă-nizm) Probable basis of most arrhythmias, requiring at least three criteria: a loop circuit, unidirectional block, and slowed conduction.

re·en·try (rē-en´trē) Return of the same impulse into a zone of recently activated heart muscle, sufficiently delayed that the zone is no longer refractory.

ref·er·ence e·lec·trode (ref´ĕr-ens ĕ-lek´trōd) One expected to have a constant potential, used with another electrode to complete an electrical circuit through a solution.

ref·er·ence range (ref´ĕr-ĕns rānj) The usual range of test values for a healthy population. SYN normal range.

ref·er·ence val·ues (ref´ĕr-ĕns val´yūz) A set of laboratory test values obtained from an individual or group in a defined state of health; replaced the so-called normal values; based on a defined state of health.

re·ferred pain (rĕ-fĕrd´ pān) Unpleasant sensation at a site other than the actual location of trauma or disease.

re·ferred sen·sa·tion (rĕ-fĕrd´ sen-sā´shŭn) Feeling perceived in one place in response to a stimulus applied in another.

re·flec·tion (rĕ-flek´shŭn) **1.** The act of reflecting. **2.** That which is reflected. **3.** In psychotherapy, a technique in which a patient's statements are repeated, restated, or rephrased so that the patient will continue to explore and expound on emotionally significant content.

re·flec·tion co·ef·fi·cient (σ) (rĕ-flek´shŭn kō´ĕ-fish´ĕnt) A measure of the relative permeability of a particular membrane to a particular solute.

R

re·flex (rē′fleks) Involuntary reaction to a stimulus applied to the periphery and transmitted to the nervous centers in the brain or spinal cord. SEE ALSO phenomenon.

re·flex arc (rē′fleks ahrk) **1.** Route followed by nerve impulses to produce of a reflex act. **2.** Neural pathway that involves both the peripheral and central nervous systems.

re·flex cough (rē′fleks kawf) One excited reflexively by irritation in some distant part, as the ear or the stomach.

re·flex dys·pep·si·a (rē′fleks dis-pep′sē-ă) Functional dyspepsia excited by reflex irritation from disease elsewhere than in the stomach or intestines.

re·flex ep·i·lep·sy (rē′fleks ep′i-lep′sē) Seizures induced by peripheral stimulation. SYN sensory precipitated epilepsy.

re·flex·o·gen·ic, re·flex·og·e·nous (rē-flek′sō-jen′ik, -fleks-oj′ĕ-nŭs) Causing a reflex.

re·flex·o·graph (rē-flek′sō-graf) An instrument for graphically recording a reflex.

re·flex·ol·o·gy (rē′flek-sol′ŏ-jē) A massage technique focusing on specific points on the feet, hands, and ears that are said to correspond through meridians to other organs or areas of the body. SYN reflex zone therapy.

re·flex·om·e·ter (rē′fleks-om′ĕ-tĕr) An instrument for measuring the force necessary to excite a reflex.

re·flex sym·pa·thet·ic dys·tro·phy (RSD) (rē′fleks sim′pă-thet′ik dis′trŏ-fē) Diffuse persistent pain usually in an extremity often associated with vasomotor disturbances, trophic changes, and limitation or immobility of joints. SEE ALSO causalgia.

re·flex symp·tom (rē′fleks simp′tŏm) Disturbance of sensation or function in an organ or part more or less remote from the morbid condition giving rise to it.

re·flex tach·y·car·di·a (rē′fleks tak′i-kahr′dē-ă) Increased heart rate in response to some stimulus conveyed through the cardiac nerves.

re·flux (rē′flŭks) *Do not confuse this word with reflux.* **1.** A backward flow. SEE ALSO regurgitation. **2.** CHEMISTRY to boil without loss of vapor because of the presence of a condenser that returns vapor as liquid.

re·flux e·soph·a·gi·tis, pep·tic e·soph·a·gi·tis (RE) (rē′flŭks ĕ-sof′ă-jī′tis, pep′tik) Inflammation of the lower esophagus from regurgitation of acid gastric contents, usually due to malfunction of the lower esophageal sphincter.

re·flux neph·rop·a·thy (rē′flŭks nefrop′ă-thē) Damaged renal parenchyma secondary to vesicoureteral reflux of infected urine. SYN reflux-associated nephropathy.

re·frac·tion (RFR) (rē-frak′shŭn) **1.** The deflection of a ray of light when it passes from one medium into another of different optic density. **2.** Determining the nature and degree of the refractive errors in the eye and correction of the same by lenses. SYN refringence.

re·frac·tion·ist (rē-frak′shŭn-ist) Someone trained to measure ocular refraction and determine the proper corrective lenses.

re·frac·tive in·dex (n) (rē-frak′tiv in′deks) The relative velocity of light in another medium compared to the velocity in air.

re·frac·tom·e·ter, re·frac·tion·om·e·ter (rē′frak-tom′ĕ-tĕr, rē-frak′shŏ-nom′ĕ-tĕr) An instrument to measure refractive degree in translucent substances. SEE ALSO refractive index.

re·frac·to·ry (rē-frak′tŏr-ē) **1.** Resistant to treatment, as of a disease. SYN intractable (1), obstinate (2). **2.** SYN obstinate (1), refrangible.

re·frac·to·ry an·e·mi·a (rē-frak′tŏr-ē ă-nē′mē-ă) Progressive anemia unresponsive to therapy other than transfusion.

re·frac·to·ry pe·ri·od (RP) (rē-frak′tŏr-ē pēr′ē-ŏd) Time after effective stimulation, during which excitable tissue fails to respond to a stimulus of threshold intensity.

re·frac·to·ry state (rē-frak′tŏr-ē stāt)

Subnormal excitability immediately following a response to previous excitation.

re·fran·gi·ble (rē-fran'ji-bĕl) SYN refractable.

re·fresh (rē-fresh') To renew, to cause to recuperate, revivify.

re·frig·er·a·tion (rē-frij'ĕr-a'shŭn) The act of cooling or reducing fever.

Ref·sum dis·ease (ref'sŭm di-zēz') A rare degenerative disorder due to a deficiency of phytanic acid α-hydroxylase. Also called Refsum syndrome.

re·fu·sion (rē-fyū'zhŭn) Return of the circulation of blood that has been temporarily cut off by ligature of a limb.

re·gen·er·a·tion (rē-jen'ĕr-a'shŭn) **1.** Reproduction or reconstitution of a lost or injured part. SYN neogenesis. **2.** A form of asexual reproduction (e.g., when a worm is divided into two or more parts, each segment is regenerated into a new individual).

reg·i·men (R) (rej'i-mĕn) *The cognate word regime is widely, and correctly, used as a synonym of regimen.* A program, including pharmacotherapy, which regulates aspects of one's lifestyle for a hygienic or therapeutic purpose; a program of treatment.

re·gion (rē'jŭn) [TA] **1.** An often arbitrarily limited portion of the surface of the body. SEE ALSO space, zone. **2.** A portion of the body having a special nervous or vascular supply, or a part of an organ having a special function. SEE ALSO area, space, spatium, zone.

re·gion·al an·es·the·si·a (rē'jŭn-ăl an'es-thē'zē-ă) Use of local anesthetic solution(s) to produce circumscribed areas of loss of sensation. SYN conduction analgesia.

re·gion·al en·ter·i·tis (rē'jŭn-ăl en'tĕr-ī'tis) Chronic inflammation of unknown cause, involving the terminal ileum and less frequently other parts of the gastrointestinal tract; characterized by patchy deep ulcers that may cause fistulas, and narrowing and thickening of the bowel by fibrosis and lymphocytic infiltration. SYN Crohn disease, distal ileitis, regional ileitis, granulomatous enteritis.

reg·is·ter (rej'is-tĕr) The file of data concerning all cases of a specified condition, such as cancer, occurring in a defined population; the register is the actual document, and the registry is the system of ongoing registration.

reg·is·tered nurse (RN, R.N.) (rej'i-stĕrd nŭrs) A health care professional who has graduated from an accredited nursing program and has been licensed by public authority to practice nursing.

reg·is·tered res·pi·ra·tor·y ther·a·pist (RRT) (rej'is-tĕrd res'pir-ă-tōr-ē thār'ă-pist) Health professional who has graduated from an accredited respiratory therapy program and has passed both theoretic and practical portions of the national credentialing examination.

reg·is·tra·tion (rej'is-trā'shŭn) The reception of external stimuli; the capacity to perform this activity.

reg·is·try (rej'is-trē) A database of patients who share a particular characteristic; common registries include those for cancer, trauma, and implants; data are used to assess the quality of care, monitor trends, and continue research.

re·gres·sion (rē-gresh'ŭn) **1.** A subsidence of symptoms. **2.** A relapse. **3.** Any retrograde movement or action. **4.** A return to a more primitive mode of behavior due to an inability to function adequately at a more adult level. **5.** The tendency of offspring of exceptional parents to possess characteristics closer to those of the general population. **6.** An unconscious defense mechanism with a return to earlier patterns of adaptation. **7.** The distribution of one random variable given particular values of other variables relevant to it.

reg·u·lar a·stig·ma·tism (reg'yū-lăr ă-stig'mă-tizm) Ocular condition in which the curvature in each meridian is equal throughout its course, and the meridians of greatest and least curvature are at right angles to each other.

reg·u·lar in·su·lin (reg'yū-lăr in'sū-lin) Rapidly acting form that a clear solution may be administered intravenously as well as subcutaneously. SYN globin insulin.

reg·u·la·tion (reg'yū-lā'shŭn) **1.** Control

R

of the rate or manner in which a process progresses or a product is formed. **2.** EXPERIMENTAL EMBRYOLOGY the power of a pregastrula embryo to continue approximately normal development after a part or parts have been manipulated or destroyed. **3.** A rule issued by a regulatory agency of government or some other recognized authority.

reg·u·la·tor gene (reg'yū-lā'tŏr jēn) Gene that produces a repressor substance that inhibits an operator gene when combined with it; prevents production of a specific protein.

reg·u·la·to·ry dis·or·der (reg'yū-lă-tōr-ē dis-ōr'dĕr) A condition, first evident in infancy and early childhood, characterized by a distinct behavioral pattern that presents with a sensory, sensorimotor, or organizational processing difficulty that interferes with a child's ability to maintain positive interactions and relationships and to make daily adaptations.

reg·u·lon (reg'yū-lon) A set of structural genes, all with the same gene regulation, with gene products involved in the same reaction pathway.

re·gur·gi·tant (rē-gŭr'ji-tănt) Regurgitating; flowing backward.

re·gur·gi·tant mur·mur (rē-gŭr'ji-tănt mŭr'mŭr) Sound due to leakage or backward flow at one of the valvular orifices of the heart.

re·gur·gi·ta·tion (rē-gŭr'ji-tā'shŭn) **1.** A backward flow, as of blood through an incompetent valve of the heart. **2.** SYN vomiting.

re·ha·bil·i·ta·tion (rē'hă-bil'i-tā'shŭn) Spontaneous or therapeutic restoration, after disease, illness, or injury, of the ability to function in a normal or near normal manner.

re·hy·dra·tion (rē'hī-drā'shŭn) The return of water to a system after its loss.

Rei·chel-Pól·ya stom·ach pro·ce·dure (rī'kel-pōl'yah stŏm'ăk prŏ-sē'jŭr) Retrocolic anastomosis of the full circumference of the open stomach to the jejunum.

re·in·fec·tion (rē'in-fek'shŭn) A second infection by the same microorganism, after recovery from or during the course of a primary infection.

re·in·force·ment (rē'in-fōrs'mĕnt) **1.** An increase of force or strength; denoting specifically the increased sharpness of the patellar reflex when the patient at the same time closes the fist tightly or pulls against the flexed fingers or contracts some other set of muscles. **2.** DENTISTRY a structural addition or inclusion used to give additional strength in function. **3.** CONDITIONING the totality of the process in which the conditioned stimulus is followed by presentation of the unconditioned stimulus that itself elicits the response to be conditioned. SEE ALSO reinforcer.

re·in·for·cer, pos·i·tive re·in·for·cer, neg·a·tive re·in·for·cer (rē'in-fōrs'ĕr, poz'i-tiv, neg'ă-tiv) In conditioning, a pleasant or satisfaction-yielding or painful or unsatisfying (negative reinforcer) stimulus, object, or stimulus event obtained on performance of a desired or predetermined operant. SEE ALSO reinforcement (3). SYN reward.

re·in·ner·va·tion (rē-in'ĕr-vā'shŭn) Restoration of nerve control of a paralyzed muscle or other effector organ by means of regrowth of nerve fibers, either spontaneously or after anastomosis.

re·in·te·gra·tion (rē-in'tĕ-grā'shŭn) In the mental health professions, the return to well-adjusted functioning following disturbances due to mental illness.

Reis-Bück·lers cor·ne·al dys·tro·phy (rīs-bĕk'lers kōr'nē-ăl dis'trŏ-fē) An autosomal dominant disorder of Bowman membrane of the cornea, characterized by a reticular haze and associated with recurrent corneal erosions.

Reis·sei·sen mus·cles (rīs'ī-sen mŭs'ĕlz) Microscopic smooth muscle fibers in the smallest bronchial tubes.

Rei·ter syn·drome (rī'ter sin'drōm) Association of urethritis, iridocyclitis, mucocutaneous lesions, and arthritis, sometimes with diarrhea.

re·jec·tion (rē-jek'shŭn) **1.** Immunologic response to incompatibility in a transplanted organ. **2.** A refusal to accept.

3. Elimination of small ultrasonic echoes from display.

re·lapse (rē'laps) Return of the manifestations of a disease after an interval of improvement. SYN recurrence (2).

re·laps·ing (rē-lap'sing) Recurring; said of a disease or its manifestations that recur after an interval of improvement.

re·laps·ing feb·rile nod·u·lar non·sup·pur·a·tive pan·ni·cu·li·tis (rē-lap'sing feb'ril nod'yū-lăr non'sŭp'yūr-ă-tiv pă-nik'yū-lī'tis) Nodular fat necrosis of a variety of causes. SYN Christian disease (2), Christian syndrome, Weber-Christian disease.

re·laps·ing fe·ver (rē-lap'sing fē'vĕr) An acute infectious disease caused by any one of a number of strains of *Borrelia*, marked by febrile attacks lasting about 6 days and separated from each other by apyretic intervals of about the same length; the microorganism is found in the blood during the febrile periods but not during the intervals.

re·laps·ing pol·y·chon·dri·tis (rē-lap'sing pol'ē-kon-drī'tis) A hereditary degenerative cartilage disease producing a bizarre form of arthritis, with collapse of the ears, the cartilaginous portion of the nose, and the tracheobronchial tree. SYN Meyenburg disease.

rel·a·tive ac·com·mo·da·tion (rel'ă-tiv ă-kom'ŏ-dā'shŭn) Quantity of accommodation required for single binocular vision for any specified distance, or for any degree of convergence.

rel·a·tive mo·lec·u·lar mass (Mr) (rel'ă-tiv mŏ-lek'yū-lăr mas) SYN molecular weight.

rel·a·tive pol·y·cy·the·mi·a (rel'ă-tiv pol'ē-sī-thē'mē-ă) Relative increase in the number of red blood cells as a result of loss of the fluid portion of the blood.

rel·a·tive risk (RR) (rel'ă-tiv risk) Ratio of the risk of disease among those exposed to a risk factor to the risk among those not exposed.

rel·a·tive sco·to·ma (rel'ă-tiv skō-tō'mă) Ocular disorder in which there is visual depression but not complete loss of light perception.

rel·a·tive spe·ci·fi·ci·ty (rel'ă-tiv spes'i-fis'i-tē) Specificity of a medical screening test as determined by comparison with the same type of test.

rel·a·tive val·ue u·nit (RVU) (rel'ă-tiv val'yū yū'nit) A numeric factor assigned to a medical service during coding based on the skill and time required to undertake such a procedure.

re·lax·ant (rē-lak'sănt) **1.** Causing relaxation; reducing tension, especially muscular tension. **2.** An agent that reduces muscular tension or produces skeletal muscle paralysis.

re·lax·ant re·ver·sal (rē-lak'sănt rē-vĕr'săl) Use of acetylcholinesterase inhibitors to terminate the action of nondepolarizing neuromuscular relaxants.

re·lax·a·tion res·ponse (rē-lak-sā'shŭn rē-spons') Integrated hypothalamic reaction in which a human being or animal experiences safety and a sense of nurturing.

re·lax·a·tion su·ture (rē'lak-sā'shŭn sū'chŭr) Stitch so arranged that it may be loosened if the tension of the wound becomes excessive.

re·lax·in (rē-lak'sin) Polypeptide hormone secreted by the corpora lutea of mammalian species during pregnancy. SYN cervilaxin, ovarian hormone, parturition-mediating factor, releasin.

re·leas·ing fac·tors, re·leas·ing hor·mone (rē-lē'sing fak'tŏrz, hŏr'mōn) **1.** Substances, usually of hypothalamic origin, capable of accelerating the rate of secretion of a given hormone by the anterior pituitary gland. **2.** Factors required in the termination phase of either RNA biosynthesis or protein biosynthesis. SYN liberins.

re·lief area (rē-lēf' ar'ē-ă) In dentistry, portion of the denture-bearing area over which the denture base is altered to reduce functional pressure.

re·lief cham·ber (rē-lēf' chām'bĕr) Recess in the impression surface of a denture to reduce or eliminate pressure from that area of the mouth.

re·line (rē'līn) In dentistry, to resurface the tissue side of a denture with new base

R

material to make it fit more accurately. SEE ALSO rebase.

REM Abbreviation for rapid eye movement.

Re·mak re·flex (rā′mahk rē′fleks) Plantar flexion of the first three toes and, sometimes, the foot with extension of the knee induced by stroking of the upper anterior surface of the thigh.

Re·mak sign (rā′mahk sīn) Dissociation of the sensations of touch and of pain in tabes dorsalis and polyneuritis.

re·min·er·al·i·za·tion (rē-min′ĕr-ăl-ī-zā′shŭn) **1.** The return to the body or a local area of necessary mineral constituents lost through disease or dietary deficiencies. **2.** DENTISTRY a process enhanced by the presence of fluoride whereby partially decalcified enamel, dentin, and cementum become recalcified by mineral replacement.

rem·i·nis·cence (rem′i-nis′ĕns) In the psychology of learning, an improvement in recall, over that shown on the last trial, of incompletely learned material after an interval without practice.

re·mis·sion (rē-mish′ŭn) **1.** Abatement or lessening in severity of the symptoms of a disease. **2.** The period during which such abatement occurs.

re·mit·tent (rē-mit′ĕnt) Characterized by temporary periods of abatement of the symptoms of a disease.

re·mit·tent fe·ver (rē-mit′ĕnt fē′vĕr) Pyrexic pattern in which temperature varies during each 24-hour period but never reaches normal.

re·mod·el·ing (rē-mod′ĕl-ing) **1.** Cyclic process by which bone maintains a dynamic steady state through sequential resorption and formation of a small amount of bone at the same site. **2.** Any process of reshaping or reorganizing. **3.** Process of changing a body part, as in plastic and reconstructive surgery. SYN remodelling.

remodelling [Br.] SYN remodeling.

re·mote mem·o·ry (rē-mōt′ mem′ŏr-y) Recall of events of long ago as opposed to recent events.

ren, gen. **re·nis,** pl. **re·nes** (ren, rē′nis, -nez) [TA] SYN kidney.

re·nal (rē′năl) SYN nephric.

re·nal ad·e·no·car·ci·no·ma (rē′năl ad′ĕ-nō-kar′si-nō′mă) Lesion arising in the renal parenchyma, usually occurring in middle-aged or older people of either gender (although more common in men). SYN clear cell carcinoma of kidney, renal cell carcinoma.

re·nal am·y·loi·do·sis (rē′năl am′i-loy-dō′sis) Amyloid kidney deposits, which may cause albuminuria and the nephrotic syndrome.

re·nal cal·cu·lus (rē′năl kal′kyū-lŭs) Stone occurring within the kidney's collecting system. SYN nephrolith.

re·nal cast (rē′năl kast) Stone formed in a renal tubule and found in the urine. SYN tube cast.

re·nal cell car·ci·no·ma (rē′năl sel kahr′si-nō′mă) SYN renal adenocarcinoma.

re·nal col·ic (rē′năl kol′ik) Sharp lower back pain that radiates down the flank and into the groin; associated with it, passage of a renal calculus through the ureter as it dilates it, causing ureteral spasms as the calculus is forced along the narrow tube; usually of sudden onset, severe and colicky, and not improved by changes in position.

re·nal cor·pus·cle (rē′năl kōr′pŭs-ĕl) The tuft of glomerular capillaries and the capsula glomeruli that encloses it. SYN malpighian corpuscles.

re·nal di·a·betes (rē′năl dī-ă-bē′tēz) SYN renal glycosuria.

re·nal fail·ure (rē′năl fāl′yŭr) Impairment of renal function, either acute or chronic, with retention of urea, creatinine, and other waste products. SYN kidney failure.

re·nal gly·co·su·ri·a (rē′năl glī′kō-syūr′ē-ă) Recurrent or persistent excretion of urinary glucose in association with blood glucose levels in the normal range.

re·nal he·ma·tu·ri·a (rē′năl hē′mă-tyūr′ē-ă) Blood disorder due to extravasation of blood into the glomerular spaces, or tubules, or pelves of the kidneys.

re·nal hy·per·ten·sion (rē′năl hī′pĕr-ten′shŭn) Hypertension secondary to kidney disease.

re·nal in·suf·fi·cien·cy (RI) (rē′năl in′sŭ-fish′ĕn-sē) Defective kidney function with hematologic accumulation of waste products.

re·nal me·dul·la (rē′năl mĕ-dŭl′ă) [TA] The inner, darker portion of the kidney parenchyma consisting of the renal pyramids.

re·nal nan·ism (rē′năl nan′izm) Infantile renal osteodystrophy.

re·nal os·te·o·dys·tro·phy (rē′năl os′tē-ō-dis′trŏ-fē) Generalized bone changes resembling osteomalacia and rickets or osteitis fibrosa, occurring in chronic renal failure.

re·nal plas·ma flow (RPF) (rē′năl plaz′mă flō) Measurement of the amount of plasma that transits the kidneys within a given duration.

re·nal ret·i·nop·a·thy (rē′năl ret′i-nop′ă-thē) Hypertensive ocular disorder associated with chronic glomerulonephritis or nephrosclerosis.

re·nal thresh·old (rē′năl thresh′ōld) The plasma concentration level of a substance below which none appears in urine.

re·nal trans·plan·ta·tion (RTx) (rē′năl trans′plan-tā′shŭn) Surgical transplantation of a kidney from a compatible donor to restore kidney function in a recipient suffering from renal failure.

re·nal tu·bu·lar ac·id·o·sis (rē′năl tū′byū-lăr as′i-dō′sis) A clinical syndrome characterized by decreased ability to acidify urine, and by low plasma bicarbonate and high plasma chloride concentrations, often with hypokalemia.

ren·i·form (ren′i-fōrm) SYN nephroid.

re·nin (rē′nin) An enzyme that converts angiotensinogen to angiotensin I. SYN angiotensinogenase.

ren·in·an·gi·o·ten·sin·al·dos·ter·one sys·tem (rē′nin-an′jē-ō-ten′sin al-dos′tĕr-ōn sis′tĕm) Hormones, renin, angiotensin, and aldosterone work together to regulate blood pressure. A sustained fall in blood pressure causes the kidney to release renin. This is converted to angiotensin in the circulation. Angiotensin then raises blood pressure directly by arteriolar constriction and stimulates the suprarenal glands to produce aldosterone that promotes sodium and water retention by kidney, such that blood volume and blood pressure increase.

re·nin·an·gi·o·ten·sin sys·tem (rē′nin-an-jē-ō-ten′sin sis′tĕm) Selective regulator of the aldosterone biosynthetic pathway that acts by increasing aldosterone production and sodium retention due to volume depletion.

reno-, reni- Combining forms denoting the kidney. SEE ALSO nephro-.

re·no·gas·tric (rē′nō-gas′trik) Relating to the kidneys and the stomach.

re·nog·ra·phy (rē-nog′ră-fē) Radiography of the kidney.

re·no·in·tes·ti·nal (rē′nō-in-tes′ti-năl) Relating to the kidneys and the intestine.

re·no·pri·val (rē′nō-prī′văl) Relating to, characterized by, or resulting from total loss of kidney function or from removal of all functioning renal tissue.

re·no·troph·ic, re·no·trop·ic (rē′nō-trō′fik, -trō′pik) Relating to any agent influencing the growth or nutrition of the kidney or to the action of such an agent. SYN nephrotrophic, nephrotropic.

re·no·vas·cu·lar (rē′nō-vas′kyū-lăr) Pertaining to the blood vessels of the kidney.

re·no·vas·cu·lar hy·per·ten·sion (rē′nō-vas′kyū-lăr hī′pĕr-ten′shŭn) Hypertension produced by renal arterial obstruction.

Ren·pen·ning syn·drome (ren′pen-ing sin′drōm) X-linked mental retardation with short stature and microcephaly not associated with the fragile X chromosome; more frequent in males.

Ren·shaw cells (ren′shaw selz) Inhibitory interneurons innervated by collaterals from motoneurons; identified physiologically and by intracellular injection technique.

Re·o·vi·rus (rē′ō-vī′rŭs) A genus of viruses currently called *Orthoreovirus* with distinct double layers of capsomeres; vertebrate hosts; recovered from children with upper respiratory tract infections; symptomatic or not.

re·pair (rē-pār′) Restoration of diseased or damaged tissues naturally by healing processes or artificially, as by surgical means.

rep·e·ti·tion-com·pul·sion (rep′ĕ-tish′ ŭn-kŏm-pŭl′shŭn) In psychoanalysis, the tendency to repeat earlier experiences or actions, in an unconscious effort to achieve belated mastery over them.

re·pet·i·tive DNA (rē-pet′ĭ-tiv) DNA segment that consists of a linear array of multiple copies of the same sequence of nucleotides.

re·place·ment (rē-plās′mĕnt) **1.** Restoration. **2.** Substitution.

re·place·ment ther·a·py (rē-plās′mĕnt thār′ă-pē) Care designed to compensate for a lack or deficiency arising from inadequate nutrition, from certain dysfunctions, or from losses; replacement may be physiologic or may entail administration of a substitute.

re·plan·ta·tion (rē′plan-tā′shŭn) Replacement of an organ or part in its original site and reestablishment of its circulation.

rep·li·ca·tion (rep′li-kā′shŭn) **1.** Execution of an experiment or study more than once to confirm the original findings, increase precision, and obtain a closer estimate of sampling error. **2.** Autoreproduction (q.v.). **3.** DNA-directed DNA synthesis.

rep·li·ca·tive form (rep′li-kă-tiv fŏrm) **1.** An intermediate stage in the replication of either DNA or RNA viral genomes that is usually double stranded. **2.** The altered, double-stranded form to which single-stranded coliphage DNA is converted after infection of a susceptible bacterium, formation of the complementary (''minus'') strand being mediated by

enzymes that were present in the bacterium before entrance of the viral (''plus'') strand.

re·po·lar·i·za·tion (rē-pō′lăr-ī-zā′shŭn) Process whereby the membrane, cell, or fiber, after depolarization, is polarized again, with positive charges.

re·press·i·ble en·zyme (rē-pres′ĭ-bĕl en′zīm) One produced continuously unless production is repressed by inhibitor excess. SEE ALSO inactive repressor.

re·pres·sion (rē-presh′ŭn) **1.** PSYCHOTHERAPY Active process of keeping out and rejecting unacceptable ideas or impulses to it. **2.** Decreased expression of some gene product.

re·pres·sor (R) (rē-pres′ŏr) Product of a regulator or repressor gene.

re·pres·sor gene (rē-pres′ŏr jēn) One that prevents a nonallele from being transcribed.

re·pro·duc·tion (rē′prō-dŭk′shŭn) **1.** The recall and presentation in the mind of the elements of a former impression. **2.** The total process by which organisms produce offspring. SYN generation (1), procreation.

re·pro·duc·tive (rē′prō-dŭk′tiv) Relating to reproduction.

re·pro·duc·tive cy·cle (rē′prō-dŭk′tiv sī′kĕl) The cycle that begins with conception and extends through gestation and parturition.

re·pro·duc·tive sys·tem (rē′prō-dŭk′ tiv sis′tĕm) SYN genital system.

rep·til·ase (rep′ti-lās) An enzyme found in the venom of *Bothrops atrox* that clots fibrinogen by splitting off its fibrinopeptide.

re·pul·sion (rĕ-pŭl′shŭn) **1.** The act of repelling or driving apart. **2.** Strong dislike. **3.** Coupling phase of genes at linked loci that are borne on opposite chromosomes.

re·quired arch length (rē-kwīrd′ ahrch length) Sum of the mesiodistal widths of the permanent teeth from first permanent molar to first permanent molar.

res·cin·na·mine (rē-sin′ă-mēn, -min) A purified ester alkaloid of species of *Rauwolfia;* related to reserpine with similar uses.

re·sect (rē-sekt′) **1.** To cut off. **2.** To excise a segment of a part.

re·sec·tion (rē-sek′shŭn) Procedure performed to remove a significant part of an organ or bodily structure; may be partial or complete. SYN excision (1).

re·sec·to·scope (rē-sek′tŏ-skōp) A special endoscopic instrument for the transurethral electrosurgical removal of lesions involving the bladder, prostate gland, uterus, or urethra.

re·ser·pine (rē-sĕr′pēn, -pin) An ester alkaloid isolated from certain species of *Rauwolfia;* decreases 5-hydroxytryptamine and catecholamine concentrations in the central nervous system and in peripheral tissues.

re·serve force (rē-zĕrv′ fōrs) Energy in an organism or any of its parts above that required for its normal functioning.

res·er·voir host (rez′ĕr-vwahr hōst) The host of an infection in which the infectious agent multiplies and develops, and on which the agent is dependent for survival in nature.

res·er·voir of in·fec·tion (rez′ĕr-vwahr in-fek′shŭn) Living or nonliving material in or on which an infectious agent multiplies and develops and is dependent on for its survival in nature. SEE ALSO fomes.

re·sid·u·al ab·scess (rē-zid′yū-ăl ab′ses) Lesion at the site of a former abscess due to persistence of microbes and pus.

re·sid·u·al cleft (rē-zid′yū-ăl kleft) Remnants of the hypophysial diverticulum that occur between the pars distalis and pars intermedia. SYN residual lumen.

re·si·du·al cyst (rē-zid′yū-ăl sist) Persistence of an apical periodontal cyst that remains after tooth extraction.

re·sid·u·al lu·men (rē-zid′yū-ăl lū′mĕn) SYN residual cleft.

re·sid·u·al ridge (rē-zid′yū-ăl rij) Portion of the processus alveolaris remaining in the edentulous mouth following resorption of the alveolar section.

re·sid·u·al schiz·o·phre·ni·a (rē-zid′ yū-ăl skits′ō-frē′nē-ă) Blunted or inappropriate affect, social withdrawal, eccentric behavior, or loose associations, but without prominent psychotic symptoms.

re·sid·u·al u·rine (rē-zid′yū-ăl yūr′in) That which remains in the bladder at the end of micturition in cases of prostatic obstruction, bladder atony, and other disorders.

res·i·due (rez′i-dū) That which remains after removal of one or more substances. SYN residuum.

re·sil·ience (rē-zil′yens) **1.** Energy (per unit of volume) released on unloading. **2.** Springiness or elasticity.

res·in (rez′in) **1.** An amorphous brittle substance consisting of the hardened secretion of a number of plants. **2.** A precipitate formed by the addition of water to certain tinctures. **3.** A broad term used to indicate organic substances insoluble in water.

re·sis·tance (rē-zis′tăns) **1.** A passive force exerted in opposition to another active force. **2.** The opposition in a conductor to the passage of a current of electricity, whereby energy is lost and heat produced. Cf. impedance (1). **3.** The opposition to flow of a fluid through one or more passageways. Cf. impedance (2). **4.** PSYCHOANALYSIS a person's unconscious defense against bringing repressed thoughts to consciousness. **5.** Ability of red blood cells to resist hemolysis and preserve their shape under varying degrees of osmotic pressure in the blood plasma. **6.** Natural or acquired ability of an organism to maintain its immunity to or to resist the effects of an antagonistic agent.

re·sis·tance form (rē-zis′tăns fōrm) Shape given to a cavity preparation that enables the dental restoration to withstand masticatory forces.

re·sis·tance-in·duc·ing fac·tor (RIF) (rē-zis′tăns-in-dūs′ing fak′tŏr) Agent from normal chick embryos that interferes with multiplication of the avian sarcoma virus.

R

re·sis·tance plas·mids (rĕ-zis'tăns plaz' midz) Plasmids carrying genes responsible for antibiotic resistance among bacteria; they may be conjugative or nonconjugative, the former possessing transfer genes lacking in the latter.

re·sis·tant starch (rĕ-zis'tănt stahrch) Dietary starch resistant to pancreatic amylase, allowing it to escape into the large bowel, where it is fermented to short-chain fatty acids by colonic microflora.

res·o·lu·tion (rez'ŏ-lū'shŭn) 1. Arrest of an inflammatory process without suppuration. 2. Optic ability to distinguish detail such as the separation of closely adjacent objects. SYN resolving power (3).

res·o·lu·tion a·cu·i·ty (rez'ŏ-lū'shŭn ă-kyū'i-tē) Detection of a target having two or more parts, often measured by using the Snellen test types.

re·sol·vent (rē-zol'vĕnt) 1. Causing resolution. 2. An agent that arrests inflammation or causes the absorption of a neoplasm.

re·solv·ing pow·er (re-zolv'ing pow'ĕr) Definition of a lens. SYN resolution (2).

res·o·nance (rez'ŏ-năns) 1. Sympathetic or forced vibration of air in the cavities above, below, in front of, or behind a source of sound. 2. The sound obtained on percussion of a part that can vibrate freely. 3. The intensification and hollow character of the voice sound obtained on auscultation over a cavity.

res·o·nant fre·quen·cy (rez'ŏ-nănt frē' kwĕn-sē) Frequency at which individual magnetic nuclei absorb or emit radiofrequency energy in magnetic resonance studies. SYN resonance (6).

re·sorb (rē-sōrb') To reabsorb; to absorb what has been excreted.

re·sorp·tion (rē-sōrp'shŭn) 1. The act of resorbing. 2. A loss of substance by lysis, or by physiologic or pathologic means.

Re·source-Based Rel·a·tive Val·ue Scale (rē'sōrs-bāst rel'ă-tiv val'yū skāl) A payment system mandated by U.S. federal law concerning Medicare's establishing a cost basis for Medicare services based on analysis of skill and time required by the health care provider for patient's care.

Re·source U·ti·li·za·tion Group (rē' sōrs yū'til-ī-zā'shŭn grŭp) One of 44 patient categories, each with a corresponding per diem reimbursement rate as mandated by Medicare.

res·pir·a·ble (res'pir-ă-bĕl) Capable of being breathed.

res·pi·ra·tion (res'pir-ā'shŭn) 1. A fundamental process of life, characteristic of both plants and animals, in which oxygen is used to oxidize organic fuel molecules, providing energy as well as carbon dioxide and water. 2. SYN ventilation (2).

res·pi·ra·tion rate (res'pir-ā'shŭn rāt) Frequency of breathing, recorded as the number of breaths per minute.

res·pi·ra·tor, ven·ti·la·tor (res'pir-ā' tŏr, ven'ti-lā'tŏr) 1. An apparatus for administering artificial respiration in cases of respiratory failure. 2. An appliance fitting over the mouth and nose, used to exclude dust, or other irritants, or of otherwise altering the air before it enters the respiratory passages. SYN inhaler (1).

res·pi·ra·to·ry (res'pir-ă-tōr-ē) Relating to respiration.

res·pi·ra·to·ry ac·i·do·sis (res'pir-ă-tōr-ē as'i-dō'sis) Acidosis caused by retention of carbon dioxide. SYN hypercapnic acidosis.

res·pi·ra·to·ry al·ka·lo·sis (res'pir-ă-tōr-ē al'kă-lō'sis) Alkalosis resulting from an abnormal loss of carbon dioxide produced by hyperventilation, either active or passive, with concomitant reduction in arterial bicarbonate concentration. SEE ALSO compensated alkalosis.

res·pi·ra·to·ry care (res'pir-ă-tōr-ē kār) An adjunctive form of health care intended to maintain or restore optimal respiratory function through the use of appropriate devices and techniques.

res·pi·ra·to·ry chain (res'pir-ă-tōr-ē chān) Sequence of energy-liberating oxidation-reduction reactions whereby electrons are accepted from reduced compounds and eventually transferred to oxygen with the formation of water.

SYN cytochrome system, electron-transport chain, electron-transport system.

res·pi·ra·to·ry dis·tress syn·drome of the new·born (res'pir-ă-tōr-ē distres' sin'drōm nū'bŏrn) An acute lung condition of newborn babies, characterized by tachypnea, nasal flaring, and respiratory grunting; occurs primarily in premature babies due to a lack of surfactant, causing alveolar collapse. SYN hyaline membrane disease.

res·pi·ra·to·ry en·ter·ic or·phan vi·rus (res'pir-ă-tōr-ē en-ter'ik ōr'făn vī'rŭs) A nonenveloped icosahedral virus with a genome that consists of double-stranded ribonucleic acid; frequently found in both the respiratory and enteric tracts.

res·pi·ra·to·ry en·zyme (res'pir-ă-tōr-ē en'zīm) A tissue enzyme that is part of an oxidation-reduction system accomplishing the conversion of substrates to carbon dioxide and water and the transfer of the electrons removed to oxygen.

res·pi·ra·to·ry gat·ing (res'pir-ă-tōr-ē gāt'ing) Any technique that derives a signal from breathing to trigger an electronic circuit.

res·pi·ra·to·ry in·suf·fi·cien·cy (res'pir-ă-tōr-ē in-sŭ-fish'ĕn-sē) Failure to adequately provide oxygen to the cells of the body and to remove excess carbon dioxide from them.

res·pi·ra·to·ry lob·ule (res'pir-ă-tōr-ē lob'yūl) SYN pulmonary acinus.

res·pi·ra·to·ry pig·ments (res'pir-ă-tōr-ē pig'mĕnts) The oxygen-carrying substances in blood and tissues.

res·pi·ra·to·ry quo·tient (RQ) (res'pir-ă-tōr-ē kwō'shĕnt) The ratio of the carbon dioxide produced during tissue metabolism to the oxygen consumed.

res·pi·ra·to·ry scle·ro·ma (res'pir-ă-tōr-ē skler-ō'mă) Rhinoscleroma in which the lesion involves the mucous membrane of the greater part or all of the upper respiratory tract.

res·pi·ra·to·ry sys·tem (RS) (res'pir-ă-tōr-ē sis'tĕm) [TA] All air passages from the nose to the pulmonary alveoli. SYN systema respiratorium [TA], apparatus respiratorius, respiratory apparatus.

res·pi·ra·to·ry ther·a·py (res'pir-ă-tōr-ē thār'ă-pē) SEE respiratory care.

res·pi·ra·to·ry tract (res'pir-ă-tōr-ē trakt) The air passages from the nose to the pulmonary alveoli, through the pharynx, larynx, trachea, and bronchi.

res·pi·rom·e·ter (res'pir-om'ĕ-tŏr) 1. An instrument for measuring the extent of the respiratory movements. 2. An instrument for measuring oxygen consumption or carbon dioxide production.

re·spon·dent con·di·tion·ing (rĕ-spon'dĕnt kŏn-dish'ŭn-ing) A type of conditioning, first studied by Pavlov, in which a previously neutral stimulus (bell sound) elicits a response (salivation) as a result of pairing it (associating it contiguously in time) a number of times with an unconditioned or natural stimulus for that response (food shown to a hungry dog).

re·sponse (rĕ-spons') 1. The reaction of a muscle, nerve, gland, or other excitable tissue to a stimulus. 2. Any act or behavior, or its constituents, which a living organism is capable of emitting.

res·ponse bi·as (rĕ-spons' bī'ăs) Systematic error due to differences in characteristics between those who choose or volunteer to take part in a study, and those who do not.

rest (rest) 1. Quiet; repose. 2. To cease work. 3. A group of poorly differentiated cells commonly believed to be cells of fetal tissue that has become displaced and lies embedded in tissue of another character. 4. DENTISTRY an extension from a prosthesis that affords vertical support for a restoration.

rest area (rest ar'ē-ă) Portion of a tooth structure or of a restoration in a tooth that is prepared to receive the positive seating of the metallic occlusal, incisal, lingual, or cingulum rest of a removable prosthesis. SYN rest seat.

re·ste·no·sis (rē'stĕ-nō'sis) Recurrence of stenosis after corrective surgery on the heart valve.

res·ti·form (res'ti-fōrm) Ropelike; referring to the restiform body, the larger (lateral) part of the inferior cerebellar peduncle.

rest·ing cell (rest′ing sel) A quiescent cell; one not undergoing mitosis.

rest·ing en·er·gy ex·pen·di·ture (rest′ing en′ĕr-jē ek-spen′di-chŭr) Energy expenditure measured under resting, although not necessarily basal conditions. *Cf.* basal metabolic rate.

rest·ing hand splint (rest′ing hand splint) A splint intended to maintain the nonfunctional hand and wrist in a neutral position of rest so as to prevent pain and muscle contracture.

rest·ing trem·or (rest′ing trem′ŏr) A coarse, rhythmic tremor, usually confined to hands and forearms, which appears when the limbs are relaxed, and disappears with active limb movements; characteristic of parkinsonism.

rest·i·tope (res′ti-tōp) The part of the T-cell receptor that associates with the class II major histocompatibility molecule.

res·ti·tu·tion (res′ti-tū′shŭn) OBSTETRICS Return of the rotated fetal head to its natural relation with the shoulders after its emergence from the vulva.

rest·less legs syn·drome (RLS) (rest′lĕs legz sin′drōm) A sense of indescribable uneasiness, twitching, aching or burning that occurs in the legs after going to bed, frequently leading to insomnia, which may be relieved temporarily by walking about; thought to be caused by inadequate circulation or as an adverse effect of some psychotropic medications.

rest of Ser·res (rest sārs) Remnant of dental lamina epithelium entrapped within the gingiva.

res·to·ra·tion (res′tŏr-ā′shŭn) DENTISTRY 1. A prosthetic restoration or appliance; a broad term applied to any inlay, crown, bridge, partial denture, or complete denture that restores or replaces lost tooth structure, teeth, or oral tissues. 2. Substance used for restoring the portion missing from a tooth due to removal of tooth decay.

re·stor·a·tive den·tis·try (rĕ-stōr′ă-tiv den′tis-trē) Individual restoration of teeth

by means of amalgam, synthetic porcelainlike materials, resins, or inlays. SEE ALSO implant, oral and maxillofacial surgery.

rest pain (rest pān) Unrelenting ischemic pain in an extremity at rest, indicating severe arterial insufficiency.

rest po·si·tion (rest pŏ-zish′ŭn) The usual position of the mandible when the patient is resting comfortably in an upright position and the condyles are in a neutral, unstrained position in the mandibular fossa. SYN physiologic rest position.

re·straint (rĕ-strānt′) PSYCHIATRY any intervention to prevent an excited or violent patient from harming self or others.

re·stric·tion (rĕ-strik′shŭn) 1. The use or action of restriction endonucleases. 2. Process by which foreign DNA that has been introduced into a prokaryotic cell becomes ineffective. 3. A limitation.

re·stric·tion en·do·nu·cle·ase (rĕ-strik′shŭn en′dō-nū′klē-ās) One of many endonucleases isolated from bacteria cut double-stranded DNA chains at specific sequences, thus inactivating a foreign (viral or other) DNA and restricting its activity. SYN restriction enzyme.

re·stric·tion map (rĕ-strik′shŭn map) Order of restriction sites along a chromosome or plasmid.

re·stric·tion site (rĕ-strik′shŭn sīt) A site in nucleic acid in which the bordering bases are of such a type as to leave them vulnerable to the cleaving action of an endonuclease. SYN cleavage site.

re·stric·tive car·di·o·my·op·a·thy (RCM) (rĕ-strik′tiv kahr′dē-ō-mī-op′ă-thē) Diverse conditions characterized by restriction of diastolic filling.

re·stric·tive ven·ti·la·to·ry de·fect (rĕ-strik′tiv ven′til-ă-tōr-ē dē′fekt) Reduction in lung volumes not explainable by obstruction of the airways; most commonly characterized physiologically by a reduction in total lung capacity (TLC).

re·sus·ci·ta·tion (rĕ-sŭs′i-tā′shŭn) Revival from potential or apparent death.

re·tained pla·cen·ta (rē-tānd′ plă-sen′tă) Incomplete separation of the placenta and its failure to be expelled at the usual time after delivery of the child. SYN incarcerated placenta.

re•tain•er (rē-tā′nĕr) **1.** Any type of clasp, attachment, or other device used to fix or stabilize a prosthesis. **2.** An appliance used to prevent the shifting of teeth following orthodontic treatment.

re•tar•da•tion (rē′tahr-dā′shŭn) The slowing or limitation of development.

re•tard•ed den•ti•tion (rē-tahrd′ĕd den-tish′ŭn) Dentition in which growth phenomena such as calcification, elongation, and eruption occur later than the average range of normal variation due to systemic metabolic dysfunction.

retch (rech) To make an involuntary effort to vomit.

retch•ing (rech′ing) Gastric and esophageal movements of vomiting without expulsion of vomitus. SYN dry vomiting.

re•te, pl. **re•ti•a** (rē′tē, -shē-ă) [TA] **1.** SYN network (1). **2.** A structure composed of a fibrous network or mesh.

re•te mi•ra•bi•le (rē′tē mē-rahb′ē-lā) [TA] A vascular network interrupting the continuity of an artery or vein.

re•ten•tion (rē-ten′shŭn) **1.** The keeping in the body of what normally belongs there. **2.** The keeping in the body of what normally should be discharged (e.g., as urine or feces). **3.** Retaining that which has been learned so that it can be used later in recall, recognition, or, if retention is partial, relearning. SEE ALSO memory. **4.** Resistance to dislodgement. **5.** DENTISTRY A passive period following treatment when a patient is wearing an appliance or appliances to maintain or stabilize the teeth in the new position into which they have been moved.

re•ten•tion cyst (rē-ten′shŭn sist) Lesion due to obstruction to the gland's excretory duct. SYN distention cyst, secretory cyst.

re•ten•tion form (rē-ten′shŭn fōrm) Shape of a cavity preparation that prevents displacement of the dental restoration by lateral or tipping forces as well as masticatory forces.

re•ten•tion groove (rē-ten′shŭn grūv) Notch forming opposing vertical constrictions in a tooth to aid retention of a dental restoration.

re•ten•tion jaun•dice (rē-ten′shŭn jawn′dis) Hepatic disorder due to insufficiency of liver function or to an excess of bile pigment production.

re•ten•tion su•ture (rē-ten′shŭn sū′chŭr) A heavy reinforcing suture placed deep within the muscles and fasciae of the abdominal wall to relieve tension on the primary suture line and thus obviate postoperative wound disruption. SYN tension suture.

re•ten•tion vom•it•ing (rē-ten′shŭn vom′it-ing) Emesis due to mechanical obstruction, usually hours after ingestion of a meal.

re•te o•va•ri•i (rē′tē ō-var′ē-ī) A transient network of cells in the developing ovary; homologous to the rete testis.

re•te•plase (r-PA, RPA) (rē′tĕ-plāz) A fibrinolytic agent that works by stimulating production of plasmin. SEE ALSO plasmin.

re•te ridge (rē′tē rij) Downward thickening of the epidermis between the dermal papillae.

re•tic•u•lar, re•tic•u•lated (rĕ-tik′yū-lăr, -lāt′ĕd) Relating to a reticulum.

re•tic•u•lar ac•ti•vat•ing sys•tem (RAS) (rĕ-tik′yū-lăr akt′i-vā′ting sis′tĕm) Physiologic term denoting that part of the brainstem reticular formation that plays a central role in the organism's bodily and behavioral alertness. SEE ALSO reticular formation. SYN nonspecific system.

re•tic•u•lar de•gen•er•a•tion (rĕ-tik′yū-lăr dĕ-jen′ĕr-ā′shŭn) Severe epidermal edema resulting in multilocular bullae.

re•tic•u•lar fi•bers (rĕ-tik′yū-lăr fī′bĕrz) The collagen (type III) fibers forming the distinctive loose connective tissue stroma of embryonic and other forms of tissue.

re•tic•u•lar for•ma•tion (rĕ-tik′yū-lăr fōr-mā′shŭn) A massive but vaguely delimited neural apparatus composed of gray and

R

white matter extending throughout the central core of the brainstem into the diencephalon. SYN formatio reticularis [TA], reticular substance (2).

re·tic·u·lar sub·stance (rĕ-tik′yū-lăr sŭb′stăns) **1.** A filamentous plasmatic material, beaded with granules, demonstrable by means of vital staining in the immature red blood cells. **2.** SYN reticular formation.

re·tic·u·lar tis·sue, ret·i·form tis·sue (rĕ-tik′yū-lăr tish′ū, ret′i-fōrm) A tissue in which the argyrophilic collagenous fibers form a network; usually has a network of reticular cells associated with the fibers.

re·tic·u·la·tion (rĕ-tik′yū-lā′shŭn) **1.** The presence or formation of a reticulum, such as that observed in red blood cells during active regeneration of blood. **2.** A chest radiographic pattern.

re·tic·u·lin (rĕ-tik′yū-lin) The chemical substance of reticular fibers, regarded as type III collagen (with its associated proteoglygans and structural glycoproteins).

re·tic·u·lo·cyte (rĕ-tik′yū-lō-sīt) A young erythrocyte that contains no nucleus but has residual ribonucleic acid. SEE ALSO reticulocyte production index, erythroblast.

re·ti·cu·lo·cyte pro·duc·tion in·dex (RPI) (rĕ-tik′yū-lō-sīt prŏ-dŭk′shŭn in′deks) A calculated value that serves as an indicator of the bone marrow response in anemia.

re·tic·u·lo·cy·to·pe·ni·a, re·ti·cu·lo·sis (rĕ-tik′yū-lō-sī′tō-pē′nē-ă) Paucity of reticulocytes in the blood.

re·tic·u·lo·cy·to·sis (rĕ-tiky′ū-lō-sī-tō′sis) An increase in the number of circulating reticulocytes above the normal, which is less than 1% of the total number of red blood cells.

re·tic·u·lo·en·do·the·li·al (rĕ-tik′yū-lō-en′dō-thē′lē-ăl) Denoting or referring to reticuloendothelium.

re·tic·u·lo·en·do·the·li·al cell (re-tik′yū-lō-en′dō-thē′lē-ăl sel) A cell of the reticuloendothelial system.

re·tic·u·lo·en·do·the·li·al sys·tem (re-tik′yū-lō-en′dō-thē′lē-ăl sis′tĕm) Collection of putative macrophages, which includes most of the true macrophages (now classified under the mononuclear phagocytic system) as well as cells lining the sinusoids of the spleen, lymph nodes, and bone marrow, and the fibroblastic reticular cells of hematopoietic tissues.

re·tic·u·lo·en·do·the·li·um (rĕ-tik′yū-lō-en′dō-thē′lē-ŭm) The cells making up the reticuloendothelial system.

re·tic·u·lo·his·ti·o·cy·to·ma (rĕ-tik′yū-lō-his′tē-ō-sī-tō′mă) A solitary skin nodule composed of glycolipid-containing multinucleated large histiocytes; multiple lesions sometimes occur in association with arthritis.

re·tic·u·lo·his·ti·o·cy·to·sis (re-tik′yū-lō-his′tē-ō-sī-tō′sis) SEE reticulosis.

re·tic·u·lo·sis (rĕ-tik′yū-lō′sis) An increase in histiocytes, monocytes, or other reticuloendothelial elements.

re·tic·u·lo·spi·nal (rĕ-tik′yū-lō-spī′năl) Pertaining to the reticulospinal tract.

re·tic·u·lo·spi·nal tract (rĕ-tik′yū-lō-spī′năl trakt) Collective term denoting a variety of fiber tracts descending to the spinal cord from the reticular formation of the pons and medulla oblongata.

re·tic·u·lum, re·tic·u·la (rĕ-tik′yū-lŭm, -ă) [TA] **1.** A fine network formed by cells, or formed of certain structures within cells or of connective tissue fibers between cells. **2.** SYN neuroglia.

ret·i·form (ret′i-fōrm) Resembling a net or network.

ret·i·na (ret′i-nă) [TA] Light-sensitive three part membrane forming the innermost layer of the eyeball.

ret·i·nac·u·lum, gen. **ret·i·nac·u·li** (ret′i-nak′yū-lŭm, -li, lă) [TA] A frenum, or a retaining band or ligament.

ret·i·nal (ret′i-năl) **1.** Relating to the retina. **2.** Retinaldehyde, most commonly referring to the all-*trans* form; participates in the visual process.

ret·i·nal·de·hyde (ret′-i-nal′dĕ-hīd) Retinol oxidized to a terminal aldehyde;

used in visual process. Also called reti-nene.

ret·i·nal de·tach·ment, de·tach·ment of ret·i·na (ret′i-năl dĕ-tach′mĕnt, ret′i-nă) Loss of apposition between the sensory retina and the retinal pigment epithelium.

ret·i·ni·tis (ret′i-nī′tis) Inflammation of the retina.

ret·i·nit·is pig·men·to·sa (ret′i-nī′tis pig-men-tō′să) Hereditary progressive neuroepithelial abiotrophy, with atrophy and pigmentary infiltration of the inner layers of the retina.

ret·i·no·blas·to·ma (ret′i-nō-blas-tō′mă) Malignant ocular neoplasm of childhood, usually occurring before the third year of life, composed of primitive retinal small round cells with deeply staining nuclei and of elongated cells forming rosettes.

ret·i·no·cho·roid·i·tis (ret′i-nō-kōr′oy-dī′tis) Inflammation of the retina extending to the choroid. SYN chorioretinitis.

ret·i·no·cho·roid·i·tis jux·ta·pa·pil·la·ris (ret′i-nō-kōr′oy-dī′tis juks′tă-pap-i-lă′ris) Inflammation close to the optic disc. SYN Jensen disease.

ret·i·no·ic ac·id (RA) (ret′i-nō′ik as′idz) Vitamin A1 acid; used topically to treat acne. SYN vitamin A1 acid.

ret·i·noid (ret′i-noyd) **1.** Resembling a resin; resinous. **2.** Resembling the retina. **3.** In plural form, term used to describe the natural forms and synthetic analogues of retinol used in skin disease.

ret·i·nol (ret′i-nol) An intermediate in the vision cycle, it also plays a role in growth and differentiation; a vitamin A1 alcohol.

ret·i·nol ac·tiv·i·ty e·quiv·a·lents (ret′i-nol ak-tiv′i-tē ē-kwiv′ă-lĕns) A measure of vitamin A activity based on the capacity of the body to convert provitamin carotenoids containing at least one unsubstituted ionone ring to retinaldehyde.

ret·i·nol-bind·ing pro·tein (ret′i-nol-bīnd′ing prō′tēn) Plasma protein that binds and transports retinol.

ret·i·no·pap·il·li·tis (ret′i-nō-pap′i-lī′tis) Inflammation of the retina extending to the optic disc.

ret·i·nop·a·thy (ret′i-nop′ă-thē) Noninflammatory degenerative retinal disease.

ret·i·nop·a·thy of pre·ma·tu·ri·ty (ret′i-nop′ă-thē prē′mă-chŭr′i-tē) Abnormal vasoproliferation in premature infants that may progress to fibroglial proliferative retinal detachment. SYN Terry syndrome.

ret·i·nos·chi·sis (ret′i-nos′ki-sis) Degenerative splitting of the retina, with cyst formation between the two layers.

ret·i·no·scope (ret′i-nŏ-skōp) An optic device used to illuminate a patient's retina during retinoscopy.

ret·i·nos·co·py (ret′i-nos′kŏ-pē) A method of determining errors of refraction by illuminating the retina and observing the rays of light emerging from the eye. SYN shadow test, skiascopy.

re·tract (rē-trakt′) To shrink, draw back, or pull apart.

re·trac·tile (rē-trak′til) Retractable; capable of being drawn back.

re·trac·tile tes·tis (rē-trak′til tes′tis) Condition with a tendency of the testis to ascend to the upper part of the scrotum or into the inguinal canal. SYN movable testis, pseudocryptorchism.

re·trac·tion (rē-trak′shŭn) **1.** A shrinking or pulling apart. **2.** Posterior movement of teeth, usually with the aid of an orthodontic appliance.

re·trac·tion syn·drome (rē-trak′shŭn sin′drōm) Retraction of the globe and pseudoptosis on attempted adduction; due to coinnervation of the horizontal recti. SYN Duane syndrome.

re·trac·tor (rē-trak′tŏr) **1.** An instrument for drawing aside the edges of a wound or for holding back structures adjacent to the operative field. **2.** A muscle that draws a part backward (e.g., the middle part of the trapezius muscle is a retractor of the scapula; the horizontal fibers of the temporalis muscle serve to retract the mandible).

R

re·trench·ment (rē-trench'mĕnt) The cutting away of superfluous tissue.

re·triev·al (rē-trē'văl) The third stage in the memory process, after encoding and storage, involving mental processes associated with bringing stored information back into consciousness. SEE ALSO memory.

ret·ro·au·ric·u·lar (ret'rō-aw-rik'yū-lăr) Posterior to the auricle.

ret·ro·bul·bar (RB) (ret'rō-bŭl'bähr) Posterior to the eyeball.

ret·ro·bul·bar neu·ri·tis (ret'rō-bŭl'bahr nūr-ī'tis) Optic neuritis without swelling of the optic disc.

ret·ro·cer·vi·cal (ret'rō-sĕr'vi-kăl) Posterior to the cervix uteri.

ret·ro·ces·sion (ret'rō-sesh'ŭn) 1. A going back; a relapse. 2. Cessation of the external symptoms of a disease followed by signs of involvement of some internal organ or part. 3. Denoting a position of the uterus or other organ farther back than is normal.

ret·ro·col·lic (ret'rō-kol'ik) Relating to the back of the neck; drawing back the head.

ret·ro·col·lic spasm (ret'rō-kol'ik spazm) Torticollis in which the spasm affects the posterior neck muscles. Also called retrocollis.

ret·ro·cur·sive (ret'rō-kŭr'siv) Running backward.

ret·ro·de·vi·a·tion (ret'rō-dē'vē-ā'shŭn) A backward bending or inclining.

ret·ro·dis·place·ment (ret'rō-dis-plās'mĕnt) Any backward displacement, such as uterine retroversion.

ret·ro·fill·ing (ret'rō-fil'ing) Placement of a sealing material into the apical foramen of a dental root from the apical end.

ret·ro·flex·ion, ret·ro·flec·tion (ret'rō-flek'shŭn) Backward bending, as of the uterus when the corpus is bent back, forming an angle with the cervix.

ret·ro·gnath·ic (ret'rog-nath'ik) *In the diphthong gn, the g is silent only at the beginning of a word.* Denoting a state in which the mandible is located posterior to its normal position in relation to the maxillae.

ret·ro·grade (RG) (ret'rō-grād) 1. Moving backward. 2. Degenerating. 3. Used in neuroscience to describe distal-proximal flow, movement, or transport in an axon toward its cell body, or degeneration of an axon proximal to a point of injury.

ret·ro·grade am·ne·si·a (ret'rō-grād am-nē'zē-ă) Lack of memory about events that occurred before the trauma or disease that caused the condition.

ret·ro·grade block (ret'rō-grād blok) Impaired conduction backward from the ventricles or atrioventricular node into the atria.

ret·ro·grade e·jac·u·la·tion (ret'rō-grād ē-jak'yū-lā'shŭn) Delivery of semen ejaculate into the bladder; seen in neurologic disease, diabetes, and occasionally after prostate surgery.

ret·ro·grade em·bo·lism (ret'rō-grād em'bŏ-lizm) Venous blockage by an embolus carried in a direction opposite to that of the normal blood current, after being diverted into a smaller vein.

ret·ro·grade her·ni·a (ret'rō-grād hĕr'nē-ă) Double loop hernia, the central loop of which lies in the abdominal cavity.

ret·ro·grade men·stru·a·tion (ret'rō-grād men'strū-ā'shŭn) Back flow of menstrual blood through the uterine tubes.

ret·ro·grade ur·og·ra·phy (ret'rō-grād yūr-og'ră-fē) Radiography of the urinary tract following injection of contrast medium directly into the bladder, ureter, or renal pelvis. SYN cystoscopic urography.

ret·ro·len·tal (ret'rō-len'tăl) Posterior to the lens of the eye. SYN retrolenticular (1).

ret·ro·len·tal fi·bro·pla·si·a (ret'rō-lent'ăl fī'brō-plā'zē-ă) A condition of premature infants, characterized by the presence of opaque tissue behind the lens, leading to retinal detachment and blindness; due to excessive concentration of oxygen.

ret•ro•mo•lar (ret′rō-mō′lăr) Distal (or posterior) to the last erupted (or present) molar tooth.

ret•ro•mo•lar pad (re′trō-mō′lăr pad) A cushioned mass of tissue, frequently pear-shaped, located on the alveolar process of the mandible behind the area of the last natural molar tooth.

ret•ro•per•i•to•ne•al (RP) (ret′rō-per′i-tŏ-nē′ăl) External or posterior to the peritoneum.

ret•ro•per•i•to•ne•al space, ret•ro•per•i•to•ne•um (ret′rō-per′i-tŏ-nēăl spăs, -tō-nē′ŭm) [TA] The space between the parietal peritoneum and the muscles and bones of the posterior abdominal wall.

ret•ro•per•i•to•ni•tis (ret′rō-per′i-tŏ-nī′tis) Inflammation of the cellular tissue behind the peritoneum.

ret•ro•pha•ryn•ge•al (ret′rō-fă-rin′jē-ăl) Behind the pharynx.

ret•ro•pha•ryn•ge•al ab•scess (ret′rō-fă-rin′jē-ăl ab′ses) Lesion arising in retropharyngeal lymph nodes, most commonly in infants.

ret•ro•pla•cen•tal (ret′rō-plă-sen′tăl) Posterior to the placenta.

ret•ro•pla•si•a (ret′rō-plă′zē-ă) Cell or tissue state in which activity is below that considered normal; associated with retrogressive changes.

ret•ro•posed (ret′rō-pōzd) Denoting retroposition.

ret•ro•po•si•tion (ret′rō-pŏ-zish′ŭn) Simple backward displacement of a structure or organ, without inclination, bending, retroversion, or retroflexion.

ret•ro•pos•on (ret′rō-pō′zon) 1. A transposition of sequences in DNA that does not originate in it but rather in a messenger ribonucleic acid transcribed back into the genomic DNA by reverse transcription. SYN retrotransposon. 2. A transposable element.

ret•ro•pu•bic (ret′rō-pyū′bik) Posterior to the pubic bone.

ret•ro•pul•sion (ret′rō-pŭl′shŭn) 1. An involuntary backward walking or running, seen in patients with parkinsonism. 2. A pushing back of any part.

ret•ro•sig•moid ap•proach (ret′rō-sig′moyd ă-prōch′) A surgical approach to the cerebellopontine angle through the occipital bone posterior to the sigmoid sinus.

ret•ro•spec•tive (ret′rō-spek′tiv) Relating to retrospection.

ret•ro•spec•tive fal•si•fi•ca•tion (ret′rō-spek′tiv fawl′si-fi-kā′shŭn) Unconscious distortion of past experience to conform to present psychological needs.

ret•ro•spon•dy•lo•lis•the•sis (ret′rō-spon′di-lō-lis-thē′sis) Slipping posteriorly of the body of a vertebra, bringing it out of line with the adjacent vertebrae.

ret•ro•ster•nal (ret′rō-stĕr′năl) Posterior to the sternum.

ret•ro•ster•nal her•ni•a (ret′rō-stĕr′năl hĕr′nē-ă) Herniation through the sternocostal foramen (foramen of Morgagni), the opening for the superior epigastric vessels. SYN Morgagni foramen hernia.

ret•ro•u•ter•ine (ret′rō-yū′tĕr-in) Posterior to the uterus.

ret•ro•ver•sion (ret′rō-vĕr′zhŭn) 1. A turning backward. 2. Condition in which the teeth are located in a more posterior position than normal.

Ret•ro•vir•i•dae (ret′rō-vir′i-dē) A family of viruses grouped in three subfamilies: Oncovirinae (human T-cell lymphotropic virus types I and II, ribonucleic acid tumor viruses), Spumavirinae (foamy viruses), and Lentivirinae (human immunodeficiency-like viruses, visna, and related agents).

ret•ro•vi•rus (ret′rō-vī′rŭs) Any virus of the family Retroviridae. A virus with RNA core genetic material; requires the enzyme reverse transcriptase to convert its RNA into proviral DNA.

re•tru•sion (rĕ-trū′zhŭn) 1. Retraction of the mandible from any given point. 2. The backward movement of the mandible.

R

re·tru·sive oc·clu·sion (rē-trū′siv ŏ-klū′zhŭn) A biting relationship in which the mandible is forcefully or habitually placed more distally than the patient's centric occlusion.

re·vac·ci·na·tion (rē′vak-si-nā′shŭn) Vaccination of an individual previously successfully vaccinated.

re·vas·cu·lar·i·za·tion (rē-vas′kyū-lăr-ī-zā′shŭn) Reestablishment of blood supply to a body part.

re·ver·ber·at·ing cir·cuit (rē-věr′běr-āt-ing sĭr′kŭt) Theory of periodic conduction through the cerebral cortex of trains of impulses traveling in circuits of neurons.

re·ver·ber·a·tion (rē-věr′běr-ā′shŭn) Multiple echoes or reflections; in ultrasonography, an artifactual image due to delay of an echo that has been reflected back and forward again before returning to the transducer.

re·verse curve (rē-věrs′ kŭrv) In dentistry, a curve of occlusion that is convex on the upward face. SYN anti-Monson curve.

re·versed co·arc·ta·tion (rē-věrst′ kō′ahrk-tā′shŭn) Aortic arch syndrome in which blood pressure in the arms is lower than in the legs.

re·verse iso·la·tion (rē-věrs′ ī′sŏ-lā′shŭn) A form of patient isolation wherein use of protective equipment is required to prevent transmission of infection to the patient.

re·verse pas·sive he·mag·glu·ti·na·tion (rē-věrs′ pas′iv hē′mă-glŭ′ti-nā′shŭn) A diagnostic technique for virus infection using agglutination by viruses of red blood cells that previously have been coated with antibody specific to the virus.

re·verse trans·crip·tase (rē-věrs′ tran-skrip′tās) RNA-dependent DNA polymerase, present in virions of RNA tumor viruses.

re·verse trans·crip·tase pol·y·mer·ase chain re·ac·tion (RT-PCR) (rē-věrs′ tran-skrip′tās pol-im′ěr-ās chān rē-ak′shŭn) A process for specific messenger ribonucleic acid (mRNA) amplification wherein reverse transcriptase added to the in vitro reaction uses mRNA as a template to produce one complimentary deoxyribonucleic acid, which is then amplified by the usual PCR.

re·ver·sion (rē-věr′zhŭn) Manifestation in an individual of certain characteristics, peculiar to a remote ancestor that have been suppressed during intermediate generations.

re·ver·tant (rē-věr′tănt) MICROBIAL GENETICS a mutant that has reverted to its former genotype or to the original phenotype by means of a suppressor mutation.

re·viv·i·fi·ca·tion (rē-viv′i-fi-kā′shŭn) **1.** Renewal of life and strength. SYN revivescence. **2.** Refreshening the edges of a wound by paring or scraping to promote healing. SYN vivification.

Reye syn·drome (RS) (rī sin′drōm) Acquired encephalopathy of young children that follows an acute febrile illness, usually influenza or varicella infection; characterized by recurrent vomiting, agitation, and lethargy, which may lead to coma with intracranial hypertension; death may result from edema of the brain; may be linked to aspirin ingestion.

Rh 1. Symbol for rhodium. **2.** Abbreviation for rhesus.

rhabdo-, rhabd- Combining forms meaning rod; rod shaped (rhabdoid).

rhab·doid (rab′doyd) Rod-shaped.

rhab·do·my·o·blast (rab′dō-mī′ō-blast) Large, round, spindle-shaped cells with deeply eosinophilic fibrillar cytoplasm that may show cross-striations.

rhab·do·my·ol·y·sis (rab′dō-mī-ol′i-sis) An acute, fulminating, potentially fatal disease of skeletal muscle that entails destruction of muscle as evidenced by myoglobinemia and myoglobinuria.

rhab·do·my·o·ma (rab′dō-mī-ō′mă) A benign neoplasm derived from striated muscle, occurring in the heart in children.

rhab·do·my·o·sar·co·ma, rhab·do·sar·co·ma (rab′dō-mī′ō-sahr-kō′mă, rab′dō-sahr-) A malignant neoplasm derived from skeletal muscle, classified as embryonal alveolar or pleomorphic.

rhab·do·sphinc·ter (rab′dō-sfingk′tĕr) A sphincter made up of striated musculature. SYN striated muscular sphincter.

Rhab·do·vir·i·dae (rab′dō-vir′i-dē) A family of rod-shaped or bullet-shaped viruses of vertebrates, insects, and plants, including rabies virus.

rha·chi·tis (ră-kī′tis) Inflammation of part of the vertebral column.

Rhad·in·o·vi·rus (ră-dē′nō-vī′rŭs) A herpesvirus genus associated with Kaposi sarcoma.

-rhage, -rrhage, -rhagia, -rrhagia Combining forms meaning excessive flow.

Rh blood group (blŭd grūp) SYN Rh factor.

rhe (rē) The absolute unit of fluidity, the reciprocal of the unit of viscosity.

-rhea, -rrhea Combining forms meaning flow or discharge.

rheg·ma (reg′mă) A rent or fissure.

rheg·ma·tog·e·nous (reg′mă-toj′ĕ-nŭs) Arising from a bursting or fractioning of an organ.

rhe·ni·um (Re) (rē′nē-ŭm) A metallic element of the platinum group.

rheo- Combining form meaning blood flow; electrical current.

rhe·o·en·ceph·a·lo·gram (rē′ō-en-sef′ă-lō-gram) Graphic registration of the changes in conductivity of tissue of the head caused by vascular factors.

rhe·o·gram (rē′ō-gram) A plot of the shear stress versus the shear rate for a fluid.

rhe·ol·o·gy (rē-ol′ŏ-jē) The study of the deformation and flow of materials.

rhe·o·stat (rheo) (rē′ō-stat) A variable resistor used to adjust the current in an electrical circuit.

rhe·os·to·sis (rē′os-tō′sis) A hypertrophying and condensing osteitis that tends to run in longitudinal streaks or columns, involves a number of the long bones.

rhe·o·tax·is (rē′ō-tak′sis) A form of positive barotaxis in which a microorganism in a fluid is impelled to move against the current flow of its medium.

Rhese pro·jec·tion (rēs prŏ-jek′shŭn) Oblique radiographic view of the skull to show the optic foramen in the lower outer quadrant of the bony orbit.

rheu·mat·ic ar·ter·i·tis (rū-mat′ik ahr′tĕr-ī′tis) That disorder resulting from rheumatic fever; Aschoff bodies are frequently found in the adventitia of small arteries, especially in the myocardium, and may lead to fibrosis and constriction of the lumens.

rheu·mat·ic car·di·tis (rū-mat′ik kahr-dī′tis) Pancarditis occurring in rheumatic fever, characterized by formation of Aschoff bodies in the cardiac, interstitial tissue; may be associated with acute cardiac failure; frequently followed by valvular scarring.

rheu·mat·ic en·do·car·di·tis (rū-mat′ik en′dō-kahr-dī′tis) Endocardial involvement as part of rheumatic heart disease, recognized clinically by valvular involvement.

rheu·mat·ic fe·ver (rū-mat′ik fē′vĕr) An inflammatory disease with pyrexia following infection of the throat with group A beta-hemolytic streptococci, occurring primarily in children and young adults; relapses are common if streptococcal infections recur; sometimes called rheumatic heart disease.

rheu·ma·tid (rū′mă-tid) Rheumatic nodules or other eruptions that may accompany rheumatism.

rheu·ma·toid (rū′mă-toyd) Resembling rheumatoid arthritis in one or more features.

rheu·ma·toid ar·thri·tis (RA) (rū′mă-toyd ahr-thrī′tis) A chronic systemic disease, occurring more often in women, which affects connective tissue; arthritis is the dominant clinical manifestation, involving many joints, especially those of the hands and feet, accompanied by thickening of articular soft tissue. SYN nodose rheumatism (1).

R

rheu·ma·toid fac·tors (RF) (rū′mă-toyd fak′tŏrz) Antibodies in the serum of patients with rheumatoid arthritis and other autoimmune and some infectious diseases.

rheu·ma·tol·o·gy (RHU) (rū′mă-tol′ŏ-jē) The medical specialty concerned with the study, diagnosis, and treatment of rheumatic conditions.

Rh fac·tor (fak′tŏr) A protein substance present in the red blood cells of most people (85%), capable of inducing intense antigenic reactions. The Rh factor was first identified in the blood of the rhesus monkey in 1940. SYN Rh blood group, Rhesus factor.

Rh-im·mune glob·u·lin (RhIG) (im-yūn′ glob′yū-lin) A concentrated solution of immunoglobulin G anti-D that is administered to an Rh-negative person who has been exposed to Rh-positive red blood cells, particularly a woman who may be carrying or has aborted an Rh-positive fetus or who has delivered an Rh-negative baby, to counteract the immunizing effect of the cells.

♺ **rhin-, rhino-** Combining forms denoting the nose.

rhi·nen·chy·sis (rī′nen-kī′sis) A nasal douche; washing out the nasal cavities.

rhin·i·on (rin′ē-on) A craniometric point: the lower end of the suture between the nasal bones.

rhi·ni·tis (rhin) (rī-nī′tis) Inflammation of the nasal mucous membrane. SYN nasal catarrh.

rhi·ni·tis ca·se·o·sa, ca·se·ous rhi·ni·tis (rī-nī′tis kā′sē-ō′să, kā′sē-ŭs) Chronic form in which the nasal cavities are more or less completely filled with foul-smelling cheesy matter.

rhi·no·an·tri·tis (rī′nō-ăn-trī′tis) Inflammation of the nasal cavities and one or both maxillary sinuses.

rhi·no·ceph·a·ly, rhi·no·ce·pha·li·a (rī′nō-sef′ă-lē, -sĕ-fā′lē-ă) Rhinencephaly; cyclopia in which the nose is represented by a fleshy protuberance arising above slitlike orbits.

rhi·no·chei·lo·plas·ty, rhi·no·chi·lo·plas·ty (rī′nō-kī′lō-plas-tē) Plastic surgery of the nose and upper lip.

rhi·nog·e·nous (rī-noj′ĕ-nŭs) Originating in the nose.

rhi·no·ky·pho·sis, rhin·ism (rī′nō-kī-fō′sis, rī′nizm) A humpback deformity of the nose.

rhi·no·la·li·a, rhi·no·pho·ni·a (rī′nō-lā′lē-ă, -fō′nē-ă) Nasalized speech.

rhi·no·lith, rhi·no·lite (rī′nō-lith, -līt) A calcareous concretion in the nasal cavity, often around a foreign body.

rhi·no·li·thi·a·sis (rī′nō-li-thī′ă-sis) The presence of a nasal calculus.

rhi·nol·o·gy (rī-nol′ŏ-jē) Medical science concerned with the nose and its diseases.

rhi·no·ma·nom·e·ter, rhi·no·an·e·mom·e·ter (rī′nō-mă-nom′ĕ-tĕr, -an′ĕ-mom′ĕ-tĕr) Device used to determine the presence and amount of nasal obstruction, and nasal air pressure, and flow relationships.

rhi·no·ma·nom·e·try (rī′nō-mă-nom′ĕ-trē) 1. Use of a rhinomanometer. 2. Measurement of nasal air flow and pressures.

rhi·no·my·co·sis (rī′nō-mī-kō′sis) Fungal infection of the nasal mucous membranes.

rhi·no·ne·cro·sis (rī′nō-nĕ-krō′sis) Necrosis of the bones of the nose.

rhi·nop·a·thy (rī-nop′ă-thē) Disease of the nose.

rhi·no·phy·ma (rī′nō-fī′mă) Nasal hypertrophy with follicular dilation, due to hyperplasia of sebaceous glands with fibrosis and increased vascularity.

rhi·no·plas·ty (rhino) (rī′nō-plas-tē) Reconstructive or cosmetic nasal surgery to correct form or function.

rhi·nor·rhe·a (rī′nōr-ē′ă) Discharge from nasal mucous membrane.

rhi·no·sal·pin·gi·tis (rī′nō-sal′pin-jī′tis) Inflammation of the mucous membrane of the nose and pharyngotympanic (auditory) tube.

rhi·no·scle·ro·ma (rī′nō-skler-ō′mă) Chronic granulomatous process involving the nose, upper lip, mouth, and upper air passages; maybe *Klebsiella*.

rhi·no·scope (rī′nŏ-skōp) A small mirror attached at a suitable angle to a rodlike handle, used in posterior rhinoscopy.

rhi·nos·co·py (rī-nos′kŏ-pē) Inspection of the nasal cavity.

rhi·no·si·nu·si·tis (rī′nō-sī′nŭs-ī′tis) Inflammation of the mucous membrane of the nose and paranasal sinuses.

rhi·no·spo·rid·i·o·sis (rī′nō-spō-rid′ē-ō′sis) Invasion of the nasal cavity or, occasionally, the conjunctiva or other superficial structures by *Rhinosporidium seeberi*.

rhi·no·ste·no·sis, rhi·no·clei·sis (rī′nō-stĕ-nō′sis, klī′sis) Nasal obstruction. SYN rhinocleisis.

rhi·not·o·my (rī-not′ŏ-mē) **1.** Any cutting operation on the nose. **2.** Operative procedure in which the nose is incised along one side so that it may be turned away to provide full vision of the nasal passages for radical sinus operations.

Rhi·no·vi·rus (rī′nō-vī′rŭs) A genus of acid-labile viruses associated with the common cold. There are more than 110 antigenic types.

rhi·no·vi·rus (RV, RhV) (rī′nō-vī′rŭs) Any virus of the genus Rhinovirus.

Rhi·pi·ceph·a·lus (rip′i-sef′ă-lŭs) A genus of inornate hard ticks consisting of about 50 species, all of which are Old World except *Rhipicephalus sanguineus*; includes important vectors of disease in humans and domestic animals.

rhizo- Combining form denoting root.

rhi·zoid (rī′zoyd) **1.** Rootlike. **2.** Irregularly branching, like a root. **3.** MYCOLOGY rootlike hyphae of fungi that arise at the nodes of the hyphae of *Rhizopus* species.

rhi·zo·mel·ic (rī′zō-mel′ik) Of or relating to the hip joint or the shoulder joint.

Rhi·zo·mu·cor (rī′zō-myū′kōr) A genus of fungi in the family Mucoraceae; a cause of mucormycosis.

Rhi·zop·o·da (rī-zop′ŏ-dă) A superclass in the subphylum Sarcodina that includes human amebae.

Rhi·zo·pus (rī′zō-pŭs) A genus of fungi some species of which cause zygomycosis in humans.

rhi·zot·o·my (rī-zot′ŏ-mē) Surgical section of the spinal nerve roots for the relief of pain or spastic paralysis. SYN radiculectomy.

Rh null syn·drome (nŭl sin′drōm) Disorder involving a lack of all Rh antigens, compensated hemolytic anemia, and stomatocytosis.

rho·do·gen·e·sis (rō′dō-jen′ĕ-sis) The production of rhodopsin by the combination of 11-*cis*-retinal and opsin in the dark.

rho·do·phy·lax·is (rō′dō-fi-lak′sis) Choroidal pigment cell action in preserving or facilitating reproduction of rhodopsin.

rho·dop·sin (rō-dop′sin) A red thermolabile protein found in the rods of the retina; it is bleached by the action of light, which converts it to opsin and all-*trans*-retinal, and is restored in the dark by rhodogenesis.

Rho·do·tor·u·la (rō′dō-tōr′yū-lă) A genus of yeasts, of questionable pathogenicity, which are generally introduced iatrogenically in prosthetic implants and into immunocompromised patients via intravenous catheters.

rhomb·en·ce·phal·ic isth·mus (romb′en-sĕ-fal′ik is′mŭs) **1.** A constriction in the embryonic neural tube delineating the mesencephalon from the rhombencephalon. **2.** The anterior portion of the rhombencephalon connecting with the mesencephalon.

rhom·ben·ceph·a·lon (romb′en-sef′ă-lon) [TA] That part of the developing brain that is the most caudal of the three primary vesicles of the embryonic neural tube. SYN hindbrain.

rhom·boid, rhom·boi·dal (rom′boyd, -boy′dăl) Resembling a rhomb, i.e., an oblique parallelogram, but having unequal sides.

rhom·boi·dal si·nus, si·nus rhom·boi·da·lis (rom-boy′dăl sī′nŭs, rom′ boy-da′lis) A dilation of the central canal of the spinal cord in the lumbar region. SYN rhombocele.

rhom·bo·mere (rom′bō-mēr) Segments of the developing neural tube in the rhombencephalon.

rhon·chal frem·i·tus (rong′kăl frem′i-tŭs) That produced by vibrations from the passage of air in bronchial tubes partially obstructed by mucous secretion.

rhon·chus, so·no·rous rhon·chus, sib·i·lant rhon·chus, pl. **rhon·chi** (rong′kŭs, son′ŏr-ŭs, sib′i-lănt, rong′kī) An added sound with a musical pitch occurring during inspiration or expiration, heard on auscultation of the chest; caused by air passing through bronchi narrowed by inflammation, spasm of smooth muscle, or presence of mucus in the lumen.

rho·ta·cism (rō′tă-sizm) Mispronunciation of the ''r'' sound.

Rhus (rūs) A genus of vines and shrubs containing various species used for their ornamental foliage. Certain poisonous species are classified as *Toxicodendron*.

rhus der·ma·ti·tis (rūs dĕr′mă-tī′tis) Contact dermatitis caused by cutaneous exposure to urushiol from species of *Toxicodendron* (*Rhus*), such as poison ivy, oak, or sumac.

rhythm (ridh′ŭm) **1.** Measured time or motion. **2.** The regular alternation of two or more different or opposite states. **3.** SYN rhythm method. **4.** Regular occurrence of an electrical event in the electroencephalogram. SEE ALSO wave. **5.** A regular sequence of heart beats.

rhythm meth·od (ridh′ŭm meth′ŏd) A natural contraceptive method that spaces sexual intercourse to avoid the fertile period of the menstrual cycle. SYN rhythm (3).

rhyt·i·dec·tom·y (rit′i-dek′tŏ-mē) Elimination of wrinkles from, or reshaping of, the face by excising any excess skin and tightening the remainder; the so-called face-lift.

rhyt·i·do·sis (rit′i-dō′sis) **1.** Facial wrinkling disproportionate to age. **2.** Laxity and wrinkling of the cornea, an indication of approaching death. SYN rutidosis.

rib (rib) Abbreviation for ribose.

rib [I–XII] (rib) One of the 24 elongated curved bones forming the main portion of the bony wall of the chest.

ribo- **1.** Prefix denoting ribose. **2.** As an italicized prefix to the systematic name of a monosaccharide, *ribo-* indicates that the configuration of a set of three consecutive CHOH groups is that of ribose.

ri·bo·fla·vin (RF, RBF) (rī′bō-flā′vin) A heat-stable factor of the vitamin B complex with isoalloxazine nucleotides that are coenzymes of the flavohydrogenases. SYN flavine, riboflavine.

ri·bo·nu·cle·ase (RNase) (rī′bō-nū′klē-ās) A transferase that catalyzes hydrolysis of ribonucleic acid.

ri·bo·nu·cle·ic ac·id (RNA) (rī′bō-nū-klē′ik as′id) A macromolecule consisting of ribonucleoside bases connected by phosphate bonds, concerned in the control of cellular chemical processes, especially protein synthesis; found in all cells, in both nuclei and cytoplasm, and in viruses.

ri·bo·nu·cle·ic ac·id pol·ym·er·ase (rī′bō-nū-klē′ik as′id po-lim′ĕr-ās) SEE nucleotidyltransferases.

ri·bo·nu·cle·o·pro·tein (RNP) (rī′bō-nū′klē-ō-prō′tēn) A combination of ribonucleic acid and protein.

ri·bo·nu·cle·o·side (rī′bō-nū′klē-ō-sīd) A nucleoside in which the sugar component is ribose; the common ribonucleosides are adenosine, cytidine, guanosine, and uridine.

ri·bo·nu·cle·o·tide (rī-bō-nū′klē-ō-tīd) A nucleotide in which the sugar component is ribose; the major ribonucleotides of ribonucleic acid are adenylic acid, cytidylic acid, guanylic acid, and uridylic acid.

ri·bose (rib) (rī′bōs) The pentose present in ribonucleic acid; epimers of D-ribose are D-arabinose, D-xylose, and L-lyxose.

ri·bo·som·al ri·bo·nu·cle·ic ac·id (RNA) (rī′bŏ-sō′măl rī′bŏ-nū-klē′ik as′ id) The RNA of ribosomes and polyribosomes.

Ric·co law (rē′kō law) For small images, light intensity × area = constant for the threshold.

rice di·et (rīs dī′ĕt) Regimen of rice, fruit, and sugar, plus vitamin and iron supplements, used to treat hypertension. SYN Kempner diet.

Rich·ter syn·drome (rik′ter sin′drōm) A high-grade lymphoma developing during chronic lymphocytic leukemia; associated with cachexia, pyrexia, and lymphomas with multinucleated tumor cells.

ri·cin (rī′sin) A highly toxic, possibly lethal, lectin and hemagglutin that occurs in castor beans.

Ric·i·nus (ris′i-nŭs) A genus of plants with one species, *Ricinus communis*, the castor oil plant, the source of castor oil. SYN castor bean.

rick·ets (rik′ĕts) Disease due to vitamin D deficiency characterized by overproduction and deficient calcification of osteoid tissue, with associated skeletal deformities, disturbances in growth, and hypocalcemia. SYN infantile osteomalacia, juvenile osteomalacia, rachitis.

Rick·ett·si·a (ri-ket′sē-ă) Bacterial genus containing (nonfilterable), often pleomorphic, coccoid to rod-shaped, gram-negative organisms that usually occur intracytoplasmically in lice, fleas, ticks, and mites; pathogenic species are parasitic in humans and other animals, causing epidemic typhus, Rocky Mountain spotted fever, rickettsialpox, and other diseases.

Rick·ett·si·a a·kar·i (ri-ket′sē-ă a-kă′ rī) Bacterial species causing human rickettsialpox, a mild, acute febrile disease.

ric·kett·si·al (ri-ket′sē-ăl) Pertaining to or caused by rickettsiae.

rick·kett·si·al·pox (ri-ket′sē-ăl-poks) Bacterial infection with *Rickettsia akari*, which is spread by mites from a reservoir in mice; a benign, self-limited febrile illness.

Rick·ett·si·a pro·wa·ze·ki·i (ri-ket′ sē-ă prō-vă-zek′ē-ī) A bacterial species causing epidemic and recrudescent typhus, transmitted by body lice; type species of the genus *Rickettsia*.

Rick·ett·si·a rick·ett·si·i (ri-ket′sē-ă ri-ket′sē-ī) Bacterial species, the agent of Rocky Mountain spotted fever, South African tick-bite fever, and other diseases in South America; transmitted by infected ixodid ticks.

ric·kett·si·o·sis (ri-ket′sē-ō′sis) Infection with rickettsiae.

ridge (rij) [TA] **1.** A linear elevation. SEE ALSO crest. **2.** DENTISTRY any linear elevation on the surface of a tooth. **3.** The remainder of the alveolar process and its soft tissue covering after the teeth are removed.

ridge ex·ten·sion (rij ek-sten′shŭn) Intraoral surgical procedure for deepening the labial, buccal, or lingual sulci; performed to increase the intraoral height of the alveolar ridge to assist denture retention.

Rie·del thy·roid·i·tis, Rie·del stru·ma (rē′del thī′roy-dī′tis, strū′mă) Rare fibrous thyroid gland induration, with adhesion to adjacent structures.

Rie·der cell leu·ke·mi·a (rē′der sel lū-kē′mē-ă) A special form of acute granulocytic leukemia in which affected tissues and the blood contain atypical myeloblasts.

Rie·der cells (rē′der selz) Abnormal myeloblasts in which the nucleus may be widely and deeply indented or may actually be a bilobate or multilobate structure; seen in acute leukemia.

Rie·gel pulse (rē′gel pŭls) One that diminishes in volume during expiration.

Rie·ger a·nom·a·ly (rē′ger ă-nom′ă-lē) Iridocorneal mesenchymal dysgenesis.

Rie·ger syn·drome (rē′ger sin′drōm) Iridocorneal mesenchymal dysgenesis combined with hypodontia or anodontia, maxillary hypoplasia, and delayed sexual development.

Riehl mel·a·no·sis (RM) (rēl mel′ă-nō′sis) Brown pigmentary condition of the exposed portions of the skin of the neck and face with melanin pigment in dermal macrophages, thought to result from photodermatitis due to materials, such as cosmetic ingredients, or oils encountered in various occupations.

right and left fi·brous rings of heart (rīt left fī′brŭs ringz hahrt) Two fibrous rings that surround atrioventricular orifices of the heart, providing attachment for the atrioventricular valve leaflets and maintaining patency of the orifices. As part of the fibrous skeleton of the heart, the fibrous rings also provide origin and insertion for the myocardium. SYN anulus fibrosus (1) [TA].

right an·te·ri·or o·blique (RAO) (rīt an-tēr′ē-ŏr ō-blēk′) Radiographic position in which the right anterior part of the body is closest to the film.

right-hand·ed (rīt-hand′ĕd) Denoting the habitual or more skillful use of the right hand for writing and most manual operations. SYN dextral.

right heart (rīt hahrt) The right atrium and right ventricle.

right liv·er (rīt liv′ĕr) Portion of the liver receiving blood from the right branches of the hepatic artery and portal vein, and from which bile is drained through the right hepatic duct; the plane of the middle hepatic vein separates right from left liver.

right low·er quad·rant of ab·do·men (RLQ) (rīt lō′ĕr kwahd′rănt ab′dŏ-mĕn) Descriptive anatomic term encompassing anything within that region of the human body (e.g., for diagnosis, charting).

right men·to·trans·verse po·si·tion (RMT) (rīt men′tō-trans-vĕrs′ pŏ-zish′ŏn) Fetal position such that the fetal chin is pointing toward the maternal right iliac fossa.

right oc·cip·it·o·pos·te·ri·or po·si·tion (ROP) (rīt ok-sip′i-tō-pos-tēr′ē-ŏr pŏ-zish′ŏn) Fetal placement such that the back of the fetal head is pointed to the right side of the back of the maternal pelvis.

right sac·ro·an·te·ri·or po·si·tion (RSA) (rīt sā′krō-an-tēr′ē-ŏr pŏ-zish′ŏn) Breech-first fetal position in which the

fetal sacrum pointing to the right side of the maternal acetabulum.

right sac·ro·trans·verse po·si·tion (RST) (rīt sā′krō-trans-vĕrs′ pŏ-zish′ŏn) Breech fetal placement such that the fetal sacrum points toward the right side of the maternal sacroiliac area.

right-to-left shunt (rīt-left shŭnt) The passage of blood from the right side of the heart into the left or from the pulmonary artery into the aorta; can occur only when right pressure exceeds left.

right up·per quad·rant (RUQ) (rīt up′ĕr kwahd′rănt) Anatomic region used in description for purposes of examination, testing, and diagnosis, as well as charting.

right ven·tric·u·lar fail·ure (rīt ventrik′yū-lăr fāl′yŭr) Congestive heart failure manifested by distention of the neck veins, enlargement of the liver, and dependent edema due to pump failure of the right ventricle.

ri·gid·i·ty (ri-jid′i-tē) **1.** Stiffness or inflexibility. SYN rigor (1). **2.** PSYCHIATRY, CLINICAL PSYCHOLOGY an aspect of personality characterized by a person's resistance to change. **3.** NEUROLOGY one type of increase in muscle tone at rest.

rig·or (rig′ŏr) **1.** SYN rigidity (1). **2.** SYN chill (2).

rig·or mor·tis (rig′ŏr mōr′tis) Stiffening of the body, from 1–7 hours after death, due to hardening of the muscular tissues in consequence of the coagulation of the myosinogen and paramyosinogen. begins. SYN postmortem rigidity.

rim (rim) A margin, border, or edge, usually circular in form.

ri·ma, gen. and pl. **ri·mae** (rī′mă, -mē) [TA] A slit or fissure, or narrow elongated opening between two symmetric parts.

ri·ma glot·ti·dis (rī′mă glot′i-dis) [TA] The interval between the true vocal cords.

ri·ma o·ris (rī′mă ōr′is) [TA] The mouth slit.

ri·ma pal·pe·bra·rum (rī′mă pal-pē-brā′rŭm) [TA] SYN palpebral fissure.

rim·u·la (rim′yū-lă) A minute slit or fissure.

ring (ring) [TA] 1. A circular band surrounding a wide central opening. SYN anulus [TA]. 2. ANATOMY Anulus. 3. The closed chain of atoms in a cyclic compound; commonly used for "cyclic" or "cycle." 4. A marginal growth on the upper surface of a broth culture of bacteria, adhering to the sides of the test tube in the form of a circle.

ring ab·scess (ring ab′ses) Acute purulent inflammation of the corneal periphery in which a necrotic area is surrounded by an anular girdle of leukocytic infiltration.

ring chro·mo·some (ring krō′mŏ-sōm) One with ends joined to form a circular structure; is abnormal in humans but normal in most bacteria.

Ring·er in·jec·tion (ring′ĕr in-jek′shŭn) Sterile solution of sodium chloride and potassium chloride; used intravenously as a fluid and electrolyte replenisher.

Ring·er so·lu·tion (ring′ĕr sŏ-lū′shŭn) 1. A solution resembling the blood serum in its salt constituents; used as a fluid and electrolyte replenisher by intravenous infusion. SEE ALSO lactated Ringer solution. 2. A salt solution usually used in combination with naturally occurring body substances or more complex, chemically defined, nutritive solutions for culturing animal cells.

ring·like cor·ne·al dys·tro·phy (ring′ lĭk kōr′nē-ăl dis′trŏ-fē) Threadlike opacities of the anterior corneal stroma, with acute, painful onset followed by decreased vision.

ring sco·to·ma (ring skō-tō′mă) An anular area of blindness in the visual field surrounding the fixation point in pigmentary degeneration of the retina and in glaucoma.

ring·worm (ring′wŏrm) SYN tinea.

Rin·ne test (R) (rin′ĕ test) Assessment used to compare the ability to hear by air conduction with the ability to hear by bone conduction.

Ri·pault sign (rē-pō′ sīn) A sign of death, consisting in a permanent change in the shape of the pupil produced by unilateral pressure on the eyeball.

rise time (rīz tīm) 1. Duration required for a pulse or echo to rise from onset to its peak amplitude; 2. Duration required for a pulse or echo to rise from 10–90% peak amplitude.

risk fac·tor (RF) (risk fak′tŏr) Characteristic statistically associated with, although not necessarily causally related to, an increased risk of morbidity or mortality.

ri·sus (rī′sŭs) *The plural of this word is* risus, *not* risi. Laughter.

Rit·ter dis·ease (rit′ĕr di-zēz′) An exfoliative dermatitis, also known as staphylococcal scalded skin syndrome (SSSS), caused by an exfoliative toxin-producing strain of *Staphylococcus aureus* characterized by the presence of large bullae and exfoliation of the epidermal layer of the skin.

Rit·ter o·pen·ing tet·a·nus (rit′ĕr ōp′ ĕn-ing tet′ă-nŭs) Contraction that occasionally occurs when a strong current, passing through a long stretch of nerve, is suddenly interrupted.

ri·val·ry (rī′văl-rē) Competition between two or more individuals or entities for the same object or goal.

Riv·e·a co·rym·bo·sa (riv′ē-ă kŏ′rim-bō′să) Mexican bindweed, ingested to produce hallucinatory and euphoric effects.

Riv·ers coc·ktail (riv′ĕrz kok′tāl) An intravenous slow injection of 1000–2000 mL of 10% dextrose in isotonic saline to which thiamine hydrochloride and 25 units of insulin are added; used in acute alcoholism.

riz·i·form (riz′i-fōrm) Resembling rice grains.

Rn Symbol for radon.

RNase-α (ahr-en-as′ al′fă) An enzyme catalyzing endonucleolytic cleavage of *O*-methylated ribonucleic acid yielding 5′-phosphomonoesters.

RNase H Abbreviation for ribonuclease H.

R

RNase P An enzyme catalyzing the endonucleolytic cleavage tRNA precursors to yield 5′-phosphomonoesters.

RNA splic·ing (splīs′ing) SYN splicing (2).

RNA virus (vī′rŭs) A group of viruses in which the core consists of RNA; a major group of animal viruses that includes the families Picornaviridae, Reoviridae, Togaviridae, Flaviviridae, Bunyaviridae, Arenaviridae, Paramyxoviridae, Retroviridae, Coronaviridae, Orthomyxoviridae, and Rhabdoviridae.

ro·bert·so·ni·an trans·lo·ca·tion (rob′ĕrt-sō′nē-ăn tranz′lō-kā′shŭn) One in which the centromeres of two acrocentric chromosomes appear to have fused, forming an abnormal chromosome consisting of the long arms of two different chromosomes. SYN centric fusion.

Rob·erts syn·drome (RS) (rob′ĕrts sin′drōm) Phocomelia or lesser degrees of hypomelia, microbrachycephaly, midfacial defect, prenatal growth deficiency, and cryptorchidism.

Rob·in·son in·dex (rob′in-sŏn in′deks) An index used to calculate heart work load. SEE ALSO double product.

Ro·cha·li·mae·a (rō-chă-lī′mē-ă) Former designation for *Bartonella* (q.v.).

rock·et im·mu·no·elec·tro·pho·re·sis (RIE) (rok′ĕt im′yū-nō-ĕ-lek′trō-fŏr-ē′sis) Quantitative method for serum proteins that involves electrophoresis of antigen into a gel containing antibody. SEE electroimmunodiffusion.

Rock·y Moun·tain spot·ted fe·ver (rok′ē mown′tăn spot′ĕd fē′vĕr) An acute infectious disease of high mortality, characterized by frontal and occipital headache, intense lumbar pain, malaise, a moderately high continuous fever, and a rash on wrists, palms, ankles, and soles from the second to the fifth day; typically contracted in the spring of the year primarily in the southeastern and Rocky Mountain regions of the United States.

ro·cu·ro·ni·um (rō′kūr-ō′nē-ŭm) Aminosteroidal-derived nondepolarizing neuromuscular blocking agent with a rapid to intermediate onset depending on dosage.

rod (rod) **1.** A slender cylindric structure or device. **2.** Photosensitive, outward-directed process of a rhodopsin-containing rod cell in the external granular layer of the retina. SYN rod cell of retina.

rod gran·ule (rod gran′yūl) Nucleus of a retinal cell connecting with one of the rods.

roent·gen (r, R) (rent′gen) The international unit of exposure dose for x-rays or gamma rays.

ro·ent·gen·e·quiv·a·lent·man (rem, REM) (rent′gen ĕ-kwiv′ă-lĕnt-man′) A unit of dose-equivalent quantity of ionizing radiation of any type that produces in human subjects the same biologic effect as one rad of x-rays or gamma rays.

roent·gen·ol·o·gy (rent′gen-ol′ŏ-jē) The study of roentgen rays in all their applications. Radiology is the preferred term in the context of medical imaging.

Roes·ler-Dress·ler in·farct (res′ler-dres′ler in′fahrkt) Myocardial infarction in dumbbell form involving the anterior and posterior left ventricle and the left side of the ventricular septum.

Ro·ger dis·ease (rō-zhă′ di-zēz′) Congenital cardiac anomaly consisting of a small, isolated, asymptomatic defect of the interventricular septum, often with a loud murmur and definite thrill. SYN maladie de Roger.

Ro·ger mur·mur (rō-zhă′ mŭr′mŭr) A loud pansystolic murmur maximal at the left sternal border, caused by a small ventricular septal defect. SYN Roger bruit.

Rog·ers sphyg·mo·ma·nom·e·ter (roj′ĕrz sfig′mō-mă-nom′ĕ-tĕr) A sphygmomanometer with an aneroid barometer gauge.

Ro·ki·tan·sky her·ni·a (rō′ki-tahn′skē hĕr′nē-ă) A separation of the muscular fibers of the bowel allowing protrusion of a sac of the mucous membrane.

ro·lan·dic ep·i·lepsy (rō-lan′dik ep′i-lep′sē) Benign, form characterized clinically by arrested speech, muscular contractions of the side of the face and arm, and epileptic discharges.

role (rōl) The pattern of behavior that a

person exhibits in relationship to significant others in his or her life; it has its roots in childhood and is influenced by significant people with whom the person has or had primary relationships.

role con·flict (rōl kon´flikt) Dilemma a person experiences when required to play two different parts that cannot be easily harmonized.

roll (rōl) **1.** Rounded or cylindric mass created by rotation of a layer of material around its own long axis. **2.** Process by which a round entity is moved by a pressure gradient.

roll·er ban·dage (rōl´ĕr ban´dăj) Strip of material of variable width, rolled into a compact cylinder to facilitate its application.

Rol·let stro·ma (rol´et strō´mă) The colorless stroma of the red blood cells.

Ro·ma·now·sky blood stain (rō-mah-nof´skē blŭd stān) Prototype of the eosin-methylene blue stains for blood smears.

Rom·berg sign, rom·berg·ism (rom´berg sīn, rom´bĕrg-izm) With feet approximated, the patient stands with eyes open and closed; if closing the eyes increases the unsteadiness, a loss of proprioceptive control is indicated, and the sign is present.

ron·geur (rōn[h]-zhur´) A strong, biting forceps for nipping away bone.

roof plate, roof·plate (rūf plāt) The thin layer of the embryonic neural tube connecting the alar plates dorsally.

room·ing-in (rūm´ing-in´) Placement of a newborn with its mother, rather than in the nursery, during the postpartum hospital stay.

room tem·per·a·ture (RT, rt) (rūm tem´pĕr-ă-chŭr) Ordinary temperature (approximately 65°F–80°F, 18.3°C–26.7°C) of the atmosphere in the laboratory.

root (rūt) [TA] **1.** The primary or beginning portion of any part, as of a nerve at its origin from the brainstem or spinal cord. SYN radix (1) [TA]. **2.** SYN root of tooth. **3.** The descending underground portion of a plant; it absorbs water and nutrients, provides support, and stores nutrients.

root am·pu·ta·tion (rūt amp´yū-tā´shŭn) Surgical removal of one or more roots of a multirooted tooth, the remaining root canal(s) usually being treated endodontically. SYN radectomy, radiectomy, radisectomy.

root a·pex (rūt ā´peks) [TA] Tip of a tooth root. SYN apex radicis dentis [TA], root tip, tip of tooth root.

root ca·nal file (rūt kă-nal´ fīl) Pointed, flexible, steel intracanal dental instrument used in rasping canal walls.

root ca·nal ther·a·py (RCT) (rūt kă-nal´ thār´ă-pē) Dental care for damaged pulp by pulp removal and sterilization and filling of the root canal.

root car·ies in·dex (rūt kar´ēz in´deks) Ratio of the number of teeth with carious lesions of the root, and/or restorations of the root, to the number of teeth with exposed root surfaces.

root of tooth (rūt tūth) [TA] That part of a tooth below the neck, covered by cementum rather than enamel, and attached by the periodontal ligament to the alveolar bone. SYN radix (2) [TA], root (2).

root sheath (rūt shēth) An epidermic layers of the hair follicle.

Ror·schach test (rōr´shahk test) Projective psychological test in which the subject reveals his or her attitudes, emotions, and personality by reporting what is seen in each of ten inkblot pictures. SYN inkblot test.

ro·sa·ce·a (rō-zā´shē-ă) Chronic vascular and follicular dilation involving the nose and contiguous portions of the cheeks with erythema, hyperplasia of sebaceous glands, and telangiectasia. SYN acne erythematosa, acne rosacea.

ro·sa·ry (rō´zăr-ē) A beadlike arrangement or structure.

rose hips (rōz hips) Fruit or berries from wild rose bushes; a rich source of vitamin C (ascorbic acid). SYN hipberries.

Ro·sen·bach law (rō´zen-bahk law) In

afflictions of the nerve trunks or nerve centers, paralysis of the flexor muscles appears later than that of the extensors.

Ro·sen·bach sign (rō′zen-bahk sīn) **1.** Loss of the abdominal reflex in cases of acute inflammation of the viscera. **2.** Liver pulsations in aortic regurgitation.

ro·se·o·la (rō′zē-ō′lă) A symmetric eruption of small, rose red, closely aggregated patches; caused by human herpesvirus type 6 and sometimes type 7. SEE ALSO exanthema subitum.

Rose po·si·tion (rōz pŏ-zish′ŏn) The patient lies supine with the head falling down over the end of the table; used in operations in the oral cavity or pharynx.

rose spots (rōz spotz) Characteristic exanthema of typhoid fever; 10–20 small pink papules on the lower trunk lasting a few days and leaving hyperpigmentation.

ro·sette (rō-zet′) **1.** The quartan malarial parasite *Plasmodium malariae* in its segmented or mature phase. **2.** A grouping of cells characteristic of neoplasms of neuroblastic or neuroectodermal origin. **3.** Roselike coiling of the uterus among certain pseudophyllidean tapeworms.

Ross pro·ce·dure (raws prŏ-sē′jŭr) Therapeutic technique for aortic valve stenosis or regurgitation in which the aortic valve is replaced with the patient's own pulmonic valve and the pulmonic valve is in turn replaced with a homograft valve.

ros·tel·lum (ros-tel′ŭm) The anterior fixed or invertible portion of the scolex of a tapeworm, frequently provided with a row (or several rows) of hooks.

ros·trad (ros′trad) **1.** In a direction toward any rostrum. **2.** Situated nearer a rostrum or the snout end of an organism in relation to a specific reference point; opposite of caudad (2).

ros·tral (ros′trăl) [TA] **1.** Relating to any rostrum or anatomic structure resembling a beak. **2.** At the head end. SYN rostralis [TA].

ros·trate (ros′trāt) Having a beak or hook.

ros·trum, pl. **ros·tra,** pl. **ros·trums** (ros′trŭm, -tră, -trŭmz) [TA] Any beak-shaped structure.

rot (rot) To decay or putrify.

ro·ta·mase (rō′tă-mās) Enzyme capable of altering the rotational conformation of a molecule.

ro·ta·mer (rō′tă-měr) An isomer differing from other conformation(s) only in rotational positioning of its parts, such as *cis-* and *trans-* forms.

ro·ta·tion (rō-tā′shŭn) **1.** Turning or movement around an axis. **2.** A recurrence in regular order of certain events, such as the symptoms of a periodic disease. **3.** In medical education and other health education progams, a period of time dedicated to a particular service or specialty. **4.** Practice of changing hours worked periodically; shift work.

ro·ta·tion flap (rō-tā′shŭn flap) A pedicle flap rotated from the donor site to an adjacent recipient area.

ro·ta·to·ry nys·tag·mus (rō′tă-tōr′ē nis-tag′mŭs) A movement of the eyes around the visual axis.

ro·ta·vi·rus (Rv, RV) (rō′tă-vī′rŭs) A group of RNA viruses of wheellike appearance, which comprise a genus, *Rotavirus*, which includes the human gastroenteritis viruses (a major cause of infant diarrhea throughout the world). SYN duovirus, gastroenteritis virus type B, infantile gastroenteritis virus, reoviruslike agent.

ro·te·none (rō′tĕ-nōn) The principal insecticidal component of derris root, used externally to treat scabies and chigger infestation.

Roth spots (rōt spots) Round white retinal spot surrounded by hemorrhage in bacterial endocarditis, and in other retinal hemorrhagic conditions.

Ro·tor syn·drome (rō-tōr′ sin′drōm) Jaundice appearing in childhood due to impaired biliary excretion.

ro·to·tome (rō′tō-tōm) A rotating cutting instrument used in arthroscopic surgery.

rough·age (rŭf′ăj) Anything in the diet

(e.g., bran) that may act as a bulk stimulant of intestinal peristalsis.

rou·leau, pl. **rou·leaux** (rū-lō′) An aggregate of erythrocytes stacked like a pile of coins.

rou·leaux for·ma·tion (rū-lō′ fōr-mā′ shŭn) Arrangement of red blood cells in fluid blood (or in diluted suspensions) with their biconcave surfaces in apposition, thereby forming groups that resemble stacks of coins. SYN pseudoagglutination (2).

round·ed at·el·ec·ta·sis, round at·el·ec·ta·sis (rownd′ĕd at′ĕ-lek′tă-sis, rownd) An area of atelectic lung caused by parenchymal infolding due to pleural fibrosis, most often from asbestos exposure.

round heart (rownd hahrt) Abnormally smooth arcuate contours of the heart on imaging due either to disease of the ventricles or to a false cardiac appearance produced by excessive pericardial fluid. SYN globular heart.

round·worm (rownd′wŏrm) A nematode member of the phylum Nematoda, commonly confined to the parasitic forms.

Rous-as·so·ci·at·ed vi·rus (RAV) (rows ă-sō′sē-āt-ĕd vī′rŭs) A leukemia virus of the leukosis-sarcoma complex that by phenotypic mixing with a defective (noninfectious) strain of Rous sarcoma virus effects production of infectious sarcoma virus with envelope antigenicity of the RAV.

Rous·sy-Lé·vy dis·ease (rū-sē′ lā-vē′ di-zēz′) Disorder consisting of a motorsensory demyelinating polyneuropathy and a coexisting essential tremor. SYN Roussy-Lévy syndrome.

Roux-en-Y an·as·to·mo·sis (rū′ŏn[h] ĕ′grek ă-nas′tŏ-mō′sis) Connection of the distal end of the divided jejunum to the stomach, bile duct, or another structure, with implantation of the proximal end into the side of the jejunum at a suitable distance usually more than 40 cm below the first anastomosis. The bowel then forms a Y-shaped pattern.

Rov·sing sign (rov′sing sīn) Pain at McBurney point induced in cases of appendicitis by pressure exerted over the descending colon.

Roy·al Col·lege of Sur·geons (roy′ăl kol′ĕj sŭr′jŏnz) British professional organization of trained medical surgeons founded in the 18th century; its members are called Mister, rather than Doctor.

Roy·al So·ci·ety (Canada) (roy′ăl sŏ-sī′ĕ-tē kan′ă-dă) Former name of honorary group now called RSC: Academies of Arts, Humanities and Sciences of Canada (in French, SRC: Académies des Arts, des Lettres et des Sciences du Canada) that includes scholars and scientists from many disciplines.

RPR test SYN rapid plasma reagin test.

-rrhagia *The diagraph rh occurring at the beginning of a syllable in a word of Greek origin is ordinarily changed to rrh when a prefix or other lexical element is placed before it, as in this terminal form, from rhexis.* Combining form denoting excessive or unusual discharge; hemorrhage.

-rrhea Suffix meaning a flowing; a flux.

Ru Symbol for ruthenium.

rub (R) (rŭb) Friction encountered in moving one body in contact with another.

rub·ber dam (RD) (rŭb′ĕr dam) **1.** In surgery, thin strips of rubber used as a surgical drain or barrier; **2.** Thin sheet of rubber with holes that is placed over teeth to isolate them from the oral cavity.

rub·ber dam clamp (rŭb′ĕr dam klamp) Springlike metal piece encircling or grasping the cervix of a tooth so shaped to prevent a rubber dam from coming off the tooth.

rub·bing al·co·hol (rŭb′ing al′kŏ-hol) Alcoholic mixture intended for external use; it usually contains 70% by volume of absolute alcohol or isopropyl alcohol; the remainder consists of water, denaturants (with and without coal tar colors), and perfume oils; used as a rubefacient for muscle and joint aches and pains.

ru·be·do (rū-bē′dō) A temporary redness of the skin.

ru·be·fa·cient (rū′bĕ-fā′shĕnt) **1.** Caus-

R

ing a reddening of the skin. **2.** A counterirritant that produces erythema when applied to the skin surface.

ru·bel·la (rū-bel′ă) An acute exanthematous disease caused by rubella virus (*Rubivirus*), with enlargement of lymph nodes, but usually with little fever or constitutional reaction; a high incidence of birth defects in children results from maternal infection during the first several months of fetal life (congenital rubella syndrome). SYN epidemic roseola.

ru·bel·la virus (rū-bel′ă vī′rŭs) An RNA virus of the genus *Rubivirus*; the agent causing rubella (German measles) in humans. SYN German measles virus.

ru·be·o·la (rū′bē-ō′lă) SYN measles (1).

ru·be·o·sis (rū′bē-ō′sis) **1.** Reddish discoloration. **2.** Neovascularization of the iris seen in ocular ischemic diseases.

ru·be·o·sis ir·i·dis di·a·be·ti·ca (rū′bē-ō′sis ī′ri-dis dī-ă-bet′i-kă) Neovascularization of the anterior surface of the iris in diabetes mellitus.

ru·bes·cent (rū-bes′ĕnt) Reddening.

ru·bid·i·um (rū-bid′ē-ŭm) An alkali element; its salts are used in medicine for the same purposes as the corresponding sodium or potassium salts.

ru·bi·do·my·cin (rū-bid′ō-mī′sin) An antibiotic used as an antineoplastic. SYN daunorubicin.

Ru·bi·vi·rus (rū′bi-vī′rŭs) A genus of viruses that includes the rubella virus.

Rub·ner laws of growth (rŭb′ner lawz grōth) Law of constant energy consumption: the rapidity of growth is proportional to the intensity of the metabolic processes.

ru·bor (rū′bōr) Redness, as one of the four signs of inflammation (r., calor, dolor, tumor) enunciated by Celsus.

ru·bra·tox·in (rū′bră-tok′sin) A mycotoxin produced by *Penicillium rubrum* and *P. purpurogenum*, which form readily on cereal grains.

ru·bric (rū′brik) Section or chapter heading, used with reference to groups of diseases.

ru·bri·cyte (rū′bri-sīt) SEE ALSO erythroblast.

ru·bro·spi·nal (rū′brō-spī′năl) Relating to the nerve fibers passing from the red nucleus to the spinal cord.

ru·di·ment (rū′di-mĕnt) **1.** An organ or structure that is incompletely developed. **2.** The first indication of a structure in the course of ontogeny. SYN rudimentum.

ru·di·men·tar·y (rū′di-men′tăr-ē) Relating to a rudiment. SYN abortive (2).

Ruf·fi·ni cor·pus·cles (rū-fē′nē kōr′pŭs-ĕlz) Sensory end structures in the subcutaneous connective tissues of the fingers, consisting of an ovoid capsule within which the sensory fiber ends with numerous collateral knobs.

ru·ga, gen. and pl. **ru·gae** (rū′gă, -jē) [TA] A fold, ridge, or crease.

ru·gi·tus (rū-jī′tŭs) A rumbling sound in the intestines. SEE ALSO borborygmus.

ru·gose, ru·gous (rū′gōs, rū′gŭs) Marked by rugae; wrinkled. SYN rugous.

ru·gos·i·ty (rū-gos′i-tē) **1.** The state of being thrown into folds or wrinkles. **2.** A ruga.

Ruhe·mann pur·ple (rū′mahn pŭr′pĕl) A blue-violet dye formed in the reaction of ninhydrin with amino acids.

rule (rūl) A principle, criterion, standard, or guideline, applied to procedures or situations in which accumulated observation is considered relevant. SEE ALSO law, principle, theorem.

rule of nines (rūl nīnz) Method used in calculating body surface area involved in burns whereby values of 9% or 18% of surface area are assigned to specific regions as follows: head and neck, 9%; anterior thorax, 18%; posterior thorax, 18%; arms, 9% each; legs, 18% each; perineum, 1%. Somewhat different values are used with children and infants.

rum (rŭm) A spirit distilled from the fermented juice of sugar cane.

ru·mi·na·tion (rū'mi-nā'shŭn) **1.** The physiologic process in ruminant animals in which coarse, hastily eaten food is regurgitated from the rumen, thoroughly rechewed, reduced to finer particles, mixed with saliva, and reswallowed. **2.** A disorder of infancy characterized by repeated regurgitation of food, with weight loss or failure to thrive, developing after a period of normal functioning. **3.** Periodic reconsideration of the same subject.

ru·mi·na·tion dis·or·der (rū'mi-nā' shŭn dis-ōr'dĕr) Mental disorder of infancy characterized by repeated regurgitation of food, usually accompanied by weight loss or failure to gain weight.

run·a·way pace·mak·er (run'ă-wā pās' māk-ĕr) Rapid heart rates over 140 per minute caused by electronic circuit instability in an implanted pulse generator.

run·ner's blad·der (rŭn'ĕrz blad'ĕr) Hematuria caused by running with an empty bladder.

run·ner's high (rŭn'ĕrz hī) Euphoria experienced by some runners and joggers as they near the end of a run. Believed to be associated with the release of endorphins produced by physical stress.

ru·pi·a (rū'pē-ă) Ulcers of late secondary syphilis, covered with yellowish or brown crusts.

rup·ture (rŭp'shŭr) **1.** SYN hernia. **2.** Break of any organ or other of the soft parts.

Rus·sell bod·ies (rŭs'ĕl bod'ēz) Small, discrete, variably sized, spheric, intracytoplasmic, acidophilic, hyaline bodies that stain deeply with fuchsin.

Rus·sell Per·i·o·don·tal In·dex (rŭs'ĕl per'ē-ŏ-don'tăl in'deks) An index that estimates the degree of periodontal disease present by measuring both bone loss around the teeth and gingival inflammation.

Rus·sell sign (rŭs'ĕl sīn) Abrasions and scars on the back of the hands of people with bulimia, usually due to manual attempts to self-induce vomiting.

Rus·sell trac·tion (rŭs'ĕl trak'shŭn) A means of applying traction to one or both legs using 5–10-lb weights per leg.

Rus·sell vi·per (rŭs'ĕl vī'pĕr) Highly venomous snake (*Vipera russellii*) of southeastern Asia.

Rus·sell vi·per ven·om (rŭs'ĕl vī'pĕr ven'ŏm) A venom derived from Russell viper (*Vipera russelli*), which acts as an intrinsic thromboplastin; used in the laboratory evaluation of deficiencies of factor X or topically to arrest local hemorrhage in hemophilia.

Rus·sian cur·rent (rŭsh'ăn kŭr'rĕnt) An electrotherapeutic modality that uses medium frequency polyphasic alternating current waveforms to strengthen muscles.

Rust phe·nom·e·non (rŭst fĕ-nom'ĕ-non) In cancer or caries of the upper cervical vertebrae, the patient will always support the head by the hands when changing from the recumbent to the sitting posture or the reverse.

rust·y spu·tum (rŭs'tē spyū'tŭm) A reddish-brown, blood-stained expectoration characteristic of pneumonococcal lobar pneumonia.

ru·the·ni·um (Ru) (rū-thē'nē-ŭm) A metallic element of the platinum group; has been used to treat ocular problems.

ru·tin (rū'tin) A flavonoid obtained from buckwheat, which causes decreased capillary fragility. SYN rutoside.

Ruysch mem·brane (roish mem'brăn) SYN choriocapillary layer.

Ruysch mus·cle (roysh mŭs'ĕl) Muscular tissue of the fundus of the uterus.

R wave (wāv) The first positive deflection of the QRS complex in the electrocardiogram.

Rx Abbreviation for recipe (℞) in a prescription. SEE prescription (2).

Ry·an stain (rī'ăn stān) Modified trichrome stain for microsporidian spores in which the chromotrope 2R is 10 times the normal concentration used in trichrome stains for stool specimens and the counterstain is aniline blue.

R

S

sa·ber-sheath tra·che·a (sā′bĕr-shēth trā′kē-ă) Tracheal collapse seen in chronic obstructive pulmonary disease.

sa·ber tib·i·a, sa·ber shin (sā′bĕr tib′ē-ă, shin) Tibial deformity in tertiary syphilis or yaws, the bone having a marked forward convexity due to formation of gummas and periostitis.

Sa·bi·a vi·rus (sā′bē-ă vī′rŭs) An arenavirus associated with hemolytic fever.

Sa·bin vac·cine (sā′bin vak-sēn′) Orally administered vaccine containing live, attenuated strains of poliovirus. SEE poliovirus vaccines.

sab·u·lous (sab′yū-lŭs) Sandy; gritty.

sa·bur·ra (să-bŭr′ă) Foulness of the stomach or mouth resulting from decomposed food.

sac (sak) 1. A pouch or bursa. SYN saccus [TA]. 2. An encysted abscess at the root of a tooth. 3. The capsule of a tumor, or envelope of a cyst. SEE ALSO sacculus.

sac·cade (sa-kahd′) A rapid movement of both eyes from one target to another; such movements allow precise scanning of the field and are necessary for smooth reading. SEE ALSO saccadic movement.

sac·cad·ic move·ment (să-kahd′ik mūv′mĕnt) 1. Quick rotation of the eyes from one fixation point to another as in reading. 2. Rapid correction movement of a jerky nystagmus, as in labyrinthine and optokinetic nystagmus.

sac·cate (sak′āt) Relating to a sac.

♻ **sacchar-** SEE saccharo-.

sac·cha·ride (sak′ă-rīd) Any substance that is either a simple sugar or a compound of such substances in glycosidic linkage to each other. Saccharides are classified as mono-, di-, tri-, and polysaccharides according to the number of monosaccharide groups composing them. SEE carbohydrate.

sac·cha·rin (SAC) (sak′ă-rin) In dilute aqueous solution it is 300–500 times sweeter than sucrose; used as a noncaloric sugar substitute. SYN benzosulfimide.

♻ **saccharo-, sacchar-, sacchari-** Combining forms denoting sugar (saccharide).

sac·cha·ro·lyt·ic (sak′ăr-ō-lit′ik) Capable of hydrolyzing or otherwise breaking down a sugar molecule.

sac·cha·ro·me·tab·o·lism (sak′ăr-ō-mĕ-tab′ŏ-lizm) Metabolism of sugar; the process of utilization of sugar in cells.

sac·ci·form, sac·cu·lar (sak′si-fōrm, sak′yū-lăr) Pouched; sac-shaped. SYN saccular.

sac·cu·lar an·eu·rysm, sac·cu·lat·ed an·eu·rysm (sak′yū-lăr an′yūr-izm, sak′yū-lā′tĕd an′yūr-izm) Saclike bulging on one side of an artery. SYN ampullary aneurysm.

sac·cu·lar gland (sak′yū-lăr gland) A single alveolar gland.

sac·cu·lat·ed (sak′yū-lāt′ĕd) SYN sacciform.

sac·cu·lat·ed pleu·ri·sy (sak′yū-lāt′ĕd plūr′i-sē) Pleurisy with the inflammatory exudate divided into separate regions by adhesions or inflammatory changes.

sac·cu·la·tion (sak′yū-lā′shŭn) 1. A structure formed by a group of sacs. 2. The formation of a sac or pouch.

sac·cule (sak′yūl) [TA] 1. The smaller of the two membranous sacs in the vestibule of the labyrinth, lying in the spheric recess. 2. The immense, bag-shaped structure formed by peptidoglycans as part of the cell wall of certain microorganisms. SYN sacculus [TA].

sac·cu·lo·co·chle·ar (sak′yū-lō-kok′lē-ăr) Relating to the sacculus and the membranous cochlea.

sac·cu·lus, gen. and pl. **sac·cu·li** (sak′yū-lŭs, -lī) [TA] SYN saccule.

sac·cus, pl. **sac·ci** (sak′ŭs, -sī) [TA] SYN sac (1).

♻ **sacr-** SEE sacro-.

sa·crad (sā′krad) In the direction of the sacrum.

sa·cral (sā′krăl) Relating to or in the neighborhood of the sacrum.

sa·cral an·es·the·si·a (sā′krăl an′es-thē′zē-ă) Regional anesthesia limited to those areas innervated by sacral sensory nerves.

sa·cral·gi·a (sā-kral′jē-ă) Pain in the sacral region. SYN sacrodynia.

sa·cral·i·za·tion (sā′krăl-ī-zā′shŭn) Lumbar development and appearance of the first sacral vertebra.

sa·cral ky·pho·sis (sā′krăl kī-fō′sis) [TA] Normal, anteriorly concave curvature of the sacrum, in which the primary curvature of the fetal embryo is maintained into maturity. SYN kyphosis sacralis [TA].

sa·crec·to·my (sā-krek′tŏ-mē) Resection of a portion of the sacrum to facilitate an operation.

sacro-, sacr- Combining forms denoting muscular substance; resemblance to flesh.

sa·cro·coc·cy·ge·al (SC) (sā′krō-kok-sij′ē-ăl) Relating to both sacrum and coccyx.

sa·cro·col·po·pex·y pro·ce·dure (sā′krō-kol′pō-peks′ē prŏ-sē′jŭr) Supporting the vaginal vault by affixing it to the periosteum sacral after hysterectomy.

sa·cro·dyn·i·a (sā′krō-din′ē-ă) SYN sacralgia.

sa·cro·il·i·ac (sac-il, SI) (sā′krō-il′ē-ak) Relating to the sacrum and the ilium.

sa·cro·il·i·ac joint, sa·cro·il·i·ac ar·tic·u·la·tion (sā′krō-il′ē-ak joynt, ahr-tik′yū-lā′shŭn) [TA] The synovial joint between the sacrum and the ilium.

sa·cro·il·i·i·tis (sā′krō-il′ē-ī′tis) Inflammation of the sacroiliac joint.

sa·cro·lum·bar (sā′krō-lŭm′bahr) SYN lumbosacral.

sa·cro·sci·at·ic (sā′krō-sī-at′ik) Relating to both sacrum and ischium.

sa·cro·spi·nal (sā′krō-spī′năl) Relating to the sacrum and the vertebral column above.

sa·cro·ver·te·bral (sā′krō-vĕr′tĕ-brăl) Relating to the sacrum and the vertebrae above.

sa·crum, pl. **sa·cra** (sā′krŭm, -kră) [TA] The segment of the vertebral column forming part of the pelvis.

sad·dle block an·es·the·si·a (sad′ĕl blok an′es-thē′zē-ă) Spinal anesthesia limited in area to the buttocks, perineum, and inner surfaces of the thighs.

sad·dle em·bo·lism (sad′ĕl em′bŏ-lizm) Straddling embolism at any vascular bifurcation, e.g., of the aorta, which occludes both common iliac arteries.

sad·dle joint (sad′ĕl joynt) [TA] Biaxial synovial joint in which double motion is effected by opposition of two surfaces, each concave in one direction and convex in the other.

sa·dism (sā′dizm) A form of perversion, often sexual in nature, in which a person finds pleasure in inflicting abuse and maltreatment. Cf. masochism, sadomasochism.

sa·do·mas·o·chism (sā′dō-mas′ŏ-kizm) A form of perversion marked by enjoyment of cruelty and humiliation, both received and dispensed.

Sae·misch sec·tion (sā′mish sek′shŭn) Transfixing the cornea beneath an ulcer and then cutting from within outward through the base.

Sae·misch ul·cer (sā′mish ŭl′sĕr) A form of creeping corneal disease, frequently accompanied by hypopyon.

safe sex (sāf seks) An umbrella term indicating sexual activity using a latex condom to avoid sexually transmitted disease and any transmission of body fluids; also called safer sex.

saf·flow·er oil (saf′low-ĕr oyl) An oil extracted from the seeds of *Carthamus tinctorius*; used in hypercholesteremia, myocardial infarction, and coronary insufficiency.

sag·it·tal (saj′i-tăl) [TA] 1. Resembling an arrow. 2. In an anteroposterior direction, referring to a sagittal plane or direction. SYN sagittalis.

sag·it·tal ax·is (saj′i-tăl ak′sis) DENTIS-

TRY the line in the frontal plane around which the working side condyle rotates during mandibular movement.

sag·it·ta·lis (saj′i-tā′lis) [TA] SYN sagittal.

sag·it·tal plane (saj′i-tăl plān) [TA] Median plane, and any other plane parallel to it is a parasagittal plane; in contemporary usage and in a broad sense, used for any plane parallel to the median, i.e., as a synonym for parasagittal.

sag·it·tal sec·tion (saj′i-tal sek′shŭn) Cross-section obtained by slicing, actually or through imaging techniques, the body or any part of the body, or any anatomic structure in the sagittal plane, i.e., in a vertical plane parallel to the median plane. SYN parasagittal section.

Saint An·tho·ny fire (sānt anth′ŏ-nē fīr) **1.** SYN ergotism. **2.** Any of several inflammations or gangrenous conditions of the skin (e.g., erysipelas).

Sak·sen·a·ea vas·i·for·mis (sak-sen′ē-ă vă-si-fōr′mis) Fungal species that causes zygomycosis; associated with localized bone and soft tissue infection, usually due to trauma.

sal·i·cyl·am·ide (SA, SAM) (sal′i-sil′ă-mīd) Amide of salicylic acid; an analgesic, antipyretic, and antiarthritic, similar in action to aspirin.

sa·lic·y·late (să-lis′i-lāt) **1.** A salt or ester of salicylic acid. **2.** To treat foodstuffs with salicylic acid as a preservative.

sa·lic·y·lat·ed (să-lis′i-lāt′ĕd) Treated by the addition of salicylic acid as a preservative.

sal·i·cyl·ic ac·id (sal′i-sil′ik as′id) A component of aspirin, derived from salicin and made synthetically; used externally as a keratolytic agent.

sal·i·cyl·ic ac·id col·lo·di·on (sal-i-sil′ik as′id ko-loy′dē-on) Keratolytic agent used to treat corns and warts.

sal·i·cyl·ism (sal′i-sil′izm) Poisoning by salicylic acid or any of its compounds.

sal·i·cy·lu·ric ac·id (sal′i-sil-yūr′ik as′id) The conjugation product of glycine with salicylic acid; excreted in urine after the administration of salicylic acid or some of its compounds.

sal·i·fi·a·ble (sal′i-fī′ă-bĕl) Capable of being made into salts; said of a base that combines with acids to make salts.

sa·line (sā′lēn) **1.** Relating to, of the nature of, or containing salt; salty. **2.** A salt solution, usually sodium chloride.

sa·line ag·glu·ti·nin (sā′lēn ă-glū′ti-nin) An antibody that causes agglutination of erythrocytes when they are suspended either in saline or in a protein medium. SYN complete antibody.

sa·line so·lu·tion (sā′lēn sŏ-lū′shŭn) A solution of any salt; specifically, isotonic or physiologic sodium chloride solution.

sa·li·va (să-lī′vă) A clear, tasteless, odorless, slightly acid (pH 6.8) viscid fluid, consisting of the secretion from the parotid, sublingual, and submandibular salivary glands and the mucous glands of the oral cavity.

sa·li·va sub·sti·tute (să-lī′vă sŭb′sti-tūt) Artificial saliva is formulated to mimic natural saliva, but does not stimulate salivary gland activity; used to treat dry mouth.

sal·i·vant (sal′i-vănt) **1.** Causing a flow of saliva. **2.** An agent that increases the flow of saliva. SYN salivator.

sal·i·var·y cal·cu·lus (sal′i-var-ē kal′kyū-lŭs) A stone in a salivary duct or gland.

sal·i·var·y di·ges·tion (sal′i-var-ē di-jes′chŭn) The conversion of starch into sugar by the action of salivary amylase.

sal·i·var·y fis·tu·la (sal′i-var-ē fis′tyū-lă) A pathologic communication between a salivary duct or gland and the cutaneous surface or the oral mucus.

sal·i·var·y gland (sal′i-var-ē gland) [TA] Any of the saliva-secreting exocrine glands of the oral cavity.

sal·i·va·tion (sal′i-vā′shŭn) Production of saliva. SEE sialorrhea.

sal·i·va·tor (sal′i-vā-tŏr) SYN salivant.

Salk vac·cine (sawk vak-sēn′) Original

poliovirus vaccine, composed of virus propagated in monkey kidney tissue culture and inactivated. SEE poliovirus vaccines.

Sal·mo·nel·la (sal′mō-nel′ă) Genus of aerobic to facultatively anaerobic bacteria containing gram-negative rods that are either motile or nonmotile; pathogenic for humans and other animals.

Sal·mo·nel·la en·ter·i·ca ser·o·var en·ter·i·ti·dis (sal′mō-nel′ă en-ter′ik-ă sěr′ō-vahr en-tĕr-ī′ti-dis) A widely distributed bacterial species that can infect humans and animals, especially rodents; causes human gastroenteritis.

Sal·mo·nel·la en·ter·i·ca se·ro·var pa·ra·ty·phi B (sal′mō-nel′ă en-ter′ik-ă sěr′ō-vahr par′ă-tī′fī) Bacterial species of two distinct strains, those that produce enteric fever, found primarily in humans, and those producing gastroenteritis in humans, also found in animal species.

Sal·mo·nel·la en·ter·i·ca se·ro·var ty·phi·mu·ri·um (sal′mō-nel′ă en-ter′ik-ă sěr′ō-vahr tī-fī-mŭr′ē-ŭm) A bacterial species causing food poisoning in humans; natural pathogen of all warmblooded animals; worldwide, most frequent cause of gastroenteritis due to *S. enterica*.

Sal·mo·nel·la en·ter·i·ca subsp. Saint-paul (sal′mō-nel′ă en-ter′i-kă sänt pawl) A variety of anaerobic bacteria, previously thought extremely rare, which caused hundreds to sicken in the summer of 2008 in more than two dozen states. Although tomatoes were likely the causative agent, suspicions were also raised about salsa, scallions, and some species of hot peppers (e.g., jalapeno). Florida and Mexico were thought to be the source of the tainted food(s).

Sal·mo·nel·la ty·phi (sal′mō-nel′ă tī′fī) A species that causes typhoid fever in humans and is transmitted in contaminated water and food. SYN typhoid bacillus.

sal·mo·nel·lo·sis (sal′mō-nĕl-ō′sis) Infection with bacteria of the genus *Salmonella*. Patients with sickle cell anemia or compromised immune systems are particularly susceptible.

salm·on patch (sam′ŏn pach) Common macular orange-pink to red vascular malformation present at or near birth on the head and neck. SYN Hutchinson patch.

sal·pin·gec·to·my (sal′pin-jek′tŏ-mē) Removal of the uterine tube.

sal·pin·gi·an (sal-pin′jē-ăn) Relating to the uterine tube or to the pharyngotympanic (auditory) tube.

sal·pin·gi·tis (sal′pin-jī′tis) Inflammation of the uterine or the pharyngotympanic (auditory) tube.

sal·pin·gi·tis isth·mi·ca no·do·sa (sal′pin-jī′tis is′mi-kă nō-dō′să) Uterine tube disorder characterized by nodular thickening of the tunica muscularis of the isthmic portion of the tube enclosing glandlike or cystic duplications of the lumen. SYN adenosalpingitis.

salpingo-, salping- Combining forms denoting a tube (usually the uterine or pharyngotympanic (auditory) tubes. SEE ALSO tubo-.

sal·pin·go·cele (sal-ping′gō-sēl) Hernia of a uterine tube.

sal·pin·gog·ra·phy (sal′ping-gog′ră-fē) Radiography of the uterine tubes after the injection of radiopaque contrast medium.

sal·pin·gol·y·sis (sal′ping-gol′i-sis) Freeing the uterine tube from adhesions.

sal·pin·go·ne·os·to·my (sal-ping′gō-nē-os′tŏ-mē) Surgical reopening of a uterine tube clubbed because of fimbrial adhesions.

sal·pin·go·o·oph·o·rec·to·my (sal-ping′gō-ō-of′ŏr-ek′tŏ-mē) Removal of the ovary and its uterine tube.

sal·pin·go·o·oph·o·ri·tis (sal-ping′gō-ō-of′ŏr-ī′tis) Inflammation of both uterine tube and ovary.

sal·pin·go·o·oph·o·ro·cele (sal-ping′gō-ō-of′ŏr-ō-sēl) Hernia of both ovary and uterine tube.

sal·pin·go·per·i·to·ni·tis (sal-ping′gō-per′i-tō-nī′tis) Inflammation of the uterine tube, perisalpinx, and peritoneum.

sal·pin·go·pex·y (sal-ping′gō-pek-sē) Operative fixation of an oviduct.

S

sal·pin·go·pha·ryn·ge·al (sal-ping′gō-fă-rin′jē-ăl) Relating to the auditory tube and pharynx.

sal·pin·go·plas·ty (sal-ping′gō-plas-tē) Surgical repair of the uterine tubes. SYN tuboplasty.

sal·pin·gor·rha·phy (sal′ping-gōr′ă-fē) Suture of the uterine tube.

sal·pin·gos·co·py (sal′ping-gos′kŏ-pē) Visualization of the intraluminal portion of the uterine tubes, usually by radiograph or with an endoscope.

sal·pin·gos·to·my (sal′ping-gos′tŏ-mē) Establishment of an artificial opening in a uterine tube primarily as surgical treatment for an ectopic pregnancy.

sal·pin·got·o·my (sal′ping-got′ŏ-mē) Incision into the uterine tube.

salt (sal) (sawlt) **1.** A compound formed by the interaction of an acid and a base, the ionizable hydrogen atoms of the acid being replaced by the positive ion of the base. **2.** Sodium chloride, the prototypical salt. **3.** A saline cathartic, especially magnesium sulfate, magnesium, citrate, or sodium phosphate; often denoted by the plural, salts.

sal·ta·to·ry spasm (sal′tă-tōr-ē spazm) A spasmodic affection of the muscles of the lower extremities. SYN Bamberger disease (1).

salt de·ple·tion (sawlt dĕ-plē′shŭn) Excessive loss of sodium chloride from the body in urine or sweat; a cause of secondary dehydration.

salt·ed plas·ma (sawl′tĕd plaz′mă) Fluid portion of blood drawn from the vessels, which is kept from coagulating by being put into a solution of sodium or magnesium sulfate. SYN salted serum.

salt fe·ver (sawlt fē′vĕr) Elevated temperature in an infant, following a rectal injection of a salt solution. SEE ALSO thirst fever.

salt·ing out (sawl′ting owt) Precipitation of a protein from its solution by full or partial saturation with sodium chloride, magnesium sulfate, or ammonium sulfate.

salt sub·sti·tute (SS) (sawlt sŭb′sti-tūt) Low-sodium food additive that tastes like salt, such as potassium chloride; useful as a dietary alternative.

sa·lu·bri·ous (să-lū′brē-ŭs) Healthful, usually in reference to climate.

sal·u·re·sis (sal′yūr-ē′sis) Excretion of sodium in the urine.

sal·u·ret·ic (sal′yūr-et′ik) Facilitating the renal excretion of sodium.

sal·vage che·mo·ther·a·py (sal′văj kē′mō-thār′ă-pē) Use of chemotherapy in a patient with recurrence of a malignancy following initial treatment, in hope of a cure or prolongation of life. SYN salvage therapy (1).

sal·vage ther·a·py (sal′văj thār′ă-pē) **1.** SYN salvage chemotherapy. **2.** Treatment designed to suppress resistant virus following combination antiviral treatment. SYN rescue therapy.

salve (sav) SYN ointment.

Salz·mann nod·u·lar cor·ne·al de·gen·er·a·tion (sahlts′mahn noj′ū-lăr kōr′nē-ăl dĕ-jen′ĕr-ā′shŭn) Large and prominent nodules of a solid, opaque material that rises from the corneal surface; occurs in chronic inflammation.

sa·mar·i·um (Sm) (să-mar′ē-ŭm) A metallic element of the lanthanide group, atomic no. 62, atomic wt. 150.36.

sam·bu·cus (sam-bū′kŭs) The dried flowers of *Sambucus canadensis* or *S. nigra* (family Caprifoliaceae), the common elder or black elder; weak laxative. SYN elder, elder flowers.

sam·ple (sam′pĕl) **1.** A specimen of a whole entity small enough to involve no threat or damage to the whole; an aliquot. **2.** A selected subset of a population. **3.** A piece or portion of a whole to demonstrate the characteristics or qualities of that whole.

sam·pling bi·as (sam′pling bī′ăs) Systematic error due to study of a nonrandom sample of a population.

Sam·ter syn·drome (sahm′ter sin′drōm) A triad of asthma, nasal polyps, and aspirin intolerance.

san·a·tive (san'ă-tiv) Having a tendency to heal.

san·a·to·ri·um, san·it·a·ri·um (san'ă-tōr'ē-ŭm, -ār'ē-ŭm) An institution for the treatment of chronic disorders and recuperation under medical supervision.

san·a·to·ry (san'ă-tōr-ē) Health-giving; conducive to health.

sand (sand) The fine granular particles of quartz and other crystalline rocks, or a gritty material resembling sand.

Sand·hoff dis·ease (sahnd'hawf di-zēz') An infantile form of G_{M2} gangliosidosis characterized by a defect in the production of hexosaminidases A and B; resembles Tay-Sachs disease, but occurs predominantly (if not entirely) in non-Jewish children.

sane (sān) Denoting sanity.

San·fi·lip·po syn·drome (san-fi-lip'pō sin'drōm) An error of mucopolysaccharide metabolism, with excretion of large amounts of heparan sulfate in the urine; characterized by severe mental retardation with hepatomegaly.

sangui-, sanguin-, sanguino- Combining forms denoting blood, bloody.

san·gui·fa·cient (sang'gwi-fā'shĕnt) SYN hemopoietic.

san·guif·er·ous (sang-gwif'ĕr-ŭs) Conveying blood. SYN circulatory (2).

san·guine (sang'gwin) SYN plethoric.

san·guin·e·ous (sang-gwin'ē-ŭs) **1.** Relating to blood; bloody. **2.** SYN plethoric.

san·guin·o·lent (sang-gwin'ō-lĕnt) Bloody; tinged with blood.

san·gui·no·pu·ru·lent (sang'gwi-nō-pyū'rŭ-lĕnt) Denoting containing blood and pus.

san·guiv·or·ous (sang-gwiv'ŏr-ŭs) Bloodsucking, as in to certain bats, and leeches.

sa·ni·es (sā'nē-ēz) A thin, blood-stained, purulent discharge.

san·i·tar·i·an (san'i-tar'ē-ăn) One who is skilled in sanitation and public health.

san·i·tar·y (sanit) (san'i-tar-ē) Healthful; conducive to health; usually in reference to a clean environment.

san·i·tar·y nap·kin (san'i-tar-ē nap'kin) Pad worn to absorb menstrual discharge.

san·i·ta·tion (sanit) (san'i-tā'shŭn) Use of measures designed to promote health and prevent disease; development and establishment of conditions in the environment favorable to health.

san·i·ti·za·tion (san'i-tī-zā'shŭn) The process of making something sanitary.

san·i·ty (san'i-tē) Soundness of mind, e-motions, and behavior; of a sound degree of mental health.

San·som sign (san'sŏm sīn) In mitral stenosis, apparent duplication of the second heart sound.

San·ti·ni boom·ing sound (sahn-tē'nē būm'ing sownd) A sonorous booming heard on auscultatation of a hydatid cyst.

sa·phe·na (să-fē'nă) SEE vein.

sa·phe·nous (SAPH) (să-fē'nŭs) *Although the correct pronunciation is as shown, the more usual pronunciation in the U.S. is saf'ĕ-nus.* Relating to or associated with a saphenous vein; denoting a number of structures in the leg.

sapo-, sapon- Combining forms meaning soap.

sap·o·na·ceous (sap'ŏ-nā'shŭs) Soapy; relating to or resembling soap.

sa·pon·i·fi·ca·tion (să-pon'i-fi-kā'shŭn) Conversion into soap, denoting the hydrolytic action of an alkali on fat, especially on triacylglycerols.

sap·o·nins (sap'ō-ninz) Glycosides of plant origin characterized by properties of foaming in water and of lysing cells; powerful surfactants; many have antibiotic activities.

sapro-, sapr- Combining forms meaning rotten, putrid, decayed.

sap·robe (sap'rōb) An organism that lives

on dead organic material. USAGE NOTE *This term is preferable to saprophyte, because bacteria and fungi are no longer regarded as plants.*

sap·ro·zo·ic (sap′rŏ-zō′ik) Living in decaying organic matter; especially certain protozoa.

Sar·ci·na (sahr′si-nă) A genus of nonmotile, strictly anaerobic bacteria containing gram-positive cocci, which divide in three perpendicular planes. Saprophytic and facultatively parasitic species occur.

sarco- Combining form denoting muscular substance or a resemblance to flesh.

sar·co·blast (sahr′kō-blast) SYN myoblast.

Sar·co·cys·tis (sahr′kō-sis′tis) A genus of protozoan parasites, related to the sporozoan genera *Eimeria*, *Isospora*, and *Toxoplasma*; abundant but rarely pathogenic; fever, severe diarrhea, abdominal pain, and weight loss have been reported in a small number of immunocompromised hosts.

sar·co·cys·to·sis (sar′kō-sis-tō′sis) Infection with protozoan parasites of the genus *Sarcocystis*.

Sar·co·di·na (sahr′kō-dī′nă) Mostly free-living amebae; a subphylum of protozoa possessing pseudopodia for movement.

sar·coi·do·sis, sar·coid (sahr′koy-dō′sis) A systemic granulomatous disease of unknown cause, especially involving the lungs with resulting fibrosis, but also involving lymph nodes, skin, liver, spleen, eyes, phalangeal bones, and parotid glands. SYN Boeck disease.

sar·co·lem·ma (sahr′kō-lem′ă) The plasma membrane of a muscle fiber.

sar·co·lem·mal, sar·co·lem·mic, sar·co·lem·mous (sahr′kō-lem′ăl, -ik, -ŭs) Relating to the sarcolemma.

sar·co·ma (sahr-kō′mă) A connective tissue neoplasm, usually highly malignant, formed by proliferation of mesodermal cells.

sar·co·ma·toid (sahr-kō′mă-toyd) Resembling a sarcoma.

sar·co·ma·to·sis (sahr′kō-mă-tō′sis) Occurrence of several sarcomatous growths on different parts of the body.

sar·co·ma·tous (sahr-kō′mă-tŭs) Relating to or of the nature of sarcoma.

sar·co·mere (sahr′kō-mēr) The segment of a myofibril between two adjacent Z lines, representing the functional unit of striated muscle.

sar·co·pe·ni·a (sahr′kō-pē′nē-ă) Progressive reduction in muscle cross-section and mass with aging.

sar·co·plasm (sahr′kō-plazm) The nonfibrillar cytoplasm of a muscle fiber.

sar·co·poi·et·ic (sahr′kō-poy-et′ik) Forming muscle.

Sar·cop·tes sca·bie·i (sahr-kop′tēz skā′bē-ī) The itch mite, varieties of which are distributed worldwide; affect humans and many animals. SEE ALSO scabies.

sar·cop·tic (sahr-kop′tik) Denotes caused by mites of the genus *Sarcoptes* or other members of the family Sarcoptidae.

sar·cop·tid (sahr-kop′tid) Common name for members of the Sarcoptidae, a family of mites that includes the genera *Sarcoptes*, *Knemidokoptes*, and *Notoedres*.

sar·co·sine (Sar) (sahr′kō-sēn) *N*-methylglycine; an intermediate in the metabolism of choline; levels elevated in certain inherited disorders.

sar·co·si·ne·mi·a (sahr′kō-si-nē′mē-ă) A disorder of amino acid metabolism due to deficiency of sarcosine dehydrogenase, causing the sarcosine level to rise in blood plasma and be excreted in the urine; some affected infants fail to thrive, are irritable, may have muscle tremors, and have retarded motor and mental development. SYN hypersarcosinemia.

sar·co·sis (sahr-kō′sis) **1.** Abnormal increase of flesh. **2.** Multiple growth of fleshy tumors. **3.** Diffuse sarcoma involving a whole organ.

sar·cos·to·sis (sahr′kos-tō′sis) Ossification of muscular tissue.

sar·co·tu·bules (sahr′kō-tū′byūlz) The continuous system of membranous tubules in striated muscle that corresponds to the smooth endoplasmic reticulum of other cells.

sar·cous (sahr′kŭs) Relating to muscular tissue; fleshy.

sar·gra·mos·tim (sahr′grä-mos′tim) A recombinant human granulocyte-macrophage colony-stimulating factor (GM-CSF); used to reduce the duration of neutropenia and incidence of infection in patients receiving myelosuppressive chemotherapy or bone marrow transplantation.

Sart·well in·cu·ba·tion mod·el (sahrt′wel ing′kyū-bā′shŭn mod′ĕl) Mathematical model based on empiric observations, showing that incubation periods for communicable diseases have a lognormal distribution.

sat·el·lite (sat′ĕ-līt) **1.** A minor structure accompanying a more important or larger one. **2.** The posterior member of a pair of gregarine gamonts in syzygy.

sat·el·lite cells (sat′ĕ-līt selz) Neuroglial cells surrounding the cell body of a neuron in the spinal, cranial, and autonomic ganglia.

sat·el·lite de·ox·y·ri·bo·nu·cle·ic a·cid (DNA) (sat′ĕ-līt dē-ok′sē-rī′bō-nū-klē′ik as′id) DNA in the satellite regions of acrocentric chromosomes.

sa·tel·li·tism (sat′ĕ-lī′tism) A state of being physiologically secondary to another system or organ.

sa·ti·e·ty cen·ter (să′shē-ĕ-tē sen′tĕr) Term referring to the region of the ventromedial nucleus in the hypothalamus; destruction in the rat leads to continuous eating and extreme obesity.

Satt·ler veil (saht′ler vāl) A diffuse edema of the corneal epithelium that may develop after wearing contact lenses.

sat·u·rat·ed fat free (sach′ŭr-āt-ĕd fat frē) A product so labeled contains, by order of the U.S. Food and Drug Administration, less than 0.5 g saturated fat per serving and 0.5 g trans-fatty acid per serving.

sat·u·rat·ed so·lu·tion (sat. sol., sat. soln.) (sach′ŭr-āt′ĕd sŏ-lū′shŭn) One that contains all of a solute capable of being dissolved in the solvent.

sat·u·ra·tion (sach′ŭr-ā′shŭn) **1.** Impregnation of one substance by another to the greatest possible extent. **2.** Neutralization. **3.** Concentration of a dissolved substance that cannot be exceeded. **4.** OPTICS SEE saturated color. **5.** Filling of all available sites on an enzyme molecule by its substrate.

sa·tu·ra·tion sound pres·sure lev·el (SSPL) (sach′ŭr-ā′shŭn sownd presh′ŭr lev′ĕl) A measure of the maximum output of a hearing aid.

sat·y·ri·a·sis (sat′ir-ī′ă-sis) Excessive sexual excitement and behavior in the male; counterpart of female nymphomania.

sau·cer·i·za·tion (saw′sĕr-ī-zā′shŭn) Excavation of tissue to form a shallow depression; performed in wound treatment to facilitate drainage from infected areas.

sax·i·tox·in (sak′si-tok′sin) A potent neurotoxin found in shellfish; cause of poisoning due to eating California sea mussels, scallops, and Alaskan butterclams.

Sb Symbol for antimony.

Sc Symbol for scandium.

scab (skab) A crust formed by coagulation of blood, pus, serum, or a combination of these, on the surface of an ulcer, erosion, or other type of wound.

scab·bard tra·che·a (skab′ărd trā′kē-ă) Tracheal deformity due to flattening and approximation of the lateral walls, producing stenosis.

sca·bi·cide (skā′bi-sīd) An agent lethal to scabies mites.

sca·bies (skā′bēz) *Scabies, a singular noun, is the name of a skin disorder, not of the mite that causes the disorder. Although the word is correctly pronounced skā′bē-ēz, the latter two syllables are usually fused in the U.S. as given here.* An eruption due to the mite *Sarcoptes scabiei* var. *hominis*; female of the species burrows into the skin, producing a vesicular eruption with intense pruritus between the fingers, on the male or female genitalia, buttocks, and elsewhere on the trunk and extremities.

scald (skawld) **1.** To burn by contact with a hot liquid or steam. **2.** The lesion resulting from such contact.

scald·ed mouth syn·drome (skawld′ĕd mowth sin′drōm) Condition in which the patient complains of a burning sensation of the oral cavity, likened to scalding caused by hot liquids; clinically the tissues appear normal; associated with angiotensin-converting enzyme inhibitors.

scale (skāl) **1.** Graduations. **2.** SYN squama. **3.** PSYCHOLOGY/PSYCHIATRY a standardized test for measuring psychological, personality, or behavioral characteristics. SEE ALSO test, score. **4.** A small, thin plate of horny epithelium, cast off from the skin. **5.** To desquamate. **6.** DENTISTRY/DENTAL HYGIENE/DENTAL ASSISTING to remove calculus from the teeth.

sca·lene (skā′lēn) **1.** Having sides of unequal length, said of a triangle so formed. **2.** One of several muscles so named. SYN scalenus.

sca·le·nec·to·my (skā′lĕ-nek′tŏ-mē) Resection of the scalene muscles.

sca·lene tu·ber·cle (skā′lēn tū′bĕr-kĕl) [TA] Small spine on the inner edge of the first rib, giving attachment to the scalenus anterior muscle, lying between and thus demarcating the grooves for the subclavian artery (anteriorly) and vein (posteriorly). SYN tuberculum musculi scaleni anterioris [TA], Lisfranc tubercle, scalene tubercle of Lisfranc, tubercle of anterior scalene muscle.

sca·le·not·o·my (skā′lĕ-not′ŏ-mē) Division or section of the anterior scalene muscle.

scal·er (skā′lĕr) **1.** An instrument to remove dental tartar. **2.** Device to count electrical impulses.

scal·ing (skāl′ing) DENTISTRY removal of accretions from the crowns and roots of teeth by use of special instruments.

scal·lop·ing (skal′ŏ-ping) A series of indentations or erosions on a normally smooth margin of a structure.

scalp (skalp) Skin and subcutaneous tissue, normally hair bearing, covering the neurocranium.

scal·pel (skalp′ĕl) A knife used in surgical dissection.

scan, scin·ti·scan (skan, sin′tĭ-skan) **1.** To survey by traversing with an active or passive sensing device. **2.** The image, record, or data obtained by scanning.

scan·di·um (Sc) (skan′dē-ŭm) A metallic element; atomic no. 21, atomic wt. 44.955910.

scan·ning (skan′ing) The act of imaging by traversing with an active or passive sensing device, often identified by the technology or device employed.

scan·ning e·lec·tron mi·cro·scope (skan′ing ĕ-lek′tron mī′krŏ-skōp) A microscope in which the object in a vacuum is scanned in a raster pattern by a slender electron beam.

scan·ning speech (skan′ing spēch) Measured or metered, often slow, speech.

Scan·zo·ni ma·neu·ver (skahn-tsō′nē mă-nū′vĕr) Forceps rotation and traction in a spiral course, with reapplication of forceps for delivery.

scapho- Prefix meaning a scapha, scaphoid.

scaph·o·ceph·a·ly (skaf′ŏ-sef′ă-lē) A form of craniosynostosis that results in a long narrow head. SYN cymbocephaly, sagittal synostosis, tectocephaly.

scaph·oid (skaf′oyd) [TA] Boat-shaped; hollowed. SEE ALSO scaphoid (bone). SYN navicular.

scaph·oid ab·do·men (skaf′oyd ab′dŏ-mĕn) A condition in which the anterior abdominal wall is sunken and presents a concave rather than a convex contour.

scap·tion (skap′shŭn) Elevation of the glenohumeral joint in the plane of the scapula, which is approximately 30 degrees of horizontal adduction from the frontal plane.

scap·u·la, gen. and pl. **scap·u·lae** (skap′ yū-lă, -lē) [TA] A large, triangular, flattened bone lying over the ribs, posteriorly on either side, articulating laterally with the clavicle at the acromioclavicular joint and the humerus at the glenohumeral joint. SYN shoulder blade.

scap·u·lar line (skap′yū-lăr līn) [TA] Vertical line passing through the inferior angle of the scapula. SYN linea scapularis [TA].

scap·u·lar re·flex (skap′yū-lăr rē′fleks) Contraction of the upper muscles of the back by stimulation between the scapulae. SYN interscapular reflex.

scap·u·lec·to·my (skap′yū-lek′tŏ-mē) Excision of the scapula.

scap·u·lo·cla·vic·u·lar (skap′yū-lō-klă-vik′yū-lăr) **1.** SYN acromioclavicular. **2.** SYN coracoclavicular.

scap·u·lo·hu·mer·al (skap′yū-lō-hyū′ měr-ăl) Relating to both scapula and humerus. SEE ALSO glenohumeral.

scap·u·lo·hu·mer·al rhythm (skap′yū-lō-hyū′měr-ăl ridh′ĕm) Coordinated rotational movement of the scapula that accompanies abduction, adduction, internal and external rotation, extension, and flexion of the humerus.

scap·u·lo·pex·y (skap′yū-lō-pek-sē) Operative fixation of the scapula to the chest wall or to the spinous process of the vertebrae.

sca·pus, pl. **sca·pi** (skā′pŭs, -pī) A shaft or stem.

scar (skahr) Fibrous tissue replacing normal tissues destroyed by injury or disease or divided after an incision.

scar car·ci·no·ma (skahr kahr′si-nō′mă) Lung cancer, usually adenocarcinoma, arising from a peripheral lung scar or associated with interstitial fibrosis in a honeycomb lung.

scar·i·fi·ca·tion (skahr′i-fi-kā′shŭn) The making of a number of superficial incisions in the skin.

scar·i·fi·ca·tor (skahr′i-fi-kā-tŏr) An instrument for scarification, consisting of close-set concealed spring-projected cutting blades that make superficial skin incisions.

scar·i·fy (skahr′i-fī) *This word has no relation, etymologically or semantically, to scar.* To produce scarification.

scar·la·ti·na (skahr′lă-tē′nă) *Avoid the misspelling scarletina.* An acute exanthematous disease, caused by infection with streptococcal organisms producing an erythrogenic toxin, marked by fever and other constitutional disturbances, and a generalized eruption of closely aggregated bright red points or small macules followed by desquamation in large scales, shreds, or sheets; mucous membrane of the mouth and fauces is usually also involved. SYN scarlet fever.

scar·la·ti·nel·la (skahr′lă-ti-nel′ă) SYN Filatov-Dukes disease.

scar·la·ti·ni·form (skahr′lă-tē′ni-fōrm) Resembling scarlatina, denoting a rash.

scar·let fever (skahr′lĕt fē′vĕr) SYN scarlatina.

scar·let red (skahr′let red) An azo dye; a dark, brownish red powder; used in medicine and in histology to stain fat in tissue sections and basic proteins at high pH. SYN Biebrich scarlet red, medicinal scarlet red, scharlach red, Sudan IV.

Scar·pa flu·id (skahr′pă flū′id) SYN endolymph.

Scar·pa meth·od (skahr′pă meth′ŏd) Cure of aneurysm by ligation of the artery at some distance above the sac.

scar·ring al·o·pe·ci·a (skahr′ing al′ō-pē′shē-ă) Hair loss in which hair follicles are irreversibly destroyed by scarring processes including trauma, burns, lupus erythematosus, and other causes. SYN cicatricial alopecia.

scato- Combining form indicating feces or excrement. SEE ALSO sterco-.

sca·tol·o·gy (skă-tol′ŏ-jē) **1.** Scientific analysis of feces, for physiologic and diagnostic purposes. SYN coprology. **2.** The study relating to the psychiatric aspects of excrement or excremental (anal) function.

sca·tos·co·py (skă-tos′kŏ-pē) Examination of the feces for purposes of diagnosis.

scav·en·ger re·cep·tor (skav′ĕn′jĕr rĕ-sep′tŏr) Receptor on macrophages that binds preferentially to oxidized low density lipoproteins, causing macrophages to internalize the low density lipoproteins.

ScD Abbreviation for Doctor of Science.

Sce·do·spor·i·um (sē-dō-spō′rē-ŭm) An imperfect fungus; anamorph of *Pseudallescheria*.

Sced·os·por·i·um ap·i·o·sper·mum (sē-dō-spō′rē-ŭm ā-pē-ō-spĕr′mŭm) Imperfect state of the fungus *Pseudallescheria boydii*; true fungi that may cause mycetoma in humans or severe infection in immunosuppressed patients.

Sche·de met·hod (shā′dĕ meth′ŏd) Filling of the defect in bone, after removal of a sequestrum or scraping away of carious material, by allowing the cavity to fill with blood that may become organized (Schede clot).

Schei·be hear·ing im·pair·ment (shī′bĕ hēr′ing im-pār′mĕnt) Hearing loss due to cochleosaccular dysplasia.

Scheie syn·drome (shā sin′drŏm) Allelic to Hurler syndrome but with a much milder phenotype; characterized by α-L-iduronidase deficiency, corneal clouding, deformity of the hands, aortic valve involvement, and normal intelligence.

sche·ma, scheme, pl. **sche·ma·ta** (skē′mă, skēm, skē′mă-tă) **1.** A plan, outline, or arrangement. **2.** In sensorimotor theory, the organized unit of cognitive experience.

sche·mat·ic (skĕ-mat′ik) Made after a definite type of formula; representing in general, but not with absolute exactness.

sche·mat·ic eye (skĕ-mat′ik ī) Representation of the optic system of an ideal normal eye in which the curvatures and indices of refraction of the refracting elements and their intervening distances are listed.

Schiff re·a·gent (shif rē-ā′jĕnt) An aqueous solution of basic fuchsin or para-

rosaniline that is decolorized by sulfur dioxide; used for aldehydes and in histochemistry to detect polysaccharides, DNA, and proteins.

Schil·der dis·ease (shil′der di-zēz′) **1.** Diffuse sclerosis or encephalitis periaxialis diffusa **2.** Leukodystrophies. SYN encephalitis periaxialis diffusa.

Schil·ler test (shil′er test) A test for nonglycogen-containing areas of the portio vaginalis of the cervix, which may be the site of early carcinoma.

Schil·ling test (shil′ing test) A procedure for determining the amount of vitamin B12 excreted in the urine.

schin·dy·le·sis (skin′di-lē′sis) [TA] A fibrous joint in which the sharp edge of one bone is received in a cleft in the edge of the other. SYN schindyletic joint, wedge-and-groove joint, wedge-and-groove suture.

Schir·mer test (shir′mĕr test) Test for tear production using a strip of filter paper; a measurement of basal and reflex lacrimal gland function.

schisto- Prefix indicating cleft, division. SEE ALSO schizo-.

schis·to·cor·mi·a (skis′tō-kōr′mē-ă) Congenital truncal clefting; fetal lower limbs are usually imperfectly developed. SYN schistosomia.

schis·to·cys·tis (skis′tō-sis′tis) Fissure of the bladder.

schis·to·cyte, schiz·o·cyte (skis′tō-sīt, skiz′ō-) A poikilocyte that owes its abnormal shape to fragmentation as the cell flows through damaged small vessels.

schis·to·cy·to·sis (skis′tō-sī-tō′sis) The occurrence of many schistocytes in the blood.

schis·to·glos·si·a (skis′tō-glos′ē-ă) Congenital fissure or cleft of the tongue.

Schis·to·so·ma (skis′tō-sō′mă) A genus of trematodes, including the blood flukes that cause schistosomiasis.

schis·to·so·mal der·ma·ti·tis (skis′tō-sōm′ăl dĕr′mă-tī′tis) A sensitization response to repeated cutaneous invasion by cercariae of bird, mammal, or human schistosomes. SYN water itch (2).

schis·to·some (skis′tō-sōm) Common name for a member of the genus *Schistosoma*.

schis·to·so·mi·a·sis (skis′tō-sō-mī′ă-sis) Infection with a species of *Schistosoma;* this chronic and debilitating disease with tissue reaction, hypertension, and liver damage.

schis·to·so·mi·a·sis hae·ma·to·bi·um (skis′tō-sō-mī′ă-sis hē′mă-tō′bē-ŭm) Infection with *Schistosoma haematobium*, the eggs of which invade the urinary tract, causing cystitis and hematuria, and possibly an increased likelihood of bladder cancer. SYN endemic hematuria.

schis·to·so·mi·a·sis man·so·ni (skis′tŏ-sō-mī′ă-sis man-sō′nī) Infection with *Schistosoma mansoni*, eggs that invade the wall of the large intestine and liver, causing irritation, and ultimately fibrosis. SYN Mansoni schistosomiasis.

schiz- SEE schizo-.

schiz·am·ni·on (skiz-am′nē-on) An amnion developing, as in the human embryo, by the formation of a cavity within the embryoblast.

schiz·ax·on (skiz-ak′son) An axon divided into two branches.

schiz·en·ceph·a·ly (skiz′en-sef′ă-lē) Abnormal divisions or clefts of the brain substance.

schizo-, schiz- Combining forms denoting split, cleft, division; schizophrenia. SEE ALSO schisto-.

schiz·o·af·fec·tive (skits′ō-ă-fek′tiv) Having mixed symptoms suggesting both schizophrenia and affective (mood) disorder.

schiz·o·af·fec·tive dis·or·der (SAD) (skit′sō-ă-fek′tiv dis-ōr′děr) Illness manifested by an enduring major depressive, manic, or mixed episode along with delusions, hallucinations, disorganized speech and behavior, and negative symptoms of schizophrenia. In the absence of a major depressive, manic, or mixed epi-

sode, there must be delusions or hallucinations for several weeks.

schiz·o·af·fec·tive psy·cho·sis (skits′ō-ă-fek′tiv sī-kō′sis) Psychotic disturbance with mixed schizophrenic and manic-depressive symptoms.

schiz·o·gen·e·sis (skits′ō-jen′ĕ-sis) Reproduction by fission. SYN fissiparity, scissiparity.

schi·zog·o·ny (skits-og′ŏ-nē) Multiple fission in which the nucleus first divides and then the cell divides into as many parts as there are nuclei; called merogony if daughter cells are merozoites, sporogony if daughter cells are sporozoites, or gametogony if daughter cells are gametes.

schiz·o·gy·ri·a (skits′ō-jī′rē-ă) Deformity of the cerebral convolutions marked by occasional interruptions of their continuity.

schiz·oid (skits′oyd) Socially isolated, withdrawn, having few (if any) friends or social relationships; resembling the personality features characteristic of schizophrenia, but in a milder form. SEE ALSO schizoid personality.

schiz·ont (skits′ont) A vegetative sporozoan trophozoite that reproduces by schizogony, producing daughter trophozoites or merozoites.

schi·zon·ti·cide (ski-zon′ti-sīd) An agent that kills schizonts.

schiz·o·nych·i·a (skits′ō-nik′ē-ă) Splitting of the nails.

schiz·o·phre·ni·a (skits′ō-frē′nē-ă) A common type of psychosis, characterized by abnormalities in perception, content of thought, and thought processes (hallucinations and delusions), and extensive withdrawal of one's interest from other people and the outside world, the investment of it being instead in one's own mental life.

schiz·o·trich·i·a (skits′ō-trik′ē-ă) A splitting of the hairs at their ends.

schiz·o·typ·al per·son·al·i·ty dis·or·der, schiz·o·typ·al per·son·al·i·ty (skits′ō-tīp′ăl pěr-sŏn-al′i-tē dis-ōr′děr) An enduring and pervasive pattern of be-

S

havior in adulthood characterized by discomfort with and reduced capacity for close relationships, cognitive or perceptual distortions, and eccentric behavior; affected people hold unusual ideas.

schlie·ren op·tics (shlēr´ĕn op´tiks) Optic system, often used in diffusion and centrifugation studies, which observes the refractive index gradient in solutions containing macromolecules.

Schmi·del an·as·to·mo·ses (shmī´dĕl ă-nas´tŏ-mō´sēz) Abnormal channels of communication between the caval and portal venous systems.

Schmidt-Lan·ter·man in·ci·sures (shmit lahn´ter-mahn in-sī´zhŭrz) Funnel-shaped interruptions in the regular structure of the myelin sheath of nerve fibers.

Schmorl nod·ule (shmōrl nod´yūl) Prolapse of the nucleus pulposus through the vertebral body endplate into the spongiosa of an adjacent vertebra.

Schnei·der first-rank symp·toms (shnī´dĕr fĭrst-rank simp´tŏms) Those symptoms that, when present, indicate that the diagnosis of schizophrenia is likely, provided that organic or toxic etiology is ruled out: delusion of control, thought broadcasting, thought withdrawal, thought insertion, hearing one's thoughts spoken aloud, auditory hallucinations that comment on one's behavior, and auditory hallucinations in which two voices carry on a conversation.

Schnitz·ler syn·drome (shnits´ler sin´drŏm) Tense, generalized chronic urticaria, joint or bone pain, and monoclonal gammopathy of kappa type.

Scho·ber test (shō´ber test) A measure of lumbar spine motion in which parallel horizontal lines are drawn 10 cm above and 5 cm below the lumbosacral junction in the erect subject; with maximum forward flexion, the distance between the lines increases at least 5 cm in normal patients but far less in patients with ankylosing spondylitis.

Schult·ze mech·a·nism (shūlt´sĕ mek´ă-nizm) Expulsion of the placenta with the fetal surface foremost.

Schult·ze sign (shūlt´sĕ sīn) In latent tet-

any, tapping the tongue causes its depression with a concave dorsum.

Schwa·bach test (shvah´bahk test) Tuning fork test in which the subject's ability to hear a tuning fork by bone conduction is compared with the examiner's ability to hear the same tuning fork by bone conduction. SEE Rinne test.

schwan·no·ma (shwah-nō´mă) A benign, encapsulated neoplasm in which the fundamental component is structurally identical to a syncytium of Schwann cells; the neoplastic cells proliferate within the endoneurium, and the perineurium forms the capsule. SEE ALSO neurofibroma. SYN neurilemmoma.

schwan·no·sis (shwah-nō´sis) A nonneoplastic proliferation of Schwann cells in the perivascular spaces of the spinal cord; seen in older patients, especially diabetics.

Schwart·ze sign (shvahrt´zĕ sīn) Vascularization of the promontory of the middle ear resulting in a rosy glow that can be seen through the tympanic membrane; a sign of otosclerosis. SEE ALSO otosclerosis. SYN promontory flush.

sci·age (sē-ahzh´) A to-and-fro, sawlike movement of the hand in massage.

sci·at·ic (sī-at´ik) **1.** Relating to or situated in the neighborhood of the ischium or hip. Ischial or sciatic. SYN ischiadic, ischial, ischiatic. **2.** Relating to sciatica.

sci·at·i·ca (sī-at´i-kă) Pain in the lower back and hip radiating down the back of the thigh into the leg, initially attributed to sciatic nerve dysfunction, but now known to usually be due to herniated lumbar disc compromising the L5 or S1 root. SEE sciatic.

sci·at·ic sco·li·o·sis (sī-at´ik skō´lē-ō´sis) Spinal disorder due to asymmetric spasms of spinal muscles usually associated with sciatica; usually listing toward one side.

sci·ence (sī´ĕns) Branch of knowledge that produces theoretic explanations of natural phenomena based on experiments and observations.

scin·ti·cis·tern·og·ra·phy (sin´ti-sis´

těrn-og′rǎ-fē) Cisternography performed with a radiopharmaceutical and recorded with a stationary imaging device.

scin·tig·ra·phy (sin-tig′rǎ-fē) A diagnostic procedure with administration of a radionuclide with an affinity for the organ or tissue of interest, followed by recording the distribution of the radioactivity with a stationary or scanning external scintillation camera.

scin·til·lat·ing sco·to·ma (sin′ti-lā′ting skō-tō′mǎ) A localized area of blindness edged by brilliantly colored shimmering lights (teichopsia). SEE ALSO fortification spectrum. SYN flittering scotoma.

scin·til·la·tion (sin′ti-lā′shŭn) 1. Flashing or sparkling; subjective sensation of sparks or flashes of light. 2. In radiation measurement, the light produced by an ionizing event in a phosphor. SEE ALSO scintillation counter.

scin·til·la·tion count·er (sin′ti-lā′shŭn kown′tĕr) Instrument used to detect and measure of radioactivity.

scin·til·la·tor (sin′ti-lā-tŏr) A substance that emits visible light when hit by a subatomic particle x-ray or gamma ray. SEE ALSO scintillation counter.

scin·ti·scan, scin·ti·gram (sin′ti-skan, -gram) The record obtained by scintigraphy. SEE ALSO scan.

scir·rhous (skir′ŭs) *Avoid the misspellings schirrous and schirrhous. Do not confuse this word with serous.* Hard; relating to a scirrhus or any hard indurated surface.

scir·rhous car·ci·no·ma (skir′ŭs kahr′si-nō′mǎ) A hard fibrous lesion due to a desmoplastic reaction by the stromal tissue. SYN fibrocarcinoma.

scis·sors gait (siz′ŏrz gāt) A manner of walking cross-legged, mimicking the motion of scissors; commonly associated with spastic paraplegia.

scis·su·ra, pl. **scis·su·rae** (shi-sūr′ǎ, -ē) 1. Cleft or fissure. 2. A splitting.

scle·ra, pl. **scle·ras,** gen. and pl. **scler·ae** (sklēr′ǎ, skēr′ē) [TA] A portion of the fibrous tunic forming the outer envelope of the eye, except for its anterior one-sixth portion, which is the cornea. SYN sclerotica.

scle·rad·e·ni·tis (sklēr′ad-ĕ-nī′tis) Inflammatory induration of a gland.

scle·ral (sklēr′ǎl) Relating to the sclera.

scle·ral ring (skēr′ǎl ring) Scleral appearance adjacent to the optic disc when retinal pigment epithelium does not extend to the optic nerve.

scle·ral spur (SS) (skēr′ǎl spŭr) [TA] Circular ridge of sclera on the internal aspect of the corneoscleral junction. SYN calcar sclerae [TA], scleral roll.

scle·rec·ta·si·a (sklēr′ek-tā′zē-ǎ) Localized bulging of the sclera.

scle·rec·to·my (sklĕr-ek′tŏ-mē) 1. Excision of a portion of the sclera. 2. Removal of the fibrous adhesions formed in chronic otitis media.

scle·re·de·ma (sklēr′ĕ-dē′mǎ) *Do not confuse this word with sclerema or scleroderma.* Hard nonpitting edema of the skin of the dorsal aspect of the upper body and limbs, giving a waxy appearance and no sharp demarcation.

scle·re·de·ma a·dul·to·rum (sklēr′ĕ-dē′mǎ ā-dŭl-tōr′ŭm) A benign spreading induration of the skin and subcutaneous tissue, possibly streptococcal, which may follow a febrile illness, with thickened skin. SYN Buschke disease.

scle·re·ma (sklēr-ē′mǎ) Induration of subcutaneous fat.

scle·ri·tis (sklēr-ī′tis) Inflammation of the sclera.

sclero-, scler- Combining forms denoting hardness (i.e., induration), sclerosis, relationship to sclera.

scle·ro·blas·te·ma (sklēr′ō-blas-tē′mǎ) The embryonic tissue entering into the formation of bone.

scle·ro·cho·roi·di·tis (sklēr′ō-kōr′oyd-ī′tis) Inflammation of the sclera and choroid.

scle·ro·cor·ne·a (sklēr′ō-kōr′nē-ǎ) 1. The cornea and sclera regarded as forming together the hard outer coat of the eye, the fibrous tunic of the eye. **2.** A congenital anomaly in which the whole or part of the cornea is opaque and resembles the sclera.

scle·ro·cor·ne·al junc·tion (sklēr'ō-kōr'nē-ăl jŭngk'shŭn) SYN corneoscleral junction.

scle·ro·dac·ty·ly, scle·ro·dac·tyl·i·a (sklēr'ō-dak'ti-lē, -dak-til'ē-ă) SYN acrosclerosis.

scle·ro·der·ma (sklēr'ō-dĕr'mă) Dermal thickening and induration due to new collagen formation, with atrophy of pilosebaceous follicles. SYN systemic scleroderma.

scleroedema [Br.] SYN scleredema.

scleroedema adultorum [Br.] SYN scleredema adultorum.

scle·rog·e·nous, scle·ro·gen·ic (sklēr-oj'ĕ-nŭs, sklēr'ō-jen'ik) Producing hard or sclerotic tissue; causing sclerosis.

scle·roid (sklēr'oyd) Indurated or sclerotic, of unusually firm texture, leathery, or of scarlike texture. SYN sclerosal, sclerous.

scle·ro·i·ri·tis (sklēr'ō-ī-rī'tis) Inflammation of both sclera and iris.

scle·ro·ker·a·ti·tis (sklēr'ō-ker'ă-tī'tis) Inflammation of the sclera and cornea.

scle·ro·ma (sklēr-ō'mă) A circumscribed indurated focus of granulation tissue in the skin or mucous membrane.

scle·ro·ma·la·ci·a (sklēr'ō-mă-lā'shē-ă) Degenerative scleral thinning seen in people with rheumatoid arthritis and other collagen disorders.

scle·ro·mere (sklēr'ō-mēr) **1.** Any metamere of the skeleton. **2.** Caudal half of a sclerotome.

scle·ro·myx·e·de·ma (sklē'rō-mik-se-dē'mă) Generalized lichen myxedematosus with diffuse thickening of the skin underlying the papules.

scle·ro·nych·i·a (sklēr'ō-nik'ē-ă) Induration and thickening of the nails.

scle·ro·o·o·pho·ri·tis (sklēr'ō-ō-of'ŏr-ī'tis) Inflammatory induration of the ovary.

scle·roph·thal·mi·a (sklēr'of-thal'mē-ă) An abnormality in which most of the normally transparent cornea resembles the opaque sclera.

scle·ro·sant (sklēr-ō'sănt) An injectable irritant used to treat varices by producing thrombi in them.

scle·rose (sklēr-ōs') To harden; to undergo sclerosis.

scle·ros·ing agent (sklĕ-rōs'ing ā'jĕnt) Compound that irritates the venous intimal epithelium; used to treat varicose veins.

scle·ros·ing he·man·gi·o·ma (sklĕ-rō'sing hē-man'jē-ō'mă) A benign lung or bronchial lesion, often subpleural, sometimes multiple, which forms hyalinized connective tissue.

scle·ros·ing ker·a·ti·tis (sklĕ-rō'sing ker'ă-tī'tis) Inflammation of the cornea complicating scleritis; characterized by opacification of the corneal stroma.

scle·ros·ing os·te·i·tis (sklĕ-rō'sing os'tē-ī'tis) Fusiform thickening or increased density of bones, of unknown cause; form of chronic nonsuppurative osteomyelitis. SYN condensing osteitis, Garré disease.

scle·ro·sis, pl. **scle·ro·ses** (sklēr-ō'sis, -sēz) **1.** SYN induration (2). **2.** In neuropathy, induration of nervous and other structures by a hyperplasia of the interstitial fibrous or glial connective tissue.

scle·ro·ste·no·sis (sklēr'ō-stĕ-nō'sis) Induration and contraction of the tissues.

scle·ros·to·my (sklēr-os'tŏ-mē) Surgical perforation of the sclera, as for the relief of glaucoma.

scle·ro·ther·a·py (sklēr'ō-thār'ă-pē) Treatment involving the injection of a sclerosing solution into vessels or tissues.

scle·rot·ic ce·men·tal mass (skle-rot'ik sĕ-men'tăl mas) Benign fibroosseous jaw lesions of unknown etiology, which present as large painless radiopaque masses. SYN florid osseous dysplasia, cemental dysplasia.

scle·ro·tome (sklĕr'ō-tōm) **1.** A knife used in sclerotomy. **2.** The group of mesenchymal cells emerging from the ventromedial part of a mesodermic somite and migrating toward the notochord.

scle·rot·o·my (sklĕr-ot'ŏ-mē) An incision through the sclera.

scle·ro·ty·lo·sis (sklĕ'rō-tī-lō'sis) Atrophic fibrosis of the skin, hypoplasia of the nails, and palmoplantar keratoderma; associated with dermatologic and gastrointestinal cancers. SYN scleroatrophy.

sco·lex, gen. and pl. **sco·li·ces** (skō'leks, -li-sēz) The head or anterior end of a tapeworm attached by suckers, and frequently by rostellar hooks, to the wall of the intestine.

scolio- Combining form meaning twisted or crooked.

sco·li·o·ky·pho·sis (skō'lē-ō-kī-fō'sis) Lateral and posterior curvature of the spine.

sco·li·om·e·ter (skō'lē-om'ĕ-tĕr) An instrument for measuring curves.

sco·li·o·sis (skō'lē-ō'sis) [TA] Abnormal lateral curvature of the vertebral column.

sco·li·ot·ic pelvis (skō'lē-ot'ik pel'vis) A deformed pelvis associated with lateral curvature of the spine.

scom·broid poi·son·ing (skom'broyd poy'zŏn-ing) Poisoning from ingestion of heat-stable toxins produced by bacterial action on inadequately preserved dark-meat fish (tuna, bonito, mackerel, albacore, skipjack); characterized by epigastric pain, nausea and vomiting, headache, thirst, difficulty in swallowing, and urticaria.

-scope Suffix meaning viewing, staring; an instrument for viewing but extended to include other methods of examination (e.g., stethoscope).

sco·pol·a·mine (skō-pol'ă-mēn, -min) An alkaloid found in the leaves and seeds of *Hyoscyamus niger*, and other solanaceous plants; exerts anticholinergic actions similar to that of atropine. SYN hyoscine.

-scopy Combining form denoting action or activity involving the use of in instrument for viewing.

scor·bu·tic (skōr-byū'tik) Relating to, suffering from, or resembling scurvy.

scor·bu·ti·gen·ic (skōr-byū'ti-jen'ik) Producing scurvy.

score (skōr) An evaluation, usually expressed numerically, of status, achievement, or condition in a given set of circumstances.

scoto- Combining form denoting darkness.

sco·to·chro·mo·gen·ic (skō'tō-krō'mŏ-jen'ik) Refers to microorganisms that produce pigment in the absence of light.

sco·to·ma, pl. **sco·to·ma·ta** (skō-tō'mă, -mă-tă) *Do not confuse this word with scotoma.* **1.** An isolated area of varying size and shape, within the visual field, in which vision is absent or depressed. **2.** A blind spot in psychological awareness.

sco·top·ic vision, sco·to·pia (skō-top'ik vizh'ŭn, skō-tō'pē-ă) Vision when the eye is dark adapted. SEE ALSO dark adaptation, dark-adapted eye. SYN night vision.

sco·top·sin (skō-top'sin) The protein moiety of the pigment in the rods of the retina.

Scott op·er·a·tion (skot op-ĕr-ā'shŭn) A jejunoileal bypass for morbid obesity using end-to-end anastomosis of the upper jejunum to the terminal ileum, with the bypassed intestine closed proximally and anastomosed distally to the colon.

scrap·ie (skrā'pē) A communicable spongiform encephalopathy of the central nervous system of sheep and goats caused by a prion; resembles Creutzfeldt-Jakob disease and kuru in humans.

scratch test (skrach test) A form of skin test in which antigen is applied through a scratch in the skin.

screen (skrēn) **1.** A sheet of any substance

S

used to shield an object from any influence. **2.** A sheet on which an image is projected. **3.** PSYCHOANALYSIS concealment, as one image or memory concealing another. SEE ALSO screen memory. **4.** To examine, evaluate. **5.** A thin layer of crystals that converts x-rays to light photons to expose film; used in a cassette to produce radiographic images on film. **6.** To examine for specified characteristics to determine whether further examination is needed.

screen·ing (skrēn'ing) **1.** To screen (5). **2.** Examination of a group of usually asymptomatic people to detect those with a high probability of having a given disease, typically by means of an inexpensive diagnostic test. **3.** In the mental health professions, initial patient evaluation that includes medical and psychiatric history, mental status evaluation, and diagnostic formulation to determine the patient's suitability for a particular treatment modality.

screen mem·o·ry (skrēn mem'ŏr-ē) In psychoanalysis, a consciously tolerable memory that unwittingly serves as a cover for another associated memory that would be emotionally painful if recalled.

screw (skrū) A helically grooved cylinder for fastening two objects together or for adjusting the position of an object resting on one end of the screw.

scro·bic·u·late (skrō-bik'yū-lăt) Pitted; marked with minute depressions.

scrof·u·la (skrof'yū-lă) Historic term for cervical tuberculous lymphadenitis.

scrof·u·lo·der·ma, scrof·u·lo·der·mi·a (skrof'yū-lō-děr'mă, -děr'mē-ă) Tuberculosis due to extension into the skin from underlying atypical mycobacterial infection. Cf. lupus vulgaris.

scroll ear (skrōl ēr) Deformity of the pinna in which it is rolled forward.

scro·tal (skrō'tăl) Relating to the scrotum. SYN oscheal.

scro·tal her·ni·a (skrō'tăl hěr'nē-ă) Complete inguinal hernia, located in the scrotum.

scro·tal tongue (skrō'tăl tŭng) SYN fissured tongue.

scro·tec·to·my (skrō-tek'tŏ-mē) Partial or total removal of the scrotum.

scro·to·plas·ty (skrō'tō-plas-tē) Surgical reconstruction of the scrotum. SYN oscheoplasty.

scro·tum, pl. **scro·ta,** pl. **scro·tums** (skrō'tŭm, -tă, -tŭmz) [TA] A musculocutaneous sac containing the testes; it is formed of skin, containing a network of nonstriated muscular fibers (the dartos or dartos fascia), which also forms the scrotal septum internally.

scrub nurse (skrŭb nŭrs) A nurse who has cleansed arms and hands, donned sterile gloves and, usually, a sterile gown, and assists an operating surgeon, primarily by passing instruments.

scur·vy (skŭr'vē) A disease marked by inanition, debility, anemia, edema of the dependent parts, a spongy condition (sometimes with ulceration) of the gums, and hemorrhages into the skin and from the mucous membranes; attributed to a diet lacking sufficient vitamin C.

scu·ti·form (skyū'ti-fōrm) Shield-shaped.

scu·tu·lum, pl. **scu·tu·la** (skyū'tyū-lŭm, -lă) A yellow, saucer-shaped crust, the characteristic lesion of favus.

scu·tum, pl. **scu·ta** (skyū'tŭm, -ă) Thin lamina.

scyb·a·lum, pl. **scyb·a·la** (sib'ă-lŭm, -lă) A hard, round mass of inspissated feces.

Se Symbol for selenium.

sea·bather's e·rup·tion (sē'bādh-ěrz ěr-ŭp'shŭn) Pruritic rash believed to result from hypersensitivity to the venom of the larval thimble jellyfish (*Linuche unguiculata*).

sea·gull mur·mur (sē'gŭl mŭr'mŭr) A cardiac sound imitating the cooing of a seagull; nearly always due to aortic stenosis or mitral regurgitation.

seal·ant (sē'lănt) **1.** A material used to effect an airtight closure. **2.** Substance applied to a damaged organ to affect homeostasis, to curtail other leakage, or to facilitate prolonged drug delivery to a limited area.

search·er (sĕr′chĕr) A sound or probe used to determine the presence of a calculus in the bladder.

sea·sick·ness (sē′sik-nĕs) A form of motion sickness caused by the movement of a floating platform, such as a ship, boat, or raft. SYN mal de mer.

sea·son·al af·fec·tive dis·or·der (SAD) (sē′zŏn′ăl ă-fek′tiv dis-ōr′dĕr) Depression that occurs at approximately the same time year after year and spontaneously remits at the same time each year. The most common type is winter depression, characterized by morning hypersomnia, low energy, increased appetite, weight gain, and carbohydrate craving, all of which remit in the spring.

seat·ed mas·sage (sē′tĕd mă-sahzh′) A massage technique that is performed while the client is fully clothed and seated, often in public settings such as offices, airports, and malls. SYN on-site massage.

sea ur·chin gran·u·loma (sē ŭr′chin gran′yū-lō′mă) Granulomatous nodules, either foreign-body type or composed of epithelioid cells, from retention of the spine of the sea urchin, occurring several months after the skin suffered the wound.

se·ba·ceous (sĕ-bā′shŭs) Relating to sebum; oily; fatty.

se·ba·ceous ad·e·no·ma (sĕ-bā′shŭs ad′ĕ-nō′mă) A benign neoplasm of sebaceous tissue, with a predominance of mature secretory sebaceous cells.

se·ba·ceous cyst (sĕ-bā′shŭs sist) Common dermal lesion containing sebum and keratin; lined by epithelium derived from the pilosebaceous follicle. SEE ALSO epidermoid cyst, pilar cyst.

se·ba·ceous horn (sĕ-bā′shŭs hōrn) Solid outgrowth from a sebaceous cyst.

se·bif·er·ous, seb·i·pa·rous (sĕ-bif′ĕr-ŭs, sĕ-bi′pă-rŭs) Producing sebaceous matter.

seb·o·lith (seb′ō-lith) A concretion in a sebaceous follicle.

seb·or·rhe·a (seb′ōr-ē′ă) Overactivity of the sebaceous glands, resulting in an excessive amount of sebum. SYN seborrhoea.

seb·or·rhe·a ca·pi·tis (seb′ōr-ē′ă kap′i-tis) Skin disorder of the scalp.

seb·or·rhe·a sic·ca (seb′ōr-ē′ă sik′ă) **1.** An accumulation on the skin, especially the scalp, of dry scales; SYN seborrhea furfuracea. **2.** SYN dandruff.

seb·or·rhe·ic bleph·a·ri·tis (seb′ōr-ē′ik blef′ăr-ī′tis) Chronic inflammation of the margins of the eyelids with erythema and white scales. SYN seborrhoeic blepharitis.

seb·or·rhe·ic der·ma·ti·tis, der·ma·ti·tis seb·or·rhe·i·ca (seb′ōr-ē′ik dĕr′mă-tī′tis, seb-ōr-rē′i-kă) A common scaly macular eruption that occurs primarily on the face, scalp (dandruff), and other areas of increased sebaceous gland secretion. SYN dyssebacia, dyssebacea, seborrheic dermatosis, Unna disease.

seb·or·rhe·ic ker·a·to·sis, ker·a·to·sis seb·or·rhe·i·ca (seb′ōr-ē′ik ker′ă-tō′sis, seb-ōr-rē′i-kă) **1.** A superficial, benign, verrucous, often pigmented, greasy lesion consisting of proliferating epidermal cells, resembling basal cells, enclosing horn cysts. **2.** SYN senile keratosis. SYN seborrhoeic keratosis.

seborrhoea [Br.] SYN seborrhea.

seborrhoea sicca [Br.] SYN seborrhea sicca.

seborrhoeic blepharitis [Br.] SYN seborrheic blepharitis.

seborrhoeic dermatitis [Br.] SYN seborrheic dermatitis.

seborrhoeic keratosis [Br.] SYN seborrheic keratosis.

se·bum (sē′bŭm) The secretion of the sebaceous glands.

sec·on·dary (sek′ŏn-dar-ē) **1.** Second in order. **2.** Caused by another condition (e.g., a secondary infection caused by antibiotic treatment for a primary infection).

sec·on·dary a·dre·no·cor·ti·cal in·suf·fi·cien·cy (sek′ŏn-dar-ē ă-drē′nō-kŏr′ti-kăl in′sŭ-fish′ĕn-sē) Condition caused by failure of adrenocorticotrophic hormone (ACTH) secretion due to anterior pituitary disease or inhibition of ACTH production resulting from exogenous steroid therapy.

sec·on·dary al·dos·ter·on·ism (sek′ŏn-dar-ē al-dos′tĕr-ōn-izm) Disorder due not to a defect intrinsic to the adrenal cortex but a stimulation of hormonal secretion caused by extraadrenal disorders; occurs in heart failure, nephrotic syndrome, cirrhosis, and hypoproteinemia.

sec·on·dar·y a·men·or·rhe·a (sek′ŏn-dar-ē ā-men′ŏr-ē′ă) Amenorrhea in which the menses appeared at puberty but subsequently ceased.

sec·on·dary am·pu·ta·tion (sek′ŏn-dar-ē am-pyū-tā′shŭn) Surgery performed after a previous amputation that failed to heal satisfactorily.

sec·on·dary am·y·loid·o·sis (sek′ŏn-dar-ē am′i-loy-dō′sis) Disorder occurring in association with another chronic inflammatory disease; organs chiefly involved are the liver, spleen, and kidneys.

sec·on·dary a·nes·thet·ic (sek′ŏn-dar-ē an′es-thet′ik) A compound that contributes to, but is not primarily responsible for, loss of sensation when two or more anesthetics are simultaneously administered.

sec·on·dar·y at·el·ec·ta·sis (sek′ŏn-dar-ē at′ĕ-lek′tă-sis) Pulmonary collapse at any age, but particularly of infants, due to hyaline membrane disease or elastic recoil of the lungs while the patient is dying from other causes.

sec·on·dary cat·a·ract (sek′ŏn-dar-ē kat′ăr-akt) **1.** One that accompanies or follows some other eye disease; SYN complicated cataract. **2.** One in the retained lens or capsule after a cataract extraction.

sec·on·dary den·tin (sek′ŏn-dar-ē den′tin) Dentin formed by normal pulp function after root end formation is complete.

sec·on·dary de·vi·a·tion (sek′ŏn-dar-ē dē′vē-ā′shŭn) Ocular deviation seen in paralysis of an ocular muscle when the paralyzed eye is used for fixation.

sec·on·dary dis·ease (sek′ŏn-dar-ē di-zēz′) **1.** Illness that follows and results from an earlier disease, injury, or event. **2.** Wasting disorder that follows successful transplantation of bone marrow into a lethally irradiated host; frequently severe and usually associated with fever, anorexia, diarrhea, dermatitis, and desquamation. SEE ALSO graft-versus-host disease.

sec·on·dar·y dys·men·or·rhe·a (sek′ŏn-dar-ē dis-men′ŏr-ē′ă) Menstrual disorder due to inflammation, infection, tumor, or anatomic factors.

sec·on·dary gain (sek′ŏn-dar-ē gān) Interpersonal or social advantages gained indirectly from illness. Cf. primary gain.

sec·on·dary hy·dro·ceph·a·lus (sek′ŏn-dar-ē hī′drō-sef′ă-lŭs) Accumulation of fluid in the cranial cavity, due to meningitis or obstruction to the venous flow.

sec·on·dary im·mune re·sponse (sek′ŏn-dar-ē i-myūn′ rĕ-spons′) SEE immune response.

sec·on·dary im·mu·no·de·fi·cien·cy (sek′ŏn-dār-ē im′yū-nō-dĕ-fish′ĕn-sē) Form with no evident defect in the lymphoid tissues, but rather hypercatabolism or loss of immunoglobulins. SYN secondary agammaglobulinemia, secondary hypogammaglobulinemia.

sec·on·dary in·fec·tion (sek′ŏn-dār-ē in-fek′shŭn) Infection, usually septic, in a person or animal already suffering another infection.

sec·on·dary pre·ven·tion (sek′ŏn-dār-ē prē-ven′shŭn) Interruption of any disease process before emergence of diagnostic findings of the disorder.

sec·on·dary pro·cess (sek′ŏn-dar-ē pros′es) PSYCHOANALYSIS Mental activity directly related to the learned and acquired functions of the ego and characteristic of conscious and preconscious mental activities; marked by logical thinking and by the tendency to delay gratification by regulation of the discharge of instinctual demands.

sec·on·dary sat·ur·a·tion (sek′ŏn-dar-ē sach′ŭr-ā′shŭn) A technique of nitrous oxide anesthesia consisting of an abrupt curtailment of the oxygen in the inhaled mixture to produce a deep plane of anesthesia.

sec·on·dary sex char·ac·ters (sĕk′ŏn-dar-ē seks kar′ăk-tĕrz) Those peculiar to the male or female that develop at puberty (e.g., men's beards and women's breasts). Also called secondary sex characteristics.

sec·on·dary sper·mat·o·cyte (sĕk′ŏn-dar-ē spĕr-mat′ō-sīt) The spermatocyte derived from a primary spermatocyte by the first meiotic division; each secondary spermatocyte produces two spermatids by the second meiotic division.

sec·ond·ar·y tu·ber·cu·lo·sis (sĕk′ŭn-dar′ē tū-bĕr′kyū-lō′sĭs) Tuberculosis found in adults and characterized by lesions near the apex of an upper lobe, which may cavitate or heal with scarring without spreading to lymph nodes; theoretically, secondary tuberculosis may be due to exogenous reinfection or to reactivation of a dormant endogenous infection.

sec·ond-de·gree burn (sĕk′ŏnd-dĕ-grē′ bŭrn) SYN partial-thickness burn.

sec·ond sight (sĕk′ŏnd sīt) Improved near vision in old people due to increased refractivity of the nucleus of the lens causing myopia. SYN senile lenticular myopia.

se·cre·ta (sĕ-krē′tă) Secretions.

se·cre·ta·go·gue, se·cre·to·go·gue (sĕ-krē′tă-gog, -ŏ-gog) An agent that promotes secretion (e.g., acetylcholine, gastrin, secretin).

se·cre·tase (sĕ-krē′tās) A proteinase that acts on amyloid precursor protein to produce peptides that do not contain the entire amyloid β protein (a major constituent of the plaques found in Alzheimer disease), are soluble, and do not precipitate to produce amyloid.

se·crete (sĕ-krēt′) To produce some physiologically active substance by a cell and to deliver it into blood, body cavity, or sap, either by direct diffusion, cellular exocytosis, or by means of a duct.

se·cre·tin (sĕ-krē′tin) A hormone, formed by the epithelial cells of the duodenum under the stimulus of acid contents from the stomach, which incites secretion of pancreatic juice; used to aid diagnosis of pancreatic exocrine disease.

se·cre·tion (sĕ-krē′shŭn) 1. Production by a cell or aggregation of cells (a gland) of a physiologically active substance and its movement out of the cell or organ in which it is formed. 2. The solid, liquid, or gaseous product of cellular or glandular activity that is stored up in or used by the organism in which it is produced. Cf. excretion.

se·cre·to·in·hib·i·tor·y (sĕ-krē′tō-in-hib′i-tōr-ē) Restraining or curbing secretion.

se·cre·tor (sĕ-krē′tŏr) A person whose bodily fluids (e.g., saliva, semen, vaginal secretions) contain a water-soluble form of the antigens of the ABO blood group.

se·cre·tor fac·tor (sĕ-krē′tŏr fak′tŏr) Capacity to secrete antigens of the ABO blood group in saliva and other body fluids.

se·cre·to·ry (sē′krĕ-tōr-ē) Relating to secretion or the secretions.

se·cre·to·ry car·ci·no·ma (sĕ-krē′tŏr-ē kahr′si-nō′mă) Breast cancer with pale-staining cells showing prominent secretory activity, as seen in pregnancy and lactation, but found mostly in children. SYN juvenile carcinoma.

se·cre·to·ry di·ar·rhe·a (sĕ-krē′tŏr-ē dī-ă-rē′ă) Voluminous watery diarrhea seen in cholera, in which the toxin stimulates intestinal secretion.

se·cre·to·ry im·mu·no·glob·u·lin A (sĕ-krē′tŏr-ē im′yū-nō-glob′yū-lin) Subclass of immunoglobulin A that is found primarily in secretions such as tears and colostrum; protected from proteolytic degradation by secretory component.

se·cre·to·ry nerve (sē′krĕ-tōr-ē nĕrv) A nerve conveying impulses that excite functional activity in a gland.

sec·ti·o, pl. **sec·ti·o·nes** (sek′shē-ō, -ō′nēz) In anatomy, a segment.

sec·tion (sek′shŭn) 1. Act of cutting. 2. Cut or division. 3. Segment or part of any organ or structure delimited from the remainder. 4. Cut surface. 5. Thin slice

S

of tissue or any material for examination under the microscope.

sec·tion·al im·pres·sion (sek´shŭn-ăl im-presh´ŭn) One that is made in sections.

sec·tor·an·o·pi·a (sek´tŏr-an-ō´pē-ă) Loss of vision in a sector of the visual field.

se·da·tion (sĕ-dā´shŭn) **1.** The act of calming, especially by the administration of a sedative. **2.** The state of being calm.

sed·a·tive (sed.) (sed´ă-tiv) **1.** Calming. **2.** Drug that quiets nervous excitement.

sed·i·ment (sed´i-mĕnt) **1.** Insoluble material that tends to sink to the bottom of a liquid. **2.** To cause formation of a sediment or deposit. SYN sedimentate.

sed·i·men·ta·tion (sed´i-mĕn-tā´shŭn) Formation of a sediment.

sed·i·men·ta·tion con·stant, sed·i·men·ta·tion co·ef·fi·cient (sed´i-mĕn-tā´shŭn kon´stănt, kō´ĕ-fish´ĕnt) Constants in the Svedberg equation for estimating the molecular weight of a protein from the rate of movement in a centrifugal field.

sed·i·men·ta·tion rate, sed rate (sed´i-mĕn-tā´shŭn rāt) The sinking velocity of blood cells; used to detect and monitor inflammatory processes in the body: an elevated rate indicates more inflammation.

sed·i·men·tom·e·ter (sed´i-mĕn-tom´ĕ-tĕr) Photographic apparatus for the automatic recording of the blood sedimentation rate.

se·dox·an·trone tri·hy·dro·chlor·ide (sē-doks´an-trōn trī´hī´drŏ-klōr´īd) A topoisomerase II inhibitor in cancer chemotherapy.

seed (sēd) **1.** The reproductive body of a flowering plant; the mature ovule. SYN semen (2). **2.** BACTERIOLOGY to inoculate a culture medium with microorganisms.

See·lig-Mül·ler sign (sē´lig-mer´ler sīn) Contraction of the pupil on the affected side in facial neuralgia.

seg·ment (seg´mĕnt) [TA] **1.** Part of an organ or other structure delimited naturally, artificially, or by invagination from the remainder. **2.** Organ territory with independent function, supply, or drainage. **3.** To divide and redivide into minute, equal parts. SEE ALSO metamere.

seg·men·tal (seg-men´tăl) Relating to a segment.

seg·men·tal at·el·ec·ta·sis (seg-men´tăl at´ĕ-lek´tă-sis) Partial collapse of one or more individual pulmonary segments.

seg·men·tal neu·ri·tis (seg-men´tăl nūr-ī´tis) **1.** Inflammation occurring at several points along the course of a nerve. **2.** Segmental demyelinating neuropathy.

seg·men·ta·tion (seg´mĕn-tā´shŭn) **1.** The act of dividing into segments. **2.** SYN cleavage (1).

seg·men·ta·tion nu·cle·us (seg´mĕn-tā´shŭn nū´klē-ŭs) **1.** Compound nucleus in the fertilized oocyte, formed by conjugation of the nuclei of the oocyte and sperm (female and male pronuclei). **2.** Zygote nucleus after it commences the first cleavage division.

seg·men·tec·to·my (seg´men-tek´tŏ-mē) Excision of a segment of any organ or gland.

seg·ment·ed cell (seg´men-tĕd sel) A polymorphonuclear leukocyte matured beyond the band cell so that two or more lobes of the nucleus occur.

seg·re·ga·tion (seg´rĕ-gā´shŭn) **1.** Removal of certain parts from a mass. **2.** Separation of contrasting characters in the offspring of heterozygotes. **3.** Separation of the paired state of genes, which occurs at the reduction division of meiosis. **4.** Progressive restriction of potencies in the zygote to the following embryo.

seg·re·ga·tion a·nal·y·sis (seg´rĕ-gā´shŭn ă-nal´i-sis) GENETICS the enumeration of progeny according to distinct and mutually exclusive phenotypes; used to test putative pattern of inheritance.

seg·re·ga·tion ra·ti·o (seg´rĕ-gā´shŭn rā´shē-ō) GENETICS proportion of progeny of a particular genotype or phenotype from actual matings of specified genotypes. The test of a mendelian hypothesis is the comparison of the segregation rate with the mendelian rate.

Sei·del sign (sī′del sīn) A sickle-shaped scotoma appearing as an upward or downward extension of the blind spot.

sei·zure (sē′zhŭr) **1.** An attack; the sudden onset of a disease or of certain symptoms. **2.** An epileptic attack. SYN convulsion (2).

Sel·din·ger tech·nique (sel′ding-er tek-nēk′) Method of percutaneous insertion of a catheter into a blood vessel or space.

se·lec·tin (sĕ-lek′tin) A cell surface molecule involved in immune adhesion and cell trafficking.

se·lec·tion co·ef·fi·cient (s) (sĕ-lek′shŭn kō′ĕ-fish′ĕnt) The proportion of progeny or potential progeny not surviving to sexual maturity.

se·lec·tive an·gi·og·ra·phy (sĕ-lek′tiv an-jē-og′ră-fē) Imaging in which visualization is improved by concentrating the contrast medium in the region to be studied by injection through a catheter positioned in a regional artery.

se·lec·tive grind·ing (sĕ-lek′tiv grīnd′ing) Modification of the occlusal forms of teeth by grinding according to a plan or by grinding at selected places marked by articulating ribbon or paper.

se·lec·tive in·at·tention (sĕ-lek′tiv in-ă-ten′shŭn) Aspect of attentiveness in which a person attempts to ignore that which generates anxiety.

se·lec·tive nor·ep·i·neph·rine re·up·take in·hib·i·tor (sĕ-lek′tiv nŏr-ep′i-nef′rin rē-up′tāk in-hib′i-tŏr) Chemical compounds that selectively, to varying degrees, inhibit reuptake of norepinephrine by the presynaptic neurons.

se·lec·tive ser·o·to·nin re·up·take in·hib·i·tor (SSRI) (sĕ-lek′tiv ser′ŏ-tō′nin rē-up′tāk in-hib′i-tŏr) A class of drugs that selectively prevent the reuptake of serotonin; widely used to treat depression.

se·lec·tiv·i·ty (sĕ-lek-tiv′i-tē) A property of a drug determined by combining its affinity at various binding sites, the knowledge of which can help predict a drug's potential for therapeutic and adverse effects.

se·le·ni·um (Se) (sĕ-lē′nē-ŭm) A metallic element chemically similar to sulfur; used in scintography of the pancreas and parathyroid glands.

se·le·no·cys·te·ine (sĕ-lē′nō-sis′tĕ-ēn) The biologically active form of selenium when attached to cysteine.

self-dif·fer·en·ti·a·tion (self′dif-ĕr-en′shē-ā′shŭn) Differentiation resulting from the action of intrinsic causes.

self-lim·it·ed dis·ease (self′lim′i-tĕd di-zēz′) Condition that resolves spontaneously with or without specific treatment.

self-reg·u·la·tion (self′reg-yū-lā′shŭn) A three-stage strategy patients are taught to use to end risky health-associated behaviors; stage 1: self-monitoring (self-observation); stage 2: self-evaluation; and stage 3: self-reinforcement.

self-re·tain·ing cath·e·ter (self′rē-tān′ing kath′ĕ-tĕr) One so constructed that it remains in the urethra and bladder until removed.

self-stim·u·la·tion (self′stim-yū-lā′shŭn) A technique for electrical stimulation of peripheral nerves, spinal cord, or brain by the patient to relieve pain.

sel·la tur·ci·ca (sel′ă tŭr′si-kă) [TA] Saddlelike bony prominence on the upper surface of the body of the sphenoid bone. SYN pars sellaris, Turkish saddle.

se·man·tics (sĕ-man′tiks) **1.** Study of the significance and development of the meaning of words. **2.** The study concerned with the relations between signs and their referents.

se·men, pl. **sem·i·na**, pl. **se·mens** (sē′mĕn, -min-ă, -mĕnz) **1.** The penile ejaculate; a thick, yellowish-white, viscid fluid containing sperms. SYN seminal fluid. **2.** SYN seed (1).

se·me·nu·ri·a (sē′mĕ-nyūr′ē-ă) The excretion of urine containing semen. SYN spermaturia, seminuria.

semi- Combining form denoting one-half; partly. Cf. hemi-.

S

sem·i·ca·nal (sem'ē-kă-nal') A half canal; a deep groove on the edge of a bone that, uniting with a similar groove or part of an adjoining bone, forms a complete canal. SYN semicanalis.

sem·i·closed an·es·the·si·a (sem'ē-klōzd an'es-thē'zē-ă) Inhalation anesthesia using a circuit in which a portion of the exhaled air is exhausted from the circuit and a portion is rebreathed following absorption of carbon dioxide.

sem·i·co·ma·tose, sem·i·co·ma, sem·i·con·scious (sem'ē-kō'mă-tōs, sem'ē-kō'mă, -kon'shŭs) An imprecise term for a state of drowsiness and inaction, in which more than ordinary stimulation may be required to evoke a response, and the response may be delayed or incomplete.

sem·i·con·duc·tor (sem'ē-kŏn-dŭk'tŏr) A metalloid that conducts electricity more easily than a true nonmetal but less easily than a metal, e.g., silicon, germanium.

sem·i·flex·ion (sem'ē-flek'shŭn) The position of a joint or segment of a limb midway between extension and flexion.

semi-Fow·ler po·si·tion (sem'ē-fowl'ěr pŏ-zish'ŭn) Placement of the patient in the inclined position, with the head of the bed elevated approximately 30 degrees. Cf. Fowler position.

sem·i·lu·nar (sem'ē-lū'năr) SYN lunar (2).

sem·i·lu·nar cusp (sem'ē-lū'năr kŭsp) One of three semilunar segments serving as the three cusps of a valve preventing regurgitation at the beginning of the aorta.

sem·i·lu·nar valve (sem'ē-lū'năr valv) [TA] A heart valve composed of a set of three semilunar cusps (valvules); hence, both the aortic and pulmonary valves are semilunar valves.

sem·i·mem·bra·nous (SM) (sem'ē-mem'bră-nŭs) Consisting partly of membrane; denoting the semimembranosus muscle.

sem·i·nal (sem'i-năl) **1.** Relating to semen. **2.** Original or influential of future developments.

sem·i·nal col·lic·u·lus (sem'i-năl kŏ-lik'yū-lŭs) [TA] Elevated portion of the urethral crest on which the two ejaculatory ducts and the prostatic utricle open.

sem·i·nal fluid (sem'i-năl flū'id) SYN semen (1).

sem·i·nal ves·i·cle (sem'i-năl ves'i-kěl) One of two folded, sacculated, glandular diverticula of the ductus deferens; one of the components of semen. SYN gonecyst, gonecystis, seminal gland.

sem·i·nif·er·ous (sem'i-nif'ěr-ŭs) Carrying or conducting semen.

sem·i·nif·er·ous ep·i·the·li·um (sem'i-nif'ěr-ŭs ep'i-thē'lē-ŭm) The epithelium lining the convoluted tubules of the testis where spermatogenesis and spermiogenesis occur.

sem·i·no·ma (sem'i-nō'mă) A radiosensitive malignant neoplasm usually arising from germ cells in the testis of young male adults that metastasizes to the paraortic lymph nodes.

sem·i·o·pen an·es·the·si·a (sem'ē-ō'pěn an'es-thē'zē-ă) Inhalation anesthesia in which a portion of inhaled gases is derived from an anesthesia circuit whereas the remainder consists of room air.

se·mi·ot·ic, se·mei·ot·ic (sě'mē-ot'ik, sē'mī-) **1.** Relating to semiotics. **2.** Relating to signs, linguistic or bodily.

sem·i·per·me·a·ble (sem'ē-pěr'mē-ă-běl) Freely permeable to water (or other solvent) but relatively impermeable to solutes.

sem·i·per·me·a·ble mem·brane (sem'ē-pěr'mē-ă-běl mem'brān) One relatively permeable to solvent but relatively impermeable to all or at least some of the solutes in either or both of the solutions separated by the membrane.

sem·i·po·lar bond (sem'ē-pō'lăr bond) A bond in which the two electrons shared by a pair of atoms belonged originally to only one of the atoms.

sem·i·prone (sem'ē-prōn') Denoting semipronation.

sem·i·re·cum·bent (sem'ē-rē-kŭm'bĕnt) Partly reclining. SYN Fowler position, semisupine position.

sem·i·sul·cus (sem'ē-sŭl'kŭs) A slight groove on the edge of a bone or other structure, which, uniting with a similar groove on the corresponding adjoining structure, forms a complete sulcus.

sem·i·su·pi·na·tion (sem'ē-sū'pi-nā'shŭn) The attitude or assumption of a partly supine position.

sem·i·su·pine (sem'ē-sū-pīn') Denoting semisupination.

sem·i·syn·thet·ic (sem'ē-sin-thet'ik) Describing the process of synthesizing a particular chemical using a naturally occurring chemical as a starting material, thus obviating part of a total synthesis.

sem·i·ten·di·no·sus (ST) (sem'ē-ten' di-nō'sŭs) SYN semitendinous.

sem·i·ten·di·nous (sem'ē-ten'di-nŭs) Descriptive of the heart's electrical axis when this is directed at approximately +60°.

se·ne·ci·o·sis (sĕ-nē'sē-ō'sis) Liver degeneration and necrosis caused by ingestion of plants of the genus *Senecio*, such as ragwort and groundsel.

se·nes·cence (sĕ-nes'ĕns) The state of being old.

se·nile (S) (sen'il) *Negative or pejorative connotations of this word may render it offensive in some contexts.* Relating to or characteristic of old age.

se·nile am·y·loi·do·sis (sen'il am'i-loy-dō'sis) Common form in very old people, usually mild and limited to the heart or seminal vesicles. SEE ALSO amyloidosis of aging.

se·nile ar·te·ri·o·scle·ro·sis (sen'il ahr-tēr'ē-ō-skler-ō'sis) A disorder similar to hypertensive arteriosclerosis, but resulting from advanced age rather than hypertension.

se·nile at·ro·phy (sen'il a'trō-fē) Wasting of tissues and organs with advancing age from decreased catabolic or anabolic processes, at times due to endocrine

changes, decreased use, or ischemia. SYN geromarasmus.

se·nile cat·a·ract (sen'il kat'ăr-akt) One occurring spontaneously in old people; mainly a cuneiform cataract, nuclear cataract, or posterior subcapsular cataract, alone or in combination.

se·nile de·men·ti·a (sen'il dĕ-men'shē-ă) Cognitive impairment first occurring in the seventh or eighth decade of life, usually due to Alzheimer disease (q.v.) or cerebrovascular impairment.

se·nile em·phy·se·ma (sen'il em'fi-sē' mă) Lung disorder consequent on the physiologic atrophy of old age.

se·nile ha·lo (sen'il hā'lō) Circumpapillary halo seen in choroidal atrophy of the aged.

se·nile he·man·gi·oma (sen'il hē-man' jē-ō'mă) Red papules caused by weakening of dermal capillary walls, which do not blanch on pressure, seen mostly in persons over 30 years of age. SYN cherry angioma, De Morgan spots.

se·nile in·vo·lution (sen'il in'vŏ-lū' shŭn) Retrogression of vital organs and psychological processes incident to aging.

se·nile ker·a·to·sis, ker·a·tosis se·ni·lis (sen'il ker'ă-tō'sis, si-nil'is) Benign flat, raised, or pedunculated lesions, colored yellow to dark brown; more usual on the trunk and increase in incidence after 40 years of age; may be known as basal cell papillomas because of their cells of origin but are not neoplastic and are not related to basal cell carcinomas. SYN seborrheic keratosis (2), keratosis seborrheica.

se·nile len·ti·go (sen'il len-tī'gō) A variably pigmented lentigo occurring on exposed skin of older white people. SYN liver spot.

se·nile me·la·no·der·ma (sen'il mel'ă-nō-dĕr'mă) Cutaneous pigmentation occurring in the aged.

se·nile plaque (sen'il plak) A spheric mass composed primarily of amyloid fibrils and interwoven neuronal processes, frequently, although not exclusively, observed in Alzheimer disease.

S

se·nile psy·cho·sis (sen'il sī-kō'sis) Mental disturbance in old age related to degenerative cerebral processes.

se·nile ret·i·nos·chi·sis (sen'il ret'i-nos'ki-sis) Degenerative ocular disorder occurring most often in the elderly and affecting the outer plexiform layer.

se·nile trem·or (sen'il trem'ŏr) An essential tremor that becomes symptomatic in the elderly.

se·nile vag·i·ni·tis (sen'il vaj'i-nī'tis) The atrophic form of the disorder resulting from withdrawal of estrogen stimulation of mucosa, often assuming the form of adhesive vaginitis.

se·nil·i·ty (sĕ-nil'i-tē) Old age; a general term for a variety of conditions seen in mental disorders occurring in old age, broken down into two broad categories, organic and psychological. SEE ALSO senile.

sen·sa·tion (sen-sā'shŭn) A feeling; translation into consciousness of stimulant effects exciting any sense organs.

sense (sens) The faculty of perceiving any stimulus.

sense of e·qui·lib·ri·um (sens ē'kwi-lib'rē-ŭm) The sense that makes possible a normal physiologic posture.

sense organs (sens ŏr'gănz) [TA] Organs of special sense, including the eye, ear, olfactory organ, taste organs, and the associated accessory structures. SYN organa sensuum.

sen·si·ble (sen'si-bĕl) **1.** Perceptible to the senses. **2.** Capable of sensation. **3.** SYN sensitive. **4.** Having reason or judgment; intelligent.

sen·si·tive (sen'si-tiv) **1.** Capable of perceiving sensations. **2.** Responding to a stimulus. **3.** Acutely perceptive of interpersonal situations. **4.** One who is readily hypnotizable. **5.** Readily undergoing a chemical change, with but slight change in environmental conditions. **6.** IMMUNOLOGY denoting: 1) a sensitized antigen; 2) a person (or animal) rendered susceptible to immunologic reactions by previous exposure to the antigen concerned. **7.** MICROBIOLOGY denoting a microorganism that is susceptible to inhibition or destruction

by a given antimicrobial agent. SYN sensible (3).

sen·si·tiv·i·ty (sen'si-tiv'i-tē) **1.** The ability to appreciate by means of one or more of the senses. **2.** State of being sensitive. **3.** CLINICAL PATHOLOGY proportion of patients with a given disease or condition in which a test intended to identify that disease or condition yields positive results. Cf. specificity (2). **4.** SYN susceptibility (2).

sen·si·tiv·i·ty train·ing group (sen'si-tiv'i-tē trān'ing grūp) Group members seek to develop self-awareness and an understanding of group processes rather than obtain therapy for an emotional disturbance. SEE ALSO encounter group.

sen·si·ti·za·tion (sen'si-tī-zā'shŭn) **1.** Immunization, especially with reference to antigens (immunogens) not associated with infection. **2.** In substance use/abuse parlance, the increased response seen to subsequent administration of the substance.

sen·si·tized cell (sen'si-tīzd sel) **1.** A cell that has combined with antibody to form a complex capable of reacting with complement components. **2.** A small, "committed," cell derived, by division and differentiation, from a transformed lymphocyte. **3.** A cell that has been either exposed to antigen or opsonized with antibodies and/or complement.

sen·so·mo·bile (sen'sō-mō'bil) Capable of movement in response to a stimulus.

sensori- Combining form denoting sensory.

sen·so·ri·al (sen-sōr'ē-ăl) Relating to the sensorium.

sen·so·ri·glan·du·lar (sen'sŏ-rē-glan'dyū-lăr) Relating to glandular secretion excited by sensory nerve stimulation.

sen·so·ri·mo·tor, sen·so·mo·tor (sen'sŏr-ē-mō'tŏr, sen'sō-) Both sensory and motor; denoting a mixed nerve with afferent and efferent fibers.

sen·so·ri·um, pl. **sen·so·ri·a**, pl. **sen·so·ri·ums** (sen-sōr'ē-ŭm, -ă, -ŭmz) **1.** An organ of sensation. **2.** The hypothetical "seat of sensation." **3.** PSYCHOLOGY consciousness; sometimes used as a generic term for the intellectual and cognitive functions.

sen·so·ri·vas·o·mo·tor (sen′sŏr-ē-vā′ sō-mō′tŏr) Denoting contraction or dilation of the blood vessels occurring as a sensory reflex. SYN sensorivascular.

sen·so·ry (sen′sŏr-ē) Relating to sensation.

sen·so·ry a·cu·i·ty lev·el (sen′sŏr-ē ă-kyū′i-tē lev′ĕl) A technique for determining air conduction thresholds with and without masking presented by bone conduction to the forehead; threshold change indicates conductive hearing loss.

sen·so·ry a·tax·i·a (sen′sŏr-ē ă-tak′sē-ă) Motor disorder due to impairment of position sense caused by lesions located at some point along the central or peripheral sensory pathways.

sen·so·ry con·flict (sen′sŏr-ē kon′flikt) A condition in which perceptions obtained through the senses of spatial orientation do not match; frequently produces nausea.

sen·so·ry de·fen·sive·ness (sen′sŏr-ē dĕ-fens′iv-nĕs) Overreaction to a nonnoxious sensory stimulus resulting in an adverse or defensive response. Types of sensory defensiveness may be associated with tactile, oral, auditory, olfactory, visual, or movement stimuli.

sen·so·ry dep·ri·va·tion (sen′sŏr-ē dep′ ri-vā′shŭn) Diminution or absence of usual external stimuli or perceptual experiences, commonly resulting in psychological distress and aberrant functioning if continued too long.

sen·so·ry ep·i·lep·sy (sen′sŏr-ē ep′i-lep′sē) Focal epilepsy initiated by a somatosensory phenomenon.

sen·so·ry nu·cle·i (sen′sŏr-ē nū′klē-ī) Group of cell bodies that receive afferent (sensory) input from the periphery.

sen·so·ry pa·ral·y·sis (sen′sŏr-ē păr-al′i-sis) Loss of sensation; anesthesia.

sen·tient (sen′chē-ĕnt) Capable of, or characterized by, sensation.

sen·ti·nel e·vent (sen′ti-nĕl ĕ-vent′) **1.** A type of clinical indicator used to monitor

and appraise the quality of care. **2.** NURSING any unexpected occurrence resulting in death, serious injury (e.g., physical, psychological, or other), or risk to the patient.

Sen·ti·nel E·vent No·ti·fi·ca·tion Sys·tem for Oc·cu·pa·tion·al Risks (SENSOR) (sen′ti-nĕl ĕ-vent′ nō′ti-fi-kā′shŭn sis′tĕm ok′yū-pā′shŭn-ăl risks) Program sponsored by the U.S. National Institute of Occupational Safety and Health in which occupational medicine clinicians report occupational diseases to the agency for follow-up and statistical analysis.

sen·ti·nel lymph node, sen·ti·nel node (sen′ti-nĕl limf nōd) The first lymph node to receive lymphatic drainage from a malignant tumor; increasingly used in operations for melanoma and breast cancer; if the sentinel node is free of metastasis, more distal nodes are also free. SEE ALSO signal lymph node.

sen·ti·nel pile (sen′ti-nĕl pīl) A circumscribed thickening of the mucous membrane at the lower end of a fissure of the anus.

sen·ti·nel tag (sen′ti-nĕl tag) Projecting edematous skin at the lower end of an anal fissure.

sep·a·rat·ing wire (sep′ăr-āt-ing wīr) Wire, usually soft brass, used to gain separation between teeth.

sep·a·ra·tion anx·i·e·ty dis·or·der (SAD) (sep-ă-rā′shŭn ang-zī′ĕ-tē dis-ŏr′dĕr) Pediatric mental disorder occurring in childhood characterized by excessive distress when the child is separated from someone to whom the child is attached, usually a parent.

sep·a·ra·tor (sep′ăr-ā-tŏr) **1.** That which divides or keeps apart two or more substances or prevents them from mingling. **2.** In dentistry, an instrument for forcing two teeth apart, so as to gain access to adjacent proximal walls. SYN segregator.

-sepsis Combining form meaning decay caused by a (specified) cause or of a (specified) sort.

sep·sis, pl. **sep·ses** (sep′sis, -sēz) Presence of various pus-forming and other pathogenic organisms, or their toxins, in blood or tissues; septicemia is a common type.

sep·sis syn·drome (sep'sis sin'drōm) Clinical evidence of acute infection with hyperthermia or hypothermia, tachycardia, tachypnea, and evidence of inadequate organ function or perfusion manifested by at least one of the following: altered mental status, hypoxemia, acidosis, oliguria, or disseminated intravascular coagulation.

sep·tal (sep'tăl) Relating to a septum.

sep·tate (sep'tāt) Having a septum; divided into compartments.

sep·tate u·ter·us (sep'tāt yū'tĕr-ŭs) A uterus divided into two cavities by an anteroposterior septum.

sep·tec·to·my (sep-tek'tŏ-mē) Operative removal of the whole or a part of a septum, specifically of the nasal septum.

♻ **septi-, septico-, sept-** Combining forms meaning seven.

sep·tic (sep'tik) Relating to or caused by sepsis.

sep·ti·ce·mi·a, blood poi·son·ing, sep·tic fe·ver (sep'ti-sē'mē-ă, blŭd poy'zŏn-ing, sep'tik fē'vĕr) A systemic disease caused by multiplication of microorganisms in circulating blood; formerly called ''blood poisoning.'' SEE ALSO pyemia. SYN septicaemia.

sep·ti·ce·mic plague (sep'ti-sē'mik plāg) Generally fatal form with intense bacteremia with symptoms of profound toxemia. SYN pestis siderans.

sep·ti·co·py·e·mi·a (sep'ti-kō-pī-ē'mē-ă) Pyemia and septicemia occurring together.

sep·tic shock (sep'tik shok) 1. Condition associated with sepsis and usually associated with abdominal and pelvic infection complicating trauma or operations. 2. Condition associated with septicemia caused by gram-negative bacteria.

sep·to·mar·gi·nal (sep'tō-mahr'ji-năl) Relating to the margin of a septum, or to both a septum and a margin.

sep·to·na·sal (sep'tō-nā'zăl) Relating to the nasal septum.

sep·to·op·tic dys·pla·si·a (sep'tō-op'tik dis-plā'zē-ă) Congenital, bilateral optic nerve hypoplasia associated with midline cerebral anomalies. SYN de Morsier syndrome.

sep·to·plas·ty (sep'tō-plas-tē) Surgery to correct defects or deformities of the nasal septum, often by alteration or partial removal of supporting structures.

sep·tos·to·my (sep-tos'tŏ-mē) Surgical creation of an artificial opening in a septum.

sep·tu·lum, pl. **sep·tu·la** (sep'tū-lŭm, -lă) A minute septum.

sep·tum, gen. **sep·ti,** pl. **sep·ta** (sep'tŭm, -tī, -tă) [TA] *The plural septa is sometimes mistaken for a singular form and wrongly pluralized as septae.* 1. A thin wall dividing two cavities or masses of softer tissue. 2. In fungi, a wall; usually a cross-wall in a hypha.

sep·tup·let (sep-tŭp'lĕt) One of seven children born at one birth.

se·que·la, gen. and pl. **se·que·lae** (sĕ-kwel'ă, -lē) A condition following as a consequence of a disease.

se·quence (sē'kwĕns) The succession, or following, of one thing or event after another.

se·ques·tra·tion (sē'kwes-trā'shŭn) 1. Formation of a sequestrum. 2. Loss of blood or of its fluid content into spaces within the body so that it is withdrawn from the circulating volume, resulting in hemodynamic impairment, and other conditions.

se·ques·trec·to·my (sē'kwes-trek'tŏ-mē) Operative removal of a sequestrum.

se·ques·trum, pl. **se·ques·tra** (sē-kwes'trŭm, -tră) Necrotic tissue, usually bone, which has become separated from the surrounding healthy tissue.

se·quoi·o·sis (sē'kwoy-ō'sis) Extrinsic allergic alveolitis caused by inhalation of fungal redwood sawdust.

Ser Abbreviation for serine and its radical.

ser·en·dip·i·ty (ser'ĕn-dip'i-tē) A knack for discovery involving a combination of accident and wisdom while pursuing something else; in science, finding one thing while looking for something else.

se·ri·al di·lu·tion (sēr'ē-ăl di-lū'shŭn) The preparation of a graded set of solutions or suspensions, each member of the set being a fixed dilution (typically 1:2) of the preceding member; used particularly in titration of antibodies in serum.

se·ri·al ex·trac·tion (sēr'ē-ăl ek-strak'shŭn) Selective removal of certain teeth during the early years of dental development to relieve crowding of anterior teeth.

se·ri·al ra·di·og·ra·phy (sēr'ē-ăl rā'dē-og'ră-fē) Making several x-ray exposures of a single region over a period of time, as in angiography.

se·ri·al sec·tion (sēr'ē-ăl sek'shŭn) One of a number of consecutive microscopic sections.

ser·ies, pl. **ser·ies** (sēr'ēz) **1.** A succession of similar objects following one another in space or time. **2.** CHEMISTRY a group of substances, either elements or compounds, having similar properties or differing from each other in composition by a constant ratio.

ser·ine (S, Ser) (sĕr'ēn) One of the amino acids occurring in proteins.

sero- Combining form denoting serum, serous.

se·ro·con·ver·sion (sēr'ō-kŏn-vĕr'zhŭn) Process by which, after exposure to the etiologic agent of a disease, blood changes from a negative to a positive serum marker for it.

se·ro·di·ag·no·sis (sēr'ō-dī'ăg-nō'sis) Diagnosis with a reaction using blood serum or other serous fluids in the body (serologic tests).

se·ro·ep·i·de·mi·ol·o·gy (sēr'ō-ep'i-dĕ'mē-ol'ŏ-jē) An epidemiologic study based on the detection of infection by serologic testing.

se·ro·fib·rin·ous (sēr'ō-fī'bri-nŭs) Denoting an exudate composed of serum and fibrin.

se·ro·fi·brous (sēr'ō-fī'brŭs) Relating to a serous membrane and a fibrous tissue.

se·ro·group (sēr'ō-grūp) **1.** A group of bacteria containing a common antigen, used to classify certain genera of bacteria. **2.** A group of antigenically closely related viral species.

se·ro·log·ic, se·ro·log·ic·al (sēr'ō-loj'ik, -ăl) Relating to serology.

se·rol·o·gy (sēr-ol'ŏ-jē) The branch of science concerned with serum, especially with specific immune or lytic serums.

se·ro·ma (sēr-ō'mă) A mass or tumefaction caused by the localized accumulation of serum within a tissue or organ.

se·ro·mem·bra·nous (sēr'ō-mem'bră-nŭs) Relating to a serous membrane.

se·ro·mu·coid (sēr'ō-myū'koyd) General term for a mucoprotein (glycoprotein) from serum.

se·ro·mu·cous (sēr'ō-myū'kŭs) Pertaining to a mixture of watery and mucinous material, such as that of certain glands.

se·ro·mu·cous gland (sēr'ō-myū'kŭs gland) **1.** Gland in which some secretory cells are serous and some mucous. **2.** Gland with cells that secrete a fluid intermediate varying between a watery and a more viscous mucoid substance. SYN glandula seromucosa.

se·ro·neg·a·tive (SN) (sēr'ō-neg'ă-tiv) Lacking an antibody of a specific type in serum.

se·ro·pos·i·tive (SP) (sēr'ō-poz'i-tiv) Containing antibody of a specific type in serum.

ser·o·prev·a·lence (ser-ō-prev'ă-lens) Prevalence of a marker as measured by results of serologic testing.

se·ro·pu·ru·lent (sēr-ō-pyūr'ŭ-lĕnt) Composed of or containing both serum and pus; denoting a discharge (seropus).

se·ro·pus (sēr'ō-pŭs) Purulent serum, i.e., pus largely diluted with serum.

se·ro·re·ver·sion (SR) (sĕ'rō-rĕ-vĕr'zhŭn) A loss in serologic reactivity; may be spontaneous or in response to therapy.

S

se•ro•sa (sĕr-ō'să) [TA] The outermost coat or serous layer of a visceral structure that lies in a body cavity (abdomen or thorax).

se•ro•san•guin•e•ous (sĕr'ō-sang-gwin'ē-ŭs) Denoting an exudate or a discharge containing both serum and blood.

se•ro•se•rous (sĕr'ō-sĕr'ŭs) **1.** Relating to two serous surfaces. **2.** Denoting a suture, as of the intestine, in which the edges of the wound are infolded so as to bring the two serous surfaces in apposition.

se•ro•si•tis (sĕr'ō-sī'tis) Inflammation of a serous membrane.

se•ros•i•ty (sĕr-os'i-tē) **1.** A serous fluid or a serum. **2.** The condition of being serous. **3.** The serous quality of a liquid.

se•ro•syn•o•vi•tis (sĕr'ō-sin'ō-vī'tis) Synovitis attended with a copious serous effusion.

se•ro•ther•a•py (sĕr'ō-thār'ă-pē) Treatment of an infectious disease by injection of an antitoxin or serum containing specific antibody.

se•ro•to•ner•gic (ser'ō-tō-nĕr'jik) Related to the action of serotonin or its precursor L-tryptophan.

ser•o•to•nin (ser'ō-tō'nin) A vasoconstrictor, liberated by platelets; inhibits gastric secretion and stimulates smooth muscle; also acts as a neurotransmitter.

se•ro•type (sĕr'ō-tīp) SYN serovar.

se•rous (sĕr'ŭs) *Do not confuse this word with scirrhous.* Relating to, containing, or producing serum or a substance having a watery consistency.

se•rous cell (sĕr'ŭs sel) A cell, especially of the salivary gland, which secretes a watery or thin albuminous fluid.

se•rous gland (sĕr'ŭs gland) One that secretes a watery substance that may or may not contain an enzyme.

se•rous in•flam•ma•tion (sĕr'ŭs in'flă-mā'shŭn) An exudative inflammation in which the exudate is predominantly fluid; relatively few cells are observed.

se•rous i•ri•tis (sĕr'ŭs ī-rī'tis) Inflammation of the iris, with a serous exudate in the anterior chamber.

se•rous men•in•gi•tis (sĕr'ŭs men'in-jī'tis) Acute form of the disease with secondary external hydrocephalus.

se•rous o•ti•tis (sĕr'ŭs ō-tī'tis) Inflammation of middle ear mucosa, often accompanied by accumulation of fluid. SYN secretory otitis media.

se•rous sy•no•vi•tis (sĕr'ŭs sin'ō-vī'tis) Inflammation of the synovial membrane with a large effusion of nonpurulent fluid.

se•ro•vac•ci•na•tion (sĕr'ō-vak'si-nā'shŭn) A process for producing mixed immunity by the injection of a serum, to secure passive immunity, and by vaccination with a modified or killed culture to acquire active immunity later.

se•ro•var (sv.) (sĕr'ō-vahr) A subdivision of a species or subspecies distinguishable from other strains based on antigenicity. SYN serotype.

ser•pig•i•nous (sĕr-pij'i-nŭs) Creeping serpentine.

ser•rate su•ture (ser'ăt sū'chŭr) One with opposing margins that present deep, saw-like indentations, as in most of the sagittal sutures.

Ser•ra•ti•a (sĕ-rā'shē-ă) A genus of motile, peritrichous, aerobic to facultatively anaerobic bacteria saprophytic on decaying plant and animal materials. The type species is *Serratia marcescens.*

ser•ra•tion (ser-ā'shŭn) **1.** The state of being serrated or notched. **2.** Any one of the processes in a serrate or dentate formation.

Ser•to•li cells (ser-tō'lē selz) Elongated cells in the seminiferous tubules that ensheathe spermatogenic cells, providing a microenvironment that supports spermiogenesis and spermatocytogenesis. SYN nurse cells.

Ser•to•li-Ley•dig cell tu•mor (ser-tō'lē-lī'dig sel tū'mŏr) An ovarian tumor composed of Sertoli and Leydig cells; may secrete androgens.

se•rum (sēr′ŭm, -ă, -ŭmz) **1.** A clear, watery fluid, especially that moistening the surface of serous membranes, or exuded in inflammation of any of those membranes. **2.** Fluid portion of the blood obtained after removal of the fibrin clot and blood cells. Sometimes a synonym for antiserum or antitoxin.

se•rum ac•cel•er•a•tor glob•u•lin (sēr′ŭm ak-sel′ĕr-ā-tŏr glob′yū-lin) A substance in serum that accelerates the conversion of prothrombin to thrombin in the presence of thromboplastin and calcium.

ser•um ag•glu•ti•nin (sēr′ŭm ă-glū′ti-nin) An antibody that coats erythrocytes. SYN incomplete antibody (2).

se•rum•al (sēr′ŭ-măl) Relating to or derived from serum.

se•rum al•bu•min (sēr′ŭm al-bū′min) The principal protein in plasma, present in blood plasma and in serous fluids. Participates in fatty acid transport and helps regulate the osmotic pressure of blood. SYN blood albumin, seralbumin.

se•rum-fast (sēr′ŭm-fast) **1.** Pertaining to a serum with little or no change in the titer of antibody, even with treatment or immunologic stimulation. **2.** Resistant to the destructive effect of sera.

se•rum shock (sēr′ŭm shok) Anaphylactic or anaphylactoid shock due to injection of antitoxin or other foreign serum.

se•rum sick•ness, se•rum re•ac•tion (sēr′ŭm sik′nĕs, rē-ak′shŭn) An immune complex disease appearing 1–2 weeks after injection of a foreign serum or serum protein, with local and systemic reactions. SYN serum disease, serum reaction.

ser•vo•mech•a•nism (sēr′vō-mek′ă-nizm) **1.** A control system using negative feedback to operate another system. **2.** A process that behaves as a self-regulatory device.

ses•a•me oil (ses′ă-mē oyl) Refined fixed oil intramuscular injections. SYN benne oil, gingili oil, teel oil.

ses•a•moid (ses′ă-moyd) **1.** Resembling in size or shape of a sesame seed. **2.** Denoting a sesamoid bone.

ses•qui•hy•drates (ses′kwi-hī′drāts) Compounds crystallizing with (nominally) 1.5 molecules of water.

ses•sile (sess) (ses′il) Having a broad base of attachment.

se•ta•ceous (sē-tā′shŭs) **1.** Having bristles. **2.** Resembling a bristle.

set•back (set′bak) Surgery to treat bilateral cleft of the palate in which the premaxilla is moved posteriorly; often accompanied by bone grafting.

set•ting sun sign (set′ing sŭn sīn) Retraction of the upper lid without upgaze so that the iris seems to ''set'' below the lower lid.

se•vere acute res•pi•ra•tory syn•drome (SARS) (sĕ-vēr′ ă-kyūt′ res′pir-ă-tōr-ē sin′drōm) Highly contagious, severe febrile respiratory illness caused by a coronavirus (SARS-CoV).

se•vere com•bined im•mu•no•de•fi•cien•cy (SCID) (sĕ-vēr′ kŏm-bīnd′ im′yū-nō-dĕ-fish′ĕn-sē) Immunodeficiency with absence of both humoral and cellular immunity with lymphopenia; characterized by thymus atrophy, lack of delayed hypersensitivity, and marked susceptibility to infections by bacteria, viruses, fungi, protozoa, and live vaccines; although bone marrow transplants have been effective, death may occur in the first year of life.

sex (seks) **1.** Biologic character or quality that distinguishes male and female as expressed by analysis of the person's gonadal, morphologic (internal and external), chromosomal, and hormonal characteristics. Cf. gender. **2.** The physiologic and psychological processes within a person that prompt behavior related to procreation or erotic pleasure.

sex cell (seks sel) A sperm or an oocyte.

sex chro•ma•tin (seks krō′mă-tin) A small, condensed mass of the inactivated X-chromosome usually located just inside the nuclear membrane of the interphase nucleus. SYN Barr chromatin body.

sex chro•mo•somes (seks krō′mŏ-sōmz) Chromosomal pair responsible for sex determination. In humans and most animals, the sex chromosomes are designated X and Y; females have two X chromosomes, males have one X and one Y chromosome.

sex de•ter•mi•na•tion (seks dĕ-tĕr′mi-nā′shŭn) Identification of the sex of a fetus in utero by identification of fetal chromosomes.

sex hor•mone-bind•ing glob•u•lin (seks hōr′mōn-bīnd′ing glob′yū-lin) Plasma β-globulin, produced by the liver, which binds testosterone and, with a weaker affinity, estrogen; serum levels in women are twice those found in men. SYN testosterone-estrogen-binding globulin.

sex hor•mones (seks hōr′mōnz) A general term covering those steroid hormones that are formed by testicular, ovarian, and adrenocortical tissues, and that are androgens or estrogens.

sex-in•flu•enced (seks-in′flū-ĕnst) Denoting a class of genetic disorders in which the same genotype has differing manifestations in the two sexes. SEE ALSO sex-influenced inheritance.

sex-in•flu•enced in•her•i•tance (seks-in′flū-ĕnst in-her′i-tăns) Inheritance that is autosomal but has a different intensity of expression in the two sexes (e.g., male pattern baldness).

sex•i•va•lent (sek′si-vā′lĕnt) Having a valence of six.

sex-lim•it•ed (seks-lim′i-tĕd) Occurring in one sex only. SEE sex-limited inheritance.

sex-lim•it•ed in•her•i•tance (seks-lim′i-tĕd in-her′i-tăns) Inheritance of a trait that can be expressed in one sex only.

sex link•age, sex-linked (seks lingk′ăj, seks′lingkt) Inheritance of a trait or a sex chromosome or gonosome. A man receives all his sex-linked genes from his mother and transmits them all to his daughters but not to his sons; a recessive sex-linked character is much more likely to be expressed in the male.

sex-linked cha•rac•ter (seks′lingkt kar′ăk-tĕr) An inherited character determined by a gene on a gonosome. SEE sex linkage, gene.

sex-link•ed in•her•i•tance (seks′lingkt in-her′i-tăns) The pattern of inheritance that may result from a mutant gene located on either the X or Y chromosome.

sex•ol•o•gy (seks-ol′ŏ-jē) The scientific study of all aspects of sex, including differentiation and dimorphism, and, particularly, sexual behavior.

sex ra•ti•o (seks rā′shē-ō) 1. The ratio of male to female progeny at some specified stage of the life cycle, notably at conception (primary), at birth (secondary), or at any stage between birth and death (tertiary). 2. The ratio of the numbers of males to females affected by a particular disease or trait.

sex•tant (seks′tănt) One of the six divisions of the dentition, the teeth of the upper and lower jaws being divided into right posterior, left posterior, and anterior.

sex•tup•let (seks-tŭp′lĕt) One of six children carried through a single pregnancy and born together.

sex•u•al de•vi•a•tion (sek′shū-ăl dē′vē-ā′shŭn) Sexual practice that is biologically atypical, considered morally wrong, or legally prohibited. SEE bestiality, pedophilia.

sex•u•al dis•or•ders (sek′shū-ăl dis′ŏr-dĕrs) Behavioral and psychophysiologic disorders in which there is symptomatic variability in sexual functioning, including either the eroticized behavior associated with sexual activity (the paraphilias) or with disturbances of desire, arousal, and orgasm.

sex•u•al gen•er•a•tion (sek′shū-ăl jen′ĕr-ā′shŭn) Reproduction by conjugation, or the union of male and female cells, as opposed to asexual generation.

sex•u•al in•fan•ti•lism (sek′shū-ăl in-fan′ti-lizm) Failure to develop secondary sexual characteristics after the normal time of puberty.

sex•u•al•i•ty (sek′shū-al′i-tē) 1. The sum of a person's sexual behaviors and tendencies, and the strength of such tendencies. 2. One's degree of sexual attractiveness. 3. The quality of having sexual functions or implications.

sex·u·al·ly   trans·mit·ted   dis·ease (STD) (sek′shū-ă-lē tranz-mit′ĕd di-zēz′) Any contagious disease acquired during sexual contact (e.g., syphilis, gonorrhea, chancroid); also called sexually transmitted infection (STI). SYN venereal disease.

sex·u·al re·pro·duc·tion (sek′shū-ăl rē′prŏ-dŭk′shŭn) Reproduction by union of male and female gametes (germ cells) to form a zygote. SYN gamogenesis, syngenesis.

Sé·za·ry syn·drome (sā-zah-rē′ sin′drŏm) Exfoliative dermatitis with intense pruritus, resulting from cutaneous infiltration by atypical mononuclear cells also found in the peripheral blood, and associated with alopecia, edema, and nail and pigmentary changes; a variant of mycosis fungoides. SYN Sézary erythroderma.

Sg Abbreviation for seaborgium.

shad·ow-cast·ing (shad′ō-kast′ing) Vacuum evaporation and deposition of a film of carbon or metals on a contoured microscopic object to allow the object to be seen in relief with an electron microscope or sometimes with a light microscope.

shaft (shaft) An elongated rodlike structure, as the part of a long bone between the epiphysial extremities. SYN diaphysis [TA].

sha·green skin (shă-grēn′ skin) An oval-shaped nevoid plaque, skin colored or occasionally pigmented, smooth or crinkled, appearing on the trunk or lower back in early childhood.

shakes (shāks) Vernacular term for a paroxysm associated with an intermittent fever and with tremor associated with alcohol (and other substance) withdrawal.

sham rage (sham rāj) Quasiemotional state, characterized by manifestations of fear and anger on trifling provocation.

shank (shangk) 1. The tibia; the shin; the leg. 2. The portion of an instrument that connects the cutting or functional portion to a handle; with rotary tools, such as burs and drills, the end that fits into the chuck.

shap·ing (shāp′ing) In operant conditioning, when the operant response is not in the organism's repertoire, a procedure in which the experimenter breaks down the response into those parts that appear most frequently, begins reinforcing them, and then slowly and successively withholds the reinforcer until more and more of the operant is emitted.

shave bi·op·sy (shāv bī′op-sē) A biopsy technique performed with a surgical blade or a razorblade; used for lesions that are elevated above the skin level or confined to the epidermis and upper dermis, or to protrusions of lesions from internal sites.

shear (shēr) The distortion of a body by two oppositely directed parallel forces. The distortion consists of a sliding over one another of imaginary planes (within the body) parallel to the planes of the forces.

sheath (shēth) 1. Any enveloping structure. SYN vagina (1). 2. The prepuce of male animals, especially of the horse. 3. A specially designed tubular instrument through which special obturators or cutting instruments can be passed, or through which blood clots, tissue fragments, or calculi can be evacuated. 4. A tube used as an orthodontic appliance, usually on molars.

Shee·han syn·drome (shē′an sin′drŏm) Hypopituitarism developing postpartum as a result of pituitary necrosis; caused by ischemia resulting from a hypotensive episode during delivery.

shell nail (shel nāl) Nail dystrophy accompanying clubbing of digits in bronchiectasis, with excessive longitudinal curvature of the nail plate and atrophy of the nail bed and underlying bone.

Shen·ton line (shen′tŏn līn) A curved line formed by the top of the obturator foramen and the inner side of the neck of the femur, normal disturbed dislocation or fracture of the joint.

Shep·herd frac·ture (shep′ĕrd frak′shūr) A fracture of the external tubercle (posterior process) of the talus.

shi·at·su (shē-aht′sū) A Japanese massage technique using direct pressure, passive and active stretching, and gentle rocking movements to restore balance in the flow of energy in the body.

Shib·ley sign (shib′lē sīn) On auscultation of the chest, the spoken sound ''e'' is heard as ''ah'' over an area of pulmonary consolidation or immediately above a pleural effusion.

shield (shēld) A protecting screen; lead sheet for protecting the operator and patient from x-rays.

shift to the left (shift left) **1.** Marked increase in the percentage of immature cells in the circulating blood, based on the premise in hematology that the bone marrow with its immature myeloid cells is on the left, whereas the circulating blood with its mature neutrophils is on the right; SYN deviation to the left. **2.** SEE maturation index.

shift to the right (shift rīt) **1.** In a differential count of white blood cells in the peripheral blood, the absence of young and immature forms. **2.** SEE maturation index.

Shi·gel·la **(Shig, S)** (shē-gel′lă) A genus of nonmotile, aerobic to facultatively anaerobic bacteria; normal habitat is the intestinal tract of humans and of higher apes; all of the species produce dysentery.

Shi·gel·la son·ne·i (shĭ-gel′lă son′ē-ī) Bacterial species causing dysentery, sometimes milder than that caused by other species. Most common pathogenic species in the U.S.

shig·el·lo·sis (shig′ĕ-lō′sis) Bacillary dysentery caused by bacteria of the genus *Shigella*, often occurring in epidemic patterns; an opportunistic infection in people with acquired immunodefiency syndrome.

shim (shim) In magnetic resonance imaging, fine adjustment of the magnetic field to improve uniformity.

shin (shin) The anterior aspect of the leg, from knee to ankle.

Shi·rod·kar op·er·a·tion (shī-rod′kahr op-ĕr-ā′shŭn) Cerclage procedure done by purse-string suturing of an incompetent cervical os with a nonabsorbent suture material.

shirt-stud ab·scess (shĭrt′stŭd ab′ses) SYN collar-button abscess.

shiv·er·ing (shiv′ĕr-ing) Trembling resulting from cold or fear. Dogs may also shiver with anticipation, in a state of excitement.

shock (shok) **1.** A sudden physical or mental disturbance. **2.** A state of profound mental and physical depression consequent to severe physical injury or an emotional disturbance. **3.** A severe disturbance of hemodynamics in which the circulatory system fails to maintain adequate perfusion of vital organs. **4.** Abnormally palpable impact, appreciated by a hand on the chest wall, of an accentuated heart sound.

shock lung (shok lŭng) In shock, the development of edema, impaired perfusion, and reduction in alveolar space so that the alveoli collapse. SYN pump lung, white lung.

shock the·ra·py, shock treat·ment (shok thār′ă-pē, trēt′mĕnt) SEE electroshock therapy.

Shone a·nom·al·y (shōn ă-nom′ă-lē) Coarctation of the aorta, subaortic stenosis, and stenosing ring of the left atrium found in association with a parachute mitral valve.

short-bow·el syn·drome, short-gut syn·drome (shōrt bow′ĕl sin′drŏm, gŭt) Malabsorption and maldigestion resulting from disease or resection of large portions of the small intestine.

short in·cre·ment sen·si·ti·v·ity in·dex (SISI) (shōrt in′krĕ-mĕnt sen′si-tiv′ i-tē in′deks) Measure of the ability to detect small (1dB) increments in intensity; with cochlear lesions, this ability exceeds normal.

short stat·ure (SS) (shōrt stach′ŭr) In pediatrics, height below the third percentile when plotted on a growth chart.

short-term mem·o·ry (STM) (shōrt-tĕrm mem′ŏr-ē) Phase of the memory process in which stimuli that have been recognized and registered are stored briefly; decay occurs rapidly, sometimes within seconds, but may be held indefinitely by using rehearsal as a holding process by which to recycle material over and over through STM. SYN temporary memory.

short wave di·a·ther·my (shōrt wāv dī′ ă-thĕr-mē) Therapeutic elevation of temperature in the tissues by means of an oscillating electric current of extremely high frequency (10–100 million Hz) and short wavelength of 3–30 meters.

shot-silk ret·i·na (shot-silk ret′i-nă) Appearance of numerous wavelike, glistening reflexes observed sometimes in the retina of a young person.

shoul·der ap·pre·hen·sion sign (shōl′ dĕr ap′prē-hen′shŭn sīn) A physical finding in which placement of the humerus in the position of abduction to 90 degrees and maximum external rotation produces anxiety and resistance in patients with a history of anterior glenohumeral instability.

shoul·der gir·dle (shōl′dĕr gĭr′dĕl) The bony ring, incomplete behind, which serves to attach and support the upper limbs; formed by the manubrium sterni, clavicles, and scapulae. SYN pectoral girdle, shoulder complex (3).

shoul·der pre·sen·ta·tion (shōl′dĕr prez′ĕn-tā′shŭn) In obstetrics, transverse presentation with the fetal shoulder as the presenting part.

show (shō) **1.** An appearance. **2.** First appearance of blood in beginning menstruation. **3.** Sign of impending labor, characterized by the discharge from the vagina of a small amount of blood-tinged mucus representing the extrusion of the mucous plug that has filled the cervical canal during pregnancy.

shunt (shŭnt) **1.** To bypass or divert. **2.** A bypass or diversion of fluid to another fluid-containing system by fistulation or a prosthetic device. SEE ALSO bypass.

shunt cy·a·no·sis (shŭnt sī′ă-nō′sis) Blue color of the entire skin or a region of the skin or mucous membrane due to a right-to-left shunt permitting unoxygenated blood to reach the left side of the circulation.

Shwach·man syn·drome, Shwach·man-Di·a·mond syn·drome (shwahk′ măn sin′drōm, dī′ă-mŏnd) Disorder characterized by sinusitis, bronchiectasis,

pancreatic insufficiency resulting in malabsorption, neutropenia with defect in neutrophile chemotaxis, short stature, and skeletal changes with radiographic findings of metaphysial flaring of long bones.

Si Abbreviation for silicon.

si·al·a·gogue, si·al·o·gogue (sī-al′ă-gog, -ŏ-gog) **1.** Promoting the flow of saliva. **2.** Agent with this action.

si·al·ic ac·ids (sī-al′ik as′idz) Esters and other *N*- and *O*-acyl derivatives of neuraminic acid.

si·a·lism (sī′ă-lizm) An excess secretion of saliva.

sialo-, sial- Combining forms denoting saliva.

si·a·lo·ad·e·nec·to·my (sī′ă-lō-ad′ĕ-nek′ tŏ-mē) Excision of a salivary gland.

si·a·lo·ad·e·not·o·my (sī′ă-lō-ad′ĕ-not′ ŏ-mē) Incision of a salivary gland.

si·a·lo·aer·oph·a·gy (sī′ă-lō-ār-of′ă-jē) A habit of frequent swallowing whereby quantities of saliva and air are taken into the stomach. SYN aerosialophagy.

si·a·lo·an·gi·ec·ta·sis (sī′ă-lō-an′jē-ek′ tă-sis) Dilation of salivary ducts.

si·a·lo·an·gi·i·tis (sī′ă-lō-an′jē-ī′tis) Inflammation of a salivary duct.

si·a·lo·do·chi·tis (sī′ă-lō-dō-kī′tis) Inflammation of the duct of a salivary gland. SYN sialoangiitis.

si·a·lo·do·cho·plas·ty (sī′ă-lō-dō′kō-plas′tē) Repair of a salivary duct.

si·a·log·e·nous (sī′ă-loj′ĕ-nŭs) Producing saliva.

si·a·log·ra·phy (sī′ă-log′ră-fē) Radiography of the salivary glands and ducts after the introduction of contrast medium into the ducts.

si·al·o·lith (sī′ă-lō-lith) A salivary calculus.

si·a·lo·li·thi·a·sis (sī′ă-lō-li-thī′ă-sis) The formation or presence of a salivary calculus.

si·a·lo·li·thot·o·my (sī'ă-lō-li-thot'ŏ-mē) Incision of a salivary duct or gland to remove a calculus.

si·a·lo·met·a·pla·si·a (sī'ă-lō-met'ă-plā'zē-ă) Squamous cell metaplasia in the salivary ducts.

si·a·lor·rhe·a (sī'ă-lōr-ē'ă) Excessive flow of saliva. SEE salivation. SYN hygrostomia, sialism, sialismus, sialosis.

si·a·los·che·sis (sī'ă-los'kĕ-sis) Suppression of the secretion of saliva.

si·a·lo·ste·no·sis (sī'ă-lō-stĕ-nō'sis) Stricture of a salivary duct.

Si·a·mese twins (sī'ă-mēz' twinz) A much publicized pair of conjoined twins born in Thailand (then Siam) in the 19th century; this term has since come into general lay usage for any type of conjoined twins.

sib (sib) A member of a sibship.

Si·ber·ian gin·seng (sī-bēr'ē-ăn jin'seng) (*Eleutherococcus senticosus*) Herbal remedy purported of value in lowering blood pressure and increasing stamina. The latter has been ruled out by results of clinical studies. SYN touch-me-not.

Si·be·ri·an tick ty·phus (sī-bēr'ē-ăn tik tī'fŭs) Tick-borne rickettsiosis caused by infection with *Rickettsia sibirica*.

sib·i·lant (sib'i-lănt) Hissing or whistling in character; a form of rhonchus.

sib·i·lant rale (sib'i-lănt rahl) A whistling sound caused by air moving through a viscid secretion narrowing the lumen of a bronchus.

sib·ling ri·val·ry (sib'ling rī'văl-rē) Jealous competition among children, especially for the attention, affection, and esteem of their parents; by extension, a factor in both normal and abnormal competitiveness throughout life.

sib·ship (sib'ship) **1.** The reciprocal state between individuals who have the same pair of parents. **2.** All progeny of one pair of parents.

si·bu·tra·mine (si-byū'tră-mēn) A serotonin and noradrenaline reuptake inhibitor used to reduce appetite to encourage weight loss.

sicklaemia [Br.] SYN sicklemia.

sick·le cell (sik'ĕl sel) An abnormal, crescentic erythrocyte characteristic of sickle cell anemia. SEE ALSO sicklemia, sickling. SYN drepanocyte.

sick·le cell a·ne·mi·a (sik'ĕl sel ă-nē'mē-ă) An autosomal dominant anemia characterized by crescentic or sickle-shaped erythrocytes and by accelerated hemolysis, due to substitution of a single amino acid (valine for glutamic acid) in the sixth position of the beta chain of hemoglobin. Homozygotes develop "crises": episodes of severe pain due to microvascular occlusions, bone infarcts, leg ulcers, and atrophy of the spleen associated with increased susceptibility to bacterial infections, especially streptococcal pneumonia. Occurs almost exclusively in blacks. SYN crescent cell anemia, sickle cell disease.

sick·le cell C dis·ease (sik'ĕl sel di-zēz') A disorder resulting from abnormal sickle-shaped erythrocytes (containing hemoglobin C and S) that appear in response to a lowering of the partial pressure of oxygen; characterized by anemia, crises due to hemolysis or vascular occlusion, chronic leg ulcers and bone deformities, and infarcts of bone or of the spleen.

sick·le cell ret·i·nop·a·thy (sik'ĕl sel ret'i-nop'ă-thē) A condition marked by dilation and tortuosity of retinal veins, and by microaneurysms and retinal hemorrhages; advanced stages may show neovascularization, vitreous hemorrhage, or retinal detachment.

sick·le cell trait (SCT) (sik'ĕl sel trāt) Heterozygous state of the gene for hemoglobin S in sickle cell anemia.

sick·le·mi·a (sik-lē'mē-ă) Presence of sickle- or crescent-shaped erythrocytes in peripheral blood; seen in sickle cell anemia and sickle cell trait. SYN sicklaemia.

sick·ling (sik'ling) Production of sickle-shaped erythrocytes in the circulation, as in sickle cell anemia.

sick si·nus syn·drome (SSS) (sik sī'

nŭs sin′drōm) Symptoms ranging from dizziness to unconsciousness due to chaotic or absent atrial activity often with bradycardia alternating with tachycardia, recurring ectopic beats including escape beats, runs of supraventricular and ventricular arrhythmias, sinus arrest, and sinuatrial block.

side chain (sīd chān) A chain of noncyclic atoms linked to a benzene ring, or to any cyclic chain compound.

side ef·fect (SE) (sīd e-fekt′) SYN adverse effect.

sidero- Combining form meaning iron.

sid·er·o·blast (SB) (sid′ĕr-ō-blast) An erythroblast containing granules of ferritin stained by the Prussian blue reaction.

sid·er·o·blas·tic a·ne·mi·a, sid·er·o·a·chres·tic a·ne·mi·a (SBA) (sid′ĕr-ō-blast′ik ă-nē′mē-ă, sid′ĕr-ō-ă-krest′ik) Refractory anemia characterized by the presence of sideroblasts in the bone marrow.

sid·er·o·cyte (sid′ĕr-ō-sīt) An erythrocyte containing granules of free iron, as detected by the Prussian blue reaction, in the blood of normal fetuses, where they constitute 0.10–4.5% of erythrocytes.

sid·er·o·fi·bro·sis (sid′ĕr-ō-fī-brō′sis) Fibrosis associated with small foci in which iron is deposited.

sid·er·o·pe·ni·a (sid′ĕr-ō-pē′nē-ă) An abnormally low level of serum iron.

sid·er·o·phil, sid·er·o·phile, sid·er·oph·i·lous (sid′ĕr-ō-fil, -fīl, -of′i-lŭs) **1.** Absorbing iron. **2.** A cell or tissue that contains iron.

sid·er·o·phore (sid′ĕr-ō-fōr) A large, extravasated, mononuclear phagocyte containing granules of hemosiderin, found in the sputum or in the lungs of people with long-standing pulmonary congestion from left ventricular failure. SYN siderophage.

sid·er·o·sil·i·co·sis (sid′ĕr-ō-sil′i-kō′sis) Silicosis due to inhalation of dust containing iron and silica.

sid·er·o·sis (sid′ĕr-ō′sis) **1.** Pneumoconiosis due to the presence of iron dust.

2. Discoloration of any part by desposition of a pigment containing iron; usually called hemosiderosis. **3.** An excess of iron in the circulating blood. **4.** Degeneration of the retina, lens, and uvea as a result of the deposition of intraocular iron.

sie·mens (S) (sē′mĕnz) The SI unit of electrical conductance.

sie·vert (Sv) (sē′vĕrt) The SI unit of ionizing radiation effective dose, equal to the absorbed dose in gray, weighted for both the quality of radiation in question and the tissue response to that radiation. SEE ALSO effective dose.

sigh (sī) **1.** An audible emotional inspiration and expiration. **2.** To perform such an act.

sight (sīt) The ability or faculty of seeing. SEE ALSO vision.

sig·ma, σ (sig′mă) **1.** The 18th letter of the Greek alphabet (σ, Σ). **2.** (σ) Denotes reflection coefficient; standard deviation; a factor in prokaryotic RNA initiation; surface tension. **3.** (Σ) Summation of a series.

sig·moid (sig′moyd) Resembling in outline the letter S or one of the forms of the Greek sigma.

sig·moid co·lon, sig·moid flex·ure (sig′moyd kō′lŏn, fleks′yūr) [TA] Colonic part describing an S-shaped curve between the pelvic brim and the third sacral segment; continuous with the rectum. SYN colon sigmoideum [TA].

sig·moi·dec·to·my (sig′moy-dek′tŏ-mē) Excision of the sigmoid colon.

sig·moid·i·tis (sig′moy-dī′tis) Inflammation of the sigmoid colon.

sig·moid kid·ney (sig′moyd kĭd′nē) Upper pole of one kidney fused with the lower pole of the other.

sig·moi·do·pex·y (sig-moy′dō-pek-sē) Operative attachment of the sigmoid colon to a firm structure to correct rectal prolapse.

sig·moi·do·proc·tos·to·my (sig-moy′dō-prok-tos′tŏ-mē) Anastomosis between the sigmoid colon and the rectum. SYN sigmoidorectostomy.

sig·moi·do·scope, sig·mo·scope (sig′ mo-y′dŏ-skōp, sig′mŏ-) An endoscope for viewing the cavity of the sigmoid colon.

sig·moi·dos·co·py (sig′moy-dos′kŏ-pē) Inspection, through an endoscope, of the interior of the sigmoid colon.

sig·moi·dos·to·my (sig′moy-dos′tŏ-mē) Establishment of an artificial anus by opening into the sigmoid colon.

sig·moi·dot·o·my (sig′moy-dot′ŏ-mē) Surgical opening of the sigmoid.

sig·moid vol·vu·lus (SV) (sig′moyd vol′vyū-lŭs) Relatively common location of volvulus, with obstruction either proximal or distal to the sigmoid segment.

sign (sīn) 1. Any abnormality indicative of disease, discoverable on examination of a patient; an objective symptom of disease, in contrast to a symptom, which is a subjective sign of disease. 2. An abbreviation or symbol. 3. PSYCHOLOGY any object or artifact that represents a specific thing or conveys a specific idea to the person who perceives it.

sig·nal lymph node, sig·nal node (sig′năl limf nōd) A firm supraclavicular lymph node, especially on the left side, sufficiently enlarged that it is palpable from the cutaneous surface; such a lymph node is so termed because it may be the first recognized presumptive evidence of a malignant neoplasm in one of the viscera. SEE ALSO sentinel lymph node. SYN Virchow node.

sig·nal trans·duc·tion in·hib·i·tor (STI) (sig′năl tranz-dŭk′shŭn in-hib′i-tŏr) Category or classification of anticancer drugs that inhibit the action of enzymes essential to the growth and survival of cancer cells while causing relatively little or no damage to noncancer cells.

sig·net-ring cell car·ci·no·ma (sig′ nĕt-ring sel kahr′si-nō′mă) Poorly differentiated adenocarcinoma composed of cells with a cytoplasmic droplet of mucus that compresses the nucleus to one side along the cell membrane; arises most frequently in the stomach, occasionally in the large bowel or elsewhere.

sig·nif·i·cant (sig) (sig-nif′i-kănt) In statistics, denoting the reliability of a finding or, conversely, the probability of the finding being the result of chance (generally less than 5%).

sign lan·guage (sīn lang′gwăj) A system of manual communication used by the deaf. True sign languages such as American Sign Language (ASL) have a complete representation of morphology, semantics, and syntax.

sil·den·a·fil (sil-den′ă-fil) Medication that relaxes the muscle in the penis, resulting in greater blood flow and erection; used to treat male impotence; potentiates the hypotensive effects of nitrates.

si·lent a·re·a (sī′lĕnt ăr′ē-ă) Any area of the cerebrum or cerebellum in which lesions cause no definite sensory or motor symptoms.

si·lent as·pir·a·tion (sī′lĕnt as′pir-ā′shŭn) Movement of a liquid or solid bolus into the trachea below the vocal cords, without clinical signs such as coughing, choking, color change, or change in respirations.

si·lent is·che·mi·a (sī′lĕnt is-kē′mē-ă) Myocardial ischemia without any of accompanying signs or symptoms of angina pectoris; can be detected by electrocardiographic and laboratory techniques. SEE ALSO silent myocardial infarction.

si·lent my·o·car·di·al in·farct·ion (sī′ lĕnt mī′ō-kahr′dē-ăl in-fahrk′shŭn) Infarct that produces none of the characteristic symptoms and signs.

sil·hou·ette sign of Fel·son (sil′ō-et′ sīn fel′sŏn) In pulmonary radiology, the obliteration of a normal air-soft tissue interface, when fluid fills the adjacent part of the lung.

sil·i·ca, sil·i·con di·ox·ide (sil′i-kă, sil′i-kŏn dī-oks′īd) The chief constituent of sand, hence of glass.

sil·i·ca gel (sil′i-kă jel) Precipitated form of silicic acid, used for adsorption of various gases.

sil·i·cate ce·ment (sil′i-kāt sĕ-ment′) Dental filling material prepared by mixing a modified phosphoric acid solution with a powdered silica alumina fluoride glass.

si·lic·ic ac·id (si-lis′ik as′id) Obtained in water as a colloid by treating silicates; precipitated silicic acid is silica gel.

sil·i·co·an·thra·co·sis (sil′i-kō-an′thră-kō′sis) Pneumoconiosis consisting of combined silicosis and anthracosis, seen in miners of hard coal.

sil·i·con (Si) (sil′i-kon) A very abundant nonmetallic element, occurring in nature as silica and silicates; in pure form, used as a semiconductor and in solar batteries.

sil·i·cone (sil′i-kōn) A polymer of organic silicon oxides, which may be a liquid, gel, or solid, depending on the extent of polymerization.

sil·i·co·pro·teino·sis (sil′i-kō-prō′tēn-ō′sis) An acute pulmonary disorder, radiographically and histologically similar to pulmonary alveolar proteinosis, resulting from relatively short exposure to high concentrations of silica dust.

sil·i·co·sis, sil·i·ca·to·sis (sil′i-kō′sis, -kă-tō′sis) Pneumoconiosis due to occupational exposure to and inhalation of silica dust over a period of years; characterized by a slowly progressive fibrosis of the lungs, which may result in impairment of lung function. SYN silicatosis.

silk (silk) The fibers or filaments obtained from the cocoon of the silkworm.

sil·ver (Ag) (sil′vĕr) L. argentum; a metallic element, atomic no. 47, atomic wt. 107.8682. Many salts have clinical applications.

sil·ver-fork frac·ture, sil·ver-fork de·for·mi·ty (sil′vĕr-fŏrk frak′shŭr, dĕ-fŏrm′i-tē) A Colles fracture of the wrist with a deformity that looks like a fork in profile.

sil·ver ni·trate (AgNO₃) (sil′vĕr nī′trāt) An antiseptic and astringent.

sil·ver sul·fa·di·a·zine (SSD) (sil′vĕr sŭl′fă-dī′ă-zēn) Derivative of sulfadiazine, used externally as a topical antibacterial agent to prevent and treat infections in burns.

si·meth·i·cone (si-meth′i-kōn) A mixture of dimethyl polysiloxanes and silica gel; an antiflatulent.

sim·i·an crease (sim′ē-ăn krēs) Single transverse palmar crease formed by fusion of the proximal and distal palmar creases, so called because of its similarity to the transverse flexion crease seen in some monkeys.

si·mi·li·a si·mil·i·bus cur·an·tur (si-mil′ē-ă si-mil′i-bŭs kū-ran′tūr) The homeopathic formula expressing the law of similars, the doctrine that any drug capable of producing morbid symptoms in the healthy will remove similar symptoms occurring as an expression of disease. Another reading of the formula, employed by Hahnemann, the founder of homeopathy, is *similia similibus curentur*, let likes be cured by likes.

Sim·monds dis·ease (sim′ŏndz di-zēz′) Anterior pituitary insufficiency due to trauma, vascular lesions, or tumors. SYN hypophysial cachexia, pituitary cachexia.

Si·mo·nart bands (sē-mō-nahr′ bandz) **1.** SYN amnionic band. **2.** Weblike band of tissue partially filling the gap between the medial and lateral portions of a cleft lip.

Si·mon po·si·tion (sē′mŏn pŏ-zish′ŏn) Placement for vaginal examination; a supine position with hips elevated, thighs and legs flexed, and thighs widely separated.

sim·ple (sim′pĕl) **1.** Not complex or compound. **2.** In anatomy, composed of a minimum number of parts. **3.** A medicinal herb.

sim·ple ab·sence (simp′ĕl ab′sĕns) A brief clouding of consciousness accompanied by the abrupt onset of 3-second spikes and waves on electroencephalography. SYN pure absence.

sim·ple ep·i·the·li·um (simp′ĕl ep′i-thē′lē-ŭm) Epithelium with one layer of cells.

sim·ple glau·co·ma, glau·co·ma sim·plex (simp′ĕl glaw-kō′mă, sim′pleks) SYN open-angle glaucoma.

sim·ple goi·ter (simp′ĕl goy′tĕr) Thyroid enlargement unaccompanied by constitu-

S

tional effects, e.g., hypo- or hyperthyroidism, commonly caused by inadequate dietary intake of iodine.

sim·ple joint (simp′ĕl joynt) [TA] A joint composed of only two bones.

sim·ple mas·tec·to·my (simp′ĕl mastek′tŏ-mē) Excision of the breast including the nipple, areola, and most of the overlying skin.

sim·ple mi·cro·scope, sin·gle mi·cro·scope (simp′ĕl mī′krŏ-skōp, sing′gĕl) A microscope that has one magnifying lens.

sim·ple par·tial sei·zure (SPS) (sim′pĕl pahr′shăl sē′zhŭr) One not associated with impairment of consciousness; seen in patients with focal epilepsy.

sim·ple pho·bi·a (simp′ĕl fō′bē-ă) SYN specific phobia.

sim·ple pro·tein (simp′ĕl prō′tēn) One that yields only α-amino acids or their derivatives by hydrolysis. Cf. conjugated protein.

sim·ple u·re·thri·tis (sim′pĕl yŭr′ĕ-thrī′tis) SYN nonspecific urethritis.

Sim·plex·vi·rus (sim′pleks-vī′rŭs) SYN herpes simplex.

Sims po·si·tion (simz pŏ-zish′ŏn) Placement to facilitate a vaginal examination, with the patient lying on her side with the lower arm behind the back, the thighs flexed, the upper one more than the lower. SYN lateral recumbent position.

sim·u·la·tor (sim′yū-lā′tŏr, tōr) *Do not confuse this word with stimulator.* An apparatus designed to produce effects simulating those of specific environmental conditions; used in experimentation and training.

si·mul·tan·ag·no·si·a (sī′mŭl-tān′ag-nō′sē-ă) Inability to recognize multiple elements in a visual presentation; i.e., one object or some elements of a scene can be appreciated but not the display as a whole.

sin·ci·put, pl. **sin·cip·i·ta,** pl. **sin·ci·puts** (sin′si-pŭt, -sip′i-tă, -pŭts) Anterior part of the head just above and including the forehead.

Sind·ing-Lar·sen-Jo·hans·son syn·drome (sin′ding-lahr′sen-yō-hahn′sŏn sin′drōm) Apophysitis of the distal pole of the patella.

sin·ew (sin′yū) SYN tendon.

sing·er's nodes (sing′ĕrz nōdz) SYN vocal fold nodules.

single nu·cle·o·tide pol·y·morph·ism (SNP) (sing′gĕl nū′klē-ō-tīd pol′ē-mōr′fizm) Naturally occurring substitution of a single nucleotide at a given location in the genome of an organism, the more interesting of which results in phenotypic variability, including alterations in the organism's physiologic responses to endogenous hormones and neurotransmitters or endogenous substances.

sin·gle pho·ton e·mis·sion com·put·ed tomography (SPECT) (sing′gĕl fō′ton ē-mi′shŭn kŏm-pyūt′ĕd tō-mog′ră-fē) Tomographic imaging of metabolic and physiologic functions in tissues, the image being formed by computer synthesis of photons of a single energy emitted by radionuclides administered in suitable form to the patient.

sin·is·ter (sin′is′tĕr) [TA] Left.

sin·is·trad (sin′is′trad) To the left.

sin·is·tral (sin′is-trăl) **1.** Relating to the left side. **2.** Denoting a left-handed person.

sin·is·tral·i·ty (sin′is-tral′i-tē) The condition of being left-handed.

sinistro- Combining form denoting left, toward the left.

sin·is·tro·cer·e·bral (sin′is-trō-ser′ĕ-brăl) Relating to the left cerebral hemisphere.

sin·is·troc·u·lar (sin′is′trok′yū-lăr) Seldom-used term denoting one who prefers the left eye in monocular work. Cf. dominant eye.

sin·is·trop·e·dal (sin′is-trop′ē-dăl) Denoting a person who uses the left leg by preference. SYN left-footed.

sin·is·tro·tor·sion (sin′is-trō-tōr′shŭn) A turning or twisting to the left. SYN levorotation (2), levotorsion (1), sinistrogyration.

Sin Nom·bre vi·rus (sēn nōm′brā vī′rŭs) A species of *Hantavirus* in North America that causes hantavirus pulmonary syndrome. SYN Four Corners virus.

si·no·pul·mo·nar·y (sī′nō-pul′mŏ-narē) Relating to the paranasal sinuses and the pulmonary airway.

sin·u·a·tri·al, si·no·a·tri·al (S-A) (sin′yū-ā′trē-ăl, sī′nō-ā′trē-ăl) Relating to the sinus venosus of the embryo, or the sinus of the venae cavae of the mature heart, and the right atrium.

sin·u·a·tri·al block, si·no·a·tri·al block (sin′yū-ā′trē-ăl blok, sī′nō-ā′trē-ăl) Blockade of an impulse leaving the sinuatrial node before it can activate atrial muscle or be propagated to the atrioventricular node. The condition is indicated on electrocardiography by the absence of some P waves.

sin·u·a·tri·al node, si·no·a·tri·al node (sin′yū-ā′trē-ăl nŏd, sī′nō-ā′trē-ăl) [TA] The mass of specialized cardiac muscle fibers that normally acts as the "pacemaker" of the cardiac conduction system; it is to be found under the epicardium at the upper end of the sulcus terminalis.

si·nu·a·trial valve (sin′yū-ā′trē-ăl valv) The valve at the sinuatrial orifice at the opening of the sinus venosus into the primordial right atrium. SYN sinoatrial valve.

si·nus, pl. **si·nus,** pl. **si·nus·es** (sī′nŭs, -ĕz) [TA] **1.** A channel for the passage of blood or lymph, without the coats of an ordinary vessel. **2.** A cavity or hollow space in bone or other tissue. **3.** A dilation in a blood vessel. **4.** A fistula or tract leading to a suppurating cavity.

si·nus ar·rest (sī′nŭs ă-rest′) Cessation of sinuatrial activity; the ventricles may continue to beat under ectopic atrial, atrioventricular junctional, or idioventricular control.

si·nus·i·tis (sī′nŭ-sī′tis) Inflammation of the mucous membrane of any sinus, especially the paranasal. SEE ALSO rhinosinusitis.

si·nu·soid (sī′nŭ-soyd) **1.** Resembling a sinus. **2.** Sinusoidal capillary; a thinwalled terminal blood vessel having a more variable and larger caliber than an ordinary capillary.

si·nus·oi·dal (sī′nŭ-soy′dăl) Relating to a sinusoid.

si·nus·ot·o·my (sī′nŭ-sot′ŏ-mē) Incision into a sinus.

si·nus pause (sī′nŭs pawz) A spontaneous interruption in the regular sinus rhythm, the pause lasting for a period that is not an exact multiple of the sinus cycle. SEE ALSO sinus arrest.

si·nus rhythm (sī′nŭs ridh′ŭm) Normal cardiac rhythm proceeding from the sinuatrial node.

si·nus tach·y·car·di·a (sī′nŭs tak′i-kahr′dē-ă) A heart rate exceeding 100 beats per minute with a normal rhythm.

si·nus ve·no·sus (sī′nŭs vē-nō′sŭs) [TA] The venosus sinus at the caudal end of the embryonic cardiac tube in which the veins from the intra- and extraembryonic circulatory arcs unite.

si·phon (sī′fŏn) A tube bent into two unequal lengths, used to remove fluid from a cavity or vessel by atmospheric pressure and gravity.

si·phon·age (sī′fŏn-ăj) Emptying of the stomach or other cavity by means of a siphon.

Sip·ple syn·drome (sip′ĕl sin′drōm) Pheochromocytoma, medullary carcinoma of the thyroid, and parathyroid adenomas.

si·re·no·me·li·a, sym·me·li·a (sī′rĕnō-mē′lē-ă, si-mē′lē-ă) Union of the legs with partial or complete fusion of the feet.

si·ri·a·sis (si-rī′ă-sis) *Do not confuse this word with sauriasis or psoriasis.* SYN sunstroke.

-sis Combining form meaning an action, process, condition, or state.

SISI test (test) Abbreviation for Short Increment Sensitivity Index test.

sis·ter (sis′tĕr) **1.** [Br.] The title of a head nurse in a public hospital or in a ward or the operating room of a hospital. **2.** Any registered nurse in private practice.

site (sīt) A place, location, or locus.

site-spe·cif·ic re·com·bi·na·tion (sīt-spĕ-sif′ik rē-kom′bi-nā′shŭn) Integration of foreign DNA into a particular site in the host genome.

♻ **sito-** Combining form denoting food or grains.

si·to·ster·ol (sī′tō-stĕr′ol) A plant-derived chemical similar to cholesterol, commonly found in wheat germ, soybeans, and corn oil. SYN beta-sitosterol.

si·to·ster·o·le·mi·a (sī′tō-stĕr′ō-lē′mē-ă) SYN phytosterolemia.

si·tus in·ver·sus vis·ce·rum (sī′tŭs in-vĕr′sŭs vis′ĕr-ŭm) Visceral transposition.

sitz bath (sits bath) Immersion of only the perineum and buttocks, with the legs being outside the tub. SYN hip bath.

SI u·nits (yū′nits) SEE International System of Units.

sixth dis·ease (siksth di-zēz′) SYN exanthema subitum.

Sjö·gren-Lars·son syn·drome (shōr′gren lahr′sŏn sin′drōm) Congenital ichthyosis in association with oligophrenia and spastic paraplegia.

Sjö·g·ren syn·drome (shōr′gren sin′drōm) Keratoconjunctivitis sicca, dryness of mucous membranes, telangiectases, or purpuric spots on the face, and bilateral parotid enlargement; seen in menopausal women and often associated with rheumatoid arthritis, Raynaud phenomenon, and dental caries.

skat·ole (skat′ōl) An indole derivative formed in the intestine by bacterial decomposition and found in fecal matter, to which it imparts its characteristic odor.

skel·e·tal (skel′ĕ-tăl) Relating to the skeleton.

skel·e·tal dys·pla·si·as (skel′ĕ-tăl dis-plā′zē-ăz) A heterogeneous group of more than 120 disorders, each of which results in numerous disturbances of the skeletal system and most of which include dwarfism.

skel·e·tal sur·vey (skel′ĕ-tăl sŭr′vā) Radiographic examination of all or selected parts of the skeleton.

skel·e·tal sys·tem (skel′ĕ-tăl sis′tĕm) [TA] Bones and cartilages of the body. SYN systema skeletale [TA].

skel·e·tal trac·tion (skel′ĕ-tăl trak′shŭn) Therapeutic pulling on a bone structure mediated through pin or wire inserted into the bone to reduce a fracture of long bones. SYN skeletal extension.

skel·e·ton (skel′ĕ-tŏn) **1.** [TA] The bony framework of the body in vertebrates (endoskeleton) or the hard outer envelope of insects (exoskeleton or dermoskeleton). **2.** All the dry parts remaining after the destruction and removal of the soft parts; this includes ligaments and cartilages as well as bones. **3.** A rigid or semirigid nonosseous structure that functions as the supporting framework of a particular structure.

skew (skyū) In statistics, departure from symmetry of a frequency distribution.

♻ **skia-** Combining form meaning shadow; superseded by radio-.

skilled nurs·ing fa·cil·i·ty (SNF) (skild nŭrs′ing fă-sil′i-tē) A nursing facility providing 24-hour nonacute nursing, medical, and rehabilitative care.

skin (skin) [TA] The membranous protective covering of the body, consisting of the epidermis and corium (dermis). SYN cutis [TA].

skin flap (skin flap) One composed of skin with or without its subjacent subcutaneous tissue.

skin graft (SG) (skin graft) Piece of skin transplanted from one part of the body to another.

skin test (skin test) A method for determining induced sensitivity (allergy) by applying an antigen (allergen) to, or inoculating it into, the skin. SYN intradermal test.

skin trac·tion (skin trak'shŭn) Limb traction with adhesive tape or other strapping applied to it.

skull (skŭl) The bones of the head collectively. In a more limited sense, the neurocranium, the bony braincase containing the brain, excluding the bones of the face (viscerocranium).

slant cul·ture (slant kŭl'chŭr) A culture made on the slanting surface of a medium solidified in a test tube inclined from the perpendicular to give a greater area than that of the lumen of the tube.

SLAP les·ion (slap lē'zhŭn) Acronymic term for the traumatic tear of the superior part of the glenoid labrum that begins posteriorly and extends anteriorly [*Superior Labrum, Anterior-Posterior*].

sleep ap·ne·a (slēp ap'nē-ă) Central and peripheral apnea during sleep, associated with frequent awakening and often with daytime sleepiness.

sleep ap·ne·a syn·drome (SAS) (slēp ap'nē-ă sin'drŏm) Disorder characterized by multiple episodes of partial or complete cessation of respiration during sleep. SYN obstructive sleep apnea syndrome.

sleep dep·ri·va·tion (slēp dep'ri-vā'shŭn) Sufficient lack of restorative sleep over a cumulative period to cause physical or psychiatric symptoms and affect routine performances of tasks.

sleep drunk·en·ness (slēp drungk'ĕn-nĕs) A half-waking condition in which the faculty of orientation is in abeyance, and under the influence of nightmarelike ideas, the person may become actively excited and violent.

sleep pa·ral·y·sis (slēp păr-al'i-sis) Brief episodic loss of voluntary movement that occurs when one is falling asleep (hypnagogic sleep paralysis) or awakening (hypnopompic sleep paralysis).

slew rate (slū rāt) In electronic pacemaker function, the maximum rate of change of an amplifier output voltage.

slide (slīd) A rectangular glass plate on which is placed an object to be examined under the microscope.

slide tra·che·o·plas·ty (slīd trā'kē-ō-plas-tē) An operation for the repair of long tracheal stenosis in which anterior and posterior sliding flaps of the tracheal wall are sutured together to reconstruct the tracheal lumen.

slid·ing e·soph·a·ge·al hi·a·tal her·ni·a (slīd'ing ĕ-sof'ă-jē'ăl hī-ā'tăl hĕr'nē-ă) Displacement of the cardioesophageal junction and the stomach through the esophageal hiatus into the mediastinum.

slid·ing flap (slīd'ing flap) A rectangular area raised in an elastic area, with its free end adjacent to a defect; the defect is covered by stretching the flap longitudinally until the end comes over it.

slid·ing her·ni·a (slīd'ing hĕr'nē-ă) One in which an abdominal viscus forms part of the sac. SYN extrasaccular hernia, parasaccular hernia, slipped hernia.

sling (sling) A supporting bandage or suspensory device.

slip·ping pat·el·la (slip'ing pă-tel'ă) Spontaneous or easily provoked dislocation of the patella.

slip·ping rib (slip'ing rib) Subluxation of a rib cartilage, with costochondral separation.

slit pores (slit pōrz) Intercellular clefts between the interdigitating pedicels of podocytes; they are part of the filtration barrier of renal corpuscles. SYN filtration slits.

Slo·cum draw·er test (slō'kŭm drŏr test) Maneuver used to determine anterior medial rotary instability (AMRI) and anterior lateral rotary instability (ALRI) of the knee.

slough (slŭf) **1.** Necrosed tissue separated from the living structure. **2.** To separate from the living tissue; said of a dead or necrosed part.

slow code (slō cōd) Intentionally tardy response to a cardiorespiratory emergency so as to reduce the likelihood of a successful resuscitation. SYN man-made death.

slow-re·act·ing subs·tance of an·a·phy·lax·is (SRS-A) (slō-rē-akt'ing sŭb'stăns an'ă-fi-lak'sis) Physiologic matter produced during shock that causes muscular contraction to a greater degree than histamine (q.v.).

slow vi·rus (slō vīˊrŭs) Virus, or a viruslike agent, etiologically associated with a disease having an incubation period of months to years with a gradual onset frequently terminating in severe illness or death.

sludge (slŭj) A muddy sediment.

slur·ry (slŭrˊē) A thin semifluid suspension of a solid in a liquid.

Sly syn·drome (slī sinˊdrōm) Disorder due to deficiency of a β-glucuronidase. SYN mucopolysaccharidosis type VII (1).

Sm Symbol for samarium.

small cal·o·rie (cal, c) (smawl kalˊŏr-ē) Quantity of energy required to raise the temperature of 1 g of water 1°C, or from 14.5–15.5°C in the case of normal or standard calorie. SYN gram calorie.

small cell car·ci·no·ma (SCC) (smawl sel kahrˊsi-nōˊmă) **1.** Anaplastic carcinoma composed of small cells. **2.** Anaplastic, highly malignant, and usually bronchogenic carcinoma composed of small ovoid cells with very scanty cytoplasm. SYN oat cell carcinoma.

small cleaved cell (SCC) (smawl klēvd sel) Lymphoid cell of follicular center cell origin that has an irregularly shaped nucleus with clumped chromatin, absent nucleoli, and one or more clefts in the nuclear membrane.

small for ges·ta·tion·al age (SGA) (smawl jes-tāˊshŭn-ăl āj) Infant whose birth weight is below the tenth percentile for gestational age.

small in·cre·ment sen·si·tiv·i·ty in·dex (SISI) (smawl inˊkrĕ-mĕnt senˊsi-tivˊi-tē inˊdeks) SEE short increment sensitivity test.

small in·tes·tine (smawl in-tesˊtin) [TA] The portion of the digestive tube between the stomach and the cecum or beginning of the large intestine; comprises duodenum, jejunum, and ileum.

small lymph·o·cyt·ic lym·pho·ma (SLL) (smawl lim-fō-sitˊik lim-fōˊmă) Low-grade non-Hodgkin lymphoma characterized by enlarged lymph nodes and other lymphoid tissue or bone marrow that are infiltrated by small lymphocytes. SYN well-differentiated lymphocytic lymphoma, white spot disease (1).

small nu·cle·ar RNA (snRNA) (smawl nūˊklē-ăr rē-komˊbi-nănt nū-klēˊik asˊid) Small RNA in the nucleus believed to have a role in RNA processing and cellular architecture.

small·pox (smawlˊpoks) An acute eruptive contagious disease caused by a poxvirus (variola); characterized by chills, fever, and an eruption of papules that become umbilicated vesicles, develop into pustules, dry, and then form scabs that, when they fall off, leave permanent indentations on the skin (pockmarks).

smear (smēr) A thin specimen for microscopic examination; usually prepared by spreading liquid or semisolid material uniformly onto a glass slide, fixing it, and staining it before examination.

smeg·ma (smegˊmă) A foul-smelling, pasty accumulation of desquamated epidermal cells and sebum that collects in moist areas of the genitalia, especially in uncircumcised males.

Smith frac·ture (smith frakˊshŭr) Reversed Colles fracture; rupture of the distal radius with displacement of the fragment toward the palmar (volar) aspect.

Smith-Lem·li-O·pitz syn·drome (smith lemˊlē ōˊpits sinˊdrōm) Mental retardation, small stature, anteverted nostrils, ptosis, male genital anomalies, and syndactyly of the second and third toes, often in breech-born babies with delayed fetal activity.

smooth cho·ri·on (smūdh kōrˊē-on) The nonvillous, membranous part of the chorion where the chorionic villi have degenerated. SYN chorion laeve.

smooth mus·cle (smūdh mŭsˊĕl) One of the muscle fibers of the internal organs, blood vessels, and hair follicles. SEE ALSO involuntary muscles.

smooth mus·cle re·lax·ant (smūdh mŭsˊĕl rē-lakˊsănt) Pharmacologic agent, such as an antispasmodic, bronchodilator, or vasodilator, which reduces the tension or tone of smooth (involuntary) muscle.

smudge cells (smŭj selz) Immature leukocytes of any type that have undergone partial breakdown during preparation of a stained smear or tissue section, because of their greater fragility; seen in chronic lymphocytic leukemia. SYN basket cell (2).

Sn Symbol for tin.

snail track de·gen·er·a·tion (snāl trak dĕ-jen'ĕr-ā'shŭn) Circumferential line of fine white dots in the peripheral retina associated with atrophic retinal holes.

snap (snap) A short, sharp click; said especially of cardiac sounds.

snap·ping hip, snap·ping hip syn·drome (snap'ing hip, sin'drōm) Condition in which the fascia lata or gluteus maximus muscle is under tension, moving over the greater trochanter of the proximal end of the femur or the iliopsoas tendon moves over the lesser trochanter and causes a click.

snare (snār) A wire-loop instrument to remove polyps and other projections, especially within a cavity.

sneeze (snēz) **1.** To expel air from the nose and mouth by an involuntary spasmodic contraction of the muscles of expiration. **2.** An act of sneezing; a reflex excited by an irritation of the mucous membrane of the nose or, sometimes, when a bright light strikes the eye.

Snel·len test type (snel'ĕn test tīp) One of a series of square black symbols employed in testing the acuity of distant vision.

sniff test (snif test) FLUOROSCOPY measurement of diaphragmatic function.

snore (snōr) **1.** A rough, rattling inspiratory noise produced by vibration of the pendulous palate, or sometimes of the vocal cords, during sleep or coma. SEE ALSO stertor, rhonchus. **2.** To breathe noisily, or with a snore.

snow·ball sam·pling (snō'bawl sam'pling) Method whereby the names of prospective interview subjects for a sta-

tistical study are obtained from subjects already interviewed for the study.

snuf·fles (snŭf'ĕlz) Obstructed nasal respiration, especially in the newborn infant, sometimes due to congenital syphilis.

SOAP (sōp) Acronym for the conceptual device used by clinicians to organize the progress notes in the problem-oriented record; *S* stands for subjective data provided by the patient, *O* for objective data gathered by health care professionals in the clinical setting, *A* for the assessment of the patient's condition, and *P* for the plan for the patient's care.

soap (sōp) The sodium or potassium salts of long-chain fatty acids; used as an emulsifier for cleansing purposes and as an excipient in the making of pills and suppositories.

so·ci·a (sō'shē-ă) An ectopic, supernumerary, or accessory portion of an organ.

so·cial·i·za·tion (SOC) (sō'shăl-ī-zā'shŭn) **1.** Learning attitudes and interpersonal and interactional skills in conformity with the values of one's society. **2.** In a group therapy setting, a way of learning to participate effectively in the group.

so·cial·ized med·i·cine (sō'shăl-īzd med'i-sin) Control of medical practice by a government agency, the practitioners being employed by the organization from which they receive standardized compensation for their services, and to which the public contributes, usually in the form of taxation rather than fee-for-service.

so·cial med·i·cine (sō'shăl med'i-sin) Specialized field of medical knowledge concentrating on the social, cultural, and economic impact of medical phenomena.

so·cial net·work ther·a·py (sō'shăl net'wŏrk thār'ă-pē) Care involving assembling all people who are emotionally or functionally important to the patient to affect a behavioral change.

so·cial pho·bi·a (sō'shăl fō'bē-ă) Persistent pattern of significant fear of a social or performance situation, manifesting in anxiety or panic on exposure to the situation or in anticipation of it.

S

so·cial psy·chi·a·try (sō′shăl sī-kī′ă-trē) An approach to psychiatric theory and practice emphasizing the cultural and sociologic aspects of mental disorders and treatment.

so·ci·o·ac·u·sis (sō′sē-ō-ă-kyū′sis) Hearing loss produced by exposure to noise outside the workplace.

so·ci·o·cen·tric (sō′sē-ō-sen′trik) Outgoing; reactive to the social or cultural milieu.

so·ci·o·gen·e·sis (sō′sē-ō-jen′ĕ-sis) The origin of social behavior from past interpersonal experiences.

so·ci·om·e·try (sō′sē-om′ĕ-trē) The study of interpersonal relationships in a group.

so·ci·op·a·thy (sō′sē-op′ă-thē) Behavioral pattern exhibited by patients with an antisocial personality disorder (q.v.).

sock·et (sok′ĕt) **1.** SYN gomphosis. **2.** Any hollow or concavity into which another part fits, as the eye socket.

so·da lime (SL) (sō′dă līm) Mixture of calcium and sodium hydroxides used to absorb carbon dioxide when rebreathing is involved.

so·di·um (Na) (sō′dē-ŭm) Alkali metal oxidizing readily in air or water; its salts are found in natural biologic systems and are extensively used in medicine and industry. SYN natrium.

so·di·um ac·e·tate (sō′dē-ŭm as′ĕ-tāt) Systemic and urinary alkalizer, expectorant, and diuretic.

so·di·um ben·zo·ate (sō′dē-ŭm ben′zō-āt) Used in chronic and acute rheumatism, as a liver function test, and as a preservative.

so·di·um bi·car·bon·ate (NaHCO₃) (sō′dē-ŭm bī-kahr′bŏ-nāt) Used as a gastric and systemic antacid, to alkalize urine, and for washes of body cavities. SYN baking soda, sodium acid carbonate, sodium hydrogen carbonate.

so·di·um bi·phos·phate (sō′dē-ŭm bī-fos′fāt) Used to increase urinary acidity. SYN primary sodium phosphate, sodium acid phosphate, sodium dihydrogen phosphate.

so·di·um bo·rate (sō′dē-ŭm bōr′āt) Used in lotions, gargles, mouthwashes, and as a detergent. SYN borax, sodium pyroborate, sodium tetraborate.

so·di·um chlo·ride (NaCl) (sō′dē-ŭm klōr′īd) Major ionic component of blood, urine, and other bodily fluids; used to make isotonic and physiologic saline solutions, to treat salt depletion, and topically for inflammatory lesions. SYN common salt.

so·di·um cit·rate (SC) (sō′dē-ŭm sit′rāt) Used as diuretic, antilithic, systemic and urinary alkalizer, expectorant, and anticoagulant (in vitro). SYN sodium acid citrate.

so·di·um fluor·ide (NaF) (sō′dē-ŭm flōr′īd) Anticaries dental prophylactic placed in tap water, and topically as a 2% solution applied to the teeth.

so·di·um hy·po·chlor·ite (NaClO) (sō′dē-ŭm hī′pō-klōr′īt) Strong oxidizer; explosive when anhydrous; used in aqueous solution household bleach and disinfectants.

so·di·um lac·tate (SL) (sō′dē-ŭm lak′tāt) A systemic and urinary alkalizer.

so·di·um lau·ryl sul·fate (sō′dē-ŭm lawr′il sŭl′fāt) A surface-active agent of the anionic type used in toothpastes.

so·di·um ni·trite (sō′dē-ŭm nī′trīt) Agent used to lower systemic blood pressure, to relieve local vasomotor spasms, and as an antidote for cyanide poisoning.

so·di·um ni·tro·prus·side (sō′dē-ŭm nī′trō-prŭs′īd) Fast acting and potent arterial and venous vasodilator used in hypertensive emergencies. SYN sodium nitroferricyanide.

so·di·um per·bo·rate (SP) (sō′dē-ŭm pĕr′bŏr-āt) Used in extemporaneous preparation of hydrogen peroxide.

so·di·um pol·y·sty·rene sul·fo·nate (sō′dē-ŭm pol′ē-stī′rēn sŭl′fŏn-nāt) Cationic exchange resin used in hyperpotassemia.

so·di·um-po·tas·si·um pump (sō′dē-ŭm pō-tas′ē-ŭm pŭmp) Membrane-bound transporter found in nearly all mammalian cells that transports potassium ions into the cytoplasm from the extracellular fluid while simultaneously transporting sodium ions out of the cytoplasm to the extracellular fluid. SYN sodium-potassium ATPase.

so·di·um pro·pi·o·nate (sō´dē-ŭm prō´pē-ŏ-nāt) Sodium salt of propionic acid; used for fungal infections of the skin, usually in combination with calcium propionate, and used as a preservative.

so·di·um pump (sō´dē-ŭm pŭmp) A biologic mechanism that uses metabolic energy from adenosine triphosphate to achieve active transport of sodium across a membrane.

so·di·um sul·fate (sō´dē-ŭm sŭl´fāt) Ingredient in many natural laxatives. SYN Glauber salt.

so·di·um tet·ra·dec·yl sul·fate (sō´dē-ŭm tet´ră-des´il sŭl´fāt) An anionic surface-active agent used for its wetting properties to enhance the surface action of certain antiseptic solutions.

so·di·um thi·o·sul·fate, so·di·um hy·po·sul·fite (sō´dē-ŭm thī´ō-sŭl´fāt, hī-pō´sŭl-fāt) An injectable compound used immediately after injection of sodium nitrate as an antidote for cyanide poisoning.

sod·o·my (sod´ŏm-ē) A term denoting sexual practices variously proscribed by law, especially bestiality, oral-genital contact, and anal intercourse. SYN buggery.

soft corn (sawft kōrn) Clavus formed by intertoe pressure; its surface is macerated and yellowish. SYN heloma molle.

soft pal·ate (sawft pal´ăt) [TA] The posterior muscular portion of the palate, forming an incomplete septum between the mouth and the oropharynx.

soft tu·ber·cle (sawft tū´bĕr-kĕl) A tubercle showing caseous necrosis.

soft wa·ter (sawft waw´tĕr) Water lacking ions that form insoluble salts with fatty acids, so that ordinary soap will lather easily in it.

so·lar chei·li·tis (sō´lăr kī-lī´tis) Mucosal atrophy with drying, crusting, and fissuring of the vermilion border of the lower lip, resulting from chronic exposure to sunlight.

so·lar e·las·to·sis (sō´lăr ĕ-las-tō´sis) Elastosis seen histologically in the sun-exposed skin of old people or in those who have chronic actinic damage.

so·lar ur·ti·ca·ri·a (sō´lăr ŭr´ti-kar´ē-ă) Skin disease due to exposure to specific light spectra (e.g., sunlight); some patients have passive-transfer antibodies, others do not.

sol·a·tion (sol-ā´shŭn) COLLOIDAL CHEM-ISTRY the transformation of a gel into a sol, as by melting gelatin.

sol·der (sod´ĕr) A fusible alloy used to unite edges or surfaces of two pieces of metal of higher melting point; hard solders, usually containing gold or silver as their main constituent, are usually used in dentistry to connect noble metal alloys.

sole (sōl) [TA] The plantar surface or underside of the foot. SYN planta [TA].

sol·i·tar·y bone cyst (sol´i-tar-ē bōn sist) A unilocular cyst containing serous fluid and lined with a thin layer of connective tissue, occurring usually in the shaft of a long bone in a child. SYN osteocystoma, unicameral bone cyst.

sol·i·tar·y lym·phoid nod·ules (sol´i-tar-ē lim´foyd nod´yūlz) Minute collections of lymphoid tissue in the mucosa of the small and large intestines, being especially numerous in the cecum and appendix.

sol·u·bil·i·ty (sol´yū-bil´i-tē) The property of being soluble.

sol·u·ble (sol´yū-bĕl) Capable of being dissolved.

sol·ute (S, SOL, solu) (sol´ūt) The dissolved substance in a solution.

so·lu·tion (sŏ-lū´shŭn) 1. Incorporation of a solid, a liquid, or a gas in a liquid or noncrystalline solid resulting in a homogeneous single phase. SEE ALSO dispersion, suspension. 2. Generally, an aqueous solution of a nonvolatile substance. 3. The termination of a disease by crisis. 4. A break, cut, or laceration of the solid tissues. SEE ALSO solution of contiguity, solution of continuity.

so·lu·tion of con·ti·gu·i·ty (sŏ-lū′shŭn kon′ti-gyū′i-tē) The breaking of contiguity; a dislocation or displacement of two normally contiguous parts.

so·lu·tion of con·ti·nu·i·ty (sŏ-lū′shŭn kon′ti-nū′i-tē) Division of bones or soft parts that are normally continuous, as by a fracture, a laceration, or an incision. SYN dieresis.

sol·vent (sol′vĕnt) A liquid that holds another substance in solution, i.e., dissolves it.

so·ma (sō′mă) 1. The axial part of the body, excluding the limbs. 2. All of an organism with the exception of the germ cells. SEE ALSO body. 3. The body of a nerve cell, from which axons and dendrites project.

so·ma·tal·gi·a (sō′mă-tal′jē-ă) 1. Pain in the body. 2. Pain due to organic causes, as opposed to psychogenic pain.

so·ma·tas·the·ni·a (sō′mat-as-thē′nē-ă) A condition of chronic physical weakness and fatigability. SYN somasthenia.

so·ma·tes·the·si·a, so·mes·the·sia (sō′mat-es-thē′zē-ă, sō′mes-) Bodily sensation, the conscious awareness of the body. SYN somataesthesia.

so·mat·ic (sō-mat′ik) 1. Relating to the soma or trunk, the wall of the body cavity, or the body in general. SYN parietal (2). 2. Relating to or involving the skeleton or skeletal (voluntary) muscle and the innervation of the latter, as distinct from the viscera or visceral (involuntary) muscle and its (autonomic) innervation. SYN parietal (3). 3. Relating to the vegetative, as distinguished from the generative, functions.

so·mat·ic cells (sō-mat′ik selz) The cells of an organism other than the germ cells.

so·mat·ic mu·ta·tion (sō-mat′ik myū-tā′shŭn) Mutation in the general body cells (as opposed to the germ cells) and hence not transmitted to progeny.

so·mat·ic nerve (sō-mat′ik nĕrv) One of the nerves of parietal sensation or voluntary motion, as distinguished from the visceral sensory, involuntary motor, and secretory nerves.

somatic nerve fibers (sō-mat′ik nĕrv fī′bĕrz) [TA] Afferent or efferent fibers distributed outside the body cavities. SYN neurofibrae somaticae [TA].

so·mat·ic re·pro·duc·tion (sō-mat′ik rē′prō-dŭk′shŭn) Asexual reproduction by fission or budding of somatic cells.

so·ma·ti·za·tion dis·or·der (SD) (sō′mă-tī-zā′shŭn dis-ōr′dĕr) Mental illness characterized by a complicated medical history and of physical symptoms referring to a variety of organ systems, but without a detectable or known organic basis. SEE conversion, hysteria.

somato-, somat-, somatico- Combining forms meaning the body, bodily.

so·mat·o·chrome (sō-mat′ō-krōm) Denoting the group of neurons or nerve cells with an abundance of cytoplasm completely surrounding the nucleus.

so·mat·o·crin·in (sō′mă-tō-krin′in) Hypothalamic growth hormone–releasing hormone (GHRH).

so·mat·o·form dis·or·der (sō′mă-tō-fōrm dis-ōr′dĕr) Conditions in which physical symptoms suggest physical disorders but not demonstrable organic findings or known physiologic mechanisms, for which positive evidence exists, suggesting that such symptoms are linked to psychological factors.

so·mat·o·gen·ic (sō′mă-tō-jen′ik) 1. Originating in the soma or body under the influence of external forces. 2. Having origin in body cells.

so·ma·to·lib·er·in (sō′mă-tō-lib′ĕr-in) A decapeptide released by the hypothalamus, which induces the release of human growth hormone (somatotropin). SYN growth hormone–releasing hormone, somatocrinin, somatotropin-releasing hormone.

so·ma·tol·o·gy (sō′mă-tol′ŏ-jē) The science concerned with the study of the body; includes both anatomy and physiology.

so·ma·to·me·din (sō′mă-tō-mē′din) A peptide synthesized in the liver, and probably in the kidney, capable of stimulating certain anabolic processes in bone and cartilage, such as synthesis of DNA, RNA, and protein, and the sulfation of mucopolysaccharides.

so•ma•to•path•ic (sō′mă-tō-path′ik) Relating to bodily or organic illness, as distinguished from mental (psychological) disorder.

so•ma•to•pause (sō′mă-tō-pawz) Decrease in growth hormone–insulinlike growth factor axis activities associated with aging.

so•mat•o•plasm (sō-mat′ō-plazm) Aggregate of all forms of specialized protoplasm entering into the composition of the body, other than germ plasm.

so•ma•to•psy•chic (sō′mă-tō-sī′kik) Relating to the body-mind relationship.

so•ma•to•psy•cho•sis (sō′mă-tō-sī-kō′sis) An emotional disorder associated with an organic disease.

so•ma•to•sen•so•ry (sō′mă-tō-sen′sŏr-ē) Sensation relating to the body's superficial and deep parts as contrasted to specialized senses such as sight.

so•ma•to•sen•so•ry au•ra (sō′mă-tō-sen′sŏr-ē awr′ă) Epileptic aura characterized by paresthesias or abdominal somatognosia of a clearly defined regional distribution. SEE ALSO aura (1).

so•ma•to•sex•u•al (sō′mă-tō-sek′shū-ăl) Denoting the somatic aspects of sexuality as distinguished from its psychosexual aspects.

so•ma•to•stat•in (sō′mă-tō-stat′in) A tetradecapeptide capable of inhibiting release of somatotropin, insulin, and gastrin. SYN growth hormone–inhibiting hormone, somatotropin release–inhibiting hormone.

so•ma•to•stat•i•no•ma (sō′mă-tō-stat′i-nō′mă) A somatostatin-secreting tumor of the pancreatic islets.

so•ma•to•ther•a•py (sō′mă-tō-thār′ă-pē) **1.** Therapy directed at physical disorders. **2.** PSYCHIATRY a variety of therapeutic interventions employing chemical or physical, as opposed to psychological, methods.

so•ma•to•top•ag•no•sis, so•ma•to•top•ag•no•si•a (sō′mă-tō-top′ag-nō′sis, -nō′zē-ă) The inability to identify any part of the body, either one's own or another's body. SYN somatagnosia.

so•ma•tot•o•py (sō′mă-tot′ŏ-pē) The topographic association of positional relationships of receptors in the body through respective nerve fibers to their terminal distribution in specific functional areas of the cerebral cortex.

so•ma•to•troph, so•ma•to•trope (sō-mat′ō-trōf, -trōp) A cell of the adenohypophysis that produces somatotropin.

so•mat•o•trop•ic (sō′mă-tō-trō′pik) Having a stimulating effect on body growth.

so•ma•to•tro•pin, so•ma•to•tro•pic hor•mone (sō-mat′ō-trō′pin, -trō′pik hōr′mōn) A protein hormone of the anterior lobe of the pituitary, produced by the acidophil cells, which promotes body growth, fat mobilization, and inhibition of glucose utilization. SYN growth hormone, pituitary growth hormone.

so•mat•o•type (sō-mat′ō-tīp) **1.** The constitutional or body type of an individual. **2.** The constitutional or body type associated with a particular personality type.

so•ma•trem (sō′mă-trem) Purified polypeptide hormone, made by recombinant DNA techniques, used in long-term treatment of children deficient in somatotropin.

so•ma•tro•pin (sō-mat′rō-pin) A drug identical with human growth hormone; used to treat growth disturbances in children or adults.

som•nam•bu•lism, som•nam•bu•lance (som-nam′byū-lizm, -byū-lăns) Disorder of sleep involving complex motor acts that occurs primarily during the first third of the night but not during rapid eye movement sleep.

som•nil•o•quence, som•nil•o•quism (som-nil′ŏ-kwĕns, -kwizm) **1.** Talking or muttering in one's sleep. **2.** SYN somniloquy.

som•nil•o•quy (som-nil′ŏ-kwē) Talking under the influence of hypnotic suggestion. SYN somniloquence (2), somniloquism.

som·nip·a·thy (som-nip′ă-thē) Any sleep disorder.

som·no·cin·e·ma·tog·ra·phy (som′nō-sin′ĕ-mă-tog′ră-fē) Recording movements during sleep.

som·no·lence, som·no·len·cy (som′nō-lĕns, -lĕn-sē) 1. Inclination to sleep. 2. Obtusion.

som·no·lent, som·no·les·cent (som′nō-lĕnt, som′nō-les′ĕnt) 1. Drowsy; sleepy; inclined to sleep. 2. In a condition of incomplete sleep; semicomatose.

So·mog·yi ef·fect, So·mog·yi phe·no·me·non (sō-mō′jē e-fekt′, fĕ-nom′ĕ-non) A rebound phenomenon of reactive hyperglycemia after relative hypoglycemia, which may be subclinical and difficult to detect. SYN posthypoglycemic hyperglycemia.

So·mog·yi u·nit (sō-mō′jē yū′nit) A measure of the level of activity of amylase in blood serum.

son·i·ca·tion (son′i-kā′shŭn) The process of disrupting biologic materials by use of sound wave energy.

son·o·lu·cent (son′ō-lū′sĕnt) In ultrasonography, containing few or no echoes. SEE anechoic.

so·no·rous rale (son′ŏr-ŭs rahl) A cooing or snoring sound often produced by vibration of viscid secretions in a large bronchus.

sop·o·rif·ic, sop·o·rif·er·ous (sop′ŏr-if′ik, -ĕr-ūs) 1. Causing sleep. SYN somniferous. 2. An agent that produces sleep.

sor·be·fa·cient (sōr′bĕ-fā′shĕnt) 1. Causing absorption. 2. An agent that causes or facilitates absorption.

sor·bic ac·id (sōr′bik as′id) A preservative obtained from berries of the rowan/mountain ash that inhibits growth of yeast and mold and is nearly nontoxic to humans.

sor·bi·tol (sorb) (sōr′bi-tol) Reduction product in the many fruits and seaweeds has many industrial and pharmaceutical uses; used as a laxative and as a sweetening agent.

sor·des (sōr′dēz) A dark crust on the lips, teeth, and gums of a person with disease-related dehydration.

sorp·tion (sōrp′shŭn) Adsorption or absorption.

Sors·by syn·drome (sorz′bē sin′drōm) Congenital macular coloboma and apical dystrophy of the extremities.

souf·fle (sū′fĕl) A soft, blowing sound heard on auscultation.

sound (sownd) 1. Vibrations produced by a sounding body, transmitted by the air or other medium, and perceived by the internal ear. 2. An elongated cylindric, usually curved, instrument of metal, used to explore body cavities. 3. Whole; healthy; not diseased or injured.

South·ern blot a·nal·y·sis (sŏdh′ĕrn blot ă-nal′i-sis) A procedure to separate and identify DNA sequences; DNA fragments are separated by electrophoresis on an agarose gel, transferred (blotted) onto a nitrocellulose or nylon membrane, and hybridized with complementary (labeled) nucleic acid probes.

soy·bean (SB) (soy′bēn) The bean of the climbing herb *Glycine soja* or *G. hispida;* rich in protein and containing little starch; used in preparing a bread for diabetic patients, in feeding formulas for infants who are unable to tolerate cow's milk, and for adults allergic to cow's milk. SYN soja, soya.

space (spās) [TA] 1. Any demarcated portion of the body, either an area of the surface, a segment of the tissues, or a cavity. SEE ALSO area, region, zone. 2. DENTISTRY SYN diastema.

space ad·ap·ta·tion syn·drome (spās ad′ap-tā′shŭn sin′drōm) Alterations in normal physiology that occur during prolonged exposure to weightlessness, unless preventive measures are taken.

space med·i·cine (SM) (spās med′i-sin) Science concerned with physiologic diseases or disturbances due to the unique conditions of space travel.

space sense (spās sens) Perception of relative positions of objects in the external world.

spar·ga·no·sis (spahr'gă-nō'sis) Infection with the plerocercoid or sparganum of a pseudophyllidean tapeworm, usually in a dermal sore resulting from application of infected flesh as a poultice; infection may also occur from ingestion of uncooked meat.

spar·ing ac·tion (spār'ing ak'shŭn) The manner in which a nonessential nutritive component, by its presence in the diet, lowers the dietary requirement for an essential component.

spasm (spazm) A sudden involuntary contraction of one or more muscle groups; includes cramps, contractures. SYN muscle spasm, spasmus.

spasmo- Combining form indicating spasm.

spas·mod·ic (spaz-mod'ik) Relating to or marked by spasm.

spas·mod·ic asth·ma (spaz-mod'ik az'mă) Asthma due to spasm of the bronchioles.

spas·mod·ic stric·ture (spaz-mod'ik strik'shŭr) One due to localized spasm of muscular fibers in the wall of the canal. SYN functional stricture, temporary stricture.

spas·mod·ic tic (spaz-mod'ik tik) Disorder in which sudden spasmodic coordinated movements of certain muscles or groups of physiologically related muscles occur at irregular intervals. SYN Henoch chorea.

spas·mod·ic tor·ti·col·lis (ST) (spaz-mod'ik tōr'ti-kol'is) Disorder of unknown cause, manifested as a restricted dystonia, localized to some of the neck muscles, especially the sternomastoid and trapezius. SYN dystonic torticollis, rotatory tic.

spas·mo·gen (spaz'mŏ-jen) A substance causing contraction of smooth muscle; e.g., histamine.

spas·mol·y·sis (spaz-mol'i-sis) The arrest of a spasm or convulsion.

spas·mo·lyt·ic (spaz'mŏ-lit'ik) 1. Relating to spasmolysis. 2. Denoting a chemical agent that relieves smooth muscle spasms.

spas·mus nu·tans (spaz'mŭs nū'tanz) Head turning and nodding with vertical, horizontal, or torsional nystagmus, appears in patients aged between 6 months and 3 years.

spas·tic (spas'tik) 1. SYN hypertonic (1). 2. Relating to spasm or to spasticity.

spas·tic a·ba·si·a (spas'tik ă-bā'zē-ă) Inability to walk due to a spastic contraction of the muscles when an attempt is made.

spas·tic a·pho·ni·a (spas'tik ă-fō'nē-ă) Voice loss due to spasmodic contraction of the laryngeal adductor muscles provoked by attempted phonation.

spas·tic co·lon (spas'tik kō'lŏn) SYN irritable bowel syndrome.

spas·tic di·ple·gi·a (spas'tik dī-plē'jē-ă) Cerebral palsy with bilateral spasticity, with the lower limbs more severely affected. Cf. flaccid paralysis. SYN Erb-Charcot disease (1), infantile diplegia, spastic spinal paralysis.

spas·tic en·tro·pi·on (spas'tik en-trō'pē-on) Eye disorder that arises from excessive contracture of the orbicularis oculi muscle.

spas·tic hem·i·ple·gi·a (spas'tik hem'i-plē'jē-ă) Hemiplegia with increased tone in the antigravity muscles of the affected side.

spas·tic·i·ty (spas-tis'i-tē) A state of increased muscular tone with exaggeration of the tendon reflexes.

spas·tic pa·ra·ple·gi·a (SP, SPG) (spas'tik par'ă-plē'jē-ă) Paresis of the lower extremities with increased muscle tone and spasmodic contraction of the muscles. SYN Erb-Charcot disease (2).

spa·tial (spā'shăl) Relating to space or a space.

spat·u·la (spach'yŭ-lă) A flat blade, used in pharmacy to spread plasters and ointments and aid in mixing ingredients with a mortar and pestle.

spat·u·late (spach'yŭ-lăt) 1. Shaped like a spatula. 2. To manipulate or mix with a spatula. 3. To incise the cut end of a tubular structure longitudinally and splay it open.

spe·cial an·at·o·my (spesh′ăl ă-nat′ŏ-mē) The composition of certain definite organs or groups of organs involved in the performance of special functions.

spe·cial·ist (spesh′ă-list) One who devotes professional attention to a particular specialty or subject area.

spe·cial·ty (spesh′ăl-tē) In health care, the particular subject area or branch of medical science to which one devotes professional attention.

spe·ci·a·tion (spē′shē-ā′shŭn) Evolutionary process by which diverse species of animals or plants are formed from a common ancestral stock.

spe·cies, pl. **spe·cies** (spē′shēz) **1.** A biologic division between the genus and a variety or the individual; a group of organisms that generally bear a close resemblance to one another in the more essential features of their organization, and that breed effectively, producing fertile progeny. **2.** A class of pharmaceutical preparations consisting of a mixture of dried plants, not pulverized, but in sufficiently fine division to be conveniently used in the making of extemporaneous decoctions or infusions, as a tea.

spe·cies-spe·cif·ic an·ti·gen (spē′shēz spĕ-sif′ik an′ti-jen) Antigenic components in tissues and fluids by means of which various species may be immunologically distinguished.

spe·cif·ic (spĕ-sif′ik) **1.** Relating to a species. **2.** Relating to an individual infectious disease. **3.** Remedy with a definite therapeutic action in relation to a particular disease or symptom.

spe·cif·ic ab·sorp·tion co·ef·fi·cient (a, α) (spĕ-sif′ik ăb-sōrp′shŭn kŏ′ĕ-fish′ĕnt) Absorbance (of light) per unit path length (usually the centimeter) and per unit of mass concentration. Cf. molar absorption coefficient. SYN absorbancy index (1), absorptivity (1), extinction coefficient, specific extinction.

spe·cif·ic dis·ease (spĕ-sif′ik di-zēz′) State produced by the action of a special pathogenic microorganism.

spe·cif·ic dy·nam·ic ac·tion (SDA) (spĕ-sif′ik dī-nam′ik ak′shŭn) Increase of heat production caused by the ingestion of food, especially of protein.

spe·cif·ic grav·i·ty (spĕ-sif′ik grav′i-tē) The weight of any body compared with that of another body of equal volume regarded as the unit.

spe·cif·ic im·mu·ni·ty (spĕ-sif′ik i-myū′ni-tē) The immune status with an altered reactivity directed solely against the antigenic determinants that stimulated it. SEE ALSO acquired immunity.

spe·ci·fi·ci·ty of train·ing prin·ci·ple (spes′i-fis′i-tē trān′ing prin′si-pĕl) EXERCISE SCIENCE concept that specific exercise elicits specific adaptations, creating specific training effects.

spe·cif·ic op·so·nin (spĕ-sif′ik op′sŏ-nin) Antibodies formed in response to stimulation by a specific antigen.

spe·cif·ic pho·bi·a (spĕ-sif′ik fō′bē-ă) Persistent pattern of significant fear of specific objects or situations, manifesting in anxiety or panic on exposure to the object or situation or in anticipation of them, which the person realizes is unreasonable or excessive and which interferes significantly with the person's functioning. SYN simple phobia.

spec·i·men (spes′i-mĕn) Sample of any substance or material obtained for testing.

spec·ta·cles (spek′tă-kĕlz) Lenses set in a frame that holds them in front of the eyes; used to correct errors of refraction or to protect the eyes. SYN eyeglasses, glasses.

spec·tral (spek′trăl) Relating to a spectrum.

spec·trin (spek′trin) A filamentous contractile protein that together with actin and other cytoskeleton proteins forms a network that gives the red blood cell membrane its shape and flexibility.

spectro- Combining form indicating a spectrum.

spec·trom·e·try (spek-trom′ĕ-trē) The procedure of observing and measuring the wavelengths of light or other electromagnetic emissions.

spec·tro·pho·tom·e·ter (spek′trō-fŏ-tom′ĕ-tĕr) An instrument for measuring the intensity of light of a definite wavelength transmitted by a substance or a solution.

spec·tro·scope (spek′trŏ-skōp) An instrument for resolving light from any luminous body into its spectrum, and for the analysis of the spectrum so formed.

spec·trum, pl. **spec·trums,** pl. **spec·tra** (spek′trŭm, -trŭmz, -tră) **1.** The range of colors presented when white light is resolved into its constituent colors by being passed through a prism or through a diffraction grating: red, orange, yellow, green, blue, indigo, and violet, arranged in increasing frequency of vibration or decreasing wavelength. **2.** The range of pathogenic microorganisms against which an antibiotic or other antibacterial agent is active.

spec·u·lum, pl. **spec·u·la** (spek′yŭ-lŭm, -lă) An instrument for enlarging the opening of any canal or cavity to facilitate inspection of its interior.

spec·u·lum for·ceps (spek′yŭ-lŭm fōr′seps) A tubular forceps for use through a speculum.

speech (spēch) Talk; the use of the voice to communicate.

SPEECH1 (spēch) Gene that when mutated causes motor dyspraxia.

speech bulb (spēch bŭlb) Vocal prosthesis used to close a cleft or other opening in the hard or soft palate, or to replace absent tissue necessary for the production of good speech.

speech cen·ters (spēch sen′tĕrz) Areas of the cerebral cortex centrally involved in speech function. SEE ALSO Broca center, Wernicke center.

speech-lan·guage path·ol·o·gist (SLP) (spēch-lang′gwăj pă-thol′ŏ-jist) A practitioner concerned with the diagnosis and rehabilitation of patients with voice, speech, and language disorders.

speech path·ol·o·gy, speech-lan·guage path·o·lo·gy (spēch pă-thol′ŏ-jē, lang′gwăj) The science concerned with functional and organic speech defects and disorders.

speech read·ing (spēch rēd′ing) Method used by people with hearing impairment of nonauditory clues as to what is being said through observing the speaker's facial expressions, lip and jaw movements, and other gestures. SYN lip reading.

sperm, pl. **sperms** (spĕrm, spĕrmz) The male gamete or sex cell that contains the genetic information to be transmitted by the male, exhibits autokinesia, and is able to effect zygosis with an oocyte. Formerly called spermatazoa.

sperma-, spermato-, spermo- Combining forms denoting semen, sperms.

sper·ma·cyt·ic sem·i·no·ma (spĕrm′ă-sit′ik sem′i-nō′mă) A relatively slow-growing, locally invasive type of testicular seminoma that does not metastasize.

sper·mat·ic (spĕr-mat′ik) Relating to the sperm or semen.

sper·mat·ic fis·tu·la (spĕr-mat′ik fis′tyū-lă) Passage communicating with the testis or any of the seminal passages.

sper·ma·tid (spĕr′mă-tid) A cell in a late stage of the development of the sperm; it is a haploid cell derived from the secondary spermatocyte and evolves by spermiogenesis into a sperm.

sper·ma·to·cele, sper·ma·to·cyst (spĕr′mă-tō-sēl, -sist) Cyst of the epididymis containing sperm.

sper·ma·to·ci·dal, sper·mi·ci·dal (spĕr′mă-tō-sī′dăl, spĕr-mi-sī′dăl) Destructive to sperms.

sper·ma·to·cyte (spĕr-mat′ō-sīt) Parent cell of a spermatid, derived by mitotic division from a spermatogonium.

sper·ma·to·gen·e·sis, sper·ma·to·cy·to·gen·e·sis, sper·ma·tog·e·ny (spĕr′mă-tō-jen′ĕ-sis, spĕr′mă-tō-sī′tō-jen′ĕ-sis, -toj′ĕ-nē) The entire process by which spermatogonial stem cells divide and differentiate into sperms. SEE ALSO spermiogenesis. SYN spermatocytogenesis.

sper·ma·to·gen·ic, sper·ma·tog·e·nous, sper·ma·to·poi·et·ic, sper·ma·to·ge·net·ic (spĕr′mă-tō-jen′ik, -toj′ĕ-nŭs, -mă-tō-poy-et′ik, -jĕ-net′ik)

Relating to spermatogenesis; sperm-producing. SYN spermatopoietic (1).

sper·ma·to·go·ni·um, sper·ma·to·gone, sper·ma·to·blast (spĕr′mă-tō-gō′nē-ŭm, -mă-tō-gōn, -mă-tō-blast) The undifferentiated male sex cell derived by mitotic division from a primordial germ cell; increasing several times in size, it becomes a primary spermatocyte.

sper·ma·toid (spĕr′mă-toyd) 1. Resembling a sperm, a sperm tail, or semen. 2. A male or flagellated form of the malarial microparasite.

sper·ma·tol·y·sis, sper·ma·tol·y·sis (spĕrm′ă-tol′i-sis, spĕr-mol′i-sis) Destruction, with dissolution, of sperms.

sper·ma·tor·rhe·a (spĕr′mă-tōr-ē′ă) An involuntary discharge of semen, without orgasm. SYN spermatorrhoea.

spermatorrhoea [Br.] SYN spermatorrhea.

sper·ma·tu·ri·a (spĕr′mă-tyūr′ē-ă) SYN semenuria.

sper·mi·cide, sper·mat·i·cide (spĕr′mi-sīd, spĕr-mat′i-sīd) An agent destructive to sperms.

sper·mi·o·gen·e·sis (spĕr′mē-ō-jen′ē-sis) Segment of spermatogenesis when immature spermatids shed much of their cytoplasm and develop a flagellum and acrosomal granule, becoming, in this process, sperms.

sphac·e·la·tion (sfas′ĕ-lā′shŭn) 1. Becoming gangrenous or necrotic. 2. Gangrene or necrosis.

sphac·e·lo·der·ma (sfas′ĕ-lō-dĕr′mă) Gangrene of the skin.

sphe·ni·on (sfē′nē-on) The tip of the sphenoidal angle of the parietal bone; a craniometric point.

♻ **spheno-** *Do not confuse this combining form with stheno-.* Wedge, wedge-shaped; the sphenoid bone.

sphe·no·bas·i·lar (sfē′nō-bas′i-lăr) Relation to the sphenoid bone and the basilar process of the occipital bone. SYN sphenooccipital.

sphe·no·ceph·a·ly (sfē′nō-sef′ă-lē) Condition characterized by a deformation of the cranium, giving it a wedge-shaped appearance.

sphe·no·eth·moi·dal re·cess (sfē′nō-eth-moy′dăl rē′ses) [TA] Small cleftlike pocket of the nasal cavity above the superior concha into which the sphenoid sinuses drain. SYN recessus sphenoethmoidalis [TA].

sphe·no·eth·moi·dec·to·my (sfē′nō-eth′moyd-ek′tŏ-mē) An operation to remove diseased tissue from the sphenoid and ethmoid sinuses.

sphe·noi·dal, sphenoid (sfē-noy′dăl) 1. Relating to the sphenoid bone. 2. Wedge-shaped. SYN sphenoid (1).

sphe·noi·di·tis (sfē′noy-dī′tis) 1. Inflammation of the sphenoid sinus. 2. Necrosis of the sphenoid bone.

sphe·noi·dot·o·my (sfē′noy-dot′ŏ-mē) Any operation on the sphenoid bone or sinus.

sphe·no·max·il·lar·y (sfē′nō-mak′si-lar′ē) Relating to the sphenoid bone and the maxilla.

sphe·no·pal·a·tine (sfē′nō-pal′ă-tīn) Relating to the sphenoid and the palatine bones.

sphe·no·pal·a·tine neu·ral·gi·a (sfēn′ō-pal′ă-tīn nūr-al′jē-ă) Pain related to the nervous system in the lower half of the face, with pain referred to the root of the nose, upper teeth, eyes, ears, mastoid, and occiput, in association with nasal congestion and rhinorrhea due to infection of the nasal sinuses, and produced by lesions of the sphenopalatine ganglion. SYN Sluder neuralgia.

sphe·no·pa·ri·e·tal (sfē′nō-pă-rī′ĕ-tăl) Relating to the sphenoid and the parietal bones.

sphere (sfēr) A ball or globular body.

♻ **sphero-** Combining form denoting spheric, a sphere.

sphe·ro·cyte (sfēr′ō-sīt) A small, spheric red blood cell.

sphe·ro·cy·to·sis (sfēr′ō-sī-tō′sis) Presence of spherelike red blood cells in the blood.

sphe·roid, sphe·roi·dal (sfēr′oyd, sfēr-oyd′ăl) Shaped like a sphere.

sphe·roi·dal joint (sfēr-oy′dăl joynt) SYN ball and socket joint.

sphe·ro·pha·ki·a (sfēr′ō-fā′kē-ă) A congenital bilateral ocular aberration in which the lenses are small, spheric, and subject to subluxation.

sphinc·ter (sfingk′tĕr) [TA] A muscle that encircles a duct, tube, or orifice in such a way that its contraction constricts the lumen or orifice. SYN sphincter muscle.

sphinc·ter·al·gi·a (sfingk′tĕr-al′jē-ă) Pain in the sphincter ani muscles.

sphinc·ter·ec·to·my (sfingk′tĕr-ek′tŏ-mē) **1.** Excision of a portion of the pupillary border of the iris. **2.** Dissecting away any sphincter muscle.

sphinc·ter·is·mus (sfingk′tĕr-iz′mŭs) Spasmodic contraction of the anal sphincter muscles.

sphinc·ter·i·tis (sfingk′tĕr-ī′tis) Inflammation of any sphincter.

sphinc·ter mus·cle (sfingk′tĕr mŭs′ĕl) [TA] SYN sphincter.

sphinc·ter of Od·di dys·func·tion (sfingk′tĕr od′ē dis-fŭngk′shŭn) Structural or functional abnormality of the sphincter of Oddi that interferes with bile drainage.

sphinc·ter·ol·y·sis (sfingk-tĕr-ol′i-sis) An operation to free the iris from the cornea in anterior synechia involving only the pupillary border.

sphinc·ter·o·plas·ty (sfingk′tĕr-ō-plas-tē) Plastic surgery of any sphincter muscle.

sphinc·ter·ot·o·my (sfingk′tĕr-ot′ŏ-mē) Incision or division of a sphincter muscle.

sphin·ga·nine (sfing′gă-nēn) Dihydrosphingosine; a precursor of sphingosine.

sphin·go·lip·id (sfing′gō-lip′id) Any lipid with a long-chain base like sphingosine, a constituent of nerve tissue.

sphin·go·lip·i·do·sis, sphin·go·lip·o·dys·tro·phy, pl. **sphin·go·lip·i·do·ses** (sfing′gō-lip′i-dō′sis, sfing′gō-lip′ō-dis′trŏ-fē, -i-dō′sēz) Collective designation for diseases characterized by abnormal sphingolipid metabolism.

sphin·go·sine (sfing′gō-sēn) The principal long-chain base found in sphingolipids.

sphyg·mic (sfig′mik) Relating to the pulse.

sphyg·mic in·ter·val (sfig′mik in′tĕr-văl) The period in the cardiac cycle when the semilunar valves are open and blood is being ejected from the ventricles into the arterial system. SYN ejection period.

sphygmo-, sphygm- Combining forms denoting a pulse.

sphyg·mo·gram (sfig′mō-gram) The graphic curve made by a sphygmograph.

sphyg·mo·graph (sfig′mō-graf) An instrument consisting of a lever, the short end of that rests on the radial artery at the wrist, its long end fitted with a stylet to record pulses on a moving ribbon of smoked paper.

sphyg·moid (sfig′moyd) Pulselike; resembling the pulse.

sphyg·mo·ma·nom·e·ter (sfig′mō-mă-nom′ĕ-tĕr) An instrument to measure arterial blood pressure indirectly, with an inflatable cuff, inflating bulb, and a gauge to show blood pressure.

sphyg·mo·scope (sfig′mŏ-skōp) An instrument by which the pulse beats are made visible by some means.

sphyg·mo·to·nom·e·ter (sfig′mō-tō-nom′ĕ-tĕr) An instrument, like the sphygmotonograph, to determine degree of blood pressure.

spi·ca ban·dage, spi·ca cast (spī′kă ban′dăj, kast) Successive strips of material applied to the body and the first part of a limb, or to the hand and a finger, which overlap slightly in a V to resemble an ear of grain.

spic·ule, spic·u·lat·ed (spik′yūl, -yū-lā-tĕd) A small, needle-shaped body.

spic·u·lum, pl. **spic·u·la** (spik′yū-lŭm, -ă) A spicule or small spike.

spi·der (spī′dĕr) An arthropod with four pairs of legs; a cephalothorax; a globose, smooth abdomen; and a complex of web-spinning spinnerets. Among the venomous spiders found in the New World are the black widow spider, red-legged widow spider, and brown recluse spider of North America.

spi·der an·gi·o·ma, spi·der tel·an·gi·ec·ta·sia (spī′dĕr an′jē-ō′mă, tel′an′jē-ek-tā′shē-ă) A telangiectatic arteriole in the skin with radiating capillary branches simulating the legs of a spider; characteristic, but not pathognomonic, of parenchymatous liver disease. SYN arterial spider, spider nevus, vascular spider.

spi·der-burst (spī′dĕr-bŭrst) Radiating dull red capillary lines on the skin of the leg, usually without any visible or palpable varicose veins, but nevertheless due to deep-seated venous dilation.

spike (spīk) **1.** A brief electrical event of 3–25 milliseconds that gives the appearance in the electroencephalogram of a rising and falling vertical line. **2.** In electrophoresis, a sharply angled upward deflection on a densitometric tracing.

spike-and-wave com·plex (spīk wāv kom′pleks) A generalized, synchronous pattern seen on an electroencephalogram, consisting of a sharply contoured fast wave followed by a slow wave.

spike po·ten·tial (spīk pŏ-ten′shăl) Main wave in the neural action potentials; followed by negative and positive afterpotentials.

spill·way (spil′wā) A groove or channel through which food may pass from the occlusal surfaces of teeth during the masticatory process. SYN sluiceway.

spi·na bi·fi·da (spī′nă bif′i-dă) Embryologic failure of fusion of one or more neural arches that will become vertebral arches.

spi·nal (spī′năl) **1.** Relating to any spine or spinous process. **2.** Relating to the vertebral column. SYN rachidial.

spi·nal ad·just·ment (spī′năl ă-jŭst′mĕnt) Manual method of specific osseous movement of the vertebrae using controlled force, direction, leverage, amplitude, and velocity; typically performed by a chiropractor. SYN adjustment (1).

spi·nal an·es·the·si·a, spi·nal an·al·ge·si·a (spī′năl an′es-thē′zē-ă, an′al-jē′zē-ă) **1.** Loss of sensation produced by injection of local anesthetic solution(s) into the spinal subarachnoid space. **2.** Loss of sensation produced by disease of the spinal cord.

spi·nal block (spī′năl blok) An obstruction to the flow of cerebrospinal fluid in the spinal subarachnoid space.

spi·nal col·umn (spī′năl kol′ŭm) SYN vertebral column.

spi·nal cord (spī′năl kōrd) [TA] The elongated cylindric portion of the cerebrospinal axis, or central nervous system, which is contained in the spinal or vertebral canal. SYN medulla spinalis.

spi·nal cord con·cus·sion (spī′năl kōrd kŏn-kŭsh′ŭn) Injury to the spinal cord due to a blow to the vertebral column with transient or prolonged dysfunction below the level of the lesion. SYN spinal concussion.

spi·nal cur·vat·ure (spī′năl kŭr′vă-chŭr) SEE kyphosis, lordosis, scoliosis.

spi·nal de·com·pres·sion (spī′năl dē′kŏm-presh′ŭn) Removal of pressure on the spinal cord as created by a tumor, cyst, hematoma, herniated nucleus pulposus, abscess, or bone.

spi·nal dys·raph·ism (spī′năl dis-rāf′izm) A general term used to describe a collection of congenital abnormalities that include defects in the vertebrae and underlying spine or nerve roots.

spi·nal fu·sion, spine fu·sion (spī′năl fyū′zhŭn, spīn) A surgical procedure to accomplish bony ankylosis between two or more vertebrae.

spi·nal gan·gli·on (spī′năl gang′glē-on) The ganglion of the posterior root of each spinal segmental nerve.

spi·nal mus·cu·lar at·ro·phy (SMA)

(spī′năl mŭs′kyū-lăr ăt′rŏ-fē) A heterogeneous group of degenerative diseases of the anterior horn cells in the spinal cord and motor nuclei of the brainstem; all are characterized by weakness.

spi·nal re·flex (spī′năl rē′fleks) A reflex arc involving the spinal cord. SEE ALSO reflex arc.

spi·nal shock (spī′năl shok) Transient depression or abolition of reflex activity below the level of an acute spinal cord injury.

spi·nal ste·no·sis (spī′năl stĕ-nō′sis) Abnormal narrowing of the spinal canal, often with compression of the spinal cord.

spi·nal tap (spī′năl tap) SYN lumbar puncture.

spi·nal tract (spī′năl trakt) Any of a multitude of fiber bundles ascending or descending in the spinal cord.

spi·nate (spī′nāt) Spined; having spines.

spin·dle (spin′dĕl) ANATOMY, PATHOLOGY any fusiform cell or structure.

spin·dle cell car·ci·no·ma (spin′dĕl sel kahr′si-nō′mă) A carcinoma composed of elongated cells, frequently a poorly differentiated squamous cell carcinoma that may be difficult to distinguish from a sarcoma.

spin·dle cell sar·co·ma (spin′dĕl sel sahr-kō′mă) Malignant neoplasm of mesenchymal origin composed of elongated, spindle-shaped cells. SYN fascicular sarcoma.

spine (spīn) [TA] **1.** A short, sharp, thornlike process of bone; a spinous process. **2.** SYN vertebral column. **3.** The bar or stay in a horse's hoof.

spinn·bar·keit (SPK, SBK) (spin′bahr-kīt) The stringy, elastic character of cervical mucus during the ovulatory period.

spino-, spin- Combining forms meaning the spine.

spi·no·ad·duc·tor re·flex (spī′nō-ad-dŭk′tŏr rē′fleks) Contraction of the adductors of the thigh on tapping the spinal column. SYN McCarthy reflexes (1).

spi·no·bul·bar (spī′nō-bŭl′bahr) SYN bulbospinal.

spi·no·cer·e·bel·lar a·tax·i·a (spī′nō-ser′ĕ-bĕl′lăr ă-tak′sē-ă) Most common hereditary ataxia, with onset in middle to late childhood, with limb ataxia, nystagmus, kyphoscoliosis, pes cavus, and pathologic spinal cord effects.

spi·no·tha·lam·ic tract (STT) (spī′nō-thă-lam′ik trakt) General term describing a large ascending fiber bundle in the ventral half of the lateral funiculus of the spinal cord, arising from cells in the posterior horn at all levels of the cord, which cross within their segments of origin in the white commissure. SYN tractus spinothalamicus.

spi·nous (spī′nŭs) Relating to, shaped like, or having a spine or spines.

spi·rad·e·no·ma (spīr′ad-ĕ-nō′mă) A benign tumor of sweat glands.

spi·ral (spī′răl) **1.** Coiled; winding around a center like a watch spring; winding and ascending like a wire spring. **2.** A structure in the shape of a coil.

spi·ral ban·dage (spī′răl ban′dăj) An oblique bandage encircling a limb, the successive turns overlapping those preceding.

spi·ral com·put·ed tom·og·ra·phy (SCT, S-CT) (spī′răl kŏm-pyū′tĕd tŏ-mog′ră-fē) Computed tomography in which the x-ray tube continuously revolves around the patient, who is simultaneously moved longitudinally. SYN helical computed tomography, helical CT, spiral CT.

spi·ral frac·ture (spī′răl frak′shŭr) A break that creates a helical line in bone.

spi·ral or·gan (spī′răl ŏr′găn) A prominent ridge of highly specialized epithelium in the floor of the cochlear duct overlying the basilar membrane of cochlea, containing one inner row and three outer rows of hair cells, or cells of Corti (the auditory receptor cells innervated by the cochlear nerve), supported by various columnar cells. SYN Corti organ.

spi·ril·lo·sis (spī′ri-lō′sis) Any disease caused by the presence of spirilla in the blood or tissues.

S

Spi·ril·lum (spī-ril′ŭm) A genus of large, rigid, helical, gram-negative bacteria that are motile by means of bipolar fascicles of flagella.

spi·ril·lum, pl. **spi·ril·la** (spī-ril′ŭm, -ă) A member of the genus *Spirillum*.

spir·it (spir′it) **1.** An alcoholic liquor stronger than wine (i.e., 15%), obtained by distillation. **2.** Any distilled liquid. **3.** An alcoholic or hydroalcoholic solution of volatile substances; some spirits are used as flavoring agents; others have medicinal value.

♻ **spiro-, spir-** **1.** Combining forms meaning coil, coil-shaped. **2.** Combining forms meaning breathing.

Spi·ro·chae·ta (spī′rō-kē′tă) Genus of motile bacteria containing gram-negative, flexible, undulating, spiral-shaped rods that may possess flagelliform, tapering ends found free living in fresh or sea water slime and are commonly also found in sewage and foul water.

spi·ro·chete (spī′rō-kēt) A vernacular term used to refer to any organism resembling a *Leptospira*, *Spirochaeta*, or *Treponema* cell.

spi·ro·che·ti·cide (spī′rō-kē′ti-sīd) An agent destructive to spirochetes.

spi·ro·che·tol·y·sis (spī′rō-kē-tol′i-sis) Destruction of spirochetes, as by chemotherapy or by specific antibodies.

spi·ro·che·to·sis (spī′rō-kē-tō′sis) Any disease caused by a spirochete.

spi·ro·gram (spī′rō-gram) The tracing made by the spirograph.

spi·ro·graph (spī′rō-graf) A device for representing graphically the depth and rapidity of respiratory movements.

spi·rom·e·ter (spī-rom′ĕ-tĕr) A gasometer used for measuring respiratory gases.

Spi·ro·me·tra (spī′rō-mē′tră) A genus of pseudophyllid tapeworms.

spi·rom·e·try (spī-rom′ĕ-trē) Making pulmonary measurements with a spirometer.

spi·ro·no·lac·tone (spī′rō-nō-lak′tōn) Diuretic that blocks aldosterone's renal tubular actions and increases urinary excretion of sodium and chloride.

spis·si·tude (spis′i-tūd) Condition of a fluid thickened almost to a solid by evaporation.

Spitz ne·vus (spits nē′vŭs) A benign, slightly pigmented or red, superficial, small skin tumor composed of spindle-shaped, epithelioid, and multinucleated cells that may appear atypical.

splanch·nec·to·pi·a (splangk′nek-tō′pē-ă) Displacement of any of the viscera.

splanch·nic an·es·the·si·a (splangk′nik an′es-thē′zē-ă) Loss of sensation in areas of the visceral peritoneum innervated by the splanchnic nerves. SYN visceral anesthesia.

splanch·nic cav·i·ty (splangk′nik kav′i-tē) The celom or one of the body cavities derived from it.

splanch·ni·cec·to·my (splangk′ni-sek′tō-mē) Resection of the splanchnic nerves and usually of the celiac ganglion as well.

splanch·nic nerve (splangk′nik nĕrv) One of the nerves supplying the viscera.

splanch·ni·cot·o·my (splangk′ni-kot′ŏ-mē) Section of a splanchnic nerve or nerves; a surgical procedure formerly used to treat hypertension.

splanch·nic wall (splangk′nik wawl) The side of one of the viscera or the splanchnopleure from which it is formed.

♻ **splanchno-, splanchn-, splanchni-** Combining forms denoting the viscera. SEE ALSO viscero-.

splanch·no·cele (splangk′nō-sēl) **1.** The primordial body cavity or celom in the embryo. **2.** Hernia of any of the abdominal viscera.

splanch·nog·ra·phy (splangk-nog′ră-fē) A description of the viscera.

splanch·no·lith (splangk′nō-lith) An intestinal calculus.

splanch·nol·o·gy (splangk-nol′ŏ-jē)

The branch of medical science dealing with the viscera. SYN splanchnologia.

splanch·nop·a·thy (splangk-nop′ă-thē) Any disease of the abdominal viscera.

splanch·no·pleure (splangk′nō-plur) The embryonic layer formed by association of the visceral layer of the lateral plate mesoderm with the endoderm.

splanch·no·scle·ro·sis (splangk′nō-skle-rō′sis) Hardening, through connective tissue overgrowth, of any of the viscera.

splanch·not·o·my (splangk-not′ŏ-mē) Dissection of the viscera by incision.

splanch·no·tribe (splangk′nō-trīb) Instrument used to occlude the intestine temporarily, before resection.

splay (splā) To lay open the end of a tubular structure by making a longitudinal incision to increase its potential diameter. SEE ALSO spatulate (3).

spleen, splen (splēn, splen) [TA] A large vascular lymphatic organ lying in the upper part of the abdominal cavity on the left side, between the stomach and diaphragm, composed of white and red pulp; a blood-forming organ in early life and later a storage organ for red corpuscles and platelets. SYN lien [TA].

sple·nec·to·my (splē-nek′tŏ-mē) Removal of the spleen.

sple·nec·to·pi·a, sple·nec·to·py (splē′nek-tō′pē-ă, splē-nek′tŏ-pē) 1. Displacement of the spleen. 2. The presence of rests of splenic tissue, usually in the region of the spleen.

splen·ic (splen′ik) Relating to the spleen. SYN lienal.

splen·ic flex·ure syn·drome (splen′ik flek′shŭr sin′drōm) Symptoms of pain, gas, bloating, and fullness experienced in the left upper abdominal quadrant, sometimes beneath the ribs, in some instances radiating upward, and in some instances producing anterior central chest pain or predominantly on the left.

splen·ic lymph fol·li·cles (splen′ik limf fol′i-kĕlz) Small, nodular masses of lymphoid tissue attached to the sides of the smaller arterial branches. SYN malpighian corpuscles.

splen·ic pulp (splen′ik pŭlp) [TA] The soft cellular substance of the spleen.

sple·ni·tis (splē-nī′tis) Inflammation of the spleen.

sple·ni·um, pl. **sple·ni·a** (splē′nē-ŭm, -ă) 1. A compress or bandage. 2. A structure resembling a bandaged part.

sple·no·cele (splē′nō-sēl) 1. SYN splenoma. 2. A splenic hernia.

sple·no·col·ic (splē′nō-kol′ik) Relating to the spleen and the colon.

sple·no·hep·a·to·meg·a·ly, sple·no·he·pa·to·me·ga·li·a (splē′nō-hep′ă-tō-meg′ă-lē, -mē-gā′lē-ă) Enlargement of both spleen and liver.

sple·noid (splē′noyd) Resembling the spleen.

sple·no·ma (splē-nō′mă) General nonspecific term for an enlarged spleen. SYN splenocele (1).

sple·no·ma·la·ci·a (splē′nō-mă-lā′shē-ă) Softening of the spleen.

sple·no·meg·a·ly, meg·a·lo·sple·ni·a, sple·no·me·ga·li·a (splē-nō-meg′ă-lē, meg-ă-lō-splē′nē-ă, splē-nō-mē-gā′lē-ă) Enlargement of the spleen.

sple·no·my·e·log·e·nous (splē′nō-mī-ĕ-loj′ĕ-nŭs) Originating in the spleen and bone marrow, denoting a form of leukemia. SYN splenomedullary.

sple·no·my·e·lo·ma·la·ci·a (splē′nō-mī′ĕ-lō′mă-lā′shē-ă) Pathologic softening of the spleen and bone marrow.

sple·no·pan·cre·at·ic (splē′nō-pan′krē-at′ik) Relating to the spleen and the pancreas. SYN lienopancreatic.

sple·nop·a·thy (splē-nop′ă-thē) Any disease of the spleen.

sple·no·pex·y, sple·no·pex·i·a (splē′nō-pek-sē, -pek′sē-ă) Suturing in place an ectopic or floating spleen. SYN splenorrhaphy (2).

sple·no·por·tog·ra·phy (splē′nō-pōr-tog′ră-fē) Introduction of radiopaque material into the spleen to obtain a radiologic visualization of the portal vessel of the portal circulation.

sple·nop·to·sis, sple·nop·to·si·a (splē′nop-tō′sis, -tō′sē-ă) *In the diphthong pt, the p is silent only at the beginning of a word.* Downward displacement of the spleen, as in a floating spleen.

sple·no·re·nal (splē′nō-rē′năl) Relating to the spleen and the kidney. SYN lienorenal, splenonephric.

sple·no·re·nal shunt (splē′nō-rē′năl shŭnt) Anastomosis of the splenic vein to the left renal vein, usually end to side, for control of portal hypertension.

sple·nor·rha·gi·a (splē′nōr-ă′jē-ă) Hemorrhage from a ruptured spleen.

sple·nor·rha·phy (splē-nōr′ă-fē) 1. Suturing of a ruptured spleen. 2. SYN splenopexy.

sple·not·o·my (splē-not′ŏ-mē) 1. Anatomy or dissection of the spleen. 2. Surgical incision of the spleen.

sple·no·tox·in (splē′nō-tok′sin) A cytotoxin specific for cells of the spleen.

splic·ing (splīs′ing) 1. Attachment of one DNA molecule to another. 2. Removal of introns from mRNA precursors and the reattachment or annealing of exons. SYN RNA splicing.

splint (splint) 1. An appliance used to prevent movement of a joint or to fixate displaced or movable parts. 2. The splint bone, or fibula.

splin·ter hem·or·rhag·es (splin′tĕr hĕm′ŏr-ăj-ĕz) Multiple tiny longitudinal subungual hemorrhages under a nail, typically seen in but not diagnostic of bacterial endocarditis and trichinelliasis.

splint·ing (splint′ing) 1. Treatment using a splint. 2. In dentistry, joining two or more teeth into a rigid unit by means of fixed or removable restorations or appliances. 3. Stiffening of a body part to avoid pain caused by movement of the part. 4. In psychiatry, the exercise by family, friends, or coworkers of the various strategies designed to minimize the impairment and increase the functional level of a person with diminished higher cortical function.

split brain (split brān) One in which the corpus callosum and usually the anterior and posterior commissures have been sectioned, usually to treat certain refractory epilepsies.

split pel·vis (split pel′vis) A pelvis in which the symphysis pubis is absent, the pelvic bones being separated; usually associated with exstrophy of the bladder.

split-thick·ness graft, split-skin graft (split-thik′nĕs graft, skin) A graft of portions of the skin, or of part of the mucosa and submucosa, but not the periosteum.

split·ting (split′ing) In chemistry, the cleavage of a covalent bond, fragmenting the molecule involved.

split·ting of heart sounds (split′ing hahrt sowndz) The production of major components of the first and second heart sounds due to contribution by the left-sided and right-sided valves.

split tol·er·ance (split tol′ĕr-ăns) Reaction to one (or more) antigen on a cell surface but no reaction to others. SYN immune deviation (1).

spo·dog·e·nous (spŏ-doj′ĕ-nŭs) Caused by waste material.

spon·dy·lal·gi·a (spond′i-lal′jē-ă) Pain in the spine.

spon·dyl·ar·thri·tis (spon′dil-ahr-thrī′tis) Inflammation of the intervertebral articulations.

spon·dy·lit·ic (spond′i-lit′ik) Relating to spondylitis.

spon·dy·li·tis (spon′di-lī′tis) Inflammation of one or more of the vertebrae.

spon·dy·li·tis de·for·mans (spon′di-lī′tis dĕ-fōrm′anz) Arthritis and osteitis deformans involving the spinal column; marked by nodular deposits at the edges of the intervertebral discs with ossification of the ligaments and bony ankylosis of the intervertebral articulations. SYN Bechterew disease, Strümpell disease (1).

spon·dy·lo·ep·i·phys·ial dys·pla·si·a (spon′di-lō-ep′i-fiz′ē-ăl dis-plā′zē-ă) Conditions characterized by growth deficiency of the vertebral column with flattening of the vertebrae or platyspondyly, lack of ossification of the epiphyses, short-trunk dwarfism with limb shortening, and sometimes other malformations.

spon·dy·lo·lis·thet·ic pel·vis (spon′di-lō-lis-thet′ik pel′vis) One with a brim that is more or less occluded by a forward dislocation of the body or one of the lumbar vertebrae. SYN Rokitansky pelvis.

spon·dy·lol·y·sis (spon′di-lol′i-sis) Degeneration or deficient development of a portion of the vertebra.

spon·dy·lop·a·thy (spon′di-lop′ă-thē) Any disease of the vertebrae or spinal column.

spon·dy·lo·py·o·sis (spon′di-lō-pī-ō′sis) Suppurative inflammation of one or more of the vertebral bodies.

spon·dy·los·chi·sis (spon′di-los′ki-sis) Embryologic failure of fusion of neural arch. SEE ALSO spina bifida.

spon·dy·lo·sis (spon′di-lō′sis) Ankylosis of the vertebrae.

spon·dyl·ous (spon′di-lŭs) Relating to a vertebra.

sponge (spŏnj) **1.** Absorbent material used to absorb fluids. **2.** A member of the phylum Porifera, the cellular endoskeleton of which is a source of commercial natural sponges.

sponge bath (spŏnj bath) A cleansing in which the body is washed with a wet sponge or cloth.

spongio- Combining form denoting sponge, sponglike, spongy.

spon·gi·o·blast (spŏn′jē-ō-blast) A neuroepithelial, filiform ependymal cell extending across the entire thickness of the wall of the brain or spinal cord; they become neuroglial and ependymal cells.

spon·gi·o·cyte (spŏn′jē-ō-sīt) **1.** A neuroglial cell. **2.** Cell in the zona fasciculata of suprarenal gland cortex containing many droplets of lipid material that, after staining with hematoxylin and eosin, show pronounced vacuolization.

spon·gi·o·sis (spŏn′jē-ō′sis) Inflammatory intercellular edema of the epidermis.

spon·gi·o·si·tis (spŏn′jē-ō-sī′tis) Inflammation of the corpus spongiosum, or corpus cavernosum urethrae.

spong·y (spŏn′jē) Resembling the commercial natural sponge. SYN spongioid.

spong·y u·re·thra (spŭn′jē yūr-ē′thră) [TA] Portion of the male urethra, which traverses the corpus spongiosum. SYN pars spongiosa urethrae masculinae [TA], pars cavernosa, penile urethra, spongy part of the male urethra.

spon·ta·ne·ous (spon-tā′nē-ŭs) Without apparent cause; said of disease processes or remissions.

spon·ta·ne·ous am·pu·ta·tion (spon-tā′nē-ŭs amp′yū-tā′shŭn) One that results from a pathologic process rather than external trauma.

spon·ta·ne·ous frac·ture (SF) (spon-tā′nē-ŭs frak′shŭr) Break occurring without any obvious external injury.

spon·ta·ne·ous gen·er·a·tion (spon-tā′nē-ŭs jen′ĕr-ā′shŭn) The false concept according to which living matter can arise by the vitalization of nonliving matter. SEE ALSO biogenesis. SYN heterogenesis (3).

spon·ta·ne·ous pha·go·cy·to·sis (spon-tā′nē-ŭs fag′ō-sī-tō′sis) Cellular action when a culture of bacteria is brought in contact with washed leukocytes in an indifferent medium.

spon·ta·ne·ous re·mis·sion (spon-tā′nē-us rē-mis′shŭn) Disappearance of symptoms without formal treatment.

spon·ta·ne·ous ver·sion (spon-tā′nē-ŭs vĕr′zhŭn) Turning of the fetus effected by the unaided contraction of the uterine muscle.

spo·rad·ic (spōr-ad′ik) **1.** Denoting a temporal pattern of disease occurrence in an animal or human population in which the disease occurs only rarely and without regularity. SEE ALSO endemic, epidemic, epizootic. **2.** Occurring irregularly, haphazardly.

spore (spōr) **1.** The asexual or sexual reproductive body of fungi or sporozoan protozoa. **2.** A cell of a plant lower in organization than the seed-bearing spermatophytic plants. **3.** A resistant form of certain species of bacteria. **4.** The highly modified reproductive body of certain protozoa, as in the phyla Microspora and Myxozoa.

spo·ri·cide (spōr′i-sīd) An agent that kills spores.

spo·ro·ag·glu·ti·na·tion (spōr′ō-ă-glū′ti-nā′shŭn) A diagnostic method in relation to the mycoses, based on the fact that the blood of patients with fungal diseases contains specific agglutinins that cause clumping of the spores of these organisms.

spo·ro·blast (spōr′ō-blast) An early stage in the development of a sporocyst before differentiation of the sporozoites. SEE ALSO oocyst, sporocyst (2).

spo·ro·cyst (spōr′ō-sist) A larval form of digenetic trematode that develops in the body of its molluscan intermediate host.

spo·rog·o·ny, spo·rog·e·ny, spo·ro·gen·e·sis (spōr-og′ŏ-nē, -oj′ĕ-nē, spōr′ō-jen′ĕ-sis) The formation of sporozoites in sporozoan protozoa, a process of asexual division within the sporoblast, which becomes the sporocyst within an oocyst.

spo·ront (spōr′ont) The zygote stage within the oocyst wall in the life cycle of coccidia.

spo·ro·phore (spōr′ō-fōr) Any specialized hyphae in fungi that give rise to spores.

spo·ro·plasm (spōr′ō-plazm) The protoplasm of a spore.

Spo·ro·thrix (spōr′ō-thriks) A genus of dimorphic imperfect fungi, including *S. schenckii*, an organism of worldwide distribution and the causative agent of sporotrichosis in humans and animals.

spo·ro·tri·cho·sis (spōr′ō-tri-kō′sis) A chronic cutaneous mycosis spread by way of the lymphatics and caused by inoculation of *Sporothrix schenckii*. SYN Schenck disease.

Spo·rot·ri·chum (spō-rot′ri-kŭm) A genus of imperfect fungi (Hyphomycetes) that are usually common contaminants.

spo·ro·zo·an (spōr′ō-zō′ăn) **1.** An individual organism of the class Sporozoea. **2.** Relating to the Sporozoea.

spo·ro·zo·ite (spōr′ō-zō′īt) A minute elongated body due to repeated division of the oocyst during sporogony. SYN germinal rod, zoite, zygotoblast.

sport (spōrt) An organism varying in whole or in part, without apparent reason, from others of its type; this variation may be transmitted to the descendants or the latter may revert to the original type.

sports med·i·cine (spōrts med′i-sin) A field of medicine that uses a holistic, comprehensive, and multidisciplinary approach to health care for those engaged in a sporting or recreational activity.

spor·u·la·tion (spōr′yū-lā′shŭn) The process by which yeasts undergo meiosis and the meiotic products are encased in spore coats.

spor·ule (spōr′yūl) A small spore.

spot (spot) **1.** SYN macula. **2.** To lose a slight amount of blood through the vagina.

spot film (spot film) Radiograph made during an examination under fluoroscopic control, with a device attached to the fluoroscope.

sprain (sprān) **1.** An injury to a ligament as a result of abnormal or excessive forces applied to a joint, but without dislocation or fracture. **2.** To cause a sprain of a joint.

Spreng·el de·for·mity (spreng′gel dĕ-fōrm′i-tē) Congenital elevation of the scapula.

spring lan·cet (spring lan′sĕt) Instrument with a handle containing a blade that is activated by a spring.

S pro·tein (prō′tēn) Major fragment produced from pancreatic ribonuclease by the limited action of subtilisin.

sprue (sprū) **1.** Primary intestinal malabsorption with steatorrhea. **2.** DENTISTRY wax or metal used to form the aperture(s) through which molten metal flows into a mold to make a casting; also, the metal that later fills the sprue hole(s).

spur cell (spŭr sel) Spiculated erythrocyte with 5–10 spiny projections of varying length distributed irregularly over cell surfaces; seen in liver disease and abetalipoproteinemia.

spur cell a·ne·mi·a (spŭr sel ă-nē′mē-ă) Blood disorder in which the red blood cells appear spiculated and are destroyed prematurely, predominantly in the spleen.

Spur·ling test (spŭr′ling test) Evaluation for cervical nerve root impingement.

spu·tum (spyū′tŭm) **1.** Expectorated matter, especially mucus or mucopurulent matter spat out in diseases of the air passages. SEE ALSO expectoration (1). **2.** An individual mass of such matter.

squa·la·mine lac·tate (skwā′lă-mēn lak′tāt) An antiangiogenic, noncytotoxic drug used to treat solid tumors.

squa·ma, pl. **squa·mae, squame** (skwā′mă, -mē, skwām) [TA] **1.** A thin plate of bone. **2.** An epidermal scale. SYN scale (2).

squa·mo·col·um·nar junc·tion (SCJ) (skwā′mō-kŏ-lŭm′năr jŭngk′shŭn) Site of transition from stratified squamous epithelium to columnar epithelium.

squa·mo·pa·ri·e·tal (skwā′mō-pă-rī′ĕ-tăl) Relating to the parietal bone and the squamous portion of the temporal bone.

squa·mous (skwā′mŭs) Relating to or covered with scales. SYN scaly, squamate.

squa·mous cell (skwā′mŭs sel) A flat, scalelike epithelial cell.

squa·mous cell car·ci·no·ma (skwā′mŭs sel kahr′si-nō′mă) A malignant neoplasm derived from stratified squamous epithelium, which may also occur in sites where only glandular or columnar epithelium is normally present.

squa·mous ep·i·the·li·um (skwā′mŭs ep′i-thē′lē-ŭm) Epithelium consisting of a single layer of cells.

squa·mous met·a·pla·si·a (skwā′mŭs met′ă-plā′zē-ă) The transformation of glandular or mucosal epithelium into stratified squamous epithelium. SYN epidermalization.

squa·mous o·don·to·gen·ic tu·mor (skwā′mŭs ō-don′tō-jen′ik tū′mŏr) A benign epithelial lesion thought to arise from the epithelial cell rests of Malassez.

squint (skwint) **1.** SYN strabismus. **2.** To narrow the interpalpebral openings of the eyelids to block light or improve focus.

squint·ing eye (skwint′ing ī) In cases of strabismus, eye not directed toward the object of regard.

squint·ing pa·tel·la (skwint′ing pă-tel′ă) A patella that is medially rotated.

Sr Symbol for strontium.

stab (stab) To pierce with a pointed instrument.

stab cul·ture (stab kŭl′chŭr) One produced by inserting an inoculating needle with inoculum down the center of a solid medium contained in a test tube.

stab drain (stab drān) An opening made into a cavity through a puncture made at a dependent part away from the wound of operation, so placed to prevent infection of the wound.

sta·bile (stā′bil) Steady; fixed. Cf. labile.

sta·ble (stā′bĕl) Steady; not varying; resistant to change. SEE ALSO stabile.

stac·ca·to speech (stă-kah′tō spēch) Abrupt utterance, each syllable being enunciated separately; noted especially in multiple sclerosis. SYN syllabic speech.

staff (staf) **1.** A specific group of workers. **2.** SYN director.

staff of Aes·cu·la·pi·us (staf es-kyū-lā′pē-ŭs) A rod with a single serpent without wings encircling it; symbol of medicine and emblem of the American Medical Association, Royal Army Medical Corps (Britain), and Royal Canadian Medical Corps. SEE ALSO caduceus.

stage (stāj) **1.** A period in the course of a disease, especially cancer. SEE ALSO period. **2.** The part of a microscope on which the microscope slide bears the object to be examined. **3.** A particular step, phase, or position in a developmental process.

stag·gers (stag′ĕrz) A form of decompression sickness in which vertigo, mental confusion, and muscular weakness are the chief symptoms.

stag·horn cal·cu·lus (stag′hōrn kal′ kyū-lŭs) Concretion in the renal pelvis, with branches extending into the infundibula and calyces.

stag·ing (stāj′ing) **1.** The determination or classification of distinct phases or periods in the course of a disease or pathologic process. **2.** The determination of the specific extent of a disease process in an individual patient.

stain (stān) **1.** To discolor. **2.** To dye. **3.** A discoloration. **4.** A dye used in histologic and bacteriologic technique. **5.** A procedure in which a dye or combination of dyes and reagents is used to color the constituents of cells and tissues.

stain·ing (stān′ing) **1.** The act of applying a stain. SEE ALSO stain. **2.** DENTISTRY modification of the color of the tooth or denture base.

stal·ag·mom·e·ter (stal′ăg-mom′ĕ-tĕr) An instrument for determining exactly the number of drops in a given quantity of liquid; used as a measure of the surface tension of a fluid.

stalk (stawk) A narrowed connection with a structure or organ.

stam·mer·ing (stam′ĕr-ing) **1.** A speech disorder characterized by hesitation and repetition of words, or by mispronunciation or transposition of certain consonants, especially *l*, *r*, and *s*. **2.** Sounds other than speech that are similar to stammering.

stan·dard (stan′dărd) Something that serves in some manner as a basis for comparison; a technical specification or written report by experts.

stan·dard bi·car·bo·nate (SBC) (stan′ dărd bī-kahr′bŏn-āt) Plasma bicarbonate concentration of a sample of whole blood that has been equilibrated at 37°C with a carbon dioxide pressure of 40mmHg and an oxygen pressure that exceeds 100 mmHg.

stan·dard de·vi·a·tion (σ, SD) (stan′ dărd dĕ′vē-ā′shŭn) **1.** Statistical index of the degree of deviation from central tendency, namely, of the variability within a distribution. **2.** A measure of dispersion or variation used to describe a characteristic of a frequency distribution.

stan·dard er·ror of dif·fer·ence (stan′ dărd er′ŏr dif′ĕr-ĕns) A statistical index of the probability that a difference between two sample means is greater than zero.

stan·dard er·ror of mea·sure·ment (SEM) (stan′dărd er′ŏr mezh′ŭr-mĕnt) A test based on error with regard to reliability. The difference between the obtained test result and the hypothetical true result. SEE ALSO standard deviation.

stan·dard er·ror of the mean (SEM) (stan′dărd er′ŏr mēn) Statistical index of the probability that a given sample mean is representative of the mean of the population from which the sample was drawn.

stan·dard pre·cau·tions (stan′dărd prĕ-kaw′shŭnz) Guidelines for the prevention of infectious diseases and nosocomial infections established by the U.S. Centers for Disease Control and Prevention; combine universal precautions and body-substance precautions for all patients regardless of diagnosis. All contact with body fluids and secretions, except sweat, are to be avoided by health care workers.

stan·dards of nurs·ing prac·tice (stan′ dărdz nŭrs′ing prak′tis) Rules or definitions of competent nursing care.

stan·dard so·lu·tion, stan·dard·ized so·lu·tion (stan′dărd sŏ-lū′shŭn, stan′ dărd-īzd) A solution of known concentration, used as a standard of comparison or analysis.

stan·nous fluor·ide (stan′ŭs flōr′īd) A preparation containing not less than 71.2% of stannous tin and not less than

22.3% nor more than 25.5% of fluoride; used in dentistry as a prophylactic against caries.

sta·pe·dec·to·my (stā′pĕ-dek′tŏ-mē) Operation to remove the stapes footplate in whole or part with replacement of the stapes superstructure (crura) by metal or plastic prosthesis.

sta·pe·di·al (stā-pē′dē-ăl) Relating to the stapes.

sta·pe·di·o·te·not·o·my (stā-pē′dē-ō-tĕ-not′ŏ-mē) Division of the tendon of the stapedius muscle.

sta·pe·di·o·ves·tib·u·lar (stā-pē′dē-ō-ves-tib′yū-lăr) Relating to the stapes and the vestibule of the ear.

sta·pe·dot·o·my (stā′pĕ-dot′ŏ-mē) A surgical technique to improve hearing in otosclerosis: a hole is made in the footplate of the stapes bone through which is placed the piston-shaped end of a prosthesis, the other end of which is attached to the long process of the incus bone.

sta·pes, pl. **sta·pe·des** (stā′pēz, stā-pē′dēz) [TA] Smallest of the three auditory ossicles; its base fits into the vestibular (oval) window, while its head is articulated with the lenticular process of the long limb of the incus.

sta·pes mo·bi·li·za·tion (stā′pēz mō′bi-lī-zā′shŭn) Operation to remobilize the footplate of the stapes to relieve conductive hearing impairment caused by its immobilization through otosclerosis or other middle ear disease.

staphylo-, staphyl- Combining forms indicating resemblance to a grape or a bunch of grapes, hence relating usually to staphylococci or to the uvula palatina.

staphylococcaemia [Br.] SYN staphylococcemia.

staph·y·lo·coc·cal bleph·a·ri·tis (staf′i-lō-kok′ăl blef′ă-rī′tis) Inflammation of the eyelids characterized by brittle, hard scales along the base of the eyelashes.

staph·y·lo·coc·cal pneu·mo·ni·a (staf′i-lō-kok′ăl nū-mō′nē-ă) Disease, usually caused by *Staphylococcus aureus*, commencing as a bronchopneumonia, and fre-quently leading to suppuration and destruction of lung tissue.

staph·y·lo·coc·cal scald·ed skin syn·drome (SSSS) (staf′i-lō-kok′ăl skawl′dĕd skin sin′drōm) Disease affecting infants in whom large areas of skin peel off, as in a partial-thickness burn, as a result of upper respiratory staphylococcal infection even though the skin lesions are sterile. SYN Lyell disease.

staph·y·lo·coc·ce·mi·a (staf′i-lō-kok-sē′mē-ă) The presence of staphylococci in the circulating blood. SYN staphylococcaemia.

Staph·y·lo·coc·cus, pl. **Staph·y·lo·coc·ci** (staf′i-lō-kok′ŭs, -kok′sī) A genus of nonmotile, non-spore-forming, aerobic to facultatively anaerobic bacteria containing gram-positive, spheric cells that divide in more than one plane to form irregular clusters; found on the skin, in skin glands, on the nasal and other mucous membranes of warm-blooded animals, and in various food products.

Staph·y·lo·coc·cus au·re·us (staf′i-lō-kok′ŭs aw′rē-ŭs) Common bacterial species found especially on nasal mucous membrane and skin (hair follicles); causes furunculosis, cellulitis, pyemia, pneumonia, osteomyelitis, other infections, and food poisoning; humans are the chief reservoir.

Staph·y·lo·coc·cus sap·ro·phy·ti·cus (staf′i-lō-kok′ŭs sap-rō-fī′ti-kŭs) A bacterial species associated with community-acquired urinary tract infections in sexually active young women; characterized in the laboratory as gram-positive cocci, but negative for catalase and coagulase.

staph·y·lol·y·sin (staf′i-lol′i-sin) 1. A hemolysin elaborated by a staphylococcus. 2. An antibody causing lysis of staphylococci.

staph·y·lo·ma (staf′i-lō′mă) A bulging of the cornea or sclera containing uveal tissue.

staph·y·lo·phar·yn·gor·rha·phy (staf′i-lō-far′in-gor′ă-fē) Surgical repair of defects in the uvula or soft palate and the pharynx. SYN palatopharyngorrhaphy.

S

starch (stahrch) A high molecular weight polysaccharide that exists in most plant tissues; used as a dusting powder, an emollient, and an ingredient in medicinal tablets.

Star·gardt dis·ease (stahr'gahrt di-zēz') Hereditary pediatric macular dystrophy with macular degeneration.

Star·ling curve (stahr'ling kŭrv) A graph in which cardiac output or stroke volume is plotted against mean atrial or ventricular end-diastolic pressure. SYN Frank-Starling curve.

Star·ling hy·poth·e·sis (stahr'ling hī-poth'ĕ-sis) The principle that net filtration through capillary membranes is proportional to the transmembrane hydrostatic pressure difference minus the transmembrane oncotic pressure difference.

Star·ling re·flex (stahr'ling rē'fleks) Tapping the volar surfaces of the fingers causes flexion of the fingers.

star·tle re·flex, star·tle re·ac·tion (stahr'tĕl rē'fleks, rē-ak'shŭn) 1. Reflex response of an infant (contraction of the limb and neck muscles) when allowed to drop a short distance through the air or when startled by a sudden noise or jolt. SYN parachute reflex. 2. SYN cochleo-palpebral reflex.

star·va·tion ac·id·o·sis (stahr-vā'shŭn as'ĭ-dō'sis) Ketoacidosis resulting from lack of food intake; leads to fat catabolism to provide energy, and subsequent release of acidic ketone bodies.

star·va·tion di·a·be·tes (stahr-vā'shŭn dī'ă-bē'tēz) After prolonged fasting, glycosuria after ingestion of carbohydrate or glucose because of reduced output of insulin and/or reduced rate of glucose metabolism with a reduced ability to form glycogen.

sta·sis (stā'sis, -sēz) Stagnation of the blood or other fluids.

sta·sis der·ma·ti·tis (stā'sis dĕr'mă-tī'tis) Erythema and scaling of the lower limbs due to impaired venous circulation; common in older women.

sta·sis ec·ze·ma (stā'sis ek'sĕ-mă) Eczematous eruption on legs due to or aggravated by venous stasis.

stat. (stat) Abbreviation for L. statim, at once, immediately.

state (stāt) A condition, situation, or status.

stat·ic sco·li·o·sis (stat'ik skō'lē-ō'sis) Lateral curvature of the spine due to inequality in length of the legs.

sta·tion (stā'shŭn) The degree of descent of the presenting part of the fetus through the maternal pelvis, as measured in relation to the ischial spines of the maternal pelvis.

sta·tis·ti·cal sig·nif·i·cance (stă-tis'ti-kăl sig-nif'i-kăns) Statistical methods allow an estimate to be made of the probability of the observed degree of association between variables, and from this the statistical significance can be expressed, commonly in terms of the p value.

sta·tis·tics (stă-tis'tiks) 1. A collection of numeric values, items of information, or other facts numerically grouped into definite classes and subject to analysis. 2. The science and art of collecting, summarizing, and analyzing data subject to random variation.

stat·o·a·cou·stic (stat'ō-ă-kū'stik) Relating to equilibrium and hearing. SYN vestibulocochlear (2).

sta·tus ep·i·lep·ti·cus (stā'tus ep-i-lep'ti-kŭs) Repeated seizure, or a seizure prolonged for at least 30 minutes; may be convulsive (tonic-clonic), nonconvulsive (absence or complex partial), partial (epilepsia partialis continuans), or subclinical (electrographic status epilepticus).

sta·tus mar·mo·ra·tus (stā'tus mahr-mōr-ā'tŭs) Congenital condition due to maldevelopment of the corpus striatum associated with choreoathetosis, in which the striate nuclei have a marblelike appearance caused by altered myelination.

Stauf·fer syn·drome (staw'fĕr sin'drōm) Abnormality of liver function test results, in the absence of metastatic disease, due to cholestasis in renal cell cancer patients.

stead·y state (sted'ē stāt) 1. A condition

obtained in moderate muscular exercise when the removal of lactic acid by oxidation keeps pace with its production, the oxygen supply being adequate, and the muscles do not rely on energy from anaerobic sources. **2.** Any condition in which the formation or introduction of substances just keeps pace with their destruction or removal so that all volumes, concentrations, pressures, and flows remain constant.

steal (stēl) Diversion of blood through alternate routes or reversed flow.

ste·a·rate (stē′ă-rāt) A salt of stearic acid.

ste·ar·ic ac·id (stē′ă-rik as′id) One of the most abundant acids found in animal lipids; used in pharmaceutical preparations, ointments, soaps, and suppositories.

ste·ar·rhe·a (stē′ă-rē′ă) SYN steatorrhea.

ste·a·ryl al·co·hol (stē′ă-ril al′kŏ-hol) An ingredient of hydrophilic ointment and hydrophilic petrolatum; also used in the preparation of creams.

ste·a·ti·tis (stē′ă-tī′tis) Inflammation of adipose tissue.

steato- Combining form denoting fat.

ste·a·to·cys·to·ma (stē′ă-tō-sis-tō′mă) A cyst with sebaceous gland cells in its wall.

ste·a·to·cys·to·ma mul·ti·plex (stē′ă-tō-sis-tō′mă mŭl′tē-pleks) Widespread, multiple, thin-walled cysts of the skin lined by squamous epithelium.

ste·a·tol·y·sis (stē′ă-tol′i-sis) The hydrolysis or emulsion of fat in the process of digestion.

ste·a·to·ne·cro·sis (stē′ă-tō-nĕ-krō′sis) SYN fat necrosis.

ste·a·top·y·ga, ste·a·to·py·gi·a (stē′ă-top′i-gă, -tō-pij′ē-ă) Excessive accumulation of fat on the buttocks.

ste·a·tor·rhe·a, ste·ar·rhe·a (stē′ă-tŏr-ē′ă, -stē′ă-rē′ă) Passage of fat in large amounts in the feces, due to failure to digest and absorb it; occurs in pancreatic disease and the malabsorption syndromes. SYN fat indigestion, stearrhea, steatorrhea.

steer·ing wheel in·ju·ry (stēr′ing wēl in′jū-rē) Trauma to the anterior chest wall caused by impact with the steering wheel during a motor vehicle accident; may include fractured sternum and ribs, cardiac contusion, tear of the aorta or other great vessels, as well as lung injuries.

steg·no·sis (steg-nō′sis) **1.** A stoppage of any of the secretions or excretions. **2.** A constriction or stenosis.

Stein-Le·ven·thal syn·drome (stīn lev′ĕn-thahl sin′drōm) SYN polycystic ovary syndrome.

Stein·mann pin (shtīn′mahn pin) Pin that is used to transfix bone for traction or fixation.

stein·stras·se (stīn′strah-sĕ) A complication of extracorporeal shock wave lithotripsy for urinary tract calculi in which stone fragments block the ureter to form a "stone street."

Stein test (stīn test) In cases of labyrinthine disease, the patient is unable to stand or to hop on one foot with eyes shut.

stel·late (stel′āt) Star-shaped.

stel·late cell (stel′āt sel) A star-shaped cell with many filaments extending radially.

stel·late hair (stel′āt hār) Hair split in several strands at the free end.

stel·late re·tic·u·lum (stel′āt rĕ-tik′yū-lŭm) A network of epithelial cells disposed in a fluid-filled compartment in the center of the enamel organ between the outer and inner enamel epithelium.

stel·lec·to·my (stel-ek′tŏ-mē) Stellate ganglionectomy.

Stell·wag sign (stel′vahg sīn) Infrequent and incomplete blinking in Graves disease.

stem (stem) A supporting structure similar to the stalk of a plant.

S

stem cell (stem sel) **1.** Any precursor cell. **2.** A cell with daughter cells that may differentiate into other cell types.

stem cell leu·ke·mi·a (stem sel lū-kē′ mē-ă) A form of blood disorder in which the abnormal cells are thought to be the precursors of lymphoblasts, myeloblasts, or monoblasts. SYN embryonal leukemia.

♻ **steno-** Combining form meaning narrowness, constriction; opposite of eury-.

sten·o·ceph·a·ly, sten·o·ceph·a·li·a (sten′ŏ-sef′ă-lē, -sē-fā′lē-ă) Marked narrowness of the head.

sten·o·cho·ri·a (sten′ŏ-kōr′ē-ă) Abnormal contraction of any canal or orifice, especially of the lacrimal ducts.

sten·o·pe·ic, sten·o·pa·ic (sten′ŏ-pē′ ik, -pā′ik) Provided with a narrow slit, as in stenopeic spectacles.

ste·no·sal mur·mur (stě-nō′săl mŭr′ mŭr) An arterial murmur due to narrowing of the vessel from pressure or organic change.

ste·nosed (stě-nōst′) Narrowed; contracted; strictured.

ste·no·sis (stě-nō′sis) A stricture of any canal, especially one of the cardiac valves.

sten·o·sto·mi·a (sten′ŏ-stō′mē-ă) Narrowness of the oral cavity.

sten·o·ther·mal (sten′ō-thěr′măl) Thermostable through a narrow temperature range.

sten·o·tho·rax (sten′ō-thōr′aks) A narrow, contracted chest.

ste·not·ic (sten-ot′ik) Narrowed; affected with stenosis.

stent (stent) **1.** Device used to maintain a bodily orifice or cavity during skin grafting, or to immobilize a skin graft after placement. **2.** Slender thread, rod, or catheter, lying within the lumen of tubular structures, used to provide support during or after their anastomosis, or to assure patency of an intact but contracted lumen.

step·page gait (step′ăj gāt) Disordered movement in which the advancing foot is lifted higher than usual so that it can clear the ground, because it cannot be dorsiflexed. SYN equine gait, high-steppage gait, steppage.

♻ **sterco-** Combining form denoting feces. SEE ALSO scato-.

ster·co·bi·lin (stěr′kō-bī′lin) A brown degradation product of hemoglobin, present in the feces.

ster·co·ra·ceous, ster·co·ral, ster·co·rous (stěr′kor-ā′shŭs, stěr-kōr′ăl, -ŭs) Relating to or containing feces.

ster·co·ra·ceous vom·it·ing (stěr′kor-ā′shŭs vom′it-ing) SYN fecal vomiting.

ster·co·ral ab·scess (stěr′kor-ăl ab′ses) A collection of pus and feces. SYN fecal abscess.

ster·co·ral ul·cer (stěr′kor-ăl ŭl′sěr) An ulcer of the colon due to pressure and irritation of retained fecal masses.

ster·cu·li·a gum (stěr-kyū′lē-ă gŭm) Dried gummy exudation from *Sterculia urens*, used as a hydrophilic laxative and to manufacture lotions and pastes.

♻ **stereo-** **1.** Combining form denoting solid. **2.** Combining form denoting spatial qualities, three-dimensionality.

ster·e·o·cam·pim·e·ter (ster′ē-ō-kam-pim′ě-těr) An apparatus for studying the central visual fields while the fellow eye holds fixation.

ster·e·o·chem·i·cal for·mu·la (ster′ē-ō-kem′i-kăl fōrm′yū-lă) Chemical formula in which the arrangement of the atoms or atomic groupings in space is indicated.

ster·e·o·chem·is·try (ster′ē-ō-kem′is-trē) Branch of chemistry concerned with the spatial three-dimensional relations of atoms in molecules.

ster·e·og·no·sis (ster′ē-og-nō′sis) *In the diphthong gn, the g is silent only at the beginning of a word.* The appreciation of the form of an object by means of touch.

ster·e·o·i·so·mer (ster′ē-ō-ī′sŏ-měr) Molecule containing the same number and kind of atom groupings as another but in a different arrangement in space, by virtue of which it exhibits different optic properties. Cf. isomer.

ster·e·o·i·som·er·ism (ster′ē-ō-ī-som′ ĕr-izm) Molecular asymmetry; form of isomerism involving different spatial arrangements of the same groups. SEE ALSO stereoisomer. SYN stereochemical isomerism.

ster·e·op·a·thy (ster′ē-op′ă-thē) Persistent stereotyped thinking.

ster·e·o·scope (ster′ē-ō-skōp) An instrument producing two horizontally separated images of the same object, providing a single image with an appearance of depth.

ster·e·o·scop·ic (ster′ē-ō-skop′ik) Relating to a stereoscope, or giving the appearance of three dimensions.

ster·e·o·scop·ic mi·cro·scope (ster′ ē-ō-skop′ik mī′krŏ-skōp) One with double eyepieces and objectives and thus independent light paths, giving a three-dimensional image.

ster·e·o·scop·ic vi·sion (ster′ē-ō-skop′ ik vizh′ŭn) The single perception of a slightly different image from each eye.

ster·e·o·tac·tic, ster·e·o·tax·ic (ster′ ē-ō-tak′tik, -sik) Relating to stereotaxis or stereotaxy.

ster·e·o·tac·tic in·stru·ment, ster·e·o·tax·ic in·stru·ment (ster′ē-ō-tak′ tik in′strŭ-mĕnt, ster′ē-ō-tak′sik) An apparatus attached to the head, used to localize an area in the brain precisely by means of coordinates related to intracerebral structures.

ster·e·o·tax·is, ster·e·otax·y (ster′ē-ō-tak′sis, -sē) **1.** Use of three-dimensional arrangement to identify nonvisualized anatomic structures. **2.** Stereotropism (q.v.), but applied more exactly when the organism as a whole, rather than a part only, reacts.

ster·e·ot·ro·pism (ster′ē-ot′rŏ-pizm) Growth or movement of a plant or animal toward (**positive stereotropism**) or away from (**negative stereotropism**) a solid body, usually applied where a part of the organism rather than the whole reacts.

ster·e·o·ty·py (ster′ē-ō-tī-pē) **1.** Maintenance of one attitude for a long period. **2.** Constant repetition of certain meaningless gestures or movements.

ster·ic (ster′ik) Pertaining to stereochemistry.

ster·ile (ster′il) *Do not confuse this word with infertile or antiseptic.* Relating to or characterized by sterility.

ster·ile cyst (ster′il sist) Hydatid lesion without brood capsules.

ste·ril·i·ty (stĕr-il′i-tē) **1.** In general, the incapability of fertilization or reproduction. **2.** Condition of being aseptic, or free from all living microorganisms and their spores.

ster·il·i·za·tion (ster′i-lī-zā′shŭn) **1.** The act or process by which an individual is rendered incapable of fertilization or reproduction. **2.** Destruction of all microorganisms in or about an object, using steam, chemical agents, high-velocity electron bombardment, or ultraviolet light radiation.

ster·il·ize (ster′i-līz) To produce sterility.

ster·il·iz·er (ster′i-lī-zĕr) An apparatus for rendering objects sterile.

ster·nal (stĕr′năl) Relating to the sternum.

ster·nal·gi·a (stĕr-nal′jē-ă) Pain in the sternum or the sternal region. SYN sternodynia.

ster·nal punc·ture (stĕr′năl pungk′shŭr) Removal of bone marrow from the manubrium by needle.

ster·ne·bra, pl. **ster·ne·brae** (stĕr′nē-bră, -brē) One of the four segments of the primordial sternum of the embryo by the fusion of which the body of the adult sternum is formed.

ster·no·cla·vic·u·lar (SC) (stĕr′nō-klă-vik′yū-lăr) Relating to the sternum and the clavicle.

ster·no·clei·do·mas·toid (stĕr′nō-klī′ dō-mas′toyd) Relating to sternum, clavicle, and mastoid process.

ster·no·cos·tal (stĕr′nō-kos′tăl) Relating to the sternum and the ribs.

S

ster·noid (stĕr′noyd) Resembling the sternum.

ster·no·mas·toid (ster′nō-mas′toyd) Relating to the sternum and the mastoid process of the temporal bone; applied to the sternocleidomastoid muscle.

ster·no·per·i·car·di·al (stĕr′nō-per′i-kahr′dē-ăl) Relating to the sternum and the pericardium.

ster·nos·chi·sis (stĕr-nos′ki-sis) Congenital cleft of the sternum.

ster·not·o·my (stĕr-not′ŏ-mē) Incision into or through the sternum.

ster·no·ver·te·bral (stĕr′nō-vĕr′tĕ-brăl) Relating to the sternum and the vertebrae; denoting the true ribs, or the seven upper ribs on either side, which articulate with the vertebrae and with the sternum.

ster·num, gen. **ster·ni**, pl. **ster·na** (stĕr′nŭm, -nī, -nă) [TA] A long, flat bone, articulating with the cartilages of the first seven ribs and with the clavicle, that forms the middle part of the anterior wall of the thorax. SYN breast bone.

ster·nu·ta·tion (stĕr′nyū-tā′shŭn) The act of sneezing.

ster·nu·ta·to·ry (ster-nyū′tă-tōr′ē) **1.** Causing sneezing. **2.** An agent that provokes sneezing. SYN ptarmic.

ster·oid (ster′oyd) **1.** Pertaining to the steroids. SYN steroidal. **2.** Generic designation for compounds closely related in structure to the steroids, such as sterols, bile acids, cardiac glycosides, and precursors of the D vitamins.

ster·oi·do·gen·e·sis (ster-oy′dō-jen′ĕ-sis) The formation of steroids; commonly referring to the biologic synthesis of steroid hormones, but not to the production of such compounds in a chemical laboratory.

ster·oid ul·cer (ster′oyd ŭl′sĕr) A lesion, usually on the leg or foot, developing from a wound in patients undergoing long-term steroid therapy.

ster·ol (ster′ol) A steroid with one OH (alcohol) group; the systematic names contain either the prefix hydroxy- or the suffix -ol, e.g., cholesterol, ergosterol.

ster·tor (stĕr′tŏr) A noisy inspiration occurring in coma or deep sleep, sometimes due to obstruction of the larynx or upper airways.

stetho-, steth- Combining forms denoting the chest.

steth·o·go·ni·om·e·ter (steth′ŏ-gō′nē-om′ĕ-tĕr) An apparatus for measuring the curvatures of the thorax.

steth·o·scope (steth′ŏ-skōp) An instrument originally devised by Laennec for aid in hearing the respiratory and cardiac sounds in the chest, but now modified in various ways and used in auscultation of any vascular or other sounds anywhere in the body.

ste·thos·co·py (stĕ-thos′kŏ-pē) **1.** Examination of the chest by means of auscultation, either mediate or immediate, and percussion. **2.** Mediate auscultation with the stethoscope.

steth·o·spasm (steth′ŏ-spazm) Spasm of the chest.

Stew·art-Holmes sign (stū′ărt hōlmz sīn) In cerebellar disease, the inability to check a movement when passive resistance is suddenly released.

sthe·ni·a (sthē′nē-ă) A condition of activity and apparent force.

sthen·ic (sthen′ik) **1.** Active; marked by sthenia; said of a fever with strong bounding pulse, high temperature, and active delirium. **2.** Pertaining to a habitus characterized by moderate overdevelopment of skeletal muscle.

stheno- Prefix indicating strength, force, power.

stib·i·al·ism (stib′ē-ăl-izm) Chronic antimonial poisoning.

stig·ma, pl. **stig·ma·ta** (stig′mă, -mă-tă) *Avoid the mispronunciation stigma′ta of the plural form.* **1.** Visible evidence of a disease. **2.** SYN follicular stigma. **3.** Any spot or blemish on the skin. **4.** A bleeding spot on the skin, which is considered a manifestation of conversion hysteria. **5.** A mark of shame or discredit.

stig·ma·ti·za·tion (stig′mă-tī-zā′shŭn)

1. Production of stigmata, especially of a hysteric nature. **2.** Debasement of a person by the attribution of a negatively toned characteristic or other stigma.

still·birth (SB) (stil′bĭrth) The birth of an infant who has died before delivery.

still·born (stil′bōrn) Born dead; denoting an infant dead at birth.

Still dis·ease (stil di-zēz′) A form of juvenile chronic arthritis (formerly juvenile rheumatoid arthritis) characterized by high fever and signs of systemic illness that can exist for months before the onset of arthritis.

Still mur·mur (stil mŭr′mŭr) Innocent musical murmur resembling the noise produced by a twanging string; almost exclusively in young children, of uncertain origin and ultimately disappearing.

stim·u·lant (stim′yū-lănt) **1.** Stimulating; exciting to action. **2.** An agent that arouses organic activity, strengthens the action of the heart, increases vitality, and promotes a sense of well-being; classified according to the parts on which it chiefly acts: cardiac, respiratory, gastric, hepatic, cerebral, spinal, vascular, or genital.

stim·u·la·tion (stim′yŭ-lā′shŭn) **1.** Arousal of the body or any of its parts to increased functional activity. **2.** Condition of being stimulated. **3.** NEUROPHYSIOLOGY application of a stimulus to a responsive structure, regardless of whether the strength of the stimulus is sufficient to produce excitation.

stim·u·lus, gen. and pl. **stim·u·li** (stim′yū-lŭs, -lī) **1.** A stimulant. **2.** That which can elicit or evoke action (response) in a muscle, nerve, gland or other excitable tissue, or cause an augmenting action on any function or metabolic process.

stim·u·lus con·trol (stim′yū-lŭs kŏn-trōl′) The use of conditioning techniques to bring the target behavior of an individual under environmental control.

sting (sting) **1.** Sharp momentary pain, most commonly produced by puncture of the skin by many species of arthropods; can also be produced by jellyfish, sea urchins, sponges, mollusks, and several species of venomous fish, such as the stingray, toadfish, rabbitfish, and catfish. **2.** The venom apparatus of a stinging animal, consisting of a chitinous spicule or bony spine and a venom gland or sac. **3.** To introduce (or the process of introducing) a venom by stinging.

stip·pled (stip′ĕld) Having a dappled or spotted appearance.

stip·pling (stip′ling) **1.** Speckling of a blood cell or other structure with fine dots when exposed to the action of a basic stain. **2.** An orange-peel appearance of the attached gingiva, which is a normal adaptive process; its absence or reduction indicates gingival disease. **3.** Roughening the surfaces of a denture base to stimulate natural gingival stippling.

stitch (stich) **1.** A sharp, sticking pain of momentary duration. **2.** A single suture. **3.** SYN suture (2).

stitch ab·scess (stich ab′ses) A purulent lesion around a suture.

St. John's wort (sānt jonz wŏrt) Any herb or shrub of the genus *Hypericum*, used to treat mild depression.

St. Lou·is en·ceph·a·li·tis virus (sānt lū′is en-sef′ă-lī′tis vī′rŭs) A group B arbovirus often causing inapparent infection but sometimes encephalitis; isolated from birds and from several mosquito species.

sto·chas·tic (stō-kas′tik) **1.** Random. **2.** RADIATION THERAPY pertaining to the effects of radiation seen in the person exposed to such radiation.

Stock·holm syn·drome (stok′hōlm sin′drōm) A form of bonding between a captive and captor in which the captive begins to identify with, and may even sympathize with, the captor.

stock vac·cine (stok vak-sēn′) A vaccine made from a stock microbial strain.

Stof·fel op·er·a·tion (stof′el op-ĕr-ā′shŭn) Division of certain motor nerves for the relief of spastic paralysis.

stoi·chi·ol·o·gy (stoy′kē-ol′-ŏ-jē) [Br.] Science of elements or principles in any branch of knowledge, especially in chemistry, cytology, or histology.

stoi·chi·om·e·try (stoy'kē-om'ĕ-trē) Determination of the relative quantities of the substances concerned in any chemical reaction.

stoke (stōk) A unit of kinematic viscosity; that of a fluid with a viscosity of 1 poise and a density of 1 g/mL; equal to 10^{-4} square meter per second.

Stokes law (stōks law) **1.** A muscle lying above an inflamed mucous or serous membrane is frequently the seat of paralysis. **2.** A relationship of the rate of fall of a small sphere in a viscous fluid. **3.** The wavelength of light emitted by a fluorescent material is longer than that of the radiation used to excite the fluorescence.

sto·ma (stō'mă) **1.** A minute opening or pore. **2.** An artificial opening between two cavities or canals, or between such and the surface of the body.

sto·ma blast (stō'mă blast) Sound produced by forceful expiration of air through a tracheal stoma.

stom·ach (stŏm'ăk) [TA] A large, irregularly piriform sac between the esophagus and the small intestine, lying just beneath the diaphragm. SYN gaster [TA], ventriculus (1).

stom·ach drops (stŏm'ăk drops) Stomachic tonic, usually tincture of gentian, alone or with other stomachics.

sto·mal (stō'măl) Relating to a stoma.

sto·ma·tal·gi·a, sto·mat·o·dyn·i·a (stō'mă-tal'jē-ă, -tō-din'ē-ă) Pain in the mouth.

sto·ma·ti·tis (stō'mă-tī'tis) Inflammation of the mucous membrane of the mouth.

sto·ma·ti·tis me·di·ca·men·to·sa (stō'mă-tī'tis med-i-kă-men-tō'să) Inflammatory alterations of the oral mucosa associated with a systemic drug allergy; lesions may consist of erythema, vesicles, bullae, ulcerations, or angioedema.

sto·ma·to·cyte (stō'mă-tō-sīt) A red blood cell that exhibits a slit or mouth-shaped pallor rather than a central one on air-dried smears; e.g., Rh null cells.

sto·ma·tog·nath·ic (stō'mă-tog-nath'ik)

In the diphthong gn, the g is silent only at the beginning of a word. Pertaining to the mouth and jaw.

sto·ma·tog·nath·ic sys·tem (stō'mă-tog-nath'ik sis'tĕm) All the structures involved in speech and in the reception, mastication, and deglutition of food.

sto·ma·tol·o·gy (stō'mă-tol'ŏ-jē) The study of the structure, function, and diseases of the mouth.

sto·ma·to·ma·la·ci·a (stō'mă-tō-mă-lā'shē-ă) Pathologic softening of oral structures.

sto·ma·to·my·co·sis (stō'mă-tō-mī-kō'sis) Oral fungal disease.

sto·ma·top·a·thy, sto·ma·to·sis (stō'mă-top'ă-thē) Any disease of the oral cavity.

sto·ma·tor·rha·gi·a (stō'mă-tōr-ā'jē-ă) Bleeding from the gums or other part of the oral cavity.

sto·mi·on (stō'mē-on) The median point of the oral slit when the lips are closed.

sto·mo·de·um, sto·ma·to·de·um (stō'mō-dē'ŭm, -mă-tō-dē'ŭm) **1.** A midline ectodermal depression ventral to the embryonic brain and surrounded by the mandibular arch. SYN stomatodeum. **2.** The anterior portion of the insect alimentary canal.

-stomy Suffix meaning artificial or surgical opening. SEE stomato-.

stone (stōn) **1.** SYN calculus. **2.** A British unit of weight for the human body, equal to 14 lb. or 6.36 kg.

stool (stūl) **1.** A discharging of the bowels. **2.** The matter discharged at one movement of the bowels. SYN evacuation (2). SYN movement (2).

stop·cock (stop'kok) A valve used to regulate flow of liquids or gases.

stor·age dis·ease (stōr'ăj di-zēz') Any accumulation of a specific substance within tissues, generally because of congenital deficiency of an enzyme necessary for further metabolism of the substance.

STORCH (stōrch) Acronym for syndrome

comprising *s*yphilis, *t*oxoplasmosis, *o*ther infections, *r*ubella, *c*ytomegalovirus infection, and *h*erpes simplex; fetal infections that can cause congenital malformations.

stor·i·form (stōr'i-fŏrm) Having a cartwheel pattern.

storm (stōrm) An exacerbation of symptoms or a crisis in the course of a disease.

stra·bis·mus (stră-biz'mŭs) A manifest lack of parallelism of the visual axes of the eyes. SYN crossed eyes, cross-eye, heterotropia, heterotropy, squint (1).

strain (strān) **1.** A population of homogeneous organisms possessing a set of defined characters. **2.** Specific host cell(s) designed or selected to optimize production of recombinant products. **3.** To make an effort to the limit of one's strength. **4.** To injure by overuse or improper use. **5.** An act of straining. **6.** Injury resulting from tensile force to muscle or tendon, especially skeletal muscles. **7.** The change in shape that a body undergoes when acted on by an external stress. **8.** To filter.

strait (strāt) A narrow passageway.

strait·jack·et (strāt'jak'ĕt) A garmentlike device with long sleeves that can be secured to restrain a violently disturbed person.

stra·mo·ni·um (stră-mō'nē-ŭm) Dried leaves and flowering or fruiting tops with branches of *Datura stramonium* or *D. tatula*; an antispasmodic used in the treatment of asthma and parkinsonism.

stran·gle (strang'gĕl) To suffocate; to compress the trachea to prevent sufficient passage of air.

stran·gu·lat·ed (strang'gyū-lāt-ĕd) Constricted so as to prevent sufficient passage of air, as through the trachea, or to cut off venous return or arterial air flow, as in the case of a hernia.

stran·gu·lat·ed her·ni·a (strang'gyū-lāt-ĕd hĕr'nē-ă) Irreducible hernia in which the circulation is arrested; gangrene occurs unless relief is prompt.

stran·gu·la·tion (strang'gyū-lā'shŭn) The act of strangulating or the condition of being strangulated.

stran·gu·ry, stran·gu·ri·a (strang'gyūr-ē, strang-gyūr'ē-ă) Difficulty in micturition in which the urine is passed only drop by drop with pain and tenesmus.

strap (strap) **1.** A strip of adhesive plaster. **2.** To apply overlapping strips of adhesive plaster.

strat·i·fied (strat'i-fīd) Arranged in the form of layers or strata.

strat·i·fied ep·i·the·li·um (strat'i-fīd ep'i-thē'lē-ŭm) Epithelium composed of a series of layers, the cells of each varying in size and shape, where only the basal layer of cells comes in contact with the basement membrane. SYN laminated epithelium.

strat·i·form fi·bro·cart·i·lage (strat'i-fŏrm fī'brō-kahr'ti-lăj) Layer of fibrocartilage in the bottom of a groove in a bone through which a tendon runs.

strat·um, gen. **stra·ta** (strā'tŭm, -tă) *The correct plural of this word is strata, not strati or stratae.* A layer of differentiated tissue, the aggregate of which forms any given structure. SEE ALSO lamina, layer.

Straus sign (strows sīn) In facial paralysis, if an injection of pilocarpine is followed by sweating on the affected side later than on the other, the lesion is peripheral.

straw·ber·ry cer·vix (straw'ber-ē sĭr'viks) Macular erythema of the uterine cervix, characteristic of vaginitis due to *Trichomonas vaginalis*.

straw·ber·ry gall·blad·der (straw'ber-ē gawl'blad-ĕr) One with mucosa dotted with yellowish cholesterol deposits contrasting with the red hyperemic background.

straw·ber·ry he·man·gi·o·ma (straw'ber-ē hē-man'jē-ō'mă) Hyperproliferation of immature capillary vessels, usually on the head and neck, present at birth or within the first 2–3 months postnatally, which commonly regresses without scar formation.

straw·ber·ry ne·vus, straw·ber·ry mark (straw'ber-ē nē'vŭs, mahrk) A small nevus vascularis resembling a strawberry in size, shape, and color; usually disappears spontaneously in early childhood. SEE ALSO capillary hemangioma.

straw·ber·ry tongue (straw′ber-ē tŭng) One with a whitish coat through which the enlarged fungiform papillae project as red points; characteristic of scarlatina and mucocutaneous lymph node syndrome.

street drug (strēt drŭg) A controlled substance taken for nonmedical purposes; includes various amphetamines, anesthetics, barbiturates, opiates, and psychoactive drugs, and many derived from natural sources (e.g., the plants *Papaver somniferum*, *Cannibis sativa*, *Amanita pantherina*, *Lophophora williamsii*). Slang names include acid (lysergic acid diethylamide), angel dust (phencyclidine), coke (cocaine), crack cocaine (rock), downers (barbiturates), grass (marijuana), hash (concentrated tetrahydrocannibinol), magic mushrooms (psilocybin), and speed (amphetamines).

street vir·us (strēt vī′rŭs) An isolate of rabies virus from a naturally infected domestic animal.

strength-du·ra·tion curve (strengkth′ dūr-ā′shŭn kŭrv) Graph relating the intensity of an electrical stimulus to the length of time it must flow to be effective. SEE chronaxie, rheobase.

strength train·ing (strengkth trān′ing) A period of training in which high levels of volume (weight resistance) with minimal rest periods resulting in muscular hypertrophy. SYN muscular strength training, strength endurance.

streph·o·sym·bo·li·a (stref′ō-sim-bō′lē-ă) **1.** Generally, the perception of objects reversed as if in a mirror. **2.** Specifically, difficulty in distinguishing written or printed letters that extend in opposite directions but are otherwise similar, such as *p* and *d*, or related kinds of mirror reversal.

strepto- Prefix meaning curved or twisted (usually relating to organisms thus described).

Strep·to·ba·cil·lus (strep′tō-bă-sil′ŭs) A genus of nonmotile, non-spore-forming, aerobic to facultatively anaerobic bacteria containing gram-negative, pleo-

morphic cells; pathogenic for rats, mice, and other mammals.

Strep·to·ba·cil·lus mo·nil·i·for·mis (strep′tō-bă-sil′ŭs mō-nil-i-fōr′mis) Bacterial species commonly found as an inhabitant of the nasopharynx of rats.

strep·to·cer·ci·a·sis (strep′tō-sĕr-sī′ă-sis) Infection of humans and higher primates with the nematode *Mansonella streptocerca*.

strep·to·coc·cal (strep′tō-kok′ăl) Relating to or caused by any organism of the genus *Streptococcus*.

strep·to·coc·cal tox·ic shock syn·drome (strep′tō-kok′ăl tok′sik shok sin′drōm) Disorder characterized by hypotension and a variety of signs and symptoms indicative of multiorgan failure including cerebral dysfunction, renal failure, acute respiratory distress syndrome, toxic cardiomyopathy, and hepatic dysfunction; usually precipitated by local infections of skin or soft tissue by streptococci.

strep·to·coc·ce·mi·a (strep′tō-kok-sē′mē-ă) The presence of streptococci in the blood. SYN strepticemia,streptosepticemia.

Strep·to·coc·cus (strep′tō-kok′ŭs) A genus of nonmotile, non-spore-forming, aerobic to facultatively anaerobic bacteria that occur in pairs or short or long chains. These organisms occur regularly in the mouth and intestines of humans and other animals, and elsewhere. Some species are pathogenic.

Strep·to·coc·cus ag·a·lac·ti·ae (strep′tō-kok′ŭs ā-gal-ak′shē-ē) A streptococcal species that is a significant cause of bacteremia, pneumonia, and meningitis in newborns.

Strep·to·coc·cus mil·ler·i (strep′tō-kok′ŭs mil′lĕr-ī) The *Streptococcus intermedius* group, found in the human oral cavity and associated with bacteremia, endocarditis, and oral and thoracic infections.

Strep·to·coc·cus pneu·mo·ni·ae (strep′tō-kok′ŭs nū-mō′nē-ē) Bacterial species of gram-positive, lancet-shaped diplococci frequently occurring in pairs or chains; normal inhabitants of the respiratory tract, and the cause of lobar pneumonia, otitis media, meningitis, sinusitis, and other infections.

Strep·to·coc·cus py·og·e·nes (strep´ tō-kok´ŭs pī-oj´ĕ-nēz) A bacterial species found in the human mouth, throat, and respiratory tract and in inflammatory exudates, bloodstream, and lesions in human diseases; sometimes found in dust from sickrooms, hospital wards, schools, theaters, and other public places; causes pus formation or even fatal septicemias.

strep·to·dor·nase (SD) (strep´tō-dōr´ nās) A "dornase" (deoxyribonuclease) obtained from streptococci; used with streptokinase to facilitate drainage in septic surgical conditions.

strep·to·ki·nase (SK) (strep´tō-kī´nās) An extracellular metalloenzyme from hemolytic streptococci that cleaves plasminogen, producing plasmin, which causes the liquefaction of fibrin; usually used in conjunction with streptodornase in the removal of clots.

strep·to·ki·nase-strep·to·dor·nase (strep´tō-kī´nās-strep´tō-dōr´nās) A purified mixture containing streptokinase, streptodornase, and other proteolytic enzymes; used by topical application or by injection into body cavities to remove clotted blood and fibrinous and purulent accumulations of exudate; thus, used in the removal of clots.

Strep·to·my·ces (strep´tō-mī´sēz) A genus of nonmotile, aerobic, gram-positive bacteria that grow in the form of a much-branched mycelium; some are parasitic on plants or animals; many produce antibiotics.

strep·to·my·cin (strep´tō-mī´sin) Antibiotic agent obtained from *Streptomyces griseus* active against the tubercle bacillus and a large number of gram-positive and gram-negative bacteria; used virtually exclusively in the treatment of tuberculosis. SYN streptomycin A.

strep·to·sep·ti·ce·mi·a (strep´tō-sep´ti-sē´mē-ă) SYN streptococcemia, streptosepticaemia.

stress (stres) **1.** Reactions of the body to forces of a deleterious nature, infections, and various abnormal states that tend to disturb its normal physiologic equilib-

rium (homeostasis). **2.** DENTISTRY the forces set up in teeth, their supporting structures, and structures restoring or replacing teeth as a result of the force of mastication. **3.** The force or pressure applied or exerted between portions of a body or bodies, generally expressed in pounds per square inch. **4.** RHEOLOGY the force in a material transmitted per unit area to adjacent layers. **5.** PSYCHOLOGY a physical or psychological stimulus such as very high heat, public criticism, or another noxious agent or experience that, when impinging on a person, produces psychological strain or disequilibrium.

stress ech·o·car·di·og·ra·phy (stres ek´ō-kahr-dē-og´rǎ-fē) Echocardiographic monitoring of a circulatory challenge, usually exercise.

stress in·oc·u·la·tion (stres i-nok´yū-lā´ shŭn) In clinical psychology, an approach intended to provide patients with cognitive and attitudinal skills that they can use to cope with stress.

stress re·ac·tion (stres rē-ak´shŭn) An acute emotional reaction related to extreme environmental stress. SYN acute situational reaction.

stress shield·ing (stres shēld´ing) Osteopenia due to removal of normal stress from the bone by an implant.

stress test (stres test) Systematic use of exercise or pharmacologic metabolic stressors to evaluate cardiovascular dynamics and evaluate the physiologic adjustments to metabolic demands that exceed the resting requirement. SYN exercise stress test.

stress ul·cer (stres ŭl´sĕr) A lesion of the duodenum in a patient with extensive superficial burns, intracranial lesions, or severe bodily injury.

stress u·ri·nar·y in·con·ti·nence (stres yūr´i-nar-ē in-kon´ti-nĕns) Leakage of urine as a result of coughing, straining, or some sudden voluntary movement.

stretch·er (strech´ĕr) A litter, usually a sheet of canvas stretched to a frame with four handles, used for transporting the sick or injured.

stretch re·cep·tors (strech rĕ-sep´tŏrz) Those sensitive to elongation, especially those in Golgi tendon organs and muscle spindles, but also those found in visceral organs.

stretch re·flex (strech rē′fleks) SYN myotactic reflex.

stri·a, gen. and pl **stri·ae** (strī′ă, -ē) [TA] **1.** A stripe, band, streak, or line, distinguished by color, texture, depression, or elevation from the tissue in which it is found. SYN striation (1). **2.** SYN striae cutis distensae.

stri·ae cu·tis dis·ten·sae (strī′ē kyū′tis dis-ten′sē) Bands of thin, wrinkled skin, initially red but becoming purple and white, which occur commonly on the abdomen, buttocks, and thighs at puberty and/or during and following pregnancy, and result from atrophy of the dermis and overextension of the skin. SYN lineae atrophicae, linear atrophy, stria (2), striae atrophicae.

stri·ae grav·i·da·rum (strī′ē grav-i-dā′rŭm) Striae cutis distensae associated with pregnancy.

stri·a·tal (strī-ā′tăl) Relating to the corpus striatum.

stri·ate bod·y (strī′āt bod′ē) The caudate and lentiform (lenticular) nuclei; the striate appearance on section is caused by slender fascicles of myelinated fibers. SYN corpus striatum [TA].

stri·at·ed duct (strī′āt-ĕd dŭkt) A type of intralobular duct found in some salivary glands that modifies the secretory product; it derives its name from extensive infolding of the basal membrane.

stri·at·ed mus·cle (strī′āt-ĕd mŭs′ĕl) Skeletal or voluntary muscle in which cross-striations occur in the fibers as a result of regular overlapping of thick and thin myofilaments.

stri·a·tion (strī-ā′shŭn) **1.** SYN stria (1). **2.** A striate appearance. **3.** The act of streaking or making striae.

stri·a·to·ni·gral (strī′ă-tō-nī′grăl) Referring to the efferent connection of the striatum with the substantia nigra.

stri·a·tum (strī-ā′tŭm) [TA] Collective name for the caudate nucleus and putamen that together with the globus pallidus or pallidum form the striate body.

stric·ture (strik′shŭr) A circumscribed narrowing or stenosis of a tube, duct, or hollow structure, such as the esophagus or urethra, usually consisting of cicatricial contracture or deposition of abnormal tissue. May be congenital or acquired.

stri·dor (strī′dŏr) A high-pitched, noisy respiration, like the blowing of the wind; a sign of respiratory obstruction, especially in the trachea or larynx.

string (string) A slender cord or cordlike structure.

strip (strip) **1.** To express the contents from a collapsible tube or canal, such as the urethra, by running a finger along it. SYN milk (4). **2.** Subcutaneous excision of a vein in its longitudinal axis, performed with a stripper. **3.** Any narrow piece, relatively long and of uniform width.

stroke (strōk) **1.** Any acute clinical event, related to impairment of cerebral circulation, which lasts longer than 24 hours. SEE ALSO cerebrovascular accident. **2.** A harmful discharge of lightning, particularly one that affects a human being. **3.** A pulsation. **4.** To pass the hand or any instrument over a surface. SEE ALSO stroking. **5.** A gliding movement over a surface. SYN apoplexy.

stroke work in·dex (strōk wŏrk in′deks) A measure of the work done by the heart with each contraction, adjusted for body surface area.

strok·ing (strōk′ing) The nonverbal fondling and nurturance accorded infants, or the nonverbal and verbal forms of acceptance, reassurance, and positive reinforcement accorded to children and adults either by a person to himself or herself or to another person to satisfy a basic biopsychological need of all developing humans; various psychopathologic conditions are believed to result when such stroking is absent or faulty.

stro·ma (strō′mă) **1.** The framework of a structure, as distinguished from the parenchyma or specific substance of the part. **2.** Aqueous phase of chloroplasts.

stro·mal cor·ne·al dys·tro·phy (strō′măl kōr′nē-ăl dis′trŏ-fē) Opacification with involvement of the middle layer of the cornea.

stro·muhr (strŏm′ur) An instrument for measuring the quantity of blood that flows per unit of time through a blood vessel.

Stron·gy·loi·des (stron′ji-loy′dēz) The threadworm, a genus of small nematode parasites commonly found in the small intestine of mammals (particularly ruminants). Human infection is chiefly by *S. stercoralis* or *S. fuelleborn*. Fatal infection in infants produces the condition known as swollen belly disease or syndrome, which causes gross abdominal distention.

stron·gy·loi·di·a·sis (stron′ji-loy-dī′ă-sis) Infection with soil-borne nematodes of the genus *Strongyloides*, considered to be a parthenogenetic parasitic female. Most serious human infections and nearly all fatalities commonly follow immunosuppression by steroids, other agents, or in AIDS.

stron·gy·lo·sis (stron′ji-lō′sis) Disease caused by infestation with nematode *Strongylus;* effects may be extreme, ranging from worm-associated inflammatory lesions and nodules to blood vessel blockage resulting in colic in horses.

Stron·gy·lus (stron′ji-lŭs) The palisade worm, a genus of nematodes parasitic in horses and other equids, and the cause of strongylosis.

stron·ti·um (Sr) (stron′shē-ŭm) A metallic element; salts of strontium are used therapeutically for their anions.

stron·ti·um 89 (⁸⁹Sr) (stron′shē-ŭm) A radioactive strontium isotope; used as a tracer in research.

struc·tur·al for·mu·la (strŭk′shŭr-ăl fŏrm′yū-lă) A formula in which the connections of the atoms and groups of atoms, as well as their kind and number, are indicated.

struc·tur·al is·o·mer·ism (strŭk′shŭr-ăl ī-som′ĕr-izm) Compound involving the same atoms in different arrangements.

struc·ture (strŭk′shŭr) **1.** Arrangement of the details of a part; manner of formation

of a part. **2.** Tissue or formation made up of different but related parts. **3.** CHEMISTRY Configuration and interconnections of the atoms in a given molecule. SYN structura.

stru·mec·to·my (strū-mek′tŏ-mē) Surgical removal of all or a portion of a goitrous tumor.

stru·mi·form (strū′mi-fŏrm) Resembling a goiter.

stru·mi·tis (strū-mī′tis) Thyroid gland inflammation, with swelling. SEE ALSO thyroiditis.

Strüm·pell phe·nom·e·non (strem′pel fĕ-nom′ĕ-non) Dorsal flexion of the great toe, sometimes of the entire foot, in a paralyzed limb when the extremity is drawn up against the body, flexing both knee and hip.

Strüm·pell re·flex (strem′pel rē′fleks) Stroking the abdomen or thigh causes flexion of the leg and adduction of the foot.

stru·vite cal·cu·lus (strū′vīt kal′kyū-lŭs) Stone in which the crystalloid component consists of magnesium ammonium phosphate; usually associated with urinary tract infection.

strych·nine (strik′nīn) An alkaloid from *Strychnos nux-vomica;* colorless crystals of intensely bitter taste, nearly insoluble in water; stimulates all parts of the central nervous system; potent chemical capable of producing acute or chronic poisoning.

Stry·ker frame (strī′kĕr frām) Device that holds the patient and permits turning in various planes without individual motion of parts.

Stu·dent *t*-test (stū′dĕnt test) A statistical significance test for assessing the difference between, or the equality of, two or more population means.

stump (stŭmp) **1.** The extremity of a limb left after amputation. **2.** The pedicle remaining after removal of the tumor attached to it.

stump can·cer (stŭmp kan′sĕr) Carcinoma of the stomach developing after

S

gastroenterostomy or gastric resection for benign disease.

stump pain (stŭmp pān) Pain in the area of an amputation.

stun (stŭn) To stupefy; to render unconscious by cerebral trauma.

stun·ned my·o·car·di·um (stŭnd mī′ō-kahr′dē-ŭm) Impaired myocardial contractile performance after a period of ischemia; ultimately reversible.

stupe (stūp) A compress or cloth wrung out of hot water, usually impregnated with turpentine or other irritant, applied to the skin surface to produce counterirritation.

stu·por (stū′pŏr) A state of impaired consciousness in which the person shows a marked reduction in reactivity to environmental stimuli; only continual stimulation arouses the person.

Sturge-Web·er syn·drome, Sturge-Ka·lisch·er-We·ber syn·drome (stŭrj vā′bĕr sin′drōm, kă-lish′ĕr) Triad of unilateral occurrence of congenital capillary malformation (flame nevus) in the distribution of the trigeminal nerve; ipsilateral leptomeningeal vascular malformations with intracranial calcification and neurologic signs; and vascular malformation of the choroid plexus, often with secondary glaucoma. SYN cephalotrigeminal angiomatosis, encephalotrigeminal angiomatosis.

stut·ter·ing (stŭt′ĕr-ing) A phonatory or articulatory disorder, characteristically beginning in childhood, sometimes accompanied by intense anxiety about the efficiency of oral communication, characterized by hesitations, repetitions, or prolongations of sounds and syllables, interjections, broken words, circumlocutions, and words produced with excess tension. SEE ALSO dysfluency.

stut·ter·ing gait (stŭt′ĕr-ing gāt) Ambulation with hesitancy in stepping.

stut·ter test (stŭt′ĕr test) Maneuver used to detect plica syndrome. The examiner palpates the patella as the patient slowly extends the knee. A stuttering or ratcheting effect between 45–60° is a positive result.

sty·lette, sty·let (stī′let, stī-let′) **1.** A flexible metallic rod inserted in the lumen of a flexible catheter to stiffen it and give it form during its passage. **2.** A slender probe. SYN style, stylus (3), stilus.

stylo- Combining form denoting the styloid process.

sty·lo·hy·al (stī′lō-hī′ăl) Relating to the styloid process of the temporal bone and to the hyoid bone.

sty·lo·hy·oid (stī′lō-hī′oyd) **1.** SYN stylohyal. **2.** Relating to the stylohyoid (muscle).

sty·loid (stī′loyd) Peg-shaped.

sty·loi·di·tis (stī′loy-dī′tis) Inflammation of a styloid process.

sty·lo·man·dib·u·lar, sty·lo·max·il·lar·y (stī′lō-man-dib′yū-lăr, stī-lō-mak′si-lar′ē) Relating to the styloid process of the temporal bone and the mandible; denoting the stylomandibular ligament. SYN stylomaxillary.

sty·lo·mas·toid (stī′lō-mas′toyd) Relating to the styloid and the mastoid processes of the temporal bone.

sty·lus, sti·lus (stī′lŭs) **1.** Any pencil-shaped structure. **2.** A pencil-shaped medicinal preparation for external application. **3.** SYN stylette.

stype (stīp) A tampon.

styp·sis (stip′sis) Application of a stringent substance to reduce blood flow.

styp·tic (stip′tik) **1.** Having an astringent or hemostatic effect. **2.** An astringent agent used topically to stop bleeding. SYN hemostyptic.

sub- Combining form denoting beneath, less than the normal or typical, inferior.

sub·ab·dom·i·nal (sŭb′ab-dom′i-năl) Below the abdomen.

sub·a·cro·mi·al (sŭb′ă-krō′mē-ăl) Beneath the acromion process.

sub·a·cro·mi·al bur·si·tis (sŭb-ă-krō′mē-ăl bŭr-sī′tis) Inflammation between the acromion above and the rotator cuff below.

sub·a·cute (sŭb′ă-kyūt′) Between acute and chronic; denoting the course of a disease of moderate duration or severity.

sub·a·cute bac·te·ri·al en·do·car·di·tis (SBE) (sŭb′ă-kyūt′ bak-tēr′ē-ăl en′dō-kahr-dī′tis) Condition usually involving cardiac valves with congenital or acquired abnormalities and usually due to α -hemolytic streptococci.

sub·a·cute care (sŭb-ă-kyūt′ kār) Therapy that does not require hospitalization.

sub·a·cute com·bined de·gen·er·a·tion of the sp·inal cord (sŭb′ă-kyūt′ kŏm′bīnd dĕ-jen′ĕr-ā′shŭn spī′năl kŏrd) A disorder of the spinal cord, such as that occurring in vitamin B12 deficiency, characterized by gliosis with spongiform degeneration of the posterior and lateral columns. SYN vitamin B12 neuropathy, Putnam-Dana syndrome.

sub·a·cute glo·mer·u·lo·neph·rit·is (sŭb′ă-kyūt′ glō-mer′yū-lō-nĕ-frī′tis) Undesirable term for glomerulonephritis with proteinuria, hematuria, and azotemia persisting for many weeks. SYN subacute nephritis.

sub·a·cute gran·u·lo·ma·tous thy·roid·i·tis (sŭb′ă-kyūt′ gran′yū-lō′mă-tŭs thī′roy-dī′tis) Thyroiditis with round cell (usually lymphocytes) infiltration, destruction of thyroid cells, epithelial giant cell proliferation, and evidence of regeneration; thought by some to be a reflection of a systemic infection and not an example of true chronic thyroiditis.

sub·ac·ute in·fec·tion (sŭb-ă-kyūt′ in-fek′shŭn) An infection in someone who appears clinically healthy.

sub·a·cute in·flam·ma·tion (sŭb′ă-kyūt′ in′flă-mā′shŭn) An inflammation with a duration between that of an acute inflammation and that of a chronic inflammation; usually persisting longer than 3–4 weeks.

sub·a·cute spon·gi·form en·ceph·a·lop·a·thy (sŭb′ă-kyūt′ spŏn′ji-fŏrm en-sef′a-lop′ă-thē) Form associated with a "slow virus," which to date has not been adequately described, is transmissible, and has a rapidly progressive, fatal course. SEE prion.

sub·al·i·men·ta·tion (sŭb′al-i-men-tā′shŭn) A condition of insufficient nourishment. SYN hypoalimentation.

sub·a·or·tic (sŭb′ā-ōr′tik) Below the aorta.

sub·a·or·tic ste·no·sis (sŭb′ā-ōr′tik stĕ-nō′sis) Congenital narrowing of the outflow tract of the left ventricle by a ring of fibrous tissue or by hypertrophy of the muscular septum below the aortic valve.

sub·ap·i·cal (sŭb-ap′i-kăl) Below the apex of any part.

sub·ap·o·neu·rot·ic (sŭb′ap-ō-nū-rot′ ik) Below an aponeurosis.

sub·a·rach·noid (SA) (sŭb′ă-rak′noyd) Underneath the arachnoid membrane.

subarachnoid haemorrhage [Br.] SYN subarachnoid hemorrhage.

sub·a·rach·noid hem·or·rhage (sŭb′ă-rak′noyd hem′ŏr-ăj) Bleeding between the middle membrane covering of the brain and the brain itself. SYN subarachnoid bleed, subarachnoid haemorrhage.

sub·ar·cu·ate (sŭb-ahr′kyū-āt) Slightly arcuate or bowed.

sub·a·re·o·lar (sŭb′ă-rē′ō-lăr) Beneath an areola.

sub·as·trag·a·lar (sŭb′ăs-trag′ă-lăr) Denotes an area beneath the talus bone.

sub·a·tom·ic (sŭb′ă-tom′ik) Pertaining to particles making up the intraatomic structure, e.g., protons, electrons, neutrons.

sub·au·ral (sŭb-awr′ăl) Below the ear.

sub·ax·il·lar·y (sŭb-ak′si-lar′ē) Below the axillary fossa. SYN infraaxillary.

sub·cal·lo·sal (sŭb′ka-lō′săl) Below the corpus callosum.

sub·cap·i·tal frac·ture (sŭb-kap′i-tăl frak′shŭr) Intracapsular fracture of the neck of the femur, at the point where the neck of the femur joins the head.

S

sub·cap·su·lar (sŭb-kap′sŭ-lăr) *Do not confuse this word with subscapular.* Beneath any capsule.

sub·cap·su·lar cat·a·ract (sŭb-kap′ sŭl-ăr kat′ăr-akt) Cataract with opacities concentrated beneath the capsule.

sub·car·ti·lag·i·nous (sŭb′kahr-ti-laj′i-nŭs) **1.** Partly cartilaginous. **2.** Beneath a cartilage.

sub·chon·dral (sŭb-kon′drăl) Beneath or below the cartilages of the ribs.

sub·cho·ri·al space (sŭb-kōr′ē-ăl spās) The part of the placenta beneath the chorionic plate; it joins with irregular channels to form marginal lakes.

sub·class (sŭb′klas) In biologic classification, a division between class and order.

sub·cla·vi·an, sub·cla·vic·u·lar (SC) (sŭb-klā′vē-ăn, -klă-vik′yū-lăr) **1.** Below the clavicle. SYN infraclavicular. **2.** Pertaining to the subclavian artery or vein.

sub·cla·vi·an steal (sŭb-klā′vē-ăn stēl) Obstruction of the subclavian artery proximal to the origin of the vertebral artery; blood flow through the vertebral artery is reversed and the subclavian artery thus ''steals'' cerebral blood, causing symptoms of vertebrobasilar insufficiency.

sub·cla·vi·an steal syn·drome (sŭb-klā′vē-ăn stēl sin′drōm) Symptoms of vertebrobasilar insufficiency resulting from subclavian steal.

sub·clin·i·cal (sŭb-klin′i-kăl) Denoting the presence of a disease without manifest symptoms; may be an early stage in the evolution of a disease.

sub·clin·i·cal di·a·be·tes (sŭb-klin′i-kăl dī′ă-bē′tēz) A form of diabetes mellitus clinically evident only under certain circumstances, such as pregnancy or extreme stress; those so afflicted may, in time, manifest more severe forms of the disease.

sub·con·junc·ti·val (sŭb′kŏn-jŭngk′ti-văl) Beneath the conjunctiva.

sub·con·scious (sŭb-kon′shŭs) **1.** Not wholly conscious. **2.** Denoting an idea

or impression present in the mind, but without conscious knowledge or realization of it.

sub·con·scious mem·o·ry (sŭb-kon′ shŭs mem′ŏr-ē) Information not immediately available for recall.

sub·con·scious·ness (sŭb-kon′shŭs-nĕs) **1.** Partial unconsciousness. **2.** The state in which mental processes take place without the conscious perception of the person.

sub·cor·a·coid (sŭb-kōr′ă-koyd) Beneath the coracoid process.

sub·cor·ne·al pus·tu·lar der·ma·to·sis (sŭb-kōr′nē-ăl pŭs′tyū-lăr dĕr′mă-tō′sis) Pruritic chronic anular eruption of sterile vesicles and pustules beneath the stratum corneum. SYN Sneddon-Wilkinson disease, subcorneal pustular dermatitis.

sub·cor·tex (sŭb-kōr′teks) Any part of the brain lying below the cerebral cortex, and not itself organized as cortex.

sub·cor·ti·cal (sŭb-kōr′ti-kăl) Relating to the subcortex; beneath the cerebral cortex.

sub·cor·ti·cal a·pha·si·a (sŭb-kōr′ti-kăl ă-fā′zē-ă) A disorder of comprehension and production of language due to damage to the basal ganglia, thalamus, or associated pathways. Symptoms vary depending on the area of subcortical damage and any related cortical damage.

sub·cos·tal (sŭb-kos′tăl) **1.** Beneath a rib or the ribs. SYN infracostal. **2.** Denoting certain arteries, veins, nerves, angles, or planes.

sub·cos·tal line (sŭb-kos′tăl rahl) Transverse line transecting the inferiormost border of the thoracic cage. SEE ALSO subcostal plane. SYN linea subcostalis.

sub·cra·ni·al (sŭb-krā′nē-ăl) Beneath or below the cranium.

sub·crep·i·tant (sŭb-krep′i-tănt) Nearly, but not frankly, crepitant; denoting a rale.

sub·crep·i·tant rale (sŭb-krep′i-tănt rahl) A fine crepitant rale.

sub·cul·ture (sŭb′kŭl-chŭr) **1.** A culture made by transferring to a fresh medium microorganisms from a previous culture; a method used to prolong the life of a particular strain where there is a tendency to degeneration in older cultures. **2.** To make a fresh culture with material obtained from a previous one.

sub·cu·ta·ne·ous (SQ, SC) (sŭb′kyū-tā′nē-ŭs) Beneath the skin. SYN hypodermic.

sub·cu·ta·ne·ous em·phy·se·ma (sŭb′kyū-tā′nē-ŭs em′fi-sē′mă) The presence of air or gas in the subcutaneous tissues. SYN pneumoderma.

sub·cu·ta·ne·ous fat ne·cro·sis (sŭb′kyū-tā′nē-ŭs fat nĕ-krō′sis) The death of subcutaneous fat tissue.

sub·cu·ta·ne·ous in·jec·tion (sŭb′kyū-tā′nē-ŭs in-jek′shŭn) Injection of fluid into loose connective tissue below the dermis. Absorption is slower than that of intramuscular injection. Common sites include outer posterior side of arm and abdomen. Usually only 0.5–1 mL fluid is given by this method.

sub·cu·ta·ne·ous mas·tec·to·my (sŭb′kyū-tā′nē-ŭs mas-tek′tŏ-mē) Excision of the breast tissues, but sparing the skin, nipple, and areola; usually followed by implantation of a prosthesis.

sub·cu·ta·ne·ous tis·sue (sŭb′kyū-tā′nē-ŭs tish′ū) [TA] A layer of loose, irregular connective tissue immediately beneath the skin and closely attached to the corium by coarse fibrous bands, the retinacula cutis.

sub·cu·ta·ne·ous wound (sŭb′kyū-tā′nē-ŭs wūnd) Trauma extending below the skin into the subcutaneous tissue, but not affecting underlying bones or organs.

sub·cu·tic·u·lar, sub·epi·der·mal, sub·epi·der·mic (sŭb′kyū-tik′yū-lăr, -epi′dĕr′măl, -mik) Beneath the cuticle or epidermis.

sub·de·lir·i·um (sŭb′dĕ-lir′ē-ŭm) A rarely used term for a slight or discontinuous delirium.

sub·del·toid (sŭb-del′toyd) Beneath the deltoid muscle.

sub·del·toid bur·si·tis (sŭb-del′toyd bŭr-sī′tis) Inflammation of the subdeltoid bursa lying between the deltoid muscle and the underlying proximal humerus and rotator cuff.

sub·der·mal (sŭb-dĕr′măl) Just under the skin.

sub·di·a·phrag·mat·ic (sŭb′dī-ă-frag-mat′ik) Beneath the diaphragm. SYN infradiaphragmatic, subphrenic.

sub·du·ral (sŭb-dūr′ăl) **1.** Deep to the dura mater. SEE spatium subdurale. **2.** Between the dura mater and the arachnoid mater.

sub·du·ral hem·or·rhage, sub·du·ral he·ma·to·ma (sŭb-dūr′ăl hem′ŏr-ăj, hē′mă-tō′mă) Extravasation of blood between the dural and arachnoidal membranes; acute and chronic forms occur.

sub·du·ral hy·gro·ma (sŭb-dūr′ăl hī-grō′mă) Accumulation in the subdural space of proteinaceous fluid, usually derived from serum, or of cerebrospinal fluid due to a tear in the arachnoid membrane.

sub·du·ral space (sŭb-dūr′ăl spās) [TA] An artificial space created by the separation of the arachnoid from the dura as the result of trauma or some pathologic process; in the healthy state, the arachnoid is tenuously attached to the dura and a naturally occurring subdural space is not present.

sub·en·do·car·di·al (SE) (sŭb′en-dō-kahr′dē-ăl) Beneath the endocardium.

sub·en·do·car·di·al con·duct·ing sys·tem of heart (sŭb′en-dō-kahr′dē-ăl kŏn-dŭkt′ing sis′tĕm hahrt) Terminal ramifications in the ventricles of the specialized conducting system of the heart. SYN Purkinje system.

sub·en·do·car·di·al lay·er (sŭb′en-dō-kahr′dē-ăl lā′ĕr) The loose connective tissue layer that joins the endocardium and myocardium.

sub·en·do·car·di·um (sŭb′en-dō-kahr′dē-ŭm) Tissue located directly under the membrane that lines the cardiac chambers.

sub·en·do·the·li·al (SE) (sŭb′en-dō-thē′lē-ăl) Below the endothelium.

sub·ep·en·dy·mo·ma (sŭb′ep-en′di-mō′mă) Discrete lobulated ependymal nodules in the walls of the anterior third or posterior fourth ventricles commonly found at autopsy.

sub·epi·car·di·um (sŭb′ep-i-kahr′dē-ŭm) Tissue located directly under the membrane that surrounds the heart.

sub·ep·i·der·mal ab·scess (sŭb′ep-i-dĕr′măl ab′ses) A microscopic lesion in the dermal layer.

sub·ep·i·the·li·al (sŭb′ep-i-thē′lē-ăl) Below the epithelium.

sub·fam·i·ly (sŭb′fam-i-lē) In biologic classification, a division between family and tribe or between family and genus.

sub·fas·ci·al (sŭb-fash′ē-ăl) Beneath a fascia.

sub·fer·til·i·ty (sŭb′fĕr-til′i-tē) Less than normal capacity for reproduction.

sub·fron·tal (sŭb-frŏn′tăl) Denotes the area below the frontal lobe.

sub·ge·nus (sŭb′jē-nŭs) In biologic classification, a division between genus and species.

sub·gin·gi·val (sŭb-jin′ji-văl) Below the gingival margin.

sub·glos·sal (sŭb-glos′ăl) Below or beneath the tongue.

sub·grun·da·tion (sŭb′grŭn-dā′shŭn) The depression of one fragment of a broken cranial bone below the other.

su·bic·u·lum, pl. **su·bic·u·la** (sŭ-bik′yū-lŭm, -lă) [TA] A support or prop.

sub·il·i·ac (sŭb-il′ē-ak) 1. Below the ilium. 2. Relating to the subilium.

sub·il·i·um (sŭb-il′ē-ŭm) The portion of the ilium contributing to the acetabulum.

sub·in·ti·mal (sŭb-in′ti-măl) Beneath the intima.

sub·in·vo·lu·tion (sŭb′in′vŏ-lū′shŭn) Arrest of the normal involution of the uterus following childbirth, with the organ remaining abnormally large.

sub·ja·cent (sŭb-jā′sĕnt) Below or beneath another part.

sub·ject (sŭb′jekt) A person or organism that is the object of research, treatment, experimentation, or dissection.

sub·jec·tive (sŭb-jek′tiv) 1. Perceived by the patient only and not evident to the examiner; said of certain symptoms, such as pain. 2. Colored by one's personal beliefs and attitudes. Cf. objective (2).

sub·jec·tive da·ta col·lec·tion (sŭb-jek′tiv dā′tă kŏ-lek′shŭn) Collecting information from a patient in the patient's words.

sub·jec·tive sen·sa·tion (sŭb-jek′tiv sen-sā′shŭn) One not readily referable to a verifiable stimulus.

sub·jec·tive symp·tom (sŭb-jek′tiv simp′tŏm) A symptom apparent only to the patient.

sub·jects (sŭb′jekts) Nonclinical participants in a medical study.

sub·ju·gal (sŭb-jū′găl) Below the zygomatic (jugal) bone.

sub·la·tion (sŭb-lā′shŭn) Detachment, elevation, or removal of a part.

sub·li·ma·tion (sŭb′li-mā′shŭn) 1. Converting a solid directly into a gas. 2. In psychoanalysis, an unconscious defense mechanism in which unacceptable instinctual drives and wishes are modified into more personally and socially acceptable channels.

sub·lime (sŭb-līm′) 1. To sublimate. 2. To undergo a process of sublimation.

sub·limed sul·fur (sŭb-limd′ sŭl′fŭr) Agent used in preparing sulfur ointment and treatment of various skin disorders. SYN flowers of sulfur.

sub·lim·i·nal (sŭb-lim′i-năl) Below the threshold of perceptions or excitation.

sub·lim·i·nal self (sŭb-lim′i-năl self) Sum of the mental processes that take place without the person's conscious knowledge. SYN subconscious mind.

sub·lin·gual ad·min·i·stra·tion of

med·i·ca·tion (sŭb-ling´gwăl ad-min´i-strā´shŭn med´i-kā´shŭn) Giving medication that is placed under the tongue.

sub·lin·gual bur·sa (sŭb-ling´gwăl bŭr´să) An inconstant serous bursa at the level of the frenulum of the tongue between the surface of the genioglossus muscle and the mucous membrane of the floor of the mouth. SYN Fleischmann bursa.

sub·lin·gual tab·let (ST) (sŭb-ling´gwăl tab´lĕt) Usually a small, flat fast-dissolving tablet intended to be inserted beneath the tongue, where the active ingredient is absorbed directly through the oral mucosa.

sub·lob·u·lar (sŭb-lob´yū-lăr) Beneath a lobule, as of the liver.

sub·lux·a·tion (sŭb´lŭk-sā´shŭn) An incomplete luxation or dislocation. SYN semiluxation.

sub·mam·ma·ry (sŭb-mam´ă-rē) **1.** Deep to the mammary gland. **2.** SYN inframammary.

sub·man·dib·u·lar (sŭb´man-dib´yū-lăr) Beneath the mandible or lower jaw. SYN inframandibular, submaxillary (2).

sub·mar·gin·al (sŭb-mahr´jin-ăl) Near the margin of any part.

sub·max·il·lar·y (sŭb-mak´si-lar-ē) **1.** SYN mandibular. **2.** SYN submandibular.

sub·men·tal (sŭb-men´tăl) **1.** Beneath the chin. **2.** Denoting a certain artery, vein, set of lymph nodes, or triangle of neck below the chin.

sub·met·a·cen·tric chro·mo·some (sŭb-met´ă-sen´trik krō´mŏ-sōm) A chromosome with the centromere so placed that it divides the chromosome into two arms of strikingly unequal length.

sub·mi·cro·scop·ic (sŭb´mī-krŏ-skop´ik) Too minute to be visible with a light microscope. SYN ultramicroscopic.

sub·mor·phous (sŭb-mōr´fŭs) Neither definitely amorphous nor definitely crystalline; denoting the structure of certain calculi.

sub·mu·co·sa (sŭb´myū-kō´să) [TA] A layer of tissue beneath a mucous membrane; the layer of connective tissue beneath the tunica mucosa. SYN tela submucosa.

sub·mu·co·sal plex·us (sŭb´myū-kō´săl plek´sŭs) A gangliated plexus of unmyelinated nerve fibers, derived chiefly from the superior mesenteric plexus, ramifying in the intestinal submucosa.

sub·mu·cous, sub·mu·co·sal (SM) (sŭb-myū´kŭs, -myū-kō´săl) Beneath a mucous membrane.

sub·mu·cous re·sec·tion (sŭb-myū´kŭs rē-sek´shŭn) Surgical procedure to correct a deviated nasal septum, in which obstructing septal cartilage or bone is removed after elevation of the investing mucoperichondrial flaps on each side.

sub·nar·cot·ic (sŭb´nahr-kot´ik) Slightly narcotic.

sub·na·sal (sŭb-nā´zăl) Under the nose.

sub·na·sal point (sŭb-nā´zăl poynt) Center of the root of the anterior nasal spine. SYN apophysary point (1), apophysial point, spinal point.

sub·neu·ral (sŭb-nūr´ăl) Below the neural axis.

sub·neu·ral ap·pa·ra·tus (sŭb-nūr´ăl ap´ă-rat´ŭs) Modified sarcoplasm in a motor end-plate.

sub·nor·mal (sŭb-nōr´măl) Below the normal standard of some quality or trait.

sub·nu·cle·us (sŭb-nū´klē-ŭs) A secondary nucleus.

sub·oc·cip·i·tal (SO) (sŭb´ok-sip´i-tăl) **1.** Below the occiput or the occipital bone. **2.** Denoting certain muscles, nerves, a nervous plexus, or triangle of the neck below the occipital bone.

sub·or·der (sŭb´ōr-dĕr) In biologic classification, a division between order and family.

sub·pap·u·lar (sŭb-pap´yū-lăr) Denoting the eruption of few and scattered papules, in which the lesions are very slightly elevated, being scarcely more than macules.

sub·pa·tel·lar (sŭb´pă-tel´ăr) **1.** Deep to the patella. **2.** SYN infrapatellar.

S

sub·per·i·car·di·al (sŭb′per-i-kar′dē-ăl) Beneath the pericardium.

sub·per·i·os·te·al (sŭb′per-ē-os′tē-ăl) Beneath the periosteum.

sub·per·i·os·te·al am·pu·ta·tion (sŭb′per-ē-os′tē-ăl amp′yū-tā′shŭn) Form of surgical removal in which the periosteum is stripped back from the bone and replaced afterward, forming a periosteal flap over the cut end. SYN periosteoplastic amputation.

sub·per·i·os·te·al frac·ture (sŭb′per-ē-os′tē-ăl frak′shŭr) Breakage beneath the periosteum, and without displacement.

sub·per·i·os·te·al im·plant (sŭb′per-ē-os′tē-ăl im′plant) Artificial dental metal appliance made to conform to the shape of a bone and placed on its surface beneath the periosteum. SEE implant denture substructure.

sub·per·i·to·ne·al (sŭb′per-i-tŏ-nē′ăl) Beneath the peritoneum.

sub·pha·ryn·ge·al (sŭb′fă-rin′jē-ăl) Below the pharynx.

sub·phren·ic (sŭb-fren′ik) SYN subdiaphragmatic.

sub·phren·ic ab·scess (sŭb-fren′ik ab′ses) Lesion directly beneath the diaphragm. SYN subdiaphragmatic abscess.

sub·phy·lum (sŭb′fī-lŭm) In biologic classification, a division between phylum and class.

sub·pleu·ral (sŭb-plūr′ăl) Beneath the pleura.

sub·pre·pu·tial (sŭb′prē-pyū′shē-ăl) Beneath the prepuce.

sub·pu·bic (sŭb-pyū′bik) Beneath the pubic arch; denoting a ligament, the arcuate pubic ligament, connecting the two pubic bones below the arch.

sub·pul·mo·nar·y (sŭb-pul′mŏ-nār′ē) Below the lungs.

sub·ret·i·nal (sŭb-ret′i-năl) **1.** Between the sensory retina and the retinal pigment epithelium. **2.** Between the retinal pigment epithelium and the choroid.

sub·scap·u·lar (sŭb-skap′yū-lăr) *Do not confuse this word with subcapsular.* **1.** Deep to the scapula. **2.** Denoting a certain artery or arterial branches, vein, nerve, fossa, or set of lymph nodes deep to the scapula. SYN infrascapular.

sub·scrip·tion (sŭb-skrip′shŭn) The part of a prescription preceding the signature giving directions for compounding.

sub·se·ro·sa (sŭb′sēr-ō′să) [TA] The layer of connective tissue beneath a serous membrane. SYN tela subserosa [TA], subserous layer.

sub·se·rous, sub·se·ro·sal (sŭb-sē′rŭs, sŭb′sē-rō′săl) Beneath a serous membrane.

sub·si·dence (sŭb′si-dĕns) Sinking or settling in bone.

sub·spi·na·le (sŭb′spī-nā′lē) In cephalometrics, the most posterior midline point on the premaxilla between the anterior nasal spine and the prosthion.

sub·spi·nous (sŭb-spī′nŭs) **1.** SYN infraspinous. **2.** Tendency to spininess.

sub·stance (sŭb′stăns) Material. SYN matter.

sub·stance a·buse (sŭb′stăns ă-byūs′) Maladaptive pattern of drug or alcohol use that may lead to social, occupational, psychological, or physical problems.

sub·stance de·pen·dence (sŭb′stăns dĕ-pen′dĕns) Pattern of behavioral, physiologic, and cognitive symptoms due to substance use or abuse; usually indicated by tolerance to the effects of the substance and withdrawal symptoms when use of the substance is terminated.

sub·stance in·tox·i·ca·tion (sŭb′stăns in-tok′si-kā′shŭn) Stimulation, excitement, or stupification related to exposure to or ingestion of a substance that physiologically affects the central nervous system (usually reversible).

sub·stance P (sŭb′stăns) A peptide neurotransmitter composed of eleven amino acid residues normally present in minute quantities in the nervous system and intestines of humans and various animals and found in inflamed tissue; primarily involved in pain transmission.

sub·stance with·draw·al (sŭb′stăns with-draw′ăl) Physiologic and psychological readjustments made during discontinuation of use of a substance previously employed to induce intoxication.

sub·stan·ti·a ni·gra (sŭb-stan′shē-ă nī′ gră) [TA] A large cell mass, crescentic on transverse section, extending forward over the dorsal surface of the crus cerebri from the rostral border of the pons into the subthalamic region; involved in the metabolic disturbances associated with parkinsonism and Huntington disease.

substantia spon·gi·o·sa (sŭb-stan′ shē-ă spŏn-jē-ō′să) [TA] Bone in which the spicules or trabeculae form a three-dimensional latticework (cancellus), with the interstices filled with embryonal connective tissue or bone marrow. SYN cancellous bone, spongy bone (1), spongy substance, trabecular bone.

sub·stan·tiv·i·ty (sŭb′stăn-tiv′i-tē) 1. Property of continuing therapeutic action despite removal of vehicle. 2. The ability of an antimicrobial agent to retain its effectiveness in the mouth for an extended period.

sub·ster·nal (sŭb-stĕr′năl) 1. Deep to the sternum. 2. SYN infrasternal.

sub·ster·nal goi·ter (sŭb-stĕr′năl goy′ tĕr) Enlargement of the thyroid gland, chiefly of the lower part of the isthmus.

sub·stit·u·ent (sŭb-stich′yū-ĕnt) A functional group that has replaced another moiety and molecular entity.

sub·sti·tu·tion (sŭb′sti-tū′shŭn) 1. In chemistry, replacement of an atom or group in a compound by another atom or group. 2. In psychoanalysis, an unconscious defense mechanism by which an unacceptable or unattainable goal or emotion is replaced by one more acceptable or attainable; the process is more acute and direct, and less subtle, than sublimation.

sub·sti·tu·tion prod·uct (sŭb′sti-tū′ shŭn prod′ŭkt) One obtained by replacing one atom or group in a molecule with another atom or group.

sub·sti·tu·tion ther·a·py (sŭb′sti-tū′ shŭn thār′ă-pē) Replacement therapy, particularly when replacement is not physiologic but entails administration of a substitute.

sub·strate (sŭb′strāt) 1. The substance acted on and changed by an enzyme. 2. The base on which an organism lives or grows.

sub·strate-lev·el phos·phor·y·la·tion (sŭb′strāt-lev′ĕl fos′fōr-i-lā′shŭn) Synthesis of adenosine triphosphate not involving electron transport coupled with oxidative phosphorylation or with photophosphorylation.

sub·stra·tum (sŭb-strā′tŭm) Any layer or stratum lying beneath another.

sub·struc·ture (sŭb′strŭk-shŭr) A tissue or structure wholly or partly beneath the surface.

sub·tar·sal (sŭb-tahr′săl) Below the tarsus.

sub·tha·lam·ic (sŭb′thă-lam′ik) Related to the subthalamus region or to the subthalamic nucleus.

sub·ten·to·ri·al (sŭb′ten-tōr′ē-ăl) Under the tentorium cerebelli.

sub·thal·a·mus (sŭb-thal′ă-mŭs) [TA] That part of the diencephalon found between the thalamus on the dorsal side and the cerebral peduncle ventrally, lateral to the dorsal half of the hypothalamus, from which it cannot be sharply delineated.

sub·tribe (sŭb′trīb) In biologic classification, a division between tribe and genus.

sub·tro·chan·ter·ic (sŭb′trō-kan-ter′ik) Below any trochanter.

sub·um·bil·i·cal (sŭb′ŭm-bil′i-kăl) Below the navel.

sub·un·gual, sub·un·gui·al (sŭb-ŭng′ gwal, -gwē-ăl) Beneath a fingernail or toenail. SYN hyponychial (1).

sub·un·gual ex·o·sto·sis (sŭb-ŭng′ gwăl eks′os-tō′sis) Painful osseous outgrowths that elevate the nail of the great toe or fingers in young people.

sub·un·gual he·ma·to·ma (sŭb-ŭng′ gwăl hē′mă-tō′mă) Collection of blood beneath a fingernail or toenail, usually due to trauma.

sub·un·gual mel·a·no·ma (sŭb-ŭng′ gwăl mel′ă-nō′mă) A melanoma beginning in the skin at the border of or beneath the nail.

S

sub·u·nit vac·cine (sŭb′yū-nit vak-sēn′) One that, through chemical extraction, is free viral nucleic acid and contains only specific protein subunits of a given virus.

sub·u·re·thral (sŭb′yūr-ē′thrăl) Beneath the male or female urethra.

sub·vag·i·nal (sŭb-vaj′i-năl) **1.** Below the vagina. **2.** On the inner side of any tubular membrane serving as a sheath.

sub·ver·te·bral (sŭb-vĕr′tĕ-brăl) Beneath, or on the ventral side, of a vertebra or the vertebral column.

sub·zy·go·mat·ic (sŭb′zī-gō-mat′ik) Below or beneath the zygomatic bone or arch.

suc·ce·da·ne·ous tooth (sŭk′sĕ-dā′nē-ŭs tūth) **1.** A permanent tooth that succeeds an exfoliated deciduous tooth. **2.** Permanent incisors, canines, and premolars.

suc·cen·tu·ri·ate (sŭk′sen-tyūr′ē-ăt) ANATOMY substituting for, or accessory to, some organ.

suc·cin·ic ac·id (sŭk-sin′ik as′id) An intermediate in the tricarboxylic acid cycle; several of its salts have been variously used in medicine.

suc·cin·i·mide (suk-sin′ă-mīd) Chemical class of drugs from which the antiepileptic agents ethosuximide, methsuximide, and phensuximide are derived. Unsubstituted succinimide has been used as an antiurolithic.

suc·ci·nyl·cho·line (sŭk′si-nil-kō′lēn) A neuromuscular relaxant used in tracheal intubation and during surgical anesthesia. SYN diacetylcholine, suxamethonium.

suc·cor·rhe·a (sŭk′ōr-ē′ă) An abnormal increase in the secretion of a digestive fluid.

suc·cus·sion sound (sŭ-kŭsh′shŭn sownd) The noise made by fluid with overlying air when shaken.

suck (sŭk) **1.** To draw a fluid through a tube by exhausting the air in front. **2.** To draw a fluid into the mouth.

suck·ing re·flex (sŭk′ing rē′fleks) Sucking movements of the lips of an infant in response to touching of the lips or surrounding area.

suck·le (sŭk′ĕl) To nurse; to feed by milk from the breast.

suck·ling (sŭk′ling) An early oral intake pattern seen in infants whose lower jaw and tongue elevate as a unit and thereby place pressure on the nipple to obtain liquid nourishment.

su·cral·fate (sū-kral′fāt) Sucrose octakis (hydrogen sulfate) aluminum complex; a polysaccharide with antipeptic activity, used to treat duodenal ulcers by providing a protective coating to allow healing.

su·crase (sū′krās) SYN sucrose α-D-glucohydrolase.

su·crose (sū′krōs) A nonreducing disaccharide made up of D-glucose and D-fructose obtained from sugar cane, *Saccharum officinarum*, from several species of sorghum, and from the sugar beet, *Beta vulgaris*. SYN saccharose.

su·crose α-D-glu·co·hy·dro·lase (sū′krōs al′fă glū′kō-hī′drŏ-lās) An enzyme found in the intestinal mucosa; a deficiency results in defective digestion of sucrose and linear α1,4-glucans. SYN sucrase.

su·cro·se·mi·a (sū′krō-sē′mē-ă) The presence of sucrose in the blood. SYN sucrosaemia.

su·cro·su·ri·a (sū′krō-syū′rē-ă) The excretion of sucrose in the urine.

suc·tion (sŭk′shŭn) The act or process of sucking. SEE ALSO aspiration (1), aspiration (2).

suc·tion cur·et·tage (sŭk′shŭn kyūr′ĕtahzh′) Abortion in which the cervix is dilated if necessary and the products of conception are removed with suction cannula. SYN dilation and suction.

suc·to·ri·al (sŭk-tōr′ē-ăl) Relating to suction, or the act of sucking; adapted for sucking.

su·da·men, pl. **su·dam·i·na** (sū-dā′mĕn, -dam′i-nă) A minute vesicle due to retention of fluid in a sweat follicle, or in the epidermis.

sud·den death (SD) (sŭd′ĕn deth) *Avoid the nonsense phrase recurrent sudden death.* Death occurring rapidly and generally unexpectedly; usually from a cardiac dysrhythmia or myocardial infarction, but also from any cause of rapid death.

sud·den in·fant death syn·drome (SIDS) (sŭd′ĕn in′fănt deth sin′drŏm) Abrupt and inexplicable death of an apparently healthy infant. SYN crib death.

Su·deck at·ro·phy (sū′dek at′rŏ-fē) Osseous wasting, commonly of the carpal or tarsal bones, following a slight injury such as a sprain. SEE ALSO complex regional pain syndrome type I. SYN acute reflex bone atrophy, Sudeck syndrome.

su·do·mo·tor (sū′dō-mō′tŏr) Denoting the autonomic (sympathetic) nerves that stimulate the sweat glands to activity.

su·do·mo·tor nerves (sū′dō-mō′tŏr nĕrvz) Those containing autonomic fibers that innervate sweat glands.

sudor- *Do not confuse this combining form with pseudo-.* Combining form denoting sweat, perspiration.

su·do·re·sis (sū′dŏr-ē′sis) Profuse sweating.

su·do·rif·ic (sū′dŏr-if′ik) Causing sweat.

su·do·rip·a·rous (sū′dŏr-ip′ă-rŭs) Secreting sweat.

suf·fo·ca·tion (sŭf′ŏ-kā′shŭn) The act or condition of suffocating or of asphyxiation.

suf·fo·ca·tive goi·ter (sŭf′ŏ-kā-tiv goy′tĕr) A goiter that by pressure causes extreme dyspnea.

suf·fu·sion (sŭ-fyū′zhŭn) **1.** The act of pouring a fluid over the body. **2.** A reddening of the surface. **3.** The condition of being wet with a fluid. **4.** SYN extravasate (2).

sug·ar (shug′ăr) Colloquial usage for sucrose; pharmaceutic forms include compressible sugar and confectioner's sugar.

sug·ar al·co·hol (shu′găr al′kŏ-hol) Polyalcohol due to reduction of the carbonyl group in a monosaccharide to a hydroxyl group.

sug·ar cat·a·ract (shu′găr kat′ă-rakt) One associated with intralenticular accumulation of pentose or hexose alcohols.

su·i·cide ges·ture (sū′i-sīd jes′chŭr) An apparent attempt at suicide by someone wishing to attract attention, gain sympathy, or achieve some goal other than self-destruction.

su·i·ci·dol·o·gy (sū′i-sī-dol′ŏ-jē) A branch of the behavioral sciences devoted to the study of the nature, causes, and prevention of suicide.

sul·bac·tam (sŭl-bak′tam) A β-lactamase inhibitor with weak antibacterial action; when used in conjunction with penicillins with little β-lactamase-inhibiting action, greatly increases their effectiveness against organisms that would ordinarily not be susceptible.

sul·cate (sŭl′kāt) Grooved; marked by a sulcus or sulci.

sul·cu·lus, pl. **sul·cu·li** (sŭl′kyū-lŭs, -lī) A small sulcus.

sul·cus, gen. and pl. **sul·ci** (sŭl′kŭs, -sī) [TA] **1.** One of the grooves or furrows on the surface of the brain, bounding the several convolutions or gyri; a fissure. **2.** Any long, narrow groove, furrow, or slight depression. **3.** A groove or depression in the oral cavity or on the surface of a tooth **4.** The healthy space between the marginal gingiva and a tooth. SYN gingival sulcus.

sul·cus sign, sul·cus test (sŭl′kŭs sīn, test) Maneuver used to determine inferior instability of the glenohumeral joint, whereby traction is applied to the humerus. If the space widens between the acromion process and humeral head to produce an indentation, a positive test result is confirmed.

sulf-, sulfo- Combining forms denoting that the compound to the name of which it is attached contains a sulfur atom. This 'f' spelling (rather than sulph-, sulpho-) is preferred by the American Chemical Society.

sul·fa·di·a·zine (SD) (sŭl′fă-dī′ă-zēn) Diazine derivative of sulfanilamide; inhibitor of bacterial folic acid synthesis, which has been highly effective against pneumococcal, staphylococcal, and streptococcal infections, against infections with *Escherichia coli* and *Kleb-*

siella pneumoniae, and in acute gonococcal arthritis.

sul·fa·meth·ox·a·zole (SMX) (sŭl´fă-me-thok´să-zōl) A sulfonamide related chemically to sulfisoxazole, with a similar antibacterial spectrum, but a slower rate of absorption and urinary excretion. Often used with trimethoprim (i.e., SMX-TMP).

sul·fa·nil·a·mide (SNM) (sŭl´fă-nil´ă-mīd) The first sulfonamide used for its chemotherapeutic effect in infections.

sul·fa·sal·a·zine (SS, SAS, SAZ, SSZ) (sŭl´fă-sal´ă-zēn) A sulfonamide (acid-azo-sulfa compound) with a marked affinity for connective tissues, especially for those rich in elastin; used in ulcerative colitis and rheumatoid arthritis. SYN salicylazosulfapyridine.

sul·fa·tase (sŭl´fă-tās) 1. Sulfuric ester hydrolase, which catalyzes hydrolysis of sulfuric esters (sulfates) to the corresponding alcohols plus inorganic sulfate. 2. SYN arylsulfatase.

sul·fate, sul·phate (SO₄) (sŭl´fāt) A salt or ester of sulfuric acid.

sulf·he·mo·glo·bi·ne·mi·a (sŭlf-hē´mŏ-glō´bi-nē´mē-ă) A morbid condition due to the presence of sulfhemoglobin in the blood; marked by a persistent cyanosis, but the blood count does not reveal any abnormality in blood cells; thought to be caused by the action of hydrogen sulfide absorbed from the intestine. SYN sulphaemoglobinaemia.

sul·fite (SO₃) (sŭl´fīt) A salt of sulfurous acid; elevated in cases of molybdenum cofactor deficiency.

sul·fite ox·i·dase (sŭl´fīt ok´si-dās) A liver oxidoreductase (hemoprotein) catalyzing reaction of inorganic sulfite ion with O₂ and water to produce sulfate ion and hydrogen peroxide. SYN sulphite oxidase.

sulf·met·he·mo·glo·bin (sŭlf´met-hē´mŏ-glō´bin) The complex formed by hydrogen sulfide (or sulfides) and ferric ion in methemoglobin.

sul·fo·bro·mo·phthal·e·in so·di·um (sŭl´fō-brō´mō-fthal´ē-in sō´dē-ŭm) Triphenylmethane derivative excreted by the liver; used in testing hepatic function. SYN bromosulfophthalein, bromsulf-ophthalein, sulphobromophthalein sodium.

sul·fone (sŭl-fōn) A compound of the general structure R′–SO₂–Rd′. SYN sulphone.

sul·fur (S) (sŭl´fŭr) An element that combines with oxygen to form sulfur dioxide and sulfur trioxide; forms sulfides; used externally to treat skin diseases. SYN sulphur.

sulfur di·ox·ide (SO₂) (sŭl´fŭr dī-ok´sīd) Colorless, nonflammable gas with a strong, suffocating odor; a powerful reducing agent used to prevent oxidative deterioration of food and medicinal products. SEE ALSO sulfurous acid. SYN sulfurous oxide.

sul·fu·ric ac·id (sŭl-fyŭr´ik as´id) H₂SO₄; Colorless, nearly odorless, heavy, oily, corrosive liquid containing 96% of the absolute acid. SYN sulphuric acid.

sul·fu·rous ac·id (sŭl´fŭr-ŭs as´id) Solution of about 6% sulfur dioxide in water; used as disinfectant and bleach; used externally for its parasiticidal effect in various skin diseases.

sulphaemoglobin [Br.] SYN sulfmethemoglobin.

sulphaemoglobinaemia [Br.] SYN sulfhemoglobinemia.

sulphatase [Br.] SYN sulfatase.

sulphite oxidase [Br.] SYN sulfite oxidase.

sulphmethaemoglobin [Br.] SYN sulfmethemoglobin.

sulphobromophthalein sodium [Br.] SYN sulfobromophthalein sodium.

sulphone [Br.] SYN sulfone.

sulphur [Br.] SYN sulfur.

sum·ma·tion (sŭm-ā´shŭn) The aggregation of a number of similar neural impulses or stimuli.

sum·ma·tion gal·lop (sŭm-ā´shŭn gal´ŏp) Rhythm in which the gallop sound is due to superimposition of third and fourth heart sounds; sometimes heard in normal subjects with tachycardia, but usually indicative of myocardial disease.

sum·mer diar·rhe·a (sŭm′ĕr dī′ă-rē′ă) Intestinal disorder of infants in hot weather, usually an acute gastroenteritis due to *Shigella* or *Salmonella*. SYN choleraic diarrhea.

Sum·ner sign (sŭm′nĕr sīn) A slight increase in tonus of the abdominal muscles, an early indication of inflammation of the appendix, stone in the kidney or ureter, or a twisted pedicle of an ovarian cyst.

sump syn·drome (sŭmp sin′drōm) A complication of side-to-side choledochoduodenostomy in which the lower end of the common bile duct at times acts as a diverticulum, resulting in stasis, trapping of food particles, and infection.

sun·down·ing (sŭn′down-ing) The onset or exacerbation of delirium during the evening or night with improvement or disappearance during the day; most often seen in the middle and later stages of dementing disorders, such as Alzheimer disease.

sun pro·tec·tion fac·tor (SPF) (sŭn prŏ-tek′shŭn fak′tŏr) The ratio of the minimal ultraviolet dose required to produce erythema with and without a sunscreen; useful sunscreens require an sun protection factor that exceeds 14.

sun·rise syn·drome (sŭn′rīz sin′drōm) Cognitive instability on arising from sleep.

sun·stroke, sun stroke (sŭn′strōk) Trauma due to heatstroke under exposure to the sun's rays, probably caused by the action of actinic rays combined with high temperature; symptoms are those of heatstroke, but often without fever.

super- Combining form properly only prefixed to words of Latin derivation, denoting in excess, above, superior, or in the upper part of; often the same usage as Latin *supra-*. Cf. hyper-.

su·per·ac·tiv·i·ty (sū′pĕr-ak-tiv′i-tē) Abnormally great activity.

su·per·an·ti·gen (sū′pĕr-an′ti-jen) An antigen that interacts with the T-cell receptor in a domain outside the antigen recognition site; interaction induces activation of larger numbers of T cells than are induced by antigens that are presented in the antigen recognition site

leading to the release of numerous cytokines. SEE ALSO antigen.

su·per·cil·i·ar·y (sū′pĕr-sil′ē-ar-ē) Relating to or in the region of the eyebrow.

su·per·cil·i·um, pl. **su·per·cil·i·a** (sū′pĕr-sil′ē-ŭm, -ă) [TA] **1.** SYN eyebrow. **2.** An individual hair of the eyebrow.

su·per·coil·ing (sū′pĕr-koyl′ing) SYN superhelicity.

su·per·e·go (sū′pĕr-ē′gō) In psychoanalysis, one of three components of the psychic apparatus in the freudian structural framework, the other two being the ego and the id.

su·per·fi·cial (sū′pĕr-fish′ăl) [TA] **1.** Cursory; not thorough. **2.** Pertaining to or situated near the surface. **3.** SYN superficialis.

su·per·fi·cial burn (sū′pĕr-fish′ăl bŭrn) A burn involving only the epidermis and causing erythema and edema without vesiculation. SYN first-degree burn.

su·per·fi·ci·a·lis (sū′pĕr-fish′ē-ā′lis) [TA] Situated nearer the surface of the body in relation to a specific reference point. SYN superficial (3).

su·per·fi·cial re·flex (sū′pĕr-fish′ăl rē′fleks) Any reflex (e.g., the abdominal or cremasteric reflex) elicited by stimulation of the skin.

su·per·fi·cial spread·ing mel·a·no·ma (sū-pĕr-fish′ăl spred′ing mel-ă-nō′mă) Primary cutaneous melanoma characterized by intraepidermal growth extending laterally beyond the site of dermal invasion.

su·per·fi·ci·es (sū′pĕr-fish′ē-ēz) Outer surface; facies.

su·per·hel·ic·i·ty (sū′pĕr-hel-is′i-tē) An attribute of native duplex DNA structure characterized by further twisting or coiling of the double helix. SYN supercoiling.

su·per·in·duce (sū′pĕr-in-dūs′) To induce or bring on in addition to something already existing.

su·per·in·fec·tion (sū′pĕr-in-fek′shŭn) A new infection in addition to one already present.

su·per·in·vo·lu·tion (sū′pĕr-in′vŏ-lū′shŭn) An extreme reduction in size of the uterus, after childbirth, to less than the normal size of the nongravid organ. SYN hyperinvolution.

su·pe·ri·or (sū-pēr'ē-ŏr) [TA] **1.** Situated above or directed upward. **2.** HUMAN ANATOMY situated nearer the vertex of the head in relation to a specific reference point; opposite of inferior. SYN cranial (2).

su·pe·ri·or·i·ty com·plex (sū-pēr'ē-ŏr'i-tē kom'pleks) Term sometimes given to compensatory behavior, e.g., aggressiveness and self-assertion.

su·per·lac·ta·tion (sū'pĕr-lak-tā'shŭn) The continuance of lactation beyond the normal period. SYN hyperlactation.

su·per·na·tant flu·id (sū'pĕr-nā'tănt flū'id) Clear fluid that, after the settling out of an insoluble liquid or solid by the action of normal gravity or of centrifugal force, takes up the upper portion of the contents of a vessel.

su·per·nu·mer·ar·y (sū'pĕr-nū'mĕr-ar-ē) Exceeding the normal number.

su·per·nu·mer·ar·y nip·ples (sū'pĕr-nū'mĕr-ar-ē nip'ĕlz) Additional nipples found in humans; they appear in two verticles lines from the armpit to the groin area and are often mistaken for moles.

su·per·nu·tri·tion (sū'pĕr-nū-trish'ŭn) Overeating leading to obesity. SYN hypernutrition.

su·per·o·lat·er·al (sū'pĕr-ō-lat'ĕr-ăl) At the side and above.

su·per·ov·u·la·tion (sū'pĕr-ov'yū-lā'shŭn) Ovulation of a supranormal number of ova; usually the result of the administration of exogenous gonadotropins.

su·per·ox·ide (sū'pĕr-oks'īd) An oxygen free radical, O_2^-, which is toxic to cells.

su·per·ox·ide dis·mu·tase (sū'pĕr-oks'īd dis'myū-tās) Enzyme that catalyzes the dismutation reaction $2O_2^{\cdot-} + 2H^+ \rightarrow H_2O_2 + O_2$; deficiency associated with amyotrophic lateral sclerosis.

su·per·sat·u·rate (sū'pĕr-sach'ŭr-āt) To make a solution hold more of a salt or other substance in solution than will dissolve when in equilibrium with that salt in the solid phase.

su·per·sat·u·rat·ed so·lu·tion (sū'pĕr-sach'ŭr-ā-tĕd sŏ-lū'shŭn) A solution containing more of the solid than the liquid would ordinarily dissolve.

su·per·scrip·tion (sū'pĕr-skrip'shŭn) The beginning of a prescription, consisting of the injunction, *recipe*, take, usually denoted by the sign ℞.

su·per·struc·ture (sū'pĕr-strŭk'shŭr) A structure above the surface.

su·per·volt·age (sū'pĕr-vōl'tăj) In radiation therapy, a descriptor for high-energy radiation exceeding 1000 V.

su·pi·nate (sū'pi-nāt) **1.** To assume, or to be placed in, a supine (face upward) position. **2.** To perform supination of the forearm or of the foot.

su·pi·na·tion (sū'pi-nā'shŭn) [TA] **1.** The condition of being supine; the act of assuming or of being placed in a supine position. **2.** Transverse plane motion at the radioulnar joint or transverse tarsal joint.

su·pine (sū-pīn') **1.** Denoting the body when lying face upward; opposite of prone. **2.** Supination of the forearm or of the foot. SYN dorsal recumbent position.

su·pine po·si·tion (sū-pīn' pŏ-zish'ŏn) Lying on one's back. SYN dorsal position.

sup·port·er (sŭ-pōrt'er) An apparatus intended to hold in place a dependent or pendulous part, prolapsed organ, or joint.

sup·port·ing a·re·a (sŭ-pōrt'ing ār'ē-ă) Portions of the maxillary and mandibular edentulous ridges considered best suited to carry the forces of mastication when the dentures are in function.

sup·port·ing treat·ment (sŭ-pōrt'ing trēt'mĕnt) Care of a patient intended to help the person sustain her or his strength.

sup·pos·i·to·ry (sŭ-poz'i-tōr-ē) A small, solid body shaped for ready introduction into one of the orifices of the body other than the oral cavity (e.g., rectum, urethra, vagina), made of a substance, usually medicated, which is solid at ordinary temperatures but melts at body temperature.

sup·pres·sant (sŭ-pres′ănt) Pharmaco-therapeutic agent that slows physical or mental activity; often denotes medication used to reduce coughing.

sup·pressed men·stru·a·tion (sŭ-prest′ men-strū-ā′shŭn) Nonappearance of menstrual bleeding from whatever cause.

sup·pres·sion (sŭ-presh′ŭn) **1.** Deliberate exclusion from conscious thought. Cf. repression. **2.** Arrest of the secretion of a fluid. **3.** Checking of an abnormal flow or discharge. SEE ALSO epistasis. **4.** The effect of a second mutation, which overwrites a phenotypic change caused by a previous mutation at a different point on the chromosome. **5.** Inhibition of vision in one eye when dissimilar images fall on corresponding retinal points.

sup·pres·sor cells (sŭ-pres′ŏr selz) Immune system cells that inhibit or help to terminate an immune response.

sup·pres·sor mu·ta·tion (sŭ-pres′ŏr myū-tā′shŭn) **1.** A mutation that alters the anticodon in a transfer RNA so that it is complementary to a termination codon, thus suppressing termination of the amino acid chain. **2.** Genetic changes such that the effect of a mutation in one place can be overcome by a second mutation in another location.

sup·pu·rant (sŭp′yū-rănt) **1.** Causing or inducing suppuration. **2.** An agent with this action.

sup·pu·ra·tion (sŭp′yŭr-ā′shŭn) The formation of pus. SYN pyogenesis, pyosis.

sup·pu·ra·tive ar·thri·tis (sŭp′yŭr-ă-tiv ahr-thrī′tis) Acute inflammation of synovial membranes, with purulent effusion into a joint, due to bacterial infection.

sup·pu·ra·tive hy·a·li·tis (sŭp′yŭr-ă-tiv hī′ă-lī′tis) Purulent vitreous humor due to exudation from adjacent structures, as in panophthalmitis.

supra- Prefix denoting a position above the part indicated by the word to which it is joined; in this sense, the same as super-; opposite of infra-.

su·pra·au·ric·u·lar (sū′pră-aw-rik′yū-lăr) Above the auricle (external part) of the ear.

su·pra·bulge (sū′pră-bŭlj) The portion of the crown of a tooth distal to its greatest circumference, with contours converging toward the occlusal surface of the tooth.

su·pra·cer·e·bel·lar (sū′pră-ser′ĕ-bel′ăr) On or above the surface of the cerebellum.

su·pra·cer·vi·cal hys·ter·ec·to·my (sū′pră-sĕr′vi-kăl his′tĕr-ek′tŏ-mē) Removal of the fundus of the uterus, leaving the cervix.

su·pra·cho·roid (sū′pră-kōr′oyd) On the outer side of the choroid of the eye.

su·pra·cla·vic·u·lar (sū′pră-kla-vik′yū-lăr) Above the clavicle, denoting some cutaneous nerves.

su·pra·con·dy·lar (sū′pră-kon′di-lăr) Above a condyle. SYN supracondyloid.

su·pra·con·dy·lar frac·ture (sū′pră-kon′di-lăr frak′shŭr) Break of the distal end of the humerus or femur located above the condylar region.

su·pra·cos·tal (sū′pră-kos′tăl) Above the ribs.

su·pra·cot·y·loid (sū′pră-kot′i-loyd) Above the cotyloid cavity, or acetabulum.

su·pra·di·a·phrag·mat·ic (sū′pră-dī′ă-frag-mat′ik) Above the diaphragm.

su·pra·duc·tion (sū′pră-dŭk′shŭn) The upward rotation of one eye.

su·pra·ep·i·con·dy·lar (sū′pră-ep′i-kon′di-lăr) Above an epicondyle.

su·pra·gin·gi·val cal·cu·lus (sū′pră-jin′ji-văl kal′kyū-lŭs) Calcified plaques adherent to tooth surfaces coronal to the free gingival margin.

su·pra·gle·noid (sū′pră-glē′noyd) Above the glenoid cavity or fossa.

su·pra·glot·ti·tis (sū′pră-glot-ī′tis) Infectious inflammation and swelling of the laryngeal tissue above the glottis, especially of the epiglottis, which becomes red and spherical leading to upper airway obstruction.

su·pra·hy·oid (sū′pră-hī′oyd) Above the hyoid bone, denoting, among other things, a group of muscles.

su·pra·lim·i·nal (sū′pră-lim′i-năl) More than just perceptible; above the threshhold for conscious awareness. Cf. sub-liminal.

su·pra·lum·bar (sū′pră-lŭm′bahr) Above the lumbar region.

su·pra·mal·le·o·lar (sū′pră-mal′ē-ō-lăr) Above a malleolus.

su·pra·mal·le·o·lar or·thot·ic (sū′pră-mal′ē-ō′lăr ōr-thot′ik) A foot orthotic that extends only above the malleoli, thus stabilizing the ankle-foot complex.

su·pra·mar·gin·al (sū′pră-mahr′jin-ăl) Above any margin.

su·pra·mas·toid (sū′pră-mas′toyd) Above the mastoid process of the temporal bone.

su·pra·max·il·lar·y (sū′pră-mak′si-lar-ē) Above the maxilla.

su·pra·men·ta·le (sū′pră-men-tā′lē) CEPH-ALOMETRICS the most posterior midline point, above the chin, on the mandibula between the infradentale and the pogonion.

su·pra·na·sal (sū′pră-nā′zăl) Above the nose.

su·pra·nor·mal ex·ci·ta·bil·i·ty (sū′pră-nōr′măl ek-sī′tă-bil′i-tē) At the end of phase three of the cardiac action potential, the successful stimulation threshold falls below (i.e., less negative than) the level necessary to produce excitation during the rest of the phase of diastole, so that an ordinary subthreshold stimulus becomes effective.

su·pra·nu·cle·ar pa·ral·y·sis (sū′pră-nū′klē-ăr păr-al′i-sis) Disorder due to lesions above the primary motor neurons.

su·pra·oc·clu·sion (sū′pră-ŏ-klū′zhŭn) An occlusal relationship in which a tooth extends beyond the occlusal plane.

su·pra·op·tic (sū′pră-op′tik) Area above the optic chiasm.

su·pra·or·bi·tal (SO) (sū′pră-ōr′bi-tăl) Above the orbit, either on the face or within the cranium; denoting numerous structures. SEE canal, foramen, notch, nerve.

su·pra·or·bit·al mar·gin (sū′pră-ōr′bi-tăl mahr′jin) The superior half of the orbital rim, which constitutes the curved superior border of the orbital opening, formed by the frontal bone.

su·pra·pa·tel·lar (SP) (sū′pră-pă-tel′ăr) Above the patella.

su·pra·pel·vic (sū′pră-pel′vik) Above the pelvis.

su·pra·phar·ma·co·log·ic (sū′pră-fahrm′ă-kŏ-loj′ik) Use of a much larger dose than the normal therapeutic level of a medication.

su·pra·pu·bic (SP) (sū′pră-pyū′bik) Above the pubic bone.

su·pra·pu·bic cath·e·ter (sū′pră-pyū′bik kath′ĕ-tĕr) Urinary drainage device inserted into the bladder through the lower abdominal wall above the symphysis pubis. Indications include urethral trauma, vaginal surgery, or long-term catheterization.

su·pra·pu·bic li·thot·o·my (sū′pră-pyū′bik li-thot′ŏ-mē) Surgery in which the bladder is entered by an abdominal incision immediately above the symphysis pubis. SYN high lithotomy.

su·pra·re·nal (sū′pră-rē′năl) **1.** Above the kidney. SYN surrenal. **2.** Pertaining to the suprarenal glands.

su·pra·re·nal gland (sū′pră-rē′năl gland) [TA] A flattened, roughly triangular body resting on the upper end of each kidney with a medulla that produces epinephrine and norepinephrine and a cortex that produces cortisol and aldosterone. SYN epinephros, paranephros.

su·pra·scap·u·lar (sū′pră-skap′yū-lăr) Above the scapula, denoting especially an artery, vein, and nerve.

su·pra·scler·al (sū′pră-skler′ăl) On the outer side of the sclera, denoting the suprascleral or perisclerotic space between the sclera and the fascia bulbi.

su·pra·sel·lar (sū′pră-sel′ăr) Above or over the sella turcica.

su·pra·spi·nal (sū′pră-spī′năl) Above the vertebral column or any spine.

su·pra·spi·na·tus syn·drome (sū′pră-spi-nā′tŭs mŭs′el) Pain on elevating the arm and tenderness on deep pressure over the supraspinatus tendon. SYN impingement syndrome, painful arc syndrome.

su·pra·spi·nous (sū′pră-spī′nŭs) Above any spine.

su·pra·ster·nal (sū′pră-stĕr′năl) Above the sternum.

su·pra·ten·to·ri·al (sū′pră-ten-tōr′ē-ăl) *Avoid the jargonistic use of this word in the sense of psychiatric or psychosomatic.* Denoting cranial contents located above the tentorium cerebelli; often used to describe functional symptoms.

su·pra·troch·le·ar (sū′pră-trok′lē-ăr) Above a trochlea.

su·pra·vag·i·nal (sū′pră-vaj′i-năl) Above the vagina, or above any sheath.

su·pra·val·var, su·pra·val·vu·lar (sū′pră-val′văr, -val′vyū-lăr) Above the valves, either pulmonary or aortic. SYN supravalvular.

su·pra·ven·tric·u·lar (sū′pră-ven-trik′yū-lăr) Above the ventricles.

su·pra·ven·tric·u·lar rhythm (sū′pră-ven-trik′yū-lăr ridh′ĕm) Heart rhythms that originate from centers above the ventricles.

su·pra·ven·tric·u·lar tach·y·car·di·a (SVT) (sū′pră-ven-trik′yū-lăr tak′i-kahr′dē-ă) Rapid heart rate due to a pacemaker anywhere above the ventricular level.

su·pra·ver·sion (sū′pră-vĕr′zhŭn) **1.** A turning (version) upward. **2.** In dentistry, position of a tooth when it is out of the line of occlusion in an occlusal direction; a deep overbite. **3.** In ophthalmology, binocular conjugate rotation upward.

su·pra·vi·tal stain (sū′pră-vī′tăl stān) Procedure in which living tissue is removed from the body; these cells are placed in a nontoxic dye solution so that their vital processes may be studied.

su·preme in·ter·cos·tal vein (sŭ-prēm′ in′tĕr-kos′tăl vān) The vein draining the first intercostal space into either the vertebral or the brachiocephalic vein.

su·preme na·sal con·cha (sŭ-prēm′ nā′zăl kong′kă) [TA] Small concha frequently present on the posterosuperior part of the lateral nasal wall; it overlies the supreme

nasal meatus. SYN concha santorini, Santorini concha.

su·ra (sūr′ă) SYN calf (1).

sur·face (sŭr′făs) [TA] The outer part of any solid. SEE superficial. SYN facies (2) [TA], face (2).

sur·face a·nat·o·my (sŭr′făs ă-nat′ŏ-mē) The study of the configuration of the surface of the body.

sur·face bi·op·sy (sŭr′făs bī′op-sē) One obtained by detaching cells from a cutaneous or mucosal surface with a spatula, cotton swab, or brush; used to diagnose cervical cancer.

sur·face ten·sion (sŭr′făs ten′shŭn) Expression of intermolecular attraction at a liquid's surface, in contact with air or another gas, a solid, or another immiscible liquid, tending to pull the liquid's molecules inward from the surface.

sur·face ther·mom·e·ter (sŭr′făs thĕr-mom′ĕ-tĕr) One in the form of a disc or strip that indicates the temperature of the portion of the skin to which it is applied.

sur·fac·tant (sŭr-fak′tănt) A surface-active agent, including substances commonly referred to as wetting agents, surface tension depressants, detergents, dispersing agents, and emulsifiers.

sur·geon (sŭr′jŏn) A physician who treats disease, injury, and deformity by operation or manipulation.

sur·geon gen·er·al (sŭr′jŏn jen′ĕr-ăl) The chief medical officer in the U.S. Army, Navy, Air Force, or Public Health Service.

sur·geon's knot (sŭr′jŏnz not) The first loop of the knot has two throws rather than a single throw. The second loop has only one throw and is placed in a square-knot fashion, leaving the free ends in the same plane as the first loop.

sur·ger·y (sŭr′jĕr-ē) **1.** The branch of medicine concerned with the treatment of disease, injury, and deformity by operation or manipulation. **2.** The performance or procedures of a surgical operation.

sur·gi·cal (sŭr′ji-kăl) Relating to surgery.

sur·gi·cal ab·do·men (sŭr′ji-kăl ab′dŏ-mĕn) SYN acute abdomen.

S

sur·gi·cal a·nat·o·my (sŭr′ji-kăl ă-nat′ŏ-mē) Applied anatomy in reference to surgical diagnosis and treatment.

sur·gi·cal an·es·the·si·a (sŭr′ji-kăl an′es-thē′zē-ă) **1.** Any anesthesia administered for the performance of an operative procedure. **2.** Loss of sensation with muscle relaxation adequate for an operative procedure.

sur·gi·cal em·phy·se·ma (sŭr′ji-kăl em′fi-sē′mă) Subcutaneous emphysema from gas trapped in the tissues by an operation or injury, frequently seen after carbon dioxide insufflation during laproscopic procedures.

sur·gi·cal in·ten·sive care u·nit (SICU) (sŭr′ji-kăl in-ten′siv kār yū′nit) Hospital unit designated for care of critically ill surgical patients.

sur·gi·cal men·o·pause (sŭr′ji-kăl men′ŏ-pawz) Clinical removal of the ovaries that brings on abrupt changes in hormone levels, which causes an immediate onset of menopause.

sur·gi·cal mi·cro·scope (sŭr′ji-kăl mī′krŏ-skōp) A binocular microscope used to obtain good visualization of fine structures in the operating field; in the standing type of microscope, a motorized zoom lens system operated by hand or foot controls provides an adjustable working distance; in headborne models, interchangeable oculars provide the magnification needed. SYN operating microscope.

sur·gi·cal path·ol·o·gy (sŭr′ji-kăl pă-thol′ŏ-jē) A field in anatomic pathology concerned with examination of tissues removed from living patients for the purpose of diagnosis of disease and guidance in the care of patients.

sur·ro·gate (sŭr′ŏ-găt) **1.** A person who functions in another's life as a substitute for some third person. **2.** A person who so reminds one of another person that one uses the first as an emotional substitute for the second.

sur·sum·ver·sion (sŭr′sŭm-vĕr′zhŭn) Rotating the eyes upward.

sur·veil·lance (sŭr-vā′lăns) **1.** The collection, collation, analysis, and dissemination of data. **2.** Ongoing scrutiny, generally using methods distinguished by practicability, uniformity, and rapidity, rather than complete accuracy.

sus·cep·ti·bil·i·ty (sŭ-sep′ti-bil′i-tē) **1.** Likelihood of an individual to develop ill effects from an external agent, such as *Mycobacterium tuberculosis*, high altitude, or ambient temperature. **2.** Likelihood that a given pathogenic microorganism will be inhibited or killed by a given microbial agent. SYN sensitivity (4).

sus·pend·ed an·i·ma·tion (sŭs-pend′ĕd an′i-mā′shŭn) Temporary state resembling death, with cessation of respiration.

sus·pen·sion (sŭs-pen′shŭn) **1.** Temporary interruption of any function. **2.** A hanging from a support. **3.** Fixation of an organ to other tissue for support. **4.** The dispersion through a liquid of a solid in finely divided particles of a size large enough to be detected by purely optic means. **5.** A class of pharmacopeial preparations of finely divided, undissolved drugs dispersed in liquid vehicles for oral or parenteral use.

sus·pen·soid, sus·pen·sion col·loid (sŭs-pen′soyd, sŭ-spen′shŭn kol′oyd) A colloidal solution in which the dispersed particles are solid and lyophobe or hydrophobe, and are therefore sharply demarcated from the fluid in which they are suspended.

sus·pen·so·ry (sŭs-pen′sŏr-ē) **1.** Supporting. **2.** A supporter applied to uplift a dependent part.

sus·ten·tac·u·lum, pl. **sus·ten·tac·u·la** (sŭs′ten-tak′yū-lŭm, -lă) A structure that serves as a stay or support to another.

Sut·ton·el·la in·dol·o·ge·nes (sŭt′ŏn-el′ă in-dō-loj′ĕ-nēz) A species that causes eye infections or endocarditis (when heart valves are present) in humans. SYN *Kingella indologenes.*

su·ture (sū′chŭr) [TA] **1.** A form of fibrous joint in which two bones formed in membrane are united by a fibrous membrane continuous with the periosteum. **2.** To unite two surfaces by sewing. SYN stitch (3). **3.** The material with which two surfaces are kept in apposition. **4.** The seam so formed.

su·tur·ing (sū′chŭr-ing) Surgically uniting two bodily surfaces by sewing them together.

Su·zanne gland (sū-zahn′ gland) Small mucous gland in the floor of the mouth.

Sved·berg u·nit (S) (sfed′berg yū′nit) A sedimentation constant of 1×10^{-13} seconds.

swab (swahb) A wad of cotton, gauze, or other absorbent material attached to the end of a stick or clamp, used to apply or remove a substance from a surface.

swad·dling (swah′dĕl-ing) Wrapping an infant snugly with arms covered in a blanket or cloth.

swage (swāj) **1.** To fuse suture thread to suture needles. **2.** To shape metal by hammering or adapting it onto a die, often by using a counterdie.

swal·low·ing re·flex (swahl′ŏ-ing rē′fleks) Swallowing (second stage) induced by stimulation of the palate, fauces, or posterior pharyngeal wall. SYN pharyngeal reflex (1).

swal·low·ing thresh·old (swah′lŏ-ing thresh′old) Start of swallow after food is chewed.

Swan-Ganz cath·e·ter (swahn ganz kath′ĕ-tĕr) Thin, flexible, flow-directed venous catheter using a balloon to carry it through the heart to a pulmonary artery.

swan-neck de·for·mi·ty (swahn′nek dĕ-fōr′mi-tē) Finger malformation with hyperextension of the proximal interphalangeal joint and flexion of the distal interphalangeal joint.

sweat (swet) **1.** Perspiration (3), especially sensible perspiration. **2.** To perspire.

sweat glands (swet glandz) [TA] The coiled glands of the skin that secrete the sweat.

sweat·ing (swet′ing) SYN perspiration (1).

sweat pore (swet pōr) The surface opening of the duct of a sweat gland. SYN pore (2).

sweat test (swet test) Test for pancreatic cystic fibrosis in which electrolytes are measured in collected sweat.

Swed·ish mas·sage (swē′dish mă-sahzh′) A manipulation technique that includes effleurage, pétrissage, friction, vibration, and tapotement; intended to improve circulation and tissue elasticity while reducing muscle tone and creating a parasympathetic response.

Swed·ish move·ments, Swed·ish gym·nas·tics (swē′dish mŭv′mentz, jim-nas′tiks) Form of kinesitherapy in which certain systematized movements of the body and limbs are regulated by resistance made by an attendant. SYN Swedish gymnastics.

swell·ing (swel′ing) **1.** An enlargement. **2.** EMBRYOLOGY a primordial elevation that develops into a fold or ridge.

swim·ming pool gran·u·lo·ma (swim′ing pūl gran-yū-lō′mă) Chronic, verrucous lesion most common on the knees. SYN fish-tank granuloma.

swine·herd's dis·ease (swīn′hĕrdz di-zēz′) Disorder due to a leptospira in those who take care of pigs or are occupied in the slaughtering or processing of pork.

swing·ing flash·light test (swing′ing flash′līt test) Assessment of retinal acuity done by measuring pupillary response to strong illumination.

Swy·er-James syn·drome (swī′ĕr jāmz sin′drōm) **1.** SYN unilateral lobar emphysema. **2.** Hyperlucency of one lung due to obliterating bronchiolitis, usually caused by adenovirus infection in childhood, with decreased size and vascularity of the lung.

Swy·er syn·drome (swī′ĕr sin′drōm) Gonadal dysgenesis in phenotypic females with XY genotype.

sy·co·ma (sī-kō′mă) **1.** A pendulous, fig-like growth. **2.** A large, soft wart.

sy·co·sis (sī-kō′sis) A pustular folliculitis, particularly of the bearded area.

Sy·den·ham cho·re·a (sid′ĕn-ham kōr-ē′ă) Postinfectious chorea appearing several months after a streptococcal infection with subsequent rheumatic fever; typically involves the distal limbs and associated with hypotonia and emotional lability.

syl·vat·ic (sil-vat′ik) Occurring in or affecting wild animals.

S

syl·vat·ic plague (sil-vat´ik plāg) Bubonic plague in rats and other wild animals.

sym·bal·lo·phone (sim-bahl´ŏ-fōn) Stethoscope with two chest pieces to lateralize sound and produce a stereophonic effect.

sym·bi·on (sim´bē-on) An organism associated with another in symbiosis.

sym·bi·o·sis (sim´bē-ō´sis) **1.** Biologic association of two or more species to their mutual benefit. Cf. commensalism, parasitism. **2.** Mutual cooperation or interdependence of two people.

sym·bi·ot·ic (sim´bē-ot´ik) Relating to symbiosis.

sym·bleph·a·ron (sim-blef´ă-ron) Adhesion of one or both eyelids to the eyeball, partial or complete, due to burns, trauma, or cicatricial pemphigoid. SEE ALSO blepharosynechia.

sym·bol (sim´bŏl) **1.** A conventional sign serving as an abbreviation. **2.** In chemistry, an abbreviation of the name of an element, radical, or compound, expressing in chemical formulas one atom or molecule of that element (e.g., H and O in H_2O). **3.** In psychoanalysis, an object or action interpreted to represent some repressed or unconscious desire.

sym·bo·li·a (sim-bō´lē-ă) The capability of recognizing the form and nature of an object by touch.

sym·bol·ism (sim´bŏl-izm) **1.** PSYCHOANALYSIS process involved in disguised representation in consciousness of unconscious or repressed contents or events. **2.** Mental state in which one regards everything that happens as indicative one's own thoughts. **3.** The description of the emotional life and experiences in abstract terms.

sym·bol·i·za·tion (sim´bŏ-lī-zā´shŭn) An unconscious mental mechanism whereby one object or idea is represented by another.

Syme am·pu·ta·tion, Syme op·er·a·tion (sīm amp´yū-tā´shŭn, op-ĕr-ā´shŭn) Surgical removal of the foot at the ankle joint; the malleoli are cut off and a flap is made with the soft parts of the heel.

sym·met·ric, sym·met·ric·al (si-met´rik, -i-kăl) Equal on either side of a central dividing line.

sym·met·ric gan·grene (si-met´rik gang-grēn´) Condition affecting the extremities of both sides of the body.

sym·me·try (sim´ĕ-trē) Equality or correspondence in form of parts distributed around a center or an axis, at the extremities or poles, or on the opposite sides of any body.

sympath-, sympatheto-, sympathico-, sympatho- Combining forms denoting the sympathetic part of the autonomic nervous system. SEE ALSO sympathetic.

sym·pa·thec·to·my, sym·pa·the·tec·to·my, sym·pa·thi·cec·to·my (sim´pă-thek´tŏ-mē, sim´pă-thĕ-tek´tŏ-mē, sim-path´i-sek´tŏ-mē) Excision of a segment of a sympathetic nerve or of one or more sympathetic ganglia.

sym·pa·thet·ic (sim´pă-thet´ik) **1.** Relating to or exhibiting sympathy. **2.** Denoting the sympathetic part of the autonomic nervous system.

sym·pa·thet·ic gan·gli·a (sim´pă-thet´ik gang´glē-ă) Those ganglia of the autonomic nervous system that receive efferent fibers originating from preganglionic visceral motor neurons in the intermediolateral cell column of thoracic and upper lumbar spinal segments (T1–L2).

sym·pa·thet·ic nerve (sim´pă-thet´ik nĕrv) One of the nerves of the sympathetic nervous system.

sym·pa·thet·ic ner·vous sys·tem (SNS) (sim´pă-thet´ik nĕr´vŭs sis´tĕm) **1.** In earlier usage, the entire autonomic nervous system. **2.** The branch of the autonomic nervous system that supplies motor control to glands, smooth muscle, and cardiac tissue, specifically in response to perceived threat, danger, or to stress. SEE ALSO autonomic division of nervous system. Cf. parasympathetic nervous system.

sym·pa·thet·ic oph·thal·mi·a (SO) (sim´pă-thet´ik of-thal´mē-ă) Serous or plastic uveitis caused by a perforating wound of the uvea followed by a similar severe reaction in the other eye that may lead to bilateral blindness. SYN transferred ophthalmia.

sym·pa·thet·ic re·sponse (sim´pă-thet´ik rē-spons´) The action in glandular smooth muscle, and cardiac tissue during perceived threat or stress. Cf. parasympathetic response.

sym·pa·thet·ic u·ve·i·tis (sim′pă-thet′ik yū′vē-ī′tis) A bilateral inflammation of the uveal tract caused by a perforating wound of one eye that injures the uvea, exposing it to the immune system.

sym·path·i·co·to·ni·a (sim-path′i-kŏtŏ′nē-ă) A condition with increased tonus of the sympathetic system and a marked tendency to vascular spasm and high blood pressure.

sym·path·i·co·trip·sy (sim-path′i-kŏtrip-sē) Operation of crushing a sympathetic ganglion.

sym·pa·thiz·ing eye (sim′pă-thīz-ing ī) Uninjured eye in sympathetic ophthalmia that becomes involved later in the disease process.

sym·pa·tho·ad·re·nal (sim′pă-thō-ă-drē′năl) Relating to the sympathetic part of the autonomic nervous system and the medulla of the suprarenal gland.

sym·pa·tho·blast (sim′pă-thō-blast) A primordial cell derived from the neural crest glia. SYN sympathetoblast, sympathicoblast.

sym·pa·tho·lyt·ic (sim′pă-thō-lit′ik) Denoting antagonism to or inhibition of adrenergic nerve activity. SEE ALSO adrenergic blocking agent, antiadrenergic.

sym·pa·tho·mi·met·ic (sim′pă-thō-mimet′ik) Denoting mimicking of action of the sympathetic system. SEE ALSO adrenomimetic. SYN sympathicomimetic.

sym·pa·thy (sim′pă-thē) 1. The mutual relation, physiologic or pathologic, between two organs, systems, or parts of the body. 2. Mental contagion. 3. An expressed sensitive appreciation or emotional concern for and sharing of the mental and emotional state of another person. Cf. empathy (1).

sym·phys·i·al, sym·phys·e·al (simfiz′ē-ăl) Grown together; relating to a symphysis; fused.

sym·phys·i·ot·o·my, sym·phys·e·ot·o·my (sim-fiz′ē-ot′ŏ-mē) Division of the pubic joint to increase the capacity of a contracted pelvis sufficiently to permit passage of a living child. SYN pelviotomy (1), pelvitomy, synchondrotomy.

sym·phy·sis (sim′fi-sis, -sēz) 1. [TA] Cartilaginous joint in which union between two bones is effected with fibrocartilage. 2. A union of any two structures. 3. A pathologic adhesion or growing together.

sym·po·di·a (sim-pō′dē-ă) Condition characterized by union of the feet.

sym·port (sim′pōrt) Coupled transport of two different molecules or ions through a membrane in the same direction by a common carrier mechanism (symporter). Cf. antiport.

symp·tom (simp′tŏm) Any morbid phenomenon or departure from the normal in structure, function, or sensation, experienced by the patient and indicative of disease. SEE ALSO phenomenon (1), sign (1), syndrome.

symp·to·mat·ic (simp′tŏ-mat′ik) Indicative; relating to or constituting the aggregate of symptoms of a disease.

symp·to·mat·ic neu·ral·gi·a (simp′tŏmat′ik nūr-al′jē-ă) Condition occurring as a symptom of some local or systemic disease not involving primarily nerve structures.

symp·to·mat·ic treat·ment (ST) (simp′tŏ-mat′ik trēt′mĕnt) Therapy aimed at relieving symptoms without necessarily affecting the basic underlying cause(s) of the symptoms.

symp·tom·a·tol·o·gy (simp′tŏ-mă-tol′ŏ-jē) *Avoid the jargonistic substitution of this word for medical history or symptoms.* 1. The science of the symptoms of disease, their production, and the indications they furnish. 2. The aggregate of symptoms of a disease.

symp·to·mat·o·lyt·ic, symp·to·mo·lyt·ic (simp′tŏ-mat′ŏ-lit′ik, -mŏ-lit′ik) Removing symptoms.

syn- Combining form meaning together, with, joined; appears as sym- before b, p, ph, or m; corresponds to L. *con-*.

synaesthesia [Br.] SYN synesthesia.

synaesthesialgia [Br.] SYN synesthesialgia.

syn·apse (sin′aps) The functional mem-

S

brane-to-membrane contact of the nerve cell with another nerve cell, an effector (muscle, gland) cell, or a sensory receptor cell. SYN synapsis.

sy·nap·sis (si-nap′sis) [TA] The point-for-point pairing of homologous chromosomes during the prophase of meiosis. SYN synaptic phase.

sy·nap·tic (si-nap′tik) **1.** Relating to a synapse. **2.** Relating to synapsis.

sy·nap·tic cleft (si-nap′tik kleft) The space about 20 nm wide between the axolemma and the postsynaptic surface. SEE ALSO synapse.

sy·nap·tic trough (si-nap′tik trawf) Depression of the surface of the striated muscle fiber that accommodates the motor endplate.

syn·ap·to·ne·mal com·plex (si-nap′tŏ-nē′măl kom′pleks) Submicroscopic structure interposed between the homologous chromosome pairs during synapsis. SYN synaptinemal complex.

syn·ap·to·some (si-nap′tŏ-sōm) Membrane-bound sac containing synaptic vesicles that breaks away from axon terminals when brain tissue is homogenized under controlled conditions.

syn·ar·thro·phy·sis (sin′ahr-thrō-fī′sis) The process of ankylosis.

syn·ar·thro·sis, pl. **syn·ar·thro·ses** (sin′ahr-thrō′sis, -sēz) [TA] Immovable or nearly immovable union of rigid components of the skeletal system. SEE articulation.

syn·can·thus (sin-kan′thŭs) Adhesion of the eyeball to orbital structures.

syn·chei·li·a, syn·chi·li·a (sin-kī′lē-ă) A more or less complete adhesion of the lips; atresia of the mouth.

syn·chei·ri·a, syn·chi·ri·a (sin-kī′rē-ă) A form of dyscheiria in which a stimulus applied to one side of the body is referred by the patient to both sides.

syn·chon·dro·se·ot·o·my (sin′kon-drŏ′sē-ot′ŏ-mē) Operation of cutting through a synchondrosis; used to treat bladder exstrophy.

syn·chon·dro·sis, pl. **syn·chon·dro·ses** (sin′kon-drŏ′sis, -sēz) [TA] A union between two bones formed either by hyaline cartilage or fibrocartilage. SYN synchondrodial joint.

syn·cho·ri·al (sin-kōr′ē-ăl) Relating to fused chorions as are found in multiple-fetus pregnancies.

syn·chro·nism (sing′krŏ-nizm) Occurrence of two or more events at the same time; the condition of being simultaneous. SYN synchronia (1).

syn·chro·nized in·ter·mit·tent man·da·to·ry ven·ti·la·tion (sing′krŏ-nīzd in′tĕr-mit′ĕnt mand′ă-tōr-ē ven′ti-lā′shŭn) Respiration in which mandatory breaths can be triggered by the patient's inspiratory effort. SEE ALSO intermittent mandatory ventilation.

syn·chro·nous (sing′krŏ-nŭs) Occurring simultaneously. SYN homochronous (1).

syn·chro·ny (sing′krŏ-nē) The simultaneous appearance of two separate events.

syn·chy·sis (sing′ki-sis) Collapse of vitreous humor collagenous framework with vitreous body liquefaction.

syn·chy·sis scin·til·lans (sing′ki-sis sin′til-lanz) An appearance of glistening spots in the eye.

syn·cli·tism (sin′kli-tizm) Condition of parallelism between the planes of the fetal head and of the pelvis, respectively.

syn·clo·nus (sin′klō-nŭs) Clonic spasm or tremor of several muscles.

syn·co·pe (sing′kŏ-pē) Loss of consciousness and postural tone caused by diminished cerebral blood flow.

syn·cy·tial (sin-sish′ăl) Relating to a syncytium.

syn·cy·tial knot (sin-sish′ăl not) A localized swelling or aggregation of syncytiotrophoblastic nuclei in the villi of the placenta during early pregnancy. SYN nuclear aggregation.

syn·cy·ti·o·tro·pho·blast (sin-sish′ē-ō-trō′fō-blast) The syncytial outer layer of the trophoblast; site of synthesis of human chorionic gonadotropin. SEE ALSO trophoblast.

syn·cy·ti·um, pl. **syn·cy·ti·a** (sin-sish´ ē-ŭm, -ă) A multinucleated protoplasmic mass formed by the secondary union of originally separate cells.

syn·dac·ty·ly, syn·dac·ty·li·a, syn· dac·tyl·ism (sin-dak´ti-lē, sin-dak-til´ ē-ă, sin-dak´ti-lizm) Any degree of webbing or fusion of fingers or toes, involving soft parts only or including bone structure. SYN symphalangy.

syn·des·mec·to·my (sin´dez-mek´tŏ-mē) Cutting away a section of a ligament.

syn·des·mec·to·pi·a (sin´dez-mek-tō´ pē-ă) Displacement of a ligament.

syn·des·mi·tis (sin´dez-mī´tis) Inflammation of a ligament.

syndesmo-, syndesm- Combining forms denoting ligament, ligamentous.

syn·des·mog·ra·phy (sin´dez-mog´ră-fē) A treatise on or description of the ligaments.

syn·des·mo·pex·y (sin-dez´mō-pek-sē) The joining of two ligaments, or attachment of a ligament in a new place.

syn·des·mo·sis, pl. **syn·des·mo·ses** (sin´dez-mō´sis, -sēz) [TA] A form of fibrous joint in which opposing surfaces that are relatively far apart are united by ligaments.

syn·des·mot·o·my (sin´dez-mot´ŏ-mē) Surgical division of a ligament.

syn·drome (sin´drōm) The combination of signs and symptoms associated with a particular morbid process, which together constitute the picture of a disease or inherited anomaly. SEE ALSO disease, disorder.

syn·drome of in·ap·pro·pri·ate se· cre·tion of an·ti·di·u·ret·ic hor· mone (SIADH) (sin´drōm in´ă-prō´prē-ăt sĕ-krē´shŭn an´tē-dī-yŭr-et´ik hŏr´mōn) A condition in which antidiuretic hormone is in excess and causes water retention, hyponatremia, and extracellular fluid volume excess.

syn·drom·ic (sin-drō´mik) Relating to a syndrome.

sy·nech·i·a, gen. and pl. **syn·ech·i·ae** (si-nek´ē-ă, -ē) Any adhesion; specifically, adhesion of an inflamed iris to the cornea (anterior synechia) or lens (posterior synechia).

syn·en·ceph·a·lo·cele (sin´en-sef´ă-lō-sēl) Protrusion of brain substance through a defect in the cranium, with adhesions preventing reduction.

sy·ner·e·sis (si-ner´ĕ-sis) **1.** The contraction of a gel by which part of the dispersion medium is squeezed out. **2.** Degeneration of the vitreous humor with loss of gel consistency to become partially or completely fluid.

syn·er·gism (sin´ĕr-jizm) Coordinated or correlated action of two or more structures, agents, or physiologic processes so that the combined action is greater than the sum of each acting separately. Cf. antagonism.

syn·er·gist (sin´ĕr-jist) A structure, agent, or physiologic process that aids the action of another. Cf. antagonist.

syn·er·gis·tic (sin´ĕr-jis´tik) **1.** Pertaining to synergism. **2.** Denoting a synergist. SYN synergic.

syn·er·gis·tic a·gent (sin´ĕr-jis´tik ā´jĕnt) A drug or agent involved in an interaction that produces effects more powerful than the sum of individual effects.

syn·er·gis·tic mus·cles (sin´ĕr-jist´ik mŭs´ĕlz) Muscles having a similar and mutually helpful function or action.

syn·es·the·si·a (sin´es-thē´zē-ă) **1.** A condition in which a stimulus, in addition to exciting the usual and normally located sensation, gives rise to a subjective sensation of different character or localization. **2.** From a neurolinguistic perspective, stimulus-response conditioning.

syn·es·the·si·al·gi·a (sin´es-thē´zē-al´jē-ă) Painful synesthesia. SYN synaesthesialgia.

syn·ga·my (sing´gă-mē) Union of the male and female gametes.

syn·ge·ne·ic (sin´jĕ-nē´ik) Relating to genetically identical individuals. SYN isogeneic, isogenic, isologous, isoplastic.

S

syn•graft (sin'graft) A tissue or organ transplanted from one member of a species to another genetically identical member, as in kidney transplantation between identical twins. SYN isogeneic graft, isograft, isologous graft, isoplastic graft, syngeneic graft.

syn•i•ze•sis (sin'i-zē'sis) **1.** Closure or obliteration of the pupil. **2.** The massing of chromatin at one side of the nucleus that occurs usually at the beginning of synapsis.

syn•ki•ne•sis, syn•ci•ne•sis, syn•ki•ne•sia (sin'ki-nē'sis, -si-nē'sis, -ki-nē'zē-ă) Involuntary movement accompanying a voluntary one.

syn•o•nych•i•a (sin'ō-nik'ē-ă) Fusion of two or more nails of the fingers or toes.

syn•op•sis (si-nop'sis) A summary; a short but comprehensive view.

syn•os•che•os (sin-os'kē-os) Partial or complete adhesion of the penis and scrotum; a malformation in hermaphroditism.

syn•os•to•sis, syn•os•te•o•sis (sin-os'tō'sis, -os-'tē-ō'sis) [TA] Osseous union between the bones forming a joint. SYN bony ankylosis, true ankylosis.

sy•no•ti•a (si-nō'shē-ă) Fusion of the auricular lobules of the external ears.

syn•o•vec•to•my (sin'ō-vek'tŏ-mē) Excision of part or all the synovial joint membrane.

sy•no•vi•al (syn) (si-nō'vē-ăl) **1.** Relating to, containing, or consisting of synovia. **2.** Relating to the membrana synovialis.

syn•o•vi•al cells (si-nō'vē-ăl selz) Fibroblastlike cells that form 1–6 epithelioid layers in the synovial membrane of joints.

syn•o•vi•al chon•dro•ma•to•sis (si-nō'vē-ăl kon-drō'mă-tō'sis) Osteocartilaginous nodules in the synovial membrane of a joint. SYN synovial osteochondromatosis.

syn•o•vi•al crypt (si-nō'vē-ăl kript) A diverticulum of the synovial membrane of a joint.

syn•o•vi•al flu•id, sy•no•vi•a (si-nō'vē-ăl flū'id, si-nō've-ă) [TA] A clear thixotropic fluid, the main function of which is to serve as a lubricant in a joint, tendon sheath, or bursa; helps nourish the avascular articular cartilage.

syn•o•vi•al her•ni•a (si-nō'vē-ăl hĕr'nē-ă) Protrusion of a fold of the stratum synoviale through a rent in the stratum fibrosum of a joint capsule.

syn•o•vi•al joint (si-nō'vē-ăl joynt) [TA] Articulation in which the opposing bony surfaces are covered with a layer of hyaline cartilage or fibrocartilage; a joint cavity contains synovial fluid, lined with synovial membrane and reinforced by a fibrous capsule and ligaments, and some degree of free movement is possible. SYN articulatio [TA], diarthrodial joint, diarthrosis, movable joint.

syn•o•vi•al lig•a•ment (si-nō'vē-ăl lig'ă-mĕnt) One of the large synovial folds in a joint.

syn•o•vi•al mem•brane (si-nō'vē-ăl mem'brān) [TA] Connective tissue membrane that lines the cavity of a synovial joint and produces synovial fluid. SYN membrana synovialis [TA], synovium.

syn•o•vi•al sar•co•ma (SS, SYS) (si-nō'vē-ăl sahr-kō'mă) Rare malignant tumor of synovial origin.

syn•o•vi•al vil•li (si-nō'vē-ăl vil'ī) [TA] Small vascular processes given off from a synovial membrane. SYN haversian gland.

syn•o•vi•o•ma (si-nō'vē-ō'mă) A tumor of synovial origin involving a joint or tendon sheath.

syn•o•vi•tis (sin'ō-vī'tis) Inflammation of a synovial membrane; in general, when unqualified, the same as arthritis.

syn•tac•tic a•pha•si•a (sin-tak'tik ă-fā'zē-ă) Neural disorder in which the words are fairly well pronounced but are spoken in short phrases or poorly constructed sentences without articles, prepositions, or conjunctions.

syn•te•ny (sin'tĕ-nē) The relationship between two genetic loci represented on the same chromosomal pair or on the same chromosome; an anatomic rather than a segregational relationship.

syn·thase (sin′thās) Trivial name used in the Enzyme Commission Report for a lyase reaction going in the reverse direction. SEE ALSO synthetase.

syn·ther·mal (sin-thĕr′măl) Having the same temperature.

syn·the·sis, pl. **syn·the·ses** (sin′thĕ-sis, -sēz) **1.** Process of building up, putting together, or composing. **2.** CHEMISTRY formation of compounds by union of simpler elements. **3.** The stage in the cell cycle in which DNA is synthesized as a preliminary to cell division.

syn·the·sis pe·ri·od (sin′thĕ-sis pēr′ē-ŏd) The period of the cell cycle when there is synthesis of DNA and histone; it occurs between gap$_1$ and gap$_2$.

syn·the·tase (sin′thĕ-tās) An enzyme catalyzing the synthesis of a specific substance.

syn·thet·ic (sin-thet′ik) Relating to or made by synthesis.

syn·thet·ic chem·is·try (sin-thet′ik kem′i-strē) Formation or building up of complex compounds by uniting simpler ones.

syn·tro·phism (sin′trō-fizm) State of mutual dependence of organs or cells of a plant or an animal.

syn·trop·ic (sin-trō′pik) Relating to syntropy.

syn·tro·py (sin′trō-pē) **1.** Tendency sometimes seen in two diseases to coalesce. **2.** Harmonious association with others. **3.** ANATOMY Similar structures inclined in one general direction.

syph·i·lid (sif′i-lid) Any of the several kinds of cutaneous and mucous membrane lesions of secondary and tertiary syphilis, but most commonly denoting the former.

syph·i·lis (sif′i-lis) An acute and chronic infectious disease caused by *Treponema pallidum* and transmitted by direct contact, usually through sexual activity.

syph·i·lit·ic a·or·ti·tis (sif′i-lit′ik ā′ōr-tī′tis) Common manifestation of tertiary syphilis, involving the thoracic aorta, where destruction of elastic tissue in the media results in dilation and aneurysm formation.

syph·i·lit·ic fe·ver (sif′i-lit′ik fē′vĕr) Elevation of temperature often present in the early roseolous stage of secondary syphilis.

syph·i·lit·ic leu·ko·der·ma (sif′i-lit′ik lū′kō-dĕr′mă) A fading of the roseola of secondary syphilis, leaving reticulated depigmented and hyperpigmented areas located chiefly on the sides of the neck. SYN melanoleukoderma colli.

syph·i·lit·ic ro·se·ola (sif′i-lit′ik rō′zē-ō′lă) Usually the first eruption of syphilis 6–12 weeks after the initial lesion.

syr·ing·ad·e·no·ma (sir′ing-ad′ĕ-nō′mă) Benign sweat gland tumor with glandular differentiation.

sy·ringe (sir-inj′) Instrument used to inject or withdraw fluids.

sy·rin·gi·tis (sir′in-jī′tis) Inflammation of the auditory tube.

sy·rin·go·bul·bi·a (si-ring′gō-bŭl′bē-ă) Fluid-filled cavity of the brainstem.

sy·rin·go·cele (si-ring′gō-sēl) **1.** SYN neural canal. **2.** A meningomyelocele in which there is a cavity in the ectopic spinal cord.

sy·rin·go·cyst·ad·e·no·ma (si-ring′gō-sist-ad′ĕ-nō′mă) A cystic benign sweat gland tumor.

sy·rin·go·en·ceph·a·lo·my·e·li·a (si-ring′gō-en-sef′ă-lō-mī-ē′lē-ă) A tubular cavity involving both brain and spinal cord and etiologically unrelated to vascular insufficiency.

sy·rin·go·ma (sir′ing-gō′mă) Benign, often multiple, sometimes eruptive neoplasm of the sweat gland ducts.

sy·rin·go·me·nin·go·cele (si-ring′gō-mĕ-ning′gō-sēl) Spina bifida cystica in which the dorsal sac consists chiefly of membranes, with very little cord substance, enclosing a cavity that communicates with a syringomyelic cavity.

S

sy·rin·go·my·e·li·a (si-ring′gō-mī-ē′lē-ă) The presence in the spinal cord of longitudinal cavities lined by dense, gliogenous tissue, which is not caused by vascular insufficiency. SYN hydrosyringomyelia, syringomyelus.

syr·up (sir′ŭp) **1.** Refined molasses. **2.** Any sweet fluid; a solution of sugar in water in any proportion. **3.** A liquid preparation of medicinal or flavoring substances in a concentrated aqueous solution of a sugar, usually sucrose.

syr·up of ip·e·cac (sir′ŭp ip′ĕ-kak) SEE ipecacuanha.

sys·tem (sis′tĕm) [TA] **1.** A consistent and complex entity composed of interrelated and interdependent parts. **2.** Any complex of structures related anatomically or functionally. **3.** The entire organism seen as a complex organization of parts. SYN systema [TA]. **4.** An organized procedure. **5.** A way of classifying (e.g., the taxonomic system). **6.** SEE health care system.

sys·te·ma (sis-tē′mă) SYN system (3).

sys·te·mat·ic name (sis′tĕ-mat′ik năm) As applied to chemical substances, a systematic name is composed of specially coined or selected words or syllables, each of which has a precisely defined chemical structural meaning, so that the structure may be derived from the name.

sys·tem·ic (sis-tem′ik) Relating to a system.

sys·tem·ic cir·cu·la·tion (sis-tem′ik sĭr′kyū-lā′shŭn) Movement of blood through the arteries, capillaries, and veins of the general system, from the left ventricle to the right atrium.

sys·tem·ic heart (sis-tem′ik hahrt) Left atrium and ventricle.

syst·em·ic in·fec·tion (sis-tem′ik in-fek′shŭn) Bodily response to a pathogen that affects the whole organism.

sys·tem·ic lu·pus er·y·the·ma·to·sus (SLE) (sis-tem′ik lū′pŭs ĕr-ith′ĕ-mă-tō′sŭs) An inflammatory connective tissue disease with variable symptoms including fever, weakness, and significant other findings. SYN disseminated lupus erythematosus.

sys·tem·ic scle·ro·sis (SSc, SS) (sis-tem′ik skler-ō′sis) **1.** Disease characterized by formation of hyalinized and thickened collagenous fibrous tissue, with thickening of the skin and adhesion to underlying tissues, dysphagia due to loss of peristalsis and submucosal fibrosis of the esophagus. SEE ALSO CREST syndrome. **2.** SYN scleroderma.

sys·tem·ic ve·nous hy·per·ten·sion (sis-tem′ik vē′nŭs hī′pĕr-ten′shŭn) Increased venous pressure ultimately leading to the right atrium.

sys·to·le (sis′tō-lē) Contraction of the heart, especially of the ventricles, by which blood is driven through the aorta and pulmonary artery to traverse the systemic and pulmonary circulations, respectively.

sys·tol·ic (sis-tol′ik) Relating to or occurring during cardiac systole.

sys·tol·ic click (SC) (sis-tol′ik klik) Sharp, thin sound heard during cardiac systole.

sys·tol·ic dys·func·tion (sis-tol′ik dis-fŭngk′shŭn) Cardiac problems during the contraction phase.

sys·tol·ic gra·di·ent (sis-tol′ik grā′dē-ĕnt) Difference in pressure during systole between two communicating cardiovascular chambers.

sys·tol·ic mur·mur (sis-tol′ik mŭr′mŭr) A sound audible during ventricular systole.

sys·tol·ic pres·sure (sis-tol′ik presh′ŭr) Intracardiac pressure during or resulting from systolic contraction of a cardiac chamber.

sys·tol·ic thrill (sis-tol′ik thril) Vibration felt over the precordium or over a blood vessel during ventricular systole.

sys·tol·ic time in·ter·vals (sis-tol′ik tīm in′tĕr-vălz) SEE electromechanical systole.

sys·trem·ma (sis-trem′ă) Muscular cramp in the calf of the leg, the contracted muscles forming a hard ball.

syz·y·gy (siz′i-jē) **1.** Association of gregarine protozoans end-to-end or in lateral pairing (without sexual fusion). **2.** Pairing of chromosomes in meiosis.

T

T₃ Symbol for 3,5,3'-triiodothyronine.

T₄ Symbol for thyroxine.

Ta Symbol for tantalum.

ta·bes (tā'bēz) Progressive wasting or emaciation.

ta·bes mes·en·te·ri·ca (tā'bēz mĕz-en-ter'i-kă) Tuberculosis of the mesenteric and retroperitoneal lymph nodes.

ta·bet·ic (tă-bet'ik) Relating to or suffering from tabes, especially tabes dorsalis.

ta·bet·ic cri·sis (tă-bet'ik krī'sis) SYN crisis (2).

ta·bet·ic neu·ro·syph·i·lis (tă-bet'ik nūr'ō-sif'i-lis) Late tertiary syphilis, seen predominantly in men; SYN myelosyphilis, posterior sclerosis, posterior spinal sclerosis, tabes dorsalis.

ta·bet·i·form (tă-bet'i-fōrm) Resembling tabes, especially tabes dorsalis.

tab·la·ture (tab'lă-chŭr) The state of division of the cranial bones into two plates separated by the diploë.

ta·ble (tā'bĕl) **1.** One of the two plates or laminae, separated by the diploë, into which the cranial bones are divided. **2.** Arrangement of data in parallel columns, showing the essential facts in a readily appreciable form. **3.** Any flat-surfaced structure.

tab·let (tab.) (tab'lĕt) Solid dosage form containing medicinal substances with or without suitable diluents. It may vary in shape, size, and weight, and may be classified according to the method of manufacture.

ta·bo·pa·re·sis (tā'bō-păr-ē'sis) A condition in which the symptoms of tabes dorsalis and general paresis are associated.

tache (tahsh) A circumscribed discoloration of the skin or mucous membrane, such as a macule or freckle.

tache blanche (tahsh blah[n]sh) SYN macula albida.

tache noire (tahsh nwahr) Characteristic lesion (the term is French for "black spot,") that can form at the site of an arthropod bite transmitting either *Rickettsia conorii* or *Orientia tsutsugamushi* to a human host.

ta·chet·ic (tă-ket'ik) Marked by bluish or brownish spots.

ta·chis·to·scope (tă-kis'tŏ-skōp) An instrument to determine the shortest time necessary for an object to be perceived.

ta·chog·ra·phy (tă-kog'ră-fē) The recording of speed or rate.

tachy- Combining form meaning rapid.

tach·y·ar·rhyth·mi·a (tak'ē-ă-ridh'mē-ă) *Do not confuse this word with tachyrhythmia.* Disturbance of cardiac rhythm, regular or irregular during physical examination.

tach·y·car·di·a (tak'i-kahr'dē-ă) Rapid heartbeat, usually over 100 beats/minute. SYN tachysystole.

tach·y·car·di·a win·dow (tak'i-kahr' dē-ă win'dō) In paroxysmal irregular heartbeat of the reentry type, the interval of time (the window) between the earliest and latest premature activation that can excite the paroxysm.

tach·y·crot·ic (tak'i-krot'ik) Relating to, causing, or characterized by a rapid pulse.

tach·y·gas·tri·a (tak'i-gas'trē-ă) Increased rate of electrical pacemaker activity in the stomach, defined as more than 4 cycles/minute for at least 1 minute. May be associated with nausea, gastroparesis, irritable bowel syndrome, and functional dyspepsia.

tach·y·phy·lax·is (tak'i-fī-lak'sis) Rapid appearance of progressive decrease in response to a given dose after repetitive administration of a pharmacologically or physiologically active substance.

tack·ler's ex·o·sto·sis (tak'lĕrz eks'os-tō'sis) Projection of the anterolateral humerus due to repeated blunt trauma, as suffered in contact sports, especially U.S. and Canadian football, where the injury occurs during blocking maneuvers.

tac·rine (tak'rēn) An anticholinesterase

agent with nonspecific stimulatory effects on the central nervous system.

tac·tile (tak'til) Relating to touch or to the sense of touch.

tac·tile an·es·the·si·a (tak'til an'es-thē'zē-ă) Loss or impairment of the sense of touch.

tac·tile cor·pus·cle (tak'til kōr'pŭs-ĕl) One of numerous oval bodies found in the papillae of the skin, especially those of the fingers and toes.

tac·tile el·e·va·tions [TA] Small areas in the skin of the palms and soles especially rich in sensory nerve endings.

tac·tile frem·i·tus (tak'til frem'i-tŭs) Vibration palpated with the hand on the chest during vocal fremitus.

tac·tile hal·lu·ci·na·tion (tak'til hă-lū'si-nā'shŭn) False perception of movement or sensation.

tac·tile hy·per·es·the·si·a (tak'til hī'pěr-es-thē'zē-ă) SYN hyperaphia.

tac·tile me·nis·cus (tak'til mě-nis'kŭs) Specialized tactile sensory nerve ending in the epidermis. SYN meniscus tactus, Merkel corpuscle, Merkel tactile cell, Merkel tactile disc.

tac·tile pa·pil·la (tak'til pă-pil'ă) One of the papillae of the dermis containing a tactile cell or corpuscle.

tac·tile sen·sa·tion (tak'til sen-sā'shŭn) Perception of a physical stimulus resulting from touch.

Tae·ni·a (tē'nē-ă) A genus of cestodes infecting carnivores with cysticerci found in tissues of various herbivores, rodents, and other animals of prey.

tae·ni·a, te·ni·a (tē'nē-ă) **1.** Coiled, bandlike anatomic structure. SEE ALSO tenia (1). **2.** Common name for a tapeworm. SYN tenia (2).

Tae·ni·a sa·gi·na·ta (tē'nē-ă saj-i-nā'tă) Beef, hookless, or unarmed tapeworm of humans.

tae·ni·a·sis (tē'nē-ī'ă-sis) Infection with cestodes of the genus *Taenia*.

Tae·ni·a so·li·um (tē'nē-ă sōl'ē-ŭm) The pork, armed, or solitary tapeworm of humans.

tail fold (tāl fōld) Ventral folding of the caudal end of the embryonic disc.

Ta·ka·ya·su ar·te·ri·tis (tah-kah-yah'sū ahr'tĕr-ī'tis) A progressive obliterative arteritis of unknown origin involving fibrosis and luminal narrowing that affects the aorta and its branches; more common in females.

take (tāk) A successful grafting operation or vaccination.

talc (talk) Native hydrous magnesium silicate; used in pharmacy as a filter aid, as a dusting powder, and in cosmetic preparations. SYN French chalk, soapstone, talcum.

tal·co·sis (tal-kō'sis) A pulmonary disorder related to silicosis, occurring in workers exposed to talc mixed with silicates.

tal·i·ped·ic (tal'i-pē'dik) Clubfooted.

tal·i·pes (tal'i-pēz) Any deformity of the foot involving the talus.

talipes cal·ca·ne·us (tal'i-pēz kal-kā'nē-ŭs) A deformity due to weakness or absence of the calf muscles, in which the axis of the calcaneus becomes vertically oriented; commonly seen in poliomyelitis. SYN calcaneus (2).

tal·i·pes e·qui·no·val·gus (tal'i-pēz ē-kwī'nō-vā'rŭs) Talipes equinus and talipes varus combined; the foot is plantiflexed, inverted, and adducted. SYN clubfoot.

talipes e·qui·nus (tal'i-pēz ē-kwīn'ŭs) Permanent extension of the foot so that only the ball rests on the ground. It is commonly combined with talipes varus.

talipes pla·nus (tal'i-pēz plā'nŭs) A condition in which the longitudinal arch is broken down, the entire sole touching the ground. SYN flatfoot, pes planus.

tal·i·pes val·gus (tal'i-pēz val'gŭs) Permanent eversion of the foot, the inner side alone of the sole resting on the ground; it is usually combined with a breaking down of the plantar arch. SYN pes valgus.

tall-man let·ters (tawl'man let'ĕrz) The use of writing in which medications with similar names (e.g., cephalosporins) have different distinguishing letters in capitals to prevent medication errors. Examples: cefaCLOR, cefADROxil, cefALEXin.

talo- Combining form denoting the talus.

ta·lo·cal·ca·ne·al, ta·lo·cal·ca·ne·an (TC) (tā'lō-kal-kā'nē-ăl, -ē-ăn) Relating to the talus and the calcaneus.

ta·lo·cru·ral (tā'lō-krūr'ăl) Relating to the talus and the bones of the leg; denoting the ankle joint.

ta·lo·fib·u·lar (tā'lō-fib'yū-lăr) Relating to the talus and the fibula.

ta·lo·na·vic·u·lar (TN) (tā'lō-nă-vik'yū-lăr) Relating to the talus and the navicular bone. SYN astragaloscaphoid, taloscaphoid.

ta·lus, gen. and pl. **ta·li** (tā'lŭs, -lī) [TA] The bone of the foot that articulates with the tibia and fibula to form the ankle joint. SYN ankle bone, ankle (3), astragalus.

Tamm-Hors·fall mu·co·pro·tein (tam hōrs'fahl myū'kō-prō'tēn) The matrix of urinary casts derived from the secretion of renal tubular cells. SYN Tamm-Horsfall protein.

tam·pon (tam'pon) **1.** A cylinder or ball of cotton wool, gauze, or other loose substance; used as a plug or pack in a canal or cavity to restrain hemorrhage, absorb secretions, or maintain a displaced organ in position. **2.** To insert such a plug or pack.

tam·po·nade, tam·pon·age (tam'pŏnād', -nazh') **1.** Pathologic compression of a joint. **2.** The insertion of a tampon.

tan·dem (tan'dĕm) **1.** A long narrow tube designed to fit inside the endocervical canal and uterine cavity **2.** Heel-to-toe placement; an assessment of balance with the heel of one foot against the toe of the other foot. SYN tandem Romberg.

tan·gen·ti·al·i·ty (tan-jen'shē-al'i-tē)

Disturbance in the associative thought process with quick shift from one topic to others; observed in bipolar disorder and schizophrenia and certain types of organic brain disorders.

tan·gle (tang'gĕl) A small irregular knot.

tan·nate (tan'āt) A salt of tannic acid.

tan·nic ac·id (tan'ik as'id) A tannin that occurs in many plants; used as a styptic and astringent and to treat diarrhea.

tan·nin (tan'in) A complex nonuniform plant constituent; used in tanning, dyeing, photography, and as clarifying agents for beer and wine.

tan·ta·lum (Ta) (tan'tă-lŭm) A heavy metal of the vanadium group; used in surgical prostheses because of its noncorrosive properties.

tan·y·cyte (tan'i-sīt) Ependymal cell found principally in the walls of the third ventricle of the brain.

tap (tap) **1.** To withdraw fluid from a cavity by means of a trocar and cannula, hollow needle, or catheter. **2.** To strike lightly with the finger or a hammerlike instrument in percussion or to elicit a tendon reflex. **3.** A light blow. **4.** An instrument to cut threads in a hole in bone before inserting a screw.

ta·pe·to·ret·i·nal (tă-pē'tō-ret'i-năl) Relating to the retinal pigment epithelium and the sensory retina.

ta·pe·to·ret·in·op·a·thy (tă-pē'tō-ret-in-op'ă-thē) Hereditary degeneration of the sensory retina and pigmentary epithelium; seen in pigmentary retinopathy, choroideremia, and other disorders.

ta·pe·tum, pl. **ta·pe·ta** (tă-pē'tŭm, -tă) [TA] **1.** In general, any membranous layer or covering. **2.** [TA] NEUROANATOMY a thin sheet of fibers in the lateral wall of the temporal and occipital horns of the lateral ventricle.

tape·worm (tāp'wŏrm) An intestinal parasitic worm, adults of which are found in the intestine of vertebrates.

Ta·pi·a syn·drome (tah'pē-ah sin'drōm) Unilateral paralysis of the larynx, the velum palati, and the tongue.

tap•i•o•ca (tap′ē-ō′kă) A starch from the root of spurges of the genus *Manihot*; easily digested, free of irritants. SYN cassava starch.

ta•pote•ment (tă-pōt′man[h]) Massage movements that involve the repetitive, regular, rhythmic striking of tissue with some part of the hand; includes beating, hacking, cupping, and tapping.

Taq pol•y•mer•ase (tak pŏ-lim′ĕr-ās) Temperature-resistant DNA polymerase isolated from *Thermus aquaticus* that can extend primers at high temperatures; used in the polymerase chain reaction.

ta•ran•tu•la (tăr-an′chū-lă) A large, hairy spider, considered highly venomous and often greatly feared; the bite, however, is usually no more harmful than a bee sting, and the creature is relatively inoffensive.

Tar•dieu ec•chy•mo•ses, Tar•dieu pe•te•chi•ae, Tar•dieu spots (tahr-dyu′ ek′ē-mō′sēz, pĕ-tē′kē-ē, spots) Subpleural and subpericardial discoloration, observed in the tissues of people who have been strangled or otherwise asphyxiated.

tar•dive (tahr′div) Late; tardy.

tar•dive dys•ki•ne•si•a (tahr′div dis′ki-nē′zē-ă) A neurologic disorder associated with involuntary repetitive movements of the facial muscles, tongue, limbs, and trunk.

tar•get (tahr′gĕt) **1.** An object fixed as a goal or point of examination. **2.** In the ophthalmometer, the mire. **3.** Anode of an x-ray tube. SEE ALSO x-ray. **4.** In molecular diagnostic assays, the nucleic acid species being studied.

tar•get cell (tahr′gĕt sel) **1.** An erythrocyte in target cell anemia, with a dark center surrounded by a light band that again is encircled by a darker ring, thus resembling a target used in practice with firearms or archery. **2.** A cell lysed by cytotoxic T lymphocytes. SYN codocyte, leptocyte, Mexican hat cell.

tar•get gland (tahr′gĕt gland) Effector that functions when stimulated by the internal secretion of another gland or by some other stimulus.

tar•get symp•tom (tahr′gĕt simp′tŏm)

An indication of disease to which treatment is most strongly focused.

Tar•lov cyst (tahr′lov sist) A perineural lesion found in the proximal radicles of the lower spinal cord.

tar•ry cyst (tahr′ē sist) A lesion filled with tarry old blood.

tar•sal (tahr′săl) Relating to a tarsus in any sense.

tar•sal bones (tahr′săl bōnz) [TA] The seven bones of the instep: talus, calcaneus, navicular, three cuneiform (wedge), and cuboid.

tar•sal tun•nel syn•drome (TTS) (tahr′ săl tŭn′ĕl sin′drōm) Disorder due to entrapment of various foot nerves in the ankle region.

tar•sec•to•my (tahr-sek′tŏ-mē) Excision of the tarsus of the foot or of a segment of the tarsus of an eyelid.

tar•si•tis (tahr-sī′tis) **1.** Inflammation of the tarsus of the foot. **2.** Inflammation of the tarsal border of an eyelid.

tar•sus (tahr′sus) The 7 instep bones.

tar•so•cla•si•a, tar•soc•la•sis (tahr′ să-klā′zē-ă, tahr-sok′lă-sis) Instrumental fracture of the tarsus, for the correction of talipes equinovarus.

tar•so•ma•la•ci•a (tahr′să-mă-lā′shē-ă) Softening of the tarsal cartilages of the eyelids.

tar•so•met•a•tar•sal (TMT) (tahr′să-met′ă-tahr′săl) Relating to the tarsal and metatarsal bones.

tar•sor•rha•phy (tahr-sōr′ă-fē) Suturing together the eyelid margins, partially or completely, to shorten the palpebral fissure or to protect the cornea in keratitis.

tar•tar (tahr′tăr) A white, brown, or yellow-brown deposit at or below the gingival margin of the teeth, chiefly hydroxyapatite in an organic matrix. SYN dental calculus (2).

tar•tar•ic ac•id (tahr-tar′ik as′id) Laxative and refrigerant; also used to manufacture various effervescing powders, tablets, and granules.

tar·trate (tahr′trāt) *Avoid the misspelling/ mispronunciation tartarate.* A salt of tartaric acid.

tas·tant (tās′tănt) Any chemical that stimulates the sensory cells in a taste bud.

taste (tāst) **1.** To perceive through the medium of the gustatory nerves. **2.** The sensation produced by a suitable stimulus applied to the gustatory nerve endings in the tongue.

taste bud (tāst bŭd) A flask-shaped cell nest located in the epithelium of vallate, fungiform, and foliate papillae of the tongue and also in the soft palate, epiglottis, and posterior wall of the pharynx.

taste cells (tāst selz) Darkly staining cells in a taste bud with long, hairlike microvilli that contain closely packed microtubules and extend into the gustatory pore. SYN gustatory cells.

taste hairs (tāst hārz) Hairlike projections of gustatory cells of taste buds.

tau·rine (tawr′īn) **1.** An aminosulfonic acid, synthesized from L-cysteine and used in a number of roles, including in the synthesis of certain bile salts. **2.** Of or pertaining to a bull.

tau·ro·cho·late (TC) (taw′rō-kō′lāt) A salt of taurocholic acid.

tau·ro·don·tism (taw′rō-don′tizm) A developmental anomaly involving molar teeth in which the bifurcation or trifurcation of the roots is very near the apex, resulting in an abnormally large and long pulp chamber with exceedingly short pulp canals.

tau·to·mer·ic (taw′tō-mer′ik) **1.** Relating to the same part. **2.** Relating to or marked by tautomerism.

tau·to·mer·ic fi·bers (taw′tō-mer′ik fī′bĕrz) Nerve fibers of the spinal cord that do not extend beyond the limits of the spinal cord segment in which they originate.

tau·tom·er·ism (taw-tom′ĕr-izm) A phenomenon in which a chemical compound

exists in two forms of different structure (isomers) in equilibrium, the two forms differing, usually, in the position of a hydrogen atom.

tax·is (tak′sis) **1.** Reduction of a hernia or of a dislocation of any part by manipulation. **2.** Systematic classification or orderly arrangement. **3.** Reaction of protoplasm to a stimulus, by virtue of which animals and plants are led to move or act in certain definite ways in relation to their environment.

tax·on, pl. **tax·a** (tak′son, -să) The name given to a particular level or grouping in a systematic classification of living things or organisms (taxonomy).

tax·on·o·my (taks-on′ŏ-mē) The systematic classification of living things or organisms. Kingdoms of living organisms are divided into groups (taxa) to show degrees of similarity or presumed evolutionary relationships, with the higher categories larger, more inclusive, and more broadly defined; the lower categories more restricted, with fewer species, and more closely related. The divisions below kingdom are, in descending order: phylum, class, order, family, genus, species, and subspecies (variety). Infra-, supra-, sub-, and super categories can be used when needed; additional categories, such as tribe, section, level, and group, are also used.

Tay·lor dis·ease (tā′lŏr di-zēz′) Diffuse idiopathic cutaneous atrophy.

Tay-Sachs dis·ease (tā saks di-zēz′) A lysosomal storage disease resulting from hexosaminidase-A deficiency. Infants present with hyperacusis and irritability, hypotonia, and failure to develop motor skills. Blindness with macular cherry-red spots and seizures are evident in the first year.

Tb Symbol for terbium.

T·binder (bīn′dĕr) Two strips of cloth at right angles; used for retaining a dressing, as on the perineum.

T-de·pen·dent an·ti·gen (dĕ-pen′dĕnt an′ti-jen) One that requires T-cell help to generate a humoral immune response by an antigen-specific cell.

Te 1. ELECTRODIAGNOSIS abbreviation denoting tetanic contraction. **2.** Symbol for tellurium.

tea (tē) **1.** The dried leaves of various genera of the family Theaceae, including *Thea* (*T. sinensis*), *Camellia*, and *Gordonia*. **2.** Infusion made by pouring boiling water on tea leaves. **3.** Any infusion or decoction made extemporaneously. SEE ALSO species (2). SYN thea.

teach·ing hos·pi·tal (tēch′ing hos′pi-tăl) A hospital that also functions as a formal center of learning for the training of physicians, nurses, and allied health personnel.

Teale am·pu·ta·tion (tēl amp′yū-tā′shŭn) **1.** Surgical removal of the forearm in its lower half, or of the thigh, with a long posterior rectangular flap and a short anterior one. **2.** Surgical removal of the leg, with a long anterior rectangular flap and a short posterior one.

tear gas, tear·gas (tēr gas, tēr′gas) A common but erroneous term for compounds that irritate the conjunctiva and cause profuse lacrimation. SEE ALSO lacrimator.

tease (tēz) To separate the structural parts of a tissue by means of a needle, to prepare it for microscopic examination.

teat (tēt) **1.** SYN nipple. **2.** SYN breast. **3.** SYN papilla.

teb·u·tate (teb′yū-tāt) USAN-approved contraction for tertiary butylacetate, $(CH_3)_3C–CH_2–CO_2^-$.

tech·ne·ti·um (Tc) (tek-nē′shē-ŭm) An artificial radioactive element, used extensively as a radiographic tracer in imaging studies of internal organs.

tech·ne·ti·um 99m (tek-nē′shē-ŭm) A radioisotope of technetium used to prepare radiopharmaceuticals for scanning the brain, parotid, thyroid, lungs, blood pool, liver, heart, spleen, kidney, lacrimal drainage apparatus, bone, and bone marrow.

tech·ni·cal (tech) (tek′ni-kăl) **1.** Relating to technique. **2.** Pertaining to some particular art, science, or trade. **3.** In connection with a chemical substance, denoting that the substance contains appreciable quantities of impurities.

tech·nique, tech·nic (tek-nēk′, tek′nik) The manner of performance, or the details, of any surgical operation, experiment, or mechanical act.

tech·nol·o·gist, tech·ni·cian (tek-nol′ŏ-jist, -nĭ′shĭn) One trained in and using the techniques of a profession, art, or science.

tec·ton·ic (tek-ton′ik) Relating to variations in structure in the eye, particularly the cornea.

tec·ton·ic ker·at·o·plast·y (tek-ton′ik ker′ă-tō-plas-tē) Corneal transplantation performed to replace lost corneal tissue to provide support.

tec·to·ri·um (tek-tōr′ē-ŭm) An overlying structure.

tec·to·spi·nal (tek′tō-spī′năl) Denoting nerve fibers passing from the mesencephalic tectum to the spinal cord.

tec·tum, pl. **tec·ta** (tek′tŭm, -tă) Any rooflike covering or structure.

TED hose (ted hōz) Elastic stockings that compress the superficial veins in the lower extremities; used in postoperative patients and others immobilized by illness to prevent thrombophlebitis by shunting blood through the deep veins of the calves and thighs. TED is an abbreviation for thromboembolic disease.

teeth·ing (tēdh′ing) Eruption or, colloquially, cutting of the teeth, especially of deciduous teeth; attendant gingival inflammation may cause a temporary painful condition.

teg·men, gen. **teg·mi·nis,** pl. **teg·mi·na** (teg′men, -mi-nis, -mi-nă) [TA] A structure that covers or roofs over a part.

teg·men·tal (teg-men′tăl) Relating to, characteristic of, or placed or oriented toward a tegmentum or tegmen.

teg·men·tal syn·drome (teg-men′tăl sin′drōm) Disorder usually due to a vascular lesion in the tegmentum; marked by contralateral hemiplegia and ipsilateral ocular paresis.

teg·men·tum, pl. **teg·men·ta** (teg-men′

tŭm, -tă) [TA] **1.** A covering structure. **2.** SYN mesencephalic tegmentum.

Teich·mann crys·tals (tīk′mahn kris′tălz) Rhombic crystals of hemin; used in microscopic detection of blood.

tei·chop·si·a (tī-kop′sē-ă) Jagged, shimmering visual sensation resembling the fortifications of a walled medieval town; scotoma of migraine.

tel-, tele-, telo- Combining forms meaning distance, end, other end.

te·la, gen. and pl. **te·lae** (tē′lă, -lē) **1.** Any thin, weblike structure. **2.** A tissue; especially one of delicate formation.

te·la e·las·ti·ca (tē′lă ē-las′ti-kă) SYN elastic tissue.

tel·al·gi·a (tel-al′jē-ă) SYN referred pain.

tel·an·gi·ec·ta·si·a (tel-an′jē-ek-tā′zē-ă) Dilation of the previously existing small or terminal vessels of a part.

tel·an·gi·ec·ta·sis, pl. **tel·an·gi·ec·ta·ses** (tel-an′jē-ek′tă-sis, -sēz) A lesion formed by a dilated capillary or terminal artery, most commonly on the skin. SEE ALSO telangiectasia.

tel·an·gi·ec·tat·ic fi·bro·ma (tel-an′jē-ek-tat′ik fī-brō′mă) A benign tumor of fibrous tissue with numerous small and large, frequently dilated, vascular channels. SYN angiofibroma.

tel·an·gi·ec·tat·ic gli·o·ma, gli·o·ma tel·an·gi·ec·to·des (tel-an′jē-ek-tat′ik glī-ō′mă, tel-an-jē-ek-tō′dēz) One in which the stroma has numerous, conspicuous, frequently dilated small blood vessels and capillaries, as well as large, endothelium-rimmed lakes of blood.

tel·an·gi·o·sis (tel-an′jē-ō′sis) Any disease of the capillaries and terminal arterioles.

tel·e·can·thus (tel′ĕ-kan′thŭs) Increased distance between the medial canthi or angles of the eyelids. SYN canthal hypertelorism.

tel·e·com·mun·i·ca·tions de·vice for the deaf (TDD, TT) (tel′ĕ-kŏ-myū′ni-kā′shŭnz dĕ-vīs′ def) Telephone accessory that transmits and receives text over standard telephone lines. Also referred to as teletypewriter (TTY) and text telephone (TT).

tel·e·di·ag·no·sis (tel′ĕ-dī′ăg-nō′sis) Detection of a disease by evaluation of data transmitted to a receiving station, a process involving patient monitoring instruments and a transfer link to a diagnostic center distant from the patient.

tel·e·med·i·cine (tel′ĕ-med′i-sin) The practice of medicine over a distance where the patient and doctor interact remotely, usually using a computer and a computer-mounted camera.

tel·e·ol·o·gy (tel′ē-ol′ŏ-jē) The philosophic doctrine according to which events, especially in biology, are explained in part by reference to final causes or end goals.

tel·e·o·mi·to·sis (tel′ē-ō-mī-tō′sis) A completed mitosis.

tel·e·op·si·a (tel′ē-op′sē-ă) An error in judging the distance of objects arising from lesions in the parietal temporal region.

tel·e·or·gan·ic (tel′ē-ōr-gan′ik) Manifesting life.

tel·e·path·ol·o·gy (tel′ē-pă-thol′-jē) Transmission of digitized images of pathology specimens over telecommunication lines for study at remote sites.

tel·e·ra·di·og·ra·phy (tel′ĕ-rā′dē-og′ră-fē) Radiography with the x-ray tube positioned 2 meters from the film, thereby securing practical parallelism of the x-rays to minimize geometric distortion. SYN teleroentgenography.

tel·e·ra·di·ol·o·gy (tel′ē-rā′dē-ol′ŏ-jē) The interpretation of digitized diagnostic images transmitted over telephone lines.

tel·e·ther·a·py (tel′ĕ-thār′ă-pē) Radiation therapy administered with the source at a distance from the body.

tel·e·type·writ·er (TTY) (tel′ĕ-tīp′rī-tĕr) SEE telecommunications device for the deaf.

tel·lu·ric (tĕ-lūr′ik) **1.** Relating to or originating in the earth. **2.** Relating to the element tellurium, especially in its 6^+ valence state.

tel·lu·ri·um (Te) (tĕ-lūr'ē-ŭm) A rare semimetallic element, atomic no. 52, atomic wt. 127.60, belonging to the sulfur group.

tel·o·den·dron (tel'ō-den'dron) The terminal arborization of an axon.

tel·o·gen (tel'ō-jen) Resting phase of hair cycle.

tel·o·gen ef·flu·vi·um (tel'ō-jen ĕ-flū'vē-ŭm) SYN postpartum alopecia.

tel·o·lec·i·thal (tel'ō-les'i-thăl) Denoting an oocyte in which a large amount of yolk accumulates at the vegetative pole.

tel·o·me·rase (TS) (tel-ō'mĕ-rās) A reverse transcriptase comprising an RNA template, which acts as a die for the TTAGGG sequence, and a catalytic protein component that is not found in normal, aging somatic cells. Telomerase mediates the repair or preservation of telomere regions (terminal sequences) of chromosomes. **2.** The aging process that takes place in normal somatic cells and the natural limit on the number of times such cells can undergo mitosis involve a sequential shortening of telomeres due to failure of terminal sequences to be replicated during mitosis.

tel·o·mere (tel'ō-mēr) The distal end of a chromosome arm; telomeres undergo dramatic changes during the progression of cancer.

tel·o·phase (tel'ō-fāz) The final stage of mitosis or meiosis, which begins when migration of chromosomes to the poles of the cell has been completed.

tem·per·ate (tem'pĕr-ăt) Moderate; restrained in the indulgence of any appetite or activity.

tem·per·ate bac·te·ri·o·phage (tem'pĕr-ăt bak-tēr'ē-ō-fāj) A bacteria-consuming virus with a genome that incorporates with, and replicates with, that of the host bacterium.

tem·plate (tem'plăt) **1.** A pattern or guide that determines the shape of a substance. **2.** Metaphorically, the specifying nature of a macromolecule, usually a nucleic

acid or polynucleotide, with respect to the primary structure of the nucleic acid or polynucleotide or protein made from it in vivo or in vitro. **3.** In dentistry, a curved or flat plate used as an aid in setting teeth. **4.** A pattern or guide that determines the specificity of antibody globulins.

tem·ple (tem'pĕl) **1.** The area of the temporal fossa on the side of the head above the zygomatic arch. **2.** The part of a spectacle frame passing from the rim backward over the ear.

tem·po·la·bile (tem'pō-lā'bῐl) Undergoing spontaneous change or destruction during the passage of time.

tem·po·ra (tem'pŏ-ră) The temples.

tem·po·ral (tem'pŏr-ăl) **1.** Relating to time; limited in time; temporary. **2.** Relating to the temple.

tem·po·ral ar·ter·i·tis (tem'pŏr-ăl ahr'tĕr-ī'tis) A subacute, granulomatous arteritis involving the external carotid arteries, especially the temporal artery; occurs in elderly people and may be manifested by constitutional symptoms, particularly severe headache, and sometimes sudden unilateral blindness. SYN cranial arteritis, giant cell arteritis, Horton arteritis.

tem·po·ral lobe (tem'pŏr-ăl lōb) [TA] The long and lowest of the major subdivisions of the cortical mantle. SYN lobus temporalis [TA].

tem·po·ral lobe ep·i·lep·sy (tem'pŏr-ăl lōb ep'i-lep'sē) Disorder with seizures originating from the temporal lobe, most commonly the mesial temporal lobe.

tem·po·ral plane (tem'pŏr-ăl plăn) [TA] A slightly depressed area on the side of the cranium, below the inferior temporal line, formed by the temporal and parietal bones, the greater wing of the sphenoid, and a part of the frontal bone.

tem·po·ro·man·dib·u·lar (tem'pŏr-ō-man-dib'yū-lăr) Relating to the temporal bone and the mandible; denoting the joint of the lower jaw. SYN temporomaxillary (2).

tem·por·o·man·di·bu·lar dis·or·der (tem'pŏr-ō-man-dib'yū-lăr dis-ōr'dĕr)

An inclusive term for all functional disturbances of the masticatory system including temporomandibular joint (TMJ) syndrome, myofacial pain–dysfunction syndrome, and temporomandibular pain-dysfunction syndrome.

tem·po·ro·man·dib·u·lar joint (TMJ) (tem′pŏr-ō-man-dib′yū-lăr joynt) [TA] The joint between the temporal bone and the mandible. SYN mandibular joint.

tem·po·ro·man·dib·u·lar joint pain dys·func·tion syn·drome (tem′pŏr-ō-man-dib′yū-lăr joynt pān dis-fŭngk′shŭn sin′drōm) SYN myofascial pain-dysfunction syndrome.

tem·po·ro·max·il·lar·y (tem′pŏ-rō-mak′si-lar-ē) **1.** Relating to the regions of the temporal and maxillary bones. **2.** SYN temporomandibular.

tem·po·ro·oc·cip·i·tal (tem′pŏ-rō-ok-sip′i-tăl) Denotes involvement of the temporal and occipital bones.

tem·po·ro·sphe·noid (tem′pŏ-rō-sfē′noyd) Relating to the temporal and sphenoid bones.

te·nac·u·lum, pl. **te·nac·u·la** (tĕ-nak′yū-lŭm, -lă) A surgical clamp to hold or grasp tissue during dissection.

te·nac·u·lum for·ceps (tĕ-nak′yū-lŭm fōr′seps) One with jaws armed with a sharp, straight hook like a tenaculum.

ten·as·cin (ten-as′in) A protein that is present in the mesenchyme that surrounds epithelia in organs undergoing development in embryos.

ten·di·ni·tis, ten·do·ni·tis (ten′di-nī′tis, ten′dō-nī′tis) Inflammation of a tendon. SYN tenonitis (2), tenontitis, tenositis.

ten·di·no·plas·ty, ten·on·to·plas·ty, ten·o·plas·ty, ten·do·plas·ty (ten′din-ō-plas-tē, ten-on′tō-, ten′ō-, ten′dō-) Reparative surgery involving tendons.

ten·di·no·sis (ten′di-nō′sis) A noninflammatory condition involving a previously injured tendon that heals with weak collagenous fibers, low weight-bearing resistance, and a high risk of future injury. SEE ALSO compartment syndrome.

ten·di·nous (ten′di-nŭs) Relating to, composed of, or resembling a tendon.

ten·di·nous arch (ten′di-nŭs ahrch) [TA] **1.** White, fibrous band attached to bone and/or muscle, arching over and thus protecting neurovascular elements passing beneath it from injurious compression. **2.** Linear thickening of the deep fascia of a muscle that provides attachment for ligaments and/or muscle fibers. SYN arcus tendineus [TA].

ten·di·nous in·ter·sec·tion (ten′di-nŭs in′tĕr-sek-shŭn) A tendinous band or partition running across a muscle. SYN inscriptio tendinea.

ten·di·nous xan·tho·ma (ten′di-nŭs zan-thō′mă) Nodule involving tendons, ligaments, and fascia, forming deep, smooth, sometimes painful nodules beneath normal-appearing freely movable skin of the extremities; associated with abnormal lipid metabolism.

♻ **tendo-** [TA] Combining form meaning a tendon. SEE ALSO teno-.

ten·dol·y·sis (ten-dol′i-sis) Release of a tendon from adhesions. SYN tenolysis.

ten·don (ten′dŏn) [TA] A nondistensible fibrous cord or band of variable length that is the part of the muscle that connects the fleshy (contractile) part of muscle with its bony attachment or other structure. SYN sinew, tendo.

ten·don cells (ten′dŏn selz) Elongated fibroblastic cells arranged in rows between the collagenous tendon fibers.

ten·don graft (TG) (ten′dŏn graft) Tendinous graft, used for transplantation or interposition.

ten·don re·flex (ten′dŏn rē′fleks) A myotatic or deep reflex in which the muscle stretch receptors are stimulated by percussing the tendon of a muscle.

ten·do·vag·i·nal (ten′dō-vaj′i-năl) Relating to a tendon and its sheath.

te·nec·to·my, ten·on·ec·to·my (tĕ-nek′tŏ-mē, ten′ō-nek-) Resection of part of a tendon.

te·nes·mus (tĕ-nez′mŭs) Painful spasm of the anal sphincter with an urgent desire to evacuate the bowel or bladder, involuntary straining, and the passage of fecal matter or urine.

ten Horn sign (ten hōrn sīn) Pain caused by gentle traction on the right spermatic cord, indicative of appendicitis.

te·ni·a, tae·ni·a, gen. and pl. **te·ni·ae** (tē′nē-ă, -ē) **1.** Any anatomic bandlike structure. Cf. *Taenia*. **2.** SYN taenia (2).

te·ni·a·cide, tae·ni·a·cide (tē′nē-ă-sīd) An agent that destroys tapeworms.

te·ni·a·sis, tae·ni·a·sis (tē-nī′ă-sis) Presence of a tapeworm in the intestine.

te·ni·o·la (tē-nē′ō-lă) A slender tenia or bandlike structure.

ten·nis thumb (ten′is thŭm) Tendinitis with calcification in the tendon of the long flexor of the thumb caused by friction and strain as in tennis playing.

♻ **teno-, tenon-, tenont-, tenonto-** Combining forms meaning tendon. SEE ALSO tendo-.

ten·o·de·sis (ten′ŏ-dē′sis) Stabilizing a joint by anchoring the tendons that move the joint.

ten·og·ra·phy (tē-nog′ră′fē) Radiography of a tendon after contrast material has been injected into the tendon sheath.

ten·ol·y·sis, ten·dol·y·sis (ten-ol′i-sis, -dol′ĭ-sis) Release of a tendon from adhesions.

ten·o·ni·tis (ten′ō-nī′tis) **1.** Inflammation of Tenon capsule or the connective tissue within Tenon space. **2.** SYN tendinitis.

ten·on·tog·ra·phy (ten′on-tog′ră-fē) A treatise on or description of the tendons.

ten·on·tol·o·gy (ten′ŏn-tol′ŏ-jē) The branch of science that has to do with the tendons.

ten·on·to·my·o·plas·ty (ten′on-tō-mī′ŏ-plas′tē) A combined tenontoplasty and myoplasty, used in the radical correction of a hernia.

ten·on·to·plas·ty (ten-on′tō-plas′tē) Reparative or plastic surgery of the tendons.

te·noph·o·ny (te-nof′ŏ-nē) A heart murmur assumed to be due to an abnormal condition of the chordae tendineae. SYN tendophony.

ten·o·phyte (ten′ŏ-fīt) Bony or cartilaginous growth in or on a tendon.

ten·o·re·cep·tor (ten′ŏ-rē-sep′tŏr) A receptor in a tendon, activated by increased tension.

ten·nor·rha·phy (tĕ-nōr′ă-fē) Suture of the divided ends of a tendon. SYN tendon suture, tenosuture.

ten·os·to·sis (ten′os-tō′sis) Ossification of a tendon.

ten·o·syn·o·vec·to·my (ten′ō-sin′-ō-vek′tŏ-mē) Excision of a tendon sheath.

ten·o·syn·o·vi·tis, ten·do·syn·o·vi·tis, ten·do·vag·i·nit·is, ten·o·vag·i·ni·tis (ten′ō-sin′-ō-vī′tis, ten′dō-, -vaj-i-nī′tis, ten′ō-vaj-i-nī′tis) Inflammation of a tendon and its enveloping sheath.

te·not·o·my, ten·dot·o·my (te-not′ŏ-mē, ten-dot′ŏ-mē) Surgical division of a tendon for relief of a deformity due to congenital or acquired shortening of a muscle.

ten·si·om·e·ter (ten′sē-om′ĕ-tĕr) A device for measuring tension.

ten·sion (ten′shŭn) **1.** The act of stretching. **2.** State of being stretched or tense. **3.** Partial pressure of a gas. **4.** Mental, emotional, or nervous strain.

ten·sion head·ache, ten·sion-type head·ache (ten′shŭn hed′āk, ten′shŭn-tīp) That associated with nervous tension and anxiety, often related to chronic scalp muscle contraction. SYN muscle contraction headache.

ten·sor, pl. **ten·so·res** (ten′sŏr, -rēz) A muscle that makes a part firm and tense.

tent (tent) **1.** Canopy used in various types of inhalation therapy to control humidity and concentration of oxygen in inspired air. **2.** Cylinder introduced into a canal or sinus to maintain its patency or to dilate it. **3.** To elevate or pick up a segment of skin, fascia, or tissue at a given point, giving it the appearance of a tent.

tent·ing of skin (tent′ing skin) A sign of dehydration; delayed return to normal appearance when the skin on the back of the hand is pinched.

ten·to·ri·um, pl. **ten·to·ri·a** (ten-tōr′ē-ŭm, -ă) [TA] A membranous cover or horizontal partition.

tep·ro·tide (tĕ′prō-tīd) A nonapeptide in which glycine is replaced by tryptophan; an angiotensin-converting enzyme inhibitor. SYN bradykinin-potentiating peptide.

tera- (**T**) **1.** Prefix used in the SI and metric system to signify one trillion. **2.** Denoting a teras. SEE ALSO terato-.

ter·as, pl. **ter·a·ta** (ter′as, -ă-tă) Embryo or fetus with deficient, redundant, misplaced, or grossly misshapen parts.

terato- Combining form indicating a teras. SEE ALSO tera- (2).

ter·a·to·blas·to·ma (ter′ă-tō-blas-tō′ mă) A tumor containing embryonic tissue differing from a teratoma in that not all germ layers are present.

ter·a·to·car·ci·no·ma (ter′ă-tō-kahr′si-nō′mă) **1.** A malignant teratoma, occurring most commonly in the testis. **2.** A malignant epithelial tumor arising in a teratoma.

ter·a·to·gen (ter′ă-tō-jen) A drug or other agent that can produce congenital anomalies or birth defects or increase the incidence of an anomaly in the population.

ter·a·to·gen·e·sis (ter′ă-tō-jen′ĕ-sis) The origin or mode of production of congenital anomalies; the disturbed growth processes involved in the production of a malformed neonate.

ter·a·to·gen·ic, ter·a·to·ge·net·ic (ter′ ă-tō-jen′ik, -jĕ-net′ik) **1.** Relating to teratogenesis. **2.** Causing congenital anomalies or birth defects.

ter·a·toid (ter′ă-toyd) Resembling a teras.

ter·a·tol·o·gy (ter′ă-tol′ŏ-jē) The branch of embryologic science concerned with the production, development, anatomy, and classification of malformed embryos or fetuses. SEE ALSO dysmorphology.

ter·a·to·ma (ter′ă-tō′mă) A neoplasm composed of multiple tissues, including tissues not normally found in the organ in which it arises.

ter·a·to·sis (ter′ă-tō′sis) An anomaly producing a teras.

ter·a·to·zo·o·sper·mi·a (ter′ă-tō-zō′ō-spĕrm′ē-ă) Condition characterized by the presence of malformed sperms in semen.

ter·bi·um (Tb) (tĕr′bē-ŭm) A metallic element of the lanthanide or rare earth series, atomic no. 65, atomic wt. 158.92534.

ter·e·bra·tion (ter′ĕ-brā′shŭn) **1.** The act of boring, or of trephining. **2.** A boring, piercing pain.

te·res, gen. **ter·e·tis,** pl. **ter·e·tes** (tĕr′ ēz, -ĕ-tis, -ĕ-tēz) Round and long; denoting certain muscles and ligaments. SEE teres minor (muscle), teres major muscle.

term (T) (tĕrm) **1.** A definite or limited period. **2.** A name or descriptive word or phrase. SEE ALSO term infant.

ter·mi·nal (tĕr′mi-năl) **1.** Relating to the end; final. **2.** Relating to the extremity or end of any body (e.g., the end of a biopolymer). **3.** A termination, extremity, end, or ending.

ter·mi·nal bar (tĕr′mi-năl bahr) Dark spots or bars (depending on the plane of section) in the lateral boundary between the apical ends of columnar epithelial cells.

ter·mi·nal hair (tĕr′mi-năl hār) A mature, pigmented, coarse hair.

ter·mi·nal res·pi·ra·to·ry u·nit (TRU) (tĕr′mi-năl res′pir-ă-tōr-ē yū′nit) All alveoli and alveolar ducts beyond the most proximal respiratory bronchiole; contains about 100 alveolar ducts and 2000 alveoli.

ter·mi·nal sac·cules (tĕr′mi-năl sak′yūlz) Thin-walled dilations (primordial alveoli) that develop at the ends of the respiratory bronchioles and develop a close relationship with the capillaries.

ter·mi·nal sac stage of lung de·vel·

op·ment (tĕr-mǐ′nǎl sak′yū-lǎr pēr′ē-ŏd lŭng dĕ-vel′ŏp-mĕnt) The period when many terminal saccules develop; their epithelium is very thin and capillaries bridge into the epithelial lining of the saccules, permitting adequate gas exchange for survival of the fetus if it is born prematurely.

ter·mi·nal web (TW) (tĕr′mǐ-nǎl web) Network of actin filaments in the apical end of columnar epithelial cells that anchor in the zonula adherens.

ter·mi·na·tion (tĕr′mǐ-nā-shŭn) **1.** Any ending. **2.** Induced end to pregnancy.

ter·mi·na·tion co·don (tĕr′mǐ-nā′shŭn kŏ′don) Trinucleotide sequence (UAA, UGA, or UAG) that specifies the end of translation or transcription. SYN termination sequence, termination signal.

term in·fant (tĕrm in′fǎnt) Baby with gestational age between 37 completed weeks (259 completed days) and 42 completed weeks (294 completed days).

Ter·mi·no·lo·gi·a An·a·to·mi·ca (TA) (tĕr-mǐ-nō-lŏ′jē-ǎ an′-ǎ-tom′i-kǎ) A system of anatomic nomenclature, consisting of about 7,500 terms, devised and approved by the International Federation of Associations of Anatomists (IFAA) and promulgated in August 1997 at São Paulo, Brazil.

ter·mi·nus, pl. **ter·mi·ni** (ter′mi-nŭs, -nī) A boundary or limit.

ter·na·ry (tĕr′nǎr-ē) Denoting or composed of three compounds, elements, molecules, or anything else.

ter·pin (ter′pin) A cyclic terpene alcohol, obtained by the action of nitric acid and dilute sulfuric acid on pine oil.

ter·race (ter′ăs) To suture in several rows, in closing a wound through a considerable thickness of tissue.

Ter·ri·en mar·gi·nal de·gen·er·a·tion (ter-rē-an[h]′ mahr′jin-ăl dĕ-jen′ĕr-ā′ shŭn) A painless, bilateral peripheral corneal thinning disorder, characterized by intact epithelium overlying areas of thinning and by irregular astigmatism.

ter·ri·to·ri·al·i·ty (ter′i-tōr′ē-al′i-tē) The tendency of individuals or groups of people to defend a particular domain or sphere of interest or influence.

Ter·son syn·drome (ter-son[h]′ sin′ drŏm) Vitreous, retinal, and subhyaloid hemorrhages associated with subarachnoid hemorrhage.

ter·tian (tĕr′shǎn) Referring to a fever that recurs at intervals of 48 hours.

ter·ti·ar·y (tĕr′shē-ăr-ē) Of or pertaining to the third of a series or type.

ter·ti·ar·y den·tin (tĕr′shē-ăr-ē den′tin) Morphologically irregular dentin formed in response to an irritant. SYN irregular dentin, irritation dentin.

ter·ti·ar·y health care (tĕr′shē-ăr-ē helth kăr) Specialized therapy in which a patient is referred from a primary or secondary health care provider; sometimes called superspeciality care.

ter·ti·ar·y pre·ven·tion (tĕr′shē-ăr-ē prē-ven′shŭn) Avoidance of sequelae of a disease process.

tes·la (T) (tes′lǎ) SI unit of magnetic flux density expressed as kg sec^{-2} A^{-1}; equal to one weber per square meter.

tes·sel·lat·ed (tes′ĕ-lāt-ĕd) Made up of small squares; checkered.

tes·sel·lat·ed fun·dus (tes′ĕ-lāt-ĕd fŭn′ dŭs) A normal fundus to which a pigmented choroid gives the appearance of dark polygonal areas between the choroidal vessels.

test (test) **1.** To prove; to try a substance; to determine the chemical nature of a substance by means of reagents. **2.** A method of examination. **3.** A statistical procedure used to determine whether a hypothesis ought to be rejected. **4.** A reagent used in undertaking a procedure. **5.** To detect, identify, or conduct a trial. SEE ALSO assay, reaction, reagent, scale, stain.

test·cross (test′kraws) Crossing of an unknown genotype to a recessive homozygote so that the phenotype of the progeny corresponds directly to the chromosomes carried by the parents of unknown genotype. SYN backcross (2).

tes·ti·cle (T) (tes'ti-kĕl) SYN testis.

tes·tic·u·lar (tes-tik'yū-lăr) Relating to the testes.

tes·tic·u·lar fem·i·ni·za·tion syn·drome (tes-tik'yū-lăr fem'i-nī-zā'shŭn sin'drōm) A type of male pseudohermaphroditism characterized by female external genitalia, incompletely developed vagina, female habitus at puberty but with scanty or absent axillary and pubic hair and amenorrhea, and testes present within the abdomen or in the inguinal canals or labia majora. SYN complete androgen insensitivity syndrome, testicular feminization.

tes·tic·u·lar self-ex·am·i·na·tion (tes-tik'yū-lăr self'eg-zam'i-nā'shŭn) Procedure for detecting tumors and other abnormalities in the testes.

tes·tis, pl. **tes·tes** (tes'tis, -tēz) [TA] One of the two male reproductive glands, normally located in the cavity of the scrotum. SYN orchis [TA], testicle.

test meal (test mēl) 1. Toast and tea, or crackers and tea, or gruel or other bland food, given to stimulate gastric secretion before withdrawal of gastric contents for analysis. 2. Administration of food containing a substance thought to be responsible for symptoms, such as an allergic reaction.

tes·tos·te·rone (tes-tos'tĕ-rōn) Most potent naturally occurring androgen, formed in greatest quantities by the interstitial cells of the testes and possibly secreted also by the ovary and adrenal cortex; used to treat hypogonadism, cryptorchism, certain carcinomas, and menorrhagia.

tes·to·tox·i·co·sis (tes'tō-tok-si-kō'sis) A G-protein mutation disease resulting in autonomous testosterone overproduction, with precocious puberty.

test tube (test tūb) A round-bottomed, cylindric vessel, made of plastic or transparent glass, in which laboratory tests involving liquids are performed.

test type (test tīp) Letters of various sizes used to test visual acuity.

tet·a·nig·e·nous (tet'ă-nij'ĕ-nŭs) Causing tetanus or tetaniform spasms.

tet·a·ni·za·tion (tet'ă-nī-zā'shŭn) 1. The act of tetanizing the muscles. 2. A condition of tetaniform spasm.

tet·a·nize (tet'ă-nīz) To stimulate a muscle by a rapid series of stimuli so that the individual muscular responses are fused into a sustained contraction.

tetano-, tetan- Combining forms denoting tetanus, tetany.

tet·a·node (tet'ă-nōd) Denoting the quiet interval between the recurrent tonic spasms in tetanus.

tet·a·noid (tet'ă-noyd) 1. Resembling or of the nature of tetanus. 2. Resembling tetany.

tet·a·nol·y·sin (tet'ă-nol'i-sin) A hemolytic principle, elaborated by *Clostridium tetani*, which seems to have no role in the etiology of tetanus.

tet·a·no·spas·min (tet'ă-nō-spaz'min) The neurotoxin of *Clostridium tetani*, which causes the characteristic signs and symptoms of tetanus.

tet·a·nus, lock·jaw (tet'ă-nŭs, lok'jaw) 1. A disease marked by painful tonic muscular contractions, caused by the neurotropic toxin (tetanospasmin) of *Clostridium tetani* acting on the central nervous system. 2. A sustained muscular contraction caused by a series of nerve stimuli repeated so rapidly that the individual muscular responses are fused, producing a sustained tetanic contraction.

tet·a·nus an·ti·tox·in (TAT) (tet'ă-nŭs an'tē-tok'sin) One specific for the toxin of *Clostridium tetani*.

tet·a·nus im·mune glob·u·lin (tet'ă-nŭs i-myūn' glob'yū-lin) Sterile solution of globulins derived from the blood plasma of adult human donors who have been immunized with tetanus toxoid. SYN tetanus immunoglobulin.

tet·a·nus tox·in (tet'ă-nŭs tok'sin) The neurotropic, heat-labile exotoxin of *Clostridium tetani* and the cause of tetanus; it is one of the most poisonous substances known, and seems to function by blocking inhibitory synaptic impulses.

tet·a·ny (tet'ă-nē) A clinical neurologic syndrome characterized by muscle twitches, cramps, and carpopedal spasm, and when severe, laryngospasm and seizures; causes include hyperventilation, hypoparathyroidism, rickets, and uremia. SYN intermittent cramp (1), intermittent tetanus.

tetra- Combining form meaning four.

tet·ra·ba·sic (tet′ră-bā′sik) Denoting an acid having four acid groups and thereby being able to neutralize 4 Eq of a base.

tet·rad (tet′rad) **1.** A group of four things having something in common. SYN tetralogy. **2.** CHEMISTRY a quadrivalent element. **3.** GENETICS a bivalent chromosome that divides into four during meiosis.

tet·ra·hy·dro·fo·lic ac·id (THFA) (tet′ră-hī-drŏ-fō′lik as′id) The active form of folic acid, which can donate four formyl groups during DNA synthesis.

tet·ral·o·gy of Fal·lot (te-tral′ŏ-jē fahl-ō′) A set of congenital cardiac defects including ventricular septal defect, pulmonic valve stenosis or infundibular stenosis, and dextroposition of the aorta so that it overrides the ventricular septum and receives venous as well as arterial blood. SYN Fallot tetrad.

tet·ra·mer (tet′ră-mĕr) A protein or a polymer with four subunits.

tet·ra·mer·ic, te·tram·er·ous (tet′ră-mer′ik, tĕ-tram′ĕr-ŭs) Having four parts, or parts arranged in groups of four, or capable of existing in four forms.

tet·ra·pa·re·sis (tet′ră-pă-rē′sis) Weakness of all four extremities. SYN quadriparesis.

tet·ra·pep·tide (tet′ră-pep′tīd) A compound of four amino acids in peptide linkage.

tet·ra·pyr·role (tet′ră-pir′ōl) A molecule containing four pyrrole nuclei; e.g., porphyrin.

tet·ra·so·mic (tet′ră-sō′mik) Relating to a cell nucleus in which one chromosome is represented four times, whereas all others are present in the normal number.

tet·ro·do·tox·in (TTX, TD) (tet′rō-dō-tok′sin) A potent neurotoxin found in the liver and ovaries of pufferfish and some newts; produces axonal blocks of the preganglionic cholinergic fibers and the somatic motor nerves.

tex·ti·form (teks′ti-fōrm) Weblike.

text tel·e·phone (TT) (tekst tel′ĕ-fōn) A device that conveys words telephonically by means of text; used by the hearing impaired.

tha·lam·ic (thă-lam′ik) Relating to the thalamus.

tha·lam·ic syn·drome (thă-lam′ik sin′drōm) Disorder produced by infarction of the posteroinferior thalamus causing transient hemiparesis, severe loss of superficial and deep sensation with preservation of crude pain in the hypalgic limbs that frequently have vasomotor or trophic disturbances. SYN Dejerine-Roussy syndrome.

thal·a·mo·cor·ti·cal (thal′ă-mō-kōr′ti-kăl) Relating to the efferent connections of the thalamus with the cerebral cortex.

thal·a·mo·len·tic·u·lar (thal′ă-mō-len-tik′yū-lăr) Relating to the thalamus, usually the dorsal, and the lenticular nucleus.

thal·a·mot·o·my (thal-ă-mot′ŏ-mē) Destruction of a selected portion of the thalamus by stereotaxy to relieve pain, involuntary movements, and other symptoms.

thal·a·mus, pl. **thal·a·mi** (thal′ă-mŭs, -mī) [TA] The large, ovoid mass of gray matter that forms the larger dorsal subdivision of the diencephalon.

thal·as·se·mi·a, thal·as·sa·ne·mi·a (thal′ă-sē′mē-ă, -ă-să-nē′mē-ă) Inherited disorders of hemoglobin metabolism with impaired synthesis of one or more of the polypeptide chains of globin.

thal·as·se·mi·a ma·jor (thal′ă-sē′mē-ă mā′jŏr) The syndrome of severe anemia due to the homozygous state of one of the thalassemia genes or one of the hemoglobin Lepore genes, with onset, in infancy or childhood, of symptoms. SYN Cooley anemia.

thal·as·se·mi·a mi·nor (thal′ă-sē′mē-ă mī′nŏr) Heterozygous state of a thalassemia gene or a hemoglobin Lepore gene; usually asymptomatic and quite variable hematologically.

tha•lid•o•mide (thă-lid′ŏ-mīd) A hypnotic drug that, if taken in early pregnancy, may cause the birth of infants with phocomelia and other defects; approved for use in the treatment of erythema nodosum leprosum and under investigational use in other clinical areas.

thal•li•um (Tl) (thal′ē-ŭm) A white metallic element used to scan the myocardium.

thal•li•um 201 (^{201}Tl) (thal′ē-ŭm) Radioisotope of thallium used widely for myocardial nuclear imaging.

thal•li•um poi•son•ing (thal′ē-ŭm poy′zŏn-ing) Condition characterized by vomiting, diarrhea, leg pains, and severe sensorimotor polyneuropathy; about 3 weeks after poisoning, temporary extensive loss of hair typically occurs; usually occurs after accidental ingestion of a rodenticide.

thanato- Combining form meaning death.

than•a•to•gno•mon•ic (than′ă-tog′nŏ-mon′ik) Of fatal prognosis.

than•a•toid (than′ă-toyd) **1.** Resembling death. **2.** Deadly.

the•a•ter (thē′ă-tĕr) **1.** A large room for lectures and demonstrations. **2.** Any operating room or suite of such rooms.

the•ca, pl. **the•cae** (thē′kă, -sē) A sheath or capsule.

the•ca fol•lic•u•li (thē′kă fŏ-lik′yū-lī) The wall of a vesicular ovarian follicle. SEE ALSO tunica externa.

the•ci•tis (thē-sī′tis) Inflammation of the sheath of a tendon.

the•co•ma (thē-kō′mă) A neoplasm derived from ovarian mesenchyme, consisting chiefly of spindle-shaped cells that frequently contain small droplets of fat.

The•den meth•od (thē′den meth′ŏd) Treatment of aneurysms or of large sanguineous effusions by compression of the entire limb with a roller bandage.

the•in•ism (thē′i-nizm) Chronic poisoning resulting from immoderate levels of tea-drinking, marked by palpitation, insomnia, nervousness, headache, and dyspepsia.

the•lar•che (thē-lahr′kē) The beginning of development of the breasts in the female.

the•lor•rha•gi•a (thē′lŏ-rā′jē-ă) Bleeding from the nipple.

T-help•er cells (Th) (hel′pĕr selz) A subset of lymphocytes that secrete various cytokines that regulate the immune response. SYN helper cells.

the•mat•ic ap•per•cep•tion test (TAT) (thē′-mat′ik ap′ĕr-sep′shŭn test) A projective psychological test in which the subject is asked to tell a story about standard ambiguous pictures depicting life situations to reveal personal attitudes and feelings.

the•nar (thē′nahr) Applied to any structure in relation to the thenar eminence or its underlying collective components.

the•o•bro•ma oil (thē′-ō-brō′mă oyl) Fat obtained from the wasted seed of *Theobroma cacao*; contains glycerides of stearic, palmitic oleic, arichidic, and linoleic acids; used as a base for suppositories and ointments and in dentistry. SYN cacao butter, cocoa butter, cacao oil.

the•o•bro•mine (thē′ō-brō′mēn) An alkaloid resembling caffeine and theophylline in its action and chemical structure, used widely as a diuretic, myocardial stimulant, dilator of coronary arteries, and smooth muscle relaxant.

the•oph•yl•line (thē-of′i-lin) An alkaloid found with caffeine in tea leaves; shares chemical and pharmacologic properties with caffeine and theobromine.

the•o•rem (thē′ŏ-rĕm) A proposition that can be proved, and so is established as a law or principle. SEE ALSO law, principle, rule.

the•o•ry (thē′ŏr-ē) A reasoned explanation of known facts or phenomena that serves as a basis of investigation. SEE ALSO hypothesis, postulate.

the•o•ther•a•py (thē′ō-thār′ă-pē) Treatment of disease by prayer or religious exercises.

thèque (tek) A nest of epidermal nevocytes.

ther·a·peu·tic (thār´ă-pyū´tik) Relating to therapeutics or to the treatment, remediating, or curing of a disorder or disease.

ther·a·peu·tic a·bor·tion (thār´ă-pyū´tik ă-bōr´shŭn) Abortion induced because of the mother's physical or mental health, or to prevent birth of a deformed child or a child conceived as the result of rape or incest.

ther·a·peu·tic com·mu·ni·ty (TC) (thār-ă-pyū´tik kŏ-myū´ni-tē) Specially structured mental hospital or community health center that provides an effective environment for behavioral changes in patients through resocialization and rehabilitation.

ther·a·peu·tic cri·sis (thār´ă-pyū´tik krī´sis) A turning point leading to positive or negative change in psychiatric treatment.

ther·a·peu·tic gain (thār´ă-pyū´tik gān) Positive response to targeted treatment; benefit.

ther·a·peu·tic in·dex (thār´ă-pyū´tik in´deks) The ratio of LD_{50} to ED_{50}, used in quantitative comparisons of drugs. SYN therapeutic ratio.

ther·a·peu·tics (thār´ă-pyū´tiks) The practical branch of medicine concerned with the treatment of disease or disorder.

ther·a·pist (thār´ă-pist) One professionally trained in the practice of a particular type of therapy.

ther·a·py (thār´ă-pē) **1.** Systematic treatment of a disease, dysfunction, or disorder. SEE ALSO therapeutic. **2.** PSYCHIATRY, CLINICAL PSYCHOLOGY psychotherapy. SEE ALSO psychotherapy, psychiatry, psychology, psychoanalysis.

ther·mal, ther·mic (therm) (thĕr´măl, -mik) Pertaining to heat.

ther·mal ar·ti·fact (thĕr´măl ahr´ti-fakt) Distortion of microscopic structure in a tissue specimen, because of heat generated by the instrument used to obtain the specimen.

ther·mal burn (thĕr´măl bŭrn) A burn caused by heat.

ther·mal·ge·si·a, ther·mo·al·ge·si·a (thĕr´măl-jē´zē-ă, thĕr´mō-al-) High sensibility to heat; pain caused by a slight degree of heat.

ther·mal·gi·a (thĕr-mal´jē-ă) Burning pain.

therm·an·al·ge·si·a, therm·o·an·al·ge·si·a (therm´an-ăl-jē´zē-ă, thĕr´mō-al-) SYN thermoanesthesia.

therm·is·tor (therm´is-tŏr) A device for determining temperature; also may be used to monitor control of temperature.

ther·mo·an·es·the·si·a, therm·an·al·ge·si·a, therm·an·es·the·si·a (thĕr´mō-an-es-thē´zē-ă, thĕrm´an-ăl-jē´zē-ă, -es-thē´zē-ă) Insensibility to heat or to temperature changes.

ther·mo·cau·te·ry (thĕr´mō-kaw´tĕr-ē) The use of an actual cautery.

ther·mo·chem·is·try (thĕr´mō-kem´is-trē) The interrelation of chemical action and heat.

ther·mo·co·ag·u·la·tion (thĕr´mō-kō-ag´yū-lā´shŭn) The process of converting tissue into a gel by heat. SYN endocoagulation.

ther·mo·cou·ple, ther·mo·coup·ler (thĕr´mō-kŭp´ĕl, -ĕr) A device for measuring slight changes in temperature.

ther·mo·dif·fu·sion (thĕr´mō-di-fyū´zhŭn) Diffusion of fluids, either gaseous or liquid, as found by fluid's temperature.

ther·mo·di·lu·tion (thĕr´mō-di-lū´shŭn) Reduction in temperature in a liquid that occurs when it is introduced into a colder liquid; the volume of the latter liquid can be calculated from the amount of rise in its temperature.

ther·mo·du·ric (thĕr´mō-dyū´rik) Resistant to the effects of exposure to high temperature; used especially with reference to microorganisms.

ther·mo·dy·nam·ics (thĕr′mō-dī-nam′iks) **1.** Physicochemical science concerned with heat and energy and their conversions of one into the other involving mechanical work. **2.** The study of the flow of heat.

ther·mo·es·the·si·a, therm·es·the·si·a (thĕr′mō-es-thē′zē-ă, thĕrm′es-thē′zē-ă) The ability to distinguish differences of temperature.

ther·mo·es·the·si·om·e·ter (thĕr′mō-es-thē′zē-om′ĕ-tĕr) An instrument for testing a subject's temperature sense, consisting of a metal disc with thermometer attached, by which the exact temperature of the disc at the time of application may be known.

ther·mo·ex·ci·to·ry (thĕr′mō-ek-sī′tŏ-rē) Stimulating the production of heat.

ther·mo·gen·e·sis (thĕr′mō-jen′ĕ-sis) Production of heat; specifically, the physiologic process of heat production in the body.

ther·mo·gram (thĕr′mō-gram) **1.** A regional temperature map of the surface of a part of the body, obtained by infrared sensing device; it measures radiant heat, and thus subcutaneous blood flow, if the environment is constant. **2.** The record made by a thermograph.

ther·mo·hy·per·al·ge·si·a (ther′mō-hī′per-al-jē′zē-ă) Excessive thermalgesia.

ther·mo·hy·per·es·the·si·a (ther′mō-hī′pĕr-es-thē′zē-ă) Very acute thermoesthesia or temperature sense; exaggerated perception of hot and cold.

ther·mo·hyp·es·the·si·a, ther·mo·hy·po·es·the·si·a (ther-mō-hīp-es-thē′zē-ă, thĕr′mō-hī′pe-) Diminished perception of temperature differences. SYN thermohypoesthesia.

ther·mo·in·hib·i·to·ry (thĕr′mō-in-hib′i-tōr-ē) Inhibiting or arresting thermogenesis.

ther·mo·in·te·gra·tor (thĕr′mō-in′tĕ-grā-tŏr) Any device for assessing the effective warmth or coldness of an environment as it might be experienced by a living organism.

ther·mo·ker·at·o·plas·ty (TKP) (ther′mō-ker′ă-tō-plas′tē) A procedure in which heat shrinks the collagen of the corneal stroma and flattens the cornea in the area of heat application.

ther·mo·la·bile (thĕr′mō-lā′bĭl) Subject to alteration or destruction by heat.

ther·mol·y·sis (thĕr-mol′i-sis) **1.** Loss of body heat by evaporation, radiation, or other causes. **2.** Chemical decomposition by heat.

ther·mo·mas·sage (thĕr′mō-mă-sahzh′) Combination of heat and massage in physical therapy.

ther·mom·e·ter (thĕr-mom′ĕ-tĕr) An instrument for indicating the temperature of any substance; usually a sealed vacuum tube containing mercury, which expands with heat and contracts with cold, its level accordingly rising or falling in the tube, with the exact degree of variation of level being indicated by a scale. SEE ALSO scale.

ther·mo·neu·tral en·vi·ron·ment (thĕr′mō-nū′trăl en-vī′rŏn-mĕnt) Ambient conditions that do not require active temperature regulation.

ther·mo·nu·cle·ar (thĕr′mō-nū′klē-ăr) Pertaining to nuclear reactions brought about by nuclear fusion.

ther·mo·phile, ther·mo·phil (thĕr′mō-fĭl, -fĭl) An organism that thrives at a temperature of 50°C or higher.

ther·mo·phore (thĕr′mō-fōr) **1.** An arrangement for applying heat to a part; consists of a water heater, a tube conveying hot water to a coil, and another tube conducting the water back to the heater. **2.** Flat bag containing salts that produce heat when moistened; a substitute for a hot-water bag or bottle.

ther·mo·plas·tic (thĕr′mō-plas′tik) Classification for materials that soften when heated and harden on cooling.

ther·mo·re·cep·tor (thĕr′mō-rē-sep′tŏr) A receptor that is sensitive to heat.

ther·mo·reg·u·la·tion (thĕr′mō-reg′yū-lā′shŭn) Temperature control, as by a thermostat.

ther·mo·reg·u·la·to·ry cen·ters (thĕr′

mō-reg′yŭ-lă-tōr-ē sen′tĕrz) Centers in the hypothalamus that control the conservation and dispersal of body heat.

ther·mo·sta·bile, ther·mo·sta·ble (thĕr′ mō-stā′bil, -stā′bĕl) Not readily subject to alteration or destruction by heat.

ther·mo·stat (ther′mō-stat) Apparatus for the automatic regulation of heat. SYN thermoregulator.

ther·mo·ste·re·sis (thĕr′mō-stĕ-rē′sis) The abstraction or deprivation of heat.

ther·mo·tax·is (thĕr′mō-tak′sis) 1. Reaction of living protoplasm to the stimulus of heat. Cf. thermotropism. 2. Regulation of the temperature of the body.

ther·mo·to·nom·e·ter (thĕr′mō-tŏ-nom′ ĕ-tĕr) Instrument to measure muscular contraction under the influence of heat.

ther·mot·ro·pism (thĕr-mot′rō-pizm) The motion by a part of an organism toward or away from a source of heat. Cf. thermotaxis.

thia- Combining form denoting replacement of carbon by sulfur in a ring or chain. Cf. thio-.

thi·a·min (thī′ă-min) A heat-labile and water-soluble vitamin contained in milk, yeast, and the germ and husk of grains; also artificially synthesized; essential for growth; a deficiency of thiamin is associated with beriberi and Wernicke-Korsakoff syndrome. SYN vitamin B1.

thi·am·i·nase (thī-am′i-nās) An enzyme present in raw fish that destroys thiamin and may produce thiamin deficiency in animals or people on a diet largely composed of raw fish. SYN thiaminase II.

thi·a·min py·ro·phos·phate (thī′ă-min pī′rō-fos′fāt) A coenzyme that aids carboxylation and has an essential role in forming acetyl CoA from pyruvate.

thi·e·mi·a (thī-ē′mē-ă) Sulfur in the circulating blood.

thi·e·nyl·al·a·nine (thī′ĕ-nil-al′ă-nēn) Compound similar to phenylalanine that inhibits growth of *Escherichia coli*.

Thiersch ca·nal·ic·u·lus (tērsh kan′ă-

lik′yŭ-lŭs) Any of numerous minute channels in newly formed reparative tissue permitting the circulation of nutritive fluids.

thigh (thī) [TA] The part of the lower limb between the hip and the knee. SYN femur (1) [TA].

thig·mes·the·si·a (thig′mes-thē′zē-ă) Sensibility to touch. SYN thigmaesthesia.

thi·mer·o·sal (thī-mer′ŏ-săl) Antiseptic used topically and as a preservative in vaccine preparations. SYN thiomersal, thiomersalate.

thin-lay·er chro·ma·tog·ra·phy (TLC) (thin-lā′ĕr krō′mă-tog′ră-fē) The investigative modality applied through a thin layer of cellulose or similar inert material supported on a glass or plastic plate.

thio- Prefix denoting the replacement of oxygen by sulfur in a compound. Cf. thia-.

thi·o·cy·a·nate (thī′ō-sī′ă-nāt) A salt of thiocyanic acid. SYN rhodanate, sulfocyanate.

thi·o·es·ter (thī′ō-es′tĕr) In enzymology, an ester where the oxygen bridging the substrate or product carbonyl carbon and the enzyme is replaced by a sulfur (usually through a Cys residue); a high-energy intermediate in many enzymes. SYN acylmercaptan.

thi·o·eth·a·nol·a·mine a·ce·tyl·trans·fer·ase (thī′ō-eth′ă-nol′ă-mēn ă-sē′til-trans′fĕr-ās) An enzyme transferring acetyl from acetyl-CoA to the sulfur atom of thioethanolamine, thus producing coenzyme A and S-acetylthioethanolamine. SYN thiotransacetylase B.

-thioic ac·id (as′id) Suffix denoting the radical –C(S)OH or –C(O)SH, the sulfur analogue of a carboxylic acid.

thi·o·ki·nase (thī′ō-kī′nās) Group term for enzymes that form acyl-CoA compounds from the corresponding fatty acids and CoA; the bond is through the sulfur atom of the CoA.

thi·ol (thī′ol) 1. The monovalent radical –SH when attached to carbon; a hydrosulfide; a mercaptan. 2. A mixture of sulfurated and sulfonated petroleum oils purified with ammonia; used in the treatment of skin diseases.

-thione Suffix denoting the radical =C=S, the sulfur analogue of a ketone, i.e., a thiocarbonyl group.

thi·on·ic (thī-on′ik) Relating to sulfur.

thi·o·sul·fate (thī′ŏ-sŭl′fāt) The anion of thiosulfuric acid; elevated in people with a molybdenum cofactor deficiency. SYN thiosulphate.

thiosulphate [Br.] SYN thiosulfate.

thi·o·xan·thene (thī′ŏ-zan′thēn) Class of tricyclic compounds used as an antipsychotic and antiemetic.

third-de·gree burn (thĭrd-dĕ′grē bŭrn) SYN full-thickness burn.

third-de·gree heartblock (thĭrd dĕ-grē′ hahrt blok) SEE atrioventricular block.

third-de·gree pro·lapse (thĭrd-dĕ-grē′ prō′laps) Form of cervical prolapse (procidentia uteri) in which the cervix protrudes well beyond the vaginal orifice.

third mo·lar tooth (thĭrd mō′lăr tūth) Eighth permanent tooth in the maxilla and mandible on each side; the most posterior tooth in human dentition. SYN dens serotinus [TA].

third spac·ing (thĭrd spās′ing) Loss of extracellular fluid from the vascular to other body compartments.

third stage of la·bor (thĭrd stāj lā′bŏr) The duration from the expulsion of the infant until the completed expulsion of the placenta and membranes.

thirst (thĭrst) A desire to drink associated with uncomfortable sensations in the mouth and pharynx.

thirst cen·ter (thĭrst sen′tĕr) Cells located in the lateral hypothalamus, which when stimulated, produce thirst.

thirst fe·ver (thĭrst fē′vĕr) An elevation of temperature in infants after reduction of fluid intake, diarrhea, or vomiting; probably caused by reduced available body water, with reduced heat loss by evaporation. SYN dehydration fever.

Thi·ry-Vel·la fis·tu·la (TVF) (tē′rē văl′ ah fis′tyū-lă) Experimental isolation of a segment of intestine in an animal. SYN Vella fistula.

thix·ot·ro·py (thik-sot′rŏ-pē) The property of certain gels of becoming less viscous when shaken or subjected to shearing forces and returning to the original viscosity on standing.

Tho·ma am·pul·la (tō-mah′ am-pul′lă) A dilation of the arterial capillary beyond the sheathed artery of the spleen.

Tho·ma laws (tō-mah′ lawz) Development of blood vessels is governed by dynamic forces acting on their walls as follows: an increase in velocity of blood flow causes dilation of the lumen; an increase in lateral pressure on the vessel wall causes it to thicken; an increase in end-pressure causes the formation of new capillaries.

Thom·as splint (tom′ăs splint) A long leg splint extending from a ring at the hip to beyond the foot, allowing traction to a fractured leg, for emergencies and transportation.

Thom·as test (tom′ăs test) Maneuver used to determine tightness of iliopsoas muscle.

tho·ra·cal·gi·a (thōr′ă-kal′jē-ă) Pain in the chest.

tho·ra·cen·te·sis (thōr′ă-sen-tē′sis) Paracentesis of the pleural cavity. SYN pleural tap, pleurocentesis, thoracocentesis.

tho·rac·ic (thōr-as′ik) Relating to the thorax.

tho·rac·ic cage (TC) (thōr-as′ik kāj) [TA] Skeleton of the thorax consisting of the thoracic vertebrae, ribs, costal cartilages, and sternum plus or minus the xiphoid. SYN compages thoracis.

tho·rac·ic con·stric·tion of e·soph·a·gus (thōr-as′ik kŏn-strik′shŭn e-sof′ă-gŭs) [TA] Normal left-sided narrowing of the esophagus, demonstrated radiographically after a barium swallow, at the T4–T5 vertebral level, where the esophagus is impressed by the left main bronchus and the arch of the aorta. SYN constrictio partis thoracicae esophagea [TA], broncho-aortic constriction, constrictio bronchoaortica esophagea, middle esophageal constriction.

tho·rac·ic duct (thōr-as´ik dŭkt) [TA] The largest lymph vessel in the body.

tho·rac·ic kid·ney (thōr-as´ik kid´nē) Ectopic kidney that partially lies above the diaphragm in the posterior mediastinum.

tho·rac·ic med·i·cine (thōr-as´ik med´i-sin) Therapy pertaining to disorders and diseases involving structures of the chest.

tho·rac·ic out·let syn·drome (TOS) (thōr-as´ik owt´lĕt sin´drōm) Collective name for several conditions attributed to compromise of blood vessels or nerve fibers (brachial plexus) at any point between the base of the neck and the axilla. SYN costoclavicular syndrome, hyperabduction syndrome, thoracic outlet compression syndrome, Wright syndrome.

tho·rac·ic spine (TS, T-spine) (thōr-as´ik spīn) Thoracic region of the vertebral column; the thoracic vertebrae [T1–T12] as a whole; that part of the vertebral column that enters into the formation of the thorax.

tho·rac·ic sple·no·sis (thōr-as´ik splē-nō´sis) Presence of splenic tissue in the thorax, resultant from combined thoracic and abdominal trauma followed by splenectomy.

♻ **thoraco-, thorac-, thoracico-** Combining forms denoting the chest (thorax).

tho·ra·co·a·cro·mi·al (thōr´ă-kō-ă-krō´mē-ăl) Relating to the acromion and the thorax; denoting especially the thoracoacromial artery. SYN acromiothoracic.

thor·a·co·ce·los·chis·is (thōr´ă-kō-sē-los´ki-sis) A congenital fissure of the trunk involving both the thoracic and abdominal cavities.

tho·ra·co·cyl·lo·sis (thōr´ă-kō-si-lō´sis) A deformity of the chest.

tho·ra·co·cyr·to·sis (thōr´ă-kō-sĭr-tō´sis) Abnormally wide curvature of the chest wall.

tho·ra·co·lum·bar (thōr´ă-kō-lŭm´bahr)

1. Relating to the thoracic and lumbar portions of the vertebral column. **2.** Relating to the origins of the sympathetic division of the autonomic nervous system. SEE ALSO autonomic division of nervous system.

thor·a·co·lum·bo·sac·ral or·tho·sis (thōr´ă-kō-lŭm´bō-sā´krăl ōr-thō´sis) An external device applied to the trunk extending from the upper portion of the thoracic spine to the pelvis; immobilizes the thoracic spine.

tho·ra·col·y·sis (thōr´ă-kol´i-sis) Breaking up of pleural adhesions.

tho·ra·com·e·ter (thōr´ă-kom´ĕ-tĕr) An instrument for measuring the circumference of the chest or its variations in respiration.

tho·ra·co·my·o·dyn·i·a (thōr´ă-kō-mī´ō-din´ē-ă) Pain in the muscles of the chest wall.

tho·ra·co·plas·ty (thōr´ă-kō-plas-tē) Surgical procedure that reduces intrathoracic space.

tho·ra·co·schi·sis (thōr´ă-kos´ki-sis) Congenital fissure of the thoracic wall, which may result in herniation of lung tissue.

tho·ra·co·scope (thō-rak´ŏ-skōp) A scope for viewing intrathoracic structures; may be video assisted.

tho·ra·co·ste·no·sis (thōr´ă-kō-stĕ-nō´sis) Narrowness of the chest.

tho·ra·co·ster·not·o·my (thōr´ă-kō-stĕr-not´ŏ-mē) Chest incision combining an intercostal incision and transsection of the sternum.

tho·ra·cos·to·my (thōr´ă-kos´tŏ-mē) Creating an opening into the thorax.

tho·ra·cos·to·my tube (thōr-ă-kos´tŏ-mē tūb) One placed through the chest wall that drains the pleural space.

tho·rax, gen. **tho·ra·cis**, pl. **tho·ra·ces** (thō´raks, thō-rā´sis, -sēz) [TA] The upper part of the trunk between the neck and the abdomen.

thought with·draw·al (TW) (thawt with-draw´ăl) Delusion that one's thoughts have been removed from one's head resulting in a diminished number of thoughts remaining.

Thr Abbreviation for threonine or its radical forms.

thread·worm (thred′wŏrm) Common name for species of the genus *Strongyloides;* sometimes applied to any of the smaller parasitic nematodes.

thread·y pulse (thred′ē pŭls) A small, fine pulse, feeling like a small cord or thread under the finger.

threat·ened a·bor·tion (TAB) (thret′ĕnd ă-bōr′shŭn) Cramplike pains with or without bleeding that may be followed by the expulsion of the fetus during the first 20 weeks of pregnancy.

three-cham·bered heart (thrē′chām′bĕrd hahrt) Congenital abnormality with a single atrium with two ventricles or a single ventricle with two atria.

three-glass test (thrē glas test) A male patient empties his bladder into a series of 3-oz test tubes, and the contents of the first and the last are examined; the first tube contains the washings from the anterior urethra, the second, material from the bladder, and the last, material from the posterior urethra, prostate, and seminal vesicles. SEE ALSO Thompson test.

three-in·ci·sion e·soph·a·gec·to·my (thrē′in-sizh′ŭn ĕ-sof′ă-jek′tŏ-mē) Removal of all or part of the esophagus using laparotomy and right chest and cervical incisions.

three-jaw chuck (thrē′jaw chŭk) A grasp pattern emerging in the 10th–12th month that involves holding an object with an opposed thumb and the index and middle fingers where the interphalangeal joints are slightly flexed. The ulnar fingers are slightly flexed to stabilize the radial side of the hand.

thre·o·nine (T, Thr) (thrē′ō-nēn) One of the naturally occurring amino acids, included in the structure of most proteins and nutritionally essential in the diet of humans and other mammals.

thresh·old (thresh′ōld) **1.** The level of intensity at which a stimulus first produces a sensation. **2.** The lower limit of perception of a stimulus. **3.** The minimal stimulus that produces excitation of any structure. **4.** SYN limen.

thresh·old dose (thresh′ōld dōs) Minimal amount of medicine needed to obtain a desired therapeutic reaction.

thresh·old of con·scious·ness (thresh′ōld kon′shŭs-nĕs) Lowest point at which a stimulus sensation can be perceived.

thresh·old trait (thresh′ōld trāt) A trait that falls into natural groups that originate not in categorically distinct causes but in whether the outcome attains critical values (e.g., gallstones may result from a categoric cause or from unusual levels of causal factors that themselves show no evidence of grouping).

thrill (thril) A vibration accompanying a cardiac or vascular murmur that can be palpated. SEE ALSO fremitus.

throat (thrōt) **1.** The fauces and pharynx. SYN gullet. **2.** The anterior aspect of the neck. **3.** Any narrowed entrance to a hollow part.

throm·bec·to·my (throm-bek′tŏ-mē) The excision of a thrombus.

throm·bin (throm′bin) **1.** An enzyme (proteinase), formed in shed blood, which converts fibrinogen into fibrin by hydrolyzing peptides (and amides and esters) of L-arginine. **2.** A sterile protein substance prepared from prothrombin of bovine origin through interaction with thromboplastin in the presence of calcium. SYN factor IIa.

throm·bin time (TT) (throm′bin tīm) Duration needed for a fibrin clot to form after the addition of thrombin to citrated plasma.

thrombo-, thromb- Combining forms meaning blood clot; coagulation; thrombin.

throm·bo·an·gi·i·tis (throm′bō-an′jē-ī′tis) Inflammation of the intima of a blood vessel, with thrombosis.

throm·bo·an·gi·i·tis ob·li·te·rans (throm′bō-an′jē-ī′tis ob-lit′ĕr-anz) Inflammation of the entire wall and connective tissue surrounding medium-sized arteries and veins, especially of the legs of young and middle-aged men; associated with thrombotic occlusion; commonly resulting in gangrene.

throm·bo·ar·ter·i·tis (throm′bō-ahr′tĕr-ī′tis) Arterial inflammation with thrombus formation.

throm·bo·cyst, throm·bo·cys·tis (throm′bō-sist, -sis′tis) A membranous sac enclosing a thrombus.

throm·bo·cyt·ic se·ries (throm′bō-sit′ik sēr′ēz) The cells of successive stages in thrombocytic (platelet) development in the bone marrow, and then into the bloodstream; examples include megakaryoblasts, promegakaryocytes, megakaryocytes, and thrombocytes.

throm·bo·cy·top·a·thy (throm′bō-sī-top′ă-thē) General term for any disorder of the coagulating mechanism that results from dysfunction of the blood platelets.

throm·bo·cy·to·pe·ni·a, throm·bo·pe·ni·a (throm′bō-sī′tō-pē′nē-ă, throm′bō-pē′nē-ă) A condition in which there is a decreased number of platelets in the circulating blood.

throm·bo·cy·to·poi·e·sis (throm′bō-sī′tō-poy-ē′sis) The process of formation of thrombocytes or platelets.

throm·bo·cy·to·sis, throm·bo·cy·the·mi·a (throm′bō-sī-tō′sis, -sī-thē′mē-ă) An increase in the number of platelets in the circulating blood. SYN thrombocythemia.

throm·bo·em·bo·lism (throm′bō-em′bŏ-lizm) Embolism from a thrombus.

throm·bo·end·ar·ter·ec·to·my (throm′bō-end′ahr-tĕr-ek′tŏ-mē) An operation that involves opening an artery, removing an occluding thrombus along with the intima and atheromatous material, and leaving a clean, fresh plane internal to the adventitia.

throm·bo·gen·e·sis (throm′bō-jen′ĕ-sis) Process of formation of a blood clot.

throm·bo·gen·ic (throm′bō-jen′ik) **1.** Relating to thrombogen. **2.** Causing thrombosis or coagulation of the blood.

throm·boid (throm′boyd) Resembling a thrombus.

throm·bo·lym·phan·gi·tis (throm′bō-lim′fan-jī′tis) Inflammation of a lymphatic vessel with the formation of a lymph clot.

throm·bol·y·sis (throm-bol′i-sis) Liquefaction or dissolving of a thrombus.

throm·bo·lyt·ic (throm′bō-lit′ik) Breaking up or dissolving a thrombus. SYN thromboclastic.

throm·bo·lyt·ic ther·a·py (throm′bō-lit′ik thār′ă-pē) Intravenous administration of an agent intended to dissolve a clot causing acute ischemia. SEE ALSO tissue plasminogen activator.

throm·bon (throm′bon) An all-inclusive term for circulating thrombocytes (blood platelets) and the cellular forms from which they arise (thromboblasts or megakaryocytes).

throm·bo·phil·i·a (throm′bō-fil′ē-ă) A disorder of the hemopoietic system with a tendency to thrombosis.

throm·bo·phle·bi·tis (throm′bō-flĕ-bī′tis) Venous inflammation with thrombus formation.

throm·bo·phle·bi·tis mi·grans (TPM) (throm′bō-flĕ-bī′tis mī′granz) Creeping or slowly advancing thrombophlebitis, appearing in first one vein and then another.

throm·bo·plas·tin (PT) (throm′bō-plas′tin) A substance present in tissues, platelets, and leukocytes necessary for the coagulation of blood. SYN platelet tissue factor, thrombozyme, zymoplastic substance.

throm·bo·poi·e·sis (throm′bō-poy-ē′sis) Precisely, the process of a clot forming in blood, but generally used with reference to the formation of blood platelets (thrombocytes).

throm·bo·poi·e·tin (throm′bō-poy′ĕ-tin) A cytokine that serves as a humoral regulator for the production of blood platelets through action on the receptor c-mp1. SYN megakaryocyte growth and development factor.

throm·bosed (throm′bōst) **1.** Clotted. **2.** Denoting a blood vessel that is the seat of thrombosis.

throm·bo·sis, pl. **throm·bo·ses** (throm-bō′sis, -sēz) Formation or presence of a thrombus; clotting within a blood vessel that may cause infarction of tissues supplied by the vessel.

throm·bos·ta·sis (throm-bos′tă-sis) Local arrest of the circulation by thrombosis.

throm·bot·ic (throm-bot′ik) Relating to, caused by, or characterized by thrombosis.

throm·bot·ic mi·cro·an·gi·op·a·thy (TMA) (throm-bot′ik mī′krō-an′jē-op′ă-thē) Thrombosis within small blood vessels, as in thrombotic thrombocytopenic purpura.

throm·bot·ic stroke (throm-bot′ik strōk) Diminished or total lack of blood flow to an area of the brain caused by a blood clot.

throm·bot·ic throm·bo·cy·to·pe·nic pur·pu·ra (throm-bot′ik throm′bō-sī′tō-pē′nik pŭr′pyūr-ă) A rapidly fatal or occasionally protracted disease with varied symptoms in addition to dermal hemorrhage, including signs of central nervous system involvement, due to formation of fibrin or platelet thrombi in arterioles and capillaries in many organs.

throm·box·ane (throm-bok′sān) The formal parent of the thromboxane class.

throm·bus, pl. **throm·bi** (throm′bŭs, -bī) A clot in the cardiovascular system formed during life from constituents of blood; may be occlusive or attached to the vessel or heart wall without obstructing the lumen. SYN blood clot.

through drain·age (thrū drān′ăj) Removal of liquid obtained by the passage of a perforated tube, open at both extremities, through a cavity.

through·put (thrū′put) A term applied to analytic instruments specifying how many tests can be performed in a given time.

thrush (thrŭsh) Infection of the oral tissues with *Candida albicans;* often an opportunistic infection in patients with AIDS or other disorders that depress the immune system.

thu·li·um (Tm) (thū′lē-ŭm) A metallic element of the lanthanide series, atomic no. 69, atomic wt. l68.93421.

thumb (thŭm) [TA] The first digit on the radial side of the hand. SYN pollex [TA].

thumb·print·ing (thŭm′print-ing) A radiographic sign of intestinal ischemia associated with hematoma formation and edema in the bowel wall; the thickened or edematous tissues encroach on theair- or contrast-filled lumen radiographically.

thun·der·clap head·ache (thŭn′dĕr-klap hed′āk) Sudden severe nonlocalizing head pain not associated with any abnormal neurologic findings; of varied etiology, including subarachnoid hemorrhage, migraine, carotid or vertebral artery dissection, and cavernous sinus thrombosis.

thy·mec·to·my (thī-mek′tŏ-mē) Removal of the thymus gland.

-thymia Suffix denoting mind, soul, emotions. SEE ALSO thymo- (2).

thy·mic (thī′mik) Relating to the thymus gland.

thy·mic a·lym·pho·pla·si·a (thī′mik ā-lim′fō-plā′zē-ă) Hypoplasia with absence of Hassall corpuscles and deficiency of lymphocytes in the thymus and usually in lymph nodes, spleen, and gastrointestinal tract.

thy·mic cor·pus·cle (thī′mik kōr′pus-ĕl) Small, spheric bodies of keratinized and usually squamous epithelial cells arranged in a concentric pattern around clusters of degenerating lymphocytes, eosinophils, and macrophages; found in the medulla of the lobules of the thymus. SYN Hassall bodies, Hassall concentric corpuscle.

thy·mi·co·lym·phat·ic (thī′mi-kō-lim-fat′ik) Relating to the thymus and the lymphatic system.

thy·mi·dine (dThd) (thī′mi-dēn) 1-(2-deoxyribosyl)thymine; one of the four major nucleosides in DNA (the others being deoxyadenosine, deoxycytidine, and deoxyguanosine). SYN deoxythymidine.

thy·mine (thī′mēn) A constituent of thymidylic acid and DNA; elevated in hyperuracil-thyminuria.

thy·mi·tis (thī-mī′tis) Inflammation of the thymus gland.

♻ **thymo-, thym-, thymi-** 1. Combining forms denoting the thymus. 2. Combining forms denoting mind, soul, emotions. SEE ALSO -thymia. 3. Combining forms denoting wart, warty.

thy·mo·cyte (thī′mō-sīt) A cell that develops in the thymus, seemingly from a stem cell of bone marrow and of fetal liver, and is the precursor of the thymus-derived lymphocyte (T lymphocyte) that affects cell-mediated (delayed type) sensitivity.

thy·mo·ki·net·ic (thī′mō-ki-net′ik) Activating the thymus gland.

thy·mol (thī′mol) A phenol present in the volatile oil of *Thymus vulgaris* (thyme), *Mentha longifolia* (horsemint), and other volatile oils; used externally and internally as an antiseptic and as a deodorizer of offensive discharges. SYN thyme camphor, thymic acid.

thy·mo·ma (thī-mō′mǎ) A neoplasm in the anterior mediastinum, originating from thymic tissue, usually benign, and frequently encapsulated; occasionally invasive, but metastases are rare.

thy·mo·poi·et·in (thī′mō-poy′ĕ-tin) Formerly called thymin; a polypeptide hormone that induces differentiation of lymphocytes to thymocytes.

thy·mo·pri·val, thy·mo·priv·ic, thy·mo·pri·vous (thī-mō-prī′văl, -priv′ik, -mop′ri-vŭs) Relating to or marked by premature atrophy or removal of the thymus.

thy·mo·sin (thī′mō-sin) A polypeptide hormone that restores T-cell function in a thymectomized animal.

thy·mus, gen. and pl. **thy·mi** (thī′mŭs, mī) [TA] A primary lymphoid organ, located in the superior mediastinum and lower part of the neck, which is necessary in early life for the normal development of immunologic function.

thy·mus-in·de·pend·ent an·ti·gen (thī′mŭs-in′dĕ-pen′dĕnt an′ti-jen) One that does not require T-helper cell activation for the host's B cells to be stimulated. Repeating polymers such as polysaccharides are examples of T-independent antigens.

♻ **thyro-, thyr-** Combining forms meaning the thyroid gland. SEE ALSO thyroid.

thy·ro·a·pla·si·a (thī′rō-ă-plā′zē-ă) A congenital defect of the thyroid gland with deficiency of its secretion.

thy·ro·ar·y·te·noid (thī′rō-ar′i-tē′noyd) Relating to the thyroid and arytenoid cartilages.

thy·ro·car·di·ac (thī′rō-kahr′dē-ak) Affecting the heart as a result of hypothyroidism or hyperthyroidism.

thy·ro·car·di·ac dis·ease (thī′rō-kahr′ dē-ak di-zēz′) Heart disease resulting from hyperthyroidism.

thy·ro·cele (thī′rō-sēl) A tumor of the thyroid gland, such as a goiter.

thy·ro·ep·i·glot·tic (thī′rō-ep′-i-glot′ik) Relating to the thyroid cartilage and the epiglottis.

thy·ro·gen·ic, thy·rog·e·nous (thī′rō-jen′ik, -roj′ĕ-nŭs) Of thyroid gland origin.

thy·ro·glob·u·lin (thī′rō-glob′yū-lin) 1. A protein that contains thyroid hormone, usually stored in the colloid within the thyroid follicles; biosynthesis of thyroid hormone entails iodination of the L-tyrosyl moieties of this protein. A defect in thyroglobulin will lead to hypothyroidism. 2. Substance obtained by fractionation of porcine thyroid glands, containing not less than 0.7% of total iodine; used as a thyroid hormone to treat hypothyroidism.

thy·ro·glos·sal (thī′rō-glos′ăl) Relating to the thyroid gland and the tongue, denoting especially an embryologic duct.

thy·ro·hy·al (thī′rō-hī′ăl) The greater cornu of the hyoid bone.

thy·ro·hy·oid (thī′rō-hī′oyd) Relating to the thyroid cartilage and the hyoid bone.

thy·roid (thī′royd) Resembling a shield; denoting a gland (thyroid gland) and a cartilage of the larynx (thyroid cartilage) having such a shape.

thy·roi·dec·to·my (thr) (thī′roy-dek′tŏ-mē) Removal of the thyroid gland.

thy·roid func·tion test (thī′royd fŭngk′shŭn test) Clinical assessments and physical examination of the thyroid gland and blood levels of thyroid hormones to determine increased or decreased thyroid function.

thy·roid gland (thī′royd gland) [TA] Endocrine gland consisting of irregularly spheroid follicles, lying in front and to the sides of the upper part of the trachea and lower part of the larynx and of horseshoe shape, with two lateral lobes connected by a narrow central portion, the isthmus; and occasionally an elongated offshoot, the pyramidal lobe, which passes upward from the isthmus in front of the larynx. SYN glandula thyroidea [TA], thyroid body, thyroidea.

thy·roid hor·mones (thī′royd hōr′mōnz) Triiodothyronine (T_3) and thyroxine (T_4), both produced by the thyroid gland; regulate basal metabolic rate.

thy·roid in·suf·fi·cien·cy (thī′royd in′sŭ-fish′ĕn-sē) Subnormal secretion of hormones by the thyroid gland. SEE ALSO hypothyroidism.

thy·roi·di·tis (thī′roy-dī′tis) Inflammation of the thyroid gland.

thy·roid sup·pres·sion test (thī′royd sŭ-presh′ŭn test) Thyroid function test used to diagnose difficult cases of hyperthyroidism, now largely replaced by the thyrotropin-releasing hormone stimulation test. SYN Werner test.

thy·ro·lib·er·in (thī′rō-lib′ĕr-in) A tripeptide hormone from the hypothalamus, which stimulates the anterior lobe of the hypophysis to release thyrotropin.

thy·ro·meg·a·ly (thī′rō-meg′ă-lē) Enlargement of the thyroid gland.

thy·ro·par·a·thy·roi·dec·to·my (thī′rō-par-ă-thī′roy-dek′tŏ-mē) Excision of thyroid and parathyroid glands.

thy·rop·to·sis (thī′rop-tō′sis) Downward dislocation of the thyroid gland.

thy·rot·o·my (thī-rot′ŏ-mē) **1.** Surgery of the thyroid gland. **2.** SYN laryngofissure.

thy·ro·tox·ic (thī′rō-tok′sik) Denoting thyrotoxicosis.

thy·ro·tox·ic cri·sis, thy·roid cri·sis (thī′rō-tok′sik krī′sis, thī′royd) Exacerbation of symptoms of hyperthyroidism; severe thyrotoxicosis; can follow shock or injury or thyroidectomy; marked by rapid pulse (140–170/minute), nausea, diarrhea, fever, loss of weight, extreme nervousness, and a sudden rise in the metabolic rate; coma and death may occur.

thy·ro·tox·ic heart dis·ease (thī′rō-tok′sik hahrt di-zēz′) Cardiac symptoms, signs, and physiologic impairment due to overactivity of the thyroid gland usually due to excessive sympathetic stimulation.

thy·ro·tox·ic my·op·a·thy (thī′rō-tok′sik mī-op′ă-thē) Extreme muscular weakness in severe thyrotoxicosis affecting muscles of limbs and trunk as well as those used in speech and swallowing. SYN dysthyroid myopathy.

thy·ro·tox·i·co·sis (thī′rō-tok′si-kō′sis) The state produced by excessive quantities of endogenous or exogenous thyroid hormone.

thy·ro·troph (thī′rō-trōf) A cell in the anterior lobe of the pituitary that produces thyrotropin.

thy·ro·tro·pic, thy·ro·tro·phic (thī′rō-trō′pik, -fik) Stimulating or nurturing the thyroid gland. SYN thyrotrophic.

thy·rot·ro·pin, thy·ro·tro·phin (thī′rō-trō′pin, -trō′fin) Glycoprotein hormone produced by the anterior lobe of the hypophysis that stimulates the growth and function of the thyroid gland; used as a diagnostic test to differentiate primary and secondary hypothyroidism.

thy·ro·tro·pin-re·leas·ing hor·mone stim·u·la·tion test, TRH-stim·u·la·

tion test (TRH-ST) (thī′rō-trō′pin rĕ-lēs′ing hōr′mōn stim′yū-lā′shŭn, test) Assessment of pituitary response to injection of thyrotropin-releasing hormone, which normally stimulates pituitary secretion of thyroid-stimulating hormone (TSH, thyrotropin), used primarily to distinguish pituitary from hypothalamic causes of thyroid disorders; does not rise in pituitary dysfunction, but does in hypothalamic disorders.

thy·rox·ine, thy·rox·in (thī-rok′sēn, -sin) Active iodine compound existing normally in the thyroid gland and extracted therefrom in crystalline form; also prepared synthetically; used to relieve hypothyroidism and myxedema.

thy·rox·ine-bind·ing glob·u·lin (TBG) (thī-rok′sēn-bīnd′ing glob′yū-lin) The α-globulin of blood with a strong binding affinity for thyroxine; triiodothyronine is bound to it much less firmly; a deficiency or excess of this protein may occur as a rare benign X-linked disorder. SYN thyroxine-binding protein (1).

Ti Symbol for titanium.

tib·i·a, gen. and pl. **tib·i·ae** (tib′ē-ă, -ē) [TA] The medial and larger of the two bones of the leg, articulating with the femur, fibula, and talus.

tib·i·al (tib′ē-ăl) [TA] Relating to the tibia or to any structure named from it; also denoting the medial or tibial aspect of the lower limb. SYN tibialis [TA].

tib·i·a·lis (tib′ē-ā′lis) [TA] SYN tibial.

tib·i·al tor·sion (tib′ē-ăl tōr′shŭn) A congenital twisting of the tibia.

♻ **tibio-** Combining form denoting the tibia.

tib·i·o·fem·o·ral (TF) (tib′ē-ō-fem′ŏ-răl) Relating to the tibia and the femur.

tib·i·o·fib·u·lar (tib′ē-ō-fib′yū-lăr) Relating to both the tibia and fibula; denotes especially the joints and ligaments between the two bones. SYN peroneotibial, tibioperoneal.

tib·i·o·tar·sal (tib′ē-ō-tahr′săl) Relating to the tarsal bones and the tibia. SYN tarsotibial.

tic (tik) Habitual, repeated contraction of certain muscles, resulting in stereotyped individualized actions that can be voluntarily suppressed for only brief periods. SYN habit chorea, habit spasm.

tic dou·lou·reux (tik dū-lū-ruh′) SYN trigeminal neuralgia.

tick (tik) Any of a variety of small, blood-sucking arachnids that may have either hard or soft shells. Ticks normally feed on wild birds, mammals, or reptiles, and transmit disease by feeding on an infected host, then later feeding on a domestic animal or human.

tick·ling (tik′ling) Denoting a peculiar itching or tingling sensation caused by excitation of surface nerves.

ti·dal (tī′dăl) Relating to or resembling the tides, alternately rising and falling.

ti·dal drain·age (tī′dăl drān′ăj) Evacuation of the urinary bladder with an intermittent filling and emptying apparatus.

ti·dal vol·ume, ti·dal air (tī′dăl vol′yūm, ār) Air inspired or expired in a single breath during regular breathing.

tide (tīd) An alternate rise and fall, ebb and flow, or an increase or decrease.

Tie·tze syn·drome (tēt′sē sin′drōm) Inflammation and painful, tender, nonsuppurative swelling of a costochondral junction.

tight junc·tion (tīt jŭngk′shŭn) An intercellular junction between epithelial cells in which the outer leaflets of lateral cell membranes fuse to form a variable number of parallel interweaving strands that greatly reduce transepithelial permeability to macromolecules, solutes, and water through the paracellular route.

tilt ta·ble (TT) (tilt tā′bĕl) Table with a top capable of being rotated on its transverse axis so that a patient lying on it can be brought into the erect position as desired; used in experimental investigation and in physical therapy.

tilt test (tilt test) Any measurement of response during tilting of the body, usually head up but also head down. The test may be monitored by catheterization, echocardiography, electrophysiologic measurements, electrocardiography, or mechanocardiography.

time con·stant (tīm kon′stănt) That part of a circuit that determines the time interval over which the rate of electrical events will be averaged; in pulmonary physiology, the factors determining rate of flow in the airways.

time-gain com·pen·sa·tion (TGC) (tīm′gān′ kom′pĕn-sā′shŭn) In ultrasonography, an increase in receiver gain with time to compensate for loss in echo amplitude with depth, usually due to attenuation. SYN attenuation compensation, depth compensation, time compensation gain, time-compensated gain, time-varied gain.

tin (Sn) (tin) A metallic element, atomic no. 50, atomic wt. 118.710. SYN stannum.

tinc·to·ri·al (tingk-tōr′ē-ăl) Relating to coloring or staining.

tinc·ture (tinct.) (tingk′shŭr) An alcoholic or hydroalcoholic solution prepared from vegetable materials or from chemical substances.

tine (tīn) **1.** In dentistry, the slender, pointed end of an explorer. **2.** An instrument used to introduce antigen, such as tuberculin into the skin, and usually containing several individual tines.

tin·e·a (tin′ē-ă) Dermatophytosis of the keratin component of hair, skin, or nails. SYN ringworm, serpigo (1).

tin·e·a bar·bae (tin′ē-ă bahr′bē) Fungal infection involving the beard. SYN tinea sycosis.

tin·e·a cap·i·tis (tin′ē-ă kap′i-tis) Common fungal scalp infection due to *Microsporum* and *Trichophyton* on or within hair shafts.

tin·e·a cor·po·ris, tin·e·a cir·ci·na·ta (tin′ē-ă kōr-pōr′is, sir′si-nă′tă) A well-defined, scaling, macular eruption of dermatophytosis that frequently forms anular lesions and may appear on any part of the body.

tin·e·a cru·ris (tin′ē-ă krūr′is) Genitocrural form of tinea imbricata including the inner side of the thighs, the perineal region, and the groin. SYN eczema marginatum, jock itch.

tin·e·a fa·ci·a·lis, tin·e·a fa·ci·ei (tin′ē-ă fā′shē-ā′lis) *Avoid the incorrect form tinea faciale.* Ringworm of the face.

tin·e·a im·bri·ca·ta (tin′ē-ă im′bri-kā′tă) Fungal eruption consisting of concentric rings of overlapping scales forming papulosquamous patches scattered over the body.

tin·e·a ke·ri·on (tin′ē-ă ker′ē-on) An inflammatory fungus infection of the scalp and beard.

tin·e·a ni·gra (tin′ē-ă nī′gră) Fungus infection due to *Exophiala werneckii*, marked by dark lesions giving a spattered appearance most common on the palms. SYN pityriasis nigra.

tin·e·a pe·dis (tin′ē-ă ped′is) Dermatophytosis of the feet, especially of the skin between the toes.

tin·e·a un·gui·um (tin′ē-ă ŭng-gwī′ŭm) Ringworm of the nails due to a dermatophyte.

tin·e·a ver·si·co·lor (tin′ē-ă vĕr′si-kŏ′lŏr) An eruption of tan or brown branny patches on the skin of the trunk, often appearing white, in contrast with hyperpigmented skin after exposure to the summer sun. SYN pityriasis versicolor.

Ti·nel sign (tē-nel′ sīn) Sense tingling, or of ''pins and needles,'' felt at the lesion site or more distally along the course of a nerve when the latter is percussed. SYN distal tingling on percussion.

ting·ling (ting′gling) A pricking type of paresthesia.

tin·ni·tus (tin′i-tŭs) *Avoid mispronunciating tin-ight′is.* A sensation of noises (ringing, whistling, booming) in the ears.

tint·ed den·ture base (tint′ĕd den′chŭr bās) One that simulates the coloring and shading of natural oral tissues.

tip·ping (tip′ing) A tooth movement in which the angulation of the long axis of the tooth is altered.

tis·sue (tish′ū) Aggregation of similar

cells or types of cells, together with any associated intercellular materials, adapted to perform one or more specific functions. There are four basic tissues in the body: 1) epithelium; 2) connective tissue, including blood, bone, and cartilage; 3) muscle; and 4) nerve.

tis·sue bank (tish′ū bangk) Repository for human tissue intended for clinical or research purposes. SEE ALSO bank.

tis·sue cul·ture (tish′ū kŭl′chŭr) The maintenance of live tissue after removal from the body, by placing in a vessel with a sterile nutritive medium.

tis·sue lymph (tish′ū limf) True lymph (i.e., lymph derived chiefly from fluid in tissue spaces, in contrast to blood lymph).

tis·sue mac·ro·phage (tish′ū mak′rō-fāj) White blood cell found in all tissues of the body that digests cellular debris and pathogens.

tis·sue plas·min·o·gen ac·ti·va·tor (tPA) (tish′ū plaz-min′ŏ-jen ak′ti-vā-tŏr) Thrombolytic serine protease catalyzing the enzymatic conversion of plasminogen to plasmin; a genetically engineered protein used as a thrombolytic agent in patients with thrombotic occlusion of a coronary or cerebral artery.

tis·sue res·pi·ra·tion (tish′ū res′pir-ā′shŭn) Blood-tissue interchange of gases. SYN internal respiration.

tis·sue ten·sion (tish′ū ten′shŭn) Theoretic condition of equilibrium or balance between the tissues and cells whereby overaction of any part is restrained by the pull of the mass.

tis·sue typ·ing (tish′ū tīp′ing) Examination and assessment of body tissues to determine compatibility of a prospective donor and recipient before organ or cell transplantation can occur.

ti·ta·ni·um (Ti) (tī-tā′nē-ŭm) A metallic element used as an implant in dental work because of its uniquely high level of biocompatibility.

ti·ta·ni·um di·ox·ide (tī-tā′nē-ŭm dī-ok′sīd) Agent used in creams and powders as a protectant against external irritations and solar rays.

ti·ter (tī′tĕr) The standard of strength of a volumetric test solution; the assay value of an unknown measure by volumetric means.

tit·il·la·tion (tit′i-lā′shŭn) The act or sensation of tickling.

ti·tra·tion (tī-trā′shŭn) Volumetric analysis by addition of definite amounts of a test solution to a solution of the substance being assayed.

tit·u·ba·tion (tit′yū-bā′shŭn) **1.** A staggering or stumbling in trying to walk. **2.** A tremor or shaking of the head, of cerebellar origin.

Tl Symbol for thallium.

TLR Abbreviation for toll-like receptors.

T lym·pho·cyte (lim′fō-sīt) A thymocyte-derived lymphocyte of immunologic importance that is responsible for cell-mediated immunity. These cells have the characteristic T_3 surface marker and may be further divided into subsets according to function, such as helper, suppressor, and cytotoxic.

T_m 1. Abbreviation for temperature midpoint (kelvin); melting point. **2.** Symbol for thulium. **3.** Abbreviation for transport maximum.

TNM stag·ing (stāj′ing) Clinicopathologic evaluation of tumors based on the extent of tumor involvement at the primary site (T, followed by a number indicating size and depth of invasion), and lymph node involvement (N) and metastasis (M), each followed by a number starting at 0 for no evident metastasis; numbers used depend on the organ involved and influence the prognosis and choice of treatment.

to·bac·co-al·co·hol am·bly·o·pi·a (tŏ-bak′ō-al′kŏ-hol am′blē-ō′pē-ă) Acquired optic neuropathy involving the maculopapillary bundle nerve fibers associated with excessive alcohol and tobacco consumption and poor nutritional status.

to·bac·co heart (tŏ-bak′ō hahrt) Cardiac irritability marked by irregular action, palpitation, and pain, believed due to heavy use of tobacco.

toco- Combining form denoting childbirth.

to·co·dy·na·graph (TKG) (tō′kō-dī′nă-graf) A recording of the force of uterine contractions. SYN tocograph.

to·co·dy·na·mom·e·ter (tō′kō-dī′nă-mom′ĕ-tĕr) An instrument for measuring the force of uterine contractions. SYN tocometer.

to·co·lyt·ic (tō′kō-lit′ik) Denoting any pharmacologic agent to arrest uterine contractions; often used to arrest premature labor contractions.

to·com·e·ter (tŏ-kom′ĕ-tĕr) SYN tocodynamometer.

α-to·coph·er·ol (tŏ-kof′ĕr-ol) One of several forms of vitamin E. A light yellow, viscous, odorless, oily liquid that deteriorates on exposure to light, is obtained from wheat germ oil or by synthesis, biologically exhibits the most vitamin E activity of the α-tocopherols, and is an antioxidant retarding rancidity by interfering with the autoxidation of fats. SYN vitamin E (1).

to·coph·er·ol (T) (tŏ-kof′ĕr-ol) **1.** A generic term for vitamin E and compounds chemically related to it, with or without biologic activity. **2.** A methylated tocol or methylated tocotrienol.

to·coph·er·ol·qui·none (TQ) (tŏ-kof′ĕr-ol-kwin′ŏn) An oxidized tocopherol. SYN tocopherylquinone.

Todd pa·ral·y·sis (tod păr-al′i-sis) Temporary inability to move (normally not more than a few days) that occurs in the limb or limbs involved in jacksonian epilepsy after a seizure. SYN Todd postepileptic paralysis.

toe (tō) [TA] One of the digits of the feet.

toe clo·nus (tō klō′nŭs) Alternating movements of flexion and extension of the great toe after forcible extension at the metatarsophalangeal joint.

to·ga·vi·rus (tō′gă-vī′rŭs) Any virus of the family Togaviridae.

toi·let (toy-let′) **1.** Cleansing of the obstetric patient after childbirth or of a wound after an operation preparatory to the ap-

plication of the dressing. **2.** DENTISTRY cavity débridement, the final step before placing a restoration in a tooth whereby the cavity is cleaned and all debris is removed.

toi·let train·ing (toy′lĕt trān′ing) Teaching a child proper control of bladder and bowel functions; psychoanalytic personality theory believes that the attitudes of both parent and child concerning this training may have important psychological implications for the child's later development.

tol·bu·ta·mide test (tol-byū′tă-mīd test) An assay to detect insulin-producing tumors.

Toldt mem·brane (tōlt mem′brān) The anterior layer of the renal fascia.

tol·er·ance (tol′ĕr-ăns) **1.** The ability to endure or be less responsive to a stimulus, especially over a period of continued exposure. **2.** The power of resisting the action of a poison or of taking a drug continuously or in large doses without injurious effects.

tol·er·ance dose (tol′ĕr-ăns dōs) Largest acceptable amount of a remedy without causing injurious symptoms.

To·lo·sa-Hunt syn·drome (tō-lō′sah-hŭnt′ sin′drōm) Cavernous sinus syndrome produced by an idiopathic granuloma.

tol·u·ene (tol′yū-ēn) A colorless liquid derived from coal tar; physical and chemical properties resemble those of benzene; used in explosives and dyes, and as a solvent. SYN methylbenzene, toluol.

To·ma sign (tō′mah sīn) Finding to distinguish between inflammatory and to noninflammatory ascites.

-tome Combining form indicating a cutting instrument.

Tom·ma·sel·li dis·ease (tom′ĕ-sel′ē di-zēz′) Hemoglobinuria and pyrexia due to quinine intoxication.

to·mo·gram, plan·o·gram, plan·i·gram (tō′mŏ-gram, plan′ŏ-, plan′i) A radiograph obtained by tomography.

to·mog·ra·phy, plan·ig·ra·phy, plan·og·ra·phy (tŏ-mog′ră-fē, plă-nig′, plă-nog′) Making a radiographic image with a selected plane with reciprocal linear or curved motion of the x-ray tube and film cassette; images of all other planes are blurred (''out of focus'') by being relatively displaced on the film. SYN planography, stratigraphy.

-tomy Suffix indicating a cutting operation. SEE ALSO -ectomy.

tone (tōn) 1. A musical sound. 2. The character of the voice expressing an emotion. 3. The tension present in resting muscles. 4. Firmness of the tissues; normal functioning of all the organs.

tone deaf·ness (tōn def′nĕs) Inability to hear differences in pitch.

tongue (tŭng) [TA] 1. A mobile mass of muscular tissue covered with mucous membrane, occupying the cavity of the mouth and forming part of its floor, constituting also by its posterior portion the anterior wall of the pharynx. It bears the organ of taste, assists in mastication and deglutition, and is the principal instrument of articulate speech. SYN lingua (1) [TA], glossa. 2. A tonguelike structure. SYN lingua (2) [TA].

tongue-thrust swal·low (tŭng′thrŭst swah′lō) Forward movement of the tongue against the teeth while swallowing.

ton·ic (ton′ik) 1. In a state of continuous unremitting action. 2. Invigorating. 3. A remedy purported to restore enfeebled function and promote vigor, qualified, according to the organ or system on which it is presumed to act, as cardiac, digestive, hematic, vascular, nervine, uterine, general, and others.

ton·ic bite re·flex (ton′ik bīt rē′fleks) An atypical oral motor pattern seen when a person bites down and cannot release the position, often accompanied by increased tension throughout the face, head, and neck.

ton·ic-clo·nic sei·zure (TCS) (ton′ik-klon′ik sē′zhŭr) One characterized by a sequence consisting of a tonic-clonic phase; when generalized, constitutes what has been known as a ''grand mal''seizure.

ton·ic con·trac·tion (ton′ik kŏn-trak′shŭn) Sustained contraction of a muscle.

ton·ic con·vul·sion (ton′ik kŏn-vŭl′shŭn) A convulsion in which muscle contraction is sustained.

ton·ic ep·i·lep·sy (ton′ik ep′i-lep′sē) An attack in which the body becomes rigid.

to·nic·i·ty (tō-nis′i-tē) 1. A state of normal tissue tension by virtue of which the parts are kept in shape, alert, and ready to function in response to a suitable stimulus. 2. The osmotic pressure or tension of a solution, usually relative to that of blood. SEE ALSO isotonicity.

ton·ic neck re·flex (ton′ik nek rē′fleks) A brainstem-level reflex that may produce positional changes of all limbs in response to active or passive head turning or to flexion/extension of the head.

ton·i·co·clon·ic, to·no·clon·ic (ton′i-kō-klon′ik, ton′ō-klon′ik) Both tonic and clonic, referring to muscular spasms.

ton·ic pu·pil (ton′ik pyū′pil) A general term for a pupil with delayed, slow, long-lasting contractions to light and to a near vision effort, often with light-near dissociation; due to denervation and aberrant reinnervation of the iris sphincter; seen in various autonomic neuropathies and in Adie syndrome.

ton·ic sei·zure (ton′ik sē′zhŭr) Attack characterized by a sustained increase in muscle tone, of abrupt or gradual onset and offset, lasting a few seconds to a minute; affected proximal muscles bilaterally frequently lead to the adoption of a certain posture.

ton·ic spasm (ton′ik spazm) A continuous involuntary muscular contraction.

ton·ic state (ton′ik stāt) Steady rigid muscle contractions with no relaxation.

tono- Combining form meaning tone, tension, pressure.

ton·o·clon·ic spasm (ton′ō-klon′ik spazm) Convulsive contraction of muscles.

ton·o·fi·bril (ton′ō-fī′bril) One of a system of fibers found in the cytoplasm of epithelial cells. SEE ALSO cytoskeleton.

to·nog·ra·phy (tō-nog′ră-fē) Continuous measurement of intraocular pressure by means of a recording tonometer, to determine the facility of aqueous outflow.

to·nom·e·ter (tō-nom′ĕ-tĕr) **1.** Instrument to determine pressure or tension. **2.** A vessel for equilibrating a liquid (e.g., blood) with a gas.

to·nom·e·try (tō-nom′ĕ-trē) **1.** Measurement of the tension of a part. **2.** Measurement of ocular tension.

ton·o·plast (tō′nō-plast) An intracellular structure or vacuole.

to·nos·cil·lo·graph (tō-nos′i-lō-graf) An instrument that produces graphic records of arterial and capillary pressures as well as of individual pulse characters.

to·no·top·ic (tō′nō-top′ik) Denoting a spatial arrangement of structures such that certain tone frequencies are transmitted, as in the auditory pathway.

to·no·trop·ic (tō′nō-trō′pik) Denoting the shortening of the resting length of a muscle.

ton·sil (ton′sil) Any collection of lymphoid tissue.

ton·sil·lar, ton·sil·lar·y (ton′si-lăr, -lar-ē) Relating to a tonsil, especially the palatine tonsil. SYN amygdaline (3).

ton·sil·lar her·ni·a·tion (ton′si-lăr hĕr′nē-ā′shŭn) Herniation of the cerebellar tonsils through the foramen magnum.

ton·sil·lec·to·my (ton′si-lek′tŏ-mē) Removal of the entire tonsil.

ton·sil·li·tis (ton′si-lī′tis) Inflammation of a tonsil, especially of the palatine tonsil.

♻ **tonsillo-** Prefix meaning tonsil.

ton·sil·lo·ad·e·noid·ec·to·my (ton′si-lō-ad′ĕ-noy-dek′tŏ-mē) Surgical removal of the tonsils and adenoid tissue.

ton·sil·lo·lith (ton-sil′ŏ-lith) A calcareous concretion in a distended tonsillar crypt.

ton·sil·lot·o·my (ton′si-lot′ŏ-mē) The cutting away of a portion or all of a hypertrophied faucial tonsil.

too nu·mer·ous to count (TNTC) (nū′mĕr-ŭs kownt) Chart marking that indicates the finding of a large number of discrete objects, usually cells in a urine specimen, the precise enumeration of which is not practicable.

tooth, pl. **teeth** (tūth, tēth) [TA] One of the hard conic structures set in the alveoli of the upper and lower jaws, used in mastication and assisting in articulation. SYN dens (1) [TA].

tooth-borne (tūth′bōrn) A term used to describe a prosthesis that depends entirely on the abutment teeth for support.

tooth-borne base (tūth′bōrn bās) Denture base restoring an edentulous area that has abutment teeth at each end for support; the tissue that it covers is not used for support.

tooth sock·et (tūth sok′ĕt) [TA] Opening in the alveolar process of the maxilla or mandible, into which each tooth fits attached by means of the periodontal ligament. SYN alveolus (4) [TA].

top·ag·no·sis (top′ag-nō′sis) Inability to localize tactile sensations. SYN topoanesthesia.

to·pal·gi·a (tō-pal′jē-ă) Pain localized in one spot; a symptom occurring in neuroses whereby localized pain, without evident organic basis, is experienced.

top·es·the·si·a (top′es-thē′zē-ă) The ability to localize a light touch applied to any part of the skin.

to·pha·ceous (tō-fā′shŭs) Sandy; gritty.

to·phus, pl. **to·phi** (tō′fŭs, -fī) **1.** SEE gouty tophus. **2.** A salivary calculus, or tartar.

top·i·cal (top′i-kăl) Relating to a definite place or locality; local.

top·i·cal an·es·the·si·a (top′i-kăl an′es-thē′zē-ă) Superficial loss of sensation in conjunctiva, mucous membranes, or skin, produced by direct application of local anesthetic solutions, ointments, or jellies.

🔃 **topo-, top-** Combining forms meaning place, topical.

topoanaesthesia [Br.] SYN topoanesthesia.

top·o·an·es·the·si·a (top′ō-an-es-thē′zē-ă) SYN topagnosis.

top·og·no·sis, top·og·no·si·a (top′og-nō′sis, -nō′zē-ă) *In the diphthong gn, the g is silent only at the beginning of a word. Do not confuse this word with topagnosis.* Recognition of the location of a sensation; in the case of touch, topesthesia.

top·o·gom·e·ter (top′ŏ-gom′ĕ-tĕr) A movable fixation target attached to the front of a keratometer, used in fitting contact lenses.

to·pog·ra·phy (tŏ-pog′ră-fē) In anatomy, the description of any part of the body, especially in relation to a definite and limited area of the surface.

to·po·i·so·mer·ase (tō′pō-ī-som′ĕr-ās) Enzyme converting one topologic version of DNA into another; acts by catalyzing the breakage and reformation of DNA phosphodiester linkages.

To·po·lan·ski sign (tō′pō-lan′skē sīn) Congestion of the pericorneal region of the eye in Graves disease.

to·pol·o·gy (tŏ-pol′ŏ-jē) The study of the dimensions of personality.

top·o·nar·co·sis (top′ō-nahr-kō′sis) A localized cutaneous anesthesia.

TORCH (tōrch) Acronym for *t*oxoplasmosis, *o*ther infections, *r*ubella, *c*ytomegalovirus infection, and *h*erpes simplex. SEE TORCH syndrome.

TORCH syn·drome (tōrch sin′drōm) Infections, seen in neonates, which have crossed the placental barrier with similar clinical manifestations, although symptoms may vary in degree and time of appearance. SEE ALSO STORCH.

Torn·waldt ab·scess (tōrn′vahlt ab′ses) Chronic suppurative infection in a Tornwaldt cyst.

Torn·waldt cyst (tōrn′vahlt sist) Inflammation or obstruction of the pharyngeal bursa or an adenoid cleft with the formation of a cyst containing pus.

to·rose, to·rous (tō′rōs, -rŭs) Bulging; knobby.

tor·pid (tōr′pid) Inactive; sluggish. SYN torpent (1).

tor·por (tōr′pŏr) **1.** Inactivity, sluggishness. **2.** Dormancy, as in hibernation. SYN torpidity.

torque (T) (tōrk) **1.** A rotatory force. **2.** In dentistry, a torsion force applied to a tooth to produce or maintain crown or root movement.

torr (tōr) SYN mmHg.

Tor·re syn·drome (tōr′ē sin′drōm) Multiple sebaceous gland adenomas associated with multiple visceral malignancies.

tor·sade de pointes (tōr-sahd′ dĕ pwahnt′) Literally, "twisting of the points," a form of ventricular tachycardia nearly always due to medications and characterized by a long QT interval and a "short-long-short" sequence in the beat preceding its onset.

tor·sion (tōr′shŭn) **1.** A twisting or rotation of a part on its long axis. **2.** Twisting of the cut end of an artery to arrest hemorrhage. **3.** Rotation of the eye around its anteroposterior axis. SEE ALSO intorsion, extorsion, dextrotorsion, levotorsion.

tor·si·ver·sion, tor·so·ver·sion (tōr′si-vĕr′zhŭn, tōr-sō-) A malposition of a tooth in which it is rotated on its long axis. SYN torsive occlusion, torsoclusion (2).

tor·so (tōr′sō) The trunk; the body without relation to head or extremities.

tor·ti·col·lis (tōr′ti-kol′is) A contraction, often spasmodic, of the muscles of the neck. SYN wryneck, wry neck.

tor·ti·pel·vis (tōr′ti-pel′vis) Twisted pelvis.

tor·u·lus, pl. **tor·u·li** (tōr′yū-lŭs, -lī) A minute elevation or papilla.

to·rus, gen. and pl. **to·ri** (tōr′ŭs, -ī) [TA]

1. A geometric figure formed by the revolution of a circle around the base of any of its arcs, such as the convex molding at the base of a pillar. **2.** A rounded swelling, such as that caused by a contracting muscle.

to·rus frac·ture (tōr'ŭs frak'shŭr) A deformity in children consisting of a local bulging caused by the longitudinal compression of the soft bone. SYN buckle fracture.

to·tal a·pha·si·a (tō'tăl ă-fā'zē-ă) SYN global aphasia.

to·tal bod·y wa·ter (TBW, TBWA) (tō'tăl bod'ē waw'tĕr) Sum of intracellular and extracellular water (volume); about 60% of body weight.

to·tal cat·a·ract (tō'tăl kat'ăr-akt) One involving the entire lens.

to·tal cleav·age (tō'tăl klē'văj) SYN holoblastic cleavage.

to·tal com·mu·ni·ca·tion (tō'tăl kŏ-myū'ni-kā'shŭn) Habilitation of patients who are deaf or hearing impaired using any or all appropriate methods to enhance communication. SYN simultaneous communication.

to·tal hip re·place·ment (THR) (tō'tăl hip rĕ-plās'mĕnt) Surgical procedure to remove the damaged or diseased joint completely and replace it with a man-made device to replace its function.

to·tal hy·per·o·pi·a (Ht) (tō'tăl hī'pĕr-ō'pē-ă) The sum of manifest hyperopia and latent hyperopia.

to·tal hys·ter·ec·to·my (tō'tăl his'tĕr-ek'tŏ-mē) Surgical removal of the uterus and cervix of the uterus.

to·tal iron-bind·ing ca·pa·ci·ty (TIBC) (tō'tăl ī'ŏrn bīnd'ing kă-pas'i-tē) An indirect method of determining the transferrin level in serum.

to·tal lung ca·pa·ci·ty (TLC) (tō'tăl lŭng kă-pas'i-tē) The inspiratory capacity plus the functional residual capacity.

to·tal pa·ren·ter·al nu·trit·ion (TPN) (tō'tăl pă-ren'tĕr-ăl nū-trish'ŭn) Feeding regimen maintained entirely by intravenous injection or other nongastrointestinal route. SEE ALSO hyperalimentation.

to·tal pe·riph·er·al re·sis·tance (tō'tăl pĕ-rif'ĕr-ăl rē-zis'tăns) That opposing blood flow in the systemic circuit; the quotient produced by dividing the mean arterial pressure by the cardiac minute-volume. SYN peripheral resistance.

to·tal thy·rox·ine test (tō'tăl thī-rok'sēn test) A blood test to determine the circulating levels of thyroxine.

to·ti·po·ten·cy, to·ti·po·tence (tō'ti-pō'tĕn-sē, tō-tip'ō-tĕns) The ability of a cell to differentiate into any type of cell and thus form a new organism or regenerate any part of an organism.

Tou·pet fun·dop·li·ca·tion (tū'pā fŭn'dō-pli-kā'shŭn) A partial posterior fundoplication, in which the stomach edge is secured to the esophagus.

Tou·rette syn·drome (tūr-et' sin'drōm) Tic disorder appearing in childhood, characterized by multiple motor and vocal tics present for longer than 1 year. Obsessive-compulsive behavior, attention-deficit disorder, and other psychiatric disorders may be associated; coprolalia and echolalia rarely occur. SYN Gilles de la Tourette syndrome.

tour·ni·quet (tūr'ni-kĕt) An instrument for temporarily arresting the flow of blood to or from a distal part by pressure applied with an encircling device.

tox·e·mi·a, tox·i·ce·mi·a (tok-sē'mē-ă, tok'si-sē'mē-ă) **1.** Clinical manifestations observed during certain infectious diseases, assumed to be caused by toxins and other noxious substances elaborated by the infectious agent. **2.** The clinical syndrome caused by toxic substances in the blood. **3.** A lay term referring to the hypertensive disorders of pregnancy.

tox·ic cat·a·ract (tok'sik kat'ăr-akt) A cataract caused by drugs or chemicals.

tox·ic dose (tok'sik dōs) Minimal dose required to produce adverse effects.

tox·ic ep·i·der·mal ne·crol·y·sis (TEN) (tok'sik ep'i-dĕr'măl nĕ-krol'i-sis) A syndrome in which a large portion of the skin becomes intensely erythematous, with epidermal necrosis and flaccid bullae, resulting from drug sensitivity or of unknown cause. SYN Lyell syndrome.

tox·ic·i·ty (tok-sis′i-tē) The state of being poisonous.

tox·ic meg·a·co·lon (tok′sik meg′ă-kō′ lŏn) Acute nonobstructive dilation of the colon, seen in fulminating ulcerative colitis and Crohn disease.

tox·ic neu·ri·tis (tok′sik nūr-ī′tis) Neuritis caused by an endogenous or exogenous toxin.

♻ **toxico-, tox-, toxi-, toxo-** Combining forms meaning poison, toxin.

Tox·i·co·den·dron (tok′si-kō-den′ dron) A genus of poisonous plants (also known as *Rhus*) with fruits and foliage that contain urushiol, which produces a contact dermatitis (rhus dermatitis); species include poison ivy (*T. radicans*), poison oak (*T. diversilobum*), and poison sumac (*T. vernix*).

tox·i·co·gen·ic (tok′si-kō-jen′ik) 1. Producing a poison. 2. Caused by a poison.

tox·i·col·o·gy (tok′si-kol′ŏ-jē) The science of poisons, including their source, chemical composition, action, tests, and antidotes.

tox·ic shock syn·drome (tok′sik shok sin′drōm) Infection with toxin-producing staphylococci, most often in the vagina of menstruating women using superabsorbent tampons but also prevalent in many soft tissue infections.

tox·ic u·nit (tok′sik yū′nit) Amount formerly synonymous with minimal lethal dose but that, because of the instability of toxins, is now measured in terms of the quantity of standard antitoxin with which the toxin combines. SYN toxin unit.

tox·in (tok′sin) 1. Noxious or poisonous substance formed or elaborated as an integral part of the cell or tissue. SEE ALSO mid-spectrum agent, biologic-warfare (BW) agent. 2. A common misnomer for poison.

tox·i·no·gen·ic (tok′si-nō-jen′ik) Producing a toxin, said of an organism.

tox·i·no·ge·nic·i·ty (tok′si-nō-jĕ-nis′i-tē) The capacity to produce toxin.

tox·i·nol·o·gy (tok′si-nol′ŏ-jē) The study of toxins, in a restricted sense, with reference to the relatively unstable proteinaceous substances of microbial, plant, or animal origins.

Tox·o·ca·ra (tok′sō-ka′ră) A genus of ascarid nematodes, chiefly found in carnivores, which causes toxocariasis.

tox·o·ca·ri·a·sis (tok′sō-kă-rī′ă-sis) Infection with nematodes of the genus *Toxocara*; parenterally migrating larvae, chiefly of *T. canis*, may cause visceral larva migrans; ocular involvement results in a solitary retinal granuloma, peripheral inflammatory masses, or chronic endophthalmitis.

tox·oid (tok′soyd) A toxin that has been treated (commonly with formaldehyde) so as to destroy its toxic property but retain its antigenicity, i.e., its capability of stimulating the production of antitoxin antibodies and thus of producing an active immunity.

tox·o·plas·mo·sis (tok′sō-plaz-mō′sis) A disease caused by the protozoan parasite *Toxoplasma gondii*, which can produce a variety of syndromes in humans.

tox·o·py·rim·i·dine (tok′sō-pi-rim′i-dēn) A product resulting from hydrolysis of thiamin by thiaminase seen in urine.

tra·bec·u·la, gen. and pl. **tra·bec·u·lae** (tră-bek′yū-lă, -lē) [TA] One of the supporting bundles of fibers traversing the substance of a structure, usually derived from the capsule or one of the fibrous septa.

tra·bec·u·lat·ed blad·der (tră-bek′yū-lā-tĕd blad′ĕr) One with thickened wall and hypertrophied muscle bundles.

tra·bec·u·lec·to·my (tră-bek′yū-lek′tŏ-mē) A filtering operation for glaucoma by creation of a fistula between the anterior chamber of the eye and the subconjunctival space.

tra·bec·u·lo·plas·ty (tră-bek′yū-lō-plas-tē) Photocoagulation of the trabecular meshwork of the eye using a laser in the treatment of glaucoma.

trace el·e·ments (trās el′ĕ-mĕnts) Elements present in minute amounts in the body (e.g., Zn, Se, V, Ni, Mg, Mn); many are essential in metabolism or to manufacture of essential compounds.

trace min·er·als (trās min′ĕr-ălz) Minerals that are essential to the body in quantities less than 100 mg/day.

trac·er (trā′sĕr) **1.** Element or compound containing atoms that can be distinguished from their normal counterparts by physical means and can thus be used to follow (trace) the metabolism of the normal substances. **2.** Colored substance (e.g., a dye) used as a tracer to follow the flow of water.

tra·che·a, pl. **tra·che·ae** (trā′kē-ă, -ē) [TA] Air tube extending from the larynx into the thorax (level of the fifth or sixth thoracic vertebra), where it bifurcates into the right and left main bronchi. SYN windpipe.

tra·che·al·gi·a (trā′kē-al′jē-ă) Pain in the trachea.

tra·che·al tube (trā′kē-ăl tūb) SYN endotracheal tube.

tra·che·i·tis, tra·chi·tis (trā′kē-ī′tis, trā-kī′tis) Inflammation of the lining membrane of the trachea. SYN trachitis.

trach·e·lism, trach·e·lis·mus (trāk′ĕ-lizm, -liz′mŭs) A bending backward of the neck.

trach·e·lo·breg·mat·ic di·am·e·ter (trāk′ĕ-lō-breg-mat′ik dī-am′ĕ-tĕr) That of the fetal head from the middle of the anterior fontanelle to the neck.

trach·e·lor·rha·phy (trā′kē-lōr′ă-fē) Repair by suture of a laceration of the cervix uteri.

♻ **tracheo-, trache-** Combining forms meaning the trachea.

tra·che·o·aer·o·cele (trā′kē-ō-ār′ō-sēl) An air cyst in the neck caused by distention of a tracheocele.

tra·che·o·bron·chi·al (trā′kē-ō-brong′kē-ăl) Relating to both trachea and bronchi.

tra·che·o·bron·chi·al tree (trā′kē-ō-brong′kē-ăl trē) A network of tubes including the trachea and bronchi.

tra·che·o·bron·chi·tis (TB) (trā′kē-ō-brong-kī′tis) Inflammation of the mucous membrane of the trachea and bronchi.

tra·che·o·bron·cho·meg·a·ly (trā′kē-ō-brong′kō-meg′ă-lē) Gross widening of the trachea and main bronchi. SYN Mounier-Kuhn syndrome.

tra·che·o·bron·chos·co·py (trā′kē-ō-brong-kos′kŏ-pē) Inspection of the interior of the trachea and bronchi.

tra·che·o·cele, tra·che·lo·cele (trā′kē-ō-sēl, -kē-lō′sēl) A protrusion of the mucous membrane through a defect in the wall of the trachea.

tra·che·o·e·soph·a·ge·al (trā′kē-ō-ĕ-sof-ā′jē-ăl) Relating to the trachea and the esophagus.

♻ **tra·che·o·e·soph·a·ge·al fis·tu·la** (trā′kē-ō-ĕ-sof-ā′jē-ăl fis′chū′lă) Neonatal gastrointestinal disorder involving a connection between the esophagus and the trachea; may result in gastric juice reflux after feeding.

tra·che·o·e·so·pha·ge·al punc·ture, tra·che·o·e·so·pha·ge·al shunt (trā′kē-ō-ĕ-sof-ā′jē-ăl pungk′shŭr, shŭnt) Surgical procedure to allow exhaled air from the lungs to enter the esophagus to produce produce speech.

tra·che·o·la·ryn·ge·al (trā′kē-ō-lă-rin′jē-ăl) Relating to the trachea and the larynx.

tra·che·o·ma·la·ci·a (trā′kē-ō-mă-lā′shē-ă) Degeneration of elastic and connective tissue of the trachea.

tra·che·o·meg·a·ly (trā′kē-ō-meg′ă-lē) An abnormally dilated trachea that may result from infection or prolonged positive pressure ventilation.

tra·che·o·path·i·a, tra·che·op·a·thy (trā′kē-ō-path′ē-ă, -op′ă-thē) Any disease of the trachea.

tra·che·o·pha·ryn·ge·al (trā′kē-ō-fă-rin′jē-ăl) Relating to both trachea and pharynx.

tra·che·oph·o·ny (trā′kē-of′ŏ-nē) The hollow vocal sound heard in auscultating over the trachea.

tra·che·o·plas·ty (trā′kē-ō-plas-tē) Surgical repair of the trachea.

tra·che·or·rha·gi·a (trā′kē-ō-rā′jē-ă) Hemorrhage from the mucous membrane of the trachea.

tra·che·os·chi·sis (trā′kē-os′ki-sis) A fissure into the trachea.

tra·che·os·co·py (trā′kē-os′kŏ-pē) Inspection of the interior of the trachea.

tra·che·o·ste·no·sis (trā′kē-ō-stĕ-nō′sis) Narrowing of the lumen of the trachea.

tra·che·os·to·my tube (trā′kē-os′tŏ-mē tūb) A curved tube used to keep the opening free after tracheotomy; may be metal or plastic.

tra·che·ot·o·my, tra·che·os·to·my (trā′kē-ot′ŏ-mē, -os′tŏ-mē) The operation of creating an opening into the trachea, usually intended to be temporary.

tra·che·ot·o·my tube (trā′kē-ot′ŏ-mē tūb) A curved tube used to keep the opening free after tracheotomy.

Tra·chi·plei·stoph·or·a (trā-kē-plī-stof′ōr-ă) A genus of microsporidia that can infect humans and cause myositis, keratoconjunctivitis, and sinusitis in the immunocompromised person.

tra·cho·ma (tră-kō′mă) Chronic inflammation and hypertrophy of the conjunctiva. SYN Egyptian ophthalmia, granular ophthalmia.

tra·cho·ma bod·ies (tră-kō′mă bod′ēz) Distinctive, complex, intracytoplasmic forms found in the conjunctival epithelial cells of patients in the acute phase of trachoma.

tra·chy·o·nych·i·a (tra′kē-ō-nik′ē-ă) Rough-surfaced nails.

trac·ing (trās′ing) Any graphic display of electrical or mechanical cardiovascular events.

tract (trakt) [TA] **1.** An elongated area; a passage or pathway. SYN tractus [TA]. **2.** An abnormal passage (e.g., a fistula or sinus communicating with an abscess cavity).

trac·tion (trak′shŭn) **1.** The act of drawing or pulling. **2.** A pulling or dragging force exerted on a limb in a distal direction.

trac·tion al·o·pe·ci·a (trak′shŭn al′ŏ-pē′shē-ă) Circumscribed or diffuse loss of hair due to repetitive traction on the hair by pulling or twisting; also occurs after excessive application of hair ''softeners'' such as permanent wave solutions or hot combs. SYN traumatic alopecia.

trac·tion di·ver·tic·u·lum (trak′shŭn dĭ′vĕr-tik′yū-lŭm) Pouch formed by the pulling force of contracting bands of adhesion, occurring mainly in the distal esophagus.

trac·tot·o·my (trak-tot′ŏ-mē) Interruption of a nerve tract in the brainstem or spinal cord.

tra·di·tion·al Chi·nese med·i·cine (TCM) (tră-di′shŭn-ăl chī-nēz′ med′i-sin) An ancient system (begun about 200 BCE) of healing; based on the concepts of balance, moderation, and harmony, from Taoism. Network of 12 channels carry life energy (qi) to organs. Symptoms represent disharmony in the balance of the flow of energy. Techniques used include herbal remedies, massage, cupping, acupuncture, and acupressure.

tra·gus, pl. **tra·gi** (trā′gŭs, -jī) [TA] A tonguelike projection of the cartilage of the auricle in front of the opening of the external acoustic meatus and continuous with the cartilage of this canal. SYN antilobium, hircus (3).

train·ing-sen·si·tive zone (trān′ing-sen′si-tiv zōn) Level of exercise heart rate, usually 65–95% of heart rate maximum or 50–85% of heart rate reserve, required to induce training improvements in aerobic fitness. SYN target heart rate range.

trait (trāt) A qualitative characteristic; a discrete attribute as contrasted with metrical character; amenable to segregation rather than quantitative analysis; an attribute of phenotype, not of genotype.

tra·ma·dol (trah′mă-dol) An analgesic drug with a mechanism of action that interacts with reuptake and/or release of norepinephrine and serotonin.

tran·ex·am·ic ac·id (tran′eks-am′ik as′ id) A competitive inhibitor of plasminogen activation and of plasmin; used in hemophilia to reduce or prevent hemorrhage.

tran·qui·liz·er (trang′kwi-lī-zĕr) A drug that promotes tranquility by calming, soothing, quieting, or pacifying with minimal sedating or depressant effects.

trans- 1. Prefix denoting across, through, beyond; opposite of *cis-*. **2.** GENETICS denoting the location of two genes on opposite chromosomes of a homologous pair. **3.** ORGANIC CHEMISTRY prefix for a form of geometric isomerism in which the atoms attached to two carbon atoms, joined by double bonds, are located on opposite sides of the molecule. **4.** BIOCHEMISTRY a prefix to a group name in an enzyme name or a reaction denoting transfer of that group from one compound to another.

trans·ac·tion·al a·nal·y·sis (tranz-ak′ shŭn-ăl ă-nal′i-sis) Psychotherapy involving understanding of the qualities of interpersonal interactions in treatment sessions.

trans·ac·yl·a·tion (tranz-as′il-ā′shŭn) The reversible transfer of acyl groups.

trans·air·way pres·sure (tranz-ār′wā presh′ŭr) The difference between the pressure at the airway opening and the pressure in the lungs.

trans·am·i·na·tion (tranz′am-i-nā′shŭn) The reaction between an amino acid and an α-keto acid through which the amino group is transferred from the former to the latter.

trans·au·di·ent (tranz-aw′dē-ĕnt) Permeable to sound waves.

trans·bron·chi·al nee·dle as·pi·ra·tion (TBNA) (trans-brong′kē-ăl nē′dĕl as′pir-ā′shŭn) Biopsy of a structure or region adjacent to a bronchus by means of a needle introduced through a bronchoscope; used in cytology and histology studies of intrathoracic and respiratory disease.

trans·cel·lu·lar trans·port (tranz-sel′ yū-lăr trans′pŏrt) Solute movement across an epithelial cell layer through the cells. Cf. paracellular transport.

trans·cel·lu·lar water (tranz-sel′yū-lăr waw′tĕr) That fraction of extracellular water in cerebrospinal, digestive, epithelial, introcular, pleural, sweat, and synovial secretions; about 1.5% of body weight.

trans·cer·vi·cal frac·ture (tranz-sĕr′vi-kăl frak′shŭr) Breakage through the femoral neck.

trans·cer·vic·al thy·mec·to·my (tranz-sĕr′vik-ăl thī-mek′tŏ-mē) Removal of the thymus gland through a cervical incision.

trans·co·bal·a·mins (trans′kō-bal′ă-minz) Substances included in ''R binder,'' the name given a family of cobalamin-binding proteins; deficiencies have been associated with low serum cobalamin levels, and can lead to megaloblastic anemia.

trans·con·dy·lar frac·ture (tranz-kon′ di-lăr frak′shŭr) Breakage through condyles of the humerus or femur.

trans·cor·ti·cal (trans-kōr′ti-kăl) Across or through the cortex of the brain, ovary, kidney, or other organ.

trans·cor·ti·cal a·pha·si·a (trans-kōr′ ti-kăl ă-fā′zē-ă) An aphasia in which the ability to imitate speech is preserved but other language abilities are impaired.

trans·cra·ni·al (tranz-krā′nē-ăl) Denotes passing through the skull.

tran·scrip·tion (tran-skrip′shŭn) **1.** Transfer of genetic code information from one kind of nucleic acid to another. **2.** Process in which medical transcriptionists convert dictated health care information into a printed document.

trans·cu·ta·ne·ous blood gas mo·ni·tor (trans-kyū-tā′nē-ŭs blŭd gas mon′ i-tŏr) A device that uses miniature electrodes applied to the skin to estimate blood oxygen and carbon dioxide tension.

trans·cu·ta·ne·ous e·lec·tric·al nerve stim·u·la·tion (TENS) (trans-kyū′tā-nē-ŭs ĕ-lek′trik-ăl nĕrv stim′yū-lā′shŭn) Noninvasive device that inhibits pain signals, thus reducing pain perception, as well as stimulating the body's own pain control mechanisms. Used for chronic pain and labor.

trans·der·mal (trans-dĕr′mal) Entering through the dermis or skin, as in administration of a drug applied to the skin in ointment or patch form. SYN topical administration.

trans·du·cer (trans-dū′sĕr) A device designed to convert energy from one form to another. SEE ALSO transduction.

trans·du·cin (tranz-dū′sin) A protein that binds guanine nucleotides, found in retinal rods and cones.

trans·duc·tant (tranz-dŭk′tănt) A cell that has acquired a new character by means of transduction; may be complete, or abortive.

trans·duc·tion (trans-dŭk′shŭn) 1. Viral transfer of genetic material from one cell to another. 2. A form of genetic bacterial recombination. 3. Conversion of energy from one form to another.

tran·sec·tion, trans·sec·tion (transek′shŭn) 1. A cross-section. 2. Cutting across.

trans·e·soph·a·ge·al echo·car·di·og·ra·phy (tranz′ē-sō-fā′jē-ăl ek′ō-kahr′dē-og′ră-fē) Recording of the echocardiogram from a swallowed transducer.

trans·eth·moi·dal (trans′eth-moy′dăl) Across or through the ethmoid bone.

trans fat·ty ac·id (tranz fa′tē as′id) Trans form of a monounsaturated fatty acid usually produced by hydrogenation of polyunsaturated plant oils during industrial processing.

trans·fer, trans·fer·ence (trans′fĕr, trans-fĕr′ĕns) 1. Process of removal or change of place. 2. A condition in which learning in one situation influences learning in another situation. 3. Shifting of symptoms from one side of the body to the other. 4. Displacement of affect from one person or one idea to another. SYN transmission.

trans·fer·ence neu·ro·sis (trans-fĕr′ĕns nūr-ō′sis) In psychoanalysis, phenomenon of the patient's developing a strong emotional relationship with the analyst, symbolizing an emotional relationship with a family figure.

trans·fer ri·bo·nu·cle·ic ac·id (tRNA) (trans′fĕr rī′bō-nū-klē′ik as′id) Cellular nucleic acid that conveys information from DNA to cellular areas that generate protein.

trans·fer·rin (trans-fer′in) A glycoprotein, found in mammalian milk and egg white, which binds and transports iron.

trans·fer·rin sat·ur·a·tion (trans-fer′in sach′ŭr-ā′shŭn) A calculation, expressed in percentages, of the amount of transferrin that is bound to iron.

trans·fix·ion (trans-fik′shŭn) A maneuver in amputation in which the knife is passed from side to side through the soft parts, close to the bone, and the muscles are then divided from within in an outward direction.

trans·fix·ion su·ture (trans-fik′shŭn sū′chŭr) 1. Criss-cross stitch so placed as to control bleeding from a tissue surface or small vessel when tied. 2. Suture used to fix the columella to the nasal septum.

trans·for·ma·tion (trans′fōr-mā′shŭn) 1. SYN metamorphosis. 2. A change of one tissue into another.

trans·form·ing growth fac·tors (TGF) (trans-fōrm′ing grōth fak′tŏrz) Two polypeptide growth factors; TGF-α stimulates growth of many epidermal and epithelial cells; TGF-β controls proliferation and differentiation in many cell types.

trans·fu·sion (trans-fyū′zhŭn) Transfer of blood or a blood component from one person (donor) to another (recipient).

trans·fu·sion hep·a·ti·tis (trans-fyū′zhŭn hep-ă-tī′tis) SYN viral hepatitis type B.

trans·fu·sion ne·phri·tis (trans-fyū′zhŭn nĕ-frī′tis) Renal failure and tubular damage resulting from the transfusion of incompatible blood.

trans·fu·sion-re·lated a·cute lung in·ju·ry (TRALI) (trans-fyū′zhŭn-rē-lā′tĕd ă-kyūt′ lŭng in′jŭr-ē) Adult respiratory distress syndrome (ARDS) occurring within 4 hours of transfusion; mechanism remains poorly understood. The prognosis is much better than with most other cases of ARDS. SEE ALSO adult respiratory distress syndrome.

trans·gene (tranz′gēn) A newly introduced gene.

trans·gen·e·sis (trans-jen′ĕ-sis) Repro- duction involving introduction of for- eign-species DNA into an ovum.

trans·glu·ta·min·ase (tranz′glū-tam′i- nās) Enzyme that catalyzes the calcium- dependent acyl transfer reaction in which the amide moiety of peptide-bound glu- taminyl residues serve as acyl donor.

tran·si·ent (trans′shĕnt, -sē-ĕnt) **1.** Short- lived; not permanent. **2.** A short-lived cardiac sound of short duration as dis- tinct from a murmur.

tran·si·ent a·can·tho·lyt·ic der·ma· **to·sis** (tran′sē-ĕnt a-kan′tho-lit′ik dĕr- mă-tō′sis) A pruritic papular thoracic eruption, with scattered lesions of the back and lateral aspects of the extremi- ties, lasting mostly weeks to months; seen predominantly in men over 40. SYN Grover disease.

tran·si·ent glo·bal am·ne·si·a (TGA) (tran′sē-ĕnt glō′băl am-nē′zē-ă) Disorder that affects mainly old people who have not sustained a recent head injury and who do not have epilepsy; characterized by the abrupt onset of the inability to form memories and the resulting bewil- derment.

tran·si·ent is·che·mic at·tack (TIA) (tran′sē-ĕnt is-kē′mik ă-tak′) Sudden focal loss of neurologic function with complete recovery usually within 24 hours.

tran·si·ent my·o·pi·a (tran′sē-ĕnt mī- ō′pē-ă) Short sightedness observed in accommodative spasm secondary to iridocyclitis or ocular contusion.

trans·il·i·ac (trans-il′ē-ak) Extending from one ilium or iliac crest or spine to the other.

trans·il·lu·mi·na·tion (tranz-i-lū′mi-nā′ shŭn) Method of examination by the pas- sage of light through tissues or a body cavity.

tran·si·tion (tran-zish′ŭn) **1.** Passage from one condition to another. **2.** In polynucleic acid, replacement of a purine base by another purine base or a pyrimidine base by a different py- rimidine.

tran·si·tion·al (tran-zish′ŭn-ăl) Relating to or marked by a transition; transitory.

tran·si·tion·al cell car·ci·no·ma (tran- zish′ŭn-ăl sel kahr′si-nō′mă) SYN uro- thelial carcinoma.

tran·si·tion·al zone (tran-zish′ŭn-ăl zōn) **1.** Equatorial region of the lens of the eye where the anterior epithelial cells become transformed into lens fibers. **2.** Portion of a scleral contact lens between the corneal and scleral sections.

trans·jug·u·lar in·tra·he·pati·c por· **to·sys·tem·ic shunt (TIPS)** (tranz- jŭg′yū-lăr in′tră-hĕ-pat′ik pōr′tō-sis-tem′ ik shŭnt) An interventional radiology procedure to relieve portal hypertension.

trans·la·tion (trans-lā′shŭn) **1.** A conver- sion into another form. **2.** The com- plex process by which messenger RNA, transfer RNA, and ribosomes effect the production of protein from amino acids. **3.** In dentistry, the movement of a tooth through alveolar bone without change in axial inclination.

trans·lo·ca·tion (t) (trans′lō-kā′shŭn) **1.** Transposition of two segments be- tween nonhomologous chromosomes due to abnormal breakage and refusion of reciprocal segments. **2.** Transport of a metabolite across a biomembrane.

trans·lu·cent (trans-lū′sĕnt) Allowing light to pass through.

trans·lu·mi·nal (tranz-lū′mi-năl) De- notes passing across the cross-sectional opening of a tube (e.g., a blood vessel).

trans·mem·brane (TM) (trans-mem′ brān) Through or across a membrane.

trans·meth·y·la·tion (trans′meth-i-lā′ shŭn) Transfer of a methyl group from one compound to another.

trans·mis·si·ble (trans-mis′i-bĕl) Capa- ble of being carried from one person to another.

trans·mis·sion (trans-mish′ŭn) **1.** SYN transfer. **2.** Conveyance of disease from one person to another. **3.** Passage of a nerve impulse across an anatomic cleft. **4.** In general, passage of energy through a material.

trans·mis·sion-based pre·cau·tions (trans-mish′ŭn-băst prē-kaw′shŭnz) Measures established by the U.S. Centers for Disease Control and Prevention to prevent transfer of highly communicable pathogens.

trans·mit·ted light (trans-mit´ĕd līt) Illumination passed through a transparent medium.

trans·mit·ter subs·tance (tranz´mit-ĕr sŭb´stăns) A protein capable of exciting or inhibiting a cell.

trans·mu·ral (trans-myū´răl) Through any wall, as of the body or of a cyst or any hollow structure.

trans·mu·ral pres·sure (trans-myūr´ăl presh´ŭr) Pressure across the wall of a cardiac chamber or of a blood vessel.

trans·mu·ta·tion (trans´myū-tā´shŭn) A change; transformation. SYN conversion (1).

trans·o·var·i·al trans·mis·sion (tranz-ō-var´ē-ăl trans-mish´ŭn) Passage of parasites or infective agents from the maternal body to eggs within the ovaries.

trans·phos·phor·y·la·tion (trans´fos-fōr-i-lā´shŭn) Reaction involving transfer of a phosphoric group from one compound to another, often with adenosine triphosphate.

tran·spi·ra·tion (trans´pir-ā´shŭn) Passage of water vapor through the skin or any membrane. SEE ALSO insensible perspiration.

trans·pla·cen·tal (trans´plă-sen´tăl) Crossing the placenta.

trans·plant, trans·plan·ta·tion (trans´plant, -plan-tā´shŭn) 1. To transfer from one part to another. 2. The tissue or organ in grafting and transplantation. SEE ALSO graft.

trans·port (trans´pōrt) 1. The movement or transference of biochemical substances in biologic systems. 2. In physical therapy, movement of patients from one area (or surface) to another.

trans·port max·i·mum (Tm) (trans´pōrt mak´si-mŭm) The maximal rate of secretion or reabsorption of a substance by the renal tubules.

trans·pos·a·ble el·e·ment (trans-pōz´ă-bĕl el´ĕ-mĕnt) A DNA sequence that can move from one location in the genome to another.

trans·po·si·tion (trans´pŏ-zish´ŭn) 1. Removal from one place to another. 2. Condition of being transposed to the wrong side of the body. 3. Positioning of teeth out of their normal sequence in an arch.

trans·po·son (trans-pō´zon) A segment of DNA that has a repeat of an insertion sequence element at each end that can migrate from one plasmid to another within the same bacterium, to a bacterial chromosome, or to a bacteriophage.

trans·res·pir·a·tor·y pres·sure (trans-res´pir-ă-tōr-ē presh´ŭr) Total pressure difference across the airways, lungs, and chest wall; the difference between the pressure at the airway opening (the mouth) and the pressure on the body surface (i.e., pressure at the airway opening − pressure at the body surface); equivalent to transairway pressure + transpulmonary pressure + transmural pressure).

trans·seg·men·tal (trans´seg-men´tăl) Across or through a segment.

trans·sep·tal (trans-sep´tăl) Across or through a septum.

trans·sex·u·al (tran-sek´shū-ăl) A person with the external genitalia and secondary sexual characteristics of one gender, but whose personal identification and psychosocial configuration are that of the opposite gender.

trans·tha·lam·ic (trans´thă-lam´ik) Passing across the thalamus.

trans·tho·rac·ic (TT) (trans´thōr-ăs´ik) Passing through the thoracic cavity.

tran·su·date (tran´sū-dāt) Any fluid that has passed through a presumably normal membrane, as a result of imbalanced hydrostatic and osmotic forces. Cf. exudate. SYN transudation (2).

trans·u·re·ter·o·u·re·ter·os·to·my (trans-yūr´ĕ-tĕr-ō-yūr´ĕ-tĕr-os´tŏ-mē) Anastomosis of the transected end of one ureter into the intact contralateral ureter, by direct or elliptic end-to-side technique. SEE ALSO ureteroureterostomy.

trans·u·re·thral (TU) (trans´yūr-ē´thrăl) Through the urethra.

trans·vag·i·nal (TV) (trans-vaj'i-năl) Across or through the vagina.

trans·vec·tor (trans-vek'tŏr) An animal that transmits a toxic substance that it does not produce, but that may be accumulated from animal (dinoflagellate) or plant (algae) sources.

trans·ve·nous (tranz-vē'nŭs) Denotes passage through a vein.

trans·verse (trans-vĕrs') [TA] Crosswise; lying across the long axis of the body or of a part. SYN transversus.

trans·verse co·lon (trans-vĕrs' kō'lŏn) [TA] The part of the colon between the right and left colic flexures.

trans·ver·sec·to·my (trans'vĕr-sek'tŏ-mē) Resection of the transverse process of a vertebra.

trans·verse fa·cial frac·ture (trans-vĕrs' fā'shăl frak'shŭr) SYN craniofacial dysjunction fracture.

trans·verse her·maph·ro·dit·ism (trans-vĕrs' hĕr-maf'rō-dit-izm) Pseudohermaphroditism in which the external genitalia are characteristic of one gender and the gonads of the other.

trans·verse hor·i·zon·tal ax·is (tranz-vĕrs' hor'i-zon'tăl ak'sis) An imaginary line around which the mandible may rotate through the horizontal plane.

trans·verse lie (trans-vĕrs' lī) That relationship in which the long axis of the fetus is transverse or at right angles to that of the mother.

trans·verse my·e·li·tis (TM) (trans-vĕrs' mī'ĕ-lī'tis) Abrupt onset inflammatory process involving almost the entire thickness of the spinal cord but of limited longitudinal extent, generally one or a few segments; of multiple etiologies, the most common being viral and post viral causes, and multiple sclerosis. SYN acute transverse myelitis.

trans·verse pal·a·tine su·ture (trans-vĕrs' pal'ă-tīn sū'chŭr) [TA] Line of union of the palatine processes of the maxillae with the horizontal plates of the palatine bones. SYN sutura palatina transversa [TA].

trans·verse plane (trans-vĕrs' plān) [TA] A plane across the body at right angles to the coronal and sagittal planes.

trans·verse pre·sen·ta·tion (trans-vĕrs' prez'ĕn-tā'shŭn) An abnormal presentation, neither head nor breech, in which the fetus lies transversely in the uterus across the axis of the parturient canal.

trans·ver·sion, trans·ver·sion mu·ta·tion (trans-vĕr'zhŭn, myū'tā-shŭn) 1. Substitution in DNA and RNA of a pyrimidine for a purine by mutation. 2. DENTISTRY eruption of a tooth in a position normally occupied by another.

trans·ver·sus (trans-ver'sŭs) [TA] SYN transverse.

trans·ves·tism, trans·ves·ti·tism (trans-ves'tizm, -ti-tizm) The practice of dressing in the clothes of the opposite sex; especially the adoption of feminine mannerisms and costume by a male. SYN transvestitism.

Tran·tas dots (trahn'tăs dots) Pale, grayish red, uneven nodules of gelatinous aspect at the limbal conjunctiva in vernal conjunctivitis.

tra·peze bar (tra-pēz' bahr) Assistive device (two cords or ropes attached to a horizontal bar) that hangs above the patient's bed; used to facilitate movement and positioning of a patient.

tra·pe·zi·al (tră-pē'zē-ăl) Relating to any trapezium.

tra·pe·zi·um, pl. **tra·pe·zi·a**, pl. **tra·pe·zi·ums** (tră-pē'zē-ŭm, -ă, -ums) 1. A four-sided geometric figure having no two sides parallel. 2. The lateral bone in the distal row of the carpus. SYN os trapezium [TA], greater multangular bone, os multangulum majus, trapezium bone.

trap·e·zoid (trap'ĕ-zoyd) [TA] 1. Resembling a trapezium. 2. A geometric figure resembling a trapezium except that two of its opposite sides are parallel.

trap·e·zoid line (trap'ĕ-zoyd līn) [TA] The area on the inferior surface of the clavicle near its lateral extremity on which the trapezoid ligament attaches.

Trapp fac·tor (trahp fak'tŏr) Last two numerals of urine's specific gravity factor;

multiplying by two gives parts per thousand in solids.

Trau·be dou·ble tone (trow′bĕ dŭ′bĕl tōn) Sound heard on auscultation over the femoral vessels in aortic and tricuspid insufficiency.

Trau·be-Her·ing curves, Trau·be-Her·ing waves (trow′bĕ-her′ing kŭrvz, wāvz) Slow oscillations in blood pressure usually extending over several respiratory cycles; related to variations in vasomotor tone.

Trau·be sign (trow′bĕ sīn) A double sound or murmur heard in auscultation over arteries (particularly the femoral arteries) in significant aortic regurgitation.

🔁 **traum-** SEE traumato-.

trau·ma, pl. **trau·ma·ta,** pl. **trau·mas** (traw′mă, -mă-tă, -măz) An injury, physical or mental.

trau·ma cen·ter (TC) (traw′mă sen′tĕr) A designated medical facility for the treatment of trauma patients.

trau·mas·the·ni·a (traw′mas-thē′nē-ă) Nervous exhaustion following an injury.

trau·mat·ic (traw-mat′ik) Relating to or caused by trauma.

trau·mat·ic a·men·or·rhe·a (traw-mat′ik ă-men′ŏr-ē′ă) Absence of menses because of endometrial scarring or cervical stenosis resulting from injury or disease. SYN Asherman syndrome.

trau·mat·ic an·es·the·si·a (traw-mat′ik an′es-thē′zē-ă) Loss of sensation resulting from nerve injury.

trau·mat·ic as·phyx·i·a (traw-mat′ik as-fik′sē-ă) Cyanotic asphyxia due to trauma; blood extravates into the skin and conjunctivae, produced by a sudden mechanical increase in venous pressure. SYN pressure stasis.

trau·mat·ic brain in·ju·ry (TBI) (traw-mat′ik brān in′jŭr-ē) An insult to the brain as the result of physical trauma or external force that may cause a diminished or altered state of consciousness and may impair cognitive, behavioral, physical, or emotional functioning. SYN acquired brain injury.

trau·mat·ic cat·a·ract (traw-mat′ik kat′ăr-akt) One caused by contusion, rupture, or a foreign body.

trau·mat·ic fe·ver (traw-mat′ik fē′vĕr) Elevation of temperature after an injury. SYN symptomatic fever, wound fever.

trau·mat·ic her·pes (traw-mat′ik hĕr′pēz) Herpes simplex infection at the site of trauma or of a burn, sometimes accompanied by temperature elevation and malaise.

trau·mat·ic neu·ro·ma (traw-mat′ik nūr-ō′mă) Nonneoplastic proliferative mass of Schwann cells and neurites that may develop at the proximal end of a severed or injured nerve. SYN amputation neuroma, false neuroma, pseudoneuroma.

🔁 **traumato-, traumat-, traum-** Combining forms meaning wound, injury.

trau·ma·to·gen·ic oc·clu·sion (traw′mă-tō-jen′ik ŏ-klū′zhŭn) Malocclusion capable of producing injury to the teeth or associated structures.

trau·ma·tol·o·gy (traw′mă-tol′ŏ-jē) The branch of surgery concerned with the injured.

trau·ma·top·a·thy (traw′mă-top′ă-thē) Any pathologic condition resulting from violence or wounds.

trau·ma·top·ne·a (traw′mă-top′nē-ă) Passage of air in and out through a wound of the chest wall.

trau·ma·to·ther·a·py (traw′mă-tō-thār′ă-pē) Treatment of trauma or the result of injury.

trav·el·er's di·ar·rhe·a (trav′ĕl-ĕrz dī′ă-rē′ă) Of sudden onset, often accompanied by abdominal cramps, vomiting, and fever, this digestive disorder occurs sporadically in travelers usually during the first week of a trip; most commonly caused by strains of enterotoxigenic *Escherichia coli.*

tray (T) (trā) A flat receptacle with raised edges.

Treach·er Col·lins syn·drome (trēch′ĕr kol′inz sin′drōm) Mandibulofacial dysostosis characterized by bone abnormalities of structures formed from the first pharyngeal arch, including downward sloping palpebral fissures, depressed cheek bones, deformed pinnae, a receding chin, and a large, fishlike mouth with dental abnormalities. SYN mandibulofacial dysostosis.

treat·ment (trēt′mĕnt) Medical or surgical management of a patient. SEE ALSO therapy, therapeutics.

Tré·lat stools (trā-lah′ stūlz) Feces that look as if stippled with eggwhite that are also streaked with blood.

Trem·a·to·da (trem′ă-tō′dă) A class in the phylum Platyhelminthes (the flatworms) consisting of flukes with a leaf-shaped body and two muscular suckers, and an acelomate parenchyma-filled body cavity.

trem·a·tode, trem·a·toid (trem′ă-tōd, -ă-toyd) 1. Common name for a fluke of the class Trematoda. 2. Relating to a fluke of the class Trematoda.

trem·or (trem′ŏr) 1. Repetitive, often regular, oscillatory movements caused by alternate, or synchronous, but irregular contraction of opposing muscle groups; usually involuntary. 2. Minute ocular movement occurring during fixation on an object. SYN trepidation (1).

trem·u·lous (trem′yū-lŭs) Characterized by tremor.

trench fe·ver (trench fē′vĕr) An uncommon rickettsial fever caused by *Bartonella quintana* and transmitted by the louse *Pediculus humanus*.

Tren·de·len·burg op·er·a·tion (tren′de-len-berg op-ĕr-ā′shŭn) Pulmonary embolectomy.

Tren·de·len·burg po·si·tion (tren′de-len-berg pŏ-zish′ŏn) A supine position on the operating table, which is inclined at varying angles so that the pelvis is higher than the head; used during and after operations in the pelvis or for shock.

Tren·de·len·burg sign, Tren·del·en·burg gait (tren′de-len-berg sīn, gāt) A physical examination finding associated with various hip abnormalities in which the pelvis sags on the side opposite the affected side during single-leg stance on the affected side; during gait, compensa-

tion occurs by leaning the torso toward the involved side during stance phase on the affected extremity.

Tren·de·len·burg symp·tom (tren′de-len-berg simp′tŏm) A waddling gait produced by paresis of the gluteal muscles.

Tren·de·len·burg test (tren′de-len-berg test) Test of the valves of the leg veins.

treph·i·na·tion, trep·a·na·tion (tref′i-nā′shŭn, trep′ă-nā′shŭn) Removal of a circular piece (''button'') of cranium by a trephine.

tre·phine, tre·pan (trē′fīn′, trĕ-pan′) A cylindric or crown saw used for the removal of a disc of bone.

trep·i·da·tion (trep′i-dā′shŭn) Anxious fear.

Trep·o·ne·ma (trep′ō-nē′mă) A genus of anaerobic bacteria consisting of cells, 3–8 mcm in length, with acute, regular, or irregular spirals and no obvious protoplasmic structure. Some species are pathogenic and parasitic for humans and other animals, generally producing local lesions in tissues.

Trep·o·ne·ma pal·li·dum (trep′ō-nē′mă pal′i-dŭm) A bacterial species that causes syphilis in humans.

trep·o·ne·mi·a·sis (trep′ŏ-nē-mī′ă-sis) Infection caused by *Treponema*.

trep·o·ne·mi·ci·dal (trep′ō-nē′mi-sī′dăl) Destructive to any species of *Treponema*. SYN antitreponemal.

tre·pop·ne·a (trē-pop′nē′ă) 1. Dyspnea relieved in the lateral recumbent position. 2. Difficult or labored breathing while lying on one side but not the other. SEE ALSO platypnea.

Tre·sil·i·an sign (trē-sil′ē-ăn sīn) Reddish prominence at the orifice of Stenson duct, noted in mumps.

♻ **tri-** Combining form meaning three. Cf. tris-.

tri·ac·e·tin (trī-as′ĕ-tin) Used as a solvent of basic dyes, as a fixative in perfumery, and as a topical antifungal agent. SYN glyceryl triacetate, triacetylglycerol.

tri·ad (trī′ad) 1. A group of three things

with something in common. **2.** The transverse tubule and the terminal cisternae on each side of it in skeletal muscle fibers.

tri·age (trē′ahzh) Medical screening of patients to determine their relative priority for treatment; the separation of a large number of casualties, in military or civilian disaster medical care, into three groups: 1) those who cannot be expected to survive even with treatment; 2) those who will recover without treatment; 3) the highest priority group, those who will not survive without treatment.

tri·al case (trī′ăl kās) In refraction, a box containing lenses for testing.

tri·al frame (trī′ăl frām) A type of spectacle frame with variable adjustments, for holding trial lenses during refraction.

tri·an·gle (trī′ang-gĕl) [TA] ANATOMY, SURGERY a three-sided area with arbitrary or natural boundaries. SEE ALSO trigonum, region.

tri·an·gle of safe·ty (trī′ang-gĕl sāf′tē) The area at the lower left sternal border where the pericardium is not covered by lung; preferred site for aspiration of pericardial fluid.

Tri·at·o·ma (trī-ă-tō′mă) A genus of insects that includes important vectors of *Trypanosoma cruzi.*

tri·a·zole (trī′ă-zōl) Member of a series of heterocyclic compounds containing three nitrogen atoms in the azole group; also used to describe of of a group of antifungal agents.

tribe (trīb) In biologic classification, an occasionally used division between the family and the genus; often the same as the subfamily.

tri·bol·o·gy (tri-bol′ŏ-jē) The study of friction and its effects in biologic systems.

tri·bra·chi·us (trī-brā′kē-ŭs) Conjoined twins exhibiting tribrachia.

TRIC (trik) Acronym for *tr*achoma and *in*clusion conjunctivitis.

tri·car·box·yl·ic ac·id cy·cle (TCA cycle) (trī-kahr-bok-sil′ik as′id sī′kĕl) With oxidative phosphorylation, the main source of energy in the mammalian body and the end toward which carbohydrate, fat, and protein metabolism is directed. SYN citric acid cycle, Krebs cycle.

tri·ceps, pl. **tri·ceps,** pl. **tri·cep·ses** (trī′seps, -sez) Three-headed; denoting especially two muscles: triceps brachii and triceps surae. SEE ALSO muscle.

tri·ceps re·flex (trī′seps rē′fleks) Sudden contraction of the triceps muscle caused by a smart tap on its tendon when the forearm hangs loosely at a right angle with the arm. SYN elbow jerk, elbow reflex.

tri·ceps skin·fold test (trī′seps skin′fōld test) A double fold of skin and subcutaneous fat measured on the triceps midway between the acromion process and the olecranon process.

tri·chi·a·sis (tri-kī′ă-sis) **1.** A condition in which the hair adjacent to a natural orifice turns inward and causes irritation. **2.** Eyelash irritation of the eye.

trich·i·lem·mo·ma, tri·cho·lem·mom·ma (trik′i-lĕ-mō′mă, -mo-mă) A benign tumor derived from outer root sheath epithelium of a hair follicle, consisting of cells with pale-staining cytoplasm containing glycogen.

tri·chi·na, pl. **tri·chi·nae** (tri-kī′nă, -nē) A larval worm of the genus *Trichinella;* the infective form in pork.

Trich·i·nel·la (trik′i-nel′ă) A nematode genus in the aphasmid group that causes trichinosis in humans and other carnivores.

trich·i·no·sis, trich·i·nel·li·a·sis, trich·i·nel·lo·sis, trich·i·ni·a·sis (trik-i-nō′sis, -nĕ-lī′ă-sis, -nel-ō′sis, trik-i-nī′ă-sis) The disease resulting from ingestion of raw or inadequately cooked pork or other meat that contains encysted larvae of the nematode parasite *Trichinella spiralis.*

trich·i·nous (trik′i-nŭs) Infected with trichina worms.

tri·chi·tis (tri-kī′tis) Inflammation of the hair bulbs.

tri·chlor·o·a·ce·tic ac·id (TCA) (trī-klōr′ō-ă-sē′tik as′id) Agent used as an astringent antiseptic in 1–5% solution or as an escharotic for venereal and other warts.

tricho-, trich-, trichi- Combining forms denoting the hair; a hairlike structure.

trich·o·be·zoar (trik′ō-bē′zōr) A hair cast in the stomach or intestinal tract. SYN hair ball, pilobezoar.

trich·o·dis·co·ma (TD) (trik′ō-dis-kō′mă) Dominantly inherited or nonfamilial elliptic parafollicular mesenchymal hamartomas.

trich·o·ep·i·the·li·o·ma (TE) (trik′ō-ep′i-thē′lē-ō′mă) Any of numerous small benign nodules, occurring mostly on the skin of the face, derived from basal cells of hair follicles enclosing small keratin cysts. SYN Brooke tumor.

trich·o·es·the·si·a (trik′ō-es-thē′zē-ă) **1.** The sensation perceived when a hair is touched. **2.** A form of paresthesia with a sensation as of a hair on the skin, on the mucous membrane of the mouth, or on the conjunctiva.

trich·o·fol·lic·u·lo·ma (trik′ō-fŏ-lik′yū-lō′mă) A usually solitary tumor or hamartoma in which multiple abortive hair follicles open into a central cyst on the skin surface.

tri·chol·o·gy (tri-kol′ŏ-jē) The study of the anatomy, growth, and diseases of the hair.

trich·o·mo·na·cide (trik′ō-mō′nă-sīd) An agent that is destructive to *Trichomonas* organisms.

trich·o·mo·nad (trik′ō-mō′nad) Common name for members of the family Trichomonadidae.

trich·o·mo·nal va·gi·ni·tis (trik′ō-mō′năl vaj′i-nī′tis) Acute variable vaginitis caused by infection with *Trichomonas vaginalis*, which does not invade tissues but provokes an intense local inflammatory reaction in the vagina, cervix, and urethra; is sexually transmitted.

Trich·o·mo·nas (TRICH, Trich) (trik′ō-mō′năs) A genus of parasitic protozoan flagellates causing trichomoniasis in humans, other primates, and birds.

Trich·o·mo·nas te·nax (trik-ō-mō′năs ten′aks) A species of parasitic protozoan flagellates that lives as a commensal in the mouth of humans and other primates.

trich·o·mo·ni·a·sis (trik′ō-mō-nī′ă-sis) Disease caused by infection with a species of protozoon of the genus *Trichomonas* or related genera.

trich·o·my·co·sis (trik′ō-mī-kō′sis) Term formerly used to mean any disease of the hair caused by a fungus; now synonymous with trichonocardiosis or trichomycosis axillaris. SYN trichomycetosis.

trich·o·no·car·di·o·sis (trik′ō-nō-kahr′dē-ō′sis) An infection of hair shafts, especially of the axillary and pubic regions, with nocardiae. Yellow, red, or black concretions develop around the infected hair shafts and contain the causative agent and, frequently, micrococci. SEE ALSO trichomycosis. SYN trichomycosis axillaris, trichonodosis.

trich·o·path·ic (trik′ō-path′ik) Relating to any disease of the hair.

tri·chop·a·thy (tri-kop′ă-thē) Any disease of the hair. SYN trichonosis, trichosis.

trich·o·pha·gi·a (trik′ō-fā′jē-ă) The eating of hair or wool.

tri·choph·a·gy (tri-kof′ă-jē) Habitual biting of the hair.

trich·o·phyt·ic (trik′ō-fit′ik) Relating to trichophytosis.

trich·o·phy·tid (tri-kof′i-tid) An eruption remote from the site of infection that is the expression of allergic response to *Trichophyton* infection.

Trich·o·ph·y·ton (tri-kof′i-ton) A genus of pathogenic fungi causing dermatophytosis in humans and animals; species attacks the hair, skin, and nails.

Trich·o·phy·ton ru·brum (tri-kof′i-ton rū′brŭm) A widely distributed refractory anthropophilic fungal species that causes persistent infections of the skin.

Tri·cho·phy·ton ton·su·rans (tri-kof′i-ton ton-sū′ranz) An anthropophilic endothrix fungal species of that causes epidemic dermatophytosis; most common cause of tinea capitis in the U.S.

Tri·cho·phy·ton vi·o·la·ce·um (tri-kof′i-ton vī-ō-lā′sē-ŭm) An anthropophilic fungal species that causes black-dot ringworm or favus infection of the scalp.

trich·o·phy·to·sis (trik′ō-fī-tō′sis) Superficial fungal infection caused by species of *Trichophyton.*

trich·opt·i·lo·sis (tri-kop′ti-lō′sis) A condition of splitting of the shaft of the hair, giving it a feathery appearance.

trich·or·rhex·is (trik′ō-rek′sis) A condition in which the hairs tend to break or split.

trich·or·rhex·is no·do·sa (trik′ō-rek′sis nō-dō′să) Congenital or acquired condition in which minute nodes are formed in the hair shafts; splitting and breaking, complete or incomplete, may occur at these points or nodes.

trich·os·chi·sis (tri-kos′ki-sis) The presence of broken or split hairs. SEE ALSO trichorrhexis.

Trich·os·po·ron (trik′ō-spōr′on) A genus of imperfect fungi that possess branching septate hyphae with arthroconidia and blastoconidia; normal in intestinal tract of humans.

tri·chos·ta·sis spi·nu·lo·sa (tri-kos′tă-sis spī-nyū-lō′să) A condition in which hair follicles are blocked with a keratin plug containing multiple vellous hairs forming pruritic papules.

trich·o·thi·o·dys·tro·phy (trik′ō-thī′ō-dis′trō-fē) Congenital brittle hair resulting from low cysteine content.

trich·o·til·lo·ma·ni·a (trik′ō-til′ō-mā′nē-ă) A compulsion to pull out one's own hair.

tri·chro·mat·ic, tri·chrom·ic (trī′krō-mat′ik, trī-krō′mik) 1. Having, or relating to, the three primary colors: red, yellow, and blue. 2. Capable of perceiving the three primary colors; having normal color vision.

tri·chro·ma·top·si·a (trī′krō-mă-top′sē-ă) Normal color vision; the ability to perceive the three primary colors.

Trich·u·ris (tri-kyūr′is) A genus of aphasmid nematodes related to the trichina worm, *Trichinella spiralis.*

Trich·u·ris trich·i·u·ra (tri-kyūr′is trī-kī-yū′ră) The whipworm of humans; a species that causes trichuriasis. Humans are the only susceptible hosts and usually acquire infection by direct finger-to-mouth contact or by ingestion of soil, water, or food that contains larvated eggs.

tri·cip·i·tal (trī-sip′i-tăl) Having three heads; denoting a triceps muscle.

tri·cor·nute (trī-kōr′nyūt) Having three cornua or horns.

tri·cro·tism (trī′krŏ-tizm) The condition of being tricrotic.

tri·cus·pid, tri·cus·pi·dal, tri·cus·pi·date (trī-kŭs′pid, -kŭs′pi-dăl, -kŭs′pi-dāt) 1. Having three points, prongs, or cusps. 2. Teeth with three tubercles or cusps.

tri·cus·pid a·tre·si·a (trī-kŭs′pid ă-trē′zē-ă) Congenital lack of the tricuspid orifice.

tri·cus·pid in·suf·fi·cien·cy (trī-kŭs′pid in′sŭ-fish′ĕn-sē) SEE valvular regurgitation.

tri·cus·pid mur·mur (trī-kŭs′pid mŭr′mŭr) Sound produced at the tricuspid orifice, either obstructive or regurgitant.

tri·cus·pid or·i·fice (trī-kŭs′pid ōr′i-fis) An atrioventricular opening that leads from the right atrium into the right ventricle of the heart.

tri·cus·pid ste·no·sis (trī-kŭs′pid stĕ-nō′sis) Pathologic narrowing of the orifice of the tricuspid valve.

tri·cus·pid valve (trī-kŭs′pid valv) [TA] Valve closing the orifice between the right atrium and right ventricle of the heart.

tri·cyc·lic an·ti·de·pres·sant (TCA) (trī-sik′lik an′tē-dĕ-pres′ănt) Chemical group of antidepressant drugs that share a three-ringed nucleus.

tri·den·tate (trī-den′tāt) Three-toothed; three-pronged.

tri·fa·cial (trī-fā′shăl) Denoting the fifth pair of cranial nerves, the trigeminal nerves.

tri·fid (trī'fid) Split into three.

tri·fo·cal (TRI) (trī'fō-kăl) Having three foci. SEE trifocal lens.

tri·fo·cal lens (trī-fō'kăl lenz) A lens with segments of three focal powers: distant, intermediate, and near.

tri·fur·ca·tion (trī'fŭr-kā'shŭn) **1.** A division into three branches. **2.** The area where the tooth roots divide into three distinct portions.

tri·gem·i·nal (trī-jem'i-năl) Relating to the fifth cranial (trigeminus) nerve. SYN trigeminus.

tri·gem·i·nal cave (trī-jĕm'i-năl kāv) The cleft in the meningeal layer of dura of the middle cranial fossa near the tip of the petrous part of the temporal bone; it encloses the roots of the trigeminal nerve and the trigeminal ganglion.

tri·gem·i·nal neu·ral·gi·a (trī-jem'i-năl nūr-al'jē-ă) Severe, paroxysmal bursts of pain in one or more branches of the trigeminal nerve. SYN Fothergill disease (1), Fothergill neuralgia, prosopalgia, prosoponeuralgia, tic douloureux, trifacial neuralgia.

tri·gem·i·nal pulse (trī-jem'i-năl pŭls) A pulse in which the beats occur in trios, a pause following every third beat. SYN pulsus trigeminus.

tri·gem·i·nal rhi·zot·o·my (trī-jem'i-năl rī-zot'ŏ-mē) Division or section of a sensory root of the fifth cranial nerve, accomplished through a subtemporal, suboccipital, or transtentorial approach.

tri·gem·i·nal rhythm (trī-jem'i-năl ridh'ŭm) A cardiac arrhythmia in which the beats are grouped in trios, usually composed of a sinus beat followed by two extrasystoles. SYN trigeminy.

trig·ger (trig'ĕr) A substance, insect, object, or agent that initiates or stimulates an action.

trig·ger point (trig'ĕr poynt) Pathologic condition characterized by a small, hypersensitive area, occurring in a predictable pattern within muscles or fascia. SYN trigger area, trigger zone.

trig·o·nal (trig'ŏ-năl) Triangular; relating to a trigonum.

tri·gone (trī'gōn) [TA] **1.** SYN trigonum. **2.** The first three dominant cusps (protocone, paracone, and metacone), taken collectively, of an upper molar tooth.

trig·o·nel·line (trig'ŏ-nel'ēn) The methyl betaine of nicotinic acid; a product of the metabolism of nicotinic acid; excreted in the urine. SYN caffearine, trigenolline.

trig·o·ni·tis (trī'gō-nī'tis) Inflammation of the urinary bladder, localized in the trigone.

trig·o·no·ceph·a·ly (trig'ŏ-nō-sef'ă-lē) Malformation with a triangular cranial configuration, due in part to premature synostosis of the cranial bones with compression of the cerebral hemispheres.

tri·go·num (trī-gō'nŭm, -nă) [TA] Any triangular area. SEE triangle. SYN trigone (1) [TA].

tri·hy·brid (trī-hī'brid) The offspring of parents that differ in three mendelian characters.

tri·lam·i·nar (trī-lam'i-năr) Having three laminae. *rae.*

tri·lo·bate, tri·lobed (trī-lō'bāt, trī'lōbd) Having three lobes.

tri·loc·u·lar (trī-lok'yū-lăr) Having three cavities or cells.

tril·o·gy (tril'ŏ-jē) A triad of related entities.

tril·o·gy of Fal·lot (tril'ŏ-jē fahl-ō') A set of congenital defects including pulmonic stenosis, atrial septal defect, and right ventricular hypertrophy. SYN Fallot triad.

tri·mes·ter (TM, TRI) (trī'mes-tĕr) A period of 3 months; one third of the length of a pregnancy.

tri·meth·o·prim (TMP) (trī-meth'ŏ-prim) An antimicrobial agent that potentiates the effect of sulfonamides and sulfones; usually used in combination with sulfamethoxazole (TMP/SMX).

tri·meth·yl·am·i·nu·ri·a (trī-meth'il-am'i-nyūr'ē-ă) Increased excretion of trimethamine in urine, sweat, and saliva, with characteristically offensive fishy body odor or breath. SYN fish-odor syndrome.

tri·mor·phous (trī-mōr′fŭs) Existing under three forms; marked by trimorphism. SYN trimorphic.

tri·ni·tro·tol·u·ene (TNT) (trī′nī-trō-tol′ yū-ēn) An explosive made by the nitrification of toluene; causes gastric and intestinal disturbances and dermatitis in workers in munition factories. SYN trinitrotoluol.

tri·ose (trī′ōs) A three-carbon monosaccharide, e.g., glyceraldehyde and dihydroxyacetone.

tri·ox·sa·len (trī-ok′să-len) An orally effective pigmenting, photosensitizing agent; used as a tanning agent and in the treatment of vitiligo.

tri·pep·tide (trī-pep′tīd) A compound containing three amino acids linked together by peptide bonds.

tri·phas·ic (trī-fā′zik) Denotes having three phases.

tri·phos·pho·pyr·i·dine nu·cle·o·tide (trī-fos′phō-pir′i-dēn nū′klē-ō-tīd) Former name for nicotinamide adenine dinucleotide phosphate.

tri·ple·gi·a (trī-plē′jē-ă) **1.** Paralysis of three limbs, both extremities on one side and one on the other. **2.** Paralysis of an upper and a lower extremity and of the face.

tri·ple point (trip′ĕl poynt) Temperature at which all three phases (i.e., solid, liquid, and gas) are in equilibrium.

tri·ple re·peat dis·or·ders (trip′ĕl rĕ-pēt′ dis-ōr′dĕrz) A group of hereditary disorders with a gene mutation on a specific chromosome produces an abnormal form of protein terminated by a long chain of amino acid glutamate repeats.

tri·ple re·sponse (trip′ĕl rĕ-spons′) **1.** Triphasic response to firm stroking of the skin. Phase 1 is the sharply demarcated erythema that follows a momentary blanching of the skin and is the result of release of histamine from the mast cells. Phase 2 is the intense red flare extending beyond the margins of the line of pressure but in the same configuration, and is the result of arteriolar dilation; also called axon flare because it is mediated by axon reflex. Phase 3 is the appearance of a line wheal in the configuration of the original stroking. **2.** A similar response due to intradermal injection of histamine.

tri·ple screen (trip′ĕl skrēn) Test of maternal serum α-fetoprotein, chorionic gonadotropin, and unconjugated estrogen for indications fetal abnormality, especially Down syndrome.

trip·let (trip′lĕt) **1.** One of three children delivered at the same birth. SYN tridymus. **2.** A set of three similar objects. SYN codon.

trip·loid (trip′loyd) Pertaining to or characteristic of triploidy.

trip·lo·pi·a (trip-lō′pē-ă) Visual defect in which three images of the same object are seen. SYN triple vision.

tri·pod frac·ture (trī′pod frak′shŭr) A facial fracture involving the three supports of the malar prominence: the arch of the zygomatic bone, the zygomatic process of the frontal bone, and the zygomatic process of the maxillary bone.

tris- Chemical prefix indicating three of the substituents that follow, independently linked. Cf. tri-.

tris·mus (triz′mŭs) Persistent contraction of the masseter muscles due to failure of central inhibition; often the initial manifestation of generalized tetanus. SYN lockjaw.

tri·so·my (trī′sō-mē) The state of an individual or cell with an extra chromosome instead of the normal pair of homologous chromosomes; in humans, the state of a cell containing 47 normal chromosomes.

tri·so·my 8 syn·drome (trī′sō-mē sin′ drōm) Full trisomy 8 is usually associated with early lethality, but most affected individuals are mosaic with craniofacial dysmorphism; short, wide neck; narrow cylindric trunk; multiple joint and digital abnormalities; and deep creases of the palms and soles.

tri·so·my 13 syn·drome (trī′sō-mē sin′ drōm) Chromosomal disorder that is usually fatal within 2 years; characterized by mental retardation, malformed ears, cleft lip or palate, microphthalmia or coloboma, small mandible, polydactyly, cardiac defects, convulsions, renal anomalies, umbilical hernia, malrotation of intestines, and dermatoglyphic anomalies. SYN Patau syndrome.

tri·so·my 18 syn·drome (trī'sō-mē sin' drōm) Chromosomal disorder that is usually fatal within 2–3 years; characterized by mental retardation, abnormal skull shape, low-set and malformed ears, small mandible, cardiac defects, short sternum, diaphragmatic or inguinal hernia, Meckel diverticulum, abnormal flexion of fingers, and dermatoglyphic anomalies.

tri·so·my 21 syn·drome (trī'sō-mē sin' drōm) SYN Down syndrome.

tri·splanch·nic (trī-splangk'nik) Relating to the three visceral cavities: skull, thorax, and abdomen.

tri·sul·cate (trī-sŭl'kāt) Marked by three grooves.

tri·ta·nom·a·ly (trī'tă-nom'ă-lē) A type of partial color blindness due to a deficiency or abnormality of blue-sensitive retinal cones.

tri·ta·no·pi·a (trī'tă-nō'pē-ă) Deficient color perception with an absence of blue-sensitive pigment in the retinal cones.

tri·ti·ceous (tri-tish'ŭs) Resembling or shaped like a grain of wheat.

tri·ton tu·mor (trī'tŏn tū'mŏr) A peripheral nerve tumor with striated muscle differentiation, seen most often in neurofibromatosis.

trit·ur·a·tion (trit'yūr-ā'shŭn) **1.** The act of reducing a drug to a fine powder and incorporating it thoroughly with sugar or milk by rubbing the two together in a mortar. **2.** Mixing of dental amalgam in a mortar and pestle or with a mechanical device.

tri·va·lence, tri·va·len·cy (trī-vā'lĕns, -lĕn-sē) The property of being trivalent.

tri·va·lent (trī-vā'lĕnt) Having the combining power (valence) of 3.

triv·i·al name (triv'ē-ăl nām) A name of a chemical, no part of which is necessarily used in a systematic sense; i.e., it gives little or no indication as to chemical structure. Such names are commonly used for drugs, hormones, proteins, and other biologicals, and by the general public (e.g., water, aspirin [in the United States], chlo-

rophyll, heme, methotrexate, folic acid, caffeine, thyroxine, epinephrine, barbital).

tro·car (trō'kahr) An instrument for withdrawing fluid from a cavity, or for use in paracentesis.

tro·chan·ter (trō-kan'tĕr) [TA] One of the bony prominences developed from independent osseous centers near the upper extremity of the femur; there are two in humans, three in the horse.

tro·che (trō'kē) A small, disc-shaped, or rhombic body composed of solidifying paste containing an astringent, antiseptic, or demulcent drug, used for local treatment of the mouth or throat; held in the mouth until dissolved. SYN lozenge, pastille (2), pastil.

troch·le·a, pl. **troch·le·ae** (trok'lē-ă, -ē) [TA] **1.** A structure serving as a pulley. **2.** A smooth articular surface of bone upon which another glides.

troch·le·ar (trok'lē-ăr) **1.** Relating to a trochlea, especially the trochlea of the superior oblique muscle of the eye. SYN trochlearis (1). **2.** SYN trochleiform.

troch·le·i·form (trok'lē-i-fōrm) Pulley-shaped. SYN trochlear (2).

tro·choid (trō'koyd) Revolving; rotating; denoting a revolving or wheellike articulation.

tro·choid joint (trō'koyd joynt) SYN pivot joint.

tro·la·mine (trō'lă-mēn) USAN-approved contraction for triethanolamine, $N(CH_2CH_2OH)_3$.

Trom·bic·u·la (trom-bik'yū-lă) The chigger mite, a genus of mites the larvae of which (chiggers, red bugs) include pests of humans and other animals, and vectors of rickettsial and, probably, viral diseases.

trom·bic·u·li·a·sis (trom-bik'yū-lī'ă-sis) Infestation by mites of the genus *Trombicula*.

Trom·bic·u·li·dae (trom-bik'yū-lī'dē) A family of mites with larvae (red bugs, rougets, harvest mites, scrub mites, or chiggers) that are parasitic on vertebrates.

Tro·pher·y·ma whip·pel·i·i (trō-fer'i-mă wi-pel'ē-ī) A gram-positive bacterium, related to Group B actinomyces, which causes Whipple disease; found in tissues of infected patients and in sewage; mode of transmission unknown.

tro·phe·sy (trō'fĕ-sē) The results of any disorder of the trophic nerves.

♻ **-trophic** Suffix denoting nutrition. Cf. -tropic.

troph·ic (trō'fik) 1. Relating to or dependent on nutrition. 2. Resulting from interruption of nerve supply.

tro·phic·i·ty (trō-fis'i-tē) A trophic influence or condition.

troph·ic syn·drome (trō'fik sin'drōm) Ulceration of a denervated area, frequently secondary to picking at the anesthetic surface.

troph·ic ul·cer (trō'fik ŭl'sĕr) Lesion resulting from cutaneous sensory denervation. SYN trophic gangrene.

♻ **tropho-, troph-** Combining forms denoting food, nutrition.

troph·o·blast (trō'fō-blast) The mesectodermal cell layer covering the blastocyst that erodes the uterine mucosa and through which the embryo receives nourishment from the mother; the cells do not enter into the formation of the embryo itself but contribute to formation of the placenta. SYN chorionic ectoderm.

troph·o·blas·tic la·cu·na (trō'fō-blas'tik lă-kū'nă) One of the spaces in the early syncytiotrophoblastic layer of the chorion before the formation of villi; in human embryos, maternal blood enters these spaces by the 10th day; with the differentiation of the chorionic villi they become intervillous spaces, sometimes called intervillous lacunae.

troph·o·blas·tic o·per·cu·lum (trō-fō-blas'tik ō-pĕr'kyū-lŭm) Mushroom-shaped fibrin plug that fills the endometrial aperture made by the implanting blastocyst.

troph·o·der·ma·to·neu·ro·sis (trō'fō-dĕr'mă-tō-nūr-ō'sis) Cutaneous trophic changes due to neural involvement.

troph·o·neu·ro·sis (trō'fō-nūr-ō'sis) A trophic disorder due to disease or injury of the nerves of the body part.

troph·o·plast (trō'fō-plast) SYN plastid (1).

troph·o·zo·ite (trō'fō-zō'īt) Ameboid, vegetative, asexual form of some Sporozoea.

♻ **-trophy** Combining form indicating growth and nourishment.

tro·pi·a (trō'pē-ă) Abnormal deviation of the eye. SEE ALSO strabismus.

♻ **-tropic** Suffix denoting a turning toward, having an affinity for. Cf. -trophic.

trop·i·cal ac·ne (trop'ik-ăl ak'nē) A severe type of acne of the entire trunk, shoulders, upper arms, buttocks, and thighs; occurs in hot, humid climates.

trop·i·cal a·ne·mi·a (trop'ik-ăl ă-nē'mē-ă) Various syndromes frequently observed in people in tropical climates, usually resulting from nutritional deficiencies or hookworm or other parasitic diseases.

trop·i·cal dis·eas·es (trop'ik-ăl di-zēz'ĕz) Infectious and parasitic diseases endemic to tropical and subtropical zones, including Chagas disease, leishmaniasis, leprosy, malaria, onchocerciasis, schistosomiasis, sleeping sickness, yellow fever, and others; often water or insect borne.

trop·i·cal med·i·cine (trop'ik-ăl med'i-sin) Branch of medicine concerned with diseases, mainly parasitic, in areas with a tropical climate.

trop·i·cal sprue, trop·i·cal di·ar·rhe·a (trop'ik-ăl sprū, dī'ă-rē'ă) A disorder that occurs in warmer climates, often associated with enteric infection and nutritional deficiency.

trop·i·cal ul·cer (trop'ik-ăl ŭl'sĕr) 1. The lesion occurring in cutaneous leishmaniasis. 2. Tropical phagedenic ulceration caused by a variety of microorganisms.

trop·ic hor·mones, troph·ic hor·mones (trop'ik hōr'mōnz, trof'ik) Hormones of the anterior lobe of the pituitary that affect the growth, nutrition, or function of other endocrine glands.

trop·ic mac·ro·cyt·ic a·ne·mi·a (trop´ ik mak´rō-sit´ik ă-nē´mē-ă) Any anemia in which the average size of circulating erythrocytes is larger than normal; including such syndromes as pernicious anemia, sprue, celiac disease, macrocytic anemia of pregnancy, anemia of diphyllobothriasis, and others.

tro·pism, pos·i·tive tro·pism, neg·a·tive tro·pism (trō´pizm, poz´i-tiv, neg´ ă-tiv) The phenomenon, observed in living organisms, of moving toward or away from a focus of light, heat, or other stimulus.

tro·po·col·la·gen (trō´pō-kol´ă-jen) The fundamental units of collagen fibrils, consisting of three helically arranged polypeptide chains.

tro·po·my·o·sin (trō´pō-mī´ŏ-sin) A fibrous protein extractable from muscle.

tro·po·nin (Tn) (trō´pō-nin) A complex of three proteins that function as regulators of muscle contraction.

trough (trawf) **1.** A long, narrow, shallow channel or depression. **2.** The lowest point in variable measurement.

trough lev·el (trawf lev´ĕl) The lowest concentration reached by a drug before the next dose is administered, as determined by therapeutic drug monitoring.

trough sign (trawf sīn) An anteromedial glenoid defect that results from posterior shoulder dislocation.

Trous·seau point (trū-sō´ poynt) A painful point, in neuralgia, at the spinous process of the vertebra below which the affected nerve arises.

Trous·seau sign (trū-sō´ sīn) In latent tetany, the occurrence of carpopedal spasm accompanied by paresthesia elicited when the upper arm is compressed.

Trous·seau syn·drome (trū-sō´ sin´ drōm) Thrombophlebitis migrans associated with visceral cancer.

Trp Abbreviation for tryptophan and its radicals.

true con·ju·gate (TC) (trū kon´jŭ-găt) [TA] Diameter that represents the shortest diameter through which the head must pass in descending into the superior strait and measures, by means of x-ray, the distance from the promontory of the sacrum to a point on the inner surface of the symphysis a few millimeters below its upper margin. SYN conjugata vera [TA], obstetric conjugate diameter, obstetric conjugate.

true her·maph·ro·di·tism (trū hĕr-maf´rō-dīt-izm) Condition in which both ovarian and testicular tissue are present; also called true intersexuality.

true lu·men (trū lū´mĕn) In a dissecting aneurysm, the channel representing the actual intima-lined artery.

true ribs [I–VII] (trū ribz) [TA] Seven upper ribs on either side; their cartilages articulate directly with the sternum. SYN costae verae [TA].

trun·cal (trŭng´kăl) Relating to the trunk of the body or to any arterial or nerve trunk, etc.

trun·cal obe·sity (trung´kăl ō-bē´si-tē) A body habitus where fat is stored is patterned in the trunk rather than on the arms, legs, or elsewhere on the body.

trun·cate (trŭng´kāt) Truncated; cut across at right angles to the long axis, or appearing to be so cut.

trun·cat·ed (trung´kāt-ĕd) Shortened.

trun·cus, gen. and pl. **trun·ci** (trungk´ŭs, trŭn´sī) [TA] SYN trunk.

trun·cus ar·te·ri·o·sus (TA) (trŭng´kŭs ahr-tē-rē-ō´sŭs) Common arterial trunk opening out of both ventricles in the embryo, later destined to be divided into aorta and pulmonary artery by development of the spiral aorticopulmonary septum.

trunk (trŭngk) [TA] **1.** The body (trunk or torso), excluding the head and extremities. **2.** A primary nerve, vessel, or collection of tissue before its division. **3.** A large collecting lymphatic vessel. SYN truncus [TA].

truss (trŭs) An appliance designed to prevent the return of a reduced hernia or the increase in size of a hernia; it consists of a pad attached to a belt kept in place by a spring or straps.

truth se·rum (trūth sēr´ŭm) Colloquialism

for a drug intravenously injected with sco-polamine to elicit information from the subject under its influence; a misnomer because the subject's revelations may or may not be factually true.

try·pan·o·ci·dal (trī-pan′ō-sī′dăl) Destructive to trypanosomes.

try·pan·o·cide (trī-pan′ō-sīd) An agent that kills trypanosomes. SYN trypanosomicid.

Try·pan·o·so·ma (trī-pan′ō-sō′mă) A genus of asexual digenetic protozoan flagellates that are parasitic in the blood plasma of many vertebrates; pathogenic species cause trypanosomiasis in humans.

tryp·sin (trip′sin) A proteolytic enzyme formed from trypsinogen in the small intestine by the action of enteropeptidase; a serine proteinase that hydrolyzes peptides, amides, and esters.

tryp·sin in·hib·i·tor (trip′sin in-hib′i-tŏr) **1.** Peptide formed from trypsinogen through hydrolysis under the catalytic influence of enteropeptidase, with trypsin also produced as a result; so called because the peptide masks or inhibits the active site of the trypsin molecule. **2.** One of the polypeptides, from various sources (e.g., human and bovine colostrum, soybeans, egg white), which inhibit the action of trypsin.

tryp·sin·o·gen, tryp·so·gen (trip-sin′ō-jen, trip′sō-jen) An inactive protein secreted by the pancreas that is converted into trypsin by the action of enteropepsidase. SYN protrypsin.

tryp·ta·mine (TA) (trip′tă-mēn, -min) A decarboxylation product of L-tryptophan that occurs in plants and certain foods. It raises the blood pressure through vasoconstrictor action, by the release of norepinephrine at postganglionic sympathetic nerve endings, and is believed to be one of the agents responsible for hypertensive episodes after therapy with monoamine oxidase inhibitors.

tryp·tic (trip′tik) Relating to trypsin, as tryptic digestion.

tryp·to·phan (trip′tŏ-fan) A nutritionally essential amino acid; the L-isomer is a component of proteins.

tryp·to·pha·nu·ria (trip′tŏ-fă-nyūr′ē-ă) Enhanced urinary excretion of tryptophan.

t test (test) SYN Student *t*-test.

T tube (tūb) Tube shaped like a T, the top of which is placed within a tubular structure such as the common bile duct and the stem placed through the skin; used for decompression.

T tu·bule (tū′byūl) The transverse tubule that passes from the sarcolemma across a myofibril of striated muscle; it is the intermediate tubule of the triad.

tu·bal (tū′băl) Relating to a tube, especially the uterine tube.

tu·bal a·bor·tion (tū′băl ă-bōr′shŭn) Extrusion of the product of conception through the fimbriated end of the oviduct or through a rupture of an oviduct; aborted ectopic pregnancy, the pregnancy having originated in a uterine tube. SYN aborted ectopic pregnancy.

tu·bal li·ga·tion (tū′băl lī-gā′shŭn) Interruption of the continuity of the uterine tubes.

tu·bal preg·nan·cy (tū′băl preg′năn-sē) Development of an impregnated ovum in the uterine tube.

tube, tub·ing (tūb, tūb′ing) [TA] **1.** A hollow cylindric structure or canal. **2.** A hollow cylinder or pipe.

tube feed·ing (tūb fēd′ing) Administering nutrition or other fluids by means of a tube inserted directly into the enteral tract when a patient is unable to swallow.

tu·ber, pl. **tu·ber·a** (tū′bĕr, -ă) **1.** [TA] A localized swelling; a knob. **2.** A short, fleshy, thick, underground stem of plants, such as the potato.

tu·ber·cle (tū′bĕr-kĕl) [TA] **1.** A nodule, especially in an anatomic, not pathologic, sense. SYN tuberculum (1) [TA]. **2.** A circumscribed, rounded, solid elevation on the skin, mucous membrane, or surface of an organ. **3.** A slight elevation from the surface of a bone giving attachment to a muscle or ligament. **4.** DENTISTRY a small elevation arising on the surface of a tooth. **5.** A granulomatous lesion due to infection by *Mycobacterium tuberculosis*.

tu·ber·cle ba·cil·lus (tū′bĕr-kĕl bă-sil′ŭs) **1.** SYN *Mycobacterium tuberculosis.* **2.** SYN *Mycobacterium bovis.*

tu·ber·cu·lar, tu·ber·cu·lat·ed, tu·ber·cu·late (tū-bĕr′kyū-lăr, -lăt-ĕd, -lāt) Pertaining to or characterized by tubercles or small nodules. Cf. tuberculous.

tu·ber·cu·lid (tū-bĕr′kyū-lid) A lesion of the skin or mucous membrane due to hypersensitivity to mycobacterial antigens disseminated from a distant site of active tuberculosis.

tu·ber·cu·lin test (tū-bĕr′kyū-lin test) A dermatologic procedure in which tuberculin or its purified protein derivative is injected into the skin; the result is read on the basis of local induration occurring in 48–72 hours.

tu·ber·cu·li·tis (tū-bĕr′kyū-lī′tis) Inflammation of any tubercle.

tu·ber·cu·lo·cele (tū-bĕr′kyū-lō-sēl) Tuberculosis of the testes.

tu·ber·cu·lo·fi·broid (tū-bĕr′kyū-lō-fī′broyd) A discrete, well-circumscribed, usually spheroidal, moderately to extremely firm encapsulated nodule formed during healing in a focus of tuberculous granulomatous inflammation.

tu·ber·cu·loid (tū-bĕr′kyū-loyd) Resembling tuberculosis or a tubercle.

tu·ber·cu·loid lep·ro·sy (tū-bĕr′kyū-loyd lep′rŏ-sē) A benign, stable, and resistant form of the disease in which the lepromin reaction is strongly positive and in which the lesions are erythematous, insensitive, infiltrated plaques with clear-cut edges. SYN smooth leprosy.

tu·ber·cu·lo·ma (tū-bĕr′kyū-lō′mă) A rounded tumorlike but nonneoplastic mass, usually in the lungs or brain, due to localized tuberculous infection.

tu·ber·cu·lo·sis (TB) (tū-bĕr′kyū-lō′sis) A specific disease caused by *Mycobacterium tuberculosis,* which may affect almost any tissue or organ of the body, with the most common seat of the disease being the lungs. A high incidence exists among injecting drug abusers.

tu·ber·cu·lo·sis cu·tis ver·ru·co·sa (tū-bĕr′kyū-lō′sis kyū′tis ver′rū-kō′să) Tuberculous skin lesion having a warty surface with a chronic inflammatory base seen on the hands in adults and lower limbs in children, with marked hypersensitivity to tuberculous antigens. SEE ALSO postmortem wart. SYN tuberculous wart.

tu·ber·cu·lo·stat·ic (tū-bĕr′kyū-lō-stat′ik) Relating to an agent that inhibits the growth of tubercle bacilli.

tu·ber·cu·lous (tū-bĕr′kyū-lŭs) Relating to or affected by tuberculosis. Cf. tubercular.

tu·ber·cu·lous ab·scess (tū-bĕr′kyū-lŭs ab′ses) An abscess caused by the tubercle bacillus. SYN cold abscess (2).

tu·ber·cu·lous lym·phad·e·ni·tis (tū-bĕr′kyū-lŭs lim-fad′ĕ-nī′tis) Disorder resulting from infection by *Mycobacterium tuberculosis;* tuberculosis of the lymph nodes. SYN tuberculosis lymphadenitis.

tu·ber·cu·lous men·in·gi·tis (TBM) (tū-bĕr′kyū-lŭs men′in-jī′tis) Inflammation of the cerebral leptomeninges marked by the presence of granulomatous inflammation; usually confined to the base of the brain and is accompanied in children by an accumulation of spinal fluid in the ventricles.

tu·ber·cu·lum, pl. **tu·ber·cu·la** (tū-bĕr′kyū-lŭm, -lă) [TA] **1.** SYN tubercle (1). **2.** A circumscribed, rounded, solid elevation on the skin, mucous membrane, or surface of an organ. **3.** A slight elevation from the surface of a bone giving attachment to a muscle or ligament.

tu·ber·cu·lum ar·thri·ti·cum (tū-bĕr′kyū-lŭm ahr-thrit′i-kŭm) **1.** SYN Heberden nodes. **2.** Any gouty concretion in or around a joint.

tu·ber·os·i·ty (tū′bĕr-os′i-tē) [TA] A large tubercle or rounded elevation, especially from the surface of a bone. SYN tuberositas.

tu·ber·ous (tū′bĕr-ŭs) Knobby, lumpy, or nodular; presenting many tubers or tuberosities.

tu·ber·ous scle·ro·sis (tū′bĕr-ŭs skler-ō′sis) Phacomatosis characterized by the formation of multisystemic hamartomas producing seizures, mental retardation, and angiofibromas of the face; the cerebral and retinal lesions are glial nodules;

other skin lesions are hypopigmented macules, shagreen patches, and periungual fibromas. SYN Bourneville disease, epiloia.

tubo- Combining form denoting tubular, a tube. SEE ALSO salpingo-.

tu·bo·ab·dom·i·nal (tū′bō-ăb-dom′i-năl) Relating to a uterine tube and the abdomen.

tu·bo·ab·dom·i·nal preg·nan·cy (tū′bō-ăb-dom′i-năl preg′năn-sē) Ectopic pregnancy occurring partly in the fimbriated end of the infundibulum of the uterine tube and partly in the abdominal cavity.

tu·bo·lig·a·men·tous (tū′bō-lig′ă-men′tŭs) Relating to the uterine tube and the broad ligament of the uterus.

tu·bo·o·var·i·an, tubo-ovarian (TO) (tū′bō-ō-var′ē-ăn) Relating to the uterine tube and the ovary.

tu·bo·o·var·i·an preg·nan·cy (tū′bō-ō-var′ē-ăn preg′năn-sē) Ectopic pregnancy occurring partly in the infundibulum of the uterine tube also involving the ovary.

tu·bo·per·i·to·ne·al (tū′bō-per′i-tŏ-nē′ăl) Relating to the uterine tubes and the peritoneum.

tu·bo·plas·ty (tū′bō-plas-tē) SYN salpingoplasty.

tu·bo·re·tic·u·lar struc·ture (tū′bō-rĕ-tik′yū-lar strŭk′shŭr) Tubules 20–30 nm in length that lie within cisterns of smooth endoplasmic reticulum; observed in connective tissue diseases such as systemic lupus erythematosus, and in various cancers and virus infections.

tu·bo·tor·sion, tu·ba·tor·sion (tū′bō-tōr-shŭn, tū′bă-) Twisting of a tubular structure.

tu·bo·tym·pan·ic, tu·bo·tym·pa·nal (tū′bō-tim-pan′ik, -tim′pă-năl) Relating to the auditory tube and the tympanic cavity of the ear.

tu·bo·u·ter·ine (tū′bō-yū′tĕr-in) Relating to a uterine tube and the uterus.

tu·bu·lar (tū′byū-lăr) Relating to or of the

form of a tube or tubule. SYN tubuliform.

tu·bu·lar ad·e·no·ma (tū′byū-lăr ad′ĕ-nō′mă) 1. Benign neoplasm composed of epithelial tissue resembling a tubular gland. 2. Dysplastic polyp of the colonic mucosa that is considered a potential precursor of adenocarcinoma.

tu·bu·lar car·ci·no·ma (tū′byū-lăr kahr′si-nō′mă) A well-differentiated form of ductal breast carcinoma with invasion of the stroma by small epithelial tubules.

tu·bu·lar vision (tū′byū-lăr vizh′ŭn) A constriction of the visual field, as though one were looking through a hollow cylinder or tube.

tu·bule (tū′byūl) [TA] A small tube.

tu·bu·lin (tū′byū-lin) A protein subunit of microtubules.

tu·bu·lo·ac·i·nar gland (tū′byū-lō-as′i-năr gland) A gland with secretory elements that are elongated acini.

tu·bu·lo·glo·mer·u·lar feed·back (tū′byū-lō-glō-mer′yū-lăr fēd′bak) A blood flow control mechanism operating in the kidneys that limits changes in glomerular filtration rate.

tu·bu·lo·in·ter·sti·tial (TI) (tū′byū-lō-in-tĕr-stish′ăl) Denotes all tubular and connective tissue elements of the kidney, except the glomerulus.

tu·bu·lo·in·ter·sti·tial neph·ri·tis (tū′byū-lō-in-tĕr-stish′ăl nĕ-frī′tis) Inflammation affecting renal tubules and interstitial tissue, with infiltration by plasma cells and mononuclear cells; seen in lupus nephritis, allograft rejection, and methicillin sensitization.

tu·bu·lor·rhex·is (tū′byū-lō-rek′sis) A pathologic process characterized by necrosis of the epithelial lining in localized segments of renal tubules, with focal rupture or loss of the basement membrane.

tuft (tŭft) A cluster, clump, or bunch, as of hairs.

tug, tug·ging (tŭg, tŭg′ing) A pulling or dragging movement or sensation.

tu·la·re·mi·a (tū′lă-rē′mē-ă) A disease caused by *Francisella tularensis* and transmitted to humans from rodents through the bite of a deer fly, and other bloodsucking insects; can also be acquired directly through the bite of an infected animal or through handling of an infected animal's carcass. SYN deerfly fever, rabbit fever, tularaemia.

Tul·li·o phe·nom·e·non (tŭ'lē-ō fĕ-nom'ĕ-non) Vertigo and nystagmus in response to high-intensity sounds, especially those of low frequency.

tu·me·fa·cient (tū'mĕ-fā'shĕnt) Causing or tending to cause swelling. SYN tumefactive.

tu·me·fac·tion (tū'mĕ-fak'shŭn) 1. A swelling. SYN tumentia. 2. SYN tumescence.

tu·me·fy (tū'mĕ-fī) To swell or to cause to swell.

tu·mes·cence, tur·ges·cence (tū-mes'ĕns, tŭr-jes') The condition of being or becoming tumid. SYN tumefaction (2), turgescence.

tu·mes·cent lip·o·suc·tion (tū-mes'ĕnt lip'ō-sŭk-shŭn) Liposuction performed after subcutaneous infusion of lidocaine solution and the use of microcannulae.

tu·mid (tū'mid) Swollen, as by congestion, edema, hyperemia.

tu·mor (tū'mŏr) 1. Any swelling or tumefaction. 2. SYN neoplasm. 3. One of the four signs of inflammation (tumor, calor, dolor, rubor) enunciated by Celsus.

tu·mor an·gi·o·gen·ic fac·tor (TAF) (tū'mŏr an'jē-ō-jen'ik fak'tŏr) A substance released by a solid tumor that induces formation of new blood vessels to supply the tumor.

tu·mor an·ti·gens (tū'mŏr an'ti-jenz) 1. Those antigens that may be frequently associated with tumors or may be specifically found on tumor cells of the same origin (tumor specific). 2. Tumor antigens may also be associated with replication and transformation by certain DNA tumor viruses, including adenoviruses and papovaviruses. SYN neoantigens.

tu·mor-as·so·ci·at·ed an·ti·gen (tū'mŏr-ă-sō'sē-ā-tĕd an'ti-jen) Antigens that are highly correlated with certain tumor cells. They are not usually found, or are found to a lesser extent, on normal cells.

tu·mor bur·den (tū'mŏr bŭr'dĕn) The total mass of tumor tissue carried by a patient with cancer.

tu·mor·i·ci·dal (tū'mŏr-i-sī'dăl) Denoting an agent destructive to tumors.

tu·mor·i·gen·e·sis (tū'mŏr-i-jen'ĕ-sis) Production of a new growth or growths.

tu·mor·i·gen·ic (tū'mŏr-i-jen'ik) Causing or producing tumors.

tu·mor in si·tu (TIS) (tū'mŏr in sit'ū) A lesion that remains localized to a given site; one that has not yet metastasized.

tu·mor ly·sis syn·drome (TLS) (tū'mŏr lī'sis sin'drōm) Hyperphosphatemia, hypocalcemia, hyperkalemia, and hyperuricemia after induction chemotherapy of malignant neoplasms.

tu·mor mark·er (tū'mŏr mahr'kĕr) A substance released into the circulation by tumor tissue; its detection in the serum indicates the presence and specific type of tumor.

tun·gi·a·sis (tŭng-gī'ă-sis) Infestation with sand fleas (*Tunga penetrans*).

tu·nic (tū'nik) Coat or covering; one of the enveloping layers of a part, especially one of the coats of a blood vessel or other tubular structure.

tu·ni·ca al·bu·gin·e·a (tū'ni-kă al-byū-jin'ē-ă) A dense white collagenous tunic surrounding a structure.

tu·ni·ca al·bu·gin·e·a of tes·tis (tū'ni-kă al-byū-jin'ē-ă tes'tis) [TA] Thick white fibrous membrane forming the outer coat or capsule of the testis. SYN tunica albuginea testis [TA], peridydimis.

tu·ni·ca ex·ter·na (tū'ni-kă eks-ter'nă) [TA] 1. The outer of two or more enveloping layers of any structure; 2. Specifically, the outer fibroelastic coat of a blood or lymph vessel.

tu·ni·ca in·ti·ma (tū'ni-kă in'ti-mă) [TA] The innermost coat of a blood or lymphatic vessel.

tu·ni·ca me·di·a (tū′ni-kă mē′dē-ă) [TA] The middle, usually muscular, coat of an artery or other tubular structure. SYN media (1).

tu·ni·ca pro·pri·a (tū′ni-kă prō′prē-ă) The special envelope of a part, as distinguished from the peritoneal or other investment common to several parts.

tu·ni·ca re·flex·a (tū′ni-kă rē-fleks′ă) The reflected layer of the tunica vasculosa testis that lines the scrotum.

tu·ni·ca vas·cu·lo·sa (tū′ni-kă vas-kyū-lō′să) Any vascular layer.

tun·ing fork (TF) (tūn′ing fōrk) Steel or magnesium-alloy instrument roughly resembling a two-pronged fork, the vibrations of the prongs which, when struck, give a musical tone of restricted bandwidth; used to test hearing and vibratory sensation.

tun·nel (tŭn′ĕl) An elongated passageway, usually open at both ends.

tur·ban tu·mor (tŭr′băn tū′mŏr) Multiple cylindromas of the scalp which, when overgrown, may resemble a turban.

tur·bid (tŭr′bid) Clouded, as by sediment or insoluble matter in a solution.

tur·bi·dim·e·ter (tŭr′bi-dim′ĕ-tĕr) An instrument for measuring turbidity.

tur·bi·dim·e·try (tŭr-bi-dim′ĕ-trē) A method for determining the concentration of a substance in a solution by the degree of cloudiness or turbidity it causes or by the degree of clarification it induces in a turbid solution.

tur·bid·i·ty (turb) (tŭr-bid′i-tē) The quality of being turbid, of losing transparency because of sediment or insoluble matter.

tur·bi·nal (tŭr′bi-năl) SYN turbinated body (1).

tur·bi·nate, tur·bi·nat·ed (tŭr′bi-nāt, -năt-ĕd) **1.** Shaped like a top. **2.** Any of the turbinated bones. SEE ALSO inferior nasal concha, middle nasal concha, superior nasal concha, supreme nasal concha.

tur·bi·nat·ed bod·y (tŭr′bi-năt-ĕd bod′ē) A concha with its covering of mucous membrane and other soft parts. SYN turbinal.

tur·bi·nec·to·my (tŭr′bi-nek′tŏ-mē) Surgical removal of a turbinated bone.

tur·bi·not·o·my (tŭr′bi-not′ŏ-mē) Incision into or excision of a turbinated body.

Türck de·gen·er·a·tion (tērk dĕ-jen′ĕr-ā′shŭn) Degeneration of a nerve fiber and its sheath distal to the point of injury or section of the axon; usually applied to degeneration within the central nervous system.

Tur·cot syn·drome (tur-kō′ sin′drōm) Rare and distinctive form of multiple intestinal polyposis associated with brain tumors.

turf toe (tŭrf tō) Sprain and subsequent inflammation of the first metatarsophalangeal joint.

tur·gor (tŭr′gŏr) Fullness.

tu·ris·ta (tū-rēs′tă) SYN Montezuma's revenge.

tur·mer·ic (tŭr′mĕr-ik) *Avoid the misspelling/mispronunciation tumeric.* **1.** Curcuma. **2.** A spice prepared from the dried rhizome of *Curcuma domestica*, used in herbal medicine for promotion of wound healing.

Turn·er tooth (tŭr′nĕr tūth) Enamel hypoplasia involving a solitary permanent tooth; related to infection in the primary tooth that preceded it or to trauma during odontogenesis.

turn·o·ver (TO) (tŭrn′ō-vĕr) The quantity of a material metabolized or processed, usually within a given length of time.

turn·o·ver num·ber (tŭrn′ō-vĕr nŭm′bĕr) The number of substrate molecules converted into product in an enzyme-catalyzed reaction under saturating conditions per unit time per unit quantity of enzyme; e.g., $k_{cat} = V_{max}/[E_{total}]$.

tus·sive frem·i·tus (tŭs′iv frem′i-tŭs) A form of palpable vibration similar to the vocal, produced by a cough.

tus·sive syn·co·pe (tŭs′iv sin′kŏ-pē) Fainting as a result of a coughing spell, caused by persistent increased intrathoracic pressure diminishing venous return to the heart, thus lowering cardiac output; most often occurs in heavy-set male smokers who have chronic bronchitis. SYN Charcot vertigo.

tu·ta·men, pl. **tu·ta·mi·na** (tū-tā´men, -mē-nă) Any defensive or protective structure.

tu·ta·mi·na oc·u·li (tū-tā´mi-nă ok´yū-lī) The eyebrows, eyelids, and eyelashes.

T wave (wāv) The next deflection in the electrocardiogram after the QRS complex; represents ventricular repolarization.

twid·dler's syn·drome (twid´lĕrz sin´drŏm) Condition in which a cardiac pacemaker wire is pulled out of position in the heart with rotation of the subcutaneous pacemaker by the patient's "twiddling."

twig (twig) One of the finer terminal branches of an artery; a small branch or small ramus.

twi·light state (twī´līt stāt) Disordered consciousness during which actions may be performed without the conscious volition of the affected person and with no memory of such actions.

twin (twin) **1.** One of two children or animals born at one birth. **2.** Double; growing in pairs. May be monozygotic or dizygotic.

twin-trans·fu·sion syn·drome (twin-tranz-fyū´zhŭn sin´drŏm) The anastomoses of blood vessels in twins with a single placenta that leads to a disproportionate amount of nutrients being received by one twin at the expense of the other.

twitch (twich) **1.** To jerk spasmodically. **2.** A momentary spasmodic contraction of a muscle fiber.

two-step ex·er·cise test (tū´step ek´sĕr-sīz test) A test used mainly for coronary insufficiency.

ty·ing for·ceps (tī´ing fōr´seps) An instrument with flat, smooth tips used in ophthalmic surgery.

ty·lec·to·my (tī-lek´tŏ-mē) Surgical removal of a localized swelling or tumor. SEE ALSO lumpectomy.

tyl·i·on, pl. **tyl·i·a** (til´ē-on, -ă) A craniometric point at the middle of the anterior edge of the prechiasmatic sulcus.

ty·lo·sis, pl. **ty·lo·ses** (tī-lō´sis, -sēz) Formation of a callosity (tyloma).

ty·lox·a·pol (tī-loks´ă-pol) A detergent and mucolytic agent used as an aerosol to liquify sputum.

tym·pa·nal (tim´pă-năl) **1.** SYN tympanic (1). **2.** Resonant. **3.** SYN tympanitic (2).

tym·pa·nec·to·my (tim´pă-nek´tŏ-mē) Excision of the tympanic membrane.

tym·pan·ic (tim-pan´ik) **1.** Relating to the tympanic cavity or membrane. SYN tympanal (1). **2.** Resonant. **3.** SYN tympanitic (2).

tym·pan·ic cells (tim-pan´ik selz) [TA] Numerous groovelike depressions in the walls of the tympanic cavity, communicating with the tubal air cells. SYN cellulae tympanicae [TA], tympanic air cells.

tym·pan·ic ther·mom·e·ter (tim-pan´ik thĕr-mom´ĕ-tĕr) An electronic thermometer that measures temperature by scanning the tympanic membrane.

tym·pa·ni·tes, tym·pa·nism (tim-pă-nī´tēz, tim´pă-nizm) Swelling of the abdomen resulting from gas in the intestinal or peritoneal cavity. SYN meteorism.

tym·pa·nit·ic (tim´pă-nit´ik) **1.** Referring to tympanites. SYN tympanous. **2.** Denoting the quality of sound elicited by percussing over the inflated intestine or a large pulmonary cavity. SYN tympanal (3), tympanic (3).

tym·pa·nit·ic res·o·nance (tim´pă-nit´ik rez´ŏ-năns) SYN tympany.

tym·pa·ni·tis (tim´pă-nī´tis) SYN myringitis.

tympano-, tympan-, tympani- Combining forms denoting eardrum, tympanites, or tympanic membrane.

tym·pa·no·cen·te·sis (tim´pă-nō-sen-tē´sis) Puncture of the tympanic membrane with a needle to aspirate middle ear fluid.

tym·pan·o·gram (tim´pă-nō-gram) A visual depiction of the relative compliance and impedance of the structures of the middle ear in response to pressure changes in the external ear canal.

tym·pa·no·mas·toi·dec·to·my (tim´pă-nō-mas´toy-dek´tŏ-mē) SYN radical mastoidectomy.

tym·pa·no·mas·toi·di·tis (tim′pă-nō-mas′toy-dī′tis) Inflammation of the middle ear and the mastoid cells.

tym·pa·nom·et·ry (tim′pă-nom′ĕ-trē) Technique that measures immittance of the middle ear at various levels of air pressure; helpful in the diagnosis of middle ear effusion, pharyngotympanic (auditory) tube function, and otitis media.

tym·pa·no·plas·ty (tim′pă-nō-plas′tē) Operative correction of a damaged middle ear.

tym·pan·o·scle·ro·sis (tim′pan-ō-skler-ō′sis) Formation of dense connective tissue in the middle ear, often causing hearing loss when the ossicles are involved.

tym·pan·os·to·my tube (tim′pan-os′tŏ-mē tūb) A small tube inserted through the tympanic membrane after myringotomy to aerate the middle ear; often used as therapy for serous otitis media.

tym·pa·not·o·my (tim′pă-not′ŏ-mē) SYN myringotomy.

tym·pan·o·ves·tib·u·lar coup·ling (tim′pă-nō-ves-tib′yū-lăr kŭp′ling) A direct or indirect coupling between the tympanic structures and a vestibular end organ; results in abnormal responsiveness of the vestibular end organ to pressure changes or sound vibrations transmitted from the tympanic structures.

tym·pa·ny (tim′pă-nē) A low-pitched, resonant, drumlike note obtained by percussing the surface of a large air-filled space. SYN tympanitic resonance.

Tyn·dall phe·nom·e·non (tin′dăl fĕ-nom′ĕ-non) Visibility of floating particles in gases or liquids when illuminated by a ray of sunlight and viewed at right angles to the illuminating ray. SYN Tyndall effect.

type (tīp) [TA] **1.** The usual form or a composite that all others of the class resemble more or less closely. SEE ALSO constitution, habitus, personality. **2.** CHEMISTRY a substance in which the arrangement of the atoms in a molecule may be taken as representative of other substances in that class. SYN typus.

type A be·ha·vior, type A per·son·al·i·ty (tīp bē-hāv′yŏr, pĕr′sŏn-al′i-tē) Behavior pattern characterized by aggressiveness, ambitiousness, restlessness, and a strong sense of time urgency.

New research has revealed that it is hostile behavior, which can be commingled with other type A traits, which is associated with increased risk for coronary heart disease.

type B be·ha·vior, type B per·son·al·i·ty (tīp bē-hāv′yŏr, pĕr′sŏn-al′i-tē) A behavior pattern characterized by the absence or obverse of type A behavior characteristics.

type cul·ture (tīp kŭl′chŭr) A type strain of microorganism preserved in a culture collection as the standard or quality-control strain.

Type 1 di·a·be·tes (tīp dī′ă-bē′tēz) Condition characterized by high blood glucose levels caused by a total lack of insulin. Occurs when the body's immune system attacks the insulin-producing beta cells in the pancreas and destroys them. The pancreas then produces little or no insulin. Type 1 diabetes develops most often in young people but can appear in adults. SYN growth-onset diabetes, juvenile-onset diabetes.

Type 2 di·a·be·tes (tīp dī′ă-bē′tēz) Condition characterized by high blood glucose levels caused by either a lack of insulin or the body's inability to use insulin efficiently. Type 2 diabetes develops most often in middle-aged and older adults but can appear in young people.

type I fa·mil·i·al hy·per·li·po·pro·teine·mi·a (tīp fă-mil′ē-ăl hī′pĕr-lip′ō-prō-tēn-ē′mē-ă) Increased hematologic lipoprotein levels characterized by the presence of large amounts of chylomicrons and triglycerides in the plasma when the patient has a normal diet, and their disappearance on a fat-free diet. It is accompanied by bouts of abdominal pain, hepatosplenomegaly, pancreatitis, and eruptive xanthomas; autosomal recessive inheritance. SYN familial fat-induced hyperlipemia.

type II fa·mil·i·al hy·per·li·po·pro·teine·mi·a (tīp fă-mil′ē-ăl hī′pĕr-lip′ō-prō-tēn-ē′mē-ă) Increased hematologic lipoprotein levels characterized by increased plasma levels of β-lipoproteins, cholesterol, and phospholipids, but normal triglycerides levels. Homozygotes have xanthomatosis and frank clinical atherosclerosis as young adults. The primary defect is a deficiency of apoprotein of very low density lipoproteins.

type III fa·mil·i·al hy·per·lip·o·pro·tein·e·mi·a (tŭp fă-mil′ē-ăl hī-pĕr-lip′ō-prō-tēn-ē′mē-ă) Increased hematologic lipoprotein levels characterized by increased plasma levels of low-density lipoprotein, β-lipoproteins, pre-β-lipoproteins, cholesterol, phospholipids, and triglycerides; frequent eruptive xanthomas and atheromatosis, particularly coronary artery disease; biochemical defect lies in apolipoproteins. SYN familial hypercholesterolemia with hyperlipemia.

type spe·cies (tŭp spē′shēz) Name of the single species or of one of the species of a genus or subgenus when the name of the genus or subgenus was originally validly published.

typh·lec·ta·sis (tif-lek′tă-sis) Dilation of the cecum.

typhlo-, typhl- **1.** Combining forms denoting the cecum. SEE ALSO ceco-. **2.** Combining forms denoting blindness.

typh·lo·dic·li·di·tis (tif′lō-dik′li-dī′tis) Inflammation of the ileocecal valve.

typh·lo·li·thi·a·sis (tif′lō-li-thī′ă-sis) Presence of fecal concretions in the cecum.

ty·phoid (tī′foyd) **1.** Typhuslike; stuporous from fever. **2.** SYN typhoid fever.

ty·phoi·dal (tī-foyd′ăl) Relating to or resembling typhoid fever.

ty·phoid car·ri·er (tī′foyd kar′ē-ĕr) One who can transmit typhoid fever virus to others without being clinically ill.

ty·phoid fe·ver (tī′foyd fē′vĕr) An acute infectious disease caused by *Salmonella typhi;* characterized by a continued fever, severe physical and mental depression, an eruption of rose-colored spots on the chest and abdomen, tympanites, often diarrhea, and sometimes intestinal hemorrhage or perforation of the bowel; average duration is 4 weeks, although aborted forms and relapses are not uncommon; the lesions are located chiefly in the lymph follicles of the intestines (Peyer patches), the mesenteric glands, and the spleen. SYN enteric fever (1), typhoid (2).

ty·phoid vac·cine (TV) (tī′foyd vak-sēn′) Suspension of *Salmonella typhi* inactivated either by heat or by chemical (acetone) with an added preservative.

ty·phus (tī′fŭs) A group of acute infectious and contagious diseases caused by rickettsiae that are transmitted by arthropods. Three main forms exist: louse borne, murine, and scrub; also called jail, camp, or ship fever.

ty·phus vac·cine (tī′fŭs vak-sēn′) Formaldehyde-inactivated suspension of *Rickettsia prowazekii* grown in embryonated eggs; effective against louse-borne (epidemic) typhus.

Tyr Abbreviation for tyrosine and its radicals.

ty·ra·mine (TYR) (tī′ră-mēn, tir′ă-) Decarboxylated tyrosine, a sympathomimetic amine having an action in some respects resembling that of epinephrine; present in ergot, mistletoe, ripe cheese, beer, red wine, and putrefied animal matter; elevated in people with tyrosinemia type II.

ty·ro·ke·to·nu·ri·a (tī′rō-kē′tō-nyūr′ē-ă) The urinary excretion of ketonic metabolites of tyrosine, such as *p*-hydroxyphenylpyruvic acid.

ty·ro·ma (tī-rō′mă) A caseous tumor.

ty·ro·sine (Tyr, Y) (tī′rō-sēn) An α-amino acid present in most proteins.

ty·ro·si·ne·mi·a (tī′rō-si-nē′mē-ă) Inherited disorders of tyrosine metabolism associated with elevated blood concentration of tyrosine, and enhanced urinary excretion of tyrosine and tyrosyl compounds. SYN hypertyrosinemia.

ty·ro·si·nu·ri·a (tī′rō-si-nyūr′ē-ă) The excretion of tyrosine in the urine.

ty·ro·sy·lu·ri·a (tī′rō-sil-yūr′ē-ă) Enhanced urinary excretion of certain metabolites of tyrosine, such as *p*-hydroxyphenylpyruvic acid; present in tyrosinosis, scurvy, pernicious anemia, and other diseases.

Tzanck test (tsahnk test) Examination of fluid from a bullous lesion for Tzanck cells. The periphery of these cells is basophilic and the nucleus is spheric and enlarged with prominent nucleoli; characteristic of lesions due to varicella, herpes zoster, herpes simplex, and pemphigus vulgaris.

U

u·bi·qui·nol (yū′bi-kwi′nol) The reduction product of a ubiquinone.

u·bi·qui·tin-pro·te·ase path·way (yū-bik′kwi-tin-prō′tē-ās path′wā) Highly selective pathway in which a small protein cofactor, ubiquitin, couples with protein substrate to catalyze proteolytic destruction by proteases.

ul·cer (ŭl′sĕr) An erosive or penetrating lesion on a cutaneous or mucosal surface, usually with inflammation. Cf. erosion. SYN ulcus.

ul·cer·ate (ŭl′sĕr-āt) To form an ulcer.

ul·cer·a·tion (ŭl-sĕr-ā′shŭn) **1.** The formation of an ulcer. **2.** An ulcer or aggregation of ulcers.

ul·cer·a·tive (ŭl′sĕr-ă-tiv) Relating to, causing, or marked by an ulcer or ulcers.

ul·cer·a·tive co·li·tis (ŭl′sĕr-ă-tiv kō-lī′tis) A chronic disease of unknown cause characterized by ulceration of the colon and rectum, with rectal bleeding, mucosal crypt abscesses, inflammatory pseudopolyps, abdominal pain, and diarrhea; frequently causes anemia, hypoproteinemia, and electrolyte imbalance.

ul·cer·o·gen·ic (ŭl′sĕr-ō-jen′ik) Ulcer-producing.

ul·cer·o·mem·bra·nous (ŭl′sĕr-ō-mem′bră-nŭs) Relating to or characterized by ulceration and the formation of a false membrane.

ul·cer·ous (ŭl′sĕr-ŭs) Relating to, affected with, or containing an ulcer.

ul·cus (ŭl′kŭs, ŭl′ser-ă) SYN ulcer.

u·le·gy·ri·a (yū′lē-jī′rē-ă) Cerebral cortex defect characterized by narrow and distorted gyri; may be congenital, but is usually due to ischemic damage.

u·ler·y·the·ma (yū′ler-i-the′mă) Scarring with erythema.

u·le·ryth·e·ma oph·ry·og·e·nes (yū′ler-i-the′mă of-rē-oj′ē-nes) Folliculitis of the eyebrows resulting in scarring and alopecia.

Ull·mann line (ŭl′mahn līn) The line of displacement in spondylolisthesis.

Ull·mann syn·drome (ŭl′mahn sin′drōm) A systemic angiomatosis due to multiple arteriovenous malformations.

ul·na (U, uln), gen. and pl. **ul·nae** (ŭl′nă, -nē) [TA] The medial and larger of the two bones of the forearm. SYN cubitus (2).

ul·nad (ŭl′nad) In a direction toward the ulna.

ul·nar, ul·na·ris (ŭl′năr, -nā′ris) [TA] Relating to the ulna, or to any of the structures (artery, nerve) named from it; relating to the ulnar or medial aspect of the upper limb.

ul·nar de·vi·a·tion (ŭl′năr dē′vē-ā′shŭn) Movement of the wrist toward the little finger side of the forearm.

ul·nar re·flex (ŭl′năr rē′fleks) Pronation and adduction of the hand caused by tapping the styloid process of the ulna.

ul·no·car·pal (ŭl′nō-kahr′păl) Relating to the ulna and the carpus, or to the ulnar side of the wrist.

ul·no·ra·di·al (ŭl′nō-rā′dē-ăl) Relating to both ulna and radius.

u·lo·der·ma·ti·tis (yū′lō-dĕr′mă-tī′tis) Inflammation of the skin with destruction of tissue and scar formation.

♻ **-ulose** Combining form for a ketose.

♻ **ultra-** Prefix meaning excess, exaggeration, beyond.

ul·tra·brach·y·ce·phal·ic (ŭl′tră-brak′ē-sĕ-fal′ik) Denoting an extremely short skull, one with a cephalic index of at least 90.

ul·tra·cen·tri·fuge (ŭl′tră-sen′tri-fyūzh) A high-speed centrifuge by means of which large molecules (e.g., of protein or nucleic acids) are caused to sediment at practicable rates.

ul·tra·di·an (ŭl-tră′dē-ăn) Relating to biologic variations or rhythms occurring in cycles more frequent than every 24 hours. Cf. circadian, infradian.

ul·tra·fil·ter (ŭl′tră-fil′tĕr) A semipermeable membrane (collodion, fish bladder, or filter paper impregnated with gels) used as a filter to separate colloids and large molecules from water and small molecules, which pass through.

ul·tra·fil·tra·tion (ŭl′tră-fil-trā′shŭn) Filtration through a semipermeable membrane or any filter that separates colloid solutions from crystalloids or separates particles of different size in a colloid mixture.

ul·tra·mi·cro·scope (ŭl′tră-mī′krŏ-skōp) A microscope that uses refracted light for visualizing objects not visible with the ordinary microscope when direct light is used.

ul·tra·mi·cro·tome (ŭl′tră-mī′krŏ-tōm) A device used in cutting sections 0.1 mcm thick, or less, for electron microscopy.

ul·tra·son·ic (US) (ŭl′tră-son′ik) Relating to energy waves similar to those of sound but of higher frequencies (above 20,000 Hz).

ul·tra·son·ic car·di·og·ra·phy (UCG, USCG) (ŭl′tră-son′ik kahr′dē-og′ră-fē) SYN echocardiography.

ul·tra·son·ic clean·ing (ŭl′tră-son′ik klēn′ing) In dentistry, the use of a high-frequency vibrating point to remove deposits from tooth structure.

ul·tra·son·ics (ŭl′tră-son′iks) The science and technology of ultrasound, its characteristics and phenomena.

ul·tra·son·ic scal·er (ŭl′tră-son′ik skā′lĕr) An ultrasonic instrument that uses high frequency vibration to remove adherent deposits from the teeth.

ul·tra·so·nog·ra·phy (ŭl′tră-sŏ-nog′ră-fē) The location, measurement, or delineation of deep structures by measuring the reflection or transmission of high-frequency or ultrasonic waves. SYN echography, sonography.

ul·tra·sound (ŭl′tră-sownd) Sound having a frequency greater than 30,000 Hz.

ul·tra·sound im·ag·ing (ŭl′tră-sownd im′ăj-ing) SEE ultrasonography.

ul·tra·struc·ture (ŭl′tră-strŭk′chŭr) Struc-

tures or particles seen with the electron microscope. SYN fine structure.

ul·tra·vi·o·let, ul·tra·vi·o·let rays (ŭl′tră-vī′ŏ-lĕt, rāz) Denoting electromagnetic rays at higher frequency than the violet end of the visible spectrum.

ul·tra·vi·o·let A (UVA) (ŭl′tră-vī′ŏ-lĕt) Ultraviolet radiation from 320–400 nm that tans skin but is very weakly carcinogenic.

ul·tra·vi·o·let B (UVB) (ŭl′tră-vī′ŏ-lĕt) Ultraviolet radiation from 290–320 nm that most effectively causes sunburning and tanning; excessive UVB exposure is a cause of cancer of fair skin.

ul·tra·vi·o·let C (UVC) (ŭl′tră-vī′ŏ-lĕt) Ultraviolet radiation from 200–290 nm; UVC in sunlight does not reach earth's surface; germicidal and mercury arc lamps may cause sunburn and photokeratitis.

ul·tra·vi·o·let ker·a·to·con·junc·ti·vi·tis (ŭl′tră-vī′ŏ-lĕt ker′ă-tō-kŏn-jŭngk′ti-vī′tis) Acute disorder resulting from exposure to intense ultraviolet irradiation.

ul·tra·vi·o·let lamp (ŭl′tră-vī′ŏ-lĕt lamp) Appliance that emits rays in the ultraviolet band of the spectrum. SEE ALSO ultraviolet.

ul·tra·vi·o·let mi·cro·scope (ŭl′tră-vī′ŏ-lĕt mī′krŏ-skōp) Device with quartz and fluorite optics that allows transmission of light waves shorter than those of the visible spectrum.

ul·tra·vi·o·let ra·di·a·tion (ŭl′tră-vī′ŏ-lĕt rā′dē-ā′shŭn) A wavelength of electromagnetic radiation that is shorter than that of visible light.

um·ber co·don (ŭm′bĕr kō′don) The termination codon UGA. SYN opal codon.

um·bil·i·cal (ŭm-bil′i-kăl) Relating to the umbilicus. SYN omphalic.

um·bil·i·cal cord (ŭm-bil′i-kăl kōrd) The definitive connecting stalk between the embryo or fetus and the placenta. SYN funiculus umbilicalis [TA], funis (1).

um·bil·i·cal fas·ci·a (ŭm-bil′i-kăl fash′

ē-ă) [TA] Thin fascial layer interposed between the transversalis fascia. SYN fascia umbilicalis [TA], umbilical prevesical fascia, umbilicovesical fascia.

um·bil·i·cal fis·tu·la (ŭm-bil´i-kăl fis´tyū-lă) Passage connecting the intestine or urachus at the umbilicus.

um·bil·i·cal her·ni·a (ŭm-bil´i-kăl hĕr´nē-ă) One in which intestine or omentum protrudes through the abdominal wall under the skin at the umbilicus. SEE ALSO omphalocele. SYN exomphalos (2), exumbilication (2).

um·bil·i·cal re·gion (ŭm-bil´i-kăl rē´jŏn) [TA] Central locus of the abdomen about the umbilicus. SYN regio umbilicalis [TA].

um·bil·i·cal ring (ŭm-bil´i-kăl ring) [TA] An opening in the linea alba through which pass the umbilical vessels in the fetus. SYN anulus umbilicalis [TA].

um·bil·i·cal ves·i·cle (ŭm-bil´i-kăl ves´i-kĕl) A saclike structure formed from the exocelomic cavity of a blastocyst.

um·bil·i·cate, um·bil·i·cat·ed (ŭm-bil´i-kāt, -kāt-ĕd) Of navel shape; pitlike; dimpled.

um·bil·i·ca·tion (ŭm-bil´i-kā´shŭn) 1. A pit or navellike depression. 2. Formation of a depression at the apex of a papule, vesicle, or pustule.

um·bil·i·cus, na·vel, gen. and pl. **um·bil·i·ci** (ŭm-bil´i-kŭs, nā´vĕl, ŭm-bil´i-sī´) [TA] The pit in the center of the abdominal wall marking the site where the umbilical cord entered in the fetus.

um·bo, gen. **um·bo·nis,** pl. **um·bo·nes** (ŭm´bō, ŭm-bō´nis, -nēz) [TA] A projecting point of a surface.

un·bal·anced trans·lo·ca·tion (ŭn-băl´ănst trans´lō-kā´shŭn) Condition due to fertilization of a gamete containing a translocation chromosome by a normal gamete; if compatible with life, the person has 46 chromosomes but a segment of the translocation chromosome is represented three times in each cell and a partial or complete trisomic state exists.

un·cal (ŭngk´ăl) Denoting or relating to the uncus.

un·ci·form (ŭn´si-fŏrm) SYN uncinate.

Un·ci·nar·i·a (ŭn´si-nar´ē-ă) A genus of nematode hookworms that infect various mammals; has been implicated in human cutaneous larva migrans.

un·ci·nate (ŭn´si-nāt) 1. Hooklike or hook-shaped. 2. Relating to an uncus or, specifically, to the uncinate gyrus (2) or a process of the pancreas or of a vertebra. SYN unciform.

un·ci·pres·sure (ŭn´si-presh´ŭr) Arrest of hemorrhage from a cut artery by pressure with a blunt hook.

un·comb·a·ble hair syn·drome (ŭn-kōm´ă-bĕl hār sin´drōm) A genetic disorder in which the hair, which is often silvery blond, is unruly and resists lying flat because of irregularly shaped hair shafts. SYN spun glass hair.

un·com·pen·sat·ed al·ka·lo·sis (ŭn-kom´pĕn-sā´tĕd al´kă-lō´sis) Disorder in which the pH of body fluids is elevated because of lack of the compensatory mechanisms of compensated alkalosis.

un·com·pet·i·tive in·hib·i·tor (ŭn´kŏm-pet´i-tiv in-hib´i-tŏr) A type of enzyme inhibitor in which the inhibiting compound only binds to the enzyme-substrate complex.

un·com·ple·ment·ed (ŭn-kom´plĕ-ment´ĕd) Not united with complement and therefore inactive.

un·con·di·tion·ed re·flex (UCR, UR) (ŭn´kŏn-dish´ŭnd rē´fleks) Instinctive reflex not dependent on previous learning or experience.

un·con·di·tion·ed re·sponse (UCR, UR) (ŭn´kŏn-dish´ŭnd rĕ-spons´) Reaction, such as salivation, which is a part of the animal or human repertoire. Cf. conditioned response.

un·con·di·tion·ed stim·u·lus (ŭn´kŏn-dish´ŭnd stim´yū-lŭs) That which elicits an unconditioned response; e.g., food is an unconditioned stimulus for salivation, which in turn is an unconditioned response in a hungry animal.

un·con·scious (ŭn-kon´shŭs) 1. Lacking awareness. 2. PSYCHOANALYSIS psychic structure comprising the drives and feelings of which one is unaware. SYN insensible (1).

un·co·ver·te·bral (ŭn'kō-vĕr'tĕ-brăl) Pertaining to or affecting the uncinate process of a vertebra.

unc·tu·ous (ŭngk'shū-ŭs) Greasy or oily.

un·cus, pl. **un·ci** (ŭng'kŭs, ŭn'sī) [TA] 1. Any hook-shaped process. 2. Anterior hooked extremity of the parahippocampal gyrus on the basomedial surface of the temporal lobe. SYN uncinate gyrus.

un·dec·y·len·ic ac·id (ŭn'des-i-len'ik as'id) One present in small amounts in sweat; used with its zinc salt in ointments. SYN zincundecate.

un·der·bite (ŭn'dĕr-bīt) A nontechnical term applied to mandibular underdevelopment or to excessive maxillary development.

un·der·cut (ŭn'dĕr-kŭt) 1. That portion of a tooth that lies between the survey line (height of contour) and the gingivae. 2. The contour of a cross-section of a residual ridge or dental arch that would prevent the insertion of a denture. 3. The contour of a flasking stone that interlocks in such a way as to prevent the separation of the parts.

un·der·drive pac·ing (ŭn'dĕr-drīv pās'ing) Electrical stimulation of the heart at a rate lower than that of an existing tachycardia; designed to capture the heart between beats.

un·der·nu·tri·tion (ŭn'dĕr-nū-trish'ŭn) A form of malnutrition resulting from a reduced supply of food or from inability to digest, assimilate, and use the necessary nutrients.

un·der·sens·ing (ŭn'dĕr-sens'ing) Nonsensing of the intracardiac atrial or ventricular depolarization signal by a pacemaker.

un·der·wa·ter weigh·ing (ŭn'dĕr-waw'tĕr wā'ing) Assessment of body volume by measuring a person's weight in air and again under water; loss in scale weight (corrected for water density) equals body volume. Body density (body mass:volume ratio) is then used to compute percent body fat. SYN hydrostatic weighing.

un·der·weight (ŭn'dĕr-wāt') A ratio of height-to-waist circumference below an acceptable range for healthy people.

un·de·scend·ed testis (ŭn'dĕ-send'ĕd tes'tis) One that has not descended into the scrotum.

un·de·ter·mined ni·tro·gen (ŭn'dĕ-tĕr'mind nī'trŏ-jĕn) The nitrogen of blood, urine, and other fluids, other than urea, uric acid, amino acids, and the like, that can be directly estimated; in blood it amounts to about 25 mg per 100 mL.

un·dif·fer·en·ti·at·ed (ŭn'dif-ĕr-en'shē-ā-tĕd) Embryonic, immature, or with no special structure or function.

un·dif·fer·en·ti·at·ed cell (ŭn-dif-ĕr-en'shē-ā-tĕd sel) Primordial cell that has not assumed the morphologic and functional characteristics it will later acquire.

un·dif·fer·en·ti·at·ed type fe·vers (ŭn'dif-fĕr-en'shē-ā'ted tīp fē'vĕrz) A term applied to illnesses resulting from infection by any one of the arboviruses pathogenic for humans, in which the only constant manifestation is fever.

un·dif·fer·en·ti·a·tion (ŭn-dif'er-en'shē-ā'shŭn) State in which cells lose normal organization and become unrecognizable.

un·dine (ŭn'dēn, -dīn) Small glass flask used in irrigation of the conjunctiva.

un·dis·placed frac·ture (ŭn'dis-plāst' frak'chŭr) Breakage of bone in which the bones remain aligned; resolution is usually accomplished with a cast, rather than surgical intervention.

un·du·late (ŭn'dyū-lăt) Having an irregular, wavy border.

un·e·qual cleav·age (ŭn-ē'kwăl klē'văj) That producing blastomeres of different sizes at the two poles.

un·e·qual pulse (ŭn-ē'kwăl pŭls) Pulses that differ in the right and left sides of the periphery.

un·es·ter·i·fied free fat·ty ac·id (FFA, UFA) (ŭn-es-ter'i-fīd frē fat'ē as´id) Those that occur in plasma due to lipolysis in adipose tissue or when plasma triacylglycerols are taken into tissues.

un·gual (ŭng´gwăl) Relating to a nail or the nails. SYN unguinal.

un·guic·u·late (ŭng-gwik´yū-lăt) Having nails or claws.

uni- Combining form denoting one, single, not paired; corresponds to G. mono-.

u·ni·ax·i·al (yū´nē-ak´sē-ăl) Having but one axis; growing chiefly in one direction.

u·ni·ax·i·al joint (yū´nē-aks´ē-ăl joynt) One in which movement is around one axis only.

u·ni·cam·er·al, u·ni·cam·er·ate (yū´ni-kam´ĕr-ăl, -kam´ĕ-răt) SYN monolocular.

u·ni·cel·lu·lar (yū´ni-sel´yū-lăr) Composed of but one cell, as in the protozoa (or protozoans).

u·ni·cel·lu·lar gland (yū´ni-sel´yū-lăr gland) A single secretory cell such as a mucous goblet cell.

u·ni·corn u·ter·us (yū´ni-kōrn yū´tĕr-ŭs) One in which only one lateral half exists, the other being undeveloped or absent.

u·ni·di·rec·tion·al block (yū´ni-dĭr-ek´shŭn-ăl blok) Block that prevents passage of an impulse when it approaches from one direction but not from the other.

u·ni·form (yū´ni-fōrm) 1. Having but one form. 2. Of the shape as another object.

u·ni·ger·mi·nal (yū´ni-jĕr´mi-năl) Relating to a single germ or zygote, e.g., monozygotic. SYN monozygous, monozygotic.

u·ni·glan·du·lar (yū´ni-gland´yū-lăr) Involving, relating to, or containing but one gland.

u·ni·lam·i·nar, u·ni·lam·i·nate (yū´ni-lam´i-năr, -lam´i-năt) Having but one layer or lamina.

u·ni·lat·e·ral (unilat) (yū´ni-lat´ĕ-răl) Confined to one side only.

u·ni·lat·er·al lo·bar em·phy·se·ma (yū´ni-lat´ĕr-ăl lō´bahr em´fi-sē´mă) A state in which the roentgenographic density of one lung (or one lobe) is markedly less than the density of the other(s) because of the presence of air trapped during expiration. SYN Swyer-James syndrome (1).

un·i·lat·er·al ne·glect (yū´ni-lat´ĕr-ăl nĕg-lekt´) Damage to one side of the brain that causes patient's inability to perceive stimuli on the opposite side of the body.

u·ni·loc·u·lar (yū´ni-lok´yū-lăr) Having but one compartment or cavity, as in a fat cell.

u·ni·loc·u·lar cyst (yū´ni-lok´yū-lăr sist) Single sac lesion.

u·ni·loc·u·lar joint (yū´ni-lok´yū-lăr joynt) Articulation in which an intraarticular disc is incomplete or absent.

u·ni·mo·lec·u·lar (yū´ni-mŏ-lek´yū-lăr) Denoting a single molecule.

u·ni·oc·u·lar (yū´nē-ok´yū-lăr) 1. Relating to one eye only. 2. Having vision in only one eye.

un·ion (yūn´yŭn) 1. Joining two or more bodies. 2. Structural adhesion or growing together of the edges of a wound. 3. Healing of a fracture represented by the development of continuity between fractured fragments.

uni·po·lar (yū´ni-pō´lăr) 1. Having but one pole. 2. Situated at one extremity only of a cell.

uni·po·lar de·pres·sion (yū´ni-pō´lăr dē-presh´ŭn) Pervasive deadened mood that occurs without a manic phase.

unique pro·vi·der iden·ti·fi·ca·tion num·ber (UPIN) (yū-nēk´ prō-vī´dĕr ī-den´ti-fi-kā´shŭn num´bĕr) Numeric designation, much like a Social Security number, which is used to determine a provider of a health care service for insurance purposes.

uni·sep·tate (yū´ni-sep´tāt) Having but one septum or partition.

U

unit (yū'nit) **1.** Single person or thing. **2.** A standard of measure, weight, or any other quality, by multiplications or fractions of which a scale or system is formed. **3.** A group of people or things considered as a whole because of mutual activities or functions. **4.** SYN international unit.

Uni·ted States A·dopt·ed Names (USAN) (yū-nī'těd stāts ǎ-dop'těd nāmz) Designation for nonproprietary names (for drugs) adopted by the USAN Council in cooperation with the manufacturers concerned; the designation USAN is applicable only to nonproprietary names coined since June 1961.

Uni·ted States Pub·lic Health Ser·vice (USPHS) (yū-nī'těd stāts pŭb'lik helth sěr'vis) A bureau of the U.S. Department of Health and Human Services, served by a corps of medical officers presided over by the Surgeon General, concerned with scientific research, domestic and insular quarantine, administration of government hospitals, publication of sanitary reports, and statistics.

u·nit fi·brils (yū'nit fī'brilz) Those that comprise a collagen fiber, ranging from 20–200 nm and averaging about 100 nm in diameter (substantially larger in tendons), with cross-striations averaging 64 nm. SYN collagen fibrils.

unit mem·brane (yū'nit mem'brān) The trilaminar structure of the plasmalemma and other intercellular membranes, when seen in cross-section with the electron microscope, composed of two electron-dense laminae separated by a less dense lamina.

unit of pen·i·cil·lin (in·ter·na·tion·al) (yū'nit pen'i-sil'in in'tĕr-nash'ŭn-ăl) The penicillin activity of 0.6 mcg of penicillin G.

uni·va·lent an·ti·body (yū'ni-vā'lěnt an'ti-bod-ē) An "incomplete" form of antibody that may coat antigen, but which according to the "lattice theory" does not have a second receptor for attachment to another molecule of antigen. SYN incomplete antibody (1).

uni·ver·sal an·ti·dote (yū'ni-věr'săl an'ti-dōt) Outdated mixture of two parts activated charcoal, one tannic acid, and one magnesium oxide administered to poisoned patients; mixture is ineffective and no longer used; activated charcoal is useful.

uni·ver·sal do·nor (yū'ni-věr'săl dō'nŏr) In blood grouping, a person belonging to group O.

uni·ver·sal pre·cau·tions (yū'ni-věr'săl prē-kaw'shŭnz) In health care, acting under the assumption that all bodily fluids may be contaminated with a contagious agent or pathogen.

uni·ver·sal re·cip·i·ent (yū'ni-věr'săl rē-sip'ē-ěnt) A patient with an AB blood type; one who can receive any other blood type.

Un·i·ver·si·ty of Wis·con·sin so·lu·tion (UW solution) (yū'ni-věr'si-tē wis-kon'sin sŏ-lū'shŭn) Normokalemic, intracellular colloid injected into vital organs during harvesting to preserve function before transplantation. SYN UW.

un·my·e·li·nat·ed (ŭn-mī'ě-li-nā-těd) Denoting nerve fibers lacking a myelin sheath.

un·my·e·li·nat·ed fi·bers (ŭn-mī'ě-li-nā-těd fī'běrz) In the central nervous system, a fiber having no myelin covering; a naked axon; in the peripheral nervous system, represented by all axons lying in troughs in a single Schwann cell (Schwann cell unit); a slow conducting fiber. SYN gray fibers, Remak fibers, nonmedullated fibers.

Un·na ne·vus (ū'nah nē'vŭs) Capillary stain on nape of neck. SYN erythema nuchae.

un·phys·i·o·log·ic (ŭn-fiz'ē-ō-loj'ik) Pertaining to conditions in the organism that are abnormal; can be used to refer to subjecting the body to abnormal amounts of substances normally present.

un·sat·ur·at·ed (ŭn-sach'ŭr-āt-ěd) **1.** Not saturated. **2.** Denoting a chemical compound in which all the affinities are not satisfied, so that still other atoms or radicals may be added to it. **3.** ORGANIC CHEMISTRY denoting compounds containing double and/or triple bonds.

un·sat·ur·at·ed fat·ty ac·id (ŭn-sach'ŭr-āt-ěd fat'ē as'id) One with a carbon chain that possesses one or more double or triple bonds; called unsaturated because it is capable of absorbing additional hydrogen.

up·per air·way (ŭp'ĕr ār'wā) Part of the respiratory tract that extends from the nares or mouth to and including the larynx.

up·per air·way ob·struc·tion (ŭp'ĕr ār'wā ŏb-strŭk'shŭn) Blockage of the throat, larynx, or trachea, in any combination.

up·per gas·tro·in·tes·tin·al ser·ies (ŭp'ĕr gas'trō-in-tes'ti-năl sĕr'ēz) Fluoroscopic-radiographic examination of the esophagus, stomach, and duodenum; a contrast medium, usually barium sulfate, is introduced.

up·per limb (UL) (ŭp'ĕr lim) [TA] Shoulder, arm, forearm, wrist, and hand. SYN membrum superius [TA], superior member [TA], superior limb, upper extremity.

up·take (UPT) (ŭp'tāk) The absorption by a tissue of some substance, food material, mineral, and its permanent or temporary retention.

u·ra·cil (U) (yūr'ă-sil) A pyrimidine (base) present in ribonucleic acid.

uraemia [Br.] SYN uremia.

uraemic coma [Br.] SYN uremic coma.

u·ra·ni·um (U) (yūr-ā'nē-ŭm) A radioactive metallic element, first substance ever shown capable of supporting a self-sustaining chain reaction.

♻ **urano-, uranisco-** Combining forms denoting the hard palate.

ura·nos·chi·sis, ura·nis·co·chasm (yūr'ă-nos'ki-sis, -nis'kō-kazm) Cleft of the hard palate.

ura·no·staph·y·lo·plas·ty, ura·no·staph·y·lor·rha·phy (yūr'ă-nō-staf'i-lō-plas'tē, -lōr'ă-fē) Repair of a cleft of both hard and soft palates. SYN uranostaphylorrhaphy.

ura·no·staph·y·los·chi·sis, ura·no·ve·lo·schi·sis (yūr'ă-nō-staf'i-los'ki-sis, -vĕ-los'ki-sis) Cleft of the soft and hard palates. SYN uranoveloschisis.

ur·ar·thri·tis (yūr'ahr-thrī'tis) Gouty inflammation of a joint.

urate (yūr'āt) A salt of uric acid.

ura·te·mia (yūr'ă-tē'mē-ă) The presence of urates, especially sodium urate, in the blood.

urate ox·i·dase (yūr'āt ok'si-dās) Copper-containing, oxygen-requiring oxidoreductase that oxidizes uric acid; used to diagnose increased uric acid levels. SYN uricase.

ura·to·sis (yūr'ă-tō'sis) Any morbid condition due to the presence of urates in the blood or tissues.

ura·tu·ri·a (yūr'ă-tyūr'ē-ă) The passage of an increased amount of urates in the urine.

Ur·ban op·er·a·tion (ŭr'băn op-ĕr-ā'shŭn) Extended radical mastectomy, including en bloc resection of internal mammary lymph nodes, part of the sternum, and costal cartilages.

♻ **ure-, urea-, ureo-** Combining forms denoting urea; urine. SEE ALSO urin-.

urea (yūr-ē'ă) Chief end product of nitrogen metabolism in mammals, formed in the liver, and excreted in normal adult human urine in the amount of about 32 g a day (about 89% of the nitrogen excreted from the body); used as a diuretic in kidney function tests and topically for various skin disorders.

urea clear·ance (yūr-ē'ă klĕr'ăns) *C* with a subscript indicating the substance removed; volume of plasma (or blood) that would be completely cleared of urea by 1 minute's excretion of urine.

urea con·cen·tra·tion test (yūr-ē'ă kon'sĕn-trā'shŭn test) A clinical assessment of the amount of urea in a liquid.

urea cy·cle (yūr-ē'ă sī'kĕl) The sequence of chemical reactions, occurring primarily in the liver, which results in the production of urea. SYN Krebs-Henseleit cycle, Krebs ornithine cycle, Krebs urea cycle.

urea frost, ure·mic frost (yūr-ē'ă frawst, yūr-ē'mik) Powdery deposits on the skin, especially the face, of urea and uric acid salts due to excretion of nitrogenous compounds in the sweat; seen in severe uremia.

ur·e·a·gen·e·sis (yūr-ē'ă-jen'ĕ-sis) Formation of urea, usually referring to the metabolism of amino acids to urea.

ur·ea ni·tro·gen (UN) (yūr-ē'ă nī'trŏ-jĕn) Portion of nitrogen in a biologic sample, such as blood or urine, which derives from its content of urea. SEE ALSO blood urea nitrogen.

Ur·e·a·plas·ma (yūr-ē'ă-plaz'mă) A genus of microaerophilic to anaerobic, nonmotile bacteria containing gram-negative, predominantly coccoidal to coccobacillary elements that are approximately 0.3 mcm in diameter, which frequently grow in short filaments. SYN T-mycoplasma.

ure·ase (yūr'ē-ās) An enzyme that catalyzes the hydrolysis of urea to carbon dioxide and ammonia; used as an antitumor enzyme.

ur·e·de·ma (yūr'ē-dē'mă) Swelling due to infiltration of urine into subcutaneous tissues.

ure·mia, ur·i·ne·mia (yūr-ē'mē-ă, -i-nē'mē) 1. An excess of urea and other nitrogenous waste in the blood. 2. The complex of symptoms due to severe persisting renal failure that can be relieved by dialysis. SYN azotemia, uraemia.

ure·mic breath (yūr-ē'mik breth) Characteristic odor in patients with chronic renal failure, variously described as "fishy," "ammoniac," and "fetid."

ure·mic co·ma (yūr-ē'mik kō'mă) A metabolic encephalopathy caused by renal failure. SYN uraemic coma.

ure·o·tel·ic (yū'rē-ō-tel'ik) Excreting nitrogen primarily in the form of urea.

ur·es·i·es·the·si·a (yūr-ē'sē-es-thē'zē-ă) The desire to urinate. SYN uriesthesia.

ure·ter (yūr'ē-tĕr) [TA] Thick-walled tube that conducts the urine from the renal pelvis to the bladder, abdominal and pelvic parts, is lined with transitional epithelium surrounded by smooth muscle, both circular and longitudinal, and is covered externally by a tunica adventitia.

ure·ter·al·gi·a (yūr-ē'tĕr-al'jē-ă) Pain in the ureter.

ure·ter·al re·im·plan·ta·tion (yūr-ē'tĕr-ăl rē'im-plan-tā'shŭn) SYN ureteroneocystostomy.

ure·ter·ec·ta·sia (yūr-ē'tĕr-ek-tā'zē-ă) Dilation of a ureter.

ure·ter·ec·to·my (yūr-ē'tĕr-ek'tŏ-mē) Excision of a segment or all of a ureter.

ure·ter·ic bud (yūr'ĕ-ter'ik bŭd) SYN metanephric diverticulum.

ur·e·ter·i·tis (yūr-ē'tĕr-ī'tis) Inflammation of a ureter.

uretero- Combining form denoting the ureter.

ur·e·ter·o·cele (yū-rē'tĕr-ō-sēl) Saccular dilation of the terminal portion of the ureter that protrudes into the lumen of the urinary bladder, probably due to a congenital stenosis of the ureteral meatus.

ur·e·ter·o·ce·lor·ra·phy (yūr-ē'tĕr-ō-sē-lōr'ă-fē) Excision and suturing of a ureterocele performed through an open cystotomy incision.

ur·e·ter·o·co·los·to·my, ur·e·ter·o·sig·moi·dos·to·my (yūr-ē'tĕr-ō-kŏ-los'tŏ-mē, -sig-moyd-os'tŏ-mē) Implantation of the ureter into the colon. SYN ureterosigmoidostomy.

ur·e·ter·o·cys·to·plas·ty (yūr-ē'tĕr-ō-sist'tŏ-plas-tē) Augmentation of the bladder using a native dilated ureter.

ur·e·ter·o·en·ter·os·to·my (yūr-ē'tĕr-ō-en'ter-os'tŏ-mē) Formation of an opening between a ureter and the intestine.

ur·e·ter·og·ra·phy (yūr-ē'tĕr-og'ră-fē) Radiography of the ureter after the direct injection of contrast medium.

ur·e·ter·o·il·e·al an·as·to·mo·sis (yūr-ē'tĕr-ō-il'ē-ăl ă-nas'tŏ-mō'sis) Connection between the ureter and an isolated segment of ileum.

ur·e·ter·o·il·e·o·ne·o·cys·tos·to·my

(yūr-ē′tĕr-ō-il′ē-ō-nē′ō-sis-tos′tŏ-mē) Restoration of the continuity of the urinary tract by anastomosis of the upper segment of a partially destroyed ureter to a segment of ileum, the lower end of which is then implanted into the bladder. SYN ileal ureter.

ur·e·ter·o·il·e·os·to·my (yūr-ē′tĕr-ō-il′ ē-os′tŏ-mē) Implantation of a ureter into an isolated segment of ileum that drains through an abdominal stoma.

ur·e·ter·o·li·thi·a·sis (yūr-ē′tĕr-ō-li-thī′ ă-sis) The formation or presence of a calculus or calculi in one or both ureters. SEE ALSO renal calculus.

ur·e·ter·o·li·thot·o·my (yūr-ē′tĕr-ō-li-thot′ŏ-mē) Removal of a stone lodged in a ureter.

ur·e·ter·ol·y·sis (yūr-ē′tĕr-ol′i-sis) Surgical freeing of the ureter from surrounding disease or adhesions.

ur·e·ter·o·ne·o·cys·tos·to·my (yūr-ē′tĕr-ō-nē′ō-sis-tos′tŏ-mē) An operation whereby a ureter is implanted into the bladder. SYN ureteral reimplantation, ureterocystostomy.

ur·e·ter·o·ne·phrec·to·my (yūr-ē′tĕr-ō-nĕ-frek′tŏ-mē) SYN nephroureterectomy.

ur·e·ter·op·a·thy (yū-rē′tĕr-op′ă-thē) Disease of the ureter.

ur·e·ter·o·pel·vic junc·tion (UPJ) (yūr-ē′tĕr-ō-pel′vik jŭngk′shŭn) Site of origin of the ureter from the renal pelvis, a common location for congenital or acquired obstruction.

ur·e·ter·o·plas·ty (yūr-ē′tĕr-ō-plas′tē) Surgical reconstruction of the ureters.

ur·e·ter·o·py·e·li·tis (yūr-ē′tĕr-ō-pī′ĕ-lī′tis) Inflammation of the pelvis of a kidney and its ureter.

ur·e·ter·o·py·e·log·ra·phy (yūr-ē′tĕr-ō-pī′ĕ-log′ră-fē) SYN pyelography.

ur·e·ter·o·py·e·lo·plas·ty, ur·e·ter·o·pel·vi·o·plas·ty (yūr-ē′tĕr-ō-pī′ĕ-lō-plas′tē, -pel′vē-ō-plas′tē) Surgical reconstruction of the ureter and of the pelvis of the kidney.

ur·e·ter·o·py·e·los·to·my (yūr-ē′tĕr-ō-pī′ĕ-los′tŏ-mē) Formation of a junction of the ureter and the renal pelvis.

ur·e·ter·o·py·o·sis (yūr-ē′tĕr-ō-pī-ō′ sis) An accumulation of pus in the ureter.

ur·e·ter·o·re·nal re·flux (yūr-ē′tĕr-ō-rē′năl rē′flŭks) Backward flow of urine from ureter into renal pelvis.

ur·e·ter·or·rha·gi·a (yūr-ē′tĕr-ō-rā′jē-ă) Hemorrhage from a ureter.

ur·e·ter·or·rha·phy (yūr-ē′tĕr-ōr′ă-fē) Suture of a ureter.

ur·e·ter·o·sig·moid an·as·to·mo·sis (yūr-ē′tĕr-ō-sig′moyd ă-nas′tŏ-mō′sis) Connection between the ureter and a segment of or entire sigmoid colon. SEE ALSO ureterocolostomy.

ur·e·ter·o·sig·moi·dos·to·my (yūr-ē′tĕr-ō-sig′moy-dos′tŏ-mē) SYN ureterocolostomy.

ur·e·ter·ot·o·my (yūr-ē′tĕr-ot′ŏ-mē) Incision and stenting of a narrow ureter.

ur·e·ter·o·ur·e·ter·os·to·my (yūr-ē′tĕr-ō-yūr-ē′tĕr-os′tŏ-mē) Establishment of an anastomosis between the two ureters or between two segments of the same ureter. SEE ALSO transureteroureterostomy.

ure·ter·o·ves·i·cal (UV) (yū-rē′tĕr-ō-ves′i-kăl) Relating to the ureter and the bladder.

ure·ter·o·ves·i·cos·to·my (yūr-ē′tĕr-ō-ves′i-kos′tŏ-mē) Surgical joining of a ureter to the bladder.

ure·thra (yūr-ē′thră) [TA] A canal leading from the bladder, discharging the urine externally. SYN urogenital canal.

ure·thral·gi·a (yūr-ē-thral′jē-ă) Pain in the urethra. SYN urethrodynia.

u·re·thral groove (yū-rē′thrăl grūv) The groove on the ventral surface of the embryonic penis that normally closes to form the penile portion of the urethra. SYN genital furrow.

ure·thral he·ma·tu·ri·a (yūr-ē′thrăl hē′mă-tyūr′ē-ă) Condition in which the site of bleeding is in the urethra.

ure·thral pa·pil·la, pa·pil·la ur·e·thra·lis (yūr-ē′thrăl pă-pil′ă, yū-rēth-rā′lis) Slight projection often present in the vestibule of the vagina marking the urethral orifice.

ure·thral syn·drome (yūr-ē′thrăl sin′drōm) Condition of uncertain etiology, characterized by urinary frequency, urgency, dysuria in the absence of specific infection, obstruction, or dysfunction. Suprapubic pain, hesitancy, and back pain may also occur. Usually seen in females.

ure·threc·to·my (yūr′ĕ-threk′tŏ-mē) Excision of a segment or of the entire urethra.

u·re·threm·or·rha·gi·a (yū-rē′threm-ŏ-rā′jē-ă) Bleeding from the urethra. SYN urethrorrhagia.

u·re·thrism (yū′rē-thrizm) Irritability or spasmodic stricture of the urethra.

ure·thri·tis (yūr′ĕ-thrī′tis) Inflammation of the urethra.

ure·thr·itis pet·ri·fi·cans (yūr′ĕ-thrī′tis pĕ-trif′i-kanz) Urethritis, sometimes of gouty origin, in which there is a deposit of calcareous matter in the wall of the urethra.

urethro-, urethr- Combining forms denoting the urethra.

ure·thro·cele (yūr-ē′thrō-sēl) Prolapse of the female urethra.

ure·thro·cu·ta·ne·ous fis·tu·la (yūr-ē′thrō-kyū-tā′nĕ-ŭs fis′tyū-lă) Passage between urethra and penile skin.

u·re·thro·cys·to·pex·y (yū-rē′thrō-sis′tŏ-pek′sē) Fixation of urethra and bladder for stress incontinence.

ure·throg·ra·phy (yū′rē-throg′ră-fē) Contrast radiography of the male or female urethra, by retrograde injection or during voiding of contrast medium in the bladder (cystourethrogram).

ure·thro·pe·nile (yū-rē′thrō-pē′nīl) Relating to the urethra and the penis.

ure·thro·per·i·ne·al (yū-rē′thrō-per′i-nē′ăl) Relating to the urethra and the perineum.

ure·thro·per·i·ne·o·scro·tal (yū-rē′thrō-per′i-nē′ŏ-skrō′tăl) Relating to the urethra, perineum, and scrotum.

ure·thro·plas·ty (yūr-ē′thrō-plas′tē) Surgical repair of the urethra, as performed to correct hypospadias, epispadias, or the effects of trauma.

ure·thro·pros·tat·ic (yū-rē′thrō-pros-tat′ik) Relating to the urethra and the prostate.

ure·thro·rec·tal (yū-rē′thrō-rek′tăl) Relating to the urethra and the rectum.

ure·thro·rrha·gi·a (yūr-ē′thrō-rā′jē-ă) SYN urethremorrhagia.

ure·thror·rha·phy (yūr′ĕ-thrōr′ă-fē) Suture of the urethra.

ure·thror·rhe·a (yūr′ĕ-thrō-rē′ă) An abnormal discharge from the urethra.

urethrorrhoea [Br.] SYN urethrorrhea.

ure·thro·scope (yūr-ē′thrō-skōp) An instrument to view the interior of the urethra.

ure·thro·scop·ic (yūr-ē′thrō-skop′ik) Relating to the urethroscope or to urethroscopy.

ure·thros·co·py (yūr-ē′thros′kŏ-pē) Inspection of the urethra with a urethroscope.

u·re·thro·stax·is (yūr-ē′thrō-stak′sis) The oozing of blood from the urethra.

ure·thro·ste·no·sis (yūr-ē′thrō-stĕ-nō′sis) Stricture of the urethra.

ure·thros·to·my (yūr′ĕ-thros′tŏ-mē) Surgical formation of a permanent opening between the urethra and the skin.

ure·thro·tome (yū-rē′thrō-tōm) An instrument for dividing a stricture of the urethra.

ure·throt·o·my (yūr′ĕ-throt′ŏ-mē) Surgical incision of a stricture of the urethra.

ure·thro·tri·gon·i·tis (yū-rē′thrō-tri′gŏ-nī′tis) Inflammation of the urethra and of the trigone of the urinary bladder.

ure·thro·vag·i·nal (yū-rē′thrō-vaj′i-năl) Relating to the urethra and the vagina.

ure·thro·ves·i·cal (yū-rē′thrō-ves′i-kăl) Relating to the urethra and bladder.

ure·thro·ves·i·co·pexy (yūr-ē′thrō-ves′i-kō-pek′sē) Surgical suspension of the urethra and bladder base to correct urinary stress incontinence.

-uretic Suffix denoting urine.

urge in·con·ti·nence, ur·gen·cy in·con·ti·nence (ŭrj in-kon′ti-nĕns, ŭr′jĕn-sē) Leakage of urine in the presence of a strong desire to void.

ur·gen·cy (ŭr′jĕn-sē) A strong desire to void.

uri-, uric-, urico- Combining forms denoting uric acid.

-uria Combining form denoting urine.

uric ac·id (yūr′ik as′id) White crystals, poorly soluble, contained in solution in urine of mammals; sometimes solidified in small masses as stones or crystals or in larger concretions as calculi; elevated levels associated with gout.

uri·co·su·ri·a (yūr′i-kō-syūr′ē-ă) Excessive amounts of uric acid in the urine.

uri·dine (yūr′i-dēn) Uracil ribonucleoside; one of the major nucleosides in RNAs; active in sugar metabolism. SYN 1-β-D-ribofuranosyluracil.

uri·dine 5′-di·phos·phate (UDP) (yūr′i-dēn dī-fos′fāt) A condensation product of uridine and pyrophosphoric acid.

uri·dine 5′-tri·phos·phate (UTP) (yūr′i-dēn trī-fos′fāt) The nucleoside esterified with triphosphoric acid at its 5′-position; the immediate precursor of uridylic acid residues in RNA.

uri·dro·sis (yūr′i-drō′sis) The excretion of urea or uric acid sweat.

uri·dyl·ic ac·id (yūr′i-dil′ik as′id) Uridine esterified by phosphoric acid. SYN uridine 5′-monophosphate.

urin-, urino- Combining forms denoting urine. SEE ALSO ure-, uro-.

uri·nal (yūr′in-ăl) A vessel into which urine is passed.

uri·nal·y·sis (yūr′in-al′i-sis) Analysis of urine.

uri·nary (yūr′i-nar-ē) Relating to urine.

uri·nary al·bu·min (yūr′i-nar-ē al-bū′min) The measurement of albumin concentration in urine that may reflect kidney dysfunction.

uri·nary cal·cu·lus (yūr′i-nar-ē kal′kyū-lŭs) Concretion in the kidney, ureter, bladder, or urethra.

uri·nary casts (yūr′i-nar-ē kasts) Casts discharged in the urine.

uri·nary fre·quen·cy (yūr′i-nar-ē frē′kwĕn-sē) Problematic increase in the urge to void.

uri·nary in·con·ti·nence (yūr′i-nar-ē in-kon′ti-nĕns) Involuntary leakage of urine.

uri·nary sand (yūr′i-nar-ē sand) Multiple small calculous particles passed in the urine of patients with nephrolithiasis; each particle is usually too small to cause significant symptoms or to be identified as a true calculus.

uri·nary sta·sis (yūr′i-nar-ē stā′sis) A cessation in urinary flow.

uri·nary tract (yūr′i-nar-ē trakt) The passage from the pelvis of the kidney to the urinary meatus through the ureters, bladder, and urethra.

uri·nary tract in·fec·tion (UTI) (yūr′i-nar-ē trakt in-fek′shŭn) Microbial infection, usually bacterial, of any part of the urinary tract.

uri·nate (yūr′i-nāt) To pass urine. SYN micturate.

uri·na·tion (yūr′i-nā′shŭn) The passing of urine. SYN miction, micturition (1), uresis.

urine (yūr′in) The fluid and dissolved substances excreted by the kidney.

urine os·mo·lal·i·ty test (yūr′in os′mō-lal′i-tē test) Assessment of the concentration of urine.

urine spe·cif·ic grav·i·ty (yūr′in spĕ-sif′ik grav′i-tē) The density of urine compared with the density of water.

u·ri·nif·er·ous tu·bule (yūr´i-nif´ĕr-ŭs tū´byūl) Functional renal unit, composed of a long convoluted portion and an intra-renal collecting duct.

u·ri·nog·e·nous, ur·og·e·nous (yūr´i-noj´ĕ-nŭs, yūr-oj´ĕ-nŭs) **1.** Producing or excreting urine. **2.** Of urinary origin.

u·ri·no·ma (yūr´i-nō´mă) A collection of extravasated urine. SYN urinary cyst.

u·ri·nom·e·ter, ur·om·e·ter (yūr´i-nom´ ĕ-tĕr, yūr-om´ĕ-tĕr) A hydrometer for determining the specific gravity of urine. SYN urogravimeter, urometer.

u·ri·nom·e·try (yūr´i-nom´ĕ-trē) The determination of the specific gravity of the urine.

u·ro·bi·lin (yūr´ō-bī´lin) Urinary pigment that gives a varying orange-red coloration to urine according to its degree of oxidation. SYN urohematin, urohematoporphyrin.

u·ro·bi·li·ne·mi·a (yūr´ō-bil´i-nē´mē-ă) The presence of urobilins in the blood.

u·ro·bi·lin·o·gen (yūr´ō-bi-lin´ō-jen) Precursor of urobilin.

u·ro·bil·i·nu·ri·a, ur·o·bil·in·o·ge·nu·ri·a (yūr´ō-bil´i-nyū´rē-ă, -i-nō-jĕ-nyūr´ē-ă) The presence in the urine of urobilins in excessive amounts, formed mainly from hemoglobin.

u·ro·cele, ur·o·sche·o·cele (yūr´ō-sēl, yūr-os´kē-ŏ-sēl) Extravasation of urine into the scrotal sac.

u·ro·che·si·a (yūr´ō-kē´zē-ă) Passage of urine from the anus.

ur·o·chrome (yūr´ō-krōm) The principal pigment of urine, a compound of urobilin and a peptide of unknown structure.

u·ro·dyn·i·a (yūr´ō-din´ē-ă) Pain on urination.

u·ro·flow·me·ter, ur·o·flo·me·ter (yūr´ō-flō´mē-tĕr) A device that measures urine flow rates during micturition.

u·ro·gen·i·tal sys·tem (yūr´ō-jen´i-tăl sis´tĕm) All organs concerned with reproduction and in the formation and discharge of urine.

ur·o·gram (yūr´ō-gram) The radiographic record obtained by urography.

ur·og·ra·phy (yūr-og´ră-fē) Radiography of any part of the urinary tract (kidneys, ureters, or bladder). SEE ALSO pyelography.

ur·o·li·thi·a·sis (yūr´ō-li-thī´ă-sis) Presence of calculi in the urinary system.

ur·o·log·ic, ur·o·log·ic·al (yūr´ō-loj´ik, -i-kăl) Relating to urology.

ur·ol·o·gy (yūr-ol´ō-jē) The medical specialty concerned with the study, diagnosis, and treatment of diseases of the genitourinary tract.

ur·on·cus (yūr-ong´kŭs) A urinary cyst.

ur·op·a·thy (yūr-op´ă-thē) Any disorder involving the urinary tract.

ur·o·phan·ic (yūr´ō-fan´ik) Appearing in urine; denoting any constituent, normal or pathologic, of urine.

ur·o·poi·e·sis (yūr´ō-poy-ē´sis) The production or secretion and excretion of urine.

ur·o·por·phy·rin (yūr´ō-pōr´fi-rin) Porphyrin excreted in the urine in porphyrinuria.

ur·o·ra·di·ol·o·gy (yūr´ō-rā´dē-ol´ō-jē) The study of the radiology of the urinary tract.

ur·os·che·sis (yūr-os´kĕ-sis) **1.** Retention of urine. **2.** Suppression of urine.

ur·os·co·py, ur·o·nos·co·py (yūr-os´ kŏ-pē, yūr´ō-nos´kŏ-pē) Examination of the urine, usually by means of a microscope.

ur·o·sep·sis (yūr´ō-sep´sis) **1.** Sepsis resulting from the decomposition of extravasated urine. **2.** Sepsis from obstruction of infected urine.

u·ro·the·li·al car·ci·no·ma (yūr´ō-thē´ lē-ăl kahr´si-nō´mă) Malignant neoplasm derived from transitional epithelium chiefly in the urinary bladder, ureters, or renal pelves.

ur·o·thor·ax (yūr´ō-thōr´aks) The presence of urine in the thoracic cavity.

ur·o·tox·ic (yūr´ō-tok´sik) Denotes something that is toxic to the bladder.

ur·so·di·ol,   **ur·so·de·ox·y·chol·ic ac·id** (ŭr´sō-dī´ōl, ŭr´sō-dō-ok´sēkŏ´lik as´id) A bile acid used to facilitate the dissolution of gallstones in patients; a potential alternative to cholecystectomy.

ur·ti·cant (ŭr´ti-kănt) Producing a wheal or other similar itching agent.

ur·ti·car·i·a (ŭr´ti-kar´ē-ă) An eruption of itching wheals, usually systemic; may be due to a state of hypersensitivity to foods or drugs, foci of infection, physical agents, or psychic stimuli. SYN hives (1), urtication (3).

ur·ti·ca·ri·a bul·lo·sa (ŭr-ti-kar´ē-ă bu-lō´să) Eruption of wheals capped with subepidermal vesicles. SYN urticaria vesiculosa.

ur·ti·ca·ri·a ma·cu·lo·sa (ŭr-ti-kar´ē-ă mak-yū-lō´să) Chronic form of urticaria with lesions of a red color and little edema.

ur·ti·ca·ri·a me·di·ca·men·to·sa (ŭr´ti-kar´ē-ă med-i-kă-men-tō´să) Urticarial form of drug eruption.

ur·ti·ca·ria pig·men·to·sa (ŭr´ti-kar´ē-ă pig-men-tō´să) Cutaneous mastocytosis resulting from an excess of mast cells in the superficial dermis, producing a chronic eruption characterized by flat or slightly elevated brownish papules that urticate when stroked.

ur·ti·cate (ŭr´ti-kāt) 1. To perform urtication. 2. Marked by the presence of wheals.

ur·ti·ca·tion (ŭr´ti-kā´shŭn) 1. A burning sensation resembling that produced by urticaria or resulting from nettle poisoning. 2. SYN urticaria.

USP unit (yū´nit) A unit as defined and adopted by the *United States Pharmacopeia.*

us·ti·lag·i·nism (ŭs´ti-laj´i-nizm) Poisoning by *Ustilago maydis* (corn smut), which produces burning, itching, hyperemia and other symptoms.

usu·al in·ter·sti·tial pneu·mo·ni·a of Lie·bow (yū´zhū-ăl in´tĕr-stish´ăl nū-mō´nē-ă lē´bō) A progressive inflammatory condition starting with diffuse alveolar damage and resulting in fibrosis and honeycombing over a variable time period.

uter·ine (yū´tĕr-in) Relating to the uterus.

uter·ine at·o·ny (yū´tĕr-in at´ŏ-nē) Failure of the myometrium to contract after delivery of the placenta; associated with excessive bleeding from the placental implantation site.

uter·ine cal·cu·lus (yū´tĕr-in kal´kyū-lŭs) A calcified myoma of the uterus.

uter·ine col·ic (yū´tĕr-in kol´ik) Painful cramps of the uterine muscle sometimes occurring at the menstrual period, or in association with uterine disease.

uter·ine con·trac·tion (yū´tĕr-in kŏn-trak´shŭn) Rhythmic activity of the myometrium associated with menstruation, pregnancy, or labor.

uter·ine in·er·ti·a, pri·mary uter·ine in·er·ti·a, sec·on·dar·y uter·ine in·er·ti·a, true uter·ine in·er·ti·a (yū´tĕr-in in-ĕr´shē-ă, prī´mar-ē, sek´ŏn-dar-ē, trū) Absence of effective uterine contractions during labor; occurs when the uterus fails to contract with sufficient force to effect continuous dilation or effacement of the cervix or descent or rotation of the fetal head, and when the uterus is easily indentable at the acme of contraction.

uter·ine souf·fle (yū´tĕr-in sū´fĕl) Blowing sound, synchronous with the cardiac systole of the mother, heard on auscultation of the pregnant uterus.

utero-, uter- Combining forms denoting the uterus. SEE ALSO hystero- (1), metr-.

uter·o·ab·dom·i·nal (yū´tĕr-ō-ăb-dom´i-năl) Relating to the uterus and the abdomen. SYN uteroventral.

u·ter·o·ab·dom·i·nal preg·nan·cy (yū´tĕr-ō-ăb-dom´i-năl preg´năn-sē) Development of the oocyte primarily in the uterus and later, in consequence of the rupture of the uterus, in the abdominal cavity.

uter·o·cer·vi·cal (yū´tĕr-ō-sĕr´vi-kăl) Relating to the cervix of the uterus.

uter·o·cys·tos·to·my (yū′tĕr-ō-sis-tos′tŏ-mē) Formation of a communication between the uterus (cervix) and the bladder.

u·ter·o·glo·bin (yū′tĕr-ō-glō′bin) Steroid-inducible homodimeric secreted protein with many biologic activities; found in blood and urine, but not in the kidneys. SYN bastokinin.

uter·o·o·var·i·an (yū′tĕr-ō-ō-var′ē-ăn) Relating to the uterus and an ovary.

uter·o·pel·vic (yū′tĕr-ō-pel′vik) Relating to the uterus and the pelvis.

uter·o·pla·cen·tal (yū′tĕr-ō-plă-sen′tăl) Relating to the uterus and the placenta.

uter·o·plas·ty (yū′tĕr-ō-plas′tē) Plastic surgery of the uterus. SYN hysteroplasty, metroplasty.

uter·o·sa·cral (yū′tĕr-ō-sā′krăl) Relating to the uterus and the sacrum.

uter·o·ton·ic (yū′tĕr-ō-ton′ik) **1.** Giving tone to the uterine muscle. **2.** An agent that overcomes relaxation of the muscular wall of the uterus.

uter·o·tub·al (yū′tĕr-ō-tū′băl) Pertaining to the uterus and the uterine tubes.

uter·o·vag·i·nal (yū′tĕr-ō-vaj′i-năl) Relating to the uterus and the vagina.

uter·o·ves·i·cal (yū′tĕr-ō-ves′i-kăl) Relating to the uterus and the urinary bladder.

uter·us, gen. and pl. **uter·i** (yū′tĕr-ŭs, -ī) [TA] The hollow muscular organ in which the blastocyst develops into a fetus. SYN metra, womb.

uter·us di·del·phys (yū′tĕr-ŭs dī-del′fis) Double uterus with double cervix and double vagina; due to failure of the paramesonephric ducts to unite during embryonic development.

ut·ri·cle (yū′tri-kĕl) **1.** A small sac or pouch. **2.** The larger of the two membranous sacs in the vestibule of the membranous labyrinth of the internal ear, lying in the elliptic recess. SYN utriculus [TA].

ut·ric·u·lar (yū-trik′yū-lăr) Relating to or resembling a utricle.

ut·ric·u·li·tis (yū-trik′yū-lī′tis) **1.** Inflammation of the internal ear. **2.** Inflammation of the prostatic utricle.

ut·ric·u·lo·sac·cu·lar (yū-trik′yū-lō-sak′yū-lăr) Relating to the utricle and the saccule of the labyrinth.

uvea (yū′vē-ă) The middle coat of the eyeball between the sclera and retina. It includes the iris and ciliary body (the anterior uvea) and the choroid.

uve·i·tis (yū′vē-ī′tis) Inflammation of the uveal tract: iris, ciliary body, and choroid.

uve·o·pa·rot·id fe·ver (yū′vē-ō-pă-rot′id fē′vĕr) Chronic enlargement of the parotid glands and inflammation of the uveal tract accompanied by a long-continued fever of low degree; a form of sarcoidosis. SYN Heerfordt disease.

uve·o·scle·ri·tis (yū′vē-ō-skler-ī′tis) Inflammation of the sclera involved by extension from the uvea.

uvi·form (yū′vi-fōrm) SYN botryoid.

uvu·la, pl. **u·vu·lae** (yū′vyū-lă, -lē) [TA] An appendant fleshy mass; a structure bearing a fancied resemblance to the palatine uvula.

uvu·lar (ū′vyū-lăr) Relating to the uvula.

uvu·lec·to·my (yū′vyū-lek′tŏ-mē) Excision of the uvula. SYN staphylectomy.

uvu·li·tis (yū′vyū-lī′tis) Inflammation of the uvula.

uvu·lo·pal·a·to·pha·ryn·go·plas·ty (yū′vyū-lō-pal′ă-tō-fă-rin′gō-plas′tē) SYN palatopharyngoplasty.

uvu·lop·to·sis, uvu·lap·to·sis (yū′vyū-lop-tō′sis, -lap-tō′sis) Relaxation or elongation of the uvula. SYN staphylodialysis, staphyloptosis.

uvu·lot·o·my (yū′vyū-lot′ŏ-mē) Any cutting operation on the uvula.

U wave (wāv) Waveform in an electrocardiographic tracing sometimes following the T wave and representing the completion of ventricular repolarization.

V

V_D Symbol for physiologic dead space.

V_max Abbreviation for maximum velocity.

V_T Symbol for tidal volume.

vac·ci·nal (vak′si-năl) Relating to vaccine or vaccination.

vac·ci·na·tion (vacc, Vx) (vak′si-nā′ shŭn) The act of administering a vaccine.

vac·cine (vak-sēn′) Any preparation intended for active immunologic prophylaxis, e.g., preparations of killed microbes of virulent strains or living microbes of attenuated strains, or microbial, fungal, plant, protozoal, or metazoan derivatives or product.

vac·cin·i·a (vak-sin′ē-ă) An infection, primarily local and limited to the site of inoculation, induced in humans by inoculation with the vaccinia virus, type species in the genus *Orthopoxvirus* to confer resistance to smallpox. SYN primary reaction, variola vaccine, variola vaccinia, variola vaccinia.

VACTERL syn·drome (vak-tĕrl′ sin′ drōm) Acronymic term for abnormalities of *v*ertebrae, *a*nus, *c*ardiovascular tree, *t*rachea, *e*sophagus, *r*enal system, and *l*imb buds associated with administration of sex steroids during early pregnancy.

vac·u·o·lar (vak′yū-ō′lăr) Relating to or resembling a vacuole.

vac·u·o·la·tion, vac·u·o·li·za·tion (vak′yū-ō-lā′shŭn, -lī-zā′shŭn) 1. Formation of vacuoles. 2. The condition of having vacuoles.

vac·u·ole (vak′yū-ōl) 1. A minute space in any tissue. 2. A clear space in the substance of a cell, sometimes degenerative, sometimes surrounding an engulfed foreign body and serving as a temporary cell stomach for the digestion of the body.

vac·u·um (vak′yūm) An empty space, one practically exhausted of air or gas.

vac·u·um pack tech·nique (vak′yūm pak tek-nēk′) Temporary closing of the abdomen by using a fenestrated plastic sheet over the intestine but under the anterior abdominal wall, followed by the placement of moistened pads with a suction catheter within the wound. The entire defect is then covered by a nonporous plastic sheet; permits drainage of the abdominal cavity by suction.

va·gal (vā′găl) Relating to the vagus nerve.

va·gal block (vā′găl blok) Injection of a substance that impedes neural perception in the vagal nerve.

va·gal tone (vā′găl tōn) The baseline level of parasympathetic impulses that control the heart rate.

va·gi·na, gen. and pl. **va·gi·nae** (vă-jī′nă, -nē) [TA] 1. SYN sheath (1). 2. The genital canal in the female, extending from the uterus to the vulva.

vag·i·nal a·tre·si·a (vaj′i-năl ă-trē′zē-ă) Congenital or acquired imperforation or occlusion of the vagina, or adhesion of the walls of the vagina. SYN colpatresia.

vag·i·nal ce·li·ot·o·my (vaj′i-năl sē′lē-ot′ŏ-mē) Opening the peritoneal cavity through the vagina.

vag·i·nal cor·ni·fi·ca·tion test (vaj′i-năl kōr′ni-fi-kā′shŭn test) Test for estrogenic activity, in which the appearance of cornified epithelial cells in a vaginal smear of a test animal indicates estrogen action.

vag·i·nal cuff (vaj′i-năl kŭf) Portion of the vaginal vault remaining open to the peritoneum following hysterectomy.

vag·i·nal hys·ter·ec·to·my (vaj′i-năl his′tĕr-ek′tŏ-mē) Removal of the uterus through the vagina.

vag·i·nal in·tra·ep·i·the·li·al ne·o·pla·si·a (VAIN, VIN) (vaj′i-năl in′tră-ep′i-thē′lē-ăl nē′ō-plā′zē-ă) Preinvasive squamous cell carcinoma (carcinoma in situ) limited to vaginal epithelium.

vag·i·nal or·i·fice (vaj′i-năl ōr′i-fis) The narrowest portion of the canal, in the floor of the vestibule posterior to the urethral orifice.

vag·i·nal plex·us (vaj′i-năl plek′sŭs) A system of nerves and blood vessels that serves the vagina.

vag·i·nal ring (vaj′i-năl ring) A silicon

ring impregnated with a drug (e.g., estrogen) designed for sustained release. SYN vaginal pouch.

vag·i·nec·to·my (vaj′i-nek′tŏ-mē) Excision of the vagina or a segment thereof. SYN colpectomy.

vag·i·nis·mus, vag·in·ism (vaj′i-niz′mŭs, -nizm) Painful spasm of the vagina preventing intercourse.

vag·i·ni·tis, pl. **vag·i·ni·ti·des** (vaj′i-nī′tis, -i-nit′i-dēz) Inflammation of the vagina.

vag·i·no·ab·dom·i·nal (vaj′i-nō-ăb-dom′i-năl) Relating to the vagina and the abdomen.

vag·i·no·dyn·i·a (vaj′i-nō-din′ē-ă) Vaginal pain. SYN colpodynia.

vag·i·no·fix·a·tion (vaj′i-nō-fik-sā′shŭn) Suturing a relaxed and prolapsed vagina to the abdominal wall. SYN colpopexy, vaginopexy.

vag·i·no·la·bi·al (vaj′i-nō-lā′bē-ăl) Relating to the vagina and the pudendal labia.

vag·i·no·my·co·sis (vaj′i-nō-mī-kō′sis) Vaginal fungal infection.

vag·i·nop·a·thy (vaj′i-nop′ă-thē) Any diseased condition of the vagina.

vag·i·no·per·i·ne·al (vaj′i-nō-per′i-nē′ăl) Relating to or involving the vagina and perineum.

vag·i·no·per·i·to·ne·al (vaj′i-nō-per′i-tŏ-nē′ăl) Relating to the vagina and the peritoneum.

vag·i·no·plas·ty (vaj′i-nō-plas′tē) Surgery involving the vagina. SYN colpoplasty.

vag·i·no·ves·i·cal (vaj′i-nō-ves′i-kăl) Relating to the vagina and the urinary bladder.

va·gi·tus u·ter·i·nus (vă-jī′tŭs yū-tĕr-ī′nŭs) Crying of the fetus while still within the uterus, possible when the membranes have been ruptured and air has entered the uterine cavity.

vago- Combining form denoting the vagus nerve.

va·gol·y·sis (vā-gol′i-sis) Surgical destruction of the vagus nerve.

va·go·lyt·ic (vā′gō-lit′ik) **1.** Pertaining to or causing vagolysis. **2.** A therapeutic or chemical agent that has inhibitory effects on the vagus nerve. **3.** Denoting an agent having such effects.

va·go·mi·met·ic (vā′gō-mi-met′ik) Mimicking the action of the efferent fibers of the vagus nerve.

va·got·o·my (vā-got′ŏ-mē) Division of the vagus nerve.

va·go·to·ni·a (vā′gō-tō′nē-ă) Archaic designation for a condition in which the parasympathetic autonomic system is reputedly overactive. SYN parasympathotonia, sympathetic imbalance.

va·go·trop·ic (vā′gō-trō′pik) Attracted by, hence acting on, the vagus nerve.

va·go·va·gal (vā′gō-vā′găl) Pertaining to a process that uses both afferent and efferent vagal nerve fibers.

va·go·va·gal re·flex (vā′gō-vā′găl rē′fleks) Bradycardia with arterial hypotension, often with supraventricular arrhythmias.

va·gus pulse (vā′gŭs pŭls) A slow pulse due to the inhibitory action of the vagus nerve on the heart.

Val Abbreviation for valine and its radicals.

va·lence, va·len·cy (vā′lĕns, -sē) The combining power of one atom of an element (or a radical), that of the hydrogen atom being the unit of comparison, determined by the number of electrons in the outer shell of the atom.

va·lence e·lec·tron (vā′lĕns ē-lek′tron) One of the electrons that take part in chemical reactions of an atom.

va·le·ric ac·id (VA) (vă-lēr′ik as′id) A monobasic aliphatic acid; distilled from valerian; some of its salts are used in medicine; found in human colon. SYN pentanoic acid.

val·gus (val′gŭs) Latin adjective describing any joint in an extremity that is deformed such that the more distal of the two bones forming the joint deviates away from the midline, as in knockknee.

val·ine (Val, V) (vă-lēn′) Nutritionally essential amino acid.

val·late (val′āt) Bordered with an elevation, as a cupped structure. SEE ALSO circumvallate.

val·late pa·pil·la (val′āt pă-pil′ă) One of several projections from the dorsum of the tongue; each papilla is surrounded by a trench called a vallum. Between the vallum and the pailla are found numerous taste buds. SYN circumvallate papillae.

val·lec·u·la, pl. **val·lec·u·lae** (vă-lek′ yū-lă, -lē) [TA] 1. A crevice or depression on any surface. 2. A sinus located between the base of the tongue and the epiglottis.

val·lec·u·lar dy·spha·gi·a (vă-lek′yū-lăr dis-fā′jē-ă) Disorder of swallowing caused by food that becomes lodged in a vallecula above the epiglottis. SYN Barclay-Baron disease.

Val·leix points (vahl′ē poynts) Various points in the course of a nerve, pressure on which is painful in cases of neuralgia. SYN tender points.

Val·sal·va leak point pres·sure (VLPP) (vahl-sahl′vă lēk poynt presh′ŭr) Abdominal pressure at which urinary incontinence may occur.

Val·sal·va ma·neu·ver (vahl-sahl′vă mă-nū′vĕr) Any forced expiratory effort (''strain'') against a closed airway, whether at the nose and mouth or at the glottis.

Val·sal·va test (vahl-sahl′vă test) Heart is monitored by electrocardiograph, pressure recording, or other methods while the patient performs the Valsalva maneuver.

val·vate (val′vāt) Relating to or provided with a valve.

valve (valv) [TA] 1. A fold of the lining membrane of a canal or other hollow organ serving to retard or prevent a reflux of fluid. 2. Any reduplication of tissue or flaplike structure resembling a valve. SEE ALSO valvule, plica. SYN valva [TA].

val·vo·plas·ty, val·vu·lo·plas·ty (val′ vō-plas-tē, val′vyū-lō-) Surgical reconstruction of a deformed cardiac valve, to relieve stenosis or incompetence.

val·vot·o·my, val·vu·lot·o·my (val-vot′ŏ-mē, val′vyū-lot′) 1. Cutting through a stenosed cardiac valve to relieve the obstruction. SYN valvulotomy. 2. Incision of a valvular structure.

val·vu·lar re·gur·gi·ta·tion (val′vyū-lăr rĕ-gŭr′ji-tā′shŭn) A leaky state of one or more of the cardiac valves, in which the valve does not close tightly and blood therefore regurgitates through it.

val·vule, val·vu·la (val′vyūl, val′vyū-lă) [TA] A valve, especially a small one.

val·vu·li·tis (val′vyū-lī′tis) Inflammation of a valve.

val·vu·lo·tome (val′vyū-lō-tōm) An instrument for sectioning a valve.

va·na·di·um (V) (vă-nā′dē-ŭm) A metallic element and bioelement; its deficiency can result in abnormal bone growth and a rise in cholesterol and triglyceride levels.

van·co·my·cin (VA) (van′kō-mī′sin) An antibiotic isolated from cultures of *Nocardia orientalis*, bactericidal against gram-positive organisms; available as the hydrochloride.

van·co·my·cin-re·sis·tant en·ter·o·coc·cus (VRE) (van′kō-mī′sin-rĕ-zis′ tănt en′tĕr-ō-kok′ŭs) A strain of enterococcal bacteria that resists therapy with vancomycin.

van den Bergh test (vahn den bĕrg test) Test for bile pigments (bilirubin) by reaction with diazotized sulfanilic acid (diazo reaction).

van der Hoeve syn·drome (vahn der hŏ′vĕ sin′drōm) A subtype of osteogenesis imperfecta in which progressive conductive hearing loss begins in childhood because of stapedial fixation.

van der Waals forc·es (vahn der valz fōrs'ĕz) Attractive forces between atoms or molecules other than electrostatic (ionic), covalent (sharing of electrons), or hydrogen bonding (sharing a proton).

va·nil·lyl·man·del·ic ac·id (VMA) (vă-nil'il-man-del'ik as'id) The major urinary metabolite of suprarenal and sympathetic catecholamines.

van·ish·ing lung syn·drome (van'i-shing lŭng sin'drōm) Progressive decrease of radiographic opacity of the lung caused by accelerated development of emphysema or rapid cystic destruction of the lung from infection.

va·por·i·za·tion (vā'pŏr-ī-zā'shŭn) **1.** Change of a solid or liquid to a vapor. **2.** Therapeutic application of a vapor.

var·i·a·bil·i·ty (var'ē-ă-bil'i-tē) **1.** The capability of being variable. **2.** In genetics, the potential or actual differences, either quantitative or qualitative, in phenotypes among individuals.

var·i·a·ble (var'ē-ă-bĕl) **1.** That which is inconstant, which can or does change, as contrasted with a constant. **2.** Deviating from the type in structure, form, physiology, or behavior.

var·i·ance (var'ē-ăns) **1.** Being variable, different, divergent, or deviate. **2.** A measure of the variation shown by a set of observations, defined as the sum of squares of deviations from the mean, divided by the number of degrees of freedom in the set of observations.

var·i·ant (var'ē-ănt) **1.** That which, or one who, is variable. **2.** Having the tendency to alter or change, exhibit variety or diversity, not conform, or differ from the usual type.

var·i·a·tion (var'ē-ā'shŭn) Deviation from type, in structure, physiology, or behavior.

var·i·ca·tion (var'i-kā'shŭn) Formation or presence of varices.

var·i·ce·al (var'i-sē'ăl) Of or pertaining to a varix.

var·i·cel·la (var'i-sel'ă) An acute contagious disease, usually in children, caused by the varicella-zoster virus. SYN chickenpox.

var·i·cel·la gan·gre·no·sa (var'i-sel'ă gang-grĕ-nō'să) Gangrenous ulceration of varicella lesions with or without secondary infection.

var·i·cel·la-zos·ter vi·rus (var'i-sel'ă-zos'tĕr vī'rŭs) A herpesvirus, morphologically identical to herpes simplex virus, which causes varicella (chickenpox) and herpes zoster. SYN chickenpox virus, herpes zoster virus, human herpesvirus 3, *Varicellovirus.*

var·i·ces (var'i-sēz) Plural of varix.

var·ic·i·form (var-is'i-fōrm) Resembling a dilated vein. SYN cirsoid.

varico- Combining form denoting a varix, varicose, varicosity.

var·i·co·bleph·a·ron (var'i-kō-blef'ă-ron) A varicosity of the eyelid.

var·i·co·cele (var'i-kō-sēl) A condition manifested by abnormal dilation of the veins of the spermatic cord, caused by incompetent valves in the internal spermatic vein.

var·i·co·ce·lec·to·my (var'i-kō-sē-lek'tŏ-mē) Operation for the correction of a varicocele by ligature and excision and by ligation of the dilated veins.

var·i·cog·ra·phy (var'i-kog'ră-fē) Radiography of the veins after injection of contrast medium into varicose veins.

var·i·com·pha·lus (var'i-kom'fă-lŭs) A swelling formed by varicose veins at the umbilicus.

var·i·co·phle·bi·tis (var'i-kō-flĕ-bī'tis) Varicose vein inflammation.

var·i·cose (var'i-kōs) Relating to, affected with, or characterized by varices or varicosis.

var·i·cose an·eu·rysm (var'i-kōs an'yūr-izm) A blood-containing sac, communicating with both an artery and a vein.

var·i·cose ul·cer (var'i-kōs ŭl'sĕr) The loss of skin surface in the drainage area of a varicose vein, usually in the leg, resulting from stasis and infection. SYN venous ulcer.

var·i·cose vein (var'i-kōs vān) Permanent dilation and tortuosity of a vein, most commonly seen in the legs, probably as a result of congenitally incomplete valves.

var·i·cos·i·ty (var'i-kos'i-tē) A varix or varicose condition.

var·i·cot·o·my (var'i-kot'ŏ-mē) An operation for varicose veins by subcutaneous incision.

va·ric·u·la (vă-rik'yū-lă) A varicose condition of the veins of the conjunctiva. SYN conjunctival varix.

var·i·cule (var'i-kyūl) A small varicose vein ordinarily seen in the skin.

var·ie·gate por·phy·ri·a (VP) (var'ĕ-gāt pōr-fir'ē-ă) Blood disorder characterized by abdominal pain and neuropsychiatric abnormalities, by dermal sensitivity to light and mechanical trauma and other findings. SYN protocoproporphyria hereditaria, royal malady, South African type porphyria.

va·ri·o·la (vă-rī'ō-lă) 1. Species type of the genus *Orthopoxvirus* that causes human smallpox. 2. Smallpox.

var·i·o·late (var'ē-ō-lāt) 1. To inoculate with smallpox. 2. Pitted or scarred, as if by smallpox.

va·ri·o·la vi·rus (var-ī'ō-lă vī'rŭs) A poxvirus of the genus *Orthopoxvirus*, the pathogen of smallpox in humans. SYN smallpox virus.

var·ix (var'iks) 1. A dilated vein. 2. An enlarged and tortuous vein, artery, or lymphatic vessel.

va·rus (var'ŭs) Descriptive of any of the paired joints of the extremities with a static angular deformity in which the bone distal to the joint deviates medially from the longitudinal axis of the proximal bone, and toward the midline of the body, when the subject is in the anatomic position. Cf. valgus.

vas, gen. **va·sis** (vas, vas'is) [TA] A duct or canal conveying any liquid, such as

blood, lymph, chyle, or semen. SEE ALSO vessel.

🌀 **vas-** (vas) Combining form indicating a vas, blood vessel. SEE ALSO vasculo-.

va·sa rec·ta ren·is (vā'să rek'tă rē'nis) [TA] Arteries penetrating and supplying the renal medulla (pyramids). SYN arteriolae rectae renis [TA], straight arteries.

va·sa va·so·rum (vā'să vă'sō-rŭm) [TA] Small arteries distributed to the outer and middle coats of the larger blood or lymph vessels, and their corresponding veins.

vas·cu·lar (vas'kyū-lăr) Relating to or containing blood vessels.

vas·cu·lar bed (vas'kyū-lăr bed) The system of minute blood vessels present in tissue.

vas·cu·lar cat·a·ract (vas'kyū-lăr kat'ăr-akt) Congenital cataract in which the degenerated lens is replaced with mesodermal tissue.

vas·cu·lar de·men·ti·a (VaD) (vas'kyū-lăr dĕ-men'shē-ă) Steplike deterioration in intellectual functions with focal neurologic signs, as the result of multiple infarctions of the cerebral hemispheres.

vas·cu·lar en·do·the·li·al growth fac·tor (VEGF) (vas'kyū-lăr en'dō-thē'lē-ăl grōth fak'tŏr) Peptide released from vascular endothelial cells and other cells in response to hypoxia, ischemia, or hypoglycemia.

vas·cu·lar·i·za·tion (vas'kyū-lăr-ī-zā'shŭn) The formation of new blood vessels in a part. SYN arterialization (3).

vas·cu·lar mur·mur (vas'kyū-lăr mŭr'mŭr) Sound originating in a blood vessel.

vas·cu·lar nerves (vas'kyū-lăr nĕrvz) [TA] Small nerve filaments that supply the wall of a blood vessel. SYN nervi vasorum [TA].

vas·cu·lar plex·us (vas'kyū-lăr plek'sŭs) [TA] Vascular network formed by frequent anastomoses between the blood vessels (arteries or veins) of a part. SYN plexus vasculosus [TA].

vas·cu·lar re·sis·tance (vas'kyū-lăr rē-zis′tăns) Resistance to flow within the smaller vessels, which is also determined by blood viscosity and the length of the vessels.

vas·cu·lar ring (vas′kyū-lăr ring) Anomalous arteries (embryonic pharyngeal arch arteries) congenitally encircling the trachea and esophagus.

vas·cu·lar sys·tem (vas′kyū-lăr sis′tĕm) The cardiovascular and lymphatic systems collectively.

vas·cu·la·ture (vas′kyū-lă-chŭr) The vascular network of an organ.

vasculo- Combining form denoting blood vessel. SEE ALSO vas-.

vas·cu·lo·gen·e·sis (vas′kyū-lō-jen′ĕ-sis) 1. Formation of the vascular system. 2. Formation of new vessels by endothelial cell progenitors.

vas·cu·lo·gen·ic im·po·tence (vas′ kyū′lo-jen′ik im′pŏ-tens) Erectile dysfunction (ED) due to alterations in the flow of blood to and from the penis.

vas·cu·lo·my·e·li·nop·a·thy (vas′kyū-lō-mī′ĕ-lin-op′ă-thē) Small cerebral vessel vasculopathy with subsequent perivascular demyelination, presumably due to circulating immune complexes.

vas·cu·lop·a·thy (vas′kyū-lop′ă-thē) Any disease affecting blood vessels.

va·sec·to·my (vas-ek′tŏ-mē) Excision of a segment of the vas deferens, performed in association with prostatectomy, or to produce sterility. SYN deferentectomy, gonangiectomy.

vas ef·fe·rens, pl. **va·sa ef·fer·en·ti·a** (vas ef′ĕr-enz, vā′să ef-ĕr-en′shē-ă) [TA] A vein carrying blood away from a part.

vas·i·form (vas′i-fŏrm) Having the shape of a vas or tubular structure.

va·so·ac·tive (vā′sō-ak′tiv) Influencing the tone and caliber of blood vessels.

va·so·ac·tive in·tes·ti·nal pol·y·pep·tide (VIP) (vā′sō-ak′tiv in-tes′ti-năl pol′ ē-pep′tīd) Hormone secreted most commonly by non-β islet cell tumors of the pancreas; increases the rate of glyco-genolysis and stimulates pancreatic bicarbonate secretion.

va·so·con·stric·tion (vā′sō-kŏn-strik′ shŭn) Reduction in the caliber of a blood vessel due to contraction of smooth muscle fibers in the tunica media.

va·so·con·stric·tive (vā′sō-kŏn-strik′ tiv) 1. Causing narrowing of the blood vessels. 2. SYN vasoconstrictor (1).

va·so·con·stric·tor (vā′sō-kŏn-strik′tŏr) 1. An agent that causes narrowing of the blood vessels. SYN vasoconstrictive (2). 2. A nerve, stimulation of which causes vascular constriction.

va·so·de·pres·sion (vā′sō-dĕ-presh′ŭn) Reduction of tone in blood vessels with vasodilation and resulting in lowered blood pressure.

va·so·de·pres·sor (vā′sō-dĕ-pres′ŏr) 1. Producing vasodepression. 2. An agent that produces vasodepression.

va·so·di·la·tion, va·so·dil·a·ta·tion (vā′sō-dī-lā′shŭn, -dil-ă-tā′shŭn) Increase in the caliber of a blood vessel due to relaxation of smooth muscle fibers in the tunica media.

va·so·di·la·tive (vā′sō-dī-lā′tiv) 1. Causing dilation of the blood vessels. 2. SYN vasodilator (1).

va·so·di·la·tor (vā′sō-dī′lā-tŏr) 1. An agent that causes dilation of the blood vessels. SYN vasodilative (2). 2. A nerve that stimulates dilation of the blood vessels.

va·so·ep·i·did·y·mos·to·my (vā′sō-ep′i-did′i-mos′tŏ-mē) Surgical anastomosis of the vasa deferentia to the epididymis, to bypass an obstruction at the level of the mid- to distal epididymis or proximal vas.

va·so·gan·gli·on (vā′sō-gang′glē-ŏn) A mass of blood vessels.

va·so·gen·ic (vā′sō-jen′ik) Denotes pertaining to blood vessels.

va·so·gen·ic shock (vā-sō-jen′ik shok) Shock due to depressed activity of the higher vasomotor centers in the brainstem and the medulla.

va·sog·ra·phy (vă-sog′ră-fē) Radiography of the vas deferens to determine patency, by injecting contrast medium into its lumen either transurethrally or by open vasotomy.

va·so·hy·per·ton·ic (vā′sō-hī′pĕr-ton′ik) Relating to increased arteriolar tension or vasoconstriction.

va·so·hy·po·ton·ic (vā′sō-hī′pō-ton′ik) Relating to reduced arteriolar tension or vasodilation.

va·so·in·hib·i·tor (vā′sō-in-hib′i-tŏr) An agent that restricts or prevents the functioning of the vasomotor nerves.

va·so·in·hib·i·tor·y (vā′sō-in-hib′i-tōr-ē) Restraining vasomotor action.

va·so·li·ga·tion (vā′sō-lī-gā′shŭn) Ligation of the vas deferens, usually after its division.

va·so·mo·tion (vā′sō-mō′shŭn) Change in the caliber of a blood vessel.

va·so·mo·tor (vā′sō-mō′tŏr) **1.** Causing dilation or constriction of the blood vessels. **2.** Denoting the nerves that have this action.

va·so·mo·tor cen·ter (VMC) (vā-sō-mō′tŏr sen′tĕr) Diffuse area of the reticular formation in the lateral medulla containing neurons that control vascular tone; consists of separate vasodepressor and vasopressor areas.

va·so·mo·tor fi·bers (vā-sō-mō′tŏr fī′bĕrz) Postganglionic visceral efferent fibers innervating the smooth muscles of vessel walls.

va·so·mo·tor nerve (vā′sō-mō′tŏr nĕrv) A motor nerve effecting or inhibiting contraction of the blood vessels.

va·so·mo·tor rhi·ni·tis (vā′sō-mō′tŏr rī-nī′tis) Congestion of nasal mucosa without infection or allergy.

va·so·mo·tor sys·tem (vā′sō-mō′tŏr sis′tĕm) The manner in which the sympathetic nervous system controls vascular smooth muscle.

va·so·neu·rop·a·thy (vā′sō-nūr-op′ă-thē) Any disease involving both the nerves and blood vessels.

va·so·oc·clu·sive cri·sis (VOCOR) (vā-sō-ŏ-klū′siv krī′sis) Painful crisis seen in patients with sickle cell anemia. SEE ALSO sickle cell anemia.

va·so·or·chi·dos·to·my (vā′sō-ōr′ki-dos′tŏ-mē) Reestablishment of the interrupted seminiferous channels by uniting the tubules of the epididymis or of the rete testis to the divided end of the vas deferens.

va·so·pa·ral·y·sis (vā′sō-păr-al′i-sis) Paralysis, atonia, or hypotonia of blood vessels.

va·so·pres·sin (vā′sō-pres′in) A nonapeptide neurohypophysial hormone related to oxytocin and vasotocin. SYN antidiuretic hormone.

va·so·pres·sor (vā′sō-pres′ŏr) **1.** Producing vasoconstriction and a rise in systemic arterial pressure. **2.** An agent that has this effect.

va·so·re·flex (vā′sō-rē′fleks) A reflex that influences the caliber of blood vessels.

va·so·re·lax·a·tion (vā′sō-rē-lak-sā′shŭn) Reduction in tension of the walls of the blood vessels.

va·so·sen·sor·y (vā′sō-sen′sŏr-ē) **1.** Relating to sensation in the blood vessels. **2.** Denoting sensory nerve fibers innervating blood vessels.

va·so·spasm (VS) (vā′sō-spazm) Contraction or hypertonia of the muscular coats of the blood vessels. SYN angiohypertonia, angiospasm.

va·so·spas·tic an·gi·na (vā′sō-spas′tik an′ji-nă) Chest pain caused by spasms in the muscular coats of the blood vessels rather than blockage of those vessels.

va·so·stim·u·lant (vā′sō-stim′yū-lănt) **1.** Exciting vasomotor action. **2.** An agent that excites the vasomotor nerves to action.

va·sos·to·my (vă-sos′tŏ-mē) Establishment of an artificial opening into the deferent duct.

va·sot·o·my, va·so·sec·tion (vă-sot′ŏ-mē, vā′sō-sek′shŭn) Incision into or division of the vas deferens

va·so·to·ni·a (vā′sō-tō′nē-ă) The tone of blood vessels. SYN angiotonia.

va·so·troph·ic (vā′sō-trō′fik) Relating to the nutrition of the blood vessels or the lymphatics.

va·so·tro·pic (vā′sō-trō′pik) Tending to act on the blood vessels.

va·so·va·gal (vā′sō-vā′găl) Relating to the action of the vagus nerve on the blood vessels.

va·so·va·gal syn·co·pe (vā′sō-vā′găl sing′kŏ-pē) Faintness or loss of consciousness due to increased vagus nerve (parasympathetic) activity.

va·so·va·sos·to·my (vā′sō-vă-sos′tŏ-mē) Surgical anastomosis of vasa deferentia to restore fertility in previously vasectomized men.

va·so·ve·sic·u·lec·to·my (vā′sō-vě-sik′yū-lek′tŏ-mē) Excision of the vas deferens and seminal vesicles.

vas·to·my (vas′tŏ-mē) Section of the vas deferens, usually with ligation.

VATER com·plex (vā′těr kom′pleks) Constellation of *v*ertebral defects, *a*nal atresia, *t*racheoesophageal fistula with *e*sophageal atresia, and *r*enal and *r*adial anomalies; associated with Fanconi anemia.

VDRL test (test) A flocculation test for syphilis, using cardiolipin-lecithin-cholesterol antigen as developed by the Venereal Disease Research Laboratory of the U.S. Public Health Service.

vec·tion (vek′shŭn) Transference of disease agents from an infected to an uninfected individual by a vector.

vec·tor (vek′tŏr) **1.** An invertebrate animal capable of transmitting an infectious agent among vertebrates. **2.** Anything having magnitude and direction. **3.** The net electrical axis of any electrocardiographic wave (usually QRS), the length of which is proportional to the magnitude of the electrical force. **4.** DNA that autonomously replicates in a cell to which another DNA segment may be inserted and be itself replicated. **5.** SYN recombinant vector. **6.** Recombinant DNA systems especially suited for production of large

quantities of specific proteins in bacterial, yeast, insect, or mammalian cell systems.

vec·tor·car·di·og·ra·phy (vek′tŏr-kahr′dē-og′ră-fē) **1.** A variant of electrocardiography in which the heart's activation currents are represented by vector loops. **2.** The study and interpretation of vectorcardiograms.

ve·cu·ro·ni·um bro·mide (ve′kyū-rō′nē-ŭm brō′mīd) A nondepolarizing neuromuscular relaxant with a relatively short duration of action.

veg·an (vē′găn) A strict vegetarian, one who consumes no animal or dairy products of any type. Cf. vegetarian.

veg·e·tal (vej′ě-tăl) Denoting the vital functions common to plants and animals, distinguished from those peculiar to animals.

veg·e·tar·i·an (vej′ě-tar′ē-ăn) One whose diet is restricted to foods of vegetable origin, excluding most animal meats. Cf. vegan.

veg·e·tar·i·an·ism (vej′ě-tār′ē-ăn-izm) The practice of following some form of vegetarian diet.

veg·e·ta·tion (vej′ě-tā′shŭn) **1.** The process of growth in plants. **2.** A condition of sluggishness, comparable to the inactivity of plant life. **3.** A growth or excrescence of any sort. **4.** Specifically, a clot, composed largely of fused blood platelets, fibrin, and sometimes microorganisms, adherent to a diseased heart orifice or valve.

veg·e·ta·tive (vej′ě-tā-tiv) **1.** Growing or functioning involuntarily or unconsciously, after the assumed manner of vegetable life; denoting especially a state of grossly impaired consciousness, in which a person is incapable of voluntary or purposeful acts and only responds reflexively to painful stimuli. **2.** Resting; not active.

veg·e·ta·tive en·do·car·di·tis, ver·ru·cous en·do·car·di·tis (vej′ě-tā-tiv en′dō-kahr-dī′tis, věr-ū′kŭs) Disorder associated with the presence of fibrinous clots (vegetations) forming on the ulcerated surfaces of the valves.

veg·e·ta·tive state (vej′ě-tā-tiv stăt) A

clinical condition with complete absence of awareness of the self and the environment, accompanied by sleep-wake cycles, but with either partial or complete preservation of hypothalamic and brainstem autonomic functions; may be transient or permanent.

ve·hi·cle (vē′i-kĕl) **1.** An excipient or a menstruum; a substance, usually without therapeutic action, used as a medium to give bulk for the administration of medicines. **2.** Substance by or on which an infectious agent passes from an infected to a susceptible host.

Veil·lo·nel·la (vā′yō-nel′ă) A genus of nonmotile, non-spore-forming, anaerobic bacteria containing small gram-negative cocci that occur as diplococci and in masses; parasitic in the mouth and in the intestinal and respiratory tracts of humans and other animals.

vein (vān) [TA] A blood vessel carrying blood toward the heart; all the veins except the pulmonary carry dark or deoxygenated blood. SYN vena [TA].

vein strip·ping (vān strip′ing) Surgical procedure to alleviate symptoms of varicose veins.

vel·a·men·tous, vel·i·form (vel′ă-men′tŭs, vel′i-fōrm) Expanded in the form of a sheet or veil.

vel·a·men·tous in·ser·tion (vel′ă-men′tŭs in-sĕr′shŭn) That of the fetal blood vessels into the placenta, in which the vessels separate before reaching the placenta and develop toward it in a fold of amnion. SYN parasol insertion.

vel·lus (vel′ŭs) **1.** Fine, nonpigmented hair covering most of the body. **2.** Any structure that is fleecy, soft, and woolly.

vel·o·car·di·o·fa·cial syn·drome (vel′ō-kahr′dē-ō-fā′shăl sin′drōm) Disorder with hypernasal speech, dysmorphic facial features, and cardiac abnormalities.

vel·o·pha·ryn·ge·al (VP) (vē′lō-făr-in′jē-ăl) Pertaining to the soft palate (velum palatinum) and the pharyngeal walls.

vel·o·pha·ryn·ge·al in·suf·fi·cien·cy (vē′lō-făr-in′jē-ăl in′sŭ-fish′ĕn-sē) Anatomic or functional deficiency in the soft palate or superior constrictor muscle, re-

sulting in the inability to achieve velopharyngeal closure.

Vel·peau ban·dage (vel-pō′ ban′dăj) Dressing that serves to immobilize an arm to the chest wall, with the forearm positioned obliquely across and upward on the front of the chest.

Vel·peau her·ni·a (vel-pō′ hĕr′nē-ă) Femoral hernia in which the intestine is in front of the blood vessels.

ve·lum, pl. **ve·la** (vē′lŭm, -lă) **1.** Any structure resembling a veil or curtain. SYN velamen. **2.** SYN caul (1). **3.** SYN greater omentum. **4.** Any serous membrane or membranous envelope or covering.

ve·na·ca·vog·ra·phy (vē′nă-kă-vog′ră-fē) Angiography of a vena cava. SYN cavography.

vene- **1.** Combining form meaning the veins, venous. SEE ALSO veno-. **2.** Combining form meaning venom.

ve·nec·ta·si·a (vē′nek-tā′zē-ă) SYN phlebectasia.

ve·nec·to·my (vē-nek′tŏ-mē) SYN phlebectomy.

ven·e·na·tion (ven′ĕ-nā′shŭn) Poisoning, as from a sting or bite.

ve·ne·re·al (vē-nēr′ē-ăl) Relating to or resulting from sexual intercourse.

ve·ne·re·al dis·ease (VD) (vĕ-nēr′ē-ăl di-zēz′) SYN sexually transmitted disease.

ve·ne·re·al lym·pho·gran·u·lo·ma, lym·pho·gran·u·lo·ma ve·ne·re·um (LGV) (vĕ-nēr′ē-ăl lim′fō-gran-yū-lō′mă, vĕ-nē′rē-ŭm) Infection usually caused by *Chlamydia trachomatis*, and generally characterized by a transient genital ulcer and inguinal adenopathy in the male; in the female, perirectal lymph nodes are involved and rectal stricture is a common occurrence. SYN Favre-Durand-Nicolas disease, lymphogranuloma inguinale, Nicolas-Favre disease, tropic bubo.

ve·ne·re·ol·o·gy (ve-nē′rē-ol′ŏ-jē) The study of venereal disease.

ven·e·sec·tion (VS, Vs) (ven´ĕ-sek´shŭn) SYN phlebotomy.

ven·i·punc·ture (VP) (ven´i-pŭngk´shŭr) The puncture of a vein.

veno-, veni- Combining forms denoting the veins. SEE ALSO vene- (1).

ve·no·gram (vē´nō-gram) 1. Radiograph of opacified veins. 2. SYN phlebogram.

ve·nog·ra·phy (vē-nog´ră-fē) Radiographic demonstration of a vein, after the injection of contrast medium. Used to demonstrate blockage of a vein. SYN phlebography (2).

ven·om (ven´ŏm) A toxin secreted by snakes, spiders, scorpions, and other cold-blooded animals.

ve·no·mo·tor (vē´nō-mō´tŏr) Altering the caliber of a vein.

ve·no·pres·sor (vē´nō-pres´ŏr) Relating to the venous blood pressure and consequently the volume of venous supply to the right side of the heart.

ve·nos·i·ty (vē-nos´i-tē) 1. A venous state; a condition in which the bulk of the blood is in the veins at the expense of the arteries. 2. The unaerated condition of venous blood.

ve·no·throm·bot·ic (vē´nō-throm-bot´ik) Denotes a blood clot that is present in the venous system.

ve·nous (vē´nŭs) Relating to a vein or to the veins.

ve·nous ad·mix·ture (vē´nŭs ad´mikschŭr) The mingling in the pulmonary circulation of arterial blood and desaturated blood resulting from ventilation-perfusion mismatching.

ve·nous an·gle (vē´nŭs ang´gĕl) 1. The junction of the internal jugular and subclavian veins. 2. NEURORADIOLOGY the angle of union of the superior thalamostriate vein (vena terminalis) with the internal cerebral vein, usually closely behind the interventricular foramen (Monro foramen).

ve·nous blood (vē´nŭs blŭd) That which has passed through the capillaries of various tissues, except the lungs, and found in the veins, the right chambers of the heart, and the pulmonary arteries; usually dark red as a result of a lower oxygen content.

ve·nous cir·cu·la·tion (vē´nŭs sĭr´kyū-lā´shŭn) The series of blood vessels that carry deoxygenated blood back to the heart.

ve·nous con·ges·tion (vē´nŭs kŏn-jes´chŭn) Venous overfilling and distention with blood due to mechanical obstruction or right ventricular failure.

ve·nous hum (vē´nŭs hŭm) Brief or continuous noise originating from the neck veins that may be confused with cardiac murmurs. SYN bruit de diable, nun's murmur.

ve·nous in·suf·fi·cien·cy (vē´nŭs in´sŭ-fish´ĕn-sē) Inadequate drainage of venous blood from a part, resulting in edema or dermatosis.

ve·nous plex·us (vē´nŭs plek´sŭs) [TA] Vascular network formed by numerous venous anastomoses. SYN plexus venosus [TA].

ve·nous pulse (vē´nŭs pŭls) A pulsation in the veins.

ve·nous star (vē´nŭs stahr) A small, red nodule formed by a dilated vein in the skin; caused by increased venous pressure.

ve·nous sta·sis (vē´nŭs stā´sis) Congestion and slowing of circulation in veins due to blockage by either obstruction or high pressure in the venous system, usually best seen in the feet and legs.

ve·nous valves (vē´nŭs valvz) Flaps present on the inside of the veins that prevent the backflow of blood between heartbeats.

ve·no·ve·nos·to·my (vē´nō-vē-nos´tŏ-mē) The formation of an anastomosis between two veins. SYN phlebophlebostomy.

ven·ter (ven´tĕr) [TA] 1. SYN abdomen. 2. SYN belly (2). 3. One of the great cavities of the body. 4. The uterus.

ven·ti·la·tion (v) (ven´ti-lā´shŭn) 1. Replacement of air or other gas in a space by fresh air or gas. **2.** Movement of gases into and out of the lungs. SYN respiration (2).

ven•ti•la•tion-per•fu•sion rate (ven´ti-lā´shŭn-pĕr-fyū´zhŭn rāt) Rate of coupling of air flow in the aveoli and blood flow through the pulmonary capillaries.

ven•ti•la•tion-per•fu•sion scan (ven´ti-lā´shŭn-pĕr-fyū´zhŭn skan) Lung function test, especially useful for pulmonary embolism, employing an inhaled radionuclide for ventilation and an intravenous radionuclide for perfusion.

ven•til•a•tor (ven´til-ā-tŏr) A mechanical device designed to perform part or all of the work of respiration.

ven•ti•la•to•ry com•pli•ance (ven´ti-lă-tōr-ē kŏm-plī´ăns) Sum of dynamic compliance of the lung and thoracic compliance.

ven•ti•la•to•ry rate (ven´ti-lă-tōr-ē rāt) Frequency of breathing.

ven•til•a•to•ry thresh•old (ven´til-ă-tōr-ē thresh´ōld) Point during exercise training at which pulmonary ventilation becomes disproportionately high with respect to oxygen consumption.

ven•trad (ven´trad) Toward the ventral aspect; opposed to dorsad.

ven•tral (ven´trăl) [TA] **1.** Pertaining to the belly or to any venter. **2.** SYN anterior (1). **3.** VETERINARY ANATOMY the undersurface of an animal; often used to indicate the position of one structure relative to another.

ven•tral as•pect (ven´trăl as´pekt) Of or pertaining to the front of the body.

ven•tral de•cu•bitus (ven´trăl dĕ-kyū´bi-tŭs) Pressure sores (decubitus ulceration) occurring in ventral locations.

ven•tral her•ni•a (ven´trăl hĕr´nē-ă) An abdominal incisional hernia.

♲ **ventri-** Combining form meaning of or pertaining to the abdomen; of or pertaining to the ventral plane.

ven•tri•cle (ven´tri-kĕl) [TA] A normal cavity. SYN ventriculus (2).

ven•tric•u•lar (ven-trik´yū-lăr) Relating to a ventricle, in any sense.

ven•tric•u•lar an•eur•ysm (VA) (ven-trik´yū-lăr an´yūr-izm) Thinning, stretching, and bulging of a weakened ventricular wall. SYN cardiac aneurysm, mural aneurysm.

ven•tric•u•lar bi•gem•i•ny (ven-trik´yū-lăr bī-jem´i-nē) Paired ventricular beats, the common form consisting of ventricular extrasystoles coupled to sinus beats.

ven•tric•u•lar cap•ture (ven-trik´yū-lăr kap´chŭr) Capture of the ventricle(s) by an impulse arising in the atria or atrioventricular junction.

ven•tric•u•lar com•plex (ven-trik´yū-lăr kom´pleks) The continuous QRST waves of each beat in the electrocardiogram.

ven•tric•u•lar es•cape (ven-trik´yū-lăr es-kāp´) A cardiac arrhythmia in which a ventricular focus usurps the pacemaker function of the sinuatrial node.

ven•tric•u•lar ex•tra•sys•to•le (ven-trik´yū-lăr eks-trä-sis´tŏ-lē) A premature contraction of the ventricle. SYN infranodal extrasystole.

ven•tric•u•lar fib•ril•la•tion (ven-trik´yū-lăr fib´ri-lă´shŭn) Coarse or fine, rapid, fibrillary movements of the ventricular muscle that replace the normal contraction. This causes failure to eject blood from the ventricle efficiently.

ven•tric•u•lar flut•ter (ven-trik´yū-lăr flŭt´ĕr) A form of rapid ventricular tachycardia in which the electrocardiographic complexes assume a regular undulating pattern without distinct QRS and T waves.

ven•tric•u•lar func•tion (ven-trik´yū-lăr fŭngk´shŭn) The pumping ability of the left side of the heart.

ven•tric•u•lar fu•sion beat (ven-trik´yū-lăr fyū´zhŭn bēt) That which occurs when the ventricles are activated partly by the descending sinus or atrioventricular junctional impulse and partly by an ectopic ventricular impulse.

ven•tric•u•lar gra•di•ent (ven-trik´yū-lär grā′dē-ĕnt) Algebraic sum of (i.e., the net electrical difference between) the area enclosed within the QRS complex and that within the T wave in the electrocardiogram.

ven·tric·u·lar hy·per·tro·phy (ven-trik′yū-lär hī-pĕr′trŏ-fē) Thickening of the ventricles, the portion of the heart that pumps blood.

ven·tric·u·lar sy·s·to·le (ven-trik′yū-lär sis′tŏ-lē) Contraction of the ventricles.

ven·tric·u·lar tach·y·car·di·a (VT, V-TACH, V tach, V-tach) (ven-trik′yū-lär tak′i-kahr′dē-ă) Paroxysmal tachycardia originating in an ectopic focus in the ventricle. SEE ALSO torsade de pointes.

ven·tric·u·li·tis (ven-trik′yū-lī′tis) Inflammation of the ventricles of the brain.

ventriculo- Prefix denoting a ventricle.

ven·tric·u·lo·a·tri·al (VA, V-A) (ven-trik′yū-lō-ā′trē-ăl) Relating to both ventricles and atria.

ven·tric·u·lo·a·tri·al shunt (ven-trik′yū-lō-ā′trē-ăl shŭnt) Surgical procedure for hydrocephalus. SYN ventriculoatriostomy.

ven·tric·u·lo·a·tri·os·to·my (ven-trik′yū-lō-ā′trē-os′tŏ-mē) SYN ventriculoatrial shunt.

ven·tric·u·lo·per·i·to·ne·al shunt (VPS, VP) (ven-trik′yū-lō-per′i-tŏ-nē′ăl shŭnt) Surgical procedure for hydrocephalus.

ven·tric·u·lo·plas·ty (ven-trik′yū-lō-plas′tē) Any surgical procedure to repair a defect of one of the ventricles of the heart.

ven·tric·u·lo·punc·ture (ven-trik′yū-lō-pŭngk′shŭr) Insertion of a needle into a ventricle.

ven·tric·u·los·co·py (ven-trik′yū-los′kŏ-pē) Direct inspection of a ventricle with an endoscope.

ven·tric·u·los·to·my (ven-trik′yū-los′tŏ-mē) Establishment of an opening in a ventricle. SEE ALSO shunt (2).

ven·tric·u·lo·sub·a·rach·noid (ven-trik′yū-lō-sŭb′ă-rak′noyd) Relating to the space occupied by the cerebrospinal fluid.

ven·tric·u·lot·o·my (ven-trik′yū-lot′ŏ-mē) Incision into a ventricle of the heart or the brain.

ven·tric·u·lus, gen. and pl. **ven·tric·u·li** (ven-trik′yū-lŭs, -lī) [TA] **1.** SYN stomach. **2.** SYN ventricle. **3.** The enlarged posterior portion of the mesenteron of the insect alimentary canal, in which digestion occurs.

ven·tri·duct (ven′tri-dŭkt) To draw toward the abdomen.

ven·tri·duc·tion (ven′tri-dŭk′shŭn) Drawing toward the abdomen or abdominal wall.

ventro- Prefix denoting ventral.

ven·tro·lat·er·al (VL) (ven′trō-lat′ĕ-răl) Both ventral and lateral.

ven·tro·me·di·al (ven′trō-mē′dē-ăl) Toward the middle of the front of the body.

ven·tro·me·di·an (ven′trō-mē′dē-ăn) Relating to the midline of the ventral surface.

Ven·tu·ri mask (VM, V-mask) (ven-tyūr′ē mask) One designed according to the Venturi principle, which allows for precise administration of specific amounts of oxygen. SYN air entrainment mask.

ven·ule (V) (ven′yūl) [TA] A venous radicle continuous with a capillary. SYN venula [TA], capillary vein.

Ve·ra·trum (vě-rā′trŭm) A genus of toxic liliaceous plants.

verb·al au·top·sy (věrb′ăl aw′top-sē) Method of obtaining as much information as possible about a deceased person by asking questions of family and others who can describe the mode of death and circumstances preceding it.

ver·big·er·a·tion (věr-bij′ĕr-ā′shŭn) Constant repetition of meaningless words or phrases; seen in schizophrenia. SYN oral stereotypy.

ver·gence (věr′jěns) Disjunctive ocular

movement in which the fixation axes are not parallel.

vermi- Combining form meaning a worm; wormlike.

ver·mi·cide (vĕr′mi-sīd) An agent that kills intestinal parasitic worms.

ver·mic·u·lar (vĕr-mik′yū-lăr) Relating to, resembling, or moving like a worm.

ver·mic·u·lar pulse (vĕr-mik′yū-lăr pŭls) A small, rapid pulse, giving a wormlike sensation to the finger.

ver·mic·u·la·tion (vĕr-mik′yū-lā′shŭn) A wormlike movement, as in peristalsis.

ver·mic·u·lose, ver·mic·u·lous (vĕr-mik′yū-lōs, -lŭs) **1.** Wormy; infected with worms or larvae. **2.** Wormlike. SEE ALSO vermiform.

ver·mi·form (vĕr′mi-fōrm) Worm shaped; resembling a worm in form. SEE ALSO lumbricoid.

ver·mi·fuge (ver′mi-fyūj) SYN anthelmintic (1).

ver·mil·ion bor·der (vĕr-mil′yŏn bōr′dĕr) Red margin of the upper and lower lips.

ver·mil·i·o·nec·to·my (vĕr-mil′yŏn-ek′tŏ-mē) Excision of the vermilion border.

ver·min (vĕr′min) Parasitic insects (e.g., lice and bedbugs); rats and other rodents.

ver·mi·na·tion (vĕr′mi-nā′shŭn) **1.** The production or breeding of worms or larvae. **2.** Infestation with vermin.

ver·mis, pl. **ver·mes** (vĕr′mis, -mēz) [TA] **1.** A worm; any structure or part resembling a worm in shape. **2.** The narrow middle zone between the two hemispheres of the cerebellum.

ver·nal con·junc·ti·vi·tis (vĕr′năl kŏn-jŭngk′ti-vī′tis) Chronic, bilateral conjunctival inflammation with photophobia and intense itching that recurs seasonally during warm weather. SYN spring ophthalmia, vernal catarrh, vernal keratoconjunctivitis.

Ver·net syn·drome (ver-nā′ sin′drŏm) Disorder characterized by paralysis of the motor components of the glossopharyngeal, vagus, and accessory cranial nerves as they lie in the posterior fossa.

ver·nix (vĕr′niks) SYN dental varnish.

ver·nix ca·se·o·sa (vĕr′niks kā-sē-ō′să) The fatty cheesy substance, consisting of desquamated epithelial cells, lanugo (downy hairs), and sebaceous matter, which covers the skin of the fetus and provides a waterproof protective cover.

ver·ru·ca, pl. **ver·ru·cae, ver·ru·ga** (vĕr-ū′kă, -kē, -gă) A flesh-colored growth characterized by circumscribed hypertrophy of the papillae of the corium, with thickening of the malpighian, granular, and keratin layers of the epidermis, caused by human *Papillomavirus*.

ver·ru·ca dig·i·ta·ta (ver-ū′kă dij-i-tā′tă) A type of wart with papillae that extend outward from the wart like fingers. SYN digitate wart.

ver·ru·ca pla·na (vĕr-ū′kă plā′nă) A smooth, flat, flesh-colored wart of small size, occurring in groups, seen especially on the face of the young; often associated with common warts of the hands, due to human *Papillomavirus*. SYN flat wart.

ver·ru·ci·form (vĕr-ū′si-fōrm) Wart shaped.

ver·ru·cous car·ci·no·ma (vĕ-rū′kŭs kahr′si-nō′mă) Well-differentiated papillary squamous cell carcinoma, especially of the oral cavity or penis.

ver·ru·cous he·man·gi·o·ma (vĕr-ū′kŭs hē-man′jē-ō′mă) A variant of the angiomatous nevus, appearing at birth or in early childhood, situated on the lower extremities with bluish-red nodules and warty surface.

ver·ru·cous hy·per·pla·si·a (vĕ-rū′kŭs hī′pĕr-plā′zē-ă) Cellular disorder of the oral mucosa.

ver·ru·cous ne·vus (vĕr-ū′kŭs nē′vŭs) Small or large, skin-colored (or darker), wartlike, often linear, lesion appearing at birth or in early childhood.

ver·ru·cous xan·tho·ma (vĕr-ū′kŭs zan-thō′mă) Histocytosis Y; a papilloma of the oral mucosa and skin.

ver·sic·o·lor (vĕr-si'kŏ-lŏr) Variegated; marked by a variety of color.

ver·sion (vĕr'zhŭn) **1.** Displacement of the uterus. **2.** Change of position of the fetus in the uterus, occurring spontaneously or effected by manipulation. **3.** SYN inclination. **4.** Conjugate rotation of the eyes in the same direction.

ver·te·bra, gen. and pl. **ver·te·brae** (vĕr'tĕ-bră, -brē) [TA] One of the segments of the spinal column; in human beings there are usually 33 vertebrae.

ver·te·bral (vĕr'tĕ-brăl) Relating to a vertebra or the vertebrae.

ver·te·bral-bas·i·lar sys·tem (vĕr'tĕ-brăl-bas'i-lăr sis'tĕm) Arterial complex comprising the two vertebral arteries joining to form the basilar artery, and their immediate branches.

ver·te·bral col·umn (vĕr'tĕ-brăl kol'ŭm) [TA] The series of vertebrae that extend from the cranium to the coccyx, providing support and forming a flexible bony case for the spinal cord. SYN columna vertebralis [TA], rachis, spinal column, spine (2).

ver·te·bral sub·lux·a·tion com·plex (vĕr'tĕ-brăl sŭb'lŭk-sā'shŭn kom'pleks) Theoretic model of vertebral motion segment dysfunction (subluxation) that incorporates the complex interaction of pathologic changes in nerves, and muscles, and in ligamentous, vascular, and connective tissues.

ver·te·bra pla·na (vĕr'tĕ-bră plā'nă) Spondylitis with reduction of vertebral body to a thin disc.

Ver·te·bra·ta (vĕr'tĕ-brā'tă) The vertebrates, consisting of those animals with a dorsal hollow nerve cord enclosed in a cartilaginous or bony spinal column; includes several classes of fishes, and the amphibians, reptiles, birds, and mammals. SYN Craniata.

ver·te·brate (vĕr'tĕ-brāt) **1.** Having a vertebral column. **2.** An animal having vertebrae.

ver·te·brec·to·my (vĕr'tĕ-brek'tŏ-mē) Resection of a vertebral body.

vertebro- Combining form denoting a vertebra, vertebral.

ver·te·bro·chon·dral, ver·te·bro·cos·tal (vĕr'tĕ-brō-kon'drăl, -kos'tal) Denoting the three false ribs (eighth, ninth, and tenth), which are connected with the vertebrae at one extremity and the costal cartilages at the other. SYN vertebrocostal (2).

ver·tex (vĕr'teks) [TA] **1.** The topmost point of the vault of the cranium. **2.** OB-STETRICS portion of the fetal head bounded by the planes of the trachelo-bregmatic and biparietal diameters.

ver·ti·cal (vert) (vĕr'ti-kăl) [TA] **1.** Relating to the vertex, or crown of the head. **2.** Perpendicular. **3.** Denoting any plane or line that passes longitudinally through the body in the anatomic position. SYN verticalis [TA].

ver·ti·cal band·ed gas·tro·plas·ty (vĕr'ti-kăl band'ĕd gas'trō-plas-tē) A surgical intervention to treat morbid obesity in which an upper gastric pouch is formed by a vertical staple line.

ver·ti·cal growth phase (vĕr'ti-kăl grōth fāz) Spread of melanoma cells from the epidermis into the dermis and later the subcutis, from which site metastasis may take place.

ver·ti·ca·lis (ver'ti-kā'lis) [TA] SYN vertical.

ver·ti·cal ny·stag·mus (vĕr'ti-kăl nis-tag'mŭs) An up-and-down oscillation of the eyes.

ver·ti·cal overlap (vĕr'ti-kăl ō'vĕr-lap) The extension of the upper teeth over the lower teeth in a vertical direction when the opposing posterior teeth are in contact in centric occlusion. SYN overbite.

ver·ti·cal plane (vĕr'ti-kăl plān) A plane that is perpendicular to the horizontal plane or ground plane.

ver·ti·cal stra·bis·mus (vĕr'ti-kăl strā-biz'mŭs) A form of strabismus in which the visual axis of one eye deviates upward or downward.

ver·ti·cal trans·mis·sion (vĕr'ti-kăl trans-mish'ŭn) **1.** Passing a virus by means of the genetic apparatus of a cell in which the viral genome is integrated. **2.** For infectious agents in general, transmission of an agent from an individual to its offspring. Cf. horizontal transmission.

ver·ti·cal ver·ti·go (vĕr´ti-kăl vĕr´ti-gō) **1.** SYN height vertigo. **2.** Dizziness experienced when standing upright.

ver·ti·go (vĕr´ti-gō) **1.** A sensation of spinning or whirling motion. **2.** Imprecisely used as a general term to describe dizziness.

ver·y low birth weight (VLBW) (ver´ē lō bĭrth wāt) Infant weighing less than 1500 g at birth. Can be due to a range of factors including interference with intrauterine growth or premature birth.

ver·y-low-den·si·ty lip·o·pro·tein (ver´ ē-lō-den´si-tē lip´ō-prō´tēn) A complex of protein and lipid in which the lipid content exceeds the protein content.

ve·si·ca, gen. and pl. **ve·si·cae** (ves´i-kă, -kē) **1.** SYN bladder. **2.** Any hollow structure or sac, normal or pathologic, containing a serous fluid.

ves·i·cal (ves´i-kăl) Relating to any bladder, but usually the urinary bladder.

ves·i·cal cal·cu·lus (ves´i-kăl kal´kyū-lŭs) A urinary calculus formed or retained in the bladder.

ves·i·cal fis·tu·la (ves´i-kăl fis´tyū-lă) Fistulous passage from the urinary bladder.

ves·i·cal he·ma·tu·ri·a (ves´i-kăl hē´ mă-tyūr´ē-ă) Form in which the site of bleeding is in the urinary bladder.

ves·i·cant (ves´i-kănt) An agent that produces a vesicle.

ves·i·cle (ves´i-kĕl) [TA] **1.** SYN vesicula. **2.** A small, circumscribed elevation of the skin containing fluid. SEE ALSO bleb, blister, bulla. **3.** A small sac containing liquid or gas.

ves·i·co·ab·dom·i·nal (ves´i-kō-ăb-dom´i-năl) Relating to the urinary bladder and the abdominal wall.

ves·i·co·cer·vi·cal (ves´i-kō-sĕr´vi-kăl)

Relating to the urinary bladder and the cervix of the uterus.

ves·i·coc·ly·sis (ves´i-kok´li-sis) Washing out, or lavage, of the urinary bladder.

ves·i·co·en·ter·ic (ves´i-kō-en-ter´ik) Denotes connection or association between between the bladder and an intestine.

ves·i·co·pros·tat·ic (ves´i-kō-pros-tat´ ik) Relating to the bladder and the prostate gland.

ves·i·co·pu·bic (ves´i-kō-pyū´bik) Relating to the bladder and the os pubis.

ves·i·co·pus·tu·lar (ves´i-kō-pŭs´tyū-lăr) Pertaining to a vesicopustule. SYN vesiculopustular (1).

ves·i·co·rec·tos·to·my (ves´i-kō-rek-tos´tō-mē) Surgical urinary tract diversion by anastomosis of the posterior bladder wall to the rectum. SYN cystorectostomy.

ves·i·co·sig·moi·dos·to·my (ves´i-kō-sig´moyd-os´tō-mē) Operative formation of a communication between the bladder and the sigmoid colon.

ves·i·co·spi·nal (ves´i-kō-spī´năl) Relating to the urinary bladder and the spinal cord.

ves·i·co·um·bil·i·cal (ves´i-kō-ŭm-bil´ i-kăl) Relating to the urinary bladder and the umbilicus. SYN omphalovesical.

ves·i·co·um·bil·i·cal lig·a·ment (ves´ i-kō-ŭm-bil´i-kăl lig´ă-mĕnt) One found between the urinary bladder and the umbilicus.

ves·i·co·u·re·ter·al (ves´i-kō-yūr-ē´tĕr-ăl) Relating to the bladder and the ureters.

ves·i·co·u·re·ter·al re·flux (ves´i-kō-yūr-ē´tĕr-ăl rē´flŭks) Backward flow of urine from bladder into ureter.

ves·i·co·u·re·thral (ves´i-kō-yūr-ē´thrăl) Relating to the bladder and the urethra.

ves·i·co·u·ter·ine (ves´i-kō-yū´tĕr-in) Relating to the bladder and the uterus.

ves·i·co·vag·i·nal (ves´i-kō-vaj´i-năl) Relating to the bladder and vagina.

ves·i·co·vag·i·nal fis·tu·la (VV, VVF) (ves′ĭ-kō-vaj′ĭ-năl fis′tyū-lă) Connection between the bladder and the vagina.

ve·sic·u·la, gen. and pl. **ve·sic·u·lae** (vĕ-sik′yū-lă, -lē) [TA] A small bladder or bladderlike structure. SYN vesicle (1) [TA].

ve·sic·u·lar (vĕ-sik′yū-lăr) **1.** Relating to a vesicle. **2.** Characterized by or containing vesicles. SYN vesiculate (2), vesiculous.

ve·sic·u·lar res·o·nance (vĕ-sik′yū-lăr rez′ŏ-năns) The sound obtained by percussion over the normal lung.

ve·sic·u·lar res·pi·ra·tion, ve·sic·u·lar breath sound (vĕ-sik′yū-lăr res′pir-ă′shŭn, brĕth sownd) The respiratory murmur heard on auscultation over the normal lung. SYN vesicular murmur.

ve·sic·u·la·tion (vĕ-sik′yū-lă′shŭn) **1.** The formation of vesicles. SYN blistering, vesication. **2.** Presence of a number of vesicles.

ve·sic·u·lec·to·my (vĕ-sik′yū-lek′tŏ-mē) Resection of a portion or all of each of the seminal vesicles.

ve·sic·u·li·form (vĕ-sik′yū-li-fōrm) Resembling a vesicle.

ve·sic·u·li·tis (vĕ-sik′yū-lī′tis) Inflammation of any vesicle.

ve·sic·u·lo·cav·er·nous (vĕ-sik′yū-lō-kav′ĕr-nŭs) **1.** An auscultatory sound having both a vesicular and a cavernous quality. **2.** The structure of certain neoplasms.

ve·sic·u·log·ra·phy (vĕ-sik′yū-log′ră-fē) Radiographic contrast study of the seminal vesicles.

ve·sic·u·lo·pap·u·lar (vĕ-sik′yū-lō-pap′yū-lăr) Pertaining to or consisting of a combination of vesicles and papules, or of papules becoming increasingly edematous with sufficient collection of fluid to form vesicles.

ve·sic·u·lo·pros·ta·ti·tis (vĕ-sik′yū-lō-pros′tă-tī′tis) Inflammation of the bladder and prostate.

ve·sic·u·lo·pus·tu·lar (vĕ-sik′yū-lō-pŭs′tyū-lăr) **1.** SYN vesicopustular. **2.** Pertaining to a mixed eruption of vesicles and pustules.

ve·sic·u·lot·o·my (vĕ-sik′yū-lot′ŏ-mē) Surgical incision of the seminal vesicles.

ve·sic·u·lo·tu·bu·lar (vĕ-sik′yū-lō-tū′byū-lăr) Denoting an auscultatory sound with both vesicular and tubular qualities.

ve·sic·u·lo·tym·pan·ic (vĕ-sik′yū-lō-tim-pan′ik) Denoting a percussion sound having both a vesicular and a tympanic quality.

ve·sic·u·lo·tym·pa·nit·ic res·o·nance (vĕ-sik′yū-lō-tim′pă-nit′ik rez′ŏ-năns) Peculiar, partly tympanitic, partly vesicular sound, obtained on percussion in cases of pulmonary emphysema. SYN bandbox resonance, wooden resonance.

Ve·si·cu·lo·vi·rus (vĕ-sik′yū-lō-vī′rŭs) Viral genus includes the vesicular stomatitis virus and related viruses.

ves·sel (ves′ĕl) [TA] A structure conveying or containing a fluid, especially a liquid. SEE ALSO vas.

ves·tib·u·lar (ves-tib′yū-lăr) **1.** Relating to a vestibule. **2.** Interpreting stimuli from the inner ear receptors regarding head position and movement.

ves·tib·u·lar func·tion (ves-tib′yū-lăr fŭngk′shŭn) The maintenance of bodily balance through structures within the inner ear.

ves·tib·u·lar hy·per·a·cu·sis (ves-tib′yū-lăr hī′pĕr-ă-kyū′sis) Abnormal sensitivity to noise in which the discomfort experienced is vestibular (e.g., vertigo, imbalance, nausea).

ves·tib·u·lar neu·ro·ni·tis (ves-tib′yū-lăr nūr′ŏ-nī′tis) Paroxysmal attack of severe vertigo, not accompanied by deafness or tinnitus, which affects young to middle-aged adults, often following a nonspecific upper respiratory infection. SYN Gerlier disease.

ves·tib·u·lar nu·cle·i (ves-tib′yū-lăr nū′klē-ī) A group of four nuclei found in the lateral region of the rhombencephalon beneath the floor of the rhomboid fossa.

ves·tib·u·lar nys·tag·mus (ves-tib′yū-lăr nis-tag′mŭs) Condition resulting from physiologic stimuli to the labyrinth that may be rotatory, caloric, compressive, or galvanic, or due to labyrinthal lesions. SYN labyrinthine nystagmus.

ves·tib·u·lar schwan·no·ma (ves-tib′yū-lăr shwah-nō′mă) A benign but life-threatening tumor arising from Schwann cells; produces hearing loss; tinnitus; vestibular disturbances; cerebellar, brainstem, and other cranial nerve signs; and increased intracranial pressure in late stages.

ves·tib·u·lar ver·ti·go (ves-tib′yū-lăr vĕr′ti-gō) The sense that a room is spinning caused by an imblance or disease state in the inner ear.

ves·ti·bule (ves′ti-byūl) [TA] **1.** A small cavity or a space at the entrance of a canal. **2.** Specifically, the central, somewhat ovoid, cavity of the osseous labyrinth communicating with the semicircular canals posteriorly and the cochlea anteriorly.

ves·tib·u·li·tis (ves-tib′yū-lī′tis) An inflammation of the vulvar vestibule and the periglandular and subepithelial stroma.

ves·tib·u·lo·oc·u·lar re·flex (VOR) (ves-tib′yū-lō-ok′yū-lăr rē′fleks) Reflexive adjustment of eye position that ensures a steady image when the head or body is moving.

ves·tib·u·lop·a·thy (ves-tib′yū-lop′ă-thē) Any abnormality of the vestibular apparatus (e.g., Ménière disease).

ves·tib·u·lo·plas·ty (ves-tib′yū-lō-plas-tē) Any of a series of surgical procedures designed to restore alveolar ridge height by lowering muscles attaching to the buccal, labial, and lingual aspects of the jaws.

ves·tib·u·lo·spi·nal re·flex (ves-tib′yū-lō-spī′năl rē′fleks) The influence of vestibular stimulation on body posture.

ves·tib·u·lot·o·my (ves-tib′yū-lot′ŏ-mē) Operation for an opening into the vestibule of the labyrinth.

ves·tib·u·lo·u·re·thral (ves-tib′yū-lō-yū-rē′thrăl) Relating to the vestibule of the vagina and urethra.

ves·tige (ves′tij) [TA] **1.** A trace or a rudimentary structure. **2.** Degenerated remains of any structure that occurs as an entity in the embryo or fetus.

ves·tig·i·al mus·cle (ves-tij′ē-ăl mŭs′ĕl) Imperfect structure in humans corresponding to a functioning muscle in the lower animals.

ves·tig·i·al or·gan (ves-tij′ē-ăl ōr′găn) Rudimentary structure in humans corresponding to a functional structure or organ in the lower animals.

vet·er·i·nar·y med·i·cine (vet′ĕr-i-nar-ē med′i-sin) The field concerned with the diseases and health of all animal species other than humans.

vi·a, pl. **vi·ae** (vī′ă, -ē) Any passage in the body.

vi·a·bil·i·ty (vī′ă-bil′i-tē) Capability of living; the state of being viable; usually connotes a fetus that has reached 500 g in weight and 20 gestational weeks (i.e., 18 weeks after fertilization).

vi·a·ble (vī′ă-bĕl) Capable of living; denoting a fetus sufficiently developed to live outside the uterus.

vi·al (VL) (vī′ăl) A small bottle or receptacle for holding liquids, including medicines. SYN phial.

Vi an·ti·gen (vē an′ti-jen) ''Virulence antigen,'' an external capsular antigen of enterobacteria formerly thought to be related to increased virulence.

vi·brat·ing line (vī′brāt-ing līn) Imaginary line across the posterior part of the palate, marking the division between the movable and immovable tissues.

vi·bra·tion (vī-brā′shŭn) A group of movements in massage that involve fine or coarse rhythmic shaking of various structures, with or without compression or traction.

vi·bra·tor (vī′brā-tŏr, tōr) An instrument used for imparting vibrations.

vi·bra·to·ry mas·sage (vī′brā-tōr-ē mă-sahzh′) Rapid tapping of a surface using a soft-tipped device. SYN seismotherapy, sismotherapy, vibrotherapeutics.

Vib·ri·o (vib′rē-ō) A genus of motile (in some instances nonmotile), non-spore-forming, aerobic, anaerobic to facultatively anaerobic, gram-negative bacteria that cause infection in humans.

Vib·ri·o al·gi·no·lyt·i·cus (vib′rē-ō al-ji-nō-lit′i-kŭs) A bacterial species associated with wound and ear infections, and with bacteremia in immunocompromised and burn patients.

Vib·ri·o cho·ler·ae (vib′rē-ō kol′ĕr-ē) A bacterial species that produces a soluble exotoxin and causes of cholera in humans. SYN comma bacillus.

Vib·ri·opa·ra·hae·mo·ly·ti·cus (vib′ rē-ō par′ă-hē-mō-lit′i-kŭs) A marine bacterial species that causes gastroenteritis and bloody diarrhea.

vib·ri·o·sis, pl. **vib·ri·o·ses** (vib′rē-ō′ sis, -sēz) Infection caused by bacteria of the genus *Vibrio*.

vi·bris·sa, gen. and pl. **vi·bris·sae** (vī-bris′ă, -ē) [TA] One of the hairs growing at the nares, or vestibule of the nose.

vi·bro·car·di·o·gram (vī′brō-kahr′dē-ō-gram) A graphic record of chest vibrations produced by hemodynamic events of the cardiac cycle.

vi·car·i·ous (vī-kar′ē-ŭs) Acting as a substitute; assumption of function or character of another person or thing.

vi·car·i·ous hy·per·tro·phy (vī-kar′ē-ŭs hī-pĕr′trō-fē) Enlargement of an organ following failure of another organ because of a functional relationship between them.

vi·car·i·ous men·stru·a·tion (vī-kar′ē-ŭs men′strū-ā′shŭn) Bleeding from any surface other than the mucous membrane of the uterine cavity, occurring periodically at the time when the normal menstruation should take place.

vi·cious ci·ca·trix (vish′ŭs sik′ă-triks) Scar, which by its contraction, causes a deformity.

vi·cious un·ion (vish′ŭs yūn′yŭn) Attachment of the ends of a broken bone resulting in a deformity or a crooked limb.

vi·dar·a·bine (vī-dar′ă-bēn) A purine nucleoside obtained from fermentation cultures of *Streptomyces antibioticus* used to treat herpes simplex infections.

vid·e·o·en·dos·co·py (vid′ē-ō-en-dos′ kŏ-pē) Endoscopy performed with an endoscope fitted with a video camera.

vid·e·o·lap·a·ros·cop·y (vid′ē-ō-lap-ă-ros′kŏ-pē) Laparoscopy augmented with a video camera with recording options.

vig·i·lance (vij′i-lăns) An attentiveness, alertness, or watchfulness for whatever may occur.

vil·lo·si·tis (vil′ō-sī′tis) Inflammation of the chorionic villi surface of the placenta. SYN villitis.

vil·los·i·ty (vi-los′i-tē) Shagginess; an aggregation of villi.

vil·lous, vil·lose (vil′ŭs, vil′ōs) *Do not confuse this adjective with the noun villus.* **1.** Relating to villi. **2.** Shaggy; covered with villi.

vil·lous ad·e·no·ma (vil′ŭs ad′ĕ-nō′mă) A solitary sessile, often large, tumor of colonic mucosa composed of mucinous epithelium covering delicate vascular projections; malignant change frequent. SYN papillary adenoma of large intestine.

vil·lous chor·i·on (vil′us kōr′ē-on) That part of chorion where the chorionic villi have persisted to form the fetal part of the placenta. SYN chorion frondosum.

vil·lous pa·pil·lo·ma (vil′ŭs pap-i-lō′ mă) Lesion composed of slender, fingerlike excrescences occurring in the bladder or large intestine, or from the choroid plexus of the cerebral ventricles. SYN villous tumor.

vil·lous pla·cen·ta (vil′ŭs plă-sen′tă) One in which the chorion forms villi.

vil·lus, gen. and pl. **vil·li** (vil′ŭs, -ī) *Do not confuse this word with the adjective villous.* **1.** A surface projection. If minute, it is termed a microvillus. **2.** An elongated dermal papilla projecting into an intraepidermal vesicle or cleft.

vi·men·tin (vī-men′tin) The major polypeptide that copolymerizes with other subunits to form the intermediate filament cytoskeleton of mesenchymal cells.

Vin·cent an·gi·na (van[h]-sawn[h]′ an′ ji-nă) Ulcerative infection of the oral soft tissues, including the tonsils and pharynx, caused by fusiform and spirochetal organisms; usually associated with necrotizing ulcerative gingivitis. Death from suffocation or sepsis may occur. SEE ALSO noma.

vin·cu·lum, pl. **vin·cu·la** (ving′kyū-lŭm, -lă) [TA] A frenum, frenulum, or ligament.

vi·nyl chlo·ride (VC) (vī′nil klōr′īd) Substance used in the plastics industry and suspected of being a potent carcinogen in humans. SYN chloroethylene.

vi·o·la·ceous (vī-ō-lā′shŭs) Denoting a purple discoloration, usually of the skin.

VIP·oma (vi-pō′mă) An endocrine tumor that produces a vasoactive intestinal polypeptide believed to cause profound cardiovascular and electrolyte changes with vasodilatory hypotension, watery diarrhea, hypokalemia, and dehydration.

vi·ral (vī′răl) Of, pertaining to, or caused by a virus.

vi·ral cys·ti·tis (vī′răl sis-tī′tis) Bladder inflammation due to a viral infection.

vi·ral gas·tro·en·ter·i·tis (VGE) (vī′răl gas′trō-en′těr-ī′tis) SEE endemic nonbacterial infantile gastroenteritis, epidemic nonbacterial gastroenteritis.

vi·ral hep·a·ti·tis type A (vī′răl hep′ă-tī′tis tīp) Viral disease with a short incubation period caused by hepatitis A virus and often transmitted by the fecal-oral route. SYN hepatitis A.

vi·ral hep·a·ti·tis type B (vī′răl hep′ă-tī′tis tīp) Viral disease with a long incubation period caused by a hepatitis B virus; usually transmitted by injection of infected blood or blood derivatives or by use of contaminated needles, lancets, or other instruments or by sexual transmission. SYN hepatitis B, transfusion hepatitis, virus B hepatitis.

vi·ral hep·a·ti·tis type C (vī′răl hep′ă-tī′tis tīp) Principal cause of non-A, non-B posttransfusion hepatitis caused by an RNA virus that is classified with the Flaviviridae family. A high percentage of patients develop chronic liver disease leading to cirrhosis and possible hepatocellular carcinoma. SYN virus C hepatitis.

vi·ral hep·a·ti·tis type D (vī′răl hep′ă-tī′tis tīp) Acute or chronic hepatitis caused by the hepatitis delta virus, a defective RNA virus requiring hepatitis B virus for replication. SYN delta hepatitis.

vi·ral load (vī′răl lōd) The plasma level of viral RNA.

vi·ral spon·gi·form en·ceph·a·lop·a·thy (vī′răl spŏn′ji-fŏrm en-sef′a-lop′ă-thē) Progressive vacuolation in dendritic and axonal processes and in neuronal cell bodies.

vi·ral ther·a·py (vī′răl thār′ă-pē) Use of genetically altered virus particles for delivering genes to specific sites for the purpose of therapy.

vi·re·mi·a (vī-rē′mē-ă) The presence of a virus in the bloodstream.

vir·gin (vĭr′jin) **1.** A person who has never had sexual intercourse. **2.** Unused; uncontaminated.

-viridae Suffix meaning a virus family.

vir·i·dans strep·to·coc·ci (vir′i-danz strep′tŏ-kok′sī) General term for any members of a family of alpha-hemolytic streptococci; found in humans, horses, and in cows and their milk. SYN *Streptococcus viridans.*

vir·ile (vir′il) Relating to the male sex.

vir·i·lism (vir′i-lizm) Possession of mature masculine somatic characteristics by a girl, woman, or prepubescent male; may be present at birth or later.

-virinae Suffix used in naming a subfamily of viruses.

vi·ri·on (vī′rē-on) The complete virus particle that is structurally intact and infectious.

vi·rol·o·gy (vī-rol′ŏ-jē) The study of viruses and of viral disease.

vir·tu·al en·dos·co·py (vĭr´chū-ăl en-dos´kŏ-pē) Computed tomographic data reconstructed in three dimensions to give information similar to that obtained with endoscopy.

vir·tu·al im·age (vĭr´chū-ăl im´ăj) Erect image formed by projection of divergent rays from an optic system. SYN direct image.

vi·ru·ci·dal, vi·ri·ci·dal (vī´rŭ-sī´dăl, vi´ri-sī´dăl) Destructive to a virus.

vir·u·lence (vir´yū-lĕns) Disease-evoking power of a pathogen.

vir·u·lif·er·ous (vir´yū-lif´ĕr-ŭs) Conveying a virus.

vi·ru·ria (vīr-yūr´ē-ă) Presence of viruses in the urine.

vi·rus shed·ding (vī´rŭs shed´ing) Excretion of virus by any route from the infected host.

vis·cer·al (vis´ĕr-ăl) Relating to the viscera.

vis·cer·al·gi·a (vis´ĕr-al´jē-ă) Pain in any viscus.

vis·cer·al lar·va mi·grans (VLM) (vis´ĕr-ăl lahr´vă mī´granz) Disease, chiefly of children, caused by ingestion of infective ova of *Toxocara canis*, less commonly by other ascarid nematodes not adapted to humans, the larvae of which hatch in the intestine, penetrate the gut wall, and wander in the viscera (chiefly the liver) for periods of up to 18–24 months; may be asymptomatic or may be marked by hepatomegaly.

vis·cer·al leish·ma·ni·a·sis (VL) (vis´ĕr-ăl lēsh´mă-nī´ă-sis) 1. Chronic disease, occurring in India, China, Pakistan, the Mediterranean littoral, the Middle East, South and Central America, Asia, and Africa caused by *Leishmania donovani* and transmitted by the bite of an appropriate species of sandfly of the genus *Phlebotomus* or *Lutzomyia*. 2. Form caused by *L. tropica*, cultured from bone marrow aspirates of some military patients following the Gulf War. SYN Assam fever, black sickness, Burdwan fever, cachectic fever, Dumdum fever, kala azar, tropic splenomegaly.

vis·cer·al nerve (vis´ĕr-ăl nĕrv) Term describing nerves conveying autonomic (general visceral efferent) fibers.

vis·cer·al obe·si·ty (vis´ĕr-ăl ō-bē´si-tē) Overweight due to excessive deposition of fat in the abdominal viscera and omentum, rather than subcutaneously, associated with dyslipidemia; poses greater risk of diabetes mellitus, hypertension, metabolic syndrome, and cardiovascular disease than peripheral obesity does. SYN abdominal obesity.

vis·cer·al pain (vis´ĕr-ăl pān) Discomfort resulting from injury or disease in an organ in the thoracic or abdominal cavity.

vis·cer·al sense (vis´ĕr-ăl sens) The perception of the existence of the internal organs. SYN splanchnesthetic sensibility.

vis·cer·al skel·e·ton (vis´ĕr-ăl skel´ĕ-tŏn) SYN visceroskeleton (2).

vis·cer·al swal·low (vis´ĕr-ăl swahl´ō) The immature swallowing pattern of an infant or a person with tongue thrust, resembling peristaltic wavelike muscular contractions observed in the gut; adult or mature swallowing is more volitional and therefore somatic.

vis·cer·o·gen·ic (vis´ĕr-ō-jen´ik) Of visceral origin; denoting a number of sensory and other reflexes.

vis·cer·o·in·hib·i·to·ry (vis´ĕr-ō-in-hib´i-tōr-ē) Restricting or arresting the functional activity of the viscera.

vis·cer·o·meg·a·ly (vis´ĕr-ō-meg´ă-lē) Abnormal enlargement of the viscera. SYN splanchnomegaly.

vis·cer·o·mo·tor, vis·cer·i·mo·tor (vis´ĕr-ō-mō´tŏr, vis´ĕr-i-) 1. Relating to or controlling movement in the viscera; denoting the autonomic nerves innervating the viscera. 2. Denoting a movement having a relation to the viscera. SYN viscerimotor.

vis·cer·o·pa·ri·e·tal (vis´ĕr-ō-pă-rī´ĕ-tăl) Relating to the viscera and the wall of the abdomen.

vis·cer·o·per·i·to·ne·al (vis´ĕr-ō-per´i-tō-nē′ăl) Relating to the peritoneum and the abdominal viscera.

vis·cer·o·pleu·ral (vis′ĕr-ō-plūr′ăl) Relating to the pleural and the thoracic viscera. SYN pleurovisceral.

vis·cer·op·to·sis, vis·cer·op·to·si·a (vis′ĕr-op-tō′sis, -tō′zē-ă) Descent of the viscera from their normal positions. SYN splanchnoptosis, splanchnoptosia.

vis·cer·o·sen·so·ry (vis′ĕr-ō-sen′sŏr-ē) Relating to the sensory innervation of internal organs.

vis·cer·o·skel·e·ton (vis′ĕr-ō-skel′ĕ-tŏn) **1.** Any bony formation in an organ; also includes, according to some anatomists, the cartilaginous rings of the trachea and bronchi. **2.** The bony framework protecting the viscera. SYN visceral skeleton.

vis·cer·o·tro·pic (vis′ĕr-ō-trō′pik) Affecting the viscera.

vis·cid·i·ty (vi-sid′i-tē) Stickiness; adhesiveness.

visc·o·can·nu·los·to·my (vis′kō-kan′ yū-los′tŏ-mē) A procedure to treat glaucoma in which viscoelastic is used to open the aqueous drainage channels.

vis·co·e·las·tic·i·ty (vis′kō-ĕ′las-tis′i-tē) The property of a viscous material that also shows elasticity.

vis·cos·i·ty (vis-kos′i-tē) In general, the resistance to flow or alteration of shape by any substance as a result of molecular cohesion.

vis·cous (vis′kŭs) Sticky; marked by high viscosity.

vis·cus, vis·cer·a (vis′kŭs, vis′ĕr-ă) An organ of the digestive, respiratory, urogenital, and endocrine systems as well as the spleen, the heart, and great vessels.

vis·i·ble spec·trum (viz′i-bĕl spek′trŭm) That part of electromagnetic radiation visible to the human eye.

vis·u·al (vis) (vizh′ū-ăl) **1.** Relating to vision. **2.** Denoting a person who learns and remembers more readily through sight than through hearing.

vis·u·al ag·no·si·a (vizh′ū-ăl ag-nō′zē-ă) Inability to recognize objects by sight.

vis·u·al an·gle (vizh′ū-ăl ang′gĕl) The angle formed at the retina by the meeting of lines drawn from the periphery of the object seen.

vis·u·al a·xis (VA) (vizh′ū-ăl ak′sis) Straight line extending from the object seen, through the center of the pupil, to the macula lutea of the retina. SYN line of vision.

vis·u·al clo·sure (viz′ū-ăl klō′zhŭr) Identification of forms or objects from incomplete presentation.

vis·u·al cor·tex (vizh′ū-ăl kōr′teks) The region of the cerebral cortex occupying the entire surface of the occipital lobe, and composed of Brodmann areas 17–19. SYN visual area.

vis·u·al cy·cle (vizh′ū-ăl sī′kĕl) Transformation of carotenoids involved in the bleaching and regeneration of the visual pigment.

vis·u·al e·voked po·ten·tial (vizh′ū-ăl ē-vōkt′ pŏ-ten′shăl) Voltage fluctuations that may be recorded from the occipital area of the scalp as the result of retinal stimulation by a light flashing at quarter-second intervals.

vis·u·al field (F) (vizh′ū-ăl fēld) The area simultaneously visible to one eye without movement.

vis·u·al-ki·net·ic dis·so·ci·a·tion (vizh′ ū-ăl ki-net′ik di-sō′sē-ā′shŭn) The neuro-linguistic programming process of removing a synesthesia from a person's internal experience. SEE ALSO neurolinguistic programming.

vis·u·al-mo·tor func·tion (vizh′yū-ăl-mō′tŏr fungk′shŭn) The synchronization of movement in response to visual stimuli.

vis·u·al or·i·en·ta·tion (vizh′ū-ăl ōr′ē-ĕn-tā′shŭn) Awareness of the location of objects in the environment and their relationship to one another and to the person viewing them.

vis·u·al path·way (vizh′ū-ăl path′wā) Neural paths and connections within the central nervous system, beginning with the retina and terminating in the occipital cortex.

vis·u·al pig·ments (vizh′yū-ăl pig′měnts) The photopigments in the retinal cones and rods that absorb light and initiate the visual process.

vis·u·al-spa·tial ag·no·si·a (vizh′ū-ăl-spā′shăl ag-nō′zē-ă) Inability to localize objects or to appreciate distance, motion, and spatial relationships; caused by lesion in the occipital lobe. Cf. simultanagnosia.

vis·u·o·au·di·tor·y (vizh′yū-ō-aw′di-tōr′ē) Relating to both vision and hearing; denoting nerves connecting the centers for these senses.

vis·u·og·no·sis (vizh′ū-og-nō′sis) Recognition and understanding of visual impressions.

vis·u·o·mo·tor, vis·u·al-mo·tor (vizh′ū-ō-mō′tŏr, vizh′yū-al-) Denoting the ability to synchronize visual information with physical movement.

vis·u·o·sen·so·ry (vizh′ū-ō-sen′sŏr-ē) Pertaining to the perception of visual stimuli.

vis·u·o·spa·tial (vizh′ū-ō-spā′shăl) Denoting the ability to comprehend and conceptualize visual representations and spatial relationships in learning and performing a task.

vi·tal ca·pa·ci·ty (VC) (vī′tăl kă-pas′i-tē) The greatest volume of air that can be exhaled from the lungs after a maximum inspiration. SYN respiratory capacity.

vi·tal in·dex (vī′tăl in′deks) The ratio of births to deaths within a population during a given time.

vi·tal signs (vī′tăl sīnz) Objective measurements of temperature, pulse, respirations, and blood pressure as a means of assessing general health and cardiorespiratory function.

vi·tal stain (vī′tăl stān) A stain applied to cells or parts of cells while they are still alive.

vi·tal sta·tis·tics (vī′tăl stă-tis′tiks) Systematically tabulated information concerning births, marriages, divorces, separations, and deaths, based on the numbers of official registrations of these vital events; the branch of statistics concerned with such data.

vi·ta·min (vīt′ă-min) Organic substance, present in minute amounts in natural foodstuffs, essential to normal metabolism; insufficient amounts may cause deficiency diseases.

vi·ta·min A (vī′tă-min) Any β-ionone derivative, except provitamin A carotenoids, possessing qualitatively the biologic activity of retinol.

vi·ta·min A1 (vī′tă-min) SYN retinol.

vi·ta·min B1 (vī′tă-min) SYN thiamin.

vi·ta·min B6 (vī′tă-min) Pyridoxine and related compounds (pyridoxal; pyridoxamine).

vi·ta·min B12 (vīt′ă-min) Generic descriptor for compounds exhibiting the biologic activity of cyanocobalamin. SYN animal protein factor, antianemic factor, antipernicious anemia factor (1), erythrocyte maturation factor, maturation factor, methylcobalamin.

vi·ta·min C (vīt′ă-min) SYN ascorbic acid.

vi·ta·min D (vīt′ă-min) Generic descriptor for all steroids exhibiting the biologic activity of ergocalciferol or cholecalciferol, the antirachitic vitamins. They promote the proper use of calcium and phosphorus, thereby favoring proper bone and tooth formation and maintenance in children.

vi·ta·min D2 (vīt′ă-min) SYN ergocalciferol.

vi·ta·min D3 (vīt′ă-min) SYN cholecalciferol.

vi·ta·min de·fi·cien·cy (vī′tă-min dĕ-fish′ĕn-sē) Low levels of essential vitamins that could lead to disease.

vi·ta·min D milk (vīt′ă-min milk) Cow's milk to which vitamin D has been added.

vi·ta·min D—re·sis·tant rick·ets (vī′tă-min rĕ-zis′tănt rik′ĕts) A form of the disease characterized by hypophosphatemia osteomalacia produced by disorders of metabolism of Vitamin D.

vi·ta·min E (vīt'ă-min) Generic descriptor of tocol and tocotrienol derivatives possessing the biologic activity of α-tocopherol.

vi·ta·min K (vīt'ă-min) Generic descriptor for compounds with the biologic activity of phylloquinone.

vit·a·min K1, vit·a·min K1(20) (vīt'ă-min) SYN phylloquinone.

vi·ta·min K2, vi·ta·min K2(30) (vīt'ă-min) SYN menaquinone-6.

vi·tel·lin (vī-tel'in) A lipophosphoprotein combined with lecithin in the yolk of egg. SYN lipovitellin, ovovitellin.

vi·tel·line (vī-tel'ēn) Relating to the vitellus.

vi·tel·lo·gen·e·sis (vī'tel-ō-jen'ĕ-sis) Formation of the yolk and its accumulation in the yolk sac.

vi·tel·lo·in·tes·tin·al cyst (vī-tel'ō-in-tes'ti-năl sist) Small red sessile or pedunculated tumor at the umbilicus in an infant; it is due to the persistence of a segment of the vitellointestinal duct. SYN umbilical cyst.

vit·i·a·tion (vish'ē-ā'shŭn) A change that impairs use or reduces efficiency.

vit·i·li·go, pl. **vit·i·lig·i·nes** (vit'i-lī'gō, -lij'nēz) The appearance on otherwise normal skin of nonpigmented white patches of varied sizes, often symmetrically distributed and usually bordered by hyperpigmented areas; hair in the affected areas is usually white. SYN acquired leukoderma.

vi·trec·to·my (vi-trek'tŏ-mē) Removal of the vitreous by means of an instrument that simultaneously removes vitreous by suction and cutting and replaces it with saline or some other fluid.

vit·re·i·tis (vit'rē-ī'tis) Inflammation of the corpus vitreum. SYN hyalitis.

♻ **vitreo-** Combining form denoting vitreous.

vit·re·o·den·tin (vit'rē-ō-den'tin) Dentin of a particularly brittle character.

vit·re·o·ret·i·nal (vit'rē-ō-ret'i-năl) Pertaining to the retina and the vitreous body.

vit·re·ous (vit'rē-ŭs) **1.** Glassy; resembling glass. **2.** SYN vitreous body.

vit·re·ous body (vit'rē-ŭs bod'ē) [TA] Transparent jellylike substance filling the interior of the eyeball behind the lens. SYN corpus vitreum [TA], hyaloid body, vitreous (2), vitreum.

vit·re·ous hu·mor (vit'rē-ŭs hyū'mŏr) [TA] The fluid component of the vitreous body.

vit·re·ous mem·brane (vit'rē-ŭs mem'brăn) A condensation of fine collagen fibers in places in the cortex of the vitreous body.

vit·re·ous table (vit'rē-ŭs tā'bĕl) Inner table of a cranial bone; more compact and harder than the outer. SYN lamina interna ossium cranii.

vit·ri·fi·ca·tion (vit'ri-fi-kā'shŭn) Conversion of dental porcelain to a glassy substance by heat and fusion.

vit·ro·nec·tin (vit'rō-nek'tin) A plasma glycoprotein involved in inflammatory and repair reactions at sites of tissue damage.

♻ **vivi-** Combining form denoting living.

viv·i·par·i·ty (viv'i-par'i-tē) The state of producing live-born offspring. SYN zoogony.

vi·vip·a·rous (vī-vip'ă-rŭs) Denotes to give birth to live young.

viv·i·sec·tion (viv'i-sek'shŭn) Any cutting operation on a living animal for purposes of experimentation.

vo·cal fold, vo·cal cord (vō'kăl fōld, kōrd) [TA] Sharp edge of a mucous membrane fold overlying the vocal ligament and stretching along either wall of the larynx from the angle between the laminae of the thyroid cartilage to the vocal process of the arytenoid cartilage. SYN plica vocalis [TA], true vocal cord.

vo·cal fold nod·ules (vō'kăl fōld nod'yūlz) Small, circumscribed beady enlargements on the vocal folds caused by overuse or abuse of the voice. SYN singer's nodes.

vo·cal frem·i·tus (vō′kăl frem′i-tŭs) Chest wall vibration, felt on palpation, produced by the spoken voice.

vo·cal fry (vō′kăl frī) Phonation at an unnaturally low frequency resulting in low-frequency popping and ticking sounds. SYN glottalization.

vo·cal res·o·nance (VR) (vō′kăl rez′ŏ-năns) The voice sounds as heard on auscultation of the chest.

vo·cal tract (vō′kăl trakt) The air passages above the glottis (including the pharynx, oral and nasal cavities, and paranasal sinuses) that contribute to the quality of the voice.

Vogt-Spiel·mey·er dis·ease (vōkt spēl′mā-yer, di-zēz′) Cerebral sphingolipidosis, late juvenile type.

voice (voys) The audible sound made by air passing out through the larynx and upper respiratory tract, the vocal folds being approximated.

voice fa·tigue syn·drome (voys fă-tēg′ sin′drōm) Weakness and loss of the voice usually toward the end of the day because of abuse by using it too long and too loudly.

void (voyd) To evacuate urine or feces.

vo·la (vō′lă) Palm of the hand or sole of the foot.

vo·lar (vō′lăr) [TA] Referring to the vola; denoting either the palm of the hand or sole of the foot.

vol·a·tile (vol., vol) (vol′ă-til) **1.** Tending to evaporate rapidly. **2.** Tending toward violence, explosiveness, or rapid change.

vol·a·tile oil (vol′ă-til oyl) A substance of oily consistency and feel, derived from a plant and containing the principles to which the odor and taste of the plant are due (essential oil). SYN ethereal oil.

vo·li·tion·al (vŏ-lish′ŭn-ăl) Intentional, as in movement or speech.

vo·li·tion·al trem·or (vŏ-lish′ŭn-ăl trem′

ŏr) **1.** One that can be arrested by a strong effort of the will. **2.** SYN intention tremor.

Volk·mann ca·nals (fŏlk′mahn kă-nalz′) Vascular canals in compact bone that, unlike those of the haversian system, are not surrounded by concentric lamellae of bone; they run for the most part transversely, perforating the lamellae of the haversian system, and connect the canals of that system.

vol·ley (vol′ē) A synchronous group of impulses induced simultaneously by artificial stimulation of either nerve fibers or muscle fibers.

volt (v, V) (vōlt) Electromotive force that will produce a current of 1 ampere in a circuit that has a resistance of 1 ohm, i.e., joule per coulomb.

Vol·to·li·ni dis·ease (vōl-tō-lē′nē di-zēz′) Infectious disease of the labyrinth, leading to meningitis in young children.

vol·ume (V) (vol′yūm) Space occupied by matter, usually expressed in units such as cubic millimeters, cubic centimeters, and liters. SEE ALSO capacity, water.

vol·ume at ATPS (vol′yūm) A volume of gas at ambient (A) temperature (T) (room temperature) and barometric pressure (P) saturated (S) with water vapor.

vol·ume at BTPS (vol′yūm) A volume of gas saturated (S) with water vapor at 37°C (body [B] temperature ([T]) and the ambient environmental barometric pressure (P).

vol·ume at STPD (vol′yūm) A volume of gas, at the standard (S) temperature (T) of 0°C and a barometric pressure (P) of 760 mmHg, and in a dry state (D).

vol·u·met·ric (vol′yū-met′rik) Relating to measurement by volume.

vol·u·met·ric flask (vol-yū-met′rik flask) Narrow-necked flask calibrated to contain or to deliver a definite amount of liquid.

vol·u·met·ric so·lu·tion (VS) (vol′yū-met′rik sŏ-lū′shŭn) A solution made by mixing measured volumes of the components.

vol·ume u·nit (VU) (vol′yūm yū′nit) Unit of a logarithmic scale for expressing the power level of a complex audio frequency electrical signal. Power in volume units equals the decibels of power above a reference level of one milliwatt.

vol·un·tar·y (vol′ŭn-tar-ē) Acting in obedience to the will.

vol·un·tar·y hos·pi·tal (vol′ŭn-tar-ē hos′pi-tăl) Facility supported in part by voluntary contributions and under the control of a local, usually self-appointed, board of managers; a nonprofit hospital. SYN philanthropic hospital.

vol·un·tar·y mus·cle (vol′ŭn-tar-ē mŭs′ĕl) One with an action under wilful control; all striated muscles, except the heart, are voluntary.

vo·lute (vō-lūt′) Rolled up; convoluted.

vol·vu·lus (vol′vyŭ-lŭs) Intestinal twisting that obstructs; if left untreated, may result in vascular compromise of the involved intestine.

vo·mer·o·na·sal (VN) (vō′měr-ō-nā′săl) Relating to the vomer and the nasal bone.

vom·it (vom′it) **1.** To eject matter from the stomach through the mouth. **2.** Vomitus; the matter so ejected.

vom·it·ing, vo·mi·tion (vom′it-ing, vō-mish′ŭn) The ejection of matter from the stomach through the esophagus and mouth. SYN emesis (1), regurgitation (2).

vom·it·ing re·flex (vom′it-ing rē′fleks) Emesis (contraction of the abdominal muscles with relaxation of the cardiac sphincter of the stomach and of the muscles of the throat) elicited by a variety of stimuli, especially one applied to the region of the fauces. SYN pharyngeal reflex (2).

von Hip·pel-Lin·dau syn·drome (fŏn hip′el-lin′dow sin′drōm) Ocular disorder associated with cerebral lesions and with kidney disease. SYN cerebroretinal angiomatosis.

von Wil·le·brand dis·ease (fahn vil′ĕ-brahnt di-zēz′) A hemorrhagic diathesis characterized by a tendency to bleed primarily from mucous membranes, prolonged bleeding time, normal platelet

count, normal clot retraction, partial and variable deficiency of factor VIIIR, and possibly a morphologic defect of platelets.

von Wil·le·brand fac·tor (vWF) (fon vil′ĕ-brahnt fak′tŏr) SEE factor VIII.

vor·tex, pl. **vor·ti·ces** (vōr′teks, -ti-sēz) **1.** SYN whorl (5). **2.** SYN vortex lentis.

vor·tex cor·ne·al dys·tro·phy (vōr′teks kōr′nē-ăl dis′trŏ-fē) A swirling pattern of abnormally pigmented corneal epithelial cells, seen in Fabry disease and in response to certain medications.

vor·tex len·tis (vōr′teks len′tis) One of the stellar figures on the surface of the lens of the eye. SYN vortex(3).

vor·ti·cose veins (vōr′ti-kōs vānz) Several veins found in the vascular tunic of the eyeball.

Vos·si·us len·tic·u·lar ring (fos′ĕ-ŭs len-tik′yŭ-lăr ring) Anular opacity found on the anterior lens capsule after contusion of the eye, due to pigment and blood.

voy·eur·ism (vwah′yur-izm) Obtaining sexual pleasure by looking at the naked body or genitals of another or at erotic acts between others.

V-pat·tern es·o·tro·pi·a (pă′těrn ē′sō-trō′pē-ă) Convergent strabismus greater in downward than in upward gaze.

V-pat·tern ex·o·tro·pi·a (pă′těrn ek′sō-trō′pē-ă) Divergent strabismus greater in upward than in downward gaze.

vul·ga·ris (vul-gā′ris) Ordinary; of the usual type.

vul·ner·a·ble pe·ri·od, vul·ner·a·ble pe·ri·od of heart (VP) (vŭl′něr-ă-běl pěr′ē-ŏd, hahrt) Moment during the cardiac cycle when stimuli are particularly likely to induce repetitive activity like tachycardia, flutter, or fibrillation that persists after the stimulus has ceased; for the ventricle, it occurs during the latter part of systole, during the relative refractory period coincident with the inscription of the latter half of the T wave of the electrocardiogram.

vul·ner·a·ble phase (vŭl′něr-ă′běl fāz)

Time in the cardiac cycle during which an ectopic impulse may lead to repetitive activity (e.g., flutter of the affected chamber).

vul·sel·la for·ceps (vŭl-sel´ă fōr´seps) A forceps with hooks at the tip of each blade.

vul·va, gen. and pl. **vul·vae** (vŭl´vă, -vē) [TA] External female genitalia, composed of the mons pubis, labia majora and minora, clitoris, vestibule of the vagina and its glands, and the opening of the urethra and of the vagina.

vul·var in·tra·ep·i·the·li·al ne·o·pla·si·a (vŭl´văr in´tră-ep´i-thē´lē-ăl nē´ō-plā´zē-ă) Preinvasive squamous cell carcinoma (carcinoma in situ) limited to vulvar epithelium.

vul·vec·to·my (vŭl-vek´tŏ-mē) Vulvar excision (partial, complete, or radical).

vul·vi·tis (vŭl-vī´tis) Inflammation of the vulva.

vulvo- Combining form denoting the vulva.

vul·vo·cru·ral (vŭl´vō-krūr´ăl) Relating to the vulva and the clitoris.

vul·vo·dyn·i·a (vŭl´vō-din´ē-ă) Chronic vulvar discomfort with complaints of burning and superficial irritation.

vul·vo·vag·i·ni·tis (vŭl´vō-vaj-i-nī´tis) Inflammation of both vulva and vagina.

V wave (wāv) A large pressure wave visible in recordings from either atrium or its incoming veins, normally produced by venous return but becoming very large when blood regurgitates through the atrioventicular valve beyond the chamber from which the recording is made.

W

Waar·den·burg syn·drome (vahr'den-burg sin'drŏm) Congenital craniofacial dysmorphism characterized by white forelock, lateral displacement of medial canthi, iris bicolored or blue, prominence of the root of the nose, hyperplasia of medial portion of eyebrows, and congenital deafness.

waist (wāst) The portion of the trunk between the ribs and the pelvis.

Wal·den·ström mac·ro·glob·u·li·ne·mi·a (vahld'ĕn-strum mak'rō-glob'yū-li-nē'mē-ă) Macroglobulinemia in old people, characterized by proliferation of cells resembling lymphocytes or plasma cells in the bone marrow, anemia, increased sedimentation rate, and hyperglobulinemia with a narrow peak in γ-globulin or β₂-globulin at about 19 S units. SYN hyperglobulinemic purpura, Waldenström purpura, Waldenström syndrome.

Wal·dron test (wawl'drŏn test) Crepitation at the patellofemoral articulation on passive extension and flexion of the knee in chondromalacia patellae.

walk·er (wawk'ĕr) A light, portable framework used for support and assistance in walking by a person with a gait impairment for which a cane or crutches are inadequate.

Walk·er chart (wawk'ĕr chahrt) A system of plotting the relative fetal and placental sizes.

walk·ing ty·phoid (wawk'ing tī'foyd) Typhoid fever of insufficient severity to curtail the patient's routine activities. SYN ambulatory typhoid, latent typhoid.

wall (wawl) 1. [TA] An investing part enclosing a cavity such as the thorax or abdomen, or covering a cell or any anatomic unit. 2. A wall, as of the thorax, abdomen, or any hollow organ. SYN paries.

Walsh pro·ce·dure (wawlsh prŏ-sē'jŭr) Anatomic (nerve-sparing) radical retropubic prostatectomy.

wan·der·ing (wahn'dĕr-ing) Moving about; not fixed; abnormally motile.

wan·der·ing pace·mak·er (wahn'dĕr-ing pās'māk'ĕr) A disturbance of the nor-

mal cardiac rhythm in which the site of the controlling pacemaker shifts from beat to beat, usually between the sinus and atrioventricular nodes, often with gradual sequential changes in P waves between upright and inverted in a given electrocardiographic lead.

Wan·gen·steen suc·tion (wang'gen-stēn sŭk'shŭn) A siphon modified so as to maintain constant negative pressure; used with a duodenal tube for the relief of gastric and intestinal distention.

War·burg the·o·ry (vahr'berg thē'ŏr-ē) Explanation for the onset of cancer that attributes it to irreversible damage to the respiratory mechanism of cells, leading to the selective multiplication of cells with increased glycolytic metabolism, both aerobic and anaerobic.

ward (wōrd) A large room or hall in a hospital containing a number of beds.

Ward·rop meth·od (wōrd'rŏp meth'ŏd) Treatment of aneurysm by ligation of the artery at some distance beyond the sac, leaving one or more branches of the artery between the sac and the ligature.

war·fa·rin (WARF) (wōr'fă-rin) An anticoagulant and rodenticide.

warm ag·glu·ti·nin (wŏrm ă-glū'ti-nin) Antibody that is more reactive at 37°C than at lower temperatures.

warm-up phe·nom·e·non (wŏrm'ŭp fĕ-nom'ĕ-non) Progressive diminution of the myotonic response of a muscle during repeated contraction of the muscle.

War·thin tu·mor (wōrth'in tū'mŏr) Benign glandular tumor arising in the parotid gland; composed of two rows of eosinophilic epithelial cells, which are often cystic and papillary. SYN adenolymphoma, papillary cystadenoma lymphomatosum.

wast·ed ven·ti·la·tion (wās'tĕd ven'ti-lā'shŭn) That part of pulmonary ventilation that is ineffective in exchanging oxygen and carbon dioxide with pulmonary capillary blood.

wast·ing (wās'ting) 1. SYN emaciation. 2. Denoting a disease characterized by emaciation.

wast·ing syn·drome (wās'ting sin'drŏm) Progressive involuntary weight loss seen in patients with HIV infection. SYN HIV wasting syndrome.

wa·ter (H₂O) (waw′tĕr) **1.** Clear, odorless, tasteless liquid, solidifying at 32°F (0°C), and boiling at 212°F (100°C), which is present in all animal and vegetable tissues and dissolves more substances than any other liquid. SEE ALSO volume. **2.** A pharmacopeial preparation of a clear, saturated aqueous solution (unless otherwise specified) of volatile oils, or other aromatic or volatile substances, prepared by processes involving distillation or solution (agitation followed by filtration).

wa·ter for in·jec·tion (waw′tĕr in-jek′shŭn) Sterile water used to dissolve or dilute materials for injection.

wa·ter-ham·mer pulse (waw′tĕr ham′ĕr pŭls) A jerky pulse with forcible impulse but immediate collapse, characteristic of aortic insufficiency. SEE ALSO Corrigan sign, Corrigan pulse. SYN cannonball pulse.

Wa·ter·house-Frid·er·ich·sen syn·drome (waw′tĕr-hows frē′der-ik-sen sin′drōm) A condition due to meningococcemia, mainly in children younger than 10 years of age, characterized by vomiting, diarrhea, and other symptoms.

wa·ter in·tox·i·ca·tion (waw′tĕr in-toks′i-kā′shŭn) Nonphysiologic state caused by excessive water intake during exercise resulting in headache, nausea, and cramping. In severe cases, it may cause seizures and even death.

wa·ters (waw′tĕrz) Colloquialism for amnionic fluid .

wa·ter·shed in·farc·tion (waw′tĕr-shed in-fahrk′shŭn) Cortical infarction in an area where the distributions of major cerebral arteries meet or overlap.

wa·ter-sol·u·ble vi·ta·mins (waw′tĕr-sol′yū-bĕl vī′tă-minz) The C- and B-complex vitamins.

wa·ter-trap stom·ach (waw′tĕr-trap stŏm′ăk) A ptotic and dilated stomach, having a relatively high pyloric outlet held up by the gastrohepatic ligament.

Wat·son-Crick he·lix (waht′sŏn-krik′ hē′liks) Helical structure assumed by two strands of deoxyribonucleic acid, held together throughout their length by hydrogen bonds between bases on opposite strands. SEE ALSO base pair. SYN DNA helix, double helix.

watt (W, w) (waht) The SI unit of electrical power.

wave (wāv) **1.** A movement of particles in an elastic body, whether solid or fluid, whereby an advancing series of alternate elevations and depressions, or expansions and condensations, is produced. **2.** The elevation of the pulse, felt by the finger, or represented graphically in the curved line of the sphygmograph. **3.** The complete cycle of changes in the level of a source of energy that is repetitively varying with respect to time. SEE ALSO rhythm.

wax (waks) **1.** A thick, tenacious substance, plastic at room temperature, secreted by bees for building the cells of their honeycomb. **2.** Any substance with physical properties similar to those of beeswax, of animal, vegetable, or mineral origin (oils, lipids, or fats that are solids at room temperature). SEE ALSO cerumen.

wax·y cast (waks′ē kast) A microscopic formed element found in the urine in renal disease.

wax·y spleen (waks′ē splēn) Amyloidosis of the spleen.

Wb Abbreviation for weber.

W chro·mo·some, X chro·mo·some, Y chro·mo·some, Z chro·mo·some (krō′mŏ-sōm) SEE sex chromosomes.

wean (wēn) To implement weaning.

wear-and-tear pig·ment (wār-tār pig′mĕnt) Lipofuscin that accumulates in aging or atrophic cells as a residue of lysosomal digestion.

web (web) A tissue or membrane bridging a space. SEE ALSO tela.

webbed fin·gers (webd fing′gĕrs) Two or more fingers united and enclosed in a common sheath of skin.

webbed neck (webd nek) The broad neck due to lateral folds of skin extending from the clavicle to the head but containing no muscles, bones, or other structures; occurs in Turner and Noonan syndromes.

webbed pe·nis (webd pē′nis) Deficient ventral skin of the penile body buried in the scrotum or tethered to the scrotal midline by a fold or web of skin. The urethra and erectile bodies are usually normal.

webbed toes (webd tōz) Syndactyly involving the toes.

web·bing (web′ing) Congenital condition apparent when adjacent structures are joined by a broad band of tissue not normally present to such a degree.

web·er (Wb) (vā′bĕr) SI unit of magnetic flux, equal to volt-seconds (V·s).

Web·er-Cock·ayne syn·drome (web′ ĕr-kok-ān′ sin′drōm) A form of epidermolysis bullosa with only the hands and feet affected. Cf. epidermolysis bullosa.

We·ber par·a·dox (vā′bĕr par′ă-doks) If a muscle is loaded beyond its power to contract, it may elongate.

We·ber syn·drome, We·ber sign (web′ ĕr sin′drōm, sīn) Midbrain tegmentum lesion characterized by ipsilateral oculomotor nerve paresis and contralateral paralysis of the extremities, face, and tongue.

We·ber test (vā′bĕr test) Test in which the stem of a vibrating tuning fork is placed on the midline of the head to ascertain in which ear the sound is heard by bone conduction.

We·ber tri·angle (vā′bĕr trī′ang-gĕl) On the sole of the foot, an area indicated by the heads of the first and fifth metatarsal bones and the center of the plantar surface of the heel.

wedge (wej) A solid body having the shape of an acute-angled triangular prism.

wedge pres·sure (wej presh′ŭr) The intravascular pressure reading obtained when a fine catheter is advanced until it completely occludes a small blood vessel or is sealed in place by inflation of a small cuff; commonly measured in the lung to estimate left atrial pressure.

wedge re·sec·tion (wej rē-sek′shŭn) Removal of a wedge-shaped portion of the ovary; used to treat virilizing disorders of ovarian origin.

Week·sel·la zo·o·hel·cum (wĕk-sel′ă zō-ō-hel′kŭm) Bacterium that produces infections in bites and scratches from dogs and cats.

weep·ing (wēp′ing) **1.** Slow discharge from a wound. **2.** Lacrimation; crying.

weep·ing ec·ze·ma (wēp′ing ĕk′sĕ-mă) Moist, eczematous dermatitis.

We·ge·ner gran·u·lo·ma·to·sis (vā′ge-ner gran′yū-lō′mă-tō′sis) A disease, occurring mainly in the fourth and fifth decades, characterized by necrotizing granulomas and ulceration of the upper respiratory tract, with purulent rhinorrhea, nasal obstruction, and other symptoms.

Wei·gert law (vī′gert law) The loss or destruction of a part or element in the organic world is likely to result in compensatory replacement and overproduction of tissue during the process of regeneration or repair.

weight (wāt) The product of the force of gravity, defined internationally as 9.81 (m/sec)/sec, × the mass of the body.

weight·less·ness (wāt′lĕs-nĕs) Psycho-physiologic effect of zero gravity, as experienced by someone falling freely in a vacuum.

Weil dis·ease (vīl di-zēz′) A form of leptospirosis generally caused by *Leptospira interrogans* serogroup *icterohaemorrhagiae*, believed to be acquired by contact with the urine of infected rats; characterized clinically by fever, jaundice, and other symptoms.

Weil-Fe·lix test, Weil-Fe·lix re·ac·tion (vīl-fā′liks test, rē-ak′shŭn) A test for the presence and type of rickettsial disease based on the agglutination of X-strains of *Proteus vulgaris* with suspected rickettsia in a patient's blood serum.

Weit·brecht for·a·men (vīt′bresht fōr-ā′mĕn) Opening in the articular capsule of the shoulder joint, communicating with the subtendinous bursa of the subscapularis muscle.

well-dif·fer·en·ti·a·ted lym·pho·cyt·ic lym·pho·ma (WDLL) (wel dif′ĕr-en′shē-ā-tĕd lim′fō-sit′ik lim-fō′mă) Essentially the same disease as chronic lymphocytic leukemia, except that lymphocytes are not increased in the peripheral blood; lymph nodes are enlarged, and other lymphoid tissue or bone marrow is infiltrated by small lymphocytes.

Wen·cke·bach block (veng′ke-bahk blok) First-degree atrioventricular block with a progressive lengthening of conduction, as manifested in prolonged P-Q interval on electrocardiography, until one QRS complex and T wave are missed.

Wen·cke·bach pe·ri·od (veng′ke-bahk pēr′ē-ŏd) A sequence of cardiac cycles in the electrocardiogram ending in a dropped beat due to atrioventricular block, the preceding cycles showing progressively lengthening P-R intervals.

Wer·ner syn·drome (ver′ner sin′drŏm) Premature aging disorder consisting of sclerodermalike skin changes, bilateral juvenile cataracts, progeria, hypogonadism, and diabetes mellitus.

Wer·nic·ke cen·ter, Wer·nic·ke a·re·a (ver′ni-kĕ sen′tĕr, ar′ē-ă) The region of the cerebral cortex thought essential for understanding and formulating coherent, propositional speech. SYN sensory speech center.

Wer·nic·ke re·ac·tion (ver′ni-kĕ rē-ak′shŭn) In hemianopia, a reaction due to damage of the optic tract, consisting of loss of pupillary constriction when the light is directed to the blind side of the retina.

Wer·nic·ke syn·drome (ver′ni-kĕ sin′drŏm) A condition frequently encountered in patients with long-term alcoholism, largely due to thiamin deficiency; characterized by disturbances in ocular motility, pupillary alterations, nystagmus, and ataxia with tremors. Also referred to as Wernicke disease and Wernicke encephalopathy.

Wes·ter·gren meth·od (ves′ter-gren meth′ŏd) A procedure for estimating the sedimentation rate in fluid blood by mixing venous blood with an aqueous solution of sodium chloride and allowing it to stand in an upright pipette.

West·ern blot a·nal·y·sis (wes′tĕrn blot ă-nal′ă-sis) A laboratory procedure used to determine the presence of antibodies and proteins. SYN blot.

Wes·tern blot test (wes′tĕrn blot test) A serum electrophoretic analysis used to identify proteins.

west·ern e·quine en·ceph·a·lo·my·e·li·tis vi·rus (wes′tĕrn ē′kwīn ensef′ă-lō-mī′ĕ-lī′tis vī′rŭs) Group A arbovirus of the genus *Alphavirus*, occurring in the western U.S. and parts of South America, usually asymptomatic in birds, but causes western equine encephalomyelitis in horses and humans following transfer by the bites of mosquitoes. SEE ALSO western equine encephalomyelitis.

West Nile fe·ver (west nīl fē′vĕr) Infection by West Nile virus. This virus is spread by mosquitoes. In mild infections, fever, headache, and muscle ache may last a few days. In severe infections, encephalitis, hyperpyrexia, stiff neck, convulsions, paralysis, and coma may last several weeks, and resulting deficits may become permanent.

West Nile vi·rus (west nīl vī′rŭs) A flavivirus found in Africa, West Asia, the Middle East, and the United States in 1999, and Canada in 2002; can infect humans, birds, mosquitoes, horses, and some other mammals.

wet dream (wet drēm) True physiologic orgasm during sleep including a nocturnal seminal emission usually accompanying a dream with sexual content.

wet gang·rene (wet gang-grēn′) Ischemic necrosis of an extremity with bacterial infection, producing cellulitis adjacent to the necrotic areas.

wet nurse (wet nŭrs) Woman who is engaged to breast-feed another woman's infant.

wet pack (WP, WPk) (wet pak) Common form of wound dressing, in which hot or cold moisture is applied.

Whar·ton jel·ly (wōr′tŏn jel′ē) Mucouslike connective tissue of the umbilical cord.

wheal (wēl) A circumscribed, evanescent papule or irregular plaque of edema of the skin, appearing as an urticarial lesion, slightly reddened, often changing in size and shape and extending to adjacent areas, and usually accompanied by intense itching. SYN hives (2), welt.

wheal-and·er·y·the·ma re·ac·tion (wēl er′i-thē′mă rē-ak′shŭn) Characteristic immediate reaction observed in an allergy skin test; within 10–15 minutes after injection of antigen, an irregular, blanched, elevated wheal appears, surrounded by an area of erythema (flare). SYN wheal-and-flare reaction.

wheeze (wēz) **1.** To breathe with difficulty and noisily. **2.** A whistling, squeaking, musical, or puffing sound made by air passing through the fauces, glottis, or narrowed tracheobronchial airways in difficult breathing.

whiff test (wif test) Procedure to find the fishy odor detectable when potassium hydroxide is applied to a sample of vaginal discharge in case of bacterial vaginosis.

whip·lash in·ju·ry (wip′lash in′jŭr-ē) An imprecise term for various injuries due to sudden and violent hyperextension of the head on the trunk, followed by hyperflexion. Can include fractures, subluxations, sprains, muscle strains, and cerebral concussion.

Whip·ple dis·ease (wip′ĕl di-zēz′) Rare disease characterized by steatorrhea, lymphadenopathy, arthritis, fever, and cough; "foamy" macrophages are found in the jejunal lamina propria; due to *Tropheryma whippleii*.

white blood cell (WBC) (wīt blŭd sel) SYN leukocyte.

white blood cell cast (wīt blŭd sel kast) Urinary stone composed of polymorphonuclear leukocytes, characteristic of tubulointerstitial disease. SYN white cell cast.

white cell (wīt sel) SYN leukocyte.

white coat hy·per·ten·sion (wīt kōt hī′pĕr-ten′shŭn) Elevations in blood pressure caused by patients' stress in clinical settings. SYN office hypertension.

white gan·grene (wīt gang-grēn) Death of a body part or tissue with accompanying whitish slough. SYN leukonecrosis.

white graft (wīt graft) Rejection of a skin allograft so acute that vascularization never occurs.

white·head (wīt′hed) **1.** SYN milium. **2.** SYN closed comedo.

White·head op·er·a·tion (wīt′hed op-ĕr-ā′shŭn) Excision of hemorrhoids by two circular incisions above and below involved veins, allowing normal mucosa to be pulled down and sutured to anal skin.

white in·farct (wīt in′fahrkt) In the placenta, intervillous fibrin with ischemic necrosis of villi.

white lim·bal gir·dle of Vogt (wīt lim′ băl gir′dĕl fōkt) Symmetric arcuate yellow-white deposits in the peripheral cornea, often seen in patients over 40 years old.

white line (wīt līn) **1.** SYN linea alba. **2.** A pale streak appearing within 30–60 seconds after stroking of the skin with a fingernail and lasting for several minutes; regarded as a sign of diminished arterial tension. SYN Sergent white line.

white mat·ter (wīt mat′ĕr) [TA] Regions of the brain and spinal cord largely composed of nerve fibers; contain few or no neuronal cell bodies or dendrites. SYN alba, white substance.

white noise (wīt noyz) Complex, rushing sound consisting of many frequencies over a wide band.

white pulp (wīt pŭlp) That part of the spleen that consists of nodules and other lymphatic concentrations.

white sponge ne·vus (wīt spŭnj nē′vŭs) Oral cavity condition characterized by soft, white or opalescent, thickened, and corrugated folds of mucous membrane. SYN familial white folded dysplasia, oral epithelial nevus.

white throm·bus (wīt throm′bŭs) Opaque dull white clot composed essentially of blood platelets. SYN pale thrombus.

white wax (wīt waks) Yellow wax that has been bleached by being rolled thinly and exposed to light and air, or bleached by chemical oxidants. Like yellow wax, used in preparing ointments, cerates, plasters, and suppositories. SYN bleached wax, white beeswax.

whit·low (wit′lō) SYN felon.

whole blood (hōl blŭd) That drawn from a selected donor under rigid aseptic precautions; contains citrate ion or heparin as an anticoagulant; used as a blood replenisher.

whoop (hūp) The loud, sonorous inspiration in pertussis with which the paroxysm of coughing terminates, due to spasm of the larynx (glottis).

whoop·ing cough (WC) (hūp′ing kawf) SYN pertussis.

Wil·der·muth ear (vil′der-mūt ēr) Auricle in which the helix is turned backward and the anthelix is prominent.

Wil·der sign (wĭl′dĕr sīn) A slight twitch of the eyeball when changing its movement from abduction to adduction or the reverse, noted in Graves disease.

wild type (wīld tīp) A gene, phenotype, or genotype that is overwhelmingly common among those possible at a locus of interest, and therefore presumably not harmful.

wild-type strain (wīld′tīp strān) One found in nature or a standard strain.

will (wil) A legal document expressing the writer's wishes for the disposal of personal property after death.

wil·low (wil′ō) A tree of the genus *Salix;* the bark of several species, especially *S. fragilis,* is a source of salicin.

Wilms tu·mor (vilmz tū′mŏr) A malignant renal tumor of young children, composed of small spindle cells and various other types of tissue. SYN nephroblastoma.

Wil·son block (wil′sŏn blok) The commonest form of right bundle-branch block, on electrocardiogram characterized in lead I by a tall, slender R wave followed by a wider S wave of lower voltage.

Wil·son dis·ease (wil′sŏn di-zēz′) **1.** A disorder of copper metabolism characterized by cirrhosis, basal ganglia degeneration, neurologic manifestations, and deposition of green or golden-brown pigment in the periphery of the cornea. SYN hepatolenticular degeneration (2),

Westphal-Strümpell disease. **2.** SYN exfoliative dermatitis. SEE ALSO Kayser-Fleischer ring.

Wil·son-Mi·ki·ty syn·drome (WMS) (wil′son mik′i-tē sin′drōm) SYN pulmonary dysmaturity syndrome.

win·dow (win′dō) SYN fenestra.

wind·pipe (wind′pīp) SYN trachea.

Win·gate test (win′gāt test) Test of maximal anaerobic power output during 30 seconds of all-out exercise on either arm-crank or leg-cycle ergometer.

wing-beat·ing trem·or (wing′bēt-ing trem′ŏr) Coarse, irregular tremor that is most prominent when the limbs are held outstretched, reminiscent of a bird's flapping its wings; seen mainly with Wilson disease (q.v.).

winged cath·e·ter (wingd kath′ĕ-tĕr) A soft rubber catheter with little flaps at each side of the beak to retain it in the bladder.

win·ter itch (win′tĕr ich) Recurrent eczema appearing with the advent of cold weather. SYN dermatitis hiemalis, frost itch, pruritus hiemalis.

wire (wīr) Slender and pliable rod or thread of metal.

wir·y pulse (wīr′ē pŭls) A small, fine, incompressible pulse.

Wis·kott-Ald·rich syn·drome (WAS) (wis′kot awl′drich sin′drōm) Immunodeficiency disorder occurring in male children characterized by thrombocytopenia, eczema, melena, and susceptibility to recurrent bacterial infections; death occurs from severe hemorrhage or overwhelming infection. SYN Aldrich syndrome.

Wiss·ler syn·drome (vis′ler sin′drōm) High intermittent fever; irregularly recurring macular and maculopapular eruption of the face, chest, and limbs, leukocytosis; arthralgia; occurs in children and adolescents, with varying duration.

with·draw·al (with-draw′ăl) **1.** The act of removal or retreat. **2.** A psychological and physical syndrome caused by the abrupt cessation of the use of a drug in a habituated person. **3.** The therapeutic process of discontinuing a drug so as to avoid withdrawal (2). **4.** A pattern of behavior observed in schizophrenia and depression, characterized by a pathologic retreat from interpersonal contact and social involvement and leading to self-preoccupation. **5.** SYN coitus interruptus.

with·draw·al symp·toms (with-draw'ăl simp'tŏmz) A group of morbid symptoms, predominantly erethistic, in an addict deprived of the accustomed addicting agent.

with·draw·al syn·drome (with-draw'ăl sin'drōm) A substance-specific syndrome that follows the cessation of, or reduction in, intake of a psychoactive substance previously used regularly. Common symptoms include anxiety, restlessness, irritability, insomnia, and impaired attention.

wob·ble (wob'ĕl) MOLECULAR BIOLOGY unorthodox pairing between the base at the 5' end of an anticodon and the base that pairs with it (in the 3' position of the codon).

Wohl·fahr·ti·a (vōl-far'tē-ă) A genus of larviparous dipterous fleshflies of which some species' larvae feed in ulcerated surfaces and flesh wounds of humans and animals.

Wol·bach·i·a (wōl-bak'ē-ă) Symbiotic bacteria in the gut of *Wuchereria bancrofti*, *Onchocerca volvulus*, and other fiarial parasites: eradication eliminates the parasitosis.

wolff·i·an cyst (vōlf'ē-ăn sist) Lesion in the broad ligament of the uterus arising from remnants of the mesonephric ducts.

wolff·i·an rest (vōlf'ē-ăn rest) Remnants of the wolffian duct in the female genital tract that give rise to cysts.

Wolff law (vōlf law) Every change in the form and the function of a bone, or in its function alone, is followed by certain definite changes in its internal architecture and secondary alterations in its external conformation.

Wolff-Par·kin·son-White syn·drome (wulf'pahrk'in-sŏn-wīt' sin'drōm) Electrocardiographic pattern sometimes associated with paroxysmal tachycardia. SYN preexcitation syndrome.

Wol·las·ton doub·let (wol'ăs-tŏn dŭb'lĕt) A combination of two planoconvex lenses in the eyepiece of a microscope designed to correct the chromatic aberration.

wood al·co·hol (wud al'kŏ-hol) SYN methyl alcohol.

wool fat (wul fat) Purified, anhydrous, fatlike substance obtained from the wool of sheep. SEE ALSO adeps lanae. SYN lanolin.

word sal·ad (wŏrd sal'ăd) A jumble of meaningless and unrelated words emitted by people with certain kinds of schizophrenia.

work con·di·tion·ing (wŏrk kŏn-dish'ŏn-ing) A treatment program focused on functional requirements of a job or employment setting, incorporating the basic components of physical conditioning such as strength, endurance, flexibility, and coordination. A component of an industrial therapy program that serves as a precursor to a work hardening program; it is undertaken after acute care or basic rehabilitation treatment has been completed.

work·ing con·tacts (wŏrk'ing kon'takts) Points of contact of artificial or natural teeth on the side of the occlusion toward which the mandible is deviated.

Work·ing Form·u·la·tion for Clin·i·cal Us·age (WF) (wŏrk'ing for'myū-lă'shŭn klin'i-kăl yū'săj) Classification of malignant lymphomas introduced by the National Cancer Institute in 1982, based on the correlation of clinical and histopathologic features of various lymphomas.

work·ing through (wŏrk'ing thrū) PSYCHOANALYSIS process of obtaining additional insight and personality changes in a patient through repeated and varied examination of a conflict or problem; includes interactions between free association, resistance, interpretation, and working out.

work·load u·nit (WLU) (wŏrk'lōd yū'nit) A unit of work used to calculate productivity (e.g., billable procedures or patient visits).

work of breath·ing (wŏrk brēdh'ing)

The total expenditure of energy necessary to accomplish the act of breathing.

World Health Or·ga·ni·za·tion (WHO) (wŏrld helth ōr′găn-ī-zā′shŭn) A unit of the United Nations devoted to international health problems.

worm (wŏrm) **1.** ANATOMY any structure resembling a worm. **2.** Term once used to designate any member of the invertebrate group or former subkingdom Vermes, a collective term no longer used taxonomically; now commonly used to designate any member of the separate phyla Annelida (the segmented or true worms), Nematoda (roundworms), and Platyhelminthes (flatworms).

wound (wūnd) **1.** Trauma to any of the tissues of the body, especially that caused by physical means and with interruption of continuity. **2.** A surgical incision.

wound bot·u·lism (wūnd bot′yū-lizm) Poisoning resulting from infection of a wound.

wound ir·ri·ga·tion (wūnd ir′i-gā′shŭn) A method of cleaning debris from a wound that involves the use of solution under pressure.

wo·ven bone (wō′věn bōn) Bony tissue characteristic of the embryonal skeleton, in which the collagen fibers of the matrix are arranged irregularly in the form of interlacing networks. SYN nonlamellar bone, reticulated bone.

Wright-Gi·em·sa stain (rīt-gē-em′ză stān) Stain used to differentiate blood cells; and in bone marrow investigations.

Wright stain (rīt stān) Mixture of eosinates of polychromed methylene blue used in staining blood smears.

Wright ver·sion (rīt věr′zhŭn) A cephalic version employed in cases of shoulder presentation when the shoulders are pushed upward while the breech is moved toward the center of the uterus by the other hand; the head is then guided into the pelvis.

wrist (rist) [TA] The proximal segment of the hand consisting of the carpal bones and the associated soft parts. SYN carpus (1) [TA].

wrist clo·nus (rist klō′nŭs) Rhythmic contractions and relaxations of the muscles of the forearm excited by a forcible passive extension of the hand.

wrist clo·nus re·flex (rist klō′nŭs rē′fleks) Sustained clonic movement of the hand induced by sudden extension of the wrist.

wrist-drop (rist drop) Paralysis of the extensors of the wrist and fingers. SYN drop hand.

wrist joint (rist joynt) Synovial articulation between the distal end of the radius and its articular disc and the proximal row of carpal bones, excluding the pisiform bone. SYN radiocarpal articulation.

wrist sign (rist sīn) In Marfan syndrome, appreciable overlap of the thumb and fifth finger when the wrist is gripped with the opposite hand.

writ·er's cramp (WC) (rī′těrz kramp) Occupational dystonia affecting chiefly the muscles of the thumb and two adjoining fingers of the writing hand, induced by excessive use of a pen or pencil. SYN dysgraphia (2), graphospasm, scrivener's palsy.

writ·ing hand (rīt′ing hand) A contraction of the hand muscles in parkinsonism, bringing the fingers somewhat into the position of holding a pen.

Wu·cher·e·ri·a (vū-ker-ē′rē-ă) A genus of filarial nematodes characterized by adult forms that live chiefly in lymphatic vessels and produce large numbers of embryos or microfilariae that circulate in the bloodstream (microfilaremia), often appearing in the peripheral blood at regular intervals.

wu·cher·e·ri·a·sis (vū′ker-ē-rī′ă-sis) Infection with worms of the genus *Wuchereria*. SEE ALSO filariasis.

Wy·burn-Ma·son syn·drome (wī′bŭrn-mā′sŏn sin′drōm) Arteriovenous malformation on the cerebral cortex, retinal arteriovenous angioma and facial nevus, usually occurring in mentally retarded people.

W

xan·the·las·ma, xan·the·las·ma pal·pe·bra·rum (zan-thĕ-laz´mă, pal-pē-brā´rŭm) Soft, yellow-orange plaques on the eyelids or medial canthus, the most common form of xanthoma.

xan·thene (zan´thēn) The basic structure of many natural products, drugs, dyes (e.g., fluorescein, pyronin, eosins), indicators, pesticides, and antibiotics.

xan·thic (zan´thik) 1. Yellow or yellowish in color. 2. Relating to xanthine.

xan·thine (zan´thēn) Oxidation product of guanine and hypoxanthine, precursor of uric acid; occurs in many organs and in the urine, occasionally forming urinary calculi.

xan·thine ox·i·dase (XO) (zan´thēn ok´si-dās) Flavoprotein containing molybdenum; also oxidizes hypoxanthine, some other purines and pterins, and aldehydes. SYN hypoxanthine oxidase, Schardinger enzyme.

xan·thi·nu·ri·a, xan·thi·u·ri·a, xan·thur·i·a (zan´thi-nyū´rē-ă, -thē-yūr´ē-ă, -thyūr´ē-ă) 1. Excretion of abnormally large amounts of xanthine in the urine. 2. A disorder [MIM*278300], characterized by urinary excretion of xanthine in place of uric acid, hypouricemia, and occasionally the formation of renal xanthine stones.

xan·thism (zan´thizm) The pigmentary anomaly in some black people, characterized by red or yellow-red hair color, copper-red skin, and often dilution of iris pigment.

♻ **xantho-, xanth-** Combining forms meaning yellow, yellowish.

xan·tho·chro·mat·ic, xan·tho·chro·mic (zan´thō-krō-mat´ik, -krō-mik) Yellow-colored.

xan·tho·chro·mi·a (zan´thō-krō´mē-ă) Patches of yellow in the skin, resembling xanthoma, but without the nodules or plates. SYN xanthoderma (1).

xan·tho·der·ma (zan´thō-dĕr´mă) 1. SYN xanthochromia. 2. Any yellow coloration of the skin.

xan·tho·gran·u·lo·ma (zan´thō-gran´yū-lō´mă) A peculiar infiltration of retroperitoneal tissue by lipid macrophages, occurring more commonly in women.

xan·tho·gran·u·lo·ma·tous cho·le·cys·ti·tis (zan´thō-gran-yū-lō´mă-tŭs kō´lē-sis-tī´tis) Chronic cholecystitis with conspicuous nodular infiltration by lipid macrophages.

xan·tho·ma (zan-thō´mă) A yellow nodule or plaque, especially of the skin, composed of lipid-laden histiocytes.

xan·tho·ma di·a·be·ti·co·rum (zan-thō´mă dī-ă-bet-i-kō´rŭm) Eruptive xanthoma associated with severe diabetes.

xan·tho·ma pla·num (zan-thō´mă plā´nŭm) A form marked by the occurrence of yellow, flat bands or minimally palpable rectangular plates in the corium.

xan·tho·ma·to·sis (zan´thō-mă-tō´sis) Widespread yellow patches, which sometimes affect mucous membranes and are sometimes associated with metabolic disturbances. SYN lipid granulomatosis, lipoid granulomatosis, xanthoma multiplex.

xan·tho·ma·to·sis bul·bi (zan´thō-mă-tō´sis bŭl´bī) Ulcerative fatty degeneration of the cornea after injury.

xan·tho·ma·tous (zan-thō´mă-tŭs) Relating to xanthoma.

xan·tho·ma tu·be·ro·sum (zan-thō´mă tū-bĕr-ō´sum) Xanthomatosis associated with familial type II, and occasionally type III, hyperlipoproteinemia.

Xan·tho·mo·nas (zan´thō-mō´nas) Aerobic, gram-negative, chemoorganotrophic, straight bacilli that exhibit motility by flagella.

Xan·tho·mo·nas mal·to·phil·i·a *Avoid the misspelling/mispronunciation maltophila.* Bacterial species found primarily in clinical specimens but also in water, milk, and frozen food. A frequent cause of infections in hospitalized and immunocompromised humans, resistant to many commonly used antibiotics.

xan·tho·phyll (zan´thō-fil) Oxygenated derivative of carotene; a yellow plant pigment, occurring also in egg yolk and corpus luteum. SYN lutein (2).

xan·thop·si·a, xan·tho·pi·a (zan-thop′sē-ă, -thŏ′pē-ă) A condition in which objects appear yellow; may occur in picric acid and santonin poisoning, in jaundice, and in digitalis intoxication.

xan·tho·sine (X, Xao) (zan′thŏ-sēn) The deamination product of guanosine (O replacing –NH₂).

xan·tho·sis (zan-thŏ′sis) A yellowish discoloration of degenerating tissues, especially seen in malignant neoplasms.

xan·thu·ren·ic ac·id (XA) (zan′thū-rēn′ik as′id) Metabolic product resulting from indoleamine 2,3-dioxygenase breakdown of tryptophan; may accumulate in human lens cells and play a role in senile-onset lens pathology, leading to lens cell apoptosis.

Xe Symbol for xenon.

xeno- Combining form meaning strange; foreign material; parasite. SEE ALSO hetero-, allo-.

xen·o·di·ag·no·sis (zen′ŏ-dī′ăg-nŏ′sis) **1.** A method of diagnosing acute or early *Trypanosoma cruzi* infection (Chagas disease) in humans. **2.** Method of biologic diagnosis based on experimental exposure of a parasite-free normal host capable of allowing the organism in question to multiply, enabling it to be more easily and reliably detected.

xen·o·ge·ne·ic, xen·og·e·nous, xen·o·gen·ic (zen′ŏ-jĕ-ne′ĭk, zĕ-noj′ĕ-nŭs, zen′ŏ-jen′ĭk) Heterologous, with respect to tissue grafts, especially when donor and recipient belong to widely separated species. Cf. allogeneic, isogenic. SYN xenogenic (2).

xen·o·graft (zen′ŏ-graft) A graft transferred from an animal of one species to one of another species. SYN heterograft, heterologous graft.

xe·nol·o·gy (ze-nol′ŏ-jē) Clinical genetic study to determine the presence of agents foreign to a bodily system.

xe·non (Xe) (ze′non) A gaseous element, present in minute proportion in the atmosphere; produces general anesthesia in concentrations of 70% vol.

xen·o·par·a·site (zen′ŏ-par′ă-sīt) An ecoparasite that becomes pathogenic in consequence of weakened resistance on the part of its host.

xen·o·pho·bi·a (zen′ŏ-fō′bē-ă) Abnormal fear of strangers or foreigners.

xen·o·pho·ni·a (zen′ŏ-fō′nē-ă) A speech defect marked by an alteration in accent and intonation.

Xen·op·syl·la (zen′op-sil′ă) *In the diphthong ps, the p is silent only at the beginning of a word.* The rat flea; a flea genus parasitic on the rat and involved in the transmission of bubonic plague. Important source of infection in epidemics, for example, in India and other regions of the world where large numbers of people live in poverty.

xen·o·tro·pic vi·rus (zen′ŏ-trō′pik vī′rŭs) A retrovirus that does not produce disease in its natural host and replicates only in tissue culture cells derived from a different species.

xero- *Avoid misspelling this combining form zero-.* Combining form meaning dry.

xe·ro·chi·li·a (zēr′ŏ-kī′lē-ă) Dryness of lips.

xe·ro·der·ma, xe·ro·der·mi·a (zēr′ŏ-dĕr′mă, -mē-ă) A mild form of ichthyosis characterized by excessive dryness of the skin due to slight thickening of the horny layer and diminished water content of the stratum corneum from decreased perspiration or exposure to wind, or low humidity; seen with aging, atopic dermatitis, and vitamin A deficiency.

xe·ro·der·ma pig·men·to·sum (zēr′ŏ-dĕr′mă pig-men-tō′sŭm) An eruption of exposed skin in childhood characterized by photosensitivity with severe sunburn in infancy and the development of numerous pigmented spots resembling freckles.

xe·ro·mam·mog·ra·phy (xero, XMM) (zē′rŏ-mam-og′ră-fē) Examination of the breast by xeroradiography.

xe·roph·thal·mi·a (zēr′of-thal′mē-ă) Excessive dryness of the conjunctiva and cornea, which lose their luster and become keratinized; may be due to local disease or to a systemic deficiency of vitamin A.

xe·ro·ra·di·o·graph (zēr´ō-rā´dē-ō-graf) The permanent record of an image made by xerography.

xe·ro·ra·di·og·ra·phy, xe·rog·ra·phy (zē´rō-rā´dē-og´ră-fē, -rog´gră-fē) Radiography using a specially coated charged plate instead of x-ray film, developing with a dry powder rather than liquid chemicals, and transferring the powder image onto paper for a permanent record.

xe·ro·sis (zēr-ō´sis) Pathologic dryness of the skin (xeroderma), the conjunctiva (xerophthalmia), or mucous membranes.

xe·ro·sto·mi·a (zēr´ō-stō´mē-ă) A dryness of the mouth, having a varied etiology, resulting from diminished or arrested salivary secretion, or asialism.

xe·rot·ic (zēr-ot´ik) Dry; affected with xerosis.

♻ **xipho-, xiph-, xiphi-** Combining forms meaning xiphoid, usually the processus xiphoideus.

xiph·o·cos·tal, xiph·i·cos·tal (zif´ō-kos´tăl, -i-kos´tăl) Relating to the xiphoid process and the ribs.

xiph·o·dyn·i·a (zif´ō-din´ē-ă) Neuralgic pain, in the region of the xiphoid cartilage. SEE ALSO hypersensitive xiphoid syndrome. SYN xiphoidalgia.

xi·phoid (zī´foyd) [TA] *Avoid the misspelling xyphoid.* Sword-shaped. SYN ensiform, gladiate, mucronate.

xi·phoi·di·tis (zī´foyd-ī´tis) Inflammation of the xiphoid process of the sternum.

xi·phoid pro·cess (zī´foyd pros´es) [TA] The cartilage at the lower end of the sternum. SYN processus xiphoideus [TA], ensiform process, xiphoid cartilage.

X-link·ed (lingkt) Pertaining to genes borne on the X chromosome. Commonly but erroneously used synonymously with sex-linked, which would also comprise Y-linked traits.

X-link·ed a·gam·ma·glob·u·li·ne·mi·a (lingkt ā-gam´ă-glob-yū-li-nē´mē-ă) B-cell immune deficiency condition, with hypo- or agammaglobulinemia; the immune deficiency becomes apparent as maternally transmitted immunoglobulin levels decline in early infancy.

X-link·ed dom·i·nant in·her·i·tance (lingkt dom´i-nănt in-her´i-tăns) A type of genetic disorder in which one copy of the gene will allow the disorder to occur.

X-link·ed hy·po·gam·ma·glob·u·lin·e·mi·a, X-link·ed in·fan·tile hy·po·gam·ma·glob·u·li·ne·mi·a (lingkt hī´pō-gam´ă-glob´yū-li-nē´mē-ă, in´făn-tīl) Congenital, primary immunodeficiency characterized by decreased numbers (or absence) of circulating B lymphocytes with corresponding decrease in immunoglobulins of the five classes; associated with marked susceptibility to infection by pyogenic bacteria (notably, pneumococci and *Haemophilus influenzae*) beginning after loss of maternal antibodies.

X-link·ed in·he·rit·ance (lingk in-her´i-tăns) Pattern of inheritance that may result from a mutant gene on an X chromosome.

X-link·ed lym·pho·pro·lif·er·a·tive syn·drome (lingkt lim´fō-prō-lif´ĕr-ă-tiv sin´drōm) An immunodeficiency and lymphoproliferative disease characterized by defective cellular or humoral immune response to Epstein-Barr virus.

X-link·ed re·ces·sive in·her·i·tance (lingkt rē-ses´iv in-her´i-tăns) A type of genetic disorder in which the disorder will occur in a male with one copy of the gene and in a female with both allelles showing the same mutation.

X-pat·tern es·o·tro·pi·a (pat´ĕrn ē´sō-trō´pē-ă) Decreasing convergence from the primary position in both upward and downward gaze.

X-pat·tern ex·o·tro·pi·a (pat´ĕrn ek´sō-trō´pē-ă) Increasing divergence from the primary position in both upward and downward gaze.

x-ray (rā) **1.** The ionizing electromagnetic radiation emitted from a highly evacuated tube, resulting from the excitation of the inner orbital electrons by the bombardment of the target anode with a stream of electrons from a heated cathode. **2.** Ionizing electromagnetic radiation produced by the excitation of the inner orbital electrons of an atom by other processes. **3.** A radiograph. SYN roentgen ray.

x-ray mi·cro·scope (rā mī′krŏ-skōp) A microscope in which images are obtained by using x-rays as an energy source that are recorded on a very fine-grained film, or the image is enlarged by projection; if film is used, it may be examined with the light microscope at fairly high magnifications.

XX Sex chromosomes found in female of the species.

XY Sex chromosomes found in the male of the species.

xy·li·tol (zī′li-tol) An optically inactive sugar alcohol; often used as a sugar substitute in diabetic diets.

xy·lol, xy·lene (zī′lol, -lēn) A volatile liquid obtained from coal tar, having physical and chemical properties similar to those of benzene; used as a solvent, in the manufacture of chemicals and synthetic fibers, and in histology as a clearing agent. SYN dimethylbenzene.

xy·lose (zī′lōs) An aldopentose, isomeric with ribose, obtained by fermentation or hydrolysis of carbohydrate.

xy·lu·lose (zī′lyū-lōs) Ketopentose that appears in the urine in cases of essential pentosuria.

xys·ma (zis′mă) Membranous shreds in the feces.

XYY syn·drome (sin′drōm) Aneuploidy with a supernumerary Y chromosome; associated with increased stature, aggressiveness, hyperactivity, mental retardation, and acne.

Y

YAG Acronym for yttrium-aluminum-garnet. SEE laser.

yaw (yaw) An individual lesion of the eruption of yaws.

Yb Symbol for ytterbium.

Y car·ti·lage, Y-shaped car·ti·lage (kahr´ti-lăj, shāpt) Connecting cartilage for the ilium, ischium, and pubis; extends through the acetabulum. SYN hypsiloid cartilage.

Y-linked in·her·i·tance (lingt in-her´ĭ-tăns) Pattern of inheritance that may result from a mutant gene located on an X-chromosome. SYN holandric inheritance.

years of po·ten·tial life lost (yĕrz pŏ-ten´shăl līf lawst) Measure of the relative impact of various diseases and lethal forces on society, computed by estimating the number of years that people would have lived if they had not died prematurely.

yeast (yēst) A general term denoting true fungi widely distributed in substrates that contain sugars (such as fruits), and in soil, animal excreta, and the vegetative parts of plants. Because of their ability to ferment carbohydrates, some yeasts are important to the brewing and baking industries.

yeast ar·ti·fi·cial chro·mo·somes (YAC) (yēst ahr´ti-fish´ăl krō´mŏ-sōmz) Yeast DNA sequences that have incorporated into them large foreign DNA fragments; the recombinant DNA is then introduced into the yeast by transformation.

yel·low (Y, Yel) (yel´ō) A color occupying a position in the spectrum between orange and green.

yel·low fe·ver (yel´ō fē´vĕr) A tropical mosquito-borne viral hepatitis, caused by one of the yellow fever viruses, with an urban form transmitted by *Aedes aegypti* and a rural, jungle, or sylvatic form from tree-dwelling mammals by various mosquitoes of the *Haemagogus* species complex; characterized by fever, slow pulse, albuminuria, jaundice, congestion of the face, and hemorrhages.

yel·low fe·ver vac·cine (YF-VAX) (yel´ō fē´vĕr vak-sēn´) **1.** Living, attenuated strain (17D) of yellow fever virus propagated in embryonized fowl eggs. **2.** Suspension of dried mouse brain infected with French neurotropic (Dakar) strain of yellow fever virus, administered topically by the scratch method; not officially recommended in the U.S. because of meningoencephalitic reactions.

yel·low fe·ver vi·rus (YFV) (yel´ō fē´vĕr vī´rŭs) An arbovirus, endemic in tropic Africa south of the Sahara and in tropic South America, occasionally spreading to countries outside these areas; causes yellow fever of humans and other primates; the virus exists in wild primates, and probably also in edentates, marsupials, and rodents.

yel·low wax (yel´ō waks) Yellowish, solid, brittle substance prepared from the honeycomb of the bee, *Apis mellifera;* used in the preparation of ointments, cerates, plasters, and suppositories.

Yer·ga·son test (yĕr´gă-sŏn test) Maneuver to diagnose bicipital tendinitis.

Yer·sin·i·a (yĕr-sin´ē-ă) A genus of motile and nonmotile, non-spore-forming bacteria containing gram-negative, unencapsulated, ovoid to rod-shaped cells; parasitic in humans and other animals.

Yer·sin·i·a en·ter·o·co·li·ti·ca (yĕr-sin´ē-ă en´tĕr-ō-kō-lit´i-kă) A bacterial species that causes yersiniosis in humans; it is found in the feces and lymph nodes of sick and healthy animals, including humans, and in material contaminated with feces.

Yer·sin·i·a pes·tis (yĕr-sin´ē-ă pes´tis) Bacterial species that causes plague in humans, rodents, cats, and many other mammals; can be transmitted by fleas, or in aerosol droplets dispersed by humans or animals manifesting a pneumonic form of plague, or by deliberate dissemination by means of an aerosol mechanism by individual people or organizations with bioterroristic intent. SYN Kitasato bacillus.

yer·sin·i·o·sis (yĕr-sin´ē-ō´sis) A common human infectious disease caused by *Yersinia enterocolitica* and marked by diarrhea, enteritis, pseudoappendicitis, ileitis, erythema nodosum, and sometimes septicemia or acute arthritis.

yield (yēld) The amount or quantity produced or returned, often measured as a percentage of the starting material.

yin/yang (yin-yang) In traditional Chinese medicine, the concept of opposing but complementary forces thought to underlie concepts of good health (e.g., heat/cold, hard/soft).

-yl Chemical suffix signifying that the substance is a radical by loss of an H atom (e.g., alkyl, methyl, phenyl) or OH group (e.g., acyl, acetyl, carbamoyl).

-ylene Chemical suffix denoting a bivalent hydrocarbon radical (e.g., methylene, $-CH_2-$) or possessing a double bond (e.g., ethylene, $CH_2=CH_2$).

yo·gurt, yo·ghurt (yō′gŭrt) Fermented, partially evaporated, whole milk prepared by maintaining it at 50°C for 12 hours after the addition of a mixed culture of *Lactobacillus bulgaricus, L. acidophilus,* and *Streptococcus lactis;* consumed as a food.

yo·him·bine (yō-him′bēn) An alkaloid, the active principle of yohimbé, the bark of *Corynanthe yohimbi;* produces a competitive blockade, of limited duration, of adrenergic α-receptors; has also been used for its alleged aphrodisiac properties.

yolk (yōk) **1.** One of the types of nutritive material stored in the oocyte for the nutrition of the embryo; particularly abundant and conspicuous in the eggs of birds. **2.** Fatty material found in the wool of sheep; when extracted and purified, it becomes lanolin.

Young-Helm·holtz the·o·ry of col·or vis·ion (yŭng helm′hōlts thē′ŏr-ē kŏl′ŏr vizh′ŭn) Idea that there are three color-perceiving elements in the retina: red, green, and blue. Perception of other colors arises from the combined stimulation of these elements; deficiency or absence of any one of these elements results in inability to perceive that color and a misperception of any other color of which it forms a part.

Young pros·tat·ic trac·tor (yŭng prostat′ik trak′tŏr) Short, straight tubular surgical instrument with blades at its tip.

yt·ter·bi·um (Yb) (i-tĕr′bē-ŭm) A metallic element of the lanthanide group; used in cisternography and in brain scans.

yt·tri·um (Y, YT) (it′rē-ŭm) A metallic element, atomic no. 39, atomic wt. 88.90585.

Z

za·fir·lu·kast (za′fir-lū′kast) A blocker of leukotriene D_4 and E_4 (LTD_4 and LTE_4) components of a slow-reacting substance of anaphylaxis (SRSA); used for prophylaxis of asthma.

Zahn in·farct (tsahn in′fahrkt) A pseudoinfarct of the liver, consisting of an area of congestion with parenchymal atrophy but no necrosis; due to obstruction of a branch of the portal vein.

zan·am·i·vir (zan-am′i-vir) An agent that inhibits neuraminidase of influenza virus.

Zar·it bur·den in·ter·view (zar′it bŭr′dĕn in′tĕr-vyū) A structured verbal interaction used to evaluate levels of stress in family members or caregivers of Alzheimer patients.

Zee·man ef·fect (tsē′mahn e-fekt′) Splitting of spectral lines into three or more symmetrically placed lines when the light source is subjected to a magnetic field.

Zeis glands (tsīs glandz) Sebaceous glands opening into the follicles of the eyelashes.

Zeit·geist (zīt′gīst) PSYCHOLOGY the climate of opinion, conventions of thought, covert influences, and unquestioned assumptions that are implicit in a given culture, the arts, or science at any time, and in which the individual person operates and thus is influenced.

Zell·we·ger syn·drome (zel′weg-ĕr sin′drōm) Metabolic disorder with neonatal onset; findings include characteristic facies, hepatomegaly, jaundice, and many others. SYN cerebrohepatorenal syndrome (CHRS).

ze·ro (zēr′ō) **1.** The figure 0, indicating the absence of magnitude, or nothing. **2.** THERMOMETRY the point from which the figures on the scale start in one or the other direction; in the Celsius and Réaumur scales, zero indicates the freezing point for distilled water; in the Fahrenheit scale, it is 32° below the freezing point of water.

ze·ro end·ex·pi·ra·to·ry pres·sure (ZEEP) (zēr′ō end′ek-spīr′ă-tōr-ē presh′ŭr) Airway pressure that, at the end of expiration, equals atmospheric pressure.

ze·ro grav·i·ty (zē′rō grav′i-tē) A physical state existing in space or at a time in flight when the centrifugal thrust of a parabolic glide or turn exactly counteracts the force of gravity.

ze·ta, ζ (zā′tă) **1.** The sixth letter of the Greek alphabet, ζ. **2.** In chemistry, denotes the sixth in a series. **3.** Symbol for electrokinetic potential.

ze·ta·crit (zā′tă-krit) The packed cell volume produced by vertical centrifugation of blood in capillary tubes, allowing controlled compaction and dispersion of red blood cells.

ze·ta po·ten·tial (zā′tă pŏ-ten′shăl) Degree of negative charge on the surface of a red blood cell.

ze·ta sed·i·men·ta·tion ra·ti·o (zā′tă sed′i-mĕn-tā′shŭn rā′shē-ō) The ratio of the zetacrit to the hematocrit, normally 0.41–0.54 (41–54%); a sensitive indicator of the erythrocyte sedimentation rate unaffected by anemia.

zeug·ma·tog·ra·phy (zūg′mă-tog′ră-fē) Term for the joining of a magnetic field and spatially defined radiofrequency field gradients to generate a two-dimensional display of proton density and relaxation times in tissues, the first nuclear magnetic resonance image.

Zie·mann dot (tsē′mahn dot) Any of numerous fine dots seen in erythrocytes in malariae malaria.

Zieve syn·drome (zēv sin′drōm) Transient jaundice, hemolytic anemia, and hyperlipemia associated with acute alcoholism in patients with cirrhosis or a fatty liver.

Zim·mer·lin at·ro·phy (tsim′er-lin at′rŏ-fē) Hereditary progressive muscular atrophy in which the atrophy begins in the upper half of the body.

Zim·mer·mann re·ac·tion (zim′er-mahn rē-ak′shŭn) Chemical reaction between an alkaline solution of *meta*-dinitrobenzene and an active methylene group (carbon-16) of 17-ketosteroids; basis of the 17-ketogenic steroid assay test. SYN Zimmermann test.

zinc (zingk) An essential bioelement; a

number of salts of zinc are used in medicine; a cofactor in many proteins.

zinc ac·e·tate (zingk as´ĕ-tāt) An emetic, styptic, and astringent.

zinc fin·ger (zingk fing´gĕr) Zinc-binding domain in a protein structure often seen in certain gene regulatory proteins.

zinc gel·a·tin (zingk jel´ă-tin) Zinc oxide, gelatin, glycerin, and purified water; used topically as a protectant.

zinc ox·ide and eu·ge·nol (zingk ok´sīd yū´jĕ-nol) Used as a base material beneath metallic dental restorations and as a temporary filling material or impression material; setting and hardening result from complex reactions between the powder and the eugenol.

zinc sul·fate (ZnSO$_4$) (zingk sŭl´fāt) Used as a local astringent to treat gonorrhea, indolent ulcers, conjunctivitis, and various skin diseases, and internally as an emetic.

zinc un·dec·y·len·ate, zinc un·dec·e·no·ate (zingk ŭn´des-i-len´āt, ŭn´des-ĕ-nō´āt) Zinc salt of undecylenic acid; used to treat fungal and other affections of the skin, including psoriasis.

zir·co·ni·um (Zr) (zĭr-kō´nē-ŭm) A metallic element widely distributed in nature, but never found in quantity in any one place.

zir·co·ni·um gran·u·lo·ma (zĭr-kō´nē-ŭm gran´yū-lō´mă) Lesion due to zirconium salts, usually occurring in the axillae, from antiperspirants containing this material, or from the application of hydrous zirconium oxide to poison ivy lesions.

Z line (līn) A cross-striation bisecting the I band of striated muscle myofibrils and serving as the anchoring point of actin filaments at either end of the sarcomere. SYN Z band.

Zn Symbol for zinc.

zo·ac·an·tho·sis (zō´ak-ăn-thō´sis) A cutaneous eruption due to introduction into the human skin of hair, bristles, or stingers, or other lower animal structures.

zo·an·thro·py (zō-an´thrŏ-pē) A delusion that one is an animal (e.g., a dog).

Zol·lin·ger-El·li·son syn·drome (ZES, ZE) (zol´in-jĕr-el´i-sŏn sin´drōm) Peptic ulceration with gastric hypersecretion and non-beta cell tumor of the pancreatic islets, sometimes associated with familial polyendocrine adenomatosis.

Zöll·ner lines (tserl´ner līnz) Figures devised to show the possibility of optic illusions; a common one consists of two parallel lines that are met by numerous short lines obliquely placed; the parallel lines then seeming to converge or diverge.

zol·pi·dem (zol´pi-dĕm) A sedative/hypnotic drug useful for treating anxiety.

zo·na, pl. **zo·nae** (zō´nă, -nē) [TA] SYN zone.

zo·na ar·cu·a·ta (zō´nă ahr´kyū-ā´tă) SYN arcuate zone.

zo·na cil·i·ar·is (zō´nă sil-ē-ā´ris) SYN ciliary zone.

zonaesthesia [Br.] SYN zonesthesia.

zo·na fas·ci·cu·la·ta (zō´nă fash-ik´yū-lā´tă) The layer of radially arranged cell cords in the cortex of the suprarenal gland, between the zona glomerulosa and zona reticularis.

zo·na glo·mer·u·lo·sa (zō´nă glō-mer-yū-lō´să) The outer layer of the cortex of the suprarenal gland just beneath the capsule; secretes aldosterone.

zo·na hem·or·rhoi·dal·is (zō´nă hem-ŏ-roy-dā´lis) SYN hemorrhoidal zone.

zo·na in·cer·ta (ZI) (zō´nă in-ser´tă) [TA] Flat, obliquely disposed plate of gray matter in the subthalamic region situated between the thalamic fasciculus (tegmental field H$_1$ of Forel) and the lenticular fasciculus (tegmental field H$_2$).

zo·na oph·thal·mi·ca (zō´nă of-thal´mik-ă) Herpes zoster in the distribution of the ophthalmic nerve.

zo·na pel·lu·ci·da (zō´nă pel-lū´sid-ă) An extracellular coat surrounding the oocyte; consists of a layer of microvilli of the oocyte, cellular processes of follicular cells, and an intervening substance

Z

rich in glycoprotein; it appears homogeneous and translucent under a light microscope. SYN pellucid zone.

zo·na ra·di·a·ta (zō′nă rā-dē-ā′tă) SYN zona striata.

zo·na re·tic·u·la·ris (zō′nă re-tik′yū-lār′is) The inner layer of the cortex of the suprarenal gland, where the cell cords anastomose in a netlike fashion.

zona stri·a·ta (zō′nă strī′ă-tă) Thickened cell membrane of the oocyte in varied forms, such as some amphibians, in which it appears radially striated under the light microscope; with the electron microscope the striations can be seen to be microvilli. SYN membrana striata, striated membrane, zona radiata.

zo·nate (zō′nāt) Zoned; ringed; having concentric layers of differing texture or pigmentation.

zo·na tec·ta (zō′nă tek′tă) SYN arcuate zone.

zone (zōn) [TA] A segment; any encircling or beltlike structure, either external or internal, longitudinal or transverse. SEE ALSO area, band, region, space, spot. SYN zona (1).

zone of equiv·a·lence (zōn ē-kwiv′ă-lens) Portion of a precipitin or agglutination curve when antibody and antigen concentrations are optimal for lattice formation.

zone of in·hib·i·tion (zōn in′hi-bish′ŭn) The area around an antibiotic disc that contains no bacterial growth.

zon·es·the·si·a (zōn′es-thē′zē-ă) A sensation as if a cord were drawn around the body, constricting it. SYN girdle sensation, strangalesthesia.

zo·nif·u·gal (zō-nif′yŭ-găl) Passing from within any region outward.

zon·ing (zōn′ing) The occurrence of a stronger reaction in a lesser amount of suspected serum, observed sometimes in serologic tests used in the diagnosis of syphilis.

zo·nip·e·tal (zō-nip′ĕ-tăl) Passing from without toward and into any region, as in mapping out an area of disturbed sensation, when the stimulus begins in a normal area and is carried into the affected region.

zon·og·ra·phy (zō-nog′ră-fē) A form of tomography with a relatively thick plane of focus; especially used in renal radiography.

zo·nu·la, pl. **zo·nu·lae** (zōn′yū-lă, -ē) SYN zonule.

zo·nu·la ad·he·rens (zōn′yū-lă ad-hē′renz) Beltlike attachment, similar to a desmosome, between columnar epithelial cells; supported by cytoplasmic filaments. SYN intermediate junction.

zo·nu·la cil·i·ar·is (zō′nyū-lă sil′ē-ār′is) [TA] SYN ciliary zonule.

zo·nu·la oc·clu·dens (ZO) (zōn′yū-lă o-klū′denz) Tight junctions formed by the fusion of integral proteins of the lateral cell membranes of adjacent epithelial cells, limiting transepithelial permeability. SYN impermeable junction, tight junction.

zo·nu·lar cat·a·ract (zō′nyū-lăr kat′ăr-akt) SYN lamellar cataract.

zo·nu·lar spaces (zō′nyū-lăr spās′ĕz) [TA] Spaces between the fibers of the ciliary zonule at the equator of the lens of the eye. SYN spatia zonularia [TA], Petit canals.

zon·ule (zō′nyūl) A small zone. SYN zonula.

zo·nu·li·tis (zō′nyū-lī′tis) Inflammation of the zonule of Zinn.

zo·nu·lol·y·sis, zo·nu·ly·sis (zō′nyū-lol′i-sis, -nyū-lī′sis) Dissolution of the zonula ciliaris by enzymes (α-chymotrypsin) to facilitate surgical removal of a cataract. SYN Barraquer method.

zoo-, zo- Combining forms denoting animal, animal life.

zoo blot a·nal·y·sis (zū blot ă-nal′i-sis) A laboratory procedure using Southern blot analysis to measure the ability of a nucleic acid probe from one species to hybridize with the DNA fragment of another species. SYN blot.

zo·o·der·mic (zō′ō-dĕr′mik) Relating to the skin of an animal.

zo•o•glea (zō′ō-glē′ă) In bacteriology, an old term for a mass of bacteria held together by a clear gelatinous substance.

zo•og•o•ny (zō-oj′ŏ-nē) SYN viviparity.

zo•o•graft (zō′ō-graft) A graft of tissue from an animal to a human.

zo•o•graft•ing (zō′ō-graft′ing) SYN zooplasty.

zo•oid (zō′oyd) **1.** Resembling an animal; an organism or object with an animalian appearance. **2.** An animal cell capable of independent existence or movement e.g., oocyte/ovum or sperm, segment of a tapeworm.

zo•ol•o•gist (zō-ol′ŏ-jist) One who specializes in zoology.

zo•ol•o•gy (Zool) (zō-ol′ŏ-jē) *Avoid the mispronunciation zū-ŏl′ō-jē.* The branch of biology that deals with animals.

zoom (zūm) The action of a varifocal lens system in a camera or microscope that maintains an object in focus while approaching it or receding from it.

zo•o•ma•ni•a (zō′ō-mā′nē-ă) An excessive, abnormal love of animals.

Zo•o•mas•ti•go•pho•re•a (zō′ō-mas′ti-gō-fōr′ē-ă) A class of flagellates found in human parasites such as the trypanosomes and trichomonads, as well as a number of other parasitic and symbiotic forms.

zo•o•no•sis (zō′ō-nō′sis) An infection or infestation shared in nature by humans and other animals that are the normal or usual host; a disease of humans acquired from an animal source. SEE ALSO anthropozoonosis.

zo•o•not•ic cu•ta•ne•ous leish•man•i•a•sis (zō′ō-not′ik kyū-tā′nē-ŭs lēsh′mă-nī′ă-sis) Cutaneous form of leishmaniasis characterized by rural distribution of human cases near infected rodents, particularly communal ground squirrels. SYN acute cutaneous leishmaniasis, rural cutaneous leishmaniasis, wet cutaneous leishmaniasis.

zo•o•not•ic po•ten•tial (zō′ō-not′ik pŏ-ten′shăl) The possibility for infections of subhuman animals to be transmissible to humans.

zo•o•par•a•site (zō′ō-par′ă-sīt) An animal parasite; an animal existing as a parasite.

zo•o•pa•thol•o•gy (zō′ō-pă-thol′ŏ-jē) The study or science of diseases of the lower animals.

zo•o•phil•i•a (zō′ō-fil′ē-ă) A paraphilia in which sexual arousal and orgasm are facilitated by engaging in sexual activities with animals. SYN zooerastia.

zo•o•phil•ic (zō′ō-fil′ik) Refers to microorganisms that prefer an animal other than humans as a host or reservoir.

zo•oph•i•lism (zō-of′i-lizm) Fondness for animals, especially to an extravagant degree.

zo•o•plas•ty (zō′ō-plas′tē) Grafting of tissue from an animal to a human. SYN zoografting.

zo•o•sper•mi•a (zō′ō-spĕr′mē-ă) The presence of live sperms in the ejaculated semen.

zo•o•tox•in (zō′ō-tok′sin) A substance, resembling the bacterial toxins in its antigenic properties, found in the fluids of certain animals.

zos•ter•i•form (zos-ter′i-fōrm) Resembling herpes zoster. SYN zosteroid.

zos•ter im•mune glob•u•lin (ZIG) (zos′tĕr i-myūn′ glob′yū-lin) Globulin fraction of pooled plasma from patients who have recovered from herpes zoster; used prophylactically for immunosuppressed children exposed to varicella and therapeutically to ameliorate varicella infection.

zos•ter•oid (zos′tĕr-oyd) Resembling herpes zoster.

Z-plas•ty (plas′tē) Surgery to elongate a contracted scar or to rotate tension 90°; the middle line of a Z-shaped incision is made along the line of greatest tension or contraction, and triangular flaps are raised on opposite sides of the two ends and transposed. SYN zigzag plasty.

Zr Symbol for zirconium.

Zuc·ker·kan·dl fas·ci·a (tsuk'ĕr-kahn-dĕl fash'ē-ă) Posterior layer of the renal fascia.

Zung Self-Rat·ing De·pres·sion Scale (zŭng self-rāt'ing dē-presh'ŭn skāl) Self-administered scale to diagnose and quantify level of depression.

zy·gal (zī'găl) Relating to a yoke shape.

zyg·i·on (Zy) (zig'ē-on) In cephalometrics and craniometrics, the most lateral point of the zygomatic arch.

♻ **zygo-, zyg-** Combining forms meaning a yoke, a joining.

zy·go·mat·ic (zī'gō-mat'ik) Relating to the zygomatic bone.

zy·go·mat·i·co·fa·cial (zī'gō-mat'i-kō-fā'shăl) Relating to the zygomatic bone and the face.

zy·go·mat·i·co·tem·po·ral (zī'gō-mat'i-kō-tem'pŏ-răl) Relating to the zygomatic and temporal bones.

zy·go·max·il·la·re (zī'gō-mak'sil-lar-ē) A craniometric point located externally at the lowest extent of the zygomaxillary suture. SYN key ridge.

Zy·go·my·ce·tes (zī'gō-mī-sē'tēz) A class of fungi characterized by sexual reproduction resulting in the formation of a zygospore, and asexual reproduction by means of nonmotile spores called sporangiospores or conidia.

zy·go·my·co·sis (zī'gō-mī-kō'sis) A fungal infection associated with *Absidia, Mortierella, Mucor,* and *Rhizopus.* SYN mucormycosis, phycomycosis.

zy·gon (zī'gon) The short crossbar connecting the branches of a zygal fissure.

zy·go·ne·ma (zī'gō-nē'mă) SYN zygotene.

zy·go·po·di·um (zī'gō-pō'dē-ŭm) The distal intermediate segment of the limb skeleton (i.e., radius and ulna, tibia and fibula).

zy·go·sis (zī-gō'sis) True conjugation or sexual union of two unicellular organisms, consisting essentially in the fusion of the nuclei of the two cells.

zy·gos·i·ty (zī-gos'i-tē) The nature of the zygotes from which twins are derived; e.g., whether by division of one zygote (monozygotic), when they will be genetically identical, or from two zygotes, when they will be genetically different.

zy·go·spore (zī'gō-spōr) Among the Phycomycetes, a thick-walled sexual spore arising from fusion of two morphologically identical structures, generally hyphal tips, bearing nuclei of opposite mating types. SYN zygosperm.

zy·gote (zī'gōt) **1.** The diploid cell resulting from union of a sperm and an oocyte. Cf. conceptus. **2.** The early embryo that develops from a fertilized oocyte.

zy·gote in·tra·fal·lo·pi·an trans·fer (zī'gōt in'tră-fă-lō'pē-ăn trans'fĕr) Implantation of a fertilized oocyte into the uterine tube.

zy·go·tene (zī'gō-tēn) The stage of prophase in meiosis in which precise point-for-point pairing of homologous chromosomes begins. SYN zygonema.

♻ **zymo-, zym-** Combining forms denoting fermentation, enzymes.

zy·mo·gen·ic (zī'mō-jen'ik) **1.** Relating to a zymogen or to zymogenesis. SYN zymogenous. **2.** Causing fermentation.

zy·mog·e·nous (zī-moj'ĕ-nŭs) Related to a zymogen, a type of proenzyme.